hydroxyzine	meperidine	metoclopramide	midazolam	morphine	nalbuphine	pentazocine	pentobarbital	prochlorperazine	promethazine	ranitidine	secobarbital	thiopental
M*	M	M	Y	M	Y	M	[illegible]	[illegible]	[illegible]	[illegible]	—	—
Y	Y	Y	Y	[illegible]	[illegible]	[illegible]	[illegible]	[illegible]	[illegible]	[illegible]	—	—
M	M	M	Y	[illegible]	[illegible]	[illegible]	[illegible]	[illegible]	[illegible]	[illegible]	[illegible]	N
Y	Y	—	Y	Y	[illegible]	[illegible]	[illegible]	[illegible]	[illegible]	—	N	—
N	M	M	N	M	[illegible]	M	N	N	N	Y	—	N
M	M	Y	Y	M	Y	M	N	M	M	Y	—	N
M	M	M	Y	M	—	M	N	M	M	Y	—	—
Y	Y	—	Y	Y	Y	N	N	Y	Y	Y	N	N
N	N	Y	N	N*	—	N	—	N	N	$M_{(5)}$	—	—
Y	M	M	Y	Y	Y	Y	N	M	M	N	—	—
M	Y	M	Y	N	—	M	N	M	M	Y	—	—
M	M	Y	Y	M	—	M	—	M	M	Y	—	—
Y	Y	Y	Y	Y	Y	—	N	N	Y	N	—	—
M	N	M	Y	Y	—	M	N	M	M*	Y	—	N
Y	—	—	Y	—	Y	—	N	Y	N*	Y	—	—
M	M	M	—	M	—	Y	N	M	M*	Y	—	—
N	N	—	N	N*	N	N	Y	N	N	N	—	Y
M	M	M	N	M*	Y	M	N	Y	M	Y	—	N
M	M	M	Y	M*	N*	M*	N	M	Y	Y	—	N
N	Y	Y	N	Y	Y	Y	N	Y	Y	Y	—	—
—	—	—	—	—	—	—	—	—	—	—	Y	—
—	—	—	—	N	—	—	Y	N	N	—	—	Y

N = Incompatible; do not mix in syringe
* = Conflicting data
— = Information about compatibility is not currently available

2011 LIPPINCOTT'S Nursing Drug Guide

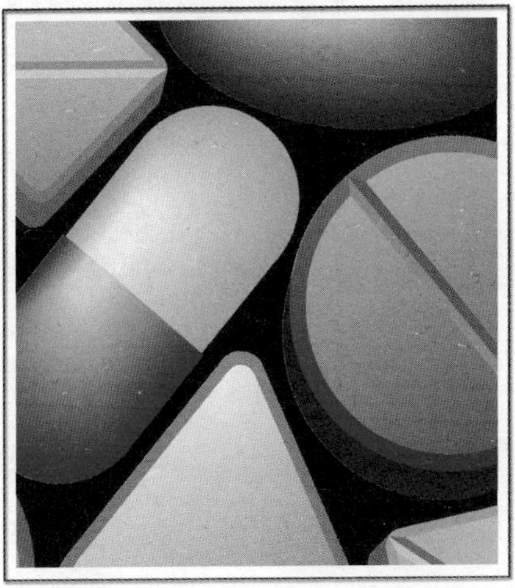

2011 LIPPINCOTT'S Nursing Drug Guide

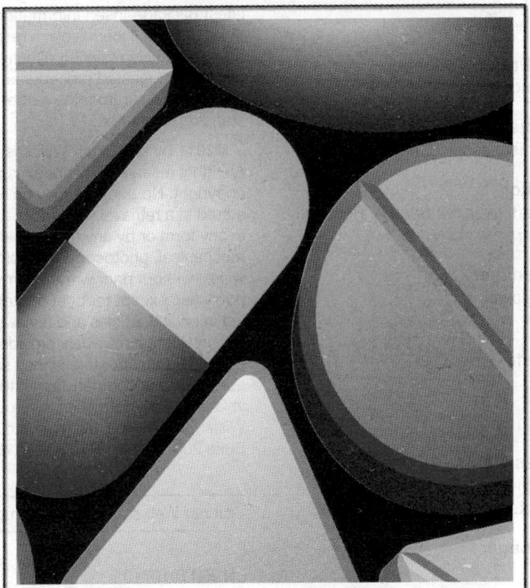

Amy M. Karch, RN, MS
Associate Professor of Clinical Nursing
University of Rochester School of Nursing
Rochester, New York

Wolters Kluwer | Lippincott Williams & Wilkins
Health
Philadelphia • Baltimore • New York • London
Buenos Aires • Hong Kong • Sydney • Tokyo

Staff

Publisher
Chris Burghardt

Clinical Director
Joan M. Robinson, RN, MSN

Product Director
David Moreau

Art Director
Elaine Kasmer

Electronic Project Manager
John Macalino

Clinical Project Manager
Beverly Ann Tscheschlog, RN, MS

Clinical Editor
Anita Lockhart, MSN, RN; Shari A. Regina-Cammon, MSN, RN, PCCN

Product Manager
Rosanne Hallowell

Editor
Karen Comerford

Copy Editor
Heather Ditch

Editorial Assistants
Megan L. Aldinger, Karen J. Kirk, Jeri O'Shea, Linda K. Ruhf

Vendor Manager
Cindy Rudy

Production and Indexing Services
Aptara, Inc.

Manufacturing Manager
Beth J. Welsh

The clinical procedures described and recommended in this publication are based on research and consultation with nursing, medical, pharmaceutical, and legal authorities. To the best of our knowledge, these procedures reflect currently accepted practice; nevertheless, they can't be considered absolute and universal recommendations. For individual application, all recommendations must be considered in light of the patient's clinical condition and, before the administration of new or infrequently used drugs, in light of the latest package-insert information. The authors and publisher disclaim responsibility for adverse effects resulting directly or indirectly from the suggested procedures, from undetected errors, or from the reader's misunderstanding of the text.

Visit our Web site at NursingDrugGuide.com

LNDG11010710
ISSN: 1081-857X
ISBN-13: 978-1-60913-237-8
ISBN-10: 1-60913-237-8
ISBN-13: 978-1-60913-234-7 (Canada)
ISBN-10: 1-60913-234-3 (Canada)

RRS1004

Contents

A quick-access full-color photoguide to pills and capsules is found between pages 746 and 747.

Consultants

Jennalie E. Blackwood, RPh, PharmD
Clinical Pharmacist
St. Louis (Mo.) College of Pharmacy

Cheryl L. Brady, RN, MSN
Assistant Professor of Nursing
Kent State University
Salem, Ohio

Lawrence Carey, PharmD
Associate Director, Physician Assistant Program
Philadelphia (Pa.) University

Peggy L. Carver, PharmD, FCCP
Associate Professor of Pharmacy
Clinical Pharmacist, Infectious Diseases
University of Michigan College of Pharmacy
University of Michigan Health System
Ann Arbor

Lauren Czosnowski, BS, PharmD, BCPS
Assistant Professor of Clinical Pharmacy
University of the Sciences in Philadelphia

Julie Ann Genuario, BS (Pharmacy)
Perdiem Pharmacist
Pottstown (Pa.) Memorial Medical Center

Tatyana Gurvich, PharmD
Clinical Geriatric Pharmacist
USC School of Pharmacy/UC Irvine Senior Center
Orange, Calif.

AnhThu Hoang, PharmD
Drug Information Pharmacist
Drug Information and Research Centre
Toronto, Ontario

James Allen Koestner, BS (Pharmacy), PharmD
Program Director—Pharmacy
Vanderbilt University Medical Center
Nashville, Tenn.

Lauren McCluggage, PharmD, BCPS
Assistant Professor of Pharmacy
Philadelphia (Pa.) College of Pharmacy

Keith M. Olsen, PharmD, FCCP, FCCM
Professor and Chair, Department of Pharmacy Practice
University of Nebraska Medical Center
Omaha

Debra A. Perlsweig, PharmD
Pharmacist
Crozer Chester Medical Center
Upland, Pa.

Christine Price, PharmD
Clinical Coordinator and PGYI Residency Director
Morton Plant Mease Health Care
Clearwater, Fla.

Michele F. Shepherd, MS, PharmD, BCPS
Clinical Specialist
Abbott Northwestern Hospital
Minneapolis, Minn.

Preface

The number of clinically important drugs increases every year, as does the nurse's responsibility for drug therapy. No nurse can memorize all the drug information needed to provide safe and efficacious drug therapy. The *2011 Lippincott's Nursing Drug Guide* provides the drug information nurses need in a concise, ready-access format. This edition was completely updated and then it was reviewed by independent clinical reviewers, including pharmacists and nurses, to ensure that nurses will have the most up-to-date and accurate information possible.

This book presents nursing considerations related to drug therapy in the format of the nursing process, a framework for applying basic pharmacologic information to patient care. It is intended for the student nurse who is just learning how to apply pharmacologic data in the clinical situation, as well as for the busy practicing professional nurse who needs a quick, easy-to-use guide to the clinical use of drugs.

This book provides broad coverage of the drugs commonly encountered by nurses and of drugs whose use commonly involves significant nursing intervention. *Anatomy of a monograph,* found at the end of this preface, explains how the information in each monograph can be used to implement the nursing process. Commonly used medical abbreviations are used throughout the book and are defined in the *Guide to abbreviations* located after *Anatomy of a monograph.* A handy guide to drug compatibility in syringes is found inside the front cover for ready access.

The first two chapters of this book provide a concise review of the nursing process and its application to pharmacologic situations, including guidelines for avoiding medication errors and concise examples of how to use the drug guide to apply the nursing process and to make a patient teaching guide. Next is a review of selected drug classifications, which provides a convenient, complete summary of the drug information pertinent to drugs in each class.

Complete drug monographs

Drug information is presented in monograph form, with the monographs arranged alphabetically by generic name. Each page of the book contains guide words at the top, much like a dictionary, to facilitate easy access to any drug. The right-hand edge of the book contains letter guides, again to facilitate finding a drug as quickly as possible.

Each drug monograph is complete in itself—that is, it includes all of the clinically important information that a nurse needs to know to give the drug safely and effectively. Every monograph begins with the drug's generic (nonproprietary) name; any alternate names follow in parentheses; an alphabetical list of the most common brand names, including common brand names found only in Canada (noted by the designation CAN); the drug's pregnancy category classification, and its schedule if it is a controlled substance. The names of drugs that are described in Appendix W, *Less commonly used drugs,* appear alphabetically in the text and are cross referenced to the index.

Preventing medication errors is a critical component of patient care. Clinical practice has revealed that some drugs are especially dangerous when involved in a medication error. The monographs for these drugs are marked with the "dangerous drug" logo to alert the nurse to use exceptional care during administration.

Each monograph provides a commonly accepted pronunciation (after *USAN* and the *USP Dictionary of Drug Names, 2009*) to help the nurse feel more comfortable discussing the drug with other members of the health care team. After the pronunciation, each monograph gives you these features:

- The clinically important drug classes of each drug are indicated to put the drug in appropriate context.
- The therapeutically useful actions of the drug are described, including, where known, the mechanism(s) by which these therapeutic effects are produced; no attempt is made to list *all* of the drug's known actions here.
- Clinical indications for the drug are listed, including important unlabeled indications not approved by the FDA, as well as orphan drug uses where appropriate. New indications for a drug are emphasized by the "New indication" logo.
- Contraindications to drug use and cautions that should be considered when using the drug are listed.
- The pharmacokinetic profile of the drug is given in table form to allow easy access to such information as half-life, peak levels, distribution, and so on, offering a quick reference on how the drug is handled by the body.
- Dosage information is listed next, including dosages for adults, pediatric patients, and geriatric patients, and dosages for indications when these differ. A listing of the available forms of each drug serves as a guide for prescribing or suggesting alternate routes of administration. Details of drug administration that must not be overlooked for the safe administration of the drug (eg, "Dilute before infusing" or "Infuse slowly over 30 min") are included in the dosage section, but other aspects of drug administration (eg, directions for reconstituting a powder for injection) are presented under *Interventions* in the next section of the monograph. If there is a treatment for the overdose of this drug, that information is indicated in *Interventions.*
- The *IV Facts* section, with a prominent logo, gives concise, important information that is needed for drugs given IV—dilution, flow rate, compatibilities—making it unnecessary to have a separate IV handbook.
- Commonly encountered adverse effects are listed by body system, with the most commonly encountered adverse effects appearing in *italics* to make it easier to assess the patient for adverse effects and to teach the patient about what to expect. Potentially life-threatening adverse effects are in **bold** for easy access. Adverse effects that have been reported, but appear less commonly or rarely, are also listed to make the drug information as complete as possible.
- Clinically important interactions are listed separately for easy access: drug-drug, drug-food, drug-lab test, drug-alternative therapy—for interferences to consider when using the drug and any nursing action that is necessary because of this interaction.
- The "Dangerous drug" heading indicates those drugs proven more likely to be involved in serious patient reactions.
- Drugs that cannot be cut, crushed, or chewed have a "Do Not Crush" (DNC) logo to immediately alert you about this caution.
- A "Black box" warning logo highlights FDA warnings regarding safe use of the drug.
- The "Warning" logo highlights important facts and potential safety issues.

Clinically focused nursing considerations

The remainder of each monograph is concerned with nursing considerations, which are presented in the format of the nursing process. The steps of the nursing process are given slightly different names by different authorities; this handbook includes: assessment (history and physical examination), interventions, and teaching points for each of the drugs presented.

"Clinical alert" provides important information about reported name confusions that have occurred with a given drug to help prevent potential medication errors.

- **Assessment:** Outlines the information that should be collected before administering the drug. This section is further divided into two subsections:

–**History:** Includes a list of those underlying conditions that constitute contraindications and cautions for use of the drug.

–**Physical:** Provides data, by organ system, that should be collected before beginning drug therapy, both to allow detection of conditions that are contraindications or cautions to the use of the drug and to provide baseline data for detecting adverse reactions to the drug and monitoring for therapeutic response.

- **Interventions:** Lists, in chronological order, those nursing activities that should be undertaken in the course of caring for a patient who is receiving the drug. This section includes interventions related to drug preparation and administration, the provision of comfort and safety measures, and drug levels to monitor, as appropriate.
- **Teaching points:** Includes specific information that is needed for teaching the patient who is receiving this drug. Proven "what to say" advice can be transferred directly to patient teaching printouts and used as a written reminder.

Evaluation

Evaluation is usually the last step of the nursing process. In all drug therapy, the patient should be evaluated for the desired effect of the drug as listed in the *Indications* section; the occurrence of adverse effects, as listed in the *Adverse effects* section; and learning following patient teaching, as described in the *Teaching points* section. These points are essential. In some cases, evaluation includes monitoring specific therapeutic serum drug levels; these cases are specifically mentioned in the *Interventions* section. The *Nursing process guidelines* chapter gives an example of how the drug monograph can be used to establish a nursing care plan, to develop a patient teaching printout, and to incorporate the nursing process into drug therapy.

Appendices

The appendices contain information that is useful to nursing practice but may not lend itself to the monograph format—alternative and complementary therapies; a guide to preventing miscommunication; a guide to patient teaching to prevent medication errors; important drug-related dietary guidelines for patient teaching; a list of drugs that interact with grapefruit juice; recommended routes of administration; new medication disposal guidelines; formulas for pediatric dosage calculations; guides to adult and pediatric immunizations; schedules of controlled substances (for U.S. and Canadian drugs); pregnancy categories (for U.S. drugs); cardiovascular guidelines—including standards for lipid levels and blood pressure monitoring; normal laboratory values; Canadian drug information, including mini-monographs of drugs that are used in Canada but not in the United States; topical drugs and corticosteroids; ophthalmic drugs; laxatives; detailed combination drug references; information about hormonal contraceptives; commonly used biologicals; and less commonly used drugs. A suggested bibliography follows the appendices.

Index

An extensive index provides a ready reference to drug information. The **generic** name of each drug is highlighted in bold. If the generic name of a drug is not known, the drug may be found quickly by using whatever name is known. *Brand names* are listed in italics, commonly used chemical names and any commonly used "jargon" name (such as IDU for idoxuridine) are in parentheses after the generic name. In addition, the index lists drugs by clinically important classes—pharmacologic and therapeutic. If you know a patient is taking an antianginal drug and don't remember the name, reviewing the list of drugs under *Antianginals* may well help you recall the name. Chlorpromazine, for example, is listed by its generic name, by all of its brand names, and by classes as an antipsychotic (a therapeutic classification), as a phenothiazine (the pharmacologic class), and as a dopaminergic blocking drug (a classification by postulated mechanism of action). The comprehensive index helps to avoid cross-referencing from within the text, which is time consuming and often confusing.

2011 Quick-access photoguide

The full-color photoguide presents nearly 400 pills and capsules, representing the most commonly prescribed generic and brand drugs. Photos of certain brands were provided by the following companies: Forest Pharmaceuticals, Inc. (Campral); Novartis Pharmaceuticals (Enablex); Sepracor, Inc. (Lunesta); Teva Pharmaceuticals (Azilect); Bayer Healthcare Pharmaceuticals (Nexavar); and Pfizer (Sutent).

What's new

The new features in the book include:

- More than 25 new drugs
- "New indication" logo to highlight new labeled indications for drugs
- "Dangerous drug" logo to identify high-risk drugs
- Expanded "Black box warnings" to help prevent medication errors
- More "Warning" logos that highlight potential complications
- Mini-monographs of commonly used Canadian drugs
- Expanded *Less commonly used drugs* appendix, which includes fertility drugs and monoclonal antibodies
- Updated nursing process section
- Logos in appropriate monographs warning about drug forms that cannot be cut, crushed, or chewed
- Expanded alternative and complementary therapies section
- Even more "Clinical alerts" to point out possible name confusion to prevent medication errors
- Continuing education tests available through NursingDrugGuide.com.

Web site access to 200 common drugs

Through the NursingDrugGuide.com Web site you will be able to access 200 of the most commonly prescribed drugs along with patient-teaching printouts, which you can use to prepare your own study aids, develop nursing care plans, and customize patient and staff teaching tools. You'll also find links to nursing organizations as well as other helpful information.

Added benefit

With this guide comes access to free monthly drug updates available to you throughout the year via the NursingDrugGuide.com Web site. Get the most recent drug information available, including the latest FDA drug approvals and advances in clinical pharmacology. In addition, you will be able to access new continuing education tests via the Web site and earn contact hours.

This 16th edition incorporates many of the suggestions and requests that have been made by the users of earlier editions of this book. It is hoped that the overall organization and concise, straightforward presentation of the material in the *2011 Lippincott's Nursing Drug Guide* will make it a readily used and clinically useful reference for the nurse who needs easily accessible information to facilitate the provision of drug therapy within the framework of the nursing process. It is further hoped that the thoroughness of the additional sections of the book will make it an invaluable resource that will replace the need for several additional references.

Amy M. Karch, RN, MS

Anatomy of a monograph

DANGEROUS DRUG ← Dangerous drug alert

vincristine sulfate (LCR, VCR) ← Generic name

*(vin **kris'** teen)* ← Pronunciation guide

Oncovin, Vincasar PFS ← Brand names

PREGNANCY CATEGORY D ← FDA pregnancy risk category

Drug classes ← Therapeutic drug class
Antineoplastic
Mitotic inhibitor

Therapeutic actions ← Action of drug on the body
Mitotic inhibitor: Arrests mitotic division at the stage of metaphase; exact mechanism of action unknown.

Indications ← Uses for the drug
Evaluation points—resolution or stabilization of those conditions

- Acute leukemia
- Hodgkin's lymphoma, non-Hodgkin's lymphoma, rhabdomyosarcoma, neuroblastoma, Wilms' tumor as part of combination therapy

Contraindications and cautions ← Conditions limiting the use of drug
Assessment points—history or physical assessment indicating these conditions

- Contraindicated with allergy to vincristine, leukopenia, acute infection, pregnancy, lactation, demyelinating form of Charcot-Marie-Tooth syndrome.
- Use cautiously with neuromuscular disease, diabetes insipidus, hepatic impairment.

Available forms ← Forms and dosages available for use
Injection—1 mg/mL

Dosages ← Recommended dose of drug for adults, pediatric patients, and special populations
Adults

1.4 mg/m^2 IV at weekly intervals. (Not to exceed 2 mg.)

Pediatric patients

1.5–2 mg/m^2 IV weekly.

- *Less than 10 kg or BSA less than 1 m^2:* 0.05 mg/kg once per wk.

Action of the body on the drug—
Assessment points (hepatic and renal function)

Nursing actions for safe and appropriate administration of the drug in IV form
Interventions—nursing actions

Effects of drug on the body—not therapeutic but can be expected
Assessment points—baselines for these systems
Nursing diagnoses—potential alterations resulting from these effects
Evaluation—presence or absence of these effects

Anticipated clinically important interactions
Assessment points—history of use of these agents, physical response
Evaluation—changes from expected therapeutic response related to drug interactions

Geriatric patients or patients with hepatic impairment
For serum bilirubin exceeding 3 mg/dL, reduce dosage by 50%.

Pharmacokinetics

Route	*Onset*	*Peak*
IV	Varies	15–30 min

Metabolism: Hepatic; $T_{1/2}$: 5 min, then 2.3 hr, then 85 hr
Distribution: Crosses placenta; enters breast milk
Excretion: Feces, urine

IV FACTS

Preparation: No further preparation required; drug should be refrigerated.
Infusion: Inject solution directly into vein or into the tubing of a running IV infusion.
Y-site incompatibility: Do not give with furosemide.

Adverse effects

- **CNS:** *Ataxia, cranial nerve manifestations;* foot drop, headache, seizures, bladder neuropathy, paresthesias, sensory impairment, *neuritic pain, muscle wasting,* SIADH, optic atrophy, transient cortical blindness, ptosis, diplopia, photophobia
- **GI:** *Constipation,* oral ulcerations, abdominal cramps, vomiting, diarrhea, intestinal necrosis
- **GU:** Acute uric acid nephropathy, polyuria, dysuria
- **Hematologic:** *Leukopenia*
- **Local:** Local irritation, cellulitis if extravasation occurs
- **Other:** *Weight loss, loss of hair,* fever, **death** with serious overdose

Interactions

✱ **Drug-drug** • Decreased serum levels and therapeutic effects of digoxin • If L-asparaginase is administered first, the hepatic clearance of vincristine may be reduced. Give vincristine 12–24 hr before L-asparaginase to minimize toxicity

✱ **Drug-food** • Decreased metabolism and risk of toxic effects if combined with grapefruit juice; avoid this combination

■ Nursing considerations

Directs nursing action to ensure safe and effective administration of this drug

Interventions—nursing actions

CLINICAL ALERT!

Confusion has occurred between vincristine and vinblastine; use extreme caution if giving either drug.

Assessment

Points to establish baselines, determine factors contraindicating drug use or requiring caution

- **History:** Allergy to vincristine, leukopenia, acute infection, neuromuscular disease, diabetes insipidus, hepatic impairment, pregnancy, lactation
- **Physical:** Weight; hair; T; reflexes, gait, sensation, cranial nerve evaluation, ophthalmic examination; mucous membranes, abdominal examination; CBC, serum sodium, LFTs, urinalysis

Interventions

Nursing actions, in chronological order, for safe and effective drug therapy

Evaluation—monitoring of these tests; effectiveness of comfort and safety measures

- Ensure that patient is not pregnant before administering; using barrier contraceptives is advised.
- Tell patient to avoid grapefruit juice while being treated with this drug.

⊗ ***Black box warning*** Do not administer IM or subcutaneously due to severe local reaction and tissue necrosis. Do not give intrathecally; drug is fatal if given intrathecally. Use extreme caution.

Black box warning logo

⊗ ***Black box warning*** Watch for irritation and infiltration; extravasation causes tissue damage and necrosis. If extravasation occurs, discontinue injection immediately and give remainder of dose in another vein. Consult with physician to arrange for hyaluronidase injection into local area, and apply heat to disperse the drug and to minimize pain.

Black box warning logo

- Arrange for wig or suitable head covering if hair loss occurs; ensure that patient's head is covered in extremes of temperature.
- Monitor urine output and serum sodium; if SIADH occurs, consult with physician, and arrange for fluid restriction and perhaps a potent diuretic.

Drug-specific teaching points to include in patient teaching program
Nursing diagnoses—deficient knowledge regarding drug therapy
Evaluation—points patient should be able to repeat

Teaching points

- Prepare a calendar of dates to return for treatment and additional therapy.
- Avoid grapefruit juice while you are using this drug.
- This drug cannot be taken during pregnancy; use birth control. If you become pregnant, consult your health care provider.
- Have regular blood tests to monitor the drug's effects.
- You may experience these side effects: Loss of appetite, nausea, vomiting, mouth sores (frequent mouth care, frequent small meals may help; maintain nutrition; request an antiemetic); constipation (bowel program may be ordered); sensitivity to light (wear sunglasses; avoid bright lights); numbness, tingling, change in style of walking (reversible; may persist for up to 6 weeks); hair loss (transient; obtain a wig or other suitable head covering; keep the head covered at extremes of temperature).
- Report change in frequency of voiding; swelling of ankles, fingers, and so forth; changes in vision; severe constipation, abdominal pain.

Guide to abbreviations

ACE	angiotensin-converting enzyme
ACT	activated clotting time
ACTH	adrenocorticotropic hormone
ADH	antidiuretic hormone
ADHD	attention-deficit hyperactivity disorder
ADLs	activities of daily living
AIDS	acquired immunodeficiency syndrome
ALL	acute lymphocytic leukemia
ALT	alanine transaminase (formerly called SGPT)
AML	acute myelogenous leukemia
ANA	anti-nuclear antibodies
ANC	absolute neutrophil count
aPTT	activated partial thromboplastin time
ARB	angiotensin II receptor blocker
ARC	AIDS-related complex
ASA	acetylsalicylic acid
AST	aspartate transaminase (formerly called SGOT)
AV	atrioventricular
bid	twice a day *(bis in die)*
BP	blood pressure
BPH	benign prostatic hypertrophy
BSP	bromsulphalein
BUN	blood urea nitrogen
C	centigrade, Celsius
CAD	coronary artery disease
cAMP	cyclic adenosine monophosphate
CBC	complete blood count
CDC	Centers for Disease Control and Prevention
CML	chronic myelogenous leukemia
CNS	central nervous system
COPD	chronic obstructive pulmonary disease
CPK	creatine phosphokinase
CPR	cardiopulmonary resuscitation
CR	controlled release
CrCl	creatinine clearance
CSF	cerebrospinal fluid
CTZ	chemoreceptor trigger zone
CV	cardiovascular
CVP	central venous pressure
CYP450	cytochrome P-450
D_5W	dextrose 5% in water
DEA	Drug Enforcement Administration
DIC	disseminated intravascular coagulopathy
dL	deciliter (100 mL)
DNA	deoxyribonucleic acid
DR	delayed release
DTP	diphtheria-tetanus-pertussis (vaccine)
DVT	deep venous thrombosis
ECG	electrocardiogram
ECT	electroconvulsive therapy
ED	erectile dysfunction
EEG	electroencephalogram
EENT	eye, ear, nose, and throat
ER	extended release
EST	electroshock therapy

F	Fahrenheit
FDA	Food and Drug Administration
5-FU	fluorouracil
5-HIAA	5-hydroxyindole acetic acid
FSH	follicle-stimulating hormone
g	gram
GABA	gamma-aminobutyric acid
GERD	gastroesophageal reflux disease
GFR	glomerular filtration rate
GGTP	gamma-glutamyl transpeptidase
GI	gastrointestinal
G6PD	glucose-6-phosphate dehydrogenase
GU	genitourinary
HCG	human chorionic gonadotropin
Hct	hematocrit
HDL	high-density lipoproteins
HF	heart failure
Hg	mercury
Hgb	hemoglobin
Hib	*Haemophilus influenzae* type b
HIV	human immunodeficiency virus
HMG-CoA	3-hydroxy-3-methylglutaryl coenzyme A
HPA	hypothalamic–pituitary axis
hr	hour
HR	heart rate
HSV	herpes simplex virus
IBS	irritable bowel syndrome
IHSS	idiopathic hypertrophic subaortic stenosis
I & O	intake and output
IM	intramuscular
INR	international normalized ratio
IOP	intraocular pressure
IPPB	intermittent (or inspiratory) positive pressure breathing
IUD	intrauterine device
IV	intravenous
JVP	jugular venous pressure
kg	kilogram
L	liter
lb	pound
LDH	lactic dehydrogenase
LDL	low-density lipoproteins
LFT	liver function test
LH	luteinizing hormone
LHRH	luteinizing hormone-releasing hormone
m	meter
MAO	monoamine oxidase
MAOI	monoamine oxidase inhibitor
mcg	microgram
mg	milligram
MI	myocardial infarction
min	minute
mL	milliliter
mo	month
MS	multiple sclerosis
ng	nanogram
NMS	neuroleptic malignant syndrome
NPO	nothing by mouth *(nihil per os)*
NSAID	nonsteroidal anti-inflammatory drug
OCD	obsessive compulsive disorder
OTC	over-the-counter
P	pulse
PABA	para-aminobenzoic acid
PAT	paroxysmal atrial tachycardia
PBI	protein-bound iodine

PCWP	pulmonary capillary wedge pressure
PDA	patent ductus arteriosus
PE	pulmonary embolus
PFT	pulmonary function test
PG	prostaglandin
pH	hydrogen ion concentration
PID	pelvic inflammatory disease
PMDD	premenstrual dysphoric disorder
PMS	premenstrual syndrome
PO	orally, by mouth *(per os)*
PRN	when required *(pro re nata)*
PSA	prostate-specific antigen
PT	prothrombin time
PTSD	post-traumatic stress disorder
PTT	partial thromboplastin time
PVCs	premature ventricular contractions
qid	four times a day *(quarter in die)*
R	respiratory rate
RAS	reticular-activating system
RBC	red blood cell
RDA	recommended dietary allowance
RDS	respiratory distress syndrome
REM	rapid eye movement
RNA	ribonucleic acid
RSV	respiratory syncytial virus
SA	sinoatrial
SBE	subacute bacterial endocarditis
sec	seconds
SIADH	syndrome of inappropriate anti-diuretic hormone secretion
SLE	systemic lupus erythematosus
SMA-12	sequential multiple analysis-12
SR	sustained release
SSRI	selective serotonin reuptake inhibitor
STD	sexually transmitted disease
Subcut.	subcutaneous
SWSD	shift-work sleep disorder
T	temperature
$T_{1/2}$	half-life
T_3	triiodothyronine
T_4	thyroxine (tetraiodothyronine)
TB	tuberculosis
TCA	tricyclic antidepressant
TIA	transient ischemic attack
tid	three times a day *(ter in die)*
URI	upper respiratory (tract) infection
US	United States
USP	United States Pharmacopeia
UTI	urinary tract infection
UV	ultraviolet
VLDL	very–low-density lipoproteins
VMA	vanillylmandelic acid
VRE	vancomycin-resistant enterococcus
WBC	white blood cell
WBCT	whole blood clotting time
wk	week
yr	year

Author's acknowledgments

I would like to thank the many people who have worked so hard to make this book possible: Students and colleagues, past and present, who have helped me learn how to make pharmacology clinically useful; the many users of past editions of the book who have taken the time to offer suggestions and provide valuable comments; Judy McCann, Chief Nursing Officer at the Ambler office of Lippincott, Williams & Wilkins; Joan Robinson and Beverly Tscheschlog, who have been so patient, supportive, and helpful; and Linda Ruhf and Karen Kirk, who continue to keep me up-to-date.

A special thanks to the amazing staff of Hastings Two, who teach all of us about patience, respect, and honor; to my students, who keep me on my toes, amused and humbled; to Sandy Harmon for sunshine, courage, and hope; to Tim, Jyoti, Mark, Tracey, Cortney, Bryan, and Kathryn for their unwavering support and encouragement; to Vikas, Nisha, Logan, and Jack for bringing the sunshine back into our lives and for teaching us all the real joy of learning and the wonders of the world; and to Hayley, Brodie, and Stanley, my harshest critics and most joyous supporters, who keep everything in perspective.

Amy M. Karch, RN, MS

Nursing Process Guidelines

The delivery of medical care is in a constant state of change and sometimes in crisis. The population is aging, resulting in more chronic disease and more complex care issues. The population is transient, resulting in unstable support systems and fewer at-home care providers and helpers. At the same time, medicine is undergoing a technological and pharmacological boom. Patients are being discharged earlier from the acute-care facility or not being admitted at all for procedures that used to be done in the hospital with follow-up support and monitoring. Patients are becoming more responsible for their own care and for following complicated medical regimens at home.

Nursing is a unique and complex science and a nurturing and caring art. Traditionally, nurses minister to and soothe the sick; currently, nursing also requires using more technical and scientific skills. Nurses have had to assume increasing responsibilities involved not only with nurturing and caring, but also with assessing, diagnosing, and intervening with patients to treat, prevent, and educate to help people cope with various health states.

The nurse deals with the whole person—the physical, emotional, intellectual, and spiritual aspects—considering the ways that a person responds to disease and treatment, and the change in lifestyle that may be required by both. The nurse is the key health care provider in a position to assess the patient (physical, social, and emotional aspects), administer therapy and medications, teach the patient how best to cope with the therapy to ensure the most effectiveness, and evaluate the effectiveness of therapy. This role requires a broad base of knowledge in the basic sciences (anatomy, physiology, nutrition, chemistry, pharmacology), the social sciences (sociology, psychology), and education (learning approaches, evaluation).

Although all nursing theorists do not completely agree on the process that defines the practice of nursing, most include certain key elements in the nursing process. These elements are the basic components of the decision-making or problem-solving process: assessment (gathering of information), diagnosis (defining that information to arrive at some conclusions), planning (developing a plan of care), intervention (eg, administration, education, comfort measures), and evaluation (determining the effects of the interventions that were performed). Using this process each time a situation arises ensures a method of coping with the overwhelming scientific and technical information. However, the unique emotional, social, and physical aspects that each patient brings to the situation can confound matters. Using the nursing process format in each instance of drug therapy will ensure that the patient receives the best, most efficient, scientifically based holistic care.

Assessment

The first step of the nursing process is the systematic, organized collection of data about the patient. Because the nurse is responsible for holistic care, these data must include information about physical, intellectual, emotional, social, and environmental factors. They will provide the nurse with information needed to plan discharge, plan educational programs, arrange for appropriate consultations, and monitor physical response to treatment or to disease. In actual clinical practice, this process never ends. The patient is not in a steady state but is dynamic, adjusting to physical, emotional, and environmental influences. Each nurse develops a unique approach to the organization of the assessment, an approach that is functional, useful, and appropriate in the clinical setting and that makes sense to that nurse and that clinical situation.

Drug therapy is a complex, integral, and important part of health care today, and the principles of drug therapy need to be incorporated into every patient assessment plan. The particular information that is needed and that should be assessed will vary with each drug, but the concepts involved are similar and are based on the principles of drug therapy. Two important areas that need to be assessed are history and physical presentation.

History

Past experiences and past illnesses and surgeries impact the actual effect of a drug.

Chronic conditions: These may be contraindications to the use of a drug or may require that caution be used or that drug dosage be adjusted.

Drug use: Prescription drugs, over-the-counter (OTC) drugs, street drugs, alcohol, nicotine, and caffeine all may have an impact on the effect of a drug. Patients often neglect to mention OTC drugs, herbal and alternative therapy, vitamin and mineral supplements, and contraceptives, not considering them actual drugs, and should be asked specifically about use of OTC drugs, herbals, supplements, contraceptives, or any drug that might be taken on a long-term basis and not mentioned.

Allergies: Past exposure to a drug or other allergen can predict a future reaction or need to use certain drugs, food, or animal products cautiously.

Level of education: This information will help to provide a basis for patient education programs and level of explanation.

Level of understanding of disease and therapy: This information also will direct the development of educational information.

Social supports: Patients are being discharged earlier than ever before and often need assistance at home to provide care and institute and monitor drug therapy.

Financial supports: The financial impact of health care and the high cost of medications need to be considered when prescribing drugs. These factors may impact a patient's ability to follow through with drug therapy.

Pattern of health care: The way that a patient seeks health care will give the nurse valuable information to include in educational information. Does this patient routinely seek physical examinations and follow-up care or wait for emergency situations?

Physical assessment

Weight: Weight is an important factor when determining if the recommended dosage of a drug is appropriate. The recommended dosage is based on the 150-lb adult male. Patients who are much lighter or much heavier will need a dosage adjustment.

Age: Patients at the extremes of the age spectrum—pediatric and geriatric—often require dosage adjustments based on the functional level of the liver and kidneys and the responsiveness of other organs.

Physical parameters related to the disease state or known drug effects: Assessment of these factors before beginning drug therapy will give a baseline level with which future assessments can be compared to determine the effects of drug therapy. The specific parameters that need to be assessed will depend on the disease process being treated and on the expected therapeutic and adverse effects of the drug therapy. Because the nurse has the greatest direct and continual contact with the patient, the nurse has the best opportunity to detect the minute changes that will determine the course of drug therapy and therapeutic success or the need for discontinuation because of adverse or unacceptable responses.

The monographs in this book include the specific parameters that need to be assessed in relation to the particular drug being discussed (see the sample monograph in the preface). This assessment provides not only the baseline information needed before giving that drug, but the data needed to evaluate the effects of that drug on the patient. The information given in this area should supplement the overall nursing assessment of the patient, which will include social, intellectual, financial, environmental, and other physical data.

Nursing diagnosis

Once data have been collected, the nurse must organize and analyze that information to arrive at a nursing diagnosis. A nursing diagnosis is simply a statement of the patient's status from a nursing perspective. This statement directs appropriate nursing interventions. A nursing diagnosis will show actual or potential alteration in patient function based on the assessment of the clinical situation. Because drug therapy is only a small part of the overall patient situation, the nursing diagnoses that are related to drug therapy must be incorporated into a total picture of the patient. In many cases the drug therapy will not present a new nursing diagnosis, but the desired effects and adverse effects related to each drug given should be considered in the identified nursing diagnoses for each patient. NANDA International (NANDA-I) produces a coded list of accepted nursing diagnoses that are updated periodically.

Interventions

The assessment and diagnosis of the patient's situation will direct specific nursing interventions. Four types of interventions are frequently involved in drug therapy: Drug administration, provision of comfort measures, monitoring the effects of drug therapy, and patient and family teaching.

Drug administration

Drug: Ensuring that the drug being administered is the correct dose of the correct drug at the correct time, and is being given to the correct patient, is standard nursing practice.

Storage: Some drugs require specific storage environments (eg, refrigeration, protection from light).

Route: Determining the best route of administration is often determined by the prescription of the drug. Nurses can often have an impact on modifying the prescribed route to determine the most efficient route and the most comfortable one for the patient based on his or her specific situation. When establishing the prescribed route, it is important to check the proper method of administering a drug by that route.

Dosage: Drug dosage may need to be calculated based on available drug form, patient body weight or surface area, or kidney function.

Preparation: Some drugs require specific preparation before administration. Oral drugs may need to be shaken or crushed; parenteral drugs may need to be reconstituted or diluted with specific solutions; topical drugs may require specific handling before administration.

Timing: Actual administration of a drug may require coordination with the administration of other drugs, foods, or physical parameters. The nurse, as the caregiver most frequently involved in administering a drug, must be aware of and juggle all of these factors and educate the patient to do this on his or her own.

Documentation: Once the nurse has assessed the patient, made the appropriate nursing diagnoses, and delivered the correct drug by the correct route, in the correct dose, and at the correct time, that information needs to be recorded in accordance with the local requirements for documenting medication administration.

Each monograph in this book contains pertinent guidelines for storage, dosage, preparation, and administration of the drug being discussed.

Comfort measures

Nurses are in the unique position to help the patient cope with the effects of drug therapy.

Placebo effect: The anticipation that a drug will be helpful (placebo effect) has been proved to have tremendous impact on the actual success of drug therapy, so the nurse's attitude and support can be a critical part of drug therapy. A back rub, a kind word, and a positive approach may be as beneficial as the drug itself.

Side effects: These interventions can be directed at decreasing the impact of the anticipated side effects of the drug and promoting patient safety. Such interventions include environmental control (eg, temperature, lighting), safety measures (eg, avoiding driving, avoiding the sun, using side rails), physical comfort (eg, skin care, laxatives, frequent meals).

Lifestyle adjustment: Some drug effects will require that a patient change his or her lifestyle to cope effectively. Diuretic users may have to rearrange the day to be near toilet facilities when the drug works. MAOI users have to adjust their diet to prevent serious drug effects.

Each monograph in this book will include a list of pertinent comfort measures appropriate to that particular drug.

Education

With patients becoming more responsible for their own care, it is essential that they have all of the information necessary to ensure safe and effective drug therapy at home. Many states now require that the patient be given written information. Key elements that need to be included in any drug education include the following:

- Name, dose, and action of drug: With many people seeing more than one health care provider, this information is important for ensuring safe and effective drug therapy.
- Timing of administration: Patients need to know specifically when to take the drug with regard to frequency, other drugs, and meals.
- Special storage and preparation instructions: Some drugs require particular handling that the patient will need to have spelled out.
- Specific OTC drugs, vitamin and mineral supplements, or alternative therapies to avoid: Many people do not consider these to be actual drugs and may inadvertently take them and cause unwanted or even dangerous drug interactions. Explaining problems will help the patient avoid these potential situations.
- Special comfort or safety measures that need to be considered: Alerting the patient to ways to cope with anticipated side effects will prevent a great deal of anxiety and noncompliance with drug therapy. The patient also may need to be alerted to the need to return for follow-up tests or evaluation.
- Safety measures: All patients need to be alerted to keep drugs out of the reach of children. They also need to be reminded to tell any health care provider whom they see that they are taking this drug. This can prevent drug-drug interactions, polypharmacy, and misdiagnosing based on drug effects.
- Specific points about drug toxicity: Warning signs of drug toxicity that the patient should be aware of should be listed. He or she can be advised to notify the health care provider if any of these effects occur.
- Specific warnings about drug discontinuation: Some drugs with a small margin of safety and drugs with particular systemic effects cannot be stopped abruptly without dangerous effects. Patients taking these drugs need to be alerted to the problem and encouraged to call immediately if they cannot take their medication for any reason (eg, illness, financial).

Each drug monograph in this book lists specific teaching points that relate to that particular drug. An example of a compact, written drug card developed from the information in the monograph is shown on page 5.

Evaluation

Evaluation is part of the continual process of patient care that leads to changes in assessment, diagnosis, and intervention. The patient is continually evaluated for therapeutic response, the occurrence of drug side effects, and the occurrence of drug-drug, drug-food, drug-laboratory test, or drug-alternative therapy interactions.

The efficacy of the nursing interventions and the education program must be evaluated. In some situations, the nurse will evaluate the patient simply by reapplying the beginning steps of the nursing process and analyzing for change. In some cases of drug therapy, particular therapeutic drug levels need to be evaluated as well.

Monographs in this book list only specific evaluation criteria, such as therapeutic serum levels, as they apply to each drug. Regular evaluation of drug effects, side effects, and the efficacy of comfort measures and education

Patient Drug Sheet: Oral Linezolid

Patient's Name: Mr. Kors
Prescriber's Name: J. Smith, ANP
Phone Number: 555-555-5555

Instructions:

1. The name of your drug is *linezolid*; the brand name is *Zyvox*. This drug is an antibiotic that is being used to treat your *pneumonia*. This drug is very specific in its action and is only indicated for your particular infection. Take the full course of your drug. Do not share this drug with other people or save tablets for future use.
2. The dose of the drug that has been prescribed for you is: *600 mg* (*1 tablet*).
3. The drug should be taken *once every 12 hours*. The best time for you to take this drug will be *8:00 in the morning and 8:00 in the evening*. Do not skip any doses. Do not take two doses at once if you forget a dose. If you miss a dose, take the dose as soon as you remember and then again in 12 hours.
4. The drug can be taken with food if GI upset is a problem. Avoid foods that are rich in tyramine (list is below) while you are taking this drug.
5. The following side effects may occur:

   Nausea, vomiting, abdominal pain (taking the drug with food and eating frequent small meals may help).

   Diarrhea (ensure ready access to bathroom facilities). Notify your health care provider if this becomes severe.
6. Do not take this drug with over-the-counter drugs or herbal remedies without first checking with your health care provider. Many of these agents can cause problems with your drug.
7. Tell any nurse, physician, or dentist who is taking care of you that you are on this drug.
8. Keep this and all medications out of the reach of children.

Notify your health care provider if any of the following occur:

Rash, severe GI problems, bloody or excessive diarrhea, weakness, tremors, increased bleeding or bruising, anxiety.

Foods high in tyramine to avoid: Aged cheeses, avocados, bananas, beer, bologna, caffeinated beverages, chocolate, liver, over-ripe fruit, pepperoni, pickled fish, red wine, salami, smoked fish, yeast, yogurt.

programs will not be specifically listed but can be deduced from information in the monograph regarding therapeutic effects and adverse effects. See *Nursing care plan: Patient receiving oral linezolid,* page 6. *Anatomy of a monograph,* in the preface, provides additional guidelines for using each section of a monograph as it applies to the nursing process.

Nursing care plan: Patient receiving oral linezolid

Assessment	Nursing diagnoses	Interventions	Evaluation
History (contraindications and cautions) Hypertension Hyperthyroidism Blood dyscrasias Hepatic dysfunction Pheochromocytoma Phenylketonuria Carcinoid syndrome Pregnancy Lactation Known allergy to linezolid **Medication History** (possible drug-drug interactions) Pseudoephedrine SSRIs MAOIs Antiplatelet drugs **Diet History** (possible drug-food interactions) Foods high in tyramine **Physical Assessment** (screen for contraindications and to establish a baseline for evaluating effects and adverse effects) **CNS:** Affect, reflexes, orientation **CV:** P, BP, peripheral perfusion **GI:** Bowel sounds, liver evaluation **Hematologic:** CBC with differential, liver function tests **Local:** Culture site of infection **Skin:** Color, lesions	Imbalanced nutrition, less than body requirements, related to GI effects Acute pain related to GI effects, headache Ineffective peripheral tissue perfusion related to bone marrow effects Deficient knowledge related to drug therapy	Safe and appropriate administration of drug: Culture infection site to ensure appropriate use of drug Provision of safety and comfort measures: • Monitor BP periodically • Monitor platelet counts before and periodically during therapy • Alleviation of GI upset • Ready access to bathroom facilities • Nutritional consult • Safety provisions if dizziness and CNS effects occur • Avoidance of tyramine-rich foods Patient teaching regarding: • Drug • Side effects to anticipate • Warnings • Reactions to report Support and encouragement to cope with disease, high cost of therapy, and side effects Provision of emergency and life-support measures in cases of acute hypersensitivity	Monitor patient for therapeutic effects of drug: Resolution of infection. If resolution does not occur, reculture site. Monitor patient for adverse effects of drug: • GI upset—nausea, vomiting, diarrhea • Liver function changes • Pseudomembranous colitis • Blood dyscrasias—changes in platelet counts • Fever • Rash • Sweating • Photosensitivity • Acute hypersensitivity reactions Evaluate effectiveness of patient teaching program: Patient can name drug, dose of drug, use of drug, adverse effects to expect, reactions to report. Monitor patient for drug-drug, drug-food interactions as appropriate. Evaluate effectiveness of life-support measures if needed.

Preventing Medication Errors

Growing numbers of patients—and drugs—bring increased risk of medication errors. Compounding this risk is the tremendous upsurge in the use of over-the-counter (OTC) drugs and herbal remedies. Physicians, pharmacists, and nurses serve as checkpoints for ensuring medication safety. A nurse is commonly the final check because nurses usually administer drugs and have responsibility for discharging patients to home to manage a potentially complicated drug regimen.

The monumental task of ensuring medication safety can be managed by consistently using the six rights of drug administration: right drug, right route, right dose, right time, right patient, and right documentation.

Right drug

- Always review a drug order before administering the drug.
- Do not assume that a computer system is always right and will protect the patient. Always double check.
- Make sure the drug name is correct. Ask for a brand name and a generic name. Because many drug names look and sound alike (note the Clinical Alerts throughout the monographs), the chance of reading the name incorrectly is greatly reduced if both generic and brand names are used.
- Avoid taking verbal or telephone orders whenever possible. If you must, have a second person listen in to verify and clarify the order.
- Abbreviations can be confusing between and even within health care facilities. Do not be afraid or embarrassed to ask the meaning of an abbreviation, even a common one. For instance, many people use hs to mean hour of sleep, others may read it as every hour. As much as possible, spell out abbreviations for clarification.
- Also, consider whether the drug makes sense for the patient's diagnosis. If you do not know or you have questions, look up the drug and ask the patient what it is being used for.

Right route

- Review the available forms of a drug to make sure the drug can be given according to the order.
- Check the routes available and the appropriateness of the route. Be familiar with the appropriate and safe technique for administration by the ordered route.
- Make sure the patient is able to take the drug by the route indicated. If you know that the patient has trouble swallowing, for example, you also know that a liquid form of the drug may be better than a tablet or capsule.
- Do not use abbreviations for routes because the danger of confusion is too great. For example, SC is often used to mean subcutaneous, but it has been misinterpreted to mean sublingual among other misinterpretations. Also, IV can be misinterpreted to mean IU, or international units.

Right dose

- Always place a 0 to the left of a decimal point, and never place a 0 to the right of a decimal point. For example, 0.5 is correct (not .5, which can be easily mistaken for 5) and 5 is correct (not 5.0, which can be easily mistaken for 50). If you see an ordered dose that starts with a decimal point, question it. And if a dose seems much too big, question that.
- Double-check drug calculations. If a dose has to be calculated for pediatric or other use, always have someone double-check the math, even if a computer did the calculations. This is especially important with drugs that have small margins of safety, such as digoxin and insulin.
- Check the measuring devices used for liquid drugs. Advise patients not to use kitchen teaspoons or tablespoons to measure drug doses.
- Do not cut tablets in half to get the correct dose without checking the warnings that come with the drug. Many drugs cannot be cut, crushed, or chewed because of the matrix systems that have been developed to prepare the drugs.

Right time

- Increased workloads, decreased nursing staffs, and constant interruptions can interfere with the delivery of medications at the right times. Even at home, patients are busy, have tight schedules, and may fail to follow a precise schedule. Ensure the timely delivery of the patient's drugs by scheduling dosage with other drugs, meals, or other consistent events to maintain the serum level.
- Teach patients the importance of timing critical drugs. Keep in mind that patients tend to take all of their daily drugs at once, in the morning, to reduce the risk of forgetting them. But with critical drugs, such as those with a small margin of safety, those that interact, and those that need meticulous spacing, you will need to stress the importance of accurate timing. As needed, make detailed medication schedules and prepare pill boxes.

Right patient

- Check the patient's identification even if you think you know who the patient is. Ask for the patient's full name, and check the patient's identification band if available.
- Review the patient's diagnosis, and verify that the drug matches the diagnosis. If a drug does not make sense for the patient's diagnosis, look it up and, if necessary, consult with the prescriber.
- Make sure all allergies have been checked before giving a drug. Serious adverse reactions can be avoided if allergies are known.
- Ask patients specifically about OTC drugs, vitamin and mineral supplements, herbal remedies, and routine drugs that they may not think to mention, such as oral contraceptives, thyroid hormones, and insulin. Serious overdoses, adverse reactions, and drug interactions can be avoided if this information is acquired early.
- Review the patient's drug regimen to prevent potential interactions between the drug you are about to give and drugs the patient already takes. If you are not sure about potential interactions, consult a drug reference.

The bottom line in avoiding medication errors is simple: "If in doubt, check it out." A strange abbreviation, a drug or dosage that is new to you, and a confusing name are all examples that signal a need for follow-up. Look up the drug in your drug guide or call the prescriber or the pharmacy to double check. Never give a drug until you have satisfied yourself that it is the right drug, given by the right route, at the right dose, at the right time, and to the right patient.

Right documentation

Document according to facility policy. Include the drug name, dose, route, and time of administration. Note special circumstances, such as the patient having difficulty swallowing or the site of the injection.

Error reporting

In recent years, the incidence of medication errors has become a frequent media headline. As the population ages and more people are taking multiple medications—and as more drugs become available—the possibilities for medication errors seem to be increasing. Institutions have adopted policies for reporting errors, which protect patients and staff and identify the need for educational programs within the institution, but it is also important to submit information about errors to national programs. These national programs, coordinated by the US Pharmacopeia (USP), help to gather and disseminate information about errors, to prevent their recurrence at other sites and by other providers. These reports might prompt the issuing of prescriber warnings to alert health care providers about potential or actual medication errors and to prevent these same errors from recurring. The reporting of actual or potential errors results in alerts and publicity about sound-alike drug names, problems with abbreviations, the need for clear writing of dosages and times, incorrect calculations, and transcribing issues.

The strongest warning that the FDA can give about potential drug problems is called a black box warning. This warning may be part of the initial drug prescribing information, if a drug is found to have potentially serious adverse effects before approval, or the warning may be added as a result of postmarketing reports of adverse effects or serious errors involving the drug. The black box warning alerts the health care provider and patient about screening to be done, adverse effects to watch for, and other drugs to avoid. The monographs in this book will highlight black box warnings to help bring attention to these reported effects and to help decrease medication errors and promote patient safety.

If you witness or participate in an actual or potential medication error, it is important to report that error to the national clearinghouse to ultimately help other professionals avoid similar errors. To help streamline the process of reporting and make it as easy as possible for professionals to participate, the USP maintains one central reporting center, from which it disseminates information to the FDA, drug manufacturers, and the Institute for Safe Medication Practices (ISMP). You can report an actual error or potential error by calling 1-800-23-ERROR, the USP Medication Errors Reporting Program. Their office will send you a mailer to fill out and return to them. Or, you can log on to www.usp.org to report an error online or to print out the form to mail or fax back to the USP. You may request to remain anonymous to all institutions to which the report is subsequently disseminated if you feel uncomfortable sharing this information. If you aren't sure about what you want to report, you may report errors to the USP through the ISMP Web site at www.ismp.org, which also offers a discussion forum on medication errors.

What kind of errors should be reported? Errors (or potential errors) such as administration of the wrong drug, strength, or dose of a drug; incorrect routes of administration; miscalculations; misuse of medical equipment; mistakes in prescribing or transcribing (misunderstanding of verbal orders); and errors resulting from sound-alike or look-alike names. In your report, you will be asked to include the following:

1. A description of the error or preventable adverse drug reaction. What went wrong?
2. Was this an actual medication accident (reached the patient) or are you expressing concern about a potential error or writing about an error that was discovered before it reached the patient?
3. Patient outcome. Did the patient suffer any adverse effects?
4. Type of practice site (eg, hospital, private office, retail pharmacy, drug company, long-term care facility)
5. Generic name (International Nonproprietary Name [INN] or official name) of all products involved
6. Brand name of all products involved
7. Dosage form, concentration or strength, and so forth
8. Where error was based on communication problem, is a sample of the order available? Are package label samples or pictures available if requested?
9. Your recommendations for error prevention.

You will also be asked to provide your name, title, facility address and e-mail, fax, or phone location if someone wants to contact you about details. You can remain anonymous and no one will contact your employer to discuss the report. The ISMP publishes case studies and publicizes warnings and alerts based on clinician reports of medication errors. Their efforts have helped to increase recognition of the many types of errors, such as those involving sound-alike names, look-alike names and packaging, instructions on equipment and delivery devices, and others.

> To report an actual or potential medication error, call 1-800-23-ERROR or log on to www.usp.org.
>
> For more information regarding warnings, error alerts, and case reports log on to www.ismp.org, www.fda.gov, or www.medwatch.gov.

Alkylating Drugs

DANGEROUS DRUG

PREGNANCY CATEGORY D

Therapeutic actions

Alkylating drugs are cytotoxic: They alkylate cellular DNA, interfering with the replication of susceptible cells and causing cell death. Their action is most evident in rapidly dividing cells.

Indications

- Palliative treatment of chronic lymphocytic leukemia; malignant lymphomas, including lymphosarcoma, giant follicular lymphoma; brain tumors; Hodgkin's lymphoma; multiple myelomas; testicular cancers; pancreatic cancer; ovarian and breast cancers
- Used as part of multiple-drug regimens

Contraindications and cautions

- Contraindicated with hypersensitivity to the drugs, concurrent radiation therapy, hematopoietic depression, pregnancy, lactation.

Adverse effects

- **CNS:** *Tremors, muscular twitching, confusion,* agitation, ataxia, flaccid paresis, hallucinations, seizures
- **Dermatologic:** *Skin rash, urticaria, alopecia,* keratitis
- **GI:** Nausea, vomiting, anorexia, **hepatotoxicity**
- **GU:** Sterility
- **Hematologic:** *Bone marrow depression,* hyperuricemia
- **Respiratory:** Bronchopulmonary dysplasia, **pulmonary fibrosis**
- **Other:** *Cancer, acute leukemia*

■ Nursing considerations

Assessment

- **History:** Hypersensitivity to drug, radiation therapy, hematopoietic depression, pregnancy, lactation
- **Physical:** T; weight; skin color, lesions; R, adventitious sounds; liver evaluation; CBC, differential, Hgb, uric acid, LFTs, renal function tests

Interventions

⊗ ***Black box warning*** Arrange for blood tests to evaluate hematopoietic function prior to and weekly during therapy; severe bone marrow suppression is possible.

- Restrict dosage within 4 wk after a full course of radiation therapy or chemotherapy because of risk of severe bone marrow depression.
- Ensure that patient is well hydrated before treatment.
- Arrange for frequent small meals and dietary consultation to maintain nutrition if GI upset occurs.
- Arrange for skin care for rashes.

⊗ ***Black box warning*** Suggest use of contraception; serious fetal abnormalities or death is possible.

Teaching points

- You may experience these side effects: Nausea, vomiting, loss of appetite (dividing dose may help; frequent small meals may help; maintain fluid intake and nutrition; drink at least 10–12 glasses of fluid each day); infertility (potentially irreversible and irregular menses to amenorrhea and aspermia; discuss feelings with your health care provider); these drugs can cause severe birth defects; use birth control methods while on these drugs.
- Report unusual bleeding or bruising; fever, chills, sore throat; cough, shortness of breath; yellowing of the skin or eyes; flank or stomach pain.

Representative drugs

altretamine
bendamustine
busulfan
carboplatin
carmustine
chlorambucil

cisplatin
cyclophosphamide
dacarbazine
estramustine
ifosfamide
lomustine
mechlorethamine
melphalan
oxaliplatin
procarbazine
streptozocin
temozolomide
thiotepa

Alpha$_1$-adrenergic Blockers

PREGNANCY CATEGORY C

Therapeutic actions

Alpha$_1$-adrenergic blockers selectively block postsynaptic alpha$_1$-adrenergic receptors, decreasing sympathetic tone on the vasculature, dilating arterioles and veins, and lowering both supine and standing BP; unlike conventional alpha-adrenergic blockers (phentolamine), they do not also block alpha$_2$ presynaptic receptors, so they do not cause reflex tachycardia. They also relax smooth muscle of bladder and prostate.

Indications

- Treatment of hypertension (alone or with other drugs)
- Treatment of BPH (alfuzosin, doxazosin, terazosin, tamsulosin)
- Unlabeled uses: Symptomatic treatment of chronic abacterial prostatitis (terazosin)

Contraindications and cautions

- Contraindicated with hypersensitivity to any alpha$_1$-adrenergic blocker, lactation.
- Use cautiously with heart failure, renal failure, pregnancy.

Adverse effects

- **CNS:** *Dizziness, headache, drowsiness, lack of energy, weakness,* nervousness, vertigo, depression, paresthesias
- **CV:** *Palpitations,* sodium and water retention, increased plasma volume, edema, dyspnea, syncope, tachycardia, orthostatic hypotension
- **Dermatologic:** Rash, pruritus, lichen planus
- **EENT:** Blurred vision, reddened sclera, epistaxis, tinnitus, dry mouth, nasal congestion
- **GI:** *Nausea,* vomiting, diarrhea, constipation, abdominal discomfort or pain
- **GU:** Urinary frequency, incontinence, impotence
- **Other:** Diaphoresis

Interactions

✱ **Drug-drug** • Severity and duration of hypotension following first dose of drug may be greater in patients receiving beta-adrenergic blockers (propranolol), verapamil

■ Nursing considerations

Assessment

- **History:** Hypersensitivity to any alpha$_1$-adrenergic blocker, heart failure, renal failure, lactation
- **Physical:** Weight; skin color, lesions; orientation, affect, reflexes; ophthalmologic examination; P, BP, orthostatic BP, supine BP, perfusion, edema, auscultation; R, adventitious sounds, status of nasal mucous membranes; bowel sounds, normal output; voiding pattern, normal output; renal function tests, urinalysis

Interventions

- Administer, or have patient take, first dose at night to lessen likelihood of first-dose syncope believed to be caused by excessive orthostatic hypotension.
- Have patient lie down, and treat supportively if syncope occurs; condition is self-limiting.
- Monitor patient for orthostatic hypotension: most marked in the morning, accentuated by hot weather, alcohol, exercise.
- Monitor edema, weight in patients with incipient cardiac decompensation; arrange to add a thiazide diuretic to the drug regimen if sodium and fluid retention, signs of impending heart failure occur.
- Provide frequent small meals, frequent mouth care if GI effects occur.
- Establish safety precautions if CNS, hypotensive changes occur (side rails, accompany patient).
- Arrange for analgesic for patients experiencing headache.

- Provide consultations to help patient cope with sexual dysfunction and priapism.

Teaching points

- Take these drugs exactly as prescribed. Take the first dose at bedtime. Do not drive a car or operate machinery for 4 hours after the first dose.
- Avoid over-the-counter drugs (nose drops, cold remedies) while taking these drugs. If you feel you need one of these preparations, consult your health care provider.
- You may experience these side effects: Dizziness, weakness may occur when changing position, in the early morning, after exercise, in hot weather, and after consuming alcohol; tolerance may occur after taking these drugs for a while, but avoid driving or engaging in tasks that require alertness while experiencing these symptoms; change position slowly, and use caution in climbing stairs; lie down if dizziness persists; GI upset (frequent small meals may help); impotence (discuss this with your health care provider); dry mouth (sucking on sugarless lozenges, ice chips may help); stuffy nose. Most of these effects will stop with continued therapy.
- Report frequent dizziness or faintness.

Representative drugs

alfuzosin
doxazosin
prazosin
silodosin
tamsulosin
terazosin

Aminoglycosides

PREGNANCY CATEGORY D

Therapeutic actions

Aminoglycosides are antibiotics that are bactericidal. They inhibit protein synthesis in susceptible strains of gram-negative bacteria, appear to disrupt the functional integrity of bacterial cell membrane, causing cell death. Oral aminoglycosides are very poorly absorbed and are used for the suppression of GI bacterial flora.

Indications

- Short-term treatment of serious infections caused by susceptible strains of *Pseudomonas* species, *Escherichia coli,* indole-positive *Proteus* species, *Providencia* species, *Klebsiella-Enterobacter-Serratia* species, *Acinetobacter* species
- Suspected gram-negative infections before results of susceptibility studies are known
- Initial treatment of staphylococcal infections when penicillin is contraindicated or when infection may be caused by mixed organisms
- Neonatal sepsis when other antibiotics cannot be used (used in combination with penicillin-type drug)
- Unlabeled uses: As part of a multidrug regimen for treatment of *Mycobacterium avium* complex (a common infection in AIDS patients) and orally for the treatment of intestinal amebiasis; adjunctive treatment of hepatic coma and for suppression of intestinal bacteria for surgery

Contraindications and cautions

- Contraindicated with allergy to any aminoglycosides, renal disease, hepatic disease, preexisting hearing loss, myasthenia gravis, parkinsonism, infant botulism, lactation.
- Use cautiously in elderly patients; patients with diminished hearing; patients with decreased renal function, dehydration, neuromuscular disorders, pregnancy.

Adverse effects

- **CNS:** *Ototoxicity,* confusion, disorientation, depression, lethargy, nystagmus, visual disturbances, headache, fever, numbness, tingling, tremor, paresthesias, muscle twitching, seizures, muscular weakness, neuromuscular blockade, apnea
- **CV:** Palpitations, hypotension, hypertension
- **GI:** Nausea, vomiting, anorexia, diarrhea, weight loss, stomatitis, increased salivation, splenomegaly
- **GU:** *Nephrotoxicity*
- **Hematologic:** Leukemoid reaction, agranulocytosis, granulocytosis, leukopenia, leukocytosis, thrombocytopenia, eosinophilia, pancytopenia, anemia, hemolytic anemia, increased or decreased reticulocyte count, electrolyte disturbances

- **Hepatic:** Hepatic toxicity, hepatomegaly
- **Hypersensitivity:** Purpura, rash, urticaria, exfoliative dermatitis, itching
- **Other:** *Superinfections, pain and irritation at IM injection sites*

Interactions

✱**Drug-drug** • Increased ototoxic and nephrotoxic effects if taken with potent diuretics and similarly toxic drugs (cephalosporins) • Increased likelihood of neuromuscular blockade if given shortly after general anesthetics, depolarizing and nondepolarizing neuromuscular junction blockers

■ Nursing considerations

Assessment

- **History:** Allergy to any aminoglycosides, renal disease, hepatic disease, preexisting hearing loss, myasthenia gravis, parkinsonism, infant botulism, lactation, diminished hearing, decreased renal function, dehydration, neuromuscular disorders
- **Physical:** Arrange culture and sensitivity tests of infection prior to therapy; renal function tests before, during, and after therapy; eighth cranial nerve function, and state of hydration, during and after therapy; LFTs, CBC; skin color, lesions; orientation, affect; reflexes, bilateral grip strength; body weight; bowel sounds

Interventions

⊗ ***Black box warning*** Monitor patient carefully for severe renal toxicity and ototoxicity; discontinue drug or adjust dosage at first indication of either.

- Arrange for culture and sensitivity testing of infected area prior to treatment.
- Monitor duration of treatment: Usual duration is 7–10 days. If no clinical response within 3–5 days, stop therapy. Prolonged treatment leads to increased risk of toxicity. If drug is used longer than 10 days, monitor auditory and renal function daily.
- Give IM dosage by deep injection.
- Ensure that patient is well hydrated before and during therapy.
- Establish safety measures if CNS, vestibular nerve effects occur (use of side rails, assistance with ambulation).
- Provide frequent small meals if nausea, anorexia occur.
- Provide comfort measures and medication for superinfections.
- Monitor drug levels periodically if used for prolonged periods.

Teaching points

- Take full course of oral drugs; drink plenty of fluids.
- You may experience these side effects: Ringing in the ears, headache, dizziness (reversible; safety measures need to be taken if severe); nausea, vomiting, loss of appetite (frequent small meals, frequent mouth care may help).
- Report pain at injection site, severe headache, dizziness, loss of hearing, changes in urine pattern, difficulty breathing, rash or skin lesions.

Representative drugs

amikacin sulfate
gentamicin
kanamycin
neomycin (oral)
streptomycin
tobramycin (parenteral)

Angiotensin-converting Enzyme (ACE) Inhibitors

PREGNANCY CATEGORY C (FIRST TRIMESTER)

PREGNANCY CATEGORY D (SECOND AND THIRD TRIMESTERS)

Therapeutic actions

ACE inhibitors block ACEs in the lungs from converting angiotensin I, activated when renin is released from the kidneys, to angiotensin II, a powerful vasoconstrictor. Blocking this conversion leads to decreased BP, decreased aldosterone secretion, a small increase in serum potassium levels, and sodium and fluid loss; increased prostaglandin synthesis also may be involved in the antihypertensive action.

Indications

- Treatment of hypertension (alone or with thiazide-type diuretics)
- Treatment of heart failure (used with diuretics and digitalis)
- Treatment of stable patients within 24 hr of acute MI to improve survival (lisinopril)
- Reduction in risk of MI, CVA, and death from CV causes (ramipril)
- Treatment of left ventricular dysfunction post-MI (captopril, trandolapril)
- Treatment of asymptomatic left ventricular dysfunction (enalapril)
- Treatment of diabetic nephropathy (captopril)
- Unlabeled uses: Renovascular hypertension, nondiabetic nephropathy, migraine prophylaxis, stroke prevention, heart failure, high risk of CAD, diabetes, chronic renal disease, scleroderma renal crisis

Contraindications and cautions

- Contraindicated with allergy to the drug, impaired renal function, heart failure, salt or volume depletion, lactation, pregnancy, history of angioedema, bilateral stenosis.

Adverse effects

- **CV:** Tachycardia, angina pectoris, **MI,** Raynaud's syndrome, heart failure, hypotension in salt- or volume-depleted patients
- **Dermatologic:** *Rash,* pruritus, alopecia, pemphigoid-like reaction, scalded mouth sensation, exfoliative dermatitis, photosensitivity
- **GI:** *Gastric irritation, aphthous ulcers,* peptic ulcers, dysgeusia, cholestatic jaundice, hepatocellular injury, anorexia, constipation
- **GU:** Proteinuria, renal insufficiency, renal failure, polyuria, oliguria, urinary frequency
- **Hematologic:** Neutropenia, agranulocytosis, thrombocytopenia, hemolytic anemia, **pancytopenia,** hyperkalemia
- **Other:** *Cough,* malaise, dry mouth, lymphadenopathy

Interactions

✱ **Drug-drug** • Increased risk of hypersensitivity reactions with allopurinol • Decreased antihypertensive effects with indomethacin

✱ **Drug-food** • Decreased absorption of selected drugs if taken with food

✱ **Drug-lab test** • False-positive test for urine acetone

■ Nursing considerations

Assessment

- **History:** Allergy to ACE inhibitors, impaired renal function, heart failure, salt or volume depletion, pregnancy, lactation
- **Physical:** Skin color, lesions, turgor; T, P, BP, peripheral perfusion; mucous membranes; bowel sounds; liver evaluation; urinalysis, LFTs, renal function tests, CBC and differential, potassium levels

Interventions

⊗ ***Black box warning*** Ensure that patient is not pregnant before beginning therapy; serious fetal effects can occur.

- Administer 1 hr before or 2 hr after meals; is affected by food in GI tract (captopril, moexipril).
- Alert surgeon and mark patient's chart that ACE inhibitor is being taken; angiotensin II formation subsequent to compensatory renin release during surgery will be blocked; hypotension may be reversed with volume expansion.
- Monitor patient closely in situations that may lead to a fall in BP due to reduction in fluid volume (excessive perspiration and dehydration, vomiting, diarrhea) because excessive hypotension may occur.
- Arrange for reduced dosage in patients with impaired renal function.
- Arrange for bowel program if constipation occurs.
- Provide frequent small meals if GI upset is severe.
- Provide frequent mouth care and oral hygiene if mouth sores, alteration in taste occur.
- Caution patient to change position slowly if orthostatic changes occur.
- Provide skin care as needed.

Teaching points

- Take these drugs 1 hour before or 2 hours after meals; do not take with food (captopril, moexipril).

- Do not stop taking the medication without consulting your health care provider.
- Be careful with any conditions that may lead to a drop in blood pressure (such as diarrhea, sweating, vomiting, dehydration); if light-headedness or dizziness occurs, consult your health care provider.
- Avoid over-the-counter drugs, especially cough, cold, allergy medications. If you need one of these, consult your health care provider.
- You may experience these side effects: GI upset, loss of appetite, change in taste perception (limited effects; if they persist or become a problem, consult your health care provider); mouth sores (frequent mouth care may help); skin rash; fast heart rate; dizziness, light-headedness (passes after a few days of therapy; if it occurs, change position slowly and limit activities requiring alertness and precision).
- Report mouth sores; sore throat, fever, chills; swelling of the hands, feet; irregular heartbeat, chest pains; swelling of the face, eyes, lips, tongue; difficulty breathing.

Representative drugs

benazepril
captopril
enalapril
enalaprilat
fosinopril
lisinopril
moexipril
perindopril
quinapril
ramipril
trandolapril

Angiotensin II Receptor Blockers (ARBs)

PREGNANCY CATEGORY C (FIRST TRIMESTER)

PREGNANCY CATEGORY D (SECOND AND THIRD TRIMESTERS)

Therapeutic actions

ARBs selectively block the binding of angiotensin II to specific tissue receptors found in the vascular smooth muscle and adrenal gland. This action blocks the vasoconstriction effect of the renin-angiotensin system as well as the release of aldosterone leading to decreased BP; may block vessel remodeling that occurs in hypertension and contributes to the development of atherosclerosis.

Indications

- Treatment of hypertension, alone or in combination with other antihypertensives
- Nephropathy in type 2 diabetes (losartan, irbesartan)
- Treatment of heart failure in patients resistant to ACE inhibitors (valsartan)
- Reduction in the risk of CVA in patients with hypertension and left ventricular hypertrophy (losartan)

Contraindications and cautions

- Contraindicated with hypersensitivity to any ARB, pregnancy (use during the second or third trimester can cause injury or even death to the fetus), lactation.
- Use cautiously with renal impairment, hypovolemia.

Adverse effects

- **CNS:** Headache, dizziness, syncope, muscle weakness, *fatigue, depression*
- **CV:** Hypotension
- **Dermatologic:** Rash, inflammation, urticaria, pruritus, alopecia, dry skin
- **GI:** Diarrhea, *abdominal pain,* nausea, constipation
- **Respiratory:** *URI symptoms,* cough, sinus disorders
- **Other:** Cancer in preclinical studies, UTIs

Interactions

✱ **Drug-drug** • Decreased effectiveness if combined with phenobarbital

■ Nursing considerations

Assessment

- **History:** Hypersensitivity to any ARB, pregnancy, lactation, renal impairment, hypovolemia
- **Physical:** Skin lesions, turgor; body T; reflexes, affect; BP; R, respiratory auscultation; renal function tests

Interventions

- Administer without regard to meals.

⊗ ***Black box warning*** Ensure that patient is not pregnant before beginning therapy; suggest the use of barrier contraception; fetal injury and deaths have been reported.

- Find an alternative method of feeding infant if ARBs are given to a nursing mother. Depression of the renin-angiotensin system in infants is potentially very dangerous.
- Alert surgeon and mark on patient's chart that an ARB is being taken. The blockage of the renin-angiotensin system after surgery can produce problems. Hypotension may be reversed with volume expansion.
- If BP control does not reach desired levels, diuretics or other antihypertensives may be added to the drug regimen. Monitor patient's BP carefully.
- Monitor patient closely in situations that may cause a decrease in BP secondary to reduction in fluid volume—excessive perspiration, dehydration, vomiting, diarrhea—excessive hypotension can occur.

Teaching points

- Take these drugs without regard to meals. Do not stop taking these drugs without consulting your health care provider.
- Use a barrier method of birth control while using these drugs; if you become pregnant or desire to become pregnant, consult with your physician.
- You may experience these side effects: Dizziness (avoid driving a car or performing hazardous tasks); nausea, abdominal pain (proper nutrition is important; consult a dietitian to maintain nutrition); symptoms of upper respiratory tract or urinary tract infection, cough (do not self-medicate, consult your health care provider if this becomes uncomfortable).
- Report fever, chills, dizziness, pregnancy.

Representative drugs

candesartan
eprosartan
irbesartan
losartan
olmesartan
telmisartan
valsartan

Antiarrhythmics

PREGNANCY CATEGORY C

Therapeutic actions

Antiarrhythmics act at specific sites to alter the action potential of cardiac cells and interfere with the electrical excitability of the heart. Most of these drugs may cause new or worsened arrhythmias (proarrhythmic effect) and must be used with caution and with continual cardiac monitoring and patient evaluation.

Indications

- Treatment of tachycardia when rapid but short-term control of ventricular rate is desirable (patients with atrial fibrillation, flutter, in perioperative or postoperative situations)
- Treatment of noncompensatory tachycardia when heart rate requires specific intervention
- Treatment of atrial arrhythmias

Contraindications and cautions

- There are no contraindications; reserve for emergency situations.
- Use cautiously during pregnancy or lactation.

Adverse effects

- **CNS:** *Light-headedness, speech disorder, midscapular pain, weakness, rigors,* somnolence, confusion
- **CV:** *Hypotension,* pallor, arrhythmias
- **GI:** *Taste perversion*
- **GU:** *Urine retention*
- **Local:** *Inflammation,* induration, edema, erythema, burning at the site of infusion
- **Other:** Fever, rhonchi, flushing

Interactions

✱ **Drug-drug** • Increased risk of drug interactions with antiarrhythmic use; monitor patients

■ Nursing considerations

Assessment

- **History:** Cardiac disease, cerebrovascular disease
- **Physical:** P, BP, ECG; orientation, reflexes; R, adventitious sounds; urinary output

Interventions

- Ensure that more toxic drug is not used in chronic settings when transfer to another drug is anticipated.
- Monitor BP, heart rate, and rhythm closely.
- Provide comfort measures for pain, rigors, fever, flushing, if patient is awake.
- Provide supportive measures appropriate to condition being treated.
- Provide support and encouragement to deal with drug effects and discomfort of IV lines.
- Monitor drug levels for procainamide and amiodarone, as indicated.

Teaching points

- Reserved for emergency use. Incorporate information about these drugs into the overall teaching program for patient. Patients maintained on oral drugs will need specific teaching.

Representative drugs

Type I

moricizine

Type IA

disopyramide
procainamide
quinidine

Type IB

lidocaine
mexiletine
phenytoin

Type IC

flecainide
propafenone

Type II

acebutolol
esmolol
propranolol

Type III

amiodarone
dofetilide
ibutilide
sotalol

Type IV

verapamil

Other

adenosine
digoxin

Anticoagulants

DANGEROUS DRUG

PREGNANCY CATEGORY C

Therapeutic actions

Oral anticoagulants interfere with the hepatic synthesis of vitamin K–dependent clotting factors (factors II, prothrombin, VII, IX, and X), resulting in their eventual depletion and prolongation of clotting times; parenteral anticoagulants interfere with the conversion of prothrombin to thrombin, blocking the final step in clot formation but leaving the circulating levels of clotting factors unaffected.

Indications

- Treatment and prevention of pulmonary embolism and venous thrombosis and its extension
- Treatment of atrial fibrillation with embolization
- Prevention of DVT
- Prophylaxis of systemic embolization after acute MI
- Prevention of thrombi following specific surgical procedures and prolonged bedrest (low–molecular-weight heparins)
- Unlabeled uses: Prevention of recurrent TIAs and MI

Contraindications and cautions

- Contraindicated with allergy to the drug; SBE; hemorrhagic disorders; TB; hepatic diseases; GI ulcers; renal disease; indwelling catheters, spinal puncture; aneurysm; diabetes; visceral carcinoma; uncontrolled hypertension; severe trauma (including recent or contemplated CNS, eye surgery, recent placement of IUD); threatened abortion, menometrorrhagia; pregnancy (oral drugs cause fetal damage and death); or lactation (heparin if anticoagulation is required).

- Use cautiously with heart failure, diarrhea, fever, thyrotoxicosis; patients with dementia, psychosis, depression.

Adverse effects

- **Bleeding:** *Hemorrhage;* GI or urinary tract bleeding (hematuria, dark stools; paralytic ileus; intestinal obstruction from hemorrhage into GI tract); petechiae and purpura, bleeding from mucous membranes; hemorrhagic infarction, vasculitis, skin necrosis of female breast; adrenal hemorrhage and resultant adrenal insufficiency; compressive neuropathy secondary to hemorrhage near a nerve
- **Dermatologic:** *Alopecia, urticaria, dermatitis*
- **GI:** *Nausea,* vomiting, anorexia, abdominal cramping, diarrhea, retroperitoneal hematoma, hepatitis, jaundice, mouth ulcers
- **GU:** Priapism, nephropathy, red-orange urine
- **Hematologic:** Granulocytosis, leukopenia, eosinophilia
- **Other:** Fever, "purple toes" syndrome

Interactions

✱ **Drug-drug** • Increased bleeding tendencies with salicylates, chloral hydrate, phenylbutazone, disulfiram, chloramphenicol, metronidazole, cimetidine, ranitidine, cotrimoxazole, sulfinpyrazone, quinidine, thyroid drugs, glucagon, danazol, erythromycin, androgens, amiodarone, cefotetan, cefazolin, cefoxitin, ceftriaxone, meclofenamate, mefenamic acid, famotidine, nizatidine, nalidixic acid • Possible decreased anticoagulation effect with barbiturates, rifampin, phenytoin, carbamazepine, vitamin K, vitamin E, cholestyramine • Altered effects of warfarin with methimazole, propylthiouracil • Increased activity and toxicity of phenytoin with oral anticoagulants

✱ **Drug-alternative therapy** • Increased risk of bleeding with chamomile, garlic, ginger, ginkgo, ginseng therapy, turmeric, horse chestnut, green tea leaf, grape seed extract, feverfew, dong quai

✱ **Drug-lab test** • Red-orange discoloration of alkaline urine may interfere with some lab tests

■ Nursing considerations

Assessment

- **History:** Allergy to the drug; SBE; hemorrhagic disorders; tuberculosis; hepatic diseases; GI ulcers; renal diseases; indwelling catheters, spinal puncture; aneurysm; diabetes; visceral carcinoma; uncontrolled hypertension; severe trauma; threatened abortion, menometrorrhagia; pregnancy; lactation; heart failure, diarrhea, fever; thyrotoxicosis; senile, psychotic, or depressed patients
- **Physical:** Skin lesions, color, T, orientation, reflexes, affect; P, BP, peripheral perfusion, baseline ECG; R, adventitious sounds; liver evaluation, bowel sounds, normal output; CBC, urinalysis, guaiac stools, PT, INR, LFTs, renal function tests, WBCT, aPTT

Interventions

- Monitor INR (warfarin) or aPTT (heparin) to adjust dosage.
- Do not change brand names once stabilized; bioavailability problems can occur.
- Evaluate patient for signs of blood loss (petechiae, bleeding gums, bruises, dark stools, dark urine).
- Establish safety measures to protect patient from injury.

⊗ ***Black box warning*** Do not give to patients receiving epidural/spinal anesthesia; risk of epidural/spinal hematoma with neurological impairment.

- Do not give patient IM injections. Monitor sites of invasive procedures; ensure prolonged compression of bleeding vessels.
- Double-check other drugs that are ordered for potential interaction: Dosage of both drugs may need to be adjusted.
- Use caution when discontinuing other medications; dosage of warfarin may need to be adjusted; carefully monitor PT and INR values.
- Keep vitamin K available in case of overdose of oral drugs; keep protamine sulfate available for parenteral drug.
- Arrange for frequent follow-up, including blood tests to evaluate drug effects.
- Evaluate for therapeutic effects: PT, 1.5–2.5 times the control value; INR, 2–3; aPTT, 1.5–2 times the control.

Teaching points

- Many factors may change your body's response to these drugs—fever, change of diet, change of environment, other medications. The dosage of the drug may have to be changed. Be sure to write down all changes prescribed.
- Do not change any medication that you are taking (adding or stopping another drug) without consulting your health care provider. Other drugs affect the way anticoagulants work; starting or stopping another drug can cause excessive bleeding or interfere with the desired effects of these drugs.
- Carry or wear a medical alert tag stating that you are using one of these drugs. This will alert medical personnel in an emergency that you are taking an anticoagulant.
- Avoid situations in which you could be easily injured—contact sports, shaving with a straight razor.
- Arrange periodic blood tests to check on the action of the drug. It is very important that you have these tests.
- Use contraceptive measures while taking these drugs; it is important that you do not become pregnant.
- You may experience these side effects: Stomach bloating, cramps (passes with time; if it becomes too uncomfortable, contact your health care provider); loss of hair, skin rash (this is a frustrating and upsetting effect; if it becomes a problem, discuss it with your health care provider); orange-red discoloration to the urine (this may be mistaken for blood; add vinegar to urine, the color should disappear).
- Report unusual bleeding (when brushing your teeth, excessive bleeding from injuries, excessive bruising), black or bloody stools, cloudy or dark urine, sore throat, fever, chills, severe headaches, dizziness, suspected pregnancy.

Representative drugs

Oral

warfarin sodium

Parenteral

argatroban
bivalirudin
desirudin
fondaparinux
heparin
lepirudin

Low–molecular-weight heparins

dalteparin
enoxaparin
tinzaparin

Antidiabetics

PREGNANCY CATEGORY C

Therapeutic actions

Oral antidiabetics include several drug types. One type, called the sulfonylureas, stimulates insulin release from functioning beta cells in the pancreas and may either improve binding between insulin and insulin receptors or increase the number of insulin receptors. Second-generation sulfonylureas (glipizide and glyburide) are thought to be more potent than first-generation sulfonylureas. Other types include drugs that increase insulin receptor sensitivity (thiazolidinediones); drugs that delay or alter glucose absorption (acarbose, miglitol); and insulin, which is used for replacement therapy.

Indications

- Adjuncts to diet and exercise to lower blood glucose in patients with type 2 (non–insulin-dependent) diabetes mellitus
- Adjuncts to insulin therapy in the stabilization of certain cases of insulin-dependent maturity-onset diabetes, reducing the insulin requirement and decreasing the chance of hypoglycemic reactions
- Replacement therapy in type 1 (insulin-dependent) diabetes mellitus and when oral drugs cannot control glucose levels in type 2 diabetes

Contraindications and cautions

- Contraindicated with allergy to sulfonylureas; diabetes complicated by fever, severe infections, severe trauma, major surgery, ketosis, acidosis, coma (insulin is indicated); type 1 diabetes, serious hepatic impairment, serious renal impairment, uremia, thyroid or endocrine impairment, glycosuria, hyperglycemia associated with primary renal disease; labor and delivery (if glipizide is used during pregnancy, discontinue drug at least 1 mo before delivery); lactation, safety not established.

Adverse effects

- **CV:** Increased risk of CV mortality
- **Endocrine:** *Hypoglycemia*
- **GI:** *Anorexia, nausea,* vomiting, *epigastric discomfort, heartburn, diarrhea*
- **Hematologic:** Leukopenia, thrombocytopenia, anemia
- **Hypersensitivity:** *Allergic skin reactions,* eczema, pruritus, erythema, urticaria, photosensitivity, fever, eosinophilia, jaundice

Interactions

✱ **Drug-drug** • Increased risk of hypoglycemia with sulfonamides, chloramphenicol, salicylates • Decreased effectiveness of both sulfonylurea and diazoxide if taken concurrently • Increased risk of hyperglycemia with rifampin, thiazides • Risk of hypoglycemia and hyperglycemia with ethanol; "disulfiram reaction" has also been reported

✱ **Drug-alternative therapy** • Increased risk of hypoglycemia with juniper berries, ginseng, garlic, fenugreek, coriander, dandelion root, celery

■ Nursing considerations

Assessment

- **History:** Allergy to sulfonylureas; diabetes complicated by fever, severe infections, severe trauma, major surgery, ketosis, acidosis, coma (insulin is indicated); type 1 diabetes, serious hepatic impairment, serious renal impairment, uremia, thyroid or endocrine impairment, glycosuria, hyperglycemia associated with primary renal disease
- **Physical:** Skin color, lesions; T; orientation, reflexes, peripheral sensation; R, adventitious sounds; liver evaluation, bowel sounds; urinalysis, BUN, serum creatinine, LFTs, blood glucose, CBC

Interventions

- Administer in appropriate relationship to meals, based on drug.
- Monitor urine or serum glucose levels to determine effectiveness of drug and dosage.
- Arrange for transfer to insulin therapy during high stress (infections, surgery, trauma).
- Arrange for use of IV glucose if severe hypoglycemia occurs as a result of overdose.
- Arrange consultation with dietitian to establish weight loss program and dietary control as appropriate.
- Arrange thorough diabetic teaching program to include disease, dietary control, exercise, signs and symptoms of hypoglycemia and hyperglycemia, avoidance of infection, hygiene.
- Provide skin care to prevent breakdown.
- Ensure access to bathroom facilities if diarrhea occurs.
- Establish safety precautions if CNS effects occur.

Teaching points

- Do not stop taking these drugs without consulting your health care provider.
- Monitor urine or blood for glucose and ketones.
- Learn to recognize symptoms of low blood sugar and have a source of glucose readily available.
- Do not use these drugs during pregnancy (except insulin).
- Avoid alcohol while on these drugs.
- Report fever, sore throat, unusual bleeding or bruising, skin rash, dark urine, light-colored stools, hypoglycemia, or hyperglycemic reactions.

Representative drugs

acarbose
chlorpropamide
exenatide
glimepiride
glipizide
glyburide
insulin
metformin
miglitol
nateglinide
pioglitazone
pramlintide
repaglinide
rosiglitazone
saxagliptin
sitagliptin

tolazamide
tolbutamide

Antifungals

PREGNANCY CATEGORY C

Therapeutic actions

Antifungals bind to or impair sterols of fungal cell membranes, allowing increased permeability and leakage of cellular components and causing the death of the fungal cell.

Indications

- Systemic fungal infections: Candidiasis, chronic mucocutaneous candidiasis, oral thrush, candiduria, blastomycosis, coccidioidomycosis, histoplasmosis, chromomycosis, paracoccidioidomycosis, dermatophytosis, ringworm infections of the skin
- Treatment of onychomycosis, pityriasis versicolor, vaginal candidiasis; topical treatment of tinea corporis and tinea cruris caused by *Trichophyton rubrum, Trichophyton mentagrophytes,* and *Epidermophyton floccosum;* treatment of tinea versicolor caused by *Malassezia furfur* (topical); and reduction of scaling due to dandruff (shampoo)

Contraindications and cautions

- Contraindicated with allergy to any antifungal, fungal meningitis, pregnancy, lactation.
- Use cautiously with hepatocellular failure (increased risk of hepatocellular necrosis).

Adverse effects

- **CNS:** Headache, dizziness, somnolence, photophobia
- **GI: Hepatotoxicity,** *nausea, vomiting,* abdominal pain
- **GU:** Impotence, oligospermia (with very high doses), **nephrotoxicity**
- **Hematologic:** Thrombocytopenia, leukopenia, hemolytic anemia
- **Hypersensitivity:** Urticaria to anaphylaxis
- **Local:** *Severe irritation, pruritus, stinging* with topical application
- **Other:** *Pruritus,* fever, chills, gynecomastia, electrolyte abnormalities (amphotericin B)

Interactions

✱ **Drug-drug** • Decreased blood levels with rifampin • Increased blood levels of cyclosporine and risk of toxicity with antifungals • Increased duration of adrenal suppression when methylprednisolone, corticosteroids are taken with antifungals

■ Nursing considerations

Assessment

- **History:** Allergy to antifungals, fungal meningitis, hepatocellular failure, pregnancy, lactation
- **Physical:** Skin color, lesions; orientation, reflexes, affect; bowel sounds, liver evaluation, LFTs; CBC and differential; culture of area involved

Interventions

⊗ ***Black box warning*** Reserve systemic antifungals for patients with progressive and potentially fatal infections because of severe toxicity.

- Arrange for culture before beginning therapy; treatment should begin prior to lab results.
- Maintain epinephrine on standby in case of severe anaphylaxis after first dose.
- Administer oral drug with food to decrease GI upset.
- Administer until infection is eradicated: candidiasis, 1–2 wk; other systemic mycoses, 6 mo; chronic mucocutaneous candidiasis often requires maintenance therapy; tinea versicolor, 2 wk of topical application.
- Discontinue treatment and consult physician about diagnosis if no improvement within 2 wk of topical application.
- Discontinue topical applications if sensitivity or chemical reaction occurs.
- Administer shampoo as follows: Moisten hair and scalp thoroughly with water; apply sufficient shampoo to produce a lather; gently massage for 1 min; rinse hair with warm water; repeat, leaving on hair for 3 min.
- Provide hygiene measures to control sources of infection or reinfection.

- Provide frequent small meals if GI upset occurs.
- Provide comfort measures appropriate to site of fungal infection.
- Arrange hepatic function tests prior to therapy and at least monthly during treatment.
- Establish safety precautions if CNS effects occur (side rails, assistance with ambulation).

Teaching points

- Take the full course of therapy. Long-term use of the drug will be needed; beneficial effects may not be seen for several weeks. Take oral drugs with meals to decrease GI upset. Apply topical drugs to affected area and surrounding area. Shampoo—moisten hair and scalp thoroughly with water; apply to produce a lather; gently massage for 1 minute; rinse with warm water; repeat, leaving on for 3 minutes. Shampoo twice a week for 4 weeks with at least 3 days between shampooing.
- Use hygiene measures to prevent reinfection or spread of infection.
- You may experience these side effects: Nausea, vomiting, diarrhea (take drug with food); sedation, dizziness, confusion (avoid driving or performing tasks that require alertness); stinging, irritation (local application).
- Report skin rash, severe nausea, vomiting, diarrhea, fever, sore throat, unusual bleeding or bruising, yellowing of skin or eyes, dark urine or pale stools, severe irritation (local applications).

Representative drugs

amphotericin B
anidulafungin
butenafine
butoconazole
caspofungin
ciclopirox
clotrimazole
econazole
fluconazole
flucytosine
griseofulvin
itraconazole
ketoconazole
micafungin
miconazole
naftifine
nystatin
oxiconazole
parconazole
posaconazole
sertaconazole
terbinafine
tolnaftate
voriconazole

Antihistamines

PREGNANCY CATEGORY B OR C

Therapeutic actions

Antihistamines competitively block the effects of histamine at peripheral H_1 receptor sites, have anticholinergic (atropine-like) and antipruritic effects.

Indications

- Relief of symptoms associated with perennial and seasonal allergic rhinitis, vasomotor rhinitis, allergic conjunctivitis, mild, uncomplicated urticaria and angioedema
- Amelioration of allergic reactions to blood or plasma
- Treatment of dermatographism
- Management of tremor in early parkinsonian syndrome and drug-induced extrapyramidal reactions
- Control of nausea, vomiting, and dizziness from motion sickness (buclizine, cyclizine, diphenhydramine, meclizine)
- Adjunctive therapy in anaphylactic reactions
- Unlabeled uses: Relief of lower respiratory conditions, such as histamine-induced bronchoconstriction in asthmatics and exercise- and hyperventilation-induced bronchospasm

Contraindications and cautions

- Contraindicated with allergy to antihistamines, pregnancy, or lactation.
- Use cautiously with narrow-angle glaucoma, stenosing peptic ulcer, symptomatic prostatic hypertrophy, asthmatic attack, bladder neck obstruction, pyloroduodenal obstruction.

Adverse effects

- **CNS:** *Depression,* nightmares, sedation
- **CV:** Arrhythmia, increase in QTc intervals
- **Dermatologic:** Alopecia, angioedema, skin eruption and itching
- **GI:** *Dry mouth, GI upset,* anorexia, increased appetite, nausea, vomiting, diarrhea, constipation
- **GU:** Galactorrhea, menstrual disorders, dysuria, hesitancy
- **Respiratory:** *Bronchospasm, cough, thickening of secretions*
- **Other:** Musculoskeletal pain, mild to moderate transaminase elevations

Interactions

✷ **Drug-drug** • Altered antihistamine metabolism with ketoconazole, troleandomycin • Increased antihistaminic anticholinergic effects with MAOIs • Additive CNS depressant effects with alcohol, CNS depressants

■ Nursing considerations

Assessment

- **History:** Allergy to any antihistamines, narrow-angle glaucoma, stenosing peptic ulcer, symptomatic prostatic hypertrophy, asthmatic attack, bladder neck obstruction, pyloroduodenal obstruction, pregnancy, lactation
- **Physical:** Skin color, lesions, texture; orientation, reflexes, affect; vision examination; R, adventitious sounds; prostate palpation; serum transaminase levels

Interventions

- Administer with food if GI upset occurs.
- Provide mouth care, sugarless lozenges for dry mouth.
- Arrange for humidifier if thickening of secretions, nasal dryness become bothersome; encourage intake of fluids.
- Provide skin care for dermatologic effects.

Teaching points

- Avoid excessive dosage.
- Take with food if GI upset occurs.
- Avoid alcohol; serious sedation could occur.
- You may experience these side effects: Dizziness, sedation, drowsiness (use caution driving or performing tasks that require alertness); dry mouth (mouth care, sucking sugarless lozenges may help); thickening of bronchial secretions, dryness of nasal mucosa (use a humidifier); menstrual irregularities.
- Report difficulty breathing, hallucinations, tremors, loss of coordination, unusual bleeding or bruising, visual disturbances, irregular heartbeat.

Representative drugs

azelastine
brompheniramine
buclizine
cetirizine
chlorpheniramine
clemastine
cyclizine
cyproheptadine
desloratadine
dimenhydrinate
diphenhydramine
fexofenadine
hydroxyzine
levocetirizine
loratadine
meclizine
promethazine

Antimetabolites

DANGEROUS DRUG

PREGNANCY CATEGORY D

Therapeutic actions

Antimetabolites are antineoplastic drugs that inhibit DNA polymerase. They are cell-cycle-phase–specific to S phase (stage of DNA synthesis), causing cell death for cells in the S phase; they also block progression of cells from G_1 to S in the cell cycle.

Indications

- Induction and maintenance of remission in acute myelocytic leukemia (higher response rate in children than in adults), chronic lymphocytic leukemia
- Treatment of acute lymphocytic leukemia, chronic myelocytic leukemia and erythroleukemia, meningeal leukemia, psoriasis and rheumatoid arthritis (methotrexate)

- Palliative treatment of GI adenocarcinoma, carcinoma of the colon, rectum, breast, stomach, pancreas
- Part of combination therapy for treatment of non-Hodgkin's lymphoma in children

Contraindications and cautions

- Contraindicated with allergy to the drug, pregnancy, lactation, premature infants.
- Use cautiously with hematopoietic depression secondary to radiation or chemotherapy; impaired liver function.

Adverse effects

- **CNS:** Neuritis, neural toxicity
- **Dermatologic:** Fever, rash, urticaria, freckling, skin ulceration, pruritus, conjunctivitis, alopecia
- **GI:** *Anorexia, nausea, vomiting, diarrhea, oral and anal inflammation or ulceration;* esophageal ulcerations, esophagitis, abdominal pain, *hepatic impairment* (jaundice), acute pancreatitis
- **GU:** Renal impairment, urine retention
- **Hematologic:** Bone marrow depression, hyperuricemia
- **Local:** Thrombophlebitis, cellulitis at injection site
- **Other:** *Fever, rash*

Interactions

✱ **Drug-drug** • Decreased therapeutic action of digoxin with cytarabine • Enhanced toxicity of 5-FU with leucovorin • Potentially fatal reactions if methotrexate is taken with various NSAIDs

■ Nursing considerations

Assessment

- **History:** Allergy to drug, hematopoietic depression, impaired hepatic function, lactation
- **Physical:** Weight; T; skin lesions, color; hair; orientation, reflexes; R, adventitious sounds; mucous membranes, liver evaluation, abdominal examination; CBC, differential; LFTs; renal function tests; urinalysis

Interventions

⊗ ***Black box warning*** Arrange for tests to evaluate hematopoietic status prior to and during therapy; serious to fatal bone marrow suppression can occur.

- Arrange for discontinuation of drug therapy if platelet count is lower than 50,000/mm^3 or polymorphonuclear granulocyte count is lower than 1,000/mm^3; consult physician for dosage adjustment.
- Monitor injection site for signs of thrombophlebitis, inflammation.
- Provide mouth care for mouth sores.
- Provide frequent small meals and dietary consultation to maintain nutrition when GI effects are severe.
- Establish safety measures if dizziness, CNS effects occur.
- Arrange for patient to obtain a wig or some other suitable head covering if alopecia occurs; ensure that head is covered in extremes of temperature.
- Protect patient from exposure to infections.
- Provide skin care.
- Arrange for comfort measures if anal inflammation, headache, or other pain associated with cytarabine syndrome occurs.
- Arrange for treatment of fever if it occurs.

Teaching points

- Keep the prepared calendar of treatment days available for your reference.
- Use birth control; these drugs may cause birth defects or miscarriages.
- Arrange to have frequent, regular medical follow-up, including frequent blood tests.
- You may experience these side effects: Nausea, vomiting, loss of appetite (medication may be ordered; frequent small meals may help; it is important to maintain nutrition); malaise, weakness, lethargy (these are all effects of the drug; consult your health care provider and avoid driving or operating dangerous machinery); mouth sores (frequent mouth care will be needed); diarrhea; loss of hair (you may wish to obtain a wig or other suitable head covering; keep the head covered in extremes of temperature); anal inflammation (consult with your health care provider; comfort measures can be ordered).
- Report black, tarry stools; fever, chills; sore throat; unusual bleeding or bruising; shortness of breath; chest pain; difficulty swallowing.

Representative drugs

capecitabine
cladribine
clofarabine
cytarabine
floxuridine
fludarabine
5-FU (fluorouracil)
gemcitabine
mercaptopurine
methotrexate
pemetrexed
pentostatin
rasburicase
thioguanine

Antimigraine Drugs (Triptans)

PREGNANCY CATEGORY C

Therapeutic actions

Triptans bind to serotonin receptors to cause vascular constrictive effects on cranial blood vessels, causing the relief of migraine in selective patients.

Indications

- Treatment of acute migraine attacks with or without aura
- Treatment of cluster headaches (sumatriptan injection)

Contraindications and cautions

- Contraindicated with allergy to any triptan, active coronary artery disease, uncontrolled hypertension, hemiplegic migraine, pregnancy.
- Use cautiously in the elderly; with lactation.

Adverse effects

- **CNS:** *Dizziness, vertigo,* headache, anxiety, malaise or fatigue, *weakness, myalgia*
- **CV:** *BP alterations, tightness or pressure in chest*
- **GI:** Abdominal discomfort, dysphagia
- **Local:** *Injection site discomfort*
- **Other:** *Tingling, warm or hot sensations, burning sensation, feeling of heaviness, pressure sensation, numbness, feeling of tightness,* feeling strange, cold sensation

Interactions

✱ **Drug-drug** • Prolonged vasoactive reactions when taken concurrently with ergot-containing drugs, MAOIs, other triptans • Risk of increased blood levels and prolonged effects with hormonal contraceptives; monitor patient very closely if this combination must be used • Risk of serious serotonin syndrome if combined with SSRIs

✱ **Drug-alternative therapy** • Increased risk of severe reaction if combined with St. John's wort

■ Nursing considerations

Assessment

- **History:** Allergy to any triptan, active coronary artery disease, uncontrolled hypertension, hemiplegic migraine, pregnancy, lactation
- **Physical:** Skin color and lesions; orientation, reflexes, peripheral sensation; P, BP; LFTs, renal function tests

Interventions

- Administer to relieve acute migraine, not as a prophylactic measure.
- Administer as prescribed—by inhalation, injection, or orally.
- Establish safety measures if CNS, visual disturbances occur.
- Provide appropriate analgesics as needed for pains related to therapy.
- Monitor injection sites—pain and redness are common—for signs of infection or irritation.
- Control environment as appropriate to help relieve migraine (eg, lighting, temperature).
- Monitor BP of patients with possible coronary artery disease; discontinue triptan at any sign of angina, prolonged high BP.

Teaching points

- Learn to use the autoinjector; injection may be repeated in not less than 1 hour if relief is not obtained; do not administer more than two injections in 24 hours (if appropriate).
- These drugs should not be taken during pregnancy; if you suspect that you are pregnant, contact your health care provider and refrain from using the drug.
- Continue to do anything that usually helps you feel better during a migraine—control lighting, noise.

- Take these drugs at first sign of a migraine.
- Contact your health care provider immediately if you experience chest pain or pressure that is severe or does not go away.
- You may experience these side effects: Dizziness, drowsiness (avoid driving or operating dangerous machinery while using these drugs); numbness, tingling, feelings of tightness or pressure.
- Report feelings of heat, flushing, tiredness, sickness, swelling of lips or eyelids.

Representative drugs

almotriptan
eletriptan
frovatriptan
naratriptan
rizatriptan
sumatriptan
zolmitriptan

Antivirals

PREGNANCY CATEGORY B or C

Therapeutic actions

Antiviral drugs inhibit viral DNA or RNA replication in the virus, preventing replication and leading to viral death.

Indications

- Initial and recurrent mucosal and cutaneous HSV-1 and HSV-2 infections in immunocompromised patients, encephalitis, herpes zoster
- HIV infections (part of combination therapy)
- Cytomegalovirus (CMV) retinitis in patients with AIDS
- Severe initial and recurrent genital herpes infections
- Treatment and prevention of influenza A respiratory tract illness
- Prevention of CMV infection in patients receiving kidney, heart, or pancreas transplant who are considered at high risk for CMV infection
- Treatment of initial HSV genital infections and limited mucocutaneous HSV infections in immunocompromised patients (ointment)
- Unlabeled uses: Treatment of herpes zoster, CMV and HSV infection following transplant, herpes simplex infections, infectious mononucleosis, varicella pneumonia, and varicella zoster in immunocompromised patients

Contraindications and cautions

- Contraindicated with allergy to drug, seizures, heart failure, renal disease, lactation.

Adverse effects

Systemic administration

- **CNS:** Headache, vertigo, depression, tremors, encephalopathic changes, fatigue
- **Dermatologic:** *Inflammation or phlebitis at injection sites,* rash, hair loss, sweating
- **GI:** *Nausea, vomiting,* diarrhea, anorexia, taste perversion
- **GU:** Crystalluria with rapid IV administration, hematuria
- **Metabolic:** Hyperglycemia, dyslipidemia

Topical administration

- **Skin:** *Transient burning at the site of application*

Interactions

✱ **Drug-drug** • Increased drug effects with probenecid • Increased nephrotoxicity with other nephrotoxic drugs

✱ **Drug-alternative therapy** • Decreased effectiveness if combined with St. John's wort

■ Nursing considerations

Assessment

- **History:** Allergy to drug, seizures, heart failure, renal disease, lactation
- **Physical:** Skin color, lesions; orientation; BP, P, auscultation, perfusion, edema; R, adventitious sounds; urinary output; BUN, creatinine clearance

Interventions

Systemic administration

- Ensure that the patient is well hydrated with IV or PO fluids.
- Provide support and encouragement to deal with disease.
- Provide frequent small meals if systemic therapy causes GI upset.
- Provide skin care, analgesics if needed for rash.

Topical administration
- Start treatment as soon as possible after onset of signs and symptoms.
- Wear a rubber glove or finger cot when applying drug.

Teaching points
Systemic administration
- Complete the full course of oral therapy, and do not exceed the prescribed dose.
- These drugs are not a cure for your disease but they should make you feel better.
- Avoid sexual intercourse if lesions are visible.
- You may experience these side effects: Nausea, vomiting, loss of appetite, diarrhea, headache, dizziness.
- Report difficulty urinating, skin rash, increased severity or frequency of recurrences.

Topical administration
- Wear rubber gloves or finger cots to apply the drug to prevent autoinoculation of other sites and transmission of the disease.
- These drugs do not cure the disease; applying the drug during symptom-free periods will not prevent recurrences.
- Avoid sexual intercourse while visible lesions are present.
- These drugs may cause burning, stinging, itching, rash; notify your health care provider if these are pronounced.

Representative drugs
abacavir
acyclovir
acyclovir sodium
adefovir
amantadine
amprenavir
atazanavir
cidofovir
darunavir
delavirdine
didanosine
docosanol
efavirenz
emtricitabine
enfuviritide
entecavir
etravirine
famciclovir
fosamprenavir
foscarnet
ganciclovir
imiquimod
indinavir
lamivudine
lopinavir
maraviroc
nelfinavir
nevirapine
oseltamivir
penciclovir
raltegravir
ribavirin
rimantadine
ritonavir
saquinavir
stavudine
tenofovir
tipranavir
valacyclovir
valganciclovir
vidarabine
zalcitabine
zanamivir
zidovudine

Barbiturates

PREGNANCY CATEGORY D

CONTROLLED SUBSTANCE C-II

Therapeutic actions
Barbiturates act as sedatives, hypnotics, and antiepileptics. They are general CNS depressants. Barbiturates inhibit impulse conduction in the ascending reticular activating system, depress the cerebral cortex, alter cerebellar function, depress motor output, and can produce excitation, sedation, hypnosis, anesthesia, and deep coma; at anesthetic doses, they have anticonvulsant activity.

Indications
- Sedatives or hypnotics for short-term treatment of insomnia
- Preanesthetic medications
- Antiepileptics, in anesthetic doses, for emergency control of certain acute seizure episodes (eg, status epilepticus, eclampsia, meningitis, tetanus, toxic reactions to strychnine or local anesthetics)

Contraindications and cautions

- Contraindicated with hypersensitivity to barbiturates, manifest or latent porphyria, marked hepatic impairment, nephritis, severe respiratory distress, respiratory disease with dyspnea, obstruction, or cor pulmonale, previous addiction to sedative-hypnotic drugs, pregnancy (causes fetal damage, neonatal withdrawal syndrome), or lactation.
- Use cautiously with acute or chronic pain (paradoxical excitement or masking of important symptoms could result), seizure disorders (abrupt discontinuation of daily doses of drug can result in status epilepticus), fever, hyperthyroidism, diabetes mellitus, severe anemia, pulmonary or cardiac disease, status asthmaticus, shock, uremia.

Adverse effects

- **CNS:** *Somnolence, agitation, confusion, hyperkinesia, ataxia, vertigo, CNS depression, nightmares, lethargy, residual sedation (hangover), paradoxical excitement, nervousness, psychiatric disturbance, hallucinations, insomnia, anxiety, dizziness, abnormal thinking*
- **CV:** *Bradycardia, hypotension, syncope*
- **GI:** *Nausea, vomiting, constipation, diarrhea, epigastric pain*
- **Hypersensitivity:** Skin rashes, angioneurotic edema, serum sickness, morbilliform rash, urticaria; rarely, exfoliative dermatitis, **Stevens-Johnson syndrome**
- **Local:** *Pain, tissue necrosis at injection site,* gangrene; arterial spasm with inadvertent intra-arterial injection; thrombophlebitis; permanent neurologic deficit if injected near a nerve
- **Respiratory:** *Hypoventilation, apnea, respiratory depression,* **laryngospasm, bronchospasm,** circulatory collapse
- **Other:** Tolerance, psychological and physical dependence; **withdrawal syndrome**

Interactions

✱ **Drug-drug** • Increased CNS depression with alcohol • Increased nephrotoxicity with methoxyflurane • Decreased effects of the following drugs given with barbiturates: oral anticoagulants, corticosteroids, oral contraceptives and estrogens, beta-adrenergic blockers (especially propranolol, metoprolol), theophylline, metronidazole, doxycycline, phenylbutazones, quinidine

■ Nursing considerations

Assessment

- **History:** Hypersensitivity to barbiturates, manifest or latent porphyria; marked hepatic impairment; nephritis; severe respiratory distress; respiratory disease with dyspnea, obstruction, or cor pulmonale; previous addiction to sedative-hypnotic drugs; acute or chronic pain; seizure disorders; pregnancy; lactation; fever, hyperthyroidism; diabetes mellitus; severe anemia; pulmonary or cardiac disease; status asthmaticus; shock; uremia
- **Physical:** Weight; T; skin color, lesions, injection site; orientation, affect, reflexes; P, BP, orthostatic BP; R, adventitious sounds; bowel sounds, normal output, liver evaluation; LFTs, renal function tests, blood and urine glucose, BUN

Interventions

- Do not administer intra-arterially; may produce arteriospasm, thrombosis, gangrene.
- Administer IV doses slowly.
- Administer IM doses deep in a muscle mass.
- Do not use parenteral dosage forms if solution is discolored or contains a precipitate.
- Monitor injection sites carefully for irritation, extravasation (IV); solutions are alkaline and very irritating to the tissues.
- Monitor P, BP, R carefully during IV administration.
- Keep resuscitative facilities available in case of respiratory depression, hypersensitivity reaction.
- Provide frequent small meals, frequent mouth care if GI effects occur.
- Use safety precautions if CNS changes occur (use side rails, accompany patient).
- Provide skin care if dermatologic effects occur.
- Provide comfort measures, reassurance for patients receiving pentobarbital for tetanus, toxic seizures.
- Offer support and encouragement to patients receiving this drug for preanesthetic medication.

- Taper dosage gradually after repeated use, especially in patients with epilepsy.

Teaching points

When giving these drugs as preanesthetic, incorporate teaching about the drug into general teaching about the procedure. Include these points:

- This drug will make you drowsy and less anxious.
- Do not try to get up after you have received this drug (request assistance if you must sit up or move about for any reason).

Outpatients

- Take these drugs exactly as prescribed. These drugs are habit forming; the drug's effectiveness in facilitating sleep disappears after a short time. Do not take these drugs longer than 2 weeks (for insomnia), and do not increase the dosage without consulting your health care provider. If the drug appears to be ineffective, consult your health care provider.
- Avoid becoming pregnant while taking these drugs. The use of hormonal contraceptives while taking these drugs is not recommended as the contraceptives lose their effectiveness.
- You may experience these side effects: Drowsiness, dizziness, hangover, impaired thinking (these effects may become less pronounced after a few days; avoid driving a car or engaging in activities that require alertness); GI upset (taking the drug with food may help); dreams, nightmares, difficulty concentrating, fatigue, nervousness (these are effects of the drug that will go away when the drug is discontinued; consult your health care provider if these become bothersome).
- Report severe dizziness, weakness, drowsiness that persists, rash or skin lesions, pregnancy.

Representative drugs

butabarbital
mephobarbital
pentobarbital
pentobarbital sodium
phenobarbital
secobarbital

Benzodiazepines

PREGNANCY CATEGORY D OR X

CONTROLLED SUBSTANCE C-IV

Therapeutic actions

Benzodiazepines are anxiolytics, antiepileptics, muscle relaxants, and sedative-hypnotics. Their exact mechanisms of action are not understood, but it is known that benzodiazepines potentiate the effects of GABA, an inhibitory neurotransmitter.

Indications

- Management of anxiety disorders, short-term relief of symptoms of anxiety
- Short-term treatment of insomnia
- Alone or as adjunct in treatment of Lennox-Gastaut syndrome (petit mal variant), akinetic and myoclonic seizures
- May be useful in patients with absence (petit mal) seizures who have not responded to succinimides; up to 30% of patients show loss of effectiveness of drug within 3 mo of therapy (may respond to dosage adjustment)
- Unlabeled use: Treatment of panic attacks, treatment of IBS, acute alcohol withdrawal syndrome, chemotherapy-induced nausea and vomiting, psychogenic catatonic depression, PMS

Contraindications and cautions

- Contraindicated with hypersensitivity to benzodiazepines, psychoses, acute narrow-angle glaucoma, shock, coma, acute alcoholic intoxication with depression of vital signs, pregnancy (risk of congenital malformations, neonatal withdrawal syndrome), labor and delivery ("floppy infant" syndrome reported), or lactation (infants become lethargic and lose weight).
- Use cautiously with impaired hepatic or renal function, debilitation.

Adverse effects

- **CNS:** *Transient, mild drowsiness initially; sedation, depression, lethargy, apathy, fatigue, light-headedness, disorientation, anger, hostility,* episodes of mania and hypomania, *restlessness, confusion, crying,* delirium,

headache, slurred speech, dysarthria, stupor, rigidity, tremor, dystonia, vertigo, euphoria, nervousness, difficulty in concentration, vivid dreams, psychomotor retardation, extrapyramidal symptoms; mild paradoxical excitatory reactions during first 2 wk of treatment
- **CV:** Bradycardia, tachycardia, CV collapse, hypertension and hypotension, palpitations, edema
- **Dermatologic:** Urticaria, pruritus, skin rash, dermatitis
- **EENT:** Visual and auditory disturbances, diplopia, nystagmus, depressed hearing, nasal congestion
- **GI:** *Constipation, diarrhea, dry mouth,* salivation, *nausea,* anorexia, vomiting, difficulty in swallowing, gastric disorders, hepatic impairment, encopresis
- **GU:** Incontinence, urine retention, changes in libido, menstrual irregularities
- **Hematologic:** Elevations of blood enzymes—LDH, alkaline phosphatase, AST, ALT; blood dyscrasias—agranulocytosis, leukopenia
- **Other:** Hiccups, fever, diaphoresis, paresthesias, muscular disturbances, gynecomastia; *drug dependence with withdrawal syndrome when drug is discontinued; more common with abrupt discontinuation of higher dosage used for longer than 4 mo*

Interactions

✱ **Drug-drug** • Increased CNS depression with alcohol • Increased effect with cimetidine, disulfiram, omeprazole, hormonal contraceptives • Decreased effect with theophylline

■ Nursing considerations

Assessment

- **History:** Hypersensitivity to benzodiazepines, psychoses, acute narrow-angle glaucoma, shock, coma, acute alcoholic intoxication with depression of vital signs, pregnancy, lactation, impaired hepatic or renal function, debilitation
- **Physical:** Skin color, lesions; T; orientation, reflexes, affect, ophthalmologic examination; P, BP; R, adventitious sounds; liver evaluation, abdominal examination, bowel sounds, normal output; CBC, LFTs, renal function tests

Interventions

- Keep addiction-prone patients under careful surveillance.
- Monitor liver function, blood counts in patients on long-term therapy.
- Ensure ready access to bathroom if GI effects occur; establish bowel program if constipation occurs.
- Provide frequent small meals, frequent mouth care if GI effects occur.
- Provide measures appropriate to care of urinary problems (protective clothing, bed changing).
- Establish safety precautions if CNS changes occur (eg, side rails, accompany patient).
- Taper dosage gradually after long-term therapy, especially in patients with epilepsy; arrange to substitute another antiepileptic.
- Monitor patient for therapeutic drug levels; levels vary with drug being used.
- Arrange for patient to wear medical alert identification indicating epilepsy and drug therapy.

Teaching points

- Take drug exactly as prescribed; do not stop taking these drugs (long-term therapy) without consulting your health care provider.
- Avoid alcohol, sleep-inducing drugs, or over-the-counter drugs.
- You may experience these side effects: Drowsiness, dizziness (may become less pronounced after a few days; avoid driving or engaging in other dangerous activities); GI upset (take drug with food); fatigue; depression; dreams; crying; nervousness; depression, emotional changes; bed wetting, urinary incontinence.
- Report severe dizziness, weakness, drowsiness that persists, rash or skin lesions, difficulty voiding, palpitations, swelling in the extremities.

Representative drugs

alprazolam
chlordiazepoxide
clonazepam
clorazepate
diazepam

estazolam
flurazepam
lorazepam
oxazepam
quazepam
temazepam
triazolam

Beta-adrenergic Blockers (β-blockers)

PREGNANCY CATEGORY C (MOST), D (ATENOLOL), B (ACEBUTOLOL, PINDOLOL, SOTALOL)

Therapeutic actions

Beta-adrenergic blockers are antianginals, antiarrhythmics, and antihypertensives. These drugs competitively block beta-adrenergic receptors in the heart and juxtaglomerular apparatus. They decrease the influence of the sympathetic nervous system on these tissues, the excitability of the heart, cardiac workload, oxygen consumption, and the release of renin; they lower BP. They have membrane-stabilizing (local anesthetic) effects that contribute to their antiarrhythmic action. They also act in the CNS to reduce sympathetic outflow and vasoconstrictor tone.

Indications

- Hypertension (alone or with other drugs, especially diuretics)
- Angina pectoris caused by coronary atherosclerosis
- Hypertrophic subaortic stenosis, to manage associated stress-induced angina, palpitations, and syncope; cardiac arrhythmias, especially supraventricular tachycardia, and ventricular tachycardias induced by digoxin or catecholamines; essential tremor, familial or hereditary
- Prevention of reinfarction in clinically stable patients when started 1–4 wk after MI
- Adjunctive therapy for pheochromocytoma after treatment with an alpha-adrenergic blocker, to manage tachycardia before or during surgery or if the pheochromocytoma is inoperable
- Prophylaxis for migraine headache (propranolol)
- Management of acute situational stress reaction (stage fright); essential tremor (propranolol)
- Unlabeled uses: Treatment of recurrent GI bleeding in cirrhotic patients, schizophrenia, tardive dyskinesia, acute panic symptoms, vaginal contraceptive, acute alcohol withdrawal

Contraindications and cautions

- Contraindicated with allergy to beta-adrenergic blockers, sinus bradycardia, second- or third-degree heart block, cardiogenic shock, heart failure, bronchial asthma, bronchospasm, COPD, pregnancy (neonatal bradycardia, hypoglycemia, and apnea have occurred in infants whose mothers received propranolol; low birth weight occurs with chronic maternal use during pregnancy), or lactation.
- Use cautiously with hypoglycemia and diabetes, thyrotoxicosis, hepatic impairment.

Adverse effects

- **Allergic reactions:** Pharyngitis, erythematous rash, fever, sore throat, laryngospasm, respiratory distress
- **CV:** *Bradycardia, heart failure, cardiac arrhythmias, sinoatrial or AV nodal block, tachycardia,* peripheral vascular insufficiency, claudication, **CVA,** pulmonary edema, hypotension
- **Dermatologic:** Rash, pruritus, sweating, dry skin
- **EENT:** Eye irritation, dry eyes, conjunctivitis, blurred vision
- **GI:** *Gastric pain, flatulence, constipation, diarrhea, nausea, vomiting,* anorexia, ischemic colitis, renal and mesenteric arterial thrombosis, retroperitoneal fibrosis, hepatomegaly, acute pancreatitis
- **GU:** *Impotence, decreased libido,* Peyronie's disease, dysuria, nocturia, frequency
- **Musculoskeletal:** Joint pain, arthralgia, muscle cramps
- **Neurologic:** Dizziness, vertigo, tinnitus, *fatigue,* emotional depression, paresthesias, sleep disturbances, hallucinations, disorientation, memory loss, slurred speech
- **Respiratory:** Bronchospasm, dyspnea, cough, bronchial obstruction, nasal stuffiness, rhinitis, pharyngitis

- **Other:** *Decreased exercise tolerance, development of antinuclear antibodies,* hyperglycemia or hypoglycemia, elevated serum transaminase, alkaline phosphatase, and LDH

Interactions

✷ **Drug-drug** • Increased effects with verapamil • Decreased effects with indomethacin, ibuprofen, piroxicam, sulindac, barbiturates • Prolonged hypoglycemic effects of insulin with beta-adrenergic blockers • Peripheral ischemia possible if combined with ergot alkaloids • Initial hypertensive episode followed by bradycardia with epinephrine • Increased "first-dose response" to prazosin with beta-adrenergic blockers • Increased serum levels and toxic effects with lidocaine, cimetidine • Increased serum levels of beta-adrenergic blockers and phenothiazines, hydralazine if the two drugs are taken concurrently • Paradoxical hypertension when clonidine is given with beta-adrenergic blockers; increased rebound hypertension when clonidine is discontinued • Decreased serum levels and therapeutic effects if taken with methimazole, propylthiouracil • Decreased bronchodilator effects of theophyllines • Decreased antihypertensive effects with NSAIDs (eg, ibuprofen, indomethacin, piroxicam, sulindac), rifampin

✷ **Drug-lab test** • Interference with glucose or insulin tolerance tests, glaucoma screening tests

■ Nursing considerations

Assessment

- **History:** Allergy to beta-adrenergic blockers, sinus bradycardia, second- or third-degree heart block, cardiogenic shock, heart failure, bronchial asthma, bronchospasm, COPD, hypoglycemia and diabetes, thyrotoxicosis, hepatic impairment, pregnancy, lactation
- **Physical:** Weight, skin color, lesions, edema, T; reflexes, affect, vision, hearing, orientation; BP, P, ECG, peripheral perfusion; R, auscultation; bowel sounds, normal output, liver evaluation; bladder palpation; LFTs, thyroid function test, blood and urine glucose

Interventions

- Do not stop drug abruptly after long-term therapy (hypersensitivity to catecholamines may have developed, causing exacerbation of angina, MI, and ventricular arrhythmias). Taper drug gradually over 2 wk with monitoring.
- Consult with physician about withdrawing drug if patient is to undergo surgery (controversial).
- Give oral drug with food to facilitate absorption.
- Provide side rails and assistance with walking if CNS, vision changes occur.
- Position patient to decrease effects of edema, respiratory obstruction.
- Space activities, and provide rest periods.
- Provide frequent small meals if GI effects occur.
- Provide comfort measures to help patient cope with eye, GI, joint, CNS, dermatologic effects.

Teaching points

- Take these drugs with meals. Do not stop taking these drugs abruptly; this can worsen the disorder being treated.
- If you have diabetes, the normal signs of hypoglycemia (sweating, tachycardia) may be blocked by these drugs; monitor your blood or urine glucose carefully; be sure to eat regular meals, and take your diabetic medication regularly.
- You may experience these side effects: Dizziness, drowsiness, light-headedness, blurred vision (avoid driving or performing hazardous tasks); nausea, loss of appetite (frequent small meals may help); nightmares, depression (notify your health care provider, who may be able to change your medication); sexual impotence (you may want to discuss this with your health care provider).
- Report difficulty breathing, night cough, swelling of extremities, slow pulse, confusion, depression, rash, fever, sore throat.

Representative drugs

acebutolol
atenolol
betaxolol
bisoprolol

esmolol
labetalol
metoprolol
nadolol
nebivolol
penbutolol
pindolol
propranolol
sotalol
timolol

Bisphosphonates

PREGNANCY CATEGORY D (PARENTERAL), C (ORAL)

Therapeutic actions

Bisphosphonates inhibit bone resorption, possibly by inhibiting osteoclast activity and promoting osteoclast cell apoptosis; this action leads to decreased release of calcium from bone and decreased serum calcium level.

Indications

- Treatment of Paget's disease of bone (oral)
- Treatment of osteoporosis (oral) (postmenopausal and in males)
- Treatment of heterotopic ossification (oral)
- Treatment of hypercalcemia of malignancy in patients inadequately managed by diet or oral hydration (parenteral)
- Treatment of hypercalcemia of malignancy, which persists after adequate hydration has been restored (parenteral)
- Prevention of new clinical fractures in patients with low-trauma hip fractures (parenteral)

Contraindications and cautions

- Contraindicated with allergy to bisphosphonates, hypocalcemia, pregnancy, lactation, severe renal impairment.
- Use cautiously in the presence of renal impairment, upper GI disease.

Adverse effects

- **CNS:** *Headache,* dizziness
- **CV:** Hypertension, chest pain
- **GI:** *Nausea, diarrhea,* altered taste, metallic taste, *abdominal pain,* anorexia, esophageal erosion
- **Hematologic:** Elevated BUN, serum creatinine, hypophosphatemia, hypokalemia, hypomagnesemia, hypocalcemia
- **Respiratory:** Dyspnea, coughing, pleural effusion
- **Skeletal:** *Increased or recurrent bone pain* (Paget's disease), focal osteomalacia, *arthralgia*
- **Other:** *Infections* (UTI, candidiasis), *fever,* progression of cancer

Interactions

✱ **Drug-drug** • Increased risk of GI distress if taken with aspirin • Decreased absorption if oral form is taken with antacids, calcium, iron, multivalent cations; separate dosing by at least 30 min • Possible increased risk of hypocalcemia if parenteral form is given with aminoglycosides, loop diuretics; if this combination is used, monitor serum calcium levels closely
✱ **Drug-food** • Significantly decreased absorption and serum levels if oral form is taken with any food; administer on an empty stomach, 2 hr before meals

■ Nursing considerations

Assessment

- **History:** Allergy to bisphosphonates, renal failure, upper GI disease, lactation, pregnancy
- **Physical:** Muscle tone, bone pain, bowel sounds, urinalysis, serum calcium, renal function tests

Interventions

- Administer oral drug with a full glass of water, 30 min to 2 hr before meals or any other medication; make sure that patient stays upright for at least 30 min after administration.
- Make sure that patient is well hydrated before and during therapy with parenteral agents.
- Monitor serum calcium levels before, during, and after therapy.
- Ensure a 3-mo rest period after treatment for Paget's disease if retreatment is required; allow 7 days between treatments for hypercalcemia of malignancy.

- Ensure adequate vitamin D and calcium intake.
- Provide comfort measures if bone pain returns.

Teaching points

- Take these drugs with a full glass of water 2 hours before meals or any other medication; stay upright for at least 30 minutes after taking these drugs.
- Periodic blood tests may be required to monitor your calcium levels.
- You may experience these side effects: Nausea, diarrhea, bone pain, headache (analgesics may help).
- Report twitching, muscle spasms, dark-colored urine, severe diarrhea, GI distress, epigastric pain.

Representative drugs

alendronate
etidronate
ibandronate
pamidronate
risedronate
tiludronate
zoledronic acid

Calcium Channel Blockers

PREGNANCY CATEGORY C

Therapeutic actions

Calcium channel blockers are antianginal and antihypertensive. They inhibit the movement of calcium ions across the membranes of cardiac and arterial muscle cells; this inhibition of transmembrane calcium flow results in the depression of impulse formation in specialized cardiac pacemaker cells, slowing of the velocity of conduction of the cardiac impulse, depression of myocardial contractility, and dilation of coronary arteries and arterioles and peripheral arterioles; these effects lead to decreased cardiac work, decreased cardiac energy consumption, and increased delivery of oxygen to myocardial cells.

Indications

- Treatment of angina pectoris caused by coronary artery spasm (Prinzmetal's variant angina), chronic stable angina (effort-associated angina), hypertension, arrhythmias (supraventricular, those related to digoxin [verapamil]), subarachnoid hemorrhage (nimodipine)
- Orphan drug use in the treatment of interstitial cystitis, hypertensive emergencies, migraines, Raynaud's syndrome
- Unlabeled uses: Treatment of preterm labor, Raynaud's phenomenon, acute ischemic stroke, vascular headaches, hypertensive emergencies

Contraindications and cautions

- Contraindicated with heart block, allergy to calcium channel blockers, sick sinus syndrome, ventricular dysfunction, pregnancy.
- Use cautiously during lactation.

Adverse effects

- **CNS:** *Dizziness, light-headedness, headache, asthenia,* fatigue, *nervousness,* sleep disturbances, blurred vision
- **CV:** *Peripheral edema, angina,* hypotension, arrhythmias, bradycardia, ***AV block,*** asystole
- **Dermatologic:** *Flushing, rash,* dermatitis, pruritus, urticaria
- **GI:** *Nausea, diarrhea, constipation,* flatulence, cramps, hepatic injury
- **Other:** *Nasal congestion, cough,* fever, chills, shortness of breath, muscle cramps, joint stiffness, sexual difficulties

Interactions

✱ **Drug-drug** • Increased effects with cimetidine, ranitidine • Increased toxicity of cyclosporine

✱ **Drug-food** • Increased serum levels when combined with grapefruit juice

■ Nursing considerations

Assessment

- **History:** Allergy to calcium channel blockers, sick sinus syndrome, heart block, ventricular dysfunction; pregnancy; lactation
- **Physical:** Skin lesions, color, edema; orientation, reflexes; P, BP, baseline ECG,

peripheral perfusion, auscultation; R, adventitious sounds; liver evaluation, normal GI output; LFTs

Interventions

- Monitor patient carefully (BP, cardiac rhythm, and output) while drug is being titrated to therapeutic dose; the dosage may be increased more rapidly in hospitalized patients under close supervision.
- Ensure that patients do not chew or divide sustained-release tablets.
- Taper dosage of beta-adrenergic blockers before beginning calcium channel blocker therapy.
- Protect drug from light and moisture.
- Ensure ready access to bathroom.
- Provide comfort measures for skin rash, headache, nervousness.
- Establish safety precautions if CNS changes occur.
- Position patient to alleviate peripheral edema.
- Provide frequent small meals if GI upset occurs.

Teaching points

- Do not chew or divide sustained-release tablets. Swallow whole.
- Avoid grapefruit juice while taking this drug.
- You may experience these side effects: Nausea, vomiting (frequent small meals may help); dizziness, light-headedness, vertigo (avoid driving, operating hazardous machinery; avoid falling); muscle cramps, joint stiffness, sweating, sexual difficulties (should stop when the drug therapy is stopped; discuss with your health care provider if these become too uncomfortable).
- Report irregular heartbeat, shortness of breath, swelling of the hands or feet, pronounced dizziness, constipation.

Representative drugs

amlodipine
clevidipine
diltiazem
felodipine
isradipine
nicardipine
nifedipine
nimodipine
nisoldipine
verapamil

Cephalosporins

PREGNANCY CATEGORY B

Therapeutic actions

Cephalosporins are antibiotics. They are bactericidal, inhibiting synthesis of bacterial cell wall, causing cell death in susceptible bacteria.

Indications

- Treatment of pharyngitis, tonsillitis caused by *Streptococcus pyogenes*; otitis media caused by *Streptococcus pneumoniae, Haemophilus influenzae, Moraxella catarrhalis, S. pyogenes;* respiratory infections caused by *S. pneumoniae, Haemophilus parainfluenzae, Staphylococcus aureus, Escherichia coli, Klebsiella, H. influenzae, S. pyogenes;* UTIs caused by *E. coli, Klebsiella pneumoniae;* dermatologic infections caused by *S. aureus, S. pyogenes, E. coli, Klebsiella, Enterobacter;* uncomplicated and disseminated gonorrhea caused by *Neisseria gonorrhea;* septicemia caused by *S. pneumoniae, S. aureus, E. coli, Klebsiella, H. influenzae;* meningitis caused by *S. pneumoniae, H. influenzae, S. aureus, Neisseria meningitidis;* bone and joint infections caused by *S. aureus*
- Perioperative prophylaxis

Contraindications and cautions

- Contraindicated with allergy to cephalosporins or penicillins, renal failure, or lactation.

Adverse effects

- **CNS:** Headache, dizziness, lethargy, paresthesias, seizures
- **GI:** *Nausea, vomiting, diarrhea, anorexia, abdominal pain, flatulence,* pseudomembranous colitis, hepatotoxicity
- **GU:** Nephrotoxicity
- **Hematologic:** Bone marrow depression; decreased WBC, platelets, Hct
- **Hypersensitivity:** Ranging from *rash, fever* to **anaphylaxis;** serum sickness reaction

- **Local:** *Pain,* abscess at injection site, *phlebitis,* inflammation at IV site
- **Other:** *Superinfections, disulfiram-like reaction with alcohol*

Interactions

✱ **Drug-drug** • Increased nephrotoxicity with aminoglycosides • Increased bleeding effects with oral anticoagulants • Disulfiram-like reaction may occur if alcohol is taken within 72 hr after cephalosporin administration
✱ **Drug-lab test** • Possibility of false results on tests of urine glucose using Benedict's solution, Fehling's solution, Clinitest tablets; urinary 17-ketosteroids; direct Coombs' test

■ Nursing considerations

Assessment

- **History:** Allergy to any cephalosporin, hepatic and renal impairment, lactation, pregnancy
- **Physical:** Skin status, LFTs, renal function tests, culture of affected area, sensitivity tests

Interventions

- Culture infected area and arrange for sensitivity tests before beginning drug therapy and during therapy if expected response is not seen.
- Administer oral drug with food to decrease GI upset and enhance absorption.
- Administer liquid drug to children who cannot swallow tablets; crushing the drug results in a bitter, unpleasant taste.
- Have vitamin K available in case hypoprothrombinemia occurs.
- Discontinue drug if hypersensitivity reaction occurs.
- Ensure ready access to bathroom and provide frequent small meals if GI complications occur.
- Arrange for treatment of superinfections.

Teaching points

Oral drug

- Take full course of therapy.
- These drugs are specific to an infection and should not be used to self-treat other problems.
- Swallow tablets whole; do not crush.
- Take the drug with food.
- Avoid drinking alcoholic beverages while taking and for 3 days after stopping this drug because severe reactions often occur (even with parenteral forms).
- You may experience these side effects: Stomach upset or diarrhea.
- Report severe diarrhea with blood, pus, or mucus; rash; difficulty breathing; unusual tiredness, fatigue; unusual bleeding or bruising; unusual itching or irritation, pain at injection site.

Representative drugs

First generation

cefadroxil
cefazolin
cephalexin

Second generation

cefaclor
cefotetan
cefoxitin
cefprozil
cefuroxime

Third generation

cefdinir
cefditoren
cefepime
cefotaxime
cefpodoxime
ceftazidime
ceftibuten
ceftizoxime
ceftriaxone

Corticosteroids

PREGNANCY CATEGORY C

Therapeutic actions

Corticosteroids enter target cells and bind to cytoplasmic receptors, initiating many complex reactions that are responsible for anti-inflammatory, immunosuppressive (glucocorticoid), and salt-retaining (mineralocorticoid) actions. Some of these actions are considered undesirable, depending on the indication for which the drug is being used.

Indications

Systemic administration

- Replacement therapy in adrenal cortical insufficiency
- Treatment of hypercalcemia associated with cancer
- Short-term management of inflammatory and allergic disorders such as rheumatoid arthritis, collagen diseases (eg, SLE), dermatologic diseases (eg, pemphigus), status asthmaticus, and autoimmune disorders
- Management of hematologic disorders—thrombocytopenic purpura, erythroblastopenia
- Treatment of trichinosis with neurologic or myocardial involvement
- Treatment of ulcerative colitis, acute exacerbations of MS, and palliation in some leukemias and lymphomas

Inhalation

- Treatment of asthma

Intra-articular or soft-tissue administration

- Treatment of arthritis, psoriatic plaques

Retention enema

- For ulcerative colitis, proctitis

Dermatologic preparations

- Relief of inflammatory and pruritic manifestations of dermatoses that are steroid-responsive

Anorectal cream, suppositories

- Relief of discomfort from hemorrhoids and perianal itching or irritation

Contraindications and cautions

- *Systemic administration:* Infections, especially tuberculosis, fungal infections, amebiasis, hepatitis B, vaccinia, or varicella, and antibiotic-resistant infections; kidney disease (predisposes to edema); liver disease, cirrhosis, hypothyroidism; ulcerative colitis with impending perforation; diverticulitis; recent GI surgery; active or latent peptic ulcer; inflammatory bowel disease (drug may cause exacerbations or bowel perforation); hypertension, heart failure; thromboembolitic tendencies, thrombophlebitis, osteoporosis, convulsive disorders, metastatic carcinoma, diabetes mellitus; lactation.
- *Retention enemas, intrarectal foam:* Systemic fungal infections; recent intestinal surgery; extensive fistulas.
- *Topical dermatologic administration:* Fungal, tubercular, herpes simplex skin infections; vaccinia, varicella; ear application when eardrum is perforated; lactation.

Adverse effects

Systemic administration

- **CNS:** *Vertigo, headache,* paresthesias, insomnia, seizures, psychosis
- **CV:** *Hypotension, shock,* hypertension and CHF secondary to fluid retention, thromboembolism, thrombophlebitis, fat embolism, cardiac arrhythmias secondary to electrolyte disturbances
- **Dermatologic:** *Thin, fragile skin; petechiae, ecchymoses,* purpura, striae, subcutaneous fat atrophy
- **Endocrine:** *Amenorrhea, irregular menses,* growth retardation, decreased carbohydrate tolerance and diabetes mellitus, cushingoid state (long-term therapy), hypothalamic-pituitary-adrenal (HPA) suppression systemic with therapy longer than 5 days
- **Eye:** Cataracts, glaucoma (long-term therapy), increased IOP
- **GI:** *Peptic or esophageal ulcer, pancreatitis,* abdominal distention, nausea, vomiting, increased appetite and weight gain (long-term therapy)
- **Hematologic:** *Sodium and fluid retention, hypokalemia,* hypocalcemia, increased blood sugar, increased serum cholesterol, decreased serum T_3 and T_4 levels
- **Hypersensitivity:** Anaphylactoid or hypersensitivity reactions
- **Musculoskeletal:** *Muscle weakness,* steroid myopathy and loss of muscle mass, osteoporosis, spontaneous fractures (long-term therapy)
- **Other:** *Immunosuppression, aggravation or masking of infections, impaired wound healing*

The following effects are related to specific routes of administration:

IM repository injections

Atrophy at injection site

Retention enema

Local pain, burning; rectal bleeding; systemic absorption and adverse effects (see above)

Inhalation

Cough, throat irritation, oral thrush

Intra-articular
Osteonecrosis, tendon rupture, infection
Intraspinal
Meningitis, adhesive arachnoiditis, conus medullaris syndrome
Intralesional therapy—head and neck
Blindness (rare)
Intrathecal administration
Arachnoiditis
Topical forms
Local burning, irritation, acneiform lesions, striae, skin atrophy

Systemic absorption can lead to HPA suppression (see above), growth retardation in children, and other systemic adverse effects. Children may be at special risk of systemic absorption because of their larger skin surface area-to-body weight ratio.

Interactions

✱ **Drug-drug** • Increased steroid blood levels if taken with hormonal contraceptives, troleandomycin • Decreased steroid blood levels if taken with phenytoin, phenobarbital, rifampin, cholestyramine • Decreased serum level of salicylates if taken with corticosteroids • Decreased effectiveness of anticholinesterases (ambenonium, edrophonium, neostigmine, pyridostigmine) if taken with corticosteroids

✱ **Drug-lab test** • False-negative nitroblue-tetrazolium test for bacterial infection (with systemic absorption) • Suppression of skin test reactions

■ Nursing considerations

Assessment

- **History:** Infections, especially TB, fungal infections, amebiasis, hepatitis B, vaccinia, varicella, and antibiotic-resistant infections; kidney disease; liver disease, cirrhosis, hypothyroidism; ulcerative colitis with impending perforation; diverticulitis; recent GI surgery; active or latent peptic ulcer; inflammatory bowel disease; hypertension, heart failure; thromboembolitic tendencies, thrombophlebitis, osteoporosis, seizure disorders, metastatic carcinoma, diabetes mellitus; lactation

  Retention enemas, intrarectal foam: Systemic fungal infections; recent intestinal surgery, extensive fistulas

  Topical dermatologic administration: Fungal, tubercular, herpes simplex skin infections; vaccinia, varicella; ear application when eardrum is perforated
- **Physical:** *Systemic administration:* Body weight, T; reflexes, affect, bilateral grip strength, ophthalmologic examination; BP, P, auscultation, peripheral perfusion, discoloration, pain or prominence of superficial vessels; R, adventitious sounds, chest X-ray; upper GI X-ray (history or symptoms of peptic ulcer), liver palpation; CBC, serum electrolytes, 2-hr postprandial blood glucose, urinalysis, thyroid function tests, serum cholesterol

  Topical, dermatologic preparations: Affected area, integrity of skin

Interventions

Systemic administration

- Administer once a day before 9 AM to mimic normal peak diurnal corticosteroid levels and minimize HPA suppression.
- Space multiple doses evenly throughout the day.
- Do not give IM injections if patient has thrombocytopenia purpura.
- Rotate sites of IM repository injections to avoid local atrophy.
- Use minimal doses for shortest duration of time to minimize adverse effects.

⊗ ***Black box warning*** Arrange to taper doses when discontinuing high-dose or long-term therapy or when transferring from systemic to inhaled corticosteroids. Monitor for signs and symptoms of adrenal insufficiency.

- Arrange for increased dosage when patient is subject to unusual stress.
- Use alternate-day maintenance therapy with short-acting corticosteroids when possible.
- Do not give live-virus vaccines with immunosuppressive doses of glucocorticoids.
- Provide skin care if patient is bedridden.
- Provide frequent small meals to minimize GI distress.

- Provide antacids between meals to help avoid peptic ulcer.
- Arrange for bed rails, other safety precautions if CNS, musculoskeletal effects occur.
- Avoid exposing patient to infection.

Inhalation

- Teach patient the proper technique for using the delivery device prescribed.

Topical dermatologic administration

- Use caution with occlusive dressings, tight or plastic diapers over affected area; these can increase systemic absorption.
- Avoid prolonged use, especially near eyes, in genital and rectal areas, on face and in skin creases.
- Provide careful wound care if lesions are present.
- Provide measures to deal with pain, discomfort on administration.

Teaching points

Systemic administration

- Take these drugs exactly as prescribed. Do not stop taking these drugs without notifying your health care provider; drug dosage must be slowly tapered to avoid problems.
- Take with meals or snacks if GI upset occurs.
- Take single daily or alternate-day doses before 9 AM; mark a calendar or use other measure as a reminder of treatment days.
- Arrange for frequent follow-up visits to your health care provider so that your response to the drug may be determined and the dosage adjusted if necessary.
- Wear a medical identification tag (if you are on long-term therapy) so that any emergency medical personnel will know that you are taking one of these drugs.
- With dosage reductions, you may experience signs of adrenal insufficiency; report fatigue, muscle and joint pains, anorexia, nausea, vomiting, diarrhea, weight loss, weakness, dizziness, low blood sugar (if you monitor blood sugar).
- You may experience these side effects: Increase in appetite, weight gain (some of the weight gain may be from fluid retention, watching calories may help); heartburn, indigestion (eat frequent small meals; use antacids between meals); increased susceptibility to infection (avoid crowded areas during peak cold or flu seasons and avoid contact with anyone with a known infection); poor wound healing (if you have an injury or wound, consult your health care provider); muscle weakness, fatigue (frequent rest periods may help).
- Report unusual weight gain, swelling of lower extremities, muscle weakness, black or tarry stools, vomiting of blood, epigastric burning, puffing of face, menstrual irregularities, fever, prolonged sore throat, cold or other infection, worsening of symptoms.

Inhalation

- Follow directions you have been given regarding proper use of the drug delivery device.

Intra-articular, intralesional administration

- Do not overuse the injected joint even if the pain is gone. Follow directions you have been given for proper rest and exercise.

Topical dermatologic administration

- Apply sparingly and rub in lightly.
- Avoid eye contact.
- Report burning, irritation, or infection of the site, worsening of the condition.
- Avoid prolonged use.

Anorectal preparations

- Maintain normal bowel function by proper diet, adequate fluid intake, and regular exercise.
- Use stool softeners or bulk laxatives if needed.
- Notify your health care provider if symptoms do not improve in 7 days, or if bleeding, protrusion, or seepage occurs.

Representative drugs

alclometasone
amcinonide
beclomethasone
betamethasone
budesonide
ciclesonide
clobetasol
clocortolone
cortisone
desonide
desoximetasone
dexamethasone
diflorasone
difluprednate

fludrocortisone
flunisolide
fluocinolone
fluocinonide
flurandrenolide
fluticasone
halcinonide
halobetasol
hydrocortisone
loteprednol
methylprednisolone
mometasone
prednicarbate
prednisolone
prednisone
rimexolone
triamcinolone

Diuretics

PREGNANCY CATEGORY B OR C

Therapeutic actions

Diuretics are divided into several subgroups. Thiazide and thiazide-related diuretics inhibit reabsorption of sodium and chloride in the distal renal tubule, increasing the excretion of sodium, chloride, and water by the kidney. Loop diuretics inhibit the reabsorption of sodium and chloride in the loop of Henle and in the distal renal tubule; because of this added effect, loop diuretics are more potent. Potassium-sparing diuretics block the effect of aldosterone on the renal tubule, leading to a loss of sodium and water and the retention of potassium; their overall effect is much weaker. Osmotic diuretics pull fluid out of the tissues with a hypertonic effect. Overall effect of diuretics is a loss of water and electrolytes from the body.

Indications

- Adjunctive therapy in edema associated with heart failure, cirrhosis, corticosteroid and estrogen therapy, renal impairment
- Treatment of hypertension, alone or in combination with other antihypertensives
- Reduction of intracranial pressure before and during neurosurgery
- Reduction of intraocular pressure in acute episodes of glaucoma when other therapies are not successful
- Unlabeled uses: Treatment of diabetes insipidus, especially nephrogenic diabetes insipidus, reduction of incidence of osteoporosis in postmenopausal women

Contraindications and cautions

- Contraindicated with fluid or electrolyte imbalances, renal or hepatic disease, gout, SLE, glucose tolerance abnormalities, hyperparathyroidism, manic-depressive disorders, or lactation.

Adverse effects

- **CNS:** *Dizziness, vertigo,* paresthesias, weakness, headache, drowsiness, fatigue
- **CV:** Orthostatic hypotension, venous thrombosis, volume depletion, cardiac arrhythmias, chest pain
- **Dermatologic:** Photosensitivity, rash, purpura, exfoliative dermatitis
- **GI:** *Nausea, anorexia, vomiting, dry mouth, diarrhea, constipation,* jaundice, hepatitis, pancreatitis
- **GU:** *Polyuria, nocturia, impotence,* loss of libido
- **Hematologic:** Leukopenia, thrombocytopenia, agranulocytosis, aplastic anemia, neutropenia, fluid and electrolyte imbalances
- **Other:** Muscle cramps and muscle spasms, fever, hives, gouty attacks, flushing, weight loss, rhinorrhea, electrolyte imbalance

Interactions

✱ Drug-drug • Increased thiazide effects and possible acute hyperglycemia with diazoxide • Decreased absorption with cholestyramine, colestipol • Increased risk of cardiac glycoside toxicity if hypokalemia occurs • Increased risk of lithium toxicity • Increased dosage of antidiabetics may be needed • Risk of hyperkalemia if potassium-sparing diuretics are given with potassium preparations or ACE inhibitors • Increased risk of ototoxicity if loop diuretics are taken with aminoglycosides or cisplatin

✱ Drug-lab test • Monitor for decreased PBI levels without clinical signs of thyroid disturbances

■ Nursing considerations

Assessment

- **History:** Fluid or electrolyte imbalances, renal or liver disease, gout, SLE, glucose tolerance abnormalities, hyperparathyroidism, bipolar disorders, lactation
- **Physical:** Orientation, reflexes, muscle strength; pulses, BP, orthostatic BP, perfusion, edema, baseline ECG; R, adventitious sounds; liver evaluation, bowel sounds; CBC, serum electrolytes, blood glucose; LFTs, renal function tests; serum uric acid, urinalysis

Interventions

- Administer with food or milk if GI upset occurs.
- Administer early in the day so increased urination will not disturb sleep.
- Ensure ready access to bathroom.
- Establish safety precautions if CNS effects, orthostatic hypotension occur.
- Measure and record regular body weights to monitor fluid changes.
- Provide mouth care and frequent small meals as needed.
- Monitor IV sites for any sign of extravasation.
- Monitor electrolytes frequently with parenteral use, periodically with chronic use.

Teaching points

- Take these drugs early in the day so sleep will not be disturbed by increased urination.
- Weigh yourself daily and record weights.
- Protect your skin from exposure to the sun or bright lights.
- If taking a potassium-sparing diuretic, avoid foods high in potassium and avoid using salt substitutes.
- Take prescribed potassium replacement, and eat foods high in potassium if taking a thiazide or loop diuretic.
- Increased urination will occur (stay close to bathroom facilities).
- Use caution if dizziness, drowsiness, or faintness occurs.
- Report rapid weight gain or loss, swelling in ankles or fingers, unusual bleeding or bruising, muscle cramps.

Representative drugs

Thiazide and related diuretics

chlorothiazide
chlorthalidone
hydrochlorothiazide
hydroflumethiazide
indapamide
methyclothiazide
metolazone

Loop diuretics

bumetanide
ethacrynic acid
furosemide
torsemide

Potassium-sparing diuretics

amiloride
spironolactone
triamterene

Osmotic diuretic

mannitol

Fluoroquinolones

PREGNANCY CATEGORY C

Therapeutic actions

Fluoroquinolones are antibacterial. They interfere with DNA replication in susceptible gram-negative bacteria, preventing cell reproduction and leading to death of bacteria.

Indications

- Treatment of infections caused by susceptible gram-negative bacteria, including *Escherichia coli, Proteus mirabilis, Klebsiella pneumoniae, Enterobacter cloacae, Proteus vulgaris, Providencia rettgeri, Morganella morganii, Pseudomonas aeruginosa, Citrobacter freundii, Staphylococcus aureus, S. epidermidis,* group D streptococci
- Unlabeled use: Treatment of patients with cystic fibrosis who have pulmonary exacerbations

Contraindications and cautions

- Contraindicated with allergy to any fluoroquinolone, pregnancy, or lactation.
- Use cautiously with renal impairment, seizures.

Adverse effects

- **CNS:** *Headache,* dizziness, insomnia, fatigue, somnolence, depression, blurred vision
- **GI:** *Nausea,* vomiting, dry mouth, *diarrhea,* abdominal pain
- **Hematologic:** Elevated BUN, AST, ALT, serum creatinine and alkaline phosphatase; decreased WBC, neutrophil count, Hct
- **Other:** Fever, rash, **photosensitivity**

Interactions

✱ **Drug-drug** • Decreased therapeutic effect with iron salts, sucralfate • Decreased absorption with antacids • Increased serum levels and toxic effects of theophyllines with fluoroquinolones

✱ **Drug-alternative therapy** • Increased photosensitivity reactions with St. John's wort

■ Nursing considerations

Assessment

- **History:** Allergy to fluoroquinolones, renal impairment, seizures, lactation
- **Physical:** Skin color, lesions; T; orientation, reflexes, affect; mucous membranes, bowel sounds; LFTs, renal function tests

Interventions

- Arrange for culture and sensitivity tests before beginning therapy.
- Continue therapy for 2 days after the signs and symptoms of infection have disappeared.
- Administer oral drug 1 hr before or 2 hr after meals with a glass of water.
- Ensure that patient is well hydrated during course of drug therapy.
- Administer antacids, if needed, at least 2 hr after dosing.
- Monitor clinical response; if no improvement is seen or a relapse occurs, repeat culture and sensitivity.
- Ensure ready access to bathroom if diarrhea occurs.
- Arrange for appropriate bowel training program if constipation occurs.
- Provide frequent small meals if GI upset occurs.
- Arrange for monitoring of environment (noise, temperature) and analgesics, for headache.
- Establish safety precautions if CNS, visual changes occur.
- Encourage patient to complete full course of therapy.

Teaching points

- Take oral drugs on an empty stomach, 1 hour before or 2 hours after meals. If you need an antacid, do not take it within 2 hours of ciprofloxacin dose.
- Drink plenty of fluids.
- You may experience these side effects: Nausea, vomiting, abdominal pain (frequent small meals may help); diarrhea or constipation (consult your health care provider); drowsiness, blurring of vision, dizziness (observe caution if driving or using hazardous equipment).
- Report rash, visual changes, severe GI problems, weakness, tremors.

Representative drugs

ciprofloxacin
gemifloxacin
levofloxacin
lomefloxacin
moxifloxacin
norfloxacin
ofloxacin

Histamine$_2$ (H_2) Antagonists

PREGNANCY CATEGORY B

Therapeutic actions

H_2 antagonists inhibit the action of histamine at the H_2 receptors of the stomach, inhibiting gastric acid secretion and reducing total pepsin output; the resultant decrease in acid allows healing of ulcerated areas.

Indications

- Short-term and maintenance treatment of active duodenal ulcer and benign gastric ulcer
- Treatment of pathologic hypersecretory conditions (Zollinger-Ellison syndrome) and erosive GERD

- Prophylaxis of stress-induced ulcers and acute upper GI bleed in critically ill patients
- Treatment of GERD, heartburn, acid indigestion, sour stomach

Contraindications and cautions

- Contraindicated with allergy to H_2 antagonists, impaired renal or hepatic function, or lactation.

Adverse effects

- **CNS:** Dizziness, somnolence, headache, confusion, hallucinations, peripheral neuropathy, symptoms of brain stem dysfunction (dysarthria, ataxia, diplopia)
- **CV:** Cardiac arrhythmias, arrest; hypotension (IV use)
- **GI:** *Diarrhea*
- **Hematologic:** Increases in plasma creatinine, serum transaminase
- **Other:** Impotence (reversible with drug withdrawal), gynecomastia (long-term treatment), rash, vasculitis, pain at IM injection site

Interactions

✱ **Drug-drug** • Increased risk of decreased white blood cell counts with antimetabolites, alkylating agents, other drugs known to cause neutropenia • Increased serum levels and risk of toxicity of warfarin-type anticoagulants, phenytoin, beta-adrenergic blockers, alcohol, quinidine, lidocaine, theophylline, chloroquine, certain benzodiazepines (alprazolam, chlordiazepoxide, diazepam, flurazepam, triazolam), nifedipine, pentoxifylline, tricyclic antidepressants, procainamide, carbamazepine when taken with H_2 antagonists

■ Nursing considerations

Assessment

- **History:** Allergy to H_2 antagonists, impaired renal or hepatic function, lactation
- **Physical:** Skin lesions; orientation, affect; pulse, baseline ECG (continuous with IV use); liver evaluation, abdominal examination, normal output; CBC, LFTs, renal function tests

Interventions

- Administer drug with food and at bedtime.
- Decrease doses in renal and hepatic impairment.
- Administer IM dose undiluted, deep into large muscle group.
- Ensure ready access to bathroom.
- Provide comfort measures for skin rash, headache.
- Establish safety measures if CNS changes occur (side rails, accompany patient).
- Arrange for regular follow-up, including blood tests to evaluate effects.

Teaching points

- Take these drugs with food and at bedtime; therapy may continue for 4–6 weeks or longer.
- Take antacids exactly as prescribed; be careful of the time.
- Inform your health care provider about your cigarette smoking habits. Cigarette smoking decreases the effectiveness of these drugs.
- Have regular medical follow-up while on this drug to evaluate your response.
- Report sore throat, fever, unusual bruising or bleeding, tarry stools, confusion, hallucinations, dizziness, muscle or joint pain.

Representative drugs

cimetidine
famotidine
nizatidine
ranitidine

HMG-CoA Inhibitors

PREGNANCY CATEGORY X

Therapeutic actions

HMG-CoA inhibitors are antihyperlipidemic. They are a fungal metabolite that inhibits the enzyme that catalyzes the first step in the cholesterol synthesis pathway in humans, resulting in a decrease in serum cholesterol, serum LDLs (associated with increased risk of CAD), and either an increase or no change in serum HDLs (associated with decreased risk of CAD).

Indications

- Adjunct to diet in the treatment of elevated total and LDL cholesterol in patients with primary hypercholesterolemia (types IIa and

IIb) whose response to dietary restriction of saturated fat and cholesterol and other nonpharmacologic measures has not been adequate
- Primary prevention of coronary events (lovastatin, pravastatin)
- Secondary prevention of CV events (fluvastatin, lovastatin, pravastatin, simvastatin)

Contraindications and cautions

- Contraindicated with allergy to HMG-CoA inhibitors, fungal byproducts, pregnancy, or lactation, concurrent gemfibrozil therapy.
- Use cautiously with impaired hepatic function, cataracts.

Adverse effects

- **CNS:** *Headache, blurred vision,* dizziness, insomnia, fatigue, muscle cramps, cataracts
- **GI:** *Flatulence, abdominal pain, cramps, constipation, nausea, vomiting,* heartburn
- **Hematologic:** Elevations of CPK, alkaline phosphatase, and transaminases
- **Musculoskeletal: Rhabdomyolysis with possible renal failure**

Interactions

✱ **Drug-drug** • Monitor patients receiving HMG-CoA inhibitors for possible severe myopathy or rhabdomyolysis if taken with cyclosporine, erythromycin, gemfibrozil, niacin
✱ **Drug-food** • Risk of increased serum levels if combined with grapefruit juice

■ Nursing considerations

Assessment

- **History:** Allergy to HMG-CoA inhibitors, fungal byproducts; impaired hepatic function; cataracts; pregnancy; lactation
- **Physical:** Orientation, affect, ophthalmologic examination; liver evaluation; lipid studies, LFTs

Interventions

- Administer drug at bedtime; highest rates of cholesterol synthesis are between midnight and 5 AM.
- Consult with dietitian about low-cholesterol diets.
- Arrange for diet and exercise consultation.
- Arrange for regular follow-up during long-term therapy.
- Provide comfort measures to deal with headache, muscle cramps, nausea.
- Arrange for periodic ophthalmologic examination to check for cataract development.
- Offer support and encouragement to deal with disease, diet, drug therapy, and follow-up.

Teaching points

- Take these drugs at bedtime.
- Institute appropriate diet changes.
- Use contraceptive measures to avoid pregnancy while using these drugs.
- Avoid grapefruit juice while taking these drugs.
- You may experience these side effects: Nausea (eat frequent small meals); headache, muscle and joint aches and pains (may lessen with time).
- Have periodic ophthalmic examinations while you are using these drugs.
- Report severe GI upset, changes in vision, unusual bleeding or bruising, dark urine or light-colored stools; muscle pain, weakness.

Representative drugs

atorvastatin
fluvastatin
lovastatin
pitavastatin
pravastatin
rosuvastatin
simvastatin

Macrolide Antibiotics

PREGNANCY CATEGORY B OR C

Therapeutic actions

Macrolides are antibiotics. They are bacteriostatic or bactericidal in susceptible bacteria; they bind to cell membranes and cause changes in protein function, leading to bacterial cell death.

Indications

- Treatment of acute infections caused by sensitive strains of *Streptococcus pneumoniae,*

Mycoplasma pneumoniae, Listeria monocytogenes, Legionella pneumophila; URIs, lower respiratory tract infections, skin and soft-tissue infections caused by group A beta-hemolytic streptococci when oral treatment is preferred to injectable benzathine penicillin; PID caused by *Neisseria gonorrhoeae* in patients allergic to penicillin; intestinal amebiasis caused by *Entamoeba histolytica;* infections in the newborn and in pregnancy that are caused by *Chlamydia trachomatis* and in adult chlamydial infections when tetracycline cannot be used; primary syphilis (*Treponema pallidum*) in penicillin-allergic patients; eliminating *Bordetella pertussis* organisms from the nasopharynx of infected individuals and as prophylaxis in exposed and susceptible individuals; superficial ocular infections caused by susceptible strains of microorganisms; prophylaxis of ophthalmia neonatorum caused by *N. gonorrhoeae* or *C. trachomatis*

- In conjunction with sulfonamides to treat URIs caused by *Haemophilus influenzae*
- Adjunct to antitoxin in infections caused by *Corynebacterium diphtheriae* and *Corynebacterium minutissimum*
- Prophylaxis against alpha-hemolytic streptococcal endocarditis before dental or other procedures in patients allergic to penicillin who have valvular heart disease and against infection in minor skin abrasions
- Unlabeled uses: Treatment of severe diarrhea associated with *Campylobacter* enteritis or enterocolitis; treatment of genital, inguinal, or anorectal lymphogranuloma venereum infection; treatment of *Haemophilus ducreyi* (chancroid); treatment of acne vulgaris and skin infections caused by sensitive microorganisms

Contraindications and cautions

- Contraindicated with allergy to any macrolide antibiotic.
- Use cautiously with hepatic impairment or lactation (secreted and may be concentrated in breast milk; may modify bowel flora of nursing infant and interfere with fever workups).

Adverse effects

- **CNS:** Reversible hearing loss, confusion, uncontrollable emotions, abnormal thinking
- **Dermatologic:** Edema, urticaria, dermatitis, angioneurotic edema
- **GI:** *Abdominal cramping, anorexia, diarrhea, vomiting,* pseudomembranous colitis, hepatotoxicity
- **Hypersensitivity:** Allergic reactions ranging from rash to **anaphylaxis**
- **Local:** *Irritation, burning, itching* at site of application
- **Other:** *Superinfections*

Interactions

✱ **Drug-drug** • Increased serum levels of digoxin • Increased effects of oral anticoagulants, theophyllines, carbamazepine • Increased therapeutic and toxic effects of corticosteroids • Increased levels of cyclosporine and risk of renal toxicity • Increased irritant effects with peeling, desquamating, or abrasive agents used with dermatologic preparations

✱ **Drug-lab test** • Interferes with fluorometric determination of urinary catecholamines • Decreased urinary estriol levels caused by inhibition of hydrolysis of steroids in the gut

■ Nursing considerations

Assessment

- **History:** Allergy to macrolides, hepatic impairment, lactation, viral, fungal, mycobacterial infections of the eye (ophthalmologic)
- **Physical:** Site of infection, skin color, lesions; orientation, affect, hearing tests; R, adventitious sounds; GI output, bowel sounds, liver evaluation; culture and sensitivity tests of infection, urinalysis, LFTs

Interventions

- Culture site of infection before therapy.
- Administer oral erythromycin base or stearate on an empty stomach, 1 hr before or 2–3 hr after meals, with a full glass of water (oral erythromycin estolate, ethylsuccinate, and certain enteric-coated tablets; see manufacturer's instructions; may be given without regard to meals).

- Administer drug around the clock to maximize therapeutic effect; scheduling may have to be adjusted to minimize sleep disruption.

⊗ ***Black box warning*** Monitor liver function in patients on prolonged therapy; serious toxicity can occur.

- Institute hygiene measures and treatment if superinfections occur.
- If GI upset occurs with oral therapy, some preparations (see previous) may be given with meals, or it may be possible to substitute one of these preparations.
- Provide frequent small meals if GI problems occur.
- Establish safety measures (accompany patient, side rails) if CNS changes occur.
- Give patient support and encouragement to continue with therapy.
- Wash affected area, rinse well, and dry before topical application.

Teaching points

- Take oral drugs on an empty stomach, 1 hour before or 2–3 hours after meals, with a full glass of water, or, as appropriate, drug may be taken without regard to meals. These drugs should be taken around the clock; schedule to minimize sleep disruption. It is important that you finish the *full course* of the drug therapy.
- Wash and rinse area and pat it dry before applying topical solutions; use fingertips or an applicator; wash hands thoroughly after application.
- You may experience these side effects: Stomach cramping, discomfort (taking the drug with meals, if appropriate, may alleviate this problem); uncontrollable emotions, crying, laughing, abnormal thinking (will end when the drug is stopped).
- Report severe or watery diarrhea, severe nausea or vomiting, dark urine, yellowing of the skin or eyes, loss of hearing, skin rash or itching.

Representative drugs

azithromycin
clarithromycin
erythromycin

Nitrates

PREGNANCY CATEGORY C

Therapeutic actions

Nitrates are antianginals. They relax vascular smooth muscle with a resultant decrease in venous return and decrease in arterial blood pressure, which reduces left ventricular workload and decreases myocardial oxygen consumption, relieving the pain of angina.

Indications

- Treatment of acute angina (sublingual, translingual, inhalant preparations)
- Prophylaxis of angina (oral sustained release, sublingual, topical, transdermal, translingual, transmucosal preparations)
- Treatment of angina unresponsive to recommended doses of organic nitrates or beta-blockers (IV preparations)
- Management of perioperative hypertension, heart failure associated with acute MI (IV preparations)
- Produce controlled hypotension during surgery (IV preparations)
- Unlabeled uses: Reduction of cardiac workload in acute MI and in heart failure (sublingual, topical); diffuse esophageal spasm without reflux

Contraindications and cautions

- Contraindicated with allergy to nitrates, angle-closure glaucoma, severe anemia, early MI, head trauma, cerebral hemorrhage, cardiomyopathy, concommitant use with phosphodiesterase type 5 (PDE5) inhibitors, pregnancy, or lactation.
- Use cautiously with hepatic or renal disease, hypotension or hypovolemia, increased intracranial pressure, constrictive pericarditis, pericardial tamponade, low ventricular filling pressure or low pulmonary capillary wedge pressure (PCWP).

Adverse effects

- **CNS:** *Headache,* apprehension, restlessness, weakness, vertigo, dizziness, faintness

- **CV:** Tachycardia, retrosternal discomfort, palpitations, **hypotension,** syncope, collapse, orthostatic hypotension, angina
- **Dermatologic:** Rash, exfoliative dermatitis, cutaneous vasodilation with flushing, pallor, perspiration, cold sweat, contact dermatitis (transdermal preparations), topical allergic reactions (topical nitroglycerin ointment)
- **GI:** Nausea, vomiting, incontinence of urine and feces, abdominal pain
- **Local:** Local burning sensation at the point of dissolution (sublingual)
- **Other:** Ethanol intoxication with high dose IV use (alcohol in diluent)

Interactions

✱ **Drug-drug** • Increased risk of hypertension and decreased antianginal effect with ergot alkaloids • Decreased pharmacologic effects of heparin • Risk of orthostatic hypotension with calcium channel-blockers • Profound hypotension with PDE5 inhibitors

✱ **Drug-lab test** • False report of decreased serum cholesterol if done by the Zlatkis-Zak color reaction

■ Nursing considerations

Assessment

- **History:** Allergy to nitrates, severe anemia, early MI, head trauma, cerebral hemorrhage, hypertrophic cardiomyopathy, hepatic or renal disease, hypotension or hypovolemia, increased intracranial pressure, constrictive pericarditis, pericardial tamponade, low ventricular filling pressure or low PCWP, pregnancy, lactation
- **Physical:** Skin color, T, lesions; orientation, reflexes, affect; P, BP, orthostatic BP, baseline ECG, peripheral perfusion; R, adventitious sounds; liver evaluation, normal output; LFTs (IV); renal function tests (IV); CBC, Hgb

Interventions

- Administer sublingual preparations under the tongue or in the buccal pouch. Encourage the patient not to swallow. Ask patient if the tablet "fizzles" or burns. Check the expiration date on the bottle; store at room temperature, protected from light. Discard unused drug 6 mo after bottle is opened (conventional tablets); stabilized tablets (*Nitrostat*) are less subject to loss of potency.
- Administer sustained-release preparations with water; tell the patient not to chew the tablets or capsules; do not crush these preparations.
- Administer topical ointment by applying it over a 6″ × 6″ area in a thin, uniform layer using the applicator. Cover area with plastic wrap held in place by adhesive tape. Rotate sites of application to decrease the chance of inflammation and sensitization; close tube tightly when finished.
- Administer transdermal systems to skin site free of hair and not subject to much movement. Shave areas that have a lot of hair. Do not apply to distal extremities. Change sites slightly to decrease the chance of local irritation and sensitization. Remove transdermal system before attempting defibrillation or cardioversion. Remove old system before applying new system.
- Administer transmucosal tablets by placing them between the lip and gum above the incisors or between the cheek and gum. Encourage patient not to swallow and not to chew the tablet.
- Administer the translingual spray directly onto the oral mucosa; preparation is not to be inhaled.
- Withdraw drug gradually; 4–6 wk recommended period for the transdermal preparations.
- Establish safety measures if CNS effects, hypotension occur.
- Keep environment cool, dim, and quiet.
- Provide periodic rest periods for patient.
- Provide comfort measures and arrange for analgesics if headache occurs.
- Maintain life support equipment on standby if overdose occurs or cardiac condition worsens.
- Provide support and encouragement to deal with disease, therapy, and needed lifestyle changes.

Teaching points

- Place sublingual tablets under your tongue or in your cheek; do not chew or swallow the tablet; the tablet should burn or "fizzle" under the tongue. Take nitroglycerin before chest pain begins, when you anticipate that your activities or situation may precipitate an attack. Do not buy large quantities; these

drugs do not store well. Keep these drugs in a dark, dry place, in a dark-colored glass bottle with a tight lid; do not combine with other drugs. You may repeat your dose every 5 minutes for a total of three tablets; if the pain is still not relieved, go to an emergency room.
- Do not chew or crush the timed-release preparations; take on an empty stomach.
- Spread a thin layer of topical ointment on the skin using the applicator. Do not rub or massage the area. Cover with plastic wrap held in place with adhesive tape. Wash your hands after application. Keep the tube tightly closed. Rotate the sites frequently to prevent local irritation.
- To use transdermal systems, you may need to shave an area for application. Apply to a slightly different area each day. Use care if changing brands; each system has a different concentration. Remove the old system before applying a new one.
- Place transmucosal tablets between the lip and gum or between the gum and cheek. Do not chew; try not to swallow.
- Spray translingual spray directly onto oral mucous membranes; do not inhale. Use 5–10 minutes before activities that you anticipate will precipitate an attack.
- Take these drugs exactly as directed; do not exceed recommended dosage.
- Do not take erectile dysfunction drugs while you are using a nitrate.
- You may experience these side effects: Dizziness, light-headedness (this may pass as you adjust to the drug; change positions slowly); headache (lying down in a cool environment and resting may help; over-the-counter preparations may not help); flushing of the neck or face (this usually passes as the drug's effects pass).
- Report blurred vision, persistent or severe headache, skin rash, more frequent or more severe angina attacks, fainting.

Representative drugs

amyl nitrite
isosorbide dinitrate
isosorbide mononitrate
nitroglycerin

Nondepolarizing Neuromuscular Junction Blockers (NMJ Blockers)

DANGEROUS DRUG

PREGNANCY CATEGORY C

Therapeutic actions

NMJ blockers interfere with neuromuscular transmission and cause flaccid paralysis by blocking acetylcholine receptors at the skeletal neuromuscular junction.

Indications

- Adjuncts to general anesthetics to facilitate endotracheal intubation and relax skeletal muscle; to relax skeletal muscle to facilitate mechanical ventilation

Contraindications and cautions

- Contraindicated with hypersensitivity to NMJ blockers and the bromide ion.
- Use cautiously with myasthenia gravis; pregnancy (teratogenic in preclinical studies; may be used in cesarean section, but reversal may be difficult if patient has received magnesium sulfate to manage preeclampsia); renal or hepatic disease, respiratory depression, altered fluid or electrolyte balance; patients in whom an increase in heart rate may be dangerous.

Adverse effects

- **CV:** *Increased heart rate*
- **Hypersensitivity:** Hypersensitivity reactions, especially rash
- **Musculoskeletal:** Profound and prolonged muscle paralysis
- **Respiratory:** *Depressed respiration, apnea,* bronchospasm

Interactions

✱ **Drug-drug** • Increased intensity and duration of neuromuscular block with some anesthetics (isoflurane, enflurane, halothane, diethyl ether), some parenteral antibiotics (aminoglycosides, clindamycin, lincomycin, bacitracin, polymyxin B), ketamine, quinine, quinidine, trimethaphan, calcium channel-blocking drugs (eg, verapamil), Mg^{2+} salts, and in hypokalemia (from K^+-depleting diuretics) • Decreased intensity of neuromuscular block with acetylcholine, cholinesterase inhibitors, K^+ salts, theophyllines, phenytoins, azathioprine, mercaptopurine, carbamazepine

■ Nursing considerations

Assessment

- **History:** Hypersensitivity to NMJ blockers and the bromide ion, myasthenia gravis, pregnancy, renal or hepatic disease, respiratory depression, altered fluid or electrolyte balance
- **Physical:** Weight, T, skin condition, hydration, reflexes, bilateral grip strength, pulse, BP, R and adventitious sounds, LFTs, renal function tests, serum electrolytes

Interventions

⊗ ***Black box warning*** Drug should be given only by trained personnel (anesthesiologists); intubation will be necessary.

- Arrange to have facilities on standby to maintain airway and provide mechanical ventilation.
- Provide neostigmine, pyridostigmine, or edrophonium (cholinesterase inhibitors) on standby to overcome excessive neuromuscular block.
- Provide atropine or glycopyrrolate on standby to prevent parasympathomimetic effects of cholinesterase inhibitors.
- Provide a peripheral nerve stimulator on standby to assess degree of neuromuscular block, as needed.
- Change patient's position frequently, and provide skin care to prevent decubitus ulcer formation when drug is used for other than brief periods.
- Monitor conscious patient for pain or distress that he may not be able to communicate.
- Reassure conscious patients frequently.

Teaching points

- Teaching points about what these drugs do and how the patient will feel should be incorporated into the overall teaching program about the procedure.

Representative drugs

atracurium
cisatracurium
pancuronium
rocuronium
tubocurarine
vecuronium

Nonsteroidal Anti-inflammatory Drugs (NSAIDs)

PREGNANCY CATEGORY B OR C

Therapeutic actions

NSAIDs have anti-inflammatory, analgesic, and antipyretic activities largely related to inhibition of prostaglandin synthesis; exact mechanisms of action are not known.

Indications

- Relief of signs and symptoms of rheumatoid arthritis, osteoarthritis, and juvenile arthritis
- Relief of mild to moderate pain
- Treatment of primary dysmenorrhea
- Fever reduction
- Reduction of number of adenomatous colorectal polyps in adults with familial adenomatous polyposis

Contraindications and cautions

- Contraindicated with allergy to salicylates or other NSAIDs (more common in patients with rhinitis, asthma, chronic urticaria, nasal polyps); CV dysfunction, hypertension; peptic ulceration, GI bleeding; pregnancy or lactation.
- Use cautiously with impaired hepatic function, impaired renal function.

Adverse effects

- **CNS:** *Headache, dizziness, somnolence, insomnia,* fatigue, tiredness, tinnitus, ophthalmologic effects
- **Dermatologic:** *Rash,* pruritus, sweating, dry mucous membranes, stomatitis
- **GI:** *Nausea, dyspepsia, GI pain,* diarrhea, vomiting, constipation, flatulence
- **GU:** Dysuria, renal impairment
- **Hematologic:** Bleeding, platelet inhibition with higher doses, neutropenia, eosinophilia, leukopenia, pancytopenia, thrombocy-

topenia, agranulocytosis, granulocytopenia, aplastic anemia, decreased Hgb or Hct, bone marrow depression, menorrhagia
- **Respiratory:** Dyspnea, hemoptysis, pharyngitis, bronchospasm, rhinitis
- **Other:** Peripheral edema, anaphylactoid reactions to **anaphylactic shock**

Interactions

✱ **Drug-drug** • Increased toxic effects of lithium with NSAIDs • Decreased diuretic effect with loop diuretics: bumetanide, furosemide, ethacrynic acid • Potential decrease in antihypertensive effect of beta-adrenergic blockers

■ Nursing considerations

Assessment

- **History:** Allergy to salicylates or other NSAIDs; CV dysfunction, hypertension; peptic ulceration, GI bleeding; impaired hepatic function; impaired renal function; pregnancy; lactation
- **Physical:** Skin color, lesions; T; orientation, reflexes, ophthalmologic evaluation, audiometric evaluation, peripheral sensation; P, BP, edema; R, adventitious sounds; liver evaluation, bowel sounds; CBC, clotting times, urinalysis, LFTs, renal function tests, serum electrolytes, stool guaiac

Interventions

⊗ ***Black box warning*** Monitor patient for CV events, GI bleed; risk may be increased.
- Administer drug with food or after meals if GI upset occurs.
- Establish safety measures if CNS, visual disturbances occur.
- Arrange for periodic ophthalmologic examination during long-term therapy.
- Arrange for discontinuation of drug if eye changes, symptoms of hepatic impairment, renal impairment occur.
- Institute emergency procedures if overdose occurs (gastric lavage, induction of emesis, supportive therapy).
- Provide comfort measures to reduce pain and to reduce inflammation.
- Provide frequent small meals if GI upset is severe.

Teaching points

- Use these drugs only as suggested. Do not exceed the prescribed dosage. Take these drugs with food or after meals if GI upset occurs.
- Avoid over-the-counter drugs while taking these drugs. Many of these drugs contain similar medications; serious overdosage can occur. If you feel you need one of these preparations, consult your health care provider.
- Avoid alcohol while taking these drugs.
- You may experience these side effects: Nausea, GI upset, dyspepsia (take with food); diarrhea or constipation; drowsiness, dizziness, vertigo, insomnia (use caution when driving or operating dangerous machinery).
- Report sore throat, fever, rash, itching, weight gain, swelling in ankles or fingers, changes in vision, black or tarry stools.

Representative drugs

celecoxib
diclofenac
diflunisal
etodolac
fenoprofen
flurbiprofen
ibuprofen
indomethacin
ketoprofen
ketorolac
meclofenamate
mefenamic acid
meloxicam
nabumetone
naproxen
oxaprozin
piroxicam
sulindac
tolmetin

Opioids

PREGNANCY CATEGORY C

CONTROLLED SUBSTANCE C-II

Therapeutic actions

Opioids act as agonists at specific opioid receptors in the CNS to produce analgesia, euphoria, sedation; the receptors mediating these effects are thought to be the same as those mediating the effects of endogenous opioids (enkephalins, endorphins).

Indications

- Relief of moderate to severe acute and chronic pain
- Preoperative medication to sedate and allay apprehension, facilitate induction of anesthesia, and reduce anesthetic dosage
- Analgesic adjunct during anesthesia
- Intraspinal use with microinfusion devices for the relief of intractable pain
- Unlabeled use: Relief of dyspnea associated with acute left ventricular failure and pulmonary edema

Contraindications and cautions

- Contraindicated with hypersensitivity to opioids, diarrhea caused by poisoning until toxins are eliminated, during labor or delivery of a premature infant (may cross immature blood–brain barrier more readily), after biliary tract surgery or following surgical anastomosis, pregnancy, or labor (can cause respiratory depression of neonate; may prolong labor).
- Use cautiously with head injury and increased intracranial pressure; acute asthma, COPD, cor pulmonale, preexisting respiratory depression, hypoxia, hypercapnia (may decrease respiratory drive and increase airway resistance); lactation (may be safer to wait 4–6 hr after administration to nurse the baby); acute abdominal conditions; CV disease, supraventricular tachycardias; myxedema; seizure disorders; acute alcoholism, delirium tremens; cerebral arteriosclerosis; ulcerative colitis; fever; kyphoscoliosis; Addison's disease; prostatic hypertrophy, urethral stricture; recent GI or GU surgery; toxic psychosis; renal or hepatic impairment.

Adverse effects

- **CNS:** *Light-headedness, dizziness, sedation,* euphoria, dysphoria, delirium, insomnia, agitation, anxiety, fear, hallucinations, disorientation, drowsiness, lethargy, impaired mental and physical performance, coma, mood changes, weakness, headache, tremor, seizures, miosis, visual disturbances, suppression of cough reflex
- **CV:** Facial flushing, peripheral circulatory collapse, tachycardia, *bradycardia,* arrhythmia, palpitations, chest wall rigidity, hypertension, hypotension, orthostatic hypotension, syncope
- **Dermatologic:** Pruritus, urticaria, laryngospasm, bronchospasm, edema
- **GI:** *Nausea, vomiting,* dry mouth, anorexia, constipation, biliary tract spasm; increased colonic motility in patients with chronic ulcerative colitis
- **GU:** Ureteral spasm, spasm of vesical sphincters, urinary retention or hesitancy, oliguria, antidiuretic effect, reduced libido or potency
- **Local:** Tissue irritation and induration (subcutaneous injection)
- **Major hazards: Respiratory depression, apnea, circulatory depression, respiratory arrest, shock, cardiac arrest**
- **Other:** *Sweating,* physical tolerance and dependence, psychological dependence

Interactions

✱ **Drug-drug** • Increased likelihood of respiratory depression, hypotension, profound sedation, or coma in patients receiving barbiturate general anesthetics

✱ **Drug-lab test** • Elevated biliary tract pressure (an effect of opioids) may cause increases in plasma amylase, lipase; determinations of these levels may be unreliable for 24 hr

■ Nursing considerations

Assessment

- **History:** Hypersensitivity to opioids; diarrhea caused by poisoning; labor or delivery of a premature infant; biliary tract surgery or surgical anastomosis; head injury and increased intracranial pressure; acute asthma, COPD, cor pulmonale, preexisting respiratory depression, hypoxia, hypercapnia; acute abdominal conditions; CV disease, supraventricular tachycardias; myxedema; seizure disorders; acute alcoholism, delirium tremens; cerebral arteriosclerosis; ulcerative colitis; fever; kyphoscoliosis; Addison's disease; prostatic hypertrophy; urethral stricture; recent GI or GU surgery; toxic psychosis; renal or hepatic impairment; pregnancy; lactation

- **Physical:** T; skin color, texture, lesions; orientation, reflexes, bilateral grip strength, affect; P, auscultation, BP, orthostatic BP, perfusion; R, adventitious sounds; bowel sounds, normal output; urinary frequency, voiding pattern, normal output; ECG; EEG; LFTs, thyroid and renal function tests

Interventions

- Caution patient not to chew or crush controlled-release preparations.
- Dilute and administer IV slowly to minimize likelihood of adverse effects.
- Direct patient to lie down during IV administration.
- Keep opioid antagonist and equipment for assisted or controlled respiration readily available during IV administration.
- Use caution when injecting IM or subcutaneously into chilled areas or in patients with hypotension or in shock; impaired perfusion may delay absorption; with repeated doses, an excessive amount may be absorbed when circulation is restored.
- Monitor injection sites for irritation, extravasation.
- Instruct postoperative patients in pulmonary toilet; drug suppresses cough reflex.
- Monitor bowel function and arrange for anthraquinone laxatives for severe constipation.
- Institute safety precautions (use side rails, assist with walking) if CNS, vision effects occur.
- Provide frequent small meals if GI upset occurs.
- Control environment if sweating, visual difficulties occur.
- Provide back rubs, positioning, and other nondrug measures to alleviate pain.
- Reassure patient about addiction liability; most patients who receive opioids for medical reasons do not develop dependence syndromes.

Teaching points

When these drugs are used as a preoperative medication, teach the patient about the drug when explaining the procedure.

- Take these drugs exactly as prescribed. Avoid alcohol, antihistamines, sedatives, tranquilizers, and over-the-counter drugs.
- Do not take any leftover medication for other disorders, and do not let anyone else take your prescription.
- You may experience these side effects: Nausea, loss of appetite (take the drug with food and lie quietly); constipation (notify your health care provider if this is severe; a laxative may help); dizziness, sedation, drowsiness, impaired visual acuity (avoid driving or performing other tasks requiring alertness, visual acuity).
- Report severe nausea, vomiting, constipation, shortness of breath or difficulty breathing, skin rash.

Representative drugs

codeine
fentanyl
hydrocodone
hydromorphone
levomethadyl
levorphanol
meperidine
methadone
morphine sulfate
opium
oxycodone
oxymorphone
propoxyphene
remifentanil
sufentanil
tramadol

Penicillins

PREGNANCY CATEGORY B

Therapeutic actions

Penicillins are antibiotics. They are bactericidal, inhibiting the synthesis of cell wall of sensitive organisms, causing cell death in susceptible organisms.

Indications

- Treatment of moderate to severe infections caused by sensitive organisms: streptococci, pneumococci, staphylococci, *Neisseria gonorrhoeae, Treponema pallidum,* meningococci, *Actinomyces israelii, Clostridium perfringens, Clostridium tetani,*

Leptotrichia buccalis (Vincent's disease), *Spirillum minus* or *Streptobacillus moniliformis, Listeria monocytogenes, Pasteurella multocida, Erysipelothrix insidiosa, Escherichia coli, Enterobacter aerogenes, Alcaligenes faecalis, Salmonella, Shigella, Proteus mirabilis, Corynebacterium diphtheriae, Bacillus anthracis*
- Treatment of syphilis, gonococcal infections
- Unlabeled use: Treatment of Lyme disease

Contraindications and cautions
- Contraindicated with allergy to penicillins, cephalosporins, other allergens.
- Use cautiously with renal disease, pregnancy, lactation (may cause diarrhea or candidiasis in the infant).

Adverse effects
- **CNS:** Lethargy, hallucinations, seizures
- **GI:** *Glossitis, stomatitis, gastritis, sore mouth,* furry tongue, black "hairy" tongue, *nausea, vomiting, diarrhea,* abdominal pain, bloody diarrhea, enterocolitis, pseudomembranous colitis, nonspecific hepatitis
- **GU:** Nephritis-oliguria, proteinuria, hematuria, casts, azotemia, pyuria
- **Hematologic:** Anemia, thrombocytopenia, leukopenia, neutropenia, prolonged bleeding time
- **Hypersensitivity:** *Rash, fever, wheezing,* **anaphylaxis**
- **Local:** *Pain, phlebitis,* thrombosis at injection site, Jarisch-Herxheimer reaction when used to treat syphilis
- **Other:** *Superinfections,* sodium overload, leading to heart failure

Interactions
✱ **Drug-drug** • Decreased effectiveness with tetracyclines • Inactivation of parenteral aminoglycosides (amikacin, gentamicin, kanamycin, neomycin, streptomycin, tobramycin) if mixed in the same solution • Risk of increased serum levels if combined with aspirin, indomethacin, diuretics, sulfonamides
✱ **Drug-lab test** • False-positive Coombs' test (IV)

■ Nursing considerations
Assessment
- **History:** Allergy to penicillins, cephalosporins, other allergens, renal disease, lactation
- **Physical:** Culture infected area; skin rashes, lesions; R, adventitious sounds; bowel sounds, normal output; CBC, LFTs, renal function tests, serum electrolytes, Hct, urinalysis; skin test with benzylpenicilloylpolylysine if hypersensitivity reactions have occurred

Interventions
- Culture infected area before beginning treatment; reculture area if response is not as expected.
- Use the smallest dose possible for IM injection to avoid pain and discomfort.
- Arrange to continue treatment for 48–72 hr after the patient becomes asymptomatic.
- Monitor serum electrolytes and cardiac status if penicillin G is given by IV infusion. Na or K preparations have been associated with severe electrolyte imbalances.
- Check IV site carefully for signs of thrombosis or local drug reaction.
- Do not give IM injections repeatedly in the same site; atrophy can occur. Monitor injection sites.
- Explain the reason for parenteral routes of administration; offer support and encouragement to deal with therapy.
- Provide frequent small meals if GI upset occurs.
- Arrange for comfort and treatment measures for superinfections.
- Provide for frequent mouth care if GI effects occur.
- Ensure that bathroom facilities are readily available if diarrhea occurs.
- Keep epinephrine, IV fluids, vasopressors, bronchodilators, oxygen, and emergency equipment readily available in case of serious hypersensitivity reaction.
- Arrange for the use of corticosteroids, antihistamines for skin reactions.

Teaching points
- You may experience these side effects: Upset stomach, nausea, vomiting (eat frequent small meals); sore mouth (provide frequent mouth care); diarrhea; pain or discomfort

at the injection site (report if very uncomfortable).
- Report unusual bleeding, sore throat, rash, hives, fever, severe diarrhea, difficulty breathing.

Representative drugs

amoxicillin
ampicillin
dicloxacillin
nafcillin
oxacillin
penicillin G benzathine
penicillin G potassium
penicillin G procaine
penicillin V
piperacillin
ticarcillin

Phenothiazines

PREGNANCY CATEGORY C

Therapeutic actions

Mechanism of action of phenothiazines is not fully understood. Antipsychotic drugs block postsynaptic dopamine receptors in the brain, but this may not be necessary and sufficient for antipsychotic activity; depresses the RAS, including the parts of the brain involved with wakefulness and emesis; anticholinergic, antihistaminic (H_1), and alpha-adrenergic blocking activity also may contribute to some of its therapeutic (and adverse) actions.

Indications

- Management of manifestations of psychotic disorders
- Control of severe nausea and vomiting, intractable hiccups

Contraindications and cautions

- Contraindicated with coma or severe CNS depression, bone marrow depression, blood dyscrasia, circulatory collapse, subcortical brain damage, Parkinson's disease, liver damage, cerebral arteriosclerosis, coronary disease, severe hypotension or hypertension, prolonged QTc interval.
- Use cautiously with respiratory disorders ("silent pneumonia" may develop); glaucoma, prostatic hypertrophy; epilepsy or history of epilepsy; breast cancer; thyrotoxicosis; peptic ulcer, decreased renal function; myelography within previous 24 hr or scheduled within 48 hr; exposure to heat or phosphorous insecticides; pregnancy; lactation; children younger than 12 yr, especially those with chickenpox, CNS infections (children are especially susceptible to dystonias that may confound the diagnosis of Reye's syndrome).

Adverse effects

- **Autonomic:** Dry mouth, salivation, nasal congestion, nausea, vomiting, anorexia, fever, pallor, flushed facies, sweating, constipation, paralytic ileus, urine retention, incontinence, polyuria, enuresis, priapism, ejaculation inhibition, male impotence
- **CNS:** *Drowsiness,* insomnia, vertigo, headache, weakness, tremor, ataxia, slurring, cerebral edema, seizures, exacerbation of psychotic symptoms, extrapyramidal syndromes—*pseudoparkinsonism; dystonias; akathisia,* tardive dyskinesias, potentially irreversible (no known treatment) **neuroleptic malignant syndrome**
- **CV:** Hypotension, orthostatic hypotension, hypertension, tachycardia, bradycardia, cardiac arrest, heart failure, cardiomegaly, **refractory arrhythmias,** pulmonary edema, prolonged QTc interval
- **EENT:** Glaucoma, *photophobia, blurred vision,* miosis, mydriasis, deposits in the cornea and lens (opacities), pigmentary retinopathy
- **Endocrine:** Lactation, breast engorgement in females, galactorrhea; syndrome of inappropriate ADH secretion; amenorrhea, menstrual irregularities; gynecomastia in males; changes in libido; hyperglycemia or hypoglycemia; glycosuria; hyponatremia; pituitary tumor with hyperprolactinemia; inhibition of ovulation, infertility, pseudopregnancy; reduced urinary levels of gonadotropins, estrogens, progestins
- **Hematologic:** Eosinophilia, leukopenia, leukocytosis, anemia; aplastic anemia; hemolytic anemia; thrombocytopenic or nonthrombocytopenic purpura; pancytopenia

- **Hypersensitivity:** Jaundice, urticaria, angioneurotic edema, laryngeal edema, photosensitivity, eczema, asthma, anaphylactoid reactions, exfoliative dermatitis
- **Respiratory:** Bronchospasm, laryngospasm, dyspnea; suppression of cough reflex and potential for aspiration (**sudden death related to asphyxia** or cardiac arrest has been reported)
- **Other:** *Urine discolored pink to red-brown*

Interactions

✱ **Drug-drug** • Additive CNS depression with alcohol • Additive anticholinergic effects and possibly decreased antipsychotic efficacy with anticholinergic drugs • Increased likelihood of seizures with metrizamide (contrast agent used in myelography) • Increased chance of severe neuromuscular excitation and hypotension if given to patients receiving barbiturate anesthetics (methohexital, phenobarbital, thiopental) • Increased risk of cardiac arrhythmias and serious adverse effects if combined with drugs that prolong the QTc interval

✱ **Drug-lab test** • False-positive pregnancy tests (less likely if serum test is used) • Increase in protein-bound iodine, not attributable to an increase in thyroxine

■ Nursing considerations

Assessment

- **History:** Coma or severe CNS depression; bone marrow depression; blood dyscrasia; circulatory collapse; subcortical brain damage; Parkinson's disease; liver damage; cerebral arteriosclerosis; coronary disease; severe hypotension or hypertension; respiratory disorders; glaucoma, prostatic hypertrophy; epilepsy or history of epilepsy; breast cancer; thyrotoxicosis; peptic ulcer, decreased renal function; myelography within previous 24 hr or myelography scheduled within 48 hr; exposure to heat or phosphorous insecticides; pregnancy; children younger than 12 yr, especially those with chickenpox, CNS infections
- **Physical:** Weight, T; reflexes, orientation, IOP; P, BP, orthostatic BP; R, adventitious sounds; bowel sounds and normal output, liver evaluation; urinary output, prostate size; CBC, urinalysis, thyroid, LFTs, renal function tests, ECG analysis

Interventions

- Obtain baseline ECG with QTc interval noted.
- Dilute oral concentrate *only* with water, saline, *7-Up,* homogenized milk, carbonated orange drink, and pineapple, apricot, prune, orange, *V-8,* tomato, or grapefruit juices; use 60 mL of diluent for each 16 mg (5 mL) of concentrate.
- Do *not* mix with beverages that contain caffeine (coffee, cola), tannics (tea), or pectinates (apple juice); physical incompatibility may result.
- Give IM injections only to seated or recumbent patients, and observe for adverse effects for a brief period afterward.
- Monitor pulse and BP continuously during IV administration.
- Do not change long-term therapy dosage more often than weekly; it takes 4–7 days to achieve steady-state plasma levels of drug.
- Avoid skin contact with oral solution; contact dermatitis has occurred.
- Arrange for discontinuation of drug if serum creatinine, BUN become abnormal or if WBC count is depressed.
- Monitor bowel function, arrange therapy for severe constipation; adynamic ileus with fatal complications has occurred.
- Monitor elderly patients for dehydration and institute remedial measures promptly; sedation and decreased sensation of thirst related to CNS effects of drug can lead to severe dehydration.
- Consult physician regarding warning of patient or patient's guardian about tardive dyskinesias.
- Consult physician about reducing dosage, using anticholinergic antiparkinsonians (controversial) if extrapyramidal effects occur.
- Provide safety measures (side rails, assist) if sedation, ataxia, vertigo, orthostatic hypotension, vision changes occur.
- Provide positioning to relieve discomfort of dystonias.
- Provide reassurance to deal with extrapyramidal effect, sexual dysfunction.

Teaching points

- Take these drugs exactly as prescribed. The full effect may require 6 weeks–6 months of therapy.
- Avoid skin contact with drug solutions.
- Avoid driving or engaging in activities requiring alertness if CNS, vision changes occur.
- Avoid prolonged exposure to sun or use a sunscreen or covering garments.
- Maintain fluid intake, and use precautions against heatstroke in hot weather.
- Report sore throat, fever, unusual bleeding or bruising, rash, weakness, tremors, impaired vision, dark urine (pink or reddish brown urine is to be expected), pale stools, yellowing of the skin or eyes.

Representative drugs

chlorpromazine
fluphenazine
perphenazine
prochlorperazine
thioridazine
trifluoperazine

Phosphodiesterase Type 5 Inhibitors

PREGNANCY CATEGORY B

Therapeutic actions

Selectively inhibits cGMP-specific phosphodiesterase type 5. The mechanism of penile erection involves the release of nitric oxide into the corpus cavernosum of the penis during sexual stimulation. Nitrous oxide activates cGMP, which causes smooth muscle relaxation allowing the flow of blood into the corpus cavernosum. Phosphodiesterase type 5 inhibitors prevent the breakdown of cGMP by phosphodiesterase, leading to increased cGMP levels and prolonged smooth muscle relaxation promoting the flow of blood into the corpus cavernosum.

Indications

- Treatment of erectile dysfunction in the presence of sexual stimulation
- Treatment of pulmonary arterial hypertension

Contraindications and cautions

- Contraindicated with allergy to any component of the drugs, for women or children; concurrent use of nitrates or alpha blockers.
- Use cautiously with hepatic or renal impairment; with anatomical deformation of the penis; with known cardiac disease (effects of sexual activity need to be evaluated); congenital prolonged QT interval; unstable angina; hypotension (systolic lower than 90); uncontrolled hypertension (higher than 170/110); severe hepatic impairment; end-stage renal disease with dialysis; hereditary degenerative retinal disorders.

Adverse effects

- **CNS:** *Headache,* abnormal vision, changes in color vision, fatigue, hearing loss
- **CV:** *Flushing,* angina, chest pain, hypertension, hypotension, **MI,** palpitation, orthostatic hypotension, tachycardia
- **GI:** *Dyspepsia,* diarrhea, abdominal pain, dry mouth, esophagitis, gastritis, GERD, nausea, abnormal LFT
- **GU:** Abnormal erection, spontaneous erection, priapism
- **Respiratory:** Rhinitis, sinusitis, dyspnea, epistaxis, pharynigitis, nasal congestion
- **Other:** Flulike symptoms, edema, pain, rash, sweating, myalgia

Interactions

✱ **Drug-drug** • Possible severe hypotension and serious cardiac events if combined with nitrates, alpha blockers; this combination is contraindicated • Possible increased levels and effects if taken with ketoconazole, itraconazole, erythromycin; monitor patient and reduce dosage as needed • Increased serum levels if combined with indinavir, ritonavir; if these drugs are being used, limit dosage • Reduced levels and effectiveness if combined with rifampin • Risk for increased cardiac effects, decreased BP, flushing if combined with alcohol; warn patient of this possibility if alcohol is used
✱ **Drug-food** • Possible increased levels if taken with grapefruit juice

■ Nursing considerations

Assessment

- **History:** Allergy to any component of the tablet, concurrent use of nitrates or alpha blockers; unstable angina; hypotension; uncontrolled hypertension; severe hepatic impairment; end-stage renal disease with dialysis; hereditary degenerative retinal disorders; anatomical deformation of the penis, cardiac disease, congenital prolonged QT interval
- **Physical:** Orientation, affect; skin color, lesions; R, adventitious sounds; P, BP, ECG, LFTs, renal function tests

Interventions

- Assure diagnosis of erectile dysfunction and determine underlying causes and other appropriate treatment.
- Advise patient that drug does not work in the absence of sexual stimulation. Limit use to once per day.
- Remind patient that drug does not protect against STDs and that appropriate measures should be taken.

⊗ ***Black box warning*** Advise patient to never take this drug with nitrates or alpha blockers; serious and even fatal complications can occur.

- Warn patient of the risk of lowered BP and dizziness if taken with alcohol.

Teaching points

- Take these drugs before anticipated sexual activity; the drug will stay in your body for up to 4 hours (sildenafil, vardenafil), or longer than 3 days (tadalafil). The drug will have no effect in the absence of sexual stimulation.
- These drugs will not protect you from sexually transmitted diseases; use appropriate precautions.
- Do not take these drugs if you are taking any nitrates or alpha blockers or other drugs for treating erectile dysfunction; serious side effects and even death can occur.
- Many drugs may interact with these drugs; consult your health care provider before taking any drug, including over-the-counter drugs and herbal therapies; dosage adjustments may be needed.
- Know that combining these drugs with alcohol could cause dizziness, loss of blood pressure, increased flushing.
- You may experience these side effects: Headache, dizziness, upset stomach, runny nose, muscle pains; these side effects should go away within a couple of hours. If side effects persist, consult your health care provider.
- Report difficult or painful urination, vision changes, hearing loss, fainting, erection that persists for longer than 4 hours (if this occurs, seek medical assistance as soon as possible).

Representative drugs

sildenafil
tadalafil
vardenafil

Selective Serotonin Reuptake Inhibitors (SSRIs)

PREGNANCY CATEGORY C

Therapeutic actions

The SSRIs act as antidepressants by inhibiting CNS neuronal uptake of serotonin and blocking uptake of serotonin with little effect on norepinephrine; they are also thought to antagonize muscarinic, histaminergic, and alpha$_1$-adrenergic receptors. The increase in serotonin levels at neuroreceptors is thought to act as a stimulant, counteracting depression and increasing motivation.

Indications

- Treatment of depression; most effective in patients with major depressive disorder
- Treatment of OCD, PTSD, social anxiety, generalized anxiety disorder, panic disorder, PMDD
- Unlabeled uses: Treatment of bulimia

Contraindications and cautions

- Contraindicated with hypersensitivity to any SSRI; pregnancy.
- Use cautiously with impaired hepatic or renal function, diabetes mellitus, lactation.

Adverse effects

- **CNS:** *Headache, nervousness, insomnia, drowsiness, anxiety, tremor, dizziness, light-headedness,* agitation, sedation, abnormal gait, seizures
- **CV:** Hot flashes, palpitations
- **Dermatologic:** *Sweating, rash, pruritus,* acne, alopecia, contact dermatitis
- **GI:** *Nausea, vomiting, diarrhea, dry mouth, anorexia, dyspepsia, constipation, taste changes,* flatulence, gastroenteritis, dysphagia, gingivitis
- **GU:** *Painful menstruation, sexual dysfunction,* frequency, cystitis, impotence, urgency, vaginitis
- **Respiratory:** *URIs, pharyngitis,* cough, dyspnea, bronchitis, rhinitis
- **Other:** *Weight loss, asthenia, fever*

Interactions

✱ **Drug-drug** • Increased therapeutic and toxic effects of TCAs with SSRIs • Decreased therapeutic effects with cyproheptadine • Risk for severe to fatal hypertensive crisis with MAOIs; avoid this combination

✱ **Drug-alternative therapy** • Increased risk of severe reaction with St. John's wort

■ Nursing considerations

Assessment

- **History:** Hypersensitivity to any SSRI; impaired hepatic or renal function; diabetes mellitus; lactation; pregnancy
- **Physical:** Weight; T; skin rash, lesions; reflexes, affect; bowel sounds, liver evaluation; P, peripheral perfusion; urinary output; LFTs, renal function tests, CBC

Interventions

- Arrange for lower dose or less frequent administration in elderly patients and patients with hepatic or renal impairment.
- Establish suicide precautions for severely depressed patients. Dispense only a small number of capsules at a time to these patients.

⊗ ***Black box warning*** Monitor children, adolescents, and young adults for suicidal thoughts and behavior, especially when changing dosage.

- Administer drug in the morning. If dose of more than 20 mg/day is needed, administer in divided doses.
- Monitor patient response for up to 4 wk before increasing dose because of lack of therapeutic effect. It frequently takes several weeks to see the desired effect.
- Provide frequent small meals if GI upset or anorexia occurs. Monitor weight loss; a nutritional consultation may be needed.
- Provide sugarless lozenges, frequent mouth care if dry mouth is a problem.
- Ensure ready access to bathroom facilities if diarrhea occurs. Establish bowel program if constipation is a problem.
- Establish safety precautions (use side rails, appropriate lighting; accompany patient) if CNS effects occur.
- Provide appropriate comfort measures if CNS effects, insomnia, rash, sweating occur.
- Encourage patient to maintain therapy for treatment of underlying cause of depression.

Teaching points

- It may take up to 4 weeks to get a full antidepressant effect from these drugs. These drugs should be taken in the morning (or in divided doses if necessary).
- Do not take these drugs during pregnancy. If you think that you are pregnant or you wish to become pregnant, consult your health care provider.
- You may experience these side effects: Dizziness, drowsiness, nervousness, insomnia (avoid driving or performing hazardous tasks); nausea, vomiting, weight loss (frequent small meals may help; monitor your weight loss—if it becomes marked, consult your health care provider); sexual dysfunction (drug effect); flulike symptoms (if severe, consult your health care provider for appropriate treatment); photosensitivity (avoid exposure to sunlight).
- Report rash, mania, seizures, severe weight loss.

Representative drugs

citalopram
desvenlafaxine
escitalopram
fluoxetine

fluvoxamine
paroxetine
sertraline
venlafaxine

Sulfonamides

PREGNANCY CATEGORY C

PREGNANCY CATEGORY D (AT TERM)

Therapeutic actions

Sulfonamides are antibiotics. They are bacteriostatic; competitively antagonize para-aminobenzoic acid, an essential component of folic acid synthesis, in susceptible gram-negative and gram-positive bacteria, causing cell death.

Indications

- Treatment of ulcerative colitis, otitis media, inclusion conjunctivitis, meningitis, nocardiosis, toxoplasmosis, trachoma, UTIs
- Management of rheumatoid arthritis, collagenous colitis, Crohn's disease

Contraindications and cautions

- Contraindicated with allergy to sulfonamides, sulfonylureas, thiazides; pregnancy (teratogenic in preclinical studies; at term, may bump fetal bilirubin from plasma protein binding sites and cause kernicterus); or lactation (risk of kernicterus, diarrhea, rash).
- Use cautiously with impaired renal or hepatic function, G6PD deficiency, porphyria.

Adverse effects

- **CNS:** Headache, peripheral neuropathy, mental depression, seizures, ataxia, hallucinations, tinnitus, vertigo, insomnia, hearing loss, drowsiness, transient lesions of posterior spinal column, transverse myelitis
- **Dermatologic:** Photosensitivity, cyanosis, petechiae, alopecia
- **GI:** Nausea, emesis, abdominal pains, diarrhea, bloody diarrhea, anorexia, pancreatitis, stomatitis, impaired folic acid absorption, hepatitis, hepatocellular necrosis
- **GU:** Crystalluria, hematuria, proteinuria, nephrotic syndrome, toxic nephrosis with oliguria and anuria, oligospermia, infertility
- **Hematologic: Agranulocytosis, aplastic anemia,** thrombocytopenia, leukopenia, hemolytic anemia, hypoprothrombinemia, methemoglobinemia, megaloblastic anemia
- **Hypersensitivity: Stevens-Johnson syndrome,** generalized skin eruptions, epidermal necrolysis, urticaria, serum sickness, pruritus, **exfoliative dermatitis, anaphylactoid reactions,** periorbital edema, conjunctival and scleral redness, photosensitization, arthralgia, allergic myocarditis, transient pulmonary changes with eosinophilia, decreased pulmonary function
- **Other:** Drug fever, chills, periarteritis nodosum

Interactions

✷ **Drug-drug** • Increased risk of hypoglycemia when tolbutamide, tolazamide, glyburide, glipizide, chlorpropamide are taken concurrently • Increased risk of folate deficiency if taking sulfonamides; monitor patients receiving folic acid carefully for signs of folate deficiency

✷ **Drug-lab test** • Possible false-positive urinary glucose tests using Benedict's method

■ Nursing considerations

Assessment

- **History:** Allergy to sulfonamides, sulfonylureas, thiazides; pregnancy; lactation; impaired renal or hepatic function; G6PD deficiency; porphyria
- **Physical:** T; skin color, lesions; culture of infected site; orientation, reflexes, affect, peripheral sensation; R, adventitious sounds; mucous membranes, bowel sounds, liver evaluation; LFTs, renal function tests, CBC and differential, urinalysis

Interventions

- Arrange for culture and sensitivity tests of infected area prior to therapy; repeat cultures if response is not as expected.
- Administer drug after meals or with food to prevent GI upset. Administer the drug around the clock.
- Ensure adequate fluid intake.

- Discontinue drug immediately if hypersensitivity reaction occurs.
- Establish safety precautions if CNS effects occur (side rails, assistance, environmental control).
- Protect patient from exposure to light (use sunscreen, protective clothing) if photosensitivity occurs.
- Provide frequent small meals if GI upset occurs.
- Provide mouth care for stomatitis.
- Offer support and encouragement to deal with side effects of drug therapy, including changes in sexual function.

Teaching points

- Complete the full course of therapy.
- Take these drugs with food or meals to decrease GI upset.
- Drink eight glasses of water per day.
- These drugs are specific to the disease being treated; do not use to self-treat any other infection.
- You may experience these side effects: Sensitivity to sunlight (use sunscreens; wear protective clothing); dizziness, drowsiness, difficulty walking, loss of sensation (avoid driving or performing tasks that require alertness); nausea, vomiting, diarrhea (ensure ready access to bathroom); loss of fertility; yellow-orange urine.
- Report blood in the urine, rash, ringing in the ears, difficulty breathing, fever, sore throat, chills.

Representative drugs

balsalazide
sulfadiazine
sulfamethoxazole (always used in combination with trimethoprim)
sulfasalazine
sulfisoxazole

Tetracyclines

PREGNANCY CATEGORY D

Therapeutic actions

Tetracyclines are antibiotics. They are bacteriostatic; inhibit protein synthesis of susceptible bacteria, preventing cell replication.

Indications

- Treatment of infections caused by rickettsiae; *Mycoplasma pneumoniae;* agents of psittacosis, ornithosis, lymphogranuloma venereum, and granuloma inguinale; *Borrelia recurrentis, Haemophilus ducreyi, Pasteurella pestis, Pasteurella tularensis, Bartonella bacilliformis, Bacteroides, Vibrio comma, Vibrio fetus, Brucella, Escherichia coli, Escherichia aerogenes, Shigella, Acinetobacter calcoaceticus, Haemophilus influenzae, Staphylococcus aureus, Diplococcus pneumoniae, Klebsiella;* when penicillin is contraindicated, infections caused by *Neisseria gonorrhoeae, Listeria monocytogenes, Treponema pallidum, Treponema pertenue, Clostridium, Bacillus anthracis, Actinomyces, Fusobacterium fusiforme, Neisseria meningitidis*
- Adjunct to amebicides in acute intestinal amebiasis
- Treatment of malaria
- Treatment of anthrax
- Treatment of acne
- Treatment of complicated urethral, endocervical, or rectal infections in adults caused by *Chlamydia trachomatis*
- Treatment of superficial ocular infections caused by susceptible strains of microorganisms
- Prophylaxis of ophthalmia neonatorum caused by *N. gonorrhoeae* or *C. trachomatis*
- Unlabeled uses: Lyme disease, carditis, facial nerve paralysis, arthritis, early syphilis, chlamydial infection, PID, epididymitis, prophylaxis after sexual assault

Contraindications and cautions

- Contraindicated with allergy to any tetracyclines, allergy to tartrazine (in 250-mg tetracycline capsules marketed under brand name *Sumycin,* pregnancy (toxic to fetus), lactation (causes damage to the teeth of infants).
- Use cautiously with hepatic or renal impairment; ocular viral, mycobacterial, or fungal infections.

Adverse effects

- **Dermatologic:** *Phototoxic reactions, rash,* **exfoliative dermatitis**

- **GI:** *Discoloring and inadequate calcification of primary teeth of fetus if used by pregnant women, discoloring and inadequate calcification of permanent teeth if used during period of dental development,* fatty liver, hepatic failure, *anorexia, nausea, vomiting, diarrhea, glossitis, dysphagia,* enterocolitis, esophageal ulcers
- **Hematologic:** Hemolytic anemia, thrombocytopenia, neutropenia, eosinophilia, leukocytosis, leukopenia
- **Hypersensitivity:** Reactions from urticaria to **anaphylaxis,** including intracranial hypertension
- **Local:** *Transient irritation, stinging, itching,* angioneurotic edema, urticaria, dermatitis, superinfections with ophthalmic or dermatologic use
- **Other:** *Superinfections,* local irritation at parenteral injection sites

Interactions

✱ **Drug-drug** • Decreased absorption with calcium salts, magnesium salts, zinc salts, aluminum salts, bismuth salts, iron, urine alkalinizers, food, dairy products, charcoal • Increased digoxin toxicity • Increased nephrotoxicity if taken with methoxyflurane • Decreased effectiveness of hormonal contraceptives (rare) with a risk of breakthrough bleeding or pregnancy • Decreased activity of penicillins

■ Nursing considerations

Assessment

- **History:** Allergy to any of the tetracyclines; allergy to tartrazine; hepatic or renal impairment, pregnancy, lactation; ocular viral, mycobacterial, or fungal infections
- **Physical:** Site of infection, skin color, lesions; R, adventitious sounds; bowel sounds, output, liver evaluation; urinalysis, BUN, LFTs, renal function tests

Interventions

- Administer oral medication on an empty stomach, 1 hr before or 2–3 hr after meals. Do not give with antacids. If antacids must be used, give them 3 hr after the dose of tetracycline.
- Culture infected area prior to drug therapy.
- Do not use outdated drugs; degraded drug is highly nephrotoxic and should not be used.
- Do not give oral drug with meals, antacids, or food.
- Provide frequent hygiene measures if superinfections occur.
- Protect patient from sunlight and bright lights if photosensitivity occurs.
- Arrange for regular renal function tests if long-term therapy is used.
- Use topical preparations of this drug only when clearly indicated. Sensitization from the topical use of this drug may preclude its later use in serious infections. Topical preparations containing antibiotics that are not ordinarily given systemically are preferable.

Teaching points

Systemic administration

- Take these drugs throughout the day for best results. These drugs should be taken on an empty stomach, 1 hour before or 2–3 hours after meals, with a full glass of water. Do not take these drugs with food, dairy products, iron preparations, or antacids.
- Take the full course of therapy prescribed; if any drug is left, discard it immediately. Never take an outdated product.
- Pregnancy may occur when taking tetracycline with hormonal contraceptives. To be sure of avoiding pregnancy, use an additional type of contraceptive while using this drug.
- Report severe cramps, watery diarrhea, rash or itching, difficulty breathing, dark urine or light-colored stools, yellowing of the skin or eyes.

Eye drop administration

- To give eye drops: Lie down or tilt your head backward and look at the ceiling. Drop suspension drug inside your lower eyelid while looking up. Close your eye, and apply gentle pressure to the inner corner of the eye for 1 minute.
- Apply ointment inside the lower eyelid; close your eyes, and roll your eyeball in all directions.
- These drugs may cause temporary blurring of vision or stinging after application.
- Notify your health care provider if stinging or itching becomes severe.
- Take the full course of therapy prescribed; discard any leftover medication.
- Apply dermatologic solution until skin is wet. Avoid eyes, nose, and mouth.

Topical administration

- You may experience transient stinging or burning; this will subside quickly; skin in the treated area may become yellow; this will wash off.
- Use cosmetics as you usually do.
- Wash area before applying (unless contraindicated); this drug may stain clothing.
- You may experience these side effects: Stomach upset, nausea; superinfections in the mouth, vagina (frequent washing may help; if it becomes severe, medication may help); sensitivity of the skin to sunlight (use protective clothing and sunscreen).
- Report worsening of condition, rash, irritation.

Representative drugs

demeclocycline
doxycycline
minocycline
tetracycline

Tricyclic Antidepressants (TCAs)

PREGNANCY CATEGORY C OR D (AMITRIPTYLINE, IMIPRAMINE, NORTRIPTYLINE)

Therapeutic actions

Mechanism of action is unknown. The TCAs are structurally related to the phenothiazine antipsychotic drugs (eg, chlorpromazine), but in contrast to them, TCAs inhibit the presynaptic reuptake of the neurotransmitters norepinephrine and serotonin; anticholinergic at CNS and peripheral receptors; the relation of these effects to clinical efficacy is unknown.

Indications

- Relief of symptoms of major depressive disorders
- Treatment of OCDs
- Unlabeled use: Treatment of obstructive sleep apnea, panic disorder, eating disorders, PMS, migraine, ADHD

Contraindications and cautions

- Contraindicated with hypersensitivity to any tricyclic drug, concomitant therapy with an MAOI, recent MI, myelography within previous 24 hr or scheduled within 48 hr, pregnancy (limb reduction abnormalities reported), or lactation.
- Use cautiously with EST; preexisting CV disorders (severe coronary heart disease, progressive heart failure, angina pectoris, paroxysmal tachycardia); angle-closure glaucoma, increased IOP, urine retention, ureteral or urethral spasm; seizure disorders (lower seizure threshold); hyperthyroidism (predisposes to CVS toxicity, including cardiac arrhythmias); impaired hepatic, renal function; psychiatric patients; schizophrenic or paranoid may exhibit a worsening of psychosis; manic-depressive disorder may shift to hypomanic or manic phase; elective surgery (discontinue as long as possible before surgery).

Adverse effects

- **CNS:** *Sedation and anticholinergic (atropine-like) effects* (dry mouth, blurred vision, disturbance of accommodation for near vision, mydriasis, increased IOP), *confusion* (especially in elderly), *disturbed concentration,* hallucinations, disorientation, decreased memory, feelings of unreality, delusions, anxiety, nervousness, restlessness, agitation, panic, insomnia, nightmares, hypomania, mania, exacerbation of psychosis, drowsiness, weakness, fatigue, headache, numbness, tingling, paresthesias of extremities, incoordination, motor hyperactivity, akathisia, ataxia, tremors, peripheral neuropathy, extrapyramidal symptoms, *seizures,* speech blockage, dysarthria, tinnitus, altered EEG
- **CV:** *Orthostatic hypotension,* hypertension, syncope, tachycardia, palpitations, MI, arrhythmias, heart block, precipitation of heart failure, CVA
- **Endocrine:** Elevated or depressed blood sugar; elevated prolactin levels; inappropriate ADH secretion
- **GI:** *Dry mouth, constipation,* paralytic ileus, *nausea,* vomiting, anorexia, epigastric distress, diarrhea, flatulence, dysphagia,

peculiar taste, increased salivation, stomatitis, glossitis, parotid swelling, abdominal cramps, black "hairy" tongue
- **GU:** Urine retention, delayed micturition, dilation of the urinary tract, gynecomastia, testicular swelling; breast enlargement, menstrual irregularity, and galactorrhea; change in libido; impotence
- **Hematologic:** Bone marrow depression, including agranulocytosis; eosinophilia; purpura; thrombocytopenia; leukopenia
- **Hypersensitivity:** Skin rash, pruritus, vasculitis, petechiae, photosensitization, edema (generalized, face and tongue), drug fever
- **Withdrawal:** Symptoms with abrupt discontinuation of prolonged therapy; nausea, headache, vertigo, nightmares, malaise
- **Other:** Nasal congestion, excessive appetite, weight change; sweating, alopecia, lacrimation, hyperthermia, flushing, chills

Interactions

✱ **Drug-drug** • Increased TCA levels and pharmacologic effects with cimetidine, fluoxetine, ranitidine • Altered response, including arrhythmias and hypertension, with sympathomimetics • Risk of severe hypertension with clonidine • Hyperpyretic crises, severe seizures, hypertensive episodes, and death with MAOIs • Decreased hypotensive activity of guanethidine

■ Nursing considerations

Assessment

- **History:** Hypersensitivity to any tricyclic drug; concomitant therapy with an MAOI; recent MI; myelography within previous 24 hr or scheduled within 48 hr; pregnancy; lactation; preexisting disorders; angle-closure glaucoma, increased IOP; urinary retention, ureteral or urethral spasm; seizure disorders; hyperthyroidism; impaired hepatic, renal function; psychiatric, manic-depressive disorder; elective surgery
- **Physical:** Weight; T; skin color, lesions; orientation, affect, reflexes, vision and hearing; P, BP, orthostatic BP, perfusion; bowel sounds, normal output, liver evaluation; urine flow, normal output; usual sexual function, frequency of menses, breast and scrotal examination; LFTs, urinalysis, CBC, ECG

Interventions

- Ensure that depressed and potentially suicidal patients have limited access to drug.
- Reduce dosage if minor side effects develop; discontinue drug if serious side effects occur.
- Arrange for CBC if patient develops fever, sore throat, or other sign of infection.
- Ensure ready access to bathroom if GI effects occur; establish bowel program for constipation.
- Provide frequent small meals, frequent mouth care if GI effects occur; provide sugarless lozenges for dry mouth.
- Establish safety precautions if CNS changes occur (side rails, assist walking).

Teaching points

- Take these drugs exactly as prescribed; do not stop taking these drugs abruptly or without consulting your health care provider.
- Avoid alcohol, sleep-inducing drugs, over-the-counter drugs.
- Avoid prolonged exposure to sunlight or sunlamps; use a sunscreen or protective garments if unavoidable.
- You may experience these side effects: Headache, dizziness, drowsiness, weakness, blurred vision (reversible; safety measures may be needed if severe; avoid driving or performing tasks requiring alertness); nausea, vomiting, loss of appetite, dry mouth (frequent small meals, mouth care, and sucking sugarless candies may help); nightmares, inability to concentrate, confusion; changes in sexual function.
- Report dry mouth, difficulty in urination, excessive sedation.

Representative drugs

amitriptyline
amoxapine
clomipramine
desipramine
doxepin
imipramine
nortriptyline
protriptyline
trimipramine

abacavir sulfate

*(ah **bak'** ah veer)*

Ziagen

PREGNANCY CATEGORY C

Drug class

Antiviral
Nucleoside reverse transcriptase inhibitor

Therapeutic actions

Nucleoside reverse transcriptase inhibitor; obstructs RNA and DNA synthesis and inhibits viral reproduction. Used in combination with other anti-HIV drugs to reduce the viral load as low as possible and decrease the chance of further viral mutation. Thought to cross the blood–brain barrier and be effective in the treatment of HIV-related dementia. There are no long-term studies on the effectiveness of this drug.

Indications

- Treatment of HIV-1 infection in combination with other antiretrovirals

Contraindications and cautions

- Contraindicated with life-threatening allergy or hypersensitivity to any component, moderate to severe hepatic impairment.
- Use cautiously with mild hepatic impairment, lactic acidosis, pregnancy, lactation.

Available forms

Tablets—300 mg; oral solution—20 mg/mL

Dosages

Adults

300 mg PO bid or 600 mg PO once daily.

Adults with mild hepatic impairment

200 mg PO bid (solution).

Pediatric patients 3 mo–16 yr

8 mg/kg PO bid; do not exceed 300 mg/dose.

Pediatric patients younger than 3 mo

Not recommended.

Pharmacokinetics

Route	*Onset*	*Peak*
Oral	Rapid	2–4 hr

Metabolism: Hepatic; $T_{1/2}$: 1–2 hr
Distribution: May cross placenta; may enter breast milk
Excretion: Urine, feces

Adverse effects

- **CNS:** *Headache, weakness, malaise, fatigue, insomnia,* dizziness, anxiety, depression
- **Dermatologic:** *Rash*
- **GI:** *Diarrhea, nausea,* anorexia, *vomiting,* dyspepsia, liver enzyme elevations, liver enlargement, **risk of severe to fatal hepatomegaly**
- **Other: Severe hypersensitivity reactions** (fever, malaise, nausea, vomiting, rash), **severe to fatal lactic acidosis,** fat redistribution, increased lipid levels

Interactions

✱ **Drug-drug** • Risk of severe toxic effects if combined with alcohol

■ Nursing considerations

Assessment

- **History:** Life-threatening allergy to any component, impaired hepatic or renal function, lactic acidosis, pregnancy, lactation
- **Physical:** T; affect, reflexes, peripheral sensation; R, adventitious sounds; bowel sounds, liver evaluation; LFTs, renal function tests

Interventions

- Administer with meals or a light snack if GI upset occurs.

⊗ ***Black box warning*** Monitor patient for signs of potentially fatal hypersensitivity reaction; give patient hypersensitivity reaction card provided by manufacturer. Advise patient to stop drug at first sign of reaction. Do not try the drug again if the patient has a hypersensitivity reaction.

⊗ ***Black box warning*** Monitor patient for lactic acidosis and severe hepatomegaly; increased risk with other antivirals.

⊗ ***Black box warning*** Patients with HLA-B*5701 allele are at high risk for hypersensitivity reactions. Screening for HLA-B*5701 allele is recommended.

- Administer the drug concurrently with other anti-HIV drugs.
- Recommend the use of barrier contraceptives while on this drug.

Teaching points

- Take drug exactly as prescribed; take missed doses as soon as possible and return to normal schedule; do not double skipped doses; take with meals or a light snack if GI upset occurs.
- This drug is not a cure for AIDS or AIDS-related complex; opportunistic infections may occur and regular medical follow-up is needed.
- Long-term effects of this drug are unknown.
- Treatment does not reduce the risk of transmission of HIV by sexual contact or blood contamination; use precautions.
- Do not drink alcohol while taking this drug.
- Use barrier contraceptives; hormonal contraceptives may not be effective.
- This drug has been connected with severe hypersensitivity reactions, which usually occur early in the use of the drug. Keep your hypersensitivity list readily available, and stop the drug if any of these effects occur.
- You may experience these side effects: Nausea, loss of appetite, diarrhea (eat frequent small meals; medication is available to control the diarrhea); dizziness, loss of feeling (take appropriate precautions).
- Report extreme fatigue, lethargy, severe headache, severe nausea, vomiting, difficulty breathing, rash, fever.

▽abarelix

See Appendix W, *Less commonly used drugs*.

▽abatacept

See Appendix W, *Less commonly used drugs*.

▽abciximab

(ab ***six'*** *ah mab)*

ReoPro

PREGNANCY CATEGORY C

Drug class

Antiplatelet
Glycoprotein IIb/IIIa inhibitor

Therapeutic actions

Interferes with platelet membrane function by inhibiting fibrinogen binding and platelet–platelet interactions; inhibits platelet aggregation and prolongs bleeding time; effect is irreversible for life of the platelet.

Indications

- Adjunct to percutaneous coronary intervention (PCI) for the prevention of acute cardiac ischemic complications in patients undergoing PCI and with unstable angina not responding to conventional therapy when PCI is planned within 24 hr; intended to be used with heparin and aspirin therapy
- Unlabeled uses: Early treatment of acute MI or acute ischemic stroke

Contraindications and cautions

- Contraindicated with allergy to abciximab; neutropenia; thrombocytopenia (fewer than 100,000 cells/mcL); hemostatic disorders; bleeding ulcer; intracranial bleeding; major trauma; vasculitis; recent major surgery; aneurysm; use of IV dextran (before or during PCI); pregnancy; severe, uncontrolled hypertension; active internal bleeding; recent (within 6 wk) GI or GU bleeding; history of stroke within 2 yr; administration of oral anticoagulants within 7 days (unless PT is 1.2 times control or less).
- Use cautiously during lactation and with concurrent use of anticoagulants, thrombolytics, or antiplatelet drugs.

Available forms

Injection—2 mg/mL

Dosages

Efficacy of abciximab has only been studied in combination with heparin and aspirin.

Adults

- *Adjunct to PCI:* 0.25 mg/kg by IV bolus 10–60 min prior to procedure, followed by continuous infusion of 0.125 mcg/kg/min (maximum dose 10 mcg/min) for 12 hr.
- *Unstable angina not responding to conventional medical therapy when PCI is planned within 24 hr:* 0.25 mg/kg by IV bolus over at least 1 min; then 10 mcg/min by IV infusion for 18–24 hr, concluding 1 hr after PCI.

Pediatric patients

Safety and efficacy not established.

Pharmacokinetics

Route	*Onset*	*Peak*
IV	Rapid	30 min

Metabolism: Cellular; $T_{1/2}$: less than 10 min, then 30 min
Distribution: Crosses placenta; may enter breast milk
Excretion: Unknown

IV FACTS

Preparation: Withdraw the necessary amount through a 0.2- or 0.22-micron filter for bolus injection. Prepare infusion by withdrawing necessary amount through filter into syringe; inject into 250 mL 0.9% sterile saline or 5% dextrose. Do not use any solution that contains visibly opaque particles; discard solution after 12 hr. Do not shake; refrigerate solution.
Infusion (as adjunct to PCI): 10–60 min before procedure give bolus of 0.25 mg/kg over at least 1 min; give continuous infusion at rate of 0.125 mcg/kg/min (to a maximum dose of 10 mcg/min) for 12 hr.
Incompatibilities: Do not mix in solution with any other medication; give through a separate IV line.

Adverse effects

- **CNS:** Dizziness, confusion, anxiety
- **CV:** Bradycardia, *hypotension,* arrhythmias, edema
- **GI:** *Nausea, vomiting*
- **Hematologic: Thrombocytopenia, bleeding**
- **Local:** *Pain, edema*
- **Respiratory:** Pneumonia, pleural effusion

■ Nursing considerations

Assessment

- **History:** Allergy to abciximab, neutropenia, thrombocytopenia, hemostatic disorders, bleeding ulcer, intracranial bleeding, severe liver disease, lactation, renal disorders, pregnancy, recent trauma or surgery
- **Physical:** Skin color, lesions; orientation; bowel sounds, normal output; CBC, LFTs, renal function tests

Interventions

- Monitor CBC count before use and frequently while initiating therapy.
- Monitor patient for signs and symptoms of bleeding.
- Arrange for concomitant aspirin and heparin therapy.
- Establish safety precautions to prevent injury and bleeding (such as using electric razor, not playing contact sports).
- Provide increased precautions against bleeding during invasive procedures—bleeding will be prolonged.
- Mark chart of any patient receiving abciximab to alert medical personnel to potential for increased bleeding in surgery or dental surgery.

Teaching points

- It may take longer than normal to stop bleeding while on this drug; avoid playing contact sports, use electrical razors, and take other precautions. Apply pressure for extended periods to bleeding sites.
- You may experience these side effects: Upset stomach, nausea.
- Report fever, chills, sore throat, rash, bruising, bleeding, dark stools or urine.

acamprosate calcium

(a kam ***pro'*** *sate)*

Campral

PREGNANCY CATEGORY C

Drug classes

Antialcoholic drug
GABA analogue

Therapeutic actions

Exact mechanism of action not understood; acts with glutamate and GABA neurotransmitter systems in the CNS to restore balance between neuronal excitation and inhibition that may be altered by chronic alcohol exposure.

Indications

- Maintenance of abstinence from alcohol in patients with alcohol dependence who are abstinent at treatment initiation as part of a comprehensive management program that includes psychosocial support

Contraindications and cautions

- Contraindicated with allergy to any component of the drug or severe renal impairment (creatinine clearance 30 mL/min or less).
- Use cautiously with pregnancy, lactation, moderate renal impairment, history of depression and suicidal thoughts.

Available forms

DR tablets—333 mg

Dosages

Adults

666 mg (two 333-mg tablets) PO tid; may be taken with meals to aid compliance. Dosage should begin as soon as possible after period of alcohol withdrawal when the patient has achieved abstinence, and should be maintained if patient relapses. Should be part of a comprehensive psychosocial treatment program.

Pediatric patients

Safety and efficacy not established.

Patients with renal impairment

Moderate impairment (creatinine clearance 30–50 mL/min): 333 mg/PO tid; severe renal impairment (creatinine clearance 30 mL/min or less): do not use acamprosate.

Pharmacokinetics

Route	*Onset*	*Peak*
Oral	Slow	3–8 hr

Metabolism: Not metabolized; $T_{1/2}$: 20–30 hr
Distribution: May cross placenta; may pass into breast milk
Excretion: Urine, unchanged

Adverse effects

- **CNS:** Anxiety, depression, dizziness, impaired judgment, insomnia, paresthesia, **suicidal thoughts**
- **GI:** Anorexia, *diarrhea,* dry mouth, flatulence, nausea
- **Respiratory:** Bronchitis, cough, dyspnea, pharyngitis, rhinitis
- **Skin:** Increased sweating, pruritus
- **Other:** Back pain, flulike symptoms, impotence, muscle aches and pains, weight gain

■ Nursing considerations

Assessment

- **History:** Allergy to any component of the drug, renal impairment, pregnancy, lactation, history of depression and suicidal thoughts, alcohol intake
- **Physical:** Skin, lesions; orientation, reflexes, affect; abdominal examination

Interventions

- Ensure that patient is abstaining from alcohol intake when treatment is initiated.
- Ensure that patient is participating in a comprehensive program, including psychological and social support, to manage abstinence from alcohol.
- Give drug three times a day with meals—timing may be helpful in aiding compliance to the regimen when the patient is managing the drug regimen at home. However, drug may be given without regard to meals.
- Instruct patient to continue to take the drug even if a relapse to alcohol consumption occurs; encourage patient to notify health care provider if a relapse occurs.
- Encourage use of barrier contraceptives during treatment with this drug; fetal abnormalities are possible.

Teaching points

- This drug is given as part of a comprehensive program to support your abstinence from alcohol; it is important that you continue that program while taking this drug.
- Take this drug three times a day; taking the drug with meals may be a helpful reminder.
- If you forget a dose, take it as soon as you remember and return to your usual regimen. Do not make up doses and do not take more than three doses in 24 hours.
- Continue to take the drug even if you relapse and drink alcohol. Notify your health care provider to discuss the renewed drinking.
- You may experience impaired judgment, impaired thinking, or impaired motor skills. You should not drive or operate hazardous machinery or sign important documents or make important decisions until you are certain that *Campral* has not affected your ability to engage in these activities safely.
- You should not take this drug during pregnancy; if you suspect that you are pregnant, or wish to become pregnant, consult your health care provider.
- You should find another method of feeding the baby if you are nursing; it is not known if this drug crosses into breast milk.
- You may experience these side effects: Flatulence, diarrhea, abdominal discomfort; depression thoughts of suicide (if this occurs, consult with your health care provider); muscle or joint aches and pains (consult your health care provider, an analgesic may be helpful).
- Report depression or thoughts of suicide, numbness or tingling, fever, severe diarrhea.

▽ acarbose

*(a **kar'** boz)*

Prandase (CAN), Precose

PREGNANCY CATEGORY B

Drug class

Alpha-glucosidase inhibitor
Antidiabetic

Therapeutic actions

Alpha-glucosidase inhibitor obtained from the fermentation process of a microorganism; delays the digestion of ingested carbohydrates, leading to a smaller increase in blood glucose following meals and a decrease in glycosylated Hgb; does not enhance insulin secretion, so its effects are additive to those of the sulfonylureas in controlling blood glucose.

Indications

- Adjunct to diet to lower blood glucose in those patients with type 2 diabetes mellitus whose hyperglycemia cannot be managed by diet alone
- Combination therapy with a sulfonylurea, metformin, or insulin to enhance glycemic control in patients who do not receive adequate control with diet and either drug alone

Contraindications and cautions

- Contraindicated with hypersensitivity to drug; diabetic ketoacidosis; cirrhosis; inflammatory bowel disease; conditions that deteriorate with increased gas in the bowel; type 1 diabetes; existence of or predisposition to intestinal obstruction; colonic ulceration.
- Use cautiously with renal impairment, pregnancy, lactation.

Available forms

Tablets—25, 50, 100 mg

Dosages

Adults

- *Monotherapy:* Initially, 25 mg PO tid with first bite of each meal. May start with 25 mg/day and gradually increase to tid if GI side effects are a problem. Increase as needed every 4–8 wk as indicated by 1-hr postprandial glucose levels or glycosylated Hgb level and tolerance. For patient 60 kg or less, maximum dosage 50 mg tid; for patient more than 60 kg, maximum dosage 100 mg tid.
- *Combination with sulfonylurea or insulin:* Blood glucose may be much lower; monitor closely and adjust dosages of each drug accordingly.

Pediatric patients

Safety and efficacy not established.

Pharmacokinetics

Route	Onset	Peak
Oral	Rapid	1 hr

Metabolism: Intestinal; $T_{1/2}$: 2 hr
Distribution: Very little
Excretion: Feces, urine

Adverse effects

- **Endocrine:** *Hypoglycemia*
- **GI:** *Abdominal pain, flatulence, diarrhea,* anorexia, nausea, vomiting
- **Hematologic:** *Leukopenia, thrombocytopenia,* anemia

Interactions

✷ **Drug-drug** • Possible decrease in digoxin levels if combined; monitor patients closely if this combination is used • Decreased effects of acarbose if taken with digestive enzymes or charcoal; avoid these combinations • Increased risk of hypoglycemia when given with other antidiabetic drugs

✷ **Drug-alternative therapy** • Increased risk of hypoglycemia if taken with juniper berries, ginseng, garlic, fenugreek, coriander, dandelion root, celery

■ Nursing considerations

Assessment

- **History:** Hypersensitivity to drug; diabetic ketoacidosis; cirrhosis; inflammatory bowel disease; existence of or predisposition to intestinal obstruction; type 1 diabetes; conditions that would deteriorate with increased gas in bowel; renal impairment; pregnancy; lactation
- **Physical:** Skin color, lesions; T; orientation, reflexes, peripheral sensation; R, adventitious sounds; liver evaluation, bowel sounds; urinalysis, BUN, blood glucose, CBC

Interventions

- Give drug tid with the first bite of each meal.
- Monitor serum glucose levels frequently to determine drug effectiveness and dosage; monitor LFTs every 3 mo for 1 year, then periodically. Oral glucose should be given if hypoglycemia occurs; sucrose absorption will be inhibited.
- Inform patient of likelihood of abdominal pain and flatulence.
- Consult with dietitian to establish weight loss program and dietary control.
- Arrange for thorough diabetic teaching program, including disease, dietary control, exercise, signs and symptoms of hypoglycemia and hyperglycemia, avoidance of infection, hygiene.

Teaching points

- Do not discontinue this drug without consulting health care provider.
- Take drug three times a day with first bite of each meal.
- Monitor blood for glucose and ketones as prescribed.
- Continue diet and exercise program established for control of diabetes.
- You may experience these side effects: Abdominal pain, flatulence, bloating.
- Report fever, sore throat, unusual bleeding or bruising, severe abdominal pain.

▽ acebutolol hydrochloride

*(a se **byoo'** toe lole)*

Apo-Acebutolol (CAN), Gen-Acebutolol (CAN), Rhotral (CAN), Sectral

PREGNANCY CATEGORY B

Drug classes

Antiarrhythmic
Antihypertensive
$Beta_1$-selective adrenergic blocker

Therapeutic actions

Blocks beta-adrenergic receptors of the sympathetic nervous system in the heart and juxtaglomerular apparatus (kidney); decreases excitability of the heart, cardiac output and oxygen consumption, and release of renin from the kidney; and lowers BP.

Indications

- Hypertension, alone or with other antihypertensive drugs, especially diuretics
- Management of ventricular premature beats

Contraindications and cautions

- Contraindicated with bradycardia (HR lower than 45 beats per min), second- or third-degree heart block (PR interval greater than 0.24 sec), cardiogenic shock, heart failure, asthma, COPD, lactation.
- Use cautiously with diabetes or thyrotoxicosis, hepatic impairment, renal failure, pregnancy, bronchospastic disease, peripheral vascular disease, anesthesia, major surgery.

Available forms

Capsules—200, 400 mg

Dosages

Adults

- *Hypertension:* Initially 400 mg/day in one or two doses PO; usual maintenance dosage range is 200 mg/day, up to 1,200 mg/day given in two divided doses.
- *Ventricular arrhythmias:* 200 mg bid PO; increase dosage gradually until optimum response is achieved (usually at 600–1,200 mg/day); discontinue gradually over 2 wk.

Pediatric patients

Safety and efficacy not established.

Geriatric patients

Because bioavailability doubles, lower doses may be required; maintain at 800 mg/day or less.

Patients with impaired renal or hepatic function

Reduce daily dose by 50% when creatinine clearance is less than 50 mL/min; reduce by 75% when creatinine clearance is less than 25 mL/min; use caution with hepatic impairment.

Pharmacokinetics

Route	Onset	Peak	Duration
Oral	Varies	3–4 hr	6–8 hr

Metabolism: Hepatic; $T_{1/2}$: 3–4 hr
Distribution: Crosses placenta; enters breast milk
Excretion: Bile, feces, urine

Adverse effects

- **Allergic reactions:** Pharyngitis, erythematous rash, fever, sore throat, *laryngospasm, respiratory distress*
- **CNS:** Dizziness, vertigo, tinnitus, *fatigue,* emotional depression, paresthesias, sleep disturbances, vision changes, hallucinations, disorientation, memory loss, slurred speech (because acebutolol is less lipid soluble than propranolol, it is less likely to penetrate the blood–brain barrier and cause CNS effects)
- **CV:** *Bradycardia, heart failure, cardiac arrhythmias, sinoatrial or AV nodal block, tachycardia,* peripheral vascular insufficiency, claudication, CVA, pulmonary edema, hypotension
- **Dermatologic:** Rash, pruritus, sweating, dry skin
- **EENT:** Eye irritation, dry eyes, conjunctivitis, blurred vision
- **GI:** *Gastric pain, flatulence, constipation, diarrhea, nausea, vomiting,* anorexia
- **GU:** *Impotence, decreased libido,* Peyronie's disease, dysuria, nocturia, frequent urination
- **Musculoskeletal:** Joint pain, arthralgia, muscle cramp
- **Respiratory: Bronchospasm,** dyspnea, cough, bronchial obstruction, nasal stuffiness, rhinitis
- **Other:** *Decreased exercise tolerance, development of antinuclear antibodies,* hyperglycemia or hypoglycemia, elevated serum transaminase

Interactions

✱ **Drug-drug** • Increased effects of both drugs if combined with calcium channel blockers • Increased risk of orthostatic hypotension with prazosin • Possible increased BP-lowering effects with aspirin, bismuth subsalicylate, magnesium salicylate • Decreased antihypertensive effects with NSAIDs, clonidine • Possible increased hypoglycemic effect of insulin

✱ **Drug-lab test** • Possible false results with glucose or insulin tolerance tests (oral)

■ Nursing considerations

Assessment

- **History:** Sinus bradycardia, second- or third-degree heart block, cardiogenic shock, heart failure, asthma, COPD, pregnancy, lactation, diabetes, or thyrotoxicosis
- **Physical:** Weight, skin condition, neurologic status, P, BP, ECG, respiratory status, renal and thyroid function tests, blood and urine glucose

Interventions

- Give with meals if needed.
- Do not discontinue drug abruptly after long-term therapy. Taper drug gradually over 2 wk with monitoring (abrupt withdrawal may cause serious beta-adrenergic rebound effects).

⊗ ***Warning*** Monitor apical pulse; do not administer if P is less than 50.

- Consult with physician about withdrawing drug if patient is to undergo surgery (withdrawal is controversial).
- Provide comfort measures for coping with drug effects.
- Provide safety precautions if CNS effects occur.

Teaching points

- Take drug with meals.
- Do not stop taking unless so instructed by your health care provider; drug must be slowly withdrawn.
- Avoid driving or dangerous activities if dizziness or weakness occurs.
- You may experience these side effects: Dizziness, lightheadedness, loss of appetite, nightmares, depression, sexual impotence.
- Report difficulty breathing, night cough, swelling of extremities, slow pulse, confusion, depression, rash, fever, sore throat.

▽acetaminophen (N-acetyl-p-aminophenol)

(a seet a ***min'*** *a fen)*

Suppositories: Acephen

Oral: Aminofen, Anacin Aspirin Free, APAP, Apacet, Apo-Acetaminophen (CAN), Atasol (CAN), Cetafen, Feverall, Genapap, Genebs, Mapap Arthritis Pain DNC, Masophen, Q-Pap, Silapap, Tylenol, Valorin

PREGNANCY CATEGORY B

Drug classes

Analgesic (nonopioid)
Antipyretic

Therapeutic actions

Antipyretic: Reduces fever by acting directly on the hypothalamic heat-regulating center to cause vasodilation and sweating, which helps dissipate heat.

Analgesic: Site and mechanism of action unclear.

Indications

- Temporary reduction of fever; temporary relief of minor aches and pains caused by common cold and influenza, headache, sore throat, toothache (patients ages 2 yr and older), backache, menstrual cramps, minor arthritis pain, and muscle aches (patients older than 12 yr)
- Unlabeled use: Prophylaxis in children and patients at risk for seizures who are receiving DTP vaccination to reduce incidence of fever and pain

Contraindications and cautions

- Contraindicated with allergy to acetaminophen.
- Use cautiously with impaired hepatic function, chronic alcoholism, pregnancy, lactation.

Available forms

Suppositories—80, 120, 325, 650 mg; chewable tablets—80 mg; tablets—325, 500 mg; ER tablets DNC—650 mg; disintegrating tablets—80, 160 mg; rapid-release tablets—500 mg; capsules—500 mg; elixir—160 mg/5 mL; liquid—160 mg/5 mL, 166.6 mg/5 mL, 500 mg/5 mL; solution—100 mg/mL, 160 mg/5 mL

Dosages

Adults and children older than 12 yr

PO or rectal suppositories

By suppository, 325–650 mg every 4–6 hr. PO, or 1,300 mg ER tablets every 8 hr. Do not exceed 3,900 mg/day.

Pediatric patients

Doses may be repeated 4–5 times/day; do not exceed five doses in 24 hr or 10 mg/kg.

PO

Age	*Dosage (mg)*
0–3 mo	40
4–11 mo	80
12–23 mo	120
2–3 yr	160
4–5 yr	240
6–8 yr	320
9–10 yr	400
11 yr	480

Rectal suppositories

Age	*Dosage*
3–11 mo	80 mg every 6 hr
12–36 mo	80 mg every 4 hr
3–6 yr	120 mg every 4–6 hr
6–12 yr	325 mg every 4–6 hr

Pharmacokinetics

Route	*Onset*	*Peak*	*Duration*
Oral	Varies	0.5–2 hr	4–6 hr

Metabolism: Hepatic; $T_{1/2}$: 1–3 hr
Distribution: Crosses placenta; enters breast milk
Excretion: Urine

Adverse effects

- **CNS:** Headache
- **CV:** Chest pain, dyspnea, **myocardial damage** when doses of 5–8 g/day are ingested daily for several weeks or when doses of 4 g/day are ingested for 1 yr
- **GI: Hepatic toxicity and failure,** jaundice
- **GU:** Acute renal failure, renal tubular necrosis
- **Hematologic:** Methemoglobinemia—cyanosis; hemolytic anemia—hematuria, anuria; neutropenia, leukopenia, pancytopenia, thrombocytopenia, hypoglycemia
- **Hypersensitivity:** Rash, fever

Interactions

✱ **Drug-drug** • Increased toxicity with long-term, excessive ethanol ingestion • Increased hypoprothrombinemic effect of oral anticoagulants • Increased risk of hepatotoxicity and possible decreased therapeutic effects with barbiturates, carbamazepine, hydantoins, rifampin, sulfinpyrazone • Possible delayed or decreased effectiveness with anticholinergics • Possible reduced absorption of acetaminophen with activated charcoal • Possible decreased effectiveness of zidovudine

✱ **Drug-lab test** • Interference with *Chemstrip G, Dextrostix,* and *Visidex II* home blood glucose measurement systems; effects vary

■ Nursing considerations

Assessment

- **History:** Allergy to acetaminophen, impaired hepatic function, chronic alcoholism, pregnancy, lactation
- **Physical:** Skin color, lesions; T; liver evaluation; CBC, LFTs, renal function tests

Interventions

- Do not exceed the recommended dosage.
- Consult physician if needed for children less than 3 yr; if needed for longer than 10 days; if continued fever, severe or recurrent pain occurs (possible serious illness).
- Reduce dosage with hepatic impairment.
- Avoid using multiple preparations containing acetaminophen. Carefully check all OTC products.
- Give drug with food if GI upset occurs.
- Discontinue drug if hypersensitivity reactions occur.
- Treatment of overdose: Monitor serum levels regularly, *N*-acetylcysteine should be available as a specific antidote; basic life support measures may be necessary.

Teaching points

- Do not exceed recommended dose; do not take for longer than 10 days unless directed by prescriber.
- Chew the chewable tablets before swallowing; dissolve dispersable tablets in mouth before swallowing; shake liquid forms well before using; do not cut, crush, or chew extended-relief forms.
- Take the drug only for complaints indicated; it is not an anti-inflammatory agent.
- Avoid the use of other over-the-counter or prescription preparations containing acetaminophen. Serious overdose can occur. If you need an over-the-counter preparation, consult your health care provider.
- Report rash, unusual bleeding or bruising, yellowing of skin or eyes, changes in voiding patterns.

acetazolamide

*(ah set a **zole'** ah mide)*

Apo-Acetazolamide (CAN), Diamox Sequels

PREGNANCY CATEGORY C

Drug classes

Antiepileptic
Antiglaucoma drug
Carbonic anhydrase inhibitor
Diuretic
Sulfonamide (nonbacteriostatic)

Therapeutic actions

Inhibits the enzyme carbonic anhydrase. This action decreases aqueous humor formation in the eye, IOP, and hydrogen ion secretion by renal tubule cells, and increases sodium, potassium, bicarbonate, and water excretion by the kidney, causing a diuretic effect. In epilepsy, carbonic anhydrase inhibition seems to retard abnormal, excessive discharge from CNS neurons.

Indications

- Adjunctive treatment of chronic open-angle glaucoma, secondary glaucoma
- Preoperative use in acute angle-closure glaucoma when delay of surgery is desired to lower IOP
- Edema caused by heart failure, drug-induced edema
- Centrencephalic epilepsy (absence, unlocalized seizures)
- Prophylaxis and treatment of acute mountain sickness

Contraindications and cautions

- Contraindicated with allergy to acetazolamide, antibacterial sulfonamides, or thiazides; chronic noncongestive angle-closure glaucomal; cirrhosis.
- Use cautiously with fluid or electrolyte imbalance (specifically decreased Na^+, decreased K^+, hyperchloremic acidosis), renal disease, hepatic disease (risk of hepatic coma if acetazolamide is given), adrenocortical insufficiency, respiratory acidosis, COPD, lactation.

Available forms

Tablets—125, 250 mg; ER capsules—500 mg; powder for injection—500 mg/vial

Dosages

Adults

- *Open-angle glaucoma:* 250 mg–1 g/day PO, usually in divided doses or ER capsules–1 capsule bid (morning and evening). Do not exceed 1 g/day.
- *Secondary glaucoma and preoperatively:* 250 mg every 4 hr or 250 mg bid PO, or 500 mg followed by 125–250 mg every 4 hr. May be given IV for rapid relief of increased IOP—500 mg IV, then 125–250 mg PO every 4 hr.
- *Diuresis in heart failure:* 250–375 mg (5 mg/kg) daily in the morning. Most effective if given on alternate days or for 2 days alternating with a day of rest.
- *Drug-induced edema:* 250–375 mg once every day or for 1 or 2 days alternating with a day of rest.
- *Epilepsy:* 8–30 mg/kg/day in divided doses. When given in combination with other antiepileptics, starting dose is 250 mg daily. SR preparation is not recommended for this use. Range of dosing: 375–1,000 mg/day.
- *Acute altitude sickness:* 500 mg–1 g/day PO in divided doses of tablets or ER capsules. For rapid ascent, the 1-g dose is recommended. When possible, begin dosing 24–48 hr

before ascent and continue for 48 hr or longer as needed while at high altitude.

Pediatric patients

- *Secondary glaucoma and preoperatively:* 5–10 mg/kg IM or IV every 6 hr, or 10–15 mg/kg/day PO in divided doses every 6–8 hr.
- *Acute glaucoma:* 5–10 mg/kg IV every 6 hr or 8–30 mg/kg/day PO or 300–900 mg/m^2/day PO in three divided doses.
- *Epilepsy:* 8–30 mg/kg/day in divided doses. When given with other antiepileptics, starting dose is 250 mg/day.
- *Drug-induced edema:* 5 mg/kg/dose PO or IV once daily in AM.

Patients with renal impairment

GFR greater than 50 mL/min, give dose every 6 hr; GFR 10–50 mL/min, give dose every 12 hr; GFR less than 10 mL/min, not effective; patients on hemodialysis, 62.5–125 mg/day after dialysis.

Pharmacokinetics

Route	*Onset*	*Peak*	*Duration*
Oral	1 hr	4 hr	6–12 hr
SR	2 hr	3–6 hr	18–24 hr
IV	1–2 min	15–18 min	4–5 hr

Metabolism: $T_{1/2}$: 5–6 hr
Distribution: Crosses placenta; enters breast milk
Excretion: Urine, unchanged

IV FACTS

Preparation: Reconstitute 500-mg vial with 5 mL of sterile water for injection; stable for 3 days if refrigerated, but use within 12 hr is recommended.
Infusion: Give over 1 min for single injection, over 4–8 hr in solution.
Incompatibilities: Do not mix with diltiazem or in multivitamin infusion.

Adverse effects

- **CNS:** Weakness, fatigue, nervousness, sedation, drowsiness, dizziness, depression, tremor, ataxia, headache, paresthesias, seizures, flaccid paralysis, transient myopia
- **Dermatologic:** Urticaria, pruritus, photosensitivity, rash, erythema multiforme (Stevens-Johnson syndrome)
- **GI:** Anorexia, nausea, vomiting, constipation, melena, hepatic insufficiency
- **GU:** Hematuria, glycosuria, *urinary frequency,* renal colic, renal calculi, crystalluria, polyuria
- **Hematologic:** Bone marrow depression
- **Other:** Weight loss, fever, acidosis

Interactions

✱ **Drug-drug** • Decreased renal excretion of quinidine, amphetamine, procainamide, TCAs • Increased excretion of salicylates, lithium • Increased risk of salicylate toxicity due to metabolic acidosis with acetazolamide

✱ **Drug-lab test** • False-positive results of tests for urinary protein

■ Nursing considerations

CLINICAL ALERT!
Name confusion has occurred between *Diamox* (acetazolamide) and *Trimox* (ampicillin); use caution.

Assessment

- **History:** Allergy to acetazolamide, antibacterial sulfonamides, or thiazides; chronic noncongestive angle-closure glaucoma; fluid or electrolyte imbalance; renal or hepatic disease; adrenocortical insufficiency; respiratory acidosis; COPD; lactation
- **Physical:** Skin color, lesions; edema, weight, orientation, reflexes, muscle strength, IOP; R, pattern, adventitious sounds; liver evaluation, bowel sounds, urinary output patterns; CBC, serum electrolytes, LFTs, renal function tests, urinalysis

Interventions

- Administer by direct IV if parenteral use is necessary; IM use is painful.
- Give with food or milk if GI upset occurs.
- Use caution if giving with other drugs with excretion inhibited by urine alkalinization.
- Make oral liquid form by crushing tablets and suspending in cherry, chocolate, raspberry, or other sweet syrup, or one tablet may be submerged in 10 mL of hot water with 1 mL of honey or syrup; do not use alcohol or glycerin as a vehicle.

- Establish safety precautions if CNS effects occur; protect patient from sun or bright lights if photophobia occurs.
- Obtain regular weight to monitor fluid changes.
- Monitor serum electrolytes and acid–base balance during course of drug therapy.

Teaching points

- Take drug with meals if GI upset occurs.
- Arrange to have intraocular pressure checked periodically.
- Weigh yourself on a regular basis, at the same time of the day and in the same clothing. Record weight on calendar.
- You may experience these side effects: Increased volume and frequency of urination; dizziness, feeling faint on arising, drowsiness, fatigue (do not engage in hazardous activities like driving a car); sensitivity to sunlight (use sunglasses; wear protective clothing or use a sunscreen when outdoors); GI upset (taking the drug with meals, eat frequent small meals).
- Report weight change of more than 3 pounds in 1 day, unusual bleeding or bruising, sore throat, dizziness, trembling, numbness, fatigue, muscle weakness or cramps, flank or loin pain, rash.

▽acetylcysteine (*N*-acetylcysteine)

*(a se teel **sis'** tay een)*

Acetadote, Mucomyst

PREGNANCY CATEGORY B

Drug classes

Antidote
Mucolytic

Therapeutic actions

Mucolytic activity: Splits links in the mucoproteins contained in respiratory mucus secretions, decreasing the viscosity of the mucus.
Antidote to acetaminophen hepatotoxicity: Protects liver cells by maintaining cell function and detoxifying acetaminophen metabolites.

Indications

- Mucolytic adjuvant therapy for abnormal, viscid, or inspissated mucus secretions in acute and chronic bronchopulmonary disease (emphysema with bronchitis, asthmatic bronchitis, tuberculosis, pneumonia, primary bronchiectasis, lung amyloidosis), in pulmonary complications of cystic fibrosis, and in tracheostomy care; pulmonary complications associated with surgery, anesthesia, posttraumatic chest conditions; diagnostic bronchial studies (oral solution only)
- To prevent or lessen hepatic injury that may occur after ingestion of a potentially hepatotoxic dose of acetaminophen; treatment must start as soon as possible; most effective if administered within 8–10 hr of ingestion, but can be given within 24 hr after ingestion; IV use approved for this indication
- Unlabeled uses: As ophthalmic solution to treat keratoconjunctivitis sicca (dry eye); as an enema to treat bowel obstruction due to meconium ileus or its equivalent; prevention of radiocontrast-induced nephrotoxicity

Contraindications and cautions

Mucolytic use

- Contraindicated with hypersensitivity to acetylcysteine; use caution and discontinue immediately if bronchospasm occurs.

Antidotal use

- No contraindications; use caution with esophageal varices, peptic ulcer.

Available forms

Solution—10%, 20%; injection—200 mg/mL

Dosages

Adult and pediatric patients

Mucolytic use

- *Nebulization with face mask, mouthpiece, tracheostomy:* 1–10 mL of 20% solution or 2–20 mL of 10% solution every 2–6 hr; the dose for most patients is 3–5 mL of the 20% solution or 6–10 mL of the 10% solution tid or qid.
- *Nebulization with tent, croupette:* Very large volumes are required, occasionally up to 300 mL, during a treatment period. The dose is the volume or solution that will maintain a very heavy mist in the tent or croupette for the desired period. Administration for

intermittent or continuous prolonged periods, including overnight, may be desirable.

Instillation

- *Direct or by tracheostomy:* 1–2 mL of a 10%–20% solution every 1–4 hr; may be introduced into a particular segment of the bronchopulmonary tree by way of a plastic catheter (inserted under local anesthesia and with direct visualization). Instill 2–5 mL of the 20% solution by a syringe connected to the catheter.
- *Percutaneous intratracheal catheter:* 1–2 mL of the 20% solution or 2–4 mL of the 10% solution every 1–4 hr by a syringe connected to the catheter.
- *Diagnostic bronchogram:* Before the procedure, give two to three administrations of 1–2 mL of the 20% solution or 2–4 mL of the 10% solution by nebulization or intratracheal instillation.

Antidotal use

- *For acetaminophen overdose:* Administer acetylcysteine immediately if 8 hr or less have elapsed since acetaminophen ingestion, using the following protocol: • If activated charcoal has been administered by lavage, charcoal may adsorb acetylcysteine and reduce its effectiveness. • Draw blood for acetaminophen plasma assay and for baseline AST, ALT, bilirubin, PT, creatinine, BUN, blood sugar, and electrolytes; if acetaminophen assay cannot be obtained or dose is clearly in the toxic range, give full course of acetylcysteine therapy; monitor hepatic and renal function, fluid and electrolyte balance. • Administer acetylcysteine PO 140 mg/kg loading dose. • See manufacturer's directions for preparation of oral dose using 10% or 20% solution and cola or other soft drink as diluent. • Administer 17 maintenance doses of 70 mg/kg every 4 hr, starting 4 hr after loading dose; administer full course of doses unless acetaminophen assay shows nontoxic level. • If patient vomits its loading or maintenance dose within 1 hr of administration, repeat that dose; if patient is persistently unable to retain oral dosing, may administer by duodenal intubation.
- *IV:* Dilute in 5% dextrose. Loading dose—150 mg/kg in 200 mL given IV over 60 min; then first maintenance dose 50 mg/kg in 500 mL IV over 4 hr followed by a second maintenance dose 100 mg/kg in 1,000 mL given IV over 16 hr. Total IV dose is 300 mg/kg over 21 hr. • Children less than 40 kg and patients who need fluid restriction should receive lowest infusion volume possible. See prescribing information for details. • Repeat blood chemistry assays as described above daily if acetaminophen plasma level is in toxic range.

Pharmacokinetics

Route	*Onset*	*Peak*	*Duration*
Oral	30–60 min	1–2 hr	Not known
Instillation, Inhalation	1 min	5–10 min	2–3 hr
IV	Immediate	5 min	2–3 hr

Metabolism: Hepatic; $T_{1/2}$: 5.6–6.25 hr
Excretion: Urine (30%)

IV FACTS

Preparation: Dilute in 5% dextrose only. Solution may change from colorless to pink or purple when the stopper is punctured. Reconstituted solution is stable 24 hr at room temperature. Discard any unused portion of the vial. Solution is preservative-free.

Infusion: Infuse loading dose over 15 min, first maintenance dose over 4 hr, second maintenance dose over 16 hr.

Incompatibilities: Do not mix with other drugs. Avoid solution contact with rubber and metals, particularly iron, copper, nickel.

Adverse effects

Mucolytic use

- **GI:** Nausea, stomatitis
- **Hypersensitivity:** Urticaria
- **Respiratory: Bronchospasm,** especially in patients with asthma
- **Other:** *Rhinorrhea*

Antidotal use

- **Dermatologic:** Rash
- **GI:** *Nausea, vomiting, other GI symptoms*
- **Other:** ***Anaphylactoid reactions***

■ Nursing considerations

CLINICAL ALERT!

Name confusion has been reported between *Mucomyst* (acetylcysteine) and *Mucinex* (guaifenesin); use caution.

Assessment

- **History:** Mucolytic use: Hypersensitivity to acetylcysteine, asthma. Antidotal use: Esophageal varices, peptic ulcer
- **Physical:** Weight, T, skin color, lesions; BP, P; R, adventitious sounds, bowel sounds, liver palpation

Interventions

Mucolytic use

- Dilute the 20% acetylcysteine solution with either normal saline or sterile water for injection; use the 10% solution undiluted. Refrigerate unused, undiluted solution, and use within 96 hr. Drug solution in the opened bottle may change color, but this does not alter safety or efficacy.
- Administer the following drugs separately, because they are incompatible with acetylcysteine solutions: Tetracyclines, erythromycin lactobionate, amphotericin B, iodized oil chymotrypsin, trypsin, hydrogen peroxide.
- Use water to remove residual drug solution on the patient's face after administration by face mask.
- Inform patient that nebulization may produce an initial disagreeable odor, but the odor will soon disappear.
- Monitor nebulizer for buildup of drug from evaporation; dilute with sterile water for injection to prevent concentrate from impeding nebulization and drug delivery.
- Establish routine for pulmonary toilet; have suction equipment on standby.

Antidotal use

- Dilute the 20% acetylcysteine solution with cola drinks or other soft drinks to a final concentration of 5%; if administered by gastric tube or Miller-Abbott tube, water may be used as diluent. Dilution minimizes the risk of vomiting.
- Prepare fresh solutions, and use within 1 hr; undiluted solution in opened vials may be kept for 96 hr.
- Treat fluid and electrolyte imbalance, hypoglycemia.
- Give vitamin K_1 if prothrombin ratio exceeds 1.5; give fresh-frozen plasma if prothrombin ratio exceeds 3.
- Do not administer diuretics.
- Monitor timing of IV doses.
- Follow acetaminophen assays carefully to determine appropriate dosage.

Teaching points

- You may experience these side effects: Increased productive cough, nausea, GI upset.
- Report difficulty breathing or nausea.

acitretin

See Appendix W, *Less commonly used drugs*.

acyclovir (acycloguanosine)

*(ay **sye'** kloe ver)*

Apo-Acyclovir (CAN), Gen-Acyclovir (CAN), ratio-Acyclovir (CAN), Zovirax

PREGNANCY CATEGORY B

Drug classes

Antiviral
Purine nucleoside analogue

Therapeutic actions

Antiviral activity; inhibits viral DNA replication.

Indications

- Initial and recurrent mucosal and cutaneous HSV-1 and HSV-2 and varicella zoster infections in immunocompromised patients
- Severe initial and recurrent genital herpes infections in immunocompromised patients
- Herpes simplex encephalitis
- Treatment of neonatal HSV infections
- Acute treatment of herpes zoster (shingles) and chickenpox (varicella)
- Ointment: Initial herpes genital infections; limited mucocutaneous HSV infections in immunocompromised patients
- Cream: Recurrent herpes labialis (cold sores) in patients 12 yr or older
- Unlabeled uses: Cytomegalovirus and HSV infection following transplant, ocular and other herpes simplex infections, varicella pneumonia, disseminated primary eczema herpeticum

Contraindications and cautions

- Contraindicated with allergy to acyclovir, seizures, heart failure, renal disease, lactation.
- Use cautiously with pregnancy.

Available forms

Tablets—400, 800 mg; capsules—200 mg; suspension—200 mg/5 mL; powder for injection—500 mg/vial, 1,000 mg/vial; injection—50 mg/mL; ointment—50 mg/g; cream—50 mg/g

Dosages

Adults

Parenteral

- *Herpes simplex:* 5–10 mg/kg infused IV over 1 hr every 8 hr for 5–10 days.

Oral

- *Initial genital herpes:* 200 mg every 4 hr five times daily (1,000 mg/day) for 10 days.
- *Long-term suppressive therapy:* 400 mg bid for up to 12 mo.
- *Intermittent therapy:* 200 mg every 4 hr five times daily for 5 days.
- *Acute herpes zoster:* 800 mg every 4 hr five times daily while awake for 7–10 days.
- *Chickenpox:* 800 mg qid for 5 days.

Pediatric patients

Parenteral

- *HSV infections in patients younger than 12 yr:* 10 mg/kg infused IV over 1 hr every 8 hr for 7 days.
- *Varicella zoster infection in patients younger than 12 yr:* 20 mg/kg IV over 1 hr every 8 hr for 7 days.
- *Shingles, HSV encephalitis in patients 3 mo to 12 yr:* 20 mg/kg IV over 1 hr every 8 hr for 10 days.
- *Neonatal HSV:* 10 mg/kg infused over 1 hr every 8 hr for 10 days.

Oral

Younger than 2 yr: Safety not established.
2 yr or older and 40 kg or less: 20 mg/kg per dose qid (80 mg/kg/day) for 5 days.
More than 40 kg: Use adult dosage.
12 yr or older: Use adult dosage.

Geriatric patients or patients with renal impairment

Oral

For creatinine clearance less than 10 mL/min, 200 mg every 12 hr. If on hemodialysis, an additional dose should be given after each dialysis session.

IV

CrCl (mL/min)	Dosage (IV)
More than 50	5 mg/kg every 8 hr
25–50	5 mg/kg every 12 hr
10–25	5 mg/kg daily
0–10	2.5 mg/kg daily

Topical

Ointment (all ages): Apply sufficient quantity to cover all lesions 6 times/day (every 3 hr) for 7 days; 1.25-cm (0.5-in) ribbon of ointment covers 2.5 cm^2 (4 in^2) surface area.
Cream (12 yr and older): Apply enough to cover all lesions 5 times/day for 4 days.

Pharmacokinetics

Route	Onset	Peak	Duration
Oral	Varies	1.5–2 hr	Not known
IV	Immediate	1 hr	8 hr
Topical	Absorption is minimal		

Metabolism: $T_{1/2}$: 2.5–5 hr
Distribution: Crosses placenta; enters breast milk
Excretion: Unchanged in urine

IV FACTS

Preparation: Reconstitute 500 mg vial in 10 mL sterile water for injection or bacteriostatic water for injection containing benzyl alcohol, 1,000 mg vial in 20 mL; concentration will be 50 mg/mL. Do not dilute drug with bacteriostatic water containing parabens. Use reconstituted solution within 12 hr; dilute IV solution to concentration of 7 mg/mL or less. Do not use biologic or colloidal fluids such as blood products or protein solutions. Warm drug to room temperature to dissolve precipitates formed during refrigeration.
Infusion: Administer by slow IV infusion of parenteral solutions; avoid bolus or rapid injection. Infuse over at least 1 hr to avoid renal damage.
Incompatibilities: Do not mix with diltiazem, dobutamine, dopamine, fludarabine, foscarnet, idarubicin, meperidine, morphine, ondansetron, piperacillin, sargramostim, vinorelbine.

Adverse effects

Systemic administration

- **CNS:** Headache, vertigo, depression, tremors, encephalopathic changes
- **Dermatologic:** *Inflammation or phlebitis at injection sites,* rash, hair loss
- **GI:** *Nausea, vomiting,* diarrhea, anorexia
- **GU:** Crystalluria with rapid IV administration, hematuria, increased BUN.

Topical administration

- **Dermatologic:** Transient burning at site of application

Interactions

Systemic administration

✱ **Drug-drug** • Increased effects with probenecid • Increased nephrotoxicity with other nephrotoxic drugs • Extreme drowsiness with zidovudine

■ Nursing considerations

Assessment

- **History:** Allergy to acyclovir, seizures, heart failure, renal disease, lactation, pregnancy
- **Physical:** Skin color, lesions; orientation; BP, P, auscultation, perfusion, edema; R, adventitious sounds; urinary output; BUN, creatinine clearance

Interventions

Systemic administration

- Ensure that the patient is well hydrated.

Topical administration

- Start treatment as soon as possible after onset of signs and symptoms.
- Wear a rubber glove or finger cot when applying drug.

Teaching points

Systemic administration

- Complete the full course of oral therapy, and do not exceed the prescribed dose.
- Oral acyclovir is not a cure for your disease but should make you feel better.
- Avoid sexual intercourse while visible lesions are present.
- You may experience these side effects: Nausea, vomiting, loss of appetite, diarrhea; headache, dizziness.
- Report difficulty urinating, rash, increased severity or frequency of recurrences.

Topical administration

- Wear rubber gloves or finger cots when applying the drug to prevent autoinoculation of other sites and transmission to others.
- This drug does not cure the disease; application during symptom-free periods will not prevent recurrences.
- Avoid sexual intercourse while visible lesions are present.
- This drug may cause burning, stinging, itching, rash; notify your health care provider if these are pronounced.

▽adalimumab

See Appendix W, *Less commonly used drugs*.

▽adefovir dipivoxil

(ah ***def'*** *o veer dye pih* ***vocks'*** *ill)*

Hepsera

PREGNANCY CATEGORY C

Drug class

Antiviral

Reverse transcriptase inhibitor

Therapeutic actions

Antiviral activity; nucleotide analogue that inhibits hepatitis B virus reverse transcriptase and causes DNA chain termination and blocked viral replication.

Indications

- Treatment of chronic hepatitis B in adults and children 12 yr and older with evidence of active viral replication and either evidence of persistent elevations in ALT or AST or histologically active disease

Contraindications and cautions

- Contraindicated with allergy to adefovir or any components of the product, lactation.
- Use cautiously with pregnancy, renal impairment, signs of lactic acidosis, risk factors for severe liver disease, the elderly.

Available forms

Tablets—10 mg

Dosages

Adults and children 12 yr and older

10 mg/day PO.

Pediatric patients

Safety and efficacy not established.

Patients with renal impairment

For creatinine clearance 30–49 mL/min, 10 mg every 48 hr; for creatinine clearance 10–29 mL/min, 10 mg every 72 hr. For hemodialysis patients, 10 mg every 7 days following dialysis. Drug not recommended for creatinine clearance less than 10 mL/min if patient is not on dialysis.

Pharmacokinetics

Route	*Onset*	*Peak*
Oral	Rapid	0.6–4 hr

Metabolism: Hepatic; $T_{1/2}$: 7.5 hr
Distribution: May cross placenta; may enter breast milk
Excretion: Urine

Adverse effects

- **CNS:** Headache, *asthenia*
- **GI:** Nausea, diarrhea, abdominal pain, flatulence, dyspepsia, **severe hepatomegaly with steatosis, sometimes fatal; exacerbation of hepatitis if therapy is discontinued,** *elevated liver enzymes*
- **GU: Nephrotoxicity,** hematuria, glycosuria
- **Metabolic: Lactic acidosis, sometimes severe,** elevated creatine kinase, elevated amylase levels
- **Other:** HIV resistance if used to treat patients with unrecognized HIV infection

Interactions

✱ **Drug-drug** • Increased risk of nephrotoxicity if combined with other drugs that cause nephrotoxicity; if this combination is used, monitor renal function closely and evaluate risks versus benefits of continuing the combination

■ Nursing considerations

Assessment

- **History:** Allergy to adefovir or any component of the drug, renal or hepatic impairment, lactic acidosis, pregnancy, lactation
- **Physical:** T; orientation, reflexes; abdominal examination, LFTs, renal function tests

Interventions

- Ensure that HIV antibody testing has been done before initiating therapy to reduce risk of emergence of HIV resistance.

⊗ ***Black box warning*** Caution patient not to run out of this drug; patients who stop taking it may develop worsened or severe hepatitis.

⊗ ***Black box warning*** Monitor patients regularly to evaluate renal function and liver enzymes; severe nephrotoxicity and hepatotoxicity can occur.

⊗ ***Black box warning*** Withdraw drug and monitor patient if patient develops signs of lactic acidosis or hepatotoxicity, including hepatomegaly and steatosis.

⊗ ***Black box warning*** HIV resistance may occur in unrecognized or untreated HIV infection; test patients for HIV infection before beginning therapy.

- Encourage women of childbearing age to use barrier contraceptives while on this drug as the effects of the drug on the fetus are not known.
- Advise women who are lactating to find another method of feeding the baby.
- Advise patient that this drug does not cure the disease and there is still a risk of transmitting the disease to others; advise the use of barrier contraceptives.

Teaching points

- Take this drug once a day.
- Take the full course of therapy as prescribed; if you miss a dose, take it as soon as you remember and then take the next dose at the usual time the next day. Do not double any doses.
- You will be asked to have an HIV antibody test if your HIV status is not known; some people with HIV who are treated with this drug develop resistant strains of HIV.
- This drug does not cure chronic hepatitis B infection; long-term effects are not yet known;

continue to take precautions as the risk of transmission is not reduced by this drug.
- Do not stop taking this drug; you may experience very serious or worsening hepatitis B if the drug is stopped after you have been taking it. Consult your health care provider if your prescription is getting low and make sure that you do not skip any doses.
- You may experience these side effects: Nausea, diarrhea, abdominal pain, headache; try to maintain nutrition and fluid intake as much as possible—eat frequent small meals.
- Report severe weakness, muscle pain, trouble breathing, dizziness, cold feelings in your arms or legs, palpitations.

▽adenosine

See Appendix W, *Less commonly used drugs*.

▽agalsidase beta

See Appendix W, *Less commonly used drugs*.

▽albumin, human (normal serum albumin)

*(al **byoo'** min)*

5%: Albuminar-5, Albutein 5%, Normal Serum Albumin 5% Solution, Plasbumin-5
20%: Plasbumin-20
25%: Albuminar-25, Albutein 25%, Normal Serum Albumin 25% Solution, Plasbumin-25

PREGNANCY CATEGORY C

Drug classes

Blood product
Plasma protein

Therapeutic actions

Normal blood protein; maintains plasma osmotic pressure and is important in maintaining normal blood volume.

Indications

- Emergency treatment of shock due to burns, trauma, surgery, and infections (20% or 25%); 5% for use in nonemergency cases
- Burns: Albumin 5% used to prevent hemoconcentration and water and protein losses in conjunction with adequate infusions of crystalloid. 20% or 25% used beyond 24 hr.
- Hypoproteinemia in nephrotic syndrome, hepatic cirrhosis, toxemia of pregnancy, postoperative patients, tuberculous patients, premature infants
- Adult respiratory distress syndrome: Albumin 20% or 25% with a diuretic may be helpful
- Cardiopulmonary bypass: Preoperative blood dilution with 20% or 25% albumin. 5% may be used as adjunct therapy.
- Acute liver failure (20% or 25%)
- Sequestration of protein-rich fluids
- Erythrocyte resuspension: Albumin 20% or 25% may be added to the isotonic suspension of washed red cells immediately before transfusion
- Acute nephrosis: Albumin 20% or 25% and loop diuretic may help to control edema repeated daily for 7–10 days
- Renal dialysis: Albumin 20% or 25% may be useful in treatment of shock and hypotension. 5% solution may be used as adjunct in hemodialysis.
- Hyperbilirubinemia and erythroblastosis fetalis: Adjunct in exchange transfusions

Contraindications and cautions

- Contraindicated with allergy to albumin; severe anemia, cardiac failure, normal or increased intravascular volume, current use of cardiopulmonary bypass.
- Use cautiously with hepatic or renal failure.

Available forms

Injection—5%, 20%, 25%

Dosages

Administer by IV infusion only; contains 130–160 mEq sodium/L.

Adults

- *Hypovolemic shock:* 5% albumin: Initial dose of 500 mL is given as rapidly as possible; additional 500 mL may be given in 30 min. Base therapy on clinical response if more than 1,000 mL is required; consider the need for whole blood. In patients with low blood volume, administer at rate of 1–2 mL/min. 20% or 25% albumin: Base therapy on clinical response. Administer as rapidly as tolerated; 1 mL/min may be given to patients with low blood volume.

- *Hypoproteinemia:* 5% albumin may be given for acute replacement of protein; if patient has edema, use 20% or 25% albumin 50–75 g/day. Do not exceed 2 mL/min. Adjust the rate of infusion based on patient response.
- *Burns:* 20% or 25% albumin can be helpful in maintaining colloid osmotic pressure; suggested regimen has not been established.
- *Hepatic cirrhosis:* 25% may be effective in temporary restoration of plasma protein levels.
- *Nephrosis:* Initial dose of 100–200 mL of 25% albumin may be repeated at intervals of 1–2 days; effects are not sustained because of the underlying problem.

Pediatric patients

- Usual rate of administration is 1/4 to 1/2 adult rate, or dosage may be calculated on basis of 0.6–1 g/kg.
- *Hypovolemic shock:* 50 mL of 5% albumin; base dosage on clinical response.
- *Hypoproteinemia:* 25 g/day of 20% or 25% albumin.
- *Hyperbilirubinemia and erythroblastosis fetalis:* 1 g/kg 1 hr before transfusion.

Pharmacokinetics

Route	*Onset*	*Peak*
IV	Immediate	End of infusion

Metabolism: Tissue; $T_{1/2}$: Unknown
Distribution: Crosses placenta; enters breast milk
Excretion: Urine

IV FACTS

Preparation: Swab stopper top with antiseptic immediately before removing seal and entering the vial. Use a 16-gauge needle or dispensing pin with vials 20 mL or larger. Inspect for particulate matter and discoloration. Store at room temperature; do not freeze. Do not dilute 5% albumin; 25% albumin may be undiluted or diluted in normal saline; if sodium restriction is required, may dilute 25% albumin with D_5W.
Infusion: Give by IV infusion slowly enough to prevent rapid plasma volume expansion 1–2 mL/min for adults, 0.25–1 mL/min for children. Give in combination with or through the same administration set as solutions of saline or carbohydrates.
Incompatibilities: Do not use with solutions containing alcohol or protein hydrolysates—precipitates may form.

Adverse effects

- **CV:** Hypotension, heart failure, pulmonary edema after rapid infusion
- **Hypersensitivity:** Fever, chills, *changes in blood pressure,* flushing, nausea, vomiting, changes in respiration, rashes

■ Nursing considerations

Assessment

- **History:** Allergy to albumin, severe anemia, heart failure, current use of cardiopulmonary bypass, hepatic failure, renal failure
- **Physical:** Skin color, lesions; T; P, BP, peripheral perfusion; R, adventitious sounds; LFTs, renal function tests, Hct, serum electrolytes

Interventions

- Give to all blood groups or types.
- Consider using whole blood; infusion provides only symptomatic relief of hypoproteinemia.
- Monitor BP; discontinue infusion if hypotension occurs.
- Stop infusion if headache, flushing, fever, changes in BP occur; treat reaction with antihistamines. If a plasma protein is still needed, try material from a different lot number.
- Monitor patient's clinical response, and adjust infusion rate accordingly.

Teaching points

- Report headache, nausea, vomiting, difficulty breathing, back pain.

albuterol sulfate

*(al **byoo'** ter ole)*

AccuNeb, ProAir HFA, Proventil, Proventil HFA, Ventolin Diskus (CAN), Ventolin HFA, Ventolin Oral Liquid (CAN), VoSpire ER DNC

PREGNANCY CATEGORY C

Drug classes

Antiasthmatic
$Beta_2$-selective adrenergic agonist
Bronchodilator
Sympathomimetic

Therapeutic actions

In low doses, acts relatively selectively at $beta_2$-adrenergic receptors to cause bronchodilation and vasodilation; at higher doses, $beta_2$ selectivity is lost, and the drug acts at $beta_2$ receptors to cause typical sympathomimetic cardiac effects.

Indications

- Relief and prevention of bronchospasm in patients with reversible obstructive airway disease or COPD
- Inhalation: Treatment of acute attacks of bronchospasm
- Prevention of exercise-induced bronchospasm
- Unlabeled use: Adjunct in treating moderate to severe hyperkalemia in dialysis patients; seems to lower potassium concentrations when inhaled by patients on hemodialysis

Contraindications and cautions

- Contraindicated with hypersensitivity to albuterol; tachyarrhythmias, tachycardia caused by digitalis intoxication; general anesthesia with halogenated hydrocarbons or cyclopropane (these sensitize the myocardium to catecholamines); unstable vasomotor system disorders; hypertension; coronary insufficiency, CAD; history of CVA; COPD patients with degenerative heart disease.
- Use cautiously with diabetes mellitus (large IV doses can aggravate diabetes and ketoacidosis); hyperthyroidism; history of seizure disorders; psychoneurotic individuals; labor and delivery (oral use has delayed second stage of labor; parenteral use of $beta_2$-adrenergic agonists can accelerate fetal heart beat and cause hypoglycemia, hypokalemia, pulmonary edema in the mother and hypoglycemia in the neonate); lactation; the elderly (more sensitive to CNS effects).

Available forms

Tablets—2, 4 mg; ER tablets DNC—4, 8 mg; syrup—2 mg/5 mL; aerosol—90 mcg/actuation; solution for inhalation—0.021%, 0.042%, 0.083%, 0.5%.

Dosages

Adults

Oral

Initially, 2 or 4 mg (1–2 tsp syrup) tid–qid PO; may cautiously increase dosage if necessary to 4 or 8 mg qid, not to exceed 32 mg/day. ER tablets, 4–8 mg q 12 hr.

Inhalation

Each actuation of aerosol dispenser delivers 90 mcg albuterol; 2 inhalations every 4–6 hr; some patients may require only 1 inhalation every 4 hr; more frequent administration or larger number of inhalations not recommended.

- *COPD:* 1 inhalation twice daily, approximately 12 hr apart.
- *Prevention of exercise-induced bronchospasm:* 2 inhalations 15 min prior to exercise.

Solution for inhalation

2.5 mg tid to qid by nebulization.

Pediatric patients

Oral, tablets

6–12 yr: 2 mg tid–qid. May be increased if needed, but do not exceed 24 mg/day. ER tablets, 4 mg q 12 hr.
12 yr and older: Use adult dosage.

Oral, syrup

Younger than 2 yr: Safety and efficacy not established.
2–6 yr: Initially 0.1 mg/kg tid, not to exceed 2 mg (1 tsp) tid; if necessary, cautiously increase stepwise to 0.2 mg/kg tid. Do not exceed 4 mg (2 tsp) tid.
6–14 yr: 2 mg (1 tsp) tid–qid; if necessary, cautiously increase dosage. Do not exceed 24 mg/day in divided doses.
Older than 14 yr: Use adult dosage.

Inhalation Solution

2–12 yr: For child 10–15 kg, use 1.25 mg bid or tid by nebulization; for child more than 15 kg, use 2.5 mg bid or tid by nebulization.

12 yr and older: Use adult dosage.

AccuNeb for patients 2–12 yr: Usual starting dose, 1.25 mg or 0.63 mg tid or qid as needed by nebulization over 5–15 min. More frequent administration is not recommended.

Geriatric patients or patients sensitive to beta-adrenergic stimulation

Restrict initial dose to 2 mg tid or qid; individualize dosage thereafter to as much as 8 mg tid–qid. Patients older than 60 yr are more likely to develop adverse effects.

Pharmacokinetics

Route	*Onset*	*Peak*	*Duration*
Oral	30 min	2–2.5 hr	4–8 hr
Inhalation	5 min	1.5–2 hr	3–8 hr

Metabolism: Hepatic; $T_{1/2}$: 2–4 hr
Distribution: Crosses placenta; enters breast milk
Excretion: Urine

Adverse effects

- **CNS:** *Restlessness, apprehension, anxiety, fear, CNS stimulation,* hyperkinesia, insomnia, tremor, drowsiness, irritability, weakness, vertigo, headache
- **CV:** *Cardiac arrhythmias,* tachycardia, palpitations, PVCs (rare), anginal pain
- **Dermatologic:** *Sweating, pallor, flushing*
- **GI:** *Nausea,* vomiting, heartburn, unusual or bad taste in mouth
- **GU:** Increased incidence of leiomyomas of uterus when given in higher than human doses in preclinical studies
- **Respiratory:** Respiratory difficulties, pulmonary edema, coughing, **bronchospasm;** paradoxical airway resistance with repeated, excessive use of inhalation preparations

Interactions

✱ **Drug-drug** • Increased sympathomimetic effects with other sympathomimetic drugs • Increased risk of toxicity, especially cardiac, when used with theophylline, aminophylline • Decreased bronchodilating effects with beta-adrenergic blockers (eg, propranolol) • Decreased effectiveness of insulin, oral hypoglycemic drugs • Decreased serum levels and therapeutic effects of digoxin

■ Nursing considerations

Assessment

- **History:** Hypersensitivity to albuterol; tachyarrhythmias, tachycardia caused by digitalis intoxication; general anesthesia with halogenated hydrocarbons or cyclopropane; unstable vasomotor system disorders; hypertension; coronary insufficiency, CAD; history of CVA; COPD patients who have developed degenerative heart disease; diabetes mellitus; hyperthyroidism; history of seizure disorders; psychoneurotic individuals; lactation
- **Physical:** Weight; skin color, T, turgor; orientation, reflexes, affect; P, BP; R, adventitious sounds; blood and urine glucose, serum electrolytes, thyroid function tests, ECG

Interventions

- Use minimal doses for minimal periods; drug tolerance can occur with prolonged use.
- Maintain a beta-adrenergic blocker (cardioselective beta-blocker, such as atenolol, should be used with respiratory distress) on standby in case cardiac arrhythmias occur.
- Prepare solution for inhalation by diluting 0.5 mL 0.5% solution with 2.5 mL normal saline; deliver over 5–15 min by nebulization.
- Do not exceed recommended dosage; administer pressurized inhalation drug forms during second half of inspiration, because the airways are open wider and the aerosol distribution is more extensive.

Teaching points

- Do not exceed recommended dosage; adverse effects or loss of effectiveness may result. Read the instructions that come with respiratory inhalant.
- Do not cut, crush, or chew ER tablets; swallow them whole.
- You may experience these side effects: Dizziness, drowsiness, fatigue, headache (use caution if driving or performing tasks that require alertness); nausea, vomiting, change in taste (eat frequent small meals); rapid heart rate, anxiety, sweating, flushing, insomnia.
- Report chest pain, dizziness, insomnia, weakness, tremors or irregular heart beat, difficulty breathing, productive cough, failure to respond to usual dosage.

▽aldesleukin

See Appendix W, *Less commonly used drugs*.

▽alefacept

See Appendix W, *Less commonly used drugs*.

▽alemtuzumab

See Appendix W, *Less commonly used drugs*.

▽alendronate sodium

*(ah **len'** dro nate)*

Co-Alendronate (CAN), Fosamax, Novo-Alendronate (CAN), PMS-Alendronate (CAN), ratio-Alendronate (CAN)

PREGNANCY CATEGORY C

Drug classes

Bisphosphonate
Calcium regulator

Therapeutic actions

Slows normal and abnormal bone resorption without inhibiting bone formation and mineralization.

Indications

- Treatment and prevention of osteoporosis in postmenopausal women
- Treatment of men with osteoporosis
- Treatment of glucocorticoid-induced osteoporosis
- Treatment of Paget's disease of bone in patients with alkaline phosphatase at least two times upper limit of normal, those who are symptomatic, those at risk for future complications
- Unlabeled uses: Osteoporosis with spinal cord injury, vitamin D intoxication

Contraindications and cautions

- Contraindicated with allergy to bisphosphonates, hypocalcemia, esophageal abnormalities, inability to stay upright for at least 30 min, and in those at risk for aspiration (oral solution).
- Use cautiously with renal impairment, upper GI disease, pregnancy, lactation.

Available forms

Tablets—5, 10, 35, 40, 70 mg; oral solution—70 mg

Dosages

Adults

- *Postmenopausal osteoporosis:* 10 mg/day PO in AM with full glass of water, at least 30 min before the first beverage, food, or medication of the day, or 70 mg PO once a week or one bottle of 70 mg oral solution once a week. Avoid lying down for 30 min after taking drug.
- *Men with osteoporosis:* 10 mg/day PO or 70 mg tablet or one bottle 70 mg oral solution once a week.
- *Prevention of osteoporosis:* 5 mg/day PO or 35 mg PO once a week.
- *Paget's disease:* 40 mg/day PO in AM with full glass of water, at least 30 min before the first beverage, food, or medication of the day for 6 mo; may retreat after 6-mo treatment-free period.
- *Glucocorticoid-induced osteoporosis:* 5 mg/day PO with calcium and vitamin D (for men and women); 10 mg/day PO for postmenopausal women not on estrogen.

Pediatric patients

Safety and efficacy not established.

Patients with renal impairment
Dosage adjustment not necessary for creatinine clearance 35–60 mL/min; not recommended if creatinine clearance less than 35 mL/min.

Pharmacokinetics

Route	*Onset*	*Duration*
Oral	Slow	Days

Metabolism: Not metabolized; $T_{1/2}$: More than 10 yr
Distribution: Crosses placenta; may enter breast milk
Excretion: Urine

Adverse effects

- **CNS:** *Headache*
- **GI:** *Nausea, diarrhea, GI irritation, pain, esophageal erosion*
- **Skeletal:** *Increased or recurrent bone pain,* focal osteomalacia

Interactions

✱ **Drug-drug** • Increased risk of GI distress with aspirin • Decreased absorption if taken with antacids, calcium, iron, multivalent cations; separate dosing by at least 30 min
✱ **Drug-food** • Significantly decreased absorption and serum levels if taken with food; separate dosing from food and beverage by at least 30 min

■ Nursing considerations

CLINICAL ALERT!
Name confusion has occurred between *Fosamax* (alendronate) and *Flomax* (tamsulosin); use caution.

Assessment

- **History:** Allergy to bisphosphonates, renal failure, upper GI disease, lactation, pregnancy
- **Physical:** Muscle tone, bone pain; bowel sounds; urinalysis, serum calcium

Interventions

⊗ ***Warning*** Give in AM with full glass of water at least 30 min before the first beverage, food, or medication of the day. Patient must stay upright for 30 min to decrease risk of potentially serious esophageal erosion.

- Monitor serum calcium levels before, during, and after therapy.
- Ensure 6-mo rest period after treatment for Paget's disease if retreatment is required.
- Ensure adequate vitamin D and calcium intake.
- Provide comfort measures if bone pain returns.

Teaching points

- Take drug in the morning with a full glass of plain water (not mineral water), at least 30 minutes before any beverage, food, or medication, and stay upright for 30 minutes and until after the first food of the day; mark calendar for once-weekly dosing.
- You may experience these side effects: Nausea, diarrhea; bone pain, headache (analgesic may help).
- Report twitching, muscle spasms, dark-colored urine, severe diarrhea, difficulty swallowing.

▽ alfuzosin hydrochloride

*(al foo **zow'** sin)*

Uroxatral DNC

PREGNANCY CATEGORY B

Drug classes

Alpha adrenergic blocker
BPH drug

Therapeutic actions

Blocks the smooth muscle alpha-1 adrenergic receptors in the prostate, prostatic capsule, prostatic urethra, and bladder neck, leading to the relaxation of the bladder and prostate and improving the flow of urine and improvement in symptoms in patients with BPH.

Indications

- Treatment of the signs and symptoms of BPH

Contraindications and cautions

- Contraindicated with allergy to any component of the product; hepatic insufficiency, pregnancy, lactation.
- Use cautiously with hypotension, renal insufficiency, prolonged QTc interval, CAD.

Available forms

ER tablets DNC—10 mg

Dosages

Adults

10 mg/day PO after the same meal each day.

Pediatric patients

Safety and efficacy not established.

Pharmacokinetics

Route	*Onset*	*Peak*
Oral	Varies	8 hr

Metabolism: Hepatic; $T_{1/2}$: 10 hr
Distribution: Crosses placenta; may enter breast milk
Excretion: Feces, urine

Adverse effects

- **CNS:** Dizziness, headache
- **CV:** Orthostatic hypotension, syncope, tachycardia, chest pain
- **GI:** Abdominal pain, dyspepsia, constipation, nausea
- **GU:** Impotence, priapism
- **Respiratory:** Cough, bronchitis, sinusitis, pharyngitis, URI
- **Other:** Fatigue, pain

Interactions

✱ **Drug-drug** • Increased serum levels and risk of adverse effects of alfuzosin if combined with CYP3A4 inhibitors, ketoconazole, itraconazole, ritonavir; use of these combinations is contraindicated • Increased risk of orthostatic hypotension and syncope if combined with antihypertensive medications; monitor patient closely and adjust antihypertensive dosage accordingly • Increased risk of adverse effects if combined with other adrenergic blockers; monitor patients closely and adjust dosages as needed

■ Nursing considerations

Assessment

- **History:** Allergy to alfuzosin, hepatic or renal impairment, CAD, prolonged QTc interval, pregnancy, lactation
- **Physical:** Body weight; skin color, lesions; orientation, affect, reflexes; P, BP, orthostatic BP; R, adventitious sounds; PSA level; voiding pattern, normal output, urinalysis

Interventions

- Ensure that patient does not have prostatic cancer before beginning treatment; check for normal PSA levels.
- Administer once a day, after the same meal each day.
- Ensure that patient does not crush, chew, or cut tablet. Tablet should be swallowed whole.
- Store tablets in a dry place, protected from light.

⊗ ***Warning*** Monitor patient carefully for orthostatic hypotension; chance of orthostatic ypotension, dizziness, and syncope are greatest with the first dose. Establish safety precautions as appropriate.

Teaching points

- Take this drug exactly as prescribed, once a day. Do not chew, crush, or cut tablets; tablets must be swallowed whole. Use care when beginning therapy; dizziness and syncope are most likely at the beginning of therapy. Change position slowly to avoid increased dizziness. Take the drug after the same meal each day. Do not take the drug on an empty stomach.
- You may experience these side effects: Dizziness, weakness (these are more likely to occur when you change position, in the early morning, after exercise, in hot weather, and when you have consumed alcohol; some tolerance may occur after you have taken the drug for a while. Avoid driving a car or engaging in tasks that require alertness while you are experiencing these symptoms; remember to change position slowly, use caution when climbing stairs, lie down for a while if dizziness persists); GI upset (eat frequent small meals); impotence (you may wish to discuss this with your health care provider); fatigue.

- Report frequent dizziness or fainting, worsening of symptoms, chest pain.

alglucosidase alfa

See Appendix W, *Less commonly used drugs*.

aliskiren

(ah liss ***kye'*** *ren)*

Tekturna

PREGNANCY CATEGORY C (FIRST TRIMESTER)

PREGNANCY CATEGORY D (SECOND AND THIRD TRIMESTERS)

Drug class

Antihypertensive
Renin inhibitor

Therapeutic actions

Directly inhibits renin, which decreases plasma renin activity and inhibits conversion of angiotensinogen to angiotensin I. Inhibition of the renin-angiotensin-aldosterone system leads to decreased blood pressure, decreased aldosterone release, and decreased sodium resorption.

Indications

- Treatment of hypertension, alone or with other antihypertensives

Contraindications and cautions

- Contraindicated with known hypersensitivity to any component of the drug, second or third trimester of pregnancy, lactation.
- Use cautiously with history of impaired renal function, hyperkalemia.

Available forms

Tablets—150, 300 mg

Dosages

Adults

150 mg/day PO. May be increased to 300 mg/day PO if needed to control blood pressure.

Pediatric patients

Safety and efficacy not established.

Patients with severe renal impairment

No dosage adjustment needed with mild to moderate renal dysfunction; caution should be used with severe dysfunction because clinical experience is limited.

Pharmacokinetics

Route	*Onset*	*Peak*
Oral	Slow	1–3 hr

Metabolism: Hepatic; $T_{1/2}$: 24 hr
Distribution: Crosses placenta; may enter breast milk
Excretion: Urine

Adverse effects

- **CNS:** Dizziness, fatigue, headache, seizures
- **CV:** Edema, hypotension
- **GI:** Diarrhea, abdominal pain, dyspepsia, GERD
- **Respiratory:** Cough, URI, **angioedema with respiratory symptoms**
- **Other:** Back pain

Interactions

✱ **Drug-drug** • Risk of decreased effectiveness of furosemide if combined with aliskiren; monitor patient closely • Risk of increased serum levels and effects of aliskiren if combined with atorvastatin, ketoconazole; monitor patient closely

■ Nursing considerations

⊗ ***Black box warning*** Use during second and third trimesters of pregnancy can cause fetal injury or death; if pregnancy occurs, discontinue drug as soon as possible.

Assessment

- **History:** Hypersensitivity to any component of the drug, second or third trimester of pregnancy, lactation, history of impaired renal function, hyperkalemia
- **Physical:** Orientation, affect; BP; R, lung sounds; abdominal examination; renal function tests, electrolytes

Interventions

- Ensure that patient is not pregnant before starting drug; suggest use of contraceptive measures.

- Monitor serum potassium level periodically.
- Monitor patients also receiving furosemide for possible loss of diuretic effects.
- Continue other antihypertensive drugs as needed to control blood pressure.

Teaching points

- Take this drug once a day, at about the same time each day. If you miss a dose, take it as soon as you remember; then resume your usual schedule the next day. Do not make up missed doses. Do not take more than one dose each day.
- Store this drug at room temperature in a dry place (not in the bathroom or near the kitchen sink). Do not share this drug with any other people; keep it out of the reach of children.
- You may also be taking other drugs to control your blood pressure; check with your health care provider, and follow your drug regimen as directed.
- This drug should not be taken during pregnancy; use of contraceptive measures is advised. If you wish to become pregnant, discuss this with your health care provider. If you become pregnant while taking *Tekturna,* stop the drug and consult with your health care provider about a different treatment for your hypertension.
- It is not known how this drug could affect a nursing baby. Because of the potential for serious adverse effects on the baby, another method of feeding should be used while you are taking this drug.
- Your health care provider will monitor your blood pressure regularly while you are taking this drug.
- You may experience low blood pressure if you are also taking diuretics, if you become dehydrated, or if you have dialysis treatments. If you feel faint or dizzy, lie down and call your health care provider right away.
- Report difficulty breathing; swelling of the face, lips, or tongue; dizziness or lightheadedness; pregnancy.

▽allopurinol

*(al oh **pure'** i nole)*

Aloprim, Apo-Allopurinol (CAN), Zyloprim

PREGNANCY CATEGORY C

Drug class

Antigout drug

Therapeutic actions

Inhibits the enzyme responsible for the conversion of purines to uric acid, thus reducing the production of uric acid with a decrease in serum and sometimes in urinary uric acid levels, relieving the signs and symptoms of gout.

Indications

- Management of the signs and symptoms of primary and secondary gout
- Management of patients with leukemia, lymphoma, and malignancies that result in elevations of serum and urinary uric acid
- Management of patients with recurrent calcium oxalate calculi whose daily uric acid excretion exceeds 800 mg/day (males) or 750 mg/day (females)
- Orphan drug use: Treatment of Chagas' disease; cutaneous and visceral leishmaniasis
- Unlabeled uses: Amelioration of granulocyte suppression with 5-FU; as a mouthwash to prevent 5-FU–induced stomatitis

Contraindications and cautions

- Contraindicated with allergy to allopurinol, blood dyscrasias.
- Use cautiously with liver disease, renal failure, lactation, pregnancy.

Available forms

Tablets—100, 300 mg; powder for injection—500 mg

Dosages

Adults

- *Gout and hyperuricemia:* 100–800 mg/day PO in divided doses, depending on the severity of the disease (200–300 mg/day is usual dose).
- *Maintenance:* Establish dose that maintains serum uric acid levels within normal limits.

- *Hyperuricosuria:* 200–300 mg/day PO; adjust dose based on 24-hr urinary urate levels.
- *Prevention of acute gouty attacks:* 100 mg/day PO; increase the dose by 100 mg at weekly intervals until uric acid levels are 6 mg/dL or less.
- *Prevention of uric acid nephropathy in certain malignancies:* 600–800 mg/day PO for 2–3 days with a high fluid intake; maintenance dose should then be established as above.
- *Recurrent calcium oxalate stones:* 200–300 mg/day PO; adjust dose based on 24-hr urinary urate determinations.
- *Parenteral:* 200–400 mg/m^2/day IV to maximum of 600 mg/day as continuous infusion or at 6-, 8-, 12-hr intervals.

Pediatric patients

- *Secondary hyperuricemia associated with various malignancies:*
  6–10 yr: 300 mg/day PO.
  Younger than 6 yr: 150 mg/day; adjust dosage after 48 hr of treatment based on serum uric acid levels.
- *Parenteral:* 200 mg/m^2/day IV as continuous infusion or at 6-, 8-, 12-hr intervals.

Geriatric patients or patients with renal impairment

For geriatric patients or for patients with creatinine clearance 10–20 mL/min, 200 mg/day; for creatinine clearance less than 10 mL/min, 100 mg/day; for creatinine clearance less than 3 mL/min, extend intervals between doses based on patient's serum uric acid levels.

Pharmacokinetics

Route	*Onset*	*Peak*
Oral	Slow	1–2 hr
IV	10–15 min	30 min

Metabolism: Hepatic; $T_{1/2}$: 1–1.5 hr, then 23–24 hr
Distribution: Crosses placenta; may enter breast milk
Excretion: Urine

IV FACTS

Preparation: Dissolve contents of each vial with 25 ml of sterile water for injection. Further dilute with NSS or D_5W to final concentration of 6 mg/ml or less. Administer within 10 hr of reconstitution.
Infusion: Administer as a continuous infusion or infused every 6, 8, or 12 hr with rate dependent on volume used.
Incompatibilities: Incompatible with many other drugs and solutions containing sodium bicarbonate. Do not mix with any other drug in same solution.

Adverse effects

- **CNS:** *Headache, drowsiness,* peripheral neuropathy, neuritis, paresthesias
- **Dermatologic: Rashes—maculopapular, scaly or exfoliative—sometimes fatal**
- **GI:** *Nausea, vomiting, diarrhea,* abdominal pain, gastritis, hepatomegaly, hyperbilirubinemia, cholestatic jaundice
- **GU:** Exacerbation of gout and renal calculi, renal failure
- **Hematologic:** Anemia, leukopenia, agranulocytosis, thrombocytopenia, aplastic anemia, bone marrow depression

Interactions

✱ **Drug-drug** • Increased risk of hypersensitivity reaction with ACE inhibitors • Increased toxicity with thiazide diuretics • Increased risk of rash with ampicillin or amoxicillin • Increased risk of bone marrow suppression with cyclophosphamide, other cytotoxic agents • Increased half-life of oral anticoagulants • Increased serum levels of theophylline • Increased risk of toxic effects with thiopurines, 6-MP (azathioprine dose and dose of 6-MP should be reduced to one-third to one-fourth the usual dose)

■ Nursing considerations

Assessment

- **History:** Allergy to allopurinol, blood dyscrasias, liver disease, renal failure, lactation
- **Physical:** Skin lesions, color; orientation, reflexes; liver evaluation, normal urinary output; normal output; CBC, LFTs, renal function tests, urinalysis

Interventions

- Administer drug following meals.
- Encourage patient to drink 2.5–3 L/day to decrease the risk of renal stone development.

- Check urine alkalinity—urates crystallize in acid urine; sodium bicarbonate or potassium citrate may be ordered to alkalinize urine.

⊗ ***Warning*** Discontinue drug at first sign of skin rash; severe to fatal skin reactions have occurred.

- Arrange for regular medical follow-up and blood tests.

Teaching points

- Take the drug after meals.
- Avoid over-the-counter medications. Many of these preparations contain vitamin C or other agents that might increase the likelihood of kidney stone formation. If you need an over-the-counter preparation, check with your health care provider.
- You may experience these side effects: Exacerbation of gouty attack or renal stones (drink 2.5–3 liters of fluids per day while on this drug); nausea, vomiting, loss of appetite (take after meals or eat frequent small meals); drowsiness (use caution while driving or performing hazardous tasks).
- Report rash; unusual bleeding or bruising; fever, chills; gout attack; numbness or tingling; flank pain, skin rash.

▽almotriptan malate

*(al moh **trip'** tan **mah'** layt)*

Axert

PREGNANCY CATEGORY C

Drug classes

Antimigraine
Serotonin selective agonist
Triptan

Therapeutic actions

Binds to serotonin receptors to cause vascular constrictive effects on cranial blood vessels, causing the relief of migraine in selective patients.

Indications

- Treatment of acute migraines with or without aura

Contraindications and cautions

- Contraindicated with allergy to almotriptan, active coronary artery disease, Prinzmetal's angina, peripheral vascular syndromes, uncontrolled hypertension, use of an ergot compound or other triptan within 24 hours, pregnancy.
- Use cautiously with hepatic or renal impairment, risk factors for CAD, lactation.

Available forms

Tablets—6.25, 12.5 mg

Dosages

Adults

6.25–12.5 mg PO as a single dose at first sign of migraine; if headache returns, may be repeated after 2 hr; do not use more than 2 doses/24 hr.

Pediatric patients

Safety and efficacy not established for patients younger than 18 yr.

Patients with hepatic or renal impairment

Starting dose—6.25 mg; do not exceed 12.5 mg/24 hr.

Pharmacokinetics

Route	*Onset*	*Peak*
Oral	Varies	1–3 hr

Metabolism: Hepatic; $T_{1/2}$: 3–4 hr
Distribution: Crosses placenta; may enter breast milk
Excretion: Feces, urine

Adverse effects

- **CNS:** *Dizziness,* headache, anxiety, malaise or fatigue, weakness, myalgia, somnolence
- **CV:** *BP alterations, tightness or pressure in chest,* arrhythmias
- **GI:** *Nausea, dry mouth,* abdominal discomfort, dysphagia
- **Other:** Tingling; cold, warm, or hot sensations; burning sensation; feeling of heaviness; pressure sensation; numbness; feeling of tightness; feeling strange

Interactions

✱ **Drug-drug** • Prolonged vasoactive reactions when taken concurrently with ergot-containing drugs, other triptans • Risk of severe effects if taken with or within 2 wk of discontinuation of an MAOI • Increased effects and possible toxicity if taken with ketoconazole and other antifungals, nefazodone, macrolide antibiotics, antivirals; monitor patient closely if this combination is used • Risk of serotonin syndrome when combined with SSRIs, other antidepressants; monitor patient carefully if combination cannot be avoided

■ Nursing considerations

Assessment

- **History:** Allergy to almotriptan, active coronary artery disease, Prinzmetal's angina, pregnancy, lactation, peripheral vascular syndromes, uncontrolled hypertension, use of an ergot compound or other triptan within 24 hr, risk factors for CAD
- **Physical:** Skin color and lesions; orientation, reflexes, peripheral sensation; P, BP; LFTs, renal function tests

Interventions

- Administer to relieve acute migraine, not as a prophylactic measure.

⊗ ***Warning*** Ensure that the patient has not taken an ergot-containing compound or other triptan within 24 hr; risk of potentially serious vasospastic events.

- Do not administer more than 2 doses in a 24-hr period.
- Establish safety measures if CNS, visual disturbances occur.
- Control environment as appropriate to help relieve migraine (lighting, temperature, noise).
- Monitor BP of patients with possible coronary artery disease; discontinue at any sign of angina, prolonged high BP, and so forth.

Teaching points

- Take drug exactly as prescribed, at the onset of headache or aura. Do not take this drug to prevent a migraine; it is only used to treat migraines that are occurring. If the headache persists after you take this drug, you may repeat the dose after 2 hours have passed.
- Do not take more than 2 doses in a 24-hour period. Do not take any other migraine medication while you are taking this drug. If the headache is not relieved, call your health care provider.
- This drug should not be taken during pregnancy; if you suspect that you are pregnant, contact your health care provider and refrain from using drug.
- Continue to do anything that usually helps you feel better during a migraine (such as controlling lighting and reducing noise).
- Contact your health care provider immediately if you experience chest pain or pressure that is severe or does not go away.
- You may experience these side effects: Dizziness, drowsiness (avoid driving or the use of dangerous machinery while on this drug), numbness, tingling, feelings of tightness or pressure.
- Report feeling hot, tired, or sick; flushing; swelling of lips or eyelids.

▽ alosetron hydrochloride

*(ah **loss'** e tron)*

Lotronex

PREGNANCY CATEGORY B

Drug classes

5-HT_3 (serotonin) antagonist
IBS drug

Therapeutic actions

Blocks 5-HT_3 (serotonin) receptors in the enteric nervous system of the GI tract; interacting with these receptors blocks visceral sensitivity, increases colonic transit time, decreases GI motility, may also decrease the perception of abdominal pain and discomfort.

Indications

- Treatment of severe diarrhea-predominant IBS in women who have chronic IBS (longer than 6 mo), have no anatomic or biochemical abnormalities of the GI tract, and who have failed to respond to conventional therapy

Contraindications and cautions

- Contraindicated with hypersensitivity to the drug, history of chronic or severe constipation or sequelae from constipation; history of intestinal obstruction, stricture, toxic megacolon, GI perforation or adhesions; history of ischemic colitis, impaired intestinal circulation, thrombophlebitis, or hypercoagulable state; history of or current Crohn's disease, ulcerative colitis, diverticulitis; inability to understand or comply with the Physician–Patient Agreement.
- Use cautiously with pregnancy, lactation, and elderly patients.

Available forms

Tablets—0.5, 1 mg

Dosages

Adults

0.5 mg PO bid for 4 wk; may be continued if drug is tolerated and symptoms of IBS are under adequate control. Dose may be increased up to 1 mg bid PO after 4 wk if well tolerated and needed.

Pediatric patients

Safety and efficacy not established for patients younger than 18 yr.

Geriatric patients or patients with hepatic impairment

These patients may be at increased risk for complications from constipation; monitor very closely.

Pharmacokinetics

Route	*Onset*	*Peak*
Oral	Rapid	1 hr

Metabolism: Hepatic; $T_{1/2}$: 1.5 hr
Distribution: Crosses placenta; enters into breast milk
Excretion: Bile, urine, feces

Adverse effects

- **CNS:** Anxiety, tremors, dreams, headache
- **Dermatologic:** Sweating, urticaria
- **GI:** Abdominal pain, nausea, *constipation,* **ischemic colitis**
- **Other:** Malaise, fatigue, pain

Interactions

✷ **Drug-drug** • Increased risk of constipation if taken with other drugs that cause decreased GI motility; if this combination cannot be avoided, monitor patient very carefully and discontinue drug at first sign of constipation or ischemic colitis • Contraindicated for use with fluvoxamine • Avoid use with fluoroquinolones, cimetidine because of risk of adverse effects

■ Nursing considerations

Assessment

- **History:** Hypersensitivity to the drug, history of chronic or severe constipation or sequelae from constipation; history of intestinal obstruction, stricture, toxic megacolon, GI perforation or adhesions; history of ischemic colitis, impaired intestinal circulation, thrombophlebitis, or hypercoagulable state; history of Crohn's disease, ulcerative colitis, diverticulitis; inability to understand or comply with the Physician–Patient Agreement, pregnancy, lactation, elderly patients
- **Physical:** Skin lesions; T; reflexes, affect; urinary output, abdominal examination; bowel patterns

Interventions

⊗ ***Black box warning*** Ensure that the patient has read and understands the Physician–Patient Agreement, which outlines the risks associated with the use of the drug, including risk for ischemic colitis, and warning signs to report.

- Ensure that the Physician–Patient Agreement is in the patient's permanent record.
- Administer drug without regard to food.
- Arrange for further evaluation of patient after 4 wk of therapy to determine effectiveness of drug; discontinue drug if symptoms are not controlled at 1 mg bid.
- Encourage the use of barrier contraceptives to prevent pregnancy while patient is using this drug.
- Maintain supportive treatment as appropriate for underlying problem.
- Provide additional comfort measures to alleviate discomfort from GI effects, headache.
- Monitor patient for any signs of constipation; discontinue drug at first sign of

constipation or ischemic colitis and alert the prescribing physician.

Teaching points

- Read and sign the Physician–Patient Agreement, which outlines the risks and benefits of therapy with this drug.
- Arrange to have regular medical follow-up while you are on this drug.
- Use barrier contraceptives while on this drug; serious adverse effects could occur during pregnancy; if you become or wish to become pregnant, consult your health care provider.
- Maintain all of the usual activities and restrictions that apply to your condition. If this becomes difficult, consult your health care provider.
- You may experience these side effects: Headache (consult your health care provider if these become bothersome, medications may be available to help); nausea, vomiting (proper nutrition is important, consult a dietician to maintain nutrition).
- Report constipation, signs of ischemic colitis—worsening abdominal pain, bloody diarrhea, blood in the stool; continuation of IBS symptoms without relief.

alpha$_1$-proteinase inhibitor

See Appendix W, *Less commonly used drugs*.

alprazolam

*(al **prah'** zoe lam)*

Alprazolam Extended Relief (DNC), Alprazolam Intensol, Apo-Alpraz (CAN), Apo-Alpraz TS (CAN), Gen-Alprazolam (CAN), Niravam, Novo-Alprazol (CAN), Xanax, Xanax TS (CAN), Xanax XR (DNC)

PREGNANCY CATEGORY D

CONTROLLED SUBSTANCE C-IV

Drug classes

Anxiolytic
Benzodiazepine

Therapeutic actions

Exact mechanisms of action not understood; main sites of action may be the limbic system and reticular formation; increases the effects of GABA, an inhibitory neurotransmitter; anxiety blocking effects occur at doses well below those necessary to cause sedation, ataxia.

Indications

- Management of anxiety disorders, short-term relief of symptoms of anxiety; anxiety associated with depression
- Treatment of panic attacks with or without agoraphobia (*Niravam, Xanax, Xanax XR*)

Contraindications and cautions

- Contraindicated with hypersensitivity to benzodiazepines, psychoses, acute narrow-angle glaucoma, shock, coma, acute alcoholic intoxication with depression of vital signs, pregnancy (crosses the placenta; risk of congenital malformations, neonatal withdrawal syndrome), labor and delivery ("floppy infant" syndrome), lactation (secreted in breast milk; infants become lethargic and lose weight).
- Use cautiously with impaired liver or renal function, debilitation.

Available forms

Tablets—0.25, 0.5, 1, 2 mg; ER tablets (DNC)—0.5, 1, 2, 3 mg; oral solution—1 mg/mL; rapidly disintegrating tablets—0.25, 0.5, 1, 2 mg

Dosages

Individualize dosage; increase dosage gradually to avoid adverse effects; decrease dosage gradually (no more than 0.5 mg q 3 days) when discontinuing drug.

Adults

- *Anxiety disorders:* Initially, 0.25–0.5 mg PO tid; adjust to maximum daily dose of 4 mg/day in divided doses at intervals of 3–4 days or extended-release form once per day in the AM once dosage is established (immediate release, intensol solution).
- *Panic disorder:* Initially, 0.5 mg PO tid; increase dose at 3- to 4-day intervals in increments of no more than 1 mg/day; ranges of 1–10 mg/day have been needed. ER tablets—Initially, 0.5–1 mg/day; dosage range, 3–6 mg/day.

Geriatric patients or patients with advanced hepatic or debilitating disease

Initially, 0.25 mg bid–tid PO; gradually increase if needed and tolerated; ER tablets—0.5 mg PO once each day; gradually increase if needed and tolerated.

Pharmacokinetics

Route	*Onset*	*Peak*	*Duration*
Oral	30 min	1–2 hr	4–6 hr

Metabolism: Hepatic; $T_{1/2}$: 6.3–26.9 hr
Distribution: Crosses placenta; enters breast milk
Excretion: Urine

Adverse effects

- **CNS:** *Transient, mild drowsiness initially; sedation, depression, lethargy, apathy, fatigue, light-headedness, disorientation, anger, hostility,* episodes of mania and hypomania, *restlessness, confusion, crying,* delirium, *headache,* slurred speech, dysarthria, stupor, rigidity, tremor, dystonia, vertigo, euphoria, nervousness, difficulty in concentration, vivid dreams, psychomotor retardation, extrapyramidal symptoms; *mild paradoxical excitatory reactions during first 2 wk of treatment*
- **CV:** Bradycardia, tachycardia, CV collapse, hypertension, hypotension, palpitations, edema
- **Dermatologic:** Urticaria, pruritus, rash, dermatitis
- **EENT:** Visual and auditory disturbances, diplopia, nystagmus, depressed hearing, nasal congestion
- **GI:** *Constipation, diarrhea, dry mouth,* salivation, *nausea,* anorexia, vomiting, difficulty in swallowing, gastric disorders, hepatic impairment
- **GU:** Incontinence, changes in libido, urine retention, menstrual irregularities
- **Hematologic:** Elevations of blood enzymes—LDH, alkaline phosphatase, AST, ALT; blood dyscrasias—agranulocytosis, leukopenia
- **Other:** Hiccups, fever, diaphoresis, paresthesias, muscular disturbances, gynecomastia. *Drug dependence with withdrawal syndrome when drug is discontinued; more common with abrupt discontinuation of higher dosage used for longer than 4 mo*

Interactions

✱ **Drug-drug** • Increased CNS depression with alcohol, other CNS depressants, propoxyphene • Increased effect with cimetidine, disulfiram, omeprazole, isoniazid, hormonal contraceptives, valproic acid • Decreased effect with carbamazepine, rifampin, theophylline • Possible increased risk of digitalis toxicity with digoxin • Decreased antiparkinson effectiveness of levodopa with benzodiazepines • Contraindicated with ketoconazole, itraconazole; serious toxicity can occur
✱ **Drug-food** • Decreased metabolism and risk of toxic effects if combined with grapefruit juice; avoid this combination
✱ **Drug-alternative therapy** • Risk of coma if combined with kava therapy • Additive sedative effects with valerian root

■ Nursing considerations

CLINICAL ALERT!
Name confusion has occurred among *Xanax* (alprazolam), *Celexa* (citalopram), and *Cerebyx* (fosphenytoin), and between alprazolam and lorazepam; use caution.

Assessment

- **History:** Hypersensitivity to benzodiazepines; psychoses; acute narrow-angle glaucoma; shock; coma; acute alcoholic intoxication with depression of vital signs; labor and delivery; lactation; impaired liver or renal function; debilitation
- **Physical:** Skin color, lesions; T; orientation, reflexes, affect, ophthalmologic examination; P, BP; liver evaluation, abdominal examination, bowel sounds, normal output; CBC, LFTs, renal function tests

Interventions

- Arrange to taper dosage gradually after long-term therapy, especially in epileptic patients.
- Do not administer with grapefruit juice or within 48 hr of grapefruit juice.
- Taper drug slowly, decrease by no more than 0.5 mg every 3 days.

Teaching points

- Take this drug exactly as prescribed; take extended-release form once a day in the morning; do not cut, crush, or chew extended-release tablets. Place the rapidly disintegrating tablet on top of your tongue, where it will disintegrate and can be swallowed with saliva.
- Do not drink grapefruit juice while on this drug.
- Do not stop taking drug (in long-term therapy) without consulting health care provider; drug should not be stopped suddenly.
- Avoid alcohol, sleep-inducing, or over-the-counter drugs.
- You may experience these side effects: Drowsiness, dizziness (these effects will be less pronounced after a few days, avoid driving a car or engaging in other dangerous activities if these occur); GI upset (take drug with food); fatigue; depression; dreams; crying; nervousness.
- Report severe dizziness, weakness, drowsiness that persists, rash or skin lesions, difficulty voiding, palpitations, swelling in the extremities.

▽alprostadil

*(al **pross'** ta dil)*

IV: Prostin VR Pediatric
Intracavernous: Caverject, Caverject Impulse, Edex, Muse

PREGNANCY CATEGORY (NOT APPLICABLE)

Drug class

Prostaglandin

Therapeutic actions

Relaxes vascular smooth muscle; the smooth muscle of the ductus arteriosus is especially sensitive to this action and will relax and stay open; this is beneficial in infants who have congenital defects that restrict pulmonary or systemic blood flow and who depend on a patent ductus arteriosus for adequate blood oxygenation and lower body perfusion. Treatment of erectile dysfunction due to neurogenic, vasculogenic, psychogenic, or mixed etiology.

Indications

- Palliative therapy to temporarily maintain the patency of the ductus arteriosus until corrective or palliative surgery can be performed in neonates with congenital heart defects who depend on a patent ductus (eg, pulmonary atresia or stenosis, tetralogy of Fallot, coarctation of the aorta)
- Treatment of erectile dysfunction (intracavernous injection)
- Unlabeled use: Peripheral vascular disease, Raynaud's disease, critical limb ischemia, peripheral angiography

Contraindications and cautions

- Contraindicated with respiratory distress syndrome (IV); conditions that might predispose to priapism, deformation of the penis, penile implants (intracavernous injection), known hypersensitivity.
- Use cautiously with patients with bleeding tendencies (drug inhibits platelet aggregation).

Available forms

Powder for injection—5, 10, 20, 40 mcg/mL; 10, 20 mcg/0.5 mL; injection (IV)—10, 20 mcg/mL; 40 mcg/2 mL (penile); 500 mcg/mL; pellets—125, 250, 500, 1,000 mcg

Dosages

Adults

Intracavernous injection

0.2–140 mcg by intracavernous injection using 0.5-in 27–30 gauge needle; may be repeated up to three times weekly with at least 24 hr between doses. Self-injection over 6-mo period has been successful. Reduce dose if erection lasts more than 1 hr.

Pellet

125, 250, 500, or 1,000 mcg based on patient response. Maximum dosage, two systems in 24 hr administered intraurethrally.

Pediatric patients

Preferred administration is through a continuous IV infusion into a large vein; may be administered through an umbilical artery catheter placed at the ductal opening. Begin infusion with 0.05–0.1 mcg/kg/min. After an increase in partial pressure of oxygen (pO_2) or in systemic BP and blood pH is achieved, reduce infusion to the lowest possible dosage that maintains the response (often achieved by reducing dosage from 0.1–0.05 to 0.025–0.01 mcg/kg/min). Up to 0.4 mcg/kg/min may be used for maintenance if required; higher dosage rates are not more effective.

Pharmacokinetics

Route	*Onset*	*Peak*
IV	5–25 min	End of infusion
Intracavernous	10 min	30–60 min
Pellet	5–10 min	30–60 min

Metabolism: Lungs, local metabolism in GU tract; $T_{1/2}$: 5–10 min
Excretion: Urine

IV FACTS

Preparation: Prepare solution by diluting 500 mcg alprostadil with sodium chloride injection or dextrose injection; dilute to volumes required for pump delivery system. Discard and prepare fresh infusion solutions every 24 hr; refrigerate drug ampules.
Infusion:

Add 500 mg Alprostadil to	*Approximate Concentration of Resulting Solution*	*Infusion Rate (mL/kg/min)*
250 mL	2 mcg/mL	0.05
100 mL	5 mcg/mL	0.02
50 mL	10 mcg/mL	0.01
25 mL	20 mcg/mL	0.005

Adverse effects

- **CNS:** *Seizures,* cerebral bleeding, hypothermia, jitteriness, lethargy, stiffness
- **CV:** *Bradycardia, flushing, tachycardia, hypotension,* **cardiac arrest,** heart block
- **GI:** Diarrhea, gastric outlet obstruction (neonates)
- **GU (with intracavernous injection):** Penile pain, rash, **fibrosis,** erection, priapism, urethral burning or bleeding
- **Hematologic:** Inhibited platelet aggregation, bleeding, anemia, DIC, hypokalemia
- **Respiratory:** *Apnea,* respiratory distress
- **Other:** Cortical proliferation of the long bones (with prolonged use, regresses after treatment is stopped), sepsis

■ Nursing considerations

CLINICAL ALERT!
Confusion has been reported with *Prostin VR Pediatric* (alprostadil), *Prostin F_2* (dinoprost—available outside US), *Prostin E_2* (dinoprostone), *Prostin 15M* (carboprost in Europe); use extreme caution.

Assessment

- **History:** Respiratory distress, bleeding tendencies
- **Physical:** T; cyanosis; skeletal development, reflexes, state of agitation, arterial pressure (using auscultation or Doppler), P, auscultation, peripheral perfusion; R, adventitious sounds, bleeding times, arterial blood gases, blood pH

Interventions

IV

- Constantly monitor arterial pressure; decrease infusion rate immediately if any fall in arterial pressure occurs.
- Regularly monitor arterial blood gases to determine efficacy of alprostadil (pO_2 in infants with restricted pulmonary flow; pH and systemic BP in infants with restricted systemic flow).

⊗ ***Black box warning*** Apnea occurs in 10%–12% of neonates treated with alprostadil, particularly those weighing less than 2 kg. Monitor respiratory status continuously, have ventilatory assistance readily available, and move the neonate often during the first hour of infusion.

Intracavernous

- Reconstitute vial with 1 mL diluent. 1 mL of solution will contain 5.4–41.1 mcg of alprostadil.
- Use solution immediately after reconstitution; do not store or freeze.
- Inject along the dorsal-lateral aspect of the proximal third of the penis using sterile technique.

Intraurethral

- Teach patient proper technique for intraurethral insertion.
- Store foil packets for pellets in the refrigerator and do not open them until ready to use.

Teaching points

IV

- Teaching about this drug should be incorporated into a total teaching program for the parents of the infant with a cyanotic congenital heart defect; specifics about the drug that they will need to know include:
- Your infant will be continually monitored and have frequent blood tests to follow the effects of the drug.
- The infant may look better, breathe easier, become fussy, and so forth, but the drug treatment is only a temporary solution, and the baby will require corrective surgery.

Intracavernous

- Learn and repeat self-injection technique. Plan for the first injection in the physician's office under supervision. Do not self-inject more than three times per week; wait at least 24 hours between injections.
- Return for regular medical follow-up and evaluation.
- You may experience these side effects: Penile pain, swelling, rash.
- Report prolonged erection, swelling, or severe pain.

Intraurethral

- If you are prescribed the pellet form for intraurethral insertion, you will need to learn proper administration technique.
- Store foil packets for pellets in the refrigerator and do not open them until ready to use.
- Do not use more than two systems in a 24-hour period.

DANGEROUS DRUG

▽alteplase, recombinant (recombinant tissue-type plasminogen activator, rt-PA)

*(al ti **plaze'**)*

Activase, Cathflo Activase

PREGNANCY CATEGORY C

Drug class

Thrombolytic enzyme
Tissue plasminogen activator (TPA)

Therapeutic actions

Human tissue enzyme produced by recombinant DNA techniques; converts plasminogen to the enzyme plasmin (fibrinolysin), which degrades fibrin clots; lyses thrombi and emboli; is most active at the site of the clot and causes little systemic fibrinolysis.

Indications

- Treatment of coronary artery thrombosis associated with acute MI; improvement of ventricular function following MI; reduction of the incidence of heart failure and mortality associated with MI *(Activase)*
- Treatment of acute, massive pulmonary embolism in adults *(Activase)*
- Treatment of acute ischemic CVA *(Activase)*
- Restoration of function to central venous access devices occluded as assessed by the ability to withdraw blood *(Cathflo Activase)*
- Unlabeled use: Treatment of unstable angina, frostbite, pleural effusion

Contraindications and cautions

- Contraindicated with allergy to TPA; active internal bleeding; recent (within 2 mo) CVA; intracranial or intraspinal surgery or neoplasm; recent major surgery, obstetric delivery, organ biopsy, or rupture of a noncompressible blood vessel; recent serious GI bleed; recent serious trauma, including CPR; SBE; hemostatic defects; cerebrovascular disease; early-onset, insulin-dependent diabetes; septic thrombosis; severe uncontrolled hypertension; subarachnoid hemorrhage; concurrent use of anticoagulants; low platelet count.
- Use cautiously with hepatic disease in elderly (more than 75 yr—risk of bleeding may be increased), pregnancy, lactation.

Available forms

Powder for injection—50, 100 mg; single use powder for injection (*Cathflo Activase*)—2 mg

Dosages

Careful patient assessment and evaluation are needed to determine the appropriate dose of this drug. Because experience is limited with this drug, careful monitoring is essential.

Adults

- *Acute MI:* For patients weighing more than 67 kg, 100 mg as a 15-mg IV bolus followed by 50 mg infused over 30 min. Then 35 mg over the next 60 min. For patients weighing 67 kg or less, 15-mg IV bolus followed by 0.75 mg/kg infused over 30 min (not to exceed 50 mg). Then 0.5 mg/kg over the next 60 min (not to exceed 35 mg). For a 3-hr infusion, 60 mg in first hr (6–10 mg as a bolus); 20 mg over second hr; 20 mg over third hr. Patients weighing less than 65 kg should receive 1.25 mg/kg over 3 hr.

⊗ ***Warning*** Do not use a total dose of 150 mg because of the increased risk of intracranial bleeding.

- *Pulmonary embolism:* 100 mg administered by IV infusion over 2 hr, followed immediately by heparin therapy.
- *Acute ischemic CVA:* 0.9 mg/kg (not to exceed 90 mg total dose) infused over 60 min with 10% given as an IV bolus over the first 1 min.
- *Restoration of function of central venous access devices (Cathflo Activase):* 2 mg in 2 mL of sterile water for injection from single use vial injected into device; may repeat after 2 hr if necessary.

Pharmacokinetics

Route	*Onset*	*Peak*	*Duration*
IV	Immediate	5–10 min	2.5–3 hr

Metabolism: Hepatic; $T_{1/2}$: 26 min
Distribution: Crosses placenta
Excretion: Liver

IV FACTS

Preparation: Do not use if vacuum is not present; add volume of the sterile water for injection provided with vial using a large bore needle and directing stream into the cake; slight foaming may occur but will dissipate after standing undisturbed for several min; reconstitute immediately before use. Do not shake. Refrigerate reconstituted solution and use within 8 hr. Do not use bacteriostatic water for injection. Reconstituted solution should be colorless or pale yellow and transparent; contains 1 mg/mL with a pH of 7.3.

Infusion: Administer as reconstituted or further dilute with an equal volume of 0.9% sodium chloride injection or 5% dextrose injection to yield 0.5 mg/mL; stable for up to 8 hr in these solutions. Avoid excessive agitation; mix by gentle swirling or slow inversion. Discard unused solution.

Incompatibilities: Do not add other medications to infusion solution; use 0.9% sodium chloride injection or 5% dextrose injection and no other solutions.

Y-site compatibility: Lidocaine.

Y-site incompatibilities: Dobutamine, dopamine, heparin, nitroglycerin.

Adverse effects

- **CV:** Cardiac arrhythmias with coronary reperfusion, hypotension
- **Hematologic:** *Bleeding*—particularly at venous or arterial access sites, GI bleeding, intracranial hemorrhage
- **Other:** Urticaria, nausea, vomiting, fever

Interactions

✱ **Drug-drug** • Increased risk of hemorrhage if used with heparin or oral anticoagulants, aspirin, dipyridamole

■ Nursing considerations

CLINICAL ALERT!

Confusion has been reported between alteplase and *Altace* (ramipril); use caution.

Assessment

- **History:** Allergy to TPA; active internal bleeding; recent (within 2 mo) obstetric delivery, organ biopsy, or rupture of a noncompressible blood vessel; recent serious GI bleed; recent serious trauma, including CPR; SBE; hemostatic defects; cerebrovascular disease; type 1 diabetes; septic thrombosis; severe uncontrolled hypertension; liver disease
- **Physical:** Skin color, T, lesions; orientation, reflexes; P, BP, peripheral perfusion, baseline ECG; R, adventitious sounds; liver evaluation, Hct, platelet count, thrombin time, aPTT, PT

Interventions

- Discontinue heparin and alteplase if serious bleeding occurs.
- Monitor coagulation studies; PT or aPTT should be less than two times control.

- Apply pressure or pressure dressings to control superficial bleeding (at invaded or disturbed areas).
- Avoid arterial invasive procedures.
- Type and cross-match blood in case serious blood loss occurs and whole-blood transfusions are required.
- Institute treatment within 6 hr of onset of symptoms for evolving MI, within 3 hr of onset of CVA.

Teaching points

- This drug can only be given IV. You will be closely monitored during drug treatment.
- Report difficulty breathing, dizziness, disorientation, headache, numbness, tingling.

altretamine

See Appendix W, *Less commonly used drugs*.

aluminum hydroxide gel

*(a **loo'** mi num)*

AlternaGEL, Amphojel, Dialume

PREGNANCY CATEGORY C

Drug class

Antacid

Therapeutic actions

Neutralizes or reduces gastric acidity, resulting in an increase in the pH of the stomach and duodenal bulb and inhibiting the proteolytic activity of pepsin, which protects the lining of the stomach and duodenum; binds with phosphate ions in the intestine to form insoluble aluminum–phosphate complexes, lowering phosphate in hyperphosphatemia and chronic renal failure; may cause hypophosphatemia in other states.

Indications

- Symptomatic relief of upset stomach associated with hyperacidity
- Hyperacidity associated with uncomplicated peptic ulcer, gastritis, peptic esophagitis, gastric hyperacidity, hiatal hernia
- Unlabeled uses: Prophylaxis of GI bleeding, stress ulcer; reduction of phosphate absorption in hyperphosphatemia in patients with chronic renal failure; suspected GERD laryngitis (adults)

Contraindications and cautions

- Contraindicated with allergy to aluminum products, gastric outlet destruction, hypertension, heart failure, hypophosphatemia, lactation.
- Use cautiously with pregnancy.

Available forms

Tablets—600 mg; capsules—500 mg; suspension—320 mg/5 mL, 450 mg/5 mL, 675 mg/5 mL; liquid—600 mg/5 mL

Dosages

Adults

Tablets and capsules: 500–1,500 mg 3–6 times/day PO between meals and at bedtime. Liquid: 5–10 mL between meals, at bedtime, or as directed.

Pediatric patients

- *General guidelines:* 5–15 mL PO every 3–6 hr or 1–3 hr after meals and at bedtime.
- *Hyperphosphatemia:* 50–150 mg/kg every 24 hr PO in divided doses every 4–6 hr; adjust dosage to normal serum phosphorus.
- *Prophylaxis of GI bleeding in critically ill infants:* 2–5 mL/dose every 1–2 hr PO.
- *Prophylaxis of GI bleeding in critically ill children:* 5–15 mL/dose every 1–2 hr PO.

Pharmacokinetics

Route	*Onset*
Oral	Varies

Metabolism: Hepatic
Distribution: Long-term use, small amounts may be absorbed systemically and cross the placenta and enter breast milk
Excretion: Feces

Adverse effects

- **GI:** *Constipation;* intestinal obstruction; decreased absorption of fluoride; accumula-

tion of aluminum in serum, bone, and CNS; rebound hyperacidity
- **Musculoskeletal:** Osteomalacia and chronic phosphate deficiency with bone pain, malaise, muscular weakness

Interactions

✱ **Drug-drug** • Do not administer other oral drugs within 1–2 hr of antacid; change in gastric pH may interfere with absorption of oral drugs • Decreased pharmacologic effect of corticosteroids, diflunisal, digoxin, fluoroquinolones, iron, isoniazid, penicillamine, phenothiazines, ranitidine, tetracyclines • Increased pharmacologic effect of benzodiazepines

■ Nursing considerations

Assessment

- **History:** Allergy to aluminum products; gastric outlet obstruction; hypertension, heart failure; hypophosphatemia; lactation
- **Physical:** Bone strength, muscle strength; P, auscultation, BP, peripheral edema; abdominal examination, bowel sounds; serum phosphorous, serum fluoride; bone X-ray is appropriate

Interventions

- Give hourly for first 2 wk when used for acute peptic ulcer; during the healing stage, give 1–3 hr after meals and at bedtime.

⊗ ***Warning*** Do not administer oral drugs within 1–2 hr of antacid administration.

- Have patient chew tablets thoroughly; follow with a glass of water.
- Monitor serum phosphorus levels periodically during long-term therapy.

Teaching points

- Take this drug between meals and at bedtime; ulcer patients need to strictly follow prescribed dosage pattern. If tablets are being used, chew thoroughly before swallowing, and follow with a glass of water.
- Do not take maximum dosage of antacids for longer than 2 weeks except under medical supervision.
- Do not take this drug with any other oral medications; absorption of those medications can be inhibited. Take other oral medications at least 1–2 hours after aluminum salt. Consult with your health care provider before using other drugs.
- Constipation may occur.
- Report constipation; bone pain, muscle weakness; coffee ground vomitus, black tarry stools; no relief from symptoms being treated.

▽ alvimopan

See Appendix W, *Less commonly used drugs.*

▽ amantadine hydrochloride

*(a **man'** ta deen)*

Endantadine (CAN), Gen-Amantadine (CAN), Symmetrel

PREGNANCY CATEGORY C

Drug classes

Antiviral
Antiparkinsonian

Therapeutic actions

May inhibit penetration of influenza A virus into the host cell; may increase dopamine release in the nigrostriatal pathway of patients with Parkinson's disease, relieving their symptoms.

Indications

- Prevention and treatment of influenza A virus respiratory infection, especially in high-risk patients
- Adjunct to late vaccination against influenza A virus, to provide interim coverage; supplement to vaccination in immunodeficient patients; prophylaxis when vaccination is contraindicated
- Treatment of Parkinson's disease and drug-induced extrapyramidal reactions

Contraindications and cautions

- Contraindicated with allergy to drug product, eczematoid rash, psychoses, lactation.
- Use cautiously with renal or hepatic disease, seizures, heart failure, pregnancy.

Available forms

Tablets—100 mg; capsules—100 mg; syrup—50 mg/5 mL

Dosages

Adults

- *Influenza A virus prophylaxis:* 200 mg/day PO or 100 mg bid PO for 10 days after exposure, for the duration of known influenza A in the community if vaccination is impossible and exposure is repeated. If used in conjunction with influenza vaccine, administer for 2–4 wk after vaccine has been given.
- *Uncomplicated influenza A virus treatment:* Same dose as above; start treatment as soon after exposure as possible, continuing for 24–48 hr after symptoms are gone.
- *Parkinsonism treatment:* 100 mg bid (up to 400 mg/day) PO when used alone; reduce in patients receiving other antiparkinsonian drugs.
- *Drug-induced extrapyramidal reactions:* 100 mg bid PO, up to 300 mg/day in divided doses has been used.

Patients with seizure disorders

100 mg/day.

Patients with renal disease

For patients on hemodialysis, 200 mg PO every 7 days. For patients with reduced creatinine clearance, use dosage as outlined below:

CrCl (mL/min)	*Dosage*
Less than 15	200 mg PO every 7 days
15–29	200 mg PO first day, then 100 mg on alternate days
30–50	200 mg PO first day, then 100 mg/day

Pediatric patients

Not recommended for children younger than 1 yr.

- *Influenza A virus prophylaxis:*
  1–9 yr: 4.4–8.8 mg/kg/day PO in one or two divided doses, not to exceed 150 mg/day.
  9–12 yr: 100 mg PO bid.
- *Influenza A virus treatment:* As above; start as soon after exposure as possible, continuing for 24-48 hr after symptoms are gone.

Geriatric patients

- *Influenza A prophylaxis treatment:* For patients older than 65 yr with no recognized renal disease, 100 mg once daily PO.
- *Parkinsonism:* 100 mg/day for patients with serious associated medical illnesses or who are using other parkinsonism drugs. May increase to 100 mg bid if necessary after 1 wk or longer.

Pharmacokinetics

Route	*Onset*	*Peak*
Oral	36–48 hr	1.5–8 hr

Metabolism: $T_{1/2}$: 10–25 hr
Distribution: Crosses placenta; enters breast milk
Excretion: Unchanged in the urine

Adverse effects

- **CNS:** *Light-headedness, dizziness, insomnia,* confusion, irritability, ataxia, psychosis, depression, hallucinations, headache, somnolence, suicidal ideation
- **CV:** HF, orthostatic hypotension, dyspnea
- **GI:** *Nausea,* anorexia, constipation, dry mouth, diarrhea
- **GU:** Urinary retention, fatigue

Interactions

✱ **Drug-drug** • Increased atropine-like side effects with anticholinergic drugs • Increased amantadine effects with hydrochlorothiazide, triamterene

■ Nursing considerations

Assessment

- **History:** Allergy to drug product, seizures, hepatic disease, eczematoid rash, psychoses, HF, renal disease, lactation
- **Physical:** Orientation, vision, speech, reflexes; BP, orthostatic BP, P, auscultation, perfusion, edema; R, adventitious sounds; urinary output; BUN, creatinine clearance

Interventions

- Do not discontinue abruptly when treating parkinsonism syndrome; parkinsonian crisis may occur.
- Be aware that the smallest amount possible should be prescribed; deaths have been reported from overdose.

Teaching points

- Mark your calendar if you are on alternating dosage schedules; it is very important to take the full course of the drug.

- You may experience these side effects: Drowsiness, blurred vision (use caution when driving or using dangerous equipment); dizziness, light-headedness (avoid sudden position changes); irritability or mood changes (common effect; if severe, drug may be changed).
- Report swelling of the fingers or ankles; shortness of breath; difficulty urinating, walking; tremors, slurred speech; thoughts of suicide.

ambenonium chloride

*(am be **noe'** nee um)*

Mytelase

PREGNANCY CATEGORY C

Drug classes

Antimyasthenic
Cholinesterase inhibitor
Parasympathomimetic (indirectly acting)

Therapeutic actions

Increases the concentration of acetylcholine at the sites of cholinergic transmission (parasympathetic neurons and skeletal muscles) and prolongs and exaggerates the effects of acetylcholine by inhibiting the enzyme acetylcholinesterase; this causes parasympathomimetic effects and facilitates transmission at the skeletal neuromuscular junction. Also has direct stimulating effects on skeletal muscle and has a longer duration of effect and fewer side effects than other agents.

Indications

- Symptomatic control of myasthenia gravis

Contraindications and cautions

- Contraindicated with hypersensitivity to anticholinesterases, intestinal or urogenital tract obstruction, peritonitis, lactation, concurrent use of atropine.
- Use cautiously with asthma, peptic ulcer, bradycardia, cardiac arrhythmias, recent coronary occlusion, vagotonia, hyperthyroidism, epilepsy, pregnancy.

Available forms

Tablets—10 mg

Dosages

Adults

5–25 mg PO tid–qid (5–75 mg per dose has been used). Start dosage with 5 mg, and gradually increase to determine optimum dosage based on optimal muscle strength and no GI disturbances; increase dose every 1–2 days. Dosage above 200 mg/day requires close supervision to avoid overdose.

Pediatric patients

Safety and efficacy not established.

Pharmacokinetics

Route	*Onset*	*Duration*
Oral	20–30 min	3–8 hr

Metabolism: $T_{1/2}$: Unknown
Distribution: Crosses placenta; enters breast milk
Excretion: Unknown

Adverse effects

Parasympathomimetic effects

- **CNS:** Seizures, dysarthria, dysphonia, drowsiness, dizziness, headache, loss of consciousness
- **CV:** *Bradycardia, cardiac arrhythmias,* AV block and nodal rhythm, **cardiac arrest,** decreased cardiac output, leading to hypotension, syncope
- **Dermatologic:** Diaphoresis, flushing
- **EENT:** *Lacrimation, miosis,* spasm of accommodation, diplopia, conjunctival hyperemia
- **GI:** *Salivation, dysphagia, nausea, vomiting, increased peristalsis, abdominal cramps,* flatulence, diarrhea
- **GU:** *Urinary frequency and incontinence,* urinary urgency
- **Respiratory:** *Increased pharyngeal and tracheobronchial secretions,* **laryngospasm, bronchospasm,** bronchiolar constriction, dyspnea

Skeletal muscle effects

- **Peripheral:** Skeletal muscle weakness, fasciculations, muscle cramps, arthralgia
- **Respiratory:** Respiratory muscle paralysis, **central respiratory paralysis**

Interactions

✱ **Drug-drug** • Decreased neuromuscular blockade of succinylcholine • Decreased effects of ambenonium and possible muscular depression with corticosteroids • Risk of severe toxicity with atropine; combination is contraindicated • Risk of toxicity if given with other anticholinesterases, antiarrhythmics, local and general anesthetics

■ Nursing considerations

Assessment

- **History:** Hypersensitivity to anticholinesterases, intestinal or urogenital tract obstruction, peritonitis, asthma, peptic ulcer, bradycardia, cardiac arrhythmias, recent coronary occlusion, vagotonia, hyperthyroidism, epilepsy, lactation
- **Physical:** Skin color, texture, lesions; reflexes, bilateral grip strength; P, auscultation, BP; R, adventitious sounds; salivation, bowel sounds, normal output; frequency, voiding pattern, normal urinary output; EEG, thyroid function tests

Interventions

- Overdose can cause muscle weakness (cholinergic crisis) that is difficult to differentiate from myasthenic weakness (use of edrophonium for differential diagnosis is recommended). The administration of atropine may mask the parasympathetic effects of anticholinesterase overdose and further confound the diagnosis.

⊗ ***Warning*** Keep atropine sulfate readily available as an antidote and antagonist in case of cholinergic crisis or hypersensitivity reaction.

- Monitor patient response carefully if increasing dosage.
- Discontinue drug and consult physician if excessive salivation, emesis, frequent urination, or diarrhea occurs.
- Arrange for decreased dosage of drug if excessive sweating, nausea, or GI upset occurs.

Teaching points

- Take this drug exactly as prescribed; does not need to be taken at night. You and your home caregiver need to know about the effects of the drug, the signs and symptoms of myasthenia gravis, the fact that muscle weakness may be related to drug overdose and to exacerbation of the disease, and that it is important to report muscle weakness promptly to your health care provider so that proper evaluation can be made.
- You may experience these side effects: Blurred vision, difficulty with far vision, difficulty with dark adaptation (use caution while driving, especially at night, or performing hazardous tasks in reduced light); increased urinary frequency, abdominal cramps (if these become a problem, notify your health care provider); sweating (avoid hot or excessively humid environments).
- Report muscle weakness, nausea, vomiting, diarrhea, severe abdominal pain, excessive sweating, excessive salivation, frequent urination, urinary urgency, irregular heartbeat, difficulty breathing.

▽ambrisentan

See Appendix W, *Less commonly used drugs*.

▽amifostine

See Appendix W, *Less commonly used drugs*.

▽amikacin sulfate

*(am i **kay'** sin)*

Amikin

PREGNANCY CATEGORY D

Drug class

Aminoglycoside

Therapeutic actions

Bactericidal: Inhibits protein synthesis in susceptible strains of gram-negative bacteria, and the functional integrity of bacterial cell membrane appears to be disrupted, causing cell death.

Indications

- Short-term treatment of serious infections caused by susceptible strains of *Pseudomonas* species, *Escherichia coli,* indole-positive and indole-negative *Proteus* species, *Providencia* species, *Klebsiella, Enter-*

obacter, and *Serratia* species, *Acinetobacter* species

- Suspected gram-negative infections before results of susceptibility studies are known (effective in infections caused by gentamicin- or tobramycin-resistant strains of gram-negative organisms)
- Initial treatment of staphylococcal infections when penicillin is contraindicated or infection may be caused by mixed organisms
- Treatment of serious infections such as bacterial septicemia (including neonatal sepsis); infections of the respiratory tract, bones, joints, CNS, skin and soft tissues; intra-abdominal infections; postoperative infections; recurrent and complicated UTIs
- Unlabeled uses: Intrathecal or intraventricular administration at 8 mg/24 hr; part of a multidrug regimen for treatment of *Mycobacterium avium* complex, a common infection in AIDS patients; aerosolized for the treatment of pneumonia or cystic fibrosis

Contraindications and cautions

- Contraindicated with allergy to any aminoglycosides, renal or hepatic disease, preexisting hearing loss, myasthenia gravis, parkinsonism, infant botulism, lactation.
- Use cautiously with elderly patients, any patient with diminished hearing, decreased renal function, dehydration, neuromuscular disorders, pregnancy.

Available forms

Injection—50 mg/mL, 250 mg/mL

Dosages

Adults and pediatric patients

15 mg/kg/day IM or IV divided into two to three equal doses at equal intervals, not to exceed 1.5 g/day. Usual course of treatment is 7–10 days. Uncomplicated infections should respond in 24–48 hr. If no clinical response is seen in 3–5 days, reevaluate therapy.

- *UTIs:* 250 mg bid IM or IV; treatment is usually required for 7–10 days. If treatment is required for longer, carefully monitor serum levels and renal and neurologic function.

Neonatal patients

Loading dose of 10 mg/kg IM or IV; then 7.5 mg/kg every 12 hr.

Geriatric patients or patients with renal failure

Reduce dosage, and carefully monitor serum drug levels and renal function tests throughout treatment; regulate dosage based on these values. If creatinine clearance is not available and patient condition is stable, calculate a dosage interval in hours for the normal dose by multiplying patient's serum creatinine by 9. Dosage guide if creatinine clearance is known: Maintenance dose every 12 hr = observed creatinine clearance ÷ normal creatinine clearance × calculated loading dose (mg). For patients on dialysis, approximately one-half of the normal dose can be administered after hemodialysis. Before peritoneal dialysis, 7.5 mg/kg is given, then drug is instilled in peritoneal dialysis at the desired concentration.

Pharmacokinetics

Route	*Onset*	*Peak*
IV	Immediate	30–90 min
IM	Varies	45–120 min

Metabolism: $T_{1/2}$: 2–3 hr
Distribution: Crosses placenta; enters breast milk
Excretion: Urine, unchanged

IV FACTS

Preparation: Prepare IV solution by adding the contents of a 500-mg vial to 100 or 200 mL of sterile diluent. Do not physically mix with other drugs. Administer amikacin separately. Prepared solution is stable in concentrations of 0.25 and 5 mg/mL for 24 hr at room temperature.
Infusion: Administer to adults or pediatric patients over 30–60 min; infuse to infants over 1–2 hr.
Compatibilities: Amikacin is stable in 5% dextrose injection; 5% dextrose and 0.2%, 0.45%, or 0.9% sodium chloride injection; lactated Ringer's injection; *Normosol M* in 5% dextrose injection; *Normosol R* in 5% dextrose injection; *Plasma-Lyte* 56 or 148 injection in D_5W.
Y-site compatibilities: May be given with enalaprilat, furosemide, magnesium sulfate, morphine, ondansetron.
Y-site incompatibility: Do not give with hetastarch.

Adverse effects

- **CNS:** *Ototoxicity,* confusion, disorientation, depression, lethargy, nystagmus, visual disturbances, headache, fever, numbness, tingling, tremor, paresthesias, muscle twitching, seizures, muscular weakness, neuromuscular blockade, apnea
- **CV:** Palpitations, hypotension, hypertension
- **GI:** *Nausea, vomiting, anorexia, diarrhea,* weight loss, stomatitis, increased salivation, splenomegaly
- **GU: Nephrotoxicity**
- **Hematologic:** Leukemoid reaction, agranulocytosis, granulocytosis, leukopenia, leukocytosis, thrombocytopenia, eosinophilia, pancytopenia, anemia, hemolytic anemia, increased or decreased reticulocyte count, electrolyte disturbances
- **Hepatic:** Hepatic toxicity; hepatomegaly
- **Hypersensitivity:** Purpura, rash, urticaria, exfoliative dermatitis, itching
- **Other:** *Superinfections, pain and irritation at IM injection sites*

Interactions

✱ **Drug-drug** • Increased ototoxic and nephrotoxic effects with potent diuretics and other similarly toxic drugs (eg, cephalosporins) • Risk of inactivation if mixed parenterally with penicillins • Increased likelihood of neuromuscular blockade if given shortly after general anesthetics, depolarizing and nondepolarizing neuromuscular junction blockers

■ Nursing considerations

CLINICAL ALERT!
Name confusion has occurred between amikacin and anakinra; use caution.

Assessment

- **History:** Allergy to any aminoglycosides, renal or hepatic disease, preexisting hearing loss, myasthenia gravis, parkinsonism, infant botulism, lactation, diminished hearing, decreased renal function, dehydration, neuromuscular disorders
- **Physical:** Arrange culture and sensitivity tests on infection prior to therapy; eighth cranial nerve function and state of hydration prior to, during, and after therapy; LFTs, renal function tests, CBC, skin color and lesions, orientation and affect, reflexes, bilateral grip strength, weight, bowel sounds

Interventions

⊠ ***Black box warning*** Monitor patient for nephrotoxicity, ototoxicity with baseline and periodic renal function and neurological examinations; risk for serious toxicity.

- Arrange for culture and sensitivity testing of infected area before treatment.

⊗ ***Warning*** Monitor duration of treatment: Usually 7–10 days. If clinical response does not occur within 3–5 days, stop therapy. Prolonged treatment leads to increased risk of toxicity. If drug is used longer than 10 days, monitor auditory and renal function daily.

- Give IM dosage by deep injection.
- Ensure that patient is well hydrated before and during therapy.

Teaching points

- This drug is only available for IM or IV use.
- You may experience these side effects: Ringing in the ears, headache, dizziness (reversible; safety measures may need to be taken if severe); nausea, vomiting, loss of appetite (eat frequent small meals, frequent mouth care may help).
- Report pain at injection site, severe headache, dizziness, loss of hearing, changes in urine pattern, difficulty breathing, rash or skin lesions.

▽ amiloride hydrochloride

*(a **mill'** oh ride)*

Midamor

PREGNANCY CATEGORY B

Drug class

Potassium-sparing diuretic

Therapeutic actions

Inhibits sodium reabsorption in the renal distal tubule, causing loss of sodium and water and retention of potassium.

Indications

- Adjunctive therapy with thiazide or loop diuretics in heart failure and in hypertension to treat hypokalemia or to prevent hypokalemia in patients who would be at high risk if hypokalemia occurred (digitalized patients, patients with cardiac arrhythmias)
- Unlabeled uses: Inhalation in the treatment of cystic fibrosis; reduction of lithium-induced polyuria without increasing lithium levels

Contraindications and cautions

- Contraindicated with allergy to amiloride, hyperkalemia, severe renal disease, diabetic nephropathy, potassium-rich diet.
- Use cautiously with renal or hepatic disease, diabetes mellitus, metabolic or respiratory acidosis, lactation, pregnancy.

Available forms

Tablets—5 mg

Dosages

Adults

- *Adjunctive therapy:* Add 5 mg/day PO to usual antihypertensive or dosage of kaliuretic diuretic; if necessary, increase dose to 10 mg/day or to 15–20 mg/day with careful monitoring of electrolytes.
- *Single-drug therapy:* Start with 5 mg/day PO; if necessary, increase to 10 mg/day or to 15–20 mg/day with careful monitoring of electrolytes.

Pediatric patients

Safety and efficacy not established.

Pharmacokinetics

Route	*Onset*	*Peak*	*Duration*
Oral	2 hr	6–10 hr	24 hr

Metabolism: Hepatic; $T_{1/2}$: 6–9 hr
Distribution: Crosses placenta; enters breast milk
Excretion: Urine, unchanged

Adverse effects

- **CNS:** *Headache,* dizziness, drowsiness, fatigue, paresthesias, tremors, confusion, encephalopathy
- **GI:** *Nausea, anorexia, vomiting, diarrhea,* dry mouth, constipation, jaundice, gas pain, GI bleeding
- **GU:** Polyuria, dysuria, *impotence,* decreased libido
- **Musculoskeletal:** *Weakness, fatigue, muscle cramps* and muscle spasms, joint pain
- **Respiratory:** Cough, dyspnea
- **Other:** Rash, pruritus, itching, alopecia, *hyperkalemia*

Interactions

✱ **Drug-drug** • Increased hyperkalemia with triamterene, spironolactone, potassium supplements, diets rich in potassium, ACE inhibitors • Reduced effectiveness of digoxin with amiloride

■ Nursing considerations

Assessment

- **History:** Allergy to amiloride, hyperkalemia, renal or liver disease, diabetes mellitus, metabolic or respiratory acidosis, lactation
- **Physical:** Skin color, lesions, edema; orientation, reflexes, muscle strength; pulses, baseline ECG, BP; R, pattern, adventitious sounds; liver evaluation, bowel sounds, urinary output patterns; CBC, serum electrolytes, blood sugar, LFTs, renal function tests, urinalysis

Interventions

⊗ ***Warning*** Monitor patient for hyperkalemia (serum potassium level greater than 5.5 mEq/L).

- Administer with food or milk to prevent GI upset.
- Administer early in the day so increased urination does not disturb sleep.
- Measure and record weight regularly to monitor mobilization of edema fluid.
- Avoid foods and salt substitutes high in potassium.
- Provide frequent mouth care and sugarless lozenges to suck.
- Arrange for regular evaluation of serum electrolytes.

Teaching points

- Take single dose early in the day so increased urination will not disturb sleep.
- Take the drug with food or meals to prevent GI upset.

- Avoid foods that are high in potassium and any flavoring that contains potassium (such as a salt substitute).
- Weigh yourself on a regular basis at the same time and in the same clothing, and record the weight on your calendar.
- You may experience these side effects: Increased volume and frequency of urination; dizziness, feeling faint on arising, drowsiness (avoid rapid position changes, hazardous activities like driving, and the use of alcohol which may intensify these problems); decrease in sexual function; increased thirst (sucking on sugarless lozenges may help; frequent mouth care also may help); avoid foods that are rich in potassium (eg, fruits, *Sanka*).
- Report loss or gain of more than 3 pounds in 1 day; swelling in your ankles or fingers; dizziness, trembling, numbness, fatigue; muscle weakness or cramps.

▽ amino acids

*(a **mee'** noe)*

Aminess 5.2%, Aminosyn, BranchAmin, FreAmine, HepatAmine, Novamine, Primene (CAN), ProcalAmine, RenAmin, Travasol, TrophAmine

PREGNANCY CATEGORY C

Drug classes
Caloric agent
Protein substrate

Therapeutic actions
Essential and nonessential amino acids provided in various combinations to supply calories and proteins and provide a protein-building and a protein-sparing effect for the body (a positive nitrogen balance).

Indications
- Provide nutrition to patients who are in a negative nitrogen balance when GI tract cannot absorb protein; when protein needs exceed the ability to absorb protein (with burns, trauma, infections); when bowel rest is needed; when tube feeding cannot supply adequate nutrition; when health can be improved or restored by replacing lost amino acids
- Treatment of hepatic encephalopathy in patients with cirrhosis or hepatitis (*HepatAmine*)
- Nutritional support of uremic patients when oral nutrition is not feasible or is impractical or insufficient

Contraindications and cautions
- Contraindicated with hypersensitivity to any component of the solution; severe electrolyte or acid–base imbalance; inborn errors in amino acid metabolism; decreased circulating blood volume; severe renal or hepatic disease; hyperammonemia; bleeding abnormalities.
- Use cautiously with hepatic or renal impairment, diabetes mellitus, heart failure, hypertension, decreased circulating blood volume.

Available forms
Many forms available for IV injections.

Dosages
Dosage must be individualized with careful observation of cardiac status and BUN and evaluation of metabolic needs. Recommended protein dietary allowances are 0.9 g/kg/day for healthy adults, 1.4–2.2 g/kg/day in healthy infants and children. Requirements increase with trauma or in those who are malnourished.
- *Hepatic encephalopathy:* 80–120 g amino acid/day; 500 mL *HepatAmine* with 500 mL 50% dextrose and electrolyte solution over 8–12 hr per day.

Adults
1–1.5 g/kg/day amino acid injection IV into a peripheral vein; 250–500 mL/day amino acid injection IV mixed with appropriate dextrose, vitamins, and electrolytes as part of a total parenteral nutrition (TPN) solution.

Pediatric patients
2–3 g/kg/day amino acid IV mixed with dextrose as appropriate.

A

Pharmacokinetics

Route	*Onset*
IV	Immediate

Metabolism: Part of normal anabolic processes
Distribution: Crosses placenta; enters breast milk
Excretion: Urine

IV FACTS

Preparation: Strict aseptic technique is required in mixing solution; use of a laminar flow hood in the pharmacy is recommended. A 0.22-micron filter should be used to block any particulate matter and bacteria. Use mixed solution immediately. If not used within 1 hr, refrigerate solution. Mixed solutions must be used within 24 hr. Use strict aseptic technique when changing bottles, catheter tubing, and so forth. Replace all IV apparatus every 24 hr. Change dressing every 24 hr to assess insertion site.
Infusion: Use a volumetric infusion pump. Infuse only if solution is absolutely clear and without particulate matter. Infuse slowly. If infusion falls behind, do not try to speed up infusion rate; serious overload could occur. Infusion rates of 20-30 mL/hr up to a maximum of 60–100 mL/hr have been used.
Incompatibilities: Do not mix with amphotericin B, ampicillin, carbenicillin, cephradine, gentamicin, metronidazole, tetracycline, ticarcillin.

Adverse effects

- **CNS:** *Headache, dizziness,* mental confusion, loss of consciousness
- **CV:** Hypertension, heart failure, **pulmonary edema,** tachycardia, *generalized flushing*
- **Endocrine:** Hypoglycemia, hyperglycemia, fatty acid deficiency, azotemia, hyperammonemia
- **GI:** *Nausea, vomiting,* abdominal pain, liver impairment, fatty liver
- **Hypersensitivity:** Fever, chills, rash, papular eruptions
- **Local:** *Pain, infection,* phlebitis, venous thrombosis, tissue sloughing at injection site

Interactions

✱ **Drug-drug** • Reduced protein-sparing effects of amino acids if taken with tetracyclines

■ Nursing considerations

Assessment

- **History:** Hypersensitivity to any component of the solution; severe electrolyte or acid–base imbalance; inborn errors in amino acid metabolism; decreased circulating blood volume; hepatic or renal disease; hyperammonemia; bleeding abnormalities; diabetes mellitus; heart failure; hypertension
- **Physical:** T, weight, height; orientation, reflexes; P, BP, edema; R, lung auscultation; abdominal examination; urinary output; CBC, platelet count, PT, electrolytes, BUN, blood glucose, uric acid, bilirubin, creatinine, plasma proteins, LFTs, renal function tests; urine glucose, osmolarity

Interventions

- Assess nutritional status before and frequently during treatment; weigh patient daily to monitor fluid load and nutritional status.
- Monitor vital signs often during infusion; monitor I&O continually during treatment.
- Observe infusion site at least daily for infection, phlebitis; change dressing using strict aseptic technique at least every 24 hr.
- Arrange to give D_5W or $D_{10}W$ for injection by a peripheral line to avoid hypoglycemia rebound if TPN infusion needs to be stopped.
- Monitor urine glucose, acetone, and specific gravity every 6 hr during initial infusion period, at least bid when the infusion has stabilized; stop solution at any sign of renal failure.
- Monitor patient for vascular overload or hepatic impairment; decrease rate of infusion or discontinue.

Teaching points

- This drug can be given only through an intravenous or central line.
- This drug helps you to build new proteins and regain strength and healing power.
- You may experience these side effects: Headache, dizziness (medication may be ordered to help); nausea, vomiting; pain at infusion site.

- Report fever, chills, severe pain at infusion site, changes in color of urine or stool, severe headache, rash.

aminocaproic acid

*(a mee noe ka **proe'** ik)*

Amicar

PREGNANCY CATEGORY C

Drug class

Systemic hemostatic drug

Therapeutic actions

Inhibits fibrinolysis by inhibiting plasminogen activator substances and by antiplasmin activity; this action prevents the breakdown of clots.

Indications

- Treatment of excessive bleeding resulting from systemic hyperfibrinolysis and urinary fibrinolysis
- Unlabeled uses: Prevention of recurrence of subarachnoid hemorrhage; management of amegakaryocytic thrombocytopenia; to decrease the need for platelet administration; to abort and treat attacks of hereditary angioneurotic edema; to reduce postoperative bleeding complications in cardiac and orthopedic procedures

Contraindications and cautions

- Contraindicated with allergy to aminocaproic acid, active intravascular clotting, cardiac disease, renal impairment, hematuria of upper urinary tract origin, hepatic impairment, lactation.
- Use cautiously with hyperfibrinolysis, pregnancy.

Available forms

Tablets—500, 1,000 mg; injection—250 mg/mL; oral solution—250 mg/mL

Dosages

Adults

- *Treatment of excessive bleeding:* Initial dose of 5 g PO or IV followed by 1–1.25 g every hr to produce and sustain plasma levels of 0.13 mg/mL; do not administer more than 30 g/day.
- *Acute bleeding:* 4–5 g IV in 250 mL of diluent during the first hour of infusion; then continuous infusion of 1 g/hr in 50 mL of diluent. Continue for 8 hr or until bleeding stops.
- *Prevention of recurrence of subarachnoid hemorrhage:* 36 g/day in six divided doses, PO or IV.
- *Amegakaryocytic thrombocytopenia:* 2–24 g/day for 3 days to 13 mo.

Pediatric patients

Safety and efficacy not established.

Pharmacokinetics

Route	*Onset*	*Peak*	*Duration*
Oral	Rapid	2 hr	Not known
IV	Immediate	Minutes	2–3 hr

Metabolism: $T_{1/2}$: 2 hr
Distribution: Crosses placenta; may enter breast milk
Excretion: Urine, unchanged

IV FACTS

Preparation: Dilute in compatible IV fluid. Rapid IV infusion undiluted is not recommended. Dilute 4 mL (1 g) of solution with 50 mL of diluent. For acute bleed, dilute 4–5 g in 250 mL diluent and give over 1 hr; then a continuous infusion of 1 g/hr given in 50 mL diluent. Store at room temperature.
Infusion: Infuse at 4–5 g the first hour of treatment, then 1 g/hr by continuous infusion; administer slowly to avoid hypotension, bradycardia, arrhythmias. Continue infusion for 8 hr or until bleeding is controlled. Undiluted, rapid injection is not recommended.
Compatibilities: Compatible with sterile water for injection, normal saline, 5% dextrose, Ringer's solution.

Adverse effects

- **CNS:** *Dizziness, tinnitus, headache,* delirium, hallucinations, psychotic reactions,

weakness, conjunctival suffusion, nasal stuffiness
- **CV:** Hypotension, cardiac myopathy, bradycardia
- **GI:** *Nausea, cramps, diarrhea,* vomiting
- **GU:** Intrarenal obstruction, renal failure, *fertility problems*
- **Hematologic:** *Elevated serum CPK,* aldolase, AST, elevated serum potassium
- **Musculoskeletal:** *Malaise,* myopathy, symptomatic weakness, fatigue
- **Respiratory:** Dyspnea, **pulmonary embolism**
- **Other:** Rash, thrombophlebitis

Interactions
✱ **Drug-drug** • Risk of hypercoagulable state with hormonal contraceptives, estrogens
✱ **Drug-lab test** • Elevation of serum K+ levels, especially with impaired renal function

■ Nursing considerations
Assessment
- **History:** Allergy to aminocaproic acid, DIC, cardiac disease, renal impairment; hematuria of upper urinary tract origin, hepatic impairment, lactation, hyperfibrinolysis
- **Physical:** Skin color, lesions; muscular strength; orientation, reflexes, affect; BP, P, baseline ECG, peripheral perfusion; liver evaluation, bowel sounds, output; clotting studies, CPK, urinalysis, LFTs, renal function tests

Interventions
- Patient on oral therapy may need up to 10 tablets the first hour of treatment and tablets around the clock during treatment.
- Orient patient and offer support if hallucinations, delirium, or psychoses occur.
- Monitor patient for signs of clotting.

Teaching points
- You may experience these side effects: Dizziness, weakness, headache, hallucinations (avoid driving or the use of dangerous machinery; take special precautions to avoid injury); nausea, diarrhea, cramps (eat frequent small meals); infertility problems (menstrual irregularities, dry ejaculation—should go away when the drug is stopped); weakness, malaise (plan activities, take rest periods as needed).
- Report severe headache, restlessness, muscle pain and weakness, blood in the urine.

▽aminolevulinic acid hydrochloride

See Appendix W, *Less commonly used drugs*.

▽aminophylline (theophylline ethylenediamine)
(am in off' i lin)

PREGNANCY CATEGORY C

Drug classes
Bronchodilator
Xanthine

Therapeutic actions
Relaxes bronchial smooth muscle, causing bronchodilation and increasing vital capacity, which has been impaired by bronchospasm and air trapping; in higher concentrations, it also inhibits the release of slow-reacting substance of anaphylaxis (SRS-A) and histamine and suppresses the response of airways to stimuli.

Indications
- Symptomatic relief or prevention of bronchial asthma and reversible bronchospasm associated with chronic bronchitis and emphysema
- As adjunct to inhaled $beta_2$ selective adrenergic agonists and systemic corticosteroids for the treatment of acute exacerbations of the symptoms and reversible airflow obstruction associated with asthma and other obstructive lung diseases
- Unlabeled uses: Respiratory stimulant in Cheyne-Stokes respiration; treatment of apnea and bradycardia in premature babies

Contraindications and cautions

- Contraindicated with hypersensitivity to any xanthine or to ethylenediamine, peptic ulcer, active gastritis.
- Use cautiously with cardiac arrhythmias, acute myocardial injury, heart failure, cor pulmonale, severe hypertension, severe hypoxemia, renal or hepatic disease, hyperthyroidism, alcoholism, labor, lactation, pregnancy.

Available forms

Tablets—100, 200 mg; injection—250 mg/10 mL

Dosages

Individualize dosage. Because of poor distribution of drug in body fat, dosing should be calculated based on ideal body weight. Base dosage adjustments on clinical response. Monitor serum theophylline levels and maintain a therapeutic range of 10–20 mcg/mL. Aminophylline is approximately 79% anhydrous theophylline by weight. To convert a theophylline dose to aminophylline, divide the theophylline dose by 0.8.

Adults

Oral

- *Acute symptoms requiring rapid theophyllinization in patients not receiving theophylline:* Initially, 300 mg PO in divided doses every 6–8 hr; after 3 days increase to 400 mg/day PO in divided doses every 6–8 hr; after 3 more days, if tolerated, 600 mg/day PO in divided doses every 6–8 hr. Dosage should then be adjusted based on the serum theophylline concentration.

Peak theophylline level	*Adjustment*
9.9 mcg/mL	Increase dose 25% if symptoms are uncontrolled and dose is tolerated; recheck levels in 3 days.
10–14.9 mcg/mL	Maintain dose and recheck at 6-mo–12-mo intervals if symptoms are controlled and dose is tolerated.
15–19.9 mcg/mL	Consider a 10% decrease in dose if current dose is tolerated to increase safety window.
20–24.9 mcg/mL	Decrease dose by 25% even if no adverse events have been reported; recheck levels in 3 days.
25–30 mcg/mL	Skip next dose and then decrease dose by 25% even if no adverse events have been reported; recheck levels in 3 days.
> 30 mcg/mL	If symptomatic for overdose, treat accordingly. Decrease dose by 50% and recheck levels in 3 days.

Pediatric patients

Children are very sensitive to CNS stimulation of theophylline; use caution in younger children unable to report minor side effects. Not recommended for children younger than 6 mo. Safety and efficacy not established for children younger than 1 yr.

Oral

Acute bronchodilation: 5 mg/kg will produce an average peak theophylline level of 5–15 mcg/mL in patients who have not received any theophylline in the previous 24 hr.

Age and weight	*Starting dose*	*After 3 days*	*After 3 more days*
Children 1–15 yr weighing less than 45 kg	12–14 mg/kg/day in divided doses every 4–6 hr, maximum 300 mg/day	16 mg/kg/day in divided doses every 4–6 hr, maximum 400 mg/day	20 mg/kg/day in divided doses every 4–6 hr, maximum 600 mg/day
Children 16 yr and older weighing more than 45 kg (adult dose)	300 mg/day in divided doses every 6–8 hr	400 mg/day in divided doses every 6–8 hr	600 mg/day in divided doses every 6–8 hr

Patients with impaired renal function
Do not exceed 16 mg/kg/day up to a maximum 400 mg/day.

Adult and pediatric patients

IV
Loading dose is 5.7 mg/kg (aminophylline) calculated on ideal body weight. Administer over 30 min. This should produce a peak serum level of 6–16 mcg/mL. Determine serum levels 30 min after administering dose. If patient has had theophylline within 24 hr, monitor levels before administering loading dose and adjust dosage accordingly.

Initial theophylline infusion rates after loading dose to target 10 mcg/mL serum level. (Divide theophylline dose by 0.8 to arrive at aminophylline dose.)

Age	*Initial infusion rate*
Neonates 24 days or younger	1 mg/kg every 12 hr
Neonates older than 24 days	1.5 mg/kg every 12 hr
Infants	mg/kg/hr = 0.008 × age in weeks + 0.21
Children 1–9 yr	0.8 mg/kg/hr
Children 9–12 yr and adolescent smokers	0.7 mg/kg/hr
Nonsmoking adolescents 12–16 yr	0.5 mg/kg/hr; do not exceed 900 mg theophylline/day
Healthy, nonsmoking adults	0.4 mg/kg/hr; do not exceed 900 mg theophylline/day
Adults older than 60 yr	0.3 mg/kg/hr; do not exceed 400 mg theophylline/day
Adults with cardiac decompensation, cor pulmonale, hepatic impairment, sepsis with multiorgan failure, shock	0.2 mg/kg/hr; do not exceed 400 mg theophylline/day; do not exceed 17 mg/hr

Infusion dosage should be adjusted based on serum theophylline levels as noted under oral dosing.

Compatibilities: Aminophylline is compatible with most IV solutions, but do not mix in solution with other drugs, including vitamins.
Y-site incompatibilities: Dobutamine, hydralazine, ondansetron.

Adverse effects

- **Serum theophylline levels less than 20 mcg/mL:** Adverse effects uncommon
- **Serum theophylline levels more than 20–25 mcg/mL:** Nausea, vomiting, diarrhea, headache, insomnia, irritability (75% of patients)
- **Serum theophylline levels more than 30–35 mcg/mL:** Hyperglycemia, hypotension, cardiac arrhythmias, **seizures,** tachycardia (more than 10 mcg/mL in premature newborns), **brain damage**
- **CNS:** Irritability (especially in children); restlessness, dizziness, muscle twitching, seizures, severe depression, stammering speech; abnormal behavior characterized by withdrawal, mutism, and unresponsiveness alternating with hyperactive periods
- **CV:** Palpitations, sinus tachycardia, ventricular tachycardia, life-threatening ventricular arrhythmias, circulatory failure
- **GI:** Loss of appetite, hematemesis, epigastric pain, gastroesophageal reflux during sleep, increased AST
- **GU:** Proteinuria, increased excretion of renal tubular cells and RBCs; diuresis (dehydration), urinary retention in men with prostate enlargement
- **Respiratory:** Tachypnea, respiratory arrest
- **Other:** Fever, flushing, hyperglycemia, SIADH, rash

Interactions

✱ **Drug-drug** • Increased effects with cimetidine, erythromycin, troleandomycin, clindamycin, lincomycin, methotrexate, diltiazem, disulfiram, enoxacin, fluvoxamine, inteferon alfa-2a, mexiletine, pentoxifylline, ticlopidine, verapamil, zileuton, influenza virus vaccine, fluoroquinolones, hormonal contraceptives • Possibly increased effects with thiabendazole, allopurinol • Increased cardiac toxicity with halothane; increased likelihood of seizures when given with ketamine; increased likelihood of adverse GI effects when given with tetracyclines • Increased or decreased effects with furosemide, levothyroxine, liothyronine, liotrix, thyroglobulin, thyroid hormones • Decreased effects in patients who are cigarette smokers (1–2 packs per day); theophylline dosage may need to be increased 50–100% • Decreased effects with phenobarbital, carbamazepine, isoproterenol, moricizine, rifamycins • Increased effects, toxicity of sympathomimetics (especially ephedrine) with theophylline preparations • Decreased effects of phenytoin and theophylline preparations when given concomitantly • Decreased effects of lithium carbonate, nondepolarizing neuromuscular blockers given with theophylline preparations • Mutually antagonistic effects of beta-blockers and theophylline preparations

✱ **Drug-food** • Elimination is increased by a low-carbohydrate, high-protein diet and by charcoal-broiled beef • Elimination is decreased by a high-carbohydrate, low-protein diet • Food may alter bioavailability and absorption of timed-release theophylline preparations, causing toxicity; these forms should be taken on an empty stomach

✱ **Drug-lab test** • Interference with spectrophotometric determinations of serum theophylline levels by furosemide, phenylbutazone, probenecid, theobromine; coffee, tea, cola beverages, chocolate, acetaminophen cause falsely high values • Alteration in assays of uric acid, urinary catecholamines, plasma free fatty acids by theophylline preparations

■ Nursing considerations

Assessment

- **History:** Hypersensitivity to any xanthine or to ethylenediamine, peptic ulcer, active gastritis, cardiac arrhythmias, acute myocardial injury, heart failure, cor pulmonale, severe hypertension, severe hypoxemia, renal or hepatic disease, hyperthyroidism, alcoholism, labor, lactation
- **Physical:** Bowel sounds, normal output; P, auscultation, BP, perfusion, ECG; R, adventitious sounds; frequency of urination, voiding, normal output pattern, urinalysis, LFTs, renal function tests; liver palpation; thyroid function tests; skin color, texture, lesions; reflexes, bilateral grip strength, affect, EEG

Interventions

- Administer to pregnant patients only when clearly needed—neonatal tachycardia, jitteriness, and withdrawal apnea observed when mothers received xanthines up until delivery.
- Give tablets, liquid dosage forms with food if GI effects occur.
- Maintain adequate hydration.
- Monitor results of serum theophylline levels carefully, and arrange for reduced dosage if serum levels exceed therapeutic range of 10–20 mcg/mL.
- Take serum samples to determine peak theophylline concentration drawn 15–30 min after an IV loading dose.
- Monitor for clinical signs of adverse effects, particularly if serum theophylline levels are not available.
- Ensure that diazepam and/or phenobarbital is readily available to treat seizures.

Teaching points

- Take this drug exactly as prescribed.
- It may be necessary to take this drug around-the-clock for adequate control of asthma attacks.
- Avoid excessive intake of coffee, tea, cocoa, cola beverages, and chocolate.
- Smoking cigarettes or other tobacco products impacts the drug's effectiveness. Try not to smoke. Notify your health care provider if smoking habits change while taking this drug.
- Frequent blood tests may be necessary to monitor the effect of this drug and to ensure safe and effective dosage; keep all appointments for blood tests and other monitoring.
- You may experience these side effects: Nausea, loss of appetite (taking this drug with food may help if taking the immediate-release or liquid dosage forms); difficulty sleeping, depression, emotional lability (reversible).
- Report nausea, vomiting, severe GI pain, restlessness, seizures, irregular heartbeat.

DANGEROUS DRUG

amiodarone hydrochloride

(a mee o' da rone)

Apo-Amiodarone (CAN), Cordarone, Gen-Amiodarone (CAN), Nexterone, Novo-Amiodarone (CAN), Pacerone, PMS-Amiodarone (CAN), ratio-Amiodarone (CAN)

PREGNANCY CATEGORY D

Drug classes

Adrenergic blocker (not used as sympatholytic drug)
Antiarrhythmic

Therapeutic actions

Type III antiarrhythmic: Acts directly on cardiac cell membrane; prolongs repolarization and refractory period; increases ventricular fibrillation threshold; acts on peripheral smooth muscle to decrease peripheral resistance.

Indications

- Only for treatment of the following documented life-threatening recurrent ventricular arrhythmias that do not respond to documented adequate doses of other antiarrhythmics or when alternative agents are not tolerated: Recurrent ventricular fibrillation, recurrent hemodynamically unstable ventricular tachycardia. Serious and even fatal toxicity has been reported with this drug; use alternative agents first; very closely monitor patient receiving this drug
- Unlabeled uses: Treatment of refractory sustained or paroxysmal atrial fibrillation and paroxysmal supraventricular tachycardia; postoperative conversion of atrial fibrillation, atrial flutter

Contraindications and cautions

- Contraindicated with hypersensitivity to amiodarone; sinus node dysfunction, heart block, cardiogenic shock, severe bradycardia; hypokalemia; lactation; sensitivity to iodine.
- Use cautiously with thyroid dysfunction, pregnancy.

Available forms

Tablets—100, 200, 400 mg; injection—50 mg/mL

Dosages

Careful patient assessment and evaluation with continual monitoring of cardiac response are necessary for titrating the dosage. Therapy should begin in the hospital with continual monitoring and emergency equipment on standby. The following is a guide to usual dosage.

Adults

Oral

Loading dose, 800–1,600 mg/day PO in divided doses for doses of 1,000 mg or more or with GI intolerance, for 1–3 wk; reduce dose to 600–800 mg/day in divided doses for 1 mo; if rhythm is stable, reduce dose to 400 mg/day in one to two divided doses for maintenance dose. Adjust to the lowest possible dose to limit side effects.

IV

1,000 mg IV over 24 hr—150 mg loading dose over 10 min, followed by 360 mg over 6 hr at rate of 1 mg/min, then 540 mg at 0.5 mg/min over the next 18 hr. After the first 24 hr, a maintenance infusion of 0.5 mg/min (720 mg/24 hr) or less can be cautiously continued for 2–3 wk. Switch to oral form as soon as possible.

Converting from IV to PO

IV dose of 720 mg/day at 0.5 mg/min: Convert to PO dose based on duration of IV therapy. Less than 1 wk—initial oral dose 800–1,600 mg; 1–3 wk—initial oral dose 600–800 mg; more than 3 wk—initial oral dose 400 mg.

Pediatric patients

Safety and efficacy not established.

Pharmacokinetics

Route	*Onset*	*Peak*	*Duration*
Oral	2–3 days	3–7 hr	6–8 hr
IV	Immediate	20 min	Infusion

Metabolism: Hepatic; $T_{1/2}$: 10 days, then 40–55 days
Distribution: Crosses placenta; enters breast milk
Excretion: Bile, feces

IV FACTS

Preparation: Do not use PVC container if infusion is to exceed 2 hr; use glass or polyolefin instead. Dilute 150 mg in 100 mL D_5W for rapid loading dose (1.5 mg/mL). Dilute 900 mg in 500 mL D_5W for slow infusions (1.8 mg/mL). Store at room temperature and use within 24 hr.

Infusion: Infuse loading dose over 10 min. Immediately follow with slow infusion of 1 mg/min or 33.3 mL/hr. Maintenance infusion of 0.5 mg/min or 16.6 mL/hr can be continued up to 96 hr. Use of an infusion pump is advised.

Incompatibilities: Do not mix with aminophylline, cefazolin, heparin, sodium bicarbonate; do not mix in solution with other drugs.

Adverse effects

- **CNS:** *Malaise, fatigue, dizziness, tremors, ataxia,* paresthesias, lack of coordination
- **CV: Cardiac arrhythmias,** heart failure, **cardiac arrest,** *hypotension*
- **EENT:** *Corneal microdeposits* (photophobia, dry eyes, halos, blurred vision); ophthalmic abnormalities including permanent blindness
- **Endocrine:** *Hypothyroidism or hyperthyroidism*
- **GI:** *Nausea, vomiting, anorexia, constipation, abnormal LFT,* **hepatotoxicity**
- **Respiratory: Pulmonary toxicity**—pneumonitis, infiltrates (shortness of breath, cough, rales, wheezes)
- **Other:** *Photosensitivity,* angioedema

Interactions

✱ **Drug-drug** • Increased digitalis toxicity with digoxin • Increased risk of rhabdomyolysis if combined with simvastatin; limit simvastatin to less than 20 mg/dose • Increased quinidine toxicity with quinidine • Increased procainamide toxicity with procainamide • Increased flecainide toxicity with amiodarone • Increased risk of arrhythmias with azole antifungals, fluoroquinolones, macrolide antibiotics, ranolazine, trazodone, cisapride, thioridazine, vardenafil, ziprasidone • Increased phenytoin toxicity with phenytoin, ethotoin • Increased bleeding tendencies with warfarin • Potential sinus arrest and heart block with beta-blockers, calcium channel blockers

✱ **Drug-lab test** • Increased T_4 levels, increased serum reverse T_3 levels

✱ **Drug-Food** • Increased risk of toxicity if oral form combined with grapefruit juice; avoid this combination

■ Nursing considerations

CLINICAL ALERT!

Name confusion has occurred with amrinone (name has now been changed to inamrinone, but confusion may still occur); use caution.

Assessment

- **History:** Hypersensitivity to amiodarone, sinus node dysfunction, heart block, severe bradycardia, hypokalemia, lactation, thyroid dysfunction, pregnancy
- **Physical:** Skin color, lesions; reflexes, gait, eye examination; P, BP, auscultation, continuous ECG monitoring; R, adventitious sounds, baseline chest X-ray; liver evaluation; LFTs, serum electrolytes, T_4, and T_3

Interventions

⊗ ***Black box warning*** Reserve use for life-threatening arrhythmias; serious toxicity, including arrhythmias, pulmonary toxicity can occur.

- Monitor cardiac rhythm continuously.
- Monitor for an extended period when dosage adjustments are made.

⊗ ***Warning*** Monitor for safe and effective serum levels (0.5–2.5 mcg/mL).

⊗ ***Warning*** Doses of digoxin, quinidine, procainamide, phenytoin, and warfarin may need to be reduced one-third to one-half when amiodarone is started.

- Give drug with meals to decrease GI problems.
- Arrange for ophthalmologic examinations; reevaluate at any sign of optic neuropathy.
- Arrange for periodic chest X-ray to evaluate pulmonary status (every 3–6 mo).
- Arrange for regular periodic blood tests for liver enzymes, thyroid hormone levels.

Teaching points

- Drug dosage will be changed in relation to response of arrhythmias; you will need to be hospitalized during initiation of drug therapy; you will be closely monitored when dosage is changed.
- Avoid grapefruit juice while on this drug.
- Have regular medical follow-up, monitoring of cardiac rhythm, chest X-ray, eye examination, blood tests.
- You may experience these side effects: Changes in vision (halos, dry eyes, sensitivity to light; wear sunglasses, monitor light exposure); nausea, vomiting, loss of appetite (take with meals; eat frequent small meals); sensitivity to the sun (use a sunscreen or protective clothing when outdoors); constipation (a laxative may be ordered); tremors, twitching, dizziness, loss of coordination (do not drive, operate dangerous machinery, or undertake tasks that require coordination until drug effects stabilize and your body adjusts to it).
- Report unusual bleeding or bruising; fever, chills; intolerance to heat or cold; shortness of breath, difficulty breathing, cough; swelling of ankles or fingers; palpitations; difficulty with vision.

▽ amitriptyline hydrochloride

*(a mee **trip'** ti leen)*

Apo-Amitriptyline (CAN)

PREGNANCY CATEGORY D

Drug class

Antidepressant
TCA; tertiary amine

Therapeutic actions

Mechanism of action unknown; TCAs inhibit the reuptake of the neurotransmitters norepinephrine and serotonin, leading to an increase in their effects; anticholinergic at CNS and peripheral receptors; sedative.

Indications

- Relief of symptoms of depression (endogenous most responsive); sedative effects may help when depression is associated with anxiety and sleep disturbance
- Unlabeled uses: Control of chronic pain (eg, intractable pain of cancer, central pain syndromes, peripheral neuropathies, postherpetic neuralgia, tic douloureux); prevention of onset of cluster and migraine headaches; treatment of pathologic weeping and laughing secondary to forebrain disease (due to MS); insomnia; fibromyalgia

Contraindications and cautions

- Contraindicated with hypersensitivity to any tricyclic drug; concomitant therapy with an MAOI; recent MI; myelography within previous 24 hr or scheduled within 48 hr; lactation.
- Use cautiously with electroshock therapy; preexisting CV disorders (severe heart disease, progressive heart failure, angina pectoris, paroxysmal tachycardia); angle-closure glaucoma, increased IOP, urinary retention, ureteral or urethral spasm; seizure disorders; hyperthyroidism; impaired hepatic, renal function; psychiatric patients (schizophrenic or paranoid patients may exhibit a worsening of psychosis with TCA therapy); patients with bipolar disorder; elective surgery (discontinue as long as possible before surgery).

Available forms

Tablets—10, 25, 50, 75, 100, 150 mg

Dosages

Adults

- *Depression, hospitalized patients:* Initially, 100 mg/day PO in divided doses; gradually increase to 200–300 mg/day as required.
- *Depression, outpatients:* Initially, 75 mg/day PO, in divided doses; may increase to 150 mg/day. Increases should be made in late afternoon or at bedtime. Total daily dosage may be administered at bedtime. Initiate single daily dose therapy with 50–100 mg at bedtime; increase by 25–50 mg as necessary to a total of 150 mg/day. Maintenance dose, 40–100 mg/day, which may be given as a single bedtime dose. After satisfactory response, reduce to lowest effective dosage. Continue therapy for 3 mo or longer to lessen possibility of relapse.
- *Chronic pain:* 75–150 mg/day PO.

Pediatric patients 12 yr and older
10 mg tid PO and then 20 mg at bedtime.
Pediatric patients younger than 12 yr
Not recommended.
Geriatric patients
10 mg tid PO and then 20 mg at bedtime.

Pharmacokinetics

Route	*Onset*	*Peak*	*Duration*
Oral	Varies	2–4 hr	2–4 wk

Metabolism: Hepatic; $T_{1/2}$: 10–50 hr
Distribution: Crosses placenta; enters breast milk
Excretion: Urine

Adverse effects

- **CNS:** *Disturbed concentration, sedation and anticholinergic (atropine-like) effects, confusion* (especially in elderly), hallucinations, disorientation, decreased memory, feelings of unreality, delusions, anxiety, nervousness, restlessness, agitation, panic, insomnia, nightmares, hypomania, mania, exacerbation of psychosis, drowsiness, weakness, fatigue, headache, numbness, tingling, paresthesias of extremities, incoordination, motor hyperactivity, akathisia, ataxia, tremors, peripheral neuropathy, extrapyramidal symptoms, seizures, speech blockage, dysarthria, tinnitus, altered EEG
- **CV:** *Orthostatic hypotension,* hypertension, syncope, tachycardia, palpitations, **MI,** arrhythmias, heart block, precipitation of heart failure, CVA
- **Endocrine:** Elevated or depressed blood sugar, elevated prolactin levels, inappropriate ADH secretion
- **GI:** *Dry mouth, constipation,* paralytic ileus, *nausea,* vomiting, anorexia, epigastric distress, diarrhea, flatulence, dysphagia, peculiar taste, increased salivation, stomatitis, glossitis, parotid swelling, abdominal cramps, black tongue, hepatitis, jaundice (rare), elevated transaminase, altered alkaline phosphatase
- **GU:** Urinary retention, delayed micturition, dilation of the urinary tract, gynecomastia, testicular swelling; breast enlargement, menstrual irregularity and galactorrhea; increased or decreased libido; impotence
- **Hematologic:** Bone marrow depression, including agranulocytosis; eosinophilia, purpura, thrombocytopenia, leukopenia
- **Hypersensitivity:** Rash, pruritus, vasculitis, petechiae, photosensitization, edema (generalized, face, tongue), drug fever
- **Withdrawal:** Symptoms on abrupt discontinuation of prolonged therapy: Nausea, headache, vertigo, nightmares, malaise
- **Other:** Nasal congestion, excessive appetite, weight change; sweating, alopecia, lacrimation, hyperthermia, flushing, chills

Interactions

✱ **Drug-drug** • Increased TCA levels and pharmacologic (especially anticholinergic) effects with cimetidine, fluoxetine • Increased TCA levels with methylphenidate, phenothiazines, hormonal contraceptives, disulfiram • Hyperpyretic crises, severe seizures, hypertensive episodes and deaths with MAOIs, furazolidone • Increased antidepressant response and cardiac arrhythmias with thyroid medication • Increased or decreased effects with estrogens • Delirium with disulfiram • Sympathetic hyperactivity, sinus tachycardia, hypertension, agitation with levodopa • Increased biotransformation of TCAs in patients who smoke cigarettes • Increased sympathomimetic (especially beta-adrenergic) effects of direct-acting sympathomimetic drugs (norepinephrine, epinephrine) • Increased anticholinergic effects of anticholinergics (including anticholinergic antiparkinsonians) • Increased response (especially CNS depression) to barbiturates • Decreased antihypertensive effect of clonidine, other antihypertensives • Decreased effects of indirect-acting sympathomimetic drugs (ephedrine)

■ Nursing considerations
Assessment

- **History:** Hypersensitivity to any tricyclic drug; concomitant therapy with an MAOI; recent MI; myelography within previous 24 hr or scheduled within 48 hr; lactation; EST; preexisting CV disorders; angle-closure glaucoma, increased IOP, urinary retention,

ureteral or urethral spasm; seizure disorders; hyperthyroidism; impaired hepatic, renal function; psychiatric patients; manic-depressive patients; elective surgery
- **Physical:** Weight; T; skin color, lesions; orientation, affect, reflexes, vision and hearing; P, BP, orthostatic BP, perfusion; bowel sounds, normal output, liver evaluation; urine flow, normal output; usual sexual function, frequency of menses, breast and scrotal examination; LFTs, urinalysis, CBC, ECG

Interventions

⊗ ***Black box warning*** Children, adolescents, and young adults have increased risk of suicidality; monitor patient carefully.
- Restrict drug access for depressed and potentially suicidal patients.
- Administer major portion of dose at bedtime if drowsiness, severe anticholinergic effects occur (note that the elderly may not tolerate single-daily-dose therapy).
- Reduce dosage if minor side effects develop; discontinue if serious side effects occur.
- Arrange for CBC if patient develops fever, sore throat, or other sign of infection.
- Be aware that drug's sedative effects may be apparent before the antidepressant effect is seen.

Teaching points

- Take drug exactly as prescribed; do not stop abruptly or without consulting your health care provider.
- Drug's sedative effects may be apparent before the antidepressant effect is seen.
- Avoid using alcohol, other sleep-inducing drugs, over-the-counter drugs.
- Avoid prolonged exposure to sunlight or sunlamps; use sunscreen or protective garments.
- You may experience these side effects: Headache, dizziness, drowsiness, weakness, blurred vision (reversible; if severe, avoid driving and tasks requiring alertness while these persist); nausea, vomiting, loss of appetite, dry mouth (eat frequent small meals; use frequent mouth care and suck on sugarless candies); nightmares, inability to concentrate, confusion; changes in sexual function.
- Report dry mouth, difficulty in urination, excessive sedation, thoughts of suicide.

▽amlodipine besylate

*(am **loe'** di peen **beh'** sah layt)*

Norvasc

Pregnancy Category C

Drug classes

Antianginal
Antihypertensive
Calcium channel blocker

Therapeutic actions

Inhibits the movement of calcium ions across the membranes of cardiac and arterial muscle cells; inhibits transmembrane calcium flow, which results in the depression of impulse formation in specialized cardiac pacemaker cells, slowing of the velocity of conduction of the cardiac impulse, depression of myocardial contractility, and dilation of coronary arteries and arterioles and peripheral arterioles; these effects lead to decreased cardiac work, decreased cardiac oxygen consumption, and in patients with vasospastic (Prinzmetal's) angina, increased delivery of oxygen to cardiac cells.

Indications

- Angina pectoris due to coronary artery spasm (Prinzmetal's variant angina)
- Chronic stable angina, alone or in combination with other drugs
- To reduce the risk of hospitalization due to angina and to reduce the need for coronary revascularization procedures in patients with angiographically documented CAD without heart failure or ejection fraction less than 40%
- Essential hypertension, alone or in combination with other antihypertensives

Contraindications and cautions

- Contraindicated with allergy to amlodipine, impaired hepatic or renal function, sick sinus syndrome, heart block (second or third degree), lactation.
- Use cautiously with heart failure, pregnancy.

Available forms

Tablets—2.5, 5, 10 mg

Dosages

Adults

Initially, 5 mg PO daily; dosage may be gradually increased over 10–14 days to a maximum dose of 10 mg PO daily.

Pediatric patients 6–17 yr

- *Hypertension:* 2.5–5 mg/day PO.

Geriatric patients or patients with hepatic impairment

Initially, 2.5 mg PO daily; dosage may be gradually adjusted over 7–14 days based on clinical assessment.

Pharmacokinetics

Route	*Onset*	*Peak*
Oral	Unknown	6–12 hr

Metabolism: Hepatic; $T_{1/2}$: 30–50 hr
Distribution: Crosses placenta; may enter breast milk
Excretion: Urine

Adverse effects

- **CNS:** *Dizziness, light-headedness, headache,* asthenia, *fatigue, lethargy*
- **CV:** *Peripheral edema,* arrhythmias
- **Dermatologic:** *Flushing,* rash
- **GI:** *Nausea,* abdominal discomfort

■ Nursing considerations

CLINICAL ALERT!
Name confusion has been reported between *Norvasc* (amlodipine) and *Navane* (thiothixene); use caution.

Assessment

- **History:** Allergy to amlodipine, impaired hepatic or renal function, sick sinus syndrome, heart block, lactation, heart failure
- **Physical:** Skin lesions, color, edema; P, BP, baseline ECG, peripheral perfusion, auscultation; R, adventitious sounds; liver evaluation, GI normal output; LFTs, renal function tests, urinalysis

Interventions

⊗ ***Warning*** Monitor patient carefully (BP, cardiac rhythm, and output) while adjusting drug to therapeutic dose; use special caution if patient has heart failure.

- Monitor BP very carefully if patient is also on nitrates.
- Monitor cardiac rhythm regularly during stabilization of dosage and periodically during long-term therapy.
- Administer drug without regard to meals.

Teaching points

- Take with meals if upset stomach occurs.
- You may experience these side effects: Nausea, vomiting (eat frequent small meals); headache (adjust lighting, noise, and temperature; medication may be ordered).
- Report irregular heartbeat, shortness of breath, swelling of the hands or feet, pronounced dizziness, constipation.

▽ammonium chloride

(ah mo' nee um)

PREGNANCY CATEGORY C

Drug classes

Electrolyte
Urinary acidifier

Therapeutic actions

Converted to urea in the liver; liberated hydrogen and chloride ions in blood and extracellular fluid lower the pH and correct alkalosis; lowers the urinary pH, producing an acidic urine that changes the excretion rate of many metabolites and drugs.

Indications

- Treatment of hypochloremic states and metabolic alkalosis
- Acidification of urine

Contraindications and cautions

- Contraindicated with renal function impairment; hepatic impairment; metabolic alkalosis due to vomiting of hydrochloric acid when it is accompanied by loss of sodium.

- Use cautiously with pregnancy, primary respiratory acidosis, high total CO_2 and buffer base, lactation.

Available forms

Injection—26.75% (5 mEq/mL)

Dosages

An oral dosage form of the drug is no longer commercially available.

Adults

Dosage is determined by patient's condition and tolerance; monitor dosage rate and amount by repeated serum bicarbonate determinations.

Pediatric patients

Safety and efficacy for injection in children have not been established.

Pharmacokinetics

Route	*Onset*	*Peak*
IV	Rapid	1–3 hr

Metabolism: Hepatic
Distribution: Crosses placenta; enters breast milk
Excretion: Urine

IV FACTS

Preparation: Add contents of one or two vials (100–200 mEq) to 500 or 1,000 mL isotonic (0.9%) sodium chloride injection. Concentration should not exceed 1%–2% ammonium chloride. Avoid excessive heat; protect from freezing. If crystals do appear, warm the solution to room temperature in a water bath prior to use.
Infusion: Do not exceed rate of 5 mL/min in adults (1,000 mL infused over 3 hr). Infuse slowly. Reduce rate in infants and children.
Incompatibilities: Do not mix with codeine, levorphanol, methadone, warfarin, dimenhydrinate, sulfadiazine, sulfisoxazole

Adverse effects

- **GI:** Severe hepatic impairment
- **Local:** *Pain or irritation at injection site,* fever, venous thrombosis, phlebitis, extravasation
- **Metabolic:** Metabolic acidosis, hypervolemia, **ammonia toxicity**—pallor, sweating, irregular breathing, retching, bradycardia, arrhythmias, twitching, seizures, coma; hypokalemia

Interactions

✱ **Drug-drug** • Decreased therapeutic levels due to increased elimination of amphetamine, methamphetamine, dextroamphetamine, ephedrine, flecainide, pseudoephedrine, methadone, mexiletine when taken with ammonium chloride • Increased effects of chlorpropamide with ammonium chloride

■ Nursing considerations

Assessment

- **History:** Renal or hepatic impairment; metabolic alkalosis due to vomiting of hydrochloric acid when it is accompanied by loss of sodium, respiratory acidosis
- **Physical:** P, BP; skin color, texture; T; injection site evaluation; LFTs, renal function tests, serum bicarbonate, urinalysis

Interventions

- Infuse IV slowly to avoid irritation; check infusion site frequently to monitor for reaction.
- Monitor IV doses for possible fluid overload.
- Monitor for acidosis (increased R, restlessness, sweating, increased blood pH); decrease infusion as appropriate. Ensure that sodium bicarbonate or sodium lactate is readily available in case of overdose.

Teaching points

- Frequent monitoring of blood tests is needed when receiving IV drugs to determine dosage and rate of drug.
- Report pain or irritation at IV site; confusion, restlessness, sweating, headache; severe GI upset, fever, chills.

▽amoxapine

(a mox' a peen)

PREGNANCY CATEGORY C

Drug classes

Anxiolytic
TCA

Therapeutic actions

Mechanism of action unknown; TCAs inhibit the reuptake of the neurotransmitters norepinephrine and serotonin, leading to an increase in their effects; anticholinergic at CNS and peripheral receptors; sedative.

Indications

- Relief of symptoms of depression in patients with neurotic or reactive depressive disorders and in those with endogenous and psychotic depression (endogenous depression most responsive)
- Treatment of depression accompanied with anxiety or agitation

Contraindications and cautions

- Contraindicated with hypersensitivity to tricyclic drugs; concomitant use with an MAOI; recent MI; myelography within previous 24 hr or scheduled within 48 hr; lactation.
- Use cautiously with EST; preexisting CV disorders (severe coronary heart disease, progressive heart failure, angina pectoris, paroxysmal tachycardia); angle-closure glaucoma, increased IOP, urinary retention, ureteral or urethral spasm; seizure disorders; hyperthyroidism; impaired hepatic, renal function; psychiatric patients (schizophrenic or paranoid patients may exhibit a worsening of psychosis); patients with bipolar disorder; elective surgery (discontinue as soon as possible before surgery), pregnancy.

Available forms

Tablets—25, 50, 100, 150 mg

Dosages

Adults

Initially, 50 mg PO bid–tid; gradually increase to 100 mg bid–tid by end of first wk if tolerated; increase above 300 mg/day only if this dosage ineffective for at least 2 wk. Hospitalized patients refractory to antidepressant therapy and with no history of seizures may be given up to 600 mg/day in divided doses; after effective dosage is established, drug may be given in a single dose at bedtime (maximum, 300 mg). Usual effective dose is 200–300 mg/day.

Pediatric patients

Not recommended for patients younger than 16 yr.

Geriatric patients

Initially, 25 mg bid–tid; if tolerated, dosage may be increased by end of first week to 50 mg bid–tid. For many elderly patients, 100–150 mg/day may be adequate; some may require up to 300 mg/day. Once effective dose is established, give as single dose at bedtime, not to exceed 300 mg.

Pharmacokinetics

Route	*Onset*	*Peak*	*Duration*
Oral	Varies	90 min	2–4 wk

Metabolism: Hepatic; $T_{1/2}$: 8–30 hr
Distribution: Crosses placenta; enters breast milk
Excretion: Urine

Adverse effects

- **CNS:** *Disturbed concentration, sedation and anticholinergic (atropine-like) effects, confusion* (especially in elderly), hallucinations, disorientation, decreased memory, feelings of unreality, delusions, anxiety, nervousness, restlessness, agitation, panic, insomnia, nightmares, hypomania, mania, exacerbation of psychosis, drowsiness, weakness, fatigue, headache, numbness, tingling, paresthesias of extremities, incoordination, motor hyperactivity, akathisia, ataxia, tremors, peripheral neuropathy, extrapyramidal symptoms, seizures, speech blockage, dysarthria, tinnitus, altered EEG
- **CV:** *Orthostatic hypotension,* hypertension, syncope, tachycardia, palpitations, **MI,** arrhythmias, heart block, precipitation of heart failure, CVA
- **Endocrine:** Elevated or depressed blood sugar, elevated prolactin levels, inappropriate ADH secretion
- **GI:** *Dry mouth, constipation,* paralytic ileus, *nausea,* vomiting, anorexia, epigastric distress, diarrhea, flatulence, dysphagia, peculiar taste, increased salivation, stomatitis, glossitis, parotid swelling, abdominal cramps, black tongue, hepatitis, jaundice (rare); elevated transaminase, altered alkaline phosphatase

- **GU:** Urinary retention, delayed micturition, dilation of the urinary tract, gynecomastia, testicular swelling in men; breast enlargement, menstrual irregularity, and galactorrhea in women; changes in libido; impotence
- **Hematologic:** Bone marrow depression
- **Hypersensitivity:** Rash, pruritus, vasculitis, petechiae, photosensitization, edema (generalized, facial, tongue), drug fever
- **Withdrawal:** Symptoms on abrupt discontinuation of prolonged therapy: Nausea, headache, vertigo, nightmares, malaise
- **Other:** Nasal congestion, excessive appetite, weight gain or loss, sweating, alopecia, lacrimation, hyperthermia, flushing, chills

Interactions

✱ **Drug-drug** • Increased TCA levels and pharmacologic (especially anticholinergic) effects with cimetidine, fluoxetine • Increased TCA levels with methylphenidate, phenothiazines, hormonal contraceptives, disulfiram, cimetidine, ranitidine • Hyperpyretic crises, severe seizures, hypertensive episodes, and deaths with MAOIs, furazolidone • Increased antidepressant response and cardiac arrhythmias with thyroid medication • Increased or decreased effects with estrogens • Delirium with disulfiram • Sympathetic hyperactivity, sinus tachycardia, hypertension, agitation with levodopa • Increased biotransformation of TCAs in patients who smoke cigarettes • Increased sympathomimetic (especially alpha-adrenergic) effects of direct-acting sympathomimetic drugs (norepinephrine, epinephrine) • Increased anticholinergic effects of anticholinergic drugs (including anticholinergic antiparkinsonians) • Increased response (especially CNS depression) to barbiturates • Decreased antihypertensive effect of clonidine, other antihypertensives

■ Nursing considerations

Assessment

- **History:** Hypersensitivity to any tricyclic drug; concomitant therapy with an MAOI; recent MI; myelography within previous 24 hr or scheduled within 48 hr; lactation; EST; preexisting CV disorders; angle-closure glaucoma, increased IOP; urinary retention, ureteral or urethral spasm; seizure disorders; hyperthyroidism; impaired hepatic, renal function; psychiatric disorders; manic-depression; elective surgery
- **Physical:** Weight; T; skin color, lesions; orientation, affect, reflexes, vision and hearing; P, BP, orthostatic BP, perfusion; bowel sounds, normal output, liver evaluation; urine flow, normal output; usual sexual function, frequency of menses, breast and scrotal examination; LFTs, urinalysis, CBC, ECG

Interventions

- Restrict drug access for depressed and potentially suicidal patients.

⊠ ***Black box warning*** Children, adolescents, and young adults have increased risk of suicidality; monitor patient carefully.

- Give most of dose at bedtime if drowsiness, severe anticholinergic effects occur (elderly patients may not tolerate single daily dose).
- Reduce dosage if minor side effects develop; discontinue if serious side effects occur.
- Arrange for CBC if patient develops fever, sore throat, or other sign of infection.
- Encourage elderly men or men with prostate problems to void before taking drug.

Teaching points

- Do not stop taking this drug abruptly or without consulting your health care provider.
- Avoid using alcohol, other sleep-inducing drugs, and over-the-counter drugs.
- Avoid prolonged exposure to sunlight or sunlamps; use a sunscreen or protective garments.
- You may experience these side effects: Headache, dizziness, drowsiness, weakness, blurred vision (reversible; safety measures may need to be taken if severe; avoid driving or tasks requiring alertness); nausea, vomiting, loss of appetite, dry mouth (eat frequent small meals, frequent mouth care, and sucking sugarless candies may help); nightmares, inability to concentrate, confusion; changes in sexual function.
- Report dry mouth, difficulty in urination, excessive sedation, thoughts of suicide.

amoxicillin trihydrate

*(a mox i **sill'** in try **high'** drayt)*

Amoxil, Amoxil Pediatric Drops, Apo-Amoxi (CAN), DisperMox, Gen-Amoxicillin (CAN), Moxatag, Novamoxin (CAN), Nu-Amoxi (CAN), Trimox

PREGNANCY CATEGORY B

Drug class
Antibiotic (penicillin–ampicillin type)

Therapeutic actions
Bactericidal: Inhibits synthesis of cell wall of sensitive organisms, causing cell death.

Indications
- Treatment of tonsillitis and pharyngitis caused by *Streptococcus pyogenes* (ER tablet)
- Infections due to susceptible strains of *Haemophilus influenzae, Escherichia coli, Proteus mirabilis, Neisseria gonorrhoeae, Streptococcus pneumoniae, Enterococcus faecalis,* streptococci, non–penicillinase-producing staphylococci
- *Helicobacter pylori* infection in combination with other agents
- Postexposure prophylaxis against *Bacillus anthracis*
- Unlabeled use: *Chlamydia trachomatis* in pregnancy, mild to moderate otitis media in children

Contraindications and cautions
- Contraindicated with allergies to penicillins, cephalosporins, or other allergens.
- Use cautiously with renal disorders, lactation.

Available forms
Chewable tablets—125, 200, 250, 400 mg; tablets—500, 875 mg; capsules—250, 500 mg; powder for oral suspension—50 mg/mL; 125 mg/5 mL, 200 mg/5 mL, 250 mg/5 mL, 400 mg/5 mL; tablets for oral suspension—200, 400 mg; ER tablets—775 mg Available in oral preparations only.

Dosages
Adults and pediatric patients weighing more than 40 kg
- *URIs, GU infections, skin and soft-tissue infections:* Mild to moderate—250 mg PO every 8 hr—500 mg PO every 12 hr; severe infection—500 mg every 8 hr or 875 mg every 12 hr.
- *Postexposure anthrax prophylaxis:* 500 mg PO tid to complete a 60-day course after 14–21 days of a fluoroquinolone or doxycycline.
- *Lower respiratory infections:* 500 mg PO every 8 hr or 875 mg PO bid.
- *Uncomplicated gonococcal infections:* 3 g amoxicillin with 1 g probenecid PO as a single dose.
- C. trachomatis *in pregnancy:* 500 mg PO tid for 7 days or 875 mg PO bid.
- *Tonsillitis or pharyngitis:* 775 mg/day PO for 10 days with food (ER tablet).
- H. pylori *infections:* 1 g bid with clarithromycin 500 mg bid and lansoprazole 30 mg bid for 14 days.

Pediatric patients 3 mo and older weighing less than 40 kg
- *URIs, GU infections, skin and soft-tissue infections:* Mild to moderate infection—20 mg/kg/day PO in divided doses every 8 hr or 25 mg/kg/day PO in divided doses every 12 hr. Severe infection—40 mg/kg/day in divided doses every 8 hr or 45 mg/kg/day PO in divided doses every 12 hr.
- *Postexposure anthrax prophylaxis:* 80 mg/kg/day PO divided into 3 doses to complete a 60-day course after 14–21 days of fluoroquinolone or doxycycline therapy.

Pediatric patients 3 mo and older
- *Mild to moderate URIs, GU infections, and skin infections:* 20 mg/kg daily in divided doses every 8 hr or 25 mg/kg in divided doses every 12 hr.
- *Acute otitis media:* 80–90 mg/kg/day PO for 10 days (severe cases) or for 5–7 days (moderate cases).
- *Gonorrhea in prepubertal children:* 50 mg/kg PO with 25 mg/kg probenecid as a single dose (probenecid contraindicated in children younger than 2 yr).
- *For lower respiratory infections, or severe URIs, GU, or skin infections:* 40 mg/kg daily

in divided doses every 8 hr or 45 mg/kg daily in divided doses every 12 hr.

Pediatric patients up to 12 wk
Up to 30 mg/kg daily in divided doses every 12 hr.

Patients with renal impairment
Do not use 875-mg tablet if GFR is less than 30 mL/min. For GFR of 10–30 mL/min, 250–500 mg every 12 hr; for GFR less than 10 mL/min, 250–500 mg every 24 hr; for hemodialysis patients, 250–500 mg every 24 hr with additional doses during and after dialysis.

Pharmacokinetics

Route	*Onset*	*Peak*	*Duration*
Oral	Varies	1 hr	6–8 hr

Metabolism: $T_{1/2}$: 1–1.4 hr
Distribution: Crosses placenta; enters breast milk
Excretion: Urine, unchanged

Adverse effects

- **CNS:** Lethargy, hallucinations, seizures
- **GI:** *Glossitis, stomatitis, gastritis, sore mouth,* furry tongue, black "hairy" tongue, *nausea, vomiting, diarrhea, abdominal pain,* bloody diarrhea, enterocolitis, pseudomembranous colitis, nonspecific hepatitis
- **GU:** Nephritis
- **Hematologic:** Anemia, thrombocytopenia, leukopenia, neutropenia, prolonged bleeding time
- **Hypersensitivity:** *Rash, fever, wheezing,* **anaphylaxis**
- **Other:** *Superinfections*—oral and rectal moniliasis, vaginitis

Interactions

✱ **Drug-drug** • Increased effect with probenecid • Decreased effectiveness with tetracyclines, chloramphenicol • Decreased efficacy of hormonal contraceptives
✱ **Drug-food** • Delayed or reduced GI absorption with food

■ Nursing considerations

Assessment

- **History:** Allergies to penicillins, cephalosporins, or other allergens; renal disorders; lactation
- **Physical:** Culture infected area; skin color, lesion; R, adventitious sounds; bowel sounds; CBC, LFTs, renal function tests, serum electrolytes, Hct, urinalysis

Interventions

- Culture infected area prior to treatment; reculture area if response is not as expected.
- Give in oral preparations only; amoxicillin is not affected by food.
- Continue therapy for at least 2 days after signs of infection have disappeared; continuation for 10 full days is recommended.
- Use corticosteroids or antihistamines for skin reactions.

Teaching points

- Take this drug around-the-clock.
- Take the full course of therapy; do not stop because you feel better.
- This antibiotic is specific for this problem and should not be used to self-treat other infections.
- You may experience these side effects: Nausea, vomiting, GI upset (eat frequent small meals); diarrhea; sore mouth (frequent mouth care may help).
- Report unusual bleeding or bruising, sore throat, fever, rash, hives, severe diarrhea, difficulty breathing.

DANGEROUS DRUG

▽ amphotericin B
(am foe ***ter'*** *i sin)*

amphotericin B desoxycholate

amphotericin B, lipid-based
Abelcet, AmBisome, Amphotec

PREGNANCY CATEGORY B

Drug class
Antifungal

Therapeutic actions
Binds to sterols in the fungal cell membrane with a resultant change in membrane permeability, an effect that can destroy fungal cells and

prevent their reproduction; fungicidal or fungistatic depending on concentration and organism.

Indications

- Reserve use for patients with progressive, potentially fatal infections: Cryptococcosis; North American blastomycosis; systemic candidiasis; disseminated moniliasis; coccidioidomycosis and histoplasmosis; mucormycosis caused by species of *Mucor, Rhizopus, Absidia, Conidiobolus, Basidiobolus;* sporotrichosis; aspergillosis
- Adjunct treatment of American mucocutaneous leishmaniasis (not choice in primary therapy)
- Treatment of aspergillosis in patients refractory to conventional therapy (*Abelcet, Amphotec*)
- Treatment of cryptococcal meningitis in HIV-infected patients (*AmBisome*)
- Treatment of invasive aspergillosis where renal toxicity precludes use of conventional amphotericin B (*Amphotec*)
- Treatment of presumed fungal infections in febrile, neutropenic patients (*AmBisome*)
- Treatment of *Aspergillis, Candida,* or *Cryptococcus* infections in patients intolerant to or refractory to conventional amphotericin B (*AmBisome*)
- Treatment of any type of progressive fungal infection that does not respond to conventional therapy
- Unlabeled use: Prophylactic to prevent fungal infections in bone marrow transplants, bladder irrigation for candidal cystitis, primary treatment of amoebic meningoencephalitis, ocular aspergillosis, treatment of severe meningitis in patients unresponsive to IV therapy (intrathecal administration)

Contraindications and cautions

- Contraindicated with allergy to amphotericin B, renal impairment, lactation (except when life-threatening and treatable only with this drug).
- Use cautiously with pregnancy.

Available forms

Injection—50 mg; suspension for injection—100 mg/20 mL; powder for injection—50, 100 mg/vial

Dosages

Adults and pediatric patients

Abelcet

Consider test dose; if tolerated, may proceed to regular dosing regimen.

- *Aspergillosis:* 5 mg/kg/day given as a single infusion at 2.5 mg/kg/hr.

Amphotec

Use test dose (10 mL of final preparation infused over 15–30 min).

- *Aspergillosis:* Initially, 3–4 mg/kg/day, may increase to 6 mg/kg/day IV. Infuse at 1 mg/kg/hr over at least 2 hr.

AmBisome

Consider test dose; if tolerated, may proceed to regular dosing regimen.

- *Presumed fungal infection in febrile neutropenic patients:* 3 mg/kg/day IV.
- *Cryptococcal meningitis in HIV:* 6 mg/kg/day IV.
- *Aspergillosis:* 3–5 mg/kg/day IV, give over more than 2 hr.
- *Leishmaniasis:* 3 mg/kg/day IV, days 1–5, 14, and 21 for immunocompetent patients; 4 mg/kg/day IV, days 1–5, 10, 17, 24, 31, and 38 for immunocompromised patients.

Pharmacokinetics

Route	*Onset*	*Peak*	*Duration*
IV	20–30 min	1–2 hr	20–24 hr

Metabolism: $T_{1/2}$: 24 hr initially and then 15 days; 173.4 hr *(Abelcet)*

Distribution: Crosses placenta; may enter breast milk

Excretion: Urine

IV FACTS

Abelcet: Shake vial gently until no yellow sediment is seen. Withdraw dose, replace needle with a 5-micron filter needle. Inject into bag containing 5% dextrose injection to a concentration of 1 mg/mL. May be further diluted. Store vials in refrigerator; stable for 48 hr once prepared if refrigerated, for 6 hr at room temperature.

Amphotec: Reconstitute with sterile water for injection. 10 mL to 50 mg/vial or 20 mL to

100 mg/vial. Dilute to 0.6 mg/mL. Refrigerate after reconstitution; use within 24 hr.
AmBisome: Add 12 mL sterile water to each vial to yield 4 mg/mL; immediately shake vial for 30 sec until yellow translucent suspension formed; draw up dose via syringe, attach 5 micron filter, and inject into appropriate volume at 5% dextrose to final concentration of 1–2 mg/mL (0.2–0.5 mg/mL for infants/small children).
Infusion: *Amphotericin B:* Protect from exposure to light if not infused within 8 hr of preparation. Infuse slowly over 6 hr.
Abelcet: Infuse at rate of 2.5 mg/kg/hr. If infusion takes more than 2 hr, remix bag by shaking.
Amphotec: Infuse at 1 mg/kg/hr over at least 2 hr; do not use an in-line filter.
AmBisome: Flush line with D_5W prior to infusion. Infuse over more than 2 hr if tolerated; stop immediately at any sign of anaphylactic reaction.
Incompatibilities: Do not mix with saline-containing solution, parenteral nutrional solutions, aminoglycosides, penicillins, phenothiazines, calcium preparations, cimetidine, metaraminol, methyldopa, polymyxin, potassium chloride, ranitidine, verapamil, clindamycin, cotrimoxazole, dopamine, dobutamine, tetracycline, vitamins, lidocaine, procaine, or heparin. **If line must be flushed, do not use heparin or saline; use D_5W.**
Y-site incompatibilities: Foscarnet, ondansetron.

Adverse effects

Systemic administration

- **CNS:** Fever (often with shaking chills), headache, malaise, generalized pain
- **GI:** *Nausea, vomiting, dyspepsia, diarrhea,* cramping, epigastric pain, anorexia
- **GU:** Hypokalemia, azotemia, hyposthenuria, renal tubular acidosis, nephrocalcinosis
- **Hematologic:** Normochromic, normocytic anemia
- **Local:** *Pain at the injection site* with phlebitis and thrombophlebitis
- **Other:** Weight loss

Interactions

✱ **Drug-drug** • Do not administer with corticosteroids unless these are needed to control symptoms • Increased risk of nephrotoxicity with other nephrotoxic antibiotics, antineoplastics, zidovudine • Increased effects and risk of toxicity of digitalis, skeletal muscle relaxants, flucytosine • Increased nephrotoxic effects with cyclosporine • Increased risk of hypokalemia with thiazide diuretics

■ Nursing considerations

CLINICAL ALERT!
Dosages between the amphotericin products are not the same and are not interchangeable. Ensure correct drug is ordered and given.

Assessment

- **History:** Allergy to amphotericin B, renal impairment, lactation
- **Physical:** Skin color, lesions; T; weight; injection site; orientation, reflexes, affect; bowel sounds, liver evaluation; LFTs, renal function tests; CBC and differential; culture of area involved

Interventions

⊗ ***Black box warning*** Reserve systemic use for progressive or potentially fatal infections; not for use in noninvasive disease; toxicity can be severe.

- Arrange for immediate culture of infection but begin treatment before lab results are returned.
- Monitor injection sites and veins for signs of phlebitis.
- Provide aspirin, antihistamines, and antiemetics, and maintain sodium balance to ease drug discomfort. Minimal use of IV corticosteroids may decrease febrile reactions. Meperidine has been used to relieve chills and fever.
- Amphotericin B products may cause severe electrolyte abnormalities, such as magnesium wasting. Monitor electrolytes often.
- Monitor renal function tests weekly; discontinue or decrease dosage of drug at any sign of increased renal toxicity.
- Continue topical administration for long-term therapy until infection is eradicated, usually 2–4 wk.
- Discontinue topical application if hypersensitivity reaction occurs.

Teaching points

- Long-term use of this drug will be needed; beneficial effects may not be seen for several weeks; the systemic form of the drug can only be given IV.
- For topical application, apply topical drug liberally to affected area after first cleansing area.
- Use good hygiene to prevent reinfection or spread of infection.
- You may experience these side effects: Nausea, vomiting, diarrhea (eat frequent small meals); discoloring, drying of the skin, staining of fabric with topical forms (washing with soap and water or cleaning fabric with standard cleaning fluid should remove stain); stinging, irritation with local application; fever, chills, muscle aches and pains, headache (medications may be ordered to help you to deal with these discomforts of the drug).
- Report pain, irritation at injection site; GI upset, nausea, loss of appetite; difficulty breathing; local irritation, burning (topical application).

ampicillin

*(am pi **sill'** in)*

ampicillin sodium

Oral: Novo-Ampicillin (CAN), Principen

PREGNANCY CATEGORY B

Drug classes

Antibiotic
Penicillin

Therapeutic actions

Bactericidal action against sensitive organisms; inhibits synthesis of bacterial cell wall, causing cell death.

Indications

- Treatment of infections caused by susceptible strains of *Shigella, Salmonella, S. typhosa, Escherichia coli, Haemophilus influenzae, Proteus mirabilis, Neisseria gonorrhoeae,* enterococci, gram-positive organisms (penicillin G–sensitive staphylococci, streptococci, pneumococci)
- Meningitis caused by *Neisseria meningitidis*
- **NEW INDICATION:** Prevention of bacterial endocarditis following dental, oral, or respiratory procedures in very high-risk patients
- Unlabeled use: Prophylaxis in cesarean section in certain high-risk patients

Contraindications and cautions

- Contraindicated with allergies to penicillins, cephalosporins, or other allergens.
- Use cautiously with renal disorders.

Available forms

Capsules—250, 500 mg; powder for oral suspension—125 mg/5 mL, 250 mg/5 mL; powder for injection—250, 500 mg, 1, 2 g

Dosages

Maximum recommended dosage, 8–14 g/day (reserve 14 g for serious infections, such as meningitis, septicemia); may be given IV, IM, or PO. Use parenteral routes for severe infections; switch to oral route as soon as possible.

Adults

- *Prevention of bacterial endocarditis for dental, oral, or upper respiratory procedures in patients at high risk:* 2 g ampicillin IM or IV within 30 min of procedure.
- *Digestive system infections:* 500 mg PO every 6 hr for 48–72 hr after patient becomes asymptomatic or eradication is evident.
- *STDs in pregnant women and patients allergic to tetracycline:* 3.5 g ampicillin PO with 1 g probenecid.
- *Prevention of infection in cesarean section:* Single IV or IM dose of 25–100 mg/kg immediately after cord is clamped.

Pediatric patients

- *Prevention of bacterial endocarditis for GI or GU surgery or instrumentation:* 50 mg/kg ampicillin IM or IV within 30 minutes of procedure. Six hours later, give 25 mg/kg ampicillin IM or IV or 25 mg/kg amoxicillin PO.
- *Prevention of bacterial endocarditis for dental, oral, or upper respiratory procedures in patients at high risk:* 50 mg/kg ampicillin IM or IV within 30 min of procedure.

Adults and pediatric patients

- *Respiratory and soft-tissue infections:* *40 kg or more:* 250–500 mg IV or IM every 6 hr.
  Less than 40 kg: 25–50 mg/kg/day IM or IV in equally divided doses at 6- to 8-hr intervals.
  20 kg or more: 250 mg PO every 6 hr.
  Less than 20 kg: 50 mg/kg/day PO in equally divided doses every 6–8 hr.
- *GI and GU infections, including women with* N. gonorrhoeae:
  More than 40 kg: 500 mg IM or IV every 6 hr.
  40 kg or less: 50 mg/kg/day IM or IV in equally divided doses every 6–8 hr.
  20 kg or more: 500 mg PO every 6 hr.
  Less than 20 kg: 100 mg/kg/day PO in equally divided doses every 6–8 hr.
- *Bacterial meningitis:* 150–200 mg/kg/day by continuous IV drip and then IM injections in equally divided doses every 3–4 hr.
- *Septicemia:* 150–200 mg/kg/day IV for at least 3 days, then IM every 3–4 hr.

Pharmacokinetics

Route	*Onset*	*Peak*	*Duration*
Oral	30 min	2 hr	6–8 hr
IM	15 min	1 hr	6–8 hr
IV	Immediate	5 min	6–8 hr

Metabolism: $T_{1/2}$: 1–2 hr
Distribution: Crosses placenta; enters breast milk
Excretion: Urine, unchanged

IV FACTS

Preparation: Reconstitute with sterile or bacteriostatic water for injection; piggyback vials may be reconstituted with sodium chloride injection; use reconstituted solution within 1 hr. Do not mix in the same IV solution as other antibiotics. Use within 1 hr after preparation because potency may decrease significantly after that.
Infusion: 125-, 250-, or 500-mg dose given over 3–5 min; 1- or 2-g dose given over 10–15 min.
IV piggyback: Administer alone or further dilute with compatible solution.
Compatibilities: Ampicillin is compatible with 0.9% sodium chloride, D_5W, or 0.45% sodium chloride solution, 10% invert sugar water, M/6 sodium lactate solution, lactated Ringer's solution, sterile water for injection. Diluted solutions are stable for 2–8 hr; check manufacturer's inserts for specifics. Discard solution after allotted time period.
Incompatibilities: Do not mix with lidocaine, verapamil, other antibiotics, dextrose solutions.
Y-site incompatibilities: Do not give with epinephrine, hydralazine, or ondansetron.

Adverse effects

- **CNS:** Lethargy, hallucinations, seizures
- **CV:** Heart failure
- **GI:** *Glossitis, stomatitis, gastritis, sore mouth,* furry tongue, black "hairy" tongue, *nausea, vomiting, diarrhea,* abdominal pain, bloody diarrhea, enterocolitis, pseudomembranous colitis, nonspecific hepatitis
- **GU: Nephritis**
- **Hematologic:** Anemia, thrombocytopenia, leukopenia, neutropenia, prolonged bleeding time
- **Hypersensitivity:** *Rash, fever, wheezing,* anaphylaxis
- **Local:** *Pain, phlebitis,* thrombosis at injection site (parenteral)
- **Other:** *Superinfections*—oral and rectal moniliasis, vaginitis

Interactions

✱ **Drug-drug** • Increased ampicillin effect with probenecid • Increased risk of rash with allopurinol • Increased bleeding effect with heparin, oral anticoagulants • Decreased effectiveness with tetracyclines, chloramphenicol • Decreased efficacy of hormonal contraceptives, atenolol with ampicillin
✱ **Drug-food** • Oral ampicillin may be less effective with food; take on an empty stomach
✱ **Drug-lab test** • False-positive Coombs' test if given IV • Decrease in plasma estrogen concentrations in pregnant women • False-positive urine glucose tests if Clinitest, Benedict's solution, or Fehling's solution is used; enzymatic glucose oxidase methods (*Clinistix, Tes-Tape*) should be used to check urine glucose

Nursing considerations

Assessment

- **History:** Allergies to penicillins, cephalosporins, or other allergens; renal disorders; lactation
- **Physical:** Culture infected area; skin color, lesion; R, adventitious sounds; bowel sounds; CBC, LFTs, renal function tests, serum electrolytes, Hct, urinalysis

Interventions

- Culture infected area before treatment; reculture area if response is not as expected.
- Check IV site carefully for signs of thrombosis or drug reaction.
- Do not give IM injections in the same site; atrophy can occur. Monitor injection sites.
- Administer oral drug on an empty stomach, 1 hr before or 2 hr after meals with a full glass of water; do not give with fruit juice or soft drinks.

Teaching points

- Take this drug around-the-clock.
- Take the full course of therapy; do not stop taking the drug if you feel better.
- Take the oral drug on an empty stomach, 1 hour before or 2 hours after meals; do not take with fruit juice or soft drinks; the oral solution is stable for 7 days at room temperature or 14 days refrigerated.
- This antibiotic is specific to your problem and should not be used to self-treat other infections.
- If you are a woman and you use a hormonal contraceptive, you should use a second form of birth control for 1–2 weeks while taking this drug.
- You may experience these side effects: Nausea, vomiting, GI upset (eat frequent small meals), diarrhea.
- Report pain or discomfort at sites, unusual bleeding or bruising, mouth sores, rash, hives, fever, itching, severe diarrhea, difficulty breathing.

▽anagrelide hydrochloride

*(an **agh'** rah lide)*

Agrylin

PREGNANCY CATEGORY C

Drug class

Antiplatelet drug

Therapeutic actions

Reduces platelet production by decreasing megakaryocyte hypermaturation; inhibits cyclic AMP and ADP collagen-induced platelet aggregation. At therapeutic doses has no effect on WBC counts or coagulation parameters; may affect RBC parameters.

Indications

- Treatment of essential thrombocythemia secondary to myeloproliferative disorders to reduce elevated platelet count and the risk of thrombosis and to improve associated symptoms, including thrombohemorrhagic events

Contraindications and cautions

- Contraindicated with known allergy to anagrelide or severe hepatic or renal impairment.
- Use cautiously with renal or hepatic disorders, pregnancy, lactation, known heart disease, thrombocytopenia.

Available forms

Capsules—0.5, 1 mg

Dosages

Adults

Initially, 0.5 mg PO qid or 1 mg PO bid. After 1 wk, reevaluate and adjust the dosage as needed. Dosage is based on platelet counts; goal is less than 600,000. Do not increase by more than 0.5 mg/day each week. Maximum dose, 10 mg/day or 2.5 mg as a single dose.

Pediatric patients

Initially, 0.5 mg/day–0.5 mg qid. Adjust to lowest effective dose to keep platelet count below 600,000/mm^3. Do not increase by more than

0.5 mg/day each week. Maximum dose, 10 mg/day or 2.5 mg in a single dose.

Patients with moderate hepatic impairment

Initially, 0.5 mg/day for at least 1 wk. Monitor patient closely. Do not increase dose by more than 0.5 mg/day in 1 wk.

Pharmacokinetics

Route	*Onset*	*Peak*
Oral	Rapid	1 hr

Metabolism: Hepatic; $T_{1/2}$: 1.3 hr
Distribution: Crosses placenta; may enter breast milk
Excretion: Feces, urine

Adverse effects

- **CNS:** Dizziness, *headaches, asthenia,* paresthesias
- **CV: Heart failure,** tachycardia, **MI, complete heart block,** atrial fibrillation, hypotension, *palpitations,* **CVA**
- **GI:** *Diarrhea, nausea, vomiting, abdominal pain,* flatulence, dyspepsia, anorexia, **pancreatitis,** ulcer
- **Hematologic:** *Thrombocytopenia,* anemia
- **Other:** Rash, purpura, edema

Interactions

✱ **Drug-food** • Risk of increased toxicity with grapefruit juice; avoid this combination

■ Nursing considerations

CLINICAL ALERT!
Confusion has been reported with *Agrylin* and *Aggrastat* (tirofiban); use caution.

Assessment

- **History:** Allergy to anagrelide, thrombocytopenia, hemostatic disorders, bleeding ulcer, intracranial bleeding, severe liver disease, lactation, renal disorders, pregnancy, known heart disease
- **Physical:** Skin color, lesions; orientation; bowel sounds, normal output; CBC, LFTs, renal function tests

Interventions

- Perform platelet counts every 2 days during the first week of therapy and at least weekly thereafter; if thrombocytopenia occurs, decrease dosage of drug and arrange for supportive therapy. During first 2 wk, also monitor CBC, LFTs, serum creatinine, BUN.
- Administer drug on an empty stomach if at all tolerated.
- Establish safety precautions to prevent injury and bleeding (eg, use an electric razor, avoid contact sports).
- Monitor BP before and periodically during therapy.
- Advise patient to use barrier contraceptives while receiving this drug; it may harm the fetus.
- Monitor patient for any sign of excessive bleeding—eg, bruises, dark stools—and monitor bleeding times.
- Mark chart of any patient receiving anagrelide to alert medical personnel of potential for increased bleeding in cases of surgery or dental surgery, invasive procedures.

Teaching points

- Take drug on an empty stomach.
- Do not drink grapefruit juice while on this drug.
- You will need frequent and regular blood tests to monitor your response to this drug.
- It may take longer than normal to stop bleeding while taking this drug, so avoid contact sports, use electric razors, and take other precautions to avoid bleeding. Apply pressure for extended periods to bleeding sites.
- Avoid pregnancy while taking this drug; it could harm the fetus; using barrier contraceptives is suggested.
- Notify any dentist or surgeon that you are taking this drug before invasive procedures.
- You may experience these side effects: Upset stomach, nausea, diarrhea, loss of appetite (eat frequent small meals).
- Report fever, chills, sore throat, rash, bruising, bleeding, dark stools or urine, palpitations, chest pain.

anakinra
*(ann **ack'** in rah)*

Kineret

PREGNANCY CATEGORY B

Drug classes
Antiarthritic
Interleukin-1 receptor antagonist

Therapeutic actions
A recombinant human interleukin-1 receptor antagonist; blocks the activity of interleukin 1 that is elevated in response to inflammatory and immune stimulation and is responsible for the degradation of cartilage due to the rapid loss of proteoglycans in rheumatoid arthritis.

Indications
- Reduction of the signs and symptoms and slowing of progression of moderately to severely active rheumatoid arthritis in patients 18 years of age and older who have failed on one or more disease-modifying antirheumatic drugs (methotrexate, sulfasalazine, hydroxychloroquine, gold, penicillamine, leflunomide, azathioprine); used alone or with disease-modifying antirheumatic drugs other than tumor necrosis factor blocking agents

Contraindications and cautions
- Contraindicated with allergy to anakinra or proteins produced by *Escherichia coli.*
- Use cautiously with immunosuppression, active infection, pregnancy, lactation, renal impairment.

Available forms
Prefilled glass syringes—100 mg/0.67 mL

Dosages
Adults
- 100 mg/day subcutaneously at approximately the same time each day.

Pediatric patients
- Safety and efficacy not established.

Patients with renal impairment
For patients with end-stage renal disease or creatinine clearance less than 30 mL/min, 100 mg every other day.

Pharmacokinetics

Route	*Onset*	*Peak*
Subcut.	Slow	3–7 hr

Metabolism: Tissue; $T_{1/2}$: 4–6 hr
Distribution: May cross placenta; may enter breast milk
Excretion: Urine

Adverse effects
- **CNS:** Headache
- **GI:** Nausea, diarrhea, abdominal pain
- **Hematologic:** Neutropenia, thrombocytopenia
- **Respiratory:** *URI, sinusitis*
- **Other:** *Injection site reactions, infections,* flulike symptoms

Interactions
✱ **Drug-drug** ⊗ ***Warning*** Increased risk of serious infections and neutropenia if combined with etanercept or other tumor necrosis factor blocking drugs; avoid this combination (if no alternative is available; use extreme caution and monitor patient closely)
- Immunizations given while on anakinra may be less effective

■ Nursing considerations

CLINICAL ALERT!
Name confusion has occurred between anakinra and amikacin; use caution.

Assessment
- **History:** Allergy to anakinra or proteins produced by *E. coli,* immunosuppression, renal impairment, pregnancy, lactation
- **Physical:** T, body weight, P, BP, R, adventitious sounds, CBC, renal function tests

Interventions
- Make sure that patient does not have an active infection before administering.

- Store the drug in the refrigerator, protected from light; use by expiration date because solution contains no preservatives.
- Administer the subcutaneous injection at about the same time each day.
- Inspect solution before injection. Do not use solution if it is discolored or contains particulate matter.
- Discard any unused portion of the drug; do not store for later use.
- Provide analgesics if headache or muscle pain are a problem.
- Monitor injection sites for erythema, ecchymosis, inflammation, and pain. Rotating sites may help to decrease severe reactions.
- Advise women of childbearing age to use a barrier form of contraception while taking this drug.
- Monitor CBC before and periodically during therapy; drug should not be given during active infections.

Teaching points

- This drug must be injected subcutaneously once each day at approximately the same time each day.
- The drug must be stored in the refrigerator, protected from light. Use the drug by the expiration date on the box; the drug contains no preservatives and will not be effective after that date. Do not use any drug that is discolored or contains particulate matter.
- You and a family member or significant other should learn the proper way to administer a subcutaneous injection, including the proper disposal of needles and syringes. Prepare a chart of injection sites to ensure that you rotate the sites. Dispose of syringes in appropriate container.
- Avoid infection while you are taking this drug; avoid crowded areas or people with known infections.
- This drug does not cure your rheumatoid arthritis, and appropriate therapies to deal with the disease should be followed.
- You may experience these side effects: Reactions at the injection site (rotating sites and applying heat may help); headache, pain (use of an analgesic may help; consult your health care provider); increased risk of infection (contact your health care provider at any sign of infection [fever, muscular aches and pains, respiratory problems] because it may be necessary to stop the drug during the infection).
- Report fever, chills, difficulty breathing, severe discomfort at injection site.

DANGEROUS DRUG

▽anastrozole

*(an **abs'** troh zol)*

Arimidex

PREGNANCY CATEGORY D

Drug class

Antiestrogen
Aromatase inhibitor

Therapeutic actions

Selective nonsteroidal aromatase inhibitor that significantly reduces serum estradiol levels with no significant effect on adrenocortical steroids or aldosterone.

Indications

- Treatment of advanced breast cancer in postmenopausal women with disease progression following tamoxifen therapy
- First-line treatment of postmenopausal women with hormone receptor positive or hormone receptor unknown locally advanced or metastatic breast cancer
- Adjuvant treatment of postmenopausal women with hormone receptor positive early breast cancer
- Unlabeled use: Male infertility

Contraindications and cautions

- Contraindicated with allergy to anastrazole, pregnancy, lactation.
- Use cautiously with hepatic or renal impairment, high cholesterol states.

Available forms

Tablets—1 mg

Dosages

Adults

1 mg PO daily.

Pediatric patients

Not recommended.

Pharmacokinetics

Route	Onset	Peak
Oral	Varies	10–12 hr

Metabolism: Hepatic; $T_{1/2}$: 50 hr
Distribution: Crosses placenta; enters breast milk
Excretion: Feces, urine

Adverse effects

- **CNS:** Depression, light-headedness, dizziness, asthenia, headache
- **CV:** Vasodilation, hypertension
- **Dermatologic:** *Hot flashes, rash*
- **GI:** *Nausea, vomiting,* food distaste, dry mouth, *pharyngitis,* constipation
- **GU:** Vaginal bleeding, vaginal pain, UTIs
- **Other:** Peripheral edema, *bone pain, back pain;* increased HDL, LDL levels

■ Nursing considerations

Assessment

- **History:** Allergy to anastrozole, hepatic or renal impairment, pregnancy, lactation, treatment profile for breast cancer, hypercholesterolemia
- **Physical:** Skin lesions, color, turgor; pelvic examination; orientation, affect, reflexes; peripheral pulses, edema; LFTs, renal function tests

Interventions

- Administer once daily without regard to meals.
- Arrange for periodic lipid profiles during therapy.
- Arrange for appropriate analgesic measures if pain and discomfort become severe.

Teaching points

- Take the drug once a day without regard to meals.
- You may experience these side effects: Bone pain; hot flashes (staying in cool temperatures may help); nausea, vomiting (eat frequent small meals); dizziness, headache, light-headedness (use caution if driving or performing tasks that require alertness); birth defects (avoid pregnancy).
- Report changes in color of stool or urine, severe vomiting, or inability to eat.

▽ anidulafungin

(an ah ***doo'*** *lah fun gin)*

Eraxis

PREGNANCY CATEGORY C

Drug classes

Antifungal
Echinocandin

Therapeutic actions

Inhibits glucan synthesis, an enzyme present in fungal cells but not human cells; this inhibition prevents the fungal cell wall from forming and results in cell death.

Indications

- Treatment of candidemia and other forms of *Candida* infections (intra-abdominal abscess, peritonitis)
- Treatment of esophageal candidiasis

Contraindications and cautions

- Contraindicated with hypersensitivity to anidulafungin or any other echinocandin, or to any component of the drug.
- Use cautiously with liver impairment, pregnancy, lactation.

Available forms

Single-use vials—50, 100 mg with diluent vial

Dosages

Adults

- Treatment of candidemia and other forms *Candida* infections: 200 mg by IV infusion on day 1, then 100 mg/day by IV infusion; generally continued for at least 14 days after the last positive culture.
- Esophageal candidiasis: 100 mg by IV infusion on day 1, then 50 mg/day by IV infusion for a minimum of 14 days and for at least 7 days following resolution of symptoms.

Pediatric patients

Safety and efficacy not established.

Pharmacokinetics

Route	Onset	Peak
IV infusion	Rapid	End of infusion

Metabolism: Degradation; $T_{1/2}$: 40–50 hr
Distribution: May cross placenta; may pass into breast milk
Excretion: Feces

IV FACTS

Preparation: Reconstitute with the diluent provided, giving a concentration of 3.33 mg/mL; then dilute with 5% dextrose injection or 0.9% sodium chloride injection to a concentration of 0.5 mg/mL. Store prepared solution at room temperature; must be used within 24 hr after dilution. Inspect solution for particulate matter or discoloration, and discard if observed.
Infusion: Infuse at no more than 1.1 mg/min.
Incompatibilities: Do not combine with any other drug or with any solution other than those listed.

Adverse effects

- **CNS:** Headache
- **CV:** Hypotension
- **GI:** Nausea, abdominal pain, vomiting, dyspepsia, elevated liver enzymes
- **Hematological:** Leukopenia, neutropenia
- **Other:** Rash, urticaria, flushing, pruritus

■ Nursing considerations

Assessment

- **History:** Hypersensitivity to anidulafungin or any other echinocandin or to any component of the drug, hepatic impairment, pregnancy, lactation
- **Physical:** Skin, BP, abdominal examination, LFTs, culture of infected area

Interventions

- Culture infected area prior to starting drug; drug can be started before results are known, but appropriate adjustments in treatment should be made when culture results are evaluated.
- Periodically monitor LFTs to make sure hepatotoxicity does not occur.
- Suggest the use of contraceptive measures while using this drug; the potential effects on a fetus are not known.
- Advise nursing mothers that another method of feeding the baby will need to be used while on this drug.
- Provide supportive measures if histamine reaction occurs; symptoms include hypotension, flushing, rash. A reaction is less likely if infusion rate does not exceed 1.1 mg/min.

Teaching points

- This drug must be given by a daily IV infusion.
- It is very important to maintain your fluid and food intake, which will help healing. Notify your health care provider if nausea or vomiting prevents this.
- You may need blood tests to evaluate the effects of the drug on your body.
- It is not known how this drug could affect a fetus, if you are pregnant or decide to become pregnant while on this drug, consult your health care provider.
- It is not known how this drug could affect a nursing baby. If you are nursing a baby, another method of feeding the baby should be selected.
- You may experience these side effects: Headache, nausea (consult your health care provider, medications may be available that could help).
- Report changes in the color of urine or stool, rash, yellowing of the skin or eyes, extreme fatigue, shortness of breath, tightness in the chest.

▽ antihemophilic factor (AHF, Factor VIII)

*(an tee hee moe **fill' ik fack'** tur)*

Advate, Alphanate, Helixate FS, Hemofil M, Humate-P, Koate-DVI, Kogenate FS, Monarc-M, Monoclate-P, Recombinate, ReFacto, Xyntha

PREGNANCY CATEGORY C

Drug class

Antihemophilic

Therapeutic actions

A normal plasma protein that is needed for the transformation of prothrombin to thrombin, the final step of the intrinsic clotting pathway.

Indications

- Treatment of classical hemophilia (hemophilia A), in which there is a demonstrated deficiency of factor VIII; provides a temporary replacement of clotting factors to correct or prevent bleeding episodes or to allow necessary surgery
- Short-term prophylaxis (*ReFacto*) to reduce frequency of spontaneous bleeding
- Surgical and/or invasive procedures in patients with von Willebrand disease in whom desmopressin is ineffective or contraindicated to control bleeding; not for major surgery (*Advate, Alphanate, Xyntha*)
- Prevention of excessive bleeding during and after surgery in certain patients with mild to moderate and severe von Willebrand disease (*Advate, Humate-P, Xyntha*)

Contraindications and cautions

- Contraindicated with antibodies to mouse, hamster, or bovine proteins or to porcine or murine factor.
- Use cautiously with pregnancy.

Available forms

IV injection—250, 500, 1,000, 1,500, 2,000, 3,000 international units/vial in numerous preparations

Dosages

Adult and pediatric patients

Administer IV using a plastic syringe; dose depends on weight, severity of deficiency, and severity of bleeding. Follow treatment carefully with factor VIII level assays.

Formulas used as a guide for dosage are:

$$\text{Expected Factor VIII increase (\% of normal)} = \frac{\text{AHF/IU given} \times 2}{\text{weight in kg}}$$

$$\text{AHF/IU required} = \text{weight (kg)} \times \text{desired factor VIII increase (\% of normal)} \times 0.5$$

- *Prophylaxis of spontaneous hemorrhage:* Level of factor VIII required to prevent spontaneous hemorrhage is 5% of normal; 30% of normal is the minimum required for hemostasis following trauma or surgery; smaller doses may be needed if treated early. *ReFacto* is given at least two times per wk for short-term prevention or to decrease the frequency of spontaneous musculoskeletal hemorrhage in patients with hemophilia.
- *Mild hemorrhage:* Do not repeat therapy unless further bleeding occurs.
- *Moderate hemorrhage or minor surgery:* 30%–50% of normal is desired for factor VIII levels; initial dose of 15–25 AHF/international units/kg with maintenance dose of 10–15 AHF/international units/kg every 8–12 hr is usually sufficient.
- *Severe hemorrhage:* Factor VIII level of 80%–100% normal is desired; initial dose of 40–50 AHF/international units/kg and a maintenance dose of 20–25 AHF/international units/kg is given every 8–12 hr.
- *Major surgery:* Dose of AHF to achieve factor VIII levels of 80%–100% of normal given an hour before surgery; repeat infusions may be necessary every 6–12 hr initially. Maintain factor VIII levels at at least 30% normal for a healing period of 10–14 days.
- *Surgery/invasive procedures:* Preoperative dose 60 international units/kg; infusion of 40–60 international units/kg at 8- to 12-hr intervals. *Children:* 75 international units/kg preoperatively; then 50–75 international units/kg infused at 8- to 12-hr intervals (*Alphanate*).
- *Dental extraction:* Factor VIII level of 60%–80% is recommended; administer 1 hr before procedure in combination with antifibrinolytic therapy.
- *Prevention of bleeding during and after surgery in patients with von Willebrand's disease:* 50–60 international units/kg IV loading dose for emergency surgery. For planned surgery, calculate as above and give 2 hr before surgery; repeat every 8–12 hr for up to 3 days (*Humate-P*).

A

Pharmacokinetics

Route	Onset
IV	Immediate

Metabolism: $T_{1/2}$: 12 hr
Distribution: Does not readily cross placenta
Excretion: Cleared from the body by normal metabolism

IV FACTS

Preparation: Reconstitute using solution provided. Refrigerate unreconstituted preparations. Before reconstitution, warm diluent and dried concentrate to room temperature. Add diluent and rotate or shake vial until completely dissolved. Do not refrigerate reconstituted preparations; give within 3 hr of reconstitution.
Infusion: Give by IV only; use a plastic syringe; solutions may stick to glass. Give preparations at a rate of 2 mL/min; can be given at up to 10 mL/min; administration of entire dose in 5–10 min is generally well tolerated.

Adverse effects

- **Allergic reactions:** Erythema, hives, fever, backache, **bronchospasm,** urticaria, chills, nausea, *stinging at the infusion site,* vomiting, headache
- **Hematologic:** Hemolysis with large or frequently repeated doses
- **Other: Hepatitis, AIDS** (risks associated with repeated use of blood products)

■ Nursing considerations

Assessment

- **History:** Antibodies to mouse, hamster, or bovine protein; porcine or murine factor; von Willebrand's disease; pregnancy
- **Physical:** Skin color, lesions; P, peripheral perfusion; R, adventitious sounds; factor VIII levels, Hct, direct Coombs' test, HIV screening, hepatitis screening

Interventions

- Monitor pulse during administration; if a significant increase occurs, reduce the rate or discontinue and consult physician.
- Monitor patient's clinical response and factor VIII levels regularly; if no response is noted with large doses, consider the presence of factor VIII inhibitors and need for anti-inhibitor complex therapy.

Teaching points

- Dosage is highly variable. All known safety precautions are taken to ensure that this blood product is pure and the risk of AIDS and hepatitis is as minimal as possible.
- Wear or carry a medical alert ID tag to alert medical emergency personnel that you require this treatment.
- Report headache; rash, itching; backache; difficulty breathing.

antihemophilic factor, recombinant

See Appendix W, *Less commonly used drugs*.

antithrombin, recombinant

See Appendix W, *Less commonly used drugs*.

antithrombin III

See Appendix W, *Less commonly used drugs*.

apomorphine

See Appendix W, *Less commonly used drugs*.

aprepitant

*(ah **pre'** pit ant)*

Emend

fosaprepitant

Emend for Injection

PREGNANCY CATEGORY B

Drug classes

Antiemetic
Substance P and neurokinin 1 receptor antagonist

Therapeutic actions

Selectively blocks human substance P and neurokinin 1 (NK1) receptors in the CNS, blocking the nausea and vomiting caused by highly emetogenic chemotherapeutic agents. Does not affect serotonin, dopamine, or corticosteroid receptors.

Indications

- In combination with other antiemetics for prevention of acute and delayed nausea and vomiting associated with initial and repeat courses of moderately or highly emetogenic cancer chemotherapy, including high-dose cisplatin
- Prevention of postoperative nausea and vomiting

Contraindications and cautions

- Contraindicated with hypersensitivity to any component of aprepitant, concurrent use of pimozide, lactation.
- Use cautiously with concomitant use of any CYP3A4 inhibitors (docetaxel, vinblastine, vincristine, ifosfamide, irinotecen, imatinib, vinorelbine, paclitaxel, etoposide), warfarin and with pregnancy, severe hepatic impairment.

Available forms

Capsules—40, 80, 125 mg; powder for injection—115 mg (fosaprepitant)

Dosages

Adults

- *Highly emetogenic cancer chemotherapy.* 125 mg PO 1 hr prior to chemotherapy (day 1) and 80 mg PO once daily in the morning on days 2 and 3; given in combination with 12 mg dexamethasone PO 30 min before chemotherapy on day 1 and 8 mg dexamethasone PO days 2 to 4 and 32 mg ondansetron IV on day 1 only.
- *Moderately emetogenic cancer chemotherapy:* 125 mg PO 1 hr before chemotherapy on day 1 with 12 mg dexamethasone PO and two 8-mg doses ondansetron PO (the first 1 hr before, the second 8 hr after chemotherapy); 80 mg PO on days 2 and 3 in the morning.
- *Postopereative nausea and vomiting:* 40 mg PO within 3 hr before induction of anesthesia.

Pediatric patients

Safety and efficacy not established.

- *Parenteral administration (fosaprepitant):* 115 mg IV 30 min before chemotherapy on day 1 of antiemetic regimen; infuse over 15 min. Use oral form on days 2 and 3.

Pharmacokinetics

Route	Onset	Peak
Oral	Rapid	4 hr

Metabolism: Hepatic metabolism, $T_{1/2}$: 9–13 hr
Distribution: Crosses placenta; enters breast milk
Excretion: Feces, urine

IV FACTS

Preparation: Inject 5 mL 0.9% sodium chloride along vial wall to prevent foaming. Swirl vial gently. Add to infusion bag containing 110 mL saline; gently invert bag two to three times. Drug is stable for 24 hr at room temperature.
Infusion: Infuse over 15 min.
Incompatibilities: Do not mix with other solutions; do not mix with divalent cations such as lactated Ringer's solution or Hartmann's solution.

Adverse effects

- **CNS:** Dizziness, *anorexia,* neuropathy, tinnitus, headache, insomnia, asthenia
- **GI:** *Constipation, diarrhea,* epigastric discomfort, gastritis, heartburn, *nausea,* vomiting, elevated ALT or AST, abdominal pain, stomatitis
- **Respiratory:** Hiccups
- **Other:** *Fatigue,* dehydration, fever, neutropenia

Interactions

✱ **Drug-drug** • Risk of increased serum levels and toxic effects of aprepitant and pimozide if combined; do not use this combination • Possible increased serum levels of docetaxel, paclitaxel, etoposide, irinotecan, ifosfamide, imatinib, vinorelbine, vinblastine, vincristine, paclitaxel; monitor patient very closely if this combination is used • Increased risk of decreased effectiveness of warfarin if combined with aprepitant; monitor patient closely and adjust warfarin dose as needed • Risk of decreased effectiveness of hormonal contraceptives if combined with aprepitant; suggest using barrier contraceptives while aprepitant is being used • Risk of altered response when aprepitant is combined with any drug that inhibits CYP3A4; use caution when adding any drug to a regimen that contains aprepitant

■ Nursing considerations

Assessment

- **History:** Hypersensitivity to any component of aprepitant, concurrent use of pimozide; lactation, concomitant use of any CYP3A4 inhibitors; pregnancy
- **Physical:** T, orientation, reflexes, affect; bowel sounds; LFT, CBC

Interventions

- Administer first dose along with dexamethasone 1 hr before beginning of chemotherapy.
- Administer additional doses of dexamethasone as well as ondansetron as indicated as part of antiemetic regimen.
- Administer within 3 hr before induction of anesthesia if used to prevent postoperative nausea and vomiting.
- Establish safety precautions (eg, side rails, assistance with ambulation, proper lighting) if CNS, visual effects occur.
- Provide appropriate analgesics for headache if needed.
- Suggest the use of barrier contraceptives to women of childbearing age.

Teaching points

- When giving drug to prevent postoperative nausea and vomiting, incorporate teaching into overall teaching plan.
- This drug is given as part of a drug regimen to alleviate the nausea and vomiting associated with your chemotherapy drug; take the first dose 1 hour before your chemotherapy and then again in the morning of days 2 and 3; you will also be taking dexamethasone and, possibly, ondansetron with this drug.
- If you miss a dose, take the drug as soon as you think of it. If you miss an entire day, consult your health care provider. Do not take two doses in the same day.
- You should avoid getting pregnant while receiving chemotherapy. Using barrier contraceptives is advised; hormonal contraceptives may be ineffective while you are taking *Emend.*
- If you are nursing a baby, another method of feeding the baby should be used.
- Tell any health care provider who is taking care of you that you are taking this drug—it may react with many other drugs; you should not add or remove any drugs from your medical regimen without checking with your health care provider.
- You may experience these side effects: Dizziness, drowsiness (if these occur, use caution if driving or performing tasks that require alertness); constipation; headache (appropriate medication will be arranged to alleviate this problem).
- Report changes in color of urine or stool, severe constipation or diarrhea, severe headache.

▽arformoterol tartrate

*(ar for **moh'** ter ol)*

Brovana

PREGNANCY CATEGORY C

Drug classes

Beta$_2$-adrenergic agonist, long-acting
Bronchodilator

Therapeutic actions

Long-acting agonist that binds to beta$_2$-adrenergic receptors in the lungs, causing bronchodilation; also inhibits release of inflammatory mediators in the lung, blocking swelling and inflammation.

Indications

- Long-term maintenance treatment of bronchoconstriction in patients with COPD, including chronic bronchitis and emphysema

Contraindications and cautions

- Contraindicated with allergy to any component of the drug, acutely deteriorating COPD, acute bronchospasm.

- Use cautiously with CV disease, convulsive disorders, thyrotoxicosis, pregnancy, lactation.

Available forms
Inhalation solution—15 mcg/2 mL

Dosages
Adults
15 mcg bid (morning and evening) by nebulization. Do not exceed total daily dose of 30 mcg.
Pediatric patients
Safety and efficacy not established.

Pharmacokinetics

Route	*Onset*	*Peak*
Inhalation	Rapid	1 hour

Metabolism: Direct conjugation; $T_{1/2}$: 26 hr
Distribution: Crosses placenta; may pass into breast milk
Excretion: Urine

Adverse effects
- **CV:** Hypertension, prolonged QT interval, tachycardia, chest pain, peripheral edema
- **GI:** Diarrhea
- **Musculoskeletal:** Leg cramps
- **Respiratory: Paradoxical bronchospasm,** dyspnea, chest congestion, sinusitis, **increase in asthma-related deaths**
- **Skin:** Rash
- **Other:** Pain, flulike symptoms

Interactions
✱ **Drug-drug** • Potential for increased toxicity if combined with MAOIs, TCAs, drugs that prolong the QT interval; use caution • Risk for decreased therapeutic effects and severe bronchospasm if combined with beta-adrenergic blockers; avoid this combination if at all possible; use a beta-specific blocker if combination must be used • Increased risk of hypokalemia if combined with non–potassium-sparing diuretics

■ Nursing considerations
Assessment
- **History:** Allergy to any component of the drug, acutely deteriorating COPD, acute bronchospasm, CV disease, convulsive disorders, thyrotoxicosis, pregnancy, lactation
- **Physical:** Skin color, lesions; R, adventitious sounds; P, BP, baseline ECG

Interventions
⊗ ***Black box warning*** Long-lasting beta agonists may increase risk for asthma-related death.
- Ensure that drug is not used to treat acute attacks or worsening or deteriorating COPD.
- Instruct patient in the proper use of nebulizer; instruct patient not to swallow or inject solution.
- Ensure that patient continues with appropriate use of other drugs to manage COPD as instructed.
- Store foil pouches in the refrigerator; use immediately after opening.
- Arrange for periodic evaluation of respiratory condition while on this drug.

Teaching points
- This drug is not for use during an acute attack, use your rescue medication if you are having an acute problem.
- You should take this drug through your nebulizer in the morning and in the evening.
- You should be aware that this type of drug is associated with an increased risk of asthma-related deaths; you should discuss this with your health care provider.
- Use this drug in your nebulizer only; do not swallow or inject this solution.
- The foil pouches should be stored in the refrigerator and protected from heat and light. Do not use after the expiration date. Use immediately after opening the foil pouch.
- Do not use any solution that is discolored or contains particles.
- Arrange for periodic evaluation of your respiratory problem while on this drug.
- It is not known if this drug could affect a fetus. If you are pregnant, or are thinking about becoming pregnant, consult with your health care provider.
- It is not known how this drug could affect a nursing baby; discuss the use of this drug during lactation with your health care provider.

- You should continue to use other medications prescribed for the treatment of your COPD as directed by your health care provider.
- Report palpitations, worsening of your COPD, tremors, nervousness.

argatroban

See Appendix W, *Less commonly used drugs*.

aripiprazole

(air eh ***pip'*** *rah zole)*

Abilify, Abilify Discmelt

PREGNANCY CATEGORY C

Drug classes

Atypical antipsychotic
Dopamine, serotonin agonist and antagonist
Psychotropic drug

Therapeutic actions

Acts as an agonist at dopamine and serotonin sites and antagonist at other serotonin receptor sites; this combination of actions is thought to be responsible for the drug's effectiveness in treating schizophrenia, though the mechanism of action is not understood.

Indications

- Treatment of schizophrenia in patients 13 yr and older
- Treatment of major depressive disorder as adjunct to antidepressant therapy
- Treatment and maintenance of acute manic and mixed episodes associated with bipolar disorders in patients 10 yr and older
- Adjunct to lithium or valproate for acute treatment of manic or mixed episodes associated with bipolar disorder in patients 10 yr and older
- Treatment of agitation associated with schizophrenia or bipolar disorder, manic or mixed (injection)
- Unlabeled use: Restless leg syndrome

Contraindications and cautions

- Contraindicated with allergy to aripiprazole, lactation.
- Use cautiously with suicidal ideation, pregnancy, cerebral vascular disease or other conditions causing hypotension, known CV disease, seizure disorders, exposure to extreme heat, Alzheimer's disease, dysphagia (risk for aspiration pneumonia), parkinsonism, elderly patients with dementia-related psychosis.

Available forms

Tablets—2, 5, 10, 15, 20, 30 mg; oral solution—1 mg/mL; orally disintegrating tablets—10, 15 mg; injection—7.5 mg/mL

Dosages

Adults

- *Schizophrenia:* 10–15 mg/day PO. Increase dose every 2 wk to maximum of 30 mg/day. Oral solution may be substituted on a mg-to-mg basis up to 25 mg of tablet. Patients taking 30-mg tablets should receive 25 mg if switched to solution.
- *Bipolar disorder:* 30 mg/day PO as one dose; maintenance dosage 15 mg/day PO. Oral solution may be substituted on a mg-to-mg basis to 25 mg. Patients taking 30-mg tablets should take 25 mg if switched to solution.
- *Major depressive disorder:* 2–15 mg/day as adjunct therapy. Dose adjustments up to 5 mg/day should occur at intervals of 1 wk or longer.
- *Agitation:* 5.25–15 mg IM; usual dose, 9.75 mg IM. Cumulative doses of up to 30 mg/day may be given.

Pediatric patients 13–17 yr

- *Schizophrenia:* Initially, 2 mg/day PO. Adjust to 5 mg/day after 2 days then to target dosage of 10 mg/day. Maximum, 30 mg/day.

Pediatric patients 10–17 yr

- *Bipolar disorder:* Initially, 2 mg/day; titrate to 5 mg/day after 2 days, then to 10 mg/day after another 2 days. Target dose, 10 mg/day; maximum dose, 30 mg/day.

Pharmacokinetics

Route	Onset	Peak
Oral	Slow	3–5 hr
IM	Rapid	1–3 hr

Metabolism: Hepatic; $T_{1/2}$: 75 hr for extensive metabolizers and 146 hr for poor metabolizers

Distribution: May cross placenta; may enter breast milk
Excretion: Urine and feces

Adverse effects

- **CNS:** Headache, anxiety, insomnia, lightheadedness, somnolence, tremor, asthenia, tardive dyskinesia, blurred vision, **seizures (potentially life-threatening),** akathisia, dizziness, restlessness
- **CV:** Orthostatic hypotension
- **Dermatologic:** Rash
- **GI:** Nausea, vomiting, constipation, diarrhea, abdominal pain, esophageal dysmotility
- **Respiratory:** Rhinitis, cough
- **Other:** Fever, **neuroleptic malignant syndrome, increased suicide risk,** development of diabetes mellitus

Interactions

✱ **Drug-drug** • Risk of serious toxic effects if combined with strong inhibitors of the CYP3A4 system (such as ketoconazole), if any of these drug are being used, initiate treatment with one-half the usual dose of aripiprazole and monitor patient closely • Potential for increased serum levels and toxicity if taken with potential CYP2D6 inhibitors—quinidine, fluoxetine, paroxetine; reduce the dose of aripiprazole to one-half the normal dose • Decreased serum levels and loss of effectiveness if combined with CYP3A4 inducers such as carbamazepine—dosage of aripiprazole should be doubled and the patient monitored closely • Risk of severe sedation, orthostatic hypotension if IM aripiprazole is combined with lorazepam injection • Risk of increased CNS depression and impairment if combined with alcohol or other CNS depressants

■ Nursing considerations

CLINICAL ALERT!
Reports have been noted of confusion of aripiprazole with proton pump inhibitors; use extreme caution.

Assessment

- **History:** Allergy to aripiprazole, lactation, suicidal ideation, pregnancy, hypotension or known CV disease, seizure disorders, exposure to extreme heat, patients with Alzheimer's disease, dysphagia, parkinsonism
- **Physical:** T, orientation, reflexes, vision; BP; R; abdominal examination

Interventions

⊠ ***Black box warning*** Elderly patients with dementia-related psychosis have an increased risk of death if given atypical antipsychotics; these drugs are not approved for treating patients with dementia-related psychosis.

⊠ ***Black box warning*** Risk of suicidal ideation increases with antidepressant drug use, especially in children, adolescents, and young adults. Observe and monitor patient accordingly.

- Dispense the least amount of drug possible to patients with suicidal ideation.
- Have patient place orally disintegrating tablet on tongue, allow to dissolve, then swallow.
- Protect patient from extremes of heat; monitor BP if overheating occurs.
- Administer drug once a day without regard to food.
- Establish baseline orientation and affect before beginning therapy.
- Ensure that patient is well hydrated while taking this drug.
- Monitor patient regularly for signs and symptoms of diabetes mellitus.
- Establish appropriate safety precautions if patient experiences adverse CNS effects.
- If a breast-feeding patient is taking this drug, suggest another method of feeding the baby.
- Advise women of childbearing age to use contraceptives while taking this drug.
- Consider switching to oral solution for patients who have difficulty swallowing.

Teaching points

- Take this drug once a day as prescribed. If you forget a dose, take the next dose as soon as you remember and then resume taking the drug the next day. Do not take more than one dose in any 24-hour period.
- If taking orally disintegrating tablet, place the tablet on your tongue, allow to dissolve,

and then swallow. It is recommended that you use no liquid to take the tablet; if you do use liquid, use the smallest amount possible.

- This drug may interact with many other medications and with alcohol. Alert any health care provider caring for you that you are taking this drug.
- This drug should not be taken during pregnancy or when nursing a baby; using barrier contraceptives is suggested.
- Make sure that you are well hydrated while taking this drug.
- You may experience these side effects: Dizziness, impaired thinking and motor coordination (use caution and avoid driving a car or performing other tasks that require alertness if you experience these effects); inability to cool body effectively (avoid extremes of heat, heavy exercise, dehydration while using this drug).
- Report severe dizziness, trembling, lightheadedness, suicidal thoughts, blurred vision.

armodafinil

(are moe ***daff'*** *ih nill)*

Nuvigil

PREGNANCY CATEGORY C

CONTROLLED SUBSTANCE C-IV

Drug class

CNS stimulant
Narcolepsy drug

Therapeutic actions

A CNS stimulant that helps to improve vigilance and decrease excessive daytime sleepiness associated with narcolepsy and other sleep disorders. May act through dopaminergic mechanisms; exact mechanism of action is not known. Not associated with the cardiac and other systemic stimulatory effects of amphetamines.

Indications

- To improve wakefulness in patients with excessive sleepiness associated with obstructive sleep apnea/hypopnea syndrome, narcolepsy, and shift work sleep disorder

Contraindications and cautions

- Contraindicated with known hypersensitivity to any component of the drug or to modafinil.
- Use cautiously with a history of psychosis, depression, mania; pregnancy, lactation; history of drug abuse or dependence.

Available forms

Tablets—50, 150, 250 mg

Dosages

Adults

- *Obstructive sleep apnea/hypopnea syndrome, narcolepsy:* 150–250 mg/day PO as a single dose in the morning.
- *Shift work sleep disorder:* 150 mg/day PO taken 1 hr before start of work shift.

Patients with severe hepatic impairment, elderly patients

Consider use of a lower dose.

Pharmacokinetics

Route	*Onset*	*Peak*
Oral	Rapid	2 hr

Metabolism: Hepatic; $T_{1/2}$: 15 hr
Distribution: May cross placenta; may enter breast milk
Excretion: Urine

Adverse effects

- **CNS:** *Headache, dizziness, insomnia,* disturbance in attention, tremor, paresthesia, anxiety, depression, agitation, nervousness
- **CV:** Tachycardia, chest pain, palpitations
- **Dermatologic:** Dermatitis, **Stevens-Johnson syndrome,** rash
- **GI:** *Nausea,* diarrhea, dry mouth, dyspepsia, constipation, vomiting, anorexia
- **GU:** Polyuria
- **Respiratory:** Dyspnea
- **Other:** Fatigue, pyrexia, flulike symptoms, dependence

Interactions

✱ **Drug-drug** • Possible decreased effectiveness of hormonal contraceptives during and up to 1 month after treatment; suggest use of barrier contraceptive • Risk of increased levels and effects of warfarin, phenytoin, omeprazole, TCAs; dosage adjustment may be needed

• Risk of decreased levels and effectiveness of cyclosporine, ethinyl estradiol, midazolam, triazolam; dosage adjustment may be needed

■ Nursing considerations

Assessment

- **History:** Hypersensitivity to any component of the drug or to modafinil, history of drug abuse or dependence, psychosis, depression, pregnancy, lactation
- **Physical:** T; skin color, lesions; orientation, affect, reflexes; bowel sounds; LFTs

Interventions

- Ensure proper diagnosis before administering drug to rule out underlying medical problems.
- Drug therapy should be part of a comprehensive program to include measures to improve sleep patterns.
- Administer once a day in the morning for narcolepsy or sleep apnea disorders; for shift work sleep disorders, have patient take tablet approximately 1 hour before shift begins.
- Establish safety precautions if CNS changes occur (dizziness, changes in thought process).

Teaching points

- This drug is a controlled substance with abuse potential; keep it in a secure place. It is illegal to sell or give this drug to other people.
- This drug should be part of an overall plan, including measures to improve your sleep habits. It is not a substitute for sleep.
- Your health care provider will run tests to accurately diagnose your sleep disorder.
- Take only your prescribed dose. Do not change your dosage or the time of day you are taking the drug without consulting your health care provider.
- Take your dose once each day in the morning if you have sleep apnea or narcolepsy. If you have shift work sleep disorder, take it 1 hour before your shift begins.
- Avoid drinking alcohol while you are taking this drug.
- This drug can decrease the effectiveness of hormonal contraceptives. The use of a barrier contraceptive is advised while you are taking this drug and for 1 month after you have stopped the drug.
- It is not known how this drug could affect a developing fetus. If you are pregnant or you wish to become pregnant, discuss this with your health care provider.
- It is not known how this drug could affect a nursing baby. if you are nursing a baby, consult with your health care provider.
- You may experience these side effects: dizziness, insomnia, nervousness, impaired thinking (do not drive a car or engage in activities that require alertness if these effects occur); headache (consult with your health care provider for possible medication to relieve this).
- Report rash; hives; peeling skin blisters; swelling of the face, eyes, lips, tongue, or throat; trouble swallowing or breathing; hoarse voice; chest pain or palpitations; thoughts of suicide; hallucinations; depression; or anxiety.

▽arsenic trioxide

See Appendix W, *Less commonly used drugs*.

▽asenapine

*(ah **sin'** ah peen)*

Saphris

PREGNANCY CATEGORY C

Drug classes

Atypical antipsychotic
Dopamine/serotonin antagonist

Therapeutic actions

Mechanism of action not fully understood; blocks dopamine and serotonin receptors in the brain and depresses the reticular activating system. Suppresses many of the negative aspects of schizophrenia, including blunted affect, social withdrawal, lack of motivation, and anger.

Indications

- Acute treatment of schizophrenia in adults
- Acute treatment of manic or mixed episodes associated with bipolar I disorder in adults

Contraindications and cautions

- Contraindicated with known hypersensitivity to any component of drug, pregnancy, lactation.

- Use cautiously in prolonged QT interval, history of seizures, diabetes, suicidal ideation.

Available forms

Sublingual tablets–5, 10 mg

Dosages

Adults

Schizophrenia: 5 mg sublingually bid
Bipolar disorder: 10 mg sublingually bid; may be decreased to 5 mg/day if needed

Pediatric patients

Safety and efficacy not established

Patients with hepatic impairment

Not recommended for patients with severe hepatic impairment, Child-Pugh C

Pharmacokinetics

Route	*Onset*	*Peak*
Sublingual	Rapid	30–90 min

Metabolism: Hepatic: $T_{1/2}$: 24 hr
Distribution: May cross placenta; may enter breast milk
Excretion: Urine and feces

Adverse effects

- **CNS:** *Dizziness, somnolence, extrapyramidal disorders, akathisia,* tremor, lethargy, blurred vision, altered thinking
- **CV:** Orthostatic hypotension, hypotension, tachycardia, prolonged QT interval
- **GI:** *Nausea,* diarrhea, dry mouth, abdominal discomfort
- **GU:** Priapism, ejaculation failure
- **Respiratory:** URI, nasal pharyngitis
- **Other:** Fatigue, lethargy, bone marrow suppression, **neuroleptic malignant syndrome (NMS),** hyperglycemia, *weight gain,* gynecomastia, galactorrhea

Interactions

✱ **Drug-drug** • Increased risk of serious cardiac arrhythmias if taken with other drugs that prolong QT interval; avoid this combination. If combination must be used, monitor patient carefully • Risk of increased effectiveness of antihypertensives if used in combination; monitor patient closely and adjust antihypertensive dosage as needed • Risk of increased CNS effects if combined with centrally acting drugs or alcohol; use caution if this combination is used • Increased risk of toxic effects of both drugs if combined with fluvoxamine; use caution

■ Nursing considerations

Assessment

- **History:** Hypersensitivity to any component of drug; pregnancy, lactation; prolonged QT interval; history of seizures; diabetes; suicidal ideation
- **Physical:** Weight; orientation, affect, reflexes; BP, P; abdominal exam; liver evaluation (LFTs); ECG, CBC, blood glucose level

Interventions

⊗ ***Black box warning*** Risk of death increases if used in elderly patients with dementia-related psychosis. Do not use for these patients; drug not approved for this use.

- Obtain baseline ECG to rule out prolonged QT interval; monitor patient periodically throughout therapy.
- Place tablet under the tongue and allow to dissolve completely, which should occur within seconds. Tell patient not to swallow tablet. Ensure that patient avoids eating and drinking for 10 minutes after administration.
- Monitor patient regularly for signs and symptoms of increased blood glucose level.
- Provide safety measures, especially early in treatment, if orthostatic hypotension occurs.
- Advise patient who is nursing to select another method of feeding the baby.
- Monitor patient for signs and symptoms of NMS (high fever, muscle rigidity, altered mental status, high or low blood pressure, diaphoresis, tachycardia); discontinue drug and support patient if these occur. Carefully consider reintroduction of drug because NMS recurrence is likely.
- Provide safety measures as needed if patient develops extrapyramidal effects or orthostatic hypotension.
- Be aware that patient may experience changes in cognitive and motor function.
- Because of risk of suicidal ideation with treatment, limit amount of drug dispensed to the smallest effective amount, to decrease chances of overdose.
- Continue other measures being used to deal with schizophrenia or bipolar disorder.

Teaching points

- Take this drug once a day, exactly as prescribed.
- If you miss a dose, take the next dose as soon as you remember. Do not take more than the prescribed amount each day.
- Avoid alcohol while taking this drug. Tell your health care provider about any other drugs, over-the-counter drugs, or herbal therapies that you are using; serious drug interactions are possible.
- If you are diabetic, monitor your blood glucose level very carefully and adjust treatment as ordered.
- It is not known how this drug could affect a fetus. If you should become pregnant while taking this drug, consult your health care provider.
- It is not known how this drug could affect a nursing baby. Because of the potential for serious adverse effects in an infant, you should use another method of feeding the baby while you are taking this drug.
- This drug may cause your blood pressure to fall when you stand up; this is called orthostatic hypotension.
- Use care when standing or changing positions, especially when starting the drug and when changing dosage.
- You may experience the following side effects: dizziness, changes in motor performance and impaired thinking (do not drive a car or engage in activities that require alertness if these effects occur), nausea, dry mouth (small frequent meals may help; sucking sugarless lozenges may also be helpful).
- Report fever accompanied by sweating, changes in mental status, muscle rigidity; heart palpitations; feeling faint; loss of consciousness; thoughts of suicide.

DANGEROUS DRUG

▽asparaginase

*(a **spare'** a gi nase)*

Elspar

PREGNANCY CATEGORY C

Drug class

Antineoplastic

Therapeutic actions

Asparaginase is an enzyme that hydrolyzes the amino acid asparagine, which is needed by some malignant cells (but not normal cells) for protein synthesis; it inhibits malignant cell proliferation by interruption of protein synthesis; maximal effect in G1 phase of the cell cycle.

Indications

- To induce remissions in children or adults with acute lymphocytic leukemia as combination therapy or as single agent when combined therapy is inappropriate or when other therapies fail

Contraindications and cautions

- Contraindicated with allergy to asparaginase, pancreatitis or history of pancreatitis, impaired hepatic function, bone marrow depression, lactation.
- Use cautiously with hyperglycemia, pregnancy, bleeding disorders, or immunosuppressed patients.

Available forms

Powder for injection—10,000 international units

Dosages

Adults and pediatric patients

- *Single-agent induction therapy:* Used only when combined therapy is inappropriate or when other therapies fail; 200 international units/kg/day IV for 28 days. Perform test dose before starting therapy.

Pediatric patients

- *Induction regimen I:* Prednisone 40 mg/m^2 per day PO in three divided doses for 15 days, followed by tapering of dosage as follows: 20 mg/m^2 for 2 days, 10 mg/m^2 for 2 days, 5 mg/m^2 for 2 days, 2.5 mg/m^2 for 2 days, and then discontinue. Vincristine sulfate 2 mg/m^2 IV once weekly on days 1, 8, 15; maximum dose should not exceed 2 mg. Asparaginase 1,000 international units/kg/day IV for 10 successive days beginning on day 22.
- *Induction regimen II:* Prednisone 40 mg/m^2 per day PO in three divided doses for 28 days, then gradually discontinue over 14 days.

Vincristine sulfate 1.5 mg/m^2 IV weekly for four doses on days 1, 8, 15, 22; maximum dose should not exceed 2 mg. Asparaginase 6,000 international units/m^2 IM on days 4, 7, 10, 13, 16, 19, 22, 25, 28.
- *Maintenance:* When remission is obtained, institute maintenance therapy; do not use asparaginase in maintenance regimen.

Pharmacokinetics

Route	*Onset*	*Peak*
IM	Varies	Unknown
IV	30–40 min	End of infusion

Metabolism: $T_{1/2}$: 8–30 hr
Distribution: Crosses placenta; may enter breast milk
Excretion: Urine

IV FACTS

Preparation: Reconstitute vial with 5 mL of sterile water for injection or sodium chloride injection. Ordinary shaking does not inactivate the drug. May be used for direct IV injection or further diluted with sodium chloride injection or 5% dextrose injection. Stable for 8 hr once reconstituted; use only when clear. Discard any cloudy solution. Gelatinous, fiber-like particles may develop with standing; filter through a 5-micron filter if desired; do not use a 0.2-micron filter because drug may lose potency.
Infusion: Infuse over not less than 30 min into an already running IV infusion of sodium chloride injection or 5% dextrose injection.

Adverse effects

- **CNS:** CNS depression, confusion, agitation, hallucinations, somnolence
- **Endocrine:** Hyperglycemia—glucosuria, polyuria
- **GI:** *Hepatotoxicity, nausea, vomiting, anorexia,* abdominal cramps, pancreatitis
- **GU:** Uric acid nephropathy, **renal toxicity**
- **Hematologic:** Bleeding problems, **bone marrow depression,** thrombosis
- **Hypersensitivity:** *Rashes, urticaria, arthralgia,* respiratory distress to **anaphylaxis**
- **Other:** Chills, fever, weight loss, **hyperthermia,** fatigue

Interactions

✱ **Drug-drug** • Increased toxicity if given IV with or immediately before vincristine or prednisone • Diminished or decreased effect of methotrexate on malignant cells if given with or immediately after asparaginase
✱ **Drug-lab test** • Inaccurate interpretation of thyroid-function tests because of decreased serum levels of thyroxine-binding globulin; levels usually return to pretreatment levels within 4 wk of the last dose of asparaginase

■ Nursing considerations

Assessment

- **History:** Allergy to asparaginase, pancreatitis or history of pancreatitis, impaired hepatic function, bone marrow depression, lactation, hyperglycemia, pregnancy, bleeding disorders
- **Physical:** Weight; T; skin color, lesions; orientation, reflexes; liver evaluation, abdominal examination; CBC, blood sugar, LFTs, renal function tests, serum amylase, clotting time, urinalysis, serum uric acid levels

Interventions

⊗ ***Black box warning*** Administer only in a hospital setting; be prepared to treat anaphylaxis with each dose.
⊗ ***Warning*** Perform an intradermal skin test prior to initial administration and if there is a week or more between doses because of risk of severe hypersensitivity reactions. To prepare skin test solution, reconstitute 10,000-international units vial with 5 mL of diluent; withdraw 0.1 mL (200 international units/mL), and inject it into a vial containing 9.9 mL of diluent, giving a solution of 20 international units/mL. Use 0.1 mL of this solution (2 international units) for the skin test. Observe site for 1 hr for a wheal or erythema that indicates allergic reaction.
- Arrange for desensitization to hypersensitivity reaction. Check manufacturer's literature for desensitization dosages, or arrange for patient to receive *Erwinia* asparaginase

(available from the National Cancer Institute).

- Arrange for lab tests (CBC, serum amylase, blood glucose, LFT, uric acid) prior to therapy and frequently during therapy; arrange to decrease dose or stop drug if severe adverse effects occur.
- For IM administration, reconstitute by adding 2 mL of sodium chloride injection to the 10,000-international units vial. Stable for 8 hr once reconstituted; use only if clear. Limit injections at each site to 2 mL; if more is required use two injection sites.

⊗ ***Warning*** Monitor for signs of hypersensitivity (eg, rash, difficulty breathing). If any occur, discontinue drug and consult with physician.

⊗ ***Warning*** Monitor for pancreatitis; if serum amylase levels rise, discontinue drug and consult with physician.

⊗ ***Warning*** Monitor for hyperglycemia—reaction may resemble hyperosmolar, nonketotic hyperglycemia. If present, discontinue drug and be ready to use IV fluids and insulin.

- Prepare a calendar for patients who must return for specific treatments and additional therapy.

Teaching points

- Use a calendar to keep track of appointments for specific treatments and additional therapy. Drug can be given only in the hospital under the direct supervision of a physician.
- Have regular blood tests to monitor the drug's effects.
- You may experience these side effects: Loss of appetite, nausea, vomiting (frequent mouth care, eat frequent small meals; good nutrition is important; dietary services are available; antiemetic may be ordered); fatigue, confusion, agitation, hallucinations, depression (reversible; use special precautions to avoid injury).
- Report fever, chills, sore throat; unusual bleeding or bruising; yellow skin or eyes; light-colored stools, dark urine; thirst, frequent urination.

▽ aspirin

(ass' pir in)

Aspergum, Bayer, Easprin, Ecotrin, Empirin, Genprin, Halfprin 81, 1/2 Halfprin, Heartline, Norwich, St. Joseph, ZORprin (DNC)

Buffered aspirin products:
Adprin-B, Alka-Seltzer, Ascriptin, Bufferin, Buffex

PREGNANCY CATEGORY D

Drug classes

Analgesic (nonopioid)
Anti-inflammatory
Antiplatelet
Antipyretic
Antirheumatic
NSAID
Salicylate

Therapeutic actions

Analgesic and antirheumatic effects are attributable to aspirin's ability to inhibit the synthesis of prostaglandins, important mediators of inflammation. Antipyretic effects are not fully understood, but aspirin probably acts in the thermoregulatory center of the hypothalamus to block effects of endogenous pyrogen by inhibiting synthesis of the prostaglandin intermediary. Inhibition of platelet aggregation is attributable to the inhibition of platelet synthesis of thromboxane A_2, a potent vasoconstrictor and inducer of platelet aggregation. This effect occurs at low doses and lasts for the life of the platelet (8 days). Higher doses inhibit the synthesis of prostacyclin, a potent vasodilator and inhibitor of platelet aggregation.

Indications

- Mild to moderate pain
- Fever
- Inflammatory conditions—rheumatic fever, rheumatoid arthritis, osteoarthritis, juvenile rheumatoid arthritis, spondyloarthropathies
- Reduction of risk of recurrent TIAs or CVA in patients with history of TIA due to fibrin platelet emboli or ischemic stroke

- Reduction of risk of death or nonfatal MI in patients with history of infarction or unstable angina pectoris or suspected acute MI
- Patients who have undergone revascularization procedures (eg, coronary artery bypass graft [CABG], percutaneous transluminal coronary angioplasty [PTCA], endarterectomy)
- Unlabeled use: Prophylaxis against cataract formation with long-term use

Contraindications and cautions

- Contraindicated with allergy to salicylates or NSAIDs (more common with nasal polyps, asthma, chronic urticaria); allergy to tartrazine (cross-sensitivity to aspirin is common); hemophilia, bleeding ulcers, hemorrhagic states, blood coagulation defects, hypoprothrombinemia, vitamin K deficiency (increased risk of bleeding).
- Use cautiously with impaired renal function; chickenpox, influenza (risk of Reye's syndrome in children and teenagers); children with fever accompanied by dehydration; surgery scheduled within 1 wk; peptic ulcer disease; gout; pregnancy (maternal anemia, antepartal and postpartal hemorrhage, prolonged gestation, and prolonged labor have been reported; readily crosses the placenta; possibly teratogenic; maternal ingestion of aspirin during late pregnancy has been associated with the following adverse fetal effects: low birth weight, increased intracranial hemorrhage, stillbirths, neonatal death); lactation.

Available forms

Tablets—81, 165, 325, 500, 650, 975 mg; SR tablets DNC—650, 800 mg; gum tablets—227.5 mg; suppositories: 120, 200, 300, 600 mg

Dosages

Available in oral and suppository forms. Also available as chewable tablets, gum; enteric coated, SR, and buffered preparations (SR aspirin is not recommended for antipyresis, short-term analgesia, or children younger than 12 yr).

Adults

- *SR forms:* 1,300 mg, then 650–1,300 mg every 8 hr; maximum, 3,900 mg/day.
- *Gum:* Chew 454 mg every 4 hr; do not exceed 3,632 mg/day.
- *Ischemic stroke, TIA:* 50–325 mg/day.
- *Angina, recurrent MI prevention:* 75–325 mg/day.
- *Suspected MI:* 160–325 mg as soon as possible; continue daily for 30 days.
- *CABG:* 325 mg 6 hr after procedure, then daily for 1 yr.
- *PTCA:* 325 mg 2 hr before procedure, then 160–325 mg/day.
- *Carotid endarterectomy:* 80 mg/day–650 mg bid started before the procedure and then continued after the procedure.
- *Spondyloarthritis:* Up to 4 g/day in divided doses.
- *Osteoarthritis:* Up to 3 g/day in divided doses.
- *Minor aches and pains:* 325–1,000 mg every 4–6 hr; maximum 4,000 mg/day.
- *Arthritis and rheumatic conditions:* 3 g/day in divided doses.
- *Acute rheumatic fever:* 5–8 g/day; modify to maintain serum salicylate level of 15–30 mg/dL.

Pediatric patients

- *Analgesic and antipyretic:* 10–15 mg/kg/dose every 4 hr, up to 60–80 mg/kg/day. Do not administer to patients with chickenpox or influenza symptoms.

Age (yr)	*Dosage (mg every 4 hr)*
2–3	162
4–5	243
6–8	324
9–10	405
11	486
12 or older	648

- *Juvenile rheumatoid arthritis:* 90–130 mg/kg per 24 hr in divided doses at 6- to 8-hr intervals. Maintain a serum level of 150–300 mcg/mL.
- *Acute rheumatic fever:* Initially, 100 mg/kg/day, then decrease to 75 mg/kg/day for 4–6 wk. Therapeutic serum salicylate level is 150–300 mcg/mL.
- *Kawasaki disease:* 80–180 mg/kg/day; very high doses may be needed during acute

febrile period; after fever resolves, dosage may be adjusted to 10 mg/kg/day.

Pharmacokinetics

Route	Onset	Peak	Duration
Oral	5–30 min	15–120 min	3–6 hr
Rectal	1–2 hr	4–5 hr	6–8 hr

Metabolism: Hepatic (salicylate); $T_{1/2}$: 15 min–12 hr
Distribution: Crosses placenta; enters breast milk
Excretion: Urine

Adverse effects

- **Acute aspirin toxicity:** Respiratory alkalosis, hyperpnea, tachypnea, hemorrhage, excitement, confusion, asterixis, pulmonary edema, seizures, tetany, metabolic acidosis, fever, coma, CV collapse, renal and respiratory failure (dose related, 20–25 g in adults, 4 g in children)
- **Aspirin intolerance:** Exacerbation of bronchospasm, rhinitis (with nasal polyps, asthma)
- **GI:** *Nausea, dyspepsia, heartburn, epigastric discomfort,* anorexia, hepatotoxicity
- **Hematologic:** *Occult blood loss, hemostatic defects*
- **Hypersensitivity:** Anaphylactoid reactions to anaphylactic shock
- **Salicylism:** *Dizziness, tinnitus, difficulty hearing, nausea,* vomiting, diarrhea, mental confusion, lassitude (dose related)

Interactions

✱ **Drug-drug** • Increased risk of bleeding with oral anticoagulants, heparin • Increased risk of GI ulceration with steroids, alcohol, NSAIDs • Increased serum salicylate levels due to decreased salicylate excretion with urine acidifiers (ammonium chloride, ascorbic acid, methionine) • Increased risk of salicylate toxicity with carbonic anhydrase inhibitors, furosemide • Decreased serum salicylate levels with corticosteroids • Decreased serum salicylate levels due to increased renal excretion of salicylates with acetazolamide, methazolamide, certain antacids, alkalinizers • Decreased absorption of aspirin with nonabsorbable antacids • Increased methotrexate levels and toxicity with aspirin • Increased effects of valproic acid secondary to displacement from plasma protein sites • Greater glucose lowering effect of sulfonylureas, insulin with large doses (more than 2 g/day) of aspirin • Decreased antihypertensive effect of captopril, beta-adrenergic blockers with salicylates; consider discontinuation of aspirin • Decreased uricosuric effect of probenecid, sulfinpyrazone • Possible decreased diuretic effects of spironolactone, furosemide (in patients with compromised renal function) • Unexpected hypotension may occur with nitroglycerin

✱ **Drug-lab test** • Decreased serum protein bound iodine (PBI) due to competition for binding sites • False-negative readings for urine glucose by glucose oxidase method and copper reduction method with moderate to large doses of aspirin • Interference with urine 5-HIAA determinations by fluorescent methods but not by nitrosonaphthol colorimetric method • Interference with urinary ketone determination by the ferric chloride method • Falsely elevated urine VMA levels with most tests; a false decrease in VMA using the Pisano method

■ Nursing considerations

Assessment

- **History:** Allergy to salicylates or NSAIDs; allergy to tartrazine; hemophilia, bleeding ulcers, hemorrhagic states, blood coagulation defects, hypoprothrombinemia, vitamin K deficiency; impaired hepatic function; impaired renal function; chickenpox, influenza; children with fever accompanied by dehydration; surgery scheduled within 1 wk; pregnancy; lactation
- **Physical:** Skin color, lesions; T; eighth cranial nerve function, orientation, reflexes, affect; P, BP, perfusion; R, adventitious sounds; liver evaluation, bowel sounds; CBC, clotting times, urinalysis, stool guaiac, LFTs, renal function tests

Interventions

⊗ ***Black box warning*** Do not use in children and teenagers to treat chickenpox or

flu symptoms without review for Reye's syndrome, a rare but fatal disorder.
- Give drug with food or after meals if GI upset occurs.
- Give drug with full glass of water to reduce risk of tablet or capsule lodging in the esophagus.
- Do not crush, and ensure that patient does not chew SR preparations.
- Do not use aspirin that has a strong vinegar-like odor.

⊗ ***Warning*** Institute emergency procedures if overdose occurs: Gastric lavage, induction of emesis, activated charcoal, supportive therapy.

Teaching points
- Take extra precautions to keep this drug out of the reach of children; this drug can be very dangerous for children.
- Use the drug only as suggested; avoid overdose. Avoid the use of other over-the-counter drugs while taking this drug. Many of these drugs contain aspirin, and serious overdose can occur.
- Take the drug with food or after meals if GI upset occurs.
- Do not cut, crush, or chew sustained-release products.
- Over-the-counter aspirins are equivalent. Price does not reflect effectiveness.
- You may experience these side effects: Nausea, GI upset, heartburn (take drug with food); easy bruising, gum bleeding (related to aspirin's effects on blood clotting).
- Report ringing in the ears; dizziness, confusion; abdominal pain; rapid or difficult breathing; nausea, vomiting, bloody stools.

▽atazanavir sulfate
*(ah **taz'** ah nah veer)*

Reyataz

PREGNANCY CATEGORY B

Drug classes
Anti-HIV drug
Antiviral
Protease inhibitor

Therapeutic actions
HIV-1 protease inhibitor; selectively inhibits processing of viral proteins in HIV-infected cells, preventing the formation of mature viruses.

Indications
- In combination with other antiretrovirals for the treatment of HIV-1 infection

Contraindications and cautions
- Contraindicated with allergy to any components of the product, lactation (HIV-infected mothers are discouraged from breast-feeding).
- Use cautiously with pregnancy; hepatic impairment; signs of lactic acidosis; risk factors for lactic acidosis, including female gender and obesity; hemophilia.

Available forms
Capsules—100, 150, 200, 300 mg

Dosages
Adults

Therapy-naïve patients: 400 mg/day PO, taken with food. If taken with didanosine, give atazanavir with food 2 hr before or 1 hr after the didanosine. If taken with efavirenz, 400 mg/day PO of atazanavir, 100 mg ritonavir and 600 mg efavirenz as a single daily dose with food; atazanavir should not be used with efavirenz without ritonavir. If taken with tenofovir, 300 mg tenofovir PO with 300 mg atazanavir PO and 100 mg ritonavir PO once daily with food.

Therapy-experienced patients: 300 mg/day PO with 100 mg ritonavir PO taken with food.

Concomitant therapy: With histamine-2 (H_2) receptor antagonists, do not exceed equivalent of 40 mg famotidine bid (for therapy-naive patients) or 20 mg famotidine bid (for therapy-experienced patients); administer 300 mg atazanavir with 100 mg ritonavir simultaneously with first dose of H_2-receptor antagonist. Administer second dose of H_2-receptor antagonist 10 hr later. With proton pump inhibitors, do not exceed equivalent of 20 mg omeprazole. Administer 12 hr prior to atazanavir for therapy-naive patients. Do not use proton pump inhibitors in therapy-experienced patients.

Pediatric patients 6–17 yr

Do not exceed recommended adult doses.

Patient type	*Body weight (kg)*	*Atazanavir dose (mg)*	*Ritonavir dose (mg)*
Therapy naïve	15 to less than 25	150	80
	25 to less than 32	200	100
	32 to less than 39	250	100
	39 or more	300	100
Therapy experienced	25 to less than 32	200	100
	32 to less than 39	250	100
	39 or more	300	100

Patients with hepatic impairment

300 mg/day PO with moderate impairment (Child-Pugh class B); do not use with severe hepatic impairment or hepatic insufficiency (Child-Pugh class C).

Patients with renal impairment

No dosage adjustment needed if patient is not on dialysis. Do not use in patients with end-stage renal disease who are on hemodialysis.

Pharmacokinetics

Route	*Onset*	*Peak*
Oral	Rapid	2–2.5 hr

Metabolism: Hepatic; $T_{1/2}$: 6.5–7.9 hr
Distribution: May cross placenta; may enter breast milk
Excretion: Feces, urine

Adverse effects

- **CNS:** *Headache,* depression, insomnia, dizziness, peripheral neurologic symptoms
- **CV:** Prolonged PR interval
- **GI:** *Nausea,* diarrhea, abdominal pain, vomiting, jaundice, **severe hepatomegaly with steatosis, sometimes fatal;** *elevated liver enzymes and bilirubin*
- **Metabolic:** Lactic acidosis, sometimes severe; hyperglycemia
- **Respiratory:** Cough
- **Other:** *Rash,* arthralgia, fever, fatigue, pain, fat redistribution, back pain

Interactions

✱ **Drug-drug** • Increased risk of severe toxicity if combined with other drugs that are metabolized via the CYP450 pathway—midazolam, triazolam, ergot derivatives, pimozide; the use of these drugs with atazanavir is contraindicated • Risk of increased toxicity of bepridil, lovastatin, simvastatin, indinavir, proton pump inhibitors, irinotecan; coadministration of atazanavir with these drugs is not recommended • Increased risk of serious adverse effects if taken with sildenafil; encourage patient to report any adverse effects to the health care provider • Risk of decreased therapeutic effects of rifampin if combined with atazanavir; this combination is not recommended • Decreased absorption of atazanavir if taken with antacids or buffered medications; if this combination is used, administer atazanavir 1 hr before or 2 hr after these drugs • Potential for increased bleeding if combined with warfarin; if this combination is used, monitor INR carefully and adjust warfarin dosage accordingly

✱ **Drug-alternative therapy** • Decreased concentrations of atazanavir and loss of therapeutic effects if combined with St. John's wort; this combination is not recommended

■ Nursing considerations

Assessment

- **History:** Allergy to any components of the product, lactation, pregnancy, hepatic impairment, signs of lactic acidosis, obesity, hemophilia
- **Physical:** T; orientation, reflexes; R, adventitious sounds; abdominal examination, LFTs

Interventions

- Ensure that HIV antibody testing has been done before initiating therapy to reduce risk of emergence of HIV resistance.
- Ensure that patient is taking this drug in combination with other antiretroviral drugs.

- Monitor patients regularly to evaluate hepatic function; establish baseline ECG to monitor P-R interval.
- Administer this drug with food.

⊗ ***Warning*** Withdraw drug and monitor patient if patient develops signs of lactic acidosis or hepatotoxicity, including hepatomegaly and steatosis.

- Encourage women of childbearing age to use barrier contraceptives while taking this drug because the effects of the drug on the fetus are not known. If drug is used in pregnancy, patient should be registered with the antiretroviral pregnancy registry.
- Advise women who are lactating to find another method of feeding the baby; HIV-infected women are advised to not breastfeed.
- Advise patient that this drug does not cure the disease and there is still a risk of transmitting the disease to others.

Teaching points

- Take this drug once a day with food and in combination with your other antiviral drugs.
- Take the drug every day; if you miss a dose, take it as soon as you remember and then take the next dose at the usual time the next day. Do not double any doses.
- Tell any other health care provider that you see that you are taking this drug; the drug interacts with many other drugs and caution may be needed; the drug also changes your ECG reading and that may be important.
- Avoid the use of St. John's wort while taking this drug; the effectiveness of this drug can be blocked.
- If you use *Viagra,* you could experience serious adverse effects with this drug; report any adverse effects to your health care provider.
- This drug does not cure your HIV infection and you will still be able to pass it to others; using condoms is advised. Women of childbearing age are discouraged from becoming pregnant while taking this drug; using barrier contraceptives is recommended.
- With some antiviral drugs, there is a redistribution of body fat—a "buffalo hump" may develop—and fat is distributed around the trunk while fat is lost in the limbs; the long-term effects of this redistribution are not known.
- You may experience these side effects: Nausea, diarrhea, abdominal pain, headache (try to maintain nutrition and fluid intake as much as possible; eat frequent small meals; and always take the drug with food).
- Report severe weakness, muscle pain, trouble breathing, dizziness, cold feelings in your arms or legs, palpitations, yellowing of the eyes or skin.

▽atenolol

*(a **ten'** o lole)*

Apo-Atenolol (CAN), Gen-Atenolol (CAN), Novo-Atenol (CAN), ratio-Atenolol (CAN), Tenormin

PREGNANCY CATEGORY D

Drug classes

Antianginal
Antihypertensive
$Beta_1$-selective adrenergic blocker

Therapeutic actions

Blocks beta-adrenergic receptors of the sympathetic nervous system in the heart and juxtaglomerular apparatus (kidney), thus decreasing the excitability of the heart, decreasing cardiac output and oxygen consumption, decreasing the release of renin from the kidney, and lowering BP.

Indications

- Treatment of angina pectoris due to coronary atherosclerosis
- Hypertension, as a step 1 agent, alone or with other drugs, especially diuretics
- Treatment of MI in hemodynamically stable patients
- Unlabeled uses: Prevention of migraine headaches; treatment of ventricular and supraventricular arrhythmias; prevention of variceal bleeding; unstable angina

Contraindications and cautions

- Contraindicated with sinus bradycardia, second- or third-degree heart block, cardiogenic shock, heart failure, pregnancy, hypersensitivity to any component of the drug.

- Use cautiously with renal failure, diabetes or thyrotoxicosis (atenolol can mask the usual cardiac signs of hypoglycemia and thyrotoxicosis), lactation, respiratory disease, heart failure (controlled by digoxin or diuretics).

Available forms

Tablets—25, 50, 100 mg

Dosages

Adults

- *Hypertension:* Initially, 50 mg PO once a day; after 1–2 wk, dose may be increased to 100 mg/day.
- *Angina pectoris:* Initially, 50 mg PO daily. If optimal response is not achieved in 1 wk, increase to 100 mg daily; up to 200 mg/day may be needed.
- *Acute MI:* 100 mg PO daily or 50 mg PO bid for 6–9 days or until discharge from the hospital.

Pediatric patients

Safety and efficacy not established.

Geriatric patients or patients with renal impairment

Dosage reduction is required because atenolol is excreted through the kidneys. For elderly patients, use initial dose of 25 mg/day PO. The following dosage is suggested for patients with renal impairment:

CrCl (mL/min)	*Half-life (hr)*	*Maximum Dosage*
15–35	16–27	50 mg/day
Less than 15	More than 27	25 mg/day

For patients on hemodialysis, give 25–50 mg after each dialysis; give only in hospital setting; severe hypotension can occur.

Pharmacokinetics

Route	*Onset*	*Peak*	*Duration*
Oral	Varies	2–4 hr	24 hr

Metabolism: $T_{1/2}$: 6–7 hr
Distribution: Crosses placenta; enters breast milk
Excretion: Bile, feces, urine

Adverse effects

- **Allergic reactions:** Pharyngitis, erythematous rash, fever, sore throat, **laryngospasm,** respiratory distress
- **CNS:** Dizziness, vertigo, tinnitus, fatigue, emotional depression, paresthesias, sleep disturbances, hallucinations, disorientation, memory loss, slurred speech
- **CV:** *Bradycardia, heart failure, cardiac arrhythmias, sinoatrial or AV nodal block, tachycardia,* peripheral vascular insufficiency, claudication, CVA, pulmonary edema, hypotension
- **Dermatologic:** Rash, pruritus, sweating, dry skin
- **EENT:** Eye irritation, dry eyes, conjunctivitis, blurred vision
- **GI:** *Gastric pain, flatulence, constipation, diarrhea, nausea, vomiting,* anorexia, ischemic colitis, renal and mesenteric arterial thrombosis, retroperitoneal fibrosis, hepatomegaly, acute pancreatitis
- **GU:** *Impotence, decreased libido,* Peyronie's disease, dysuria, nocturia, frequent urination
- **Musculoskeletal:** Joint pain, arthralgia, muscle cramps
- **Respiratory: Bronchospasm,** dyspnea, cough, bronchial obstruction, nasal stuffiness, rhinitis, pharyngitis (less likely than with propranolol)
- **Other:** *Decreased exercise tolerance, development of antinuclear antibodies,* hyperglycemia or hypoglycemia, elevated serum transaminase, alkaline phosphatase, and LDH

Interactions

✱ **Drug-drug** • Increased effects with verapamil, anticholinergics, quinidine • Increased risk of orthostatic hypotension with prazosin • Increased risk of lidocaine toxicity with atenolol • Possible increased BP-lowering effects with aspirin, bismuth subsalicylate, magnesium salicylate, sulfinpyrazone, hormonal contraceptives • Decreased antihypertensive effects with NSAIDs, clonidine • Decreased antihypertensive and antianginal effects of atenolol with ampicillin, calcium salts • Possible increased hypoglycemic effect of insulin

✱ **Drug-lab test** • Possible false results with glucose or insulin tolerance tests

■ Nursing considerations

Assessment

- **History:** Sinus bradycardia, second- or third-degree heart block, cardiogenic shock, heart failure, renal failure, diabetes or thyrotoxicosis, lactation, pregnancy
- **Physical:** Baseline weight, skin condition, neurologic status, P, BP, ECG, respiratory status, renal and thyroid function tests, blood and urine glucose, cholesterol, triglycerides

Interventions

⊗ ***Warning*** Do not discontinue drug abruptly after long-term therapy (hypersensitivity to catecholamines may have developed, causing exacerbation of angina, MI, and ventricular arrhythmias). Taper drug gradually over 2 wk with monitoring.

- Consult physician about withdrawing drug if patient is to undergo surgery (withdrawal is controversial).

Teaching points

- Take drug with meals if GI upset occurs.
- Do not stop taking this drug unless told to do so by a health care provider.
- Avoid driving or dangerous activities if dizziness or weakness occurs.
- You may experience these side effects: Dizziness, light-headedness, loss of appetite, nightmares, depression, sexual impotence.
- Report difficulty breathing, night cough, swelling of extremities, slow pulse, confusion, depression, rash, fever, sore throat.

▽ atomoxetine hydrochloride

*(at oh **mox' ah** teen)*

Strattera

PREGNANCY CATEGORY C

Drug class

Selective norepinephrine reuptake inhibitor

Therapeutic actions

Selectively blocks the reuptake of norepinephrine at the neuronal synapse. The mechanism by which this action has a therapeutic effect in ADHD is not understood.

Indications

- Treatment of ADHD as part of a total treatment program

NEW INDICATION: Unlabeled use: Treatment of obesity

Contraindications and cautions

- Contraindicated with hypersensitivity to atomoxetine or constituents of *Strattera;* use of MAOIs within the past 14 days; narrow-angle glaucoma.
- Use cautiously with hypertension, tachycardia, CV or cerebrovascular disease, pregnancy, lactation, severe hepatic impairment.

Pharmacokinetics

Route	*Onset*	*Peak*
Oral	Rapid	1–2 hr

Metabolism: Hepatic; $T_{1/2}$: 5 hr
Distribution: May cross placenta; may enter breast milk
Excretion: Feces, urine

Available forms

Capsules—10, 18, 25, 40, 60, 80, 100 mg

Dosages

Adults and children over 70 kg

40 mg/day PO, increase after a minimum of 3 days to a target total daily dose of 80 mg PO given as a single dose in the morning or two evenly divided doses, in the morning and late afternoon or early evening; after 2–4 additional wk, total dosage may be increase to a maximum of 100 mg/day if needed.

Pediatric patients weighing 70 kg or less

Initially, 0.5 mg/kg/day PO; increase after a minimum of 3 days to a target total daily dose of approximately 1.2 mg/kg/day PO as a single daily dose in the morning; may be given in two evenly divided doses in the morning and late afternoon or early evening. Do not exceed 1.4 mg/kg or 100 mg/day, whichever is less.

Patients with hepatic impairment

For moderate hepatic impairment (Child-Pugh class B), reduce dose to 50% of the normal dose;

for severe hepatic impairment (Child-Pugh class C), reduce dose to 25% of the normal dose.

Adverse effects

- **CNS:** Aggression, irritability, crying, somnolence, dizziness, *headache,* mood swings, *insomnia,* **possible suicidal ideation in children, adolescents, and young adults**
- **CV:** Palpitations
- **Dermatologic:** Dermatitis, increased sweating
- **GI:** *Dry mouth, nausea,* dyspepsia, flatulence, *decreased appetite, constipation, upper abdominal pain, vomiting*
- **GU:** Urinary hesitation, urinary retention, dysmenorrhea, erectile problems
- **Respiratory:** *Cough,* rhinorrhea, sinusitis
- **Other:** Fever, rigors, sinusitis, weight loss, myalgia, fatigue

Interactions

✱ **Drug-drug** • Possible increased serum levels if combined with potent CYP2D6 inhibitors—paroxetine, fluoxetine, quinidine; monitor and adjust dosage of atomoxetine to 0.5 mg/kg/day with a target dose of 1.2 mg/kg/day for children less than 70 kg or 40 mg/day with a target dose of 80 mg/day for children more than 70 kg or adults • Risk of neuroleptic malignant syndrome if combined with MAOIs; do not combine with an MAOI and do not give atomoxetine within 14 days of using an MAOI; do not start MAOI within 2 wk after discontinuing atomoxetine

■ Nursing considerations

Assessment

- **History:** Hypersensitivity to atomoxetine or constituents of *Strattera;* use of MAOIs within the past 14 days; narrow-angle glaucoma, hypertension, tachycardia, CV or cerebrovascular disease, pregnancy, lactation
- **Physical:** Height, weight, T; skin color, lesions; orientation, affect; P, BP, auscultation; R, adventitious sounds; bowel sounds, normal output

Interventions

⊠ ***Black box warning*** Adolescents and children have an increased risk of suicidality when treated with atomoxetine. Monitor patient closely, and alert caregivers of risk.

- Ensure proper diagnosis before administering to children for behavioral syndromes; drug should not be used until other causes and concomitants of abnormal behavior (learning disability, EEG abnormalities, neurologic deficits) are ruled out.
- Ensure that drug is being used as part of an overall treatment program including education and psychosocial interventions.
- Arrange to interrupt drug dosage periodically in children being treated for behavioral disorders to determine if symptoms recur at an intensity that warrants continued drug therapy.
- Monitor growth and weight of children on long-term atomoxetine therapy.
- Administer drug before 6 PM to prevent insomnia if that is a problem.
- Monitor BP early in treatment, particularly with adult patients.
- Arrange for consult with school nurse for school-age patients receiving this drug.
- For women of childbearing age who are using this drug, suggest using contraceptives.

Teaching points

- Take this drug exactly as prescribed. It can be taken once a day in the morning; if adverse effects are a problem, the drug can be taken in two evenly divided doses in the morning and in the late afternoon or early evening.
- Do not open capsule; swallow it whole.
- Take drug before 6 PM to avoid nighttime sleep disturbance.
- Avoid the use of alcohol and over-the-counter drugs, including nose drops, cold remedies, and herbal therapies while taking this drug; some of these products cause dangerous effects. If you think that you need one of these preparations, consult your health care provider.
- The effects of this drug on the unborn baby are not known; women of childbearing age are advised to use contraceptives.
- You may experience these side effects: Dizziness, insomnia, moodiness (these effects may become less pronounced after a few days; avoid driving a car or engaging in activities

that require alertness if these occur; notify your health care provider if these are pronounced or bothersome); headache (analgesics may be available to help) loss of appetite, dry mouth (eat frequent small meals and suck on sugarless lozenges); thoughts of suicide (if you are a minor, report this to your parents or health care provider).
- Report palpitations, dizziness, weight loss, severe dry mouth and difficulty swallowing, pregnancy, thoughts of suicide.

▽ atorvastatin calcium

*(ah **tor'** va stah tin)*

Lipitor

PREGNANCY CATEGORY X

Drug classes

Antihyperlipidemic
HMG-CoA reductase inhibitor

Therapeutic actions

Inhibits HMG-CoA reductase, the enzyme that catalyzes the first step in the cholesterol synthesis pathway, resulting in a decrease in serum cholesterol, serum LDLs (associated with increased risk of CAD), and increases serum HDLs (associated with decreased risk of CAD); increases hepatic LDL recapture sites, enhances reuptake and catabolism of LDL; lowers triglyceride levels.

Indications

- Adjunct to diet in treatment of elevated total cholesterol, serum triglycerides, and LDL cholesterol and to increase HDL-C in patients with primary hypercholesterolemia (types IIa and IIb) and mixed dyslipidemia and primary dysbetalipoproteinemia, whose response to dietary restriction of saturated fat and cholesterol and other nonpharmacologic measures has not been adequate
- To reduce total cholesterol and LDL-C in patients with homozygous familial hypercholesterolemia as adjunct to lipid-lowering treatments
- Reduction of risk of MI and stroke in patients with type 2 diabetes and in those with multiple risk factors for CAD (such as age 55 or older, smoking, hypertension, low HDL-C, family history of early CAD) but no clinical evidence of CAD
- Adjunct to diet to treat elevated serum triglyceride levels (Fredrickson Type IV)
- Adjunct to diet in treatment of boys and postmenarchal girls ages 10–17 with heterozygous familial cholesterolemia if diet alone is not adequate to control lipid levels and LDL-C levels are 190 mg/dL or greater or if LDL-C level is 160 mg/dL or greater and there is a family history of premature CV disease or the child has two or more risk factors for the development of coronary disease
- Reduction of risk of MI, fatal and nonfatal stroke, revascularization procedures, heart failure, hospitalization, and angina in patients with clinically evident CAD
- Prevention of CV disease in adults without clinically evident coronary disease but with multiple risk factors for CAD; to reduce the risk of MI and risk for revascularization procedures and angina

Contraindications and cautions

- Contraindicated with allergy to atorvastatin, fungal byproducts, active hepatic disease, or unexplained and persistent elevations of transaminase levels, pregnancy, lactation.
- Use cautiously with impaired endocrine function, history of liver disease, alcoholism.

Available forms

Tablets—10, 20, 40, 80 mg

Dosages

Adults

Initially, 10–20 mg PO once daily without regard to meals; if more than 45% reduction in LDL is needed, may start with 40 mg daily; for maintenance, 10–80 mg PO daily. May be combined with bile acid–binding resin. Check lipid levels every 2–4 wk; adjust dose as needed.

Pediatric patients 10–17 yr

Initially, 10 mg PO daily. Maximum, 20 mg/day; do not change dose at intervals less than 4 wk.

Pharmacokinetics

Route	*Onset*	*Peak*
Oral	Slow	1–2 hr

Metabolism: Hepatic and cellular; $T_{1/2}$: 14 hr
Distribution: Crosses placenta; enters breast milk
Excretion: Bile

Adverse effects

- **CNS:** *Headache,* asthenia
- **GI:** *Flatulence, abdominal pain, cramps, constipation, nausea,* dyspepsia, heartburn, **liver failure**
- **Respiratory:** Sinusitis, pharyngitis
- **Other: Rhabdomyolysis with acute renal failure,** arthralgia, myalgia, infections, cataracts

Interactions

✱ **Drug-drug** • Possible severe myopathy or rhabdomyolysis with erythromycin, cyclosporine, niacin, fibric acid derivatives, antifungals, clarithromycin, diltiazem, cimetidine, protease inhibitors, other HMG-CoA reductase inhibitors; limit dose to 10 mg/day with cyclosporine; limit dose to 20 mg/day with clarithromycin or protease inhibitors • Increased digoxin levels with possible toxicity if taken together; monitor digoxin levels • Increased estrogen levels with hormonal contraceptives; monitor patients on this combination
✱ **Drug-food** • Decreased metabolism and risk of toxic effects if combined with grapefruit juice; avoid this combination

■ Nursing considerations

CLINICAL ALERT!
Name confusion has been reported between written orders for *Lipitor* (atorvastatin) and *Zyrtec* (cetirizine). Use extreme caution.

Assessment

- **History:** Allergy to atorvastatin, fungal byproducts; active hepatic disease; acute serious illness; pregnancy, lactation
- **Physical:** Orientation, affect, muscle strength; liver evaluation, abdominal examination; lipid studies, LFTs, renal function tests

Interventions

- Obtain LFTs as a baseline and periodically during therapy; discontinue drug if AST or ALT levels increase to 3 times normal levels.

⊗ ***Warning*** Withhold atorvastatin in any acute, serious condition (severe infection, hypotension, major surgery, trauma, severe metabolic or endocrine disorder, seizures) that may suggest myopathy or serve as risk factor for development of renal failure.

- Ensure that patient has tried cholesterol-lowering diet regimen for 3–6 mo before beginning therapy.
- Administer drug without regard to food, but at same time each day.
- Atorvastatin may be combined with a bile acid-binding agent. Do not combine with other HMG-CoA reductase inhibitors or fibrates.
- Consult dietitian about low-cholesterol diets.

⊗ ***Warning*** Ensure that patient is not pregnant and has appropriate contraceptives available during therapy; serious fetal damage has been associated with this drug.

Teaching points

- Take this drug once a day, at about the same time each day, preferably in the evening; may be taken with food. Do not drink grapefruit juice while taking this drug.
- Institute appropriate dietary changes.
- Arrange to have periodic blood tests while you are taking this drug.
- Alert any health care provider that you are taking this drug; it will need to be discontinued if acute injury or illness occurs.
- Do not become pregnant while you are taking this drug; use barrier contraceptives. If you wish to become pregnant or think you are pregnant, consult your health care provider.
- You may experience these side effects: Nausea (eat frequent small meals); headache, muscle and joint aches and pains (may lessen over time).
- Report muscle pain, weakness, tenderness; malaise; fever; changes in color of urine or stool; swelling.

▽atovaquone

(a toe' va kwon)

Mepron

PREGNANCY CATEGORY C

Drug class

Antiprotozoal

Therapeutic actions

Directly inhibits enzymes required for nucleic acid and ATP synthesis in protozoa; effective against *Pneumocystis carinii*.

Indications

- Prevention and acute oral treatment of mild to moderate *P. carinii* pneumonia (PCP) in patients who are intolerant to trimethoprim-sulfamethoxazole

Contraindications and cautions

- Contraindicated with development or history of potentially life-threatening allergic reactions to any of the components of the drug.
- Use cautiously with severe PCP infections, the elderly, lactation, hepatic impairment.

Available forms

Suspension—750 mg/5 mL

Dosages

Adults and patients 13–16 yr

- *Prevention of PCP:* 1,500 mg PO daily with a meal.
- *Treatment of PCP:* 750 mg PO bid with food for 21 days.

Pediatric patients younger than 13 yr

Safety and efficacy not established.

Geriatric patients

Use caution, and evaluate patient response regularly.

Pharmacokinetics

Route	*Onset*	*Peak*	*Duration*
Oral	Varies	1–8 hr	3–5 days

Metabolism: $T_{1/2}$: 2.2–2.9 days
Distribution: Crosses placenta; may enter breast milk
Excretion: Feces

Adverse effects

- **CNS:** Dizziness, *insomnia, headache,* depression
- **Dermatologic:** *Rash,* pruritus, sweating, dry skin
- **GI:** Constipation, *diarrhea, nausea, vomiting,* anorexia, abdominal pain, oral monilia infections
- **Other:** *Fever,* elevated liver enzymes, hyponatremia, increased cough, dyspnea, flu-like syndrome, sweating

Interactions

✱ **Drug-drug** • Decreased effects if taken with rifamycins

✱ **Drug-food** • Markedly increased absorption of atovaquone when taken with food

■ Nursing considerations

Assessment

- **History:** History of potentially life-threatening allergic reactions to any components of the drug, severe PCP infections, elderly, lactation
- **Physical:** T, skin condition, neurologic status, abdominal evaluation, serum electrolytes, LFTs

Interventions

- Give drug with meals.
- Ensure that this drug is taken for 21 days as treatment.

Teaching points

- Take drug with food; food increases the absorption of the drug.
- You may experience these side effects: Dizziness, insomnia, headache (medication may be ordered); nausea, vomiting (eat frequent small meals); diarrhea or constipation (consult your health care provider for appropriate treatment); superinfections (therapy may be ordered); rash (good skin care may help).
- Report fever, mouth infection, severe headache, severe nausea or vomiting, rash.

▽atropine sulfate
(a' troe peen)

Parenteral and oral preparations: AtroPen, Sal-Tropine

Ophthalmic solution: Atropine Sulfate S.O.P., Isopto Atropine Ophthalmic

PREGNANCY CATEGORY C

Drug classes
Anticholinergic
Antidote
Antimuscarinic
Antiparkinsonian
Belladonna alkaloid
Diagnostic agent (ophthalmic preparations)
Parasympatholytic

Therapeutic actions
Competitively blocks the effects of acetylcholine at muscarinic cholinergic receptors that mediate the effects of parasympathetic postganglionic impulses, depressing salivary and bronchial secretions, dilating the bronchi, inhibiting vagal influences on the heart, relaxing the GI and GU tracts, inhibiting gastric acid secretion (high doses), relaxing the pupil of the eye (mydriatic effect), and preventing accommodation for near vision (cycloplegic effect); also blocks the effects of acetylcholine in the CNS.

Indications
Systemic administration
- Antisialagogue for preanesthetic medication to prevent or reduce respiratory tract secretions
- Treatment of parkinsonism; relieves tremor and rigidity
- Restoration of cardiac rate and arterial pressure during anesthesia when vagal stimulation produced by intra-abdominal traction causes a decrease in pulse rate, lessening the degree of AV block when increased vagal tone is a factor (eg, some cases due to cardiac glycosides)
- Relief of bradycardia and syncope due to hyperactive carotid sinus reflex
- Relief of pylorospasm, hypertonicity of the small intestine, and hypermotility of the colon
- Relaxation of the spasm of biliary and ureteral colic and bronchospasm
- Relaxation of the tone of the detrusor muscle of the urinary bladder in the treatment of urinary tract disorders
- Control of crying and laughing episodes in patients with brain lesions
- Treatment of closed head injuries that cause acetylcholine release into CSF, EEG abnormalities, stupor, neurologic signs
- Relaxation of uterine hypertonicity
- Management of peptic ulcer
- Control of rhinorrhea of acute rhinitis or hay fever
- Antidote (with external cardiac massage) for CV collapse from overdose of parasympathomimetic (cholinergic) drugs (choline esters, pilocarpine), or cholinesterase inhibitors (eg, physostigmine, isoflurophate, organophosphorus insecticides)
- Antidote for poisoning by certain species of mushroom (eg, *Amanita muscaria*)

Ophthalmic preparations
- Diagnostically to produce mydriasis and cycloplegia-pupillary dilation in acute inflammatory conditions of the iris and uveal tract

Contraindications and cautions
- Contraindicated with hypersensitivity to anticholinergic drugs.

Systemic administration
- Contraindicated with glaucoma, adhesions between iris and lens; stenosing peptic ulcer; pyloroduodenal obstruction; paralytic ileus; intestinal atony; severe ulcerative colitis; toxic megacolon; symptomatic prostatic hypertrophy; bladder neck obstruction; bronchial asthma; COPD; cardiac arrhythmias; tachycardia; myocardial ischemia; impaired metabolic, hepatic, or renal function; myasthenia gravis.
- Use cautiously with Down syndrome, brain damage, spasticity, hypertension, hyperthyroidism, pregnancy, lactation.

Ophthalmic solution
- Contraindicated with glaucoma or tendency to glaucoma.

Available forms

Tablets—0.4 mg; injection—0.05, 0.1, 0.3, 0.4, 0.5, 0.8, 1, 2 mg/mL; ophthalmic ointment—1%; ophthalmic solution—0.5%, 1%, 2%; auto-injector—0.25, 0.5, 1, 2 mg

Dosages

Adults

Systemic administration

0.4–0.6 mg PO, IM, IV, or subcutaneously.

- *Hypotonic radiography:* 1 mg IM.
- *Surgery:* 0.5 mg (0.4–0.6 mg) IM (or subcutaneously or IV) prior to induction of anesthesia; during surgery, give IV; reduce dose to less than 0.4 mg with cyclopropane anesthesia.
- *Bradyarrhythmias:* 0.4–1 mg (up to 2 mg) IV every 1–2 hr as needed.
- *Antidote:* For poisoning due to cholinesterase inhibitor insecticides, give large doses of at least 2–3 mg parenterally, and repeat until signs of atropine intoxication appear; for rapid type of mushroom poisoning, give in doses sufficient to control parasympathetic signs before coma and CV collapse intervene. Auto-injector provides rapid administration.

Ophthalmic solution

- *For refraction:* Instill 1–2 drops into eye 1 hr before refracting.
- *For uveitis:* Instill 1–2 drops into eye tid.

Pediatric patients

Systemic administration

Refer to the following table:

Weight	Dose (mg)
7–16 lb (3.2–7.3 kg)	0.1
16–24 lb (7.3–10.9 kg)	0.15
24–40 lb (10.9–18.1 kg)	0.2
40–65 lb (18.1–29.5 kg)	0.3
65–90 lb (29.5–40.8 kg)	0.4
> 90 lb (> 40.8 kg)	0.4–0.6

- *Surgery:* For infants weighing less than 5 kg, 0.04 mg/kg; infants weighing more than 5 kg, 0.03 mg/kg. Repeat every 4–6 hr as needed.
- *Bradyarrhythmias:* 0.01–0.03 mg/kg IV.
- *Antidote:*
  90 lb or more: 2 mg auto-injector.
  40–90 lb: 1-mg auto-injector.
  15–40 lb: 0.5 mg auto-injector.
  Less than 15 lb: Individualized doses of 0.25 mg.

Geriatric patients

More likely to cause serious adverse reactions, especially CNS reactions, in elderly patients; use with caution.

Pharmacokinetics

Route	Onset	Peak	Duration
IM	10–15 min	30 min	4 hr
IV	Immediate	2–4 min	4 hr
Subcut.	Varies	1–2 hr	4 hr
Topical	5–10 min	30–40 min	7–14 days

Metabolism: Hepatic; $T_{1/2}$: 2.5 hr

Distribution: Crosses placenta; enters breast milk

Excretion: Urine

IV FACTS

Preparation: Give undiluted or dilute in 10 mL sterile water.

Infusion: Give direct IV; administer 1 mg or less over 1 min.

Adverse effects

Systemic administration

- **CNS:** Blurred vision, mydriasis, cycloplegia, photophobia, increased IOP, headache, flushing, nervousness, weakness, dizziness, insomnia, mental confusion or excitement (after even small doses in the elderly), nasal congestion
- **CV:** *Palpitations, bradycardia* (low doses), *tachycardia* (higher doses)
- **GI:** *Dry mouth, altered taste perception, nausea,* vomiting, dysphagia, heartburn, constipation, bloated feeling, **paralytic ileus,** gastroesophageal reflux
- **GU:** *Urinary hesitancy and retention;* impotence
- **Other:** *Decreased sweating and predisposition to heat prostration,* suppression of lactation

Ophthalmic preparations

- **Local:** Transient stinging
- **Systemic:** Systemic adverse effects, depending on amount absorbed

Interactions

✱ **Drug-drug** • Increased anticholinergic effects with other drugs that have anticholinergic activity—certain antihistamines, certain antiparkinsonians, TCAs, MAOIs • Decreased antipsychotic effectiveness of haloperidol with atropine • Decreased effectiveness of phenothiazines, but increased incidence of paralytic ileus • If cholinesterase inhibitors and atropine are given together, opposing effects will render both drugs ineffective

■ Nursing considerations

Assessment

- **History:** Hypersensitivity to anticholinergics; glaucoma; adhesions between iris and lens; stenosing peptic ulcer, pyloroduodenal obstruction, paralytic ileus, intestinal atony, severe ulcerative colitis, toxic megacolon, symptomatic prostatic hypertrophy, bladder neck obstruction, bronchial asthma, COPD, cardiac arrhythmias, myocardial ischemia, impaired metabolic, liver, or renal function, myasthenia gravis, Down syndrome, brain damage, spasticity, hypertension, hyperthyroidism, lactation
- **Physical:** Skin color, lesions, texture; T; orientation, reflexes, bilateral grip strength; affect; ophthalmic examination; P, BP; R, adventitious sounds; bowel sounds, normal GI output; normal urinary output, prostate palpation; LFTs, renal function tests, ECG

Interventions

- Ensure adequate hydration; provide environmental control (temperature) to prevent hyperpyrexia.
- Have patient void before taking medication if urinary retention is a problem.

Teaching points

When used preoperatively or in other acute situations, incorporate teaching about the drug with teaching about the procedure; the ophthalmic solution is mainly used acutely and will not be self-administered by the patient; the following apply to oral medication for outpatients:

- Take as prescribed, 30 minutes before meals; avoid excessive dosage.
- Avoid hot environments; you will be heat intolerant, and dangerous reactions may occur.
- You may experience these side effects: Dizziness, confusion (use caution driving or performing hazardous tasks); constipation (ensure adequate fluid intake, proper diet); dry mouth (sugarless lozenges, frequent mouth care may help; may be transient); blurred vision, sensitivity to light (reversible; avoid tasks that require acute vision; wear sunglasses in bright light); impotence (reversible); difficulty in urination (empty the bladder prior to taking drug).
- Report rash; flushing; eye pain; difficulty breathing; tremors, loss of coordination; irregular heartbeat, palpitations; headache; abdominal distention; hallucinations; severe or persistent dry mouth; difficulty swallowing; difficulty in urination; constipation; sensitivity to light.

auranofin

See Appendix W, *Less commonly used drugs*.

azacitidine

See Appendix W, *Less commonly used drugs*.

azathioprine

*(ay za **thye'** oh preen)*

Azasan, Imuran

PREGNANCY CATEGORY D

Drug class

Immunosuppressant

Therapeutic actions

Suppresses cell-mediated hypersensitivities and alters antibody production; exact mechanisms of action in increasing homograft survival and affecting autoimmune diseases not clearly understood.

Indications

- Renal homotransplantation: Adjunct for prevention of rejection
- Rheumatoid arthritis: Use only with adults meeting criteria for classic rheumatoid arthritis and not responding to conventional management

- Unlabeled use: Treatment of chronic ulcerative colitis, myasthenia gravis, Behçet's syndrome, Crohn's disease, clinically definite MS (alone or in combination with other drugs)

Contraindications and cautions

- Contraindicated with allergy to azathioprine; rheumatoid arthritis patients previously treated with alkylating agents, increasing their risk for neoplasia; pregnancy.
- Use cautiously with bone marrow suppression, hepatic impairment, lactation, serious infection.

Available forms

Tablets—50, 75, 100 mg; injection—100 mg/vial

Dosages

Adults

- *Renal homotransplantation:* Initially, 3–5 mg/kg/day PO or IV as a single dose on the day of transplant; for maintenance, use 1–3 mg/kg/day PO. Do not increase dose to decrease risk of rejection.
- *Rheumatoid arthritis:* Usually given daily; initial dose is 1 mg/kg PO given as a single dose or bid. Dose may be increased at 6–8 wk and thereafter by steps at 4-wk intervals. Dose increments should be 0.5 mg/kg/day up to a maximum dose of 2.5 mg/kg/day. Once patient is stabilized, dose should be decreased to lowest effective dose; decrease in 0.5-mg/kg increments. Patients who do not respond in 12 wk are probably refractory.

Pediatric patients

Safety and efficacy not established.

Geriatric patients or patients with renal impairment

Lower doses may be required because of decreased rate of excretion and increased sensitivity to the drug.

Pharmacokinetics

Route	*Onset*	*Peak*
Oral	Varies	1–2 hr
IV	Immediate	30–45 min

Metabolism: Hepatic; $T_{1/2}$: 5 hr
Distribution: Crosses placenta; may enter breast milk
Excretion: Urine

IV FACTS

Preparation: Add 10 mL sterile water for injection and swirl until a clear solution results; use within 24 hr. Further dilution into sterile saline or dextrose is usually made for infusion.
Infusion: Infuse over 30–60 min; can range from 5 min–8 hr for the daily dose.

Adverse effects

- **GI:** *Nausea, vomiting,* hepatotoxicity (especially in homograft patients)
- **Hematologic:** *Leukopenia, thrombocytopenia, macrocytic anemia*
- **Other: Serious infections** (fungal, bacterial, protozoal infections secondary to immunosuppression), *carcinogenesis* (increased risk of neoplasia, especially in homograft patients)

Interactions

✱ **Drug-drug** • Increased effects with allopurinol; reduce azathioprine to one-third to one-fourth the usual dose • Reversal of the neuromuscular blockade of nondepolarizing neuromuscular junction blockers (atracurium, pancuronium, tubocurarine, vecuronium) with azathioprine

■ Nursing considerations

Assessment

- **History:** Allergy to azathioprine; rheumatoid arthritis patients previously treated with alkylating agents; pregnancy or male partners of women trying to become pregnant; lactation
- **Physical:** T; skin color, lesions; liver evaluation, bowel sounds; LFTs, renal function tests, CBC

Interventions

- Give drug IV if oral administration is not possible; switch to oral route as soon as possible.
- Administer in divided daily doses or with food if GI upset occurs.

⊗ ***Black box warning*** Monitor blood counts regularly; severe hematologic effects may require the discontinuation of therapy; increases risk of neoplasia.

Teaching points

- Take drug in divided doses with food if GI upset occurs.

- Avoid infections; avoid crowds or people who have infections. Notify your physician at once if you are injured.
- Notify your health care provider if you think you are pregnant or wish to become pregnant, or if you are a man whose sexual partner wishes to become pregnant.
- You may experience these side effects: Nausea, vomiting (take drug in divided doses or with food), diarrhea, rash.
- Report unusual bleeding or bruising, fever, sore throat, mouth sores, signs of infection, abdominal pain, severe diarrhea, darkened urine or pale stools, severe nausea and vomiting.

▽ azithromycin

*(ay zi thro **my'** sin)*

Zithromax, Zmax

PREGNANCY CATEGORY B

Drug class

Macrolide antibiotic

Therapeutic actions

Bacteriostatic or bactericidal in susceptible bacteria.

Indications

- Treatment of lower respiratory infections: Acute bacterial exacerbations of COPD due to *Haemophilus influenzae, Moraxella catarrhalis, Streptococcus pneumoniae;* community-acquired pneumonia due to *S. pneumoniae, H. influenzae*
- Treatment of lower respiratory infections: Streptococcal pharyngitis and tonsillitis due to *Streptococcus pyogenes* in those who cannot take penicillins
- Treatment of genital ulcer disease caused by *Haemophilus ducreyi* (chancroid) in men
- Treatment of uncomplicated skin infections due to *Staphylococcus aureus, S. pyogenes, Streptococcus agalactiae*
- Treatment of nongonococcal urethritis and cervicitis due to *Chlamydia trachomatis;* treatment of PID
- Treatment of otitis media caused by *H. influenzae, M. catarrhalis, S. pneumoniae* in children older than 6 mo
- Treatment of pharyngitis and tonsillitis caused by *S. pyogenes* in children older than 2 yr who cannot use first-line therapy
- Prevention and treatment of disseminated *Mycobacterium avium* complex (MAC) in patients with advanced HIV infection
- Treatment of patients with mild to moderate acute bacterial sinusitis caused by *H. influenzae, M. catarrhalis, S. pneumoniae* (*Zmax*)
- Treatment of mild to moderate community-acquired pneumonia caused by *Chlamydophila pneumoniae, H. influenzae, Mycoplasma pneumoniae, S. pneumoniae* (*Zmax*)
- Unlabeled uses: Uncomplicated gonococcal infections caused by *N. gonorrhoeae,* gonococcal pharyngitis caused by *N. gonorrhoeae,* chlamydial infections caused by *C. trachomatis,* prophylaxis after sexual attack, babesiosis, early Lyme disease, granuloma inguinale, treatment of cholera in adults

Contraindications and cautions

- Contraindicated with hypersensitivity to azithromycin, erythromycin, or any macrolide antibiotic.
- Use cautiously with gonorrhea or syphilis, pseudomembranous colitis, hepatic or renal impairment, lactation.

Available forms

Tablets–250, 500, 600 mg; powder for injection—500 mg; injection—2.5 g; powder for oral suspension–100 mg/5 mL, 200 mg/5 mL, 1 g/packet; bottles for oral suspension—2 g to be reconstituted with 60 mL water (*Zmax*)

Dosages

Adults

- *Mild to moderate acute bacterial exacerbations of COPD, pneumonia, pharyngitis and tonsillitis (as second-line), uncomplicated skin and skin structure infections:* 500 mg PO single dose on first day, followed by 250 mg PO daily on days 2–5 for a total dose of 1.5 g or 500 mg/day PO for 3 days.

- *Nongonococcal urethritis, genital ulcer disease, and cervicitis due to* C. trachomatis: A single 1-g PO dose.
- *Gonococcal urethritis and cervicitis:* A single dose of 2 g PO.
- *Disseminated MAC infections:* For prevention, 1,200 mg PO taken once weekly. For treatment, 600 mg/day PO with etambutol.
- *Acute sinusitis:* 500 mg/day PO for 3 days or a single 2-g dose of *Zmax*.
- *Mild to moderate acute bacterial sinusitis, community acquired pneumonia:* 2 g PO as a single dose (*Zmax*).
- *Community-acquired pneumonia:* 500 mg IV daily for at least 2 days; then 500 mg PO for a total of 7–10 days.
- *PID:* 500 mg IV daily for 1–2 days; then 250 mg/day PO for a total of 7 days.

Pediatric patients

- *Otitis media:* Initially, 10 mg/kg PO as a single dose, then 5 mg/kg on days 2–5 or 30 mg/kg PO as a single dose.
- *Community-acquired pneumonia:* 10 mg/kg PO as a single dose on first day, then 5 mg/kg PO on days 2–5.
- *Pharyngitis or tonsillitis:* 12 mg/kg/day PO on days 1–5 (maximum of 500 mg/day).
- *Acute sinusitis:* 10 mg/kg/day PO for 3 days.

Pharmacokinetics

Route	*Onset*	*Peak*	*Duration*
Oral	Varies	2.5–3.2 hr	24 hr

Metabolism: $T_{1/2}$: 11–48 hr
Distribution: Crosses placenta; enters breast milk
Excretion: Bile, urine—unchanged

IV FACTS

Preparation: Add 4.8 mL sterile water for injection to 500-mg vial. Shake until drug is dissolved; may be further diluted in 0.9% normal saline; 0.45% normal saline, D_5W in water, 5% dextrose in lactated Ringer's solution, 1/2 or 1/3 normal saline, lactated Ringer's solution, *Normosol-M or Normosol-R* in 5% dextrose. Drug is stable for 24 hr at room temperature or for 7 days refrigerated.
Infusion: Infuse over 60 minutes or longer. Guidelines: 1 mg/mL solution over 3 hr; 2 mg/mL over 1 hr.

Adverse effects

- **CNS:** Dizziness, headache, vertigo, somnolence, fatigue
- **GI:** *Diarrhea, abdominal pain, nausea,* dyspepsia, flatulence, vomiting, melena, pseudomembranous colitis
- **Other:** *Superinfections,* **angioedema,** rash, photosensitivity, vaginitis

Interactions

✱ **Drug-drug** • Decreased serum levels and effectiveness of azithromycin with aluminum and magnesium-containing antacids • Possible increased effects of theophylline • Possible increased anticoagulant effects of warfarin
✱ **Drug-food** • Food greatly decreases the absorption of azithromycin

■ Nursing considerations

Assessment

- **History:** Hypersensitivity to azithromycin, erythromycin, or any macrolide antibiotic; gonorrhea or syphilis, pseudomembranous colitis, hepatic or renal impairment, lactation
- **Physical:** Site of infection; skin color, lesions; orientation, GI output, bowel sounds, liver evaluation; culture and sensitivity tests of infection, urinalysis, LFTs, renal function tests

Interventions

- Culture site of infection before therapy.
- Administer on an empty stomach 1 hr before or 2–3 hr after meals. Food affects the absorption of this drug.
- Prepare *Zmax* by adding 60 mL water to bottle, shake well.
- Counsel patients being treated for STDs about appropriate precautions and additional therapy.

Teaching points

- Take the full course prescribed. Do not take with antacids. Tablets and oral suspension can be taken with or without food.
- Prepare *Zmax* by adding 60 mL (¼ cup) water to bottle, shake well, drink all at once.
- You may experience these side effects: Stomach cramping, discomfort, diarrhea; fatigue, headache (medication may help); additional infections in the mouth or vagina (consult your health care provider for treatment).

- Report severe or watery diarrhea, severe nausea or vomiting, rash or itching, mouth sores, vaginal sores.

aztreonam

(az' tree oh nam)

Azactam

PREGNANCY CATEGORY B

Drug class
Monobactam antibiotic

Therapeutic actions
Bactericidal: Interferes with bacterial cell wall synthesis, causing cell death in susceptible gram-negative bacteria, ineffective against gram-positive and anaerobic bacteria.

Indications
- Treatment of UTIs, lower respiratory infections, skin and skin-structure infections, septicemia, intra-abdominal infections and gynecologic infections caused by susceptible strains of *Escherichia coli, Enterobacter, Serratia, Proteus, Salmonella, Providencia, Pseudomonas, Citrobacter, Haemophilus, Neisseria, Klebsiella*
- Adjunct to surgery in managing infections caused by susceptible organisms (especially gram-negative aerobic pathogens)
- Unlabeled use: 1 g IM for treatment of acute uncomplicated gonorrhea as alternative to spectinomycin in penicillin-resistant gonococci

Contraindications and cautions
- Contraindicated with allergy to aztreonam.
- Use cautiously with immediate hypersensitivity reaction to penicillins or cephalosporins, renal and hepatic disorders, lactation.

Available forms
Powder for injection—500 mg, 1 g, 2 g

Dosages
Available for IV and IM use only; maximum recommended dose, 8 g/day.

Adults
- *UTIs:* 500 mg–1 g every 8–12 hr.
- *Moderately severe systemic infection:* 1–2 g every 8–12 hr.
- *Severe systemic infection:* 2 g every 6–8 hr.

Pediatric patients 9 mo and older
- *Mild to moderate infections:* 30 mg/kg every 8 hr.
- *Moderate to severe infections:* 30 mg/kg every 6–8 hr.

Maximum recommended dose, 120 mg/kg/day.

Geriatric patients or patients with renal impairment
Reduce dosage by one-half in patients who have estimated creatinine clearances between 10 and 30 mL/min/1.73m^2 after an initial loading dose of 1 or 2 g. For patients on hemodialysis, give 500 mg, 1 g, or 2 g initially; maintenance dose should be one-fourth the usual initial dose at fixed intervals of 6, 8, or 12 hr. In serious or life-threatening infections, give an additional one-eighth of the initial dose after each hemodialysis session.

Pharmacokinetics

Route	Onset	Peak	Duration
IM	Varies	60–90 min	6–8 hr
IV	Immediate	30 min	6–8 hr

Metabolism: $T_{1/2}$: 1.5–2 hr
Distribution: Crosses placenta; enters breast milk
Excretion: Urine

IV FACTS
Preparation: After adding diluent to container, shake immediately and vigorously. Constituted solutions are not for multiple-dose use; discard any unused solution. Solution should be colorless to light straw yellow, or it may be slightly pink.
IV injection: Reconstitute contents of 15-mL vial with 6–10 mL sterile water for injection. Inject slowly over 3–5 min directly into vein or into IV tubing of compatible IV infusion.
IV infusion: Reconstitute contents of 100-mL bottle to make a final concentration of 20 mg/mL or less (add at least 50 mL of one of the following solutions per gram of aztreonam): 0.9%

sodium chloride injection, Ringer's injection, lactated Ringer's injection, 5% or 10% dextrose injection, 5% dextrose and 0.2%, 0.45%, or 0.09% sodium chloride, sodium lactate injection, *Ionosol B with 5% Dextrose, Isolyte E, Isolyte E with 5% Dextrose, Isolyte M with 5% Dextrose, Normosol-R, Normosol-R and 5% Dextrose, Normosol-M and 5% Dextrose,* 5% and 10% mannitol injection, lactated Ringer's and 5% dextrose injection, *Plasma-Lyte M and 5% Dextrose, 10% Travert Injection, 10% Travert and Electrolyte no. 1, 2, or 3 Injection.* Use reconstituted solutions promptly after preparation; those prepared with sterile water for injection or sodium chloride injection should be used within 48 hr if stored at room temperature and within 7 days if refrigerated. Administer over 20–60 min. If giving into IV tubing that is used to administer other drugs, flush tubing with delivery solution before and after aztreonam administration.

Incompatibilities: Do not mix with nafcillin sodium, cephradine, metronidazole; other admixtures are not recommended because data are not available.

Y-site incompatibility: Vancomycin.

Adverse effects

- **Dermatologic:** *Rash, pruritus*
- **GI:** *Nausea, vomiting, diarrhea,* transient elevation of AST, ALT, LDH
- **Hypersensitivity: Anaphylaxis**
- **Local:** *Local phlebitis or thrombophlebitis* at IV injection site, swelling or discomfort at IM injection site
- **Other:** Superinfections

■ Nursing considerations

Assessment

- **History:** Allergy to aztreonam, immediate hypersensitivity reaction to penicillins or cephalosporins, renal and hepatic disorders, lactation
- **Physical:** Skin color, lesions; injection sites; T; GI mucous membranes, bowel sounds, liver evaluation; GU mucous membranes; culture and sensitivity tests of infected area; LFTs, renal function tests

Interventions

- Arrange for culture and sensitivity tests of infected area before therapy. In acutely ill patients, therapy may begin before test results are known. If therapeutic effects are not noted, reculture area.
- For IM administration, reconstitute contents of 15-mL vial with at least 3 mL of diluent per gram of aztreonam. Appropriate diluents are sterile water for injection, bacteriostatic water for injection, 0.9% sodium chloride injection, bacteriostatic sodium chloride injection. Inject deeply into a large muscle mass. Do not mix with any local anesthetic.

⊗ ***Warning*** Discontinue drug and provide supportive measures if hypersensitivity reaction or anaphylaxis occurs.

- Monitor injection sites and provide comfort measures.
- Provide treatment and comfort measures if superinfections occur.
- Monitor patient's nutritional status, and provide small, frequent meals and mouth care if GI effects or superinfections interfere with nutrition.

Teaching points

- This drug can be given only IM or IV.
- You may experience these side effects: Nausea, vomiting, diarrhea.
- Report pain, soreness at injection site; difficulty breathing; mouth sores.

▽ bacitracin

*(bass i **tray'** sin)*

Oral: Altracin

Powder for injection: Baci-IM, BaciJect (CAN)

Ophthalmic: AK-Tracin

Topical ointment: Baciguent (CAN)

PREGNANCY CATEGORY C

Drug class

Antibiotic

Therapeutic actions

Antibacterial; inhibits cell wall synthesis of susceptible bacteria, primarily staphylococci, causing cell death.

Indications

- IM: Pneumonia and empyema caused by susceptible strains of staphylococci in infants
- Ophthalmic preparations: Superficial ocular infections involving the conjuctiva or cornea caused by susceptible strains of staphylococci
- Topical ointment: Prophylaxis of minor skin abrasions; treatment of superficial infections of the skin caused by susceptible staphylococci
- Orphan drug use (oral preparation): Antibiotic-associated pseudomembranous enterocolitis

Contraindications and cautions

- Contraindicated with allergy to bacitracin, renal disease (IM use), lactation.
- Use cautiously with pregnancy, dehydration.

Available forms

Powder for injection—50,000 units; ophthalmic ointment—500 units/g; topical ointment—500 units/g

Dosages

Adults and pediatric patients

Ophthalmic

Administration and dosage vary depending on the product used. See the product's package insert.

Topical

Apply to affected area one to three times per day; cover with sterile bandage if needed. Do not use longer than 1 wk.

IM

Infants weighing less than 2.5 kg: 900 units/kg/day IM in two to three divided doses. *Infants weighing more than 2.5 kg:* 1,000 units/kg/day IM in two to three divided doses.

Pharmacokinetics

Route	*Onset*	*Peak*	*Duration*
IM	Rapid	1–2 hr	12–14 hr

Metabolism: Hepatic; $T_{1/2}$: 6 hr
Distribution: Crosses placenta; enters breast milk
Excretion: Urine

Adverse effects

- **GI:** Nausea, vomiting
- **GU:** *Nephrotoxicity*
- **Local:** *Pain at injection site* (IM); *contact dermatitis* (topical ointment); *irritation, burning, stinging, itching, blurring of vision* (ophthalmic preparations)
- **Other:** Superinfections

Interactions

✱ **Drug-drug** • Increased neuromuscular blockade and muscular paralysis with anesthetics, nondepolarizing neuromuscular blocking drugs, drugs with neuromuscular blocking activity • Increased risk of respiratory paralysis and renal failure with aminoglycosides

■ Nursing considerations

Assessment

- **History:** Allergy to bacitracin, renal disease, lactation
- **Physical:** Site of infection; skin color, lesions; normal urinary output; urinalysis, serum creatinine, renal function tests

Interventions

- For IM use, reconstitute 50,000-unit vial with 9.8 mL 0.9% sodium chloride injection with 2% procaine hydrochloride; reconstitute the 10,000-unit vial with 2 mL of diluent (resulting concentration of 5,000 units/mL). Do not use diluents containing parabens; precipitates can form. Refrigerate unreconstituted vials. Reconstituted solutions are stable for 1 wk, refrigerated.
- For topical application, cleanse the area before applying new ointment.
- Culture infected area before therapy.
- Ensure adequate hydration to prevent renal toxicity.

⊗ ***Black box warning*** During IM therapy, monitor renal function tests daily; risk of serious renal toxicity.

Teaching points

- Give ophthalmic preparation as follows: Tilt head back; place medication inside the eyelid and close eyes; gently hold the inner corner of the eye for 1 minute. Do not touch tube to eye. For topical application, cleanse area being treated before applying new ointment; cover with sterile bandage (if possible).

- You may experience these side effects: Superinfections (frequent hygiene measures, medications may help); transient burning, stinging, or blurring of vision (ophthalmic).
- Report rash or skin lesions; change in urinary voiding patterns; changes in vision, severe stinging, or itching (ophthalmic).

baclofen

(bak' loe fen)

Apo-Baclofen (CAN), Gen-Baclofen (CAN), Kemstro, Lioresal, Lioresal Intrathecal, PMS-Baclofen (CAN), ratio-Baclofen (CAN)

PREGNANCY CATEGORY C

Drug class
Centrally acting skeletal muscle relaxant

Therapeutic actions
Precise mechanism not known; GABA analogue but does not appear to produce clinical effects by actions on GABA-minergic systems; inhibits both monosynaptic and polysynaptic spinal reflexes; CNS depressant.

Indications
- Alleviation of signs and symptoms of spasticity resulting from MS, particularly for the relief of flexor spasms and concomitant pain, clonus, muscular rigidity (for patients with reversible spasticity to aid in restoring residual function); treatment of severe spasticity (intrathecal route)
- Spinal cord injuries and other spinal cord diseases—may be of some value (oral)
- Unlabeled uses: Trigeminal neuralgia (tic douloureux); may be beneficial in reducing spasticity in cerebral palsy in children (intrathecal use); intractable hiccups unresponsive to other therapies, alcohol and opiate withdrawal (oral)

Contraindications and cautions
- Contraindicated with hypersensitivity to baclofen; skeletal muscle spasm resulting from rheumatic disorders.
- Use cautiously with stroke, cerebral palsy, Parkinson's disease, seizure disorders, lactation, pregnancy.

Available forms
Tablets—10, 20 mg; intrathecal—0.05 mg/mL, 10 mg/20 mL, 10 mg/5 mL; oral disintegrating tablets—10, 20 mg

Dosages
Adults
Oral

Individualize dosage; start at low dosage and increase gradually until optimum effect is achieved (usually 40–80 mg/day). The following dosage schedule is suggested: 5 mg PO tid for 3 days; 10 mg tid for 3 days; 15 mg tid for 3 days; 20 mg tid for 3 days. Thereafter, additional increases may be needed, but do not exceed 80 mg/day (20 mg qid); use lowest effective dose. If benefits are not evident after a reasonable trial period, gradually withdraw the drug.

Intrathecal

Refer to manufacturer's instructions on pump implantation and initiation of long-term infusion. Testing is usually done with 50 mcg/mL injected into intrathecal space over 1 min. Patient is observed for 4–8 hr, then dose of 75 mcg/1.5 mL is given; patient is observed for 4–8 hr; a final screening bolus of 100 mcg/2 mL is given 24 hr later if the response is still not adequate. Patients who do not respond to this dose are not candidates for the implant. Maintenance dose is determined by monitoring patient response for doses ranging from 22–1,400 mcg/day. Smallest dose possible to achieve muscle tone without adverse effects is desired.

Pediatric patients
Safety for use in children younger than 12 yr not established; orphan drug use to decrease spasticity in children with cerebral palsy is being studied.

Geriatric patients or patients with renal impairment
Dosage reduction may be necessary; monitor closely (drug is excreted largely unchanged by the kidneys).

Pharmacokinetics

Route	Onset	Peak	Duration
Oral	1 hr	2 hr	4–8 hr
Intrathecal	30–60 min	4 hr	4–8 hr

Metabolism: Hepatic; $T_{1/2}$: 3–4 hr
Distribution: Crosses placenta; enters breast milk
Excretion: Urine

Adverse effects

- **CNS:** *Transient drowsiness, dizziness, weakness, fatigue, confusion, headache, insomnia*
- **CV:** *Hypotension,* palpitations
- **GI:** Nausea, constipation
- **GU:** *Urinary frequency,* dysuria, enuresis, impotence
- **Other:** Rash, pruritus, ankle edema, excessive perspiration, weight gain, nasal congestion, increased AST, elevated alkaline phosphatase, elevated blood sugar

Interactions

✱ **Drug-drug** • Increased CNS depression with alcohol, other CNS depressants

■ Nursing considerations

Assessment

- **History:** Hypersensitivity to baclofen, skeletal muscle spasm resulting from rheumatic disorders, stroke, cerebral palsy, Parkinson's disease, seizure disorders, lactation, pregnancy
- **Physical:** Weight; T; skin color, lesions; orientation, affect, reflexes, bilateral grip strength, visual examination; P, BP; bowel sounds, normal GI output, liver evaluation; normal urinary output; LFTs, renal function tests, blood and urine glucose

Interventions

- Patients given implantable device for intrathecal delivery need to learn about the programmable delivery system, frequent checks; how to adjust dose and programming.
- Give with caution to patients whose spasticity contributes to upright posture or balance in locomotion or whenever spasticity is used to increase function.

⊗ ***Black box warning*** Taper dosage gradually to prevent hallucinations, possible psychosis, rhabdomyolysis, or other serious effects; abrupt discontinuation can cause serious reactions.

Teaching points

- Take this drug exactly as prescribed. Do not stop taking this drug without consulting your health care provider; abrupt discontinuation may cause hallucinations or other serious effects.
- Avoid alcohol, sleep-inducing, or over-the-counter drugs because these could cause dangerous effects.
- Do not take this drug during pregnancy. If you decide to become pregnant or find that you are pregnant, consult your health care provider.
- You may experience these side effects: Drowsiness, dizziness, confusion (avoid driving or engaging in activities that require alertness); nausea (eat frequent small meals); insomnia, headache, painful or frequent urination (effects reversible; will go away when the drug is discontinued).
- Report frequent or painful urination, constipation, nausea, headache, insomnia, or confusion that persists or is severe.

▽ balsalazide disodium

*(bal **sal'** a zyde)*

Colazal

PREGNANCY CATEGORY B

Drug class

Anti-inflammatory

Therapeutic actions

Mechanism of action is unknown; thought to be direct, delivered intact to the colon; a local anti-inflammatory effect occurs in the colon where balsalazide is converted to mesalamine (5-ASA), which blocks cyclooxygenase and inhibits prostaglandin production in the colon.

Indications

- Treatment of mildly to moderately active ulcerative colitis

Contraindications and cautions

- Contraindicated with hypersensitivity to salicylates or mesalamine.
- Use cautiously with renal impairment, pregnancy, lactation.

Available forms

Capsules—750 mg

Dosages

Adults

Three 750-mg capsules PO tid for a total daily dose of 6.75 g. Continue for up to 12 wk.

Pediatric patients 5–17 yr

Three 750-mg capsules PO tid (6.75 g/day) with or without food for 8 wk, or one 750 mg capsule PO tid (2.25 g/day) with or without food for 8 wk.

Pharmacokinetics

Route	*Onset*	*Peak*
Oral	Varies	1–2 hr

Metabolism: Hepatic; $T_{1/2}$: Unknown
Distribution: Crosses placenta; may enter breast milk
Excretion: Feces and urine

Adverse effects

- **CNS:** *Headache, fatigue, malaise, depression,* dizziness, asthenia, insomnia
- **GI:** *Abdominal pain, cramps, vomiting, discomfort; gas; flatulence; nausea; diarrhea, dyspepsia,* bloating, hemorrhoids, rectal pain, constipation, diarrhea, dry mouth
- **Other:** *Flulike symptoms, rash,* fever, cold, back pain, peripheral edema, *arthralgia*

■ Nursing considerations

CLINICAL ALERT!

Name confusion has occurred between *Colazal* (balsalazide) and *Clozaril* (clozapine). Serious effects have occurred; use extreme caution.

Assessment

- **History:** Hypersensitivity to salicylates; renal impairment; pregnancy, lactation
- **Physical:** T, hair status; reflexes, affect; abdominal examination, rectal examination; urinary output, renal function tests

Interventions

- Administer with meals. May be given for up to 12 wk.
- Monitor patients with renal impairment for possible adverse effects.
- Ensure ready access to bathroom facilities if diarrhea occurs.
- Offer support and encouragement to deal with GI discomfort, CNS effects.
- Arrange for appropriate measures to deal with headache, arthralgia, GI problems.
- Provide small, frequent meals if GI upset is severe.
- Maintain all therapy (such as dietary restrictions, reduced stress) necessary to support remission of the ulcerative colitis.

Teaching points

- Take the drug with meals in evenly divided doses.
- Maintain all of the usual restrictions and therapy that apply to your colitis. If this becomes difficult, consult your health care provider.
- You may experience these side effects: Abdominal cramping, discomfort, pain, diarrhea (ensure ready access to bathroom facilities, taking the drug with meals may help), headache, fatigue, fever, flulike symptoms (consult health care provider if these become bothersome, medications may be available to help); rash, itching (skin care may help; consult your health care provider if this becomes a problem).
- Report severe diarrhea, malaise, fatigue, fever, blood in the stool.

basiliximab

See Appendix W, *Less commonly used drugs*.

BCG intravesical

See Appendix W, *Less commonly used drugs*.

beclomethasone dipropionate

*(be kloe **meth'** a sone)*

Apo-Beclomethasone (CAN), Beconase AQ, Gen-Beclo AQ (CAN), Propaderm (CAN), QVAR, ratio-Beclomethasone AQ (CAN)

PREGNANCY CATEGORY C

Drug classes

Corticosteroid
Glucocorticoid
Hormone

Therapeutic actions

Anti-inflammatory effects; local administration into lower respiratory tract or nasal passages maximizes beneficial effects on these tissues while decreasing the likelihood of adverse corticosteroid effects from systemic absorption.

Indications

- Maintenance treatment of asthma as prophylactic therapy in patients 5 yr and older
- Respiratory inhalant use: Control of bronchial asthma that requires corticosteroids along with other therapy
- Intranasal use: Relief of symptoms of seasonal or perennial rhinitis that respond poorly to other treatments; prevention of recurrence of nasal polyps following surgical removal

Contraindications and cautions

- Respiratory inhalant therapy: Contraindicated with acute asthmatic attack, status asthmaticus. Use caution with systemic fungal infections (may cause exacerbations), allergy to any ingredient, lactation.
- Intranasal therapy: Use caution with untreated local infections (may cause exacerbations); nasal septal ulcers, recurrent epistaxis, nasal surgery or trauma (interferes with healing); lactation.

Available forms

Inhalation aerosol—40 mcg/actuation, 80 mcg/actuation; nasal spray—0.042%

Dosages

Respiratory inhalant use

Adults and children 12 yr and older

40–160 mcg bid. Do not exceed 320 mcg/bid.

Pediatric patients 5–11 yr

40 mcg bid. Do not exceed 80 mcg bid.

Pediatric patients younger than 5 yr

Do not use.

Intranasal therapy

Each actuation delivers 42 mcg. Discontinue therapy after 3 wk if no significant symptomatic improvement.

Adults and children 12 yr and older

One to two inhalations (42–84 mcg) in each nostril bid (total dose 168–336 mcg/day).

Pediatric patients 6–11 yr

One inhalation in each nostril bid. Total dose 168 mcg. With more severe symptoms, may increase to two inhalations in each nostril bid (336 mcg).

Pharmacokinetics

Route	*Onset*	*Peak*
Inhalation	Rapid	1–2 wk

Metabolism: Lungs, GI, and liver; $T_{1/2}$: 3–15 hr

Distribution: Crosses placenta; may enter breast milk

Excretion: Feces

Adverse effects

Respiratory inhalant use

- **Endocrine:** Cushing's syndrome with overdose, suppression of HPA function due to systemic absorption
- **Local:** *Oral, laryngeal, pharyngeal irritation,* fungal infections

Intranasal use

- **Local:** Nasal irritation, fungal infections
- **Respiratory:** *Epistaxis, rebound congestion,* perforation of the nasal septum, anosmia
- **Other:** *Headache, nausea,* urticaria

■ Nursing considerations

Assessment

- **History:** Acute asthmatic attack, status asthmaticus; systemic fungal infections; allergy to any ingredient; lactation; untreated local infections, nasal septal ulcers, recurrent epistaxis, nasal surgery or trauma
- **Physical:** Weight, T; P, BP, auscultation; R, adventitious sounds; chest radiograph before respiratory inhalant therapy; examination of nares before intranasal therapy

Interventions

⊗ ***Black box warning*** Taper systemic steroids carefully during transfer to inhalational steroids; deaths resulting from adrenal insufficiency have occurred during and after transfer from systemic to aerosol steroids.

- Use decongestant nose drops to facilitate penetration of intranasal steroids if edema or excessive secretions are present.

Teaching points

- This respiratory inhalant has been prescribed to prevent asthmatic attacks, not for use during an attack.
- Allow at least 1 minute between puffs (respiratory inhalant); if you also are using an inhalational bronchodilator (albuterol, levalbuterol, metaproterenol, epinephrine), use it several minutes before using the steroid aerosol.
- Rinse your mouth after using the respiratory inhalant aerosol.
- Use a decongestant before the intranasal steroid, and clear your nose of all secretions if nasal passages are blocked; intranasal steroids may take several days to produce full benefit.
- Use this product exactly as prescribed; do not take more than prescribed, and do not stop taking the drug without consulting your health care provider. The drug must not be stopped abruptly but must be slowly tapered.
- You may experience these side effects: Local irritation (use the device correctly), headache (consult your health care provider for treatment).
- Report sore throat or sore mouth.

▽ benazepril hydrochloride

(ben a' za pril)

Lotensin

PREGNANCY CATEGORY C (FIRST TRIMESTER)

PREGNANCY CATEGORY D (SECOND AND THIRD TRIMESTERS)

Drug classes

ACE inhibitor
Antihypertensive

Therapeutic actions

Blocks ACE from converting angiotensin I to angiotensin II, a potent vasoconstrictor, leading to decreased BP, decreased aldosterone secretion, a small increase in serum potassium levels, and sodium and fluid loss; increased prostaglandin synthesis also may be involved in the antihypertensive action.

Indications

- Treatment of hypertension alone or in combination with thiazide-type diuretics
- Unlabeled uses: nondiabetic neuropathy, heart failure, post MI, diabetes, chronic kidney disease, recurrent stroke prevention

Contraindications and cautions

- Contraindicated with allergy to benazepril or other ACE inhibitors, second or third trimester of pregnancy.
- Use cautiously with impaired renal function, immunosuppression, hypotension, heart failure, salt or volume depletion, lactation, first trimester of pregnancy, hyperkalemia.

Available forms

Tablets—5, 10, 20, 40 mg

Dosages

Adults

Initial dose, 10 mg PO daily. Maintenance dose, 20–40 mg/day PO, single or two divided doses. Patients using diuretics should discontinue them 2–3 days prior to benazepril therapy. If BP is not controlled, add diuretic slowly. If diuretic cannot be discontinued, begin benazepril therapy with 5 mg. Maximum dose, 80 mg.

Pediatric patients (6 yr and older)

0.1–0.6 mg/kg/day. Starting dose for monotherapy—0.2 mg/kg/day. Do not exceed 0.6 mg/kg/day (40 mg daily).

Patients with renal impairment

For creatinine clearance less than 30 mL/min (serum creatinine greater than 3 mg/dL), 5 mg PO daily. Dosage may be gradually increased until BP is controlled, up to a maximum of 40 mg/day.

Pharmacokinetics

Route	*Onset*	*Peak*	*Duration*
Oral	0.5–1 hr	3–4 hr	24 hr

Metabolism: Hepatic; $T_{1/2}$: 10–11 hr
Distribution: Crosses placenta; enters breast milk
Excretion: Urine

Adverse effects

- **CNS:** Dizziness, fatigue, headache, somnolence
- **CV:** Angina pectoris, hypotension in salt- or volume-depleted patients, palpitations
- **Dermatologic:** Rash, pruritus, diaphoresis, flushing, **Stevens-Johnson syndrome**
- **GI:** *Nausea,* abdominal pain, vomiting, constipation
- **Respiratory:** *Cough,* asthma, bronchitis, dyspnea, sinusitis
- **Other:** Angioedema, impotence, decreased libido, asthenia, myalgia, arthralgia

Interactions

✱ **Drug-drug** • Increased risk of hypersensitivity reactions with allopurinol • Increased coughing with capsaicin • Decreased antihypertensive effects with indomethacin and other NSAIDs • Increased lithium levels and neurotoxicity may occur if combine • Increased risk of hyperkalemia with potassium-sparing diuretics or potassium supplements

■ Nursing considerations

Assessment

- **History:** Allergy to benazepril or other ACE inhibitors, impaired renal function, heart failure, salt or volume depletion, lactation, pregnancy
- **Physical:** Skin color, lesions, turgor; T; P, BP, peripheral perfusion; mucous membranes, bowel sounds, liver evaluation; urinalysis, LFTs, renal function tests, CBC and differential

Interventions

⊗ ***Warning*** Alert surgeon: Note use of benazepril on patient's chart; the angiotensin II formation subsequent to compensatory renin release during surgery will be blocked; hypotension may be reversed with volume expansion.

- Monitor patient for possible drop in BP secondary to reduction in fluid volume (excessive perspiration and dehydration, vomiting, diarrhea) because excessive hypotension may occur.

⊗ ***Black box warning*** Ensure that patient is not pregnant; fetal abnormalities and death have occurred if used during second or third trimester. Encourage use of contraceptive measures.

- Reduce dosage in patients with impaired renal function.

Teaching points

- Do not stop taking the medication without consulting your health care provider.
- Be careful with any conditions that may lead to a drop in blood pressure (such as diarrhea, sweating, vomiting, dehydration); if light-headedness or dizziness occurs, consult your health care provider.
- You should not become pregnant while on this drug. Serious fetal abnormalities could occur; use of contraceptives is advised.
- You may experience these side effects: GI upset, loss of appetite (transient effects; if persistent, consult health care provider); lightheadedness (transient; change position slowly, and limit activities to those that do not require alertness and precision); dry cough (irritating but not harmful; consult your health care provider).

- Report mouth sores; sore throat, fever, chills; swelling of the hands, feet; irregular heartbeat, chest pains; swelling of the face, eyes, lips, tongue, difficulty breathing, persistent cough.

DANGEROUS DRUG

bendamustine hydrochloride

(ben' dah moos' teen)

Treanda

PREGNANCY CATEGORY D

Drug classes
Antineoplastic
Alkylating agent

Therapeutic actions
Cytotoxic; alkylates DNA and RNA and inhibits several enzymatic processes, leading to cell death.

Indications
- Treatment of chronic lymphocytic leukemia (CLL)
- **NEW INDICATION:** Treatment of indolent B-cell non-Hodgkin lymphoma that has progressed during or within 6 mo of rituxima therapy or a rituximab-containing regimen

Contraindications and cautions
- Contraindicated with known hypersensitivity to bendamustine or mannitol, pregnancy, lactation, moderate or severe hepatic impairment, severe renal impairment.
- Use cautiously in patients with moderate renal impairment, mild hepatic impairment.

Available forms
Single-use vials—100 mg

Dosages
Adults
- *CLL*: 100 mg/m^2 IV over 30 min on days 1 and 2 of a 28-day cycle for up to 6 cycles; dosage may need to be lowered based on patient response and drug toxicity.
- *Non-Hodgkin lymphoma:* 120 mg/m^2 IV on days 1 and 2 of a 21-day cycle for up to 8 cycles; dosage may need to be adjusted based on patient response.

Pediatric patients
Safety and efficacy not established.

Patients with hepatic or renal impairment
Use caution with mild or moderate dysfunction; do not use with severe dysfunction.

Pharmacokinetics

Route	*Onset*	*Peak*
IV	Rapid	End of infusion

Metabolism: Hepatic; $T_{1/2}$: 3 hr
Distribution: Crosses placenta; may enter breast milk
Excretion: Feces

IV FACTS
Preparation: Reconstitute 100-mg vial with 20 mL sterile water for injection; solution should be clear yellow with concentration of 5 mg/mL. Withdraw desired dose and transfer immediately to 500 mL 0.9% sodium chloride injection within 30 min of reconstitution; thoroughly mix bag. Drug is stable for 24 hr if refrigerated, 3 hr at room temperature.
Infusion: Administer complete infusion over 30 min (CLL) or 60 min for non-Hodgkin lymphoma.
Incompatibilities: Do not mix in solution with any other medications. Administer only with sterile water for injection diluent and 0.9% sodium chloride injection.

Adverse effects
- **Dermatologic:** Rash to **toxic skin reactions,** pruritus
- **GI:** *Diarrhea, nausea, vomiting*
- **Hematologic:** *Myelosuppression,* hyperuricemia
- **Respiratory:** Nasopharyngitis, cough
- **Other:** *Infusion reaction,* tumor lysis syndrome, *infections, fever, fatigue,* chills, weight loss

Interactions

✱ **Drug-drug** • Concurrent use of CYP1A2 inhibitors (fluvoxamine, ciprofloxacin) or inducers (omeprazole, nicotine) can lead to treatment failure or increased toxicity; an alternative treatment should be considered

■ Nursing considerations

Assessment

- **History:** Hypersensitivity to mannitol or bendamustine, pregnancy, lactation, hepatic or renal impairment
- **Physical:** T; skin color, lesions; R, adventitious sounds; GI exam, renal function tests, LFTs

Interventions

- Monitor hematopoietic function before therapy and weekly during therapy to monitor patient response and ensure dosage is reduced when needed.
- Review safety precautions for bone marrow suppression with patient, such as avoiding infections and injuries and arranging rest periods throughout the day.
- Monitor patient carefully during infusion; severe infusion reactions have been reported. Antihistamines, antipyretics and corticosteroids may be needed if reactions do occur. Consider discontinuing drug if severe reactions occur.
- Monitor patient for tumor lysis syndrome, especially during the first cycle; provide appropriate fluid volume, monitor electrolytes, and consider prophylactic allopurinol for high-risk patients.
- Assess skin regularly. If skin reactions occur and become severe or progressive, drug may need to be stopped.

Teaching Points

- Mark your calendar with the days you will need to have IV infusions.
- You will need to have regular blood tests, including tests right before your infusion, to monitor the drug's effects on your body and determine the dose you will need.
- You may feel tired because your red blood cell count is decreased. Plan rest periods during the day.
- You may experience increased bruising and bleeding because your platelet count is decreased. Try to avoid activities that could lead to injury.
- You are susceptible to infection because your white blood cell count is decreased. Avoid crowded places, people with known infections, and digging in the dirt (unless you are wearing gloves).
- This drug could harm a fetus. You should use contraceptive measures while you are on this drug. If you become pregnant, notify your health care provider immediately.
- It is not known how this drug could affect a nursing baby. Because of the potential for serious adverse effects to the baby, another method of feeding the baby should be used while you are on this drug.
- You may experience these side effects: Nausea, vomiting (small, frequent meals may help; medication may be available to relieve these symptoms), diarrhea (medications may also help this symptom), rash.
- Report rash of any kind, any signs of infection (fever, fatigue, muscle aches and pains), significant bleeding, shortness of breath, swelling of the face, persistent or severe nausea, vomiting, or diarrhea.

▽ benzonatate

(ben zoe' na tate)

Benzonatate Softgels (DNC), Tessalon (DNC), Tessalon Perles (DNC)

PREGNANCY CATEGORY C

Drug class

Antitussive (nonopioid)

Therapeutic actions

Related to the local anesthetic tetracaine; anesthetizes the stretch receptors in the respiratory passages, lungs, and pleura, hampering their activity and reducing the cough reflex at its source.

Indications

- Symptomatic relief of nonproductive cough
- Unlabeled use: May be used to reduce cough reflex during procedures (ie, endoscopy)

Contraindications and cautions

- Contraindicated with allergy to benzonatate or related compounds (tetracaine); lactation.
- Use cautiously with pregnancy.

Available forms

Capsules—100, 200 mg

Dosages

Adults and pediatric patients 10 yr and older

100–200 mg PO tid; up to 600 mg/day may be used.

Pharmacokinetics

Route	*Onset*	*Duration*
Oral	15–20 min	3–8 hr

Metabolism: Hepatic; $T_{1/2}$: 2–4 hr
Distribution: Crosses placenta; may enter breast milk
Excretion: Urine

Adverse effects

- **CNS:** *Sedation, headache, mild dizziness,* hallucinations, nasal congestion, sensation of burning in the eyes
- **Dermatologic:** Pruritus, skin eruptions
- **GI:** *Constipation, nausea,* GI upset
- **Other:** Vague "chilly" feeling, numbness in the chest

■ Nursing considerations

Assessment

- **History:** Allergy to benzonatate or related compounds (tetracaine); lactation, pregnancy
- **Physical:** Nasal mucous membranes; skin color, lesions; orientation, affect; adventitious sounds

Interventions

⊗ ***Warning*** Administer orally; caution patient not to chew or break capsules but to swallow them whole; choking could occur if drug is released in the mouth.

Teaching points

- Swallow the capsules whole; do not chew or break capsules because numbness of the throat and mouth could occur, and swallowing could become difficult.
- You may experience these side effects: Rash, itching (skin care may help); constipation, nausea, GI upset; sedation, dizziness (avoid driving or tasks that require alertness).
- Report restlessness, tremor, difficulty breathing, constipation, rash, bizarre behavior.

benztropine mesylate

***(benz'** troe peen)*

Apo-Benztropine (CAN), Cogentin

PREGNANCY CATEGORY C

Drug class

Antiparkinsonian (anticholinergic type)

Therapeutic actions

Has anticholinergic activity in the CNS that is believed to help normalize the hypothesized imbalance of cholinergic and dopaminergic neurotransmission in the basal ganglia of the brain of a parkinsonism patient. Reduces severity of rigidity and, to a lesser extent, akinesia and tremor; less effective overall than levodopa; peripheral anticholinergic effects suppress secondary symptoms of parkinsonism, such as drooling.

Indications

- Adjunct in the therapy of parkinsonism (postencephalitic, arteriosclerotic, and idiopathic types)
- Control of extrapyramidal disorders (except tardive dyskinesia) due to neuroleptic drugs (phenothiazines)

Contraindications and cautions

- Contraindicated with hypersensitivity to benztropine; glaucoma, especially angle-closure glaucoma; pyloric or duodenal obstruction, stenosing peptic ulcers, achalasia (megaesophagus); prostatic hypertrophy or bladder neck obstructions; myasthenia gravis.
- Use cautiously with tachycardia, cardiac arrhythmias, hypertension, hypotension, hepatic or renal impairment, alcoholism, chronic illness, work in hot environments; hot weather; lactation, Alzheimer's disease, pregnancy.

Available forms

Tablets—0.5, 1, 2 mg; injection—1 mg/mL

Dosages

Adults

- *Parkinsonism:* Initially, 0.5–1 mg PO at bedtime; a total daily dose of 0.5–6 mg given at bedtime or in two to four divided doses is usual. Increase initial dose in 0.5-mg increments at 5- to 6-day intervals to the smallest amount necessary for optimal relief. Maximum daily dose, 6 mg. May be given IM or IV in same dosage as oral. When used with other drugs, gradually substitute benztropine for all or part of them and gradually reduce dosage of the other drug.
- *Drug-induced extrapyramidal symptoms:* For acute dystonic reactions, initially, 1–2 mg IM (preferred) or IV to control condition; may repeat if parkinsonian effect begins to return. After that, 1–4 mg PO daily or bid to prevent recurrences. Some patients may require higher doses.
- *Extrapyramidal disorders occurring early in neuroleptic treatment:* 1–2 mg PO bid to tid. Withdraw drug after 1 or 2 wk to determine its continued need; reinstitute if disorder reappears.

Pediatric patients

Safety and efficacy not established.

Geriatric patients

Strict dosage regulation may be necessary; patients older than 60 yr often develop increased sensitivity to the CNS effects of anticholinergic drugs.

Pharmacokinetics

Route	*Onset*	*Duration*
Oral	1 hr	6–10 hr
IM, IV	15 min	6–10 hr

Metabolism: Hepatic; $T_{1/2}$: Unknown
Distribution: Crosses placenta; enters breast milk
Excretion: Unknown

IV FACTS

Preparation: Give undiluted. Store in tightly covered, light-resistant container. Store at room temperature.

Injection: Administer direct IV at a rate of 1 mg over 1 min.

Adverse effects

Peripheral anticholinergic effects

- **CV:** Tachycardia, palpitations, hypotension, orthostatic hypotension
- **Dermatologic:** Rash, urticaria, other dermatoses
- **EENT:** *Blurred vision,* mydriasis, diplopia, increased intraocular tension, angle-closure glaucoma
- **GI:** *Dry mouth, constipation,* dilation of the colon, paralytic ileus, *nausea,* vomiting, epigastric distress
- **GU:** *Urinary retention, urinary hesitancy,* dysuria, difficulty achieving or maintaining an erection
- **Other:** Flushing, decreased sweating, elevated temperature

CNS effects, characteristic of centrally acting anticholinergic drugs

- **CNS:** Disorientation, confusion, memory loss, hallucinations, psychoses, agitation, nervousness, delusions, delirium, paranoia, euphoria, excitement, light-headedness, dizziness, depression, drowsiness, weakness, giddiness, paresthesia, heaviness of the limbs
- **Other:** Muscular weakness, muscular cramping; inability to move certain muscle groups (high doses), numbness of fingers

Interactions

✱ **Drug-drug** • Paralytic ileus, sometimes fatal, when given with other anticholinergic drugs, or drugs that have anticholinergic properties (phenothiazines, TCAs) • Additive adverse CNS effects (toxic psychosis) with other drugs that have CNS anticholinergic properties (TCAs, phenothiazines) • Possible masking of the development of persistent extrapyramidal symptoms, tardive dyskinesia, in patients on long-term therapy with antipsychotic drugs (phenothiazines, haloperidol) • Decreased therapeutic efficacy of antipsychotic drugs (phenothiazines, haloperidol), possibly due to central antagonism

■ Nursing considerations
Assessment
- **History:** Hypersensitivity to benztropine; glaucoma; pyloric or duodenal obstruction, stenosing peptic ulcers, achalasia; prostatic hypertrophy or bladder neck obstructions; myasthenia gravis; cardiac arrhythmias, hypertension, hypotension; hepatic or renal impairment; alcoholism, chronic illness, people who work in hot environments; lactation, pregnancy
- **Physical:** Weight; T; skin color, lesions; orientation, affect, reflexes, bilateral grip strength, visual examination including tonometry; P, BP, orthostatic BP; adventitious sounds; bowel sounds, normal output, liver evaluation; normal urinary output, voiding pattern, prostate palpation; LFTs, renal function tests

Interventions
- Decrease dosage or discontinue temporarily if dry mouth makes swallowing or speaking difficult.
- Do not give to patients on cholinesterase inhibitors. Benztropine directly counteracts the effects of these drugs.

⊗ ***Warning*** Give with caution and reduce dosage in hot weather. Drug interferes with sweating and body's ability to maintain heat equilibrium; provide sugarless lozenges or ice chips to suck for dry mouth.

- Give with meals if GI upset occurs; give before meals for dry mouth; give after meals if drooling or nausea occurs.
- Ensure patient voids before receiving each dose if urinary retention is a problem.

Teaching points
- Take this drug exactly as prescribed.
- Avoid alcohol, sedatives, and over-the-counter drugs (could cause dangerous effects).
- You may experience these side effects: Drowsiness, dizziness, confusion, blurred vision (avoid driving or engaging in activities that require alertness and visual acuity); nausea (eat frequent small meals); dry mouth (suck sugarless lozenges or ice chips); painful or difficult urination (empty bladder immediately before each dose); constipation (maintain adequate fluid intake and exercise regularly); use caution in hot weather (you are susceptible to heat prostration).
- Report difficult or painful urination, constipation, rapid or pounding heartbeat, confusion, eye pain, or rash.

B

▽beractant (natural lung surfactant)
*(ber **ak'** tant)*

Survanta

PREGNANCY CATEGORY UNKNOWN

Drug class
Lung surfactant

Therapeutic actions
A natural bovine compound containing lipids and apoproteins that reduce surface tension and allow expansion of the alveoli; replaces the surfactant missing in the lungs of neonates suffering from respiratory distress syndrome (RDS).

Indications
- Prophylactic treatment of infants at risk of developing RDS; infants with birth weights less than 1,250 g or infants with birth weights more than 1,250 g who have evidence of pulmonary immaturity
- Rescue treatment of premature infants who have developed RDS

Contraindications and cautions
- Because beractant is used as an emergency drug in acute respiratory situations, the benefits usually outweigh any possible risks.

Available forms
Suspension—25 mg/mL suspended in 0.9% sodium chloride injection

Dosages
Pediatric patients
Accurate determination of birth weight is essential for correct dosage. Beractant is instilled into the trachea using a catheter inserted into the endotracheal tube.

- *Prophylactic treatment:* Give first dose of 100 mg phospholipids/kg birth weight (4 mL/kg) soon after birth. After determining the needed dose, inject one-quarter of the dose into the endotracheal tube over 2–3 sec. Remove the catheter and ventilate the baby. Repeat the procedure to give the remaining one-quarter dose. A repeat dose may be given no sooner than 6 hr after previous dose if infant remains intubated and requires at least 30% inspired oxygen to maintain a partial pressure of arterial oxygen of 80 mm Hg or less. Four doses can be administered in the first 48 hr of life.
- *Rescue treatment:* Administer 100 mg phospholipids/kg birth weight (4 mL/kg) intratracheally. Administer the first dose as soon as possible after the diagnosis of RDS is made and patient is on the ventilator. Repeat doses can be given based on clinical improvement and blood gases. Administer subsequent doses no sooner than every 6 hr.

Pharmacokinetics

Route	*Onset*	*Peak*
Intratracheal	Immediate	Hours

Metabolism: Normal surfactant metabolic pathways; $T_{1/2}$: Unknown
Distribution: Lung tissue

Adverse effects

- **CNS:** Seizures
- **CV:** *Patent ductus arteriosus,* **intraventricular hemorrhage, hypotension, bradycardia**
- **Hematologic:** Hyperbilirubinemia, thrombocytopenia
- **Respiratory: Pneumothorax, pulmonary air leak, pulmonary hemorrhage, apnea,** pneumomediastinum, emphysema
- **Other:** *Sepsis, nonpulmonary infections*

■ Nursing considerations

Assessment

- **History:** Time of birth, exact birth weight
- **Physical:** Skin T, color; R, adventitious sounds, oximeter, endotracheal tube position and patency, chest movement; ECG, P, BP, peripheral perfusion, arterial pressure (desirable); oxygen saturation, blood gases, CBC; muscular activity, facial expression, reflexes

Interventions

- Monitor ECG and transcutaneous oxygen saturation continually during administration.
- Ensure that endotracheal tube is in the correct position, with bilateral chest movement and lung sounds.
- Have staff view manufacturer's teaching video before regular use to cover all the technical aspects of administration.
- Suction the infant immediately before administration, but do not suction for 1 hr after administration unless clinically necessary.
- Inspect vial for discoloration. Vial should contain off-white to brown liquid. Gently mix. Warm to room temperature before using—20 min standing or 8 min warmed by hand. Do not use other warming methods.
- Store drug in refrigerator. Protect from light. Enter drug vial only once. Discard remaining drug after use. Unopened, unused vials warmed to room temperature may be returned to refrigerator within 8 hr of warming.
- Insert 5 French catheter into the endotracheal tube; do not instill into the mainstem bronchus.
- Instill dose slowly; inject one-fourth dose over 2–3 sec; remove catheter and reattach infant to ventilator for at least 30 sec or until stable; repeat procedure administering one-fourth dose at a time.
- Do not suction infant for 1 hr after completion of full dose; do not flush catheter.
- Continually monitor patient's color, lung sounds, ECG, oximeter, and blood gas readings during administration and for at least 30 min after.

Teaching points

- Details of drug effects and administration are best incorporated into parents' comprehensive teaching program.

B

betamethasone
*(bay ta **meth'** a sone)*

betamethasone
Topical dermatologic ointment, cream, lotion, gel

betamethasone dipropionate
*(dye proh **py'** oh nayt)*

Topical dermatologic ointment, cream, lotion, aerosol: Diprolene, Diprolene AF, Diprosone, Maxivate, Taro-Sone (CAN)

betamethasone sodium phosphate
Systemic, including IV and local injection: Betnesol (CAN)

betamethasone sodium phosphate and acetate
Systemic, IM, and local intra-articular, intralesional, intradermal injection: Celestone Soluspan

betamethasone valerate
*(val **ayr'** ayt)*

Topical dermatologic ointment, cream, lotion: Betaderm (CAN), Beta-Val, Luxiq, Prevex B (CAN), Psorion Cream, Valisone

PREGNANCY CATEGORY C

Drug classes
Corticosteroid (long acting)
Glucocorticoid
Hormone

Therapeutic actions
Binds to intracellular corticosteroid receptors, thereby initiating many natural complex reactions that are responsible for its anti-inflammatory and immunosuppressive effects.

Indications
Systemic administration
- Hypercalcemia associated with cancer
- Short-term management of inflammatory and allergic disorders, such as rheumatoid arthritis, collagen diseases (eg, SLE), dermatologic diseases (eg, pemphigus), status asthmaticus, and autoimmune disorders
- Hematologic disorders: Thrombocytopenia purpura, erythroblastopenia
- Ulcerative colitis, acute exacerbations of MS, and palliation in some leukemias and lymphomas
- Trichinosis with neurologic or myocardial involvement

Intra-articular or soft-tissue administration
- Arthritis, psoriatic plaques, and so forth

Dermatologic preparations
- Relief of inflammatory and pruritic manifestations of steroid-responsive dermatoses

Contraindications and cautions
Systemic (oral and parenteral) administration
- Contraindicated with infections, especially tuberculosis, fungal infections, amebiasis, vaccinia and varicella, and antibiotic-resistant infections, lactation.

All forms
- Use cautiously with kidney or liver disease, hypothyroidism, ulcerative colitis with impending perforation, diverticulitis, active or latent peptic ulcer, inflammatory bowel disease, heart failure, hypertension, thromboembolic disorders, osteoporosis, seizure disorders, diabetes mellitus.

Available forms
Syrup—0.6 mg/5 mL; injection—4 mg, 3 mg betamethasone sodium phosphate with 3 mg betamethasone acetate; ointment—0.1%, 0.05%; cream—0.01%, 0.05%, 0.1%; lotion—0.1%, 0.05%; gel—0.05%

Dosages
Adults

Systemic administration
Individualize dosage, based on severity and response. Give daily dose before 9 AM to minimize adrenal suppression. Reduce initial dosage in small increments until the lowest

dose that maintains satisfactory clinical response is reached. If long-term therapy is needed, alternate-day therapy with a short-acting corticosteroid should be considered. After long-term therapy, withdraw drug slowly to prevent adrenal insufficiency.

- *Oral (betamethasone):* Initial dosage, 0.6–7.2 mg/day.
- *IV (betamethasone sodium phosphate):* Initial dosage, up to 9 mg/day.
- *IM (betamethasone sodium phosphate; betamethasone sodium phosphate and acetate):* Initial dosage, 0.5–9 mg/day. Dosage range is one-third to one-half oral dose given every 12 hr. In life-threatening situations, dose can be in multiples of the oral dose.

Intrabursal, intra-articular, intradermal, intralesional (betamethasone sodium phosphate and acetate)

0.25–2 mL intra-articular, depending on joint size; 0.2 mL/cm^3 intradermally, not to exceed 1 mL/wk; 0.25–1 mL at 3- to 7-day intervals for disorders of the foot.

Topical dermatologic cream, ointment (betamethasone dipropionate)

Apply sparingly to affected area daily or bid.

Pediatric patients

Systemic administration

Individualize dosage on the basis of severity and response rather than by formulae that correct adult doses for age or weight. Carefully observe growth and development in infants and children on prolonged therapy.

Pharmacokinetics

Route	*Onset*	*Duration*
Systemic	Varies	3 days

Metabolism: Hepatic; $T_{1/2}$: 36–54 hr
Distribution: Crosses placenta; enters breast milk
Excretion: Urine, unchanged

IV FACTS

Preparation: No further preparation needed.
Infusion: Infuse by direct IV injection over 1 min or into the tubing of running IV of dextrose or saline solutions.

Adverse effects

- **CNS:** *Vertigo, headache,* paresthesias, insomnia, seizures, psychosis, cataracts, increased IOP, glaucoma (in long-term therapy)
- **CV:** Hypotension, shock, hypertension, and heart failure secondary to fluid retention, thromboembolism, thrombophlebitis, fat embolism, cardiac arrhythmias
- **Electrolyte imbalance:** *Na^+ and fluid retention,* hypokalemia, hypocalcemia
- **Endocrine:** Amenorrhea, irregular menses, growth retardation, decreased carbohydrate tolerance, diabetes mellitus, cushingoid state (long-term effect), increased blood sugar, increased serum cholesterol, decreased T_3 and T_4 levels, HPA suppression with systemic therapy longer than 5 days
- **GI:** Peptic or esophageal ulcer, pancreatitis, abdominal distention, nausea, vomiting, *increased appetite, weight gain (long-term therapy)*
- **Musculoskeletal:** Muscle weakness, steroid myopathy, loss of muscle mass, osteoporosis, spontaneous fractures (long-term therapy)
- **Other:** *Immunosuppression, aggravation, or masking of infections; impaired wound healing;* thin, fragile skin; petechiae, ecchymoses, purpura, striae; subcutaneous fat atrophy; hypersensitivity or anaphylactoid reactions

Effects related to various local routes of steroid administration

- **Intra-articular:** Osteonecrosis, tendon rupture, infection
- **Intralesional therapy:** Blindness when applied to face and head
- **Topical dermatologic ointments, creams, sprays:** *Local burning, irritation,* acneiform lesions, striae, skin atrophy, skin infections

Interactions

✱ **Drug-drug** • Risk of severe deterioration of muscle strength in myasthenia gravis patients receiving ambenonium, edrophonium, neostigmine, pyridostigmine • Decreased steroid blood levels with barbiturates, phenytoin, rifampin • Decreased effectiveness of salicylates with betamethasone

⁕ **Drug-lab test** • False-negative nitroblue-tetrazolium test for bacterial infection • Suppression of skin test reactions

■ Nursing considerations

Assessment

- **History:** (systemic administration): Infections, fungal infections, amebiasis, vaccinia and varicella, and antibiotic-resistant infections; kidney or liver disease; hypothyroidism; ulcerative colitis with impending perforation; diverticulitis; active or latent peptic ulcer; inflammatory bowel disease; heart failure; hypertension; thromboembolic disorders; osteoporosis; seizure disorders; diabetes mellitus; lactation
- **Physical:** Baseline weight, T, reflexes and grip strength, affect and orientation, P, BP, peripheral perfusion, prominence of superficial veins, R and adventitious sounds, serum electrolytes, blood glucose

Interventions

Systemic use

- Give daily dose before 9 AM to mimic normal peak corticosteroid blood levels.
- Increase dosage when patient is subject to stress.
- Taper doses when discontinuing high-dose or long-term therapy.
- Do not give live-virus vaccines with immunosuppressive doses of corticosteroids.

Topical dermatologic preparations

- Examine area for infections and skin integrity before application.
- Administer cautiously to pregnant patients; topical corticosteroids have caused teratogenic effects and can be absorbed from systemic site.

⊗ ***Warning*** Use caution when occlusive dressings or tight diapers cover affected area; these can increase systemic absorption of the drug.

- Avoid prolonged use near eyes, in genital and rectal areas, and in skin creases.

Teaching points

Systemic use

- Do not stop taking the oral drug without consulting your health care provider.
- Take single dose or alternate-day doses before 9 AM.
- Avoid exposure to infections; ability to fight infections is reduced.
- Wear a medical alert tag so emergency care providers will know that you are on this medication.
- You may experience these side effects: Increase in appetite, weight gain (counting calories may help); heartburn, indigestion (eat frequent small meals; take antacids); poor wound healing (consult your health care provider); muscle weakness, fatigue (frequent rest periods will help).
- Report unusual weight gain, swelling of the extremities, muscle weakness, black or tarry stools, fever, prolonged sore throat, colds or other infections, worsening of original disorder.

Intrabursal, intra-articular therapy

- Do not overuse joint after therapy, even if pain is gone.

Topical dermatologic preparations

- Apply sparingly; do not cover with tight dressings.
- Avoid contact with the eyes.
- Report irritation or infection at the site of application.

▽ betaxolol hydrochloride

*(beh **tax'** oh lol)*

Ophthalmic: Betoptic, Betoptic S

Oral: Kerlone

PREGNANCY CATEGORY C

Drug classes

Antiglaucoma drug
Antihypertensive
$Beta_1$-selective adrenergic blocker

Therapeutic actions

Blocks beta-adrenergic receptors of the sympathetic nervous system in the heart and juxtaglomerular apparatus (kidney), decreasing the excitability of the heart, decreasing cardiac output and oxygen consumption, decreasing the release of renin from the kidney, and lowering BP. Decreases IOP by decreasing the secretion of aqueous humor.

Indications

- Oral: Hypertension, used alone or with other antihypertensive agents, particularly thiazide-type diuretics
- Ophthalmic: Treatment of ocular hypertension and open-angle glaucoma alone or in combination with other antiglaucoma drugs

Contraindications and cautions

- Contraindicated with sinus bradycardia, second- or third-degree heart block, cardiogenic shock, heart failure.
- Use cautiously with renal failure, diabetes, or thyrotoxicosis (betaxolol masks the cardiac signs of hypoglycemia and thyrotoxicosis), lactation, pregnancy.

Available forms

Tablets—10, 20 mg; ophthalmic solution (0.5%)—5.6 mg/mL; ophthalmic suspension (0.25%)—2.8 mg/mL

Dosages

Adults

Oral

Initially, 10 mg PO daily, alone or added to diuretic therapy. Full antihypertensive effect is usually seen in 7–14 days. If desired response is not achieved, dose may be doubled.

Ophthalmic

One or two drops bid to affected eye or eyes.

Pediatric patients

Safety and efficacy not established.

Geriatric patients or patients with severe renal impairment; patients undergoing dialysis

Oral

Consider reducing initial dose to 5 mg PO daily.

Pharmacokinetics

Route	*Onset*	*Peak*	*Duration*
Oral	30–60 min	2 hr	12–15 hr
Ophthalmic	≤ 30 min	2 hr	12 hr

Metabolism: Hepatic; $T_{1/2}$: 14–22 hr
Distribution: Crosses placenta; enters breast milk
Excretion: Urine

Adverse effects

Oral form

- **Allergic reactions:** Pharyngitis, erythematous rash, fever, sore throat, laryngospasm, respiratory distress
- **CNS:** Dizziness, vertigo, tinnitus, fatigue, emotional depression, paresthesias, sleep disturbances, hallucinations, disorientation, memory loss, slurred speech
- **CV:** *Bradycardia, heart failure, cardiac arrhythmias, sinoatrial or AV nodal block, tachycardia,* peripheral vascular insufficiency, claudication, stroke, **pulmonary edema,** hypotension
- **Dermatologic:** Rash, pruritus, sweating, dry skin
- **EENT:** Eye irritation, dry eyes, conjunctivitis, blurred vision
- **GI:** *Gastric pain, flatulence, constipation, diarrhea, nausea, vomiting,* anorexia, ischemic colitis, renal and mesenteric arterial thrombosis, retroperitoneal fibrosis, hepatomegaly, acute pancreatitis
- **GU:** *Impotence, decreased libido,* Peyronie's disease, dysuria, nocturia, frequent urination
- **Musculoskeletal:** Joint pain, arthralgia, muscle cramp
- **Respiratory: Bronchospasm,** dyspnea, cough, bronchial obstruction, nasal stuffiness, rhinitis, pharyngitis (less likely than with propranolol)
- **Other:** *Decreased exercise tolerance, development of ANA,* hyperglycemia or hypoglycemia, elevated serum transaminase, alkaline phosphatase, and LDH

Betaxolol ophthalmic solution

- **CNS:** Insomnia, depressive neurosis
- **Local:** *Brief ocular discomfort, occasional tearing, itching, decreased corneal sensitivity,* corneal staining, keratitis, photophobia

Interactions

✱ **Drug-drug** • Increased effects with verapamil, anticholinergics • Increased risk of orthostatic hypotension with prazosin • Possible increased antihypertensive effects with aspirin, bismuth subsalicylate, magnesium salicylate, sulfinpyrazone, hormonal contraceptives • Decreased antihypertensive effects with NSAIDs • Possible increased hypoglycemic effect of insulin with betaxolol

✱ Drug-lab test • Possible false results with glucose or insulin tolerance tests

■ Nursing considerations

Assessment

- **History:** Sinus bradycardia, second- or third-degree heart block, cardiogenic shock, heart failure, renal failure, diabetes or thyrotoxicosis, lactation, pregnancy
- **Physical:** Baseline weight, skin condition, neurologic status, P, BP, ECG, R, renal and thyroid function tests, blood and urine glucose

Interventions

⊗ ***Warning*** Do not discontinue drug abruptly after long-term therapy (hypersensitivity to catecholamines may develop, exacerbating angina, MI, and ventricular arrhythmias). Taper drug gradually over 2 wk with monitoring.

- Consult with physician about withdrawing drug if patient is to undergo surgery (withdrawal is controversial).
- With ophthalmic use, protect eye from injury if corneal sensitivity is lost.

Teaching points

- Administer eye drops as instructed to minimize systemic absorption of the drug.
- Take oral drug as prescribed.
- Do not stop taking unless told to do so by a health care provider.
- Avoid driving or dangerous activities if dizziness or weakness occurs.
- You may experience these side effects: Dizziness, light-headedness, loss of appetite, nightmares, depression, sexual impotence.
- Report difficulty breathing, night cough, swelling of extremities, slow pulse, confusion, depression, rash, fever, sore throat; eye pain or irritation (ophthalmic).

▽ bethanechol chloride

*(beh **than'** e kole)*

PMS-Bethanechol (CAN), Urecholine

PREGNANCY CATEGORY C

Drug class

Parasympathomimetic

Therapeutic actions

Acts at cholinergic receptors in the urinary bladder (and GI tract) to mimic the effects of acetylcholine and parasympathetic stimulation; increases the tone of the detrusor muscle and causes the emptying of the urinary bladder; not destroyed by the enzyme cholinesterase, so effects are more prolonged than those of acetylcholine.

Indications

- Acute postoperative and postpartum nonobstructive urinary retention and neurogenic atony of the urinary bladder with retention
- Unlabeled use: Reflux esophagitis, gastroesophageal reflux (pediatric use)

Contraindications and cautions

- Contraindicated with unusual sensitivity to bethanechol or tartrazine, hyperthyroidism, peptic ulcer, latent or active asthma, bradycardia, vasomotor instability, coronary artery disease, epilepsy, parkinsonism, hypotension, obstructive uropathies or intestinal obstruction, recent surgery on GI tract or bladder.
- Use cautiously with lactation, pregnancy.

Available forms

Tablets—5, 10, 25, 50 mg

Dosages

Determine and use the minimum effective dose; larger doses may increase side effects.

Adults

10–50 mg PO three or four times a day. Initial dose of 5–10 mg with gradual increases hourly until desired effect is seen; or until 50 mg has been given.

Pediatric patients

Safety and efficacy not established for children.

Pharmacokinetics

Route	*Onset*	*Peak*	*Duration*
Oral	30–90 min	60–90 min	1–6 hr

Metabolism: Unknown
Distribution: Crosses placenta; may enter breast milk
Excretion: Unknown

B

Adverse effects
- **CV:** Transient heart block, **cardiac arrest,** orthostatic hypotension (with large doses)
- **GI:** *Abdominal discomfort, salivation, nausea, vomiting,* involuntary defecation, abdominal cramps, diarrhea, belching
- **GU:** Urinary urgency
- **Respiratory:** Dyspnea
- **Other:** Malaise, headache, *sweating, flushing*

Interactions
✱ **Drug-drug** • Increased cholinergic effects with other cholinergic drugs, cholinesterase inhibitors • Critical drop in BP may occur if taken with ganglionic blockers

■ Nursing considerations
Assessment
- **History:** Unusual sensitivity to bethanechol or tartrazine, hyperthyroidism, peptic ulcer, latent or active asthma, bradycardia, vasomotor instability, CAD, epilepsy, parkinsonism, hypotension, obstructive uropathies or intestinal obstruction, recent surgery on GI tract or bladder, lactation, pregnancy
- **Physical:** Skin color, lesions; T; P, rhythm, BP; bowel sounds, urinary bladder palpation; bladder tone evaluation, urinalysis

Interventions
- Administer on an empty stomach (1 hr before or 2 hr after meals) to avoid nausea and vomiting.
- Monitor response to establish minimum effective dose.

⊗ ***Warning*** Keep atropine readily available to reverse overdose or severe response.

- Monitor bowel function, especially in elderly patients who may become impacted or develop serious intestinal problems.

Teaching points
- Take this drug on an empty stomach (1 hour before or 2 hours after meals) to avoid nausea and vomiting.
- Dizziness, light-headedness, or fainting may occur when getting up from sitting or lying down.
- You may experience these side effects: Increased salivation, sweating, flushing, abdominal discomfort.
- Report diarrhea, headache, belching, substernal pressure or pain, dizziness.

▽ bevacizumab
See Appendix W, *Less commonly used drugs*.

▽ bexarotene
See Appendix W, *Less commonly used drugs*.

▽ bicalutamide
See Appendix W, *Less commonly used drugs*.

▽ biperiden
(bye ***per'*** *i den)*

biperiden hydrochloride (oral)

biperiden lactate (injection)

Akineton

PREGNANCY CATEGORY C

Drug class
Antiparkinsonian

Therapeutic actions
Anticholinergic activity in the CNS that is believed to help normalize the hypothesized imbalance of cholinergic and dopaminergic neurotransmission in the basal ganglia in the brain of a parkinsonism patient. Reduces severity of rigidity, and to a lesser extent, akinesia and tremor characterizing parkinsonism; less effective overall than levodopa; peripheral anticholinergic effects suppress secondary symptoms of parkinsonism, such as drooling.

Indications

- Adjunct in the therapy of parkinsonism (postencephalitic, arteriosclerotic, and idiopathic types)
- Relief of symptoms of extrapyramidal disorders that accompany phenothiazine therapy

Contraindications and cautions

- Contraindicated with hypersensitivity to benztropine; glaucoma, especially angle-closure glaucoma; pyloric or duodenal obstruction, stenosing peptic ulcers, achalasia (megaesophagus); prostatic hypertrophy or bladder neck obstructions; myasthenia gravis.
- Use cautiously with tachycardia, cardiac arrhythmias, hypertension, hypotension, hepatic or renal impairment, alcoholism, chronic illness, people who work in a hot environment; hot weather; lactation; Alzheimer's disease, pregnancy.

Available forms

Tablets—2 mg

Dosages

Adults

- *Parkinsonism:* 2 mg PO three to four times a day; individualize dosage. Maximum, 16 mg/day (8 tablets).
- *Drug-induced extrapyramidal disorders:* 2 mg PO daily to tid.

Pediatric patients

Safety and efficacy not established.

Geriatric patients

Strict dosage regulation may be necessary; patients older than 60 yr often develop increased sensitivity to the CNS effects of anticholinergic drugs.

Pharmacokinetics

Route	Onset	Peak
Oral	1 hr	60–90 min

Metabolism: Hepatic; $T_{1/2}$: 18.4–24.3 hr
Distribution: Crosses placenta; enters breast milk
Excretion: Unknown

Adverse effects

- **CNS:** *Disorientation, confusion,* memory loss, hallucinations, psychoses, agitation, *nervousness,* delusions, delirium, paranoia, euphoria, excitement, *light-headedness, dizziness,* depression, drowsiness, weakness, giddiness, paresthesia, heaviness of the limbs (centrally acting anticholinergic effects)
- **CV:** Tachycardia, palpitations, hypotension, orthostatic hypotension (peripheral anticholinergic effects)
- **Dermatologic:** Rash, urticaria, other dermatoses
- **EENT:** *Blurred vision, mydriasis,* diplopia, increased intraocular tension, angle-closure glaucoma
- **GI:** *Dry mouth, constipation,* dilation of the colon, paralytic ileus, acute suppurative parotitis, nausea, vomiting, epigastric distress
- **GU:** *Urinary retention, urinary hesitancy,* dysuria, difficulty achieving or maintaining an erection
- **Other:** *Flushing, decreased sweating,* elevated temperature, muscular weakness, muscular cramping

Interactions

✱ **Drug-drug** • Paralytic ileus, sometimes fatal, with other anticholinergics, with drugs that have anticholinergic properties (phenothiazines, TCAs) • Additive adverse CNS effects (toxic psychosis) with drugs that have CNS anticholinergic properties (phenothiazines, TCAs) • Possible masking of extrapyramidal symptoms, tardive dyskinesia, in long-term therapy with antipsychotics (phenothiazines, haloperidol) • Decreased therapeutic efficacy of antipsychotics (phenothiazines, haloperidol), possibly due to central antagonism

■ Nursing considerations

Assessment

- **History:** Hypersensitivity to benztropine; glaucoma; pyloric or duodenal obstruction, stenosing peptic ulcers, achalasia; prostatic hypertrophy or bladder neck obstructions; myasthenia gravis; cardiac arrhythmias, hypertension, hypotension; hepatic or renal impairment; alcoholism, chronic illness, work in hot environment; lactation
- **Physical:** Body weight; T; skin color, lesions; orientation, affect, reflexes, bilateral

grip strength, visual examination, including tonometry; P, BP, orthostatic BP; adventitious sounds; bowel sounds, normal output, liver evaluation; normal urinary output, voiding pattern, prostate palpation; LFTs, renal function tests

Interventions

- Decrease dosage or discontinue temporarily if dry mouth makes swallowing or speaking difficult.

⊗ ***Warning*** Give with caution, and reduce dosage in hot weather. Drug interferes with sweating and ability of body to maintain heat equilibrium; anhidrosis and fatal hyperthermia have occurred.

- Give with meals if GI upset occurs; give before meals to patients with dry mouth; give after meals if drooling or nausea occurs.
- Ensure that patient voids just before receiving each dose of drug if urinary retention is a problem.

Teaching points

- Take this drug exactly as prescribed.
- Avoid the use of alcohol, sedative, and over-the-counter drugs (can cause dangerous effects).
- You may experience these side effects: Drowsiness, dizziness, confusion, blurred vision (avoid driving or engaging in activities that require alertness and visual acuity); nausea (eat frequent small meals); dry mouth (suck sugarless lozenges or ice chips); painful or difficult urination (empty the bladder immediately before each dose); constipation (maintain adequate fluid intake and exercise regularly); use caution in hot weather (you are susceptible to heat prostration).
- Report difficult or painful urination; constipation; rapid or pounding heartbeat; confusion, eye pain, or rash.

▽bismuth subsalicylate

(bis' mith sub sah lih' sih late)

Bismatrol, Bismatrol Extra Strength, Kao-Tin, Kaopectate, Kaopectate Children's, Kaopectate Extra Strength, Maalox Total Stomach Relief, Peptic Relief, Pepto-Bismol, Pepto-Bismol Maximum Strength, Pink Bismuth

PREGNANCY CATEGORY C

Drug class

Antidiarrheal

Therapeutic actions

Adsorbent actions remove irritants from the intestine; forms a protective coating over the mucosa and soothes the irritated bowel lining.

Indications

- To control diarrhea, gas, upset stomach, indigestion, heartburn, nausea
- To reduce the number of bowel movements and help firm stool
- To control traveler's diarrhea
- Unlabeled use: Prevention of traveler's diarrhea; treatment of chronic infantile diarrhea

Contraindications and cautions

- Contraindicated with allergy to any components or to aspirin or other salicylates.
- Use cautiously with pregnancy, lactation.

Available forms

Caplets—262 mg; chewable tablets—262 mg; liquid—87 mg/5 mL, 130 mg/15 mL, 262 mg/15 mL, 524 mg/15 mL; suspension—525 mg/15 mL; tablets— 262 mg

Dosages

Adults and children 12 yr and older

2 tablets or 30 mL PO, repeat every 30 min–1 hr as needed, up to eight doses per 24 hr.

- *Traveler's diarrhea:* 1 ounce every 30 min for a total of 8 doses.

Pediatric patients 9–11 yr
One tablet or 15 mL (1 tablespoon) PO.
Pediatric patients 6–8 yr
Two-thirds tablet or 10 mL (2 teaspoons) PO.
Pediatric patients 3–5 yr
One-third tablet or 5 mL (1 teaspoon) PO.
Pediatric patients younger than 3 yr
Dosage not established.

Pharmacokinetics

Route	*Onset*
Oral	Varies

Metabolism: Hepatic; $T_{1/2}$: Unknown
Distribution: Crosses placenta
Excretion: Urine

Adverse effects
- **GI:** *Darkening of the stool,* impaction in infants or debilitated patients
- **Salicylate toxicity:** Ringing in the ears, rapid respirations

Interactions
✱ **Drug-drug** • Increased risk of salicylate toxicity with aspirin-containing products • Increased toxic effects of methotrexate, valproic acid if taken with salicylates • Use caution with drugs used for diabetes • Decreased effectiveness with corticosteroids • Decreased absorption of oral tetracyclines • Decreased effectiveness of sulfinpyrazone with salicylates
✱ **Drug-lab test** • May interfere with radiologic examinations of GI tract; bismuth is radiopaque

■ Nursing considerations
Assessment
- **History:** Allergy to any components
- **Physical:** T; orientation, reflexes; R and depth of respirations; abdominal examination, bowel sounds; serum electrolytes; acid-base levels

Interventions
- Shake liquid well before administration; have patient chew tablets thoroughly or dissolve in mouth; do not swallow whole.
- Discontinue drug if any sign of salicylate toxicity (ringing in the ears) occurs.

Teaching points
- Take this drug as prescribed; do not exceed prescribed dosage. Shake liquid well before using. Chew tablets thoroughly or let them dissolve in your mouth; do not swallow whole.
- Darkened stools may occur.
- Do not take this drug with other drugs containing aspirin or aspirin products; serious overdose can occur.
- Report fever or diarrhea that does not stop after 2 days, ringing in the ears, rapid respirations.

B

▽bisoprolol fumarate
*(bis **oh'** pro lole **few'** mah rate)*

Apo-Bisoprolol (CAN), Zebeta

PREGNANCY CATEGORY C

Drug classes
Antihypertensive
$Beta_1$-selective adrenergic blocker

Therapeutic actions
Blocks beta-adrenergic receptors (primarily $beta_1$) of the sympathetic nervous system in the heart and juxtaglomerular apparatus (kidney), thus decreasing the excitability of the heart, decreasing cardiac output and oxygen consumption, decreasing the release of renin from the kidney, and lowering BP.

Indications
- Management of hypertension, used alone or with other antihypertensives

Contraindications and cautions
- Contraindicated with sinus bradycardia, second- or third-degree heart block, cardiogenic shock, heart failure.
- Use cautiously with renal failure, diabetes or thyrotoxicosis (bisoprolol can mask the usual cardiac signs of hypoglycemia and thyrotoxicosis), pregnancy, lactation, and in those with bronchospastic disease.

Available forms
Tablets—5, 10 mg

Dosages

Adults

Initially, 5 mg PO daily, alone or added to diuretic therapy; 2.5 mg may be appropriate; up to 20 mg PO daily has been used.

Pediatric patients

Safety and efficacy not established.

Patients with renal or hepatic impairment

Initially, 2.5 mg PO; adjust, and use extreme caution in dose titration.

Pharmacokinetics

Route	*Onset*	*Peak*	*Duration*
Oral	30–60 min	2 hr	12–15 hr

Metabolism: Hepatic; $T_{1/2}$: 9–12 hr
Distribution: Crosses placenta; may enter breast milk
Excretion: Urine

Adverse effects

- **Allergic reactions:** Pharyngitis, erythematous rash, fever, sore throat, **laryngospasm,** respiratory distress
- **CNS:** Dizziness, vertigo, tinnitus, *fatigue,* emotional depression, paresthesias, sleep disturbances, hallucinations, disorientation, memory loss, slurred speech
- **CV:** *Bradycardia, heart failure, cardiac arrhythmias, sinoatrial or AV nodal block, tachycardia,* peripheral vascular insufficiency, claudication, stroke, **pulmonary edema,** hypotension
- **Dermatologic:** Rash, pruritus, sweating, dry skin
- **EENT:** Eye irritation, dry eyes, conjunctivitis, blurred vision
- **GI:** *Gastric pain, flatulence, constipation, diarrhea, nausea, vomiting,* anorexia, ischemic colitis, renal and mesenteric arterial thrombosis, retroperitoneal fibrosis, hepatomegaly, acute pancreatitis
- **GU:** *Impotence, decreased libido,* Peyronie's disease, dysuria, nocturia, frequent urination
- **Musculoskeletal:** Joint pain, arthralgia, muscle cramp
- **Respiratory: Bronchospasm,** dyspnea, cough, bronchial obstruction, nasal stuffiness, rhinitis, pharyngitis (less likely than with propranolol)
- **Other:** *Decreased exercise tolerance, development of antinuclear antibodies,* hyperglycemia or hypoglycemia, elevated serum transaminase, alkaline phosphatase, and LDH

Interactions

✱ **Drug-drug** • Increased effects with verapamil, anticholinergics • Increased risk of orthostatic hypotension with prazosin • Possible increased BP-lowering effects with aspirin, bismuth subsalicylate, magnesium salicylate, sulfinpyrazone, hormonal contraceptives • Decreased antihypertensive effects with NSAIDs • Possible increased hypoglycemic effect of insulin • Possible masking of hypoglycemic symptoms in patients with diabetes

✱ **Drug-lab test** • Possible false results with glucose or insulin tolerance tests

■ Nursing considerations

CLINICAL ALERT!
Name confusion has occurred between *Zebeta* (bisoprolol) and *DiaBeta* (glyburide); use caution.

Assessment

- **History:** Sinus bradycardia, cardiac arrhythmias, cardiogenic shock, heart failure, renal failure, diabetes or thyrotoxicosis, pregnancy, lactation
- **Physical:** Baseline weight, skin condition, neurologic status, P, BP, ECG, R, LFTs, renal function tests, blood and urine glucose

Interventions

⊗ ***Warning*** Do not discontinue drug abruptly after long-term therapy (hypersensitivity to catecholamines may have developed, causing exacerbation of angina, MI, and ventricular arrhythmias). Taper drug gradually over 2 wk with monitoring.

- Be aware that half-life can be up to 21 hr in patients with cirrhosis.
- Consult with physician about withdrawing drug if patient is to undergo surgery (withdrawal is controversial).

B

Teaching points
- Do not stop taking this drug unless instructed to do so by a health care provider.
- Avoid over-the-counter medications.
- Avoid driving or dangerous activities if dizziness or weakness occurs.
- You may experience these side effects: Dizziness, light-headedness, loss of appetite, nightmares, depression, sexual impotence.
- Report difficulty breathing, night cough, swelling of extremities, slow pulse, confusion, depression, rash, fever, sore throat.

bivalirudin

See Appendix W, *Less commonly used drugs*.

DANGEROUS DRUG

bleomycin sulfate

*(blee oh **mye'** sin)*

BLM, Blenoxane

PREGNANCY CATEGORY D

Drug classes
Antibiotic
Antineoplastic

Therapeutic actions
Inhibits DNA, RNA, and protein synthesis in susceptible cells, preventing cell division; cell cycle phase-specific agent with major effects in G2 and M phases.

Indications
- Palliative treatment of squamous cell carcinoma, lymphomas, testicular carcinoma, alone or with other drugs
- Treatment of malignant pleural effusion and prevention of recurrent pleural effusions
- Unlabeled uses: Mycosis fungoides, osteosarcoma, AIDS-related Kaposi sarcoma, germ cell tumors, sclerosis of pleural effusions, palliative treatment of children with lymphomas

Contraindications and cautions
- Contraindicated with allergy to bleomycin sulfate; lactation, pregnancy.
- Use cautiously with pulmonary disease; hepatic or renal impairment.

Available forms
Powder for injection—15, 30 units

Dosages
Adults
Treat lymphoma patients with 2 units or less for the first two doses; if no acute anaphylactoid reaction occurs, use the regular dosage schedule:
- *Squamous cell carcinoma, non-Hodgkin's lymphoma, testicular carcinoma:* 0.25–0.5 unit/kg IV, IM, or subcutaneously, once or twice weekly.
- *Hodgkin's lymphoma:* 0.25–0.5 unit/kg IV, IM, or subcutaneously once or twice weekly. After a 50% response, give maintenance dose of 1 unit/day or 5 units/wk, IV or IM. Response should be seen within 2 wk (Hodgkin's lymphoma, testicular tumors) or 3 wk (squamous cell cancers). If no improvement is seen by then, it is unlikely to occur.
- *Malignant pleural effusion:* 60 units dissolved in 50–100 mL 0.9% saline solution, given via thoracostomy tube.

Pediatric patients
Safety and efficacy not established.

Pharmacokinetics

Route	*Onset*	*Peak*
IV	Immediate	10–20 min
IM, Subcut.	15–20 min	30–60 min

Metabolism: Hepatic; $T_{1/2}$: 2 hr
Distribution: May cross placenta; may enter breast milk
Excretion: Urine

IV FACTS
Preparation: Dissolve contents of 15- or 30-unit vial with 5 or 10 mL physiologic saline, sterile water for injection, or bacteriostatic water for injection. Do not use D_5W or dextrose-containing diluents; stable for 24 hr at room temperature in saline solution. Powder should be refrigerated.
Infusion: Infuse slowly over 10 min.
Incompatibilities: Incompatible in solution with aminophylline, ascorbic acid, carbenicillin, diazepam, hydrocortisone, methotrexate, mitomycin, nafcillin, penicillin G, terbutaline.

Adverse effects

- **Dermatologic:** *Rash, striae, vesiculation, hyperpigmentation, skin tenderness, hyperkeratosis, nail changes, alopecia, pruritus*
- **GI:** Hepatic toxicity, *stomatitis, vomiting,* anorexia, weight loss
- **GU:** Renal toxicity
- **Hypersensitivity:** Idiosyncratic reaction similar to anaphylaxis: Hypotension, mental confusion, fever, chills, wheezing (lymphoma patients, 1% occurrence)
- **Respiratory:** *Dyspnea, rales, pneumonitis,* **pulmonary fibrosis**
- **Other:** *Fever, chills*

Interactions

✱ **Drug-drug** • Decreased serum levels and effectiveness of digoxin and phenytoin • Increased risk of pulmonary toxicity if combined with oxygen use

■ Nursing considerations

Assessment

- **History:** Allergy to bleomycin sulfate, pregnancy, lactation, pulmonary disease, hepatic or renal impairment
- **Physical:** T; skin color, lesions; weight; R, adventitious sounds; liver evaluation, abdominal status; PFTs, urinalysis, LFTs, renal function tests, chest radiograph

Interventions

- Reconstitute for IM or subcutaneous use by dissolving contents of 15-unit vial in 1–5 mL, 30-unit vial with 2–10 mL of sterile water for injection, sodium chloride for injection, bacteriostatic water for injection.
- Label drug solution with date and hour of preparation; check label before use. Stable at room temperature for 24 hr in 0.9% sodium chloride; discard after that time.

⊗ ***Black box warning*** Monitor pulmonary function regularly and chest radiograph weekly or biweekly to monitor onset of pulmonary toxicity; consult physician immediately if changes occur. Risk is markedly increased with doses over 400 units/day.

- Arrange for periodic monitoring of LFTs and renal function tests.
- Advise women of childbearing age to avoid pregnancy while on this drug.

⊗ ***Black box warning*** Be alert for rare, severe idiosyncratic reaction including fever, chills, hypertension in lymphoma patients.

Teaching points

- This drug has to be given by injection. Mark calendar with dates for injection.
- This drug may cause fetal harm; using a barrier contraceptive is advised.
- You may experience these side effects: Rash, skin lesions, loss of hair, changes in nails (you may want to invest in a wig, skin care may help); loss of appetite, nausea, mouth sores (try frequent mouth care, eat frequent small meals; maintain good nutrition).
- Report difficulty breathing, cough, yellowing of skin or eyes, severe GI upset, fever, chills.

▽ bortezomib

See Appendix W, *Less commonly used drugs.*

▽ bosentan

*(bow **sen'** tan)*

Tracleer

PREGNANCY CATEGORY X

Drug classes

Endothelin receptor antagonist
Pulmonary antihypertensive
Vasodilator

Therapeutic actions

Specifically blocks receptor sites for endothelin ET_A and ET_B in the endothelium and vascular smooth muscles; these endothelins are elevated in plasma and lung tissue of patients with pulmonary arterial hypertension.

Indications

- Treatment of pulmonary arterial hypertension in patients with World Health Organization class III or class IV symptoms, to improve exercise ability and to decrease the rate of clinical worsening
- Unlabeled uses: Improvement of microcirculatory blood flow in splanchnic organs during septic shock; prevention of Reynaud's

phenomenon; prevention of digital ulcers in systemic sclerosis

Contraindications and cautions

- Contraindicated with allergy to bosentan, severe liver impairment, pregnancy, lactation.
- Use cautiously with hepatic impairment, anemia.

Available forms

Tablets—62.5, 125 mg

Dosages

Adults

62.5 mg PO bid for 4 wk. Then, for patients weighing 40 kg or more, maintenance dose is 125 mg PO bid. For patients weighing less than 40 kg, but older than 12 yr, maintenance dose is 62.5 mg PO bid. Administer in the morning and evening.

Pediatric patients

Safety and efficacy not established.

Patients with hepatic impairment

Avoid use in moderate to severe hepatic impairment; reduce dosage and monitor patients closely with mild hepatic impairment.

Pharmacokinetics

Route	*Onset*	*Peak*
Oral	Varies	3–5 hr

Metabolism: Hepatic; $T_{1/2}$: 5 hr
Distribution: Crosses placenta; may enter breast milk
Excretion: Bile

Adverse effects

- **CNS:** *Headache,* fatigue
- **CV:** *Flushing, edema, hypotension,* palpitations
- **EENT:** *Nasopharyngitis*
- **GI:** Liver injury, dyspepsia
- **Hematologic:** Decreased Hgb level, decreased Hct
- **Skin:** Pruritus

Interactions

✱ **Drug-drug** • Potential for decreased effectiveness of hormonal contraceptives; advise using barrier contraceptives • Bosentan serum concentrations increased with cyclosporine A, and cyclosporine A concentrations decrease by 50% with bosentan; avoid this combination • Decreased serum levels of statins if combined with bosentan; if the combination is used, patients should have serum cholesterol levels monitored regularly • Increased risk of liver damage if combined with glyburide; avoid this combination • Increased bosentan concentrations with ketoconazole and tacrolimus; monitor patients for adverse effects

■ Nursing considerations

Assessment

- **History:** Allergy to bosentan, severe liver impairment, anemia, pregnancy, lactation
- **Physical:** Skin color and lesions, orientation, BP, LFTs, CBC, Hgb level, pregnancy test

Interventions

⊗ ***Black box warning*** Make sure that the patient is not pregnant before initiating therapy and that patient will conform to use of a nonhormonal, barrier contraceptive while using this drug.

⊗ ***Black box warning*** Obtain baseline and then monthly liver enzyme levels; dosage reduction or drug withdrawal is indicated at signs of elevated liver enzymes.

⊗ ***Warning*** Obtain baseline Hgb level and then repeat at 1 and 3 mo, then every 3 mo. If Hgb drops, the situation should be evaluated and appropriate action taken.

- Do not administer to any patient taking cyclosporine or glyburide.
- Administer in the morning and in the evening with or without food.

⊗ ***Warning*** Monitor patients who are discontinuing bosentan; dose may need to be tapered to avoid sudden worsening of disease.

- Provide analgesics as appropriate for patients who develop headache.
- Monitor patient's functional level to note improvement in exercise tolerance.
- Maintain other measures used to treat pulmonary arterial hypertension.

Teaching points

- Take drug exactly as prescribed, in the morning and the evening.
- This drug should not be taken during pregnancy; serious fetal abnormalities have occurred. A negative pregnancy test will be required before the drug is started. The use of

barrier contraceptives is advised; hormonal contraceptives may not be effective.
- Keep a chart of your exercise tolerance to help monitor improvement in your condition.
- Continue your usual procedures for treating your pulmonary arterial hypertension.
- You will need monthly blood tests to evaluate the effect of this drug on your liver and your hemoglobin.
- You may experience these side effects: Headache (analgesics may be available that will help); stomach upset (taking the drug with food may help).
- Report swelling, changes in color of urine or stool, yellowing of the eyes or skin.

▽botulinum toxin type A

(bot' yoo lin um)

Botox, Botox Cosmetic

PREGNANCY CATEGORY C

Drug class
Neurotoxin

Therapeutic actions
Blocks neuromuscular transmission by binding to receptor sites on the motor nerve terminals and inhibiting the release of acetylcholine; this blocking results in localized muscle denervation, which causes local muscle paralysis; this denervation can lead to muscle atrophy and reinnervation if the muscle develops new acetylcholine receptors.

Indications
- Temporary improvement in the appearance of moderate to severe glabellar lines—associated with corrugator or procerus muscle activity in adults 65 yr and younger (*Botox Cosmetic*)
- Treatment of cervical dystonia in adults to decrease severity of abnormal head position and neck pain (*Botox* only)
- Treatment of severe primary axillary hyperhidrosis that is not adequately managed with topical agents (*Botox* only)
- Treatment of strabismus and blepharospasm associated with dystonia in patients 12 yr and older (*Botox* only)
- Unlabeled uses: Achalasia, cosmetic improvement of facial lines and wrinkles, gustatory sweating, hand dystonia, tension headache, palmar hyperhidrosis, sialorrhea

Contraindications and cautions
- Contraindicated with hypersensitivity to any component of the drug, active infection at the injection site area.
- Use cautiously with peripheral neuropathic diseases (amyotrophic lateral sclerosis [ALS], motor neuropathies), neuromuscular disorders such as myasthenia gravis, inflammation in the injection area, lactation, pregnancy, known CV disease.

Available forms
Powder for injection—100 units/vial

Dosages
Adults
- *Glabellar lines:* Total of 20 units (0.5 mL solution) injected as divided doses of 0.1 mL into each of five sites—two in each corrugator muscle, and one in the procerus muscle; injections usually need to be repeated every 3–4 mo to maintain effect.
- *Cervical dystonia:* 236 units (range 198–300 units) divided among affected muscles and injected into each muscle in patients with known tolerance. In patients without prior use, 100 units or less, then adjust dosage based on patient response.
- *Primary axillary hyperhidrosis:* 50 units per axilla injected intradermally 0.1–0.2 mL aliquots at multiple sites (10–15), approximately 2 cm apart. Repeat as needed.
- *Blepharospasm associated with dystonia:* 1.25–2.5 units injected into the medial and lateral pretarsal orbicularis oculi of the lower lid and upper lid. Repeat approximately every 3 mo.
- *Strabismus associated with dystonia:* 1.25–50 units in any one muscle.

Pharmacokinetics
Not absorbed systemically

Adverse effects

- **CNS:** *Headache,* blepharoptosis, transient ptosis, *dizziness*
- **CV:** Arrhythmias, **MI** (patients with preexisting disease), hypertension
- **GI:** Nausea, difficulty swallowing, dyspepsia, tooth disorder
- **Respiratory:** Pneumonia, bronchitis, sinusitis, pharyngitis, UTI
- **Other:** Redness, edema, and pain at injection site, *flulike symptoms,* paralysis of facial muscles, facial pain, infection, skin tightness, ecchymosis, **anaphylactic reactions**

Interactions

✱ **Drug-drug** • Risk for additive effects if combined with aminoglycosides or other drugs that interfere with neuromuscular transmission—neuromuscular junction blockers, lincosamides, quinidine, magnesium sulfate, anticholinesterases, succinylcholine, polymyxin; use extreme caution if this combination is used

■ Nursing considerations

Assessment

- **History:** Hypersensitivity to any component of the drug; active infection in the injection site area, pregnancy, peripheral neuropathic diseases (ALS, motor neuropathies), neuromuscular disorders such as myasthenia gravis, inflammation in the injection area, lactation, known CV disease
- **Physical:** T; reflexes; R, respiratory auscultation, assessment of injection site and muscle function

Interventions

⊗ ***Black box warning*** Drug is not for the treatment of muscle spasticity; toxin may spread from injection area and cause signs and symptoms of botulism (CNS alterations, trouble speaking and swallowing, loss of bladder conrol). Use only for approved indications.

- Store vials in the refrigerator before reconstitution.
- Reconstitute with 0.9% sterile, preservative-free saline as indicated for each use using a 21-gauge needle. Inject saline into vial; gently rotate vial to reconstitute and label vial with time and date of reconstitution. Reconstituted solution may be refrigerated but must be used within 4 hr. Discard after that time.
- Inspect vial for particulate matter or discoloration before use.
- Check manufacturer's guidelines for appropriate needle-gauge for each use.

⊗ ***Warning*** Ensure that epinephrine is readily available in case of anaphylactic reaction to the drug.

- Inform the patient that the effect of the drug may not be seen for 1 or 2 days, with the full effect taking up to a week. The effect usually lasts 3–4 mo. Do not administer the drug more often than every 3–4 mo.
- Advise patient not to become pregnant while this drug is being used; advise using contraceptives.

Teaching points

- This drug will be injected into your muscles to block the contraction of particular muscles.
- The effects of the drug may not be apparent for 1–2 days and may not be fully apparent for a week. The effects of the drug persist for 3–4 months.
- Avoid pregnancy while using this drug, the effects on the fetus are not known. If you become pregnant or desire to become pregnant, consult your health care provider. Using contraceptives is advised.
- You may experience these side effects: Pain, redness at injection site, and headache (analgesics may be helpful), drooping of the eyelid (this is usually transient), nausea, flu-like symptoms.
- Report difficulty swallowing, facial paralysis; difficulty speaking; difficulty breathing; persistent pain, redness, or swelling at injection site.

▽botulinum toxin type B

See Appendix W, *Less commonly used drugs*.

bromocriptine mesylate

*(broe moe **krip'** teen **mess'** ah late)*

Apo-Bromocriptine (CAN), Cycloset, Parlodel, Parlodel SnapTabs

PREGNANCY CATEGORY B

Drug classes

Antiparkinsonian
Dopamine receptor agonist
Semisynthetic ergot derivative

Therapeutic actions

Parkinsonism: Acts as an agonist directly on postsynaptic dopamine receptors of neurons in the brain, mimicking the effects of the neurotransmitter dopamine, which is deficient in parkinsonism. Unlike levodopa, bromocriptine does not require biotransformation by the nigral neurons that are deficient in parkinsonism patients; thus, bromocriptine may be effective when levodopa has begun to lose its efficacy.
Hyperprolactinemia: Acts directly on postsynaptic dopamine receptors of the prolactin-secreting cells in the anterior pituitary, mimicking the effects of prolactin inhibitory factor, inhibiting the release of prolactin and galactorrhea. Also restores normal ovulatory menstrual cycles in patients with amenorrhea or galactorrhea, and inhibits the release of growth hormone in patients with acromegaly.
Diabetes: Stimulates CNS dopamine activity, which improves glycemic control; exact mechanism of action not known, but these patients may have decreased dopamine activity as part of their metabolic syndrome.

Indications

- Treatment of postencephalitic or idiopathic Parkinson's disease; may provide additional benefit in patients currently maintained on optimal dosages of levodopa with or without carbidopa, beginning to deteriorate or develop tolerance to levodopa, and experiencing "end of dose failure" on levodopa therapy; may allow reduction of levodopa dosage and decrease the dyskinesias and "on-off" phenomenon associated with long-term levodopa therapy
- Short-term treatment of amenorrhea or galactorrhea associated with hyperprolactinemia due to various etiologies, excluding demonstrable pituitary tumors
- Treatment of hyperprolactinemia associated with pituitary adenomas to reduce elevated prolactin levels, cause shrinkage of macroprolactinomas; may be used to reduce the tumor mass before surgery
- Female infertility associated with hyperprolactinemia in the absence of a demonstrable pituitary tumor
- Acromegaly; used alone or with pituitary irradiation or surgery to reduce serum growth hormone level
- **NEW INDICATION:** Treatment of type 2 diabetes as monotherapy or in combination with other antidiabetics
- Unlabeled uses: Neuroleptic malignant syndrome, cocaine addiction, cyclical mastalgia

Contraindications and cautions

- Contraindicated with hypersensitivity to bromocriptine or any ergot alkaloid; severe ischemic heart disease or peripheral vascular disease; pregnancy, lactation.
- Use cautiously with history of MI with residual arrhythmias (atrial, nodal, or ventricular); renal or hepatic disease, history of peptic ulcer (fatal bleeding ulcers have occurred in patients with acromegaly treated with bromocriptine).

Available forms

Capsules—5 mg; tablets—0.8, 2.5 mg

Dosages

Adults and pediatric patients 15 yr and older

Give drug with food; individualize dosage; increase dosage gradually to minimize side effects; adjust dosage carefully to optimize benefits and minimize side effects.

- *Hyperprolactinemia:* Initially, 1.25–2.5 mg PO daily; an additional 2.5-mg tablet may be added as tolerated every 2–7 days until optimal response is achieved; therapeutic dosage range is 2.5–15 mg/day.

- *Acromegaly:* Initially, 1.25–2.5 mg PO for 3 days at bedtime; add 1.25–2.5 mg as tolerated every 3–7 days until optimal response is achieved. Evaluate patient monthly, and adjust dosage based on growth hormone levels. Usual dosage range is 20–30 mg/day; do not exceed 100 mg/day; withdraw patients treated with pituitary irradiation for a yearly 4- to 8-wk reassessment period.
- *Parkinson's disease:* 1.25 mg PO bid; assess every 2 wk, and adjust dosage carefully to ensure lowest dosage producing optimal response. If needed, increase dosage by increments of 2.5 mg/day every 14–28 days; do not exceed 100 mg/day.
- *Type 2 diabetes:* 0.8 mg/day PO in the morning; increase by 1 tablet per wk to maximum daily dose of 6 tablets (4.8 mg) or until maximum tolerated dose between 2 and 6 tablets/day (*Cycloset*).

Pediatric patients

Safety for use in patients younger than 16 yr not established.

Pharmacokinetics

Route	*Onset*	*Peak*	*Duration*
Oral	Varies	1–3 hr	14 hr

Metabolism: Hepatic; $T_{1/2}$: 3 hr (initial phase), 45–50 hr (terminal phase)
Excretion: Bile

Adverse effects

Hyperprolactinemic indications

- **CNS:** Dizziness, fatigue, light-headedness, nasal congestion, drowsiness, headache, CSF rhinorrhea in patients who have had transsphenoidal surgery, pituitary radiation
- **CV:** Hypotension
- **GI:** *Constipation, diarrhea, nausea, vomiting, abdominal cramps*

Physiologic lactation

- **CNS:** Headache, dizziness, nausea, vomiting, fatigue, syncope
- **CV:** Hypotension
- **GI:** Diarrhea, cramps

Acromegaly

- **CNS:** Nasal congestion, digital vasospasm, drowsiness
- **CV:** Exacerbation of Raynaud's syndrome, *orthostatic hypotension*
- **GI:** *Nausea, constipation, anorexia,* indigestion, dry mouth, vomiting, GI bleeding

Parkinson's disease

- **CNS:** Abnormal involuntary movements, hallucinations, confusion, "on-off" phenomenon, dizziness, drowsiness, faintness, asthenia, visual disturbance, ataxia, insomnia, depression, vertigo
- **CV:** *Hypotension, shortness of breath*
- **GI:** *Nausea, vomiting, abdominal discomfort, constipation*

Interactions

✱ **Drug-drug** • Increased serum bromocriptine levels and increased pharmacologic and toxic effects with erythromycin • Decreased effectiveness with phenothiazines for treatment of prolactin-secreting tumors • Increased bromocriptine adverse effects if combined with sympathomimetics

■ Nursing considerations

Assessment

- **History:** Hypersensitivity to bromocriptine or any ergot alkaloid; severe ischemic heart disease or peripheral vascular disease; pregnancy; history of MI with residual arrhythmias; hepatic, renal disease; history of peptic ulcer, lactation
- **Physical:** Skin T (especially fingers), color, lesions; nasal mucous membranes; orientation, affect, reflexes, bilateral grip strength, vision examination, including visual fields; P, BP, orthostatic BP, auscultation; R, depth, adventitious sounds; bowel sounds, normal output, liver evaluation; LFTs, renal function tests, CBC with differential

Interventions

- Evaluate patients with amenorrhea or galactorrhea before drug therapy begins; syndrome may result from pituitary adenoma that requires surgical or radiation procedures.
- Arrange to administer drug with food.
- Taper dosage in patients with Parkinson's disease if drug must be discontinued.
- Monitor hepatic, renal, and hematopoietic function periodically during therapy.

Teaching points

- Take drug exactly as prescribed with food; take the first dose at bedtime while lying down.
- If taking this drug for diabetes, take once a day in the morning. Continue diet and exercise program. You may also be taking other antidiabetic drugs.
- Do not discontinue drug without consulting health care provider (patients with macroadenoma may experience rapid growth of tumor and recurrence of original symptoms).
- Use barrier contraceptives while taking this drug (amenorrhea or galactorrhea); pregnancy may occur before menses, and the drug is contraindicated in pregnancy (estrogen contraceptives may stimulate a prolactinoma).
- You may experience these side effects: Drowsiness, dizziness, confusion (avoid driving or engaging in activities that require alertness); nausea (take the drug with meals, eat frequent small meals); dizziness or faintness when getting up (change position slowly, be careful climbing stairs); headache, nasal stuffiness (medication may help).
- Report fainting; light-headedness; dizziness; uncontrollable movements of the face, eyelids, mouth, tongue, neck, arms, hands, or legs; mental changes; irregular heartbeat or palpitations; severe or persistent nausea or vomiting; coffee-ground vomitus; black tarry stools; vision changes (macroadenoma); any persistent watery nasal discharge (hyperprolactinemic).

▽ brompheniramine maleate (parabromdylamine maleate)

*(brome fen **ir'** a meen **mal'** ee ate)*

BroveX, BroveX CT, J-Tan, Lodrane XR, LoHist 12 Hour (DNC), P-Tex, VaZol

PREGNANCY CATEGORY C

Drug class

Antihistamine (alkylamine type)

Therapeutic actions

Competitively blocks the effects of histamine at H_1-receptor sites; has anticholinergic (atropine-like), antipruritic, and sedative effects.

Indications

- Symptomatic relief of symptoms associated with perennial and seasonal allergic rhinitis—runny nose, sneezing, itching nose and throat, watery eyes
- Temporary relief of sneezing and runny nose due to common cold; treatment of allergic and nonallergic pruritic symptoms; mild urticaria and angioedema; amelioration of allergic reactions to blood or plasma; adjunctive therapy in anaphylactic reactions (*VaZol*)

Contraindications and cautions

- Contraindicated with allergy to any antihistamines, allergy to tartrazine (*BroveX CT*), third trimester of pregnancy (newborn or premature infants may have severe reactions).
- Use cautiously with lactation, narrow-angle glaucoma, stenosing peptic ulcer, symptomatic prostatic hypertrophy, asthma attack, bladder neck obstruction, pyloroduodenal obstruction. Use cautiously in the elderly (this population is extremely sensitive to anticholinergic side effects of this drug).

Available forms

Chewable tablets—12 mg; ER tablets (DNC)—6 mg; ER capsules (DNC)—12 mg; drops—1 mg; liquid—2 mg/5 mL; oral suspension—4 mg/5 mL, 8 mg/5 mL, 10 mg/5 mL, 12 mg/5 mL

Dosages

Adults and pediatric patients 12 yr and older

ER tablets: 6–12 mg PO every 12 hr. Chewable tablets: 12–24 mg PO every 12 hr, maximum 48 mg/day. ER capsules: 12–24 mg/day PO. Oral suspension (*BroveX*): 5–10 mL (12–24 mg) PO every 12 hr; maximum 48 mg/day. Oral liquid: 10 mL (4 mg) PO 4 times/day. Oral suspension (*Lodrane XR*): 5 mL PO every 12 hr; do not exceed 2 doses/day.

Pediatric patients 6–12 yr

ER tablets: 6 mg PO every 12 hr. Chewable tablets: 6–12 mg PO every 12 hr, maximum 24 mg/day. ER capsules: 12 mg/day PO. Oral liquid: 5 mL (2 mg) PO 4 times/day. Oral suspension (*BroveX*): 5 mL (12 mg) PO every 12 hr; maximum 24 mg/day. Oral suspension (*Lodrane XR*): 2.5 mL PO every 12 hr; up to 5 mL/day.

Pediatric patients 2–6 yr

Chewable tablets: 6 mg PO every 12 hr; maximum 12 mg/day. Oral liquid: 2.5 mL (1 mg) PO 4 times/day. Oral suspension (*BroveX*): 2.5 mL (6 mg) PO every 12 hr up to 12 mg/day. Oral suspension (*Lodrane XR*): 1.25 mL PO every 12 hr; maximum 2.5 mg/day.

Pediatric patients 12 mo–2 yr

Oral suspension: 1.25 mL (3 mg) PO every 12 hr up to 2.5 mL (6 mg)/day. Oral liquid: Titrate dose based on 0.5 mg/kg/day PO in equally divided doses four times/day.

Geriatric patients

More likely to cause dizziness, sedation, syncope, toxic confusional states, and hypotension in elderly patients; use with caution.

Pharmacokinetics

Route	*Onset*	*Peak*	*Duration*
Oral	15–30 min	1–2 hr	4–6 hr

Metabolism: Hepatic; $T_{1/2}$: 12–35 hr
Distribution: Crosses placenta; enters breast milk
Excretion: Urine

Adverse effects

- **CNS:** *Drowsiness, sedation, dizziness, faintness, disturbed coordination,* fatigue, confusion, restlessness, excitation, nervousness, tremor, headache, blurred vision, diplopia, vertigo, tinnitus, acute labyrinthitis, hysteria, tingling, heaviness and weakness of the hands
- **CV:** Hypotension, palpitations, bradycardia, tachycardia, extrasystoles
- **GI:** *Epigastric distress,* anorexia, increased appetite and weight gain, nausea, vomiting, diarrhea or constipation
- **GU:** Urinary frequency, dysuria, urinary retention, early menses, decreased libido, impotence
- **Hematologic:** Hemolytic anemia, hypoplastic anemia, thrombocytopenia, leukopenia, agranulocytosis, pancytopenia
- **Hypersensitivity:** Urticaria, rash, **anaphylactic shock,** photosensitivity
- **Respiratory:** *Thickening of bronchial secretions,* chest tightness, wheezing, nasal stuffiness, dry mouth, dry nose, dry throat, sore throat

Interactions

✱ Drug-drug • Increased sedation with alcohol, other CNS depressants • Increased and prolonged anticholinergic (drying) effects with MAOIs

■ Nursing considerations

Assessment

- **History:** Allergy to any antihistamines, tartrazine, narrow-angle glaucoma, stenosing peptic ulcer, symptomatic prostatic hypertrophy, asthmatic attack, bladder neck obstruction, pyloroduodenal obstruction, third trimester of pregnancy, lactation
- **Physical:** Skin color, lesions, texture; orientation, reflexes, affect; vision examination; P, BP; R, adventitious sounds; bowel sounds; prostate palpation; CBC with differential

Interventions

- Give orally with food if GI upset occurs.

Teaching points

- Take as prescribed; avoid excessive dosage; take with food if GI upset occurs. Swallow extended-release forms whole; do not cut, crush, or chew them.
- Avoid alcohol while on this drug; serious sedation could occur.
- Oral liquid and oral suspensions differ in strength; do not use interchangeably.
- You may experience these side effects: Dizziness, sedation, drowsiness (use caution if driving or performing tasks that require alertness); epigastric distress, diarrhea or constipation (take with meals); dry mouth (frequent mouth care, sucking sugarless lozenges may help); thickening of bronchial secretions, dryness of nasal mucosa (try a humidifier).
- Report difficulty breathing, hallucinations, tremors, loss of coordination, unusual bleeding or bruising, visual disturbances, irregular heartbeat.

budesonide

*(byoo **des'** oh nide)*

Inhalation: Entocort (CAN), Pulmicort Flexhaler, Pulmicort Respules, Rhinocort Aqua, Rhinocort Turbuhaler (CAN)

Oral: Entocort EC (DNC)

PREGNANCY CATEGORY B, C (ORAL)

Drug class

Corticosteroid

Therapeutic actions

Anti-inflammatory effect; local administration into nasal passages maximizes beneficial effects on these tissues, while decreasing the likelihood of adverse effects from systemic absorption.

Indications

- *Rhinocort Aqua:* Management of symptoms of seasonal or perennial allergic rhinitis in adults and children
- *Respules/Flexhaler:* Maintenance treatment of asthma as prophylactic therapy in adults and children age 6 yr and older and for patients requiring corticosteroids for asthma
- Inhalation suspension: Maintenance treatment and prophylaxis therapy of asthma in children 12 mo–8 yr
- Oral: Treatment and maintenance of clinical remission for up to 3 mo of mild to moderate active Crohn's disease involving the ileum or ascending colon

Contraindications and cautions

Inhalation

- Contraindicated with hypersensitivity to drug or for relief of acute asthma or bronchospasm.
- Use cautiously with TB, systemic infections, lactation.

Oral

- Contraindicated with hypersensitivity to drug, lactation.
- Use cautiously with TB, hypertension, diabetes mellitus, osteoporosis, peptic ulcer disease, glaucoma, cataracts, family history of diabetes or glaucoma, other conditions in which glucocorticosteroids may have unwanted effects.

Nasal

- Contraindicated with hypersensitivity to drug, nasal infections, nasal trauma, nasal septal ulcers, recent nasal surgery.
- Use cautiously with lactation, TB, systemic infection.

Available forms

Spray—32 mcg/actuation; dry powder for inhalation (*Pulmicort Flexhaler*)—90 mcg (delivers 80 mcg), 180 mcg (delivers 160 mcg); inhalation suspension—0.25 mg/2 mL, 0.5 mg/2 mL, 1 mg/2 mL; capsules (DNC)—3 mg

Dosages

Nasal inhalation

Adults and patients 6 yr and older

Initial dose, 64 mcg/day given as 1 spray (32 mcg) in each nostril once daily. After desired clinical effect is achieved, reduce dosage to the smallest dose possible to maintain the control of symptoms. Maximum daily dose for patients older than 12 yr is 256 mcg/day given as 4 sprays per nostril once daily. Patients 6 to younger than 12 yr should not exceed 128 mcg/day (given as 2 sprays per nostril once daily). Generally takes 3–7 days to achieve maximum clinical effect.

Pulmicort Flexhaler

Adults

360 mcg bid; maximum dose, 720 mcg bid.

Pediatric patients 6 yr and older

180 mcg bid; maximum dose, 360 mcg bid.

Pulmicort Respules

Pediatric patients 12 mo–8 yr

0.5–1 mg once daily or in two divided doses using jet nebulizer.

Oral

Adults

9 mg/day PO taken in the morning for up to 8 wk. Recurrent episodes may be retreated for 8-wk periods. Maintenance treatment, 6 mg/day PO for up to 3 mo, then taper until cessation is complete.

Pediatric patients younger than 6 yr

Safety and efficacy not established.

Patients with hepatic impairment
Monitor patients very closely for signs of hypercorticism; reduced dosage should be considered with these patients.

Pharmacokinetics

Route	*Onset*	*Peak*	*Duration*
Intranasal, inhaled	Immediate	Rapid	8–12 hr
Oral	Slow	0.5–10 hr	Unknown

Metabolism: Hepatic; $T_{1/2}$: 2–3.6 hr (oral); $T_{1/2}$: 2.8 hr (inhalation)
Distribution: Crosses placenta; may enter breast milk
Excretion: Urine

Adverse effects

- **CNS:** *Headache, dizziness,* lethargy, *fatigue,* paresthesias, nervousness
- **Dermatologic:** Rash, edema, pruritus, alopecia
- **Endocrine:** HPA suppression, Cushing's syndrome with overdosage and systemic absorption
- **GI:** Nausea, dyspepsia, dry mouth
- **Local:** *Nasal irritation,* fungal infection
- **Respiratory:** Epistaxis, rebound congestion, *pharyngitis, cough*
- **Other:** Chest pain, asthenia, moon face, acne, bruising, *back pain*

Interactions

Oral use
✱ **Drug-drug** • Increased risk of corticosteroid toxic effects if combined with ketoconazole, itraconazole, ritonavir, indinavir, saquinavir, erythromycin, or other known CYP3A4 inhibitors; if drugs must be used together, decrease dosage of budesonide and monitor patient closely
✱ **Drug-food** • Risk of increased toxic effects if combined with grapefruit juice; avoid this combination

■ Nursing considerations

Assessment

- **History:** Untreated local nasal infections, nasal trauma, septal ulcers, recent nasal surgery, lactation
- **Physical:** BP, P, auscultation; R, adventitious sounds; examination of nares

Interventions

Inhalation
⊗ ***Black box warning*** Taper systemic steroids carefully during transfer to inhalational steroids; deaths from adrenal insufficiency have occurred.

- Arrange for use of decongestant nose drops to facilitate penetration if edema, excessive secretions are present.
- Use spray within 6 mo of opening. Shake well before each use.
- Store *Pulmicort Respules* upright and protected from light; gently shake before use; open envelopes should be discarded after 2 wk.
- Store *Flexhaler* tightly closed at room temperature. Do not remove or twist mouthpiece. Do not immerse in water or use liquid to clean *Flexhaler*.

Nasal inhalation

- Prime pump eight times before first use. If not used for 2 consecutive days, reprime with 1 spray or until fine mist appears. If not used for more than 14 days, rinse applicator and reprime with 2 sprays or until fine mist appears.

Oral

- Make sure patient does not cut, crush, or chew capsules; they must be swallowed whole.
- Administer the drug once each day, in the morning; have patient avoid drinking grapefruit juice.
- Encourage patient to complete full 8 wk of drug therapy.

⊗ ***Warning*** Monitor patient for signs of hypercorticism—acne, bruising, moon face, swollen ankles, hirsutism, skin striae, buffalo hump—which could indicate need to decrease dosage.

Teaching points

Inhalation

- Do not use more often than prescribed; do not stop without consulting your health care provider.
- It may take several days to achieve good effects; do not stop if effects are not immediate.
- Use decongestant nose drops first if nasal passages are blocked.

- Store *Pulmicort Respules* upright, protect from light; discard open envelopes after 2 weeks; gently shake before use.
- Store *Flexhaler* at room temperature. Keep tightly closed. Do not immerse in water and do not use liquid to clean the device. Do not twist or remove mouthpiece.
- You may experience these side effects: Local irritation (use your device correctly), dry mouth (suck sugarless lozenges).
- Prime the pump eight times before its first use. If it is not used for 2 consecutive days, reprime it with 1 spray or until a fine mist appears. If it is not used for more than 14 days, rinse the applicator off and reprime it with 2 sprays or until fine mist appears.
- Report sore mouth, sore throat, worsening of symptoms, severe sneezing, exposure to chickenpox or measles, eye infections.

Oral

- Take the drug once a day in the morning. Do not cut, crush, or chew the capsules, they must be swallowed whole.
- If you miss a day, take the capsules as soon as you remember them. Take the next day's capsules at the regular time. Do not take more than three capsules in a day.
- Take the full course of the drug therapy (8 weeks in most cases).
- Do not take this drug with grapefruit juice; avoid grapefruit juice entirely while using this drug.
- You may experience these side effects: Dizziness, headache (avoid driving or operating dangerous machinery if these effects occur); nausea, flatulence (small, frequent meals may help; try to maintain your fluid and food intake).
- Report chest pain, ankle swelling, respiratory infections, increased bruising.

▽bumetanide

*(byoo **met'** a nide)*

Bumex, Burinex (CAN)

PREGNANCY CATEGORY C

Drug class
Loop (high-ceiling) diuretic

Therapeutic actions
Inhibits the reabsorption of sodium and chloride from the proximal and distal renal tubules and the loop of Henle, leading to a natriuretic diuresis.

Indications
- Edema associated with heart failure, hepatic and renal disease (including nephrotic syndrome)
- Unlabeled use: Treatment of adult nocturia (not effective in men with BPH)

Contraindications and cautions
- Contraindicated with allergy to bumetanide or sulfonamides; electrolyte depletion; anuria, severe renal failure; hepatic coma, lactation.
- Use cautiously with SLE; gout; diabetes mellitus; pregnancy.

Available forms
Tablets—0.5, 1, 2 mg; injection—0.25 mg/mL

Dosages
Adults
Oral

0.5–2 mg/day PO in a single dose; may repeat at 4- to 5-hr intervals up to a maximum daily dose of 10 mg. Intermittent dosage schedule of drug and rest days is 3–4 on/1–2 off, which is most effective with edema.

Parenteral

0.5–1 mg IV or IM. Give over 1–2 min. Dose may be repeated at intervals of 2–3 hr if response is not sufficient. Do not exceed 10 mg/day.

Pediatric patients
Not recommended for patients younger than 18 yr.

Geriatric patients or patients with renal impairment
Initiate at lower dose and consider decreased renal, hepatic, and cardiac function.

Pharmacokinetics

Route	Onset	Peak	Duration
Oral	30–60 min	1–2 hr	4–6 hr
IV	Minutes	15–30 min	30–60 min

Metabolism: $T_{1/2}$: 60–90 min
Distribution: Crosses placenta; may enter breast milk
Excretion: Urine

IV FACTS

Preparation: May be given direct IV or diluted in solution with D_5W, 0.9% sodium chloride, or lactated Ringer's solution. Discard unused solution after 24 hr.
Injection: Give by direct injection slowly, over 1–2 min; do not exceed 10 mg/day.

Adverse effects

- **CNS:** *Asterixis, dizziness,* vertigo, paresthesias, confusion, fatigue, nystagmus, *weakness, headache, drowsiness,* fatigue, blurred vision, tinnitus, irreversible hearing loss
- **CV:** *Orthostatic hypotension,* volume depletion, cardiac arrhythmias, thrombophlebitis
- **GI:** *Nausea, anorexia, vomiting, diarrhea,* gastric irritation and pain, dry mouth, acute pancreatitis, jaundice
- **GU:** *Polyuria, nocturia,* glycosuria, renal failure
- **Hematologic:** *Hypokalemia,* leukopenia, anemia, thrombocytopenia
- **Local:** *Pain, phlebitis at injection site*
- **Other:** Muscle cramps and muscle spasms, weakness, arthritic pain, fatigue, hives, photosensitivity, rash, pruritus, sweating, nipple tenderness

Interactions

✱ **Drug-drug** • Decreased diuresis and natriuresis with NSAIDs and probenecid • Increased risk of cardiac glycoside toxicity (secondary to hypokalemia) • Increased risk of ototoxicity if taken with aminoglycoside antibiotics, cisplatin

■ Nursing considerations

Assessment

- **History:** Allergy to bumetanide, electrolyte depletion, anuria, severe renal failure, hepatic coma, SLE, gout, diabetes mellitus, lactation
- **Physical:** Skin color, lesions; edema; orientation, reflexes, hearing; pulses, baseline ECG, BP, orthostatic BP, perfusion; R, pattern, adventitious sounds; liver evaluation, bowel sounds; urinary output patterns; CBC, serum electrolytes (including calcium), blood glucose, LFTs, renal function tests, uric acid, urinalysis

Interventions

- Give with food or milk to prevent GI upset.
- Mark calendars or use reminders if intermittent therapy is best for treating edema.
- Give single dose early in day so increased urination will not disturb sleep.
- Avoid IV use if oral use is possible.

⊗ ***Black box warning*** Arrange to monitor serum electrolytes, hydration, and hepatic function during long-term therapy; water and electrolyte depletion can occur.

- Provide diet rich in potassium or supplemental potassium.

Teaching points

- Record alternate day or intermittent therapy on a calendar or dated envelopes.
- Take the drug early in the day so increased urination will not disturb sleep; take with food or meals to prevent GI upset.
- Weigh yourself on a regular basis, at the same time and in the same clothing; record the weight on your calendar.
- You may experience these side effects: Increased volume and frequency of urination; dizziness, feeling faint on arising, drowsiness (avoid rapid position changes; hazardous activities, such as driving; and alcohol consumption); sensitivity to sunlight (use sunglasses, sunscreen, wear protective clothing); increased thirst (suck sugarless lozenges; use frequent mouth care); loss of body potassium (a potassium-rich diet, or supplement will be needed).
- Report weight change of more than 3 pounds in 1 day; swelling in ankles or fingers; unusual bleeding or bruising; nausea, dizziness, trembling, numbness, fatigue; muscle weakness or cramps.

DANGEROUS DRUG

buprenorphine hydrochloride

*(byoo pre **nor'** feen)*

Buprenex, Subutex

PREGNANCY CATEGORY C

CONTROLLED SUBSTANCE C-III

Drug class

Opioid agonist-antagonist analgesic

Therapeutic actions

Acts as an agonist at specific opioid receptors in the CNS to produce analgesia; also acts as an opioid antagonist; exact mechanism of action not understood.

Indications

- Parenteral: Relief of moderate to severe pain
- Oral: Treatment of opioid dependence, preferably used as induction treatment

Contraindications and cautions

- Contraindicated with hypersensitivity to buprenorphine.
- Use cautiously with physical dependence on opioid analgesics (withdrawal syndrome may occur); compromised respiratory function; increased intracranial pressure (buprenorphine may elevate CSF pressure; may cause miosis and coma, which could interfere with patient evaluation), myxedema, Addison's disease, toxic psychosis, prostatic hypertrophy or urethral stricture, acute alcoholism, delirium tremens, kyphoscoliosis, biliary tract dysfunction (may cause spasm of the sphincter of Oddi), hepatic or renal impairment, lactation, pregnancy.

Available forms

Injection—0.324 mg/mL (equivalent to 0.3 mg); sublingual tablets (*Subutex*)—2, 8 mg

Dosages

Adults and pediatric patients older than 13 yr

Parenteral

- *Relief of pain:* 0.3 mg IM or by slow (over 2 min) IV injection. May repeat once, 30–60 min after first dose; repeat every 6 hr as needed. If necessary, nonrisk patients may be given up to 0.6 mg by deep IM injection.

Oral

- *Opioid dependence:* 12–16 mg/day sublingually (*Subutex*), used as induction with switch to *Suboxone* (buprenorphine/naloxone combination) for maintenance.

Pediatric patients (2–12 yr)

2–6 mcg/kg of body weight IM or slow IV injection every 4–6 hr.

Geriatric or debilitated patients

Reduce dosage to one-half usual adult dose.

Pharmacokinetics

Route	Onset	Peak	Duration
Oral	15 min	1 hr	6 hr
IV	10 min	30–45 min	6 hr

Metabolism: Hepatic; $T_{1/2}$: 2–3 hr
Distribution: Crosses placenta; may enter breast milk
Excretion: Feces

IV FACTS

Preparation: May be diluted with isotonic saline, lactated Ringer's solution, 5% dextrose and 0.9% saline, 5% dextrose. Protect from light and excessive heat.
Injection: Administer slowly over 2 min.
Compatibilities: Compatible IV with scopolamine HBr, haloperidol, glycopyrrolate, droperidol and hydroxyzine HCl.
Incompatibilities: Do not mix with diazepam and lorazepam.

Adverse effects

- **CNS:** *Sedation, dizziness or vertigo, headache,* confusion, dreaming, psychosis, euphoria, weakness, fatigue, nervousness, slurred speech, paresthesia, depression, malaise, hallucinations, depersonalization, coma, tremor, dysphoria, agitation, seizures, tinnitus

- **CV:** *Hypotension,* hypertension, tachycardia, bradycardia, Wenckebach's block
- **Dermatologic:** *Sweating,* pruritus, rash, pallor, urticaria
- **EENT:** *Miosis,* blurred vision, diplopia, conjunctivitis, visual abnormalities, amblyopia
- **GI:** *Nausea, vomiting,* dry mouth, constipation, flatulence
- **Local:** Injection site reaction
- **Respiratory:** *Hypoventilation,* dyspnea, cyanosis, apnea

Interactions

✱ Drug-drug • Potentiation of effects of buprenorphine with other opioid analgesics, phenothiazines, tranquilizers, barbiturates, general anesthetics, benzodiazepines

■ Nursing considerations

Assessment

- **History:** Hypersensitivity to buprenorphine, physical dependence on opioid analgesics, compromised respiratory function, increased intracranial pressure, myxedema, Addison's disease, toxic psychosis, prostatic hypertrophy or urethral stricture, acute alcoholism, delirium tremens, kyphoscoliosis, biliary tract dysfunction, hepatic or renal impairment, lactation, pregnancy
- **Physical:** Skin color, texture, lesions; orientation, reflexes, bilateral grip strength, affect; pupil size, vision; pulse, auscultation, BP; R, adventitious sounds; bowel sounds, normal output, liver palpation; prostate palpation, normal urine output; LFTs, renal, thyroid, adrenal function tests

Interventions

⊗ ***Warning*** Keep opioid antagonist and facilities for assisted or controlled respiration readily available in case respiratory depression occurs.

- Have the patient hold sublingual tablets (*Subutex*) beneath the tongue until they dissolve; these tablets should not be swallowed. Place all tablets for a single dose under patient's tongue at once; if not possible, place two tablets at a time.
- Instruct patient being treated for opioid dependence that CNS depression and death can occur with overdose of these drugs, or if this drug is combined with sedatives, alcohol, tranquilizers, antidepressants, or benzodiazepines.
- Manage overdose by providing ventilation and support.

Teaching points

- Hold sublingual tablets under the tongue until they dissolve. Do not swallow these tablets. If possible, place all tablets for a single dose under the tongue at once; if not possible, place two tablets at a time.
- Inform all health care or emergency workers that you are opioid dependent and using this drug for maintenance; serious effects could occur if certain drugs are used with this drug.
- Avoid combining *Subutex* with any alcohol, antidepressants, sedatives, benzodiazepines, or tranquilizers; serious CNS depression could occur. Do not crush and inject these tablets.
- Overdose with *Subutex* can result in coma and death; use this drug exactly as prescribed.
- You may experience these side effects: Dizziness, sedation, drowsiness, impaired visual acuity (avoid driving, performing other tasks that require alertness); nausea, loss of appetite (lie quietly, eat frequent small meals).
- Report severe nausea, vomiting, palpitations, shortness of breath or difficulty breathing, urinary difficulty.

▽ bupropion

(byoo ***proe'*** *pee on)*

bupropion hydrobromide

Aplenzin (DNC)

bupropion hydrochloride

Budeprion SR (DNC),
Wellbutrin, Wellbutrin SR (DNC),
Budeprion XL (DNC),
Wellbutrin XL (DNC), Zyban

PREGNANCY CATEGORY C

Drug classes

Antidepressant
Smoking deterrent

Therapeutic actions

The neurochemical mechanism of the antidepressant effect of bupropion is not understood; it is chemically unrelated to other antidepressant agents; it is a weak blocker of neuronal uptake of serotonin and norepinephrine and inhibits the reuptake of dopamine to some extent.

Indications

- Treatment of major depressive disorder
- Aid to smoking cessation treatment (*Zyban*)
- Prevention of major depressive episodes in patients with seasonal affective disorder (*Wellbutrin XL*)
- Unlabeled uses: treatment of neuropathic pain, ADHD, weight loss

Contraindications and cautions

- Contraindicated with hypersensitivity to bupropion; history of seizure disorder, bulimia or anorexia, head trauma, CNS tumor (increased risk of seizures); treatment with MAOIs; lactation.
- Use cautiously with renal or liver disease; heart disease, history of MI, pregnancy.

Available forms

Tablets—75, 100 mg; SR tablets DNC—100, 150, 200 mg; ER tablets DNC—150, 200, 300 mg; 174, 348, 522 mg (*Aplenzin*)

Dosages

Adults

- *Depression:* 300 mg PO given as 100 mg tid; begin treatment with 100 mg PO bid; if clinical response warrants, increase to 300 mg/day (given as 100 mg tid) 3 days after beginning treatment. If 4 wk after treatment, no clinical improvement is seen, dose may be increased to 150 mg PO tid (450 mg/day). Do not exceed 150 mg in any one dose. Discontinue drug if no improvement occurs at the 450-mg/day level. *SR:* 150 mg PO bid; allow at least 8 hr between doses. *ER:* Initially, 150 mg/day PO as a once-a-day dose; range 300–450 mg/day. *ER (Aplenzin):* 174–348 mg/day PO.
- *Smoking cessation:* 150 mg (*Zyban*) PO daily for 3 days, then increase to 300 mg/day in two divided doses at least 8 hr apart. Treat for 7–12 wk.
- *Seasonal affective disorder:* 150 mg (*Wellbutrin XL*) PO daily in the morning; may increase after 1 wk to 300 mg/day PO. Begin in autumn and taper off (150 mg/day for 2 wk before discontinuation) in early spring.

Pediatric patients

Safety and efficacy in patients younger than 18 yr not established.

Patients with impaired renal function

Bupropion is excreted through the kidneys; use with caution, and monitor patients carefully.

Patients with impaired hepatic function

Consider reduced dose or frequency in patients with mild or moderate impairment. For those with severe impairment, do not exceed 75 mg/day (*Wellbutrin*), 100 mg/day or 150 mg every other day (*Wellbutrin SR*), or 150 mg every other day (*Wellbutrin XL* and *Zyban*).

Pharmacokinetics

Route	Onset	Peak	Duration
Oral	Varies	2 hr	8–12 hr
SR Oral	Varies	3 hr	16–20 hr
ER Oral	Varies	5 hr	15–25 hr

Metabolism: Hepatic; $T_{1/2}$: 14 hr; 21 hr (*Wellbutrin SR*)
Distribution: May cross placenta; may enter breast milk
Excretion: Feces, urine

Adverse effects

- **CNS:** *Agitation,* dizziness, *insomnia, headache, migraine, tremor,* ataxia, incoordination, seizures, mania, alterations in libido, hallucinations, visual disturbances
- **CV:** *Tachycardia,* edema, ECG abnormalities, chest pain, shortness of breath
- **Dermatologic:** Rash, alopecia, dry skin
- **GI:** *Dry mouth, constipation,* nausea, vomiting, stomatitis
- **GU:** Nocturia, vaginal irritation, testicular swelling
- **Other:** *Weight loss,* flulike symptoms

Interactions

✱ **Drug-drug** • Increased risk of adverse effects with levodopa • Increased risk of toxicity with MAOIs • Increased risk of seizures with drugs that lower seizure threshold, including alcohol

■ Nursing considerations

Assessment

- **History:** Hypersensitivity to bupropion, history of seizure disorder, bulimia or anorexia, head trauma, CNS tumor, treatment with MAOI, renal or hepatic disease, heart disease, lactation
- **Physical:** Skin, weight; orientation, affect, vision, coordination; P, rhythm, auscultation; R, adventitious sounds; bowel sounds, condition of mouth

Interventions

- Give drug three times a day for depression; do not administer more than 150 mg in any one dose. Administer SR forms twice a day with at least 8 hr between doses. Administer ER forms once a day. Caution patient not to cut, crush, or chew ER or SR forms.
- Increase dosage slowly to reduce the risk of seizures.
- Administer 100-mg immediate-release tablets four times a day for depression, with at least 6 hr between doses, if patient is receiving more than 300 mg/day; use combinations of 75-mg tablets to avoid giving more than 150 mg in any single dose.
- Arrange for patient evaluation after 6 wk.
- Discontinue MAOI therapy for at least 14 days before beginning bupropion.
- Monitor hepatic and renal function tests in patients with a history of hepatic or renal impairment.
- Have patient quit smoking within first 2 wk of treatment for smoking cessation; may be used with transdermal nicotine.

⊠ ***Black box warning*** Monitor response and behavior; suicide is a risk in depressed patients, children, adolescents, and young adults. Serious mental health events, including changes in behavior, depression, and hostility, have been reported.

Teaching points

- Take this drug in equally divided doses three to four times a day as prescribed for depression. Take sustained-release forms twice a day, at least 8 hours apart. Do not combine doses or make up missed doses. Take once a day, or divided into two doses at least 8 hours apart for smoking cessation. Do not cut, crush, or chew ER or SR forms.
- Avoid or limit the use of alcohol while on this drug. Seizures can occur if these are combined.
- May be used with transdermal nicotine; most effective for smoking cessation if combined with behavioral support program.
- You may experience these side effects: Dizziness, lack of coordination, tremor (avoid driving or performing tasks that require alertness); dry mouth (use frequent mouth care, suck sugarless lozenges); headache, insomnia (consult your health care provider if these become a problem; do not self-medicate); nausea, vomiting, weight loss (eat frequent small meals).
- Report dark urine, light-colored stools; rapid or irregular heartbeat; hallucinations; severe headache or insomnia; thoughts of suicide; fever, chills, sore throat.

▽ buspirone hydrochloride

*(byoo **spye'** rone)*

Apo-Buspirone (CAN), BuSpar, CO Buspirone (CAN), Gen-Buspirone (CAN), PMS-Buspirone (CAN)

PREGNANCY CATEGORY B

Drug class

Anxiolytic

Therapeutic actions

Mechanism of action not known; lacks antiseizure, sedative, or muscle relaxant properties; binds serotonin receptors, but the clinical significance is unclear.

Indications

- Management of anxiety disorders or short-term relief of symptoms of anxiety
- Unlabeled use: Decreasing the symptoms (aches, pains, fatigue, cramps, irritability) of PMS

Contraindications and cautions

- Contraindicated with hypersensitivity to buspirone; marked liver or renal impairment; lactation.
- Use cautiously with pregnancy, mild renal or hepatic impairment.

Available forms

Tablets—5, 7.5, 10, 15, 30 mg

Dosages

Adults

Initially, 15 mg/day PO (7.5 mg bid). Increase dosage 5 mg/day at intervals of 2–3 days to achieve optimal therapeutic response. Do not exceed 60 mg/day. Divided doses of 20–30 mg/day have been used.

Pediatric patients

Safety and efficacy for patients younger than 18 yr not established.

Pharmacokinetics

Route	*Onset*	*Peak*
Oral	7–10 days	40–90 min

Metabolism: Hepatic; $T_{1/2}$: 3–11 hr
Distribution: May enter breast milk
Excretion: Urine

Adverse effects

- **CNS:** *Dizziness, headache, nervousness, insomnia, light-headedness,* excitement, dream disturbances, drowsiness, decreased concentration, anger, hostility, confusion, depression, tinnitus, blurred vision, numbness, paresthesia, incoordination, tremor, depersonalization, dysphoria, noise intolerance, euphoria, akathisia, fearfulness, loss of interest, dissociative reaction, hallucinations, suicidal ideation, seizures, altered taste and smell, involuntary movements, slowed reaction time
- **CV:** Nonspecific chest pain, tachycardia or palpitations, syncope, hypotension, hypertension
- **GI:** *Nausea, dry mouth, vomiting, abdominal or gastric distress, diarrhea,* constipation, flatulence, anorexia, increased appetite, salivation, irritable colon, rectal bleeding
- **GU:** Urinary frequency, urinary hesitancy, dysuria, increased or decreased libido, menstrual irregularity, spotting
- **Respiratory:** Hyperventilation, shortness of breath, chest congestion
- **Other:** Musculoskeletal aches and pains, sweating, clamminess, sore throat, nasal congestion

Interactions

✱ **Drug-drug** • Give with caution to patients taking alcohol, other CNS depressants • Decreased effects with fluoxetine • Increased serum levels of buspirone if taken with erythromycin, itraconazole; decrease buspirone dose to 2.5 mg and monitor closely if these combinations are used • Risk of increased haloperidol levels if combined • Risk of marked hypertension if combined with MAOIs

✱ **Drug-food** • Risk of increased serum levels and toxicity if taken with grapefruit juice

■ Nursing considerations

Assessment

- **History:** Hypersensitivity to buspirone, marked liver or renal impairment, lactation
- **Physical:** Weight; T; skin color, lesions; mucous membranes, throat color, lesions, orientation, affect, reflexes, vision examination; P, BP; R, adventitious sounds; bowel sounds, normal GI output, liver evaluation; normal urinary output, voiding pattern; LFTs, renal function tests, urinalysis, CB and differential

Interventions

- Provide sugarless lozenges or ice chips if dry mouth or altered taste occurs.
- Arrange for analgesic for headache or musculoskeletal aches.

Teaching points

- Take this drug exactly as prescribed.
- Avoid the use of alcohol, sleep-inducing, or over-the-counter drugs and grapefruit juice; these could cause dangerous effects.
- You may experience these side effects: Drowsiness, dizziness, light-headedness (avoid driving or operating complex machinery); GI upset (eat frequent small meals); dry mouth

(suck ice chips or sugarless candies); dreams, nightmares, difficulty concentrating or sleeping, confusion, excitement (reversible; will stop when the drug is discontinued).

- Report abnormal involuntary movements of facial or neck muscles, motor restlessness; sore or cramped muscles; abnormal posture; yellowing of the skin or eyes.

DANGEROUS DRUG

busulfan

*(byoo **sul'** fan)*

Busulfex, Myleran

PREGNANCY CATEGORY D

Drug classes

Alkylating drug
Antineoplastic

Therapeutic actions

Cytotoxic: Interacts with cellular thiol groups causing cell death; cell cycle nonspecific.

Indications

- Tablets: Palliative treatment of chronic myelogenous leukemia; less effective in patients without the Philadelphia chromosome (Ph1); ineffective in the blastic stage
- Injection: In combination with cyclophosphamide as conditioning regimen prior to allogenic hematopoietic progenitor cell transplant for CML
- **NEW INDICATION:** Oral: Other myeloproliferative disorders, including severe thrombocytosis and polycythemia vera, myelofibrosis; bone marrow transplantation

Contraindications and cautions

- Contraindicated with allergy to busulfan, history of resistance to busulfan, chronic lymphocytic leukemia, acute leukemia, blastic phase of chronic myelogenous leukemia, hematopoietic depression, pregnancy, lactation.
- Use cautiously with bone marrow suppression, history of seizure disorders, hepatic impairment.

Available forms

Tablets—2 mg; injection—6 mg/mL

Dosages

Adults

Oral

- *Remission induction:* 4–8 mg total dose PO daily. Continue until WBC has dropped to 15,000/mm^3; WBC may continue to fall for 1 mo after drug is discontinued. Normal WBC count is usually achieved in approximately 12–20 wk in most cases.
- *Maintenance therapy:* Resume treatment with induction dosage when WBC count reaches 50,000/mm^3. If remission is shorter than 3 mo, maintenance therapy of 1–3 mg PO daily is advised to keep hematologic status under control.

Parenteral

- *Conditioning regimen:* 0.8 mg/kg of ideal body weight or actual body weight, whichever is lower, as a 2-hr infusion every 6 hr for 4 consecutive days (16 doses) via central venous catheter.

Pediatric patients

Oral

Children may be dosed at 60 mcg/kg/day *or* 1.8 mg/m^2/day (body surface) for remission induction.

Pharmacokinetics

Route	*Onset*	*Peak*	*Duration*
Oral, IV	30 min–2 hr	2–3 hr	4 hr

Metabolism: Hepatic; $T_{1/2}$: 2.5 hr
Distribution: Crosses placenta; enters breast milk
Excretion: Urine

IV FACTS

Preparation: Dilute to 10 times the busulfan volume using 0.9% sodium chloride injection or D_5W. Use enclosed filter when withdrawing drug from ampule. Final concentration should be greater than or equal to 0.5 mg/mL. Use strict aseptic technique. Always add busulfan to the diluent. Mix by inverting bag several times. Stable at room temperature for 8 hr, then discard.
Infusion: Use an infusion pump to deliver total dose over 2 hr. Flush catheter with 5 mL D_5W

or 0.9% sodium chloride before and after each dose. Infusion must be completed within 8 hr.
Incompatibilities: Do not infuse with any other solution or drugs.

Adverse effects

- **CNS:** Seizures
- **CV:** Hypertension, tachycardia, thrombosis
- **Dermatologic:** *Hyperpigmentation,* urticaria, **Stevens-Johnson syndrome,** erythema nodosum, alopecia, porphyria cutanea tarda, excessive dryness and fragility of the skin with anhidrosis
- **EENT:** Cataracts (with prolonged use)
- **Endocrine:** *Amenorrhea, ovarian suppression, menopausal symptoms,* interference with spermatogenesis, testicular atrophy, syndrome resembling adrenal insufficiency (weakness, fatigue, anorexia, weight loss, nausea, vomiting, melanoderma)
- **GI:** Dryness of the oral mucous membranes and cheilosis; *nausea, vomiting*, abdominal pain, anorexia
- **GU:** Hyperuricemia
- **Hematologic:** *Leukopenia, thrombocytopenia, anemia,* **pancytopenia** (prolonged)
- **Respiratory: Pulmonary dysplasia**
- **Other:** Cancer

■ Nursing considerations

Assessment

- **History:** Allergy to or history of resistance to busulfan, chronic lymphocytic leukemia, acute leukemia, blastic phase of chronic myelogenous leukemia, hematopoietic depression, pregnancy, lactation, hepatic impairment, seizure disorders
- **Physical:** Weight; skin color, lesions, turgor; earlobe tophi; eye examination; bilateral hand grip; R, adventitious sounds; mucous membranes; CBC, differential; urinalysis; serum uric acid; PFTs; bone marrow examination if indicated

Interventions

⊗ ***Black box warning*** Arrange for blood tests to evaluate bone marrow function prior to therapy as well as weekly during and for at least 3 wk after therapy has ended. Severe bone marrow suppression is possible.

⊗ ***Warning*** Arrange for respiratory function tests before beginning therapy, periodically during therapy, and periodically after busulfan therapy has ended, to monitor for pulmonary dysplasia.

- Reduce dosage in cases of bone marrow depression.
- Give at the same time each day.
- Suggest barrier contraceptive use during therapy.

⊗ ***Warning*** Ensure patient is hydrated before and during therapy; alkalinization of the urine or allopurinol may be needed to prevent adverse effects of hyperuricemia.

- Monitor patient for cataracts.
- Administer IV busulfan through a central venous catheter.
- Premedicate patient receiving IV busulfan with phenytoin to decrease occurrence of seizures.
- Medicate patient receiving IV busulfan with antiemetics prior to the first dose and on a fixed schedule through the administration regimen.

Teaching points

Oral drug

- Take drug at the same time each day.
- Drink 10–12 glasses of fluid each day.
- Have regular medical follow-up, including blood tests, to monitor effects of the drug.
- Consider using barrier contraceptives. This drug has been known to cause fetal damage.
- You may experience these side effects: Darkening of the skin, rash, dry and fragile skin (skin care suggestions will be outlined for you to help to prevent skin breakdown); weakness, fatigue (consult with health care provider if pronounced); loss of appetite, nausea, vomiting, weight loss (eat frequent small meals); amenorrhea in women, change in sperm production in men (may affect fertility).
- Report unusual bleeding or bruising; fever, chills, sore throat; stomach, flank, or joint pain; cough, shortness of breath.

butabarbital sodium (secbutabarbital, secbutobarbitone)

*(byoo ta **bar'** bi tal)*

Butisol Sodium

Pregnancy Category D

Controlled Substance C-III

Drug classes

Barbiturate (intermediate acting)
Sedative-hypnotic

Therapeutic actions

General CNS depressant; barbiturates inhibit impulse conduction in the ascending reticular activating system, depress the cerebral cortex, alter cerebellar function, depress motor output, and can produce excitation (especially with subanesthetic doses in the presence of pain), sedation, hypnosis, anesthesia, deep coma.

Indications

- Short-term use as a sedative and hypnotic

Contraindications and cautions

- Contraindicated with hypersensitivity to barbiturates, tartrazine (in 30-, 50-mg tablets, and elixir marketed as *Butisol Sodium);* manifest or latent porphyria; marked liver impairment; nephritis; severe respiratory distress, respiratory disease with dyspnea, obstruction, or cor pulmonale; previous addiction to sedative-hypnotic drugs.
- Use cautiously with acute or chronic pain (may cause paradoxical excitement or mask important symptoms); seizure disorders (abrupt discontinuation of daily doses can result in status epilepticus); lactation (can cause drowsiness in nursing infants); fever, hyperthyroidism, diabetes mellitus, severe anemia, pulmonary or cardiac disease, status asthmaticus, shock, uremia; impaired liver or kidney function, debilitation, pregnancy.

Available forms

Tablets—15, 30, 50 mg; elixir—30 mg/5 mL

Dosages

Adults

- *Daytime sedation:* 15–30 mg PO three to four times a day.
- *Hypnotic:* 50–100 mg PO at bedtime. Drug loses effectiveness within 2 wk and should not be used longer than that.
- *Preanesthetic sedation:* 50–100 mg PO 60–90 min before surgery. It is not considered safe to administer oral medication when a patient is NPO for surgery or anesthesia.

Pediatric patients

- *Preanesthetic sedation:* 2–6 mg/kg; maximum dose 100 mg. Use caution: Barbiturates may produce irritability, excitability, inappropriate tearfulness, and aggression.

Geriatric patients or patients with debilitating disease or hepatic or renal impairment

Reduce dosage and monitor closely; may produce excitement, depression, or confusion.

Pharmacokinetics

Route	Onset	Peak	Duration
Oral	45–60 min	3–4 hr	6–8 hr

Metabolism: Hepatic; $T_{1/2}$: 50–100 hr
Distribution: Crosses placenta; enters breast milk
Excretion: Urine

Adverse effects

- **CNS:** *Somnolence, agitation, confusion, hyperkinesia, ataxia, vertigo, CNS depression, nightmares, lethargy, residual sedation (hangover), paradoxical excitement, nervousness, psychiatric disturbance, hallucinations, insomnia, anxiety, dizziness, thinking abnormality*
- **CV:** *Bradycardia, hypotension, syncope*
- **GI:** *Nausea, vomiting, constipation, diarrhea, epigastric pain*
- **Hypersensitivity:** Rashes, angioneurotic edema, serum sickness, morbilliform rash, urticaria; rarely, exfoliative dermatitis, **Stevens-Johnson syndrome**
- **Respiratory:** *Hypoventilation, apnea, respiratory depression,* **laryngospasm, bronchospasm, circulatory collapse**
- **Other: Anaphylaxis, angioedema,** tolerance, psychological and physical dependence; **withdrawal syndrome**

Interactions

✱ **Drug-drug** • Increased CNS depression with alcohol • Increased risk of nephrotoxicity with methoxyflurane • Decreased effects of theophyllines, oral anticoagulants, beta-blockers, doxycycline, corticosteroids, hormonal contraceptives and estrogens, metronidazole, phenylbutazones, quinidine, carbamazepine

■ Nursing considerations

Assessment

- **History:** Hypersensitivity to barbiturates, tartrazine, manifest or latent porphyria; marked liver impairment, nephritis, respiratory disease; previous addiction to sedative-hypnotic drugs, acute or chronic pain, seizure disorders, fever, hyperthyroidism, diabetes mellitus, severe anemia, cardiac disease, shock, uremia, debilitation, pregnancy, lactation
- **Physical:** Weight; T; skin color, lesions; orientation, affect, reflexes; P, BP, orthostatic BP; R, adventitious sounds; bowel sounds, normal output, liver evaluation; LFTs, renal function tests, blood and urine glucose, BUN

Interventions

- Monitor responses and blood levels if any of the interacting drugs (see Interactions) are given with butabarbital; suggest alternatives to hormonal contraceptives.

⊗ ***Warning*** Keep resuscitative equipment readily available in case of respiratory depression or hypersensitivity reaction.

- Taper dosage gradually after repeated use, especially in epileptic patients.

Teaching points

- This drug will make you drowsy and less anxious.
- Try not to get up after you have received this drug (request assistance to sit up or move about).

Outpatients taking this drug

- Take this drug exactly as prescribed.
- This drug is habit-forming; its effectiveness in facilitating sleep stops after a short time. Do not take drug longer than 2 weeks (for insomnia), and do not increase the dosage without consulting your health care provider.
- Consult the care provider if the drug appears to be ineffective.
- Avoid alcohol, sleep-inducing, or over-the-counter drugs; they may cause dangerous effects.
- Use an alternative to hormonal contraceptives; avoid becoming pregnant while taking this drug.
- You may experience these side effects: Drowsiness, dizziness, hangover, impaired thinking (less pronounced after a few days; avoid driving or dangerous activities); complex sleep disorders; GI upset (take the drug with food); nightmares, difficulty concentrating, fatigue, nervousness (reversible, will go away when drug is discontinued).
- Report severe dizziness, weakness, drowsiness that persists, rash or skin lesions, pregnancy, complex sleep-related behaviors.

DANGEROUS DRUG

butorphanol tartrate

*(byoo **tor'** fa nole)*

Stadol

PREGNANCY CATEGORY C (DURING PREGNANCY)

PREGNANCY CATEGORY D (DURING LABOR AND DELIVERY)

CONTROLLED SUBSTANCE C-IV

Drug class

Opioid agonist-antagonist analgesic

Therapeutic actions

Acts as an agonist at opioid receptors in the CNS to produce analgesia, sedation (therapeutic effects), but also acts to cause hallucinations (adverse effect); has low abuse potential.

Indications

- Relief of moderate to severe pain when use of an opioid analgesic is appropriate
- For preoperative or preanesthetic medication, to supplement balanced anesthesia, and to relieve prepartum pain (parenteral)

- Nasal spray: Relief of migraine headache pain and relief of moderate to severe pain

Contraindications and cautions

- Contraindicated with hypersensitivity to butorphanol or benzethonium chloride preservative, physical dependence on an opioid analgesic, pregnancy, lactation.
- Use cautiously with bronchial asthma, COPD, respiratory depression, anoxia, increased intracranial pressure, acute MI, ventricular failure, coronary insufficiency, hypertension, biliary tract surgery, renal or hepatic impairment, geriatric patients.

Available forms

Injection—1 mg/mL, 2 mg/mL; nasal spray—10 mg/mL

Dosages

Adults

IM

Usual single dose is 2 mg every 3–4 hr; patient must be able to remain recumbant. Dosage range is 1–4 mg every 3–4 hr; single doses should not exceed 4 mg.

- *Preoperative:* 2 mg IM, 60–90 min before surgery.

IV

Usual single dose is 1 mg every 3–4 hr. Dosage range is 0.5–2 mg every 3–4 hr.

- *Balanced anesthesia:* 2 mg IV shortly before induction or 0.5–1 mg IV in increments during anesthesia.

IV or IM

- *Labor:* 1–2 mg IV or IM at full term during early labor; repeat every 4 hr. Use alternative analgesia for pain associated with delivery or if delivery is expected within 4 hr.

Nasal

- *Relief of pain:* 1 mg (1 spray per nostril). May repeat in 60–90 min if adequate relief is not achieved. May repeat two-dose sequence every 3–4 hr.

Pediatric patients

Not recommended for patients younger than 18 yr.

Geriatric patients or patients with renal or hepatic impairment

Parenteral

Use one-half the usual dose at least 6 hr apart. Monitor patient response.

Nasal

Initially, 1 mg. Allow 90–120 min to elapse before a second dose is given.

Pharmacokinetics

Route	*Onset*	*Peak*	*Duration*
IV	Rapid	0.5–1 hr	3–4 hr
IM	10–15 min	0.5–1 hr	3–4 hr
Nasal	15 min	1–2 hr	4–5 hr

Metabolism: Hepatic; $T_{1/2}$: 2.1–9.2 hr
Distribution: Crosses placenta; enters breast milk
Excretion: Feces, urine

IV FACTS

Preparation: May be given undiluted. Store at room temperature. Protect from light.
Injection: Administer direct IV over 3–5 min.
Compatibilities: Do not mix in solution with dimenhydrinate or pentobarbital.
Y-site compatibility: Enalaprilat.

Adverse effects

- **CNS:** Sedation, clamminess, sweating, headache, vertigo, floating feeling, dizziness, lethargy, confusion, light-headedness, nervousness, unusual dreams, agitation, euphoria, hallucinations
- **CV:** Palpitation, increase or decrease in BP
- **Dermatologic:** Rash, hives, pruritus, flushing, warmth, sensitivity to cold
- **EENT:** Diplopia, blurred vision
- **GI:** *Nausea,* dry mouth
- **Respiratory:** Slow, shallow respiration

Interactions

✱ **Drug-drug** • Potentiation of effects of butorphanol when given with barbiturate anesthetics

■ Nursing considerations

Assessment

- **History:** Hypersensitivity to butorphanol, physical dependence on a narcotic analgesic, pregnancy, lactation, bronchial asthma, COPD, increased intracranial pressure, acute MI, ventricular failure, coronary insufficiency, hypertension, biliary tract surgery, renal or hepatic impairment

- **Physical:** Orientation, reflexes, bilateral grip strength, affect; pupil size, vision; pulse, auscultation, BP; R, adventitious sounds; bowel sounds, normal output; LFTs, renal function tests

Interventions
- Ensure that opioid antagonist facilities for assisted or controlled respiration is readily available during parenteral administration.

Teaching points
- You may experience these side effects: Dizziness, sedation, drowsiness, impaired visual acuity (avoid driving, performing other tasks that require alertness); nausea, loss of appetite (lie quietly, eat frequent small meals).
- Report severe nausea, vomiting, palpitations, shortness of breath or difficulty breathing, nasal lesions or discomfort (nasal spray).

C1-Inhibitor (human)

See Appendix W, *Less commonly used drugs*.

caffeine
*(kaf **een'**)*

Caffedrine, Enerjets, Fastlene, Keep Alert, Keep Going, Molie, NoDoz, Overtime, Stay Awake, Valentine, Vivarin

caffeine citrate
CAFCIT

PREGNANCY CATEGORY C

Drug classes
Analeptic
CNS stimulant
Xanthine

Therapeutic actions
Increases calcium permeability in sarcoplasmic reticulum, promotes the accumulation of cAMP, and blocks adenosine receptors; stimulates the CNS, cardiac activity, gastric acid secretion, and diuresis.

Indications
- An aid in staying awake and restoring mental awareness
- Adjunct to analgesic formulations
- IM: Possibly an analeptic in conjunction with supportive measures to treat respiratory depression associated with overdose with CNS depressants
- Caffeine citrate: Short-term treatment of apnea of prematurity in infants between 28 and 33 wk gestation
- Unlabeled uses: Headache, obesity, alcohol intoxication, postprandial hypotension

Contraindications and cautions
- Contraindicated with duodenal ulcers, diabetes mellitus, lactation.
- Use cautiously with pregnancy, renal or hepatic impairment, depression, CV disease.

Available forms
Tablets—200 mg; capsules—200 mg; lozenges—75 mg; injection—250 mg/mL; caffeine citrate injection and oral solution—20 mg/mL

Dosages
20 mg caffeine citrate = 10 mg caffeine base; use caution.

Adults
100–200 mg PO every 3–4 hr as needed.
- *Respiratory depression:* 500 mg–1 g caffeine and sodium benzoate (250–500 mg caffeine) IM; do not exceed 2.5 g/day; may be given IV in severe emergency situation.

Pediatric patients
- *Neonatal apnea:* 20 mg/kg IV over 30 min followed 24 hours later by 5 mg/kg/day IV over 10 min or PO as maintenance *(CAFCIT)*.

Pharmacokinetics

Route	Onset	Peak
Oral	15 min	15–45 min
IV	Immediate	End of infusion

Metabolism: Hepatic; $T_{1/2}$: 3–7.5 hr, 100 hr (neonates)
Distribution: Crosses placenta; enters breast milk
Excretion: Urine

IV FACTS

Preparation: Dissolve 10 g caffeine citrate powder in 250 mL sterile water for injection USP to 500 mL; filter and autoclave. Final concentration is 10 mg/mL caffeine base (20 mg/mL caffeine citrate). Stable for 3 mo. Or dissolve 10 mg caffeine powder and 10.9 g citric acid powder in bacteriostatic water for injection, USP to 1 L. Sterilize by filtration. *CAFCIT:* 60 mg/3 mL vial may be diluted to achieve desired dose.

Infusion: IV single dose of 500 mg caffeine may be given slowly over 2 min in emergency situations; not recommended. *CAFCIT:* Give 20 mg/kg as a single dose over 30 min; maintain with infusion of 5 mg/kg/day.

Adverse effects

- **CNS:** *Insomnia, restlessness, excitement,* nervousness, tinnitus, muscular tremor, headaches, light-headedness
- **CV:** *Tachycardia,* hypertension, extrasystoles, palpitations
- **GI:** Nausea, vomiting, diarrhea, stomach pain
- **GU:** *Diuresis*
- **Other:** Withdrawal syndrome: Headache, anxiety, muscle tension

Interactions

✱ **Drug-drug** • Increased CNS effects of caffeine with cimetidine, hormonal contraceptives, disulfiram, ciprofloxacin, mexiletine • Decreased effects of caffeine while smoking • Increased serum levels of theophylline, clozapine with caffeine

✱ **Drug-food** • Decreased absorption of iron if taken with or 1 hr after coffee or tea

✱ **Drug-alternative therapy** • Avoid concomitant administration with guarana, ma huang, or ephedra; may cause additive effects

✱ **Drug-lab test** • Possible false elevations of serum urate, urine VMA, resulting in false-positive diagnosis of pheochromocytoma or neuroblastoma

■ Nursing considerations

Assessment

- **History:** Depression, duodenal ulcer, diabetes mellitus, lactation, pregnancy
- **Physical:** Neurologic status, P, BP, ECG, normal urinary output, abdominal examination, blood glucose

Interventions

⊗ ***Warning*** Do not stop the drug abruptly after long-term use to avoid withdrawal reactions.

- Monitor diet for caffeine-containing foods that may contribute to overdose.
- Parents of infants being treated with caffeine citrate for apnea should have drug information incorporated into the overall teaching plan.

Teaching points

- Do not stop taking this drug abruptly; withdrawal symptoms may occur.
- Avoid foods high in caffeine (coffee, tea, cola, chocolate), which may cause symptoms of overdose.
- Avoid driving or dangerous activities if dizziness, tremors, or restlessness occur.
- Consult your health care provider if fatigue continues.
- You may experience these side effects: Diuresis, restlessness, insomnia, muscular tremors, light-headedness; nausea, abdominal pain.
- Report abnormal heart rate, dizziness, palpitations.

▽ calcitonin

(kal si toe' nin)

calcitonin, salmon

Apo-Calcitonin (CAN), Calcimar, Caltine (CAN), Fortical, Miacalcin, Miacalcin Nasal Spray, Osteocalcin, Salmonine

PREGNANCY CATEGORY C (SALMON)

Drug classes

Hormone
Calcium regulator

Therapeutic actions

The calcitonins are polypeptide hormones secreted by the thyroid; salmon calcitonin appears to be a chemically identical polypeptide to human calcitonin but with greater potency per milligram and longer duration; inhibits bone resorption; lowers elevated serum calcium in children and patients with Paget's disease; increases the excretion of filtered phosphate, calcium, and sodium by the kidney.

Indications

- Treatment of Paget's disease
- Treatment of postmenopausal osteoporosis in conjunction with adequate calcium and vitamin D intake to prevent loss of bone mass
- Treatment of hypercalcemia, emergency treatment (injection only)

Contraindications and cautions

- Contraindicated with allergy to salmon calcitonin or fish products, lactation.
- Use cautiously with renal insufficiency, osteoporosis, pernicious anemia.

Available forms

Injection—200 units/mL; nasal spray—200 units/actuation

Dosages

Adults

Calcitonin, salmon

- *Skin testing:* 0.1 mL of a 10 units/mL solution injected subcutaneously.
- *Paget's disease:* Initial dose, 100 units/day IM or subcutaneously. For maintenance, 50 units/day or every other day. Actual dose should be determined by patient response.
- *Postmenopausal osteoporosis:* 100 units every other day IM or subcutaneously, with supplemental calcium (calcium carbonate, 1.5 g/day) and vitamin D (400 units/day) or 200 units intranasally daily, alternating nostrils daily.
- *Hypercalcemia:* Initial dose, 4 units/kg every 12 hr IM or subcutaneously. If response is not satisfactory after 1–2 days, increase to 8 units/kg every 12 hr; if response remains unsatisfactory after 2 more days, increase to 8 units/kg every 6 hr.

Pediatric patients

Safety and efficacy not established.

Pharmacokinetics

Route	*Onset*	*Peak*	*Duration*
IM, Subcut.	15 min	16–25 min	8–24 hr
Nasal	Rapid	31–39 min	8–24 hr

Metabolism: Renal; $T_{1/2}$: 43 min (salmon), 1 hr (human)
Distribution: May enter breast milk
Excretion: Urine

Adverse effects

- **Dermatologic:** *Flushing of face or hands, rash*
- **GI:** *Nausea, vomiting*
- **GU:** *Urinary frequency*
- **Local:** *Local inflammatory reactions at injection site*, nasal irritation (nasal spray)

■ Nursing considerations

Assessment

- **History:** Allergy to salmon calcitonin or fish products, lactation, osteoporosis, pernicious anemia, renal disease
- **Physical:** Skin lesions, color, T; muscle tone; urinalysis, serum calcium, serum alkaline phosphatase and urinary hydroxyproline excretion

Interventions

⊗ ***Warning*** Give skin test to patients with any history of allergies; salmon calcitonin is a protein, and risk of allergy is significant. Prepare solution for skin test as follows: Withdraw 0.05 mL of the 200 units/mL solution into a tuberculin syringe. Fill to 1 mL with sodium chloride injection. Mix well. Discard 0.9 mL, and inject 0.1 mL (about 1 unit) subcutaneously into the inner aspect of the forearm. Observe after 15 min; the presence of a wheal or more than mild erythema indicates a positive response.

- Ensure that parenteral calcium is readily available in case hypocalcemic tetany develops.
- Monitor serum alkaline phosphatase and urinary hydroxyproline excretion prior to therapy and during first 3 mo and every 3–6 mo during long-term therapy.
- Periodically examine urine sediment for casts in patients on chronic therapy.

⊗ ***Warning*** Inject doses of more than 2 mL IM, not subcutaneously; use multiple injection sites.

- Refrigerate nasal spray until activated, then store at room temperature.

Teaching points

- This drug is given IM or subcutaneously; you or a significant other must learn how to do this at home. Refrigerate the drug vials. Dispose of needles and syringes in an appropriate container.
- For intranasal use, alternate nostrils daily; notify health care provider if significant nasal irritation occurs.
- Before first use, activate spray by holding bottle upright and depressing the two white side arms toward bottle six times, until a faint spray appears.
- You may experience these side effects: Nausea, vomiting (this passes); irritation at injection site (rotate sites); flushing of the face or hands, rash.
- Report twitching, muscle spasms, dark urine, hives, rash, difficulty breathing.

▽ calcium salts

(kal si' uhm)

calcium carbonate

Apo-Cal (CAN), Calcite 500 (CAN), Caltrate, Chooz, Equilet, Os-Cal, Oyst-Cal
PMS-Calcium (CAN), Tums

calcium chloride

calcium glubionate

Calcionate, Calciquid

calcium gluconate

Cal-G

calcium lactate

Cal-Lac

PREGNANCY CATEGORY C

Drug classes

Antacid
Electrolyte

Therapeutic actions

Essential element of the body; helps maintain the functional integrity of the nervous and muscular systems; helps maintain cardiac function, blood coagulation; is an enzyme cofactor and affects the secretory activity of endocrine and exocrine glands; neutralizes or reduces gastric acidity (oral use).

Indications

- Dietary supplement when calcium intake is inadequate
- Treatment of calcium deficiency in tetany of the newborn, acute and chronic hypoparathyroidism, pseudohypoparathyroidism, postmenopausal and senile osteoporosis, rickets, osteomalacia
- Prevention of hypocalcemia during exchange transfusions
- Adjunctive therapy for insect bites or stings, such as black widow spider bites; sensitivity reactions, particularly when characterized by urticaria; depression due to overdose of magnesium sulfate; acute symptoms of lead colic
- Calcium chloride: Combats the effects of hyperkalemia as measured by ECG, pending correction of increased potassium in the extracellular fluid
- Improves weak or ineffective myocardial contractions when epinephrine fails in cardiac resuscitation, particularly after open heart surgery
- Calcium carbonate: Symptomatic relief of upset stomach associated with hyperacidity; hyperacidity associated with peptic ulcer, gastritis, peptic esophagitis, gastric hyperacidity, hiatal hernia
- Calcium carbonate: Prophylaxis of GI bleeding, stress ulcers, and aspiration pneumonia; possibly useful
- Unlabeled use: Treatment of hypertension in some patients with indices suggesting calcium "deficiency"; treatment of premenstrual syndrome (calcium glubionate)

Contraindications and cautions

- Contraindicated with allergy to calcium, renal calculi, hypercalcemia, ventricular fibrillation during cardiac resuscitation and patients with the risk of existing digitalis toxicity.
- Use cautiously with renal impairment, pregnancy, lactation.

Available forms

Tablets—250, 500, 650, 975 mg, 1 g, 1.25 g, 1.5 g; powder—2,400 mg; injection—10%, 1.1 g/5 mL; syrup—1.8 g/5 mL

Dosages

Adults

Calcium carbonate or lactate

- *RDA:*
  14–18 yr: 1,300 mg/day
  19–50 yr: 1,000 mg/day
  Older than 50 yr: 1,200 mg/day
  Pregnant or lactating
    14–18 yr: 1,300 mg/day
    19–50 yr: 1,000 mg/day
- *Dietary supplement:* 500 mg–2 g PO, bid–qid.
- *Antacid:* 0.5–2 g PO calcium carbonate as needed.

Calcium chloride

For IV use only. 1 g contains 272 mg (13.6 mEq) calcium.

- *Hypocalcemic disorders:* 500 mg–1 g at intervals of 1–3 days; response may dictate more frequent injections.
- *Magnesium intoxication:* 500 mg promptly. Observe patient for signs of recovery before giving another dose.
- *Hyperkalemic ECG disturbances of cardiac function:* Adjust dosage according to ECG response.
- *Cardiac resuscitation:* 500 mg–1 g IV or 200–800 mg into the ventricular cavity.

Calcium gluconate

IV infusion preferred. 1 g contains 90 mg (4.5 mEq) calcium. 0.5–2 g as required; daily dose 1–15 g.

Pediatric patients

Calcium carbonate or lactate

- *RDA:*
  0–6 mo: 210 mg/day
  7–12 mo: 270 mg/day
  1–3 yr: 500 mg/day
  4–8 yr: 800 mg/day
  9–13 yr: 1,300 mg/day

Calcium gluconate

500 mg/kg/day IV given in divided doses.

Pharmacokinetics

Route	*Onset*	*Peak*
Oral	3–5 min	N/A
IV	Immediate	3–5 min

Metabolism: Hepatic; $T_{1/2}$: 1–3 hr
Distribution: Crosses placenta; enters breast milk
Excretion: Feces, urine

IV FACTS

Preparation: Warm solutions to body temperature; use a small needle inserted into a large vein to decrease irritation.
Infusion: Infuse slowly, 0.5–2 mL/min. Stop infusion if patient complains of discomfort; resume when symptoms disappear. Repeated injections are often necessary.
Incompatibilities: Avoid mixing calcium salts with carbonates, phosphates, sulfates, tartrates, amphotericin, cefazolin, clindamycin, dobutamine, prednisolone.

Adverse effects

- **CV:** *Slowed heart rate, tingling, "heat waves"* (rapid IV administration); *peripheral vasodilation, local burning, drop in BP* (calcium chloride injection)
- **Local:** *Local irritation,* severe necrosis, sloughing and abscess formation (IM, subcutaneous use of calcium chloride)
- **Metabolic:** Hypercalcemia (*anorexia, nausea, vomiting, constipation,* abdominal pain, dry mouth, thirst, polyuria), *rebound hyperacidity* and milk-alkali syndrome (hypercalcemia, alkalosis, renal damage with calcium carbonate used as an antacid)

Interactions

✱ **Drug-drug** • Decreased serum levels of oral tetracyclines, oral fluoroquinolones, salicylates, iron salts with oral calcium salts; give these drugs at least 1 hr apart • Increased serum levels of quinidine and possible toxicity with calcium salts • Antagonism of effects of verapamil with calcium • Decreased effect of thyroid hormone replacement; space doses 2 hr apart if this combination is used

✱ **Drug-food** • Decreased absorption of oral calcium when taken concurrently with oxalic acid (found in rhubarb and spinach), phytic acid (bran and whole cereals), phosphorus (milk and dairy products)

✱ **Drug-lab test** • False-negative values for serum and urinary magnesium

■ Nursing considerations

Assessment

- **History:** Allergy to calcium; renal calculi; hypercalcemia; ventricular fibrillation during cardiac resuscitation; digitalis toxicity, renal impairment, pregnancy, lactation
- **Physical:** Injection site; P, auscultation, BP, peripheral perfusion, ECG; abdominal examination, bowel sounds, mucous membranes; serum electrolytes, urinalysis

Interventions

- Give drug hourly for first 2 wk when treating acute peptic ulcer. During healing stage, administer 1–3 hr after meals and at bedtime.
- Do not administer oral drugs within 1–2 hr of antacid administration.
- Have patient chew antacid tablets thoroughly before swallowing; follow with a glass of water or milk.
- Give calcium carbonate antacid 1 and 3 hr after meals and at bedtime.

⊗ ***Warning*** Avoid extravasation of IV injection; it irritates the tissues and can cause necrosis and sloughing. Use a small needle in a large vein.

- Have patient remain recumbent for a short time after IV injection.
- Administer into ventricular cavity during cardiac resuscitation, not into myocardium.
- Warm calcium gluconate if crystallization has occurred.
- Monitor serum phosphorus levels periodically during long-term oral therapy.
- Monitor cardiac response closely during parenteral treatment with calcium.

Teaching points

Parenteral

- Report any pain or discomfort at the injection site as soon as possible.

Oral

- Take drug between meals and at bedtime. Ulcer patients must take drug as prescribed. Chew tablets thoroughly before swallowing, and follow with a glass of water or milk.
- Do not take with other oral drugs. Absorption of those medications can be blocked; take other oral medications at least 1–2 hours after calcium carbonate.
- You may experience these side effects: Constipation (can be medicated), nausea, GI upset, loss of appetite (special dietary consultation may be necessary).
- Report loss of appetite, nausea, vomiting, abdominal pain, constipation, dry mouth, thirst, increased voiding.

▽ calfactant (DDPC, natural lung surfactant)

*(cal **fak'** tant)*

Infasurf

Drug class

Lung surfactant

Therapeutic actions

A natural bovine compound containing lipids and apoproteins that reduce surface tension, allowing expansion of the alveoli; replaces the surfactant missing in the lungs of neonates suffering from RDS.

Indications

- Prophylactic treatment of infants at risk of developing RDS; infants less than 29 wk gestation
- Rescue treatment of premature infants up to 72 hr of age who have developed RDS and require endotracheal intubation; best if started within 30 min after birth

Contraindications and cautions

- Because calfactant is used as an emergency drug in acute respiratory situations, the benefits usually outweigh any possible risks.

Available forms

Intratracheal suspension—35 mg/mL

Dosages

Infants

Accurate determination of birth weight is essential for determining appropriate dosage. Calfactant is instilled into the trachea using a catheter inserted into the endotracheal tube.

- *Prophylactic treatment:* Instill 3 mL/kg of birth weight as soon after birth as possible, administered as two doses of 1.5 mL/kg each.
- *Rescue treatment:* Instill 3 mL/kg of birth weight in two doses of 1.5 mL/kg each. Repeat doses of 3 mL/kg of birth weight up to a total of three doses 12 hr apart.

Pharmacokinetics

Route	*Onset*	*Peak*
Intratracheal	Immediate	Hours

Metabolism: Normal surfactant metabolic pathways; $T_{1/2}$: less than 24 hr
Distribution: Lung tissue
Excretion: Unknown

Adverse effects

- **CNS: Seizures, intracranial hemorrhage**
- **CV: Patent ductus arteriosus, intraventricular hemorrhage,** *hypotension, bradycardia*
- **Hematologic:** *Hyperbilirubinemia, thrombocytopenia*
- **Respiratory: Pneumothorax,** *pulmonary air leak,* **pulmonary hemorrhage** (more often seen with infants weighing less than 700 g), *apnea,* pneumomediastinum, emphysema
- **Other:** *Sepsis, nonpulmonary infections*

■ Nursing considerations

Assessment

- **History:** Time of birth, exact birth weight
- **Physical:** T, color; R, adventitious sounds, oximeter, endotracheal tube position and patency, chest movement; ECG, P, BP, peripheral perfusion, arterial pressure (desirable); oxygen saturation, blood gases, CBC; muscular activity, facial expression, reflexes

Interventions

- Arrange for appropriate assessment and monitoring of critically ill infant.
- Monitor ECG and transcutaneous oxygen saturation continually during administration.
- Ensure that endotracheal tube is in the correct position, with bilateral chest movement and lung sounds.
- Do not dilute or mix calfactant with any other drugs or solutions. Administer as provided. Warm unopened vials to room temperature. Gently swirl to mix contents.
- Suction the infant immediately before administration; but do not suction for 2 hr after administration unless clinically necessary.
- Store drug in refrigerator. Protect from light. Enter drug vial only once. Discard remaining drug after use. Avoid repeated warmings to room temperature.
- Administer through a side-port adapter into the endotracheal tube or insert 5 French feeding catheter into the endotracheal tube; do not instill into the mainstream bronchus.
- Two attendants, one to instill drug and one to monitor, are needed. Administer total dose in two aliquots of 1.5 mL/kg each. After each instillation, position infant on either right or left side dependent. Administer while continuing ventilation over 20–30 breaths for each aliquot, with small bursts timed during inspiration cycles. A pause followed by evaluation of respiratory status and repositioning should separate the two aliquots. May repeat doses of 3 mL/kg up to a total of three doses 12 hr apart.
- Endotracheal suctioning and/or reintubation is sometimes needed if signs of airway obstruction occur after surfactant.

⊗ ***Warning*** Continually monitor patient color, lung sounds, ECG, oximeter and blood gas readings during administration and for at least 30 min following administration.

- Maintain appropriate interventions for critically ill infant.
- Offer support and encouragement to parents.

Teaching points

- Parents of the critically ill infant will need a comprehensive teaching and support program. Details of drug effects and administration are best incorporated into the comprehensive program.

canakinumab

See Appendix W, *Less commonly used drugs*.

candesartan cilexetil

*(can dah **sar' tan**)*

Atacand

PREGNANCY CATEGORY C (FIRST TRIMESTER)

PREGNANCY CATEGORY D (SECOND AND THIRD TRIMESTERS)

Drug classes

Angiotensin II receptor antagonist
Antihypertensive

Therapeutic actions

Selectively blocks the binding of angiotensin II to specific tissue receptors found in vascular smooth muscle and adrenal gland; this action blocks the vasoconstriction effect of the renin–angiotensin system as well as the release of aldosterone leading to decreased BP.

Indications

- Treatment of hypertension, alone or in combination with other antihypertensives
- Treatment of heart failure (New York Heart Association class II–IV, ejection fraction 40% or less) to reduce risk of CV death and to reduce hospitalization for heart failure; may be combined with an ACE inhibitor

Contraindications and cautions

- Contraindicated with hypersensitivity to candesartan, pregnancy (use during the second or third trimester can cause injury or even death to the fetus), lactation.
- Use cautiously with renal impairment, hypovolemia.

Available forms

Tablets—4, 8, 16, 32 mg

Dosages

Adults

- *Hypertension:* Usual starting dose, 16 mg PO daily. Can be administered in divided doses bid with a total daily dose of 32 mg/day. Dose range: 8–32 mg a day.
- *Heart failure:* 4 mg/day PO; may be doubled at 2 wk intervals to achieve target dose of 32 mg/day PO as a single dose.

Pediatric patients

Safety and efficacy not established.

Pharmacokinetics

Route	*Onset*	*Peak*
Oral	Rapid	3–4 hr

Metabolism: Hepatic; $T_{1/2}$: 9 hr
Distribution; Crosses placenta; enters breast milk
Excretion: Feces, urine

Adverse effects

- **CNS:** *Headache, dizziness,* syncope, muscle weakness
- **CV:** Hypotension
- **Dermatologic:** Rash, inflammation, urticaria, pruritus, alopecia, dry skin
- **GI:** *Diarrhea, abdominal pain, nausea,* constipation, dry mouth, dental pain
- **Respiratory:** *URI symptoms,* cough, sinus disorders
- **Other:** Cancer in preclinical studies, back pain, fever, gout

■ Nursing considerations

Assessment

- **History:** Hypersensitivity to candesartan, pregnancy, lactation, renal impairment, hypovolemia
- **Physical:** Skin lesions, turgor; T; reflexes, affect; BP; R, respiratory auscultation; renal function tests

Interventions

- Administer without regard to meals.

⊗ ***Black box warning*** Ensure that patient is not pregnant before beginning therapy, suggest the use of barrier birth control while using candesartan; fetal injury and deaths have been reported. When pregnancy is detected, discontinue candesartan as soon as possible.

- Find an alternate method of feeding the baby for a nursing mother. Depression of the renin-angiotensin system in infants is potentially very dangerous.

⊗ ***Warning*** Alert surgeon and mark patient's chart with notice that candesartan is being taken. The blockage of the renin-angiotensin system following surgery can produce problems. Hypotension may be reversed with volume expansion.

- If BP control does not reach desired levels, diuretics or other antihypertensives may be added to candesartan. Monitor patient's BP carefully.
- Monitor patient closely in any situation that may lead to a decrease in BP secondary to reduction in fluid volume—excessive perspiration, dehydration, vomiting, diarrhea—excessive hypotension can occur.

Teaching points

- Take this drug without regard to meals. Do not stop taking this drug without consulting your health care provider.
- Use a barrier method of birth control while on this drug; if you become pregnant or desire to become pregnant, consult your health care provider.
- Maintain your fluid intake, especially in situations that could cause loss of fluids, such as diarrhea, vomiting, or excessive sweating.
- You may experience these side effects: Dizziness (avoid driving a car or performing hazardous tasks); headache (medications may be available to help); nausea, vomiting, diarrhea (proper nutrition is important, consult with your dietitian to maintain nutrition); symptoms of URI, cough (do not self-medicate, consult your health care provider if this becomes uncomfortable).
- Report fever, chills, dizziness, pregnancy.

DANGEROUS DRUG

▽capecitabine

*(kap ah **seat'** ah been)*

Xeloda

PREGNANCY CATEGORY D

Drug classes

Antimetabolite
Antineoplastic

Therapeutic actions

A prodrug of 5-fluorouridine that is readily converted to 5-FU; inhibits thymidylate synthetase, leading to inhibition of DNA and RNA synthesis and cell death.

Indications

- Treatment of breast cancer in patients with metastatic breast cancer resistant to both paclitaxel and doxorubicin or doxorubicin-equivalent chemotherapy
- Treatment of breast cancer in combination with docetaxel in patients with metastatic disease after failure with anthracycline chemotherapy
- Treatment of metastatic colorectal cancer as first-time treatment when treatment with fluoropyrimidine therapy is preferred
- Adjuvant post-surgery treatment of patients with Dukes C colon cancer who have undergone complete resection of the primary tumor who are candidates for single oral agent chemotherapy

Contraindications and cautions

- Contraindicated with allergy to 5-FU; pregnancy; lactation; severe renal impairment, concomitant warfarin therapy.
- Use cautiously with renal or hepatic impairment, severe diarrhea or intestinal disease, coronary artery disease, bleeding disorders (adverse cardiac effects are more common).

Available forms

Tablets—150, 500 mg

Dosages

Adults

- *Breast and colorectal cancer:* Starting dose, 2,500 mg/m^2/day PO in two divided doses 12 hr apart within 30 min after a meal for 2 wk followed by a 1-wk rest period; given in 3-wk cycles.
- *Adjuvant post-surgery Dukes C colon cancer:* 1,250 mg/m^2 PO twice daily, morning

and evening within 30 min after a meal, for 2 wk, followed by 1 wk rest, given as 3-wk cycles for a total of 8 cycles (24 wk).

Pediatric patients

Safety and efficacy not established.

Geriatric patients or patients with hepatic impairment

These patients may be more sensitive to the toxic effects of the drug. Monitor closely and decrease dosage as needed to avoid toxicity.

Patients with renal impairment

For creatinine clearance 51–80 mL/min, no adjustment recommended, but monitor carefully; for creatinine clearance 30–50 mL/min, reduce dosage by 75%; for creatinine clearance less than 30 mL/min, use is contraindicated.

- *Patients on concurrent therapy with docetaxel:* Severe toxicity may result, as manifested by NCIC grade 2–4 toxicity criteria; monitor/adjust doses of both drugs as needed.

Pharmacokinetics

Route	*Onset*	*Peak*
Oral	Rapid	1.5 hr

Metabolism: Hepatic and cellular; $T_{1/2}$: 45 min

Distribution: Crosses placenta; may enter breast milk

Excretion: Lungs, urine

Adverse effects

- **CNS:** Fatigue, paresthesias, headache, dizziness, insomnia
- **CV: MI,** angina, arrhythmias, ECG changes
- **Dermatologic:** *Hand-and-foot syndrome* (numbness, dysesthesias, tingling, pain, swelling, blisters, pain), *dermatitis,* nail disorders
- **GI: Diarrhea,** *anorexia, nausea, vomiting, cramps, constipation, stomatitis*
- **Hematologic:** *Leukopenia, thrombocytopenia,* anemia
- **Other:** Fever, edema, myalgia

Interactions

✱ **Drug-drug** ⊗ ***Warning*** Increased capecitabine levels and toxicity, with possibility of death, when combined with leucovorin; avoid this combination.

⊠ ***Black box warning*** Increased risk of excessive bleeding and even death if combined with warfarin anticoagulants; avoid this combination. If the combination must be used, INR and prothrombin levels should be monitored very closely and anticoagulant dose adjusted as needed.

- Increased capecitabine levels when taken with antacids • Increased phenytoin levels if taken together; consider reduction of phenytoin dose

■ Nursing considerations

Assessment

- **History:** Allergy to 5-FU; impaired hepatic or renal function; pregnancy; lactation; diarrhea, intestinal disease, coronary disease, warfarin therapy
- **Physical:** Weight; T; skin lesions, color; orientation, reflexes, affect, sensation; P, BP, cardiac rhythm, peripheral perfusion; mucous membranes, liver evaluation, abdominal examination; CBC, differential; LFTs, renal function tests

Interventions

- Evaluate renal function before starting therapy to ensure accurate dosage.
- Always administer drug with food, within 30 min of a meal. Have patient swallow drug with water.
- Monitor for toxicities, especially if used with docetaxel; dosage may need to be adjusted based on toxicity.

⊗ ***Warning*** Arrange for discontinuation of drug therapy if any sign of toxicity occurs—severe nausea, vomiting, diarrhea, hand-and-foot syndrome, stomatitis.

- Monitor nutritional status and fluid and electrolyte balance when GI effects occur; provide supportive care and fluids as needed; loperamide may be helpful for severe diarrhea.
- Provide frequent mouth care for stomatitis or mouth sores.

⊗ ***Warning*** Arrange for frequent small meals and dietary consultation to maintain nutrition when GI effects are severe.

- Protect patient from exposure to infection; monitor temperature and CBC regularly.
- Suggest use of barrier contraceptives while patient is using this drug; serious birth defects can occur.
- Monitor for toxicities, especially if used with docetaxel; dosage may need to be adjusted, based on toxicity.

Teaching points

- Take this drug every 12 hours, within 30 minutes of a meal; always take the drug after you have eaten and have food in your stomach. Swallow the tablets with water.
- Prepare a calendar of treatment days to follow. The drug is given in 3-week cycles.
- Arrange to have frequent, regular medical follow-up, including frequent blood tests to follow the effects of the drug on your body.
- Avoid pregnancy while taking this drug; using barrier contraceptives is advised. This drug can cause serious birth defects if taken during pregnancy.
- You may experience these side effects: Nausea, vomiting, loss of appetite (medication may be ordered to help; eat frequent small meals; it is very important to maintain your nutrition while you are taking this drug); mouth sores (frequent mouth care will be needed); diarrhea (have ready access to bathroom facilities if this occurs).
- Report fever, chills, sore throat; chest pain; mouth sores; pain or tingling in hands or feet; severe nausea, vomiting or diarrhea (more than five episodes of any of these per day); dizziness.

capreomycin

*(kap ree oh **mye'** sin)*

Capastat Sulfate

PREGNANCY CATEGORY C

Drug classes

Antibiotic
Antituberculotic ("third line")

Therapeutic actions

Polypeptide antibiotic; mechanism of action against *Mycobacterium tuberculosis* unknown.

Indications

- Treatment of pulmonary tuberculosis that is not responsive to first-line antituberculosis agents but is sensitive to capreomycin in conjunction with other antituberculosis agents

Contraindications and cautions

- Contraindicated with allergy to capreomycin; preexisting auditory impairment.
- Use cautiously with lactation, renal impairment, pregnancy.

Available forms

Powder for injection—1 g/10 mL

Dosages

Always give in combination with other antituberculotics.

Adults

1 g daily (not to exceed 20 mg/kg/day) IM or IV for 60–120 days, followed by 1 g IM two to three times weekly for 12–24 mo. Can also give IV infusion after further dilution in 100 mL 0.9% sodium chloride and infuse over 60 min.

Pediatric patients

15 mg/kg/day IM or IV (maximum 1 g) has been recommended.

Geriatric patients or patients with renal impairment

CrCl (mL/min)	*Dose (mg/kg) at These Intervals* 24 hr	48 hr	72 hr
0–9	1.29	2.58	3.87
10	2.43	4.87	7.3
20	3.58	7.16	10.7
30	4.72	9.45	14.2
40	5.87	11.7	–
50	7.01	14	–
60	8.16	–	–
80	10.4	–	–
100	12.7	–	–
110	13.9	–	–

Pharmacokinetics

Route	*Onset*	*Peak*	*Duration*
IM	20–30 min	1–2 hr	8–12 hr

Metabolism: $T_{1/2}$: 4–6 hr
Distribution: Crosses placenta; may enter breast milk
Excretion: Urine

IV FACTS

Preparation: Dissolve vial contents in 2 mL 0.9% sodium chloride and allow 3 min for full dissolution. Further dilute in 100 mL 0.9% sodium chloride.

Infusion: Infuse over 60 min.

Adverse effects

- **CNS:** *Ototoxicity*
- **GI:** Hepatic impairment
- **GU:** *Nephrotoxicity*
- **Hematologic:** Leukocytosis, leukopenia, eosinophilia, hypokalemia
- **Hypersensitivity:** Urticaria, rashes, fever
- **Local:** Pain, induration at injection sites, sterile abscesses

Interactions

✱ **Drug-drug** • Increased nephrotoxicity and ototoxicity if used with similarly toxic drugs • Increased risk of peripheral neuromuscular blocking action with nondepolarizing muscle relaxants (atracurium, pancuronium, tubocurarine, vecuronium)

■ Nursing considerations

Assessment

- **History:** Allergy to capreomycin; renal insufficiency; auditory impairment; lactation, pregnancy
- **Physical:** Skin color, lesions; T; orientation, reflexes, affect, audiometric measurement, vestibular function tests; liver evaluation; LFTs, renal function tests, CBC, serum K^+

Interventions

- Arrange for culture and sensitivity studies before use.
- Administer this drug only when other forms of therapy have failed.
- Administer only in conjunction with other antituberculotics to which the mycobacteria are susceptible.
- Prepare solution by dissolving in 2 mL of 0.9% sodium chloride injection or sterile water for injection; allow 2–3 min for dissolution. To administer 1 g, use entire vial—if less than 1 g is needed, see the manufacturer's instructions for dilution. Reconstituted solution may be stored for 24 hr refrigerated. Solution may acquire a straw color and darken with time; this is not associated with loss of potency. Can also give IV infusion after further dilution in 100 mL 0.9% sodium chloride and infuse over 60 min.
- Administer by deep IM injection into a large muscle mass.

⊗ ***Black box warning*** Arrange for audiometric testing and assessment of vestibular function, renal function tests, and serum potassium before and at regular intervals during therapy; risk of renal failure, auditory damage is severe.

⊗ ***Black box warning*** Be aware that safety of drug has not been established in children or pregnant women.

Teaching points

- This drug can be given by IM injection or IV infusion.
- Take this drug regularly; avoid missing doses. You must not discontinue this drug without first consulting your health care provider.
- Arrange to have regular, periodic medical checkups, including blood tests.
- You may experience these side effects: Loss of hearing, dizziness, vertigo (avoid injury).
- Report rash, loss of hearing, decreased urine output, palpitations.

captopril

(kap' toe pril)

Apo-Capto (CAN), Capoten, Gen-Captopril (CAN), PMS-Captopril (CAN)

PREGNANCY CATEGORY C (FIRST TRIMESTER)

PREGNANCY CATEGORY D (SECOND AND THIRD TRIMESTERS)

Drug classes

ACE inhibitor
Antihypertensive

Therapeutic actions

Blocks ACE from converting angiotensin I to angiotensin II, a powerful vasoconstrictor, leading to decreased BP, decreased aldosterone secretion, a small increase in serum potassium levels, and sodium and fluid loss; increased prostaglandin synthesis also may be involved in the antihypertensive action.

Indications

- Treatment of hypertension alone or in combination with thiazide-type diuretics
- Treatment of heart failure in patients unresponsive to conventional therapy; used with diuretics and cardiac glycosides
- Treatment of diabetic nephropathy
- Treatment of left ventricular dysfunction after MI
- Unlabeled uses: Management of hypertensive crises; treatment of rheumatoid arthritis; diagnosis of anatomic renal artery stenosis, hypertension related to scleroderma renal crisis; diagnosis of primary aldosteronism, idiopathic edema; Bartter's syndrome; Raynaud's syndrome

Contraindications and cautions

- Contraindicated with allergy to captopril, history of angioedema, second or third trimester of pregnancy.
- Use cautiously with renal impairment, heart failure, salt or volume depletion, history of renal artery stenosis, lactation.

Available forms

Tablets—12.5, 25, 50, 100 mg

Dosages

Adults

- *Hypertension:* 25 mg PO bid or tid; if satisfactory response is not noted within 1–2 wk, increase dosage to 50 mg bid–tid; usual range is 25–150 mg bid–tid PO with a mild thiazide diuretic. Do not exceed 450 mg/day.
- *Heart failure:* Initially, 6.25–12.5 mg PO tid in patients who may be salt or volume depleted. Usual initial dose, 25 mg PO tid; maintenance dose, 50–100 mg PO tid. Do not exceed 450 mg/day. Use in conjunction with diuretic and cardiac glycoside therapy.
- *Left ventricular dysfunction after MI:* 50 mg PO tid, starting as early as 3 days post-MI. (Initial dose of 6.25 mg, then 12.5 mg tid, increasing slowly to 50 mg tid.)
- *Diabetic nephropathy:* Reduce dosage; suggested dose is 25 mg PO tid.

Pediatric patients

Safety and efficacy not established.

Geriatric patients and patients with renal impairment

Excretion is reduced in renal failure; use smaller initial dose; adjust at smaller doses with 1- to 2-wk intervals between increases; slowly adjust to smallest effective dose. Use a loop diuretic with renal impairment.

Pharmacokinetics

Route	*Onset*	*Peak*
Oral	15 min	30–90 min

Metabolism: $T_{1/2}$: 2 hr
Distribution: Crosses placenta; enters breast milk
Excretion: Urine

Adverse effects

- **CV:** *Tachycardia,* angina pectoris, heart failure, **MI,** Raynaud's syndrome, hypotension in salt- or volume-depleted patients
- **Dermatologic:** Alopecia, *rash, pruritus,* scalded mouth sensation, pemphigoidlike reaction, exfoliative dermatitis, photosensitivity
- **GI:** *Gastric irritation, aphthous ulcers, peptic ulcers, dysgeusia,* cholestatic jaundice, hepatocellular injury, anorexia, constipation
- **GU:** *Proteinuria,* renal insufficiency, renal failure, polyuria, oliguria, urinary frequency
- **Hematologic:** Neutropenia, agranulocytosis, thrombocytopenia, hemolytic anemia, **pancytopenia**
- **Other:** *Cough,* malaise, dry mouth, lymphadenopathy

Interactions

✱ **Drug-drug** • Increased risk of hypersensitivity reactions with allopurinol • Decreased antihypertensive effects with indomethacin • Increased captopril effects with probenecid
✱ **Drug-food** • Decreased absorption of captopril with food
✱ **Drug-lab test** • False-positive test for urine acetone

■ Nursing considerations

Assessment

- **History:** Allergy to captopril, history of angioedema, impaired renal function, heart failure, salt or volume depletion, pregnancy, lactation
- **Physical:** Skin color, lesions, turgor; T; P, BP, peripheral perfusion; mucous membranes, bowel sounds, liver evaluation; urinalysis, LFTs, renal function tests, CBC and differential

Interventions

- Administer 1 hr before meals.

⊠ ***Black box warning*** Ensure that patient is not pregnant before beginning treatment. Encourage use of contraceptives; if pregnancy is detected, stop drug.

⊗ ***Warning*** Alert surgeon and mark patient's chart with notice that captopril is being taken; the angiotensin II formation subsequent to compensatory renin release during surgery will be blocked; hypotension may be reversed with volume expansion.

- Monitor patient for drop in BP secondary to reduction in fluid volume (due to excessive perspiration, dehydration, vomiting, or diarrhea); excessive hypotension may occur.
- Reduce dosage in patients with impaired renal function.

Teaching points

- Take drug 1 hour before meals; do not take with food. Do not stop taking drug without consulting your health care provider.
- Watch for drop in blood pressure (occurs most often with diarrhea, sweating, vomiting, or dehydration); if light-headedness or dizziness occurs, consult your health care provider.
- Severe fetal damage can occur if captopril is taken during pregnancy. Use of contraceptives is advised; if pregnancy should occur, stop drug and notify health care provider.
- Avoid over-the-counter medications, especially cough, cold, or allergy medications that may contain ingredients that will interact with ACE inhibitors. Consult your health care provider.
- You may experience these side effects: cough, GI upset, loss of appetite, change in taste perception (limited effects, will pass); mouth sores (frequent mouth care may help); rash; fast heart rate; dizziness, light-headedness (usually passes after the first few days; change position slowly, and limit activities to those that do not require alertness and precision).
- Report mouth sores; sore throat; fever; chills; swelling of the hands or feet; irregular heartbeat; chest pains; swelling of the face, eyes, lips, or tongue; difficulty breathing.

▽ carbamazepine

(kar ba ***maz'*** *e peen)*

Apo-Carbamazepine (CAN), Carbatrol DNC, Epitol, Equetro DNC, Gen-Carbamazepine CR (CAN) DNC, PMS-Carbamazepine (CAN), Tegretol, Tegretol-XR DNC

PREGNANCY CATEGORY D

Drug class

Antiepileptic

Therapeutic actions

Mechanism of action not understood; antiepileptic activity may be related to its ability to inhibit polysynaptic responses and block post-tetanic potentiation. Drug is chemically related to the TCAs.

Indications

- Refractory seizure disorders: Partial seizures with complex symptoms (psychomotor, temporal lobe epilepsy), generalized tonic-clonic (grand mal) seizures, mixed seizure patterns or other partial or generalized seizures. Reserve for patients unresponsive to other agents with seizures difficult to control or who are experiencing marked side effects, such as excessive sedation
- Trigeminal neuralgia (tic douloureux): Treatment of pain associated with true trigeminal neuralgia; also beneficial in glossopharyngeal neuralgia
- Treatment of acute manic and mixed episodes associated with bipolar 1 disorder (*Equetro*)
- Unlabeled uses: Certain psychiatric disorders, including schizoaffective illness, resistant schizophrenia, and dyscontrol

syndrome associated with limbic system dysfunction; alcohol withdrawal (800–1,000 mg/day); restless leg syndrome (100–300 mg/day at bedtime); non-neuritic pain syndrome (600–1,400 mg/day)

Contraindications and cautions

- Contraindicated with hypersensitivity to carbamazepine or TCAs, history of bone marrow depression, concomitant use of MAOIs, lactation, pregnancy.
- Use cautiously with history of adverse hematologic reaction to any drug (increased risk of severe hematologic toxicity), glaucoma or increased IOP; history of cardiac, hepatic, or renal damage; psychiatric patients (may activate latent psychosis).

Available forms

Tablets—200 mg; chewable tablets—100 mg; ER tablets (DNC)—100, 200, 400 mg; ER capsules (DNC)—100, 200, 300 mg; suspension—100 mg/5 mL

Dosages

Individualize dosage; a low initial dosage with gradual increase is advised.

Adults

- *Epilepsy:* Initial dose, 200 mg PO bid on the first day; increase gradually by up to 200 mg/day in divided doses every 6–8 hr, until best response is achieved. *Suspension:* 100 mg PO qid. Do not exceed 1,200 mg/day in patients older than age 15; doses up to 1,600 mg/day have been used in adults (rare). For maintenance, adjust to minimum effective level, usually 800–1,200 mg/day.
- *Trigeminal neuralgia:* Initial dose, 100 mg PO bid on the first day; may increase by up to 200 mg/day, using 100-mg increments every 12 hr as needed. Do not exceed 1,200 mg/day. For maintenance, control of pain can usually be maintained with 400–800 mg/day (range 200–1,200 mg/day). Attempt to reduce the dose to the minimum effective level or to discontinue the drug at least once every 3 mo. *Suspension:* Start at 50 mg PO qid; increase by 50 mg PO qid as needed to maximum dose.
- *Combination therapy:* When added to existing antiepileptic therapy, do so gradually while other antiepileptics are maintained or discontinued.
- *Bipolar 1 disorder:* 200–600 mg/day PO in divided doses; may be increased in 200 mg/day increments. Do not exceed 1,600 mg/day (*Equetro*).

Pediatric patients older than 12 yr

Use adult dosage. Do not exceed 1,000 mg/day in patients 12–15 yr; 1,200 mg/day in patients older than 15 yr.

Pediatric patients 6–12 yr

Initial dose, 100 mg PO bid on the first day. Increase gradually by adding 100 mg/day at 6- to 8-hr intervals until best response is achieved. Do not exceed 1,000 mg/day. Dosage also may be calculated on the basis of 20–30 mg/kg/day in divided doses tid–qid.

Pediatric patients younger than 6 yr

Optimal daily dose, less than 35 mg/kg/day.

Geriatric patients

Use caution; may cause confusion, agitation.

Pharmacokinetics

Route	Onset	Peak
Oral	Slow	4–5 hr
ER oral	Slow	3–12 hr

Metabolism: Hepatic; $T_{1/2}$: 25–65 hr, then 12–17 hr

Distribution: Crosses placenta; enters breast milk

Excretion: Feces, urine

Adverse effects

- **CNS:** *Dizziness, drowsiness, unsteadiness,* disturbance of coordination, confusion, headache, fatigue, visual hallucinations, depression with agitation, behavioral changes in children, talkativeness, speech disturbances, abnormal involuntary movements, paralysis and other symptoms of cerebral arterial insufficiency, peripheral neuritis and paresthesias, tinnitus, hyperacusis, blurred vision, transient diplopia and oculomotor disturbances, nystagmus, scattered punctate cortical lens opacities, conjunctivitis, ophthalmoplegia, fever, chills; SIADH, suicidal ideation

- **CV:** Heart failure, increased hypertension, hypotension, syncope and collapse, edema, primary thrombophlebitis, thrombophlebitis reccurence, aggravation of CAD, arrhythmias and AV block; **CV complications**
- **Dermatologic:** Pruritic and erythematous rashes, urticaria, **Stevens-Johnson syndrome,** photosensitivity reactions, alterations in pigmentation, exfoliative dermatitis, alopecia, diaphoresis, erythema multiforme and nodosum, purpura, aggravation of lupus erythematosus
- **GI:** *Nausea, vomiting,* gastric distress, abdominal pain, diarrhea, constipation, anorexia, dryness of mouth or pharynx, glossitis, stomatitis; abnormal LFT, cholestatic and hepatocellular jaundice, **hepatitis, massive hepatic cellular necrosis with total loss of intact liver tissue**
- **GU:** Urinary frequency, acute urinary retention, oliguria with hypertension, renal failure, azotemia, impotence, proteinuria, glycosuria, elevated BUN, microscopic deposits in urine
- **Hematologic: Hematologic disorders** (severe bone marrow suppression)
- **Respiratory:** Pulmonary hypersensitivity characterized by fever, dyspnea, pneumonitis or pneumonia

Interactions

✱ **Drug-drug** • Increased serum levels and manifestations of toxicity with erythromycin, troleandomycin, cimetidine, danazol, isoniazid, propoxyphene, verapamil; dosage of carbamazepine may need to be reduced (reductions of about 50% recommended with erythromycin) • Increased CNS toxicity with lithium • Increased risk of hepatotoxicity with isoniazid (MAOI qualities); because of the chemical similarity of carbamazepine to the TCAs and because of the serious adverse interaction of TCAs and MAOIs, discontinue MAOIs for minimum of 14 days before carbamazepine administration • Decreased absorption with charcoal • Decreased serum levels and decreased effects of carbamazepine with barbiturates • Increased metabolism but no loss of seizure control with phenytoin, primidone • Increased metabolism of phenytoin, valproic acid • Decreased anticoagulant effect of warfarin, oral anticoagulants; dosage of warfarin may need to be increased during concomitant therapy but decreased if carbamazepine is withdrawn • Decreased effects of nondepolarizing muscle relaxants, haloperidol • Decreased antimicrobial effects of doxycycline

C

■ Nursing considerations

Assessment

- **History:** Hypersensitivity to carbamazepine or TCAs; history of bone marrow depression; concomitant use of MAOIs; history of adverse hematologic reaction to any drug; glaucoma or increased IOP; history of cardiac, hepatic, or renal damage; psychiatric history; lactation; pregnancy
- **Physical:** Weight; T; skin color, lesions; palpation of lymph glands; orientation, affect, reflexes; ophthalmologic examination (including tonometry, funduscopy, slit lamp examination); P, BP, perfusion; auscultation; peripheral vascular examination; R, adventitious sounds; bowel sounds, normal output; oral mucous membranes; normal urinary output, voiding pattern; CBC including platelet, reticulocyte counts and serum iron; LFTs, urinalysis, BUN, thyroid function tests, EEG

Interventions

- Use only for classifications listed. Do not use as a general analgesic. Use only for epileptic seizures that are refractory to other safer agents.
- Give drug with food to prevent GI upset.
- Do not mix suspension with other medications or elements—precipitation may occur.

⊗ ***Warning*** Reduce dosage, discontinue, or substitute other antiepileptic medication gradually. Abrupt discontinuation of all antiepileptic medication may precipitate status epilepticus.

⊗ ***Warning*** There is an increased risk of suicidal ideation with antiepileptic administration. Caution patient and monitor accordingly.

- Suspension will produce higher peak levels than tablets—start with a lower dose given more frequently.
- Ensure that patient swallows ER tablets whole—do not cut, crush, or chew. *Equetro* capsules may be opened and contents sprinkled over soft food, such as 1 tsp applesauce.
- Arrange for frequent LFTs; discontinue drug immediately if hepatic impairment occurs.

Black box warning Arrange for patient to have CBC, including platelet, reticulocyte counts, and serum iron determination, before initiating therapy; repeat weekly for the first 3 mo of therapy and monthly thereafter for at least 2–3 yr. Discontinue drug if there is evidence of marrow suppression, as follows:

Erythrocytes	Less than 4 million/mm^3
Hct	Less than 32%
Hgb	Less than 11 gm/dL
Leukocytes	Less than 4,000/mm^3
Platelets	Less than 100,000/mm^3
Reticulocytes	Less than 0.3% (20,000/mm^2)
Serum iron	Less than 150 g/100 mL

- Arrange for frequent eye examinations, urinalysis, and BUN determinations.
- Arrange for frequent monitoring of serum levels of carbamazepine and other antiepileptics given concomitantly, especially during the first few weeks of therapy. Adjust dosage on basis of data and clinical response.
- Counsel women who wish to become pregnant; advise the use of barrier contraceptives.
- Evaluate for therapeutic serum levels (usually 4–12 mcg/mL).

Teaching points

- Take drug with food as prescribed. Swallow extended-release tablets whole; do not cut, crush, or chew them. If using *Equetro* capsules, they may be opened and contents sprinkled over soft food, such as 1 teaspoon of applesauce.
- Do not discontinue this drug abruptly or change dosage, except on the advice of your physician.
- Avoid alcohol, sleep-inducing, or over-the-counter drugs; these could cause dangerous effects.
- Arrange for frequent checkups, including blood tests, to monitor your response to this drug. Keep all appointments for checkups.
- Use contraceptives at all times; if you wish to become pregnant, you should consult your physician.
- Wear a medical alert tag at all times so that any emergency medical personnel will know that you have epilepsy and are taking antiepileptic medication.
- You may experience these side effects: Drowsiness, dizziness, blurred vision (avoid driving or performing other tasks requiring alertness or visual acuity); GI upset (take the drug with food or milk, eat frequent small meals).
- Report bruising, unusual bleeding, abdominal pain, yellowing of the skin or eyes, pale feces, darkened urine, impotence, central nervous system disturbances, edema, fever, chills, sore throat, mouth ulcers, rash, pregnancy, thoughts of suicide.

DANGEROUS DRUG

carboplatin

(kar' boe pla tin)

Paraplatin

PREGNANCY CATEGORY D

Drug classes

Alkylating drug
Antineoplastic

Therapeutic actions

Cytotoxic: Heavy metal that produces cross-links within and between strands of DNA, thus preventing cell replication; cell cycle nonspecific.

Indications

- Initial treatment of advanced ovarian carcinoma in combination with other antineoplastics
- Palliative treatment of patients with ovarian carcinoma recurrent after prior chemotherapy, including patients who have been treated with cisplatin
- Unlabeled uses: Alone or with other agents to treat small-cell lung cancer, squamous cell cancer of the head and neck, endometrial cancer, relapsed or refractory acute leukemia, seminoma of testicular cancer

Contraindications and cautions

- Contraindicated with history of severe allergic reactions to carboplatin, cisplatin, platinum compounds, mannitol; severe bone marrow depression; lactation.

- Use cautiously in renal impairment, pregnancy, history of neuropathic disorders.

Available forms

Powder for injection—50, 150, 450 mg; injection—10 mg/mL

Dosages

Adults

- *As a single agent:* 360 mg/m^2 IV on day 1 every 4 wk. Do not repeat single doses of carboplatin until the neutrophil count is at least 2,000/mm^3 and the platelet count is at least 100,000/mm^3. These adjustments of dosage can be used: For platelets more than 100,000 and neutrophils more than 2,000, use dosage 125% of prior course; for platelets 50,000–100,000 and neutrophils 500–2,000, no adjustment in dosage; for platelets less than 50,000 and neutrophils less than 500—dosage 75% of previous course. Doses of more than 125% are not recommended. May also be given at 300 mg/m^2 in combination with cyclophosphamide.

Pediatric patients

Safety and efficacy not established.

Geriatric patients and patients with renal impairment

Increased risk of bone marrow depression with renal impairment. Use caution.

CrCl (mL/min)	*Dose (mg/m^2 on Day 1)*
41–59	250
16–40	200
15 or less	No data available

Pharmacokinetics

Route	*Onset*	*Duration*
IV	Rapid	48–96 hr

Metabolism: $T_{1/2}$: 1.2–2 hr, then 2.6–5.9 hr
Distribution: Crosses placenta; may enter breast milk
Excretion: Urine

IV FACTS

Preparation: Immediately before use, reconstitute the contents of each vial with sterile water for injection, D_5W, or sodium chloride injection. For a concentration of 10 mg/mL, combine 50-mg vial with 5 mL of diluent, 150-mg vial with 15 mL of diluent, or 450-mg vial with 45 mL of diluent. Carboplatin can be further diluted using D_5W or sodium chloride injection. Store unopened vials at room temperature. Protect from exposure to light. Reconstituted solution is stable for 8 hr at room temperature. Discard after 8 hr. Do not use needles of IV administration sets that contain aluminum; carboplatin can precipitate and lose effectiveness when in contact with aluminum.
Infusion: Administer by slow infusion lasting at least 15 min.

Adverse effects

- **CNS:** *Peripheral neuropathies,* ototoxicity, visual disturbances, change in taste perception
- **GI:** *Vomiting, nausea, abdominal pain, diarrhea, constipation*
- **GU:** *Increased BUN or serum creatinine*
- **Hematologic: Bone marrow depression;** *decreased serum sodium, magnesium, calcium, potassium*
- **Hypersensitivity:** *Anaphylactic-like reaction,* rash, urticaria, erythema, pruritus, **bronchospasm**
- **Other:** *Pain, alopecia, asthenia,* **cancer**

Interactions

✱ **Drug-drug** • Decreased potency of carboplatin and precipitate formation in solution using needles or administration sets containing aluminum

■ Nursing considerations

Assessment

- **History:** Severe allergic reactions to carboplatin, cisplatin, platinum compounds, mannitol; severe bone marrow depression; renal impairment; pregnancy, lactation
- **Physical:** Weight, skin, and hair evaluation; eighth cranial nerve evaluation; reflexes; sensation; CBC, differential; renal function tests; serum electrolytes; serum uric acid; audiogram

Interventions

⊗ ***Black box warning*** Evaluate bone marrow function before and periodically during therapy. Do not give next dose if bone marrow depression is marked. Consult physician for dosage.

⊗ ***Black box warning*** Ensure that epinephrine, corticosteroids, and antihistamines are readily available in case of anaphylactic-like reactions, which may occur within minutes of administration.

- Arrange for an antiemetic if nausea and vomiting are severe.

Teaching points

- This drug can only be given IV. Prepare a calendar of treatment days.
- Use contraceptives while taking this drug. This drug may cause birth defects or miscarriages.
- Have frequent, regular medical follow-up, including frequent blood tests to monitor drug effects.
- You may experience these side effects: Nausea, vomiting (medication may be ordered; eat frequent small meals); numbness, tingling, loss of taste, ringing in ears, dizziness, loss of hearing; rash, loss of hair (you can use a wig or scarves).
- Report loss of hearing, dizziness; unusual bleeding or bruising; fever, chills, sore throat; leg cramps, muscle twitching; changes in voiding patterns; difficulty breathing.

carboprost tromethamine

(kar' boe prost)

Hemabate

PREGNANCY CATEGORY C

Drug classes

Abortifacient
Prostaglandin

Therapeutic actions

Stimulates the myometrium of the gravid uterus to contract in a manner that is similar to the contractions of the uterus during labor, thus evacuating the contents of the gravid uterus.

Indications

- Termination of pregnancy 13–20 wk from the first day of the last menstrual period
- Evacuation of the uterus in instance of missed abortion or intrauterine fetal death in the second trimester
- Postpartum hemorrhage due to uterine atony unresponsive to conventional methods

Contraindications and cautions

- Contraindicated with allergy to prostaglandin preparations; acute PID; active cardiac, hepatic, pulmonary, renal disease.
- Use cautiously with history of asthma; hypotension; hypertension; CV, adrenal, renal, or hepatic disease; anemia; jaundice; diabetes; epilepsy; scarred uterus; cervicitis, infected endocervical lesions; acute vaginitis.

Available forms

Injection—250 mcg/mL

Dosages

Adults

- *Abortion:* Initially, 250 mcg (1 mL) IM; give 250 mcg IM at 1.5- to 3.5-hr intervals, depending on uterine response; may be increased to 500 mcg if uterine contractility is inadequate after several 250-mcg doses; do not exceed 12 mg total dose or continuous administration over 2 days.
- *Refractory postpartum uterine bleeding:* 250 mcg IM as one dose; in some cases, multiple doses at 15- to 90-min intervals may be used; do not exceed a total dose of 2 mg (8 doses).

Pharmacokinetics

Route	*Onset*	*Peak*
IM	15 min	2 hr

Metabolism: Hepatic and lung; $T_{1/2}$: 8 hr
Distribution: Crosses placenta; may enter breast milk
Excretion: Urine

Adverse effects

- **CNS:** Headache, paresthesias, *flushing,* anxiety, weakness, syncope, dizziness
- **CV:** *Hypotension,* arrhythmias, chest pain

- **GI:** Vomiting, diarrhea, *nausea*
- **GU:** Endometritis, **perforated uterus, uterine rupture,** uterine or vaginal pain, incomplete abortion
- **Respiratory:** Coughing, dyspnea
- **Other:** Chills, diaphoresis, backache, breast tenderness, eye pain, skin rash, pyrexia

■ Nursing considerations

Assessment

- **History:** Allergy to prostaglandin preparations; acute PID; active cardiac, hepatic, pulmonary, renal disease; history of asthma; hypotension; hypertension; anemia; jaundice; diabetes; epilepsy; scarred uterus; cervicitis, infected endocervical lesions; acute vaginitis
- **Physical:** T; BP, P, auscultation; R, adventitious sounds; bowel sounds, liver evaluation; vaginal discharge, pelvic examination, uterine tone; LFTs, renal function tests, WBC, urinalysis, CBC

Interventions

- Refrigerate unopened vials.
- Administer a test dose of 100 mcg (0.4 mL) prior to abortion if indicated.
- Administer by deep IM injection.
- Arrange for pretreatment or concurrent treatment with antiemetics and antidiarrheals to decrease the incidence of GI side effects.

⊗ ***Warning*** Ensure that abortion is complete or that other measures are used to complete the abortion if drug effects are not sufficient.

- Monitor T, using care to differentiate prostaglandin-induced pyrexia from postabortion endometritis pyrexia.
- Monitor uterine tone and vaginal discharge during procedure and several days after to assess drug effects and recovery.
- Ensure adequate hydration throughout procedure.

Teaching points

- Several IM injections may be required to achieve desired effect.
- You may experience these side effects: Nausea, vomiting, diarrhea, uterine or vaginal pain, fever, headache, weakness, dizziness.
- Report severe pain, difficulty breathing, palpitations, eye pain, rash.

▽ carisoprodol (isomeprobamate)

*(kar eye soe **proe'** dol)*

Soma

PREGNANCY CATEGORY C

Drug class

Centrally acting skeletal muscle relaxant

Therapeutic actions

Precise mechanism not known; chemically related to meprobamate, an anxiolytic; has sedative properties; also found in animal studies to inhibit interneuronal activity in descending reticular formation and spinal cord; does not directly relax tense skeletal muscles.

Indications

- Relief of discomfort associated with acute, painful musculoskeletal conditions as an adjunct to rest, physical therapy, and other measures

Contraindications and cautions

- Contraindicated with allergic or idiosyncratic reactions to carisoprodol, meprobamate (reported cross-reactions with meprobamate); acute intermittent porphyria, suspected porphyria, lactation.
- Use cautiously with renal or hepatic impairment, pregnancy.

Available forms

Tablets—350 mg

Dosages

Adults and children older than 12 yr

350 mg PO tid–qid; take last dose at bedtime for a maximum of 2–3 wk.

Pediatric patients

Not recommended for children younger than 12 yr.

Geriatric patients or patients with hepatic or renal impairment

Dosage reduction may be necessary; monitor closely.

Pharmacokinetics

Route	Onset	Peak	Duration
Oral	30 min	1–2 hr	4–6 hr

Metabolism: Hepatic; $T_{1/2}$: 8 hr
Distribution: May cross placenta; enters breast milk
Excretion: Urine

Adverse effects

- **CNS:** *Dizziness, drowsiness, vertigo, ataxia, tremor, agitation, irritability*
- **CV:** Tachycardia, orthostatic hypotension, facial flushing
- **GI:** Nausea, vomiting, hiccups, epigastric distress
- **Hypersensitivity: Allergic or idiosyncratic reactions** (seen with first to fourth dose in patients new to drug)—rash, erythema multiforme, pruritus, eosinophilia, fixed drug eruption; asthmatic episodes, fever, weakness, dizziness, angioneurotic edema, smarting eyes, hypotension, **anaphylactoid shock**

■ Nursing considerations

Assessment

- **History:** Allergic or idiosyncratic reactions to carisoprodol, meprobamate; acute intermittent porphyria, suspected porphyria; lactation
- **Physical:** T; skin color, lesions; orientation, affect; P, BP, orthostatic BP; bowel sounds, liver evaluation; LFTs, renal function tests, CBC

Interventions

⊗ ***Warning*** Monitor patient for potentially serious idiosyncratic reactions—most likely with first few doses.

- Reduce dose with hepatic impairment.
- Provide safety measures if CNS effects occur.
- Drug may be habit forming. Monitor patient.

Teaching points

- Take this drug exactly as prescribed; do not take a higher dosage; take with food if GI upset occurs.
- Avoid alcohol, sleep-inducing, or over-the-counter drugs; these could cause dangerous effects; if you feel you need one of these preparations, consult your health care provider.
- You may experience these side effects: Drowsiness, dizziness, vertigo (avoid driving or activities that require alertness); dizziness when you get up or climb stairs (avoid sudden changes in position, use caution climbing stairs); nausea (take drug with food, eat frequent small meals); insomnia, headache, depression (transient effects).
- Report rash, severe nausea, dizziness, insomnia, fever, difficulty breathing.

DANGEROUS DRUG

▽ carmustine (BCNU)

*(car **mus'** teen)*

BiCNU, Gliadel

PREGNANCY CATEGORY D

Drug classes

Alkylating agent, nitrosourea
Antineoplastic

Therapeutic actions

Cytotoxic: Alkylates DNA and RNA and inhibits several enzymatic processes, leading to cell death.

Indications

- Palliative therapy alone or with other agents (injection) for brain tumors: Glioblastomas, brainstem glioma, medullablastoma, astrocytoma, ependymoma, metastatic brain tumors
- Hodgkin's lymphoma and non-Hodgkin's lymphomas (as secondary therapy)
- Multiple myeloma (with prednisone)
- Adjunct to surgery for the treatment of recurrent glioblastoma as implantable wafer after removal of tumor (wafer)
- Treatment of newly diagnosed high-grade malignant glioma as adjunct to surgery and radiation (wafer)
- Unlabeled use: Treatment of mycosis fungoides (topical), cutaneous T-cell lymphoma

Contraindications and cautions

- Contraindicated with allergy to carmustine.
- Use cautiously with radiation therapy, chemotherapy, hematopoietic depression, impaired renal or hepatic function, pregnancy (teratogenic and embryotoxic), lactation.

Available forms

Powder for injection—100 mg; wafer (*Gliadel*)—7.7 mg

Dosages

⊗ ***Black box warning*** Do not give doses more often than every 6 wk because of delayed bone marrow toxicity.

Adults and pediatric patients

IV

As single agent in untreated patients, 150–200 mg/m² IV every 6 wk as a single dose or in divided daily injections (75–100 mg/m² on 2 successive days). Do not repeat dose until platelets exceed 100,000/mm³, leukocytes exceed 4,000/mm³. Adjust dosage after initial dose based on hematologic response, as follows:

Leukocytes	*Platelets*	*Percentage of Prior Dose to Give*
More than 4,000	More than 100,000	100%
3,000–3,999	75,000–99,999	100%
2,000–2,999	25,000–74,999	70%
Less than 2,000	Less than 25,000	50%

Wafer

Implanted in resection cavity as part of a surgical procedure; up to 8 wafers at a time.

Pharmacokinetics

Route	*Onset*	*Peak*
IV	Immediate	15 min
Wafer	Absorbed locally	Unknown

Metabolism: Hepatic; $T_{1/2}$: 15–30 min
Distribution: Crosses placenta; may enter breast milk
Excretion: Lungs, urine

IV FACTS

Preparation: Reconstitute with 3 mL of supplied sterile diluent, then add 27 mL of sterile water for injection to the alcohol solution; resulting solution contains 3.3 mg/mL of carmustine in 10% ethanol, pH is 5.6–6; may be further diluted with 5% dextrose injection. Refrigerate unopened vials. Protect reconstituted solution from light; lacking preservatives, solution decomposes with time, but is stable for 8 hr at room temperature. Check vials before use for absence of oil film residue; if present, discard vial.
Infusion: Administer reconstituted solution by IV drip over 1–2 hr; shorter infusion time may cause intense pain and burning. Stability of dextrose-diluted solutions at a concentration of 0.2 mg/mL is 8 hr at room temperature.
Incompatibility: Do not add to sodium bicarbonate.

Adverse effects

- **CNS:** Ocular toxicity—nerve fiber-layer infarcts, retinal hemorrhage
- **GI:** *Nausea, vomiting, stomatitis, hepatotoxicity*
- **GU:** Renal toxicity—decreased renal size, azotemia, **renal failure**
- **Hematologic:** *Myelosuppression, leukopenia, thrombocytopenia, anemia* (delayed for 4–6 wk)
- **Respiratory:** *Pulmonary infiltrates,* **pulmonary fibrosis**
- **Other:** *Local burning at site of injection;* intense flushing of the skin, suffusion of the conjunctiva with rapid IV infusion; **cancer**

Interactions

✱ **Drug-drug** • Increased toxicity and myelosuppression with cimetidine • Decreased serum levels of digoxin, phenytoin • Risk of corneal and epithelial damage with mitomycin

■ Nursing considerations

Assessment

- **History:** Allergy to carmustine; radiation therapy; chemotherapy; hematopoietic depression; impaired renal or hepatic function; pregnancy; lactation
- **Physical:** T; weight; ophthamologic examination; R, adventitious sounds; mucous membranes, liver evaluation; CBC, differential; urinalysis, LFTs, renal function tests; PFTs

Interventions

⊗ ***Black box warning*** Evaluate hematopoietic function before therapy and weekly during and for at least 6 wk after therapy to monitor for bone marrow suppression.

- Do not give full dosage within 2–3 wk after a full course of radiation therapy or chemotherapy because of the risk of severe bone marrow depression; reduced dosage may be needed.

⊗ ***Black box warning*** Monitor patient for pulmonary toxicity and delayed toxicity, which can occur years after therapy; even death can occur. Cumulative doses of 1,400 mg/m^2 increase the risk.

- Unopened foil pouches of wafer may be kept at ambient room temperature for a maximum of 6 hr.
- Reduce dosage in patients with depressed bone marrow function.
- Arrange for pretherapy medicating with antiemetic to decrease the severity of nausea and vomiting.
- Monitor injection site for any adverse reaction; accidental contact of carmustine with the skin can cause burning and hyperpigmentation of the area.
- Monitor ophthalmologic status.
- Monitor urine output for volume and any sign of renal failure.
- Monitor LFTs, renal function tests, and PFTs.

Teaching points

- This drug can only be given IV or implanted during surgery.
- Maintain your fluid intake and nutrition.
- Use birth control; this drug can cause severe birth defects.
- You may experience these side effects: Nausea, vomiting, loss of appetite (an antiemetic may be ordered; eat frequent small meals); increased susceptibility to infection (avoid exposure to infection by avoiding crowded places; avoid injury).
- Report unusual bleeding or bruising, fever, chills, sore throat, stomach or flank pain, changes in vision, difficulty breathing, shortness of breath, burning or pain at IV injection site.

▽ carteolol hydrochloride

*(**kar'** tee oh lol)*

Cartrol

PREGNANCY CATEGORY C

Drug classes

Antihypertensive
Beta blocker

Therapeutic actions

Blocks beta-adrenergic receptors of the sympathetic nervous system in the heart and juxtaglomerular apparatus (kidney), thus decreasing the excitability of the heart, decreasing cardiac output and oxygen consumption, decreasing the release of renin from the kidney, and lowering BP.

Indications

- Management of hypertension, alone or with other drugs
- Reduction of IOP in chronic open-angle glaucoma (ophthalmic solution)

Contraindications and cautions

- Contraindicated with sinus bradycardia (HR 45 beats per min or less), second- or third-degree heart block (PR interval more than 0.24 sec), cardiogenic shock, heart failure, asthma, COPD, lactation, hypersensitivity to beta blockers.
- Use cautiously with diabetes or thyrotoxicosis, hepatic impairment, renal failure, pregnancy.

Available forms

Tablets—2.5, 5 mg; ophthalmic solution—1%

Dosages

Adults

Oral

Initially, 2.5 mg as a single daily oral dose, alone or with a diuretic. If inadequate, gradually increase to 5–10 mg as a single daily dose. Doses of more than 10 mg are not likely to produce further benefit and may decrease response. For maintenance, 2.5–5 mg PO daily.

Ophthalmic

1 drop in affected eye or eyes bid.

Pediatric patients

Safety and efficacy not established.

Geriatric patients or patients with impaired renal function

Oral

Because bioavailability increases twofold, lower doses may be required. For creatinine clearance greater than 60 mL/min, administer every 24 hr; creatinine clearance of 20–60 mL/min, administer every 48 hr; creatinine clearance less than 20 mL/min, administer every 72 hr.

Pharmacokinetics

Route	*Onset*	*Peak*	*Duration*
Oral	Varies	1–3 hr	24–48 hr

Metabolism: Hepatic; $T_{1/2}$: 6 hr
Distribution: Crosses placenta; may enter breast milk
Excretion: Urine

Adverse effects

- **Allergic:** Pharyngitis, erythematous rash, fever, sore throat, **laryngospasm,** respiratory distress
- **CNS:** Dizziness, vertigo, tinnitus, fatigue, emotional depression, paresthesias, sleep disturbances, hallucinations, disorientation, memory loss, slurred speech (carteolol is less lipid-soluble than propranolol; it is less likely to penetrate the blood–brain barrier and cause CNS effects)
- **CV:** *Bradycardia, heart failure, cardiac arrhythmias, sinoatrial or AV nodal block, tachycardia,* peripheral vascular insufficiency, claudication, CVA, pulmonary edema, hypotension
- **Dermatologic:** Rash, pruritus, sweating, dry skin
- **EENT:** Eye irritation, dry eyes, conjunctivitis, blurred vision
- **GI:** *Gastric pain, flatulence, constipation, diarrhea, nausea, vomiting,* anorexia
- **GU:** *Impotence, decreased libido,* Peyronie's disease, dysuria, nocturia, frequent urination
- **Musculoskeletal:** Joint pain, arthralgia, muscle cramps
- **Respiratory: Bronchospasm,** dyspnea, cough, bronchial obstruction, nasal stuffiness, rhinitis
- **Other:** *Decreased exercise tolerance, development of antinuclear antibodies,* hyperglycemia or hypoglycemia, elevated serum transaminase

Interactions

✱ **Drug-drug** • Increased effects with verapamil • Decreased effects of theophyllines and carteolol if taken concurrently • Increased risk of orthostatic hypotension with prazosin • Possible increased BP-lowering effects with aspirin, bismuth subsalicylate, magnesium salicylate, sulfinpyrazone • Decreased antihypertensive effects with NSAIDs, clonidine • Possible increased hypoglycemic effect of insulin • Initial hypertensive episode followed by bradycardia if combined with epinephrine • Peripheral ischemia and possible gangrene if combined with ergot alkaloids

✱ **Drug-lab test** • Monitor for possible false results with glucose or insulin tolerance tests

■ Nursing considerations

Assessment

- **History:** Arrhythmias, cardiogenic shock, heart failure, asthma, COPD, pregnancy, lactation, diabetes or thyrotoxicosis
- **Physical:** Weight, skin condition, neurologic status, P, BP, ECG, respiratory status, renal and thyroid function tests, blood and urine glucose

Interventions

- Give carteolol (oral) once a day. Monitor response and maintain at lowest possible dose.

⊗ ***Warning*** Do not discontinue drug abruptly after long-term therapy (hypersensitivity to catecholamines may have developed, causing exacerbation of angina, MI, and ventricular arrhythmias); taper drug gradually over 2 wk with monitoring.

- Consult with physician about withdrawing drug if patient is to undergo surgery (withdrawal is controversial).
- Monitor IOP of patients receiving eye drops; if pressure not controlled, institute concomitant therapy.

C

Teaching points

- Follow instructions for instillation of eyedrops carefully.
- Do not stop taking this drug unless told to do so by a health care provider.
- Avoid driving or dangerous activities if dizziness or weakness occurs.
- You may experience these side effects: Loss of appetite, nightmares, depression, sexual impotence. (Discuss these side effects with your health care provider if they become a concern.)
- Report difficulty breathing, night cough, swelling of extremities, slow pulse, confusion, depression, rash, fever, sore throat.

carvedilol

(kar vah' da lol)

Apo-Carvedilol (CAN), Coreg, Coreg CR, PMS-Carvedilol (CAN), ratio-Carvedilol (CAN)

PREGNANCY CATEGORY C

Drug classes

Alpha- and beta-adrenergic blocker
Antihypertensive

Therapeutic actions

Competitively blocks alpha-, beta-, and beta$_2$-adrenergic receptors and has some sympathomimetic activity at beta$_2$-receptors. Both alpha and beta blocking actions contribute to the BP-lowering effect; beta blockade prevents the reflex tachycardia seen with most alpha-blocking drugs and decreases plasma renin activity. Significantly reduces plasma renin activity.

Indications

- Hypertension, alone or with other oral drugs, especially diuretics
- Treatment of mild to severe heart failure of ischemic or cardiomyopathic origin with digitalis, diuretics, ACE inhibitors
- Left ventricular dysfunction (LVD) after MI
- Unlabeled uses: Angina (25–50 mg bid)

Contraindications and cautions

- Contraindicated with decompensated heart failure, bronchial asthma, heart block, cardiogenic shock, hypersensitivity to carvedilol, pregnancy, lactation.
- Use cautiously with hepatic impairment, peripheral vascular disease, thyrotoxicosis, diabetes, anesthesia, major surgery.

Available forms

Tablets—3.125, 6.25, 12.5, 25 mg; CR capsules—10, 20, 40, 80 mg

Dosages

Adults

- *Hypertension:* 6.25 mg PO bid; maintain for 7–14 days, then increase to 12.5 mg PO bid if needed to control BP. Do not exceed 50 mg/day.
- *Heart failure:* Monitor patient very closely, individualize dose based on patient response. Initial dose, 3.125 mg PO bid for 2 wk, may then be increased to 6.25 mg PO bid. Do not increase doses at intervals shorter than 2 wk. Maximum dose, 25 mg PO bid in patients weighing less than 85 kg or 50 mg PO bid in patients weighing more than 85 kg.
- *LVD following MI:* 6.25 mg PO bid; increase after 3–10 days to target dose of 25 mg bid.

For conversion from tablets to CR capsules, follow these instructions. For dosage of 6.25 mg daily (3.125 mg bid), give 10 mg CR capsules once daily. For 12.5 mg (6.25 mg bid), give 20 mg CR capsules once daily. For 25 mg (12.5 mg bid), give 40 mg CR capsules once daily. For 50 mg (25 mg bid), give 80 mg CR capsules once daily.

Pediatric patients

Safety and efficacy not established.

Patients with hepatic impairment

Do not administer to any patient with severe hepatic impairment.

Pharmacokinetics

Route	Onset	Peak	Duration
Oral	Rapid	30 min	8–10 hr

Metabolism: Hepatic; $T_{1/2}$: 7–10 hr

Distribution: Crosses placenta; may enter breast milk
Excretion: Bile, feces

Adverse effects
- **CNS:** *Dizziness, vertigo, tinnitus, fatigue,* emotional depression, paresthesias, sleep disturbances
- **CV:** *Bradycardia,* orthostatic hypertension, heart failure, cardiac arrhythmias, pulmonary edema, *hypotension*
- **GI:** *Gastric pain, flatulence, constipation, diarrhea,* **hepatic failure**
- **Respiratory:** *Rhinitis,* pharyngitis, dyspnea
- **Other:** *Fatigue,* back pain, infections

Interactions
✱ **Drug-drug** • Increased effectiveness of antidiabetics; monitor blood glucose and adjust dosages appropriately • Increased effectiveness of clonidine; monitor patient for potential severe bradycardia and hypotension • Increased serum levels of digoxin; monitor serum levels and adjust dosage accordingly • Increased plasma levels of carvedilol with rifampin • Potential for dangerous conduction system disturbances with verapamil or diltiazem; if this combination is used, closely monitor ECG and BP
✱ **Drug-food** • Slowed rate of absorption but not decreased effectiveness with food

■ Nursing considerations
Assessment
- **History:** Heart failure, bronchial asthma, heart block, cardiogenic shock, hypersensitivity to carvedilol, pregnancy, lactation, hepatic impairment, peripheral vascular disease, thyrotoxicosis, diabetes, anesthesia or major surgery
- **Physical:** Baseline weight, skin condition, neurologic status, P, BP, ECG, respiratory status, LFTs, renal and thyroid function tests, blood and urine glucose

Interventions
⊗ ***Warning*** Do not discontinue drug abruptly after chronic therapy (hypersensitivity to catecholamines may have developed, causing exacerbation of angina, MI, and ventricular arrhythmias); taper drug gradually over 2 wk with monitoring.

- Consult with physician about withdrawing drug if patient is to undergo surgery (withdrawal is controversial).
- Give with food to decrease orthostatic hypotension and adverse effects.
- Monitor for orthostatic hypotension and provide safety precautions.
- Monitor diabetic patient closely; drug may mask hypoglycemia or worsen hyperglycemia.

⊗ ***Warning*** Monitor patient for any sign of hepatic impairment (pruritus, dark urine or stools, anorexia, jaundice, pain); arrange for LFTs and discontinue drug if tests indicate liver injury. Do not restart carvedilol.

Teaching points
- Take drug with meals.
- Do not stop taking drug unless instructed to do so by a health care provider.
- Avoid use of over-the-counter medications.
- If you are diabetic, promptly report changes in glucose level.
- You may experience these side effects: Depression, dizziness, light-headedness (avoid driving or performing dangerous activities; getting up and changing positions slowly may help ease dizziness), decreased tears with contact lenses.
- Report difficulty breathing, swelling of extremities, changes in color of stool or urine, very slow heart rate, continued dizziness.

▽ caspofungin acetate

See Appendix W, *Less commonly used drugs*.

▽ cefaclor
(sef' a klor)

Apo-Cefaclor (CAN), Ceclor, Ceclor Pulvules, Cefaclor (ONE), Raniclor

PREGNANCY CATEGORY B

Drug classes
Antibiotic
Cephalosporin (second generation)

Therapeutic actions
Bactericidal: Inhibits synthesis of bacterial cell wall, causing cell death.

Indications
- Lower respiratory infections caused by *Streptococcus pneumoniae, Haemophilus influenzae, Streptococcus pyogenes*
- URIs caused by *S. pyogenes*
- Dermatologic infections caused by *Staphylococcus aureus*
- UTIs caused by *Escherichia coli, Proteus mirabilis, Klebsiella,* coagulase-negative staphylococci
- Otitis media caused by *S. pneumoniae, H. influenzae, S. pyogenes,* staphylococci
- ER tablets: Acute exacerbations of chronic bronchitis, secondary infections of acute bronchitis, pharyngitis, and tonsillitis due to *S. pyogenes;* uncomplicated skin infections
- Unlabeled use: Acute uncomplicated UTI in select patients, single 2-g dose

Contraindications and cautions
- Contraindicated with allergy to cephalosporins or penicillins.
- Use cautiously with renal failure, lactation, pregnancy.

Available forms
Capsules—250, 500 mg; chewable tablets—125, 187, 250, 375 mg; ER tablets (DNC)—375, 500 mg; powder for oral suspension—125 mg/5 mL, 187 mg/5 mL, 250 mg/5 mL, 375 mg/5 mL

Dosages
Adults
250 mg PO every 8 hr or 375–500 mg every 12 hr for 7–10 days; dosage may be doubled in severe cases. **Do not exceed 4 g/day.**

Pediatric patients
20 mg/kg per day PO in divided doses every 8 hr; in severe cases 40 mg/kg/day may be given. **Do not exceed 1 g/day.**
- *Otitis media and pharyngitis:* Total daily dosage may be divided and administered every 12 hr.

Pharmacokinetics
Route	*Peak*	*Duration*
Oral	30–60 min	8–10 hr

Metabolism: $T_{1/2}$: 30–60 min
Distribution: Crosses the placenta; enters breast milk
Excretion: Urine, unchanged

Adverse effects
- **CNS:** Headache, dizziness, lethargy, paresthesias
- **GI:** *Nausea, vomiting, diarrhea, anorexia, abdominal pain, flatulence,* **pseudomembranous colitis,** hepatotoxicity
- **GU:** Nephrotoxicity
- **Hematologic:** Bone marrow depression
- **Hypersensitivity:** *Ranging from rash to fever* to **anaphylaxis;** serum sickness reaction
- **Other:** *Superinfections*

Interactions
✱ **Drug-drug** • Increased nephrotoxicity with aminoglycosides • Increased bleeding effects with oral anticoagulants • Decreased serum level of ER form if taken with antacids; separate by at least 2 hr
✱ **Drug-lab test** • Possibility of false results on tests of urine glucose using Benedict's solution, Fehling's solution, Clinitest tablets; urinary 17-ketosteroids; direct Coombs' test

■ Nursing considerations
Assessment
- **History:** Penicillin or cephalosporin allergy, pregnancy or lactation
- **Physical:** Renal function tests, respiratory status, skin status, culture and sensitivity tests of infected area

Interventions
- Culture infection site before drug therapy.
- Give drug with meals or food to decrease GI discomfort. Ensure that patient swallows ER tablets whole; do not cut, crush, or allow patient to chew them.
- Refrigerate suspension after reconstitution, and discard after 14 days.

- Discontinue drug if hypersensitivity reaction occurs.
- Give patient yogurt or buttermilk in case of diarrhea.
- Arrange for oral vancomycin for serious colitis that fails to respond to discontinuation of drug.

Teaching points

- Take this drug with meals or food.
- Complete the full course of this drug, even if you feel better.
- Do not cut, crush, or chew ER form; swallow tablets whole.
- This drug is prescribed for this particular infection; do not self-treat any other infection.
- You may experience these side effects: Stomach upset, loss of appetite, nausea (take drug with food); diarrhea; headache, dizziness.
- Report severe diarrhea with blood, pus, or mucus; rash or hives; difficulty breathing; unusual tiredness or fatigue; unusual bleeding or bruising.

cefadroxil

(sef a ***drox'*** *ill)*

Apo-Cefadroxil (CAN), Duricef

PREGNANCY CATEGORY B

Drug classes

Antibiotic
Cephalosporin (first generation)

Therapeutic actions

Bactericidal: Inhibits the formation of bacterial cell wall, causing the cell's death.

Indications

- UTIs caused by *Escherichia coli, Proteus mirabilis, Klebsiella* species
- Pharyngitis, tonsillitis caused by group A beta-hemolytic streptococci
- Skin and skin structure infections caused by staphylococci, streptococci

Contraindications and cautions

- Contraindicated with allergy to cephalosporins or penicillins.
- Use cautiously with renal failure, lactation, pregnancy.

Available forms

Capsules—500 mg; tablets—1,000 mg; powder for oral suspension—125 mg/5 mL, 250 mg/5 mL, 500 mg/5 mL

Dosages

Adults

- *UTIs:* 1–2 g/day PO in single dose or two divided doses for uncomplicated lower UTIs. For all other UTIs, 2 g/day in two divided doses.
- *Skin and skin-structure infections:* 1 g/day PO in single dose or two divided doses.
- *Pharyngitis, tonsillitis caused by group A beta-hemolytic streptococci:* 1 g/day PO in single dose or two divided doses for 10 days.

Pediatric patients

- *UTIs, dermatologic infections:* 30 mg/kg per day PO in divided doses every 12 hr.
- *Pharyngitis, tonsillitis caused by group A beta-hemolytic streptococci:* 30 mg/kg/day in single or two divided doses, continue for 10 days.

Geriatric patients or patients with impaired renal function

1 g PO loading dose, followed by 500 mg PO at these intervals:

CrCl (mL/min)	Interval (hr)
25–50	12
10–25	24
0–10	36

Pharmacokinetics

Route	Peak	Duration
Oral	1.5–2 hr	20–22 hr

Metabolism: $T_{1/2}$: 78–96 min
Distribution: Crosses the placenta; enters breast milk
Excretion: Urine

Adverse effects

- **CNS:** Headache, dizziness, lethargy, paresthesias
- **GI:** *Nausea, vomiting, diarrhea, anorexia, abdominal pain, flatulence,* **pseudomembranous colitis,** hepatotoxicity

- **GU:** Nephrotoxicity
- **Hematologic: Bone marrow depression**
- **Hypersensitivity:** Ranging from *rash* to *fever* to **anaphylaxis;** serum sickness reaction
- **Other:** *Superinfections*

Interactions

✱ **Drug-drug** • Decreased bactericidal activity if used with bacteriostatic agents • Increased serum levels of cephalosporins if used with probenecid • Increased nephrotoxicity with aminoglycosides

✱ **Drug-lab test** • False-positive urine glucose using Benedict's solution, Fehling's solution, Clinitest tablets • False-positive direct Coombs' test • Falsely elevated urinary 17-ketosteroids

■ Nursing considerations

Assessment

- **History:** Penicillin or cephalosporin allergy, pregnancy or lactation, renal failure
- **Physical:** Renal function tests, respiratory status, skin status, culture and sensitivity tests of infected area

Interventions

- Culture infection site before drug therapy.
- Give drug with meals or food to decrease GI discomfort.
- Refrigerate suspension after reconstitution, and discard after 14 days; shake refrigerated suspension well before using.
- Discontinue if hypersensitivity reaction occurs.
- Give the patient yogurt or buttermilk in case of diarrhea.

⊗ ***Warning*** Arrange for oral vancomycin for serious colitis that fails to respond to discontinuation of drug.

Teaching points

- Take this drug only for this infection; do not use to treat other problems; complete the full course of therapy, even if you feel better.
- Refrigerate the suspension, and discard unused portion after 14 days; shake suspension well before each use.
- You may experience these side effects: Stomach upset, loss of appetite, nausea (take drug with food), diarrhea, headache, dizziness.
- Report severe diarrhea with blood, pus, or mucus; rash; difficulty breathing; unusual tiredness, fatigue; unusual bleeding or bruising.

▽ cefdinir

(sef' din er)

Omnicef

PREGNANCY CATEGORY B

Drug classes

Antibiotic
Cephalosporin (third generation)

Therapeutic actions

Bactericidal: Inhibits synthesis of bacterial cell wall, causing cell death.

Indications

Adults and adolescents

- Community-acquired pneumonia caused by *Haemophilus influenzae, Haemophilus parainfluenzae, Streptococcus pneumoniae, Moraxella catarrhalis*
- Acute exacerbations of chronic bronchitis caused by *H. influenzae, H. parainfluenzae, S. pneumoniae, M. catarrhalis*
- Acute maxillary sinusitis caused by *H. influenzae, S. pneumoniae, M. catarrhalis*
- Pharyngitis and tonsillitis caused by *Streptococcus pyogenes*
- Uncomplicated skin and skin structure infections caused by *Staphylococcus aureus, S. pyogenes*

Pediatric patients

- Acute bacterial otitis media caused by *H. influenzae, S. pneumoniae, M. catarrhalis*
- Pharyngitis and tonsillitis caused by *S. pyogenes*
- Uncomplicated skin and skin-structure infections caused by *S. aureus, S. pyogenes*

Contraindications and cautions

- Contraindicated with allergy to cephalosporins or penicillins.
- Use cautiously with renal failure, lactation, pregnancy.

Available forms

Capsules—300 mg; oral suspension—125 mg/5 mL; 250 mg/5 mL

Dosages

Adults and adolescent patients

- *Community-acquired pneumonia, uncomplicated skin or skin-structure infections:* 300 mg PO every 12 hr for 10 days.
- *Acute exacerbation of chronic bronchitis, acute maxillary sinusitis, pharyngitis, or tonsillitis:* 300 mg every 12 hr PO for 10 days or 600 mg every 24 hr PO for 10 days.

Pediatric patients 6 mo–12 yr

- *Otitis media, acute maxillary sinusitis, pharyngitis, tonsillitis:* 7 mg/kg every 12 hr PO or 14 mg/kg every 24 hr PO for 10 days up to maximum dose of 600 mg/day.
- *Skin and skin-structure infections:* 7 mg/kg PO every 12 hr for 10 days.

Patients with renal impairment

For adults with creatinine clearance less than 30 mL/min, 300 mg PO daily. For patients on dialysis, 300 mg PO every other day; start with 300 mg PO at the end of dialysis and then every other day.

Pediatric patients with renal impairment

For creatinine clearance less than 30 mL/min, 7 mg/kg (up to 300 mg) once daily.

Pharmacokinetics

Route	*Peak*	*Duration*
Oral	60 min	8–10 hr

Metabolism: $T_{1/2}$: 100 min
Distribution: Crosses the placenta, enters breast milk
Excretion: Urine, unchanged

Adverse effects

- **CNS:** Headache, dizziness, lethargy, paresthesias
- **GI:** *Nausea, vomiting, diarrhea, anorexia, abdominal pain, flatulence,* **pseudomembranous colitis,** hepatotoxicity
- **GU:** Nephrotoxicity
- **Hematologic:** Bone marrow depression
- **Hypersensitivity:** Ranging from *rash* to *fever* to **anaphylaxis;** serum sickness reaction
- **Other:** *Superinfections*

C

Interactions

✱ **Drug-drug** • Increased nephrotoxicity with aminoglycosides • Increased bleeding effects if taken with oral anticoagulants • Interferes with absorption of cefdinir if taken with antacids containing magnesium or aluminum or with iron supplements; separate by at least 2 hr

✱ **Drug-lab test** • Possibility of false results on tests of urine glucose using Benedict's solution, Fehling's solution, Clinitest tablets; urinary 17-ketosteroids; direct Coombs' test

■ Nursing considerations

Assessment

- **History:** Penicillin or cephalosporin allergy; pregnancy or lactation, renal failure
- **Physical:** Renal function tests, respiratory status, skin status; culture and sensitivity tests of infected area

Interventions

- Arrange for culture and sensitivity tests of infected area before beginning drug therapy and during therapy if infection does not resolve.
- Reconstitute oral suspension by adding 38 mL water to the 60 mL bottle, 63 mL water to the 100 mL bottle; shake well before each use. Store at room temperature. Discard after 10 days.
- Give drug with meals; arrange for small, frequent meals if GI complications occur. Separate antacids or iron supplements by 2 hr from the cefdinir dose.
- Arrange for treatment of superinfections if they occur.

Teaching points

- Take this drug with meals or food. Store suspension at room temperature, shake well before each use; discard any drug after 10 days.
- Complete the full course of this drug, even if you feel better before the course of treatment is over.

- This drug is prescribed for this particular infection; do not self-treat any other infection with this drug.
- You may experience these side effects: Stomach upset, loss of appetite, nausea (taking the drug with food may help); diarrhea (stay near bathroom facilities); headache, dizziness.
- Report severe diarrhea with blood, pus, or mucus; rash or hives; difficulty breathing; unusual tiredness, fatigue; unusual bleeding or bruising.

▽ cefditoren pivoxil

(sef' di tore en)

Spectracef

PREGNANCY CATEGORY B

Drug classes

Antibiotic
Cephalosporin

Therapeutic actions

Bactericidal. Inhibits synthesis of susceptible gram-negative and gram-positive bacterial cell wall, causing cell death. Effective in the presence of beta-lactamases, including penicillinases and cephalosporinases.

Indications

- Acute exacerbations of chronic bronchitis caused by *Haemophilus influenzae, Haemophilus parainfluenzae, Streptococcus pneumoniae, Moraxella catarrhalis*
- Community-acquired pneumonia caused by *H. influenzae, H. parainfluenzae, S. pneumoniae, M. catarrhalis*
- Pharyngitis and tonsillitis caused by *Streptococcus pyogenes*
- Uncomplicated skin and skin-structure infections caused by *Staphylococcus aureus, S. pyogenes*

Contraindications and cautions

- Contraindicated with allergy to cephalosporins or penicillins, carnitine deficiencies, milk protein hypersensitivities, renal failure, lactation.
- Use cautiously with renal or hepatic impairment, pregnancy.

Available forms

Tablets—200 mg

Dosages

Adults and patients older than 12 yr

- *Uncomplicated skin or skin-structure infections; pharyngitis or tonsillitis:* 200 mg PO bid for 10 days.
- *Acute exacerbation of chronic bronchitis, community-acquired pneumonia:* 400 mg PO bid for 10 days (chronic bronchitis) or 14 days (pneumonia).

Patients with renal impairment

For creatinine clearance 30–49 mL/min, 200 mg PO bid; creatinine clearance less than 30 mL/min, 200 mg PO daily.

Pharmacokinetics

Route	*Peak*	*Duration*
Oral	1.5–3 hr	8–10 hr

Metabolism: $T_{1/2}$: 100–115 min
Distribution: Crosses the placenta; enters breast milk
Excretion: Urine, primarily unchanged

Adverse effects

- **CNS:** Headache, dizziness, lethargy, paresthesias, nervousness
- **GI:** *Nausea, vomiting, diarrhea,* anorexia, *abdominal pain,* **pseudomembranous colitis,** hepatotoxicity
- **GU:** Nephrotoxicity, vaginitis, urinary frequency
- **Hematologic:** Bone marrow depression, carnitine deficiency with long-term use
- **Hypersensitivity:** Ranging from *rash* to *fever* to **anaphylaxis;** serum sickness reaction
- **Other:** *Superinfections*

Interactions

✱ **Drug-drug** • Increased bleeding effects if taken with oral anticoagulants • Interference with absorption of cefditoren if taken with antacids containing magnesium or aluminum or with histamine$_2$-receptor antagonists; separate by at least 2 hr if concomitant use is necessary

✱ **Drug-lab test** • Possibility of false results on tests of urine glucose using Benedict's solution, Fehling's solution, Clinitest tablets; urinary 17-ketosteroids; direct Coombs' test

■ Nursing considerations

Assessment

- **History:** Penicillin or cephalosporin allergy, carnitine deficiency, milk protein hypersensitivity, renal or hepatic impairment, pregnancy, lactation
- **Physical:** Renal function tests, respiratory status, skin status, culture and sensitivity tests of infected area, GI function, orientation, affect

Interventions

- Arrange for culture and sensitivity tests of infected area before therapy and during therapy if infection does not resolve.
- Do not administer for longer than 10 days; risk of carnitine deficiency with prolonged use.

⊗ ***Warning*** Do not administer drug to patients with hypersensitivity to sodium caseinate or milk protein; this is not lactose intolerance.

- Give drug with meals; arrange for small, frequent meals if GI complications occur. Separate antacids or histamine$_2$-receptor antagonists by 2 hr from the cefditoren dose.
- Arrange for treatment of superinfections if they occur.

Teaching points

- Take this drug with meals or food.
- Complete the full course of this drug, even if you feel better before the course of treatment is over.
- This drug is prescribed for this particular infection; do not self-treat any other infection with this drug.
- Do not take this drug with antacids or histamine$_2$-receptor antagonists because they decrease absorption.
- You may experience these side effects: Stomach upset, loss of appetite, nausea (taking the drug with food may help); diarrhea (stay near bathroom facilities); headache, dizziness.
- Report severe diarrhea with blood, pus, or mucus; rash or hives; difficulty breathing; unusual tiredness, fatigue; unusual bleeding or bruising.

C

▽ cefepime hydrochloride

(sef' ah peem)

Maxipime

PREGNANCY CATEGORY B

Drug classes

Antibiotic

Cephalosporin (third generation)

Therapeutic actions

Bactericidal: Inhibits synthesis of bacterial cell wall, causing cell death.

Indications

- UTIs caused by *Escherichia coli, Proteus mirabilis, Klebsiella* species, including *Klebsiella pneumoniae*
- Pneumonia caused by *Streptococcus pneumoniae, Pseudomonas aeruginosa, K. pneumoniae, Enterobacter*
- Uncomplicated skin and skin-structure infections caused by *Staphylococcus aureus* group or *Streptococcus pyogenes*
- Empiric therapy for febrile neutropenic patients
- Complicated intra-abdominal infections in combination with metronidazole

Contraindications and cautions

- Contraindicated with allergy to cephalosporins or penicillins.
- Use cautiously with renal failure, lactation, pregnancy.

Available forms

Powder for injection—500 mg; 1, 2 g

Dosages

Adults

0.5–2 g IV or IM every 12 hr.

- *Mild to moderate UTI:* 0.5–1 g IM or IV every 12 hr for 7–10 days.
- *Severe UTI:* 2 g IV every 12 hr for 10 days.

CrCl (mL/min)	*Recommended Maintenance Schedule*			
More than 60 (Normal recommended schedule)	500 mg every 12 hr	1 g every 12 hr	2 g every 12 hr	2 g every 8 hr
30–60	500 mg every 24 hr	1 g every 24 hr	2 g every 24 hr	2 g every 12 hr
11–29	500 mg every 24 hr	500 mg every 24 hr	1 g every 24 hr	2 g every 24 hr
Less than 11	250 mg every 24 hr	250 mg every 24 hr	500 mg every 24 hr	1 g every 24 hr
CAPD	500 mg every 48 hr	1 g every 48 hr	2 g every 48 hr	2 g every 48 hr
Hemodialysis*	1 g on day 1, then 500 mg every 24 hr thereafter			1 g every 24 hr

*On hemodialysis days, cefepime should be administered following hemodialysis. Whenever possible, cefepime should be administered at the same time each day.

- *Moderate to severe pneumonia:* 1–2 g IV every 12 hr for 10 days.
- *Moderate to severe skin infections:* 2 g IV every 12 hr for 10 days.
- *Empiric therapy for febrile neutropenic patients:* 2 g IV every 8 hr for 7 days.
- *Complicated intra-abdominal infections:* 2 g IV every 12 hr for 7–10 days.

Pediatric patients older than 2 mo, weighing less than 40 kg

50 mg/kg/day dose IV or IM every 12 hr for 7–10 days depending on severity of infection. If treating febrile neutropenia, give every 8 hr.

Geriatric patients or patients with impaired renal function

Use recommended adult starting dose and then maintenance dose as shown in the table at the top of the page.

Pharmacokinetics

Route	*Onset*	*Peak*	*Duration*
IM	30 min	1.5–2 hr	10–12 hr
IV	Immediate	5 min	10–12 hr

Metabolism: $T_{1/2}$: 102–138 min
Distribution: Crosses placenta; enters breast milk
Excretion: Urine, unchanged

IV FACTS

Preparation: Dilute with 50–100 mL 0.9% sodium chloride, 5% and 10% dextrose injection, M/6 sodium lactate injection, 5% dextrose and 0.9% sodium chloride injection, lactated Ringer's and 5% dextrose injection, *Normosol-R, Normosol-M and D_5W* injection. Diluted solution is stable for 24 hr at room temperature or up to 7 days if refrigerated. Protect from light.
Infusion: Infuse slowly over 30 min.
Incompatibilities: Do not mix with ampicillin, metronidazole, vancomycin, gentamicin, tobramycin, or aminophylline. If concurrent therapy is needed, administer each drug separately. If possible, do not give any other drug in same solution as cefepime.

Adverse effects

- **CNS:** Headache, dizziness, lethargy, paresthesias
- **GI:** *Nausea, vomiting, diarrhea, anorexia, abdominal pain, flatulence,* **pseudomembranous colitis,** hepatotoxicity
- **GU:** Nephrotoxicity
- **Hematologic:** Bone marrow depression
- **Hypersensitivity:** Ranging from *rash* to *fever* to **anaphylaxis;** serum sickness reaction
- **Other:** *Superinfections, pain,* abscess (redness, tenderness, heat, tissue sloughing), inflammation at injection site, *phlebitis, disulfiram-like reaction with alcohol*

Interactions

✱ **Drug-drug** • Increased nephrotoxicity with aminoglycosides; monitor renal function tests • Increased bleeding effects with oral anticoagulants; reduced dosage may be needed • Increased toxicity if combined with alcohol; avoid this combination during and for 3 days after completing therapy

✱ **Drug-lab test** • False reports of urine glucose using Benedict's solution, Fehling's solution, Clinitest tablets; urinary 17-ketosteroids; direct Coombs' test

■ Nursing considerations
Assessment
- **History:** Penicillin or cephalosporin allergy; pregnancy, lactation
- **Physical:** Renal function tests, respiratory status, skin status; culture and sensitivity tests of infection area, injection site

Interventions
- Culture infected area and arrange for sensitivity tests before beginning therapy.
- Reconstitute for IM use with 0.9% sodium chloride, 5% dextrose injection, 0.5% or 1% lidocaine HCl or bacteriostatic water with parabens or benzyl alcohol. Reserve IM use for mild to moderate UTIs due to *E. coli.*
- Have vitamin K available in case hypoprothrombinemia occurs.

Teaching points
- Do not drink alcohol while taking this drug and for 3 days after drug has been stopped; severe reactions may occur.
- You may experience these side effects: Stomach upset, loss of appetite, nausea (take drug with food); diarrhea (stay near bathroom); headache, dizziness.
- Report severe diarrhea, difficulty breathing, unusual tiredness or fatigue, pain at injection site.

▽ cefotaxime sodium
(sef oh ***taks'*** *eem)*

Claforan

PREGNANCY CATEGORY B

Drug classes
Antibiotic
Cephalosporin (third generation)

Therapeutic actions
Bactericidal: Inhibits synthesis of bacterial cell wall, causing cell death.

Indications
- Lower respiratory infections caused by *Streptococcus pneumoniae, Staphylococcus aureus, Klebsiella* species, *Haemophilus influenzae, Escherichia coli, Proteus mirabilis, Enterobacter* species, *Serratia marcescens, Streptococcus pyogenes*
- UTIs caused by *Enterococcus* species, *S. epidermidis, S. aureus, Citrobacter* species, *Enterobacter* species, *E. coli, Klebsiella* species, *P. mirabilis, Proteus* species, *S. marcescens*
- Gynecologic infections caused by *S. epidermidis, Enterococcus* species, *E. coli, P. mirabilis, Bacteroides* species, *Clostridium* species, *Peptococcus* species, *Peptostreptococcus* species, streptococci; and uncomplicated gonorrhea caused by *N. gonorrhoeae*
- Dermatologic infections caused by *S. aureus, E. coli, Serratia* species, *Proteus* species, *Klebsiella* species, *Enterobacter* species, *Pseudomonas, S. marcescens, Bacteroides* species, *Peptococcus* species, *Peptostreptococcus* species, *P. mirabilis, S. epidermidis, S. pyogenes, Enterococcus* species
- Septicemia caused by *E. coli, Klebsiella* species, *S. marcescens*
- Peritonitis and intra-abdominal infections caused by *E. coli, Peptostreptococcus* species, *Bacteroides* species, *Peptococcus* species, *Klebsiella* species
- CNS infections caused by *E. coli, H. influenzae, Neisseria meningitidis, S. pneumoniae, K. pneumoniae*
- Bone and joint infections caused by *S. aureus*
- Perioperative prophylaxis

Contraindications and cautions
- Contraindicated with allergy to cephalosporins or penicillins.
- Use cautiously with renal failure, lactation, pregnancy.

Available forms
Powder for injection—500 mg, 1, 2 g; injection—1, 2 g

Dosages
Adults
2–8 g/day IM or IV in equally divided doses every 6–8 hr. Do not exceed 12 g/day.

- *Gonorrhea:* 0.5–1 g IM in a single injection.
- *Disseminated infection:* 1–2 g IV every 8 hr.
- *Perioperative prophylaxis:* 1 g IV or IM 30–90 min before surgery.
- *Cesarean section:* 1 g IV after cord is clamped and then 1 g IV or IM at 6 and 12 hr.

Pediatric patients 1 mo–12 yr weighing less than 50 kg

50–180 mg/kg/day IV or IM in four to six divided doses.

Pediatric patients 1–4 wk

50 mg/kg IV every 8 hr.

Pediatric patients 0–1 wk

50 mg/kg IV every 12 hr.

Geriatric patients or patients with reduced renal function

For creatinine clearance less than 20 mL/min, reduce dosage by half.

Pharmacokinetics

Route	*Onset*	*Peak*	*Duration*
IV	Immediate	5 min	18–24 hr
IM	5–10 min	30 min	18–24 hr

Metabolism: $T_{1/2}$: 1 hr

Distribution: Crosses the placenta; enters breast milk

Excretion: Urine

IV FACTS

Preparation: Reconstitute for intermittent IV injection with 1 or 2 g with 10 mL sterile water for injection. Reconstitute vials for IV infusion with 10 mL of sterile water for injection. Reconstitute infusion bottles with 50 or 100 mL of 0.9% sodium chloride injection or 5% dextrose injection. Drug solution may be further diluted with 50–100 mL of 5% or 10% dextrose injection; 5% dextrose and 0.2%, 0.45%, or 0.9% sodium chloride injection; lactated Ringer's solution; 0.9% sodium chloride injection; sodium lactate injection (M/6); 10% invert sugar. Reconstituted solution is stable for 24 hr at room temperature or 5 days if refrigerated. Powder and reconstituted solution darken with storage.

Infusion: Inject slowly into vein over 3–5 min or over a longer time through IV tubing; give intermittent IV infusions over 20–30 min. If administered with aminoglycosides, administer at different sites.

Incompatibilities: Do not mix in solutions with aminoglycoside solutions.

Y-site incompatibility: Hetastarch.

Adverse effects

- **CNS:** Headache, dizziness, lethargy, paresthesias
- **GI:** *Nausea, vomiting, diarrhea, anorexia, abdominal pain, flatulence,* **pseudomembranous colitis,** hepatotoxicity
- **GU:** Nephrotoxicity
- **Hematologic: Bone marrow depression**—decreased WBC count, decreased platelets, decreased Hct
- **Hypersensitivity:** *Ranging from rash* to *fever* to **anaphylaxis;** serum sickness reaction
- **Local:** *Pain,* abscess at injection site, *phlebitis,* inflammation at IV site
- **Other:** *Superinfections, disulfiram-like reaction with alcohol*

Interactions

✱ **Drug-drug** • Increased nephrotoxicity with aminoglycosides • Increased bleeding effects with oral anticoagulants • Risk of severe toxicity if combined with alcohol; avoid this combination during and for 3 days after completing therapy

✱ **Drug-lab test** • Possibility of false results on tests of urine glucose using Benedict's solution, Fehling's solution, Clinitest tablets; urinary 17-ketosteroids; direct Coombs' test

■ Nursing considerations

Assessment

- **History:** Hepatic and renal impairment, lactation, pregnancy
- **Physical:** Skin status, LFTs, renal function tests, culture of affected area, sensitivity tests

Interventions

- Culture infection site, and arrange for sensitivity tests before and during therapy if expected response is not seen.

- Reconstitution of drug varies by size of package; see manufacturer's directions for details.
- Reconstitute drug for IM use with sterile water or bacteriostatic water for injection; divide doses of 2 g and administer at two different sites by deep IM injection.
- Discontinue if hypersensitivity reaction occurs.

Teaching points

- Avoid alcohol while taking this drug and for 3 days after because severe reactions often occur.
- You may experience these side effects: Stomach upset, diarrhea.
- Report severe diarrhea, difficulty breathing, unusual tiredness or fatigue, pain at injection site.

cefoxitin sodium

(se fox' i tin)

Mefoxin

PREGNANCY CATEGORY B

Drug classes

Antibiotic
Cephalosporin (second generation)

Therapeutic actions

Bactericidal: Inhibits synthesis of bacterial cell wall, causing cell death.

Indications

- Lower respiratory infections caused by *Streptococcus pneumoniae, Staphylococcus aureus,* streptococci, *Escherichia coli, Klebsiella, Haemophilus influenzae, Bacteroides*
- Skin and skin structure infections caused by *S. aureus, Staphylococcus epidermidis,* streptococci, *E. coli, Proteus mirabilis, Klebsiella, Bacteroides, Clostridium, Peptococcus, Peptostreptococcus*
- UTIs caused by *E. coli, P. mirabilis, Klebsiella, Morganella morganii, Proteus rettgeri, Proteus vulgaris, Providencia*
- Uncomplicated gonorrhea caused by *Neisseria gonorrhoeae*
- Intra-abdominal infections caused by *E. coli, Klebsiella, Bacteroides, Clostridium*
- Gynecologic infections caused by *E. coli, N. gonorrhoeae, Bacteroides, Clostridium, Peptococcus, Peptostreptococcus,* group B streptococci
- Septicemia caused by *S. pneumoniae, S. aureus, E. coli, Klebsiella, Bacteroides*
- Bone and joint infections caused by *S. aureus*
- Perioperative prophylaxis

C

Contraindications and cautions

- Contraindicated with allergy to cephalosporins or penicillins.
- Use cautiously with renal failure, lactation, pregnancy.

Available forms

Powder for injection—1, 2 g; injection—1 g/50 mL, 2 g/50 mL in D_5W

Dosages

Adults

1–2 g IM or IV every 6–8 hr, depending on the severity of the infection.

- *Uncomplicated gonorrhea:* 2 g IM with 1 g oral probenecid.
- *Uncomplicated lower respiratory infections, UTIs, skin infections:* 1 g every 6–8 hr IV.
- *Moderate to severe infections:* 1 g every 4 hr IV to 2 g every 6–8 hr IV.
- *Severe infections:* 2 g every 4 hr IV or 3 g every 6 hr IV.
- *Perioperative prophylaxis:* 2 g IV or IM 30–60 min prior to initial incision and every 6 hr for 24 hr after surgery.
- *Cesarean section:* 2 g IV as soon as the umbilical cord is clamped, followed by 2 g IM or IV at 4 and 8 hr, then every 6 hr for up to 24 hr.
- *Transurethral prostatectomy:* 1 g prior to surgery and then 1 g every 8 hr for up to 5 days.

Pediatric patients 3 mo or older

80–160 mg/kg/day IM or IV in divided doses every 4–6 hr. Do not exceed 12 g/day.

- *Prophylactic use:* 30–40 mg/kg per dose IV or IM every 6 hr.

Geriatric patients or patients with impaired renal function

IV loading dose of 1–2 g. If patient is on hemodialysis, give loading dose after session. Maintenance dosages are as follows:

CrCl (mL/min)	Maintenance Dosage
30–50	1–2 g every 8–12 hr
10–29	1–2 g every 12–24 hr
5–9	0.5–1 g every 12–24 hr
Less than 5	0.5–1 g every 24–48 hr

Pharmacokinetics

Route	Onset	Peak	Duration
IV	Immediate	5 min	6–8 hr
IM	5–10 min	20–30 min	6–8 hr

Metabolism: $T_{1/2}$: 45–60 min
Distribution: Crosses the placenta; enters breast milk
Excretion: Urine

IV FACTS

Preparation: For IV intermittent administration, reconstitute 1 or 2 g with 10–20 mL sterile water for injection. For continuous IV infusion, add reconstituted solution to 5% dextrose injection, 0.9% sodium chloride injection, 5% dextrose and 0.9% sodium chloride injection, or 5% dextrose injection with 0.02% sodium bicarbonate solution. Store dry powder in cool, dry area. Powder and reconstituted solution darken with storage. Infusion bottles stable for 24 hr at room temperature; reconstituted vials stable for 6 hr at room temperature.
Infusion: For intermittent administration, slowly inject over 3–5 min, or give over longer time through IV tubing; discontinue other solutions temporarily. If given with aminoglycosides, give each at a different site.
Incompatibilities: Do not mix aminoglycosides and cefoxitin in the same IV solution.
Y-site incompatibility: Hetastarch.

Adverse effects

- **CNS:** Headache, dizziness, lethargy, paresthesias
- **GI:** *Nausea, vomiting, diarrhea, anorexia, abdominal pain, flatulence,* **pseudomembranous colitis,** hepatotoxicity
- **GU:** Nephrotoxicity
- **Hematologic: Bone marrow depression—**decreased WBC count, decreased platelets, decreased Hct
- **Hypersensitivity:** Ranging from *rash* to *fever* to **anaphylaxis,** serum sickness reaction
- **Local:** *Pain,* abscess at injection site, *phlebitis,* inflammation at IV site
- **Other:** *Superinfections, disulfiram-like reaction with alcohol*

Interactions

✱ **Drug-drug** • Increased nephrotoxicity with aminoglycosides • Increased bleeding effects with oral anticoagulants • Disulfiram-like reaction may occur if alcohol is taken during or within 72 hr after cefoxitin administration
✱ **Drug-lab test** • Possibility of false results on tests of urine glucose using Benedict's solution, Fehling's solution, Clinitest tablets; urinary 17-ketosteroids; direct Coombs' test

■ Nursing considerations

Assessment

- **History:** Hepatic and renal impairment, lactation, pregnancy
- **Physical:** Skin status, LFTs, renal function tests, culture of affected area, sensitivity tests

Interventions

- Culture infection site, and arrange for sensitivity tests before and during therapy if expected response is not seen.
- Reconstitute each gram for IM use with 2 mL sterile water for injection or with 2 mL of 0.5% lidocaine HCl solution (without epinephrine) to decrease pain at injection site. Inject deeply into large muscle group.
- Dry powder and reconstituted solutions darken slightly at room temperature.
- Have vitamin K available in case hypoprothrombinemia occurs.
- Discontinue if hypersensitivity reaction occurs.

Teaching points

- Avoid alcohol while taking this drug and for 3 days after because severe reactions often occur.
- You may experience these side effects: Stomach upset, diarrhea.
- Report severe diarrhea, difficulty breathing, unusual tiredness or fatigue, pain at injection site.

cefpodoxime proxetil

*(sef poe **docks'** eem)*

Vantin

PREGNANCY CATEGORY B

Drug classes

Antibiotic
Cephalosporin (third generation)

Therapeutic actions

Bactericidal: Inhibits synthesis of bacterial cell wall, causing cell death.

Indications

- Lower respiratory infections, including community-acquired pneumonia, caused by *Streptococcus pneumoniae, Haemophilus influenzae*
- URIs, including acute maxillary sinusitis, caused by *Streptococcus pyogenes, H. influenzae, Moraxella catharrhalis*
- **NEW INDICATION:** Uncomplicated skin and skin structure infections caused by *Staphylococcus aureus, S. pyogenes*
- UTIs caused by *Escherichia coli, Proteus mirabilis, Klebsiella, Staphylococcus saprophyticus*
- Otitis media caused by *S. pneumoniae, H. influenzae, M. catarrhalis*
- STD caused by *Neisseria gonorrhoeae*

Contraindications and cautions

- Contraindicated with allergy to cephalosporins or penicillins.
- Use cautiously with renal failure, lactation, pregnancy.

Available forms

Tablets—100, 200 mg; granules for oral suspension—50 mg/5 mL, 100 mg/5 mL

Dosages

Adults

100–400 mg every 12 hr PO depending on severity of infection; continue for 7–14 days.

Pediatric patients

5 mg/kg per dose PO every 12 hr; do not exceed 100–200 mg per dose; continue for 10 days.

- *Acute otitis media:* 10 mg/kg/day PO divided every 12 hr; do not exceed 400 mg/day; continue for 5 days.

Geriatric patients or patients with renal impairment

For creatinine clearance less than 30 mL/min, increase dosing interval to every 24 hr. For patient on hemodialysis, give dose three times weekly after session.

Pharmacokinetics

Route	*Peak*	*Duration*
Oral	30–60 min	16–18 hr

Metabolism: $T_{1/2}$: 120–180 min
Distribution: Crosses the placenta; enters breast milk
Excretion: Renal, unchanged

Adverse effects

- **CNS:** Headache, dizziness, lethargy, paresthesias
- **GI:** *Nausea, vomiting, diarrhea, anorexia, abdominal pain, flatulence,* **pseudomembranous colitis,** hepatotoxicity
- **GU:** Nephrotoxicity
- **Hematologic: Bone marrow depression**
- **Hypersensitivity:** *Ranging from rash* to *fever* to **anaphylaxis;** serum sickness reaction
- **Other:** *Superinfections*

Interactions

✱ **Drug-drug** • Increased nephrotoxicity with aminoglycosides • Increased bleeding effects with oral anticoagulants

✱ **Drug-food** • Increased absorption and increased effects of cefpodoxime if taken with food

✱ **Drug-lab test** • Possibility of false results on tests of urine glucose using Benedict's solution, Fehling's solution, Clinitest tablets; urinary 17-ketosteroids; direct Coombs' test

■ Nursing considerations

Assessment

- **History:** Penicillin or cephalosporin allergy, pregnancy or lactation, renal failure
- **Physical:** Renal function tests, respiratory status, skin status; culture and sensitivity tests of infected area

Interventions

- Culture infection site before drug therapy.
- Give drug with meals or food to enhance absorption.
- Store reconstituted solution in refrigerator. Shake well before using; use within 14 days, then discard.
- Discontinue drug if hypersensitivity reaction occurs.
- Give the patient yogurt or buttermilk in case of diarrhea.
- Arrange for oral vancomycin for serious colitis that fails to respond to discontinuation.

Teaching points

- Take this drug with food.
- Complete the full course of this drug even if you feel better.
- If using suspension, store in refrigerator and shake well before each use. Discard after 14 days.
- This drug is prescribed for this particular infection; do not self-treat any other infection.
- You may experience these side effects: Stomach upset, loss of appetite, nausea (take drug with food); diarrhea; headache, dizziness.
- Report severe diarrhea with blood, pus, or mucus; rash or hives; difficulty breathing; unusual tiredness, fatigue; unusual bleeding or bruising.

▽ cefprozil

*(sef **pro'** zil)*

Cefzil

PREGNANCY CATEGORY B

Drug classes

Antibiotic
Cephalosporin (second generation)

Therapeutic actions

Bactericidal: Inhibits synthesis of bacterial cell wall, causing cell death.

Indications

- Pharyngitis or tonsillitis caused by *Streptococcus pyogenes*
- Secondary bacterial infection of acute bronchitis and exacerbation of chronic bronchitis caused by *Streptococcus pneumoniae, Haemophilus influenzae, Moraxella catarrhalis*
- Dermatologic infections caused by *Staphylococcus aureus, S. pyogenes*
- Otitis media caused by *S. pneumoniae, H. influenzae, M. catarrhalis*
- Acute sinusitis caused by *S. pneumoniae, S. aureus, H. influenzae, M. catarrhalis*

Contraindications and cautions

- Contraindicated with allergy to cephalosporins or penicillins.
- Use cautiously with renal failure, lactation, pregnancy.

Available forms

Tablets—250, 500 mg; powder for suspension—125 mg/5 mL, 250 mg/5 mL

Dosages

Adults

250–500 mg PO every 12–24 hr. Continue treatment for 10 days.

Pediatric patients

Acute sinusitis, otitis media

- *6 mo–12 yr:* 7.5–15 mg/kg PO every 12 hr for 10 days.

Pharyngitis, tonsillitis
- *2–12 yr:* 7.5 mg/kg PO every 12 hr; continue treatment for 10 days.

Skin and skin structure infection
- *2–12 yr:* 20 mg/kg PO once daily; continue treatment for 10 days.

Geriatric patients or patients with renal impairment

For creatinine clearance of 30–120 mL/min, use standard dose; for creatinine clearance of 0–30 mL/min, use 50% of standard dose.

Pharmacokinetics

Route	*Peak*	*Duration*
Oral	6–10 hr	24–28 hr

Metabolism: $T_{1/2}$: 78 min
Distribution: Crosses the placenta, enters breast milk
Excretion: Urine, unchanged

Adverse effects
- **CNS:** Headache, dizziness, lethargy, paresthesias
- **GI:** *Nausea, vomiting, diarrhea, anorexia, abdominal pain, flatulence,* **pseudomembranous colitis,** hepatotoxicity
- **GU:** Nephrotoxicity
- **Hematologic: Bone marrow depression**
- **Hypersensitivity:** Ranging from *rash* to *fever* to **anaphylaxis;** serum sickness reaction
- **Other:** *Superinfections*

Interactions
✱ **Drug-drug** • Increased nephrotoxicity with aminoglycosides • Increased bleeding effects if taken with oral anticoagulants

✱ **Drug-lab test** • Possibility of false results on tests of urine glucose using Benedict's solution, Fehling's solution, Clinitest tablets; urinary 17-ketosteroids; direct Coombs' test

■ Nursing considerations
Assessment
- **History:** Penicillin or cephalosporin allergy, pregnancy or lactation, renal failure
- **Physical:** Renal function tests, respiratory status, skin status, culture and sensitivity tests of infected area

Interventions
- Culture infection site before drug therapy.
- Give drug with food to decrease GI discomfort.
- Refrigerate suspension after reconstitution, and discard after 14 days.
- Discontinue if hypersensitivity reaction occurs.
- Give the patient yogurt or buttermilk in case of diarrhea.
- Arrange for oral vancomycin for serious colitis that fails to respond to discontinuation.

Teaching points
- Take this drug with food.
- Complete the full course of this drug, even if you feel better.
- This drug is prescribed for this particular infection; do not use it to self-treat any other infection.
- You may experience these side effects: Stomach upset, loss of appetite, nausea (take drug with food); diarrhea; headache, dizziness.
- Report severe diarrhea with blood, pus, or mucus; rash or hives; difficulty breathing; unusual tiredness, fatigue; unusual bleeding or bruising.

ceftazidime
*(sef **taz'** i deem)*

Ceptaz, Fortaz, Tazicef, Tazidime

PREGNANCY CATEGORY B

Drug classes
Antibiotic
Cephalosporin (third generation)

Therapeutic actions
Bactericidal: Inhibits synthesis of bacterial cell wall, causing cell death.

Indications
- Lower respiratory infections caused by *Pseudomonas aeruginosa,* other *Pseudomonas, Streptococcus pneumoniae, Staphylococcus aureus, Klebsiella, Haemophilus influenzae, Proteus mirabilis, Escherichia coli, Enterobacter, Serratia, Citrobacter*

- UTIs caused by *P. aeruginosa, Enterobacter, E. coli, Klebsiella, P. mirabilis, Proteus*
- Gynecologic infections caused by *E. coli*
- Skin and skin structure infections caused by *P. aeruginosa, S. aureus, E. coli, Serratia, Proteus, Klebsiella, Enterobacter, Streptococcus pyogenes*
- Septicemia caused by *P. aeruginosa, E. coli, Klebsiella, H. influenzae, Serratia, S. pneumoniae, S. aureus*
- Intra-abdominal infections caused by *E. coli, S. aureus, Bacteroides, Klebsiella*
- CNS infections caused by *H. influenzae, Neisseria meningitidis*
- Bone and joint infections caused by *P. aeruginosa, Klebsiella, Enterobacter, S. aureus*

Contraindications and cautions

- Contraindicated with allergy to cephalosporins or penicillins.
- Use cautiously with renal failure, lactation, pregnancy.

Available forms

Powder for injection—500 mg, 1, 2 g; injection—1, 2 g

Dosages

Adults

Usual dose, 1 g (range 250 mg–2 g) every 8–12 hr IM or IV. Do not exceed 6 g/day. Dosage will vary with infection.

- *UTI:* 250–500 mg IV or IM every 8–12 hr.
- *Pneumonia, skin and skin structure infections:* 500 mg–1 g IV or IM every 8 hr.
- *Bone and joint infections:* 2 g IV every 12 hr.
- *Gynecologic, intra-abdominal, life-threatening infections, meningitis:* 2 g IV every 8 hr.

Pediatric patients 1 mo–12 yr

30–50 mg/kg IV every 8 hr. Do not exceed 6 g/day.

Pediatric patients 0–4 wk

30 mg/kg IV every 12 hr.

Geriatric patients or patients with reduced renal function

Loading dose of 1 g IV, followed by:

CrCl (mL/min)	*Dosage*
31–50	1 g every 12 hr
16–30	1 g every 24 hr
6–15	500 mg every 24 hr
5 or less	500 mg every 48 hr

Pharmacokinetics

Route	*Onset*	*Peak*	*Duration*
IV	Rapid	1 hr	24–28 hr
IM	30 min	1 hr	24–28 hr

Metabolism: $T_{1/2}$: 114–120 min
Distribution: Crosses the placenta; enters breast milk
Excretion: Urine

IV FACTS

Preparation: Reconstitute drug for direct IV injection with sterile water for injection. Reconstituted solution is stable for 24 hr at room temperature for *Fortaz* and *Tazidime,* or 18 hr at room temperature for *Ceptaz* and *Tazicef* or 7 days if refrigerated. For 500-mg vial, mix with 5 mL diluent; resulting concentration, 11 mg/mL. For 1-g vial, mix with 5 (10) mL diluent; resulting concentration, 180 (100) mg/mL. For 2-g vial, mix with 10 mL diluent; resulting concentration, 170–180 mg/mL.
Infusion: For IV, reconstitute 1- or 2-g infusion pack with 100 mL sterile water for injection; infuse slowly. For direct injection, slowly over 3–5 min. For infusion, over 30 min. If patient is also receiving aminoglycosides, administer at separate sites.
Incompatibilities: Do not mix with sodium bicarbonate injection or aminoglycoside solutions.

Adverse effects

- **CNS:** Headache, dizziness, lethargy, paresthesias
- **GI:** *Nausea, vomiting, diarrhea, anorexia, abdominal pain, flatulence,* **pseudomembranous colitis,** hepatotoxicity
- **GU:** Nephrotoxicity
- **Hematologic: Bone marrow depression**—decreased WBC count, decreased platelets, decreased Hct

- **Hypersensitivity:** Ranging from *rash* to *fever* to **anaphylaxis;** serum sickness reaction
- **Local:** *Pain,* abscess at injection site; *phlebitis,* inflammation at IV site
- **Other:** *Superinfections, disulfiram-like reaction with alcohol*

Interactions

✷ **Drug-drug** • Increased nephrotoxicity with aminoglycosides • Increased bleeding effects with oral anticoagulants • Disulfiram-like reaction if combined with alcohol during or for 3 days after completion of therapy

✷ **Drug-lab test** • Possibility of false results on tests of urine glucose using Benedict's solution, Fehling's solution, Clinitest tablets; urinary 17-ketosteroids; direct Coombs' test

■ Nursing considerations

Assessment

- **History:** Hepatic and renal impairment, lactation, pregnancy
- **Physical:** Skin status, LFTs, renal function tests, culture of affected area, sensitivity tests

Interventions

- Culture infection site, and arrange for sensitivity tests before and during therapy if expected response is not seen.
- Reconstitute drug for IM use with sterile water or bacteriostatic water for injection or with 0.5% or 1% lidocaine HCl injection to reduce pain; inject deeply into large muscle group.

⊗ ***Warning*** Do not mix with aminoglycoside solutions. Administer these drugs separately.

- Powder and reconstituted solution darken with storage.
- Have vitamin K available in case hypoprothrombinemia occurs.
- Discontinue if hypersensitivity reaction occurs.

Teaching points

- Avoid alcohol while taking this drug and for 3 days after because severe reactions often occur.
- You may experience these side effects: Stomach upset or diarrhea.
- Report severe diarrhea, difficulty breathing, unusual tiredness or fatigue, pain at injection site.

▽ceftibuten

*(sef ta **byoo'** ten)*

Cedax

PREGNANCY CATEGORY B

Drug classes

Antibiotic
Cephalosporin (third generation)

Therapeutic actions

Bactericidal: Inhibits synthesis of bacterial cell wall, causing cell death.

Indications

- Acute bacterial exacerbations of chronic bronchitis due to *Haemophilus influenzae, Moraxella catarrhalis, Streptococcus pneumoniae*
- Acute bacterial otitis media due to *H. influenzae, M. catarrhalis, Streptococcus pyogenes*
- Pharyngitis and tonsillitis due to *S. pyogenes*

Contraindications and cautions

- Contraindicated with allergy to cephalosporins or penicillins.
- Use cautiously with renal failure; lactation, pregnancy.

Available forms

Capsules—400 mg; oral suspension—90 mg/5 mL

Dosages

Adults

400 mg PO daily for 10 days.

Pediatric patients

9 mg/kg/day PO for 10 days to a maximum daily dose of 400 mg/day.

Patients with renal impairment

CrCl (mL/min)	*Dose*
More than 50	9 mg/kg or 400 mg PO every 24 hr
30–49	4.5 mg/kg or 200 mg PO every 24 hr
5–29	2.25 mg/kg or 100 mg PO every 24 hr

Pharmacokinetics

Route	*Peak*	*Duration*
Oral	30–60 min	8–10 hr

Metabolism: $T_{1/2}$: 30–60 min
Distribution: Crosses placenta; enters breast milk
Excretion: Urine, unchanged

Adverse effects

- **CNS:** Headache, dizziness, lethargy, paresthesias
- **GI:** *Nausea, vomiting, diarrhea, anorexia, abdominal pain, flatulence,* **pseudomembranous colitis,** hepatotoxicity
- **GU:** Nephrotoxicity
- **Hematologic: Bone marrow depression**
- **Hypersensitivity:** Ranging from *rash* to *fever* to **anaphylaxis;** serum sickness reaction
- **Other:** *Superinfections*

Interactions

✱ **Drug-drug** • Increased nephrotoxicity with aminoglycosides • Increased bleeding effects with oral anticoagulants • Disulfiram-like reaction may occur if alcohol is taken within 72 hr after administration

✱ **Drug-lab test** • Possibility of false results on tests of urine glucose using Benedict's solution, Fehling's, Clinitest tablets; urinary 17-ketosteroids; direct Coombs' test

■ Nursing considerations

Assessment

- **History:** Allergy to penicillin or cephalosporin; pregnancy, lactation, renal failure
- **Physical:** Renal function tests, respiratory status, skin status; culture and sensitivity tests of infection

Interventions

- Culture infection site before beginning drug therapy.
- Give capsules with meals to decrease GI discomfort; suspension must be given on an empty stomach at least 2 hr before or 1 hr after meals.
- Refrigerate suspension after reconstitution; shake vigorously before use and discard after 14 days.
- Discontinue drug if hypersensitivity reaction occurs.
- Give patient yogurt or buttermilk in case of diarrhea.
- Arrange for treatment of superinfections.
- Reculture infection if patient fails to respond.

Teaching points

- Take capsules with meals or food; suspension must be taken on an empty stomach, at least 2 hours before or 1 hour after meals.
- Refrigerate suspension; shake vigorously after use and discard after 14 days.
- Complete the full course of this drug, even if you feel better before the course of treatment is over.
- Avoid alcohol while taking this drug and for 3 days after completion of therapy; serious reactions can occur.
- This drug is prescribed for this particular infection; do not use it to self-treat any other infection.
- You may experience these side effects: Stomach upset, loss of appetite, nausea (take drug with food); diarrhea; headache, dizziness.
- Report severe diarrhea with blood, pus, or mucus; rash or hives; difficulty breathing; unusual tiredness, fatigue; unusual bleeding or bruising.

▽ ceftizoxime sodium

(sef ti ***zox'*** *eem)*

Cefizox

Pregnancy Category B

Drug classes
Antibiotic
Cephalosporin (third generation)

Therapeutic actions
Bactericidal: Inhibits synthesis of bacterial cell wall, causing cell death.

Indications
- Lower respiratory infections caused by *Streptococcus pneumoniae, Staphylococcus aureus, Klebsiella, Haemophilus influenzae, Escherichia coli, Proteus mirabilis, Enterobacter, Serratia, Bacteroides*
- UTIs caused by *S. aureus, Citrobacter, Enterobacter, E. coli, Klebsiella, Pseudomonas aeruginosa, Proteus vulgaris, Proteus rettgeri, Proteus mirabilis, Morganella morganii, Serratia marcescens, Enterobacter*
- Uncomplicated cervical and urethral gonorrhea caused by *Neisseria gonorrhoeae*
- PID caused by *N. gonorrhoeae, E. coli, Streptococcus agalactiae*
- Intra-abdominal infections caused by *E. coli, Staphylococcus epidermidis, Streptococcus* (except enterococci), *Enterobacter, Klebsiella, Bacteroides, Peptococcus, Peptostreptococcus*
- Skin and skin structure infections caused by *S. aureus, E. coli, Klebsiella, Enterobacter, Bacteroides, Peptococcus, Peptostreptococcus, P. mirabilis, S. epidermidis, Streptococcus pyogenes*
- Septicemia caused by *E. coli, Klebsiella, S. pneumoniae, S. aureus, Bacteroides, Serratia*
- Bone and joint infections caused by *S. aureus, Streptococcus* (excluding enterococci), *P. mirabilis, Bacteroides, Peptococcus, Peptostreptococcus*
- Meningitis caused by *H. influenzae,* some cases caused by *S. pneumoniae*
- Mixed infections caused by aerobic gram-negative and mixtures of organisms resistant to other cephalosporins, aminoglycosides, or penicillins

Contraindications and cautions
- Contraindicated with allergy to cephalosporins or penicillins.
- Use cautiously with renal failure, lactation, pregnancy.

Available forms
Powder for injection—500 mg, 1, 2 g; injection in D_5W—1 g/50 mL, 2 g/50 mL

Dosages
Adults
Usual dose, 500 mg–2 g (range 500 mg–4 g) IM or IV every 8–12 hr. Do not exceed 12 g/day. Dosage will vary with infection.
- *Gonorrhea:* Single 1-g IM dose.
- *Uncomplicated UTIs:* 500 mg every 12 hr IM or IV.
- *PID:* 2 g every 8 hr IV.
- *Life-threatening infections:* 3–4 g every 8 hr IV.

Pediatric patients 6 mo and older
50 mg/kg every 6–8 hr; up to 200 mg/kg/day in severe infections. Do not exceed maximum adult dose.

Geriatric patients or patients with reduced renal function
Initial dose of 500 mg–1 g IM or IV followed by:

CrCl (mL/min)	Usual Dosage	Maximum Dosage
50–79	500 mg every 8 hr	0.75–1.5 g every 8 hr
5–49	250–500 mg every 12 hr	0.5–1 g every 12 hr
0–4	500 mg every 48 hr or 250 mg every 24 hr	0.5–1 g every 48 hr or 0.5 g every 24 hr

Pharmacokinetics

Route	Onset	Peak	Duration
IV	Rapid	1 hr	18–24 hr
IM	30 min	1 hr	18–24 hr

Metabolism: $T_{1/2}$: 84–114 min
Distribution: Crosses the placenta; enters breast milk
Excretion: Urine

IV FACTS
Preparation: Dilute reconstituted solution for IV infusion with 50–100 mL of 5% or 10% dextrose injection; 5% dextrose and 0.2%,

0.45%, or 0.9% sodium chloride injection; lactated Ringer's injection; Ringer's injection; 0.9% sodium chloride injection; invert sugar 10% in sterile water for injection; 5% sodium bicarbonate in sterile water for injection; or 5% dextrose in lactated Ringer's injection if reconstituted with 4% sodium bicarbonate injection.

Package Size	*Diluent to Add*	*Volume*	*Resulting Concentration*
1-g vial	10 mL	10.7 mL	95 mg/mL
2-g vial	20 mL	21.4 mL	95 mg/mL

Piggyback vials should be reconstituted with 50–100 mL of any of the above solutions. Shake well, and administer as a single dose with primary IV fluids. Reconstituted solution is stable for 24 hr at room temperature or 4 days if refrigerated; discard solution after allotted time.
Infusion: If given with aminoglycosides, give each antibiotic at a different site. For direct injection, administer slowly over 3–5 min directly or through tubing. For infusion, give over 30 min.
Incompatibilities: Do not mix aminoglycosides and ceftizoxime in the same IV solution.

Adverse effects

- **CNS:** Headache, dizziness, lethargy, paresthesias
- **GI:** *Nausea, vomiting, diarrhea, anorexia, abdominal pain, flatulence,* **pseudomembranous colitis,** hepatotoxicity
- **GU:** Nephrotoxicity
- **Hematologic: Bone marrow depression**—decreased WBC count, decreased platelets, decreased Hct
- **Hypersensitivity:** Ranging from *rash* to *fever* to **anaphylaxis;** serum sickness reaction
- **Local:** *Pain,* abscess at injection site, *phlebitis,* inflammation at IV site
- **Other:** *Superinfections, disulfiram-like reaction with alcohol*

Interactions

✱ **Drug-drug** • Increased nephrotoxicity with aminoglycosides • Increased bleeding effects with oral anticoagulants • Risk of disulfiram-like reaction with alcohol; avoid this combination during and for 3 days after completion of therapy
✱ **Drug-lab test** • Possibility of false results on tests of urine glucose using Benedict's solution, Fehling's solution, Clinitest tablets; urinary 17-ketosteroids; direct Coombs' test

■ Nursing considerations

Assessment

- **History:** Hepatic and renal impairment, lactation, pregnancy
- **Physical:** Skin status, LFTs, renal function tests, culture of affected area, sensitivity tests

Interventions

- Culture infection site, and arrange for sensitivity tests before and during therapy if expected response is not seen.
- Divide and administer IM doses of 2 g at two different sites by deep IM injection.
- Give each antibiotic at a different site, if given as part of combination therapy with aminoglycosides.
- Discontinue if hypersensitivity reaction occurs.
- Have vitamin K available in case hypoprothrombinemia occurs.

Teaching points

- Avoid alcohol while taking this drug and for 3 days after because severe reactions often occur.
- You may experience these side effects: Stomach upset or diarrhea.
- Report severe diarrhea, difficulty breathing, unusual tiredness or fatigue, pain at injection site.

▽ceftriaxone sodium

*(sef try **ax'** ohn)*

Rocephin

PREGNANCY CATEGORY B

Drug classes

Antibiotic
Cephalosporin (third generation)

C

Therapeutic actions

Bactericidal: Inhibits synthesis of bacterial cell wall, causing cell death.

Indications

- Lower respiratory infections caused by *Streptococcus pneumoniae, Staphylococcus aureus, Klebsiella, Haemophilus influenzae, Escherichia coli, Proteus mirabilis, Enterobacter aerogenes, Serratia marcescens, Haemophilus parainfluenzae, Streptococcus* (excluding enterococci)
- **NEW INDICATION:** Acute bacterial otitis media caused by *S. pneumoniae, H. influenzae, Moraxella catarrhalis*
- UTIs caused by *E. coli, Klebsiella, Proteus vulgaris, Proteus mirabilis, Morganella morganii*
- Gonorrhea caused by *Neisseria gonorrhoeae*
- Intra-abdominal infections caused by *E. coli, Klebsiella pneumoniae*
- PID caused by *N. gonorrhoeae*
- Skin and skin structure infections caused by *S. aureus, Klebsiella, Enterobacter cloacae, P. mirabilis, Staphylococcus epidermidis, Pseudomona aeruginosa, Streptococcus* (excluding enterococci)
- Septicemia caused by *E. coli, S. pneumoniae, H. influenzae, S. aureus, K. pneumoniae*
- Bone and joint infections caused by *S. aureus, Streptococcus* (excluding enterococci), *P. mirabilis, S. pneumoniae, E. coli, K. pneumoniae, Enterobacter*
- Meningitis caused by *H. influenzae, S. pneumoniae, Neisseria meningitidis*
- Perioperative prophylaxis for patients undergoing coronary artery bypass surgery and in contaminated or potentially contaminated surgical procedures (eg, vaginal or abdominal hysterectomy)
- Unlabeled use: Treatment of Lyme disease in doses of 2 g IV daily for 14–28 days

Contraindications and cautions

- Contraindicated with allergy to cephalosporins or penicillins.
- Use cautiously with renal failure, lactation, pregnancy.

Available forms

Powder for injection—2 g; injection—1, 2 g

Dosages

Adults

1–2 g/day IM or IV once a day or in equal divided doses bid. Do not exceed 4 g/day.

- *Gonorrhea:* Single 250-mg IM dose.
- *Meningitis:* 2 g IV every 12 hr, or 50–100 mg/kg every 12 hr for 4–14 days. Do not exceed 4 g/day.
- *Perioperative prophylaxis:* Give 1 g IV 30–120 min before surgery.

Pediatric patients

50–75 mg/kg/day IV or IM in divided doses every 12 hr. Do not exceed 2 g/day.

- *Meningitis:* 100 mg/kg/day IV or IM in divided doses every 12 hr for 7–14 days. Do not exceed 4 g/day. Loading dose of 80–100 mg/kg may be used.

Pharmacokinetics

Route	*Onset*	*Peak*	*Duration*
IV	Rapid	Immediate	15–18 hr
IM	30 min	1.5–4 hr	15–18 hr

Metabolism: $T_{1/2}$: 5–10 hr

Distribution: Crosses the placenta; enters breast milk

Excretion: Bile, urine

IV FACTS

Preparation: Dilute reconstituted solution for IV infusion with 50–100 mL of 5% or 10% dextrose injection, 5% dextrose and 0.45% or 0.9% sodium chloride injection, 0.9% sodium chloride injection, 10% invert sugar, 5% sodium bicarbonate, *FreAmine 111, Normosol-M in 5% Dextrose, Ionosol-B in 5% Dextrose,* 5% or 10% mannitol, sodium lactate.

Package Size	*Diluent to Add*	*Resulting Concentration*
250-mg vial	2.4 mL	100 mg/mL
500-mg vial	4.8 mL	100 mg/mL
1-g vial	9.6 mL	100 mg/mL
2-g vial	19.2 mL	100 mg/mL
Piggyback 1 g	10 mL	
Piggyback 2 g	20 mL	

Stability of reconstituted and diluted solution depends on diluent, concentration and type of container (eg, glass, PVC); check manufacturer's inserts for specific details. Protect drug from light.

Infusion: Administer by intermittent infusion over 15–30 min. Do not mix ceftriaxone with any other antimicrobial drug.
Incompatibilities: Do not mix aminoglycosides and ceftriaxone in the same IV solution.

Adverse effects

- **CNS:** Headache, dizziness, lethargy, paresthesias
- **GI:** *Nausea, vomiting, diarrhea, anorexia, abdominal pain, flatulence,* **pseudomembranous colitis,** hepatotoxicity
- **GU:** Nephrotoxicity
- **Hematologic: Bone marrow depression**—decreased WBC count, decreased platelets, decreased Hct
- **Hypersensitivity:** *Ranging from rash* to *fever* to **anaphylaxis;** serum sickness reaction
- **Local:** *Pain,* abscess at injection site; *phlebitis,* inflammation at IV site
- **Other:** *Superinfections, disulfiram-like reaction with alcohol*

Interactions

✱ **Drug-drug** • Increased nephrotoxicity with aminoglycosides • Increased bleeding effects with oral anticoagulants • Disulfiram-like reaction may occur if alcohol is taken within 72 hr after ceftriaxone administration
✱ **Drug-lab test** • Possibility of false results on tests of urine glucose using Benedict's solution, Fehling's solution, Clinitest tablets; urinary 17-ketosteroids; direct Coombs' test

■ Nursing considerations

Assessment

- **History:** Hepatic and renal impairment, lactation, pregnancy
- **Physical:** Skin status, LFTs, renal function tests, culture of affected area, sensitivity tests

Interventions

- Culture infection site, and arrange for sensitivity tests before and during therapy if expected response is not seen.
- Reconstitute for IM use with sterile water for injection, 0.9% sodium chloride solution, 5% dextrose solution, bacteriostatic water with 0.9% benzyl alcohol, or 1% lidocaine solution (without epinephrine); inject deeply into a large muscle group.
- Check manufacturer's inserts for specific details. Stability of reconstituted and diluted solution depends on diluent, concentration and type of container (eg, glass, PVC).
- Protect drug from light.

⊗ ***Warning*** Do not mix ceftriaxone with any other antimicrobial drug.

- Monitor ceftriaxone blood levels in patients with severe renal impairment and in patients with renal and hepatic impairment.
- Have vitamin K available in case hypoprothrombinemia occurs.
- Discontinue if hypersensitivity reaction occurs.

Teaching points

- Avoid alcohol while taking this drug and for 3 days after because severe reactions often occur.
- You may experience these side effects: Stomach upset or diarrhea.
- Report severe diarrhea, difficulty breathing, unusual tiredness or fatigue, pain at injection site.

▽ cefuroxime
(se fyoor ***ox'*** *eem)*

cefuroxime axetil
Ceftin (DNC)

cefuroxime sodium
Zinacef

PREGNANCY CATEGORY B

Drug classes

Antibiotic
Cephalosporin (second generation)

Therapeutic actions

Bactericidal: Inhibits synthesis of bacterial cell wall, causing cell death.

Indications

Oral (cefuroxime axetil)

- Pharyngitis, tonsillitis caused by *Streptococcus pyogenes*
- Otitis media caused by *Streptococcus pneumoniae, S. pyogenes, Haemophilus influenzae, Moraxella catarrhalis*
- Acute bacterial maxillary sinusitis caused by *S. pneumoniae, H. influenzae*
- Lower respiratory infections caused by *S. pneumoniae, Haemophilus parainfluenzae, H. influenzae*
- UTIs caused by *Escherichia coli, Klebsiella pneumoniae*
- Uncomplicated gonorrhea (urethral and endocervical)
- Skin and skin structure infections, including impetigo caused by *Streptococcus aureus, S. pyogenes*
- Treatment of early Lyme disease

Parenteral (cefuroxime sodium)

- Lower respiratory infections caused by *S. pneumoniae, S. aureus, E. coli, Klebsiella pneuemoniae, H. influenzae, S. pyogenes*
- Dermatologic infections caused by *S. aureus, S. pyogenes, E. coli, K. pneuemoniae, Enterobacter*
- UTIs caused by *E. coli, K. pneumoniae*
- Uncomplicated and disseminated gonorrhea caused by *N. gonorrhoeae*
- Septicemia caused by *S. pneumoniae, S. aureus, E. coli, K. pneumoniae, H. influenzae*
- Meningitis caused by *S. pneumoniae, H. influenzae, S. aureus, N. meningitidis*
- Bone and joint infections due to *S. aureus*
- Perioperative prophylaxis
- Treatment of acute bacterial maxillary sinusitis in patients 3 mo–12 yr

Contraindications and cautions

- Contraindicated with allergy to cephalosporins or penicillins.
- Use cautiously with renal failure, lactation, pregnancy.

Available forms

Tablets DNC—125, 250, 500 mg; suspension—125 mg/5 mL, 250 mg/5 mL; powder for injection—750 mg, 1.5 g; injection—750 mg, 1.5 g

Dosages

Oral

Adults and patients 12 yr and older

250 mg bid. For severe infections, may be increased to 500 mg bid. Treat for up to 10 days.

- *Uncomplicated UTIs:* 250 mg bid. Treat for 7–10 days.
- *Uncomplicated gonorrhea:* 1,000 mg once as a single dose.

Pediatric patients younger than 12 yr

125 mg bid.

- *Acute otitis media:*
  3 mo–12 yr: 250 mg PO bid for 10 days in children who can swallow tablets whole. Or, 30 mg/kg/day (maximum, 1 g/day) in two divided doses for 10 days (oral solution).
- *Pharyngitis or tonsillitis:*
  3 mo–12 yr: 125 mg PO every 12 hr for 10 days in children who can swallow tablets whole. Or, 20 mg/kg/day (maximum, 500 mg/day) in two divided doses for 10 days (oral solution).
- *Acute sinusitis:*
  3 mo–12 yr: 250 mg PO bid for 10 days in children who can swallow tablets whole. Or, 30 mg/kg/day (maximum, 1 g/day) in two divided doses for 10 days (oral solution).
- *Impetigo:*
  3 mo–12 yr: 30 mg/kg/day (maximum, 1 g/day) in two divided doses for 10 days (oral suspension).

Parenteral

Adults

750 mg–1.5 g IM or IV every 8 hr, depending on severity of infection, for 5–10 days.

- *Uncomplicated gonorrhea:* 1.5 g IM (at two different sites) with 1 g of oral probenecid.
- *Perioperative prophylaxis:* 1.5 g IV 30–60 min prior to initial incision; then 750 mg IV or IM every 8 hr for 24 hr after surgery.

Pediatric patients older than 3 mo

50–100 mg/kg/day IM or IV in divided doses every 6–8 hr.

- *Bacterial meningitis:* 200–240 mg/kg/day IV in divided doses every 6–8 hr.

Pediatric patients with impaired renal function

Adjust adult dosage for renal impairment by weight or age of child.

Geriatric patients or adults with impaired renal function

CrCl (mL/min)	*Dosage*
More than 20	750 mg–1.5 g every 8 hr
10–20	750 mg every 12 hr
Less than 10	750 mg every 24 hr

Pharmacokinetics

Route	*Onset*	*Peak*	*Duration*
IV	Rapid	Immediate	18–24 hr
IM	20 min	30 min	18–24 hr
Oral	Varies	2 hr	18–24 hr

Metabolism: $T_{1/2}$: 1–2 hr
Distribution: Crosses the placenta; enters breast milk
Excretion: Urine

IV FACTS

Preparation: Preparation of parenteral drug solutions and suspensions differs for different starting preparations and different brand names; check the manufacturer's directions carefully. Reconstitute parenteral drug with sterile water for injection, D_5W, 0.9% sodium chloride, or any of the following, which also may be used for further dilution: 0.9% sodium chloride, 5% or 10% dextrose injection, 5% dextrose and 0.45% or 0.9% sodium chloride injection, or 1/6 M sodium lactate injection. Stability of solutions depends on diluent and concentration: Check manufacturer's specifications.

⊗ ***Warning*** Do not mix with IV solutions containing aminoglycosides. Powder form, solutions, and suspensions darken during storage.

Infusion: Inject slowly over 3–5 min directly into vein for IV administration, or infuse over 30 min; may be given by continuous infusion. Give aminoglycosides and cefuroxime at different sites.

Incompatibilities: Do not mix aminoglycosides and cefuroxime in the same IV solution.

Adverse effects

- **CNS:** Headache, dizziness, lethargy, paresthesias
- **GI:** *Nausea, vomiting, diarrhea, anorexia, abdominal pain, flatulence,* **pseudomembranous colitis,** hepatotoxicity
- **GU:** Nephrotoxicity
- **Hematologic: Bone marrow depression** (decreased WBC, decreased platelets, decreased Hct)
- **Hypersensitivity:** *Ranging from rash* to *fever* to **anaphylaxis;** serum sickness reaction
- **Local:** *Pain,* abscess at injection site, *phlebitis,* inflammation at IV site
- **Other:** *Superinfections, disulfiram-like reaction with alcohol*

Interactions

✱ **Drug-drug** • Increased nephrotoxicity with aminoglycosides • Increased bleeding effects with oral anticoagulants • Risk of disulfiram-like reaction with alcohol; avoid this combination during and for 3 days after completion of therapy

✱ **Drug-lab test** • Possibility of false results on tests of urine glucose using Benedict's solution, Fehling's solution, Clinitest tablets; urinary 17-ketosteroids; direct Coombs' test

■ Nursing considerations

Assessment

- **History:** Hepatic and renal impairment, lactation, pregnancy
- **Physical:** Skin status, LFTs, renal function tests, culture of affected area, sensitivity tests

Interventions

- Culture infection site, and arrange for sensitivity tests before and during therapy if expected response is not seen.
- Give oral drug with food to decrease GI upset and enhance absorption.
- Give oral tablets to children who can swallow tablets; crushing the drug results in a bitter, unpleasant taste. Use solution for children who cannot swallow tablets.
- Have vitamin K available in case hypoprothrombinemia occurs.
- Discontinue if hypersensitivity reaction occurs.

Teaching points

Oral drug

- Take full course of therapy even if you are feeling better.
- This drug is specific for this infection and should not be used to self-treat other problems.
- Swallow tablets whole; do not crush them. Take the drug with food.
- Store solution in the refrigerator. Shake well before each use.
- You may experience these side effects: Stomach upset or diarrhea.
- Report severe diarrhea with blood, pus, or mucus; rash; difficulty breathing; unusual tiredness, fatigue; unusual bleeding or bruising; unusual itching or irritation.

Parenteral drug

- Avoid alcohol while taking this drug and for 3 days after because severe reactions often occur.
- You may experience these side effects: Stomach upset or diarrhea.
- Report severe diarrhea, difficulty breathing, unusual tiredness or fatigue, pain at injection site.

celecoxib

*(sell ah **cocks'** ib)*

Celebrex

PREGNANCY CATEGORY C (FIRST AND SECOND TRIMESTER)

PREGNANCY CATEGORY D (THIRD TRIMESTER)

Drug classes

Analgesic (nonopioid)
NSAID
Specific COX-2 enzyme inhibitor

Therapeutic actions

Analgesic and anti-inflammatory activities related to inhibition of the COX-2 enzyme, which is activated in inflammation to cause the signs and symptoms associated with inflammation; does not affect the COX-1 enzyme, which protects the lining of the GI tract and has blood clotting and renal functions.

Indications

- Acute and long-term treatment of signs and symptoms of rheumatoid arthritis and osteoarthritis
- Reduction of the number of colorectal polyps in familial adenomatous polyposis (FAP)
- Management of acute pain
- Treatment of primary dysmenorrhea
- Relief of signs and symptoms of ankylosing spondylitis
- Relief of signs and symptoms of juvenile rheumatoid arthritis

NEW INDICATION: Unlabeled uses: Treatment of preterm labor; prevention of colorectal cancer; adjunctive therapy in schizophrenia

Contraindications and cautions

- Contraindicated with allergies to sulfonamides, celecoxib, NSAIDs, or aspirin; significant renal impairment; perioperative pain post CABG surgery; pregnancy (third trimester); lactation.
- Use cautiously with impaired hearing, hepatic and CV conditions.

Available forms

Capsules—50, 100, 200, 400 mg

Dosages

Adults

Initially, 100 mg PO bid; may increase to 200 mg/day PO bid as needed.

- *Acute pain, dysmenorrhea:* 400 mg, then 200 mg PO bid.
- *FAP:* 400 mg PO bid.
- *Ankylosing spondylitis:* 200 mg/day PO; after 6 wk, a trial of 400 mg/day may be tried for 6 wk; if no effect is seen, suggest another therapy.

Pediatric patients 2 yr and older

10 kg or 25 kg or less: 50 mg capsule PO bid.
More than 25 kg: 100 mg capsule PO bid.

Patients with hepatic impairment

Reduce dosage by 50%.

Pharmacokinetics

Route	Onset	Peak
Oral	Slow	3 hr

Metabolism: Hepatic; $T_{1/2}$: 11 hr

Distribution: Crosses placenta; may enter breast milk
Excretion: Bile, urine

Adverse effects

- **CNS:** *Headache, dizziness, somnolence, insomnia,* fatigue, tiredness, dizziness, tinnitus, ophthalmologic effects
- **CV: MI, CVA**
- **Dermatologic:** *Rash,* pruritus, sweating, dry mucous membranes, stomatitis
- **GI:** Nausea, abdominal pain, *dyspepsia,* flatulence, GI bleed
- **Hematologic:** Neutropenia, eosinophilia, leukopenia, pancytopenia, thrombocytopenia, agranulocytosis, granulocytopenia, aplastic anemia, decreased Hgb or Hct, bone marrow depression, menorrhagia
- **Other:** Peripheral edema, **anaphylactoid reactions** to **anaphylactic shock**

Interactions

✱ **Drug-drug** • Increased risk of bleeding if taken concurrently with warfarin. Monitor patient closely and reduce warfarin dose as appropriate • Increased lithium levels and toxicity • Increased risk of GI bleeding with long-term alcohol use, smoking

■ Nursing considerations

CLINICAL ALERT!
Name confusion has occurred between *Celebrex* (celecoxib), *Celexa* (citalopram), *Xanax* (alprazolam), and *Cerebyx* (fosphenytoin); use caution.

Assessment

- **History:** Renal impairment, impaired hearing, allergies, hepatic and CV conditions, lactation, pregnancy
- **Physical:** Skin color and lesions; orientation, reflexes, ophthalmologic and audiometric evaluation, peripheral sensation; P, edema; R, adventitious sounds; liver evaluation; CBC, LFTs, renal function tests; serum electrolytes

Interventions

⊗ ***Black box warning*** Be aware that patient may be at increased risk for CV events, GI bleeding; monitor accordingly.

- Administer drug with food or after meals if GI upset occurs.
- Establish safety measures if CNS or visual disturbances occur.
- Arrange for periodic ophthalmologic examination during long-term therapy.

⊗ ***Warning*** If overdose occurs, institute emergency procedures—gastric lavage, induction of emesis, supportive therapy.

- Provide further comfort measures to reduce pain (eg, positioning, environmental control) and to reduce inflammation (eg, warmth, positioning, rest).

Teaching points

- Take drug with food or meals if GI upset occurs.
- Take only the prescribed dosage; do not increase dosage.
- You may experience these side effects: Dizziness, drowsiness (avoid driving or the use of dangerous machinery while taking this drug).
- Report sore throat, fever, rash, itching, weight gain, swelling in ankles or fingers; changes in vision.

▽cellulose sodium phosphate (CSP)

See Appendix W, *Less commonly used drugs*.

▽cephalexin

*(sef a **lex'** in)*

Apo-Cephalex (CAN), Keflex, Novo-Lexin (CAN), Nu-Cephalex (CAN)

PREGNANCY CATEGORY B

Drug classes

Antibiotic
Cephalosporin (first generation)

Therapeutic actions
Bactericidal: Inhibits synthesis of bacterial cell wall, causing cell death.

Indications
- Respiratory tract infections caused by *Streptococcus pneumoniae,* group A beta-hemolytic streptococci
- Skin and skin structure infections caused by staphylococcus, streptococcus
- Otitis media caused by *S. pneumoniae, Haemophilus influenzae,* streptococcus, staphylococcus, *Moraxella catarrhalis*
- Bone infections caused by staphylococcus, *Proteus mirabilis*
- GU infections caused by *Escherichia coli, P. mirabilis, Klebsiella*

Contraindications and cautions
- Contraindicated with allergy to cephalosporins or penicillins.
- Use cautiously with renal failure, lactation, pregnancy.

Available forms
Capsules—250, 333, 500, 750 mg; tablets—250, 500 mg; oral suspension—125 mg/5 mL, 250 mg/5 mL

Dosages
Adults
1–4 g/day in divided doses; 250 mg PO every 6 hr usual dose.
- *Skin and skin structure infections:* 500 mg PO every 12 hr. Larger doses may be needed in severe cases; do not exceed 4 g/day.

Pediatric patients
25–50 mg/kg/day PO in divided doses.
- *Skin and skin structure infections:* Divide total daily dose, and give every 12 hr. Dosage may be doubled in severe cases.
- *Otitis media:* 75–100 mg/kg/day PO in four divided doses.

Pharmacokinetics

Route	*Peak*	*Duration*
Oral	60 min	8–10 hr

Metabolism: $T_{1/2}$: 50–80 min
Distribution: Crosses the placenta, enters breast milk
Excretion: Urine

Adverse effects
- **CNS:** Headache, dizziness, lethargy, paresthesias
- **GI:** *Nausea, vomiting, diarrhea, anorexia, abdominal pain, flatulence,* **pseudomembranous colitis,** hepatotoxicity
- **GU:** Nephrotoxicity
- **Hematologic: Bone marrow depression**
- **Hypersensitivity:** *Ranging from rash* to *fever* to **anaphylaxis;** serum sickness reaction
- **Other:** *Superinfections*

Interactions
✱ **Drug-drug** • Increased nephrotoxicity with aminoglycosides • Increased bleeding effects with oral anticoagulants • Disulfiram-like reaction may occur if alcohol is taken within 72 hr after cephalexin administration
✱ **Drug-lab test** • Possibility of false results on tests of urine glucose using Benedict's solution, Fehling's solution, Clinitest tablets; urinary 17-ketosteroids; direct Coombs' test

■ Nursing considerations
Assessment
- **History:** Penicillin or cephalosporin allergy, pregnancy, or lactation
- **Physical:** Renal function tests, respiratory status, skin status; culture and sensitivity tests of infected area

Interventions
- Arrange for culture and sensitivity tests of infection before and during therapy if infection does not resolve.
- Give drug with meals; arrange for small, frequent meals if GI complications occur.
- Refrigerate suspension, discard after 14 days.

Teaching points
- Take this drug with food. Refrigerate suspension; discard any drug after 14 days.
- Complete the full course of this drug even if you feel better.
- This drug is prescribed for this particular infection; do not self-treat any other infection.
- You may experience these side effects: Stomach upset, loss of appetite, nausea (take drug with food); diarrhea; headache, dizziness.

- Avoid alcohol while taking cephalexin and for 3 days after completion of therapy.
- Report severe diarrhea with blood, pus, or mucus; rash or hives; difficulty breathing; unusual tiredness, fatigue; unusual bleeding or bruising.

certolizumab

See Appendix W, *Less commonly used drugs*.

cetirizine hydrochloride

(se teer' i zeen)

Reactine (CAN), Zyrtec, Zyrtec Allergy, Zyrtec Children's Allergy, Zyrtec Children's Hives Relief, Zyrtec Hives Relief

PREGNANCY CATEGORY B

Drug class

Antihistamine

Therapeutic actions

Potent specific histamine (H_1) receptor antagonist; inhibits histamine release and eosinophil chemotaxis during inflammation, leading to reduced swelling and decreased inflammatory response.

Indications

- Management of seasonal and perennial allergic rhinitis, allergies, hay fever
- Treatment of chronic, idiopathic urticaria
- Treatment of year-round allergic rhinitis and chronic idiopathic urticaria in infants older than 6 mo
- Unlabeled uses: To decrease wheal response and pruritus of mosquito bites; possible use in allergic asthma

Contraindications and cautions

- Contraindicated with allergy to any antihistamines, hydroxyzine.
- Use cautiously with narrow-angle glaucoma, stenosing peptic ulcer, symptomatic prostatic hypertrophy, asthmatic attack, bladder neck obstruction, pyloroduodenal obstruction (avoid use or use with caution as condition may be exacerbated by drug effects); lactation.

Available forms

Tablets—5, 10 mg; chewable tablets—5, 10 mg; oral solution—1 mg/mL

Dosages

Adults and children 6 yr and older

10 mg/day PO or 5 mg PO bid; maximum dose 10 mg/day.

Pediatric patients 6–11 yr

5 or 10 mg PO daily.

Pediatric patients 2–6 yr

2.5 mg PO once daily to a maximum 5 mg/day.

Pediatric patients 6 mo–2 yr

2.5 mg (one-half tsp) PO once daily. In children 1 yr and older, may increase to maximum 5 mg daily given as one-half tsp (2.5 mL) every 12 hr.

Patients with hepatic or renal impairment, elderly patients

5 mg PO daily.

Pharmacokinetics

Route	*Onset*	*Peak*	*Duration*
Oral	Rapid	1 hr	24 hr

Metabolism: Hepatic; $T_{1/2}$: 7–10 hr
Distribution: Crosses placenta; enters breast milk
Excretion: Feces, urine

Adverse effects

- **CNS:** *Somnolence, sedation*
- **CV:** Palpitation, edema, dizziness
- **GI:** Nausea, diarrhea, abdominal pain, constipation, dry mouth
- **Respiratory: Bronchospasm,** pharyngitis
- **Other:** Fever, photosensitivity, rash, myalgia, arthralgia, angioedema, fatigue

■ Nursing considerations

CLINICAL ALERT!

Name confusion has occurred between *Zyrtec* (cetirizine) and *Zyprexa* (olanzapine) and between *Zyrtec* (cetirizine) and *Zantac* (ranitidine); use caution.

Assessment
- **History:** Allergy to any antihistamines, hydroxyzine; narrow-angle glaucoma, stenosing peptic ulcer, symptomatic prostatic hypertrophy, asthmatic attack, bladder neck obstruction, pyloroduodenal obstruction; lactation
- **Physical:** Skin color, lesions, texture; orientation, reflexes, affect; vision examination; R, adventitious sounds; prostate palpation; renal and hepatic function tests

Interventions
- Give without regard to meals.
- Provide oral solution form or chewable tablets for pediatric use if needed.
- Arrange for use of humidifier if thickening of secretions, nasal dryness become bothersome; encourage adequate intake of fluids.
- Provide skin care for urticaria.

Teaching points
- Take this drug without regard to meals.
- You may experience these side effects: Dizziness, sedation, drowsiness (use caution if driving or performing tasks that require alertness); thickening of bronchial secretions, dry nasal mucosa (humidifier may help).
- Report difficulty breathing, hallucinations, tremors, loss of coordination, irregular heartbeat.

cetrorelix acetate

See Appendix W, *Less commonly used drugs*.

cetuximab

See Appendix W, *Less commonly used drugs*.

cevimeline hydrochloride

See Appendix W, *Less commonly used drugs*.

charcoal, activated
(char' kole)

OTC: Actidose-Aqua, Actidose with Sorbitol, CharcoAid, CharcoAid 2000, Liqui-Char

PREGNANCY CATEGORY C

Drug class
Antidote

Therapeutic actions
Adsorbs toxic substances swallowed into the GI tract, inhibiting GI absorption; maximum amount of toxin absorbed is 100–1,000 mg/g charcoal.

Indications
- Emergency treatment in poisoning by most drugs and chemicals

Contraindications and cautions
- Contraindicated with poisoning or overdosage of cyanide, mineral acids, alkalies.
- Use cautiously; not effective with ethanol, methanol, and iron salts.

Available forms
Powder—15, 30, 40, 120, 240 g; liquid—208 mg/mL, 12.5 g/60 mL, 15 g/75 mL, 15 g/120 mL, 25 g/120 mL, 30 g/120 mL, 50 g/240 mL; suspension—15, 30 g; granules—15 g

Dosages
Adults
50–60 g or 1 g/kg PO or approximately 5–10 times the amount of poison ingested, as an oral suspension; administer as soon as possible after poisoning.
- *Gastric dialysis:* 20–40 g every 6 hr for 1–2 days for severe poisonings; for optimum effect, administer within 30 min of poisoning.

Pediatric patients 1–12 yr
Weighing more than 32 kg: 50–60 g.
Weighing16–32 kg: 25–30 g.
Weighing less than 16 kg and younger than 1 yr: Not recommended.

Pharmacokinetics
Not absorbed systemically
Excretion: Feces

Adverse effects
- **GI:** *Vomiting* (related to rapid ingestion of high doses), *constipation, diarrhea,* black stools

Interactions
✱ **Drug-drug** • Adsorption and inactivation of laxatives with activated charcoal • Decreased effectiveness of other medications because of adsorption by activated charcoal
✱ **Drug-food** • Decreased adsorptive capacity if taken with milk, ice cream, or sherbet

■ Nursing considerations

CLINICAL ALERT!
Name confusion can occur between *Actidose* (charcoal) and *Actos* (pioglitazone); use caution.

Assessment
- **History:** Poisoning or overdosage of cyanide, mineral acids, alkalies, ethanol, methanol, and iron salts
- **Physical:** Stools, bowel sounds

Interventions
- Repeat dose if patient vomits shortly after administration.
- Give drug to conscious patients only.
- Take measures to prevent aspiration of charcoal powder; fatalities have occurred.
- Give drug as soon after poisoning as possible; most effective results are seen if given within 30 min.
- Prepare suspension of powder in 6–8 oz of water; taste may be gritty and disagreeable. Sorbitol is added to some preparations to improve taste; diarrhea more likely with these preparations.
- Store in closed containers; activated charcoal adsorbs gases from the air and will lose its effectiveness with prolonged exposure to air.
- Ensure that life-support equipment is readily available for poisoning and overdose.

Teaching points
- Drink 6–8 glasses of liquid per day to avoid constipation.
- You may experience these side effects: Black stools, diarrhea, constipation.

▽ chenodiol
See Appendix W, *Less commonly used drugs*.

DANGEROUS DRUG

▽ chloral hydrate
*(klor al **hye'** drate)*

Aquachloral Supprettes, Chloral Hydrate-Odan (CAN), Somnote (DNC)

PREGNANCY CATEGORY C

CONTROLLED SUBSTANCE C-IV

Drug class
Sedative-hypnotic (nonbarbiturate)

Therapeutic actions
Mechanism by which CNS is affected is not known; hypnotic dosage produces mild cerebral depression and quiet, deep sleep; does not depress REM sleep, produces less hangover than most barbiturates and benzodiazepines.

Indications
- Nocturnal sedation
- Preoperative sedation to lessen anxiety and induce sleep without depressing respiration or cough reflex
- Adjunct to opiates and analgesics in postoperative care and control of pain
- Prevention or suppression of alcohol-withdrawal symptoms (rectal form)

Contraindications and cautions
- Contraindicated with hypersensitivity to chloral derivatives, allergy to tartrazine (in 324-mg and 648-mg suppositories marketed as *Aquachloral Supprettes*), severe cardiac disease, gastritis, gastric or duodenal ulcers; hepatic or renal impairment, lactation.

- Use cautiously with acute intermittent porphyria (may precipitate attacks).

Available forms

Capsules ONC—500 mg; syrup—250 mg/5 mL, 500 mg/5 mL; suppositories—325, 500, 650 mg

Dosages

Adults

Single doses or daily dose should not exceed 2 g.

- *Hypnotic:* 500 mg–1 g PO or rectally 15–30 min before bedtime or 30 min before surgery. It is not usually considered safe practice to give oral medication to patients who are NPO for anesthesia or surgery.
- *Sedative:* 250 mg PO or rectally tid after meals.
- *Alcohol withdrawal:* 500 mg–1 g rectally, repeated at 6-hr intervals as needed.

Pediatric patients

- *Hypnotic:* 50 mg/kg/day PO up to 1 g per single dose; may be given in divided doses.
- *Sedative:* 25 mg/kg/day PO up to 500 mg per single dose; may be given in divided doses.

Pharmacokinetics

Route	*Onset*	*Peak*	*Duration*
Oral, rectal	30–60 min	1–3 hr	4–8 hr

Metabolism: Hepatic; $T_{1/2}$: 7–10 hr
Distribution: Crosses placenta; enters breast milk
Excretion: Bile, urine

Adverse effects

- **CNS:** *Somnambulism, disorientation, incoherence, paranoid behavior,* excitement, delirium, drowsiness, staggering gait, ataxia, light-headedness, vertigo, nightmares, malaise, mental confusion, headache, hallucinations
- **Dermatologic:** *Skin irritation;* allergic rashes including hives, erythema, eczematoid dermatitis, urticaria
- **GI:** Gastric irritation, nausea, vomiting, **gastric necrosis** (following intoxicating doses), flatulence, diarrhea, unpleasant taste
- **Hematologic:** Leukopenia, eosinophilia
- **Other:** Physical, psychological dependence; tolerance; withdrawal reaction; hangover

Interactions

✱ **Drug-drug** • Additive CNS depression with alcohol, other CNS depressants • Mutual inhibition of metabolism with alcohol • Complex effects on oral (warfarin) anticoagulants given with chloral hydrate; monitor prothrombin levels and adjust warfarin dosage whenever chloral hydrate is instituted or withdrawn from drug regimen

✱ **Drug-lab test** • Interference with the copper sulfate test for glycosuria, fluorometric tests for urine catecholamines, and urinary 17-hydroxycorticosteroid determinations (when using the Reddy, Jenkins, and Thorn procedure)

■ Nursing considerations

Assessment

- **History:** Hypersensitivity to chloral derivatives, allergy to tartrazine, severe cardiac disease, gastritis, hepatic or renal impairment, acute intermittent porphyria, lactation
- **Physical:** Skin color, lesions; orientation, affect, reflexes; P, BP, perfusion; bowel sounds, normal output, liver evaluation; LFTs, renal function tests, CBC and differential, stool guaiac test

Interventions

- Give capsules with a full glass of liquid; ensure that patient swallows capsules whole; give syrup in half glass of water, fruit juice, or ginger ale.
- Supervise dose and amount of drug prescribed for patients who are addiction prone or alcoholic; give least amount feasible to patients who are depressed or suicidal.
- Withdraw gradually over 2 wk if patient has been maintained on high doses for weeks or months; if patient has built up high tolerance, withdrawal should occur in a hospital, using supportive therapy similar to that for barbiturate withdrawal; fatal withdrawal reactions have occurred.
- Reevaluate patients with prolonged insomnia; therapy for the underlying cause (eg, pain, depression) is preferable to prolonged use of sedative-hypnotic drugs.

Teaching points

- Take this drug exactly as prescribed: Swallow capsules whole with a full glass of liquid

(take syrup in half glass of water, fruit juice, or ginger ale).
- Do not discontinue the drug abruptly. Consult your health care provider if you wish to discontinue the drug.
- Avoid alcohol, sleep-inducing, or over-the-counter drugs; these could cause dangerous effects.
- You may experience these side effects: Drowsiness, dizziness, light-headedness (avoid driving or performing tasks requiring alertness); GI upset (eat frequent small meals); sleep-walking, nightmares, confusion (use caution: close doors, keep medications out of reach so inadvertent overdose does not occur while confused).
- Report rash, coffee ground vomitus, black or tarry stools, severe GI upset, fever, sore throat.

DANGEROUS DRUG

chlorambucil

*(klor **am'** byoo sil)*

Leukeran

PREGNANCY CATEGORY D

Drug classes
Alkylating drug, nitrogen mustard derivative
Antineoplastic

Therapeutic actions
Cytotoxic: Alkylates cellular DNA, interfering with the replication of susceptible cells.

Indications
- Palliative treatment of chronic lymphocytic leukemia; malignant lymphomas, including lymphosarcoma; giant follicular lymphoma; and Hodgkin's lymphoma
- Unlabeled uses: Ovarian and testicular carcinoma, Waldenstrom's macroglobulinemia, non-Hodgkin's lymphoma, polycythemia vera

Contraindications and cautions
- Contraindicated with allergy to chlorambucil; cross-sensitization with melphalan, pregnancy.
- Use cautiously with radiation therapy, chemotherapy, myelosuppression, lactation.

Available forms
Tablets—2 mg

Dosages
Individualize dosage based on hematologic profile and response.

Adults
- *Initial dose and short-course therapy:* 0.1–0.2 mg/kg per day PO for 3–6 wk; single daily dose may be given.
- *Chronic lymphocytic leukemia (alternate regimen):* 0.4 mg/kg PO every 2 wk, increasing by 0.1 mg/kg with each dose until therapeutic or toxic effect occurs.
- *Maintenance dose:* 0.03–0.1 mg/kg/day PO. Do not exceed 0.1 mg/kg/day. Short courses of therapy are safer than continuous maintenance therapy; base dosage and duration on patient response and bone marrow status.

Pediatric patients
Safety and efficacy not established.

Pharmacokinetics

Route	Onset	Peak	Duration
Oral	Varies	1 hr	15–20 hr

Metabolism: Hepatic; $T_{1/2}$: 60–90 min
Distribution: Crosses placenta; enters breast milk
Excretion: Urine

Adverse effects
- **CNS:** Tremors, muscular twitching, confusion, agitation, ataxia, flaccid paresis, hallucinations, seizures
- **Dermatologic:** Rash, urticaria, *alopecia*, keratitis, **Stevens-Johnson syndrome, erythema multiforme**
- **GI:** *Nausea, vomiting, stomatitis,* anorexia, **hepatotoxicity,** jaundice (rare)
- **GU:** *Sterility* (especially in prepubertal or pubertal males and adult men; amenorrhea can occur in females)
- **Hematologic: Bone marrow depression,** hyperuricemia
- **Respiratory:** Bronchopulmonary dysplasia, pulmonary fibrosis
- **Other:** Cancer, **acute leukemia**

■ Nursing considerations

CLINICAL ALERT!
Name confusion has occurred between *Leukeran* (chlorambucil), *Myleran* (busulfan), *Alkeran* (melphalan), and leucovorin; use caution.

Assessment

- **History:** Allergy to chlorambucil, cross-sensitization with melphalan (rash), radiation therapy, chemotherapy, hematopoietic depression, pregnancy, lactation
- **Physical:** T; weight; skin color, lesions; R, adventitious sounds; liver evaluation; CBC, differential, Hgb, uric acid, LFTs

Interventions

⊠ ***Black box warning*** Arrange for blood tests to evaluate hematopoietic function before and weekly during therapy. Severe bone marrow suppression can occur.

⊠ ***Black box warning*** This drug is carcinogenic. Monitor patient regularly.

- Do not give full dosage within 4 wk after a full course of radiation therapy or chemotherapy because of risk of severe bone marrow depression.
- Ensure that patient is well hydrated before treatment.

⊠ ***Black box warning*** Ensure that patient is not pregnant before beginning therapy; encourage use of barrier contraceptives because this drug is teratogenic. This drug may also cause infertility.

⊗ ***Warning*** Monitor uric acid levels; ensure adequate fluid intake, and prepare for appropriate treatment of hyperuricemia if it occurs.

- Divide single daily dose if nausea and vomiting occur with large single dose.

Teaching points

- Take this drug once a day and take it with food. If nausea and vomiting occur, consult health care provider about dividing the dose.
- You may experience these side effects: Nausea, vomiting, loss of appetite (dividing dose, eat frequent small meals; maintain your fluid intake and nutrition; drink at least 10–12 glasses of fluid each day); infertility (from irregular menses to complete amenorrhea; men may stop producing sperm—may be irreversible; discuss with your health care provider); severe birth defects—use barrier contraceptives; cancer—follow all suggested screening protocols.
- Report unusual bleeding or bruising, fever, chills, sore throat; cough, shortness of breath, yellow skin or eyes, flank or stomach pain.

C

▽ chloramphenicol

*(klor am **fen'** i kole)*

chloramphenicol sodium succinate

PREGNANCY CATEGORY C

Drug class

Antibiotic

Therapeutic actions

Bacteriostatic effect against susceptible bacteria; prevents cell replication.

Indications

Systemic

- Serious infections for which no other antibiotic is effective
- Acute infections caused by *Salmonella typhi*
- Serious infections caused by *Salmonella, Haemophilus influenzae*, rickettsiae, lymphogranuloma—psittacosis group
- Cystic fibrosis regimen

Contraindications and cautions

- Contraindicated with allergy to chloramphenicol.
- Use cautiously with renal failure, hepatic failure, G6PD deficiency, intermittent porphyria, pregnancy (may cause gray syndrome in premature infants and newborns), lactation.

Available forms

Powder for injection—100 mg/mL

Dosages

Systemic

⊠ ***Black box warning*** Severe and sometimes fatal blood dyscrasias (in adults) and severe and sometimes fatal gray syndrome (in newborns and premature infants) may occur. Use should be restricted to situations in which no other antibiotic is effective. Serum levels should be monitored at least weekly to minimize risk of toxicity (therapeutic concentrations: peak, 10–20 mcg/mL; trough, 5–10 mcg/mL).

Adults

50 mg/kg/day IV in divided doses every 6 hr up to 100 mg/kg/day in severe cases.

Pediatric patients

50–100 mg/kg/day IV in divided doses every 6 hr.

- *Meningitis:* 50–100 mg/kg/day IV in divided doses every 6 hr.
- *Neonates:*
  - Less than 2 kg and/or younger than 7 days: 25 mg/kg daily.
  - Older than 7 days and more than 2 kg: 50 mg/kg/day in divided doses every 12 hr.
- *Infants and children with immature metabolic processes:* 25 mg/kg/day IV (monitor serum concentration carefully).

Geriatric patients or patients with renal or hepatic failure

Use serum concentration of the drug to adjust dosage.

Pharmacokinetics

Route	*Onset*	*Peak*	*Duration*
IV	20–30 min	1 hr	48–72 hr

Metabolism: Hepatic; $T_{1/2}$: 1.5–4 hr
Distribution: Crosses placenta; enters breast milk
Excretion: Urine

IV FACTS

Preparation: Dilute with 10 mL of sterile water for injection, or 5% dextrose injection.
Infusion: Administer as a 10% solution over 3–5 min, single-dose infusion over 30–60 min.

Adverse effects

Systemic

- **CNS:** Headache, mild depression, mental confusion, delirium
- **GI:** Nausea, vomiting, glossitis, stomatitis, diarrhea
- **Hematologic: Blood dyscrasias**
- **Other:** Fever, macular rashes, urticaria, **anaphylaxis; gray baby syndrome** (seen in neonates and premature infants—abdominal distention, pallid cyanosis, vasomotor collapse, irregular respirations), **superinfections**

Interactions

✱ **Drug-drug** • Increased serum levels and drug effects of warfarin, phenytoins, tolbutamide, glipizide, glyburide, tolazamide with chloramphenicol • Decreased hematologic response to iron salts, vitamin B_{12} with chloramphenicol • Risk of increased bone marrow suppression if taken with other drugs that suppress bone marrow

■ Nursing considerations

Assessment

- **History:** Allergy to chloramphenicol, renal or hepatic failure, G6PD deficiency, intermittent porphyria, pregnancy, lactation
- **Physical:** Culture infection; orientation, reflexes, sensation; R, adventitious sounds; bowel sounds, output, liver evaluation; urinalysis, BUN, CBC, LFTs, renal function tests

Interventions

Systemic administration

- Culture infection site before beginning therapy.

⊗ ***Warning*** Do not give this drug IM because it is ineffective.

⊗ ***Black box warning*** Monitor hematologic data carefully, especially with long-term therapy by any route of administration. Serious and fatal blood dyscrasias have occurred.

- Reduce dosage in patients with renal or hepatic disease.
- Monitor serum levels periodically as indicated in dosage section.
- Change to another antibiotic as soon as possible.

Teaching points

- This drug can only be given IV.
- You may experience these side effects: Nausea, vomiting; diarrhea (reversible); headache

(request medication); confusion (avoid driving or operating machinery); superinfections (good hygiene may help; medications are available if severe).

- Report sore throat, tiredness, unusual bleeding or bruising (even as late as several weeks after you finish the drug), numbness, tingling, pain in the extremities, pregnancy; discomfort at IV site.

▽ chlordiazepoxide (metaminodiazepoxide hydrochloride)

*(klor dye az e **pox'** ide)*

Apo-Chlordiazepoxide (CAN), Librium

PREGNANCY CATEGORY D

CONTROLLED SUBSTANCE C-IV

Drug classes

Anxiolytic
Benzodiazepine

Therapeutic actions

Exact mechanisms of action not understood; acts mainly at subcortical levels of the CNS; main sites of action may be the limbic system and reticular formation; potentiates the effects of GABA.

Indications

- Management of anxiety disorders or for short-term relief of symptoms of anxiety
- Acute alcohol withdrawal; may be useful in symptomatic relief of acute agitation, tremor, delirium tremens, hallucinosis
- Preoperative relief of anxiety and tension

Contraindications and cautions

- Contraindicated with hypersensitivity to benzodiazepines, psychoses, acute narrow-angle glaucoma, shock, coma, acute alcoholic intoxication with depression of vital signs, pregnancy (increased risk of congenital malformations, neonatal withdrawal syndrome), labor and delivery ("floppy infant" syndrome reported), lactation (infants may become lethargic and lose weight).
- Use cautiously with hepatic or renal impairment, debilitation and in geriatric patients who are at increased risk for mental status changes.

Available forms

Capsules—5, 10, 25 mg; powder for injection—100 mg/ampule

Dosages

Adults

Individualize dosage; increase dosage cautiously to avoid adverse effects.

Oral

- *Anxiety disorders:* 5 or 10 mg, up to 20 or 25 mg, tid–qid, depending on severity of symptoms.
- *Preoperative apprehension:* 5–10 mg tid–qid on days preceding surgery.
- *Alcohol withdrawal:* Parenteral form usually used initially. If given orally, initial dose is 50–100 mg, followed by repeated doses as needed up to 300 mg/day; then reduce to maintenance levels.

Parenteral

- *Severe anxiety:* Initially, 50–100 mg IM or IV; then 25–50 mg tid–qid if necessary, or switch to oral dosage form.
- *Preoperative apprehension:* 50–100 mg IM 1 hr prior to surgery.
- *Alcohol withdrawal:* Initially, 50–100 mg IM or IV; repeat in 2–4 hr if necessary. Up to 300 mg may be given in 6 hr; do not exceed 300 mg/24 hr.

Pediatric patients

Oral

Younger than 6 yr: Not recommended.
Older than 6 yr: Initially, 5 mg bid–qid; may be increased in some children to 10 mg bid–tid.

Parenteral

12–18 yr: 25–50 mg IM or IV.

Geriatric patients or patients with debilitating disease

5 mg PO bid–qid; 25–50 mg IM or IV.

Pharmacokinetics

Route	Onset	Peak	Duration
Oral	Varies	1–4 hr	48–72 hr
IM	10–15 min	15–30 min	48–72 hr
IV	Immediate	3–30 min	48–72 hr

Metabolism: Hepatic; $T_{1/2}$: 24–48 hr

Distribution: Crosses placenta; enters breast milk
Excretion: Urine

IV FACTS

Preparation: Add 5 mL sterile physiologic saline or sterile water for injection to contents of ampule; agitate gently until drug is dissolved.
Infusion: Administer IV doses slowly over 1 min. Change patients on IV therapy to oral therapy as soon as possible.

Adverse effects

- **CNS:** *Transient, mild drowsiness initially; sedation, depression, lethargy, apathy, fatigue, light-headedness, disorientation, restlessness, confusion,* crying, delirium, headache, slurred speech, dysarthria, stupor, rigidity, tremor, psychomotor retardation, extrapyramidal symptoms; *mild paradoxical excitatory reactions during first 2 wk of treatment* (especially in psychiatric patients, aggressive children, and those with high dosage), visual and auditory disturbances, diplopia, nystagmus, depressed hearing, nasal congestion
- **CV:** Bradycardia, tachycardia, CV collapse, hypertension and hypotension, palpitations, edema
- **Dependence:** *Drug dependence with withdrawal syndrome* when drug is discontinued (more common with abrupt discontinuation of higher dosage used for longer than 4 mo)
- **Dermatologic:** Urticaria, pruritus, skin rash, dermatitis
- **GI:** *Constipation, diarrhea,* dry mouth, salivation, nausea, anorexia, vomiting, difficulty in swallowing, gastric disorders, hepatic impairment, jaundice
- **GU:** *Incontinence, urinary retention, changes in libido,* menstrual irregularities
- **Hematologic:** Decreased Hct, blood dyscrasias
- **Other:** Phlebitis and thrombosis at IV injection sites, hiccups, fever, diaphoresis, paresthesias, muscular disturbances, gynecomastia, pain, burning, and redness after IM injection

Interactions

✱ **Drug-drug** • Increased CNS depression with alcohol, omeprazole • Increased pharmacologic effects with cimetidine, disulfiram, hormonal contraceptives • Decreased sedative effects with theophylline, aminophylline, dyphylline, smoking

✱ **Drug-alternative therapy** • Risk of increased CNS effects with kava

■ Nursing considerations

Assessment

- **History:** Hypersensitivity to benzodiazepines; psychoses; acute narrow-angle glaucoma; shock; coma; acute alcoholic intoxication; pregnancy; lactation; impaired hepatic or renal function, debilitation
- **Physical:** Skin color, lesions; T; orientation, reflexes, affect, ophthalmologic examination; P, BP; R, adventitious sounds; liver evaluation, abdominal examination, bowel sounds, normal output; CBC, LFTs, renal function tests

Interventions

⊗ ***Warning*** Do not administer intra-arterially; arteriospasm or gangrene may result.

- Reconstitute solutions for IM injection only with 2 mL special diluent provided; do not use diluent if it is opalescent or hazy; prepare injection immediately before use, and discard any unused solution.
- Do not use drug solutions made with physiologic saline or sterile water for injection for IM injections because of pain.
- Give IM injection slowly into upper outer quadrant of the gluteus muscle; monitor injection sites.
- Do not use small veins (dorsum of hand or wrist) for IV injection.
- Monitor P, BP, R carefully during IV administration.
- Keep patients receiving parenteral benzodiazepines in bed for 3 hr; do not permit ambulatory patients to drive following an injection.

⊗ ***Warning*** Reduce dosage of opioid analgesics in patients receiving IV benzodiazepines; doses should be reduced by at least one-third or totally eliminated.

- Monitor LFTs, renal function tests, and CBC at intervals during long-term therapy.

⊗ ***Warning*** Taper dosage gradually after long-term therapy, especially in epileptic patients.

- Advise use of barrier contraceptives; serious fetal abnormalities have been reported.

Teaching points

- Take drug exactly as prescribed.
- Do not stop taking this drug (long-term therapy) without consulting your health care provider. Avoid alcohol, sleep-inducing, or over-the-counter drugs.
- Avoid becoming pregnant while taking this drug; serious adverse effects could occur. Using barrier contraceptives is suggested.
- You may experience these side effects: Drowsiness, dizziness (transient; avoid driving or engaging in other dangerous activities); GI upset (take drug with water); depression, dreams, emotional upset, crying.
- Report severe dizziness, weakness, drowsiness that persists, rash or skin lesions, palpitations, swelling of the extremities, visual changes, difficulty voiding, smoking (can decrease effectiveness).

▽ chloroquine phosphate

(klo' ro kwin)

Aralen Phosphate

PREGNANCY CATEGORY NOT ESTABLISHED

Drug classes

4-aminoquinoline
Amebicide
Antimalarial

Therapeutic actions

Inhibits protozoal reproduction and protein synthesis. Mechanism of anti-inflammatory action in rheumatoid arthritis is not known.

Indications

- Treatment of extraintestinal amebiasis
- Prophylaxis and treatment of acute attacks of malaria caused by susceptible strains of *Plasmodia*
- Unlabeled uses: Treatment of rheumatoid arthritis (150 mg PO daily) and discoid lupus erythematosus

Contraindications and cautions

- Contraindicated with allergy to chloroquine and other 4-aminoquinolines.
- Use cautiously with porphyria, psoriasis, retinal disease, hepatic disease, G6PD deficiency, alcoholism, lactation, pregnancy.

Available forms

Tablets—250, 500 mg

Dosages

⊗ ***Warning*** Dosage is often expressed as chloroquine base.

Adults

- *Amebiasis:* 1 g (600 mg base)/day PO for 2 days; then 500 mg (300 mg base)/day for 2–3 wk.
- *Malaria:* For suppression, 300 mg base PO once a week on the same day for 2 wk before exposure and continuing until 4–8 wk after exposure. For acute attack, initially 600 mg base PO; then 300 mg 6–8 hr, 24 hr, 48 hr after the initial dose for a total dose of 1.5 g in 3 days.

Pediatric patients

- *Amebiasis:* Not recommended.
- *Malaria:* For suppression, 5 mg base/kg PO once a week on the same day for 2 wk before exposure and continuing until 6–8 wk after exposure. For acute attack, 10 mg base/kg PO initially; then 5 mg base/kg 6 hr later and on days 2 and 3. Do not exceed 10 mg base/kg/day or 300 mg/base/day.

Pharmacokinetics

Route	*Onset*	*Peak*	*Duration*
Oral	Varies	1–2 hr	1 wk

Metabolism: Hepatic; $T_{1/2}$: 70–120 hr
Distribution: May cross placenta; enters breast milk
Excretion: Urine

Adverse effects

- **CNS:** *Visual disturbances,* possibly permanent retinal changes (blurring of vision, difficulty in focusing), ototoxicity, muscle weakness

- **CV:** Hypotension, ECG changes
- **Dermatologic**: Skin eruptions, pruritus, hair loss
- **GI:** *Nausea, vomiting, diarrhea,* loss of appetite, abdominal pain
- **Hematologic:** Blood dyscrasias, hemolysis in patients with G6PD deficiency

Interactions

✱ **Drug-drug** • Increased effects of chloroquine with cimetidine • Decreased GI absorption of both drugs with magnesium trisilicate

■ Nursing considerations

Assessment

- **History:** Allergy to chloroquine and other 4-aminoquinolines, porphyria, psoriasis, retinal disease, hepatic disease, G6PD deficiency, alcoholism, lactation, pregnancy
- **Physical:** Reflexes, muscle strength, auditory and ophthalmologic screening; BP, ECG; liver palpation; CBC, G6PD in deficient patients, LFTs

Interventions

- Administer with meals if GI upset occurs.
- Schedule weekly, same-day therapy on a calendar.

⊗ ***Warning*** Double check pediatric doses; children are very susceptible to overdosage.

- Arrange for ophthalmologic examinations during long-term therapy.

Teaching points

- Take full course of drug therapy. Take drug with meals if GI upset occurs. Mark your calendar with the days you should take your drug for malarial prophylaxis.
- Arrange to have regular ophthalmologic examinations if long-term use is indicated.
- You may experience these side effects: Stomach pain, loss of appetite, nausea, vomiting, or diarrhea.
- Report blurring of vision, loss of hearing, ringing in the ears, muscle weakness, fever.

▽ chlorothiazide

*(klor oh **thye'** a zide)*

Diuril

chlorothiazide sodium

Sodium Diuril

PREGNANCY CATEGORY C

Drug class

Thiazide diuretic

Therapeutic actions

Inhibits reabsorption of sodium and chloride in distal renal tubule, increasing the excretion of sodium, chloride, and water by the kidney.

Indications

- Adjunctive therapy in edema associated with heart failure, cirrhosis, corticosteroid, and estrogen therapy, renal impairment
- Treatment of hypertension, alone or with other antihypertensives
- Unlabeled uses: Treatment of diabetes insipidus, especially nephrogenic diabetes insipidus; reduction of incidence of osteoporosis in postmenopausal women, calcium nephrolithiasis

Contraindications and cautions

- Contraindicated with anuria, renal failure, allergy to thiazide diuretics or other sulfonamide drugs, hepatic coma.
- Use cautiously with fluid or electrolyte imbalances, renal or liver disease, gout, SLE, glucose tolerance abnormalities, hyperparathyroidism, bipolar disorder, lactation, pregnancy.

Available forms

Tablets—250, 500 mg; oral suspension—250 mg/5 mL; powder for injection—500 mg

Dosages

Note: Dosage should be individualized according to patient response, and the lowest possible dose should be used.

Adults

- *Edema:* 0.5–2 g daily PO or IV (if patient unable to take PO), daily in one or two doses.
- *Hypertension:* 0.5–2 g/day PO as a single or divided dose; adjust dosage to BP response, giving up to 2 g/day in divided doses. IV use is not recommended.

Pediatric patients

10–20 mg/kg/day PO in a single dose or two doses.

Pediatric patients 2–12 yr

375 mg–1 g PO in two divided doses.

Pediatric patients 2 yr or younger

125–375 mg PO in two divided doses.

Pediatric patients younger than 6 mo

Up to 30 mg/kg per day PO in two doses. IV use not recommended.

Pharmacokinetics

Route	*Onset*	*Peak*	*Duration*
Oral	2 hr	3–6 hr	6–12 hr
IV	15 min	30 min	2 hr

Metabolism: $T_{1/2}$: 45–120 min
Distribution: Crosses placenta; enters breast milk
Excretion: Urine

IV FACTS

Preparation: Dilute vial for parenteral solution with 18 mL sterile water for injection. Never add less than 18 mL. Discard diluted solution after 24 hr.
Infusion: Administer slowly. Switch to oral drug as soon as possible.
Compatibilities: Compatible with dextrose and sodium chloride solutions.
Incompatibilities: Do not give parenteral solution with whole blood or blood products.

Adverse effects

- **CNS:** *Dizziness, vertigo,* paresthesias, weakness, headache, drowsiness, fatigue
- **CV:** Orthostatic hypotension, venous thrombosis, volume depletion, cardiac arrhythmias, chest pain
- **Dermatologic:** Photosensitivity, rash, purpura, exfoliative dermatitis
- **GI:** *Nausea, anorexia, vomiting, dry mouth, diarrhea, constipation,* jaundice, hepatitis, pancreatitis
- **GU:** *Polyuria, nocturia, impotence,* loss of libido, renal failure
- **Hematologic:** Leukopenia, thrombocytopenia, agranulocytosis, aplastic anemia, neutropenia, fluid and electrolyte imbalances
- **Other:** Muscle cramps and muscle spasms, fever, hives, gouty attacks, flushing, weight loss, rhinorrhea, electrolyte imbalances

Interactions

✱ Drug-drug • Increased thiazide effects and chance of acute hyperglycemia with diazoxide • Decreased absorption with cholestyramine • Increased risk of cardiac glycoside toxicity if hypokalemia occurs • Increased risk of lithium toxicity • Increased dosage of antidiabetics may be needed • Possible potentiation of hypotension with alcohol, opioids • Potentiation of hypokalemia with corticosteroids
✱ Drug-lab test • Monitor for decreased PBI levels without clinical signs of thyroid disturbances

■ Nursing considerations

Assessment

- **History:** Fluid or electrolyte imbalances, renal or liver disease, gout, SLE, glucose tolerance abnormalities, hyperparathyroidism, manic-depressive disorders, lactation
- **Physical:** Orientation, reflexes, muscle strength; pulses, BP, orthostatic BP, perfusion, edema, baseline ECG; R, adventitious sounds; liver evaluation, bowel sounds; CBC, serum electrolytes, blood glucose, LFTs, renal function tests, serum uric acid, urinalysis

Interventions

- Administer with food or milk if GI upset occurs.
- Do not administer drug IM or subcutaneously.
- Administer early in the day, so increased urination will not disturb sleep.
- Measure and record weight to monitor fluid changes.

Teaching points

- Take drug early in the day, so your sleep will not be disturbed by increased urination.

- Weigh yourself daily, and record weights.
- Protect skin from exposure to the sun or bright lights.
- Increased urination will occur; you may want to plan activities accordingly.
- You may experience these side effects: Dizziness, drowsiness, or feeling faint (use caution).
- Report rapid weight change of more than 3 pounds a day, swelling in ankles or fingers, unusual bleeding or bruising, muscle cramps.

chlorpheniramine maleate

*(klor fen **ir'** a meen **mal'** ee ate)*

Aller-Chlor; Allergy; Allergy Relief; Chlo-Amine; Chlor-Trimeton Allergy 4 hr, 8 hr, and 12 hr; ED-CHLOR-TAN (DNC); Efidac 24 (DNC); Pediatan, QDALL-AR (DNC)

PREGNANCY CATEGORY B

Drug class

Antihistamine (alkylamine type)

Therapeutic actions

Competitively blocks the effects of histamine at H_1-receptor sites; has atropine-like, antipruritic, and sedative effects.

Indications

- Symptomatic relief of symptoms associated with perennial and seasonal allergic rhinitis; vasomotor rhinitis; allergic conjunctivitis

Contraindications and cautions

- Contraindicated with allergy to any antihistamines, narrow-angle glaucoma, stenosing peptic ulcer, symptomatic prostatic hypertrophy, asthmatic attack, bladder neck obstruction, pyloroduodenal obstruction, third trimester of pregnancy, lactation.
- Use cautiously in pregnancy, geriatric patients.

Available forms

Chewable tablets—2 mg; tablets—4 mg; ER tablets (DNC)—8, 12, 16 mg; syrup—2 mg/5 mL; SR capsules (DNC)—8, 12 mg, ER capsules (DNC)—12 mg; caplets—8 mg

Dosages

Adults and children older than 12 yr

Tablets or syrup

4 mg PO every 4–6 hr; do not exceed 24 mg in 24 hr.

SR

8–12 mg PO at bedtime or every 8–12 hr during the day; do not exceed 24 mg in 24 hr.

ER (Efidac 24)

16 mg with liquid PO every 24 hr.

ER capsules

12 mg/day PO; do not exceed 24 mg/day.

Caplets

8 mg/day PO every 12 hr.

Pediatric patients

Tablets or syrup

Age 2–younger than 6 yr: 1 mg every 4–6 hr PO; do not exceed 4 mg in 24 hr.

6–12 yr: 2 mg every 4–6 hr PO; do not exceed 12 mg in 24 hr.

SR

Younger than 6 yr: Not recommended.

6–12 yr: 8 mg PO at bedtime or during the day.

Geriatric patients

More likely to cause dizziness, sedation, syncope, toxic confusional states, and hypotension in elderly patients; use with caution.

Pharmacokinetics

Route	Onset	Peak
Oral	0.5–6 hr	2–6 hr

Metabolism: Hepatic; $T_{1/2}$: 12–15 hr

Distribution: Crosses placenta; may enter breast milk

Excretion: Urine

Adverse effects

- **CNS:** *Drowsiness, sedation, dizziness, disturbed coordination,* fatigue, confusion, restlessness, excitation, nervousness, tremor, headache, blurred vision, diplopia, vertigo, tinnitus, acute labyrinthitis, hysteria, tingling, heaviness and weakness of the hands

- **CV:** Hypotension, palpitations, bradycardia, tachycardia, extrasystoles
- **GI:** *Epigastric distress,* anorexia, increased appetite and weight gain, nausea, vomiting, diarrhea, or constipation
- **GU:** Urinary frequency, dysuria, urinary retention, early menses, decreased libido, impotence
- **Hematologic:** Hemolytic anemia, aplastic anemia, thrombocytopenia, leukopenia, agranulocytosis, pancytopenia
- **Respiratory:** *Thickening of bronchial secretions,* chest tightness, wheezing, nasal stuffiness, dry mouth, dry nose, dry throat, sore throat
- **Other:** Urticaria, rash, anaphylactic shock, photosensitivity, excessive perspiration, chills

Interactions

✱ **Drug-drug** • Increased depressant effects with alcohol, other CNS depressants

■ Nursing considerations

Assessment

- **History:** Allergy to any antihistamines; narrow-angle glaucoma, stenosing peptic ulcer, symptomatic prostatic hypertrophy, asthmatic attack, bladder neck obstruction, pyloroduodenal obstruction, pregnancy, lactation
- **Physical:** Skin color, lesions, texture; orientation, reflexes, affect; vision examination; P, BP; R, adventitious sounds; bowel sounds; prostate palpation; CBC with differential

Interventions

- Administer with food if GI upset occurs.
- Caution patient not to crush or chew SR or ER preparations.
- Arrange for periodic blood tests during prolonged therapy.

Teaching points

- Take as prescribed; avoid excessive dosage. Take with food if GI upset occurs; do not cut, crush, or chew the sustained-release or extended-release preparations.
- Avoid over-the-counter drugs; many contain ingredients that could cause serious reactions if taken with this antihistamine.
- Avoid alcohol; serious sedation may occur.
- You may experience these side effects: Dizziness, sedation, drowsiness (use caution driving or performing tasks that require alertness); epigastric distress, diarrhea, or constipation (take with meals; consult your health care provider if severe); dry mouth (frequent mouth care, sucking sugarless lozenges may help); thickening of bronchial secretions, dryness of nasal mucosa (use a humidifier).
- Report difficulty breathing; hallucinations, tremors, loss of coordination; unusual bleeding or bruising; visual disturbances; irregular heartbeat.

▽ chlorpromazine hydrochloride

*(klor **proe'** ma zeen)*

Novo-Chlorpromazine (CAN)

PREGNANCY CATEGORY C

Drug classes

Antiemetic
Antipsychotic
Anxiolytic
Dopaminergic blocker
Phenothiazine

Therapeutic actions

Mechanism not fully understood; antipsychotic drugs block postsynaptic dopamine receptors in the brain; depress those parts of the brain involved with wakefulness and emesis; anticholinergic, antihistaminic (H_1), and alpha-adrenergic blocking.

Indications

- Management of manifestations of psychotic disorders; control of manic phase of manic-depressive illness
- Relief of preoperative restlessness and apprehension
- Adjunct in treatment of tetanus
- Acute intermittent porphyria therapy
- Severe behavioral problems in children
- Therapy for combativeness, hyperactivity
- Control of nausea and vomiting and intractable hiccups

Contraindications and cautions

- Contraindicated with allergy to chlorpromazine, comatose or severely depressed states, bone marrow depression, circulatory collapse, subcortical brain damage, Parkinson's disease, liver damage, cerebral or coronary arteriosclerosis, severe hypotension or hypertension.

- Use cautiously with respiratory disorders; glaucoma; epilepsy or history of epilepsy; peptic ulcer or history of peptic ulcer; decreased renal function; prostate hypertrophy; breast cancer; thyrotoxicosis; myelography within 24 hr or scheduled within 48 hr, lactation; exposure to heat, phosphorous insecticides; children with chickenpox, CNS infections (makes children more susceptible to dystonias, confounding the diagnosis of Reye's syndrome or other encephalopathy; antiemetic effects of drug may mask symptoms of Reye's syndrome, encephalopathies).

Available forms

Tablets—10, 25, 50, 100, 200 mg; suppository—100 mg; injection—25 mg/mL

Dosages

Full clinical antipsychotic effects may require 6 wk to 6 mo of therapy.

Adults

- *Excessive anxiety, agitation in psychiatric patients:* 25 mg IM; may repeat in 1 hr. Increase dosage gradually in inpatients, up to 400 mg every 4–6 hr. Switch to oral dosage as soon as possible, 25–50 mg PO tid for outpatients; up to 2,000 mg/day PO for inpatients. Initial oral dosage, 10 mg tid–qid PO or 25 mg PO bid–tid; increase daily dosage by 20–50 mg semiweekly until optimum dosage is reached (maximum response may require months); doses of 200–800 mg/day PO are not uncommon in discharged mental patients.
- *Surgery:* Preoperatively, 25–50 mg PO 2–3 hr before surgery or 12.5–25 mg IM 1–2 hr before surgery; intraoperatively, 12.5 mg IM, repeated in 30 min or 2 mg IV repeated every 2 min up to 25 mg total to control vomiting (if no hypotension occurs); postoperatively, 10–25 mg PO every 4–6 hr or 12.5–25 mg IM repeated in 1 hr (if no hypotension occurs).
- *Acute intermittent porphyria:* 25–50 mg PO or 25 mg IM tid–qid until patient can take oral therapy.
- *Tetanus:* 25–50 mg IM tid–qid, usually with barbiturates, or 25–50 mg IV diluted and infused at rate of 1 mg/min.
- *Antiemetic:* 10–25 mg PO every 4–6 hr; 50–100 mg rectally every 6–8 hr; 25 mg IM. If no hypotension, give 25–50 mg every 3–4 hr. Switch to oral dose when vomiting ends.
- *Intractable hiccups:* 25–50 mg PO tid–qid. If symptoms persist for 2–3 days, give 25–50 mg IM; if inadequate response, give 25–50 mg IV in 500–1,000 mL of saline with BP monitoring and administer to patient flat in bed.

Pediatric patients

Generally not used in children younger than 6 mo.

- *Psychiatric outpatients:* 0.5 mg/kg PO every 4–6 hr; 1 mg/kg rectally every 6–8 hr; 0.5 mg/kg IM every 6–8 hr, not to exceed 40 mg/day (up to 5 yr) or 75 mg/day (5–12 yr).
- *Surgery:* Preoperatively, 0.5 mg/kg PO 2–3 hr before surgery or 0.5 mg/kg IM 1–2 hr before surgery; intraoperatively, 0.25 mg/kg IM or 1 mg (diluted) IV, repeated at 2-min intervals up to total IM dose; postoperatively, 0.5 mg/kg PO every 4–6 hr or 0.5 mg/kg IM, repeated in 1 hr if no hypotension.
- *Psychiatric inpatients:* 50–100 mg/day PO; maximum of 40 mg/day IM for children up to 5 yr; maximum of 75 mg/day IM for children 5–12 yr.
- *Tetanus:* 0.5 mg/kg IM every 6–8 hr or 0.5 mg/min IV, not to exceed 40 mg/day for children up to 23 kg; 75 mg/day for children 23–45 kg.
- *Antiemetic:* 0.55 mg/kg PO every 4–6 hr; 1.1 mg/kg rectally every 6–8 hr or 0.55 mg/kg IM every 6–8 hr. Maximum IM dosage, 40 mg/day for children up to 5 yr or 75 mg/day for children 5–12 yr.

Geriatric patients

Start dosage at one-fourth to one-third that given in younger adults and increase more gradually.

Pharmacokinetics

Route	Onset	Peak	Duration
Oral	30–60 min	2–4 hr	4–6 hr
IM	10–15 min	15–20 min	4–6 hr

Metabolism: Hepatic, $T_{1/2}$: 2 hr, then 30 hr
Distribution: Crosses placenta; enters breast milk
Excretion: Urine

IV FACTS

Preparation: Dilute drug for IV injection to a concentration of 1 mg/mL or less.
Injection: Reserve IV injections for hiccups, tetanus, or use during surgery. Administer at a rate of 1 mg/min for adults, 0.5 mg/min for children.
Incompatibilities: Precipitate or discoloration may occur when mixed with morphine, meperidine, cresols.

Adverse effects

- **CNS:** *Drowsiness,* insomnia, *vertigo,* headache, weakness, tremors, ataxia, slurring, cerebral edema, seizures, exacerbation of psychotic symptoms, *extrapyramidal syndromes,* **neuroleptic malignant syndrome,** tardive dyskinesia
- **CV:** *Hypotension, orthostatic hypotension,* hypertension, tachycardia, bradycardia, cardiac arrest, heart failure, cardiomegaly, refractory arrhythmias, pulmonary edema
- **EENT:** Nasal congestion, glaucoma, *photophobia, blurred vision,* miosis, mydriasis, deposits in the cornea and lens, pigmentary retinopathy
- **Endocrine:** Lactation; breast engorgement in females; galactorrhea; SIADH; amenorrhea; menstrual irregularities; gynecomastia; changes in libido; hyperglycemia; inhibition of ovulation; infertility; pseudopregnancy; reduced urinary levels of gonadotropins, estrogens, and progestins
- **GI:** *Dry mouth, salivation, nausea, vomiting, anorexia, constipation,* paralytic ileus, incontinence
- **GU:** *Urinary retention,* polyuria, incontinence, priapism, ejaculation inhibition, male impotence, urine discolored pink to red-brown
- **Hematologic:** Eosinophilia, leukopenia, leukocytosis, anemia, **aplastic anemia,** hemolytic anemia, thrombocytopenic or nonthrombocytopenic purpura, pancytopenia, elevated serum cholesterol
- **Hypersensitivity:** Jaundice, *urticaria,* angioneurotic edema, laryngeal edema, photosensitivity, eczema, asthma, anaphylactoid reactions, exfoliative dermatitis, contact dermatitis
- **Respiratory: Bronchospasm, laryngospasm,** dyspnea, suppression of cough reflex and potential aspiration
- **Other:** Fever, heatstroke, pallor, flushed facies, sweating, *photosensitivity*

Interactions

✷ **Drug-drug** • Additive anticholinergic effects and possibly decreased antipsychotic efficacy with anticholinergic drugs • Additive CNS depression, hypotension if given preoperatively with barbiturate anesthetics, alcohol, meperidine • Additive effects of both drugs if taken concurrently with beta blockers • Increased risk of tachycardia, hypotension with epinephrine, norepinephrine • Decreased hypotension effect with guanethidine
✷ **Drug-lab test** • False-positive pregnancy tests (less likely if serum test is used) • Increase in protein-bound iodine, not attributable to an increase in thyroxine • False positive on PKU test

■ Nursing considerations

CLINICAL ALERT!
Name confusion has occurred between chlorpromazine, chlorpropamide, and clomipramine; use caution.

Assessment

- **History:** Allergy to chlorpromazine; comatose or severely depressed states; bone marrow depression; circulatory collapse; subcortical brain damage, Parkinson's disease; liver damage; cerebral or coronary arteriosclerosis; severe hypotension or hypertension; respiratory disorders; glaucoma; epilepsy or history of epilepsy; peptic ulcer or history of peptic ulcer; decreased renal function; prostate hypertrophy; breast cancer; thyrotoxicosis; myelography within 24 hr or scheduled within 48 hr; lactation; exposure to heat, phosphorous insecticides; children with chickenpox; CNS infections

- **Physical:** T, weight; skin color, turgor; reflexes, orientation, IOP, ophthalmologic examination; P, BP, orthostatic BP, ECG; R, adventitious sounds; bowel sounds, normal output, liver evaluation; prostate palpation, normal urine output; CBC; urinalysis; thyroid, LFTs, renal function tests; EEG

Interventions

- Do not give by subcutaneous injection; give slowly by deep IM injection into upper outer quadrant of buttock.
- Keep patient recumbent for 30 min after injection to avoid orthostatic hypotension.
- If giving drug via continuous infusion for intractable hiccups, keep patient flat in bed during infusion and monitor BP.
- Avoid skin contact with parenteral drug solutions due to possible contact dermatitis.
- Patient or the patient's guardian should be advised about the possibility of tardive dyskinesias.

⊗ ***Warning*** Be alert to potential for aspiration because of suppressed cough reflex.

- Monitor renal function tests; discontinue if serum creatinine or BUN becomes abnormal.
- Monitor CBC; discontinue if WBC count is depressed.
- Consult with physician about dosage reduction or use of anticholinergic antiparkinsonian drugs (controversial) if extrapyramidal effects occur.
- Withdraw drug gradually after high-dose therapy; possible gastritis, nausea, dizziness, headache, tachycardia, insomnia after abrupt withdrawal.
- Monitor elderly patients for dehydration; sedation and decreased sensation of thirst; CNS effects can lead to dehydration, hemoconcentration, and reduced pulmonary ventilation; promptly institute remedial measures.
- Avoid epinephrine as vasopressor if drug-induced hypotension occurs.

Teaching points

- Take drug exactly as prescribed. Avoid over-the-counter drugs and alcohol unless you have consulted your health care provider.
- Use caution in hot weather; risk of heatstroke; keep up fluid intake, and do not overexercise in a hot climate.
- You may experience these side effects: Drowsiness (avoid driving or operating dangerous machinery; avoid alcohol, which increases drowsiness); sensitivity to the sun (avoid prolonged sun exposure, wear protective garments or use a sunscreen); pink or reddish brown urine (expected effect); faintness, dizziness (change position slowly; use caution climbing stairs; usually transient).
- Report sore throat, fever, unusual bleeding or bruising, rash, weakness, tremors, impaired vision, dark urine, pale stools, yellowing of the skin and eyes.

▽ chlorpropamide

See Appendix W, *Less commonly used drugs*.

▽ chlorthalidone

*(klor **thal'** i done)*

Apo-Chlorthalidone (CAN), Hygroton, Thalitone

PREGNANCY CATEGORY B

Drug class

Thiazide-like diuretic

Therapeutic actions

Inhibits reabsorption of sodium and chloride in distal renal tubule, increasing excretion of sodium, chloride, and water by the kidney.

Indications

- Adjunctive therapy in edema associated with heart failure, cirrhosis, corticosteroid and estrogen therapy, renal impairment
- Hypertension, alone or with other antihypertensives

Contraindications and cautions

- Contraindicated with anuria, renal failure, allergy to any thiazides or sulfonamides, hepatic coma.

- Use cautiously with fluid or electrolyte imbalances, renal or hepatic disease, gout, SLE, glucose tolerance abnormalities, hyperparathyroidism, manic-depressive disorders, lactation, pregnancy.

Available forms

Tablets—15, 25, 50, 100 mg

Dosages

Adults

- *Edema:* 30–60 mg/day PO or 60 mg every other day; up to 120 mg/day.
- *Hypertension:* Initiate with 15 mg/day; if response is insufficient, increase to 30 mg/day, then 45–50 mg/day PO. Add a second antihypertensive if additional control is needed based on patient response. Increases in serum uric acid and decreases in serum potassium are dose-related over the 15- to 50-mg/day range and beyond.

Pediatric patients

Safety and efficacy not established.

Pharmacokinetics

Route	*Onset*	*Peak*	*Duration*
Oral	2–3 hr	2–6 hr	24–72 hr

Metabolism: Eliminated primarily as unchanged drug; $T_{1/2}$: 40–60 hr
Distribution: Crosses placenta; enters breast milk
Excretion: Urine

Adverse effects

- **CNS:** *Dizziness, vertigo,* paresthesias, weakness, headache, drowsiness, fatigue
- **CV:** Orthostatic hypotension, venous thrombosis, volume depletion, cardiac arrhythmias, chest pain
- **Dermatologic:** Photosensitivity, rash, purpura, exfoliative dermatitis
- **GI:** *Nausea, anorexia, vomiting, dry mouth, diarrhea, constipation,* jaundice, hepatitis, pancreatitis
- **GU:** *Polyuria, nocturia, impotence,* loss of libido
- **Hematologic:** Leukopenia, thrombocytopenia, agranulocytosis, aplastic anemia, neutropenia, fluid and electrolyte imbalances
- **Other:** Muscle cramps and muscle spasms, fever, hives, gouty attacks, flushing, weight loss

Interactions

✱ **Drug-drug** • Increased thiazide effects and chance of acute hyperglycemia with diazoxide • Decreased absorption with cholestyramine, colestipol • Increased risk of cardiac glycoside toxicity if hypokalemia occurs • Increased risk of lithium toxicity • Increased dosage of antidiabetics may be needed
✱ **Drug-lab test** • Decreased PBI levels without clinical signs of thyroid disturbances

■ Nursing considerations

Assessment

- **History:** Fluid or electrolyte imbalances, renal or hepatic disease, gout, SLE, glucose tolerance abnormalities, hyperparathyroidism, bipolar disorder, lactation, allergy to thiazides or sulfonamides, pregnancy
- **Physical:** Skin color and lesions; orientation, reflexes, muscle strength; pulses, BP, orthostatic BP, perfusion, edema, baseline ECG; R, adventitious sounds; liver evaluation, bowel sounds; CBC, serum electrolytes, blood glucose, LFTs, renal function tests, serum uric acid, urinalysis

Interventions

⊗ ***Warning*** Differentiate between *Thalitone* and other preparations; dosage varies.

- Give with food or milk if GI upset occurs.
- Administer early in the day, so increased urination will not disturb sleep.
- Mark calendars or other reminders of drug days for outpatients on every other day or 3-to 5-day/wk therapy.
- Measure and record weight to monitor fluid changes.

Teaching points

- Take drug early in the day, so your sleep will not be disturbed by increased urination.
- Weigh yourself daily, and record weights.
- Protect skin from exposure to the sun or bright lights.
- Increased urination will occur.
- You may experience these side effects: Dizziness, drowsiness, feeling faint (use caution).
- Report rapid weight change, swelling in ankles or fingers, unusual bleeding or bruising, muscle cramps.

chlorzoxazone

(klor zox' a zone)

Paraflex, Parafon Forte DSC, Remular-S

PREGNANCY CATEGORY C

Drug class
Skeletal muscle relaxant (centrally acting)

Therapeutic actions
Precise mechanism not known; has sedative properties; acts at spinal and supraspinal levels of the CNS to depress reflex arcs involved in producing and maintaining skeletal muscle spasm.

Indications
- Relief of discomfort associated with acute, painful musculoskeletal conditions, adjunct to rest, physical therapy, and other measures

Contraindications and cautions
- Contraindicated with allergic or idiosyncratic reactions to chlorzoxazone.
- Use cautiously with history of allergies or allergic drug reactions, lactation, pregnancy.

Available forms
Tablets—250, 500 mg

Dosages
Adults
Usual dose, 250 mg PO tid–qid; painful conditions may require 500 mg PO tid–qid; may increase to 750 mg tid–qid; reduce dosage as improvement occurs.

Pediatric patients
Safety and efficacy not established.

Pharmacokinetics

Route	*Onset*	*Peak*	*Duration*
Oral	30–60 min	1–2 hr	3–4 hr

Metabolism: Hepatic; $T_{1/2}$: 60 min
Distribution: Crosses placenta; may enter breast milk
Excretion: Urine

Adverse effects
- **CNS:** *Dizziness, light-headedness, drowsiness,* malaise, overstimulation
- **GI:** *GI disturbances,* GI bleeding (rare)
- **GU:** Urine discoloration (orange to purple-red)
- **Hypersensitivity:** Rashes, petechiae, ecchymoses, angioneurotic edema, **anaphylaxis** (rare)

Interactions
✱ **Drug-drug** • Additive CNS effects with alcohol, other CNS depressants

■ Nursing considerations
Assessment
- **History:** Allergic or idiosyncratic reactions to chlorzoxazone; history of allergies or allergic drug reactions; lactation, pregnancy
- **Physical:** Skin color, lesions; orientation; liver evaluation; LFTs

Interventions
⊗ ***Warning*** Discontinue if signs or symptoms of hepatic impairment or allergic reaction (urticaria, redness, or itching) occur.
- Institute rest, physical therapy, and other measures to relieve discomfort.

Teaching points
- Take this drug exactly as prescribed; do not take a higher dosage.
- Avoid alcohol, sleep-inducing, or over-the-counter drugs; these could cause dangerous effects.
- You may experience these side effects: Drowsiness, dizziness, light-headedness (avoid driving or engaging in activities that require alertness); nausea (take with food and eat frequent small meals); discolored urine (expected effect).
- Report rash, severe nausea, coffee-ground vomitus, black or tarry stools, pale stools, yellow skin or eyes, difficulty breathing.

cholestyramine

*(koe **less'** tir a meen)*

Cholestyramine Light, PMS-Cholestyramine (CAN), Prevalite, Questran, Questran Light

PREGNANCY CATEGORY C

Drug classes
Antihyperlipidemic
Bile acid sequestrant

Therapeutic actions
Binds bile acids in the intestine, allowing excretion in the feces; as a result, cholesterol is oxidized in the liver to replace the bile acids lost; serum cholesterol and LDL are lowered.

Indications
- Adjunctive therapy: Reduction of elevated serum cholesterol in patients with primary hypercholesterolemia (elevated LDL)
- Pruritus associated with partial biliary obstruction
- Unlabeled uses: Antibiotic-induced pseudomembranous colitis, chlordecone (*Kepone*) pesticide poisoning to bind the poison in the intestine, treatment of thyroid hormone overdose, treatment of digitalis toxicity

Contraindications and cautions
- Contraindicated with allergy to bile acid sequestrants, tartrazine (tartrazine sensitivity occurs often with allergies to aspirin); complete biliary obstruction.
- Use cautiously with abnormal intestinal function, pregnancy, lactation.

Available forms
Powder for suspension—4 g/5.5, 5.7, 6.4, or 9 g powder

Dosages
Adults

Initially, 4 g one to two times per day PO. In patients with constipation, start with 4 g once/day. Individualize dose based on response. For maintenance, 8–16 g/day divided into two doses. Increase dose gradually with periodic assessment of lipid/lipoprotein levels at intervals of at least 4 wk. Maximum dose 6 packets or scoopfuls. May be administered 1–6 doses/day. Dosage may be as high as 36 g every day.

Pediatric patients

240 mg/kg/day in 2–3 divided doses, not to exceed 8 g/day. Dose is based on anhydrous cholestyramine resin. Optimal dose schedule has not been established.

C

Pharmacokinetics
Not absorbed systemically
Excretion: Feces

Adverse effects
- **CNS:** Headache, anxiety, vertigo, dizziness, fatigue, syncope, drowsiness
- **Dermatologic:** Rash and irritation of skin, tongue, perianal area
- **GI:** *Constipation* to *fecal impaction, exacerbation of hemorrhoids,* abdominal cramps, pain, flatulence, anorexia, heartburn, nausea, vomiting, steatorrhea
- **GU:** Hematuria, dysuria, diuresis
- **Hematologic:** *Increased bleeding tendencies related to vitamin K malabsorption,* vitamins A and D deficiencies, reduced serum and red cell folate, hyperchloremic acidosis
- **Other:** Osteoporosis, backache, muscle and joint pain, arthritis, fever

Interactions
✱ **Drug-drug** • Decreased or delayed absorption with warfarin, thiazide diuretics, digitalis preparations, thyroid, corticosteroids • Malabsorption of fat-soluble vitamins with cholestyramine

■ Nursing considerations
Assessment
- **History:** Allergy to bile acid sequestrants, tartrazine; complete biliary obstruction; abnormal intestinal function; lactation, pregnancy
- **Physical:** Skin lesions, color, T; orientation, affect, reflexes; P, auscultation, baseline ECG, peripheral perfusion; liver evaluation, bowel sounds; lipid studies, LFTs, clotting profile

Interventions
- Mix contents of one packet or one level scoop of powder with 2–6 fluid oz of beverage (water, milk, fruit juices, noncarbonates), highly

fluid soup, pulpy fruits (applesauce, pineapple); do not give drug in dry form.
- Administer drug before meals.

⊗ ***Warning*** Monitor intake of other oral drugs due to risk of binding in the intestine and delayed or decreased absorption, give oral medications 1 hr before or 4–6 hr after the cholestyramine.
- Alert patient about potentially high cost of drug.

Teaching points
- Take drug before meals; do not take the powder in the dry form; mix one packet or one scoop with 2–6 ounces of fluid—water, milk, juice, noncarbonated drinks, highly fluid soups, cereals, pulpy fruits such as applesauce or pineapple.
- Take other medications 1 hour before or 4–6 hours after cholestyramine.
- You may experience these side effects: Constipation (ask about measures that may help); nausea, heartburn, loss of appetite (eat frequent small meals); dizziness, drowsiness, vertigo, fainting (avoid driving and operating dangerous machinery); headache, muscle and joint aches and pains (may lessen with time).
- Report unusual bleeding or bruising, severe constipation, severe GI upset, chest pain, difficulty breathing, rash, fever.

▽ choline magnesium trisalicylate

See Appendix W, *Less commonly used drugs*.

▽ chorionic gonadotropin (human chorionic gonadotropin, HCG)

*(kor e **awn** ick goe **nad'** oh troe pin)*

Choron 10, Gonic, Novarel, Pregnyl, Profasi

PREGNANCY CATEGORY X

Drug class
Hormone

Therapeutic actions
A human placental hormone with actions identical to pituitary LH; stimulates production of testosterone and progesterone.

Indications
- Prepubertal cryptorchidism not due to anatomic obstruction
- Treatment of selected cases of hypogonadotropic hypogonadism in males
- Induction of ovulation in the anovulatory, infertile woman in whom the cause of anovulation is secondary and not due to primary ovarian failure and who has been pretreated with human menotropins

Contraindications and cautions
- Contraindicated with known sensitivity to chorionic gonadotropin, precocious puberty, prostatic carcinoma or androgen-dependent neoplasm, pregnancy.
- Use cautiously with epilepsy, migraine, asthma, cardiac or renal disease, lactation.

Available forms
Powder for injection—5,000, 10,000, 20,000 units/vial with 10 mL diluent

Dosages
Patients older than 4 yr

For IM use only; individualize dosage; the following dosage regimens are suggested:
- *Prepubertal cryptorchidism not due to anatomic obstruction:* 4,000 USP units IM, three times per week for 3 wk; 5,000 USP units IM, every second day for 4 injections; 15 injections of 500–1,000 USP units over 6 wk; 500 USP units three times per week for 4–6 wk; if not successful, start another course 1 mo later, giving 1,000 USP units/injection.
- *Hypogonadotropic hypogonadism in males:* 500–1,000 USP units, IM three times per week for 3 wk; followed by the same dose twice a week for 3 wk; 1,000–2,000 USP units IM three times per week; 4,000 USP units three times per week for 6–9 mo; reduce

dosage to 2,000 USP units three times per week for an additional 3 mo.
- *Induction of ovulation and pregnancy:* 5,000–10,000 units IM, 1 day following the last dose of menotropins.

Pediatric patients
Safety and efficacy in children younger than 4 yr have not been established.

Pharmacokinetics

Route	*Onset*	*Peak*
IM	2 hr	6 hr

Metabolism: Hepatic; $T_{1/2}$: 23 hr
Distribution: Crosses placenta; may enter breast milk
Excretion: Urine

Adverse effects
- **CNS:** *Headache, irritability, restlessness,* depression, fatigue
- **CV:** Edema, arterial thromboembolism
- **Endocrine:** *Precocious puberty, gynecomastia,* ovarian hyperstimulation (sudden ovarian enlargement, ascites, rupture of ovarian cysts, multiple births)
- **Other:** *Pain at injection site,* **ovarian malignancy**

■ Nursing considerations
Assessment
- **History:** Sensitivity to chorionic gonadotropin, precocious puberty, prostatic carcinoma or androgen-dependent neoplasm, epilepsy, migraine, asthma, cardiac or renal disease, lactation, pregnancy
- **Physical:** Skin texture, edema; prostate examination; injection site; sexual development; orientation, affect, reflexes; R, adventitious sounds; P, auscultation, BP, peripheral edema; liver evaluation; renal function tests

Interventions
⊠ ***Black box warning*** Be aware that this drug has no known effect on fat metabolism and is not for treatment of obesity.
- Prepare solution for injection using manufacturer's instructions; brand and concentrations vary.

⊗ ***Warning*** Discontinue at any sign of ovarian overstimulation, and have patient admitted to the hospital for observation and supportive measures.
- Provide comfort measures for CNS effects, pain at injection site.

Teaching points
- This drug can only be given IM. Prepare a calendar with a treatment schedule.
- You may experience these side effects: Headache, irritability, restlessness, depression, fatigue (reversible; if uncomfortable, consult your health care provider).
- Report pain at injection site, severe headache, restlessness, swelling of ankles or fingers, difficulty breathing, severe abdominal pain.

▽ chorionic gonadotropin alfa

See Appendix W, *Less commonly used drugs.*

▽ cidofovir

See Appendix W, *Less commonly used drugs.*

▽ cilostazol
*(sill **abs'** tah zoll)*

Pletal

PREGNANCY CATEGORY C

Drug class
Antiplatelet

Therapeutic actions
Reversibly inhibits platelet aggregation induced by a variety of stimuli including ADP, thrombin, collagen, shear stress, epinephrine, and arachidonic acid by inhibiting cAMP phosphodiesterase III; produces vascular dilation in vascular beds with a specificity for femoral beds; seems to have no effect on renal arteries.

Indications
- Reduction of symptoms of intermittent claudication allowing increased walking distance

Contraindications and cautions

- Contraindicated with allergy to cilostazol, heart failure of any severity (decreased survival rates have occurred), active bleeding, hemostatic disorders.
- Use cautiously with pregnancy, lactation, renal dysfunction.

Available forms

Tablets—50, 100 mg

Dosages

Adults

100 mg PO bid taken at least 30 min before or 2 hr after breakfast and dinner. Response may not be noted for 2–4 wk and may take up to 12 wk.

Pediatric patients

Safety and efficacy not established.

Pharmacokinetics

Route	*Onset*	*Peak*
Oral	Gradual	4–6 hr

Metabolism: Hepatic; $T_{1/2}$: 11–13 hr
Distribution: Crosses placenta; may enter breast milk
Excretion: Urine

Adverse effects

- **CNS:** *Dizziness, headaches*
- **CV:** Heart failure, tachycardia, *palpitations*
- **GI:** *Diarrhea, nausea, flatulence, dyspepsia*
- **Respiratory:** Cough, pharyngitis, *rhinitis*
- **Other:** Peripheral edema, infection, back pain

Interactions

✱ **Drug-drug** • Increased serum levels and risk of toxic effects of cilostazol if combined with macrolide antibiotics, diltiazem, azole antifungals (itraconazole, ketoconazole), or omeprazole; if this combination is used, consider decreasing cilostazol dose to 50 mg bid and monitor patient closely • Smoking decreased cilostazol exposure by 20%
✱ **Drug-food** • Increased absorption if taken with high-fat meal; administer drug at least 30 min before or 2 hr after meals • Increased serum levels and risk of adverse effects if combined with grapefruit juice; avoid grapefruit juice if taking this drug

■ Nursing considerations

Assessment

- **History:** Allergy to cilostazol, heart failure, lactation, CV disorders, pregnancy
- **Physical:** Skin color, lesions; orientation; bowel sounds, normal output; P, BP; R, adventitious sounds; CBC, LFTs, renal function tests

Interventions

⊠ ***Black box warning*** Do not administer to patients with heart failure; decreased survival has been reported.

- Administer drug on an empty stomach, at least 30 min before or 2 hr after breakfast and dinner.
- Encourage patient to avoid the use of grapefruit juice.
- Establish baseline walking distance to monitor drug effectiveness.

⊗ ***Warning*** Establish safety precautions to prevent injury and bleeding (eg, tell patient to use an electric razor, avoid contact sports).

- Advise patient to use barrier contraceptives while receiving this drug; potentially, it could harm the fetus.
- Encourage patient to continue therapy; results may not be seen for 2–4 wk and in some cases may take up to 12 wk.
- Advise patient that the CV risks associated with this drug are not known; potentially serious CV effects have occurred in laboratory animals but drug has been successfully used in patients with CAD.

Teaching points

- Take drug on an empty stomach at least 30 minutes before or 2 hours after breakfast and dinner.
- Avoid drinking grapefruit juice while you are taking this drug.
- The therapeutic effects of this drug may not be seen for 2–4 weeks and may take up to 12 weeks.
- Avoid pregnancy while taking this drug; it could potentially harm the fetus. Use barrier

contraceptives; notify your health care provider immediately if you think you are pregnant.
- You may experience these side effects: Upset stomach, nausea, diarrhea, loss of appetite (eat frequent small meals).
- Report fever, chills, sore throat, palpitations, chest pain, edema or swelling, difficulty breathing, fatigue, bleeding, or bruising.

cimetidine

*(sye **met'** i deen)*

Apo-Cimetidine (CAN), Gen-Cimetidine (CAN), Nu-Cimet (CAN), Tagamet, Tagamet HB, Tagamet HB Suspension

PREGNANCY CATEGORY B

Drug class
Histamine$_2$ (H_2) antagonist

Therapeutic actions
Inhibits the action of histamine at the H_2 receptors of the stomach, inhibiting gastric acid secretion and reducing total pepsin output.

Indications
- Short-term treatment and maintenance of active duodenal ulcer
- Short-term treatment of benign gastric ulcer
- Treatment of pathologic hypersecretory conditions (Zollinger-Ellison syndrome)
- Prophylaxis of stress-induced ulcers and acute upper GI bleeding in critical patients
- Treatment of erosive GERD
- OTC use: Relief of symptoms of heartburn, acid indigestion, sour stomach
- Unlabeled use: Part of multidrug regimen for *Helicobacter pylori*

Contraindications and cautions
- Contraindicated with allergy to cimetidine.
- Use cautiously with impaired renal or hepatic function, lactation, pregnancy.

Available forms
Tablets—200, 300, 400, 800 mg; liquid—300 mg/5 mL; injection—150 mg/mL; injection premixed—300 mg/50 mL

Dosages
Adults
- *Active duodenal ulcer:* 800 mg PO at bedtime or 300 mg PO qid with meals and at bedtime or 400 mg PO bid; continue for 4–6 wk unless healing is demonstrated by endoscopy. For intractable ulcers, 300 mg IM or IV every 6–8 hr.
- *Maintenance therapy for duodenal ulcer:* 400 mg PO at bedtime.
- *Active benign gastric ulcer:* 300 mg PO qid with meals and at bedtime or 800 mg at bedtime. Treat for 8 wk.
- *Pathologic hypersecretory syndrome:* 300 mg PO qid with meals and at bedtime, or 300 mg IV or IM every 6 hr. Individualize doses as needed; do not exceed 2,400 mg/day.
- *Erosive GERD:* 1,600 mg PO in divided doses bid–qid for 12 wk.
- *Prevention of upper GI bleeding:* Continuous IV infusion of 50 mg/hr. Do not treat beyond 7 days.
- *Heartburn, acid indigestion:* 200 mg as symptoms occur; up to 4 tablets/24 hr. Do not take maximum dose for more than 2 wk.

Pediatric patients
Not recommended for children younger than 12 yr.

Geriatric patients or patients with impaired renal function
Accumulation may occur. Use lowest dose possible, 300 mg PO or IV every 12 hr; may be increased to every 8 hr if patient tolerates it and levels are monitored; if creatinine clearance is less than 30 mL/min, give 25 mg/hr IV for prevention of upper GI bleed.

Pharmacokinetics

Route	*Onset*	*Peak*
Oral	Varies	1–1.5 hr
IV, IM	Rapid	1–1.5 hr

Metabolism: Hepatic; $T_{1/2}$: 2 hr
Distribution: Crosses placenta; enters breast milk
Excretion: Urine

IV FACTS
Preparation: For IV injections, dilute in 0.9% sodium chloride injection, 5% or 10% dextrose injection, lactated Ringer's solution, 5% sodium bicarbonate injection to a volume of 20 mL.

Solution is stable for 48 hr at room temperature. For IV infusions, dilute 300 mg in at least 50 mL of 5% dextrose injection or one of above listed solutions.

Infusion: Inject by direct injection over not less than 5 min; by infusion, slowly over 15–20 min.

Incompatibilities: Incompatible with aminophylline, barbiturate in IV solutions; pentobarbital sodium and pentobarbital sodium and atropine in the same syringe.

Adverse effects

- **CNS:** *Dizziness, somnolence, headache, confusion, hallucinations,* peripheral neuropathy; symptoms of brain stem dysfunction (dysarthria, ataxia, diplopia)
- **CV:** Cardiac arrhythmias, **cardiac arrest,** hypotension (IV use)
- **GI:** *Diarrhea*
- **Hematologic:** Increases in plasma creatinine, serum transaminase
- **Other:** *Impotence* (reversible), gynecomastia (in long-term treatment), rash, vasculitis, pain at IM injection site

Interactions

✱ **Drug-drug** • Increased risk of decreased white blood cell counts with antimetabolites, alkylating agents, other drugs known to cause neutropenia • Increased serum levels and risk of toxicity of warfarin-type anticoagulants, phenytoin, beta-adrenergic blocking agents, alcohol, quinidine, lidocaine, theophylline, chloroquine, certain benzodiazepines (alprazolam, chlordiazepoxide, diazepam, flurazepam, triazolam), nifedipine, pentoxifylline, TCAs, procainamide, carbamazepine when taken with cimetidine

■ Nursing considerations

Assessment

- **History:** Allergy to cimetidine, impaired renal or hepatic function, lactation
- **Physical:** Skin lesions; orientation, affect; pulse, baseline ECG (continuous with IV use); liver evaluation, abdominal examination, normal output; CBC, LFTs, renal function tests

Interventions

- Give drug with meals and at bedtime.
- Decrease doses in patients with renal and hepatic impairment.
- Administer IM dose undiluted deep into large muscle group.
- Arrange for regular follow-up, including blood tests to evaluate effects.

Teaching points

- Take drug with meals and at bedtime; therapy may continue for 4–6 weeks or longer.
- Take antacids as prescribed and at recommended times.
- Inform your health care provider about your cigarette smoking habits. Cigarette smoking decreases the drug's effectiveness.
- Have regular medical follow-up care to evaluate your response to drug.
- Tell your health care providers about all medications, over-the-counter drugs, or herbs you take; this drug may interact with many of these.
- Report sore throat, fever, unusual bruising or bleeding, tarry stools, confusion, hallucinations, dizziness, muscle or joint pain.

▽ cinacalcet hydrochloride

*(sin ah **kal'** set)*

Sensipar (DNC)

PREGNANCY CATEGORY C

Drug classes

Calcimimetic
Calcium-lowering drug

Therapeutic actions

Increases the sensitivity to extracellular calcium of the calcium-sensing receptors on the surface of the chief cell of the parathyroid gland, resulting in a decrease in parathyroid hormone secretion. The drop in parathyroid hormone level leads to a decrease in serum calcium levels.

Indications

- Secondary hyperparathyroidism in patients receiving dialysis for chronic renal disease
- Treatment of hypercalcemia in patients with parathyroid carcinoma

Contraindications and cautions

- Contraindicated with allergy to any component of the drug, lactation.
- Use cautiously with a history of seizure disorders, moderate to severe hepatic impairment, pregnancy.

Available forms

Tablets DNC—30, 60, 90 mg

Dosages

Adults

- *Secondary hyperparathyroidism:* 30 mg/day PO; monitor serum calcium and phosphorous levels within 1 wk after starting therapy and intact parathyroid hormone levels within 1–4 wk of starting therapy to adjust dosage to therapeutic level. May increase dose 30 mg every 2–4 wk to a maximum dose of 180 mg/day. May be combined with vitamin D and phosphate binders.
- *Hypercalcemia associated with parathyroid carcinoma:* Initially 30 mg PO bid to maintain calcium levels within a normal range; may adjust dosage every 2–4 wk in sequential dosages of 60 mg bid, then 90 mg bid to a maximum dosage of 90 mg tid to qid.

Pediatric patients

Safety and efficacy not established.

Pharmacokinetics

Route	Onset	Peak
Oral	Slow	2–6 hr

Metabolism: Hepatic; $T_{1/2}$: 30–40 hr
Distribution: May cross placenta; may pass into breast milk
Excretion: Urine

Adverse effects

- **CNS:** Asthenia, *dizziness,* **seizures**
- **CV:** Chest pain, hypertension
- **GI:** Anorexia, diarrhea, *nausea, vomiting*
- **Other:** Adynamic bone disease, hypocalcemia, *myalgia*

Interactions

✱ **Drug-drug** • Risk of increased amitriptyline levels if used concomitantly; monitor patient • Risk of increased serum levels of flecainide, vinblastine, thioridazine, TCAs; if this combination is used, monitor patient and adjust dosage accordingly • Risk of increased serum levels of cinacalet and resulting hypocalcemia if combined with ketoconazole, erythromycin, itraconazole; monitor serum calcium levels carefully and adjust dosage accordingly

■ Nursing considerations

Assessment

- **History:** Allergy to any component of the drug, pregnancy, lactation, history of seizure disorders, moderate to severe hepatic impairment
- **Physical:** Orientation, reflexes; BP; abdominal examination; LFTs, renal function tests; serum calcium, phosphorous levels, intact parathyroid hormone levels

Interventions

- Monitor serum calcium levels before and regularly during therapy.
- Administer with food or shortly after a meal; ensure that patient does not cut, crush or chew the tablet.
- Suggest alternate method of feeding the baby if patient is lactating; it is not known if this drug passes into breast milk, but it does cross in animal studies.
- Monitor patient's nutritional status as nausea, vomiting, and diarrhea are common.

Teaching points

- Take this drug with food or shortly after a meal.
- Do not cut, crush, or chew this tablet; it must be swallowed whole.
- If you miss a dose, take the dose as soon as you remember. Take the next dose the next day; do not make up or double doses.
- If you are taking this drug with hemodialysis, you will also be taking vitamin D and phosphate binders.
- If you are nursing a baby, choose a different method of feeding the baby while you are on this drug.

C

- You will need to have regular follow-ups, including blood tests to monitor your calcium levels while you are on this drug.
- You may experience these side effects: Dizziness, drowsiness (avoid driving or use of dangerous machinery while on this drug); nausea, vomiting, loss of appetite (it is important to try to maintain your nutrition and fluid intake; if this becomes a problem, consult your health care provider); confusion, hallucinations (it might help to know that this is a drug effect; consult your health care provider if this becomes a problem).
- Report muscle cramping, tingling, pain; fever, flulike symptoms.

ciprofloxacin

*(si proe **flox'** a sin)*

Apo-Ciprofloxacin (CAN), Ciloxan, Cipro, Cipro HC Otic, Cipro I.V., Cipro XR (DNC), Co Ciprofloxacin (CAN), Gen-Ciprofloxacin (CAN), PMS-Ciprofloxacin (CAN), Proquin XR (DNC), ratio-Ciprofloxacin (CAN)

PREGNANCY CATEGORY C

Drug classes

Antibacterial
Fluoroquinolone

Therapeutic actions

Bactericidal; interferes with DNA replication in susceptible bacteria preventing cell reproduction.

Indications

- For the treatment of infections caused by susceptible gram-negative bacteria, including *Escherichia coli, Proteus mirabilis, Klebsiella pneumoniae, Enterobacter cloacae, Proteus vulgaris, Proteus rettgeri, Morganella morganii, Pseudomonas aeruginosa, Citrobacter freundii, Staphylococcus aureus, Staphylococcus epidermidis,* group D streptococci
- Treatment of uncomplicated UTIs caused by *E. coli, K. pneumoniae* as a one-time dose in patients at low risk of nausea, diarrhea (*Proquin XR*)
- Otic: Treatment of acute otitis externa
- Treatment of chronic bacterial prostatitis
- IV: Treatment of nosocomial pneumonia caused by *Haemophilus influenzae, K. pneumoniae*
- Oral: Typhoid fever
- Oral: STDs caused by *Neisseria gonorrheae*
- Prevention of anthrax following exposure to anthrax bacilla (prophylactic use in regions suspected of using germ warfare)
- Acute sinusitis: Caused by *H. influenzae, Streptococcus pneumoniae,* or *Moraxella catarrhalis*
- Lower respiratory tract infections: Caused by *E. coli, Klebsiella, Enterobacter species, P. mirabilis, P. aeruginosa, H. influenzae, Haemophilus parainfluenzae, S. pneumoniae*
- Unlabeled use: Cystic fibrosis in patients who have pulmonary exacerbations, gastroenteritis in children, mycobacterial infection, traveler's diarrhea

Contraindications and cautions

- Contraindicated with allergy to ciprofloxacin, norfloxacin or other fluoroquinolones, pregnancy, lactation.
- Use cautiously with renal impairment, seizures, tendinitis or tendon rupture associated with fluoroquinolone use.

Available forms

Tablets—100, 250, 500, 750 mg; ER tablets (DNC)—500, 1,000 mg; injection—200, 400 mg; microcapsules for suspension—250, 500 mg; ophthalmic ointment—3.33 mg/g; ophthalmic solution—3.5 mg/mL; otic suspension—2 mg/mL

Dosages

Adults

- *Uncomplicated UTIs:* 250 mg PO every 12 hr for 3 days or 500 mg PO daily (ER tablets) for 3 days. *Proquin XR*—500 mg PO as a single dose.

- *Mild to moderate UTIs:* 250 mg every 12 hr PO for 7–14 days or 200 mg IV every 12 hr for 7–14 days.
- *Complicated UTIs:* 500 mg every 12 hr PO for 7–14 days or 400 mg IV every 12 hr or 1,000 mg (ER tablets) PO daily every 7–14 days.
- *Chronic bacterial prostatitis:* 500 mg PO every 12 hr for 28 days or 400 mg IV every 12 hr for 28 days.
- *Infectious diarrhea:* 500 mg every 12 hr PO for 5–7 days.
- *Anthrax postexposure:* 500 mg PO every 12 hr for 60 days or 400 mg IV every 12 hr for 60 days.
- *Respiratory infections:* 500–750 mg PO every 12 hr or 400 mg IV every 8–12 hr for 7–14 days.
- *Acute sinusitis:* 500 mg PO every 12 hr or 400 mg IV every 12 hr for 10 days.
- *Acute uncomplicated pyelonephritis:* 1,000 mg ER tablets PO daily every 7–14 days.
- *Bone, joint, skin infections:* 500–750 mg PO every 12 hr or 400 mg IV every 8–12 hr for 4–6 wk.
- *Nosocomial pneumonia:* 400 mg IV every 8 hr for 10–14 days.
- *Ophthalmic infections caused by susceptible organisms not responsive to other therapy:* 1 or 2 drops per eye daily or bid or ½ inch ribbon of ointment into conjunctival sac tid on first 2 days, then apply ½ inch ribbon bid for next 5 days.
- *Acute otitis externa:* 4 drops in infected ear, tid–qid.

Pediatric patients

⊗ ***Warning*** Drug produced lesions of joint cartilage in immature experimental animals. *Inhalational anthrax:* 15 mg/kg/dose PO every 12 hr for 60 days or 10 mg/kg/dose IV every 12 hr for 60 days; do not exceed 500 mg/dose PO or 400 mg/dose IV.

Patients with impaired renal function

For creatinine clearance of 30–50 mL/min, give 250–500 mg PO every 12 hr. For creatinine clearance of 5–29 mL/min, give 250–500 mg PO every 18 hr or 200–400 mg IV every 18–24 hr. For patients on hemodialysis, give 250–500 mg every 24 hr, after dialysis.

Pharmacokinetics

Route	*Onset*	*Peak*	*Duration*
Oral	Varies	60–90 min	4–5 hr
IV	10 min	30 min	4–5 hr

Metabolism: Hepatic; $T_{1/2}$: 3.5–4 hr
Distribution: Crosses placenta; enters breast milk
Excretion: Bile, urine

IV FACTS

Preparation: Dilute to a final concentration of 1–2 mg/mL with 0.9% sodium chloride injection or 5% dextrose injection. Stable up to 14 days refrigerated or at room temperature.
Infusion: Administer slowly over 60 min.
Incompatibilities: Discontinue the administration of any other solutions during ciprofloxacin infusion. Incompatible with aminophylline, amoxicillin, clindamycin, heparin in solution.

Adverse effects

- **CNS:** *Headache,* dizziness, insomnia, fatigue, somnolence, depression, blurred vision, hallucinations, ataxia, nightmares
- **CV:** Arrhythmias, hypotension, angina
- **EENT:** Dry eye, eye pain, keratopathy
- **GI:** *Nausea,* vomiting, dry mouth, *diarrhea,* abdominal pain
- **GU:** Renal failure
- **Hematologic:** Elevated BUN, AST, ALT, serum creatinine and alkaline phosphatase; decreased WBC count, neutrophil count, Hct
- **Other:** Fever, rash

Interactions

✱ Drug-drug • Decreased therapeutic effect with iron salts, sucralfate • Decreased absorption with antacids, didanosine • Increased serum levels and toxic effects of theophyllines if taken concurrently with ciprofloxacin • Increased effects of coumarin or its derivatives • Increased risk of seizures with foscarnet

✱ Drug-alternative therapy • Increased risk of severe photosensitivity reactions if combined with St. John's wort

■ Nursing considerations

Assessment

- **History:** Allergy to ciprofloxacin, norfloxacin or other quinolones; renal impairment; seizures; lactation
- **Physical:** Skin color, lesions; T; orientation, reflexes, affect; mucous membranes, bowel sounds; LFTs, renal function tests

Interventions

⊗ ***Black box warning*** Risk of tendinitis and tendon rupture exists; risk is higher in patients older than 60 yr; those on steroids; and those with renal, heart, or lung transplant.

- Arrange for culture and sensitivity tests before beginning therapy.
- Continue therapy for 2 days after signs and symptoms of infection are gone.
- Be aware that *Proquin XR* is not interchangeable with other forms.
- Ensure that patient swallows ER tablets whole; do not cut, crush, or chew.
- Ensure that patient is well hydrated.
- Give antacids at least 2 hr after dosing.
- Monitor clinical response; if no improvement is seen or a relapse occurs, repeat culture and sensitivity.
- Encourage patient to complete full course of therapy.

Teaching points

- If an antacid is needed, take it at least 2 hours before or after dose. Swallow ER tablets whole; do not cut, crush, or chew them.
- Take *Proquin XR* with the main meal of the day.
- Do not touch tip of eye ointment or solution as this may contaminate the product.
- Drink plenty of fluids while you are taking this drug.
- You may experience these side effects: Nausea, vomiting, abdominal pain (eat frequent small meals); diarrhea or constipation; drowsiness, blurring of vision, dizziness (use caution if driving or using dangerous equipment).
- Report rash, visual changes, severe GI problems, weakness, tremors.

DANGEROUS DRUG

▽ cisplatin (CDDP)

(sis' pla tin)

Platinol-AQ

PREGNANCY CATEGORY D

Drug classes

Alkylating drug
Antineoplastic
Platinum agent

Therapeutic actions

Cytotoxic: Heavy metal that inhibits cell replication by alkylating DNA; cell cycle nonspecific.

Indications

- Metastatic testicular tumors: Combination therapy with bleomycin sulfate and vinblastine sulfate after surgery or radiotherapy
- Metastatic ovarian tumors: As single therapy in resistant patients or in combination therapy with doxorubicin or cyclophosphamide after surgery or radiotherapy
- Advanced bladder cancer: Single agent for transitional cell bladder cancer no longer amenable to surgery or radiotherapy
- Unlabeled uses: Lung cancer; endometrial cancer; osteogenic sarcoma; liver cancer; breast cancer; squamous cell carcinoma of the head, neck, cervix; brain tumor; esophageal cancer; carcinoma of adrenal cortex

Contraindications and cautions

- Contraindicated with allergy to cisplatin, platinum-containing products; hematopoietic depression; impaired renal function; hearing impairment; pregnancy; lactation.
- Use cautiously with hepatic impairment, peripheral vascular disease.

Available forms

Injection—1 mg/mL

Dosages

Dose is often given in combination with another chemotherapeutic drug.

Adults

- *Metastatic testicular tumor:*
  Remission induction: Cisplatin, 20 mg/m^2 per day IV for 5 consecutive days (days 1–5) every 3 wk for three courses of therapy; bleomycin, 30 units IV weekly (day 2 of each wk) for 12 consecutive doses; vinblastine, 0.15–0.2 mg/kg IV twice weekly (days 1 and 2) every 3 wk for four courses.
  Maintenance: Vinblastine, 0.3 mg/kg IV every 4 wk for 2 yr.
- *Metastatic ovarian tumors:* 75–100 mg/m^2 IV once every 4 wk. For combination therapy, administer sequentially: Cisplatin, 50–100 mg/m^2 IV once every 3–4 wk; cyclophosphamide, 600 mg/m^2 IV once every 4 wk.
- *Advanced bladder cancer:* 50–70 mg/m^2 IV once every 3–4 wk; in heavily pretreated (radiotherapy or chemotherapy) patients, give an initial dose of 50 mg/m^2 repeated every 4 wk. Do not give repeated courses until serum creatinine is lower than 1.5 mg/dL or BUN is lower than 25 mg/dL or until platelets exceed 100,000/mm^3 and WBCs exceed 4,000/mm^3. Do not give subsequent doses until audiometry indicates hearing is within normal range.

Pharmacokinetics

Route	Onset	Peak	Duration
IV	8–10 hr	18–23 days	30–35 days

Metabolism: Hepatic; $T_{1/2}$: 25–49 min, then 58–73 hr
Distribution: Crosses placenta; enters breast milk
Excretion: Urine

IV FACTS

Preparation: Available solution contains 1 mg/mL cisplatin; stable for 28 days protected from light or 7 days under room light at room temperature—do not refrigerate. Dilute drug in 1–2 L of 5% dextrose in one-half or one-third normal saline containing 37.5 g mannitol.
Infusion: Hydrate patient with 1–2 L of fluid infused for 8–12 hr before drug therapy; infuse dilute drug over 6–8 hr.

Adverse effects

- **CNS:** *Ototoxicity,* peripheral neuropathies, seizures, loss of taste
- **GI:** *Nausea, vomiting, anorexia,* liver impairment
- **GU:** *Nephrotoxicity,* dose limiting
- **Hematologic:** *Leukopenia, thrombocytopenia, anemia,* hypomagnesemia, hypocalcemia, hypokalemia, hypophosphatemia, hyperuricemia
- **Hypersensitivity: Anaphylactic-like reactions,** facial edema, bronchoconstriction, tachycardia, hypotension (treat with epinephrine, corticosteroids, antihistamines)

Interactions

✱ **Drug-drug** • Additive ototoxicity with furosemide, bumetanide, ethacrynic acid • Decreased serum levels of phenytoins with cisplatin • Additive nephrotoxicity with aminoglycosides

■ Nursing considerations

Assessment

- **History:** Allergy to cisplatin, platinum-containing products; hematopoietic depression; impaired renal function; hearing impairment; pregnancy, lactation
- **Physical:** Weight; eighth cranial nerve evaluation; reflexes; sensation; CBC, differential; renal function tests; serum electrolytes; serum uric acid; audiogram

Interventions

⊗ ***Warning*** Arrange for tests to evaluate serum creatinine, BUN, creatinine clearance, magnesium, calcium, and potassium levels before initiating therapy and before each subcourse of therapy. Do not give if there is evidence of nephrotoxicity.

⊠ ***Black box warning*** Arrange for audiometric testing before beginning therapy and prior to subsequent doses. Do not give dose if audiometric acuity is outside normal limits.

⊠ ***Black box warning*** Monitor renal function; severe toxicity related to dose is possible.

⊠ ***Black box warning*** Have epinephrine and corticosteroids available in case the patient has anaphylaxis-like reactions.

⊗ ***Warning*** Do not use needles of IV sets containing aluminum parts; can cause precipitate and loss of drug potency. Use gloves while preparing drug to prevent contact with the skin or mucosa; contact can cause skin reactions. If contact occurs, wash area immediately with soap and water.

- Maintain adequate hydration and urinary output for the 24 hr following drug therapy.
- Use of prophylactic antiemetics is required (ondansetron).
- Monitor uric acid levels; if markedly increased, allopurinol may be ordered.
- Monitor electrolytes and maintain by supplements.

Teaching points

- This drug can only be given IV. Prepare a calendar of treatment days.
- Use birth control; drug may cause birth defects or miscarriages.
- Have frequent, regular medical follow-up care, including frequent blood tests, to monitor drug effects.
- You may experience these side effects: Nausea, vomiting (medication may be ordered; eat frequent small meals); numbness, tingling, loss of taste, ringing in the ears, dizziness, loss of hearing (reversible).
- Report loss of hearing, dizziness; unusual bleeding or bruising, fever, chills, sore throat, leg cramps, muscle twitching, changes in voiding patterns.

▽ citalopram hydrobromide

(si ***tal'*** *oh pram hi dro* ***broh'*** *myde)*

Apo-Citalopram (CAN) DNC, Celexa DNC, Co Citalopram (CAN) DNC, Gen-Citalopram (CAN) DNC, PMS-Citalopram (CAN) DNC, ratio-Citalopram (CAN) DNC

PREGNANCY CATEGORY C

Drug classes

Antidepressant
SSRI

Therapeutic actions

Potentiates serotonergic activity in the CNS by inhibiting neuronal reuptake of serotonin, resulting in antidepressant effect, with little effect on norepinephrine or dopamine reuptake.

Indications

- Treatment of depression, particularly effective in major depressive disorders
- Unlabeled uses: OCD, panic disorder, PMDD, social phobia, trichotillomania, PTSD

Contraindications and cautions

- Contraindicated with MAOI use; allergy to drug or any component of the drug or other SSRIs; concomitant use of pimozide.
- Use cautiously with renal or hepatic impairment, pregnancy, and lactation, and in patients who are elderly or suicidal.

Available forms

Tablets DNC—10, 20, 40 mg; oral solution—2 mg/mL

Dosages

Adults

Initially, 20 mg/day PO as a single daily dose. May be increased to 40 mg/day if needed no less than an interval of 1 wk.

Pediatric patients

Safety and efficacy not established.

Geriatric patients or patients with renal or hepatic impairment

20 mg/day PO as a single dose; increase to 40 mg/day only if clearly needed and patient is not responding.

Pharmacokinetics

Route	*Onset*	*Peak*
Oral	Slow	2–4 hr

Metabolism: Hepatic; $T_{1/2}$: 35 hr
Distribution: Crosses placenta; enters breast milk
Excretion: Urine

Adverse effects

- **CNS:** *Somnolence, dizziness, insomnia, tremor,* nervousness, headache, anxiety, paresthesia, blurred vision

- **CV:** Palpitations, vasodilation, orthostatic hypotension, hypertension
- **Dermatologic:** *Sweating,* rash, redness
- **GI:** *Nausea, dry mouth,* constipation, diarrhea, anorexia, flatulence, vomiting
- **GU:** *Ejaculatory disorders*
- **Respiratory:** Sinusitis, URI, cough, rhinitis

Interactions

✱ **Drug-drug** • Increased citalopram levels and toxicity if taken with MAOIs; ensure that patient has been off the MAOI for at least 14 days before administering citalopram • Increased citalopram levels with azole antifungals, macrolides • Possible severe adverse effects if combined with TCAs, erythromycin; use caution • Possible increased effects of beta blockers; monitor patient and reduce beta blocker dose as needed • Possible increased bleeding with warfarin; monitor patient carefully • Risk of prolonged QT interval and potentially fatal cardiac arrhythmias if combined with pimozide; avoid this combination • Risk of serotonin syndrome with linezolid • Increased citalopram levels with cimetidine
✱ **Drug-alternative therapy** • Increased risk of severe reaction if combined with St. John's wort

■ Nursing considerations

CLINICAL ALERT!
Name confusion has occurred between *Celexa* (citalopram), *Celebrex* (celecoxib), *Xanax* (alprazolam), and *Cerebyx* (fosphenytoin); use caution.

Assessment

- **History:** MAOI use; allergy to drug or any component of the drug; renal or hepatic impairment, the elderly, pregnancy, lactation, suicidal tendencies
- **Physical:** Orientation, reflexes; P, BP, perfusion; bowel sounds, normal output; urinary output; liver evaluation; LFTs, renal function tests

Interventions

⊠ ***Black box warning*** Be aware of increased risk of suicidality in children, adolescents, and young adults; monitor accordingly.

- Administer once a day, in the morning; may be taken with food if desired.
- Encourage patient to continue use for 4–6 wk, as directed, to ensure adequate levels to affect depression.
- Limit amount of drug given in prescription to potentially suicidal patients.
- Establish appropriate safety precautions if patient experiences adverse CNS effects.
- Institute appropriate therapy for patient suffering from depression.

Teaching points

- Take this drug exactly as directed, and as long as directed; it may take a few weeks to realize the benefits of the drug. The drug may be taken with food if desired. Do not cut, crush, or chew tablets.
- This drug should not be taken during pregnancy or when nursing a baby; use of barrier contraceptives is suggested.
- You may experience these side effects: Drowsiness, dizziness, tremor (use caution and avoid driving a car or performing other tasks that require alertness if you experience daytime drowsiness); GI upset (eat frequent small meals, perform frequent mouth care); alterations in sexual function (it may help to know that this is a drug effect, and will pass when drug therapy is ended).
- Report severe nausea, vomiting; palpitations; blurred vision; excessive sweating; thoughts of suicide.

DANGEROUS DRUG

▽cladribine (CdA, 2-chlorodeoxyadenosine)

(kla' dri been)

Leustatin

PREGNANCY CATEGORY D

Drug classes

Antimetabolite
Antineoplastic
Purine analogue

Therapeutic actions
Blocks DNA synthesis and repair, causing cell death in active and resting lymphocytes and monocytes.

Indications
- Treatment of active hairy cell leukemia
- Unlabeled uses: Advanced cutaneous T-cell lymphomas, chronic lymphocytic leukemia, non-Hodgkin's lymphomas, acute myeloid leukemia, autoimmune hemolytic anemia, mycosis fungoides, Sézary syndrome

Contraindications and cautions
- Contraindicated with hypersensitivity to cladribine or any components, pregnancy, lactation.
- Use cautiously with active infection, myelosuppression, debilitating illness, renal or hepatic impairment.

Available forms
IV solution—1 mg/mL

Dosages
Adults
Single course given by continuous IV infusion of 0.09 mg/kg/day for 7 days.
Pediatric patients
Safety and efficacy not established.

Pharmacokinetics

Route	*Onset*	*Peak*
IV	Rapid	8–10 hr

Metabolism: Hepatic; $T_{1/2}$: 5.4 hr
Distribution: Crosses placenta; may enter breast milk
Excretion: Urine

IV FACTS
Preparation: Prepare daily dose by adding calculated dose to 500-mL bag of 0.9% sodium chloride injection. Stable for 24 hr at room temperature. Prepare 7-day infusion using aseptic technique, and add calculated dose to 100 mL bacteriostatic, 0.9% sodium chloride injection (0.9% benzyl alcohol preserved) through a sterile 0.22-mcg filter. Store unopened vials in refrigerator; protect from light. Vials are single-use only, discard after use.
Infusion: Infuse daily dose slowly over 24 hr. 7-day dose should be infused continuously over the 7-day period. Stable for 7 days in CADD medication cassettes.
Incompatibilities: Do not mix with any other solutions, drugs, or additives. Do not infuse through IV line with any other drug or additive.

Adverse effects
- **CNS:** *Fatigue, headache,* dizziness, insomnia, **neurotoxicity**
- **CV:** Tachycardia, edema
- **Dermatologic:** *Rash,* pruritus, pain, erythema, petechiae, purpura
- **GI:** *Nausea, anorexia, vomiting, diarrhea, constipation,* abdominal pain
- **GU: Nephrotoxicity**
- **Hematologic:** *Neutropenia,* **myelosuppression,** anemia, thrombocytopenia, *lymphopenia*
- **Local:** *Injection site redness, swelling, pain;* thrombosis, phlebitis
- **Respiratory:** *Cough, abnormal breath sounds,* shortness of breath
- **Other:** *Fever, chills,* asthenia, diaphoresis, myalgia, arthralgia, **infection,** cancer

■ Nursing considerations
Assessment
- **History:** Allergy to cladribine or any component, renal or hepatic impairment, myelosuppression, infection, pregnancy, lactation
- **Physical:** Weight, skin condition, neurologic status, abdominal examination, P, respiratory status, LFTs, renal function tests, CBC, uric acid levels

Interventions
⊗ ***Warning*** Use disposable gloves and protective garments when handling cladribine. If drug contacts skin or mucous membranes, wash immediately with copious amounts of water.
- Ensure continuous infusion of drug over 7 days.
- Alert patients of childbearing age to drug's severe effects on fetus; advise using birth control during and for several weeks after treatment.

Black box warning Monitor complete hematologic profile and LFTs and renal function tests before and frequently during treatment. Consult with physician at first sign of toxicity; consider delaying or discontinuing dose if neurotoxicity or renal toxicity occurs.

Teaching points

- This drug must be given continuously for 7 days.
- Frequent monitoring of blood tests is needed during the treatment and for several weeks thereafter to assess the drug's effect.
- Using barrier contraceptives is advised during therapy and for several weeks following therapy.
- You may experience these side effects: Fever, headache, rash, nausea, vomiting, fatigue, pain at injection site.
- Report numbness or tingling, severe headache, nausea, rash, extreme fatigue, edema, pain or swelling at injection site.

clarithromycin

(klar ith' ro my sin)

Biaxin, Biaxin XL DNC

PREGNANCY CATEGORY C

Drug class

Macrolide antibiotic

Therapeutic actions

Inhibits protein synthesis in susceptible bacteria, causing cell death.

Indications

- Treatment of URIs caused by *Streptococcus pyogenes, Streptococcus pneumoniae*
- Treatment of lower respiratory infections caused by *Mycoplasma pneumoniae, S. pneumoniae, Haemophilus influenzae, Moraxella catarrhalis*
- Treatment of skin and skin structure infections caused by *Staphylococcus aureus, S. pyogenes*
- Treatment and prevention of disseminated mycobacterial infections due to *Mycobacterium avium* and *Mycobacterium intracellulare*
- Treatment of active duodenal ulcer associated with *Helicobacter pylori* in combination with proton pump inhibitor
- Treatment of acute otitis media, acute maxillary sinusitis due to *H. influenzae, M. catarrhalis, S. pneumoniae*
- Treatment of mild to moderate community-acquired pneumonia

Contraindications and cautions

- Contraindicated with hypersensitivity to clarithromycin, erythromycin, or any macrolide antibiotic.
- Use cautiously with colitis, hepatic or renal impairment, pregnancy, lactation.

Available forms

Tablets—250, 500 mg; granules for suspension—125, 250 mg/5 mL; ER tablets DNC—500 mg

Dosages

Adults

- *Pharyngitis, tonsillitis; pneumonia due to* S. pneumoniae, M. pneumoniae; *skin or skin structure infections; lower respiratory infections due to* S. pneumoniae, M. catarrhalis: 250 mg PO every 12 hr for 7–14 days.
- *Acute maxillary sinusitis, acute otitis media, lower respiratory infections caused by* H. influenzae: 500 mg PO every 12 hr for 7–14 days.
- *Mycobacterial infections:* 500 mg PO bid.
- *Duodenal ulcers:* 500 mg PO tid plus omeprazole 40 mg PO every AM for 14 days, then omeprazole 20 mg PO every AM for 14 days.
- *Community-acquired pneumonia:* 250 mg PO every 12 hr for 7–14 days or 1,000 mg PO of ER tablets every 24 hr for 7 days.

Pediatric patients

Usual dosage, 15 mg/kg/day PO divided every 12 hr for 10 days.

- *Mycobacterial infections:* 7.5 mg/kg PO bid, up to 500 mg PO bid.

Geriatric patients or patients with impaired renal function

Decrease dosage or prolong dosing intervals as appropriate. If creatinine clearance is less than 30 mL/min, halve the dose or double the interval.

Pharmacokinetics

Route	Onset	Peak
Oral	Varies	2 hr

Metabolism: Hepatic; $T_{1/2}$: 3–7 hr
Distribution: Crosses placenta; enters breast milk
Excretion: Urine

Adverse effects

- **CNS:** Dizziness, headache, vertigo, somnolence, fatigue
- **GI:** *Diarrhea, abdominal pain, nausea,* dyspepsia, flatulence, vomiting, melena, pseudomembranous colitis, abnormal taste
- **Other:** *Superinfections,* increased PT, decreased WBC count

Interactions

✱ Drug-drug • Increased serum levels and effects of carbamazepine, theophylline, lovastatin, phenytoin
✱ Drug-food • Food decreases the rate of absorption of clarithromycin but does not alter effectiveness • Decreased metabolism and risk of toxic effects if combined with grapefruit juice; avoid this combination

■ Nursing considerations

Assessment

- **History:** Hypersensitivity to clarithromycin, erythromycin, or any macrolide antibiotic; pseudomembranous colitis, hepatic or renal impairment, lactation, pregnancy
- **Physical:** Site of infection; skin color, lesions; orientation, GI output, bowel sounds, liver evaluation; culture and sensitivity tests of infection, urinalysis, LFTs, renal function tests

Interventions

- Culture infection site before therapy.
- Do not cut or crush, and ensure that patient does not chew ER tablets.
- Monitor patient for anticipated response.
- Administer without regard to meals; administer with food if GI effects occur.

Teaching points

- Take drug with food if GI effects occur. Take the full course of therapy. Do not drink grapefruit juice while taking this drug.
- Shake suspension before use; do not refrigerate; do not cut, crush, or chew extended-release tablets; swallow them whole.
- You may experience these side effects: Stomach cramping, discomfort, diarrhea; fatigue, headache (medication may be ordered); additional infections in the mouth or vagina (consult your health care provider for treatment).
- Report severe or watery diarrhea, severe nausea or vomiting, rash or itching, mouth sores, vaginal sores.

clemastine fumarate

(klem' as teen)

Dayhist-1, Tavist Allergy

PREGNANCY CATEGORY B

Drug class

Antihistamine

Therapeutic actions

Blocks the effects of histamine at H_1-receptor sites; has atropine-like, antipruritic, and sedative effects.

Indications

- Symptomatic relief of symptoms associated with perennial and seasonal allergic rhinitis; vasomotor rhinitis; allergic conjunctivitis
- Mild, uncomplicated urticaria and angioedema

Contraindications and cautions

- Contraindicated with allergy to any antihistamines, third trimester of pregnancy, lactation.
- Use cautiously with narrow-angle glaucoma, stenosing peptic ulcer, symptomatic prostatic hypertrophy, asthmatic attack, bladder neck obstruction, pyloroduodenal obstruction.

Available forms
Tablets—1.34, 2.68 mg; syrup—0.67 mg/5 mL

Dosages
Adults and children older than 12 yr
- *Allergic rhinitis:* 1.34 mg PO bid. Do not exceed 8.04 mg/day (syrup); 2.68 mg/day (tablets).
- *Urticaria or angioedema:* 2.68 mg PO daily–tid. Do not exceed 8.04 mg/day.

Pediatric patients 6–12 yr
- *Allergic rhinitis (syrup only):* 0.67 mg PO as syrup bid. Do not exceed 4.02 mg/day.
- *Urticaria or angioedema (syrup only):* 1.34 mg PO as syrup bid. Do not exceed 4.02 mg/day.

Pediatric patients younger than 6 yr
Safety and efficacy not established.

Geriatric patients
More likely to cause dizziness, sedation, syncope, toxic confusional states, and hypotension in elderly patients; use with caution.

Pharmacokinetics

Route	*Onset*	*Peak*	*Duration*
Oral	15–30 min	1–2 hr	12 hr

Metabolism: Hepatic; $T_{1/2}$: 3–4 hr
Distribution: Crosses placenta; enters breast milk
Excretion: Urine

Adverse effects
- **CNS:** *Drowsiness, sedation, dizziness, disturbed coordination,* fatigue, confusion, restlessness, excitation, nervousness, tremor, headache, blurred vision, diplopia, vertigo, tinnitus, acute labyrinthitis, hysteria, tingling, heaviness and weakness of the hands
- **CV:** Hypotension, palpitations, bradycardia, tachycardia, extrasystoles
- **GI:** *Epigastric distress,* anorexia, increased appetite and weight gain, nausea, vomiting, diarrhea or constipation
- **GU:** Urinary frequency, dysuria, urinary retention, early menses, decreased libido, impotence
- **Hematologic:** Hemolytic anemia, aplastic anemia, thrombocytopenia, leukopenia, agranulocytosis, pancytopenia
- **Respiratory:** *Thickening of bronchial secretions,* chest tightness, wheezing, nasal stuffiness, dry mouth, dry nose, dry throat, sore throat
- **Other:** Urticaria, rash, **anaphylactic shock,** photosensitivity, excessive perspiration, chills

C

Interactions
✱ **Drug-drug** • Increased depressant effects with alcohol, other CNS depressants • Increased and prolonged anticholinergic (drying) effects with MAOIs; avoid this combination

■ Nursing considerations
Assessment
- **History:** Allergy to any antihistamines; narrow-angle glaucoma, stenosing peptic ulcer, symptomatic prostatic hypertrophy, asthmatic attack, bladder neck obstruction, pyloroduodenal obstruction; lactation, pregnancy
- **Physical:** Skin color, lesions, texture; orientation, reflexes, affect; vision examination; P, BP; R, adventitious sounds; bowel sounds; prostate palpation; CBC with differential

Interventions
- Administer with food if GI upset occurs.
- Administer syrup form if patient is unable to take tablets; children 6–12 yr should receive only syrup form.
- Monitor patient response, adjust to lowest possible effective dose.

Teaching points
- Take drug as prescribed; avoid excessive dosage.
- Take with food if GI upset occurs.
- Avoid alcohol; serious sedation could occur.
- You may experience these side effects: Dizziness, sedation, drowsiness (use caution if driving or performing tasks that require alertness); epigastric distress, diarrhea, or constipation (take with meals; consult your health care provider as needed); dry mouth (frequent mouth care, sucking sugarless lozenges may help); thickening of bronchial secretions, dryness of nasal mucosa (use a humidifier).

- Report difficulty breathing, hallucinations, tremors, loss of coordination, unusual bleeding or bruising, visual disturbances, irregular heartbeat.

clevidipine butyrate

*(klev **id'** ih peen)*

Cleviprex

PREGNANCY CATEGORY C

Drug classes
Calcium channel blocker
Antihypertensive

Therapeutic actions
Blocks the influx of calcium in the arterial smooth muscle, leading to arterial muscle relaxation and decreased vascular resistance, which lowers BP; does not affect preload or cardiac filling pressure, showing no effect on venous vessels.

Indications
- BP reduction when oral therapy is not possible or is not desirable

Contraindications and cautions
- Contraindicated with known hypersensitivity to any component of the drug, soy, or egg products; defective lipid metabolism; acute pancreatitis; severe aortic stenosis.
- Use cautiously with heart failure, pregnancy, lactation.

Available forms
Single-use vials—0.5 mg/mL

Dosages
Adults
- Initially, give IV infusion of 1–2 mg/hr; titrate quickly by doubling the dose every 90 sec to achieve desired BP. Maintenance dose is usually 4–6 mg/hr. Maximum dose, 21 mg/hr per 24–hr period.

Pediatric patients
- Safety and efficacy not established.

Pharmacokinetics

Route	*Onset*	*Peak*
IV	Rapid	End of infusion

Metabolism: Blood and tissues; $T_{1/2}$: 15 min
Distribution: May cross placenta; may enter breast milk
Excretion: Blood and tissues

IV FACTS
Preparation: Maintain strict sterile technique; product contains phospholipids, which can support microbial growth. Administer within 4 hr of puncturing the stopper; discard any unused drug. Invert vial several times to dispense drug. Drug should appear milky; inspect for any particulate matter, which indicates a contaminated product. Do not dilute. May be administered with water for injection, sodium chloride (0.9%) injection, 5% dextrose injection, 5% dextrose in 0.9% sodium chloride, 5% dextrose in lactated Ringer's solution, lactated Ringer's injection, 10% amino acids.
Infusion: Monitor patient's BP and cardiac status continuously. Infuse using a controlled infusing device that allows for calibrated titration.
Incompatibilities: Do not administer in the same line as any other medications.

Adverse effects
- **CNS:** *Headache*
- **CV: Hypotension,** reflex tachycardia, hypertension, heart failure
- **GI:** *Nausea, vomiting*

■ Nursing considerations
Assessment
- **History:** Known hypersensitivity to any component of the drug, soy, or egg products; defective lipid metabolism; acute pancreatitis; severe aortic stenosis; heart failure; pregnancy; lactation
- **Physical:** Orientation, affect; BP, P, peripheral perfusion, auscultation

Interventions
- Continuously monitor BP and cardiac status during administration; titrate drug accordingly to achieve desired BP.

- Be aware that drug does not protect from rebound affect of beta blocker discontinuation; if patient has been maintained on a beta blocker, drug should be tapered to avoid rebound tachycardia and hypertension.
- Patient should be switched to an oral antihypertensive as appropriate to maintain BP control. If patient is not started on an oral antihypertensive, be prepared for effects of rebound hypertension for at least 8 hr after discontinuation of clevidipine.
- Be aware that drug should be handled using strict sterile technique because drug contains phospholipids that can support microbial growth.
- Use drug within 4 hr of puncturing the stopper.

Teaching points

- This drug must be given IV to regulate your high blood pressure. You will be continuously monitored and the dosage will be adjusted to achieve the desired blood pressure.
- You will need to have regular medical follow-up appointments with your health care provider to monitor your hypertension. Oral medications may be ordered to maintain a safe blood pressure.
- You may experience these side effects: Headache (medications may be available to help); nausea and vomiting (frequent small meals may help, medication may be available to relieve these symptoms).
- Report changes in vision, swelling of the ankles or legs, changes in orientation or alertness, difficulty breathing, fast heart rate.

▽clindamycin

*(klin da **mye'** sin)*

clindamycin hydrochloride

Oral: Cleocin, Dalacin C (CAN)

clindamycin palmitate hydrochloride

Oral: Cleocin Pediatric, Dalacin C Flavored Granules (CAN)

clindamycin phosphate

Oral, parenteral, topical dermatologic solution for acne, vaginal preparation: Cleocin T, Cleocin Vaginal Ovules, Clinda-Derm (CAN), Clindagel, ClindaMax, Clindesse, Clindets, Dalacin C Phosphate (CAN), Dalacin Vaginal Cream (CAN), Dalacin T (CAN), Evoclin

PREGNANCY CATEGORY B

Drug class

Lincosamide antibiotic

Therapeutic actions

Inhibits protein synthesis in susceptible bacteria, causing cell death.

Indications

- Systemic administration: Serious infections caused by susceptible strains of anaerobes, streptococci, staphylococci, pneumococci; reserve use for penicillin-allergic patients or when penicillin is inappropriate; less toxic antibiotics (erythromycin) should be considered
- Parenteral: Treatment of septicemia caused by staphylococci, streptococci; acute hematogenous osteomyelitis; adjunct to surgical treatment of chronic bone and joint infections due to susceptible organisms; do not use to treat meningitis; does not cross the blood–brain barrier.
- Topical dermatologic solution: Treatment of acne vulgaris
- Vaginal preparation: Treatment of bacterial vaginosis

Contraindications and cautions

Systemic administration

- Contraindicated with allergy to clindamycin, lactation.
- Use cautiously in newborns and infants due to benzyl alcohol content (associated with gasping syndrome) and in patients with tartrazine sensitivity or hepatic or renal impairment.

Topical dermatologic solution, vaginal preparation

- Contraindicated with allergy to clindamycin or lincomycin.
- Use caution with history of regional enteritis or ulcerative colitis; history of antibiotic-associated colitis.

Available forms

Capsules—75, 150, 300 mg; granules for oral solution—75 mg/5 mL; injection—150 mg/mL, 300 mg/12 mL, 600 mg/14 mL, 900 mg/16 mL, 300, 600, 900 mg/50 mL; topical gel—1%; topical lotion—1%; topical suspension—1%; vaginal cream—2%; vaginal suppository—100 mg

Dosages

Adults

Oral

150–300 mg every 6 hr, up to 300–450 mg every 6 hr in more severe infections.

Parenteral

600–2,700 mg/day in two to four equal doses; up to 4.8 g/day IV or IM may be used for life-threatening situations.

Vaginal

One applicator (100 mg clindamycin phosphate) intravaginally, preferably at bedtime for 7 consecutive days; or insert vaginal suppository, preferably at bedtime for 3 days for *Cleocin Vaginal Ovules*.

Topical

Apply a thin film to affected area bid.

Pediatric patients

Oral

For clindamycin hydrochloride, 8–16 mg/kg/day (serious infections) or 16–20 mg/kg/day (more serious infections) in three or four equal doses. For clindamycin palmitate hydrochloride, 8–25 mg/kg/day in three or four equal doses; for children weighing less than 10 kg, use 37.5 mg tid as the minimum dose.

Parenteral

Neonates: 15–20 mg/kg/day in three or four equal doses.
Older than 1 mo: 20–40 mg/kg/day in three or four equal doses or 350 mg/m^2/day to 450 mg/m^2/day.

Geriatric patients or patients with renal failure

Reduce dose, and monitor patient carefully.

Pharmacokinetics

Route	Onset	Peak	Duration
Oral	Varies	1–2 hr	8–12 hr
IM	20–30 min	1–3 hr	8–12 hr
IV	Immediate	Minutes	8–12 hr

Metabolism: Hepatic; $T_{1/2}$: 2–3 hr
Distribution: Crosses placenta; enters breast milk
Excretion: Feces, urine
Topical: Minimal systemic absorption

IV FACTS

Preparation: Store unreconstituted product at room temperature. Reconstitute by adding 75 mL of water to 100-mL bottle of palmitate in two portions. Shake well; do not refrigerate reconstituted solution. Reconstituted solution is stable for 2 wk at room temperature. Dilute reconstituted solution to a concentration of 300 mg/50 mL or more of diluent using 0.9% sodium chloride injection, 5% dextrose injection, or lactated Ringer's solution. Do not exceed 18 mg/mL. Solution is stable for 16 days at room temperature.

Infusion: ⊗ ***Warning*** Do not administer more than 1,200 mg in a single 1-hr infusion. Infusion rates: 300 mg in 50 mL diluent, 10 min; 600 mg in 50 mL diluent, 20 min; 900 mg in 50–100 mL diluent, 30 min; 1,200 mg in 100 mL diluent, 40 min. Do not infuse faster than 30 mg/min; rapid infusion can cause cardiac arrest.

Incompatibilities: Do not mix with calcium gluconate, ampicillin, phenytoin, barbiturates, aminophylline, and magnesium sulfate. May be mixed with sodium chloride, dextrose, calcium, potassium, vitamin B complex, kanamycin, gentamicin, penicillin, carbenicillin. Incompatible in syringe with tobramycin.

Adverse effects

Systemic administration

- **CV:** Hypotension, **cardiac arrest** (with rapid IV infusion)

- **GI:** Severe colitis, including **pseudomembranous colitis,** *nausea, vomiting, diarrhea, abdominal pain, esophagitis, anorexia,* jaundice, hepatic function changes
- **Hematologic:** Neutropenia, leukopenia, agranulocytosis, eosinophilia
- **Hypersensitivity:** *Rashes,* urticaria to anaphylactoid reactions
- **Local:** *Pain following injection,* induration and sterile abscess after IM injection, thrombophlebitis after IV use

Topical dermatologic solution

- **CNS:** Fatigue, headache
- **Dermatologic:** *Contact dermatitis, dryness,* gram-negative folliculitis
- **GI:** Pseudomembranous colitis, diarrhea, bloody diarrhea; abdominal pain, sore throat
- **GU:** Urinary frequency

Vaginal preparation

- **GU:** Cervicitis, vaginitis, vulvar irritation

Interactions

Systemic administration

✱ **Drug-drug** • Increased neuromuscular blockade with neuromuscular blocking agents • Decreased GI absorption with kaolin, aluminum salts

■ Nursing considerations

Assessment

- **History:** Allergy to clindamycin, history of asthma or other allergies, allergy to tartrazine (in 75- and 150-mg capsules); hepatic or renal impairment; lactation; history of regional enteritis or ulcerative colitis; history of antibiotic-associated colitis
- **Physical:** Site of infection or acne; skin color, lesions; BP; R, adventitious sounds; bowel sounds, output, liver evaluation; complete blood count, LFTs, renal function tests

Interventions

Systemic administration

- Culture infection site before therapy.
- Administer oral drug with a full glass of water or with food to prevent esophageal irritation.
- Do not give IM injections of more than 600 mg; inject deep into large muscle to avoid serious problems.
- Do not use for minor bacterial or viral infections.

⊗ ***Black box warning*** Be aware that serious to fatal colitis can occur up to several wk after completion of therapy; reserve use, and monitor patient closely.

- Monitor LFTs and renal function tests, and blood counts with prolonged therapy.

Topical dermatologic administration

- Keep solution away from eyes, mouth, and abraded skin or mucous membranes; alcohol base will cause stinging. Shake well before use.
- Keep cool tap water available to bathe eye, mucous membranes, abraded skin inadvertently contacted by drug solution.

Vaginal preparation

- Give intravaginally, preferably at bedtime.

Teaching points

Systemic administration

- Take oral drug with a full glass of water or with food.
- Take full prescribed course of oral drug. Do not stop taking without notifying your health care provider.
- You may experience these side effects: Nausea, vomiting (eat frequent small meals); superinfections in the mouth, vagina (use frequent hygiene measures, request treatment if severe).
- Report severe or watery diarrhea, abdominal pain, inflamed mouth or vagina, skin rash or lesions.

Topical dermatologic administration

- Apply thin film of acne solution to affected area twice daily, being careful to avoid eyes, mucous membranes, abraded skin; if solution contacts one of these areas, flush with lots of cool water.
- Report abdominal pain, diarrhea.

Vaginal preparation

- Use vaginal preparation for 7 or 3 consecutive days, preferably at bedtime. Refrain from sexual intercourse during treatment with this product.
- Report vaginal irritation, itching; diarrhea, no improvement in complaint being treated.

▽ clofarabine

See Appendix W, *Less commonly used drugs.*

clomiphene citrate
(kloe' mi feen)

Clomid, Milophene, Serophene

PREGNANCY CATEGORY X

Drug classes
Fertility drug
Hormone

Therapeutic actions
Binds to estrogen receptors, decreasing the number of available estrogen receptors, which gives the hypothalamus and pituitary the false signal to increase FSH and LH secretion, resulting in ovarian stimulation.

Indications
- Treatment of ovulatory failure in patients with normal liver function and normal endogenous estrogen levels, whose partners are fertile and potent
- Unlabeled use: Treatment of male infertility

Contraindications and cautions
- Contraindicated with known sensitivity to clomiphene, liver disease, uterine fibroids, abnormal vaginal bleeding of undetermined origin, ovarian cyst, uncontrolled thyroid or adrenal dysfunction, organic intracranial lesions, pregnancy.
- Use cautiously with lactation.

Available forms
Tablets—50 mg

Dosages
Adults
- *Treatment of ovulatory failure:*
  Initial therapy: 50 mg/day PO for 5 days started anytime there has been no recent uterine bleeding or about the fifth day of the cycle if uterine bleeding does occur.
  Second course: If ovulation does not occur after the first course, administer 100 mg/day PO for 5 days; start this course as early as 30 days after the previous one.
  Third course: Repeat second course regimen; if patient does not respond to three courses of treatment, further treatment is not recommended.
- *Male infertility:* 50–400 mg/day PO for 2–12 mo (controversial).

Pharmacokinetics

Route	*Onset*	*Duration*
Oral	5–8 days	6 wk

Metabolism: Hepatic; $T_{1/2}$: 5 days
Distribution: Crosses placenta
Excretion: Feces

Adverse effects
- **CNS:** Visual symptoms (blurring, spots, flashes), nervousness, insomnia, dizziness, light-headedness, photophobia, diplopia
- **CV:** *Vasomotor flushing*
- **GI:** *Abdominal discomfort, distention, bloating, nausea, vomiting*
- **GU:** Uterine bleeding, *ovarian enlargement,* **ovarian overstimulation,** birth defects in resulting pregnancies
- **Other:** *Breast tenderness*

Interactions
✱ **Drug-lab test** • Increased levels of serum thyroxine, thyroxine-binding globulin

■ Nursing considerations

CLINICAL ALERT!
Name confusion has occurred between *Serophene* (clomiphene) and *Sarafem* (fluoxetine); use caution.

Assessment
- **History:** Sensitivity to clomiphene, liver disease, uterine fibroids, abnormal vaginal bleeding of undetermined origin, ovarian cyst, pregnancy, thyroid or adrenal dysfunction, intracranial lesions
- **Physical:** Skin color, T; affect, orientation, ophthalmologic examination; abdominal examination, pelvic examination, liver evaluation; urinary estrogens and estriol levels (women); LFTs

Interventions

- Complete a pelvic examination before each treatment to rule out ovarian enlargement, pregnancy, and other uterine difficulties.
- Check urine estrogen and estriol levels before therapy; normal levels indicate appropriate patient selection.
- Refer patient for complete ophthalmic examination; if visual symptoms occur, discontinue drug.

⊗ ***Warning*** Discontinue drug at any sign of ovarian overstimulation, admit patient to hospital for observation and supportive measures.

- Provide women with calendar of treatment days and explanations about signs of estrogen and progesterone activity; caution patient that 24-hr urine collections will be needed periodically; timing of intercourse is important for achieving pregnancy.
- Alert patient to risks and hazards of multiple births.
- Explain failure to respond after three courses of therapy probably means drug will not help, and treatment will be discontinued.

Teaching points

- Prepare a calendar showing the treatment schedule, plotting ovulation.
- There is an increased incidence of multiple births in women using this drug.
- You may experience these side effects: Abdominal distention; flushing; breast tenderness; dizziness, drowsiness, light-headedness, visual disturbances (use caution driving or performing tasks that require alertness).
- Report bloating, stomach pain, blurred vision, yellow skin or eyes, unusual bleeding or bruising, fever, chills, visual changes.

▽ clomipramine hydrochloride

*(kloe **mi'** pra meen)*

Anafranil, Apo-Clomipramine (CAN), Co Clomipramine (CAN), Gen-Clomipramine (CAN)

PREGNANCY CATEGORY C

Drug class

TCA (tertiary amine)

Therapeutic actions

Mechanism unknown; inhibits the presynaptic reuptake of the neurotransmitters norepinephrine and serotonin; anticholinergic at CNS and peripheral receptors.

Indications

- Treatment of obsessions and compulsions in patients with OCD, whose obsessions or compulsions cause marked distress, are time-consuming, or interfere with social or occupational functioning
- Unlabeled uses: Panic disorders, PMS

Contraindications and cautions

- Contraindicated with hypersensitivity to any tricyclic drug, concomitant therapy with an MAOI, patients in the acute recovery phase following MI, myelography within previous 24 hr or scheduled within 48 hr, lactation.
- Use cautiously with allergy to dibenzazepines, ECT, preexisting CV disorders (eg, severe coronary heart disease, progressive heart failure, angina pectoris, paroxysmal tachycardia); angle-closure glaucoma, increased IOP, urinary retention, ureteral or urethral spasm; seizure disorders; hyperthyroidism; impaired hepatic, renal function; psychiatric patients (schizophrenic or paranoid patients may exhibit a worsening of psychosis with TCA therapy); patients with bipolar disorder; elective surgery; pregnancy; lactation.

Available forms

Capsules—25, 50, 75 mg

Dosages

Adults

- *Initial treatment:* 25 mg PO daily; gradually increase as tolerated to approximately 100 mg during the first 2 wk. Then increase gradually over the next several weeks to a maximum dose of 250 mg/day. At maximum dose, give once a day at bedtime to minimize sedation.
- *Maintenance therapy:* Adjust to maintain the lowest effective dosage, and periodically assess need for treatment. Effectiveness after 10 wk has not been documented.

Pediatric patients

- *Initial treatment:* 25 mg PO daily; gradually increase as tolerated during the first 2 wk to a maximum of 3 mg/kg or 100 mg, whichever is smaller. Administer in divided doses with meals to reduce GI side effects. Then increase dosage to a daily maximum of 3 mg/kg or 200 mg, whichever is smaller. At maximum, give once a day at bedtime to minimize sedation.

- *Maintenance therapy:* Adjust dosage to maintain lowest effective dosage, and periodically assess patient to determine the need for treatment. Effectiveness after 10 wk has not been documented.

Pharmacokinetics

Route	*Onset*	*Duration*
Oral	Slow	1–6 wk

Metabolism: Hepatic; $T_{1/2}$: 19–37 hr
Distribution: Crosses placenta; enters breast milk
Excretion: Bile, feces, urine

Adverse effects

- **CNS:** *Sedation and anticholinergic (atropine-like) effects; confusion* (especially in elderly), *disturbed concentration, dizziness, tremor,* hallucinations, disorientation, decreased memory, feelings of unreality, delusions, anxiety, nervousness, restlessness, agitation, panic, insomnia, nightmares, hypomania, mania, *asthenia,* aggressive reaction
- **CV:** *Orthostatic hypotension,* hypertension, syncope, tachycardia, palpitations, **MI,** arrhythmias, heart block, precipitation of heart failure, CVA
- **Endocrine:** Hyperglycemia or hypoglycemia; elevated prolactin levels; inappropriate ADH secretion
- **GI:** *Dry mouth, constipation,* paralytic ileus, *nausea,* vomiting, anorexia, epigastric distress, diarrhea, flatulence, dysphagia, peculiar taste, increased salivation, stomatitis, parotid swelling, abdominal cramps, black tongue, *eructation*
- **GU:** Urinary retention, delayed or frequent micturition, dilation of the urinary tract, gynecomastia, testicular swelling; breast enlargement, *menstrual irregularity* and galactorrhea in women; increased or decreased libido; *impotence,* painful ejaculation
- **Hematologic:** Bone marrow depression, including agranulocytosis; eosinophilia, purpura, thrombocytopenia, leukopenia, anemia
- **Hypersensitivity:** Skin rash, pruritus, vasculitis, petechiae, photosensitization, edema (generalized, facial, tongue), drug fever
- **Withdrawal:** Symptoms on abrupt discontinuation of prolonged therapy—nausea, headache, vertigo, nightmares, malaise
- **Other:** *Nasal congestion, laryngitis,* excessive appetite, weight change; sweating hyperthermia, flushing, chills

Interactions

✷ **Drug-drug** • Increased TCA levels and pharmacologic effects with cimetidine • Increased TCA levels with fluoxetine, methylphenidate, phenothiazines, hormonal contraceptives, disulfiram • Hyperpyretic crises, severe seizures, hypertensive episodes and deaths when MAOIs, furazolidone, clonidine are given with TCAs; don't give within 14 days before or after an MAOI • Increased antidepressant response and cardiac arrhythmias when given with thyroid medication • Increased anticholinergic effects of anticholinergic drugs when given with TCAs • Increased response to alcohol, barbiturates, benzodiazepines, other CNS depressants with TCAs • Decreased effects of indirect-acting sympathomimetic drugs (ephedrine) with TCAs • Risk of arrhythmias if combined with fluoroquinolones • Decreased levels with drugs that induce CYP450 (such as rifampin, phenytoin)

✷ **Drug-alternative therapy** • Clomipramine levels reduced with St. John's wort

■ Nursing considerations

CLINICAL ALERT!
Name confusion has occurred between clomipramine and chlorpromazine; use caution.

Assessment

- **History:** Hypersensitivity to any tricyclic drug; concomitant therapy with an MAOI; myelography within previous 24 hr or scheduled within 48 hr; lactation; ECT; preexisting CV disorders; angle-closure glaucoma,

increased IOP, urinary retention, ureteral or urethral spasm; seizure disorders; hyperthyroidism, impaired hepatic, renal function; psychiatric patients; elective surgery, pregnancy
- **Physical:** Weight; T; skin color, lesions; orientation, affect, reflexes, vision and hearing; P, BP, orthostatic BP, perfusion; bowel sounds, normal output, liver evaluation; urine flow, normal output; usual sexual function, frequency of menses, breast and scrotal examination; LFTs, urinalysis, CBC, ECG

Interventions

⊗ ***Black box warning*** Increased risk of suicidal thinking and behavior in children, adolescents, and young adults; use caution, and monitor patient.
- Limit depressed and potentially suicidal patients' access to drug.
- Administer in divided doses with meals to reduce GI side effects while increasing dosage to therapeutic levels.
- Give maintenance dose once daily at bedtime to decrease daytime sedation.
- Reduce dose if minor side effects develop; discontinue drug if serious side effects occur.
- Arrange for CBC if patient develops fever, sore throat, or other signs of infection.

Teaching points

- Take this drug as prescribed; do not stop taking abruptly or without consulting your health care provider.
- Avoid alcohol, sleep-inducing drugs, and over-the-counter drugs.
- Avoid prolonged exposure to sun or sunlamps; use a sunscreen or protective garments if exposure to sun is unavoidable.
- You may experience these side effects: Headache, dizziness, drowsiness, weakness, blurred vision (reversible; take safety measures if severe; avoid driving or performing tasks that require alertness); nausea, vomiting, loss of appetite, dry mouth (eat frequent small meals; practice frequent mouth care; and suck sugarless candies); nightmares, inability to concentrate, confusion; changes in sexual function.
- Report dry mouth, difficulty urinating, excessive sedation.

▽ clonazepam

*(kloe **na'** ze pam)*

Apo-Clonazepam (CAN), CO Clonazepam (CAN), Gen-Clonazepam (CAN), Klonopin, Klonopin Wafers, PMS-Clonazepam (CAN), ratio-Clonazepam (CAN), Rivotril (CAN)

PREGNANCY CATEGORY D

CONTROLLED SUBSTANCE C-IV

Drug classes

Antiepileptic
Benzodiazepine

Therapeutic actions

Exact mechanisms not understood; benzodiazepines potentiate the effects of GABA, an inhibitory neurotransmitter.

Indications

- Used alone or as adjunct in treatment of Lennox-Gastaut syndrome (petit mal variant), akinetic and myoclonic seizures; may be useful in patients with absence (petit mal) seizures who have not responded to succinimides; up to 30% of patients show loss of anticonvulsant activity of drug, often within 3 mo of therapy (may respond to dosage adjustment)
- Treatment of panic disorder with or without agoraphobia
- Unlabeled uses: Periodic leg movements during sleep; hypokinetic dysarthria; acute manic episodes; multifocal tic disorders; neuralgias; adjunct in managing schizophrenia

Contraindications and cautions

- Contraindicated with hypersensitivity to benzodiazepines, psychoses, acute narrow-angle glaucoma, shock, coma, acute alcoholic intoxication with depression of vital signs; pregnancy (risk of congenital malformations, neonatal withdrawal syndrome), labor and delivery ("floppy infant" syndrome), lactation (infants become lethargic and lose weight).
- Use cautiously with hepatic or renal impairment, debilitation; elderly patients.

Available forms

Tablets—0.5, 1, 2 mg; orally disintegrating tablets—0.125, 0.25, 0.5, 1, 2 mg

Dosages

Individualize dosage; increase dosage gradually to avoid adverse effects; drug is available only in oral dosage forms.

Adults

Seizure disorders: Initial dose should not exceed 1.5 mg/day PO divided into three doses; increase in increments of 0.5–1 mg PO every 3 days until seizures are adequately controlled or until side effects preclude further increases. Maximum recommended dosage is 20 mg/day.

Panic disorders: Initial dose 0.25 mg PO bid; gradually increase to a target dose of 1 mg/day.

Pediatric patients at least 10 yr or 30 kg

Initially, 0.01–0.03 mg/kg/day PO; do not exceed 0.05 mg/kg/day PO, given in two or three doses. Increase dosage by not more than 0.25–0.5 mg every third day until a daily maintenance dose of 0.1–0.2 mg/kg has been reached, unless seizures are controlled by lower dosage or side effects preclude increases. Whenever possible, divide daily dose into three equal doses, or give largest dose at bedtime.

Pharmacokinetics

Route	Onset	Peak	Duration
Oral	Varies	1–2 hr	Weeks

Metabolism: Hepatic; $T_{1/2}$: 18–50 hr
Distribution: Crosses placenta; enters breast milk
Excretion: Urine

Adverse effects

- **CNS:** *Transient, mild drowsiness initially; sedation, depression, lethargy, apathy, fatigue, light-headedness, disorientation, anger, hostility,* episodes of mania and hypomania, restlessness, confusion, crying, delirium, suicidal ideation, headache, slurred speech, dysarthria, stupor, rigidity, tremor, dystonia, vertigo, euphoria, nervousness, difficulty in concentration, vivid dreams, psychomotor retardation, extrapyramidal symptoms; *mild paradoxical excitatory reactions during first 2 wk of treatment*
- **CV:** Bradycardia, tachycardia, **CV collapse,** hypertension and hypotension, palpitations, edema
- **Dermatologic:** Urticaria, pruritus, rash, dermatitis
- **EENT:** Visual and auditory disturbances, diplopia, nystagmus, depressed hearing, nasal congestion
- **GI:** *Constipation, diarrhea, dry mouth,* salivation, *nausea,* anorexia, vomiting, difficulty in swallowing, gastric disorders, encoporesis
- **GU:** Incontinence, urinary retention, changes in libido, menstrual irregularities
- **Hematologic:** Elevations of blood enzymes—LDH, alkaline phosphatase, AST, ALT; blood dyscrasias: agranulocytosis, leukopenia
- **Other:** Hiccups, fever, diaphoresis, paresthesias, muscular disturbances, gynecomastia. Drug dependence with withdrawal syndrome when drug is discontinued; more common with abrupt discontinuation of higher dosage used for longer than 4 mo

Interactions

✱ **Drug-drug** • Increased CNS depression with alcohol and other CNS depressants • Increased effect with cimetidine, disulfiram, omeprazole, hormonal contraceptives • Decreased effect with theophylline • Risk of increased digoxin levels and toxicity; monitor patient carefully

■ Nursing considerations

CLINICAL ALERT!
Name confusion has occurred between *Klonopin* (clonazepam) and clonidine; use caution.

Assessment

- **History:** Hypersensitivity to benzodiazepines; psychoses; acute narrow-angle glaucoma; shock; coma; acute alcoholic intoxication; pregnancy; lactation; hepatic or renal impairment, debilitation

- **Physical:** Skin color, lesions; T; orientation, reflexes, affect, ophthalmologic examination; P, BP; R, adventitious sounds; liver evaluation, abdominal examination, bowel sounds, normal output; CBC, LFTs, renal function tests

Interventions

- Monitor addiction-prone patients carefully because of their predisposition to habituation and drug dependence.
- Monitor patient for suicidal ideation.
- Monitor liver function and blood counts periodically in patients on long-term therapy.

⊗ ***Warning*** Taper dosage gradually after long-term therapy, especially in patients with epilepsy; substitute another antiepileptic.

- Monitor patient for therapeutic drug levels: 20–80 nanograms/mL.
- If patient has epilepsy, arrange for patient to wear medical alert identification indicating patient has epilepsy and is receiving drug therapy.

Teaching points

- Take drug exactly as prescribed; do not stop taking drug (long-term therapy) without consulting your health care provider.
- Avoid alcohol, sleep-inducing, or over-the-counter drugs.
- Avoid pregnancy; serious adverse effects can occur. Using barrier contraceptives is advised while taking this drug.
- It is advisable to wear or carry a medical alert identification indicating your diagnosis and drug therapy.
- You may experience these side effects: Drowsiness, dizziness (may become less pronounced; avoid driving or engaging in other dangerous activities); GI upset (take drug with food); fatigue; dreams; crying; nervousness; depression, emotional changes; bedwetting, urinary incontinence.
- Report severe dizziness, weakness, drowsiness that persists, rash or skin lesions, difficulty voiding, palpitations, swelling in the extremities, thoughts of suicide.

▽clonidine hydrochloride

(kloe' ni deen)

Antihypertensives: Apo-Clonidine (CAN), Catapres, Catapres-TTS
Transdermal preparations: Dixarit (CAN), Duraclon
Analgesic: Duraclon

PREGNANCY CATEGORY C

Drug classes

Antihypertensive
Central analgesic
Sympatholytic (centrally acting)

Therapeutic actions

Stimulates CNS $alpha_2$-adrenergic receptors, inhibits sympathetic cardioaccelerator and vasoconstrictor centers, and decreases sympathetic outflow from the CNS.

Indications

- Hypertension, used alone or as part of combination therapy
- Treatment of severe pain in cancer patients in combination with opiates; epidural more effective with neuropathic pain (*Duraclon*)
- Unlabeled uses: Tourette syndrome; migraine, decreases severity and frequency; menopausal flushing, decreases severity and frequency of episodes; chronic methadone detoxification; rapid opiate detoxification (in doses up to 17 mcg/kg/day); alcohol and benzodiazepine withdrawal treatment; management of hypertensive "urgencies" (oral clonidine "loading" is used; initial dose of 0.2 mg then 0.1 mg every hour until a dose of 0.7 mg is reached or until BP is controlled); atrial fibrillation; attention deficit hyperactivity disorder; post-herpetic neuralgia, smoking cessation (transdermal)

Contraindications and cautions

- Contraindicated with hypersensitivity to clonidine or any adhesive layer components of the transdermal system.
- Use cautiously with severe coronary insufficiency, recent MI, cerebrovascular disease; chronic renal failure; pregnancy, lactation.

Available forms

Tablets—0.1, 0.2, 0.3 mg; transdermal—0.1, 0.2, 0.3 mg/24 hr; epidural injection—100 mcg/mL

Dosages

Adults

Oral therapy

Individualize dosage. Initial dose is 0.1 mg bid; for maintenance dosage, increase in increments of 0.1 or 0.2 mg to reach desired response. Common range is 0.2–0.6 mg/day, in divided doses; maximum dose is 2.4 mg/day. Minimize sedation by slowly increasing daily dosage; giving majority of daily dose at bedtime.

Transdermal system

Apply to a hairless area of intact skin of upper arm or torso once every 7 days. Change skin site for each application. If system loosens while wearing, apply adhesive overlay directly over the system to ensure adhesion. Start with the 0.1-mg system (releases 0.1 mg/24 hr); if, after 1–2 wk, desired BP reduction is not achieved, add another 0.1-mg system, or use a larger system. Dosage of more than two 0.3-mg systems does not improve efficacy. Antihypertensive effect may only begin 2–3 days after application; therefore, when substituting transdermal systems, a gradual reduction of prior dosage is advised. Remove old system before applying new one. Previous antihypertensive medication may have to be continued, particularly with severe hypertension.

Epidural

- *Pain management:* 30 mcg/hr by continuous epidural infusion.

Pediatric patients

Safety and efficacy not established.

Pharmacokinetics

Route	*Onset*	*Peak*	*Duration*
Oral	30–60 min	3–5 hr	24 hr
Transdermal	Slow	2–3 days	7 days
Epidural	Rapid	19 min	Variable

Metabolism: Hepatic; $T_{1/2}$: 12–16 hr, 19 hr (transdermal system); 48 hr (epidural)
Distribution: Crosses placenta; enters breast milk
Excretion: Urine

Adverse effects

- **CNS:** *Drowsiness, sedation, dizziness,* headache, fatigue that tend to diminish within 4–6 wk, dreams, nightmares, insomnia, hallucinations, delirium, nervousness, restlessness, anxiety, depression, retinal degeneration
- **CV:** Heart failure, orthostatic hypotension, palpitations, tachycardia, bradycardia, Raynaud's phenomenon, ECG abnormalities manifested as Wenckebach period or ventricular trigeminy
- **Dermatologic:** Rash, angioneurotic edema, hives, urticaria, hair thinning and alopecia, pruritus, dryness, itching or burning of the eyes, pallor
- **GI:** *Dry mouth, constipation,* anorexia, malaise, nausea, vomiting, parotid pain, parotitis, mild transient abnormalities in LFTs
- **GU:** Impotence, sexual dysfunction, nocturia, difficulty in micturition, urinary retention
- **Other:** Weight gain, transient hyperglycemia or elevated serum creatine phosphokinase level, gynecomastia, weakness, muscle or joint pain, cramps of the lower limbs, dryness of the nasal mucosa, fever

Transdermal system

- **CNS:** Drowsiness, fatigue, headache, lethargy, sedation, insomnia, nervousness
- **GI:** *Dry mouth,* constipation, nausea, change in taste, dry throat
- **GU:** Impotence, sexual dysfunction
- **Local:** *Transient localized skin reactions,* pruritus, erythema, allergic contact sensitization and contact dermatitis, localized vesiculation, hyperpigmentation, edema, excoriation, burning, papules, throbbing, blanching, generalized macular rash

Interactions

✷ **Drug-drug** • Decreased antihypertensive effects with TCAs (imipramine) • Paradoxical hypertension with propranolol; also greater withdrawal hypertension when abruptly discontinued and patient is taking beta-adrenergic blocking agents • Additive sedation with CNS depressants, alcohol

Nursing considerations

CLINICAL ALERT!
Name confusion has occurred between clonidine and *Klonopin* (clonazepam); use caution.

Assessment

- **History:** Hypersensitivity to clonidine or adhesive layer components of the transdermal system; severe coronary insufficiency, recent MI, cerebrovascular disease; chronic renal failure; lactation, pregnancy
- **Physical:** Body weight; T; skin color, lesions, T; mucous membranes color, lesions; breast examination; orientation, affect, reflexes; ophthalmologic examination; P, BP, orthostatic BP, perfusion, edema, auscultation; bowel sounds, normal output, liver evaluation, palpation of salivary glands; normal urinary output, voiding pattern; LFTs, ECG

Interventions

⊗ ***Warning*** Do not discontinue use abruptly; discontinue therapy by reducing the dosage gradually over 2–4 days to avoid rebound hypertension, tachycardia, flushing, nausea, vomiting, cardiac arrhythmias (hypertensive encephalopathy and death have occurred after abrupt cessation of clonidine).

- Do not discontinue transdermal therapy prior to surgery; monitor BP carefully during surgery; have other BP-controlling drugs readily available.
- Continue oral clonidine therapy to within 4 hr of surgery then resume as soon as possible thereafter.

⊗ ***Black box warning*** Epidural route is not recommended for obstetric, postpartum, or perioperative pain because of the risk of hemodynamic instability.

- Store epidural injection at room temperature; discard any unused portions.
- Reevaluate therapy if clonidine tolerance occurs; giving concomitant diuretic increases the antihypertensive efficacy of clonidine.
- Monitor BP carefully when discontinuing clonidine; hypertension usually returns within 48 hr.

⊗ ***Warning*** Remove transdermal patch before defibrillation to prevent arcing. Remove system if patient is having an MRI.

- Assess compliance with drug regimen in a supportive manner with pill counts, or other methods.

Teaching points

- Take this drug exactly as prescribed. Do not miss doses. Do not discontinue the drug unless instructed by your health care provider. Do not discontinue abruptly; life-threatening adverse effects may occur. If you travel, take an adequate supply of drug.
- Use the transdermal system as prescribed; refer to directions in package insert, or contact your health care provider with questions. Be sure to remove old systems before applying new ones. System must be removed if you are going to have an MRI; inform technician that you are using this system.
- Attempt lifestyle changes that will reduce your blood pressure: Stop smoking and using alcohol; lose weight; restrict intake of salt; exercise regularly.
- Use caution with alcohol. Your sensitivity may increase while using this drug.
- You may experience these side effects: Drowsiness, dizziness, light-headedness, headache, weakness (often transient; observe caution driving or performing other tasks that require alertness or physical dexterity); dry mouth (sucking on sugarless lozenges or ice chips may help); GI upset (eat frequent small meals); dreams, nightmares (reversible); dizziness, light-headedness when you change position (get up slowly; use caution climbing stairs); impotence, other sexual dysfunction, decreased libido (discuss with your health care provider); breast enlargement, sore breasts; palpitations.
- Report urinary retention, changes in vision, blanching of fingers, rash.

▽ clopidogrel bisulfate

*(cloe **pid'** oh grel)*

Plavix

PREGNANCY CATEGORY B

Drug classes

Adenosine diphosphate (ADP) receptor antagonist
Antiplatelet

Therapeutic actions

Inhibits platelet aggregation by blocking ADP receptors on platelets, preventing clumping of platelets.

Indications

- Treatment of patients at risk for ischemic events—recent MI, recent ischemic CVA, peripheral artery disease
- Treatment of patients with acute coronary syndrome
- Unlabeled use: As loading dose with aspirin to prevent adverse cardiac events in coronary stent implantation

Contraindications and cautions

- Contraindicated with allergy to clopidogrel, active pathological bleeding such as peptic ulcer or intracranial hemorrhage, lactation.
- Use cautiously with bleeding disorders, recent surgery, hepatic impairment, pregnancy.

Available forms

Tablets—75 mg

Dosages

Adults

- *Recent MI, CVA, or established peripheral arterial disease:* 75 mg PO daily.
- *Acute coronary syndrome:* 300 mg PO loading dose, then 75 mg/day PO with aspirin, given at a dose from 75–325 mg once daily.

Pharmacokinetics

Route	*Onset*	*Peak*	*Duration*
Oral	Varies	1 hr	2 hr

Metabolism: Hepatic; $T_{1/2}$: 8 hr
Distribution: Crosses placenta; enters breast milk
Excretion: Bile, feces, urine

Adverse effects

- **CNS:** *Headache, dizziness,* weakness, syncope, flushing
- **CV:** Hypertension, edema
- **Dermatologic:** *Rash,* pruritus
- **GI:** Nausea, GI distress, constipation, diarrhea, **GI bleed**
- **Other:** Increased bleeding risk

Interactions

✱ **Drug-drug** • Increased risk of GI bleeding with NSAIDs, monitor patient carefully • Increased risk of bleeding with warfarin; monitor carefully

■ Nursing considerations

Assessment

- **History:** Allergy to clopidogrel, pregnancy, lactation, bleeding disorders, recent surgery, hepatic impairment, peptic ulcer
- **Physical:** Skin color, T, lesions; orientation, reflexes, affect; P, BP, orthostatic BP, baseline ECG, peripheral perfusion; R, adventitious sounds

Interventions

- Provide frequent small meals if GI upset occurs (not as common as with aspirin).
- Provide comfort measures and arrange for analgesics if headache occurs.
- Monitor patient for increased bleeding; limit invasive procedures.

Teaching points

- Take daily as prescribed. May be taken with meals.
- You may experience these side effects: Dizziness, light-headedness (this may pass as you adjust to the drug); headache (lie down in a cool environment and rest; over-the-counter preparations may help); nausea, gastric distress (eat frequent small meals); prolonged bleeding (alert dentists and health care providers of this drug use).
- Report rash, chest pain, fainting, severe headache, abnormal bleeding or bruising.

▽ clorazepate dipotassium

(klor az' e pate)

Apo-Clorazepate (CAN),
Tranxene-SD,
Tranxene-SD Half Strength,
Tranxene-T-tab

PREGNANCY CATEGORY D

CONTROLLED SUBSTANCE C-IV

Drug classes
Antiepileptic
Anxiolytic
Benzodiazepine

Therapeutic actions
Exact mechanisms not understood; benzodiazepines potentiate the effects of GABA, an inhibitory neurotransmitter; anxiolytic effects occur at doses well below those necessary to cause sedation, ataxia.

Indications
- Management of anxiety disorders or for short-term relief of symptoms of anxiety
- Symptomatic relief of acute alcohol withdrawal
- Adjunctive therapy for partial seizures

Contraindications and cautions
- Contraindicated with hypersensitivity to benzodiazepines; psychoses; acute narrow-angle glaucoma; shock; coma; acute alcoholic intoxication with depression of vital signs; pregnancy (risk of congenital malformations, neonatal withdrawal syndrome); labor and delivery ("floppy infant" syndrome); lactation (infants tend to become lethargic and lose weight).
- Use cautiously with impaired liver or renal function, debilitation; elderly patients.

Available forms
Tablets—3.75, 7.5, 15 mg; ER tablets—11.25, 22.5 mg

Dosages
Individualize dosage; increase dosage gradually to avoid adverse effects. Drug is available only in oral forms.

Adults
- *Anxiety:* Usual dose is 30 mg/day PO in divided doses tid; adjust gradually within the range of 15–60 mg/day; also may be given as a single daily dose at bedtime with a maximum starting dose of 15 mg. For maintenance, give the 22.5-mg PO tablet in a single daily dose as an alternate form for patients stabilized on 7.5 mg PO tid; do not use to initiate therapy; the 11.25-mg tablet may be given as a single daily dose.
- *Adjunct to antiepileptic medication:* Maximum initial dose is 7.5 mg PO tid. Increase dosage by no more than 7.5 mg every wk, do not exceed 90 mg/day.
- *Acute alcohol withdrawal:* Day 1: 30 mg PO initially, then 30–60 mg in divided doses. Day 2: 45–90 mg PO in divided doses. Day 3: 22.5–45 mg PO in divided doses. Day 4: 15–30 mg PO in divided doses. Thereafter, gradually reduce dose to 7.5–15 mg/day PO, and stop as soon as condition is stable.

Pediatric patients
- *Adjunct to antiepileptic medication:*
  Older than 12 yr: Use adult dosage.
  9–12 yr: Maximum initial dose is 7.5 mg PO bid; increase dosage by no more than 7.5 mg every wk, and do not exceed 60 mg/day.
  Younger than 9 yr: Not recommended.

Geriatric patients or patients with debilitating disease
- *Anxiety:* Initially, 7.5–15 mg/day PO in divided doses. Adjust as needed and tolerated.

Pharmacokinetics

Route	Onset	Peak	Duration
Oral	Fast	1–2 hr	Days

Metabolism: Hepatic; $T_{1/2}$: 40–50 hr
Distribution: Crosses placenta; enters breast milk
Excretion: Urine

Adverse effects
- **CNS:** *Transient, mild drowsiness initially; sedation, depression, lethargy, apathy, fatigue, light-headedness, disorientation, anger, hostility,* episodes of mania and hypomania, restlessness, confusion, crying, delirium, *headache,* slurred speech, dysarthria, stupor, rigidity, tremor, dystonia, vertigo, euphoria, nervousness, difficulty in concentration, vivid dreams, psychomotor retardation, extrapyramidal symptoms; *mild paradoxical excitatory reactions during first 2 wk of treatment*
- **CV:** Bradycardia, tachycardia, **CV collapse,** hypertension and hypotension, palpitations, edema
- **Dermatologic:** Urticaria, pruritus, rash, dermatitis
- **EENT:** Visual and auditory disturbances, diplopia, nystagmus, depressed hearing, nasal congestion

- **GI:** *Constipation, diarrhea, dry mouth,* salivation, *nausea,* anorexia, vomiting, difficulty in swallowing, gastric disorders, hepatic impairment, encopresis
- **GU:** Incontinence, urinary retention, changes in libido, menstrual irregularities
- **Hematologic:** Elevations of blood enzymes—LDH, alkaline phosphatase, AST, ALT; blood dyscrasias—agranulocytosis, leukopenia
- **Other:** Hiccups, fever, diaphoresis, paresthesias, muscular disturbances, gynecomastia; drug dependence with withdrawal syndrome is common with abrupt discontinuation of higher dosage used for longer than 4 mo

Interactions

✱ **Drug-drug** • Increased CNS depression with alcohol and other CNS depressants • Increased effect with cimetidine, disulfiram, omeprazole, hormonal contraceptives • Decreased effect with theophylline • Risk of increased digoxin levels and toxicity; monitor patient carefully

✱ **Drug-alternative therapy** • Increased CNS effects with kava

■ Nursing considerations

CLINICAL ALERT!

Name confusion has occurred between clorazepate and clofibrate; use caution.

Assessment

- **History:** Hypersensitivity to benzodiazepines; psychoses; acute narrow-angle glaucoma; shock; coma; acute alcoholic intoxication; pregnancy; lactation; renal or hepatic impairment; debilitation
- **Physical:** Skin color, lesions; T; orientation, reflexes, affect, ophthalmologic examination; P, BP; R, adventitious sounds; liver evaluation, abdominal examination, bowel sounds, normal output; CBC, LFTs, renal function tests

Interventions

⊗ ***Warning*** Taper dosage gradually after long-term therapy, especially in epileptics.

- Arrange for patients with epilepsy to wear medical alert identification, indicating disease and medication usage.
- Because of increased risk of suicide, monitor patient for suicidal ideation.

Teaching points

- Take drug exactly as prescribed; do not stop taking drug (long-term therapy) without consulting your health care provider.
- Avoid alcohol, sleep-inducing, or over-the-counter drugs.
- Avoid pregnancy while taking this drug; use of barrier contraceptives is advised. If you become pregnant, do not stop the drug; contact your health care provider.
- You may experience these side effects: Drowsiness, dizziness (may be transient; avoid driving a car or engaging in other dangerous activities); GI upset (take with food); fatigue; depression; dreams; crying; nervousness; depression, emotional changes; bed-wetting, urinary incontinence.
- Report severe dizziness, weakness, drowsiness that persists, rash or skin lesions, difficulty voiding, palpitations, swelling in the extremities, thoughts of suicide.

clotrimazole

(kloe ***trim'*** *a zole)*

Oral, Topical use only: Mycelex Troche

Vaginal preparations: Canesten Vaginal (CAN), Gyne-Lotrimin 3, Gyne-Lotrimin 3 Combination Pack, Mycelex-7, Mycelex-7 Combination Pack

Topical preparations: Canesten Topical (CAN), Clotrimaderm (CAN), Cruex, Desenex, Fungoid, Lotrimin AF, Lotrimin Ultra

PREGNANCY CATEGORY B (TOPICAL, VAGINAL FORMS)

PREGNANCY CATEGORY C (ORAL TROCHE)

Drug class
Antifungal

Therapeutic actions
Fungicidal and fungistatic: Binds to fungal cell membrane with a resultant change in membrane permeability, allowing leakage of intracellular components, causing cell death.

Indications
- Troche: Treatment of oropharyngeal candidiasis; prevention of oropharyngeal candidiasis in immunocompromised patients receiving radiation, chemotherapy, or steroid therapy
- Vaginal preparations: Local treatment of vulvovaginal candidiasis (moniliasis)
- Topical preparations: Topical treatment of tinea pedia, tinea cruris, tinea corporis due to *Trichophyton rubrum, Trichophyton mentagrophytes, Epidermophyton floccosum, Microsporum canis;* candidiasis due to *Candida albicans;* tinea versicolor due to *Malassezia furfur*

Contraindications and cautions
- Contraindicated with allergy to clotrimazole or components used in preparation. Vaginal products contraindicated in girls younger than 12 yr.
- Use vaginal and topical preparations cautiously with pregnancy, lactation.
- Use oral troche only when benefits to mother outweigh risk to fetus.

Available forms
Vaginal suppositories—100, 200 mg; vaginal cream, solution, lotion—1%, 2%; topical cream, solution, lotion—1%; oral troche—10 mg

Dosages
Adults and children 2 yr and older
Oral troche
For treatment, dissolve slowly in the mouth five times daily for 14 days. For prevention, tid for the duration of chemotherapy or radiation therapy or until steroids are reduced to maintenance levels.
Topical
Gently massage into affected and surrounding skin areas bid in the morning and evening for 7 days. Relief is usually noted during first week of therapy; therapy 2–4 wk.
Vaginal suppository
100-mg suppository intravaginally at bedtime for 7 consecutive nights; 200-mg suppository for 3 consecutive nights.
Vaginal preparation, cream
One applicator (5 g/day), preferably at bedtime for 3–7 consecutive days.

Pharmacokinetics
Action is primarily local; pharmacokinetics are not known.

Adverse effects
Troche
- **GI:** *Nausea, vomiting, abnormal LFTs*

Vaginal
- **Dermatologic:** Rash
- **GI:** *Lower abdominal cramps,* bloating (elevated AST), unpleasant mouth sensations
- **GU:** *Slight urinary frequency; burning or irritation in the sexual partner*

Topical
- **Local:** Erythema, stinging, blistering, peeling, edema, pruritus, urticaria, general skin irritation

■ Nursing considerations

CLINICAL ALERT!
Name confusion has occurred between clotrimazole and co-trimoxazole; use caution.

Assessment
- **History:** Allergy to clotrimazole or components used in preparation, pregnancy, lactation
- **Physical:** Skin color, lesions, area around lesions; bowel sounds; culture of area involved, LFTs

Interventions
- Culture fungus involved before therapy.
- Have patient dissolve troche slowly in mouth.
- Insert vaginal suppository into vagina at bedtime for 3–7 consecutive nights. Provide sanitary napkin to protect clothing from stains.
- Administer vaginal cream high into vagina using the applicator supplied with the

product. Administer for 3–7 consecutive nights, even during menstrual period.

- Cleanse affected area before topical application. Do not apply to eyes or near eyes.
- Monitor response to drug therapy. If no response is noted, arrange for more cultures to determine causative organism.
- Ensure that patient receives full course of therapy to eradicate the fungus and prevent recurrence.
- Discontinue topical or vaginal administration if rash or sensitivity occurs.
- Supervise children younger than 12 yr using topical products.

Teaching points

- Take the full course of drug therapy, even if symptoms improve. Continue during menstrual period if vaginal route is being used. Long-term use of the drug may be needed; beneficial effects may not be seen for several weeks. Vaginal creams should be inserted high into the vagina. Troche preparation should be allowed to dissolve slowly in the mouth. Apply topical preparation by gently massaging into the affected area.
- Use hygiene measures to prevent reinfection or spread of infection.
- With vaginal use, refrain from sexual intercourse, or advise partner to use a condom to avoid reinfection. Use a sanitary napkin to prevent staining of clothing.
- You may experience these side effects: Nausea, vomiting, diarrhea (oral use); irritation, burning, stinging (local).
- Report worsening of the condition being treated, local irritation, burning (topical), rash, irritation, pelvic pain (vaginal), nausea, GI distress (oral administration).

▽ clozapine

*(**kloe'** za peen)*

Apo-Clozapine (CAN), Clozaril, FazaClo, Gen-Clozapine (CAN)

PREGNANCY CATEGORY B

Drug classes

Antipsychotic
Dopaminergic blocker

Therapeutic actions

Mechanism not fully understood: Blocks dopamine receptors in the brain, depresses the RAS; anticholinergic, antihistaminic (H_1), and alpha-adrenergic blocking activity may contribute to some of its therapeutic (and adverse) actions. Clozapine produces fewer extrapyramidal effects than other antipsychotics.

Indications

- Management of severely ill schizophrenics who are unresponsive to standard antipsychotic drugs
- Reduction of the risk of recurrent suicidal behavior in patients with schizophrenia or schizoaffective disorder (not orally disintegrating tablet)

Contraindications and cautions

- Contraindicated with allergy to clozapine, myeloproliferative disorders, history of clozapine-induced agranulocytosis or severe granulocytopenia, severe CNS depression, comatose states, history of seizure disorders, lactation, therapy with other drugs that cause bone marrow suppression.
- Use cautiously with CV disease, narrow-angle glaucoma, pregnancy.

Available forms

Tablets—25, 100 mg; orally disintegrating tablets—12.5, 25, 50, 100 mg

Dosages

Adults

- *Initial therapy:* 12.5 mg PO once or twice daily. If using orally disintegrating tablets, begin with one half (12.5 mg) of a 25-mg tablet and destroy the remaining half. Continue to 25 mg PO daily or bid; then gradually increase with daily increments of 25–50 mg/day, if tolerated, to a dose of 300–450 mg/day by the end of second week. Adjust later dosage no more often than twice weekly in increments of less than 100 mg. Do not exceed 900 mg/day.

- *Maintenance:* Maintain at the lowest effective dose for remission of symptoms.
- *Discontinuation of therapy:* Gradual reduction over a 2-wk period is preferred. If abrupt discontinuation is required, carefully monitor patient for signs of acute psychotic symptoms.
- *Reinitiation of treatment:* Follow initial dosage guidelines, use extreme care; increased risk of severe adverse effects with re-exposure.

Pediatric patients

Safety and efficacy in patients younger than 16 yr not established.

Pharmacokinetics

Route	*Onset*	*Peak*	*Duration*
Oral	Varies	1–6 hr	Weeks

Metabolism: Hepatic; $T_{1/2}$: 4–12 hr
Distribution: Crosses placenta; enters breast milk
Excretion: Feces, urine

Adverse effects

- **CNS:** *Drowsiness, sedation, seizures, dizziness, syncope, headache,* tremor, disturbed sleep, nightmares, restlessness, agitation, increased salivation, sweating, tardive dyskinesia, neuroleptic malignant syndrome
- **CV:** *Tachycardia, hypotension,* hypertension, ECG changes, **potentially fatal myocarditis**
- **GI:** *Nausea, vomiting, constipation,* abdominal discomfort, dry mouth
- **GU:** Urinary abnormalities
- **Hematologic:** Leukopenia, **agranulocytosis**
- **Other:** *Fever,* weight gain, rash, development of diabetes mellitus

Interactions

✱ **Drug-drug** • Increased therapeutic and toxic effects with cimetidine, caffeine, other CYP450 inhibitors • Decreased therapeutic effect with phenytoin, ethotoin, other CYP450 inducers

■ Nursing considerations

CLINICAL ALERT!
Name confusion has occurred with *Clozaril* (clozapine) and *Colazal* (balsalazide); dangerous effects could occur. Use caution.

Assessment

- **History:** Allergy to clozapine, myeloproliferative disorders, history of clozapine-induced agranulocytosis or severe granulocytopenia, severe CNS depression, comatose states, history of seizure disorders, CV disease, narrow-angle glaucoma, lactation, pregnancy
- **Physical:** T, weight; reflexes, orientation, IOP, ophthalmologic examination; P, BP, orthostatic BP, ECG; R, adventitious sounds; bowel sounds, normal output, liver evaluation; prostate palpation, normal urine output; CBC, urinalysis, LFTs, renal function tests, EEG

Interventions

⊗ ***Black box warning*** Use only when unresponsive to conventional antipsychotic drugs; risk of serious CV and respiratory effects.

- Obtain clozapine through the *Clozaril* Patient Assistance Program. For more information, call 1-800-448-5938.
- Dispense only 1 wk supply at a time.
- Monitor WBC count carefully prior to first dose.

⊗ ***Black box warning*** Monitor WBC count weekly during treatment and for 4 wk thereafter. Dosage must be adjusted based on WBC count. Potentially fatal agranulocytosis has been reported.

⊗ ***Black box warning*** Elderly patients with dementia-related psychosis are at increased risk for death; drug is not approved for these patients.

- Monitor T. If fever occurs, rule out underlying infection, and consult physician for comfort measures.

⊗ ***Black box warning*** Monitor for seizures; with history of seizures, risk increases as dose increases.

- Monitor elderly patients for dehydration. Institute remedial measures promptly; sedation and decreased thirst related to CNS effects can lead to dehydration.
- Monitor patient regularly for signs and symptoms of diabetes mellitus.
- Encourage voiding before taking drug to decrease anticholinergic effects of urinary retention.
- Follow guidelines for discontinuation or reinstitution of the drug.

- Educate patient on seriousness of potential agranulocytosis.

Teaching points

- Weekly blood tests will be taken to determine safe dosage; dosage will be increased gradually to achieve most effective dose. Only 1 week of medication can be dispensed at a time and will depend on your white blood cell count. Do not take more than your prescribed dosage. Do not make up missed doses; instead contact your health care provider. Do not stop taking this drug suddenly; gradual reduction of dosage is needed to prevent side effects.
- If you think you are pregnant or wish to become pregnant, contact your health care provider.
- You may experience these side effects: Drowsiness, dizziness, sedation, seizures (avoid driving or performing tasks that require concentration); dizziness, faintness on arising (change positions slowly); increased salivation (reversible); constipation (consult your health care provider for correctives); fast heart rate (rest, take your time).
- Report lethargy, weakness, fever, sore throat, malaise, mouth ulcers, and flulike symptoms.

coagulation factor VIIa (recombinant)

See Appendix W, *Less commonly used drugs*.

DANGEROUS DRUG

codeine phosphate

(koe' deen)

PREGNANCY CATEGORY C (DURING PREGNANCY)

PREGNANCY CATEGORY D (DURING LABOR)

CONTROLLED SUBSTANCE C-II

Drug classes

Antitussive
Opioid agonist analgesic

Therapeutic actions

Acts at opioid receptors in the CNS to produce analgesia, euphoria, sedation; acts in the medullary cough center to depress cough reflex.

Indications

- Relief of mild to moderate pain in adults and children
- Suppression of coughing induced by chemical or mechanical irritation of the respiratory system

Contraindications and cautions

- Contraindicated with hypersensitivity to opioids, physical dependence on an opioid analgesic (drug may precipitate withdrawal).
- Use cautiously with pregnancy, labor, lactation, bronchial asthma, COPD, respiratory depression, anoxia, increased intracranial pressure, acute MI, ventricular failure, coronary insufficiency, hypertension, biliary tract surgery, renal or hepatic impairment.

Available forms

Tablets—15, 30, 60 mg; oral solution—15 mg/5 mL; injection—15, 30 mg/mL

Dosages

Adults

Analgesic

15–60 mg PO, IM, IV or subcutaneously every 4–6 hr; do not exceed 360 mg/24 hr.

Antitussive

10–20 mg PO every 4–6 hr; do not exceed 120 mg/24 hr.

Pediatric patients

Contraindicated in premature infants.

Analgesic

1 yr and older: 0.5 mg/kg or 15 mg/m^2 IM or subcutaneously every 4–6 hr.

Antitussive

2–6 yr: 2.5–5 mg PO every 4–6 hr; do not exceed 12–18 mg/day based on age.
6–12 yr: 5–10 mg PO every 4–6 hr; do not exceed 60 mg/24 hr.

Geriatric patients or impaired adults

Use caution; respiratory depression may occur in elderly, the very ill, or those with respiratory problems. Reduced dosage may be necessary.

Pharmacokinetics

Route	*Onset*	*Peak*	*Duration*
Oral, IM, IV	10–30 min	30–60 min	4–6 hr

Metabolism: Hepatic; $T_{1/2}$: 3 hr
Distribution: Crosses placenta; enters breast milk
Excretion: Urine

IV FACTS

Preparation: Protect vials from light.
Infusion: Administer slowly over 5 min by direct injection or into running IV tubing.

Adverse effects

- **CNS:** *Sedation, clamminess, sweating, headache, vertigo, floating feeling, dizziness, lethargy, confusion, light-headedness,* nervousness, unusual dreams, agitation, euphoria, hallucinations, delirium, insomnia, anxiety, fear, disorientation, impaired mental and physical performance, coma, mood changes, weakness, tremor, seizures
- **CV:** Palpitation, increase or decrease in BP, circulatory depression, **cardiac arrest, shock,** tachycardia, bradycardia, arrhythmia
- **Dermatologic:** Rash, hives, pruritus, flushing, warmth, sensitivity to cold
- **EENT:** Diplopia, blurred vision
- **GI:** *Nausea, vomiting,* dry mouth, anorexia, *constipation,* biliary tract spasm
- **GU:** Ureteral spasm, spasm of vesical sphincters, urinary retention or hesitancy, oliguria, antidiuretic effect, reduced libido or potency
- **Local:** Phlebitis following IV injection, pain at injection site; tissue irritation and induration (subcutaneous injection)
- **Respiratory:** Slow, shallow respiration; apnea; suppression of cough reflex; **laryngospasm; bronchospasm**
- **Other:** Physical tolerance and dependence, psychological dependence

Interactions

✱ **Drug-drug** • Additive CNS effects when given with CNS depressants • Potentiation of effects of codeine with barbiturate anesthetics; decrease dose of codeine when coadministering

✱ **Drug-lab test** • Elevated biliary tract pressure may increase plasma amylase, lipase; determinations of these levels may be unreliable for 24 hr after administration of opioids

■ Nursing considerations

CLINICAL ALERT!
Name confusion has occurred between codeine and *Cardene* (nicardipine); use caution.

Assessment

- **History:** Hypersensitivity to codeine, physical dependence on an opioid analgesic, pregnancy, labor, lactation, bronchial asthma, COPD, increased intracranial pressure, acute MI, ventricular failure, coronary insufficiency, hypertension, biliary tract surgery, renal or hepatic impairment
- **Physical:** Orientation, reflexes, bilateral grip strength, affect; pupil size, vision; pulse, auscultation, BP; R, adventitious sounds; bowel sounds, normal output; LFTs, renal function tests

Interventions

- Give to nursing women 4–6 hr before scheduled feeding to minimize drug in milk.
- Use the smallest effective dose for the shortest period.

⊗ ***Warning*** Nursing mothers should monitor infants for evidence of overdose (increased sleepiness, difficulty breathing, limpness) and seek medical help immediately if it occurs.

⊗ ***Warning*** During parenteral administration, ensure that opioid antagonist and facilities for assisted or controlled respirations are readily available.

- Use caution when injecting subcutaneously into chilled body areas or in patients with hypotension or in shock; impaired perfusion may delay absorption; with repeated doses, an excessive amount may be absorbed when circulation is restored.

⊗ **Warning** Do not use IV in children.

- Instruct postoperative patients in pulmonary toilet; drug suppresses cough reflex.
- Monitor bowel function, arrange for stimulant laxatives to be given regularly, and initiate bowel training program if severe constipation occurs.

Teaching points

- Take drug exactly as prescribed.
- Do not take any leftover drug for other disorders, and do not let anyone else take it.
- If you are nursing a baby, take drug 4 to 6 hours before scheduled feeding. Monitor baby for increased sleepiness or difficulty breathing.
- You may experience these side effects: Dizziness, sedation, drowsiness, impaired visual acuity (avoid driving and performing other tasks that require alertness); nausea, loss of appetite (lie quietly, eat frequent small meals); constipation (use a laxative).
- Report severe nausea, vomiting, palpitations, constipation, shortness of breath or difficulty breathing.

colchicine

(kol' chih seen)

Colcrys

PREGNANCY CATEGORY C

Drug class

Antigout drug

Therapeutic actions

Exact mechanism of action unknown; decreases deposition of uric acid, inhibits kinin formation and phagocytosis, and decreases inflammatory reaction to urate crystal deposition.

Indications

- Treatment and prophylaxis of acute gout flares in adults
- Treatment of familial Mediterranean fever in adults and children 4 yr and older

Contraindications and cautions

- Contraindicated with hypersensitivity to colchicine, concurrent use of cyclosporine, ranolazine, or strong to moderate CYP3A4 inhibitors in presence of hepatic or renal impairment.
- Use cautiously with hepatic or renal impairment, pregnancy, lactation, and in elderly patients.

Available forms

Tablets—0.6 mg

Dosages

Adults

Acute gout flares: 1.2 mg PO at first sign of gout flare, followed by 0.6 mg 1 hour later. Maximum recommended dosage is 1.8 mg over a 1-hour period.

Prophylaxis of gout flares: 0.6 mg/day PO, to maximum of 1.2 mg/day PO.

Familial Mediterranean fever: 1.2–2.4 mg/day PO in one or two divided doses; increase or decrease in 0.3-mg increments as needed.

Pediatric patients

Treatment and prophylaxis of acute gout flares: Safety and efficacy not established.

Familial Mediterranean fever: 4–6 yr: 0.3–1.8 mg/day PO; 6–12 yr: 0.9–1.8 mg/day PO; older than 12 yr: use adult dosage. May be given as one dose or in two divided doses.

Patients with hepatic impairment

Acute gout flares: For mild to moderate impairment, no dosage adjustment is needed. For severe impairment, dosage should be the same but should not be repeated more often than once every 2 wk.

Familial Mediterranean fever: Monitor patient closely. Consider dosage reduction with careful monitoring.

Patients with renal impairment

Acute gout flares: For mild to moderate impairment, no dosage adjustment is needed. For severe impairment (CrCl less than 30 mL/min), dosage adjustment is not needed, but do not repeat more than once every 2 wk. For patient on dialysis, give 0.6 mg as a single dose; do not repeat more than once every 2 wk.

Familial Mediterranean fever: For mild to moderate impairment, consider dosage reduction; monitor patient closely. For severe impairment, start with 0.3 mg/day and increase with careful monitoring. Patients on dialysis should receive a total dose of 0.3 mg/day.

Pharmacokinetics

Route	*Onset*	*Peak*
Oral	Slow	1-2 hr

Metabolism: Hepatic; $T_{1/2}$: 26–31 hr
Distribution: Crosses placenta; may enter breast milk
Excretion: Urine, bile

Adverse effects

- **CNS:** Peripheral neuropathy
- **Dermatologic:** Alopecia, rash, purpura, dermatoses
- **GI:** *Nausea, diarrhea, vomiting, abdominal pain,* dyspepsia
- **GU:** Azoospermia, oligospermia
- **Hematologic: Bone marrow suppression,** elevated AST and ALT, aplastic anemia
- **Other:** Myopathy, muscle pain, weakness, **rhabdomyolysis**

Interactions

✱ **Drug-drug** • Increased risk of serious toxic effects, including fatalities if combined with cyclosporine, ranolazine; this combination is contraindicated but if combination must be used, monitor patient closely and limit dose to maximum of 0.6 mg/day • Significant increase in serum colchicine level and toxicity if combined with atazanavir, clarithromycin, indinavir, itraconazole, ketoconazole, nefazodone, nelfinavir, ritonavir, saquinavir, telithromycin; this combination is contraindicated but if combination must be used, monitor patient closely and limit dose to 0.6 mg followed by 0.3 mg in 1 hour (for gout), repeat no earlier than every 3 days; 0.6 mg/day (for familial Mediterranean fever) • Risk of significant increase in colchicine plasma level and toxicity with amprenavir, aprepitant, diltiazem, erythromycin, fluconazole, fosamprenavir, verapamil; these combinations are contraindicated, but if combination must be used, limit dose to 1.2 mg (for gout), repeat no earlier than every 3 days; 1.2 mg/day (for familial Mediterranean fever) • Risk of altered pharmacokinetics or pharmacodynamics if combined with atorvastatin, digoxin, fibrates, fluvastatin, gemfibrozil, pravastatin, simvastatin; weigh benefit versus risk in use of these combinations and carefully monitor patient for muscle pain or weakness

✱ **Drug-food** • Risk of serious adverse effects if combined with grapefruit juice; avoid this combination

■ Nursing considerations

Assessment

- **History:** Hypersensitivity to components of drug; blood dyscrasias; serious GI, hepatic or renal disorders; pregnancy; lactation
- **Physical:** T; skin color, lesions; orientation, reflexes; P, BP; liver evaluation, normal bowel output; normal urine output; CBC, LFTs, renal function tests, urinalysis

Interventions

- Obtain baseline and periodic liver and renal function tests, serum uric acid levels, CBC.
- Administer drug as prescribed. Do not make up missed doses.
- Encourage patient to avoid grapefruit juice.
- Check patient's complete drug list and ensure that interacting drugs are not being used, and that appropriate dosage adjustments have been considered.
- Monitor patient for relief of pain and signs and symptoms of acute gout flair. Begin therapy at first sign of acute flare for best therapeutic effect.
- Monitor GI effects; antidiarrheal medication may be needed.

Teaching points

- Take this drug exactly as prescribed. If taking this drug for gout, take it at the first sign of an acute flare; then take the second dose 1 hour later.
- If you are taking this drug for familial Mediterranean fever and forget a dose, take the next dose at the regular time. Do not attempt to make up or double doses.
- Do not drink grapefruit juice while you are taking drug; serious adverse effects could occur.

C

- Continue to take this drug as prescribed; do not discontinue this drug without consulting your health care provider.
- Keep a record of all drugs, herbs, and over-the-counter medications you are taking and review it with your health care provider. This drug interacts with many of these drugs and serious complications could occur. Your health care provider may need to adjust the dosages of these drugs for your safety.
- This drug can suppress the activity of your bone marrow, resulting in lower than normal red blood cells (you may feel fatigued), platelets (you may bleed more than normal), and white blood cells (you may have increased susceptibility to infections).
- You may experience these side effects: Nausea, vomiting, diarrhea, abdominal pain (small, frequent meals may help; consult your health care provider if abdominal pain becomes too uncomfortable), loss of hair (which is reversible), rash
- You will need periodic medical exams and blood tests to evaluate the effects of this drug.
- Report severe diarrhea, muscle pain or weakness, tingling or numbness in the fingers or toes, persistent gout attacks, extreme fatigue, unusual bleeding or bruising, fever and chills, signs of infection.

▽ colesevelam hydrochloride

*(koe leh **seve'** eh lam)*

WelChol

PREGNANCY CATEGORY B

Drug classes

Antihyperlipidemic
Bile acid sequestrant

Therapeutic actions

Binds bile acids in the intestine allowing excretion in the feces; as a result, cholesterol is oxidized in the liver to replace the bile acids lost; serum cholesterol and LDLs are lowered.

Indications

- Reduction of elevated LDLs as adjunct to diet and exercise in patients with primary hypercholesterolemia; used alone or in conjunction with an HMG-CoA reductase inhibitor
- As adjunct to diet and exercise to improve glycemic control in adults with type 2 diabetes
- **NEW INDICATION:** Adjunct to diet and exercise to reduce LDL in boys and postmenarchal girls ages 10–17 yr with familial hypercholesterolemia not responsive to diet alone

Contraindications and cautions

- Contraindicated with allergy to bile acid sequestrants; complete biliary obstruction; intestinal obstruction; lactation.
- Use cautiously with difficulty swallowing; GI motility disorders; major GI tract surgery; patients susceptible to fat-soluble vitamin deficiency, pregnancy.

Available forms

Tablets—625 mg; oral suspension—1.875-, 3.75-g packets

Dosages

Adults

- *Monotherapy for hyperlipidemia:* 3 tablets bid PO with meals or 6 tablets daily PO with a meal; do not exceed 7 tablets/day.
- *Combination therapy with an HMG-CoA inhibitor:* 3 tablets PO bid with meals or 6 tablets once a day PO with a meal; do not exceed 6 tablets/day.
- *Type 2 diabetes:* 6 tablets/day PO or 3 tablets PO bid.

Pediatric patients 10–17 yr

- *Familial hypercholesterolemia:* 1.8 g PO bid or 3.7 g/day PO oral suspension

Pharmacokinetics

Not absorbed systemically
Excretion: Feces

Adverse effects

- **CNS:** Headache, anxiety, vertigo, dizziness, fatigue, syncope, drowsiness

- **GI:** *Constipation to fecal impaction,* exacerbation of hemorrhoids, abdominal cramps, pain, flatulence, nausea, vomiting, diarrhea, heartburn
- **GU:** Hematuria, dysuria, diuresis
- **Hematologic:** Increased bleeding tendencies related to vitamin K malabsorption, vitamin A and D deficiencies, reduced serum and red cell folate, hyperchloremic acidosis
- **Other:** Osteoporosis, backache, muscle and joint pain, arthritis, fever, pharyngitis

Interactions

✱ **Drug-drug** • Malabsorption of fat-soluble vitamins if taken concurrently with cholestyramine • Decreased absorption of oral drugs; take other oral drugs 1 hr before or 4–6 hr after colesevelam • Decreased bioavailability of SR verapamil

■ Nursing considerations

Assessment

- **History:** Allergy to bile acid sequestrants; complete biliary obstruction; intestinal obstruction; pregnancy; lactation; difficulty swallowing, GI motility disorders; major GI tract surgery; susceptibility to fat-soluble vitamin deficiency
- **Physical:** Skin lesions, color, T; orientation, affect, reflexes; P, auscultation, baseline ECG, peripheral perfusion; liver evaluation, bowel sounds; lipid studies, LFTs, clotting profile

Interventions

- Monitor serum cholesterol, LDLs, triglycerides, and serum glucose before starting treatment and periodically during treatment.
- For hyperlipidemia, administer drug with meals. For type 2 diabetes, administer once or twice a day.
- Store at room temperature; protect from moisture.
- Mix oral suspension packet with 4–8 oz of water; do not use dry. Administer with meals.
- Establish bowel program to deal with constipation.
- Monitor nutritional status and arrange for consults if needed.
- Consult with dietitian regarding low-cholesterol diets and provide information regarding exercise programs.
- Ensure that patients with type 2 diabetes follow diet and exercise regimen.
- Arrange for regular follow-up during long-term therapy.

C

Teaching points

- If this drug was prescribed for hyperlipidemia, take drug with meals. If drug was prescribed for type 2 diabetes, take drug once or twice per day.
- Take this drug at least 1 hour before or 4–6 hours after other drugs.
- Continue to follow your low-fat or diabetic diet and participate in an exercise program.
- If using the oral solution, mix entire content of packet with 4–8 ounces of water. Take with meals. Do not use dry.
- Plan to return for periodic blood tests to evaluate the effectiveness of this drug.
- You may experience these side effects: Constipation (this may resolve, or other measures may need to be taken to alleviate this problem); nausea, heartburn, loss of appetite (eat frequent small meals); dizziness, drowsiness, vertigo, fainting (avoid driving and operating dangerous machinery until you know how this drug affects you); headache, muscle and joint aches and pains (this may decrease over time; if it becomes bothersome, consult your health care provider).
- Report unusual bleeding or bruising, severe constipation, severe GI upset, chest pain, difficulty breathing, rash, fever.

▽ colestipol hydrochloride

*(koe **les'** ti pole)*

Colestid

PREGNANCY CATEGORY C

Drug classes

Antihyperlipidemic
Bile acid sequestrant

Therapeutic actions

Binds bile acids in the intestine to form a complex that is excreted in the feces; as a result, cholesterol is lost, oxidized in the liver, and serum cholesterol and LDL are lowered.

Indications
- Adjunctive therapy: Reduction of elevated serum cholesterol in patients with primary hypercholesterolemia (elevated LDL)
- Unlabeled uses: Digitalis toxicity, hyperoxaluria, relief of pruritus associated with biliary obstruction, adjunctive treatment of hyperthyroidism, binding of *Clostridium difficile* toxin

Contraindications and cautions
- Contraindicated with allergy to bile acid sequestrants, complete biliary obstruction.
- Use cautiously with abnormal intestinal function, pregnancy, lactation.

Available forms
Tablets—1 g; granules—5-g packets, 5 g/7.5 g powder

Dosages
Adults
- For suspension, 5–30 g/day PO once or in divided doses two to four times/day. Start with 5 g daily or bid PO, and increase in 5-g/day increments at 1- to 2-mo intervals. For tablets, 2–16 g/day PO in 1–2 divided doses; initially, 2 g once or twice daily; increasing in 2-g increments at 1- to 2-mo intervals.

Pediatric patients
Safety and efficacy not established.

Pharmacokinetics
Not absorbed systemically
Excretion: Feces

Adverse effects
- **CNS:** *Headache,* anxiety, vertigo, dizziness, fatigue, syncope, drowsiness
- **Dermatologic:** Rash and irritation of skin, tongue, perianal area
- **GI:** *Constipation* to fecal impaction, *exacerbation of hemorrhoids,* abdominal cramps, *abdominal pain,* flatulence, anorexia, heartburn, nausea, vomiting, steatorrhea
- **GU:** Hematuria, dysuria, diuresis
- **Hematologic:** Increased bleeding tendencies related to vitamin K malabsorption, vitamin A and D deficiencies, hyperchloremic acidosis
- **Other:** Osteoporosis, chest pain, backache, muscle and joint pain, arthritis, fever

Interactions
✱ **Drug-drug** • Decreased serum levels or delayed absorption of thiazide diuretics, digitalis preparations • Malabsorption of fat-soluble vitamins • Decreased absorption of oral drugs; administer 1 hr before or 4–6 hr after colestipol

■ Nursing considerations
Assessment
- **History:** Allergy to bile acid sequestrant, complete biliary obstruction, abnormal intestinal function, pregnancy, lactation
- **Physical:** Skin lesions, color, T; orientation, affect, reflexes; P, auscultation, baseline ECG, peripheral perfusion; liver evaluation, bowel sounds; lipid studies, LFTs, clotting profile

Interventions
- Do not administer drug in dry form. Mix in liquids, soups, cereals, or pulpy fruits; add the prescribed amount to a glassful (90 mL) of liquid; stir until completely mixed. The granules will not dissolve. May be mixed with carbonated beverages, slowly stirred in a large glass. Rinse the glass with a small amount of additional beverage to ensure that the entire dose has been taken.
- Make sure that patient swallows tablets whole; do not cut, crush, or chew them. Tablets should be taken with plenty of fluids.
- Administer drug before meals.

⊗ ***Warning*** Monitor administration of other oral drugs for binding in the intestine and delayed or decreased absorption. Give them 1 hr before or 4–6 hr after the colestipol.

- Arrange for regular follow-up care during long-term therapy.
- Alert patient and concerned others about the high cost of drug.

Teaching points
- Take drug before meals. Do not take the powder in the dry form. Mix in liquids, soups,

cereals, or pulpy fruit; add the prescribed amount to a glassful of the liquid; stir until completely mixed. The granules will not dissolve; rinse the glass with a small amount of additional liquid to ensure that you receive the entire dose of the drug. Or, carbonated beverages may be used; mix by slowly stirring in a large glass. If taking tablet form, swallow tablet whole with plenty of fluids; do not cut, crush, or chew it.
- This drug may interfere with the absorption of other oral medications. Take other oral medications 1 hour before or 4–6 hours after colestipol.
- You may experience these side effects: Constipation (transient, if it persists, request correctives); nausea, heartburn, loss of appetite (eat frequent small meals); dizziness, drowsiness, vertigo, fainting (avoid driving and operating dangerous machinery); headache, muscle and joint aches and pains (may decrease with time).
- Report unusual bleeding or bruising, severe constipation, severe GI upset, chest pain, difficulty breathing, rash, fever.

▽corticotropin (ACTH, adrenocorticotropin, corticotrophin)

*(kor ti koe **troe'** pin)*

Repository injection: H.P. Acthar Gel

PREGNANCY CATEGORY C

Drug classes

Anterior pituitary hormone
Diagnostic agent

Therapeutic actions

Stimulates the adrenal cortex to synthesize and secrete adrenocortical hormones.

Indications

- Allergic states unresponsive to conventional treatments
- Therapy of some glucocorticoid-sensitive disorders
- Nonsuppurative thyroiditis
- Hypercalcemia associated with cancer
- Acute exacerbations of MS
- Tuberculous meningitis with subarachnoid block
- Trichinosis with neurologic or myocardial involvement
- Rheumatic, collagen, dermatologic, allergic, ophthalmologic, respiratory, hematologic, edematous, and GI diseases
- Palliative management of leukemias, lymphomas
- Unlabeled use: Treatment of infantile spasms

Contraindications and cautions

- Contraindicated with adrenocortical insufficiency or hyperfunction; infections, especially systemic fungal infections, ocular herpes simplex; scleroderma, osteoporosis; recent surgery; heart failure, hypertension; allergy to pork or pork products (corticotropin is isolated from porcine pituitaries); liver disease; ulcerative colitis with impending perforation; recent GI surgery; active or latent peptic ulcer; inflammatory bowel disease; hypothyroidism; pregnancy, lactation.
- Use cautiously with mental disturbances, diabetes, diverticulitis, renal impairment, myasthenia gravis.

Available forms

Repository injection—80 units/mL

Dosages

Adults

- *Therapy:* 40–80 units IM or subcutaneously every 24–72 hr; when indicated, gradually reduce dosage by increasing intervals between injections or decreasing the dose injected, or both.
- *Acute exacerbations of MS:* 80–120 units/day IM for 2–3 wk.

Pediatric patients

Use only if necessary, and only intermittently and with careful observation. Prolonged use will inhibit skeletal growth.

- *Infantile spasms:* 20–40 units/day or 80 units every other day IM for 3 mo or 1 mo after cessation of seizures.

Pharmacokinetics

Route	*Onset*	*Peak*	*Duration*
IM, Subcut.	Rapid	1 hr	2–4 hr

Metabolism: $T_{1/2}$: 15 min
Distribution: Does not cross placenta; may enter breast milk

Adverse effects

- **CNS:** Seizures, vertigo, *headaches,* pseudotumor cerebri, *euphoria, insomnia, mood swings, depression,* psychosis, intracerebral hemorrhage, reversible cerebral atrophy in infants, cataracts, increased IOP, glaucoma
- **CV:** *Hypertension,* heart failure, necrotizing angiitis
- **Endocrine:** Growth retardation, decreased carbohydrate tolerance, diabetes mellitus, cushingoid state, *secondary adrenocortical and pituitary unresponsiveness*
- **GI:** Peptic or esophageal ulcer, pancreatitis, abdominal distention
- **GU:** *Amenorrhea, irregular menses*
- **Hematologic:** *Fluid and electrolyte disturbances,* negative nitrogen balance
- **Hypersensitivity: Anaphylactoid** or hypersensitivity reactions
- **Musculoskeletal:** *Muscle weakness,* steroid myopathy, loss of muscle mass, osteoporosis, spontaneous fractures
- **Other:** *Impaired wound healing, petechiae, ecchymoses, increased sweating, thin and fragile skin, acne, immunosuppression and masking of signs of infection,* activation of latent infections, including tuberculosis, fungal, and viral eye infections, pneumonia, abscess, septic infection, GI and GU infections

Interactions

✱ **Drug-drug** • Decreased effects with barbiturates • Decreased effects of anticholinesterases with corticotropin; profound muscular depression is possible • Decreased effectiveness of insulin, antidiabetics; monitor patient closely and increase dosage as needed

✱ **Drug-lab test** • Suppression of skin test reactions

■ Nursing considerations

Assessment

- **History:** Adrenocortical insufficiency or hyperfunction; infections, ocular herpes simplex; scleroderma, osteoporosis; recent surgery; heart failure, hypertension; allergy to pork or pork products; liver disease: cirrhosis; ulcerative colitis; diverticulitis; active or latent peptic ulcer; inflammatory bowel disease, lactation; diabetes mellitus; hypothyroidism, pregnancy
- **Physical:** Weight, T; skin color, integrity; reflexes, bilateral grip strength, ophthalmologic examination, affect, orientation; P, BP, auscultation, peripheral perfusion, status of veins; R, adventitious sounds, chest X-ray; upper GI X-ray (peptic ulcer symptoms), liver palpation; CBC, serum electrolytes, 2-hr postprandial blood glucose, thyroid function tests, urinalysis

Interventions

- Verify adrenal responsiveness (increased urinary and plasma corticosteroid levels) to corticotropin before therapy; use the administrative route proposed for treatment.
- Administer only by IM or subcutaneous injection.
- Use minimal doses for minimal duration to minimize adverse effects.
- Taper doses when discontinuing high-dose or long-term therapy.
- Administer a rapidly acting corticosteroid before, during, and after stress when patients are on long-term therapy.
- Do not give patients receiving corticotropins live virus vaccines.

Teaching points

- Avoid immunizations with live vaccines.
- Diabetics may require an increased dosage of insulin or oral hypoglycemic drug; consult your health care provider.
- Take antacids between meals to reduce heartburn.
- Avoid exposure to people with contagious diseases. This drug masks signs of infection and decreases resistance to infection; wash hands carefully after touching contaminated surfaces.
- Report unusual weight gain, swelling of lower extremities, muscle weakness, abdominal pain, seizures, headache, fever, prolonged sore throat, cold or other infection, worsening of symptoms for which drug is being taken.

cosyntropin

See Appendix W, *Less commonly used drugs*.

cromolyn sodium

See Appendix W, *Less commonly used drugs*.

cyanocobalamin, intranasal

*(sigh' an oh coh **ball'** a min)*

CaloMist Nasal Spray, Nascobal

PREGNANCY CATEGORY C

Drug class
Synthetic vitamin

Therapeutic actions
Intranasal gel that allows absorption of vitamin B_{12}, which is essential to cell growth and reproduction, hematopoiesis, and nucleoprotein and myelin synthesis, and has been associated with fat and carbohydrate metabolism and protein synthesis.

Indications
- Maintenance of patients in hematologic remission after IM vitamin B_{12} therapy for pernicious anemia, inadequate secretion of intrinsic factor, dietary deficiency, malabsorption, competition by intestinal bacteria or parasites, or inadequate utilization of vitamin B_{12}
- Maintenance of effective therapeutic levels of vitamin B_{12} in patients with HIV, AIDS, MS, and Crohn's disease

Contraindications and cautions
- Contraindicated with hypersensitivity to cobalt, vitamin B_{12}, or any component of drug.
- Use cautiously with pregnancy or lactation, Leber's disease, nasal lesions, or URIs.

Available forms
Intranasal gel—500 mcg/0.1 mL; spray—25 mcg/0.1 mL, 500 mcg/0.1 mL

Dosages
Adults

One spray (500 mcg) in one nostril, once per wk (*Nascobal*). One spray (25 mcg) in each nostril once per day for a total of 50 mcg; may be increased to bid if needed (*CaloMist Nasal Spray*).

Pediatric patients

Safety and efficacy not established.

Pharmacokinetics

Route	Onset	Peak
Nasal	Slow	1–2 hr

Metabolism: $T_{1/2}$: Unknown
Distribution: May cross placenta, may enter breast milk
Excretion: Urine

Adverse effects
- **CNS:** *Headache*
- **Hematologic:** Bone marrow suppression
- **Local:** *Rhinitis, nasal congestion*
- **Other:** Fever, pain, local irritation

Interactions
✱ **Drug-drug** • Decreased effectiveness may be seen with antibiotics, methotrexate, colchicine, para-aminosalicylic acid, excessive alcohol use

■ Nursing considerations
Assessment
- **History:** Pregnancy or lactation, Leber's disease, nasal lesions or URIs; history of pernicious anemia, vitamin B_{12} deficiency, dates of IM cyanocobalamin therapy
- **Physical:** State of nasal mucous membranes; serum vitamin B_{12} levels, CBC, potassium level

Interventions
- Confirm diagnosis before administering; ensure that patient is hemodynamically stable after IM therapy.
- Monitor serum vitamin B_{12} levels before starting, 1 mo after starting, and every 3–6 mo during therapy.
- Do not administer if nasal congestion, rhinitis, or URI is present.
- Evaluate patient response and consider need for folate or iron replacement.

Teaching points

- Take drug as prescribed, one spray in one nostril once a week (*Nascobal*) or one spray in each nostril once a day (*CaloMist*).
- Periodic blood tests will be needed to monitor your response to this drug.
- Take drug 1 hour before or 1 hour after ingestion of hot foods or liquids because hot foods can cause nasal secretions and interfere with absorption.
- Do not administer if you have nasal congestion, rhinitis, or upper respiratory tract infection; consult your health care provider.
- You may experience these side effects: Headache (analgesics may help), nausea (eat frequent small meals).
- Report nasal pain, nasal sores, fatigue, weakness, easy bruising.

cyclizine

(sye' kli zeen)

Marezine

PREGNANCY CATEGORY B

Drug classes

Anticholinergic
Antiemetic
Antihistamine
Anti–motion-sickness drug

Therapeutic actions

Reduces sensitivity of the labyrinthine apparatus; peripheral anticholinergic effects may contribute to efficacy.

Indications

- Prevention and treatment of nausea, vomiting, dizziness associated with motion sickness

Contraindications and cautions

- Contraindicated with allergy to cyclizine.
- Use cautiously with pregnancy, lactation, narrow-angle glaucoma, stenosing peptic ulcer, symptomatic prostatic hypertrophy, bronchial asthma, bladder neck obstruction, pyloroduodenal obstruction, cardiac arrhythmias; postoperative patients (hypotensive effects may be confusing and dangerous).

Available forms

Tablets—50 mg

Dosages

Adults

50 mg PO 30 min before exposure to motion; repeat every 4–6 hr. Do not exceed 200 mg in 24 hr.

Pediatric patients 6–12 yr

25 mg PO up to three times a day.

Geriatric patients

More likely to cause dizziness, sedation, syncope, toxic confusional states, and hypotension in elderly patients; use with caution.

Pharmacokinetics

Route	Onset	Peak	Duration
Oral	30–60 min	60–90 min	4–6 hr

Metabolism: Hepatic; $T_{1/2}$: 2–3 hr
Distribution: Crosses placenta; enters breast milk
Excretion: Unknown

Adverse effects

- **CNS:** *Drowsiness, confusion,* euphoria, nervousness, restlessness, insomnia and excitement, seizures, vertigo, tinnitus, blurred vision, diplopia, auditory and visual hallucinations
- **CV:** Hypotension, palpitations, tachycardia
- **Dermatologic:** Urticaria, drug rash
- **GI:** *Dry mouth, anorexia, nausea,* vomiting, diarrhea or constipation, cholestatic jaundice
- **GU:** *Urinary frequency, difficult urination,* urinary retention
- **Respiratory:** Respiratory depression, dry nose and throat

Interactions

✱ **Drug-drug** • Increased depressant effects with alcohol, other CNS depressants

■ Nursing considerations

Assessment

- **History:** Allergy to cyclizine, narrow-angle glaucoma, stenosing peptic ulcer, symptomatic prostatic hypertrophy, bronchial asthma, bladder neck obstruction, pyloroduodenal obstruction, cardiac arrhythmias, recent surgery, lactation
- **Physical:** Skin color, lesions, texture; orientation, reflexes, affect; vision examination; P, BP; R, adventitious sounds; bowel sounds; prostate palpation; CBC

Interventions

- Monitor elderly patients carefully for adverse effects.

Teaching points

- Take drug as prescribed; avoid excessive dosage.
- Use before motion sickness occurs; antimotion sickness drugs work best if used prophylactically.
- Avoid alcohol; serious sedation could occur.
- You may experience these side effects: Dizziness, sedation, drowsiness (use caution driving or performing tasks that require alertness); epigastric distress, diarrhea or constipation (take drug with food); dry mouth (practice frequent mouth care, suck sugarless lozenges); thickening of bronchial secretions, dryness of nasal mucosa (consider another type of motion sickness remedy).
- Report difficulty breathing, hallucinations, tremors, loss of coordination, unusual bleeding or bruising, visual disturbances, irregular heartbeat.

▽ cyclobenzaprine hydrochloride

(sye kloe ***ben'*** *za preen)*

Amrix, Apo-Cyclobenzaprine (CAN), Flexeril, Gen-Cyclobenzaprine (CAN), PMS-Cyclobenzaprine (CAN), ratio-Cyclobenzaprine (CAN)

PREGNANCY CATEGORY B

Drug class

Skeletal muscle relaxant (centrally acting)

Therapeutic actions

Precise mechanism not known; does not directly relax tense skeletal muscles but appears to act mainly at brain stem levels or in the spinal cord.

Indications

- Relief of discomfort associated with acute, painful musculoskeletal conditions, as adjunct to rest, physical therapy
- Unlabeled use: Adjunct in the management of fibrositis syndrome

Contraindications and cautions

- Contraindicated with hypersensitivity to cyclobenzaprine, acute recovery phase of MI, arrhythmias, heart block or conduction disturbances, heart failure, hyperthyroidism.
- Use cautiously with urinary retention, angle-closure glaucoma, increased IOP, lactation, mild hepatic impairment.

Available forms

Tablets—5, 7.5, 10 mg; ER capsules—15, 30 mg

Dosages

Adults

5 mg PO tid, up to 10 mg PO tid. Do not exceed 60 mg/day; do not use longer than 2 or 3 wk. For ER capsules, 15 mg once/day; some patients need 30 mg/day.

Pediatric patients

Safety and efficacy in patients younger than 15 yr not established.

Pharmacokinetics

Route	*Onset*	*Peak*	*Duration*
Oral	1 hr	4–6 hr	12–24 hr

Metabolism: Hepatic; $T_{1/2}$: 1–3 days, 18 hr (range 8–37 hr)

Distribution: Crosses placenta; may enter breast milk

Excretion: Urine

Adverse effects

- **CNS:** *Drowsiness, dizziness,* fatigue, asthenia, blurred vision, headache, nervousness, confusion
- **CV:** Arrhythmias, **MI**

C

- **GI:** *Dry mouth,* nausea, constipation, dyspepsia, unpleasant taste, liver toxicity
- **GU:** Frequency, urinary retention

Interactions

✱ **Drug-drug** • Additive CNS effects with alcohol, barbiturates, other CNS depressants, MAOIs, TCAs; avoid concomitant use • Risk of hyperpyretic crisis and seizures if given within 14 days of MAOIs • Increased risk of seizures with tramadol

■ Nursing considerations

Assessment

- **History:** Hypersensitivity to cyclobenzaprine, acute recovery phase of MI, arrhythmias, heart failure, hyperthyroidism, urinary retention, angle-closure glaucoma, increased IOP, lactation
- **Physical:** Orientation, affect, ophthalmic examination (tonometry); bowel sounds, normal GI output; prostate palpation, normal voiding pattern; thyroid function tests

Interventions

- Arrange for analgesics if headache occurs.

Teaching points

- Take this drug exactly as prescribed. Do not take a higher dosage.
- Avoid alcohol, sleep-inducing, or over-the-counter drugs; these may cause dangerous effects.
- You may experience these side effects: Drowsiness, dizziness, blurred vision (avoid driving or engaging in activities that require alertness); dyspepsia (take drug with food, eat frequent small meals); dry mouth (suck sugarless lozenges or ice chips).
- Report urinary retention or difficulty voiding, pale stools, yellow skin or eyes.

DANGEROUS DRUG

▽ cyclophosphamide

*(sye kloe **foss'** fa mide)*

Procytox (CAN)

PREGNANCY CATEGORY D

Drug classes

Alkylating drug
Antineoplastic
Nitrogen mustard derivative

Therapeutic actions

Cytotoxic: Interferes with the replication of susceptible cells. Not specific to cell cycle. Immunosuppressive: Lymphocytes are especially sensitive to drug effects.

Indications

- Treatment of malignant lymphomas, multiple myeloma, leukemias, mycosis fungoides, neuroblastoma, adenocarcinoma of the ovary, retinoblastoma, carcinoma of the breast; used concurrently or sequentially with other antineoplastic drugs
- Treatment of minimal change nephrotic syndrome in children
- Unlabeled uses: Severe rheumatologic conditions, Wegener's granulomatosis, steroid-resistant vasculitis, SLE

Contraindications and cautions

- Contraindicated with allergy to cyclophosphamide, allergy to tartrazine (in tablets marketed as *Cytoxan*), pregnancy, lactation.
- Use cautiously with radiation therapy; tumor cell infiltration of the bone marrow; adrenalectomy with steroid therapy; infections, especially varicella-zoster; hematopoietic depression, impaired hepatic or renal function.

Available forms

Tablets—25, 50 mg; injection—500 mg, 1 g, 2 g

Dosages

Consult current chemotherapeutic reference for appropriate protocol, and individualize dosage based on hematologic profile and response.

Adults

- *Induction therapy:* 40–50 mg/kg IV given in divided doses over 2–5 days or 1–5 mg/kg/day PO.

- *Maintenance therapy:* 1–5 mg/kg/day PO, 10–15 mg/kg IV every 7–10 days, or 3–5 mg/kg IV twice weekly.

Pediatric patients

- *Minimal change nephrotic syndrome:* 2.5–3 mg/day PO for 60–90 days.

Pharmacokinetics

Route	*Onset*	*Peak*
Oral	Varies	1 hr
IV	Rapid	15–30 min

Metabolism: Hepatic; $T_{1/2}$: 3–12 hr
Distribution: Crosses placenta; enters breast milk
Excretion: Urine

IV FACTS

Preparation: Add sterile water for injection or bacteriostatic water for injection to the vial, and shake gently. Use 25 mL for 500-mg vial, 50 mL for 1-g vial, 100 mL for 2-g vial. Prepared solutions may be injected IV, IM, intraperitoneally, intrapleurally. Use within 24 hr if stored at room temperature or within 6 days if refrigerated. If bacteriostatic water for injection is not used, use within 6 hr.
Infusion: Infuse in 5% dextrose injection, 5% dextrose and 0.9% sodium chloride injection; infuse over 15 min or longer (infusion can be painful).

Adverse effects

- **CV:** Cardiotoxicity
- **Dermatologic:** *Alopecia,* darkening of skin and fingernails
- **GI:** *Anorexia, nausea, vomiting, diarrhea, stomatitis*
- **GU:** *Hemorrhagic cystitis,* bladder fibrosis, hematuria to potentially fatal **hemorrhagic cystitis,** increased urine uric acid levels, infertility
- **Hematologic:** *Leukopenia,* thrombocytopenia, anemia
- **Respiratory:** Interstitial pulmonary fibrosis
- **Other:** SIADH, immunosuppression secondary to malignancy

Interactions

✱ **Drug-drug** • Prolonged apnea with succinylcholine: Metabolism is inhibited by cyclophosphamide • Decreased serum levels and therapeutic activity of digoxin • Myelosuppressive effects are enhanced with coadministration of allopurinol • Increased anticoagulant effects with anticoagulants • Increased cardiac effects with doxorubicin • Reduced activity of cyclophosphamide with chloramphenicol
✱ **Drug-food** • Decreased metabolism and risk of toxic effects if combined with grapefruit juice; avoid this combination

■ Nursing considerations

Assessment

- **History:** Allergy to cyclophosphamide, allergy to tartrazine, radiation therapy, chemotherapy, tumor cell infiltration of the bone marrow, adrenalectomy with steroid therapy, infections, hematopoietic depression, impaired hepatic or renal function, pregnancy, lactation
- **Physical:** T; weight; skin color, lesions; hair; P, auscultation, baseline ECG; R, adventitious sounds; mucous membranes, liver evaluation; CBC, differential; urinalysis; LFTs, renal function tests

Interventions

- Arrange for blood tests to evaluate hematopoietic function before therapy and weekly during therapy.

⊗ ***Warning*** Do not give full dosage within 4 wk after a full course of radiation therapy due to the risk of severe bone marrow depression; reduced dosage may be needed.

- Arrange for reduced dosage in patients with impaired renal or hepatic function.

⊗ ***Warning*** Ensure that patient is well hydrated before treatment to reduce risk of cystitis.

- Prepare oral solution by dissolving injectable cyclophosphamide in aromatic elixir. Refrigerate in a glass container and use within 14 days.
- Give tablets on an empty stomach. If severe GI upset occurs, tablet may be given with food.
- Counsel male patients not to father a child during or immediately after therapy; infant cardiac and limb abnormalities have occurred.
- Make sure that antiemetics have been ordered before each dose.

Teaching points

- Take drug on an empty stomach. If severe GI upset occurs, the tablet may be taken with food. Do not drink grapefruit juice while taking this drug.
- Try to maintain your fluid intake and nutrition (drink at least 10–12 glasses of fluid each day).
- Both men and women should use birth control during and after drug use; this drug can cause severe birth defects.
- You may experience these side effects: Nausea, vomiting, loss of appetite (take drug with food, eat frequent small meals); darkening of the skin and fingernails; loss of hair (obtain a wig or other head covering prior to hair loss; head must be covered in extremes of temperature).
- Report unusual bleeding or bruising, fever, chills, sore throat, cough, shortness of breath, blood in the urine, painful urination, rapid heartbeat, swelling of the feet or hands, stomach or flank pain.

▽ cycloserine

(sye kloe ser' een)

Seromycin Pulvules

PREGNANCY CATEGORY C

Drug classes

Antibiotic
Antituberculotic (third line)

Therapeutic actions

Inhibits cell wall synthesis in susceptible strains of gram-positive and gram-negative bacteria and in *Mycobacterium tuberculosis,* causing cell death.

Indications

- Treatment of active pulmonary and extrapulmonary (including renal) TB that is not responsive to first-line antituberculotics in conjunction with other antituberculotics
- UTIs caused by susceptible bacteria

Contraindications and cautions

- Contraindicated with allergy to cycloserine, epilepsy, depression, severe anxiety or psychosis, severe renal insufficiency, excessive concurrent use of alcohol, lactation.
- Use cautiously with pregnancy.

Available forms

Capsules—250 mg

Dosages

Adults

Initial dose, 250 mg bid PO at 12-hr intervals for first 2 wk; monitor serum levels (above 30 mcg/mL is generally toxic). Maintenance dose, 500 mg–1 g/day PO in divided doses monitored by blood levels. Do not exceed 1 g/day.

Pediatric patients

Safety and efficacy not established.

Pharmacokinetics

Route	*Onset*	*Peak*	*Duration*
Oral	Varies	4–8 hr	48–72 hr

Metabolism: $T_{1/2}$: 10 hr
Distribution: Crosses placenta; enters breast milk
Excretion: Feces, urine

Adverse effects

- **CNS:** *Drowsiness, somnolence, headache, tremor, vertigo, confusion,* disorientation, loss of memory, psychoses (possibly with suicidal tendencies), hyperirritability, aggression, paresis, hyperreflexia, paresthesias, seizures, coma
- **Dermatologic:** Rash
- **Hematologic:** Elevated serum transaminase levels

■ Nursing considerations

CLINICAL ALERT!
Name confusion has occurred among cycloserine, cyclosporine, and cyclophosphamide; use caution.

Assessment

- **History:** Allergy to cycloserine, epilepsy, depression, severe anxiety or psychosis, severe

renal insufficiency, excessive concurrent use of alcohol, lactation, pregnancy
- **Physical:** Skin color, lesions; orientation, reflexes, affect, EEG; liver evaluation; LFTs

Interventions
- Arrange for culture and sensitivity studies before use.
- Give this drug only when other therapy has failed, and only in conjunction with other antituberculotics, when treating TB.
- Arrange for follow-up of LFTs, renal function tests, hematologic tests, and serum drug levels.
- Consult with physician regarding the use of antiepileptics, sedatives, or pyridoxine if CNS effects become severe.
- Discontinue drug, and notify physician if rash or severe CNS reactions occur.

Teaching points
- Avoid excessive alcohol consumption while on this drug.
- Take this drug regularly; avoid missing doses. Do not discontinue this drug without first consulting your health care provider.
- Avoid taking with a high-fat meal.
- Have regular, periodic medical checkups, including blood tests to evaluate the drug's effects.
- You may experience these side effects: Drowsiness, tremor, disorientation (use caution operating a car or dangerous machinery); depression, personality change, numbness, tingling.
- If you experience trouble breathing or if signs or symptoms of heart failure occur, notify your health care provider immediately, especially if you are receiving more than 1 to 1.5 g per day.
- Report rash, headache, tremors, shaking, confusion, dizziness.

▽cyclosporine (cyclosporin A)

(sye' kloe spor een)

Gengraf, Neoral, Sandimmune

PREGNANCY CATEGORY C

Drug class
Immunosuppressant

Therapeutic actions
Exact mechanism of immunosuppressant is not known; specifically and reversibly inhibits immunocompetent lymphocytes in the G0 or G1 phase of the cell cycle; inhibits T-helper and T-suppressor cells, lymphokine production, and release of interleukin-2 and T-cell growth factor.

Indications
- Prophylaxis for organ rejection in kidney, liver, and heart transplants in conjunction with adrenal corticosteroids
- Treatment of chronic rejection in patients previously treated with other immunosuppressive agents (*Sandimmune*)
- *Neoral, Gengraf:* Alone, or in combination with methotrexate for treatment of patients with severe active rheumatoid arthritis
- *Neoral, Gengraf:* Treatment of recalcitrant, plaque psoriasis in non–immune-compromised adults
- Unlabeled use: Aplastic anemia; resistant leukemias; other procedures, including pancreas, bone marrow, lung transplants; Crohn's disease, SLE

Contraindications and cautions
- Contraindicated with allergy to cyclosporine or polyoxyethylated castor oil, lactation.
- Use cautiously with impaired renal function, malabsorption, pregnancy, uncontrolled hypertension.

Available forms
Capsules—25, 100 mg; soft gel capsules for microemulsion—25, 100 mg; oral solution—100 mg/mL; IV solution—50 mg/mL

Dosages
Adults and pediatric patients

Neoral, Gengraf, and *Sandimmune* are not bioequivalent—do not interchange. Concentrations should be monitored when switching because of variable bioavailability.

Oral
- *Organ rejection:* 15 mg/kg/day PO (*Sandimmune*) initially given 4–12 hr prior to transplantation; continue dose postoperatively

for 1–2 wk, then taper by 5% per wk to a maintenance level of 5–10 mg/kg/day.
- *Rheumatoid arthritis:* 2.5 mg/kg/day (*Neoral, Gengraf*) PO in divided doses bid; may increase up to 4 mg/kg/day. If no benefit after 16 wks, discontinue drug.
- *Psoriasis:* 2.5 mg/kg/day (*Neoral, Gengraf*) PO divided bid for 4 wk, then may increase up to 4 mg/kg/day. If no satisfactory response after 6 wk at 4 mg/kg/day, discontinue drug.

Parenteral

Patients unable to take oral solution preoperatively or postoperatively may be given IV infusion (*Sandimmune*) at one-third the oral dose (ie, 5–6 mg/kg/day given 4–12 hr prior to transplantation, administered as a slow infusion over 2–6 hr). Continue this daily dose postoperatively. Switch to oral drug as soon as possible.

Pharmacokinetics

Route	*Onset*	*Peak*
Oral	Varies	3.5 hr
IV	Rapid	1–2 hr

Metabolism: Hepatic; $T_{1/2}$: 10–27 hr (*Sandimmune*), 5–18 hr (*Neoral, Gengraf*)
Distribution: Crosses placenta; enters breast milk
Excretion: Bile, urine

IV FACTS

Preparation: Dilute IV solution immediately before use. Dilute 1 mL concentrate in 20–100 mL of 0.9% sodium chloride injection or 5% dextrose injection. Discard unused infusion solutions after 24 hr.
Infusion: Give in a slow IV infusion over 2–6 hr.
Incompatibility: Do not mix with magnesium sulfate.

Adverse effects

- **CNS:** *Tremor,* seizures, headache, paresthesias
- **CV:** *Hypertension*
- **GI: Hepatotoxicity,** *gum hyperplasia, diarrhea,* nausea, vomiting, anorexia
- **GU:** *Renal impairment,* nephrotoxicity
- **Hematologic:** Leukopenia, *hyperkalemia, hypomagnesemia,* hyperuricemia
- **Other:** *Hirsutism, acne,* lymphomas, infections, elevated serum creatinine and BUN

Interactions

✱ **Drug-drug** • Increased risk of nephrotoxicity with other nephrotoxic agents (aminoglycosides, amphotericin B, acyclovir) • Increased risk of digoxin toxicity • Risk of severe myopathy or rhabdomyolysis with HMG-CoA reductase inhibitors • Increased risk of toxicity if taken with SSRIs, diltiazem, metoclopramide, nicardipine, amiodarone, androgens, azole antifungals, colchicine, hormonal contraceptives, foscarnet, macrolides, metoclopramide • Increased plasma concentration of cyclosporine with ketoconazole • Decreased therapeutic effect with hydantoins, rifampin, phenobarbital, carbamazepine, orlistat

✱ **Drug-food** • Increased serum levels and adverse effects if combined with grapefruit juice • Decreased absorption of *Neoral* if taken with a high-fat meal

✱ **Drug-alternate therapy** • Decreased cyclosporine levels with use of St. John's wort

■ Nursing considerations

CLINICAL ALERT!

Name confusion has been associated with cyclosporine, cycloserine, and cyclophosphamide; use caution.

Assessment

- **History:** Allergy to cyclosporine or polyoxyethylated castor oil, impaired renal function, malabsorption, lactation
- **Physical:** T; skin color, lesions; BP, peripheral perfusion; liver evaluation, bowel sounds, gum evaluation; LFTs, renal function tests, CBC

Interventions

- Mix oral solution with milk, chocolate milk, or orange juice at room temperature. Stir well, and administer at once. Do not allow mixture to stand before drinking. Use a glass container, and rinse with more diluent to ensure that the total dose is taken.

- Use parenteral administration only if patient is unable to take the oral solution; transfer to oral solution as soon as possible. *Sandimmune* must be taken with corticosteroids.
- Do not refrigerate oral solution; store at room temperature and use within 2 mo after opening.

⊗ ***Black box warning*** Monitor patient for infections, malignancies; risks are increased.

⊗ ***Black box warning*** Monitor LFTs and renal function tests prior to and during therapy; marked decreases in function may require dosage adjustment or discontinuation.

⊗ ***Black box warning*** Monitor BP; heart transplant patients may require concomitant antihypertensive therapy.

Teaching points

- Dilute solution with milk, chocolate milk, or orange juice at room temperature; drink immediately after mixing. Rinse the glass with the solution to ensure that all of the dose is taken. Store solution at room temperature. Use solution within 2 months of opening the bottle.
- Do not drink grapefruit juice while taking this drug.
- Do not take with high-fat meals or within 30 minutes of high-fat meals.
- Avoid infection; avoid crowds or people who have infections. Notify your health care provider at once if you injure yourself.
- This drug should not be taken during pregnancy. Use of barrier contraceptives is advised. If you think that you are pregnant or you want to become pregnant, discuss this with your health care provider.
- Have periodic blood tests to monitor your response to drug effects.
- Do not discontinue this medication without your health care provider's advice.
- You may experience these side effects: Nausea, vomiting (take the drug with food); diarrhea; rash; mouth sores (practice frequent mouth care).
- Report unusual bleeding or bruising, fever, sore throat, mouth sores, tiredness.

▽ cyproheptadine hydrochloride

(si proe ***hep'*** *ta deen)*

PREGNANCY CATEGORY B

Drug class

Antihistamine (piperidine type)

Therapeutic actions

Blocks the effects of histamine at H_1 receptor sites; has atropine-like, antiserotonin, antipruritic, sedative, and appetite-stimulating effects.

Indications

- Relief of symptoms associated with perennial and seasonal allergic rhinitis; vasomotor rhinitis; allergic conjunctivitis; mild, uncomplicated urticaria and angioedema; amelioraton of allergic reactions to blood or plasma; dermatographism; adjunctive therapy in anaphylactic reactions
- Treatment of cold urticaria
- Unlabeled use: Treatment of vascular cluster headaches, appetite stimulation, treatment of nightmares associated with PTSD

Contraindications and cautions

- Contraindicated with allergy to any antihistamines, third trimester of pregnancy, newborns, premature infants.
- Use cautiously with narrow-angle glaucoma, stenosing peptic ulcer, symptomatic prostatic hypertrophy, asthmatic attack, bladder neck obstruction, pyloroduodenal obstruction, lactation.

Available forms

Tablets—4 mg; syrup—2 mg/5 mL

Dosages

Adults

For initial therapy, 4 mg tid PO. For maintenance therapy, 4–20 mg/day in three divided doses PO; do not exceed 0.5 mg/kg/day.

Pediatric patients

0.25 mg/kg/day PO or 8 mg/m^2.

Pediatric patients 2–6 yr

2 mg PO bid or tid; do not exceed 12 mg/day.

C

Pediatric patients 7–14 yr
4 mg PO bid or tid; do not exceed 16 mg/day.
Geriatric patients
More likely to cause dizziness, sedation, syncope, toxic confusional states, and hypotension in elderly patients; use with caution.

Pharmacokinetics

Route	*Onset*	*Peak*	*Duration*
Oral	15–30 min	1–2 hr	4–6 hr

Metabolism: Hepatic; $T_{1/2}$: 3–4 hr
Distribution: Crosses placenta; enters breast milk
Excretion: Urine

Adverse effects

- **CNS:** *Drowsiness, sedation, dizziness, disturbed coordination,* fatigue, confusion, restlessness, excitation, nervousness, tremor, headache, blurred vision, diplopia, vertigo, tinnitus, acute labyrinthitis, hysteria, tingling, heaviness and weakness of the hands
- **CV:** Hypotension, palpitations, bradycardia, tachycardia, extrasystoles
- **GI:** *Epigastric distress,* anorexia, increased appetite and weight gain, nausea, vomiting, diarrhea or constipation
- **GU:** Urinary frequency, dysuria, urinary retention, early menses, decreased libido, impotence
- **Hematologic:** Hemolytic anemia, hypoplastic anemia, thrombocytopenia, leukopenia, agranulocytosis, pancytopenia
- **Respiratory:** *Thickening of bronchial secretions,* chest tightness, wheezing, nasal stuffiness, dry mouth, dry nose, dry throat, sore throat
- **Other:** Urticaria, rash, **anaphylactic shock,** photosensitivity, excessive perspiration, chills

Interactions

✱ **Drug-drug** • Subnormal pituitary-adrenal response to metyrapone • Decreased effects of fluoxetine • Increased and prolonged anticholinergic (drying) effects if taken with MAOIs • Increased sedation with alcohol, CNS depressants

■ Nursing considerations

Assessment

- **History:** Allergy to any antihistamines; narrow-angle glaucoma, stenosing peptic ulcer, symptomatic prostatic hypertrophy, asthmatic attack, bladder neck obstruction, pyloroduodenal obstruction; lactation, pregnancy
- **Physical:** Skin color, lesions, texture; orientation, reflexes, affect; vision examination; P, BP; R, adventitious sounds; bowel sounds; prostate palpation; CBC with differential

Interventions

- Administer with food if GI upset occurs.
- Give syrup form if unable to take tablets.
- Monitor patient response, and adjust dosage to lowest possible effective dose.

Teaching points

- Take as prescribed; avoid excessive dosage.
- Take drug with food if GI upset occurs.
- Avoid alcohol; serious sedation could occur.
- You may experience these side effects: Dizziness, sedation, drowsiness (use caution if driving or performing tasks that require alertness); epigastric distress, diarrhea, or constipation (take drug with meals); dry mouth (practice frequent mouth care, suck sugarless lozenges); thickening of bronchial secretions, dryness of nasal mucosa (use humidifier).
- Report difficulty breathing, hallucinations, tremors, loss of coordination, unusual bleeding or bruising, visual disturbances, irregular heartbeat.

DANGEROUS DRUG

▽ cytarabine (cytosine arabinoside)

*(sye **tare'** a been)*

Cytosar-U, DepoCyt, Tarabine PFS

PREGNANCY CATEGORY D

Drug classes

Antimetabolite
Antineoplastic

C

Therapeutic actions

Inhibits DNA polymerase; cell cycle phase specific—S phase (stage of DNA synthesis); also blocks progression of cells from G1 to S.

Indications

- Induction and maintenance of remission in AML (higher response rate in children than in adults)
- Treatment of acute lymphocytic leukemia in adults and children; treatment of chronic myelocytic leukemia and erythroleukemia
- Intrathecal use: Treatment of meningeal leukemia
- Liposomal: Treatment of lymphomatous meningitis
- In combination therapy: Treatment of non-Hodgkin's lymphoma in children
- Unlabeled uses: Hodgkin's lymphoma, bone marrow transplantation

Contraindications and cautions

- Contraindicated with allergy to cytarabine, active meningeal infection (liposomal).
- Use cautiously with hematopoietic depression secondary to radiation or chemotherapy; hepatic impairment, pregnancy, lactation, premature infants.

Available forms

Powder for injection—100, 500 mg, 1, 2 g; injection—20 mg/mL, 100 mg/mL, 10 mg/mL (liposomal)

Dosages

Doses vary based on protocol; consult a current chemotherapy reference.

Adults

- *AML induction of remission:* 100–200 mg/m^2 per day by continuous infusion for 5 days for a total dose of 1,000 mg/m^2; repeat every 2 wk. Individualize dosage based on hematologic response.
- *Maintenance of AML:* Use same dosage and schedule as induction; often a longer rest period is allowed.
- *ALL:* Dosage similar to AML.
- *Intrathecal use for meningeal leukemia:* 5 mg/m^2 to 75 mg/m^2 once daily for 4 days or once every 4 days. Most common dose is 30 mg/m^2 every 4 days until CSF is normal, followed by one more treatment.
- *Treatment of lymphomatous meningitis:* 50 mg liposomal cytarabine intrathecal every 14 days for two doses; then every 14 days for three doses; repeat every 28 days for four doses.
- *Refractory acute leukemia:* 3 g/m^2 IV over 2 hr every 12 hr for 4–12 doses (repeated at 2- to 3-wk intervals).

Pediatric patients

- *Remission induction and maintenance of AML:* Calculate dose by body weight or surface area.
- *ALL:* Same dosage as AML.

Intrathecal

(Has been used as treatment of meningeal leukemia and prophylaxis in newly diagnosed patients): Cytarabine, 30 mg/m^2 every 4 days until CSF is normal; hydrocortisone sodium succinate, 15 mg/m^2; methotrexate, 15 mg/m^2.

Combination therapies

For persistent leukemias, give at 2- to 4-wk intervals.

Cytarabine: 100 mg/m^2/day by continuous IV infusion, days 1–10. *Doxorubicin:* 30 g/m^2/day by IV infusion over 30 min, days 1–3.

Cytarabine: 100 mg/m^2/day by IV infusion over 30 min every 12 hr, days 1–7. *Thioguanine:* 100 mg/m^2 PO every 12 hr, days 1–7. *Daunorubicin:* 60 mg/m^2/day by IV infusion, days 5–7.

Cytarabine: 100 mg/m^2/day by continuous infusion, days 1–7. *Doxorubicin:* 30 mg/m^2/day by IV infusion, days 1–3. *Vincristine:* 1.5 mg/m^2/day by IV infusion, days 1 and 5. *Prednisone:* 40 mg/m^2/day by IV infusion every 12 hr, days 1–5.

Cytarabine: 100 mg/m^2/day by continuous infusion, days 1–7. *Daunorubicin:* 45 mg/m^2/day by IV push, days 1–3.

Pharmacokinetics

Route	Onset	Peak	Duration
IV	Rapid	20–60 min	12–18 hr

Metabolism: Hepatic; $T_{1/2}$ in plasma: 1–3 hr; $T_{1/2}$ in CSF: 2 hr:

Distribution: Crosses placenta; may enter breast milk

Excretion: Urine

IV FACTS

Preparation: Reconstitute 100-mg vial with 5 mL of bacteriostatic water for injection with benzyl alcohol 0.9%; resultant solution contains 20 mg/mL cytarabine. Reconstitute 500-mg vial with 10 mL of the above; resultant solution contains 50 mg/mL cytarabine. Reconstitute 1 g vial and 2 g vial with 10 mL, 20 mL of the above respectively; resultant solution contains 100 mg/mL cytarabine. Store at room temperature for up to 48 hr. Discard solution if a slight haze appears. Can be further diluted with water for injection, D_5W, or sodium chloride injection; stable for 8 days.
Infusion: Administer by IV infusion over at least 30 min, IV injection over 1–3 min for each 100 mg, or subcutaneously; patients can usually tolerate higher doses when given by rapid IV injection. There is no clinical advantage to any particular route.
Incompatibilities: Do not mix with insulin, heparin, penicillin G, oxacillin, nafcillin, 5-FU.

Adverse effects

- **CNS:** Neuritis, neural toxicity
- **Dermatologic:** Fever, rash, urticaria, freckling, skin ulceration, pruritus, conjunctivitis, alopecia
- **GI:** *Anorexia, nausea, vomiting, diarrhea, oral and anal inflammation or ulceration;* esophageal ulcerations, esophagitis, abdominal pain, hepatic impairment (jaundice), acute pancreatitis
- **GU:** Renal impairment, urine retention
- **Hematologic:** Bone marrow depression, hyperuricemia, *leukopenia, thrombocytopenia,* anemia
- **Local:** *Thrombophlebitis,* cellulitis at injection site
- **Other:** Cytarabine syndrome (fever, myalgia, bone pain, occasional chest pain, maculopapular rash, conjunctivitis, malaise, which is sometimes responsive to corticosteroids), *fever, rash,* arachnoiditis (liposomal preparation)

Interactions

✱ **Drug-drug** • Decreased therapeutic action of digoxin if taken with cytarabine

■ Nursing considerations

Assessment

- **History:** Allergy to cytarabine, hematopoietic depression, impaired liver function, lactation, pregnancy
- **Physical:** Weight; T; skin lesions, color; hair; orientation, reflexes; R, adventitious sounds; mucous membranes, liver evaluation, abdominal exam; CBC, differential; LFTs, renal function tests; urinalysis

Interventions

- Evaluate hematopoietic status before and frequently during therapy.

⊗ ***Warning*** Discontinue drug therapy if platelet count is less than 50,000/mm³ or neutrophil count is less than 1,000/mm³; consult physician for dosage adjustment.

- Use Elliott's B solution for diluent, similar to CSF, for intrathecal use. Administer within 4 hr after withdrawal from vial; contains no preservatives. Do not use in-line filters; inject directly into CSF.
- Use caution to avoid skin contact with liposomal form; use liposomal form within 4 hr of withdrawing from vial.
- Make sure antiemetics are ordered before each dose.
- Give comfort measures for anal inflammation, headache, other pain associated with cytarabine syndrome.

Teaching points

- Prepare a calendar of treatment days. Drug must be given IV, subcutaneously, or intrathecally.
- Use birth control; this drug may cause birth defects or miscarriages.
- Have frequent, regular medical follow-up care, including blood tests to assess drug's effects.
- You may experience these side effects: Nausea, vomiting, loss of appetite (medication may be ordered; eat frequent small meals; maintain nutrition); malaise, weakness, lethargy (reversible; avoid driving or operating dangerous machinery); mouth sores (practice frequent mouth care); diarrhea; loss of hair (obtain a wig or other head covering; keep the head covered in extreme temperatures); anal inflammation (use comfort measures).

- Report black, tarry stools; fever; chills; sore throat; unusual bleeding or bruising; shortness of breath; chest pain; difficulty swallowing.

DANGEROUS DRUG

dacarbazine (DTIC, imidazole carboxamide)

*(da **kar'** ba zeen)*

DTIC-Dome

PREGNANCY CATEGORY C

Drug class
Antineoplastic

Therapeutic actions
Cytotoxic: Exact mechanism of action unknown; inhibits DNA and RNA synthesis, causing cell death; cell cycle nonspecific.

Indications
- Metastatic malignant melanoma
- Hodgkin's disease—second-line therapy in combination with other drugs
- Unlabeled uses: Malignant pheochromocytoma with cyclophosphamide and vincristine; metastatic soft tissue sarcoma; alone or in combination therapy for Kaposi's sarcoma; alone or in combination for the treatment of neuroblastomas

Contraindications and cautions
- Contraindicated with allergy to dacarbazine, lactation.
- Use cautiously with impaired hepatic function, bone marrow depression, pregnancy, lactation; choose another method of feeding a baby.

Available forms
Powder for injection—100, 200 mg

Dosages
- *Adult and pediatric malignant melanoma:* 2–4.5 mg/kg/day IV for 10 days, repeated at 4-wk intervals or 250 mg/m^2 per day IV for 5 days, repeated every 3 wk.
- *Adult Hodgkin's disease:* 150 mg/m^2 per day for 5 days in combination with other drugs, repeated every 4 wk or 375 mg/m^2 on day 1 in combination with other drugs, repeated every 15 days.

Pharmacokinetics

Route	*Onset*	*Duration*
IV	15–20 min	6–8 hr

Metabolism: Hepatic; $T_{1/2}$: 19 min then 5 hr
Distribution: Crosses placenta; enters breast milk
Excretion: Urine

IV FACTS
Preparation: Reconstitute 100-mg vials with 9.9 mL and the 200-mg vials with 19.7 mL of sterile water for injection; the resulting solution contains 10 mg/mL of dacarbazine. Reconstituted solution may be further diluted with 5% dextrose injection or 0.9% sodium chloride injection and administered as an IV infusion. Reconstituted solution is stable for 72 hr if refrigerated, 8 hr at room temperature. If further diluted, solution is stable for 24 hr if refrigerated or 8 hr at room temperature. Protect reconstituted solution from light.
Infusion: Infuse slowly over 30–60 min; avoid extravasation.
Incompatibility: Do not combine with hydrocortisone sodium succinate.

Adverse effects
- **Dermatologic:** *Photosensitivity,* erythematous and urticarial rashes, alopecia
- **GI:** *Anorexia, nausea, vomiting,* hepatotoxicity, **hepatic necrosis**
- **Hematologic: Leukopenia, thrombocytopenia**
- **Hypersensitivity: Anaphylaxis**
- **Local:** *Local tissue damage and pain if extravasation occurs*
- **Other:** Facial flushing and paresthesias, flulike symptoms, cancer

■ Nursing considerations
Assessment
- **History:** Allergy to dacarbazine, impaired hepatic function, bone marrow depression, lactation, pregnancy

- **Physical:** Weight; T; skin color, lesions; hair; mucous membranes, liver evaluation; CBC, LFTs, renal function tests

Interventions

⊗ ***Black box warning*** Arrange for lab tests (liver function; WBC, RBC, platelet counts) before and frequently during therapy; serious bone marrow suppression, hepatotoxicity may occur.

⊗ ***Warning*** Give IV only; avoid extravasation into the subcutaneous tissues during administration because tissue damage and severe pain may occur.

- Apply hot packs to relieve pain locally if extravasation occurs.
- Restrict oral intake of fluid and foods for 4–6 hr before therapy to alleviate nausea and vomiting.
- Consult with physician for antiemetic if severe nausea and vomiting occur. Phenobarbital and prochlorperazine may be used. Assure patient that nausea usually subsides after 1–2 days.

Teaching points

- Prepare a calendar for treatment days and additional therapy.
- Have regular blood tests to monitor drug's effects.
- You may experience these side effects: Loss of appetite, nausea, vomiting (frequent mouth care, eat frequent small meals; maintain good nutrition; consult a dietitian; antiemetic available); rash; loss of hair (reversible; obtain a wig or other suitable head covering; keep head covered in extreme temperature); sensitivity to UV light (use a sunscreen and protective clothing); increased risk of infection (avoid crowded areas, people with known infections).
- Report fever, chills, sore throat, unusual bleeding or bruising, yellow skin or eyes, light-colored stools, dark urine, pain or burning at IV injection site.

▽ daclizumab

See Appendix W, *Less commonly used drugs*.

DANGEROUS DRUG

▽ dactinomycin (actinomycin D, ACT)

(dak ti noe ***mye'*** *sin)*

Cosmegen

PREGNANCY CATEGORY D

Drug classes

Antibiotic
Antineoplastic

Therapeutic actions

Cytotoxic: Inhibits synthesis of messenger RNA, causing cell death; cell cycle nonspecific.

Indications

- Wilms' tumor, rhabdomyosarcoma, Ewing's sarcoma, in combination therapy
- Testicular cancer (metastatic nonseminomatous) in combination
- Gestational trophoblastic neoplasia, as monotherapy or in combination
- Palliative treatment or adjunct to tumor resection via isolation-perfusion technique for solid malignancies

Contraindications and cautions

- Contraindicated with allergy to dactinomycin; chickenpox, herpes zoster (severe, generalized disease and death could result); pregnancy; lactation.
- Use cautiously with bone marrow suppression, radiation therapy, and patients with reduced renal and hepatic function.

Available forms

Powder for injection—500 mcg

Dosages

⊗ ***Warning*** Individualize dosage. Toxic reactions are frequent, limiting the amount of the drug that can be given. Give drug in short courses.

Adults

Do not exceed 15 mcg/kg/day or 400–600 mcg/m^2 per day for 5 days. Calculate dosage for obese or edematous patients on the basis of surface area as an attempt to relate dosage to lean body mass.

- *Nonseminomatous testicular carcinoma:* 1,000 mcg/m^2 IV on day 1 of a combination regimen.
- *Gestational trophoblastic neoplasia:* 12 mcg/kg/day IV for 5 days when used as monotherapy. When used as part of a combination regimen, can give 500 mcg IV on days 1 and 2.
- *Isolation-perfusion technique:* 50 mcg/kg for lower extremity or pelvis; 35 mcg/kg for upper extremity. Use lower dose for obese patients or when previous chemotherapy or radiation therapy has been used.

Pediatric patients

Do not give to children younger than 6 mo. 15 mcg/kg/day IV for 5 days; do not exceed 15 mcg/kg/day or 400–600 mcg/m^2/day for 5 days.

Pharmacokinetics

Route	*Onset*	*Duration*
IV	Rapid	9 days

Metabolism: Hepatic; $T_{1/2}$: 36 hr
Distribution: Crosses placenta; may enter breast milk
Excretion: Feces, urine

IV FACTS

Preparation: Reconstitute by adding 1.1 mL of sterile water for injection (without preservatives) to vial, creating a 500 mcg/mL concentration solution. Discard any unused portion. Highly toxic—handle and administer cautiously. Avoid inhalation of dust or vapors and contact with mucous membranes, especially the eyes. Protective equipment should be worn when handling.
Infusion: Add to IV infusions of 5% dextrose or to sodium chloride, or inject into IV tubing of a running IV infusion. Direct drug injection without infusion requires two needles, one sterile needle to remove drug from vial and another for the direct IV injection. Do not inject into IV lines with cellulose ester membrane filters; drug may be partially removed by filter. Inject over 2–3 min; infuse slowly over 20–30 min. Protect from light.

Adverse effects

- **Dermatologic:** *Alopecia, skin eruptions,* acne, erythema, increased pigmentation of previously irradiated skin
- **GI:** *Cheilitis, dysphagia, esophagitis,* ulcerative stomatitis, pharyngitis, *anorexia, abdominal pain, diarrhea,* GI ulceration, proctitis, nausea, vomiting, **hepatotoxicity**
- **GU:** Renal abnormalities
- **Hematologic:** *Anemia,* **aplastic anemia, agranulocytosis, leukopenia, thrombocytopenia, pancytopenia, reticulopenia**
- **Local:** *Tissue necrosis at sites of extravasation*
- **Other:** *Malaise, fever, fatigue, lethargy, myalgia,* hypocalcemia, **death,** increased incidence of second primary tumors with radiation

Interactions

✱ **Drug-lab test** • Inaccurate bioassay procedure results for determination of antibacterial drug levels

■ Nursing considerations

CLINICAL ALERT!
Name confusion has been reported between dactinomycin and daptomycin. Use extreme caution.

Assessment

- **History:** Allergy to dactinomycin; chickenpox, herpes zoster; bone marrow suppression, prior chemotherapy, radiation therapy; pregnancy, lactation
- **Physical:** T; skin color, lesions; weight; hair; local injection site; mucous membranes, abdominal examination; CBC, LFTs, renal function tests, urinalysis

Interventions

⊗ ***Black box warning*** Use strict handling procedures; drug is extremely toxic to skin and eyes.

- Do not give IM or subcutaneously; severe local reaction and tissue necrosis occur; IV use only.

⊗ ***Black box warning*** Monitor injection site for extravasation, burning, or stinging. Discontinue infusion immediately, apply cold compresses to the area, and restart in another vein. Local infiltration with injectable corticosteroid and flushing with saline may lessen reaction.

- Monitor response, including CBC, often at start of therapy; adverse effects may require a decrease in dose or discontinuation of the drug; consult physician.
- Adverse effects may not occur immediately, may be worst 1–2 wk after therapy.

Teaching points

- Prepare a calendar for therapy days.
- Have regular medical follow-up, including blood tests to monitor the drug's effects.
- Adverse effects of the drug may not occur immediately; may be 1 week after therapy before maximal effects.
- You may experience these side effects: Rash, skin lesions, loss of hair (obtain a wig; use skin care); loss of appetite, nausea, mouth sores (frequent mouth care, eat frequent small meals; maintain good nutrition; consult a dietitian; antiemetic may be ordered).
- Report severe GI upset, diarrhea, vomiting, fever, burning or pain at injection site, unusual bleeding or bruising, severe mouth sores, sore throat, GI lesions.

DANGEROUS DRUG

▽dalteparin

(dahl' tep ah rin)

Fragmin

PREGNANCY CATEGORY B

Drug classes

Anticoagulant
Antithrombotic
Low–molecular-weight heparin

Therapeutic actions

Low–molecular-weight heparin that inhibits thrombus and clot formation by blocking factor Xa, factor IIa, preventing the formation of clots.

Indications

- Treatment of unstable angina and non–Q-wave MI for the prevention of complications in patients on aspirin or standard therapy
- Prevention of DVT, which may lead to pulmonary embolism, following abdominal or hip replacement surgery
- Extended treatment of symptomatic venous thromboembolism, DVT, or pulmonary embolism to reduce the recurrence of venous thromboembolism in patients with cancer
- Unlabeled use: Systemic anticoagulation in venous and arterial thromboembolic complications; prophylaxis of DVT in situations that may lead to PE

Contraindications and cautions

- Contraindicated with hypersensitivity to dalteparin, heparin, pork products, or benzyl alcohol; severe thrombocytopenia; uncontrolled bleeding; use of unstable angina dosage in patients undergoing regional anesthesia; pregnancy.
- Use cautiously with lactation; history of GI bleed; severe hepatic or renal impairment; recent childbirth or surgery; history of heparin-induced thrombocytopenia; severe and uncontrolled hypertension, spinal tap, spinal/epidural anesthesia.

Available forms

Injection (prefilled syringes)—2,500 international units/0.2 mL, 5,000 international units/0.2 mL, 7,500 international units/0.3 mL, 10,000 international units/mL, 12,500 international units/0.5 mL, 15,000 international units/0.6 mL, 18,000 international units/0.72 mL.

Dosages

Adults

- *Unstable angina:* 120 international units/kg subcutaneously every 12 hr with aspirin therapy for 5–8 days; not to exceed 10,000 international units every 12 hr.
- *DVT prophylaxis, abdominal surgery:* 2,500 international units subcutaneously given 1–2 hr before surgery and repeated once daily for 5–10 days after surgery; high-risk patients, 5,000 international units subcutaneously starting the evening before surgery; then daily for 5–10 days.

- *Hip replacement surgery:* 5,000 international units subcutaneously the evening before surgery *or* 2,500 international units within 2 hr before surgery *or* 2,500 international units 4–8 hr after surgery; then, 5,000 international units subcutaneously each day for 5–10 days or up to 14 days.
- *Extended treatment of venous thromboembolism:*
  Month 1: 200 international units/kg/day subcutaneously; do not exceed 18,000 international units/day
  Months 2–6: 150 international units/kg/day subcutaneously; do not exceed 18,000 international units/day.

Pediatric patients

Safety and efficacy not established.

Patients with thrombocytopenia on extended treatment

Reduce daily dose by 2,500 international units until platelet count exceeds 100,000/mm^3. If platelet count is less than 50,000/mm^3, discontinue drug.

Patients with renal insufficiency on extended treatment

If creatinine clearance is less than 30 mL/min, target anti-Xa range is 0.5–1.5 international units/mL; after at least 3–4 doses have been given, draw blood 4–6 hr after dose

Pharmacokinetics

Route	*Onset*	*Peak*	*Duration*
Subcut.	20–60 min	3–5 hr	2–12 hr

Metabolism: $T_{1/2}$: 4.5 hr
Distribution: May cross placenta, may enter breast milk
Excretion: Urine

Adverse effects

- **Hematologic: Hemorrhage,** *bruising,* thrombocytopenia
- **Hepatic:** Elevated concentrations of AST, ALT
- **Hypersensitivity:** Chills, fever, urticaria, asthma
- **Other:** Fever; pain; local irritation, hematoma, erythema at site of injection; risk of spinal or epidural hematoma if used with spinal/epidural anesthesia or spinal tap, skin necrosis

Interactions

✱ **Drug-drug** • Increased bleeding tendencies with oral anticoagulants or platelet inhibitors; clopidogrel, ticlopidine, salicylates • Risk of severe bleeding with heparin; avoid this combination

✱ **Drug-lab test** • Increased AST, ALT levels

✱ **Drug-alternative therapy** • Increased risk of bleeding if combined with chamomile, garlic, ginger, ginkgo, and ginseng therapy, high-dose vitamin E

■ Nursing considerations

Assessment

- **History:** Recent surgery or injury; sensitivity to heparin, pork products, either low–molecular-weight heparins or enoxaparin, tinzaparin, benzyl alcohol; lactation, pregnancy; history of GI bleed; renal or hepatic impairment
- **Physical:** Peripheral perfusion, R, stool guaiac test, PTT or other tests of blood coagulation, platelet count, LFTs, renal function tests

Interventions

⊗ ***Black box warning*** Carefully monitor patients with spinal epidural anesthesia; risk of spinal hematoma and paralysis.

- Give 1–2 hr before abdominal surgery.
- Do not give dalteparin by IM injection.
- Administer by deep subcutaneous injection; patient should be lying down; alternate administration between the left and right anterolateral and left and right posterolateral abdominal wall. Introduce the whole length of the needle into a skin fold at a 45 degree and 90 degree angle held between the thumb and forefinger; hold the skin fold throughout the injection.
- Cannot be used interchangeably (unit for unit) with other low–molecular-weight heparin or unfractionated heparin.
- Apply pressure to all injection sites after needle is withdrawn; inspect injection sites for signs of hematoma.
- Do not massage injection sites.
- Do not mix with other injections or infusions.
- Store at room temperature; fluid should be clear, colorless to pale yellow.

D

- Alert all health care providers that patient is on dalteparin.
- If thromboembolic episode should occur despite therapy, discontinue and initiate appropriate therapy.

⊗ ***Warning*** Keep protamine sulfate (dalteparin antidote) readily available in case of overdose.

- Treatment of overdose: Protamine sulfate (1% solution). Administer 1 mg of protamine per 100 antifactor Xa international units of dalteparin. Give very slowly IV over 10 min.

Teaching points

- This drug must be given by a parenteral route (not orally). You or your caregiver need to learn to administer the drug subcutaneously, and to safely dispose of syringes.
- Periodic blood tests are needed to monitor response.
- Avoid injury while using this drug—use an electric razor, avoid potentially injurious activities.
- Report nose bleed, bleeding of the gums, unusual bruising, black or tarry stools, cloudy or dark urine, abdominal or lower back pain, severe headache, light-headedness, or dizziness.

dantrolene sodium

(dan' troe leen)

Dantrium, Dantrium Intravenous

PREGNANCY CATEGORY C

Drug class

Skeletal muscle relaxant (direct acting)

Therapeutic actions

Relaxes skeletal muscle within the skeletal muscle fiber, probably by interfering with the release of calcium from the sarcoplasmic reticulum; does not interfere with neuromuscular transmission or affect the surface membrane of skeletal muscle.

Indications

- Oral: Control of clinical spasticity resulting from upper motor neuron disorders, such as spinal cord injury, CVA, cerebral palsy, or MS; not indicated for relief of skeletal muscle spasm resulting from rheumatic disorders; continued long-term administration is justified if use significantly reduces painful or disabling spasticity (clonus); significantly reduces the intensity or degree of nursing care required; rids the patient of problematic manifestation of spasticity
- Oral: Preoperatively to prevent or attenuate the development of malignant hyperthermia in susceptible patients who must undergo surgery or anesthesia; after a malignant hyperthermia crisis to prevent recurrence
- Parenteral (IV): Management of the fulminant hypermetabolism of skeletal muscle characteristic of malignant hyperthermia crisis; preoperative prevention of malignant hyperthermia
- Unlabeled use: Exercise-induced muscle pain

Contraindications and cautions

- Contraindicated with active hepatic disease; spasticity used to sustain upright posture, balance in locomotion or to gain or retain increased function; lactation.
- Use cautiously with female patients and patients older than 35 yr (increased risk for potentially fatal, hepatocellular disease); impaired pulmonary function; severely impaired cardiac function due to myocardial disease; history of previous liver disease or impairment.
- Malignant hyperthermia is a medical emergency that would override contraindications and cautions.

Available forms

Capsules—25, 50, 100 mg; powder for injection—20 mg/vial

Dosages

Adults

Oral

- *Chronic spasticity:* Titrate and individualize dosage; establish a therapeutic goal before therapy, and increase dosage until maximum performance compatible with the dysfunction is achieved. Initially, 25 mg daily; increase to 25 mg tid for 7 days; then increase to 50 mg tid and to 100 mg tid if necessary. Most patients will respond to 400 mg/day or less; maintain each dosage level for 4–7 days to evaluate response. Discontinue drug after 45 days if benefits are not evident.

- *Preoperative prophylaxis of malignant hyperthermia:* 4–8 mg/kg/day PO in three to four divided doses for 1–2 days prior to surgery; give last dose about 3–4 hr before scheduled surgery with a minimum of water. Adjust dosage to the recommended range to prevent incapacitation due to drowsiness and excessive GI irritation.
- *Postcrisis follow-up:* 4–8 mg/kg/day PO in four divided doses for 1–3 days to prevent recurrence.

Parenteral

- *Treatment of malignant hyperthermia:* Discontinue all anesthetics as soon as problem is recognized. Give dantrolene by continuous rapid IV push beginning at a minimum dose of 1 mg/kg and continuing until symptoms subside or a maximum cumulative dose of 10 mg/kg has been given. If physiologic and metabolic abnormalities reappear, repeat regimen. Give continuously until symptoms subside.
- *Preoperative prophylaxis of malignant hyperthermia:* 2.5 mg/kg IV 1 hr before surgery infused over 1 hr.

Pediatric patients

Safety for use in children younger than 5 yr not established. Since adverse effects may appear only after many years, weigh benefits and risks of long-term use carefully.

Oral

- *Chronic spasticity:* Use an approach similar to that for the adult. Initially, 0.5 mg/kg once daily for 7 days, followed by 0.5 mg/kg tid for 7 days; then 1 mg/kg tid for 7 days; then 2 mg/kg tid if necessary. Do not exceed dosage of 100 mg qid.
- *Malignant hyperthermia:* Dosage orally and IV is same as adult.

Pharmacokinetics

Route	*Onset*	*Peak*	*Duration*
Oral	Slow	4–6 hr	8–10 hr
IV	Rapid	5 hr	6–8 hr

Metabolism: Hepatic; $T_{1/2}$: 9 hr (oral), 4–8 hr (IV)

Distribution: Crosses placenta; enters breast milk

Excretion: Urine

IV FACTS

Preparation: Add 60 mL of sterile water for injection (without bacteriostatics) to each vial; shake until solution is clear. Use within 6 hr; store at room temperature and protect from light.

Infusion: Administer by rapid continuous IV push. Administer continuously until symptoms subside; prophylactic doses infused over 1 hr.

Incompatibilities: Dantrolene sodium is not compatible with 5% dextrose or 0.9% sodium chloride or bacteriostatic water for injection.

D

Adverse effects

Oral

- **CNS:** *Drowsiness, dizziness, weakness, general malaise, fatigue,* speech disturbance, seizure, headache, light-headedness, visual disturbance, diplopia, alteration of taste, insomnia, mental depression, mental confusion, increased nervousness
- **CV:** Tachycardia, erratic BP, phlebitis, heart failure
- **Dermatologic:** Abnormal hair growth, acnelike rash, pruritus, urticaria, eczematoid eruption, sweating, photosensitivity
- **GI:** *Diarrhea,* constipation, GI bleeding, anorexia, dysphagia, gastric irritation, abdominal cramps, **hepatitis**
- **GU:** Increased urinary frequency, hematuria, crystalluria, difficult erection, urinary incontinence, nocturia, dysuria, urinary retention
- **Hematologic:** Aplastic anemia, leukopenia, thrombocytopenia
- **Other:** Myalgia, backache, chills and fever, feeling of suffocation, respiratory depression

Parenteral

- None of the above reactions with short-term IV therapy for malignant hyperthermia

Interactions

✱ **Drug-drug** • Risk of hyperkalemia, myocardial depression if combined with verapamil

■ Nursing considerations

Assessment

- **History:** Active hepatic disease; spasticity used to sustain upright posture and balance in locomotion or to gain and retain increased function; female patient and patients older than 35 yr; impaired pulmonary function; severely impaired cardiac function; history of previous liver disease; lactation, pregnancy
- **Physical:** T; skin color, lesions; orientation, affect, reflexes, bilateral grip strength, vision; P, BP, auscultation; adventitious sounds; bowel sounds, normal GI output; prostate palpation, normal output, voiding pattern; urinalysis, LFTs

Interventions

⊗ ***Warning*** Monitor IV injection sites, and ensure that extravasation does not occur—drug is very alkaline and irritating to tissues.

⊗ ***Warning*** Ensure that all appropriate measures are used to treat malignant hyperthermia: Discontinue triggering drugs, monitor and provide for increased oxygen requirements, manage metabolic acidosis and electrolyte imbalance, use cooling measures if necessary.

- Establish a therapeutic goal before beginning long-term oral therapy to gain or enhance ability to engage in therapeutic exercise program, use of braces, transfer maneuvers.
- Withdraw oral drug for 2–4 days to confirm therapeutic benefits; clinical impression of exacerbation of spasticity would justify use of this potentially dangerous drug.
- Discontinue if diarrhea is severe; it may be possible to reinstitute drug at a lower dose.

⊠ ***Black box warning*** Have liver function tests done periodically; arrange to discontinue at first sign of abnormality; early detection of liver abnormalities may permit reversion to normal function. Hepatotoxicity is possible.

Teaching points

Preoperative prophylaxis of malignant hyperthermia

- Call for assistance if you wish to get up; do not move about alone; this drug can cause drowsiness.
- Report GI upset; a dosage change is possible; eat frequent small meals.

Long-term oral therapy for spasticity

- Take this drug exactly as prescribed; do not take a higher dosage.
- Avoid alcohol, sleep-inducing, or over-the-counter drugs; these could cause dangerous effects.
- You may experience these side effects: Drowsiness, dizziness, blurred vision (avoid driving or engaging in activities that require alertness); diarrhea; nausea (take with food, eat frequent small meals); difficulty urinating, increased urinary frequency, urinary incontinence (empty bladder just before taking medication); headache, malaise (an analgesic may be allowed); photosensitivity (avoid sun and ultraviolet light or use sunscreens, protective clothing).
- Report rash, itching, bloody or black tarry stools, pale stools, yellowish discoloration of the skin or eyes, severe diarrhea.

dapsone

See Appendix W, *Less commonly used drugs*.

daptomycin

*(dap toe **mye'** sin)*

Cubicin

PREGNANCY CATEGORY B

Drug class

Cyclic lipopeptide antibiotic

Therapeutic actions

Binds to bacterial cell membranes, causing a rapid depolarization of membrane potential. The loss of membrane potential leads to the inhibition of protein, DNA, and RNA synthesis, which results in bacterial cell death.

Indications

- Treatment of complicated skin and skin structure infections caused by susceptible

strains of the following gram-positive bacteria: *Staphylococcus aureus* (including methicillin-resistant strains), *Streptococcus pyogenes, Streptococcus agalactiae, Streptococcus dysgalactiae,* and *Enterococcus faecalis* (vancomycin-susceptible strains only)
- Treatment of *S. aureus* bloodstream infections, including right-sided endocarditis caused by methicillin-susceptible and methicillin-resistant *S. aureus*

Contraindications and cautions
- Contraindicated with known allergy to daptomycin.
- Use cautiously with pregnancy, lactation, renal impairment.

Available forms
Powder for injection—500 mg/vial

Dosages
Adults
Skin and skin structure infections: 4 mg/kg IV given over 30 min in 0.9% sodium chloride injection every 24 hr for 7–14 days.
Bacteremia: 6 mg/kg/day IV over 30 min for for 2–6 wk or longer.
Pediatric patients
Safety and efficacy not established.
Patients with renal impairment
For patients with creatinine clearance less than 30 mL/min or for those on dialysis, give 4 mg/kg IV once every 48 hr (6 mg/kg for *S. aureus* bloodstream infections).

Pharmacokinetics

Route	Onset	Peak
IV	Rapid	30 min

Metabolism: Hepatic; $T_{1/2}$: 8–9 hr
Distribution: May cross placenta; may enter breast milk
Excretion: Urine

IV FACTS
Preparation: Reconstitute with 10 mL (500-mg vial) 0.9% sodium chloride injection; further dilute with 0.9% sodium chloride injection for infusion. Final concentration should not exceed 20 mg/mL. Reconstituted and diluted solution is stable for 12 hr at room temperature, up to 48 hr if refrigerated; date bag to ensure that solution is discarded after that time; solution should be clear and free of particulate matter.
Infusion: Infuse over 30 min.
Compatibilities: Compatible with 0.9% sodium chloride injection, lactated Ringer's.
Incompatibilities: Do not mix with dextrose solutions; do not mix in solution with any other drugs, if a line is used for several drugs, flush the line with compatible fluids between drugs.

Adverse effects
- **CNS:** *Headache, insomnia,* dizziness
- **CV:** Hypotension, hypertension
- **GI:** *Constipation, nausea, diarrhea, vomiting,* dyspepsia, **pseudomembranous colitis**
- **Respiratory:** Dyspnea
- **Other:** *Injection site reactions,* fever, *rash,* pruritus, arthralgia, limb pain, **myopathy,** *superinfections,* anemia

Interactions
✱ Drug-drug • Potential for increased effects of oral anticoagulants if combined; monitor patient closely and adjust dosage as needed • Risk of altered effects of both drugs if combined with tobramycin; if this combination is used, monitor patient very closely • Increased risk of myopathy if combined with HMG-CoA inhibitors; consider discontinuing the HMG-CoA inhibitor while daptomycin is being used

■ Nursing considerations

CLINICAL ALERT!
Name confusion has been reported between dactinomycin and daptomycin. Use extreme caution.

Assessment
- **History:** Allergy to daptomycin, renal impairment, pregnancy, lactation
- **Physical:** Site of infection, skin color, lesions; orientation, affect; GI output, bowel sounds; orientation, affect; culture and sensitivity tests of infection, renal function tests

D

Interventions

- Culture site of infection before beginning therapy.
- Monitor CPK levels weekly to assess for myopathy.

⊗ ***Warning*** Discontinue drug and provide supportive care for any patient developing signs of pseudomembranous colitis.

⊗ ***Warning*** Discontinue drug with any unexplained signs of myopathy (muscle pain or weakness) or with increasing levels of CPK. Consider discontinuing any other drugs that are associated with myopathy (HMG-CoA inhibitors) while daptomycin is being used.

- Monitor renal function in patients before beginning therapy.
- Institute appropriate hygiene measures and arrange treatment if superinfections occur.
- If GI upset occurs, provide small, frequent meals; encourage patient to maintain fluid intake and nutrition.
- Establish safety measures (eg, accompany patient, use side rails) if CNS changes occur.

Teaching points

- This drug will be given IV over 30 minutes once a day for 7–14 days or longer.
- You may experience these side effects: Nausea, diarrhea, discomfort (eat frequent small meals); headache (analgesics may be available to help; consult your health care provider); dizziness (ask for help when you are walking); reaction at the injection site (if this becomes painful, notify your health care provider).
- Report severe or watery diarrhea, skin rash, muscle pain or weakness.

▽ darbepoetin alfa

*(dar bah poe **e'** tin)*

Aranesp

PREGNANCY CATEGORY C

Drug class

Erythropoiesis-stimulating hormone

Therapeutic actions

An erythropoietin-like glycoprotein hormone produced by recombinant DNA technology; stimulates RBC production in the bone marrow in the same manner as naturally occurring erythropoietin, a hormone released into the bloodstream in response to renal hypoxia.

Indications

- Treatment of anemia associated with chronic renal failure, including during dialysis
- Treatment of chemotherapy-induced anemia in patients with nonmyeloid malignancies
- Unlabeled use: Anemia associated with malignancy

Contraindications and cautions

- Contraindicated with uncontrolled hypertension or hypersensitivity to any component of the drug.
- Use cautiously with hypertension, pregnancy, lactation.

Available forms

Polysorbate solution for injection—25, 40, 60, 100, 150, 200, 300, 500 mcg/mL; 25 mcg/0.42 mL; 40 mcg/0.4 mL; 60 mcg/0.3 mL; 100 mcg/0.5 mL; 150 mcg/0.3 or 0.75 mL; 200 mcg/0.4 mL; 300 mcg/0.6 mL

Dosages

Adults

- *Starting dose:* 0.45 mcg/kg IV or subcutaneously once per wk. Dosage may be adjusted no more frequently than once per mo. Target Hgb level is 12 g/dL. Adjust dosage by 25% at a time to achieve that level. Avoid rapid increase in Hgb.
- *Switching from epoetin alfa:*

Epoetin Alfa Dose in Units/wk	*Darbepoetin Alfa Dose in mcg/wk*
Less than 2,500	6.25
2,500–4,999	12.5
5,000–10,999	25
11,000–17,999	40
18,000–33,999	60
34,000–89,999	100
90,000 or more	200

Patients who were receiving epoetin two to three times per week should receive darbepoetin once per wk. Patients who were receiving epoetin once per wk should receive darbepoetin once every 2 wk.

- *Chemotherapy-induced anemia:* 2.25 mcg/kg subcutaneously once per wk; adjust to maintain acceptable Hgb levels. Or 500 mcg by subcutaneous injection once every 3 wk; adjust dosage to maintain Hgb level at 12 g/dL.

Pediatric patients

Safety and efficacy not established.

Patients with chronic renal failure

IV administration should be used instead of subcutaneous injection. Dosage should start slowly and be increased based on Hgb levels; check Hgb levels weekly until stable, then monthly.

Pharmacokinetics

Route	*Peak*	*Duration*
Subcut.	34 hr	24–72 hr
IV	14 hr	24–72 hr

Metabolism: Serum; $T_{1/2}$: 21 hr (IV), 49 hr (subcutaneously)
Distribution: May cross placenta; enters breast milk
Excretion: Urine

IV FACTS

Preparation: Administer as provided; no additional preparation needed. Enter vial only once; discard any unused solution. Refrigerate. Do not shake vial. Inspect for any discoloring or precipitates before use.
Infusion: Administer by direct IV injection or into tubing of running IV.
Incompatibilities: Do not mix with any other drug solution.

Adverse effects

- **CNS:** *Headache, fatigue, asthenia,* dizziness, **seizure,** TIA, **CVA**
- **CV:** *Hypertension, edema, hypotension,* chest pain, arrhythmias, chest pain, **MI**
- **GI:** *Nausea, vomiting, diarrhea, abdominal pain*
- **Respiratory:** *URI, dyspnea, cough*
- **Other:** *Arthralgias, myalgias,* limb pain, clotting of access line, pain at injection site, **development of anti-erythropoetin antibodies with subsequent pure red cell aplasia and extreme anemia**

■ Nursing considerations

Assessment

- **History:** Hypertension; hypersensitivity to any component of product, pregnancy, lactation
- **Physical:** Reflexes, affect, BP, P, R, adventitious sounds, urinary output, renal function tests, CBC, hemoglobin, Hct, iron levels, electrolytes

Interventions

⊗ ***Warning*** Ensure chronic, renal nature of anemia or response to chemotherapy. Darbepoetin is not intended as a treatment of severe anemia and is not a substitute for emergency transfusion.

⊠ ***Black box warning*** Risk of death and serious CV events increases if hemoglobin target exceeds 12 g/dL. Use lowest level of any drug needed to increase hemoglobin to lowest level needed to avoid transfusion.

⊠ ***Black box warning*** Risk of DVT is higher in patients who receive erythropoietin-stimulating agents preoperatively to decrease need for transfusion; note that darbepoetin is not approved for this use.

⊠ ***Black box warning*** Risk of death or tumor progression increases when drug is used in cancer patients with Hgb target range exceeding 12 g/dL. Monitor Hgb closely in these patients.

- Prepare solution by gently mixing. Do not shake; shaking may denature the glycoprotein. Use only one dose per vial; do not reenter the vial. Discard unused portions.
- Patients with chronic renal failure on hemodialysis should receive this drug IV, not by subcutaneous injection, to decrease the risk of developing anti-erythropoetin antibodies.
- Do not administer with any other drug solution.
- Administer dose once weekly. If administered independent of dialysis, administer into venous access line. If patient is not on dialysis, administer IV or subcutaneously.

- Evaluate chemotherapy patients for once-every-3-wk treatment program.
- Monitor access lines for signs of clotting.
- Arrange for Hct or Hgb reading before administration of each dose to determine appropriate dosage. Do not exceed Hgb target of 12 g/dL. If patient fails to respond within 4 wk of therapy, evaluate patient for other causes of the problem.
- Evaluate iron stores before and periodically during therapy. Supplemental iron may be needed.
- Monitor patient for sudden loss of response and severe anemia with low reticulocyte count; hold drug and check patient for anti-erythropoetin antibodies. If antibodies are present, discontinue drug permanently and do not switch to any other erythropoetic agent; cross-sensitivity can occur.
- Monitor diet and assess nutrition; arrange for nutritional consult as necessary.
- Establish safety precautions (eg, siderails, environmental control, lighting) if CNS effects occur.
- Maintain seizure precautions during administration.
- Provide additional comfort measures, as necessary, to alleviate discomfort from GI effects, headache.
- Offer support and encouragement to deal with chronic disease and need for prolonged therapy and testing.

Teaching points

- The drug will need to be given once a week or once every 3 wk, as prescribed, and can only be given IV or subcutaneously or into a dialysis access line. Prepare a schedule of administration dates. You and a significant other should learn to administer subcutaneous injections. Dispose of needles and syringes properly.
- Keep appointments for blood tests; frequent blood tests will be needed to determine the effects of the drug on your blood count and to determine the appropriate dosage needed.
- Maintain all of the usual activities and restrictions that apply to your chronic renal failure. If this becomes difficult, consult your health care provider.
- You may experience these side effects: Dizziness (avoid driving a car or performing hazardous tasks); headache, fatigue, joint pain (consult your health care provider if these become bothersome; medications may be available to help); nausea, vomiting, diarrhea (proper nutrition is important; consult with your dietitian to maintain nutrition and ensure ready access to bathroom facilities); upper respiratory infection, cough (consult your health care provider if this occurs).
- Report difficulty breathing, numbness or tingling, chest pain, seizures, severe headache.

▽ darifenacin hydrobromide

*(da ree **fen'** ah sin high droh **broh'** myde)*

Enablex (DNC)

PREGNANCY CATEGORY C

Drug classes

Muscarinic receptor antagonist
Urinary antispasmodic

Therapeutic actions

Counteracts smooth muscle spasm of the urinary tract by relaxing the detrusor and other smooth muscles through action at the muscarinic parasympathetic receptors.

Indications

- Treatment of overactive bladder with symptoms of urge urinary incontinence, urgency and urinary frequency

Contraindications and cautions

- Contraindicated with allergy to drug or any component of the drug, urinary retention, gastric retention, uncontrolled narrow-angle glaucoma.
- Use cautiously with bladder outflow obstruction, GI obstructive disorders, decreased GI motility, controlled narrow-angle glaucoma, reduced hepatic function, pregnancy, lactation.

Available forms

ER tablets DNC—7.5, 15 mg

Dosages

Adults

7.5 mg/day PO taken with liquid and swallowed whole. May be increased to 15 mg/day PO as early as week 2, if needed for patient response.

Pediatric patients

Safety and efficacy not established.

Patients with moderate hepatic impairment

Do not exceed 7.5 mg/day PO.

Patients with severe hepatic impairment

Not recommended.

Pharmacokinetics

Route	*Onset*	*Peak*
Oral	Slow	6.5–7.5 hr

Metabolism: Hepatic; $T_{1/2}$: 13–19 hr
Distribution: May cross placenta; may enter breast milk
Excretion: Feces, urine

Adverse effects

- **CNS:** Dizziness, asthenia, headache
- **EENT:** Dry eyes, blurred vision
- **GI:** *Dry mouth, constipation,* nausea, dyspepsia, abdominal pain, diarrhea
- **GU:** UTI, urinary retention
- **Other:** Flulike symptoms

Interactions

✱ **Drug-drug** • Risk of increased serum levels and toxic effects if combined with clarithromycin, ketoconazole, itraconazole, ritonavir, nelfinavir, clarithromycin, nefazadone; if this combination is used, monitor patient and do not exceed 7.5 mg/day darifenacin • Risk of increased toxic effects of flecainide, thioridazine, TCAs; monitor patient closely and use caution if this combination is used • Risk of increased anticholinergic adverse effects (dry mouth, constipation, blurred vision) if combined with anticholinergic drugs; monitor patient carefully if this combination is used

■ Nursing considerations

Assessment

- **History:** Allergy to drug or any component of the drug; urinary retention, gastric retention, uncontrolled narrow-angle glaucoma, bladder outflow obstruction, GI obstructive disorders, decreased GI motility, reduced renal or hepatic function, pregnancy, lactation
- **Physical:** Orientation, affect, reflexes, ophthalmic examination, ocular pressure measurement; P; bowel sounds, oral mucous membranes; LFTs

Interventions

- Arrange for definitive treatment of underlying medical conditions that may be causing overactive bladder.
- Ensure that patient swallows tablet whole; do not cut, crush, or allow patient to chew tablet.
- Provide sugarless lozenges for patient to suck and frequent mouth care if dry mouth is a serious problem.
- Provide small, frequent meals if GI upset occurs.
- Establish bowel program if constipation is a problem.
- Arrange for ophthalmic examination before beginning therapy and periodically during therapy.
- Establish safety precautions if CNS effects occur.

Teaching points

- Take drug once a day with water. Swallow whole, do not cut, crush, or chew tablet. Take with or without food.
- Be aware that this drug is meant to relieve the symptoms you are experiencing; other medications may be used to treat the cause of the symptoms.
- You may not be able to sweat normally while on this drug, use caution in any situation that could lead to overheating.
- Consult your health care provider if you become pregnant or wish to become pregnant, it is not known if this drug affects the fetus.
- If you are nursing a baby, another method of feeding the baby should be used while you are on this drug.

D

- You may experience these side effects: Dry mouth, GI upset (sucking on sugarless lozenges and frequent mouth care may help); drowsiness, blurred vision (avoid driving or performing tasks that require alertness while on this drug); constipation (medication may be available to help).
- Report inability to void, fever, blurring of vision, severe constipation.

darunavir

See Appendix W, *Less commonly used drugs*.

dasatinib

See Appendix W, *Less commonly used drugs*.

daunorubicin citrate

See Appendix W, *Less commonly used drugs*.

decitabine

See Appendix W, *Less commonly used drugs*.

deferasirox

See Appendix W, *Less commonly used drugs*.

deferoxamine mesylate

See Appendix W, *Less commonly used drugs*.

degarelix

See Appendix W, *Less commonly used drugs*.

delavirdine mesylate

*(dell ah **vur'** den)*

Rescriptor

PREGNANCY CATEGORY C

Drug classes

Antiviral
Nonnucleoside reverse transcriptase inhibitor

Therapeutic actions

Nonnucleoside inhibitor of HIV reverse transcriptase; binds directly to HIV's reverse transcriptase and blocks RNA-dependent and DNA-dependent DNA polymerase activities.

Indications

- Treatment of HIV-1 infection in combination with other appropriate retroviral drugs when therapy is warranted; not intended as a monotherapy because resistant virus emerges rapidly

Contraindications and cautions

- Contraindicated with life-threatening allergy to any component.
- Use cautiously with compromised or impaired liver function, pregnancy, lactation.

Available forms

Tablets—100, 200 mg

Dosages

Adults and patients older than 16 yr

400 mg PO tid used in combination with appropriate antiretroviral drugs.

Pediatric patients

Not recommended for patients younger than 16 yr.

Pharmacokinetics

Route	*Onset*	*Peak*
Oral	Rapid	1 hr

Metabolism: Hepatic; $T_{1/2}$: 2–11 hr
Distribution: May cross placenta; may enter breast milk
Excretion: Urine, feces

Adverse effects

- **CNS:** *Headache,* insomnia, myalgia, *asthenia,* malaise, dizziness, paresthesia, somnolence, fatigue

- **GI:** *Nausea,* GI pain, *diarrhea,* anorexia, vomiting, dyspepsia, increased liver enzymes
- **Skin:** *Rash,* pruritus, maculopapular rash, nodules, urticaria
- **Other:** Anemia, arthralgia, breast enlargement, fat redistribution

Interactions

✱ Drug-drug ⊗ ***Warning*** Potentially serious or life-threatening adverse effects may occur in combination with antiarrhythmics, clarithromycin, dapsone, rifabutin, benzodiazepines, calcium channel blockers, ergot derivatives, indinavir, saquinavir, quinidine or warfarin; avoid these combinations if at all possible; if the combination cannot be avoided, monitor patient very closely and decrease dosage as appropriate.

✱ Drug-alternative therapy • Possible loss of antiviral response with St. John's wort; avoid this combination

■ Nursing considerations

Assessment

- **History:** Life-threatening allergy to any component, impaired liver function, pregnancy, lactation
- **Physical:** Skin rashes, lesions, texture; T; affect, reflexes, peripheral sensation; bowel sounds, LFTs, CBC and differential

Interventions

- Arrange to monitor hematologic indices and liver function periodically during therapy.
- Monitor patient for signs of opportunistic infections that will need to be treated appropriately.

⊗ ***Black box warning*** Administer the drug concurrently with appropriate antiretroviral drugs; not for monotherapy.

- Disperse tablets in water before administration; add four 100-mg tablets to at least 3 oz water; allow to stand for a few minutes, stir until a uniform dispersion occurs; have patient drink immediately. Rinse glass and have patient drink rinse; the 200-mg tablets are not readily soluble in water.
- Offer support and encouragement to deal with the diagnosis; explain that this drug must be taken in combination with other drugs and that the long-term effects of the use of this drug are not known.

Teaching points

- Take drug as prescribed; take with other prescribed drugs; do not change dose or alter routine without consulting your health care provider. If also taking antacids, take at least 1 hour apart.
- Disperse four 100-mg tablets in 3 ounces of water; let stand, then stir and drink immediately, rinse glass with water and drink rinse; the 200-mg tablets are not readily soluble in water.
- These drugs are not a cure for AIDS or AIDS-related complex; opportunistic infections may occur and regular medical care should be sought to deal with the disease.
- Frequent blood tests are needed during the course of treatment; results of blood counts may indicate a need for decreased dosage or discontinuation of the drug for a specific time.
- This drug may interact with several other drugs; alert any health care provider that you are on this drug. If you are taking antacids, take them at least 1 hour apart from delavirdine.
- Delavirdine does not reduce the risk of transmission of HIV to others by sexual contact or blood contamination; use appropriate precautions.
- You may experience these side effects: Nausea, loss of appetite, change in taste (eat frequent small meals); headache, fever, muscle aches (an analgesic may help; consult your health care provider); rash (skin care will be important).
- Report use of any prescription or over-the-counter drugs or dietary supplements to your physician or pharmacist.
- Report rash, severe headache, severe nausea, vomiting, changes in color of urine or stool, fatigue.

demeclocycline hydrochloride (demethylchlortetracycline hydrochloride)

*(dem e kloe **sye'** kleen)*

Declomycin

PREGNANCY CATEGORY D

Drug classes

Antibiotic
Tetracycline antibiotic

Therapeutic actions

Bacteriostatic: Inhibits protein synthesis of susceptible bacteria, preventing cell reproduction.

Indications

- Infections caused by susceptible strains of rickettsiae; *Mycoplasma pneumoniae;* agents of psittacosis, ornithosis, lymphogranuloma venereum, and granuloma inguinale; *Borrelia recurrentis; Haemophilus ducreyi; Pasteurella pestis; P. tularensis; Bartonella bacilliformis; Bacteroides; Vibrio comma; Vibrio fetus; Brucella; Escherichia coli; Enterobacter aerogenes; Shigella; Acinetobacter calcoaceticus; Haemophilus influenzae; Klebsiella; Diplococcus pneumoniae; Staphylococcus aureus; Streptococcus pyogenes; Streptococcus pneumoniae; Mycoplasma* bacteria
- When penicillin is contraindicated, infections caused by *Neisseria gonorrhoeae, Treponema pallidum, T. pertenue, Listeria monocytogenes, Clostridium, Bacillus anthracis, Fusobacterium fusiforme, Actinomyces, Neisseria meningitidis*
- As an adjunct to amebicides in acute intestinal amebiasis
- Treatment of acne or uncomplicated urethral, endocervical, or rectal infections in adults caused by *Chlamydia trachomatis*

Contraindications and cautions

- Contraindicated with allergy to tetracyclines; pregnancy, lactation; in children during tooth-forming years.
- Use cautiously with renal or hepatic impairment.

Available forms

Tablets—150, 300 mg

Dosages

Adults

- *General guidelines:* 150 mg PO qid or 300 mg PO bid.
- *Gonococcal infection:* 600 mg PO then 300 mg every 12 hr for 4 days to a total of 3 g.
- *Streptococcal infections:* Treat for at least 10 days.

Pediatric patients 8 yr and older

3–6 mg/lb/day (6.6–13.2 mg/kg/day) PO in two to four divided doses.

Pediatric patients younger than 8 yr

Not recommended.

Pharmacokinetics

Route	*Onset*	*Peak*	*Duration*
Oral	Varies	3–4 hr	18–20 hr

Metabolism: Hepatic; $T_{1/2}$: 12–16 hr
Distribution: Crosses placenta; enters breast milk
Excretion: Feces, urine

Adverse effects

- **Dental:** *Discoloring and inadequate calcification of primary teeth of fetus if used by pregnant women, discoloring and inadequate calcification of permanent teeth if used during period of dental development*
- **Dermatologic:** *Phototoxic reactions, rash,* exfoliative dermatitis (especially frequent and severe with this tetracycline)
- **GI:** Fatty liver, **liver failure,** *anorexia, nausea, vomiting, diarrhea, glossitis,* dysphagia, enterocolitis, esophageal ulcer
- **Hematologic: Hemolytic anemia, thrombocytopenia, neutropenia, eosinophilia, leukocytosis, leukopenia**
- **Other:** Superinfections, nephrogenic diabetes insipidus syndrome (polyuria, polydipsia, weakness) in patients being treated for SIADH

Interactions

✷ **Drug-drug** • Decreased absorption with antacids, iron, alkali • Increased digoxin toxicity • Increased nephrotoxicity with methoxyflurane • Decreased activity of penicillin • Possibly decreased effectiveness of hormonal contraceptives

✷ **Drug-food** • Decreased effectiveness of demeclocycline if taken with food, dairy products

✷ **Drug-lab test** • Interference with culture studies for several days following therapy

■ Nursing considerations

Assessment

- **History:** Allergy to tetracyclines, renal or hepatic impairment, pregnancy, lactation
- **Physical:** Skin status, R and adventitious sounds, GI function and liver evaluation, urinary output and concentration, urinalysis and BUN, LFTs, renal function tests; culture infected area before beginning therapy

Interventions

- Give on an empty stomach; if severe GI upset occurs, give with food.
- Give with a full 8-oz glass of water.
- Discontinue drug if diabetes insipidus occurs in SIADH patients.
- Recommend the use of barrier contraceptives while on this drug; fetal abnormalities can occur.

Teaching points

- Take drug throughout the day for best results; take on an empty stomach, 1 hour before or 1 hour after meals, unless GI upset occurs; then it can be taken with food.
- Use of contraceptive measures is advised while on this drug. Hormonal contraceptives may not be effective; fetal harm has been reported.
- You may experience these side effects: Sensitivity to sunlight (use protective clothing and sunscreen), diarrhea.
- Report rash, itching; difficulty breathing; dark urine or light-colored stools; severe cramps; increased thirst, increased urination, weakness (SIADH patients).

▽ denileukin diftitox

See Appendix W, *Less commonly used drugs*.

▽ desipramine hydrochloride

*(dess **ip'** ra meen)*

Apo-Desipramine (CAN), Norpramin, PMS-Desipramine (CAN), ratio-Desipramine (CAN)

PREGNANCY CATEGORY C

D

Drug classes

Antidepressant
TCA (secondary amine)

Therapeutic actions

Mechanism of action unknown; inhibits the presynaptic reuptake of the neurotransmitters norepinephrine and serotonin; anticholinergic at CNS and peripheral receptors; sedating.

Indications

- Relief of symptoms of depression (endogenous depression most responsive)
- Unlabeled uses: Treatment of eating disorders, chronic urticaria, diabetic neuropathy, ADHD, enuresis, alcohol dependence

Contraindications and cautions

- Contraindicated with hypersensitivity to any tricyclic drug, concomitant therapy with an MAOI, recent MI, myelography within previous 24 hr or scheduled within 48 hr.
- Use cautiously with ECT; preexisting CV disorders (eg, severe coronary heart disease, progressive heart failure, angina pectoris, paroxysmal tachycardia; possibly increased risk of serious CVS toxicity with TCAs); angle-closure glaucoma, increased IOP, urinary retention, ureteral or urethral spasm (anticholinergic effects of TCAs may exacerbate these conditions); seizure disorders (TCAs lower the seizure threshold); hyperthyroidism (predisposes to CVS toxicity, including cardiac arrhythmias); impaired hepatic, renal function; psychiatric patients (schizophrenic or paranoid patients may exhibit a worsening of psychosis with TCA therapy); manic-depressive patients (may shift to hypomanic or manic phase); elective surgery (TCAs should be discontinued as long as possible before surgery), pregnancy, lactation.

Available forms

Tablets—10, 25, 50, 75, 100, 150 mg

Dosages

Adults

- *Depression:* 100–200 mg/day PO as single dose or in divided doses initially. May gradually increase to 300 mg/day. Do not exceed 300 mg/day. Patients requiring 300 mg/day should generally have treatment initiated in a hospital. Continue a reduced maintenance dosage for at least 2 mo after a satisfactory response has been achieved.

Pediatric patients

Not recommended in children younger than 12 yr.

Geriatric patients and adolescents

Initially, 25–100 mg/day PO; dosages more than 100–150 mg are not recommended.

Pharmacokinetics

Route	Onset	Peak	Duration
Oral	Varies	2–4 hr	3–4 days

Metabolism: Hepatic; $T_{1/2}$: 12–24 hr
Distribution: Crosses placenta; enters breast milk
Excretion: Urine

Adverse effects

- **CNS:** *Sedation and anticholinergic effects, confusion* (especially in elderly), *disturbed concentration,* hallucinations, disorientation, decreased memory, feelings of unreality, delusions, anxiety, nervousness, restlessness, agitation, panic, insomnia, nightmares, hypomania, mania, exacerbation of psychosis, drowsiness, weakness, fatigue, headache, numbness, tingling, paresthesias of extremities, incoordination, motor hyperactivity, akathisia, ataxia, tremors, peripheral neuropathy, extrapyramidal symptoms, *seizures,* speech blockage, dysarthria, tinnitus, altered EEG, **CVA**
- **CV:** *Orthostatic hypotension,* hypertension, syncope, tachycardia, palpitations, **MI,** arrhythmias, heart block, precipitation of heart failure
- **Endocrine:** Elevated or depressed blood sugar; elevated prolactin levels; SIADH secretion
- **GI:** *Dry mouth, constipation,* paralytic ileus, *nausea,* vomiting, anorexia, epigastric distress, diarrhea, flatulence, dysphagia, peculiar taste, increased salivation, stomatitis, glossitis, parotid swelling, abdominal cramps, black tongue
- **GU:** Urinary retention, delayed micturition, dilation of the urinary tract, gynecomastia, testicular swelling in men; breast enlargement, menstrual irregularity and galactorrhea in women; increased or decreased libido; impotence
- **Hematologic: Bone marrow depression**
- **Hypersensitivity:** Rash, pruritus, vasculitis, petechiae, photosensitization, edema (generalized or of face and tongue), drug fever
- **Withdrawal:** Symptoms on abrupt discontinuation of prolonged therapy—nausea, headache, vertigo, nightmares, malaise
- **Other:** Nasal congestion, excessive appetite, weight gain or loss; sweating (paradoxical effect in a drug with prominent anticholinergic effects), alopecia, lacrimation, hyperthermia, flushing, chills

Interactions

✱ **Drug-drug** • Increased TCA levels and pharmacologic (especially anticholinergic) effects with cimetidine, fluoxetine • Increased serum levels and risk of bleeding with oral anticoagulants • Altered response, including arrhythmias and hypertension with sympathomimetics, quinolones • Risk of severe hypertension with clonidine • Hyperpyretic crises, severe seizures, hypertensive episodes, and deaths when MAOIs are given with TCAs

■ Nursing considerations

Assessment

- **History:** Hypersensitivity to any tricyclic drug; concomitant therapy with an MAOI; recent MI; myelography within previous 24 hr or scheduled within 48 hr; lactation; ECT; preexisting CV disorders; angle-closure

glaucoma, increased IOP, urinary retention, ureteral or urethral spasm; seizure disorders; hyperthyroidism; impaired hepatic, renal function; psychiatric patients; elective surgery; pregnancy, lactation
- **Physical:** Body weight; T; skin color, lesions; orientation, affect, reflexes, vision and hearing; P, BP, orthostatic BP, perfusion; bowel sounds, normal output, liver evaluation; urine flow, normal output; usual sexual function, frequency of menses, breast and scrotal examination; LFTs, urinalysis, CBC, ECG

Interventions

⊠ ***Black box warning*** Risk of suicidality in children, adolescents, and young adults; monitor patient, and inform caregivers.

⊗ ***Warning*** For depressed and potentially suicidal patients, limit access to drug.
- Give major portion of dose at bedtime if drowsiness or severe anticholinergic effects occur.
- Reduce dosage if minor side effects develop; contact health care provider if serious side effects occur.
- Monitor elderly patients for possibly increased adverse effects.
- Arrange for CBC if patient develops fever, sore throat, or other sign of infection.

Teaching points
- Take drug exactly as prescribed; do not stop taking this drug abruptly or without consulting your health care provider.
- Avoid alcohol and other sleep-inducing and over-the-counter drugs while taking this drug.
- Avoid prolonged exposure to sunlight or sunlamps; use a sunscreen or protective garments with prolonged exposure to sunlight.
- You may experience these side effects: Headache, dizziness, drowsiness, weakness, blurred vision (reversible; if severe, avoid driving or performing tasks that require alertness); nausea, vomiting, loss of appetite, dry mouth (eat frequent small meals, frequent mouth care, and sucking sugarless candies may help); nightmares, inability to concentrate, confusion; changes in sexual function.
- Report dry mouth, difficulty in urination, excessive sedation, suicidal thoughts.

▽desirudin

See Appendix W, *Less commonly used drugs*.

▽desloratadine

*(dess lor **at'** a deen)*

Clarinex, Clarinex Reditabs

PREGNANCY CATEGORY C

Drug class
Antihistamine (nonsedating type)

Therapeutic actions
Competitively blocks the effects of histamine at peripheral H_1-receptor sites.

Indications
- Relief of nasal and non-nasal symptoms of seasonal allergic rhinitis in patients 2 yr and older
- Treatment of chronic idiopathic urticaria and perennial allergies caused by indoor and outdoor allergens in patients 6 mo and older

Contraindications and cautions
- Contraindicated with allergy to desloratadine, loratadine, or any components of the product; lactation.
- Use cautiously with hepatic or renal impairment or pregnancy.

Available forms
Tablets—5 mg; rapidly disintegrating tablets—2.5, 5 mg; syrup—2.5 mg/5 mL

Dosages
Adults and children 12 yr and older

5 mg/day PO or 2 tsp (5 mg/10 mL) syrup PO once daily.

Pediatric patients 6–11 yr

1 tsp syrup (2.5 mg/5 mL) PO once daily, or 2.5-mg rapidly disintegrating tablet PO once daily.

Pediatric patients 12 mo–5 yr

1/2 tsp syrup (1.25 mg/2.5 mL) PO once daily.

Pediatric patients 6–11 mo

2 mL syrup (1 mg) PO once daily.

D

Patients with hepatic or renal impairment
5 mg PO every other day.

Pharmacokinetics

Route	*Onset*	*Peak*	*Duration*
Oral	1 hr	3 hr	24 hr

Metabolism: Hepatic; $T_{1/2}$: 27 hr
Distribution: May cross placenta; enters breast milk
Excretion: Feces, urine

Adverse effects

- **CNS:** Somnolence, nervousness, dizziness, fatigue
- **CV:** Tachycardia
- **GI:** *Dry mouth,* nausea
- **Respiratory:** Bronchospasm, pharyngitis, dry throat
- **Other:** Flulike symptoms, hypersensitivity

■ Nursing considerations

Assessment

- **History:** Allergy to desloratadine, loratadine, other antihistamines; hepatic or renal impairment; pregnancy; lactation
- **Physical:** T, orientation, reflexes, affect, R, adventitious sounds, LFTs, renal function tests

Interventions

- Administer without regard to meals.
- Arrange for use of humidifier if thickening of secretions, throat dryness become bothersome; encourage adequate intake of fluids.
- Provide sugarless lozenges to suck and regular mouth care if dry mouth is a problem.
- Provide safety measures if CNS effects occur.

Teaching points

- Take this drug exactly as prescribed, with or without food.
- Place rapidly disintegrating tablets on tongue immediately after opening blister pack; administer with or without water.
- You may experience these side effects: Dizziness, fatigue (use caution if driving or performing tasks that require alertness); dry throat, thickening of bronchial secretions, dryness of nasal mucosa (use of a humidifier may help if this becomes a problem); dry mouth (sucking on sugarless lozenges and frequent mouth care may help).
- Report difficulty breathing, tremors, palpitations.

▽desmopressin acetate (1-deamino-8-D-arginine vasopressin)

*(des moe **press' in**)*

Apo-Desmopressin (CAN), DDAVP, Octostim (CAN), Stimate

PREGNANCY CATEGORY B

Drug class

Hormone

Therapeutic actions

Synthetic analogue of human ADH; promotes resorption of water in the renal tubule; increases levels of clotting factor VIII.

Indications

- *DDAVP:* Neurogenic diabetes insipidus (not nephrogenic in origin; intranasal and parenteral); hemophilia A (with factor VIII levels exceeding 5%; parenteral); von Willebrand's disease (type I; parenteral)
- *Stimate:* Treatment of hemophilia A (with factor VIII levels exceeding 5%), von Willebrand's disease (type I)
- Unlabeled use (intranasal): Treatment of chronic autonomic failure

Contraindications and cautions

- Contraindicated with allergy to desmopressin acetate; type II von Willebrand's disease.
- Use cautiously with vascular disease or hypertension, lactation, water intoxication, fluid and electrolyte imbalance, pregnancy.

Available forms

Tablets—0.1, 0.2 mg; nasal solution—0.1 mg/mL, 1.5 mg/mL; injection—4 mcg/mL

Dosages

Adults

- *Diabetes insipidus:* 0.1–0.4 mL/day intranasally as a single dose or divided into two to three doses; 0.5–1 mL/day subcutaneously or IV, divided into two doses, adjusted to achieve a diurnal water turnover pattern, or 0.05 mg PO bid—adjust according to water turnover pattern.

- *Hemophilia A or von Willebrand's disease:* 0.3 mcg/kg diluted in 50 mL sterile physiologic saline; infuse IV slowly over 15–30 min. If needed preoperatively, infuse 30 min before the procedure. Determine need for repeated administration based on patient response. Intranasal—1 spray per nostril, 2 hr preoperatively for a total dose of 300 mcg.

Pediatric patients

- *Diabetes insipidus:* For patients 3 mo–12 yr, 0.05–0.3 mL/day intranasally as a single dose or divided into two doses; or 0.05 mg PO daily—adjust according to water turnover pattern.
- *Hemophilia A or von Willebrand's disease:* For patients weighing 10 kg or less, 0.3 mcg/kg diluted in 10 mL of sterile physiologic saline. Infuse IV slowly over 15–30 min.

Pharmacokinetics

Route	*Onset*	*Peak*	*Duration*
Oral	1 hr	60–90 min	7 hr
IV, Subcut.	30 min	90–120 min	Varies
Nasal	15–60 min	1–5 hr	5–21 hr

Metabolism: $T_{1/2}$: 7.8 min then 75.5 min (IV); 1.5–2.5 hr (oral); 3.3–3.5 hr (nasal)
Distribution: May cross placenta; may enter breast milk
Excretion: Unknown

IV FACTS

Preparation: Use drug as provided; refrigerate vial.
Infusion: Administer by direct IV injection over 1 min; infuse for hemophilia A or von Willebrand's disease over 15–30 min. May dilute in normal saline solution.

Adverse effects

- **CNS:** Transient headache
- **CV:** Slight elevation of BP, facial flushing (with high doses)
- **GI:** Nausea, mild abdominal cramps
- **GU:** Vulval pain
- **Local:** *Local erythema, swelling, burning pain* (parenteral injection)
- **Other:** Fluid retention, water intoxication, hyponatremia (rare)

Interactions

✱ **Drug-drug** • Risk of increased antidiuretic effects if combined with carbamazepine, chlorpropamide • Increased risk of hyponatremia related to increased fluid intake if used with TCAs or SSRIs; monitor patient closely and limit fluid intake

■ Nursing considerations

Assessment

- **History:** Allergy to desmopressin acetate; type II von Willebrand's disease; vascular disease or hypertension; lactation, pregnancy
- **Physical:** Nasal mucous membranes; skin color; P, BP, edema; R, adventitious sounds; bowel sounds, abdominal examination; urine volume and osmolality, plasma osmolality; factor VIII coagulant activity, skin bleeding times, factor VIII coagulant levels, factor VIII antigen and ristocetin cofactor levels (as appropriate)

Interventions

- Refrigerate nasal solution and injection.
- Administer intranasally by drawing solution into the rhinal tube or flexible calibrated plastic tube supplied with preparation. Insert one end of tube into nostril; blow on the other end to deposit solution deep into nasal cavity. Administer to infants, young children, or obtunded adults by using an air-filled syringe attached to the plastic tube. Spray form also available.
- Monitor condition of nasal passages during long-term therapy; inappropriate administration can lead to nasal ulcerations.

⊗ ***Warning*** Monitor patients with CV diseases carefully for cardiac reactions.

⊗ ***Warning*** Monitor patient for signs of hyponatremia, which could lead to seizures. Hold drug when patient has fluid or electrolyte disturbances. If using tablets, limit fluid intake 1 hr before and up to 8 hr after dosing.

- Arrange to individualize dosage to establish a diurnal pattern of water turnover; estimate response by adequate duration of sleep and adequate, not excessive, water turnover.

- Monitor P and BP during infusion for hemophilia A or von Willebrand's disease. Monitor clinical response and lab reports to determine effectiveness of therapy and need for more desmopressin or use of blood products.

Teaching points

- *Stimate* pump must be primed before first use; prime pump by pressing down on pump four times. Discard after 25 doses. Administer intranasally by drawing solution into the rhinal tube or flexible calibrated plastic tube supplied with preparation. Insert one end of tube into nostril; blow on the other end to deposit solution deep into nasal cavity. Review proper administration technique for nasal use.
- You may experience these side effects: GI cramping, facial flushing, headache, nasal irritation (proper administration may decrease these problems).
- Report drowsiness, listlessness, headache, shortness of breath, heartburn, abdominal cramps, vulval pain, severe nasal congestion or irritation.

desvenlafaxine

(des ven la fax' een)

Pristiq DNC

PREGNANCY CATEGORY C

Drug classes

Serotonin-norepinephrine reuptake inhibitor
Antidepressant

Therapeutic actions

Potentiates the neurotransmitter activity in the CNS; inhibits serotonin and norepinephrine reuptake at the nerve synapse, leading to prolonged stimulation at the neuroreceptor; this action is thought to decrease the signs and symptoms of depression.

Indications

- Treatment of major depressive disorder in adults

Contraindications and cautions

- Contraindicated with known hypersensitivity to any component of the drug or venlafaxine, with use of an MAOI, or within 14 days of stopping an MAOI.
- Use cautiously with hypertension, glaucoma, abnormal bleeding, use of drugs that alter coagulation, vascular disease, lipid disorders, renal impairment, lung disease, pregnancy, lactation.

Available forms

ER tablets DNC—50, 100 mg

Dosages

Adults

50 mg/day PO with or without food; range, 50–400 mg/day.

Pediatric patients

Safety and efficacy not established.

Patients with severe renal dysfunction

50 mg PO every other day.

Pharmacokinetics

Route	*Onset*	*Peak*
Oral	Slow	7.5 hr

Metabolism: Hepatic; $T_{1/2}$: 11 hr
Distribution: May cross placenta, enter breast milk
Excretion: Urine

Adverse effects

- **CNS:** *Dizziness, headache,* somnolence, tremor, paresthesia, *insomnia,* anxiety, nervousness, irritability, abnormal dreams, **suicidal ideation,** vision impairment, tinnitus, glaucoma, activation of bipolar symptoms
- **CV:** Palpitations, increased BP, tachycardia
- **GI:** *Nausea, dry mouth, diarrhea, constipation, vomiting, decreased appetite*
- **Respiratory: Interstitial lung disease, eosinophilic pneumonia**
- **Other:** *Fatigue, hyperhidrosis,* rash, yawning, increased bleeding, increased cholesterol and triglyceride levels

Interactions

✷ **Drug-drug** • Risk of serious adverse reactions if combined with MAOIs; wait 14 days after stopping MAOI before beginning desvenlafaxine, allow 7 days from stopping desvenlafaxine before beginning MAOI • Risk of serotonin syndrome if combined with other drugs that increase serotonin levels; monitor patient closely • Increased risk of bleeding if combined with other drugs that affect coagulation (NSAIDs, aspirin, warfarin); monitor patient closely and adjust dosage as needed • Potential for increased impairment of mental ability if combined with alcohol or other CNS drugs; monitor patient closely • Risk of increased toxicity if combined with venlafaxine; avoid this combination

✷ **Drug-alternative therapy** • Increased risk of serotonin syndrome if combined with St. John's Wort; avoid this combination

■ Nursing considerations

Assessment

- **History:** Hypersensitivity to any component of the drug or venlafaxine, current use of an MAOI or use of an MAOI within 14 days, hypertension, glaucoma, abnormal bleeding or the use of drugs that alter coagulation, vascular disease, lipid disorders, renal impairment, lung disease, pregnancy, lactation
- **Physical:** T; skin—color, lesions; orientation, affect, sensory examination, eye pressure; P, BP; abdominal examination; R, adventitious sounds

Interventions

⊗ ***Black box warning*** Monitor patient for suicidal ideation, especially when beginning therapy or changing dosage; high risk in children, adolescents, and young adults. Drug is not approved for use in pediatric patients.

- Limit amount of drug available to patient because of increased risk of suicidal ideation.
- Give with food if GI upset occurs.
- Instruct patient to swallow tablet whole; do not cut, crush, or chew.
- Do not administer with an MAOI or within 14 days of stopping an MAOI; allow 7 days after stopping desvenlafaxine before starting an MAOI.
- Monitor patients with glaucoma, hypertension, CV disease, SIADH for potential exacerbation of these problems.
- Inform patient that it may take several weeks to see the effects of this drug.
- Avoid suddenly stopping drug; taper gradually.
- Tell patient that the matrix of the drug may be seen in the stool; assure patient that the active drug has been absorbed.
- Advise women of childbearing age to use contraception.
- Encourage nursing mothers to find a different method of feeding the baby while on this drug.

Teaching points

- Take this drug about the same time each day; swallow the tablet whole; do not cut, crush or chew the tablets.
- If you miss a dose, take it as soon as you remember. If it is almost time for the next dose, just skip the missed dose. Do not make up doses. Do not take more than one dose a day.
- Do not stop taking this drug suddenly; if you are running low on tablets, contact your health care provider about a refill. Your health care provider will reduce the dose over time if the drug is to be stopped.
- It may take several weeks before you see the effects of this drug; keep taking the drug as prescribed.
- You may notice something in your stool that looks like your tablet. This is the empty shell of the tablet; the medicine has already been absorbed into your system.
- Do not use St. John's Wort while on this drug; serious adverse effects could occur.
- Do not drive or operate dangerous machinery until you know how this drug affects you.
- Avoid drinking alcohol while on this drug.
- It is not known whether this drug affects an unborn baby. Use contraceptive measures while on this drug. If you wish to become pregnant, discuss this with your health care provider. If you become pregnant while taking this drug, consult with your health care provider.
- It is not known how this drug affects a nursing baby. Because of the potential for adverse effects on an infant, another method of feeding the baby should be used while you are on this drug.
- Your health care provider may monitor your eye pressure, blood pressure, and various blood tests while you are on this drug.

- There is a risk of suicidal thoughts, especially when starting the drug or adjusting the dose. Be alert for these thoughts. Call your health care provider if you have any suicidal thoughts or increased depression or anxiety.
- You may experience these side effects: Dry mouth, nausea (eating frequent small meals and sucking sugarless lozenges may help); dizziness, tremor, changes in ability to concentrate (do not drive a car or operate dangerous machinery until you know how this drug will affect you); constipation (medication may be available to help).
- Report suicidal thoughts, behavioral changes, difficulty breathing, increased bleeding, hallucinations, fever.

dexamethasone
(dex a ***meth'*** *a sone)*

dexamethasone
Oral, topical dermatologic aerosol and gel, ophthalmic suspension: Aeroseb-Dex, Apo-Dexamethasone (CAN), Decadron, Decaspray, Dexasol, DexPak TaperPak, Maxidex Ophthalmic, ratio-Dexamethasone (CAN)

dexamethasone sodium phosphate
IV, IM, intra-articular, intralesional injection; respiratory inhalant; intranasal steroid; ophthalmic solution and ointment; topical dermatologic cream: Cortastat, Dalalone, Decadron Phosphate, Decaject, Dexasone, Hexadrol Phosphate, PMS-Dexamethasone (CAN)

Pregnancy Category C

Drug classes
Corticosteroid
Glucocorticoid
Hormone

Therapeutic actions
Enters target cells and binds to specific receptors, initiating many complex reactions that are responsible for its anti-inflammatory and immunosuppressive effects.

Indications
- Hypercalcemia associated with cancer
- Short-term management of various inflammatory and allergic disorders, such as rheumatoid arthritis, collagen diseases (SLE), dermatologic diseases (pemphigus), status asthmaticus, and autoimmune disorders
- Hematologic disorders: Thrombocytopenic purpura, erythroblastopenia
- Trichinosis with neurologic or myocardial involvement
- Ulcerative colitis, acute exacerbations of MS, and palliation in some leukemias and lymphomas
- Cerebral edema associated with brain tumor, craniotomy, or head injury
- Testing adrenocortical hyperfunction
- Unlabeled uses: Antiemetic for cisplatin-induced vomiting, diagnosis of depression
- Intra-articular or soft-tissue administration: Arthritis, psoriatic plaques
- Respiratory inhalant: Control of bronchial asthma requiring corticosteroids in conjunction with other therapy
- Intranasal: Relief of symptoms of seasonal or perennial rhinitis that responds poorly to other treatments
- Dermatologic preparations: Relief of inflammatory and pruritic manifestations of dermatoses that are steroid-responsive
- Ophthalmic preparations: Inflammation of the lid, conjunctiva, cornea, and globe

Contraindications and cautions
- Contraindicated with infections, especially tuberculosis, fungal infections, amebiasis, vaccinia and varicella, and antibiotic-resistant infections, allergy to any component of the preparation used.
- Use cautiously with renal or hepatic disease; hypothyroidism, ulcerative colitis with impending perforation; diverticulitis; active or latent peptic ulcer; inflammatory bowel

disease; heart failure, hypertension, thromboembolic disorders; osteoporosis; seizure disorders; diabetes mellitus; lactation.

Available forms

Tablets—0.25, 0.5, 0.75, 1, 1.5, 2, 4, 6 mg; elixir—0.5 mg/5 mL; oral solution concentrate—0.5 mg/0.5 mL; injection—4 mg/mL, 8 mg/mL, 10 mg/mL, 16 mg/mL, 20 mg/mL, 24 mg/mL; aerosol—84 mcg/actuation; ophthalmic solution—0.1%; ophthalmic suspension—0.1%; ophthalmic ointment—0.05%; topical ointment—0.05%; topical cream—0.05%, 0.1%; topical aerosol—0.01%, 0.04%

Dosages

Adults

Systemic administration

Individualize dosage based on severity of condition and response. Give daily dose before 9 AM to minimize adrenal suppression. If long-term therapy is needed, alternate-day therapy with a short-acting steroid should be considered. After long-term therapy, withdraw drug slowly to avoid adrenal insufficiency. For maintenance therapy, reduce initial dose in small increments at intervals until the lowest clinically satisfactory dose is reached.

Oral (dexamethasone)

0.75–9 mg/day.

- *Suppression test for Cushing's syndrome:* 1 mg at 11 PM; assay plasma cortisol at 8 AM the next day. For greater accuracy, give 0.5 mg every 6 hr for 48 hr, and collect 24-hr urine to determine 17-hydroxycorticosteroid (17-OHCS) excretion.
- *Suppression test to distinguish Cushing's syndrome due to ACTH excess from that resulting from other causes:* 2 mg every 6 hr for 48 hr. Collect 24-hr urine to determine 17-OHCS excretion.

IV or IM (dexamethasone sodium phosphate)

0.5–9 mg/day.

- *Cerebral edema:* 10 mg IV and then 4 mg IM every 6 hr until cerebral edema symptoms subside; change to oral therapy, 1–3 mg tid, as soon as possible and taper over 5–7 days.

Pediatric patients

Individualize dosage based on severity of condition and response, rather than by strict adherence to formulas that correct adult doses for age or body weight. Carefully observe growth and development in infants and children on long-term therapy.

IV

- *Unresponsive shock:* 1–6 mg/kg as a single IV injection (as much as 40 mg initially followed by repeated injections every 2–6 hr has been reported).

(dexamethasone sodium phosphate)

0.4–6 mg (depending on joint or soft-tissue injection site).

Respiratory inhalant (dexamethasone sodium phosphate)

84 mcg released with each actuation.

Adults

3 inhalations tid–qid, not to exceed 12 inhalations/day.

Pediatric patients

2 inhalations tid–qid, not to exceed 8 inhalations/day.

Intranasal (dexamethasone sodium phosphate)

Each spray delivers 84 mcg dexamethasone.

Adults

2 sprays (168 mcg) into each nostril bid–tid, not to exceed 12 sprays (1,008 mcg)/day.

Pediatric patients

1 or 2 sprays (84–168 mcg) into each nostril bid, depending on age, not to exceed 8 sprays (672 mcg). Arrange to reduce dose and discontinue therapy as soon as possible.

Topical dermatologic preparations

Adults and pediatric patients

Apply sparingly to affected area bid–qid.

Ophthalmic solutions, suspensions

Adults and pediatric patients

Instill 1 or 2 drops into the conjunctival sac every 1 hr during the day and every 2 hr during the night; after a favorable response, reduce dose to 1 drop every 4 hr and then 1 drop tid–qid.

D

Ophthalmic ointment

Adults and pediatric patients

Apply a thin coating in the lower conjunctival sac tid–qid; reduce dosage to bid and then qid after improvement.

Pharmacokinetics

Route	Onset	Peak	Duration
Oral	Slow	1–2 hr	2–3 days
IM	Rapid	30–60 min	2–3 days
IV	Rapid	30–60 min	2–3 days

Metabolism: Hepatic; $T_{1/2}$: 110–210 min
Distribution: Crosses placenta; may enter breast milk
Excretion: Urine

IV FACTS

Preparation: No preparation required.
Infusion: Administer by slow, direct IV injection over 1 min.
Incompatibilities: Do not combine with daunorubicin, doxorubicin, metaraminol, vancomycin.

Adverse effects

Adverse effects depend on dose, route, and duration of therapy.

Systemic administration

- **CNS: Seizures,** *vertigo, headaches,* pseudotumor cerebri, *euphoria, insomnia, mood swings, depression,* psychosis, intracerebral hemorrhage, reversible cerebral atrophy in infants, cataracts, IOP, glaucoma
- **CV:** *Hypertension,* heart failure, necrotizing angiitis
- **Endocrine:** Growth retardation, decreased carbohydrate tolerance, diabetes mellitus, cushingoid state, *secondary adrenocortical and pituitary unresponsiveness*
- **GI:** Peptic or esophageal ulcer, pancreatitis, abdominal distention
- **GU:** *Amenorrhea, irregular menses*
- **Hematologic:** *Fluid and electrolyte disturbances,* negative nitrogen balance, increased blood sugar, glycosuria, increased serum cholesterol, decreased serum T_3 and T_4 levels
- **Hypersensitivity:** Anaphylactoid or hypersensitivity reactions
- **Musculoskeletal:** *Muscle weakness,* steroid myopathy, loss of muscle mass, osteoporosis, spontaneous fractures
- **Other:** *Impaired wound healing; petechiae; ecchymoses; increased sweating; thin and fragile skin; acne; immunosuppression and masking of signs of infection;* activation of latent infections, including TB, fungal, and viral eye infections; pneumonia; abscess; septic infection; GI and GU infections

Intra-articular

- **Musculoskeletal:** Osteonecrosis, tendon rupture, infection

Intralesional therapy

- **CNS:** Blindness (when used on face and head—rare)

Respiratory inhalant

- **Endocrine:** Suppression of HPA function due to systemic absorption
- **Respiratory:** Oral, laryngeal, pharyngeal irritation
- **Other:** Fungal infections

Intranasal

- **CNS:** Headache
- **Dermatologic:** Urticaria
- **Endocrine:** Suppression of HPA function due to systemic absorption
- **GI:** Nausea
- **Respiratory:** Nasal irritation, fungal infections, epistaxis, rebound congestion, perforation of the nasal septum, anosmia

Topical dermatologic ointments, creams, sprays

- **Endocrine:** Suppression of HPA function due to systemic absorption, growth retardation in children (children may be at special risk for systemic absorption because of their large skin surface area to body weight ratio)
- **Local:** Local burning, irritation, acneiform lesions, striae, skin atrophy

Ophthalmic preparations

- **Endocrine:** Suppression of HPA function due to systemic absorption; more common with long-term use
- **Local:** Infections, especially fungal; glaucoma, cataracts with long-term use

Interactions

✷ **Drug-drug** • Decreased effects of anticholinesterases with corticotropin; profound muscular depression is possible • Decreased steroid blood levels with phenytoin, phenobarbital, rifampin • Decreased serum levels of salicylates with dexamethasone and increased risk of gastric ulceration

✷ **Drug-lab test** • False-negative nitroblue-tetrazolium test for bacterial infection • Suppression of skin test reactions

■ Nursing considerations

Assessment

- **History for systemic administration:** Active infections; renal or hepatic disease; hypothyroidism, ulcerative colitis; diverticulitis; active or latent peptic ulcer; inflammatory bowel disease; heart failure, hypertension, thromboembolic disorders; osteoporosis; seizure disorders; diabetes mellitus; lactation
- **History for ophthalmic preparations:** Acute superficial herpes simplex keratitis, fungal infections of ocular structures; vaccinia, varicella, and other viral diseases of the cornea and conjunctiva; ocular TB
- **Physical for systemic administration:** Baseline body weight, T; reflexes, and grip strength, affect, and orientation; P, BP, peripheral perfusion, prominence of superficial veins; R and adventitious sounds; serum electrolytes, blood glucose
- **Physical for topical dermatologic preparations:** Affected area for infections, skin injury

Interventions

- For systemic administration, do not give drug to nursing mothers; drug may be secreted in breast milk.

⊗ ***Warning*** Give daily doses before 9 AM to mimic normal peak corticosteroid blood levels.

- Increase dosage when patient is subject to stress.
- Monitor blood glucose levels; dietary restrictions may be needed.
- Taper doses when discontinuing high-dose or long-term therapy.
- Do not give live virus vaccines with immunosuppressive doses of corticosteroids.
- For respiratory inhalant, intranasal preparation, do not use respiratory inhalant during an acute asthmatic attack or to manage status asthmaticus.
- Do not use intranasal product with untreated local nasal infections, epistaxis, nasal trauma, septal ulcers, or recent nasal surgery.

⊗ ***Warning*** Taper systemic steroids carefully during transfer to inhalational steroids; adrenal insufficiency deaths have occurred.

- For topical dermatologic preparations, use caution when occlusive dressings, tight diapers cover affected area; these can increase systemic absorption.
- Avoid prolonged use near the eyes, in genital and rectal areas, and in skin creases.

Teaching points

Systemic administration

- Do not stop taking the oral drug without consulting your health care provider.
- Avoid exposure to infection.
- Report unusual weight gain, swelling of the extremities, muscle weakness, black or tarry stools, fever, prolonged sore throat, colds or other infections, worsening of this disorder.

Intra-articular administration

- Do not overuse joint after therapy, even if pain is gone.

Respiratory inhalant, intranasal preparation

- Do not use more often than prescribed.
- Do not stop using this drug without consulting your health care provider.
- Use the inhalational bronchodilator drug before using the oral inhalant product when using both.
- Administer decongestant nose drops first if nasal passages are blocked.

Topical

- Apply the drug sparingly.
- Avoid contact with eyes or skin around eyes.
- Report any irritation or infection at the site of application.

Ophthalmic

- Administer as follows: Lie down or tilt head backward and look at ceiling. Warm tube of ointment in hand for several minutes. Apply one-fourth to one-half inch of ointment, or drop suspension inside lower eyelid while looking up. After applying ointment, close eyelids and roll eyeball in all directions. After

D

instilling eye drops, release lower lid, but do not blink for at least 30 seconds; apply gentle pressure to the inside corner of the eye for 1 minute. Do not close eyes tightly, and try not to blink more often than usual; do not touch ointment tube or dropper to eye, fingers, or any surface.

- Wait at least 10 minutes before using any other eye preparations.
- Eyes will become more sensitive to light (use sunglasses).
- Report worsening of the condition, pain, itching, swelling of the eye, failure of the condition to improve after 1 week.

▽dexchlorpheniramine maleate DNC

(dex klor fen ***ir'*** *a meen)*

PREGNANCY CATEGORY B

Drug class

Antihistamine (alkylamine type)

Therapeutic actions

Blocks the effects of histamine at H_1-receptor sites, has atropine-like, antipruritic, and sedative effects.

Indications

- Relief of symptoms associated with perennial and seasonal allergic rhinitis; vasomotor rhinitis; allergic conjunctivitis; mild, uncomplicated urticaria and angioedema; amelioration of allergic reactions to blood or plasma; dermatographism; adjunctive therapy in anaphylactic reactions

Contraindications and cautions

- Contraindicated with allergy to antihistamines, narrow-angle glaucoma, stenosing peptic ulcer, symptomatic prostatic hypertrophy, asthmatic attack, bladder neck obstruction, pyloroduodenal obstruction, MAOI use, third trimester of pregnancy, lactation.
- Use cautiously with pregnancy.

Available forms

ER tablets DNC—4, 6 mg; syrup—2 mg/5 mL

Dosages

Adults and children older than 12 yr

4–6 mg at bedtime PO or every 8–10 hr PO during the day.

Pediatric patients 6–12 yr

4 mg PO once daily at bedtime.

Geriatric patients

More likely to cause dizziness, sedation, syncope, toxic confusional states, and hypotension in elderly patients; use with caution.

Pharmacokinetics

Route	*Onset*	*Peak*
Oral	15–30 min	3 hr

Metabolism: Hepatic; $T_{1/2}$: 12–15 hr
Distribution: May cross placenta; may enter breast milk
Excretion: Urine

Adverse effects

- **CNS:** *Drowsiness, sedation, dizziness, disturbed coordination,* fatigue, confusion, restlessness, excitation, nervousness, tremor, headache, blurred vision, diplopia, vertigo, tinnitus, acute labyrinthitis, hysteria, tingling, heaviness and weakness of the hands
- **CV:** Hypotension, palpitations, bradycardia, tachycardia, extrasystoles
- **GI:** *Epigastric distress,* anorexia, increased appetite and weight gain, nausea, vomiting, diarrhea or constipation
- **GU:** Urinary frequency, dysuria, urinary retention, early menses, decreased libido
- **Hematologic:** Hemolytic anemia, hypoplastic anemia, **thrombocytopenia, leukopenia, agranulocytosis, pancytopenia**
- **Respiratory:** *Thickening of bronchial secretions,* chest tightness, wheezing, nasal stuffiness, dry mouth, dry nose, dry throat, sore throat
- **Other:** Urticaria, rash, **anaphylactic shock,** photosensitivity, excessive perspiration

Interactions

✱ **Drug-drug** • Increased depressant effects with alcohol, other CNS depressants

■ Nursing considerations
Assessment
- **History:** Allergy to any antihistamines; narrow-angle glaucoma, stenosing peptic ulcer, symptomatic prostatic hypertrophy, asthmatic attack, bladder neck obstruction, pyloroduodenal obstruction, pregnancy, lactation
- **Physical:** Skin color, lesions, texture; orientation, reflexes, affect; vision examination; P, BP; R, adventitious sounds; bowel sounds; prostate palpation; CBC with differential

Interventions
- Administer with food if GI upset occurs.
- Have patient swallow tablets whole—do not cut, crush, or chew.
- Monitor patient response, and adjust dosage to lowest possible effective dose.

Teaching points
- Take as prescribed; avoid excessive dosage. Take with food if GI upset occurs; do not crush or chew the tablets; swallow whole.
- Avoid alcohol; serious sedation can occur.
- You may experience these side effects: Dizziness, sedation, drowsiness (use caution driving or performing tasks that require alertness); epigastric distress, diarrhea, or constipation (take with meals); dry mouth (frequent mouth care, sucking sugarless lozenges may help); thickening of bronchial secretions, dryness of nasal mucosa (use a humidifier).
- Report difficulty breathing; hallucinations, tremors, loss of coordination; unusual bleeding or bruising; visual disturbances; irregular heartbeat.

▽ dexlansoprazole
(decks' lan soh' pray zol)

Kapidex (DNC)

PREGNANCY CATEGORY B

Drug classes
Antisecretory drug
Proton pump inhibitor

Therapeutic actions
Gastric acid pump inhibitor that suppresses gastric acid secretion by specific inhibition of the hydrogen-potassium ATPase enzyme system at the secretory surface of the gastric parietal cells; blocks the final step in acid production.

Indications
- Healing of all grades of erosive esophagitis
- Maintenance of healing of erosive esophagitis
- Treatment of heartburn associated with nonerosive gastroesophageal reflux disease (GERD)

Contraindications and cautions
- Contraindicated with hypersensitivity to components of drug, lactation.
- Use cautiously with pregnancy.

Available forms
DR capsules (DNC)—30, 60 mg

Dosages
Adults
Healing of erosive esophagitis: 60 mg/day PO for up to 8 wk.
Maintenance of healing of erosive esophagitis: 30 mg/day PO.
GERD: 30 mg/day PO for up to 4 wk.
Pediatric patients
Safety and efficacy not established.

Pharmacokinetics
Route	Onset	Peak
Oral	Rapid	1–2 hr, then 4–5 hr

Metabolism: Hepatic; $T_{1/2}$: 1–2 hr
Distribution: May cross placenta; may enter breast milk
Excretion: Urine and feces

Adverse effects
- **CNS:** Headache, dizziness, insomnia, taste changes
- **GI:** Nausea, *diarrhea,* vomiting, abdominal pain
- **Respiratory:** URI
- **Other:** Fatigue

Interactions
✱ **Drug-drug** • Decreased absorption of atazanavir with resultant loss of effectiveness; avoid this combination • Potential interference

with absorption of drugs that require acidic gastric fluids (ampicillin, digoxin, iron salts, ketoconazole); monitor patient accordingly
- Potential increased effects of warfarin when taken with proton pump inhibitors; if this combination is used, monitor INR regularly and adjust warfarin dosage as needed

■ Nursing considerations

Assessment

- **History:** Hypersensitivity to components of drug; pregnancy, lactation
- **Physical:** Orientation, affect; abdominal exam; respiratory auscultation

Interventions

- Administer without regard to food.
- Capsule should be swallowed whole. Do not cut, crush, or allow patient to chew capsule. If patient cannot swallow capsule, it can be opened and the contents sprinkled over 1 tablespoon of applesauce and swallowed immediately.
- Advise patient to select another method of feeding the baby if nursing.

Teaching points

- Take this drug once a day, with or without food.
- Capsule should be swallowed whole. Do not cut, crush, or chew capsule. If you cannot swallow the capsule, it can be opened and the contents sprinkled over 1 tablespoon of applesauce and swallowed immediately.
- If you miss a dose, take the next dose as soon as you remember.
- It is not known how this drug affects a fetus. If you should become pregnant while taking this drug, consult your health care provider.
- It is not known how this drug affects a nursing baby. Because of the potential for serious adverse effects in an infant, another method of feeding the baby should be used while you are taking this drug.
- You may experience these side effects: Dizziness, headache (do not drive a car or engage in activities that require alertness if these effects occur); diarrhea, nausea, vomiting, abdominal pain (these effects may lessen over time; consult your health care provider if they are too uncomfortable).
- Report persistent or increasing pain, severe diarrhea or vomiting.

▽dexmedetomidine hydrochloride

See Appendix W, *Less commonly used drugs*.

▽dexmethylphenidate hydrochloride

*(decks meth ill **fen'** i date)*

Focalin, Focalin XR (DNC)

PREGNANCY CATEGORY C

CONTROLLED SUBSTANCE C-II

Drug class

CNS stimulant

Therapeutic actions

Mild cortical stimulant with CNS actions similar to those of the amphetamines; is thought to block the reuptake of norepinephrine and dopamine, increasing their concentration in the synaptic cleft; mechanism of effectiveness in hyperkinetic syndromes is not understood.

Indications

- Treatment of ADHD in patients 6 yr and older as part of a total treatment program

Contraindications and cautions

- Contraindicated with hypersensitivity to dexmethylphenidate or methylphenidate; marked anxiety, tension, and agitation; glaucoma; motor tics, family history or diagnosis of Tourette syndrome; use of MAOIs within the past 14 days.
- Use cautiously with psychosis, seizure disorders; heart failure, recent MI, hyperthyroidism; drug dependence, alcoholism, severe depression of endogenous or exogenous origin; as treatment of normal fatigue states; pregnancy, lactation.

Available forms
Tablets—2.5, 5, 10 mg; ER capsules DNC—5, 10, 15, 20 mg

Dosages
Adults and children 6 yr and older
Individualize dosage. Administer orally twice a day, at least 4 hr apart, without regard to meals. Starting dose, 2.5 mg PO bid; may increase as needed in 2.5- to 5-mg increments to a maximum dose of 10 mg PO bid. ER capsules, initially 5 mg/day for children; increase in 5-mg increments to 20 mg/day; start adults at 10 mg/day; increase in 10-mg increments to 20 mg/day.
- *Patients already on methylphenidate:* Start dose at one-half the methylphenidate dose with a maximum dose of 10 mg PO bid.

Pediatric patients younger than 6 yr
Safety and efficacy not established.

Pharmacokinetics

Route	Onset	Peak
Oral	Varies	1–1.5 hr

Metabolism: Hepatic; $T_{1/2}$: 2.2 hr
Distribution: May cross placenta; may enter breast milk
Excretion: Urine

Adverse effects
- **CNS:** *Nervousness, insomnia,* dizziness, headache, dyskinesia, chorea, drowsiness, Tourette's syndrome, toxic psychosis, blurred vision, accommodation difficulties
- **CV:** Increased or decreased pulse and blood pressure; *tachycardia,* angina, arrhythmias, palpitations
- **Dermatologic:** Skin rash, loss of scalp hair
- **GI:** *Anorexia, nausea, abdominal pain;* weight loss, abnormal liver function
- **Hematologic:** Leukopenia, anemia
- **Other:** Fever, tolerance, psychological dependence, abnormal behavior with abuse

Interactions
✱ Drug-drug ⊗ *Warning* Risk of severe hypertensive crisis if combined with MAOIs; do not administer dexmethylphenidate with or within 14 days of an MAOI.
- Possible increased serum levels of warfarin, phenobarbital, phenytoin, primidone, TCAs, some SSRIs; if any of these drugs are used with dexmethylphenidate, monitor the patient closely and decrease dose of the other drugs as needed • Risk of adverse effects if combined with pressor drugs (dopamine, epinephrine) or antihypertensives; monitor patients closely

■ Nursing considerations
Assessment
- **History:** Hypersensitivity to dexmethylphenidate or methylphenidate; marked anxiety, tension, and agitation; glaucoma; motor tics, family history or diagnosis of Tourette's syndrome; severe depression of endogenous or exogenous origin; seizure disorders; hypertension; drug dependence, alcoholism, emotional instability; pregnancy, lactation
- **Physical:** Body weight, height, T, skin color, lesions, orientation, affect, ophthalmic examination (tonometry), P, BP, auscultation, R, adventitious sounds, bowel sounds, normal output, CBC with differential, platelet count, baseline ECG (as indicated)

Interventions
- Ensure proper diagnosis before administering to children for behavioral syndromes. Drug should not be used until other causes and concomitants of abnormal behavior (learning disability, EEG abnormalities, neurologic deficits) are ruled out.

⊗ *Black box warning* Use caution with history of substance dependence or alcoholism; dependence, severe depression, psychotic reactions possible with withdrawal.
- Arrange to interrupt drug dosage periodically in children being treated for behavioral disorders to determine if symptoms recur at an intensity that warrants continued drug therapy.
- Monitor growth of children on long-term dexmethylphenidate therapy.

⊗ *Warning* Arrange to dispense the least feasible amount of drug at any one time to minimize risk of overdose.
- Administer drug before 6 PM to prevent insomnia if that is a problem.
- Ensure that ER capsules are swallowed whole or contents are sprinkled over a spoonful of applesauce and taken immediately.

D

- Arrange to monitor CBC and platelet counts periodically in patients on long-term therapy.
- Monitor BP frequently early in treatment.
- Arrange for consult with school nurse of school-age patients receiving this drug.

Teaching points

- Take this drug exactly as prescribed. It is taken two times a day, at least 4 hours apart.
- Take immediate-release tablets before 6 PM to avoid nighttime sleep disturbance.
- Take extended-release capsules in the morning.
- Swallow extended-release capsules whole; do not cut, crush, or chew. Capsules can be opened and contents sprinkled over applesauce and taken immediately.
- This drug is a controlled substance and should be stored securely and safely out of the reach of children.
- Avoid the use of alcohol and over-the-counter drugs, including nose drops and cold remedies, while taking this drug; some over-the-counter drugs could cause dangerous effects. If you feel that you need one of these preparations, consult your health care provider.
- You may experience these side effects: Nervousness, restlessness, dizziness, insomnia, impaired thinking (these effects may become less pronounced after a few days, avoid driving a car or engaging in activities that require alertness if these occur, notify your health care provider if these are pronounced or bothersome); headache, loss of appetite, dry mouth.
- Report nervousness, insomnia, palpitations, vomiting, skin rash, depression.

dexpanthenol (dextro-pantothenyl alcohol)

(dex ***pan'*** *the nole)*

Ilopan

PREGNANCY CATEGORY C

Drug class

GI stimulant

Therapeutic actions

Mechanism is unknown; is the alcohol analog of pantothenic acid, a cofactor in the synthesis of the neurotransmitter acetylcholine; acetylcholine is the transmitter released by parasympathetic postganglionic nerves; the parasympathetic nervous system provides stimulation to maintain intestinal function.

Indications

- Prophylactic use immediately after major abdominal surgery to minimize paralytic ileus, intestinal atony causing abdominal distention
- Treatment of intestinal atony causing abdominal distention; postoperative or postpartum retention of flatus; postoperative delay in resumption of intestinal motility; paralytic ileus
- Topical treatment of mild eczema, dermatosis, bee stings, diaper rash, chafing

Contraindications and cautions

- Contraindicated with allergy to dexpanthenol, hemophilia, ileus due to mechanical obstruction.
- Use cautiously in pregnancy, lactation.

Available forms

Injection—250 mg/mL; topical cream—2%

Dosages

Adults

IM

- *Prevention of postoperative adynamic ileus:* 250–500 mg IM; repeat in 2 hr, then every 6 hr until danger of adynamic ileus has passed.
- *Treatment of adynamic ileus:* 500 mg IM; repeat in 2 hr, then every 6 hr as needed.

IV

500 mg diluted in IV solutions.

Topical

Apply once or twice daily to affected areas.

Pediatric patients

Safety and efficacy not established.

Pharmacokinetics

Route	*Onset*	*Peak*
IM	Rapid	4 hr

Metabolism: Hepatic; $T_{1/2}$: Unknown
Distribution: May cross placenta; may enter breast milk
Excretion: Feces, urine

IV FACTS

Preparation: Dilute with bulk solutions of glucose or lactated Ringer's.
Infusion: Infuse slowly over 3–6 hr. Do not administer by direct IV injection.

Adverse effects

- **CV:** *Slight drop in BP*
- **Dermatologic:** Itching, tingling, red patches of skin, generalized dermatitis, urticaria
- **GI:** *Intestinal colic* (30 min after administration), *nausea, vomiting; diarrhea*
- **Respiratory:** Dyspnea

■ Nursing considerations

Assessment

- **History:** Allergy to dexpanthenol, hemophilia, ileus due to mechanical obstruction, lactation
- **Physical:** Skin color, lesions, texture; P, BP; bowel sounds, normal output

Interventions

- Monitor BP carefully during IV administration.

Teaching points

Teaching about this drug should be incorporated into the overall postoperative or postpartum teaching. Intestinal colic may occur within 30 minutes of administration.

- You may experience these side effects: Nausea, vomiting, diarrhea, itching, rash.
- Report difficulty breathing, severe itching, or rash.

dexrazoxane

See Appendix W, *Less commonly used drugs*.

dextran, high–molecular-weight

(dex' tran)

Dextran 70, Dextran 75, Gentran 70, Gentran 75, Macrodex

PREGNANCY CATEGORY C

Drug class

Plasma volume expander (nonbacteriostatic)

Therapeutic actions

Synthetic polysaccharide used to approximate the colloidal properties of albumin.

Indications

- Adjunctive therapy for treatment of shock or impending shock due to hemorrhage, burns, surgery, or trauma; to be used only in emergency situations when blood or blood products are not available

Contraindications and cautions

- Contraindicated with allergy to dextran (dextran 1 can be used prophylactically in patients known to be allergic to clinical dextran); marked hemostatic defects (risk for increased bleeding effects); severe cardiac congestion; renal failure, anuria, or oliguria.
- Use cautiously in pregnancy and lactation.

Available forms

Injection—6% dextran 75 in 0.9% sodium chloride, 6% dextran 70 in 0.9% sodium chloride, 6% dextran 75 in 5% dextrose, 6% dextran 70 in 5% dextrose

Dosages

Adults

500–1,000 mL, given at a rate of 20–40 mL/min IV as an emergency procedure. Do not exceed 20 mL/kg the first 24 hr of treatment.

Pediatric patients

Determine dosage by body weight or surface area of the patient. Do not exceed 20 mL/kg IV total dose.

Patients with renal impairment

Decrease dose for creatinine clearance less than 30 mL/min.

Pharmacokinetics

Route	Onset	Peak	Duration
IV	Minutes	Minutes	12–24 hr

Metabolism: Hepatic; $T_{1/2}$: 24 hr
Distribution: May cross placenta; may enter breast milk
Excretion: Urine

IV FACTS

Preparation: Administer in unit provided. Discard any partially used containers. Do not use unless the solution is clear.
Infusion: Infuse at rate of 20–40 mL/min.

Adverse effects

- **GI:** Nausea, vomiting
- **Hematologic:** *Hypervolemia, coagulation problems*
- **Hypersensitivity:** Urticaria, nasal congestion, wheezing, tightness of chest, mild hypotension (antihistamines may be helpful in relieving these symptoms), anaphylactoid reaction
- **Local:** Infection at injection site, extravasation
- **Other:** Fever, joint pains

Interactions

✱ **Drug-lab test** • Falsely elevated blood glucose assays • Interference with bilirubin assays in which alcohol is used, with total protein assays using biuret reagent • Blood typing and cross-matching procedures using enzyme techniques may give unreliable readings; draw blood samples before giving infusion of dextran

■ Nursing considerations

Assessment

- **History:** Allergy to dextran; marked hemostatic defects; severe cardiac congestion; renal failure or anuria; pregnancy
- **Physical:** T; skin color, lesions; P, BP, peripheral edema; R, adventitious sounds; urinalysis, LFTs, renal function tests, clotting times, PT, PTT, Hgb, Hct, urine output

Interventions

- Administer by IV infusion only; monitor rates based on patient response.
- Do not give more than recommended dose.
- Use only clear solutions. Discard partially used containers; solution contains no bacteriostat.

⊗ ***Warning*** Monitor patients carefully for any sign of hypervolemia or the development of heart failure; supportive measures may be needed.

Teaching points

- Report difficulty breathing, rash, unusual bleeding or bruising, pain at IV site.

▽ dextran, low-molecular-weight

(dex' tran)

Dextran 40, Gentran 40, 10% LMD, Rheomacrodex

PREGNANCY CATEGORY C

Drug class

Plasma volume expander (nonbacteriostatic)

Therapeutic actions

Synthetic polysaccharide used to approximate the colloidal properties of albumin.

Indications

- Adjunctive therapy for treatment of shock or impending shock due to hemorrhage, burns, surgery, or trauma when blood or blood products are not available
- Priming fluid in pump oxygenators during extracorporeal circulation
- Prophylaxis against DVT and PE in patients undergoing procedures known to be associated with a high incidence of thromboembolic complications, such as hip surgery

Contraindications and cautions

- Contraindicated with allergy to dextran (dextran 1 can be used prophylactically in patients known to be allergic to clinical dextran); marked hemostatic defects; severe cardiac congestion; renal failure, anuria, or oliguria.
- Use cautiously with pregnancy, lactation.

Available forms

Injection—10% *Dextran 40* in 0.9% sodium chloride, 10% *Dextran 40* in 5% dextrose

Dosages

Adults

- *Adjunctive therapy in shock:* Total dosage of 20 mL/kg IV in first 24 hr. The first 10 mL/kg should be infused rapidly, and the remaining dose administered slowly. Beyond 24 hr, total daily dosage should not exceed 10 mL/kg. Do not continue therapy for more than 5 days.
- *Hemodiluent in extracorporeal circulation:* Generally 10–20 mL/kg are added to perfusion circuit. Do not exceed a total dosage of 20 mL/kg.
- *Prophylaxis therapy for DVT, PE:* 500–1,000 mL IV on day of surgery, continue treatment at dose of 500 mL/day for an additional 2–3 days. Thereafter, based on procedure and risk, 500 mL may be administered every second to third day for up to 2 wk.

Pediatric patients

Total dose should not exceed 20 mL/kg.

Pharmacokinetics

Route	Onset	Peak	Duration
IV	Immediate	Minutes	12 hr

Metabolism: Hepatic; $T_{1/2}$: 3 hr
Distribution: Crosses placenta; enters breast milk
Excretion: Urine

IV FACTS

Preparation: Protect from freezing. Use in units provided; no further preparation necessary.
Infusion: Administer first 10 mL/kg rapidly, remainder of solution slowly over 8–24 hr, monitoring patient response.

Adverse effects

- **CV:** Hypotension, anaphylactoid shock, *hypervolemia*
- **GI:** Nausea, vomiting
- **Hypersensitivity:** Ranging from mild cutaneous eruptions to generalized urticaria
- **Local:** Infection at site of injection, extravasation, venous thrombosis or phlebitis
- **Other:** Headache, fever, wheezing

Interactions

✱ **Drug-lab test** • Falsely elevated blood glucose assays • Interference with bilirubin assays in which alcohol is used, with total protein assays using biuret reagent • Blood typing and cross-matching procedures using enzyme techniques may give unreliable readings; draw blood samples before giving infusion of dextran

■ Nursing considerations

Assessment

- **History:** Allergy to dextran; marked hemostatic defects; severe cardiac congestion; renal failure or anuria; lactation, pregnancy
- **Physical:** T; skin color, lesions; P, BP, peripheral edema; R, adventitious sounds; urinalysis, LFTs, renal function tests, clotting times, PT, PTT, Hgb, Hct, urine output

Interventions

- Administer by IV infusion only; monitor rates based on patient response. Do not administer more than recommended dose.
- Monitor urinary output carefully; if no increase in output is noted after 500 mL of dextran, discontinue drug until diuresis can be induced by other means.

⊗ ***Warning*** Monitor patient for hypervolemia or development of heart failure; slow rate or discontinue drug if rapid CVP increase occurs.

Teaching points

- Report difficulty breathing, rash, unusual bleeding or bruising, pain at IV site.

▽ dextroamphetamine sulfate

*(dex troe am **fet'** a meen)*

Dexedrine Spansule (DANGER), DextroStat

PREGNANCY CATEGORY C

CONTROLLED SUBSTANCE C-II

Drug classes

Amphetamine
CNS stimulant

Therapeutic actions

Acts in the CNS to release norepinephrine from nerve terminals; in higher doses also releases dopamine; suppresses appetite; increases alertness, elevates mood; often improves physical performance, especially when fatigue and sleep deprivation have caused impairment; efficacy in hyperkinetic syndrome, ADHD in children appears paradoxical and is not understood.

Indications

- Narcolepsy
- Adjunct therapy for abnormal behavioral syndrome in children (ADHD, hyperkinetic syndrome) that includes psychological, social, educational measures

Contraindications and cautions

- Contraindicated with hypersensitivity to sympathomimetic amines, tartrazine (*Dextro-Stat*); advanced arteriosclerosis, symptomatic CV disease, moderate to severe hypertension, hyperthyroidism, glaucoma, agitated states.
- Use cautiously with history of drug abuse; pregnancy; lactation.

Available forms

Tablets—5, 10 mg; ER capsules DNC—5, 10, 15 mg

Dosages

Adults

- *Narcolepsy:* Start with 10 mg/day PO in divided doses; increase in increments of 10 mg/day at weekly intervals. If insomnia or anorexia occurs, reduce dose. Usual dosage is 5–60 mg/day PO in divided doses. Give first dose on awakening, additional doses (one or two) every 4–6 hr; long-acting forms can be given once a day.

Pediatric patients

- *Narcolepsy:*
  6–12 yr: Condition is rare in children younger than 12 yr; when it does occur, initial dose is 5 mg/day PO. Increase in increments of 5 mg at weekly intervals until optimal response is obtained.
  12 yr and older: Use adult dosage.
- *ADHD:*
  Younger than 3 yr: Not recommended.
  3–5 yr: 2.5 mg/day PO. Increase in increments of 2.5 mg/day at weekly intervals until optimal response is obtained.
  6 yr and older: 5 mg PO daily–bid. Increase in increments of 5 mg/day at weekly intervals until optimal response is obtained. Dosage will rarely exceed 40 mg/day. Give first dose on awakening, additional doses (one or two) every 4–6 hr. Long-acting forms may be used once a day.

Pharmacokinetics

Route	*Onset*	*Peak*	*Duration*
Oral	Rapid	1–5 hr	8–10 hr

Metabolism: Hepatic; $T_{1/2}$: 12 hr
Distribution: May cross placenta; enters breast milk
Excretion: Urine

Adverse effects

- **CNS:** *Overstimulation, restlessness, dizziness, insomnia,* dyskinesia, euphoria, dysphoria, tremor, headache, psychotic episodes
- **CV:** *Palpitations, tachycardia, hypertension*
- **Dermatologic:** Urticaria
- **Endocrine:** Reversible elevations in serum thyroxine with heavy use
- **GI:** *Dry mouth, unpleasant taste, diarrhea,* constipation, anorexia and weight loss
- **GU:** Impotence, changes in libido
- **Other:** Tolerance, psychological dependence, social disability with abuse

Interactions

✱ **Drug-drug** ⊗ ***Warning*** Hypertensive crisis and increased CNS effects if given within 14 days of MAOIs; do not give dextroamphetamine to patients who are taking or who have recently taken MAOIs.
• Decreased duration of effects if taken with urinary alkalinizers (acetazolamide, sodium bicarbonate), furazolidone • Decreased effects if taken with urinary acidifiers • Decreased efficacy of antihypertensive drugs given with amphetamines

■ Nursing considerations

Assessment

- **History:** Hypersensitivity to sympathomimetic amines, tartrazine; advanced arteriosclerosis, symptomatic CV disease, moderate to severe hypertension, hyperthyroidism, glaucoma, agitated states, history of drug abuse; lactation, pregnancy, use of MAOI in the last 14 days
- **Physical:** Weight; T; skin color, lesions; orientation, affect, ophthalmic examination (tonometry); P, BP, auscultation; R, adventitious sounds; bowel sounds, normal output; thyroid function tests, blood and urine glucose, baseline ECG

Interventions

- Ensure proper diagnosis before administering to children for behavioral syndromes: Drug should not be used until other causes (learning disability, EEG abnormalities, neurologic deficits) are ruled out.

⊗ ***Black box warning*** Be aware that drug has a high abuse potential; avoid prolonged use, and prescribe sparingly.

⊗ ***Black box warning*** Misuse may cause sudden death or serious CV events; increased risk with heart problems or structural heart anomalies.

- Interrupt drug dosage periodically in children being treated for behavioral disorders to determine if symptomatic response still validates drug therapy.
- Monitor growth of children on long-term amphetamine therapy.
- Dispense the lowest feasible dose to minimize risk of overdosage; drug should be stored in a light-resistant container.
- Ensure that patient swallows ER capsules whole; do not cut, crush, or allow patient to chew them.
- Give drug early in the day to prevent insomnia.
- Monitor BP frequently early in therapy.

Teaching points

- Take this drug exactly as prescribed. Do not increase the dosage without consulting your health care provider. If the drug appears ineffective, consult your health care provider.
- Do not crush or chew extended-release or long-acting capsules.
- Take drug (especially sustained-release forms) early in the day to avoid insomnia.
- This drug is a controlled substance; store it in a secure location and safely out of the reach of children.
- Avoid pregnancy while taking this drug. This drug can cause harm to the fetus.
- You may experience these side effects: Nervousness, restlessness, dizziness, insomnia, impaired thinking (may diminish in a few days; avoid driving or engaging in activities that require alertness); headache, loss of appetite, dry mouth.
- Report nervousness, insomnia, dizziness, palpitations, anorexia, GI disturbances.

▽ dextromethorphan hydrobromide

*(dex troe meth **or'** fan)*

Balminil DM (CAN), Buckley's Cough Mixture, Creo-Terpin, Delsym, DexAlone, Hold DM, Koffex (CAN), Novahistex DM (CAN), PediaCare Infants Long-Acting Cough, Robitussin Childrens (CAN), Robitussin CoughGels, Sucrets 8 Hour Cough Suppressant, Theraflu Thin Strips Long-Acting Cough, Triaminic Thin Strips Long-Acting Cough, Trocal, Vicks 44 Cough Relief

PREGNANCY CATEGORY C

Drug class

Nonopioid antitussive

Therapeutic actions

Lacks analgesic and addictive properties; controls cough spasms by depressing the cough center in the medulla; analogue of codeine.

Indications

- Control of nonproductive cough

Contraindications and cautions

- Contraindicated with hypersensitivity to any component (check label of products for flavorings, vehicles); sensitivity to bromides; cough that persists for more than 1 wk, tends

to recur, is accompanied by excessive secretions, high fever, rash, nausea, vomiting, or persistent headache (dextromethorphan should not be used; patient should consult a physician).
- Use cautiously with lactation, pregnancy.

Available forms
Gelcaps—15, 30 mg; lozenges—7.5, 10 mg; liquid—5 mg/5 mL, 10 mg/15 mL, 15 mg/5 mL, 30 mg/5 mL; syrup—5 mg/5 mL, 7.5 mg/5 mL, 10 mg/5 mL, 20 mg/5 mL; sustained-action liquid—30 mg/5 mL; oral disintegrating strips—7.5, 15 mg; freezer pops—7.5 mg/pop

Dosages
Adults and children 12 yr and older

Gelcaps

30 mg every 6–8 hr. Do not exceed 120 mg/day.

Lozenges

5–15 mg every 1–4 hr up to 120 mg/day.

Liquid, syrup, strips

10–20 mg every 4 hr or 30 mg every 6–8 hr up to 120 mg/day.

ER suspension

60 mg every 12 hr up to 120 mg/day.

Pediatric patients (6–11 yr)

Lozenges

5–10 mg every 1–4 hr up to 60 mg/day. Do not give to children younger than 6 yr unless directed by a physician.

Liquid, syrup, strips

15 mg every 6–8 hr up to 60 mg/day.

Freezer pop

2 pops every 6–8 hr.

Pediatric patients (2–6 yr)

Liquid, syrup, strips

7.5 mg every 6–8 hr up to 30 mg/day.

Freezer pop

1 pop every 6–8 hr.

Pharmacokinetics

Route	*Onset*	*Peak*	*Duration*
Oral	15–30 min	2 hr	3–6 hr

Metabolism: Hepatic; $T_{1/2}$: 2–4 hr
Distribution: May cross placenta; enters breast milk
Excretion: Urine

Adverse effects
- **Respiratory: Respiratory depression (with overdose)**

Interactions
✱ **Drug-drug** • Concomitant MAOI use may cause hypotension, fever, nausea, myoclonic jerks, and coma; avoid this combination

■ Nursing considerations
Assessment
- **History:** Hypersensitivity to any component; sensitivity to bromides; cough that persists for more than 1 wk or is accompanied by excessive secretions, high fever, rash, nausea, vomiting, or persistent headache; lactation, pregnancy
- **Physical:** T; R, adventitious sounds

Interventions
- Ensure drug is used only as recommended. Coughs may be symptomatic of a serious underlying disorder that should be diagnosed and properly treated; drug may mask symptoms of serious disease.

Teaching points
- Take this drug exactly as prescribed. Do not take more than recommended or for longer than recommended.
- Be cautious when using over-the-counter products; may contain the same ingredients and overdose can occur.
- Report continued or recurring cough, cough accompanied by fever, rash, persistent headache, nausea, vomiting.

▽ diazepam
*(dye **az'** e pam)*

Apo-Diazepam (CAN), Diastat AcuDial, Diazemuls (CAN), Diazepam Intensol, Valium

PREGNANCY CATEGORY D

CONTROLLED SUBSTANCE C-IV

Drug classes
Antiepileptic
Anxiolytic

Benzodiazepine
Skeletal muscle relaxant (centrally acting)

Therapeutic actions

Exact mechanisms of action not understood; acts mainly at the limbic system and reticular formation; may act in spinal cord and at supraspinal sites to produce skeletal muscle relaxation; potentiates the effects of GABA, an inhibitory neurotransmitter; anxiolytic effects occur at doses well below those necessary to cause sedation, ataxia; has little effect on cortical function.

Indications

- Management of anxiety disorders or for short-term relief of symptoms of anxiety
- Acute alcohol withdrawal; may be useful in symptomatic relief of acute agitation, tremor, delirium tremens, hallucinosis
- Muscle relaxant: Adjunct for relief of reflex skeletal muscle spasm due to local pathology (inflammation of muscles or joints) or secondary to trauma; spasticity caused by upper motoneuron disorders (cerebral palsy and paraplegia); athetosis, stiff-man syndrome
- Parenteral: Treatment of tetanus
- Antiepileptic: Adjunct in status epilepticus and severe recurrent convulsive seizures (parenteral); adjunct in seizure disorders (oral)
- Preoperative (parenteral): Relief of anxiety and tension and to lessen recall in patients prior to surgical procedures, cardioversion, and endoscopic procedures
- Rectal: Management of selected, refractory patients with epilepsy who require intermittent use to control bouts of increased seizure activity
- Unlabeled use: Treatment of night terrors

Contraindications and cautions

- Contraindicated with hypersensitivity to benzodiazepines; psychoses, acute narrow-angle glaucoma, shock, coma, acute alcoholic intoxication; pregnancy (cleft lip or palate, inguinal hernia, cardiac defects, microcephaly, pyloric stenosis when used in first trimester; neonatal withdrawal syndrome reported in newborns); lactation.
- Use cautiously with elderly or debilitated patients; impaired liver or renal function; and in patients with history of substance abuse.

Available forms

Tablets—2, 5, 10 mg; oral solution—1 mg/mL, 5 mg/mL; rectal pediatric gel—2.5, 5, 10 mg; injection—5 mg/mL

Dosages

Individualize dosage; increase dosage cautiously to avoid adverse effects.

Adults

Oral

- *Anxiety disorders, skeletal muscle spasm, seizure disorders:* 2–10 mg bid–qid.
- *Alcohol withdrawal:* 10 mg tid–qid first 24 hr; reduce to 5 mg tid–qid, as needed.

Rectal

0.2 mg/kg; treat no more than one episode every 5 days. May give a second dose in 4–12 hr.

Parenteral

Usual dose is 2–20 mg IM or IV. Larger doses may be required for some indications (tetanus). Injection may be repeated in 1 hr.

- *Anxiety:* 2–10 mg IM or IV; repeat in 3–4 hr if necessary.
- *Alcohol withdrawal:* 10 mg IM or IV initially, then 5–10 mg in 3–4 hr if necessary.
- *Endoscopic procedures:* 10 mg or less, up to 20 mg IV just before procedure or 5–10 mg IM 30 min prior to procedure. Reduce or omit dosage of opioids.
- *Muscle spasm:* 5–10 mg IM or IV initially, then 5–10 mg in 3–4 hr if necessary.
- *Status epilepticus:* 5–10 mg, preferably by slow IV. May repeat every 5–10 min up to total dose of 30 mg. If necessary, repeat therapy in 2–4 hr; other drugs are preferable for long-term control.
- *Preoperative:* 10 mg IM.
- *Cardioversion:* 5–15 mg IV 5–10 min before procedure.

Pediatric patients

Oral

Older than 6 mo: 1–2.5 mg PO tid–qid initially. Gradually increase as needed and tolerated. Can be given rectally if needed.

Rectal

Younger than 2 yr: Not recommended.
2–5 yr: 0.5 mg/kg.
6–11 yr: 0.3 mg/kg.
Older than 12 yr: 0.2 mg/kg; may give a second dose in 4–12 hr.

Parenteral

Maximum dose of 0.25 mg/kg IV administered over 3 min; may repeat after 15–30 min. If no relief of symptoms after three doses, adjunctive therapy is recommended.

- *Tetanus (older than 1 mo):* 1–2 mg IM or IV slowly every 3–4 hr as necessary.
- *Tetanus (5 yr and older):* 5–10 mg IV every 3–4 hr.
- *Status epilepticus (older than 1 mo–younger than 5 yr):* 0.2–0.5 mg slowly IV every 2–5 min up to a maximum of 5 mg.
- *Status epilepticus (5 yr and older):* 1 mg IV every 2–5 min up to a maximum of 10 mg; repeat in 2–4 hr if necessary.

Geriatric patients or patients with debilitating disease

2–2.5 mg PO daily–bid or 2–5 mg parenteral initially; reduce rectal dose. Gradually increase as needed and tolerated; use cautiously.

Pharmacokinetics

Route	*Onset*	*Peak*	*Duration*
Oral	30–60 min	1–2 hr	3 hr
IM	15–30 min	30–45 min	3 hr
IV	1–5 min	30 min	15–60 min
Rectal	Rapid	1.5 hr	3 hr

Metabolism: Hepatic; $T_{1/2}$: 20–80 hr

Distribution: Crosses placenta; enters breast milk

Excretion: Urine

IV FACTS

Preparation: Do not mix with other solutions; do not mix in plastic bags or tubing.

Infusion: Inject slowly into large vein, 1 mL/min at most; for children, give over at least 3 min; do not inject intra-arterially; if injected into IV tubing, inject as close to vein insertion site as possible.

Incompatibilities: Do not mix with other solutions; do not mix with any other drugs.

Y-site incompatibilities: Atracurium, heparin, foscarnet, pancuronium, potassium, vecuronium.

Adverse effects

- **CNS:** *Transient, mild drowsiness initially; sedation, depression, lethargy, apathy, fatigue, light-headedness, disorientation, restlessness, confusion,* crying, delirium, headache, slurred speech, dysarthria, stupor, rigidity, tremor, dystonia, vertigo, euphoria, nervousness, difficulty in concentration, vivid dreams, psychomotor retardation, extrapyramidal symptoms; *mild paradoxical excitatory reactions during first 2 wk of treatment,* visual and auditory disturbances, diplopia, nystagmus, depressed hearing, nasal congestion
- **CV:** *Bradycardia, tachycardia,* CV collapse, hypertension and hypotension, palpitations, edema
- **Dependence:** *Drug dependence with withdrawal syndrome* when drug is discontinued (common with abrupt discontinuation of higher dosage used for longer than 4 mo); IV diazepam: 1.7% incidence of fatalities; oral benzodiazepines ingested alone; no well-documented fatal overdoses
- **Dermatologic:** Urticaria, pruritus, skin rash, dermatitis
- **GI:** *Constipation; diarrhea,* dry mouth; salivation; nausea; anorexia; vomiting; difficulty in swallowing; gastric disorders; elevations of blood enzymes—LDH, alkaline phosphatase, AST, ALT; hepatic impairment; jaundice
- **GU:** *Incontinence, urinary retention, changes in libido,* menstrual irregularities
- **Hematologic:** Decreased Hct, blood dyscrasias
- **Other:** Phlebitis and thrombosis at IV injection sites, hiccups, fever, diaphoresis, paresthesias, muscular disturbances, gynecomastia; pain, burning, and redness after IM injection

Interactions

✱ **Drug-drug** • Increased CNS depression with alcohol, omeprazole • Increased pharmacologic effects of diazepam if combined with cimetidine, disulfiram, hormonal contraceptives • Decreased effects of diazepam with theophyllines, ranitidine

■ Nursing considerations

Assessment

- **History:** Hypersensitivity to benzodiazepines; psychoses, acute narrow-angle glaucoma, shock, coma, acute alcoholic intoxication; elderly or debilitated patients; impaired liver or renal function; pregnancy, lactation

- **Physical:** Weight; skin color, lesions; orientation, affect, reflexes, sensory nerve function, ophthalmologic examination; P, BP; R, adventitious sounds; bowel sounds, normal output, liver evaluation; normal output; LFTs, renal function tests, CBC

Interventions

⊗ ***Warning*** Do not administer intra-arterially; may produce arteriospasm, gangrene.

- Change from IV therapy to oral therapy as soon as possible.
- Do not use small veins (dorsum of hand or wrist) for IV injection.
- Reduce dose of opioid analgesics with IV diazepam; dose should be reduced by at least one-third or eliminated.
- Carefully monitor P, BP, respiration during IV administration.

⊗ ***Warning*** Maintain patients receiving parenteral benzodiazepines in bed for 3 hr; do not permit ambulatory patients to operate a vehicle following an injection.

- Monitor EEG in patients treated for status epilepticus; seizures may recur after initial control, presumably because of short duration of drug effect.
- Monitor liver and renal function, CBC during long-term therapy.
- Taper dosage gradually after long-term therapy, especially in epileptic patients.
- Arrange for epileptic patients to wear medical alert ID indicating that they are epileptics taking this medication.
- Discuss risk of fetal abnormalities with patients desiring to become pregnant.

Teaching points

- Take this drug exactly as prescribed. Do not stop taking this drug (long-term therapy, antiepileptic therapy) without consulting your health care provider.
- Caregiver should learn to assess seizures, administer rectal form, and monitor patient.
- Use of barrier contraceptives is advised while on this drug; if you become or wish to become pregnant, consult your health care provider.
- It is advisable to wear a medical alert ID indicating your diagnosis and treatment (as antiepileptic).
- You may experience these side effects: Drowsiness, dizziness (may lessen; avoid driving or engaging in other dangerous activities); GI upset (take drug with food); dreams, difficulty concentrating, fatigue, nervousness, crying (reversible).
- Report severe dizziness, weakness, drowsiness that persists, rash or skin lesions, palpitations, swelling of the ankles, visual or hearing disturbances, difficulty voiding.

▽ diazoxide

*(di az **ok'** side)*

Oral: Proglycem

Parenteral: Hyperstat IV

PREGNANCY CATEGORY C

Drug classes

Antihypertensive
Glucose-elevating drug (oral)

Therapeutic actions

Increases blood glucose by decreasing insulin release and decreasing glucose. Decreases BP by relaxing arteriolar smooth muscle.

Indications

- Oral: Management of hypoglycemia due to hyperinsulinism in infants and children and to inoperable pancreatic islet cell malignancies
- Parenteral: Short-term use in malignant and nonmalignant hypertension, used primarily in hospital

Contraindications and cautions

- Contraindicated with allergy to thiazides or other sulfonamide derivatives; pregnancy, lactation, functional hypoglycemia.
- Use extreme caution with decreased cardiac reserve, decreased renal function, gout or hyperuricemia when using oral diazoxide; compensatory hypertension, dissecting aortic aneurysm, pheochromocytoma, decreased cerebral or cardiac circulation, labor and delivery (IV use may stop uterine contractions and cause neonatal hyperbilirubinemia,

thrombocytopenia) when using parenteral diazoxide.

Available forms

Capsules—50 mg; oral suspension—50 mg/mL; injection—15 mg/mL

Dosages

Adults

Oral

3–8 mg/kg/day PO in two to three divided doses every 8–12 hr. Starting dose, 3 mg/kg/day in three equal doses every 8 hr.

Parenteral

1–3 mg/kg (maximum dose, 150 mg) undiluted and rapidly by IV injection in a bolus dose within 30 sec; repeat bolus doses every 5–15 min until desired decrease in BP is achieved. Repeat doses every 4–24 hr until oral antihypertensive medications can be started. Treatment is seldom needed for longer than 4–5 days and should not be continued for longer than 10 days.

Pediatric patients

Oral

Infants and newborns: 8–15 mg/kg/day PO in two to three doses every 8–12 hr. Starting dose, 10 mg/kg/day in three equal doses every 8 hr.

Children: 3–8 mg/kg/day PO in two to three doses every 8–12 hr. Starting dose, 3 mg/kg/day in three equal doses every 8 hr.

Pharmacokinetics

Route	Onset	Peak	Duration
Oral	1 hr	8 hr	N/A
IV	30–60 sec	5 min	2–12 hr

Metabolism: Hepatic; $T_{1/2}$: 21–45 hr

Distribution: Crosses placenta; may enter breast milk

Excretion: Urine

IV FACTS

Preparation: Do not mix or dilute solution. Protect from light.

Infusion: Inject directly as rapid bolus, over 30 sec or less; maximum of 150 mg in one injection.

Y-site incompatibilities: Do not give with hydralazine, propranolol.

Adverse effects

- **CNS:** Cerebral ischemia, headache, hearing loss, blurred vision, apprehension, **cerebral infarction, coma, seizures,** paralysis, *dizziness, weakness,* altered taste sensation
- **CV:** *Hypotension* (managed by Trendelenburg position or sympathomimetics), occasional hypertension, angina, **MI,** cardiac arrhythmias, palpitations, *heart failure secondary to fluid and sodium retention*
- **Dermatologic:** Hirsutism, rash
- **GI:** *Nausea, vomiting,* **hepatotoxicity,** anorexia, parotid swelling, constipation, diarrhea, acute pancreatitis
- **GU:** Renal toxicity
- **Hematologic: Thrombocytopenia,** decreased Hgb, decreased Hct
- **Local:** Pain at IV injection site
- **Metabolic:** Hyperglycemia, glycosuria, ketoacidosis, nonketotic hyperosmolar coma, hyperuricemia
- **Respiratory:** Dyspnea, choking sensation

Interactions

✱ **Drug-drug** • Increased therapeutic and toxic effects of diazoxide if taken concurrently with thiazides • Increased risk of hyperglycemia if taken concurrently with chlorpropamide, glipizide, glyburide, tolazamide, tolbutamide • Decreased serum levels and effectiveness of hydantoins taken concurrently with diazoxide

✱ **Drug-lab test** • Hyperglycemic and hyperuricemic effects of diazoxide prevent testing for disorders of glucose and xanthine metabolism • False-negative insulin response to glucagon

■ Nursing considerations

Assessment

- **History:** Allergy to thiazides or other sulfonamide derivatives; pregnancy; lactation; functional hypoglycemia, decreased cardiac reserve, decreased renal function, gout or hyperuricemia; compensatory hypertension, dissecting aortic aneurysm, pheochromocytoma; decreased cerebral or cardiac circulation; pregnancy
- **Physical:** Body weight, skin integrity, swelling or limited motion in joints, earlobes;

P, BP, edema, peripheral perfusion; R, pattern, adventitious sounds; intake and output; CBC, blood glucose, serum electrolytes and uric acid, urinalysis, urine glucose and ketones, LFTs, renal function tests

Interventions

- Monitor intake and output and weigh patient daily at the same time to check for fluid retention.
- Check urine glucose and ketones daily.

⊗ ***Warning*** Have insulin and oral hypoglycemic agents readily available in case hyperglycemic reaction occurs.

⊗ ***Warning*** Have dopamine and norepinephrine readily available in case of severe hypotensive reaction.

Oral

- Decrease dose in renal disease.
- Protect oral drug suspensions from light.
- Reassure patient that hirsutism will resolve when drug is discontinued.

Parenteral

⊗ ***Warning*** Monitor BP closely during administration until stable and then every 30 min–1 hr.

- Protect drug from freezing and light.
- Patient should remain supine for 1 hr after last injection or 8–10 hr if given with furosemide.

Teaching points

Oral

- Check urine or blood daily for glucose and ketones; report elevated levels.
- Weigh yourself daily at the same time and with the same clothes, and record the results.
- Excessive hair growth may appear on your forehead, back, or limbs; growth will end after drug is stopped.
- Report weight gain of more than 5 pounds in 2–3 days, increased thirst, nausea, vomiting, confusion, fruity odor on breath, abdominal pain, swelling of extremities, difficulty breathing, bruising, bleeding.

Parenteral

- Report increased thirst, nausea, headache, dizziness, hearing or vision changes, difficulty breathing, pain at injection site.

▽diclofenac

*(dye **kloe'** fen ak)*

diclofenac epolamine

Flector

diclofenac potassium

Apo-Diclo Rapide (CAN), Cambia, Cataflam, Novo-Difenac-K (CAN), Voltaren Rapide (CAN), Zipsor

diclofenac sodium

Apo-Diclo (CAN), Apo-Diclo SR (CAN) DNC, Novo-Difenac (CAN), Novo-Difenac SR (CAN), Nu-Diclo (CAN), Nu-Diclo SR (CAN) DNC, PMS-Diclofenac (CAN), PMS-Diclofenac SR (CAN) DNC, Solaraze, Voltaren, Voltaren Ophtha (CAN), Voltaren-XR DNC

PREGNANCY CATEGORY C (FIRST AND SECOND TRIMESTERS)

PREGNANCY CATEGORY D (THIRD TRIMESTER)

Drug classes

Analgesic (nonopioid)
Anti-inflammatory
Antipyretic
NSAID

Therapeutic actions

Inhibits prostaglandin synthetase to cause antipyretic and anti-inflammatory effects; the exact mechanism is unknown.

Indications

- Acute or long-term treatment of mild to moderate pain, including dysmenorrhea
- Rheumatoid arthritis
- Acute treatment of migraine headache with or without aura (*Cambia*)
- Osteoarthritis
- Ankylosing spondylitis
- Treatment of actinic keratosis in conjunction with sun avoidance

- Topical treatment of acute pain due to minor strains, sprains, contusions (*Flector*)
- Ophthalmic: Postoperative inflammation from cataract extraction

Contraindications and cautions

- Contraindicated with allergy to NSAIDs, significant renal impairment, pregnancy, lactation.
- Use cautiously with impaired hearing, allergies, hepatic, CV, GI conditions, and in elderly patients.

Available forms

Tablets—50 mg; DR tablets (DNC)—25, 50, 75 mg; ER tablets (DNC)—100 mg; liquid-filled capsules—25 mg; packet for oral solution—50 mg; topical gel—3%; ophthalmic solution—0.1%; transdermal patch—180 mg

Dosages

Adults

Oral

- *Pain, including dysmenorrhea:* 50 mg tid PO; initial dose of 100 mg may help some patients (*Cataflam*).
- *Osteoarthritis:* 100–150 mg/day PO in divided doses (*Voltaren*); 50 mg bid–tid PO (*Cataflam*).
- *Rheumatoid arthritis:* 150–200 mg/day PO in divided doses (*Voltaren*); 50 mg bid–tid PO (*Cataflam*).
- *Ankylosing spondylitis:* 100–125 mg/day PO. Give as 25 mg qid, with an extra 25-mg dose at bedtime (*Voltaren*); 25 mg qid PO with an additional 25 mg at bedtime if needed (*Cataflam*).

NEW INDICATION: *Acute migraine:* 50-mg packet mixed in 30–60 mL water as single dose at onset of headache (*Cambia*).

NEW INDICATION: *Treatment of mild to moderate pain:* 25 mg liquid-filled capsule PO qid (*Zipsor*). *Not interchangeable with other forms of diclofenac.*

Topical

- *Actinic keratosis:* Cover lesion with gel and smooth into skin; do not cover with dressings or cosmetics (*Solaraze*).

Transdermal patch

1 patch applied to most painful area bid. Use lowest effective dose for shortest time; do not apply to damaged or broken skin (*Flector*).

Ophthalmic

1 drop to affected eye qid starting 24 hr after surgery for 2 wk.

Pediatric patients

Safety and efficacy not established.

Pharmacokinetics

Route	Onset	Peak	Duration
Oral (sodium)	Varies	2–3 hr	12–15 hr
Oral (potassium)	Rapid	20–120 min	12–15 hr

Metabolism: Hepatic; $T_{1/2}$: 1.5–2 hr
Distribution: Crosses placenta; may enter breast milk
Excretion: Feces, urine

Adverse effects

- **CNS:** *Headache, dizziness,* somnolence, insomnia, fatigue, tiredness, tinnitus, ophthalmic effects
- **Dermatologic:** Rash, pruritus, sweating, dry mucous membranes, stomatitis
- **GI:** *Nausea, dyspepsia, GI pain, diarrhea,* vomiting, *constipation,* flatulence, GI bleed
- **GU:** Dysuria, renal impairment
- **Hematologic:** Bleeding, platelet inhibition with higher doses
- **Other:** Peripheral edema, **anaphylactoid reactions to fatal anaphylactic shock**

Interactions

✱ **Drug-drug** • Increased serum levels and increased risk of lithium toxicity • Increased risk of bleeding with anticoagulants; monitor patient closely

■ Nursing considerations

Assessment

- **History:** Renal impairment; impaired hearing; allergies; hepatic, CV, and GI conditions; lactation, pregnancy
- **Physical:** Skin color and lesions; orientation, reflexes, ophthalmologic and audiometric evaluation, peripheral sensation;

P, edema; R, adventitious sounds; liver evaluation; CBC, clotting times, renal function tests, LFTs; serum electrolytes, stool guaiac

Interventions

⊗ ***Black box warning*** Be aware that patient may be at increased risk for CV events, GI bleed, renal insufficiency; monitor accordingly.

- Administer drug with food or after meals if GI upset occurs. Ensure that patient does not cut, crush, or chew ER or DR tablets. Mix packets for oral suspension in 30–60 mL water.
- Arrange for periodic ophthalmologic examination during long-term therapy.

⊗ ***Warning*** Institute emergency procedures if overdose occurs (gastric lavage, induction of emesis, supportive therapy).

⊗ ***Warning*** Liquid-filled capsules (*Zipsor*) are not interchangeable with other forms of diclofenac.

Teaching points

- Take drug with food or meals if GI upset occurs. Do not cut, crush, or chew delayed-release or extended-release tablets.
- Mix packets for oral solution in 30 to 60 mL water. Take at first sign of a migraine.
- Take only the prescribed dosage.
- You may experience these side effects: Dizziness or drowsiness (avoid driving or using dangerous machinery while using this drug).
- Report sore throat, fever, rash, itching, weight gain, swelling in ankles or fingers, changes in vision; black, tarry stools.

dicyclomine hydrochloride

(dye sye' kloe meen)

Bentyl, Bentylol (CAN), Byclomine, Dibent, Dilomine, Or-Tyl

PREGNANCY CATEGORY B

Drug classes

Anticholinergic
Antimuscarinic
Antispasmodic
Parasympatholytic

Therapeutic actions

Direct GI smooth muscle relaxant; competitively blocks the effects of acetylcholine at muscarinic cholinergic receptors that mediate the effects of parasympathetic postganglionic impulses, thus relaxing the GI tract.

D

Indications

- Treatment of functional bowel or IBS (irritable colon, spastic colon, mucous colitis)

Contraindications and cautions

- Contraindicated with glaucoma; adhesions between iris and lens, stenosing peptic ulcer, pyloroduodenal obstruction, paralytic ileus, intestinal atony, severe ulcerative colitis, toxic megacolon, symptomatic prostatic hypertrophy, bladder neck obstruction, bronchial asthma, COPD, cardiac arrhythmias, tachycardia, myocardial ischemia; impaired metabolic, liver, or renal function, myasthenia gravis; lactation, pregnancy.
- Use cautiously with Down syndrome, brain damage, spasticity, hypertension, hyperthyroidism.

Available forms

Capsules—10, 20 mg; tablets—20 mg; syrup—10 mg/5 mL; injection—10 mg/mL

Dosages

Adults

Oral

The only effective dose is 160 mg/day PO divided into four equal doses; however, begin with 80 mg/day divided into four equal doses; increase to 160 mg/day unless side effects limit dosage.

Parenteral

80 mg/day IM in four divided doses; do not give IV.

Pediatric patients

Not recommended.

Geriatric patients

Use caution; more prone to side effects.

Pharmacokinetics

Route	*Onset*	*Duration*
Oral	1–2 hr	4 hr

Metabolism: Hepatic; $T_{1/2}$: 9–10 hr

Distribution: May cross placenta; enters breast milk
Excretion: Urine

Adverse effects

- **CNS:** *Blurred vision,* mydriasis, cycloplegia, photophobia, increased IOP
- **CV:** Palpitations, tachycardia
- **GI:** *Dry mouth, altered taste perception, nausea, vomiting, dysphagia,* heartburn, constipation, bloated feeling, paralytic ileus, gastroesophageal reflux
- **GU:** *Urinary hesitancy and retention,* impotence
- **Local:** *Irritation at site of IM injection*
- **Other:** Decreased sweating and predisposition to heat prostration, suppression of lactation

Interactions

✱ **Drug-drug** • Decreased effectiveness of all antipsychotic medications when used in combination with dicyclomine • Increased anticholinergic effects when administered with TCAs, amantadine • Possible increased effect of atenolol and digoxin

■ Nursing considerations

Assessment

- **History:** Glaucoma; adhesions between iris and lens, stenosing peptic ulcer, pyloroduodenal obstruction, paralytic ileus, intestinal atony, severe ulcerative colitis, toxic megacolon, symptomatic prostatic hypertrophy, bladder neck obstruction, bronchial asthma, COPD, cardiac arrhythmias, myocardial ischemia; impaired metabolic, liver, or renal function, myasthenia gravis; Down syndrome, brain damage, spasticity, hypertension, hyperthyroidism; lactation, pregnancy
- **Physical:** Bowel sounds, normal output; normal urinary output, prostate palpation; R, adventitious sounds; pulse, BP; IOP, vision; bilateral grip strength, reflexes; liver palpation, LFTs, renal function tests; skin color, lesions, texture

Interventions

- IM use is temporary; switch to oral form as soon as feasible.
- Ensure adequate hydration; control environmental temperature to prevent hyperpyrexia.
- Have patient void before each drug dose if urinary retention is a problem.
- Monitor lighting to minimize discomfort of photophobia.
- Do not give IV.

Teaching points

- Take drug exactly as prescribed.
- Avoid hot environments while taking this drug (heat intolerance may lead to dangerous reactions).
- You may experience these side effects: Constipation (ensure adequate fluid intake, proper diet); dry mouth (sugarless lozenges, frequent mouth care may help; may lessen with time); blurred vision, sensitivity to light (transient effects; avoid tasks that require acute vision; wear sunglasses); impotence (reversible); difficulty in urination (empty bladder immediately before taking drug).
- Report rash, flushing, eye pain, difficulty breathing, tremors, loss of coordination, irregular heartbeat, palpitations, headache, abdominal distention, hallucinations, severe or persistent dry mouth, difficulty swallowing, difficulty in urination, severe constipation, sensitivity to light.

▽ didanosine (ddI, dideoxyinosine)

*(dye **dan'** oh seen)*

Videx, Videx EC (DNC)

PREGNANCY CATEGORY B

Drug class

Antiviral

Therapeutic actions

A synthetic nucleoside that inhibits replication of HIV, leading to viral death.

Indications

- Treatment of patients with HIV infection in combination with other antiretroviral drugs (*Videx*)

- Treatment of adults with advanced HIV infection who would require once-daily therapy with didanosine (*Videx EC*)

Contraindications and cautions

- Contraindicated with allergy to any component of the formulation, lactation.
- Use cautiously with impaired hepatic or renal function; history of alcohol abuse; pregnancy.

Available forms

DR capsules DNC—125, 200, 250, 400 mg; powder for oral solution—2, 4 g

Dosages

Adults

DR capsules

- 60 kg or greater: 400 mg/day PO.
- 25–60 kg: 250 mg/day PO.
- 20–25 kg: 200 mg/day PO.

Powder for oral solution

- 60 kg or greater: 200 mg PO bid.
- Less than 60 kg: 125 mg PO bid.

Pediatric patients

Older than 8 mo: 120 mg/m^2 bid using buffered formulation or pediatric powder.
2 wk–8 mo: 100 mg/m^2 bid.
DR capsule can be used following adult dosage, based on weight.

Patients with renal impairment

For creatinine clearance of 60 mL/min or more, usual dose. For creatinine clearance of 30–59 mL/min, 125–200 mg/day. For creatinine clearance of 10–29 mL/min, 100–130 mg/day. For creatinine clearance less than 10 mL/min, 75–100 mg/day.

Pharmacokinetics

Route	*Peak*	*Onset*
Oral	15–90 min	Varies

Metabolism: Hepatic; $T_{1/2}$: 1.6 hr
Distribution: May cross placenta; may enter breast milk
Excretion: Urine

Adverse effects

- **CNS:** Headache, pain, anxiety, confusion, nervousness, twitching, depression, peripheral neuropathy
- **Dermatologic:** Rash, pruritus
- **GI:** *Nausea, vomiting,* **hepatotoxicity,** *abdominal pain,* diarrhea, **pancreatitis,** stomatitis, oral thrush, melena, dry mouth, elevated bilirubin
- **Hematologic:** *Hemopoietic depression*
- **Other:** Chills, fever, infections, dyspnea, myopathy, elevated uric acid, **lactic acidosis**

D

Interactions

✱ **Drug-drug** • Decreased effectiveness of tetracycline, fluoroquinolone antibiotics • Increased effect of *Videx* when combined with allopurinol • Changed concentrations for either drug when combined with ganciclovir • Decreased effect of *Videx* when combined with methadone • Decreased effect of azole antifungals

✱ **Drug-food** • Decreased absorption and effectiveness of didanosine if taken with food

■ Nursing considerations

Assessment

- **History:** Allergy to any components of formulation, impaired hepatic or renal function, lactation, history of alcohol abuse, pregnancy
- **Physical:** Weight; T; skin color, lesions; orientation, reflexes, muscle strength, affect; abdominal examination; CBC, pancreatic enzymes, LFTs, renal function tests

Interventions

- Arrange for lab tests (CBC, SMA-12) before and frequently during therapy; monitor for bone marrow depression.
- Administer drug on an empty stomach, 1 hr before or 2 hr after meals.
- Ensure patient swallows *Videx EC* whole; do not cut, crush, or chew.

⊗ ***Black box warning*** Monitor patient for signs of pancreatitis—abdominal pain, elevated enzymes, nausea, vomiting. Stop drug, resume only if pancreatitis has been ruled out.

⊗ ***Black box warning*** Monitor patients with hepatic impairment; decreased doses may be needed if toxicity occurs. Fatal liver toxicity with lactic acidosis has been reported.

Teaching points

- Take drug on an empty stomach, 1 hour before or 2 hours after meals.
- Pediatric solution should be reconstituted by the pharmacy. Shake admixture thoroughly.

Store tightly closed in the refrigerator. If taking a delayed-release capsule, it must be swallowed whole; do not cut, crush, or chew it.
- Have regular blood tests and physical examinations to monitor drug's effects and progress of disease.
- You may experience these side effects: Loss of appetite, nausea, vomiting (frequent mouth care, frequent small meals may help); rash; chills, fever; headache.
- Report abdominal pain, nausea, vomiting, cough, sore throat, change in color of urine or stools.

diflunisal (DNC)

(dye floo' ni sal)

Apo-Diflunisal (CAN) (DNC)

PREGNANCY CATEGORY C

Drug classes

Analgesic (nonopioid)
Anti-inflammatory
Antipyretic
NSAID

Therapeutic actions

Exact mechanism of action not known: Inhibition of prostaglandin synthetase, the enzyme that breaks down prostaglandins, may account for its antipyretic and anti-inflammatory effects.

Indications

- Acute or long-term treatment of mild to moderate pain
- Rheumatoid arthritis
- Osteoarthritis

Contraindications and cautions

- Contraindicated with allergy to diflunisal, salicylates or other NSAIDs; with pregnancy, lactation; for treatment of perioperative pain following coronary artery bypass graft (CABG) surgery.
- Use cautiously with CV dysfunction, peptic ulceration, GI bleeding, impaired hepatic or renal function, and in elderly patients.

Available forms

Tablets (DNC)—500 mg

Dosages

Adults

- *Mild to moderate pain:* 1,000 mg PO initially, followed by 500 mg every 8–12 hr PO.
- *Osteoarthritis or rheumatoid arthritis:* 500–1,000 mg/day PO in two divided doses; maintenance dosage should not exceed 1,500 mg/day.

Pediatric patients

Safety and efficacy not established.

Pharmacokinetics

Route	*Onset*	*Peak*	*Duration*
Oral	30–60 min	2–3 hr	12 hr

Metabolism: Hepatic; $T_{1/2}$: 8–12 hr
Distribution: Crosses placenta; enters breast milk
Excretion: Urine

Adverse effects

- **CNS:** *Headache, dizziness, somnolence, insomnia,* fatigue, tiredness, dizziness, tinnitus, ophthalmologic effects
- **Dermatologic:** *Rash,* pruritus, sweating, dry mucous membranes, stomatitis
- **GI:** *Nausea, dyspepsia, GI pain, diarrhea,* vomiting, constipation, flatulence
- **GU:** Dysuria, renal impairment
- **Hematologic:** Bleeding, platelet inhibition with higher doses
- **Other:** Peripheral edema, **anaphylactoid reactions to anaphylactic shock**

Interactions

✱ **Drug-drug** • Decreased absorption with antacids (especially aluminum salts) • Decreased serum diflunisal levels with multiple doses of aspirin • Possible increased acetaminophen levels if combined

■ Nursing considerations

Assessment

- **History:** Allergy to diflunisal, salicylates or other NSAIDs, CV dysfunction, peptic ulceration, GI bleeding, impaired hepatic or renal function, lactation, pregnancy

- **Physical:** Skin color, lesions; T; orientation, reflexes, ophthalmologic evaluation; P, BP, edema; R, adventitious sounds; liver evaluation, bowel sounds; CBC, clotting times, urinalysis, LFTs, renal function tests

Interventions

⊠ ***Black box warning*** Be aware that patient may be at increased risk for CV events, GI bleeding; monitor accordingly.

- Give drug with food or after meals if GI upset occurs.
- Do not crush, and ensure that patient does not chew tablets.

⊗ ***Warning*** Institute emergency procedures if overdose occurs—gastric lavage, induction of emesis, supportive therapy.

⊠ ***Black box warning*** Do not use drug to treat perioperative pain following CABG surgery.

- Arrange for ophthalmologic examination if patient offers any eye complaints.

Teaching points

- Take the drug only as recommended to avoid overdose.
- Take the drug with food or after meals if GI upset occurs. Swallow the tablet whole; do not cut, chew, or crush it.
- You may experience these side effects: Nausea, GI upset, dyspepsia (take drug with food); diarrhea or constipation; dizziness, vertigo, insomnia (use caution if driving or operating dangerous machinery).
- Report eye changes, unusual bleeding or bruising, swelling of the feet or hands, difficulty breathing, severe GI pain.

DANGEROUS DRUG

digoxin

(di jox' in)

Lanoxin

PREGNANCY CATEGORY C

Drug classes

Cardiac glycoside
Cardiotonic

Therapeutic actions

Increases intracellular calcium and allows more calcium to enter the myocardial cell during depolarization via a sodium–potassium pump mechanism; this increases force of contraction (positive inotropic effect), increases renal perfusion (seen as diuretic effect in patients with heart failure), decreases heart rate (negative chronotropic effect), and decreases AV node conduction velocity.

Indications

- Heart failure
- Atrial fibrillation

Contraindications and cautions

- Contraindicated with allergy to cardiac glycosides, ventricular tachycardia, ventricular fibrillation, heart block, sick sinus syndrome, IHSS, acute MI, renal insufficiency and electrolyte abnormalities (decreased K^+, decreased Mg^{2+}, increased Ca^{2+}).
- Use cautiously with pregnancy and lactation.

Available forms

Tablets—0.125, 0.25 mg; injection—0.25 mg/mL; pediatric injection—0.1 mg/mL

Dosages

Patient response is quite variable. Evaluate patient carefully to determine the appropriate dose.

Adults

Loading dose, 0.75–1.25 mg PO or 0.125–0.25 mg IV. Maintenance dose, 0.125–0.25 mg/day PO.

Pediatric patients

Loading dose:

	Oral (mcg/kg)	*IV (mcg/kg)*
Premature	20–30	15–25
Neonate	25–35	20–30
1–24 mo	35–60	30–50
2–5 yr	30–40	25–35
5–10 yr	20–35	15–30
Older than 10 yr	10–15	8–12

Maintenance dose, 20%–30% of loading dose in divided daily doses. Usually 0.125–0.5 mg/day PO; 20%–30% for premature infants.

Geriatric patients with impaired renal function

CrCl (mL/min)	*Dose*
10–25	0.125 mg/day
26–49	0.1875 mg/day
50–79	0.25 mg/day

Pharmacokinetics

Route	*Onset*	*Peak*	*Duration*
Oral	30–120 min	2–6 hr	6–8 days
IV	5–30 min	1–5 hr	4–5 days

Metabolism: Some hepatic; $T_{1/2}$: 30–40 hr
Distribution: May cross placenta; enters breast milk
Excretion: Urine, unchanged

IV FACTS

Preparation: Give undiluted or diluted in fourfold or greater volume of sterile water for injection, 0.9% sodium chloride injection, 5% dextrose injection. Use diluted product promptly. Do not use if solution contains precipitates.
Infusion: Inject slowly over 5 min or longer.
Incompatibility: Do not mix with dobutamine.

Adverse effects

- **CNS:** *Headache, weakness,* drowsiness, visual disturbances, mental status change
- **CV:** *Arrhythmias*
- **GI:** *GI upset,* anorexia

Interactions

✱ **Drug-drug** • Increased therapeutic and toxic effects of digoxin with thioamines, verapamil, amiodarone, quinidine, erythromycin, cyclosporine (a decrease in digoxin dosage may be necessary to prevent toxicity; when the interacting drug is discontinued, an increase in the digoxin dosage may be necessary) • Increased incidence of cardiac arrhythmias with potassium-losing (loop and thiazide) diuretics • Increased absorption or increased bioavailability of oral digoxin, leading to increased effects with tetracyclines, erythromycin • Decreased therapeutic effects with thyroid hormones, metoclopramide, penicillamine • Decreased absorption of oral digoxin if taken with cholestyramine, charcoal, colestipol, antineoplastics (bleomycin, cyclophosphamide, methotrexate) • Increased or decreased effects of oral digoxin (adjust the dose of digoxin during concomitant therapy) with oral aminoglycosides

✱ **Drug-alternative therapy** • Increased risk of digoxin toxicity if taken with ginseng, hawthorn, or licorice therapy • Decreased absorption with psyllium • Decreased serum levels with St. John's Wort

■ Nursing considerations

Assessment

- **History:** Allergy to cardiac glycosides, ventricular tachycardia, ventricular fibrillation, heart block, sick sinus syndrome, IHSS, acute MI, renal insufficiency, decreased K^+, decreased Mg^{2+}, increased Ca^{2+}, pregnancy, lactation
- **Physical:** Weight; orientation, affect, reflexes, vision; P, BP, baseline ECG, cardiac auscultation, peripheral pulses, peripheral perfusion, edema; R, adventitious sounds; abdominal percussion, bowel sounds, liver evaluation; urinary output; electrolyte levels, LFTs, renal function tests

Interventions

⊗ ***Warning*** Monitor apical pulse for 1 min before administering; hold dose if pulse lower than 60 beats/min in adult or lower than 90 beats/min in infant; retake pulse in 1 hr. If adult pulse remains lower than 60 beats/min or infant pulse remains lower than 90 beats/min, hold drug and notify prescriber. Note any change from baseline rhythm or rate.

- Check dosage and preparation carefully.
- Avoid IM injections, which may be very painful.
- Follow diluting instructions carefully, and use diluted solution promptly.
- Avoid giving with meals; taking this drug with food will delay absorption and alter drug pharmacokinetics.
- Have emergency equipment ready; have K^+ salts, lidocaine, phenytoin, atropine, and cardiac monitor readily available in case toxicity develops.

⊗ ***Warning*** Monitor for therapeutic drug levels: 0.5–2 ng/mL.

Teaching points

- Do not stop taking this drug without notifying your health care provider.
- Take pulse at the same time each day, and record it on a calendar (normal pulse for you is ____; call your health care provider if your pulse rate falls below _____.)
- Weigh yourself every other day with the same clothing and at the same time. Record this on the calendar.
- Do not start taking any prescription or over-the-counter products without talking to your health care provider. Some combinations may increase the risk of digoxin toxicity and may put you at risk of adverse reactions.
- Wear or carry a medical alert tag stating that you are on this drug.
- Have regular medical checkups, which may include blood tests, to evaluate the effects and dosage of this drug.
- Report slow or irregular pulse, rapid weight gain, loss of appetite, nausea, diarrhea, vomiting, blurred or "yellow" vision, unusual tiredness and weakness, swelling of the ankles, legs or fingers, difficulty breathing.

▽ digoxin immune fab (bovine; digoxin-specific antibody fragments)

(di jox' in)

Digibind, DigiFab

PREGNANCY CATEGORY C

Drug class

Antidote

Therapeutic actions

Antigen-binding fragments (fab) derived from specific antidigoxin antibodies; binds molecules of digoxin, making them unavailable at the site of action; fab-fragment complex accumulates in the blood and is excreted by the kidneys.

Indications

- Treatment of potentially life-threatening digoxin toxicity (serum digoxin level exceeding 10 nanograms/mL, serum K^+ exceeding 5 mEq/L in setting of digoxin toxicity)

Contraindications and cautions

- Contraindicated with allergy to sheep products.
- Use cautiously with pregnancy or lactation.

Available forms

Powder for injection—38 mg/vial (*Digibind*), 40 mg/vial (*DigiFab*)

Dosages

Adults and pediatric patients

Dosage is determined by serum digoxin level or estimate of the amount of digoxin ingested. If no estimate is available and serum digoxin levels cannot be obtained, use 800 mg (20 vials *DigiFab*) or 760 mg (20 vials *Digibind*), which should treat most life-threatening ingestions in adults and children.

Digibind

- Estimated fab fragment dose based on amount of digoxin ingested:

Estimated Number of 0.25-mg Tablets or 0.2-mg Capsules Ingested	*Dose (No. of Vials of Digibind)*
25	10
50	20
75	30
100	40
150	60
200	80

- Estimated fab fragments dose based on serum digoxin concentration (*Digibind*):

	Wt	*Serum Digoxin Concentration (ng/mL)*						
	(kg)	*1*	*2*	*4*	*8*	*12*	*16*	*20*
Pediatric patients (dose in mg)	1	0.4	1	1.5	3	5	6	8
	3	1	2	5	9	14	18	23
	5	2	4	8	15	23	30	38
	10	4	8	15	30	46	61	76
	20	8	15	30	61	91	122	152
Adults (dose in vials)	40	0.5	1	2	3	5	7	8
	60	0.5	1	3	5	7	10	12
	70	1	2	3	6	9	11	14
	80	1	2	3	7	10	13	16
	100	1	2	4	8	12	16	20

DigiFab

- Estimated fab fragment dose based on amount of digoxin ingested:

Estimated Number of 0.25-mg Tablets or 0.2-mg Capsules Ingested	*Dose (Number of Vials of DigiFab)*
25	10
50	20
75	30
100	40
150	60
200	80

- Estimated fab fragments dose based on serum digoxin concentration (*DigiFab*):

	Wt (kg)	*Serum Digoxin Concentration (ng/mL)* 1	2	4	8	12	16	20
Pediatric patients **(dose in mg)***	1	0.4	1	1.5	3	5	6.5	8
	3	1	2.5	5	10	14	19	24
	5	2	4	8	16	24	32	40
	10	4	8	16	32	48	64	80
	20	8	16	32	64	96	128	160
Adults **(dose in vials)**	40	0.5	1	2	3	5	7	8
	60	0.5	1	3	5	7	10	12
	70	1	2	3	6	9	11	14
	80	1	2	3	7	10	13	16
	100	1	2	4	8	12	16	20

* Dilution of reconstituted vial to 1 mg/mL is desirable.

Equations also are available for calculating exact dosage from serum digoxin concentrations.

Pharmacokinetics

Route	*Onset*	*Duration*
IV	15–30 min	4–6 hr

Metabolism: $T_{1/2}$: 15–20 hr
Distribution: May cross placenta; may enter breast milk
Excretion: Urine

IV FACTS

Preparation: Dissolve the contents in each vial with 4 mL of sterile water for injection. Mix gently to give an approximate isosmotic solution with a protein concentration of 10 mg/mL (*DigiFab*) or 9.5 mg/mL (*Digibind*). Use reconstituted solution promptly. Store in refrigerator for up to 4 hr. Discard after that time. Reconstituted solution may be further diluted with sterile isotonic saline.
Infusion: Administer IV over 30 min. Use a 0.22-micron filter for *Digibind*; administer as a bolus injection if cardiac arrest is imminent.

Adverse effects

- **CV:** *Low cardiac output states,* heart failure, rapid ventricular response in patients with atrial fibrillation
- **Hematologic:** Hypokalemia due to reactivation of Na^+, K^+, ATPase
- **Hypersensitivity:** Allergic reactions: Drug fever to **anaphylaxis**

■ Nursing considerations

Assessment

- **History:** Allergy to sheep products, digoxin drug history, lactation, pregnancy
- **Physical:** P, BP, auscultation, baseline ECG, serum digoxin levels, serum electrolytes

Interventions

⊗ ***Warning*** Check dosage carefully before administering. The two available brand names have slightly different recommended doses. Distinguish between *Digibind* and *DigiFab.*

- Arrange for serum digoxin concentration determinations before administration when possible.
- Monitor patient's cardiac response to digoxin overdose and therapy—cardiac rhythm, serum electrolytes, T, BP.
- Keep life-support equipment and emergency drugs (IV inotropes) readily available for severe overdose.

⊗ ***Warning*** Do not redigitalize patient until digoxin immune-fab has been cleared from the body; several days to a week or longer in cases of renal insufficiency. Serum digoxin levels will be very high and will be unreliable for up to 3 days after administration.

Teaching points

- Report muscle cramps, dizziness, palpitations.

▽ dihydroergotamine mesylate

See Appendix W, *Less commonly used drugs*.

▽ diltiazem hydrochloride

(dil tye' a zem)

Apo-Diltiaz (CAN), Apo-Diltiaz CD (CAN) DNC, Apo-Diltiaz SR (CAN) DNC, Cardizem, Cardizem CD DNC, Cardizem LA DNC, Cartia XT DNC, Dilacor XR DNC, Dilt-CD DNC, Dilt-XR DNC, Diltia XT DNC, Diltzac DNC, Gen-Diltiazem (CAN), Gen-Diltiazem CD (CAN) DNC, Novo-Diltiazem (CAN), Novo-Diltiazem CD (CAN) DNC, Nu-Diltiaz (CAN), Nu-Diltiaz-CD (CAN) DNC, ratio-Diltiazem (CAN), Taztia XT DNC, Tiazac DNC

PREGNANCY CATEGORY C

Drug classes

Antianginal
Antihypertensive
Calcium channel blocker

Therapeutic actions

Inhibits the movement of calcium ions across the membranes of cardiac and arterial muscle cells, resulting in the depression of impulse formation in specialized cardiac pacemaker cells, slowing of the velocity of conduction of the cardiac impulse, depression of myocardial contractility, and dilation of coronary arteries and arterioles and peripheral arterioles; these effects lead to decreased cardiac work, decreased cardiac energy consumption, and in patients with vasospastic (Prinzmetal's) angina, increased delivery of oxygen to myocardial cells.

Indications

- Angina pectoris due to coronary artery spasm (Prinzmetal's variant angina)
- Effort-associated angina; chronic stable angina in patients not controlled by beta-adrenergic blockers, nitrates
- ER and SR forms only: Essential hypertension
- Parenteral: Paroxysmal supraventricular tachycardia, atrial fibrillation, atrial flutter

Contraindications and cautions

- Contraindicated with allergy to diltiazem, impaired hepatic or renal function, sick sinus syndrome, heart block (second or third degree), severe hypertension, cardiogenic shock, acute MI with cardiogenic shock (oral), lactation.

Available forms

Tablets—30, 60, 90, 120 mg; ER capsules DNC—60, 90, 120, 180, 240, 300, 360, 420 mg; ER tablets DNC—120, 180, 240, 300, 360, 420 mg; injection—5 mg/mL; powder for injection—25 mg

Dosages

Evaluate patient carefully to determine the appropriate dose of this drug.

Adults

Initially, 30 mg PO qid before meals and at bedtime; gradually increase dose at 1- to 2-day intervals to 180–360 mg PO in three to four divided doses.

ER

Cardizem CD and Cartia XT: 180–240 mg daily PO for hypertension; 120–180 mg daily PO for angina.

Cardizem LA: 120–540 mg daily PO for hypertension; 180-360 mg/day PO for chronic, stable angina. May be given with nitroglycerin or nitrate therapy.

Dilacor XR, Diltia XT, Dilt-CD, and Dilt-XR: 180–240 mg daily PO as needed; up to 480 mg has been used.

Tiazac: 120–240 mg daily PO for hypertension—once daily dose; 120–180 mg PO once daily for angina.

IV

Direct IV bolus: 0.25 mg/kg (20 mg for the average patient); second bolus of 0.35 mg/kg.

Continuous IV infusion: 5–10 mg/hr with increases up to 15 mg/hr; may be continued for up to 24 hr.

Pediatric patients

Safety and efficacy not established.

Pharmacokinetics

Route	*Onset*	*Peak*
Oral	30–60 min	2–3 hr
ER	30–60 min	6–11 hr
IV	Immediate	2–3 min

Metabolism: Hepatic; $T_{1/2}$: 3.5–6 hr; 5–7 hr (ER)
Distribution: May cross placenta; enters breast milk
Excretion: Urine

IV FACTS

Preparation: For continuous infusion, transfer to normal saline, D_5W, D_5W/0.45% sodium chloride as below. Mix thoroughly. Use within 24 hr. Keep refrigerated.

Diluent Volume (mL)	*Quantity of Injection*	*Final Concentration (mg/mL)*	*Dose (mg/hr)*	*Infusion Rate (mL/hr)*
100	125 mg	1	10	10
	(25 mL)	—	15	15
250	250 mg	0.83	10	12
	(50 mL)	—	15	18
500	250 mg	0.45	10	22
	(50 mL)	—	15	33

Infusion: Administer bolus dose over 2 min. For continuous infusion, rate of 10 mg/hr is the recommended rate. Do not use continuous infusion longer than 24 hr.
Incompatibility: Do not mix in the same solution with furosemide solution.

Adverse effects

- **CNS:** *Dizziness, light-headedness, headache, asthenia,* fatigue
- **CV:** *Peripheral edema,* hypotension, arrhythmias, *bradycardia, AV block,* **asystole**
- **Dermatologic:** *Flushing,* rash
- **GI:** *Nausea,* hepatic injury, reflux

Interactions

✱ **Drug-drug** • Increased serum levels and toxicity of cyclosporine if taken with diltiazem • Possible depression of myocardial contractility, AV conduction if combined with beta blockers; use caution and monitor patient closely
✱ **Drug-food** • Decreased metabolism and increased risk of toxic effects if taken with grapefruit juice; avoid this combination

■ Nursing considerations

Assessment

- **History:** Allergy to diltiazem, impaired hepatic or renal function, sick sinus syndrome, heart block, lactation, pregnancy
- **Physical:** Skin lesions, color, edema; P, BP, baseline ECG, peripheral perfusion, auscultation; R, adventitious sounds; liver evaluation, normal output; LFTs, renal function tests, urinalysis

Interventions

- Monitor patient carefully (BP, cardiac rhythm, and output) while drug is being titrated to therapeutic dose; dosage may be increased more rapidly in hospitalized patients under close supervision.
- Monitor BP carefully if patient is on concurrent doses of nitrates.
- Monitor cardiac rhythm regularly during stabilization of dosage and periodically during long-term therapy.
- Ensure patient swallows ER or SR preparations whole; do not cut, crush, or chew.

Teaching points

- Swallow extended-release and long-acting preparations whole; do not cut, crush, or chew; do not drink grapefruit juice while using this drug.
- You may experience these side effects: Nausea, vomiting (eat frequent small meals); headache (regulate light, noise, and temperature; medicate if severe).
- Report irregular heart beat, shortness of breath, swelling of the hands or feet, pronounced dizziness, constipation.

▽ dimenhydrinate

*(dye men **hye'** dri nate)*

Oral preparations: Apo-Dimenhydrinate (CAN), Children's Dramamine, Dimetabs, Dramamine, Gravol (CAN), Triptone
Parenteral preparations: Dinate, Dramanate, Dymenate

PREGNANCY CATEGORY B

Drug classes

Anticholinergic
Antihistamine
Anti–motion-sickness drug

Therapeutic actions

Antihistamine with antiemetic and anticholinergic activity; depresses hyperstimulated labyrinthine function; may block synapses in the vomiting center; peripheral anticholinergic effects may contribute to anti–motion-sickness efficacy.

Indications

- Prevention and treatment of nausea, vomiting, or vertigo of motion sickness

Contraindications and cautions

- Contraindicated with allergy to dimenhydrinate or its components, lactation.
- Use cautiously with narrow-angle glaucoma, stenosing peptic ulcer, symptomatic prostatic hypertrophy, bronchial asthma, bladder neck obstruction, pyloroduodenal obstruction, cardiac arrhythmias, pregnancy.

Available forms

Tablets—50 mg; chewable tablets—50 mg; injection—50 mg/mL; liquid—12.5 mg/4 mL, 12.5 mg/5 mL; 15.62 mg/5 mL

Dosages

Adults

Oral

50–100 mg every 4–6 hr PO; for prophylaxis, first dose should be taken 30 min before exposure to motion. Do not exceed 400 mg in 24 hr.

Parenteral

50 mg IM as needed; 50 mg in 10 mL sodium chloride injection given IV over 2 min.

Pediatric patients 6–12 yr

25–50 mg PO every 6–8 hr, not to exceed 150 mg/day.

Pediatric patients 2–6 yr

Up to 25 mg PO every 6–8 hr, not to exceed 75 mg/day.

Pediatric patients younger than 2 yr

Only on advice of physician; 1.25 mg/kg IM qid, not to exceed 300 mg/day.

Neonates

Contraindicated.

Geriatric patients

Can cause dizziness, sedation, syncope, confusion, and hypotension in elderly patients; use with caution.

Pharmacokinetics

Route	Onset	Peak	Duration
Oral	15–30 min	2 hr	3–6 hr
IM	20–30 min	1–2 hr	3–6 hr
IV	Immediate	1–2 hr	3–6 hr

Metabolism: Hepatic; $T_{1/2}$: Unknown
Distribution: May cross placenta; enters breast milk
Excretion: Urine

IV FACTS

Preparation: Dilute 50 mg in 10 mL sodium chloride injection.
Infusion: Administer by direct IV injection over 2 min.
Incompatibilities: Do not combine with tetracycline, thiopental.
Y-site incompatibilities: Do not mix with aminophylline, heparin, hydrocortisone, hydroxyzine, phenobarbital, phenytoin, prednisolone, promethazine.

Adverse effects

- **CNS:** *Drowsiness, confusion, nervousness, restlessness, headache, dizziness, vertigo, lassitude, tingling, heaviness and weakness of hands; insomnia* and excitement (especially in children), hallucinations, seizures, **death,** blurring of vision, diplopia
- **CV:** Hypotension, palpitations, tachycardia
- **Dermatologic:** Urticaria, drug rash, photosensitivity
- **GI:** Epigastric distress, anorexia, nausea, vomiting, diarrhea or constipation; dryness of mouth, nose, and throat
- **GU:** Urinary hesitancy, urinary retention
- **Respiratory:** Nasal stuffiness, chest tightness, thickening of bronchial secretions
- **Other: Anaphylaxis;** in geriatric patients may cause mental status changes, excessive sedation, constipation; in men, may cause urinary retention

Interactions
✱ **Drug-drug** • Increased depressant effects with alcohol, other CNS depressants

■ Nursing considerations
Assessment
- **History:** Allergy to dimenhydrinate or its components, lactation, narrow-angle glaucoma, stenosing peptic ulcer, symptomatic prostatic hypertrophy, bronchial asthma, bladder neck obstruction, pyloroduodenal obstruction, cardiac arrhythmias
- **Physical:** Skin color, lesions, texture; orientation, reflexes, affect; vision examination; P, BP; R, adventitious sounds; bowel sounds; prostate palpation; CBC

Interventions
⊗ ***Warning*** Keep epinephrine 1:1,000 readily available when using parenteral preparations; hypersensitivity reactions, including anaphylaxis, have occurred.

Teaching points
- Take drug as prescribed; avoid excessive dosage.
- Drug works best if taken before motion sickness occurs.
- Avoid alcohol; serious sedation could occur.
- You may experience these side effects: Dizziness, sedation, drowsiness (use caution if driving or performing tasks that require alertness); epigastric distress, diarrhea or constipation (take drug with food); dry mouth (use frequent mouth care, suck sugarless lozenges); thickening of bronchial secretions, dryness of nasal mucosa (try another motion sickness remedy).
- Report difficulty breathing, hallucinations, tremors, loss of coordination, unusual bleeding or bruising, visual disturbances, irregular heartbeat.

▽ dimercaprol

See Appendix X, *Less commonly used drugs*.

▽ dinoprostone (prostaglandin E_2)

*(dye noe **prost'** ohn)*

Cervidil, Prepidil, Prostin E2

PREGNANCY CATEGORY C

Drug classes
Abortifacient
Prostaglandin

Therapeutic actions
Stimulates the myometrium of the pregnant uterus to contract, similar to the contractions of the uterus during labor, thus evacuating the contents of the uterus.

Indications
- Termination of pregnancy 12–20 wk from the first day of the last menstrual period
- Evacuation of the uterus in the management of missed abortion or intrauterine fetal death up to 28 wk gestational age
- Management of nonmetastatic gestational trophoblastic disease (benign hydatidiform mole)
- Initiation of cervical ripening before induction of labor

Contraindications and cautions
- Contraindicated with allergy to prostaglandin preparations; acute PID; active cardiac, hepatic, pulmonary, renal disease; women in whom prolonged uterine contractions are inappropriate (eg, caesarean delivery, uterine surgery, fetal distress, obstetric emergency).
- Use cautiously with history of asthma; hypotension; hypertension; CV, adrenal, renal, or hepatic disease; anemia; jaundice; diabetes; epilepsy; scarred uterus; cervicitis, infected endocervical lesions, acute vaginitis.

Available forms
Vaginal suppository—20 mg; vaginal gel—0.5 mg; vaginal insert—10 mg

Dosages

Adults

- *Termination of pregnancy:* Insert one suppository (20 mg) high into the vagina; keep supine for 10 min after insertion. Additional suppositories may be given at 3- to 5-hr intervals based on uterine response and tolerance. Do not give longer than 2 days.
- *Cervical ripening:* Give 0.5 mg gel via provided cervical catheter with patient in the dorsal position and cervix visualized using a speculum. Repeat dose may be given if no response in 6 hr. Wait 6–12 hr before beginning oxytocin IV to initiate labor. Insert: Place one insert transversely in the posterior fornix of the vagina. Keep patient supine for 2 hr; one insert delivers 0.3 mg/hr over 12 hr. Remove, using retrieval system, at onset of active labor or 12 hr after insertion.

Pharmacokinetics

Route	*Onset*	*Peak*	*Duration*
Intravaginal	10 min	30–45 min	2–3 hr

Metabolism: Tissue; $T_{1/2}$: 5–10 hr
Distribution: May cross placenta; may enter breast milk
Excretion: Urine

Adverse effects

- **CNS:** *Headache,* paresthesias, anxiety, weakness, syncope, dizziness
- **CV:** *Hypotension,* arrhythmias, chest pain
- **Fetal:** Abnormal heart rates
- **GI:** *Vomiting, diarrhea, nausea*
- **GU:** Endometritis, perforated uterus, uterine rupture, uterine or vaginal pain, incomplete abortion
- **Respiratory:** Coughing, dyspnea
- **Other:** Chills, diaphoresis, backache, breast tenderness, eye pain, skin rash, pyrexia

■ Nursing considerations

CLINICAL ALERT!

Name confusion has occurred among *Prostin VR Pediatric* (alprostadil), *Prostin FZ* (dinoprost—available outside the US), *Prostin E$_2$* (dinoprostone), and *Prostin 15* (carboprost in Europe). Confusion has also been reported with Prepidil (dinoprostone) and bepridil. Use extreme caution.

Assessment

- **History:** Allergy to prostaglandin preparations; acute PID; active cardiac, hepatic, pulmonary, renal disease; history of asthma; hypotension; hypertension; anemia; jaundice; diabetes; epilepsy; scarred uterus; cervicitis, infected endocervical lesions, acute vaginitis
- **Physical:** T; BP, P, auscultation; R, adventitious sounds; bowel sounds, liver evaluation; vaginal discharge, pelvic examination, uterine tone; LFTs, renal function tests, WBC, urinalysis, CBC

Interventions

- Store suppositories in freezer; bring to room temperature before insertion.
- Store cervical gel in refrigerator. Gel is stable for 24 mo at 2°–8°C
- Arrange for pre- or concurrent treatment with antiemetic and antidiarrheal drugs to decrease the incidence of GI side effects.
- Ensure that abortion is complete or that other measures are used to complete the abortion if drug effects are not sufficient.
- Monitor temperature, using care to differentiate prostaglandin-induced pyrexia from postabortion endometritis pyrexia.
- Give gel using aseptic technique via cervical catheter to patient in dorsal position. Patient should remain in this position 15–30 min.
- Monitor uterine tone and vaginal discharge throughout procedure and several days after the procedure.
- Ensure adequate hydration throughout procedure.
- Be prepared to support patient through labor (cervical ripening). Give oxytocin infusion 6–12 hr after dinoprostone.

Teaching points

- If you have never had a vaginal suppository, a health care provider will explain the procedure. You will need to lie down for 10 minutes after insertion.
- You will need to stay on your side for 15–30 minutes after injection of gel.
- You may experience these side effects: Nausea, vomiting, diarrhea, uterine or vaginal pain, fever, headache, weakness, dizziness.
- Report severe pain, difficulty breathing, palpitations, eye pain, rash.

diphenhydramine hydrochloride

(dye fen ***bye'*** *dra meen)*

Oral: Allerdryl (CAN), AllerMax Caplets, Banophen, Banophen Allergy, Benadryl Allergy, Diphen AF, Diphenhist, Diphenhist Captabs, Genahist, Siladryl

Oral prescription preparations: Benadryl

Parenteral preparations: Benadryl

PREGNANCY CATEGORY B

Drug classes

Antihistamine
Anti–motion-sickness drug
Antiparkinsonian
Cough suppressant
Sedative-hypnotic

Therapeutic actions

Competitively blocks the effects of histamine at H_1-receptor sites, has atropine-like, antipruritic, and sedative effects.

Indications

- Relief of symptoms associated with perennial and seasonal allergic rhinitis; vasomotor rhinitis; allergic conjunctivitis; mild, uncomplicated urticaria and angioedema; amelioration of allergic reactions to blood or plasma; dermatographism; adjunctive therapy in anaphylactic reactions
- Active and prophylactic treatment of motion sickness
- Nighttime sleep aid
- Parkinsonism (including drug-induced parkinsonism and extrapyramidal reactions), in the elderly intolerant of more potent drugs, for milder forms of the disorder in other age-groups, and in combination with centrally acting anticholinergic antiparkinsonian drugs
- Syrup formulation: Suppression of cough due to colds or allergy

Contraindications and cautions

- Contraindicated with allergy to antihistamines, third trimester of pregnancy, lactation.
- Use cautiously with narrow-angle glaucoma, stenosing peptic ulcer, symptomatic prostatic hypertrophy, asthmatic attack, bladder neck obstruction, pyloroduodenal obstruction, pregnancy; elderly patients who may be sensitive to anticholinergic effects.

Available forms

Capsule soft gels—25 mg; capsules—25, 50 mg; tablets—25, 50 mg; chewable tablets—12.5 mg; elixir—12.5 mg/5 mL; syrup—12.5 mg/5 mL; liquid—12.5 mg/5 mL; injection—10, 50 mg/mL; solution—12.5 mg/5 mL

Dosages

Adults

Oral

25–50 mg every 4–6 hr PO, not to exceed 300 mg/24 hr.

- *Motion sickness:* Give full dose prophylactically 30 min before exposure to motion, and repeat before meals and at bedtime.
- *Nighttime sleep aid:* 25–50 mg PO at bedtime.
- *Cough suppression:* 25 mg every 4 hr PO, not to exceed 150 mg in 24 hr.

Parenteral

10–50 mg IV or deep IM or up to 100 mg if required. Maximum daily dose is 400 mg.

Pediatric patients

Oral

2–6 yr: 12.5–25 mg PO every 12 hr.
6–12 yr: 12.5–25 mg tid–qid PO or 5 mg/kg/day PO or 150 mg/m^2 per day PO. Maximum daily dose, 300 mg.

- *Motion sickness:* Give full dose prophylactically 30 min before exposure to motion and repeat before meals and at bedtime.
- *Cough suppression:*
  2–6 yr: 6.25 mg every 4 hr, not to exceed 25 mg in 24 hr.
  6–12 yr: 12.5 mg every 4 hr PO, not to exceed 75 mg in 24 hr.

Parenteral

5 mg/kg/day or 150 mg/m^2 per day IV or by deep IM injection. Maximum daily dose is 300 mg divided into four doses.

Geriatric patients

More likely to cause dizziness, sedation, syncope, toxic confusional states, and hypotension in elderly patients; use with caution.

Pharmacokinetics

Route	*Onset*	*Peak*	*Duration*
Oral	15–30 min	1–4 hr	4–7 hr
IM	20–30 min	1–4 hr	4–8 hr
IV	Rapid	30–60 min	4–8 hr

Metabolism: Hepatic; $T_{1/2}$: 2.5–7 hr
Distribution: May cross placenta; may enter breast milk
Excretion: Urine

IV FACTS

Preparation: No additional preparation required.
Infusion: Administer slowly each 25 mg over 1 min by direct injection or into tubing of running IV.
Incompatibilities: Do not combine with amobarbital, amphotericin B, hydrocortisone, phenobarbital, phenytoin, thiopental.
Y-site incompatibility: Do not mix with foscarnet.

Adverse effects

- **CNS:** *Drowsiness, sedation, dizziness, disturbed coordination,* fatigue, confusion, restlessness, excitation, nervousness, tremor, headache, blurred vision, diplopia
- **CV:** Hypotension, palpitations, bradycardia, tachycardia, extrasystoles
- **GI:** *Epigastric distress,* anorexia, increased appetite and weight gain, nausea, vomiting, diarrhea or constipation
- **GU:** Urinary frequency, dysuria, urinary retention, early menses, decreased libido, impotence
- **Hematologic: Hemolytic anemia, hypoplastic anemia, thrombocytopenia, leukopenia, agranulocytosis, pancytopenia**
- **Respiratory:** *Thickening of bronchial secretions,* chest tightness, wheezing, nasal stuffiness, dry mouth, dry nose, dry throat, sore throat
- **Other:** Urticaria, rash, **anaphylactic shock,** photosensitivity, excessive perspiration

Interactions

✱ **Drug-drug** • Possible increased and prolonged anticholinergic effects with MAOIs • Risk of increased sedation with alcohol, CNS depressants; avoid this combination

■ Nursing considerations

Assessment

- **History:** Allergy to any antihistamines, narrow-angle glaucoma, stenosing peptic ulcer, symptomatic prostatic hypertrophy, asthmatic attack, bladder neck obstruction, pyloroduodenal obstruction, third trimester of pregnancy, lactation
- **Physical:** Skin color, lesions, texture; orientation, reflexes, affect; vision examination; P, BP; R, adventitious sounds; bowel sounds; prostate palpation; CBC with differential

Interventions

- Administer with food if GI upset occurs.
- Administer syrup form if patient is unable to take tablets.
- Monitor patient response, and arrange for adjustment of dosage to lowest possible effective dose.

Teaching points

- Take as prescribed; avoid excessive dosage.
- Take with food if GI upset occurs.
- Avoid alcohol; serious sedation could occur.
- These side effects may occur: Dizziness, sedation, drowsiness (use caution driving or performing tasks requiring alertness); epigastric distress, diarrhea or constipation (take drug with meals); dry mouth (use frequent mouth care, suck sugarless lozenges); thickening of bronchial secretions, dryness of nasal mucosa (use a humidifier).
- Report difficulty breathing, hallucinations, tremors, loss of coordination, unusual bleeding or bruising, visual disturbances, irregular heartbeat.

dipyridamole

See Appendix W, *Less commonly used drugs*.

disopyramide phosphate

(dye soe ***peer'*** *a mide)*

Norpace, Norpace CR (DNC), Rythmodan (CAN), Rythmodan-LA (CAN) (DNC)

PREGNANCY CATEGORY C

Drug class

Antiarrhythmic

Therapeutic actions

Type 1a antiarrhythmic: Decreases rate of diastolic depolarization, decreases automaticity, decreases the rate of rise of the action potential, prolongs the refractory period of cardiac muscle cells.

Indications

- Treatment of ventricular arrhythmias considered to be life-threatening
- Unlabeled use: Treatment of paroxysmal supraventricular tachycardia

Contraindications and cautions

- Contraindicated with cardiogenic shock, allergy to disopyramide, cardiac conduction abnormalities (eg, Wolff-Parkinson-White syndrome, sick sinus syndrome, heart block, prolonged QT interval).
- Use cautiously with heart failure, hypotension, cardiac myopathies, urinary retention, glaucoma, myasthenia gravis, renal or hepatic disease, potassium imbalance, pregnancy, lactation.

Available forms

Capsules—100, 150 mg; CR capsules (DNC)—100, 150 mg; ER tablets (DNC)—150 mg (CAN)

Dosages

Evaluate patient carefully and monitor cardiac response closely to determine the correct dosage for each patient.

Adults

400–800 mg/day PO given in divided doses every 6 hr or every 12 hr if using the CR products.

- *Rapid control of ventricular arrhythmias:* 300 mg PO (immediate release). If no response within 6 hr, give 200 mg PO every 6 hr; may increase to 250–300 mg every 6 hr if no response in 48 hr.
- *Patients with cardiomyopathy:* No loading dose, 100 mg PO every 6–8 hr (immediate release).

Pediatric patients

Give in equal, divided doses every 6 hr PO, adjusting the dose to the patient's need.

Age	*Daily Dosage (mg/kg)*
Younger than 1 yr	10–30
1–4 yr	10–20
4–12 yr	10–15
12–18 yr	6–15

Patients with renal impairment

Loading dose of 150 mg PO may be given, followed by 100 mg at the intervals shown.

Creatinine Clearance (mL/min)	*Interval*
30–40	Every 8 hr
15–30	Every 12 hr
Less than 15	Every 24 hr

Pharmacokinetics

Route	*Onset*	*Peak*	*Duration*
Oral	30–60 min	2 hr	1.5–8.5 hr

Metabolism: Hepatic; $T_{1/2}$: 4–10 hr
Distribution: Crosses placenta; enters breast milk
Excretion: Urine

Adverse effects

- **CNS:** Dizziness, fatigue, headache, *blurred vision*
- **CV:** Heart failure, hypotension, cardiac conduction disturbances
- **GI:** *Dry mouth, constipation,* nausea, abdominal pain, gas
- **GU:** *Urinary hesitancy and retention, impotence*
- **Other:** *Dry nose, eyes, and throat; rash; itching; muscle weakness; malaise; aches and pains*

Interactions

✱ **Drug-drug** • Decreased disopyramide plasma levels if used with phenytoins, rifampin • Risk of increased disopyramide effects with antiarrhythmics, erythromycin, quinidine

■ Nursing considerations

Assessment

- **History:** Allergy to disopyramide, heart failure, hypotension, Wolff-Parkinson-White syndrome, sick sinus syndrome, heart block, cardiac myopathies, urinary retention, glaucoma, myasthenia gravis, renal or hepatic disease, potassium imbalance, labor or delivery, lactation, pregnancy
- **Physical:** Weight; orientation, reflexes; P, BP, auscultation, ECG, edema; R, adventitious sounds; bowel sounds, liver evaluation; urinalysis, LFTs, renal function tests, blood glucose, serum K^+

Interventions

⊗ ***Black box warning*** Monitor patient for possible refractory arrhythmias that can be life-threatening; reserve use for life-threatening arrhythmias.

- Check that patients with supraventricular tachyarrhythmias have been digitalized before starting disopyramide.
- Reduce dosage in patients weighing less than 110 lb.
- Reduce dosage in patients with hepatic or renal failure.
- Monitor patients with severe refractory tachycardia, who may be given up to 1,600 mg/day continuously.
- Make a pediatric suspension form (1–10 mg/mL) by adding contents of the immediate-release capsule to cherry syrup, if desired. Store in amber glass bottle, and refrigerate. Shake well before using. Stable for 1 mo.
- Take care to differentiate the CR form from the immediate-release preparation. Ensure that patient swallows CR form whole; do not cut, crush, or chew.
- Monitor BP, orthostatic pressure.

⊗ ***Warning*** Evaluate for safe and effective serum levels (2–8 mcg/mL).

Teaching points

- You will require frequent monitoring of cardiac rhythm and blood pressure.
- Swallow controlled-release capsules whole; do not cut, crush, or chew.
- Take missed dose as soon as possible, unless within 4 hours of next dose. Do not double up on next dose.
- Do not stop taking this drug for any reason without consulting your health care provider.
- Return for regular follow-up visits to check your heart rhythm and blood pressure.
- You may experience these side effects: Dry mouth (try frequent mouth care, suck sugarless lozenges); constipation (laxatives may be ordered); difficulty voiding (empty the bladder before taking drug); muscle weakness or aches and pains.
- Report swelling of fingers or ankles, difficulty breathing, dizziness, urinary retention, severe headache or visual changes.

▽ disulfiram

(dye ***sul'*** *fi ram)*

Antabuse

PREGNANCY CATEGORY C

Drug classes

Antialcoholic drug
Enzyme inhibitor

Therapeutic actions

Inhibits the enzyme aldehyde dehydrogenase, blocking oxidation of alcohol and allowing acetaldehyde to accumulate to concentrations in the blood 5–10 times higher than normally achieved during alcohol metabolism; accumulation of acetaldehyde produces the highly unpleasant reaction described below that deters consumption of alcohol.

Indications

- Aids in the management of selected chronic alcoholics who want to remain in a state of enforced sobriety

Contraindications and cautions

- Contraindicated with allergy to disulfiram or other thiuram derivatives used in pesticides and rubber vulcanization, severe myocardial disease or coronary occlusion; psychoses, current or recent treatment

with metronidazole, paraldehyde, alcohol, alcohol-containing preparations (eg, cough syrups), pregnancy.
- Use cautiously with diabetes mellitus, hypothyroidism, epilepsy, cerebral damage, chronic and acute nephritis, hepatic cirrhosis or impairment.

Available forms

Tablets—250 mg

Dosages

Black box warning Never administer to an intoxicated patient or without patient's knowledge. Do not administer until patient has abstained from alcohol for at least 12 hr.

Adults

- *Initial dosage:* Administer maximum of 500 mg/day PO in a single dose for 1–2 wk. If a sedative effect occurs, administer at bedtime or decrease dosage.
- *Maintenance regimen:* 125–500 mg/day PO. Do not exceed 500 mg/day. Continue use until patient fully recovers socially and has basis for permanent self-control.
- *Trial with alcohol (do not give to anyone older than 50 yr):* After 1–2 wk of therapy with 500 mg/day PO, a drink of 15 mL of 100-proof whiskey or its equivalent is taken slowly. Dose may be repeated once, if patient is hospitalized and support facility is available.

Pharmacokinetics

Route	Onset	Peak	Duration
Oral	Slow	12 hr	1–2 wk

Metabolism: Hepatic; $T_{1/2}$: Unclear
Distribution: Crosses placenta; enters breast milk
Excretion: Feces, lungs

Adverse effects

Disulfiram with alcohol

- **CNS:** Throbbing headaches, syncope, weakness, vertigo, confusion, seizures, unconsciousness, throbbing in head and neck
- **CV:** Flushing, chest pain, palpitations, tachycardia, hypotension, **arrhythmias, CV collapse, acute heart failure, MI**
- **Dermatologic:** Sweating
- **EENT:** Blurred vision
- **GI:** Nausea, copious vomiting, thirst
- **Respiratory:** Respiratory difficulty, dyspnea, hyperventilation
- **Other: Death**

Disulfiram alone

- **CNS:** *Drowsiness, fatigability, headache,* restlessness, peripheral neuropathy, optic or retrobulbar neuritis
- **Dermatologic:** *Skin eruptions,* acneiform eruptions, allergic dermatitis
- **GI:** *Metallic or garliclike aftertaste,* **hepatotoxicity**

Interactions

✷ **Drug-drug** • Increased serum levels and risk of toxicity of phenytoin and its congeners, diazepam, chlordiazepoxide • Increased therapeutic and toxic effects of theophyllines and caffeine • Increased PT caused by disulfiram may lead to a need to adjust dosage of oral anticoagulants • Severe alcohol-intolerance reactions with any alcohol-containing liquid medications (eg, elixirs, tinctures) • Acute toxic psychosis with metronidazole

■ Nursing considerations

Assessment

- **History:** Allergy to disulfiram or other thiuram derivatives; severe myocardial disease or coronary occlusion; psychoses; current or recent treatment with metronidazole, paraldehyde, alcohol, alcohol-containing preparations (eg, cough syrups, tonics); diabetes mellitus, hypothyroidism, epilepsy, cerebral damage, chronic and acute nephritis, hepatic cirrhosis or impairment; pregnancy
- **Physical:** Skin color, lesions; thyroid palpation; orientation, affect, reflexes; P, auscultation, BP; R, adventitious sounds; liver evaluation; LFTs, renal function tests, CBC, SMA-12

Interventions

- Do not administer until patient has abstained from alcohol for at least 12 hr.
- Administer orally; tablets may be crushed and mixed with liquid beverages.
- Monitor LFTs before, in 10–14 days, and every 6 mo during therapy to evaluate for hepatic impairment.
- Monitor CBC, SMA-12 before and every 6 mo during therapy.

- If patient reports ability to drink alcohol while on this drug, assume noncompliance. Directly observe drug ingestion.
- Inform patient about the seriousness of disulfiram–alcohol reaction and the potential consequences of alcohol use. Disulfiram should not be taken for at least 12 hr after alcohol ingestion, and a reaction may occur up to 2 wk after disulfiram therapy is stopped; all forms of alcohol must be avoided.
- Arrange for treatment with antihistamines if skin reaction occurs.

⊗ ***Warning*** Institute supportive measures if disulfiram-alcohol reaction occurs; oxygen, carbon dioxide combination, massive doses of vitamin C IV, ephedrine have been used.

Teaching points

- Take drug daily; if drug makes you dizzy or tired, take it at bedtime. Tablets may be crushed and mixed with liquid.
- Abstain from forms of alcohol (beer, wine, liquor, vinegars, cough mixtures, sauces, aftershave lotions, liniments, colognes, liquid medications). Using alcohol while taking this drug can cause severe, unpleasant reactions—flushing, copious vomiting, throbbing headache, difficulty breathing, even death.
- Wear or carry a medical ID while you are taking this drug to alert any medical emergency personnel that you are taking it.
- Have periodic blood tests while taking drug to evaluate its effects on the liver.
- You may experience these side effects: Drowsiness, headache, fatigue, restlessness, blurred vision (use caution driving or performing tasks that require alertness); metallic aftertaste (transient).
- Report unusual bleeding or bruising, yellowing of skin or eyes, chest pain, difficulty breathing, ingestion of any alcohol.

DANGEROUS DRUG

▽ dobutamine hydrochloride

(doe' byoo ta meen)

PREGNANCY CATEGORY B

Drug classes

Beta$_1$-selective adrenergic agonist
Sympathomimetic

Therapeutic actions

Positive inotropic effects are mediated by beta$_1$-adrenergic receptors in the heart; increases the force of myocardial contraction with relatively minor effects on heart rate, arrhythmogenesis; has minor effects on blood vessels.

Indications

- For inotropic support in the short-term treatment of adults with cardiac decompensation due to depressed contractility, resulting from either organic heart disease or from cardiac surgical procedures
- Investigational use in children with congenital heart disease undergoing diagnostic cardiac catheterization, to augment CV function

Contraindications and cautions

- Contraindicated with IHSS; hypovolemia (dobutamine is not a substitute for blood, plasma, fluids, electrolytes, which should be restored promptly when loss has occurred and in any case before treatment with dobutamine); acute MI (may increase the size of an infarct by intensifying ischemia); general anesthesia with halogenated hydrocarbons or cyclopropane, which sensitize the myocardium to catecholamines; pregnancy.
- Use cautiously with diabetes mellitus, lactation; allergy to sulfites, more common in asthmatic patients.

Available forms

Injection—12.5 mg/mL; injection in 5% dextrose injection—1 mg/mL, 2 mg/mL, 4 mg/mL

Dosages

Administer only by IV infusion using an infusion pump or other device to control the rate of flow. Titrate on the basis of the patient's hemodynamic and renal response. Close monitoring is necessary.

Adults

2.5–10 mcg/kg/min IV is usual rate to increase cardiac output; rarely, rates up to 40 mcg/kg/min are needed.

Pediatric patients

Safety and efficacy not established. When used investigationally in children undergoing cardiac catheterization (see above), doses of 2 and 7.75 mcg/kg/min were infused for 10 min.

Pharmacokinetics

Route	Onset	Peak	Duration
IV	1–2 min	Up to 10 min	Length of infusion

Metabolism: Hepatic; $T_{1/2}$: 2 min
Distribution: May cross placenta; may enter breast milk
Excretion: Urine

IV FACTS

Preparation: Dilute vials to at least 50 mL with 5% dextrose injection, 0.9% sodium chloride injection, or sodium lactate injection. Store final diluted solution in glass or Viaflex container at room temperature. Stable for 24 hr. Do not freeze. (Drug solutions may exhibit a pink color that increases with time; this indicates oxidation of the drug, not a loss of potency up to 24 hr.)
Infusion: May be administered through common IV tubing with dopamine, lidocaine, tobramycin, nitroprusside, potassium chloride, or protamine sulfate. Titrate rate based on patient response—P, BP, rhythm; use of an infusion pump is suggested.
Incompatibilities: Do not mix drug with alkaline solutions, such as 5% sodium bicarbonate injection; do not mix with hydrocortisone sodium succinate, cefazolin, penicillin, sodium ethacrynate; sodium heparin.
Y-site incompatibilities: Do not mix with acyclovir, alteplase, aminophylline, foscarnet.

Adverse effects

- **CNS:** *Headache*
- **CV:** *Increase in HR, increase in systolic BP, increase in ventricular ectopic beats (PVCs),* anginal pain, palpitations, shortness of breath
- **GI:** *Nausea*

Interactions

✱ **Drug-drug** • Increased effects with TCAs (eg, imipramine), furazolidone, methyldopa

■ Nursing considerations

CLINICAL ALERT!
Name confusion has occurred between dobutamine and dopamine; use caution.

Assessment

- **History:** IHSS, hypovolemia, acute MI, general anesthesia with halogenated hydrocarbons or cyclopropane, diabetes, lactation, pregnancy
- **Physical:** Weight, skin color, T; P, BP, pulse pressure, auscultation; R, adventitious sounds; urine output; serum electrolytes, Hct, ECG

Interventions

- Arrange to digitalize patients who have atrial fibrillation with a rapid ventricular rate before giving dobutamine—dobutamine facilitates AV conduction.

⊗ ***Warning*** Monitor urine flow, cardiac output, pulmonary wedge pressure, ECG, and BP closely during infusion; adjust dose and rate accordingly.

Teaching points

- Used only in acute emergencies; teaching depends on patient's awareness and emphasizes need for the drug.

DANGEROUS DRUG

docetaxel

*(dohs eh **tax'** ell)*

Taxotere

PREGNANCY CATEGORY D

Drug class

Antineoplastic

Therapeutic actions

Inhibits the normal dynamic reorganization of the microtubule network that is essential for dividing cells; leads to cell death in rapidly dividing cells.

Indications

- Treatment of patients with locally advanced or metastatic breast cancer after failure of prior chemotherapy
- Treatment of non–small-cell lung cancer after failure with platinum-based chemotherapy, with metastases
- First-line treatment of unresectable, locally advanced, or metastatic non–small-cell lung cancer in patients who have not received prior chemotherapy when used in combination with cisplatin
- Treatment of androgen-independent metastatic prostate cancer with prednisone
- Adjuvant post-surgery treatment of patients with operable node-positive breast cancer in combination with doxorubicin and cyclophosphamide
- Induction treatment of patients with locally advanced squamous cell carcinoma of the head and neck, in combination with cisplatin and 5-FU, before the patient undergoes chemoradiotherapy or radiotherapy
- Treatment of advanced gastric adenocarcinoma in patients who have not received chemotherapy for advanced disease with cisplatin and 5-FU
- Unlabeled uses: Esophageal, ovarian, small-cell lung, urothelial cancers

Contraindications and cautions

- Contraindicated with hypersensitivity to docetaxel or drugs using polysorbate 80; bone marrow depression with neutrophil counts less than 1,500 cells/mm^2, lactation, pregnancy.
- Use cautiously with hepatic impairment, history of treatment with platinum-based chemotherapy.

Available forms

Injection—20 mg/0.5 mL, 80 mg/2 mL

Dosages

Adults

- *Breast cancer:* 60–100 mg/m^2 IV infused over 1 hr every 3 wk.
- *Non–small-cell lung cancer:* 75 mg/m^2 IV over 1 hr every 3 wk.
- *First-line treatment of non–small-cell lung cancer:* 75 mg/m^2 of *Taxotere* given over 1 hr followed by 75 mg/m^2 cisplatin IV given over 30–60 min every 3 wk.
- *Androgen-independent metastatic prostate cancer:* 75 mg/m^2 IV every 3 wk as a 1-hr infusion with 5 mg prednisone PO bid constantly throughout therapy. Premedicate with dexamethasone 8 mg PO 12 hr, 3 hr, and 1 hr before docetaxel infusion. Reduce dosage to 60 mg/m^2 if febrile neutropenia, severe or cumulative cutaneous reactions, moderate neurosensory signs or symptoms, or neutrophil count less than 500 mm^3 occurs for longer than 1 wk. Stop therapy if reactions continue with reduced dose.
- *Operable node-positive breast cancer:* 75 mg/m^2 IV given 1 hr after doxorubicin 50 mg/m^2 and cyclophosphamide 500 mg/m^2 every 3 wk for 6 courses. Adjust dosage based on neutrophil count.
- *Induction for squamous cell cancer of the head and neck before radiotherapy:* 75 mg/m^2 as a 1-hr IV infusion followed by cisplatin 75 mg/m^2 IV over 1 hr on day 1, followed by 5-FU 750 mg/m^2/day IV for 5 days. Repeat every 3 wk for four cycles before radiotherapy starts.
- *Induction for squamous cell cancer of the head and neck before chemoradiotherapy:* 75 mg/m^2 as a 1-hr IV infusion, followed by cisplatin 100 mg/m^2 as a 30-min–3-hr infusion followed by 5-FU 1,000 mg/m^2/day as a continuous infusion on days 1–4. Administer every 3 wk for three cycles before chemoradiotherapy starts. If GI toxicity occurs, consider reducing dosage of 5-FU, docetaxol, or both.
- *Advanced gastric adenocarcinoma:* 75 mg/m^2 IV as a 1-hr infusion followed by cisplatin 75 mg/m^2 IV as a 1- to 3-hr infusion (both on day 1), followed by 5-FU 750 mg/m^2/day IV as a 24-hr infusion for 5 days. Repeat cycle every 3 wk.

Pediatric patients

Safety and efficacy not established.

Pharmacokinetics

Route	Onset	Duration
IV	Slow	20–24 hr

Metabolism: Hepatic; $T_{1/2}$: 36 min and 11.1 hr

Distribution: Crosses placenta; may enter breast milk
Excretion: Feces, urine

IV FACTS

Preparation: Dilute concentrate with provided diluent; resultant concentration is 10 mg/mL. Stand vials at room temperature for 5 min before diluting; stable at room temperature for 8 hr; refrigerate unopened vials, protect from light; avoid use of PVC infusion bags and tubing. Final dilution: Add to 250 mL normal saline solution or 5% dextrose injection; final concentration is 0.3–0.74 mg/mL. Premedicate patient with oral corticosteroids before beginning infusion.
Infusion: Administer over 1 hr.

Adverse effects

- **CNS:** Neurosensory disturbances, including paresthesias, pain, *asthenia*
- **CV:** Sinus tachycardia, hypotension, arrhythmias, **fluid retention**
- **GI:** *Nausea, vomiting, diarrhea, stomatitis,* constipation
- **Hematologic: Bone marrow depression,** *infection*
- **Other:** *Hypersensitivity reactions, myalgia, arthralgia, alopecia*

Interactions

✱ **Drug-drug** • Possible increase in effectiveness and toxicity with cyclosporine, ketoconazole, erythromycin; avoid these combinations • Avoid giving live vaccines within 3 mo of administration because of immunosuppression

■ Nursing considerations

CLINICAL ALERT!
Name confusion has occurred between *Taxotere* (docetaxel) and *Taxol* (paclitaxel). Serious adverse effects can occur; use extreme caution.

Assessment

- **History:** Hypersensitivity to docetaxel, polysorbate 80; bone marrow depression; hepatic impairment, pregnancy, lactation
- **Physical:** Neurologic status, T; P, BP, peripheral perfusion; abdominal examination, mucous membranes; LFTs, CBC

Interventions

⊠ ***Black box warning*** Do not give drug unless blood counts are within acceptable parameters (neutrophils exceed 1,500 cells/m^2).
⊗ ***Warning*** Handle drug with great care; wearing gloves is recommended; if drug comes into contact with skin, wash immediately with soap and water.
⊗ ***Warning*** Premedicate patient before administration with oral corticosteroids (eg, dexamethasone 16 mg/day PO for 3 days starting 1 day before docetaxel administration) to reduce severity of fluid retention.

- Monitor BP and P during administration.
- Arrange for blood counts before and regularly during therapy.
- Monitor patient's neurologic status frequently during treatment; provide safety measures as needed.

⊠ ***Black box warning*** Do not give with hepatic impairment; increased risk of toxicity and death. Monitor LFTs carefully.
⊠ ***Black box warning*** Monitor patient for hypersensitivity reactions, possibly severe; do not give with history of hypersensitivity.
⊠ ***Black box warning*** Monitor patient carefully for fluid retention and treat accordingly.

Teaching points

- This drug is given IV once every 3 weeks; mark calendar with days to return for treatment.
- You may experience these side effects: Nausea and vomiting (if severe, antiemetics may be helpful; eat frequent small meals); weakness, lethargy (take frequent rest periods); increased susceptibility to infection (avoid crowds, exposure to many people or diseases); numbness and tingling in fingers or toes (avoid injury to these areas; use care if performing tasks that require precision); loss of hair (arrange for a wig or other head covering; keep the head covered at extremes of temperature).
- Report severe nausea and vomiting; fever, chills, sore throat; unusual bleeding or bruising; numbness or tingling in fingers or toes; fluid retention or swelling.

dofetilide

(doe fe' ti lyed)

Tikosyn

PREGNANCY CATEGORY C

Drug class

Antiarrhythmic

Therapeutic actions

Selectively blocks potassium channels, widening the QRS complex and prolonging the action potential; has no effect on calcium channels or cardiac contraction; Class III antiarrhythmic.

Indications

- Conversion of atrial fibrillation or flutter to normal sinus rhythm
- Maintenance of normal sinus rhythm in patients with atrial fibrillation or flutter of more than 1-week's duration who have been converted to sinus rhythm

Contraindications and cautions

- Contraindicated with hypersensitivity to dofetilide, ibutilide; second- or third-degree AV heart block; prolonged QT intervals; lactation.
- Use cautiously with ventricular arrhythmias, renal impairment, severe hepatic impairment, pregnancy.

Available forms

Capsules—125, 250, 500 mcg

Dosages

Adults

Dosage is based on ECG response and creatinine clearance. For creatinine clearance greater than 60 mL/min, 500 mcg bid PO; for creatinine clearance 40–60 mL/min, 250 mcg bid PO; for creatinine clearance 20–less than 40 mL/min, 125 mcg bid PO; for creatinine clearance less than 20 mL/min, use is contraindicated.

Pediatric patients

Not recommended.

Pharmacokinetics

Route	*Onset*	*Peak*
Oral	Varies	2–3 hr

Metabolism: Hepatic; $T_{1/2}$: 10 hr
Distribution: May cross placenta, may enter breast milk
Excretion: Feces, urine

Adverse effects

- **CNS:** *Headache, fatigue,* light-headedness, dizziness, tingling in arms, numbness
- **CV: Ventricular arrhythmias,** hypotension, hypertension
- **GI:** Nausea, flatulence, diarrhea

Interactions

✱ **Drug-drug** ⊗ ***Warning*** Increased risk of serious to life-threatening arrhythmias with disopyramide, quinidine, procainamide, amiodarone, sotalol; do not give together • Increased risk of proarrhythmias if given with phenothiazines, TCAs, antihistamines • Increased risk of serious adverse effects if given with verapamil, cimetidine, trimethoprim, ketoconazole; do not use these combinations

■ Nursing considerations

Assessment

- **History:** Hypersensitivity to dofetilide, ibutilide; second- or third-degree AV heart block, time of onset of atrial arrhythmia; prolonged QT intervals; pregnancy; lactation; ventricular arrhythmias
- **Physical:** Orientation, BP, P, auscultation, ECG, R, adventitious sounds, renal function tests

Interventions

- Dofetilide is only available to those who have completed a *Tikosyn* education program.
- Determine time of onset of arrhythmia and timing of conversion to sinus rhythm before beginning therapy (for maintenance).

⊗ ***Black box warning*** Monitor patient's ECG before and periodically during administration; monitor continually for at least 3 days. Dosage may be adjusted based on the maintenance of sinus rhythm. Risk of induced arrhythmias exist.

- Monitor serum creatinine prior to and every 3 mo during treatment; periodically monitor potassium, magnesium levels.
- Do not attempt electroconversion within 24 hr of starting therapy; if then successful, closely monitor patient for 3 days.
- Provide appointments for continued follow-up including ECG monitoring; tendency to revert to the atrial arrhythmia after conversion increases with length of time patient was in the abnormal rhythm.

Teaching points

- This drug should be taken twice a day at the same time each day. It will help to keep your heart in a normal rhythm.
- If you miss a dose, skip the dose and resume regular dosing schedule. Do not double up on doses.
- Arrange for follow-up medical evaluation, including ECG, which is important to monitor the effect of this drug on your heart.
- These side effects may occur: Headache, fatigue, dizziness, light-headedness (avoid driving a car or operating dangerous equipment if these effects occur).
- Report chest pain, difficulty breathing, numbness or tingling, palpitations.

▽ dolasetron mesylate

(doe laz' e tron)

Anzemet

PREGNANCY CATEGORY B

Drug classes

Antiemetic
Serotonin receptor blocker

Therapeutic actions

Selectively binds to serotonin receptors in the CTZ, blocking the nausea and vomiting caused by the release of serotonin by mucosal cells during chemotherapy, radiotherapy, or surgical invasion (an action that stimulates the CTZ and causes nausea and vomiting).

Indications

- Prevention and treatment of nausea and vomiting associated with emetogenic chemotherapy
- Prevention of postoperative nausea and vomiting
- Injection only: Treatment of postoperative nausea and vomiting
- Unlabeled use: Treatment and prevention of radiation therapy–induced nausea and vomiting

Contraindications and cautions

- Contraindicated with allergy to dolasetron or any of its components; markedly prolonged QTc interval, second- or third-degree AV block.
- Use cautiously in any patient at risk of developing prolongation of cardiac conduction intervals, especially QT interval (congenital QT syndrome, hypokalemia, hypomagnesemia), pregnancy, lactation.

Available forms

Tablets—50, 100 mg; injection—12.5 mg/0.625 mL, 20 mg/mL

Dosages

Adults

100 mg PO within 1 hr before chemotherapy or within 2 hr before surgery; or 1.8 mg/kg IV about 30 min before chemotherapy or 100 mg IV injection. For prevention of postoperative nausea and vomiting, 12.5 mg IV about 15 min before stopping anesthesia. For treatment of postoperative nausea and vomiting, 12.5 mg IV as soon as needed.

Pediatric patients 2–16 yr

1.8 mg/kg PO using tablets or injection diluted in apple or apple-grape juice within 1 hr before chemotherapy; for prevention of postoperative nausea and vomiting, 1.2 mg/kg PO using tablets or injection diluted in apple or apple-grape juice within 2 hr before surgery; or 1.8 mg/kg IV for chemotherapy-induced nausea and vomiting about 30 min before chemotherapy; up to a maximum of 100 mg; 0.35 mg/kg IV about 15 min before stopping anesthesia to prevent postoperative nausea and vomiting; 0.35 mg/kg IV as soon as needed to treat postoperative nausea and vomiting; up to a maximum of 12.5 mg per dose.

Pediatric patients younger than 2 yr
Not recommended.

Pharmacokinetics

Route	*Onset*	*Peak*
Oral	Rapid	1–2 hr
IV	Immediate	End of infusion

Metabolism: Hepatic; $T_{1/2}$: 3.5–5 hr
Distribution: May cross placenta; may enter breast milk
Excretion: Feces, urine

IV FACTS

Preparation: Dilute in 50 mL 5% dextrose injection, 0.9% sodium chloride injection, 5% dextrose and 0.45% sodium chloride injection, lactated Ringer's, 10% mannitol; 3% sodium chloride injection; do not mix in any alkaline solution, precipitates may form. Stable at room temperature for 24 hr, or 48 hr if refrigerated, after dilution.
Infusion: Up to 100 mg may be administered IV undiluted over 30 sec or infuse diluted over up to 15 min.
Incompatibilities: Dilute only in recommended solutions. IV infusion line should be flushed before and after administration.

Adverse effects

- **CNS:** *Headache, dizziness,* somnolence, drowsiness, sedation, *fatigue*
- **CV:** *Tachycardia,* ECG changes
- **GI:** *Diarrhea,* constipation, abdominal pain
- **Other:** Fever, pruritus, injection site reaction

Interactions

✱ **Drug-drug** • Possible cardiac arrhythmias with drugs that cause ECG interval prolongation • Potential for severe toxic reaction with high-dose anthracycline therapy • Decreased levels if combined with rifampin

■ Nursing considerations

Assessment

- **History:** Allergy to dolasetron, pregnancy, lactation, QTc prolongation, hypokalemia, hypomagnesemia, pregnancy, lactation
- **Physical:** Orientation, reflexes, affect; BP; P, baseline ECG

Interventions

- If patient is unable to swallow tablets, dilute injection in apple or apple-grape juice; dosage remains the same; solution is stable for 2 hr at room temperature.
- Provide mouth care, sugarless lozenges to suck to help alleviate nausea.
- Obtain baseline ECG and periodically monitor ECG in any patient at risk for QTc prolongation.
- Provide appropriate analgesics for headache.

Teaching points

- This drug may be given IV or orally when you are receiving your chemotherapy; it will help decrease nausea and vomiting.
- You may experience these side effects: Dizziness, drowsiness (use caution if driving or performing tasks that require alertness), diarrhea; headache (appropriate medication will be arranged to alleviate this problem).
- Report severe headache, fever, numbness or tingling, palpitations, fainting episodes, change in color of stools or urine.

donepezil hydrochloride

*(doe **nep'** ah zill)*

Aricept, Aricept ODT

PREGNANCY CATEGORY C

Drug classes

Alzheimer's disease drug
Cholinesterase inhibitor

Therapeutic actions

Centrally acting reversible cholinesterase inhibitor leading to elevated acetylcholine levels in the cortex, which slows the neuronal degradation that occurs in Alzheimer's disease.

Indications

- Treatment of dementia of the Alzheimer's type, including severe dementia
- Unlabeled uses: Possible treatment for vascular dementia; improvement of memory in MS patients

Contraindications and cautions

- Contraindicated with allergy to donepezil.
- Use cautiously with sick sinus syndrome, GI bleeding, seizures, asthma, pregnancy, lactation.

Available forms

Tablets—5, 10 mg; orally disintegrating tablets—5, 10 mg; oral solution—1 mg/mL

Dosages

Adults

5 mg PO daily at bedtime for mild to moderate disease. May be increased to 10 mg daily after 4–6 wk. 10 mg PO daily for severe disease.

Pediatric patients

Safety and efficacy not established.

Pharmacokinetics

Route	*Onset*	*Peak*
Oral	Varies	3–4 hr

Metabolism: Hepatic; $T_{1/2}$: 70 hr
Distribution: May cross placenta; may enter breast milk
Excretion: Feces, urine

Adverse effects

- **CNS:** *Insomnia, fatigue,* dizziness, confusion, ataxia, somnolence, tremor, agitation, depression, anxiety, abnormal thinking
- **CV:** Bradycardia
- **Dermatologic:** *Rash,* flushing, purpura
- **GI:** *Nausea, vomiting, diarrhea, dyspepsia, anorexia, abdominal pain,* flatulence, constipation, **hepatotoxicity**
- **Other:** *Muscle cramps*

Interactions

✱ **Drug-drug** • Increased effects and risk of toxicity with theophylline, cholinesterase inhibitors • Decreased effects of anticholinergics • Increased risk of GI bleeding with NSAIDs • Decreased efficacy with anticholinergics

■ Nursing considerations

CLINICAL ALERT!
Name confusion has occurred between *Aricept* (donepezil) and *Aciphex* (rabeprazole); use caution.

Assessment

- **History:** Allergy to donepezil, pregnancy, lactation, sick sinus syndrome, GI bleeding, seizures, asthma
- **Physical:** Orientation, affect, reflexes; BP, P; abdominal examination; renal function tests, LFTs

Interventions

- Administer at bedtime each day.
- Provide small, frequent meals if GI upset is severe.
- Place orally disintegrating tablet on tongue; allow to dissolve and follow with water.
- Notify surgeons that patient is on donepezil; exaggerated muscle relaxation may occur if succinylcholine-type drugs are used.

Teaching points

- Take this drug exactly as prescribed, at bedtime.
- Place orally disintegrating tablet on your tongue; allow it to dissolve and then drink water.
- This drug does not cure the disease but is thought to slow down the degeneration associated with the disease.
- Continue taking this drug if no change in symptoms is noted.
- Arrange for regular blood tests and follow-up visits while adjusting to this drug.
- You may experience these side effects: Nausea, vomiting (eat frequent small meals); insomnia, fatigue, confusion (use caution if driving or performing tasks that require alertness).
- Report severe nausea, vomiting, changes in stool or urine color, diarrhea, changes in neurologic functioning, yellowing of eyes or skin.

DANGEROUS DRUG

▽ dopamine hydrochloride

(doe' pa meen)

PREGNANCY CATEGORY C

Drug classes

Alpha-adrenergic agonist
$Beta_1$-selective adrenergic agonist

Dopaminergic drug
Sympathomimetic

Therapeutic actions

Drug acts directly and by the release of norepinephrine from sympathetic nerve terminals; dopaminergic receptors mediate dilation of vessels in the renal and splanchnic beds, which maintains renal perfusion and function; alpha receptors, which are activated by higher doses of dopamine, mediate vasoconstriction, which can override the vasodilating effects; $beta_1$ receptors mediate a positive inotropic effect on the heart.

Indications

- Correction of hemodynamic imbalances present in the shock syndrome due to MI, trauma, endotoxic septicemia, open heart surgery, renal failure, and chronic cardiac decompensation in heart failure
- Poor perfusion of vital organs
- Low cardiac output
- Hypotension
- Unlabeled uses: COPD, heart failure, RDS in infants

Contraindications and cautions

- Contraindicated with pheochromocytoma, tachyarrhythmias, ventricular fibrillation, hypovolemia (dopamine is not a substitute for blood, plasma, fluids, electrolytes, which should be restored promptly when loss has occurred), general anesthesia with halogenated hydrocarbons or cyclopropane, which sensitize the myocardium to catecholamines.
- Use cautiously with atherosclerosis, arterial embolism, Raynaud's disease, cold injury, frostbite, diabetic endarteritis, Buerger's disease (monitor color and temperature of extremities), pregnancy, lactation.

Available forms

Injection—40, 80, 160 mg/mL; injection in 5% dextrose—80, 160, 320 mg/100 mL

Dosages

Dilute before using; administer only by IV infusion, using an infusion pump to control the rate of flow. Titrate on the basis of patient's hemodynamic and renal response. Close monitoring is necessary. In titrating to desired systolic BP response, optimum administration rate for renal response may be exceeded, thus necessitating a reduction in rate after hemodynamic stabilization.

Adults

- *Patients likely to respond to modest increments of cardiac contractility and renal perfusion:* Initially, 2–5 mcg/kg/min IV.
- *Patients who are more seriously ill:* Initially, 5 mcg/kg/min IV. Increase in increments of 5–10 mcg/kg/min up to a rate of 20–50 mcg/kg/min. Check urine output frequently if doses exceed 16 mcg/kg/min.

Pediatric patients

Safety and efficacy not established.

Pharmacokinetics

Route	*Onset*	*Peak*	*Duration*
IV	1–2 min	10 min	Length of infusion

Metabolism: Hepatic; $T_{1/2}$: 2 min
Distribution: May cross placenta; may enter breast milk
Excretion: Urine

IV FACTS

Preparation: Prepare solution for IV infusion as follows: Add 200–400 mg dopamine to 250–500 mL of one of the following IV solutions: 0.9% sodium chloride solution; 5% dextrose injection; 5% dextrose and 0.45% or 0.9% sodium chloride solution; 5% dextrose in lactated Ringer's solution; sodium lactate (1/6 Molar) injection; lactated Ringer's injection. Commonly used concentrations are 800 mcg/mL (200 mg in 250 mL) and 1,600 mcg/mL (400 mg in 250 mL). The 160-mg/mL concentrate may be preferred in patients with fluid retention. Protect drug solutions from light; drug solutions should be clear and colorless.
Infusion: Determine infusion rate based on patient response.
Incompatibilities: Do not mix with other drugs; do not add to 5% sodium bicarbonate or other alkaline IV solutions, oxidizing drugs, or iron salts because drug is inactivated in alkaline solution (solutions become pink to violet).

Y-site incompatibilities: Do not give with acyclovir, alteplase, amphotericin B.

Adverse effects

- **CNS:** Headache, anxiety
- **CV:** *Ectopic beats, tachycardia, anginal pain, palpitations, hypotension, vasoconstriction, dyspnea,* bradycardia, hypertension, widened QRS
- **GI:** *Nausea, vomiting*
- **Other:** Piloerection, azotemia, gangrene with prolonged use

Interactions

✱ **Drug-drug** • Increased effects with MAOIs, TCAs (imipramine) • Increased risk of hypertension with furazolidone, methyldopa • Seizures, hypotension, bradycardia when infused with phenytoin

■ Nursing considerations

CLINICAL ALERT!

Name confusion has occurred between dopamine and dobutamine; use caution.

Assessment

- **History:** Pheochromocytoma, tachyarrhythmias, ventricular fibrillation, hypovolemia, general anesthesia with halogenated hydrocarbons or cyclopropane, occlusive vascular disease, pregnancy, labor, and delivery
- **Physical:** Body weight; skin color, T; P, BP, pulse pressure; R, adventitious sounds; urine output; serum electrolytes, Hct, ECG

Interventions

⊗ ***Warning*** Exercise extreme caution in calculating and preparing doses; dopamine is a very potent drug; small errors in dosage can cause serious adverse effects. Drug should always be diluted before use if not prediluted.

- Reduce initial dosage to one-tenth of usual dose in patients who have been on MAOIs.
- Administer into large veins of the antecubital fossa in preference to veins in hand or ankle.

⊠ ***Black box warning*** To prevent sloughing and necrosis after extravasation, infiltrate area with 10–15 mL saline containing 5–10 mg phentolamine. Do so as soon as possible after extravasation occurs.

- Monitor urine flow, cardiac output, and BP closely during infusion.

Teaching points

- Drug is used only in acute emergency; teaching will depend on patient's awareness and will relate mainly to patient's status and monitors, rather than to drug. Instruct patient to report any pain at injection site.

▽ doripenem

*(door ih **pen'** em)*

Doribax

PREGNANCY CATEGORY B

Drug class

Carbapenem antibiotic

Therapeutic actions

Drug inhibits synthesis of bacterial cell wall and causes cell death in susceptible cells. Structure and action are similar to those of beta lactams.

Indications

- Treatment of complicated intra-abdominal infections caused by *Escherichia coli, Klebsiella pneumoniae, Pseudomonas aeruginosa, Bacteroides caccea, Bacteroides fragilis, Bacteroides thetaiotaomicron, Bacteroides uniformis, Bacteroides vulgatus, Streptococcus intermedius, Streptococcus constellatus, Peptostreptococcus micros*
- Treatment of complicated UTI, including pyelonephritis, caused by *E. coli, K. pneumoniae, Proteus mirabilis, P. aeruginosa, Acinetobacter baumannii*

Contraindications and cautions

- Contraindicated with hypersensitivity to any component of this drug or drugs in this class; history of anaphylactic reaction to beta-lactams.
- Use cautiously with sodium valproate therapy, pregnancy, lactation.

Available forms
Single-use vials—500 mg

Dosages
Adults
500 mg IV over 1 hr every 8 hr for 5–14 days (intra-abdominal infection) or for 10 days (UTI or pyelonephritis).

Patients with renal impairment
If creatinine clearance is equal to or greater than 30 and equal to or less than 50 mL/min, 250 mg IV every 8 hr; if creatinine clearance is greater than 10 and less than 30 mL/min, 250 mg IV every 12 hr.

Pharmacokinetics

Route	*Onset*	*Peak*	*Duration*
IV	Rapid	End of infusion	Length of infusion

Metabolism: Hepatic; $T_{1/2}$: 1 hr
Distribution: Does not cross placenta; may enter breast milk
Excretion: Unchanged in urine

IV FACTS
Preparation: Constitute vial with 10 mg sterile water for injection or 0.9% sodium chloride injection; gently shake to from a suspension (concentration is 50 mg/mL). Add suspension to 100 mL normal saline solution or 5% dextrose; gently shake until clear. Infusion concentration is 4.5 mg/mL. If using normal saline solution, drug stays stable for 8 hr at room temperature or 24 hr refrigerated; if using 5% dextrose, stable for 4 hr at room temperature or 24 hr refrigerated. Do not freeze.
Infusion: Infuse over 1 hr.
Incompatibility: Do not mix with or add to solutions containing any other drugs.

Adverse effects
- **CNS:** *Headache*
- **GI:** *Nausea,* diarrhea, including *C. difficile* diseases
- **Other:** *Rash, phlebitis,* superinfection, hypersensitivity reaction

Interactions
✱ **Drug-drug** • Risk for significant reduction in serum valproic acid level and risk of seizures if combined; alternative antibiotic treatment should be considered • Increased serum doripenem level if combined with probenecid; avoid this combination

■ Nursing considerations
Assessment
- **History:** Hypersensitivity to doripenem, its components, drugs of this class, or beta lactams; pregnancy, lactation
- **Physical:** T, orientation, abdominal examination

Interventions
- Obtain culture and sensitivity tests to ensure appropriate use of the drug.
- Ensure that patient is not controlling seizures with valproic acid therapy; serious drug interaction and seizures could occur.
- Do not administer by inhalation; serious pneumonitis has occurred.
- Administer IV every 8 hr for full length of prescribed dose to prevent emergence of resistant strains of bacteria.
- Monitor injection site for possible phlebitis.
- Encourage women of childbearing age to use barrier contraceptives while on this drug because effects of drug on fetus are not known.
- Advise lactating women to find another method of feeding; potential effects on the baby are not known.
- Monitor patient for possible *C. difficile* diarrhea. Provide fluid and electrolyte management, protein supplements, and antibiotic treatment as needed. Monitor patient for up to 2 mo after therapy.

Teaching points
- This drug is given by IV infusion every 8 hours for 5–14 days, depending on your infection and your response to the drug; it is important to complete the full course of drug therapy.
- If you are being treated as an outpatient and miss a dose, contact your health care provider immediately.
- It is not known how this drug could affect a nursing baby. If you are nursing a baby, another method of feeding the baby should be selected.
- It is not known how this drug could affect a fetus, if you are pregnant or decide to become

pregnant while on this drug, consult your health care provider.
- You may experience these side effects: Headache (consult your health care provider, medication may be available to help); nausea (frequent small meals may help); diarrhea (if it becomes severe, contact your health care provider immediately); irritation and inflammation at the injection site.
- Report difficulty breathing; severe or persistent rash, redness, or pain at the injection site; severe diarrhea.

dornase alfa

See Appendix W, *Less commonly used drugs*.

doxapram hydrochloride

(docks' a pram)

Dopram

PREGNANCY CATEGORY B

Drug classes

Analeptic
Respiratory stimulant

Therapeutic actions

Stimulates the peripheral carotid chemoreceptors to cause an increase in tidal volume and slight increase in respiratory rate; this stimulation also has a pressor effect.

Indications

- To stimulate respiration in patients with drug-induced postanesthesia respiratory depression or apnea; also used to "stir up" patients in combination with oxygen postoperatively
- To stimulate respiration, hasten arousal in patients experiencing drug-induced CNS depression
- As a temporary measure in hospitalized patients with acute respiratory insufficiency superimposed on COPD
- Unlabeled use: Treatment of apnea of prematurity when methylxanthines have failed, obstructive sleep apnea, laryngospasm secondary to tracheal extubation

Contraindications and cautions

- Contraindicated with newborns (contains benzyl alcohol), epilepsy, incompetence of the ventilatory mechanism, flail chest, hypersensitivity to doxapram, head injury, pneumothorax, acute bronchial asthma, pulmonary fibrosis, severe hypertension, CVA.
- Use cautiously with pregnancy, lactation.

Available forms

Injection—20 mg/mL

Dosages

Adults

- *Postanesthetic use:* Single injection of 0.5–1 mg/kg IV; do not exceed 1.5 mg/kg as a total single injection or 2 mg/kg when given as multiple injections at 5-min intervals.

Infusion

250 mg in 250 mL of dextrose or sodium chloride solution; initiate at 5 mg/min until response is seen; maintain at 1–3 mg/min; recommended total dose is 300 mg or 4 mg/kg.

- *COPD associated with acute hypercapnia:* Mix 400 mg in 180 mL of IV infusion; start infusion at 1–2 mg/min (0.5–1 mL/min); check blood gases, and adjust rate accordingly. Do not use for longer than 2 hr. Maximum of 3 mg/min.
- *Management of drug-induced CNS depression:*

Intermittent injection

Priming dose of 1–2 mg/kg IV; repeat in 5 min. Repeat every 1–2 hr until patient awakens; if relapse occurs, repeat at 1–2 hr intervals.

Intermittent IV infusion

Priming dose of 1–2 mg/kg IV; if no response, infuse 250 mg in 250 mL of dextrose or saline solution at a rate of 1–3 mg/min, discontinue at end of 2 hr if patient awakens; repeat in 30 min–2 hr if relapse occurs; do not exceed 3 g/day.

Pediatric patients

Do not give to children younger than 12 yr.

Pharmacokinetics

Route	*Onset*	*Peak*	*Duration*
IV	20–40 sec	1–2 min	5–12 min

Metabolism: Hepatic; $T_{1/2}$: 2.4–4.1 hr

Distribution: May cross placenta; may enter breast milk
Excretion: Urine

IV FACTS

Preparation: Add 250 mg doxapram to 250 mL of 5% or 10% dextrose or 0.9% sodium chloride solution.
Infusion: Initiate infusion at 5 mg/min; once response is seen, 1–3 mg/min is satisfactory.
Incompatibilities: Do not mix in alkaline solutions—precipitate or gas may form; aminophylline, sodium bicarbonate, thiopental.

Adverse effects

- **CNS:** Headache, dizziness, apprehension, disorientation, pupillary dilation, *increased reflexes,* hyperactivity, **seizures,** muscle spasticity, clonus, pyrexia, flushing sweating
- **CV:** Arrhythmias, chest pain, tightness in the chest, *increased BP*
- **GI:** Nausea, vomiting, diarrhea
- **GU:** Urinary retention, spontaneous voiding, proteinuria
- **Hematologic:** Decreased Hgb, Hct
- **Respiratory:** Cough, dyspnea, tachypnea, laryngospasm, **bronchospasm,** hiccups, rebound hypoventilation, hyperventilation

Interactions

✱ **Drug-drug** • Increased pressor effect with sympathomimetics, MAOIs • Increased effects with halothane, cyclopropane, enflurane (delay treatment for at least 10 min after discontinuance of anesthesia) • Possible masked residual effects of muscle relaxants if combined with doxapram • Risk of increased muscle activity, agitation with aminophylline, theophylline; use caution

■ Nursing considerations

Assessment

- **History:** Epilepsy, incompetence of the ventilatory mechanism, flail chest, hypersensitivity to doxapram, head injury, pneumothorax, acute bronchial asthma, pulmonary fibrosis, severe hypertension, CVA, lactation, pregnancy
- **Physical:** T; skin color; weight; R, adventitious sounds; P, BP, ECG; reflexes; urinary output; arterial blood gases, CBC

Interventions

- Administer IV only.

⊗ ***Warning*** Monitor injection site for extravasation. Discontinue, and restart in another vein if extravasation occurs; apply cold compresses.

- Monitor patient carefully until fully awake—P, BP, ECG, reflexes and respiratory status. Patients with COPD should have arterial blood gases monitored during drug use.
- Do not use longer than 2 hr.

⊗ ***Warning*** Discontinue drug and notify physician if deterioration, sudden hypotension, or dyspnea occurs.

Teaching points

- Drug is used in emergency; patient teaching should be general and include procedure and drug.

▽ doxazosin mesylate

*(dox **ay'** zoe sin **mess'** ah late)*

Cardura, Cardura XL ONC

PREGNANCY CATEGORY C

Drug classes

Alpha-adrenergic blocker
Antihypertensive

Therapeutic actions

Reduces total peripheral resistance through alpha-blockade, causing an antihypertensive effect. The degree of smooth muscle tone in prostate/bladder neck is also mediated by alpha receptors. Its blockade reduces urethral resistance and relieves obstructions.

Indications

- Treatment of mild-to-moderate hypertension, alone or as part of combination therapy
- Treatment of BPH

Contraindications and cautions

- Contraindicated with lactation.
- Use cautiously with allergy to doxazosin, heart failure, renal failure, pregnancy, hepatic impairment.

Available forms

Tablets—1, 2, 4, 8 mg; ER tablets (DNC)—4, 8 mg

Dosages

Adults

- *Hypertension:* Initially, 1 mg daily PO, given once daily. For maintenance, 2, 4, 8, or 16 mg daily PO, given once a day; dose may be increased every 2 wk. Do not use ER tablets.
- *BPH:* Initially: 1 mg PO daily; for maintenance, may increase to 2 mg, 4 mg, 8 mg daily, adjusted at 1–2 wk intervals. For ER tablets, 4 mg PO once daily at breakfast; may be increased after 3–4 wk to maximum of 8 mg/day PO.

Pediatric patients

Safety and efficacy not established.

Pharmacokinetics

Route	Onset	Peak
Oral	Varies	2–3 hr

Metabolism: Hepatic; $T_{1/2}$: 22 hr
Distribution: Crosses placenta; enters breast milk
Excretion: Bile, feces, urine

Adverse effects

- **CNS:** *Headache, fatigue, dizziness, postural dizziness, lethargy, vertigo,* asthenia, anxiety, paresthesia, insomnia, eye pain, conjunctivitis
- **CV:** *Tachycardia, palpitations, edema, orthostatic hypotension,* chest pain
- **GI:** *Nausea, dyspepsia, diarrhea,* abdominal pain, flatulence, constipation
- **GU:** *Sexual dysfunction,* increased urinary frequency
- **Other:** Dyspnea, increased sweating, rash, rhinitis, muscle cramps

Interactions

✱ **Drug-drug** • Increased hypotensive effects if taken with alcohol, nitrates, other antihypertensives

■ Nursing considerations

Assessment

- **History:** Allergy to doxazosin, heart failure, renal failure, hepatic impairment, lactation, pregnancy
- **Physical:** Weight; skin color, lesions; orientation, affect, reflexes; ophthalmologic examination; P, BP, orthostatic BP, supine BP, perfusion, edema, auscultation; R, adventitious sounds, status of nasal mucous membranes; bowel sounds, normal output; voiding pattern, normal output; renal function tests, urinalysis

Interventions

- Ensure that patient does not cut, crush, or chew ER tablets.
- Monitor edema, weight in patients with incipient cardiac decompensation, and arrange to add a thiazide diuretic to the drug regimen if sodium and fluid retention, signs of impending heart failure occur.

⊗ ***Warning*** Monitor patient carefully with first dose; chance of orthostatic hypotension, dizziness and syncope are great with the first dose. Establish safety precautions.

- Monitor signs and symptoms of BPH to adjust dosage.

Teaching points

- Take this drug exactly as prescribed, once a day. Do not cut, crush, or chew extended-release tablets. Dizziness or syncope may occur at beginning of therapy. Change position slowly to avoid increased dizziness. Taking your first dose at bedtime may decrease excessive dizziness.
- You may experience these side effects: Dizziness, weakness (when changing position, in the early morning, after exercise, in hot weather, and after consuming alcohol; some tolerance may occur after a while; avoid driving or engaging in tasks that require alertness; change position slowly, use caution in climbing stairs, lie down if dizziness persists); GI upset (eat frequent small meals); impotence; stuffy nose; most of these effects gradually disappear with continued therapy.
- Report frequent dizziness or fainting.

doxepin hydrochloride
(dox' e pin)

Apo-Doxepin (CAN), Sinequan, Zonalon

PREGNANCY CATEGORY C

Drug classes
Antidepressant
TCA (tertiary amine)

Therapeutic actions
Mechanism of action unknown; TCAs inhibit the reuptake of the neurotransmitters norepinephrine and serotonin, leading to an increase in their effects; anticholinergic at CNS and peripheral receptors; sedative.

Indications
- Relief of symptoms of depression (endogenous depression most responsive); sedative effects may help depression associated with anxiety and sleep disturbance
- Treatment of depression in patients with bipolar disorder, psychotic depressive disorders
- Treatment of anxiety
- Treatment of pruritus in adults with atopic dermatitis, lichen chronicus (5% topical cream)
- Unlabeled uses: Neuropathy, neurogenic pain

Contraindications and cautions
- Contraindicated with hypersensitivity to any tricyclic drug; concomitant therapy with an MAOI; recent MI; myelography within previous 24 hr or scheduled within 48 hr; lactation, pregnancy.
- Use cautiously with EST; preexisting CV disorders (severe coronary heart disease, progressive heart failure, angina pectoris, paroxysmal tachycardia); angle-closure glaucoma, increased IOP, urinary retention, ureteral or urethral spasm; seizure disorders; hyperthyroidism; impaired hepatic, renal function; psychiatric patients (schizophrenic or paranoid patients may exhibit a worsening of psychosis); patients with bipolar disorder; patients with suicidal ideation (overdose may be fatal); elective surgery (TCAs should be discontinued as long as possible before surgery); geriatric patients (may be more sensitive to drug and adverse effects).

Available forms
Capsules—10, 25, 50, 75, 100, 150 mg; oral concentrate—10 mg/mL; cream—30-g, 40-g tubes

Dosages
Adults
- *Mild to moderate anxiety or depression:* Initially, 25 mg tid PO; individualize dosage. Usual optimum dosage is 75–150 mg/day; alternatively, total daily dosage, up to 150 mg, may be given at bedtime.
- *More severe anxiety or depression:* Initially, 50 mg tid PO; if needed, may gradually increase to 300 mg/day. Dose may be taken all at once at bedtime.
- *Mild symptomatology or emotional symptoms accompanying organic disease:* 25–50 mg PO is often effective.
- *Pruritus:* Apply cream four times/day at least 3–4 hr apart for 8 days. Do not cover dressing.

Pediatric patients
Not recommended for children younger than 12 yr.

Pharmacokinetics
Route	Onset	Peak
Oral	Varies	4 hr

Metabolism: Hepatic; $T_{1/2}$: 8–25 hr
Distribution: Crosses placenta; enters breast milk
Excretion: Urine

Adverse effects
- **CNS:** *Sedation and anticholinergic (atropine-like) effects; confusion* (especially in elderly), *disturbed concentration,* hallucinations, disorientation, decreased memory, feelings of unreality, delusions, anxiety, nervousness, restlessness, agitation, panic, insomnia, nightmares, hypomania, mania, exacerbation of psychosis, drowsiness, weakness, fatigue, headache, numbness, tingling, paresthesias of extremities, incoordination, motor hyperactivity, akathisia, ataxia, tremors, peripheral neuropathy,

extrapyramidal symptoms, seizures, speech blockage, dysarthria, tinnitus, altered EEG
- **CV:** *Orthostatic hypotension,* hypertension, syncope, tachycardia, palpitations, **MI,** arrhythmias, heart block, precipitation of heart failure, CVA
- **Endocrine:** Elevated or depressed blood sugar; elevated prolactin levels; inappropriate ADH secretion
- **GI:** *Dry mouth, constipation,* paralytic ileus, *nausea,* vomiting, anorexia, epigastric distress, diarrhea, flatulence, dysphagia, peculiar taste, increased salivation, stomatitis, glossitis, parotid swelling, abdominal cramps, black tongue, hepatitis, jaundice (rare), elevated transaminase, altered alkaline phosphatase
- **GU:** Urinary retention, delayed micturition, dilation of the urinary tract, gynecomastia, testicular swelling; breast enlargement, menstrual irregularity and galactorrhea; changes in libido; impotence
- **Hematologic:** Bone marrow depression, including agranulocytosis; eosinophilia, purpura, thrombocytopenia, leukopenia
- **Hypersensitivity:** Rash, pruritus, vasculitis, petechiae, photosensitization, edema (generalized or of face and tongue), drug fever
- **Withdrawal:** Symptoms on abrupt discontinuation of prolonged therapy: Nausea, headache, vertigo, nightmares, malaise
- **Other:** Nasal congestion, excessive appetite, weight gain or loss; sweating (paradoxical effect in a drug with prominent anticholinergic effects), alopecia, lacrimation, hyperthermia, flushing, chills

Interactions

✱ **Drug-drug** • Increased TCA levels and pharmacologic (especially anticholinergic) effects with cimetidine, fluoxetine • Increased TCA levels (due to decreased metabolism) with methylphenidate, phenothiazines, hormonal contraceptives, disulfiram • Hyperpyretic crises, severe seizures, hypertensive episodes, and deaths with MAOIs • Increased antidepressant response and cardiac arrhythmias with thyroid medication • Increased or decreased effects with estrogens • Delirium with disulfiram • Sympathetic hyperactivity, sinus tachycardia, hypertension, agitation with levodopa • Increased biotransformation of TCAs in patients who smoke cigarettes • Increased sympathomimetic (especially alpha-adrenergic) effects of direct-acting sympathomimetic drugs (norepinephrine, epinephrine), due to inhibition of uptake into adrenergic nerves • Increased anticholinergic effects of anticholinergic drugs (including anticholinergic antiparkinsonian drugs) • Increased response (especially CNS depression) to barbiturates • Increased CNS suppression with alcohol or other CNS depressants; avoid this combination • Decreased antihypertensive effect of clonidine, other antihypertensives (because the uptake of the antihypertensive drug into adrenergic neurons is inhibited) • Decreased effects of indirect-acting sympathomimetic drugs (ephedrine) because of inhibition of uptake into adrenergic nerves

■ Nursing considerations

CLINICAL ALERT!

Name confusion has occurred between *Sinequan* (doxepin) and saquinavir; use caution.

Assessment

- **History:** Hypersensitivity to any tricyclic drug; concomitant therapy with an MAOI; recent MI; myelography within previous 24 hr or scheduled within 48 hr; lactation; EST; preexisting CV disorders; angle-closure glaucoma, increased IOP, urinary retention, ureteral or urethral spasm; seizure disorders; hyperthyroidism; impaired hepatic, renal function; psychiatric treatment; bipolar disorder; elective surgery; pregnancy
- **Physical:** Weight; T; skin color, lesions; orientation, affect, reflexes, vision and hearing; P, BP, orthostatic BP, perfusion; bowel sounds, normal output, liver evaluation; urine flow, normal output; usual sexual function, frequency of menses, breast and scrotal examination; LFTs, urinalysis, CBC, ECG

Interventions

⊗ ***Black box warning*** Risk of suicidality in children, adolescents, and young adults increases. Monitor patient accordingly.

⊗ ***Warning*** Limit drug access with depressed and potentially suicidal patients.

- Give most of dose at bedtime if drowsiness or severe anticholinergic effects occur.
- Dilute oral concentrate with approximately 120 mL of water, milk, or fruit juice just prior to administration; do not prepare or store bulk dilutions.
- Expect clinical antianxiety response to be rapidly evident, although antidepressant response may require 2–3 wk.
- Reduce dosage if minor side effects develop; discontinue the drug if serious side effects occur.
- Arrange for CBC if patient develops fever, sore throat, or other sign of infection during therapy.

Teaching points

- Take drug exactly as prescribed; do not stop abruptly or without consulting the health care provider.
- Avoid alcohol, sleep-inducing drugs, over-the-counter drugs.
- Avoid prolonged exposure to sunlight or sunlamps; use a sunscreen or protective garments for exposure to sunlight.
- You may experience these side effects: Headache, dizziness, drowsiness, weakness, blurred vision (reversible; safety measures will be needed if severe; avoid driving or performing tasks that require alertness while these persist); nausea, vomiting, loss of appetite, dry mouth (eat frequent small meals; frequent mouth care and sucking sugarless candies may help); nightmares, inability to concentrate, confusion; changes in sexual function, suicidal thoughts.
- Report dry mouth, difficulty in urination, excessive sedation, suicidal thoughts.

doxercalciferol

See Appendix W, *Less commonly used drugs*.

DANGEROUS DRUG

doxorubicin hydrochloride

*(dox oh **roo'** bi sin)*

Adriamycin PFS, Adriamycin RDF, Doxil

PREGNANCY CATEGORY D

Drug classes

Antibiotic
Antineoplastic

Therapeutic actions

Cytotoxic: Binds to DNA and inhibits DNA synthesis in susceptible cells, causing cell death.

Indications

- To produce regression in the following neoplasms: ALL, AML, Wilms' tumor, neuroblastoma, soft tissue and bone sarcoma, breast carcinoma, ovarian carcinoma, transitional cell bladder carcinoma, thyroid carcinoma, Hodgkin's and non-Hodgkin's lymphomas, bronchogenic carcinoma
- Liposomal form: Treatment of AIDS-related Kaposi's sarcoma, ovarian cancer that has progressed or recurred after platinum-based chemotherapy

Contraindications and cautions

- Contraindicated with allergy to doxorubicin hydrochloride, malignant melanoma, kidney carcinoma, large bowel carcinoma, brain tumors, CNS metastases, myelosuppression, cardiac disease (may predispose to cardiac toxicity), pregnancy, lactation.
- Use cautiously with impaired hepatic function, previous courses of doxorubicin or daunorubicin therapy (may predispose to cardiac toxicity), prior mediastinal irradiation, concurrent cyclophosphamide therapy (predispose to cardiac toxicity).

Available forms

Powder for injection—10, 20, 50, 100, 150 mg; injection (aqueous)—2 mg/mL; preservative-free injection—2 mg/mL; injection (lipid)—2 mg/mL; liposomal—20-mg, 50-mg injectables

Dosages

Adults

60–75 mg/m^2 as a single IV injection administered at 21-day intervals. Alternate schedule: 30 mg/m^2 IV on each of 3 successive days, repeated every 4 wk.

Liposomal form

For AIDS-related Kaposi's sarcoma, 20 mg/m^2 IV every 3 wk starting with initial rate of 1 mg/min. If no adverse effects, increase rate to complete dose in 1 hr.

For ovarian cancer, initially 50 mg/m^2 IV at 1 mg/min; if no adverse effects, complete infusion in 1 hr. Repeat every 4 wk.

Patients with elevated bilirubin

For serum bilirubin 1.2–3 mg/100 mL, use 50% of normal dose. For serum bilirubin exceeding 3 mg/100 mL, use 25% of normal dose.

Pharmacokinetics

Route	*Onset*	*Peak*	*Duration*
IV	Rapid	2 hr	24–36 hr

Metabolism: Hepatic; $T_{1/2}$: 12 min, then 3.3 hr, then 29.6 hr

Distribution: May cross placenta; enters breast milk

Excretion: Bile, feces, urine

IV FACTS

Preparation: Reconstitute the 10-mg vial with 5 mL, the 50-mg vial with 25 mL of 0.9% sodium chloride to give a concentration of 2 mg/mL doxorubicin. Reconstituted solution is stable for 7 days at room temperature and normal light or 15 days if refrigerated. Protect from sunlight. Liposomal form: Dilute dose to maximum of 90 mg in 250 mL of 5% dextrose injection; do not use in-line filters; refrigerate and use within 24 hr.

Infusion: Administer slowly into tubing of a freely running IV infusion of sodium chloride injection or 5% dextrose injection; attach the tubing to a butterfly needle inserted into a large vein; avoid veins over joints or in extremities with poor perfusion. Rate of administration will depend on the vein and dosage; do not give in less than 3–5 min; red streaking over the vein and facial flushing are often signs of too-rapid administration. Liposomal form: Single dose infused over 30 min; rapid infusion increases risk of reaction.

Incompatibilities: Do not mix with heparin, dexamethasone sodium phosphatase (a precipitate forms and the IV solution must not be used), aminophylline, and 5-FU (doxorubicin decomposes) denoted by a color change from red to blue-purple.

Y-site incompatibilities: Do not give with furosemide, heparin.

Adverse effects

- **CV: Cardiac toxicity,** heart failure, phlebosclerosis
- **Dermatologic:** *Complete but reversible alopecia,* hyperpigmentation of nailbeds and dermal creases, facial flushing
- **GI:** *Nausea, vomiting, mucositis,* anorexia, diarrhea
- **GU:** *Red urine*
- **Hematologic:** *Myelosuppression,* hyperuricemia due to cell lysis
- **Hypersensitivity:** Fever, chills, urticaria, **anaphylaxis**
- **Local: Severe local cellulitis,** vesication and tissue necrosis if extravasation occurs
- **Other:** Carcinogenesis (documented in experimental models)

Interactions

✱ **Drug-drug** • Decreased serum levels and actions of digoxin if taken concurrently with doxorubicin

■ Nursing considerations

CLINICAL ALERT!

Name confusion has been reported between conventional doxorubicin and liposomal doxorubicin; use caution.

Assessment

- **History:** Allergy to doxorubicin hydrochloride, malignant melanoma, kidney carcinoma, large bowel carcinoma, brain tumors, CNS metastases, myelosuppression, cardiac disease, impaired hepatic function, previous courses of doxorubicin or daunorubicin therapy, prior mediastinal irradiation, concurrent cyclophosphamide therapy, lactation, pregnancy
- **Physical:** T; skin color, lesions; weight; hair; nailbeds; local injection site; auscultation, peripheral perfusion, pulses, ECG; R, adventitious sounds; liver evaluation, mucous membranes; CBC, LFTs, uric acid levels

Interventions

- Do not give IM or subcutaneously because severe local reaction and tissue necrosis occur.

⊗ ***Black box warning*** Monitor injection site for extravasation and for reports of burning or stinging. If these events occur, discontinue administration and restart in another vein. Local subcutaneous extravasation: Local infiltration with corticosteroid may be ordered; flood area with normal saline; apply cold compress to area. If ulceration begins, arrange consultation with plastic surgeon.

⊗ ***Black box warning*** Monitor patient's response frequently at beginning of therapy: Serum uric acid level, cardiac output (listen for S_3); CBC changes may require a decrease in the dose; consult with physician; risk of heart failure, myelosuppression, liver damage. Record doses received to monitor total dosage; toxic effects are often dose-related, as total dose approaches 550 mg/m^2.

- Ensure adequate hydration during the course of therapy to prevent hyperuricemia.

Teaching points

- Prepare a calendar of days to return for drug therapy.
- Avoid pregnancy while using this drug; using barrier contraceptives is advised.
- Arrange for regular medical follow-up, including blood tests.
- You may experience these side effects: Rash, skin lesions, loss of hair, changes in nails (you may want to obtain a wig before hair loss occurs; skin care may help); loss of appetite, nausea, mouth sores (frequent mouth care, eat frequent small meals; try to maintain good nutrition; a dietitian may be able to help; an antiemetic may be ordered); red urine (transient).
- Report difficulty breathing, sudden weight gain, swelling, burning or pain at injection site, unusual bleeding or bruising.

▽ doxycycline

(dox i sye' kleen)

Adoxa, Apo-Doxy (CAN), Atridox, Doryx, Doxy 100, Doxy 200, Doxycin (CAN), Monodox, Nu-Doxycycline (CAN), Oracea, Periostat, Vibramycin, Vibra-Tabs

PREGNANCY CATEGORY D

Drug classes

Tetracycline antibiotic

Therapeutic actions

Bacteriostatic: Inhibits protein synthesis of susceptible bacteria, causing cell death.

Indications

- Infections caused by rickettsia; *Mycoplasma pneumoniae;* agents of psittacosis, ornithosis, lymphogranuloma venereum, and granuloma inguinale; *Borrelia recurrentis; Haemophilus ducreyi; Pasteurella pestis; Pasteurella tularensis; Bartonella bacilliformis; Bacteroides; Vibrio comma; Vibrio fetus; Brucella; Escherichia coli; Enterobacter aerogenes; Shigella; Acinetobacter calcoaceticus; Haemophilus influenzae, Klebsiella, Streptococcus pneumoniae, Staphylococcus aureus*
- When penicillin is contraindicated, infections caused by *Neisseria gonorrhoeae, Treponema pallidum, Treponema pertenue, Listeria monocytogenes, Clostridium, Bacillus anthracis, Chlamydia psittaci, Chlamydia trachomatis*
- Oral tetracyclines used for acne, uncomplicated adult urethral, endocervical, or rectal infections caused by *C. trachomatis*
- Acute intestinal amebiasis
- Reduction of incidence and progression of disease following exposure to anthrax
- Malaria prophylaxis for malaria due to *Plasmodium falciparum* for short-term use in travelers
- Treatment of inflammatory lesions (papules and pustules) of rosacea in adults; not for generalized erythema of rosacea
- Treatment of periodontal disease as an adjunct to scaling and root planing
- Unlabeled uses: Prevention of traveler's diarrhea commonly caused by enterotoxigenic *E. coli;* Lyme disease; CDC-recommended treatment of STDs, including granuloma inguinale, syphilis, chlamydial infections in patients older than 8 yr, pelvic inflammatory disease, epididymitis, and sexual assault prophylaxis

Contraindications and cautions

- Contraindicated with allergy to tetracyclines.
- Use cautiously with renal or hepatic impairment, pregnancy, lactation.

Available forms

Tablets—20, 50, 75, 100 mg; DR tablets—75, 100 mg; capsules—50, 100 mg; coated pellets, capsules—75, 100 mg; powder for oral suspension—25 mg; syrup—50 mg/5 mL; powder for injection—100, 200 mg; injection—42.5 mg

Dosages

Adults

- *Rosacea:* 40 mg/day PO in the morning with a full glass of water, on an empty stomach, for up to 9 mo.

Adults and pediatric patients older than 8 yr and weighing more than 45 kg

200 mg IV in one or two infusions (each over 1–4 hr) on the first treatment day, followed by 100–200 mg/day IV, depending on the severity of the infection, or 200 mg PO on day 1, followed by 100 mg/day PO.

- *Primary or secondary syphilis:* 100 mg PO bid for 14 days.
- *Acute gonococcal infection:* 200 mg PO, then 100 mg at bedtime, followed by 100 mg bid for 3 days; or 300 mg PO followed by 300 mg in 1 hr.
- *Traveler's diarrhea:* 100 mg/day PO as prophylaxis.
- *Malaria prophylaxis:* 100 mg PO daily.
- *Anthrax prophylaxis:* 100 mg PO bid for 60 days.
- *CDC recommendations for STDs:* 100 mg bid PO for 7–28 days, depending on disease being treated.
- *Periodontal disease:* 20 mg PO bid, following scaling and root planing.

Pediatric patients older than 8 yr and weighing less than 45 kg

4.4 mg/kg, IV in one or two infusions, followed by 2.2–4.4 mg/kg/day IV in one or two infusions; or 4.4 mg/kg, PO in two divided doses the first day of treatment, followed by 2.2–4.4 mg/kg/day on subsequent days.

- *Lyme disease:* 100 mg PO bid for 14–21 days.
- *Malaria prophylaxis:* 2 mg/kg/day PO, up to 100 mg/day.
- *Anthrax prophylaxis:* 2.2 mg/kg PO bid for 60 days.

Geriatric patients or patients with renal failure

IV doses of doxycycline may not be as toxic as other tetracyclines in these patients.

Pharmacokinetics

Route	Onset	Peak
Oral	Varies	1.5–4 hr
IV	Rapid	End of infusion

Metabolism: $T_{1/2}$: 15–25 hr
Distribution: Crosses placenta; enters breast milk
Excretion: Feces, urine

IV FACTS

Preparation: Prepare solution of 10 mg/mL, reconstitute with 10 mL (100-mg vial): 20 mL (200-mg vial) of sterile water for injection; dilute further with 100–1,000 mL (100-mg vial) or 200–2,000 mL (200-mg vial) of sodium chloride injection, 5% dextrose injection, Ringer's injection, 10% invert sugar in water, lactated Ringer's injection, 5% dextrose in lactated Ringer's, Normosol-M in D_5W, Normosol-R in D_5W, or Plasma-Lyte 56 or 148 in 5% Dextrose. If mixed in lactated Ringer's or 5% dextrose in lactated Ringer's, infusion must be completed within 6 hr after reconstitution; otherwise, may be stored up to 72 hr if refrigerated and protected from light, but infusion should then be completed within 12 hr; discard solution after that time.
Infusion: Infuse slowly over 1–4 hr.

Adverse effects

- **Dental:** *Discoloring and inadequate calcification of primary teeth of fetus if used by pregnant women, discoloring and inadequate calcification of permanent teeth if used during period of dental development*
- **Dermatologic:** *Phototoxic reactions, rash,* **exfoliative dermatitis** (more frequent and more severe with this tetracycline than with any others)
- **GI:** Fatty liver, **liver failure,** *anorexia, nausea, vomiting, diarrhea, glossitis,* dysphagia, enterocolitis, esophageal ulcer
- **Hematologic: Hemolytic anemia, thrombocytopenia, neutropenia, eosinophilia,** leukocytosis, **leukopenia**

- **Local:** Local irritation at injection site
- **Other:** Superinfections, nephrogenic diabetes insipidus syndrome

Interactions

✱ **Drug-drug** • Decreased absorption with antacids, iron, alkali • Decreased therapeutic effects with barbiturates, carbamazepine, phenytoins • Increased digoxin toxicity with doxycycline • Increased nephrotoxicity with methoxyflurane • Decreased activity of penicillins
✱ **Drug-food** • Decreased effectiveness of doxycycline if taken with food, dairy products
✱ **Drug-lab test** • Interference with culture studies for several days following therapy

■ Nursing considerations

Assessment

- **History:** Allergy to tetracyclines, renal or hepatic impairment, pregnancy, lactation
- **Physical:** Skin status, R and sounds, GI function and liver evaluation, urinary output and concentration, urinalysis and BUN, LFTs, renal function tests; culture infected area before beginning therapy

Interventions

- Patients on long-term treatment for rosacea should be given drug in the morning, on an empty stomach, with a full glass of water.
- Administer the oral medication without regard to food or meals; if GI upset occurs, give with meals; patients being treated for periodontal disease should receive tablet at least 1 hr before morning and evening meals.
- Protect patient from light and sun exposure.

Teaching points

- Take drug throughout the day for best results; if GI upset occurs, take drug with food. If being treated for periodontal disease, take at least 1 hour before morning and evening meals. If being treated for rosacea, take first thing in the morning, on an empty stomach, with a full glass of water.
- Avoid pregnancy while taking this drug; using barrier contraceptives is advised.
- You may experience these side effects: Sensitivity to sunlight (wear protective clothing, use sunscreen), diarrhea.
- Report rash, itching, difficulty breathing, dark urine or light-colored stools, pain at injection site.

▽dronabinol (delta-9-tetrahydrocannabinol, delta-9-THC)

*(droe **nab'** i nol)*

Marinol

Pregnancy Category C

Controlled Substance C-III

Drug classes

Antiemetic
Appetite stimulant

Therapeutic actions

Principal psychoactive substance in marijuana; has complex CNS effects; mechanism of action as antiemetic is not understood.

Indications

- Treatment of nausea and vomiting associated with cancer chemotherapy in patients who have failed to respond adequately to conventional antiemetic treatment (should be used only under close supervision by a responsible individual because of potential to alter the mental state)
- Treatment of anorexia associated with weight loss in patients with AIDS for appetite stimulation

Contraindications and cautions

- Contraindicated with allergy to dronabinol or sesame oil vehicle in capsules, nausea and vomiting arising from any cause other than cancer chemotherapy, lactation.
- Use cautiously with hypertension; heart disease; manic, depressive, schizophrenic patients (dronabinol may unmask symptoms of these disease states); pregnancy; history of substance abuse; seizures.

Available forms

Capsules—2.5, 5, 10 mg

Dosages

Adults and pediatric patients

- *Antiemetic:* Initially, 5 mg/m^2 PO 1–3 hr prior to the administration of chemotherapy. Repeat dose every 2–4 hr after chemotherapy is given, for a total of four to six doses per day. If the 5 mg/m^2 dose is ineffective and there are no significant side effects, increase dose by 2.5 mg/m^2 increments to a maximum of 15 mg/m^2 per dose.
- *Appetite stimulation:* Initially, give 2.5 mg PO bid before lunch and supper. May reduce dose to 2.5 mg/day as a single evening or bedtime dose; up to 10 mg PO bid (not recommended for pediatric use).

Pharmacokinetics

Route	*Onset*	*Peak*	*Duration*
Oral	30–60 min	2–4 hr	4–6 hr

Metabolism: Hepatic; $T_{1/2}$: 25–36 hr
Distribution: May cross placenta; enters breast milk
Excretion: Bile, feces, urine

Adverse effects

- **CNS:** *Drowsiness; elation, laughing easily, heightened awareness, "high" dizziness; anxiety; muddled thinking; perceptual difficulties; impaired coordination; irritability, depression; weird feeling, weakness, sluggishness, headache; unsteadiness, hallucinations, memory lapse;* paresthesia, visual distortions; ataxia; paranoia, depersonalization; disorientation, confusion; tinnitus, nightmares, speech difficulty
- **CV:** Tachycardia, orthostatic hypotension; syncope
- **Dependence:** Psychological and physical dependence; tolerance to CNS and subjective effects after 30 days of use; withdrawal syndrome (irritability, insomnia, restlessness, hot flashes, sweating, rhinorrhea, loose stools, hiccups, anorexia) beginning 12 hr and ending 96 hr after discontinuation of high doses of the drug
- **Dermatologic:** Facial flushing, perspiring
- **GI:** *Dry mouth,* nausea, vomiting
- **GU:** Decrease in pregnancy rate, spermatogenesis when doses higher than those used clinically were given in preclinical studies

Interactions

✱ **Drug-drug** • Do not give with ritonavir, alcohol, sedatives, hypnotics, other psychotomimetic substances • Increased tachycardia, hypertension, drowsiness with anticholinergics, antihistamines, TCAs • Use caution if combined with dofetilide

■ Nursing considerations

Assessment

- **History:** Allergy to dronabinol or sesame oil vehicle in capsules; nausea and vomiting arising from any cause other than cancer chemotherapy; hypertension; heart disease; manic, depressive, schizophrenic disorders; lactation; pregnancy; seizures; substance abuse
- **Physical:** Skin color, texture; orientation, reflexes, bilateral grip strength, affect; P, BP, orthostatic BP; status of mucous membranes

Interventions

- Store capsules in refrigerator.
- Limit prescriptions to the minimum necessary for a single cycle of chemotherapy because of abuse potential.
- Warn patient about drug's profound effects on mental status and abuse potential before giving drug; patient needs full information regarding the use of this drug.
- Warn patient about drug's potential effects on mood and behavior to prevent panic in case these occur.
- Patient should be supervised by a responsible adult while taking drug; monitor during the first cycle of chemotherapy in which dronabinol is used to determine how long patient will need supervision.

⊗ ***Warning*** Discontinue drug if psychotic reaction occurs; observe patient closely until evaluated and counseled; patient should participate in decision about further use of drug, perhaps at lower dosage.

Teaching points

- Take drug exactly as prescribed; a responsible adult should be with you at all times while you are taking this drug.
- Avoid alcohol, sedatives, and over-the-counter drugs, including nose drops and cold remedies, while you are taking this drug.

- You may experience these side effects: Mood changes (euphoria, feeling "high" or weird, laughing, anxiety, depression, hallucinations, memory lapse, impaired thinking); weakness, faintness (change position slowly to avoid injury); dizziness, drowsiness (do not drive or perform tasks that require alertness if you experience these effects).
- Report bizarre thoughts, uncontrollable behavior or thought processes, fainting, dizziness, irregular heartbeat.

▽ dronedarone

(droh ***neh'*** *dah roan)*

Multaq

PREGNANCY CATEGORY X

Drug class

Antiarrhythmic

Therapeutic actions

Mechanism of action is not clear. Has properties of all antiarrhythmic classes; affects action potential of cardiac cells to alter conduction.

Indications

- To reduce risk of cardiovascular hospitalization in patients with paroxysmal or persistent atrial fibrillation or atrial flutter with a recent episode of either and associated cardiovascular risk factors (age older than 70 yr, hypertension, diabetes, prior CVA, left atrial diameter 50 mm or more, left ventricular ejection factor less than 40%) who are in sinus rhythm or will be cardioverted

Contraindications and cautions

- Contraindicated with hypersensitivity to components of drug, class IV heart failure or recent acute failure requiring hospitalization or referral to a specialized heart failure clinic, second- or third-degree heart block, sick sinus syndrome, pulse rate less than 50, concomitant use of drugs or herbs that prolong QT interval, prolonged QT interval, severe hepatic impairment, concurrent use of CYP3A inhibitors, pregnancy, lactation.
- Use cautiously with mild to moderate hepatic impairment, hypokalemia, hypomagnesemia, mild to moderate heart failure.

Available forms

Tablets—400 mg

Dosages

Adults

400 mg PO bid with morning and evening meal.

Pediatric patients

Safety and efficacy not established.

Pharmacokinetics

Route	*Onset*	*Peak*
Oral	Slow	3–6 hr

Metabolism: Hepatic; $T_{1/2}$: 13–19 hr
Distribution: Crosses placenta; enters breast milk
Excretion: Feces

Adverse effects

- **CV:** Bradycardia, *prolonged QT interval,* **heart failure**
- **GI:** *Nausea, diarrhea,* vomiting, abdominal pain, dyspepsia
- **Other:** *Asthenic conditions,* hypokalemia, hypomagnesemia, *rash*

Interactions

✱ **Drug-drug** • Increased risk of serious arrhythmias if combined with other antiarrhythmics; avoid this combination • Risk of digoxin toxicity if combined with dronedarone; cut digoxin dose in half and monitor patient closely • Risk of calcium channel blocker toxicity if combined; start with low dose of calcium channel blocker and monitor patient closely to verify effects and tolerability • Risk of serious bradycardia with beta blockers; start beta blocker with low dose and monitor patient closely • Risk of serious toxicity with CYP3A inhibitors (clarithromycin, itraconazole, ketoconazole, nefazodone, ritonavir; this combination is contraindicated • Decreased effectiveness with CYP3A inducers (phenobarbital, phenytoin, rifampin); avoid this combination • Increased serum levels of sirolimus, tacrolimus; adjust dosage and monitor patient closely • Risk of increased serum statins levels;

adjust dosage accordingly and monitor patient closely

✱ **Drug-food** • Risk of serious adverse effects if combined with grapefruit juice; avoid this combination

✱ **Drug-alternative therapy** • Risk of serious arrhythmia if combined with St. John's wort; avoid this combination

■ Nursing considerations

Assessment

- **History:** Hypersensitivity to components of drug, heart failure or recent acute heart failure requiring hospitalization or referral to a specialized heart failure clinic, second- or third-degree heart block, sick sinus syndrome, pulse rate less than 50, concomitant use of drugs or herbs that prolong the QT interval, prolonged QT interval, hepatic impairment, concurrent use of CYP3A inhibitors, hypokalemia, hypomagnesemia, pregnancy, lactation
- **Physical:** Skin color, lesions; P, BP, ECG with QT evaluation, heart sounds, peripheral exam for edema; abdominal exam; LFTs; serum electrolytes

Interventions

- Obtain baseline and periodic ECGs to monitor for QT interval prolongation.
- Ensure that patient does not have serious heart failure; closely monitor patient with mild to moderate heart failure for worsening of condition.
- Administer drug twice a day with morning and evening meal. Do not make up missed doses.
- Encourage patient to avoid grapefruit juice.
- Check patient's complete drug list and ensure that interacting drugs are not being used, and that appropriate dosage adjustments have been considered.
- Advise patient to use contraceptive measures; drug can cause serious fetal abnormalities.
- Advise patient to select another method of feeding the baby if nursing.
- Arrange for regular monitoring of heart rhythm, cardiac status.

Teaching points

- Take this drug twice a day with your morning and evening meal.
- If you forget a dose, take the next dose at the regular time. Do not attempt to make up or double doses.
- Do not drink grapefruit juice or use St. John's wort while taking this drug; serious adverse effects could occur.
- Continue to take this drug as prescribed, even if you are feeling well; you may be feeling well because the drug is working.
- Keep a record of all drugs, herbs, and over-the-counter medications you are taking and review it with your health care provider. This drug interacts with many of these drugs and serious complications could occur. Your health care provider may need to adjust the dosages of these drugs for your safety.
- This drug can cause serious harm to a fetus. The use of contraceptive measures is advised. If you become pregnant or wish to become pregnant, discuss this with your health care provider.
- This drug appears in breast milk and could seriously affect a baby. If you are nursing, use another method of feeding the baby.
- You may experience these side effects: Nausea, vomiting, diarrhea, abdominal pain (small, frequent meals may help; consult your health care provider if abdominal pain becomes too uncomfortable), slow heart rate (you should learn to take your pulse; contact your health care provider if your heart rate becomes markedly slower), rash.
- You will need periodic ECGs to monitor the effects of this drug on your atrial arrhythmias.
- Report shortness of breath, wheezing; difficulty sleeping because of breathing problems; rapid weight gain of 5 pounds or more; swelling in the feet or legs; the need to prop yourself up with many pillows to sleep at night; extreme fatigue.

▽ droperidol

See Appendix W, *Less commonly used drugs*.

DANGEROUS DRUG

drotrecogin alfa (activated)

*(drow tra **coh'** gin)*

Xigris

PREGNANCY CATEGORY C

Drug classes

Anti-sepsis agent
Human activated protein

Therapeutic actions

A human activated protein that exerts an antithrombotic effect by inhibiting factors Va and VIIIa; may also have indirect profibrinolytic activity. May exert an anti-inflammatory effect by inhibiting human necrosis factor production by monocytes, blocking leukocyte adhesion to cells, and limiting thrombin-induced inflammatory responses within the microvascular endothelium. Mechanism of action in severe sepsis is not completely understood but thought to be a combination of the above effects leading to a decrease in the complex organ failure associated with sepsis.

Indications

- Reduction of mortality in adult patients with severe sepsis (sepsis with acute organ dysfunction) who have a high risk of death

Contraindications and cautions

- Contraindicated with allergy to drotrecogin, active internal bleeding, hemorrhagic CVA within the last 3 mo; intracranial or intraspinal surgery or severe head trauma within the last 2 mo; trauma with an increased risk of life-threatening bleeding; presence of an epidural catheter; intracranial neoplasm or mass lesion or evidence of cerebral herniation.
- Use cautiously with known bleeding disorders; recent use of thrombolytic (within 3 days) or anticoagulant (within 7 days); GI bleeding within the last 6 wk; recent use of aspirin (more than 650 mg/day) or other platelet inhibitors (within 7 days); chronic, severe hepatic disease; pregnancy; lactation.

Available forms

Single-use vials—5, 20 mg

Dosages

Adults

24 mcg/kg/hr by IV infusion for a total of 96 hr; do not exceed 24 mcg/kg/hr.

Pediatric patients

Safety and efficacy not established for patients younger than 18 yr.

Pharmacokinetics

Route	*Onset*	*Peak*
IV	Minutes	Length of infusion

Metabolism: Plasma; $T_{1/2}$: Unknown
Distribution: May cross placenta; may enter breast milk
Excretion: Unknown

IV FACTS

Preparation: Protect from heat and light. Reconstitute 5-mg vial with 2.5 mL sterile water for injection; 20-mg vials with 10 mL sterile water for injection (resulting solution contains 2 mg/mL). Add the diluent slowly and avoid shaking or inverting the vial; gently swirl until the powder is completely dissolved. Dilute reconstituted solution with 0.9% sodium chloride injection; inject solution slowly against the side of the infusion bag. Avoid agitation. Gently invert bag to mix; do not transport in a mechanical delivery system. Reconstituted solution must be used within 3 hr; diluted solution must be used within 14 hr at room temperature. May store in refrigerator for up to 12 hours. Total in-use time should not exceed 24 hr. If particulate matter is present or solution is discolored, discard solution.
Infusion: Infuse via a dedicated line at a rate of 24 mcg/kg/hr; do not administer by bolus or IV push injection.
Incompatibilities: Do not mix with any other drug solution; can be mixed in solution only with 0.9% sodium chloride injection, lactated Ringer's injection, dextrose, or dextrose and saline mixtures. Always administer via a separate line.

Adverse effects
- **CNS:** Intracranial bleeding
- **GI:** GI bleeding, intra-abdominal bleeding, retroperitoneal bleeding
- **GU:** GU bleeding
- **Hematologic: Bleeding**
- **Other:** Skin or soft-tissue bleeding, intrathoracic bleeding

Interactions
✱ **Drug-drug** • Increased risk for bleeding to severe bleeding if combined with other drugs that affect coagulation (eg, platelet inhibitors, anticoagulants); if this combination is used, monitor patient very closely for hemorrhagic effects and discontinue drug as appropriate
✱ **Drug-lab test** • False-low clotting factor values using aPTT assay; avoid this test, and use PT for monitoring drug effects

■ Nursing considerations
Assessment
- **History:** Allergy to drotrecogin, active internal bleeding, hemorrhagic CVA within the last 3 mo, intracranial or intraspinal surgery or severe head trauma within the last 2 mo, trauma with an increased risk of life-threatening bleeding, presence of an epidural catheter, intracranial neoplasm or mass lesion or evidence of cerebral herniation, known bleeding disorders, recent thrombolytic (3 days) or anticoagulant (7 days) therapy, GI bleeding within the last 6 wk, recent use of aspirin or other platelet inhibitors (7 days), chronic severe hepatic disease, pregnancy, lactation
- **Physical:** T, body weight, skin color, lesions, P, R, BP, GI, cardiac and respiratory evaluation, PT

Interventions
- Obtain a baseline and regular PT level to evaluate effects of drug on coagulopathy; do not rely on aPTT assays.
- Arrange for packed RBC availability when drug is started.
- Discontinue drug 2 hr before any invasive procedure with inherent bleeding risk; once hemostasis has been achieved, restarting of drug may be considered—12 hr after major invasive procedure or immediately if uncomplicated, minor procedure.

⊗ ***Warning*** Stop drotrecogin immediately if clinically significant bleeding occurs. Reevaluate use of this and other drugs that affect coagulation before resuming therapy.
- Continue monitoring and other supportive measures being used to treat the sepsis.
- Ensure that IV bag is covered with UV protectant bag.
- Do not administer for longer than 96 hr.
- Monitor patient closely for any signs of bleeding and take appropriate steps to limit blood loss.

Teaching points
Many patients with severe sepsis are not cognizant; patients should be told what they are being given and what effects they may experience.
- This drug must be given IV; you will be monitored very closely.
- Bleeding may occur as a result of this drug.
- You will be closely followed with blood tests to monitor the effects of this drug on your blood.

▽ duloxetine hydrochloride
*(do **locks'** ah teen)*

Cymbalta (DNC)

PREGNANCY CATEGORY C

Drug classes
Antidepressant
Serotonin and norepinephrine reuptake inhibitor

Therapeutic actions
Inhibits neuronal serotonin and norepinephrine reuptake in the CNS resulting in a potentiation of serotonin and norepinephrine effects with resultant antidepressive effects.

Indications

- Treatment of major depressive disorder
- Management of neuropathic pain associated with diabetic peripheral neuropathy
- Treatment of generalized anxiety disorder
- Treatment of fibromyalgia
- Unlabeled uses: Stress incontinence

Contraindications and cautions

- Contraindicated with allergy to any component of drug, concurrent use of MAOIs, uncontrolled narrow-angle glaucoma, lactation, concurrent substantial alcohol use, end-stage renal disease, hepatic impairment.
- Use cautiously with pregnancy, history of mania, history of seizures, controlled narrow-angle glaucoma.

Available forms

DR capsules DNC—20, 30, 60 mg

Dosages

Adults

- *Major depressive disorder:* 20 mg PO bid; up to 60 mg/day given once a day or 30 mg bid has been used; may be increased in 30-mg increments to a maximum of 120 mg/day.
- *Switching from an MAOI:* Allow at least 14 days to elapse between discontinuing the MAOI and beginning duloxetine.
- *Switching to an MAOI:* Allow at least 5 days to elapse between discontinuing duloxetine and starting an MAOI.
- *Diabetic neuropathic pain:* 60 mg/day PO taken as a single dose, without regard to food.
- *Generalized anxiety disorder:* 60 mg/day PO; may be increased in 30-mg increments to maximum of 120 mg/day.
- *Fibromyalgia:* 30 mg/day PO for 1 wk; then increase to 60 mg/day.

Pharmacokinetics

Route	*Peak*	*Duration*
Oral	2 hr	6 hr

Metabolism: Hepatic; $T_{1/2}$: 8–17 hr
Distribution: May cross placenta; may enter breast milk
Excretion: Feces, urine

Adverse effects

- **CNS:** *Dizziness,* somnolence, tremor, blurred vision, *insomnia,* anxiety, suicidal ideation, agitation, irritability
- **CV:** Increased BP, increased heart rate
- **GI:** *Nausea, dry mouth, constipation, diarrhea,* **hepatoxicity,** vomiting, decreased appetite
- **GU:** Decreased libido, abnormal orgasm, erectile dysfunction, delayed ejaculation, dysuria
- **Other:** Hot flushes, *fatigue, increased sweating,* rash

D

Interactions

✱ **Drug-drug** • Risk of increased serum levels and toxic effects if combined with fluvoxamine; avoid this combination • Risk of bleeding if taken with NSAIDs, aspirin, warfarin • Risk of serotonin syndrome if combined with other SSRIs, triptans, linezolid, lithium, tramadol; avoid these combinations • Risk of higher serum levels if combined with paroxetine, fluoxetine, quinidine; use caution • Risk of increased levels of TCAs, phenothiazines, propafenone, flecainide if combined with duloxetine; monitor patient closely and adjust dosage as needed • Risk of serious to potentially fatal reactions if combined with MAOIs; avoid this combination and make sure patient has not had an MAOI for at least 14 days before beginning duloxetine • Risk of toxicity if combined with alcohol; avoid this combination

✱ **Drug-alternative therapy** • Risk of serotonin syndrome if combined with St. John's wort; avoid this combination

■ Nursing considerations

Assessment

- **History:** Allergy to any component of the drug, concurrent use of MAOIs, narrow-angle glaucoma, lactation, concurrent substantial alcohol use, end-stage renal disease, hepatic impairment, pregnancy, history of mania, history of seizures
- **Physical:** Skin lesions, orientation, reflexes, affect; BP, P; abdominal examination

Interventions

- Ensure that patient is not taking an MAOI and has not taken one in at least 14 days before starting therapy.
- Monitor patient for signs of hepatotoxicity—darkened urine, right upper quadrant pain, flulike symptoms, elevated liver enzymes—especially if the patient uses alcohol excessively or has a history of liver impairment.

⊗ ***Black box warning*** Monitor patient for increased depression, including agitation, irritability, and increased suicidal ideation, especially when beginning therapy or changing dosage; especially likely with children, adolescents, and young adults. Provide appropriate interventions and protection. Drug is not approved for pediatric use.

- Ensure that patient swallows capsules whole; they should not be cut, crushed, or chewed, nor should the capsule be opened and the contents sprinkled on food.
- Instruct the patient not to consume considerable amounts of alcohol while on this drug; occurrence of liver damage is much greater when combined with alcohol; if the patient cannot refrain from alcohol intake, a different antidepressant should be used.
- Encourage the use of barrier contraceptives during treatment with this drug: fetal abnormalities are possible.
- Help the patient find another method of feeding the baby if lactating.
- Arrange to taper the drug when discontinuing; tapering decreases the risk of adverse events.

Teaching points

- Take this drug two times a day; it may be taken with or without food; if taking for diabetic neuropathy, take once a day.
- If you forget a dose, take it as soon as you remember and return to your usual regimen. Do not make up doses and do not take more than two doses in 24 hours.
- Swallow the capsule whole; do not cut, crush, chew, or sprinkle the contents of the capsule on food.
- Be aware that this drug should not be taken during pregnancy; if you suspect that you are pregnant, or wish to become pregnant, consult your health care provider.
- You should find another method of feeding the baby if you are nursing; it is not known if this drug crosses into breast milk.
- Do not stop this drug abruptly; it should be tapered slowly to decrease adverse effects.
- You may experience impaired judgment, impaired thinking, or impaired motor skills. You should not drive or operate hazardous machinery or sign important documents or make important decisions until you are certain that *Cymbalta* has not affected your ability to engage in these activities safely.
- You may experience these side effects: Dry mouth, diarrhea, abdominal discomfort, nausea (sucking on sugarless lozenges may help; consult your health care provider if this becomes a problem); depression, thoughts of suicide (you and your family should discuss this possibility and they should be on the alert for signs that this is happening; if this occurs, consult your health care provider); changes in libido or sexual response (discuss this with your health care provider).
- Report depression or thoughts of suicide, changes in color of stool or urine, sexual dysfunction, agitation, fever, hallucinations, rapid heart rate.

▽dutasteride

(du tas' teh ride)

Avodart (DNC)

PREGNANCY CATEGORY X

Drug classes

Androgen hormone inhibitor
BPH drug

Therapeutic actions

Inhibits the intracellular enzyme (5 alpha-reductase) that converts testosterone into a potent androgen (DHT); does not affect androgen receptors in the body; the prostate gland is dependent on DHT for its development and maintenance.

Indications

- Treatment of symptomatic BPH in men with an enlarged prostate gland
- In combination with tamsulosin for treatment of symptomatic BPH in men with enlarged prostate gland

Contraindications and cautions

- Contraindicated with allergy to any component of the product, other 5-alpha-reductase inhibitors, women, children, pregnancy, lactation.
- Use cautiously with hepatic impairment.

Available forms

Capsule DNC—0.5 mg

Dosages

Adults

0.5 mg/day PO. Swallow whole.

- *Combination therapy with tamsulosin:* 0.5 mg/day PO with tamsulosin 0.4. mg/day PO.

Pediatric patients

Contraindicated in pediatric patients.

Pharmacokinetics

Route	Peak	Duration
Oral	2–3 hr	Unknown

Metabolism: Hepatic; $T_{1/2}$: 5 wk
Distribution: Crosses placenta; may enter breast milk (but not indicated for use in women)
Excretion: Feces

Adverse effects

- **GI:** Abdominal upset
- **GU:** Impotence, decreased libido, decreased volume of ejaculation
- **Other:** Breast enlargement, breast tenderness

Interactions

✱ **Drug-drug** • Possible increased serum levels with ketoconazole, ritonavir, verapamil, diltiazem, cimetidine, ciprofloxacin

✱ **Drug-lab test** • Decreased PSA levels; false decrease in PSA does not mean that patient is free of risk of prostate cancer

■ Nursing considerations

Assessment

- **History:** Allergy to any component of the product or other 5 alpha-reductase inhibitors, hepatic impairment, pregnancy, lactation
- **Physical:** Liver evaluation, abdominal examination; LFTs, renal function tests, normal urine output, prostate examination

Interventions

- Assess patient to ensure that problem is BPH and that other disorders (eg, prostate cancer, infection, strictures, hypotonic bladder) have been ruled out.
- Administer without regard to meals; ensure that the patient swallows capsules whole; do not cut, crush, or chew capsules.
- Arrange for regular follow-up, including prostate examination, PSA levels, and evaluation of urine flow.
- Monitor urine flow and output. Increase in urine flow may not occur in all patients.

⊗ ***Warning*** Do not allow pregnant women to handle dutasteride capsules because of risk of absorption, which could adversely affect the fetus.

⊗ ***Warning*** Caution patient that if his sexual partner is or may become pregnant, she should be protected from his semen, which contains dutasteride and could adversely affect the fetus. The patient should use a condom or discontinue dutasteride therapy.

- Caution patient that he will not be able to donate blood until at least 6 mo after the last dose of dutasteride.
- Alert patient that libido may be decreased as well as volume of ejaculate; these effects are usually reversible when the drug is stopped.
- Provide counseling to help patient deal with effects on sexuality.

Teaching points

- Take this drug without regard to meals. Swallow the capsule whole; do not cut, crush, or chew capsules. If you miss a dose, take the capsule as soon as you remember and take the next dose the following day. Do not take more than one capsule each day.

D

- Arrange to have regular medical follow-up while you are on this drug to evaluate your response.
- This drug has serious adverse effects on unborn babies; do not allow a pregnant woman to handle the drug; if your sexual partner is or may become pregnant, protect her from exposure to your semen by using a condom; you may need to discontinue the drug if this is not acceptable.
- You will not be able to donate blood until at least 6 months after your last dose of dutasteride to prevent inadvertently giving dutasteride to a pregnant woman in a blood transfusion.
- You may experience these side effects: Loss of libido, impotence, decreased amount of ejaculate (these effects are usually reversible when the drug is stopped).
- Report inability to void, groin pain, sore throat, fever, weakness.

▽ dyphylline (dihydroxypropyl theophyllin)

(dye' fi lin)

Dylix, Lufyllin, Lufyllin-400

PREGNANCY CATEGORY C

Drug classes

Bronchodilator
Xanthine

Therapeutic actions

A theophylline derivative that is not metabolized to theophylline; relaxes bronchial smooth muscle, causing bronchodilation and increasing vital capacity, which has been impaired by bronchospasm and air trapping; at high doses it also inhibits the release of slow-reacting substance of anaphylaxis and histamine.

Indications

- Symptomatic relief or prevention of bronchial asthma and reversible bronchospasm associated with chronic bronchitis and emphysema

Contraindications and cautions

- Contraindicated with hypersensitivity to any xanthine or to ethylenediamine, peptic ulcer, active gastritis.
- Use cautiously with cardiac arrhythmias, acute myocardial injury, heart failure, cor pulmonale, severe hypertension, severe hypoxemia, renal or hepatic disease, hyperthyroidism, alcoholism, pregnancy, lactation.

Available forms

Tablets—200, 400 mg; elixir—100 mg/15 mL

Dosages

Individualize dosage based on clinical responses with monitoring of serum dyphylline levels; serum theophylline levels do not measure dyphylline; equivalence of dyphylline to theophylline is not known.

Adults

Up to 15 mg/kg, PO every 6 hr.

Pediatric patients

Safety and efficacy not established.

Geriatric patients or impaired adults

Use cautiously in elderly men and with cor pulmonale, heart failure, or renal disease.

Pharmacokinetics

Route	*Peak*	*Duration*
Oral	1 hr	6 hr

Metabolism: Hepatic; $T_{1/2}$: 2 hr
Distribution: Crosses placenta; enters breast milk
Excretion: Urine

Adverse effects

- **CNS:** *Headache, insomnia,* irritability; restlessness, dizziness, muscle twitching, seizures, severe depression, stammering speech; abnormal behavior: Withdrawal, mutism, and unresponsiveness alternating with hyperactivity; brain damage, **death**
- **CV:** Palpitations, sinus tachycardia, ventricular tachycardia, life-threatening ventricular arrhythmias, circulatory failure, hypotension
- **GI:** *Nausea, vomiting, diarrhea,* loss of appetite, hematemesis, epigastric pain, gastroesophageal reflux during sleep, increased AST

- **GU:** Proteinuria, increased excretion of renal tubular cells and RBCs; diuresis (dehydration), urinary retention in men with prostate enlargement
- **Respiratory:** Tachypnea, respiratory arrest
- **Other:** Fever, flushing, hyperglycemia, SIADH, rash

Interactions

✱ **Drug-drug** • Increased effects with probenecid, mexiletine • Increased cardiac toxicity with halothane • Decreased effects of benzodiazepines, nondepolarizing neuromuscular blockers • Mutually antagonistic effects of beta blockers and dyphylline

■ Nursing considerations

Assessment

- **History:** Hypersensitivity to any xanthine or to ethylenediamine, peptic ulcer, active gastritis, cardiac arrhythmias, acute myocardial injury, heart failure, cor pulmonale, severe hypertension, severe hypoxemia, renal or hepatic disease, hyperthyroidism, alcoholism, labor, lactation
- **Physical:** Bowel sounds, normal output; P, auscultation, BP, perfusion, ECG; R, adventitious sounds; frequency, voiding, normal output pattern, urinalysis, renal function tests; liver palpation, LFTs; thyroid function tests; skin color, texture, lesions; reflexes, bilateral grip strength, affect, EEG

Interventions

- Give with food if GI effects occur.
- Monitor patient carefully for clinical signs of adverse effects.
- Keep diazepam readily available to treat seizures.

Teaching points

- Take this drug exactly as prescribed (around the clock for adequate control of asthma attacks).
- Avoid excessive intake of coffee, tea, cocoa, cola beverages, and chocolate.
- Keep all appointments for monitoring of response to this drug.
- You may experience these side effects: Nausea, loss of appetite (take with food); difficulty sleeping, depression, emotional lability.
- Report nausea, vomiting, severe GI pain, restlessness, seizures, irregular heartbeat.

▽eculizumab

See Appendix W, *Less commonly used drugs*.

▽edetate calcium disodium (calcium EDTA)

(ed' e tate)

Calcium Disodium Versenate

PREGNANCY CATEGORY B

Drug class

Antidote

Therapeutic actions

Calcium in this compound is easily displaced by heavy metals, such as lead, to form stable complexes that are excreted in the urine; edetate disodium has strong affinity to calcium, lowering calcium levels and pulling calcium out of extracirculatory stores during slow infusion.

Indications

- Acute and chronic lead poisoning and lead encephalopathy

Contraindications and cautions

- Contraindicated with sensitivity to EDTA preparations, anuria, increased intracranial pressure (rapid IV infusion).
- Use cautiously with cardiac disease, heart failure, lactation, renal impairment, pregnancy.

Available forms

Injection—200 mg/mL

Dosages

Effective by IV, IM routes; IM route is safest in children and patients with lead encephalopathy.

Adults and pediatric patients

- *Lead poisoning:* For blood levels 20–70 mcg/dL, 1,000 mg/mg^2/day IV or IM for 5 days. Interrupt therapy for 2–4 days; follow with another 5 days of treatment if indicated. For blood levels higher than 70 mcg/dL, combine with dimercaprol therapy.

Pharmacokinetics

Route	*Onset*	*Peak*
IM, IV	1 hr	24–48 hr

Metabolism: $T_{1/2}$: 20–60 min (IV), 90 min (IM)
Distribution: May cross placenta; may enter breast milk
Excretion: Urine

IV FACTS

Preparation: *Lead poisoning:* Dilute the 5 mL ampule with 250–500 mL of 0.9% sodium chloride or 5% dextrose solution. *Pediatric:* Dissolve dose in a sufficient volume of 5% dextrose injection or 0.9% sodium chloride injection to bring the final concentration to not more than 3%.
Infusion: *Lead poisoning:* Infuse the total daily dose over 4–24 hr. *Pediatric:* Infuse over 3 hr or more. Do not exceed the patient's cardiac reserve.

Adverse effects

- **CNS:** Headache, transient circumoral paresthesia, numbness
- **CV:** Heart failure, blood pressure changes, thrombophlebitis
- **GI:** *Nausea, vomiting, diarrhea* (edetate disodium)
- **GU:** Renal tubular necrosis
- **Hematologic:** *Electrolyte imbalance* (hypocalcemia, hypokalemia, hypomagnesemia, altered blood sugar)

Interactions

✱ **Drug-drug** • Decreased effectiveness of zinc insulin with edetate calcium disodium; suggest use of other insulin preparation

■ Nursing considerations

Assessment

- **History:** Sensitivity to EDTA preparations; anuria; increased intracranial pressure; cardiac disease, heart failure, lactation, pregnancy
- **Physical:** Pupillary reflexes, orientation; P, BP; urinalysis, BUN, serum electrolytes

Interventions

⊠ ***Black box warning*** Reserve use for serious conditions that require aggressive therapy; serious toxicity can occur.

- Administer IM or IV.
- Avoid excess fluids in patients with lead encephalopathy and increased intracranial pressure; for these patients, mix edetate calcium disodium 20% solution with procaine to give a final concentration of 0.5% procaine, and administer IM.
- Establish urine flow by IV infusion prior to first dose to those dehydrated from vomiting. Once urine flow is established, restrict further IV fluid. Stop EDTA when urine flow ceases.
- Arrange for periodic BUN and serum electrolyte determinations before and during each course of therapy. Stop drug if signs of increasing renal damage occur.
- Do not administer in larger than recommended doses.

⊗ ***Warning*** Keep patient supine for a short period because of the possibility of orthostatic hypotension.

Teaching points

- Prepare a schedule of rest and drug days.
- Arrange for periodic blood tests during the course of therapy.
- Constant monitoring of heart rhythm may be needed during drug administration.
- Report pain at injection site, difficulty voiding, markedly decreased urine production.

▽ edrophonium chloride

*(ed roe **foe'** nee um)*

Reversol

PREGNANCY CATEGORY C

Drug classes

Antidote
Cholinesterase inhibitor (anticholinesterase)

Diagnostic agent
Muscle stimulant

Therapeutic actions
Increases the concentration of acetylcholine at the sites of cholinergic transmission; prolongs and exaggerates the effects of acetylcholine by reversibly inhibiting the enzyme acetylcholinesterase, facilitating transmission at the skeletal neuromuscular junction.

Indications
- Differential diagnosis and adjunct in evaluating treatment of myasthenia gravis
- Antidote for nondepolarizing neuromuscular junction blockers (curare, tubocurarine) after surgery

Contraindications and cautions
- Contraindicated with hypersensitivity to anticholinesterases, intestinal or urogenital tract obstruction, peritonitis, sulfite sensitivity, lactation.
- Use cautiously with asthma, peptic ulcer, bradycardia, cardiac arrhythmias, recent coronary occlusion, vagotonia, hyperthyroidism, epilepsy, pregnancy near term.

Available forms
Injection—10 mg/mL

Dosages
Adults
IM
- *Differential diagnosis of myasthenia gravis:* If veins are inaccessible, inject 10 mg IM. Patients who demonstrate cholinergic reaction (see table) should be retested with 2 mg IM after 30 min to rule out false-negative results.

IV
- *Differential diagnosis of myasthenia gravis:* Prepare tuberculin syringe containing 10 mg edrophonium with IV needle. Inject 2 mg IV in 15–30 sec; leave needle in vein. If no reaction occurs after 45 sec, inject the remaining 8 mg. If a cholinergic reaction (parasympathomimetic effects, muscle fasciculations, or increased muscle weakness) occurs after 2 mg, discontinue the test, and administer atropine sulfate 0.4–0.5 mg IV. May repeat test after 30 min.
- *Evaluation of treatment requirements in myasthenia gravis:* 1–2 mg IV 1 hr after oral intake of the treatment drug. Responses are summarized below:

Response to Edrophonium Test	*Myasthenia (Under-treated)*	*Cholinergic (Over-treated)*
Muscle strength: ptosis, diplopia, respiration, limb strength	Increased	Decreased
Fasciculations: orbicularis oculi facial and limb muscles	Absent	Present or absent
Side reactions: lacrimation, sweating, salivating, nausea, vomiting, diarrhea, abdominal cramps	Absent	Severe

- *Edrophonium test in crisis:* Secure controlled respiration immediately if patient is apneic, then administer test. If patient is in cholinergic crisis, administration of edrophonium will increase oropharyngeal secretions and further weaken respiratory muscles. If crisis is myasthenic, administration of edrophonium will improve respiration, and patient can be treated with longer-acting IV anticholinesterase medication. To administer the test, draw up no more than 2 mg edrophonium into the syringe. Give 1 mg IV initially. Carefully observe cardiac response. If after 1 min this dose does not further impair the patient, inject the remaining 1 mg. If after a 2-mg dose no clear improvement in respiration occurs, discontinue all anticholinesterase drug therapy, and control ventilation by tracheostomy and assisted respiration.
- *Antidote for nondepolarizing neuromuscular junction blockers:* 10 mg given slowly IV over 30–45 sec so that onset of cholinergic reaction can be detected; repeat when necessary. Maximal dose for any patient is 40 mg.

Pediatric patients
IV
- *Differential diagnosis of myasthenia gravis:*
  Infants: 0.5 mg.
  Child weighing 34 kg or less: 1 mg.
  Child weighing more than 34 kg: 2 mg.

E

If child does not respond in 45 sec, dose may be titrated up to 5 mg in child less than 34 kg, up to 10 mg in child more than 34 kg, given in increments of 1 mg every 30–45 sec.

IM

- *Differential diagnosis of myasthenia gravis: Child weighing 34 kg or less:* 2 mg. *Child weighing more than 34 kg:* 5 mg. A delay of 2–10 min occurs until reaction.

Pharmacokinetics

Route	*Onset*	*Duration*
IM	2–10 min	5–30 min
IV	30–60 sec	5–20 min

Metabolism: $T_{1/2}$: 5–10 min
Distribution: May cross placenta; may enter breast milk
Excretion: Unknown

IV FACTS

Preparation: No preparation is required.
Infusion: Rate of infusion varies with reason for administration; see Dosages.

Adverse effects

Parasympathomimetic effects

- **CV:** *Bradycardia, cardiac arrhythmias,* AV block and nodal rhythm, **cardiac arrest;** decreased cardiac output, leading to hypotension, syncope
- **Dermatologic:** Diaphoresis, flushing
- **EENT:** *Lacrimation, miosis,* spasm of accommodation, diplopia, conjunctival hyperemia
- **GI:** *Salivation, dysphagia, nausea, vomiting, increased peristalsis, abdominal cramps,* flatulence, diarrhea
- **GU:** *Urinary frequency and incontinence,* urinary urgency
- **Respiratory:** *Increased pharyngeal and tracheobronchial secretions,* laryngospasm, bronchospasm, bronchiolar constriction, dyspnea

General effects

- **CNS:** Seizures, dysarthria, dysphonia, drowsiness, dizziness, headache, loss of consciousness
- **Dermatologic:** Rash, urticaria, **anaphylaxis**
- **Local:** Thrombophlebitis after IV use
- **Peripheral:** Skeletal muscle weakness, fasciculations, muscle cramps, arthralgia
- **Respiratory:** Respiratory muscle paralysis, central respiratory paralysis

Interactions

✱ **Drug-drug** • Risk of profound muscular depression refractory to anticholinesterases if given concurrently with corticosteroids, succinylcholine

■ Nursing considerations

Assessment

Administering edrophonium for diagnostic purposes is generally supervised by a neurologist or other physician skilled and experienced in dealing with myasthenic patients; administering edrophonium to reverse neuromuscular blocking drugs is generally supervised by an anesthesiologist. Any nurse participating in the care of a patient receiving anticholinesterases should keep these points in mind.

- **History:** Hypersensitivity to anticholinesterases; intestinal or urogenital tract obstruction, peritonitis, lactation, asthma, peptic ulcer, cardiac arrhythmias, recent coronary occlusion, vagotonia, hyperthyroidism, epilepsy, pregnancy near term
- **Physical:** Bowel sounds, normal output; frequency, voiding pattern, normal output; R, adventitious sounds; P, auscultation, BP; reflexes, bilateral grip strength, EEG; thyroid function tests; skin color, texture, lesions

Interventions

- Administer IV slowly with constant monitoring of patient's response.
- Overdosage with anticholinesterase drugs can cause muscle weakness (cholinergic crisis) that is difficult to differentiate from myasthenic weakness; edrophonium is used to help make this diagnostic distinction. The administration of atropine may mask the parasympathetic effects of anticholinesterases and confound the diagnosis.

⊗ ***Warning*** Keep atropine sulfate readily available as an antidote and antagonist to edrophonium.

Teaching points

- The patient should know what to expect during diagnostic test with edrophonium (patients receiving drug to reverse neuromuscular blockers will not be aware of drug effects and do not require specific teaching about the drug).

efalizumab

See Appendix W, *Less commonly used drugs*.

efavirenz

(eff ah vye' renz)

Sustiva DNG

PREGNANCY CATEGORY D

Drug classes

Antiviral
Non-nucleoside reverse transcriptase inhibitor

Therapeutic actions

A non-nucleoside reverse transcriptase inhibitor shown to be effective in suppressing the HIV virus in adults and children.

Indications

- Treatment of HIV and AIDS in adults and children when used in combination with other antiretroviral drugs

Contraindications and cautions

- Contraindicated with life-threatening allergy to any component, lactation.
- Use cautiously with hepatic impairment, hypercholesterolemia, psychiatric disorders, pregnancy.

Available forms

Capsules DNG—50, 200 mg; tablets DNG—600 mg

Dosages

Adults

600 mg PO daily in conjunction with a protease inhibitor or other nucleoside reverse transcriptase inhibitor. In combination with voriconazole 400 mg PO every 12 hr: 300 mg/day PO.

Pediatric patients 3 yr and older

Dosage is based on weight of child as follows:

Weight (kg)	*Daily Dosage (mg)*
10– less than 15	200 PO
15– less than 20	250 PO
20– less than 25	300 PO
25– less than 32.5	350 PO
32.5– less than 40	400 PO
40 or more	600 PO

Pediatric patients younger than 3 yr

Not recommended.

Pharmacokinetics

Route	*Onset*	*Peak*
Oral	Varies	3–5 hr

Metabolism: Hepatic; $T_{1/2}$: 52–76 hr
Distribution: Crosses placenta; may enter breast milk
Excretion: Urine

Adverse effects

- **CNS:** *Headache,* insomnia, *drowsiness, asthenia,* malaise, *dizziness,* paresthesia, somnolence, impaired concentration, depression, suicidal ideation
- **GI:** *Nausea, diarrhea,* anorexia, vomiting, dyspepsia, liver impairment
- **Other:** Increased cholesterol, *rash*

Interactions

✱ **Drug-drug** ⊗ ***Warning*** Possible severe adverse effects if taken with astemizole, cisapride, pimozide, bepridil, midazolam, rifabutin, triazolam, ergot derivatives; avoid these combinations, which are contraindications • Possible increased hepatic impairment if combined with alcohol or hepatotoxic drugs; avoid this combination • Decreased levels of voriconazole if combined; adjust dosages of both drugs • Decreased effectiveness of indinavir, saquinavir; consider dosage adjustments • Decreased serum levels of efavirenz if combined with rifampin • Risk of increased levels of ritonavir when combined • Risk of decreased methadone levels and withdrawal symptoms of methadone if taken with efavirenz

✱ **Drug-food** • Decreased absorption and therapeutic effects if taken with a high-fat meal; avoid taking with food

✱ **Drug-lab test** • False-positive urine cannabinoid test

✱ **Drug-alternative therapy** • Decreased effectiveness of efavirenz with St. John's wort; avoid this combination

■ Nursing considerations

Assessment

- **History:** Life-threatening allergy to any component, impaired hepatic function, pregnancy, lactation, hypercholesterolemia
- **Physical:** Skin rashes, lesions, texture; body T; affect, reflexes, peripheral sensation; bowel sounds, liver evaluation; LFTs, CBC and differential, serum cholesterol

Interventions

- Arrange to monitor hematologic indices every 2 wk during therapy.
- Ensure that patient is taking this drug as part of a combination therapy program.

⊗ ***Warning*** Administer the drug at bedtime for the first 2–4 wk of therapy to minimize the CNS effects of the drug.

- Monitor patient for signs of opportunistic infections that will need to be treated appropriately.
- Administer the drug once a day, with meals if GI effects occur. Avoid high-fat meals.
- Provide comfort measures to help patient to cope with drug's effects—environmental control (temperature, lighting), back rubs, mouth care.
- Recommend patient use barrier contraceptives while taking this drug; serious fetal deformities have occurred.
- Establish safety precautions if CNS effects occur, especially likely during the first few days of treatment.
- Offer support and encouragement to the patient to deal with the diagnosis as well as the effects of drug therapy.

Teaching points

- Take drug once a day. Take the drug at bedtime to cut down some of the unpleasant effects of the drug. You may take the drug with meals if GI upset is a problem. Avoid taking this drug with high-fat meals. Be sure to take your other drugs regularly along with the efavirenz. Do not break tablets; swallow them whole.
- Efavirenz is not a cure for AIDS or HIV; opportunistic infections may occur and regular medical care should be sought to deal with the disease.
- Efavirenz does not reduce the risk of transmission of HIV to others by sexual contact or blood contamination; use appropriate precautions.
- Use barrier contraceptives while you are taking this drug; serious fetal deformities can occur. If you wish to become pregnant, consult your health care provider.
- Report any medications or herbs you are taking to your health care provider; avoid St. John's wort while taking this drug.
- You may experience these side effects: Nausea, loss of appetite, GI upset (eat frequent small meals; consult your health care provider if this becomes severe); dizziness, drowsiness (this is more likely at the beginning of drug therapy; avoid driving and operating machinery if these occur).
- Report extreme fatigue, lethargy, severe headache, severe nausea, vomiting, difficulty breathing, rash, depression, changes in color of stools, thoughts of suicide.

▽ eletriptan hydrobromide

*(ell ah **trip'** tan)*

Relpax

PREGNANCY CATEGORY C

Drug classes

Antimigraine drug
5-HT receptor selective agonist
Triptan

Therapeutic actions

Binds to serotonin receptors to cause vascular constrictive effects on cranial blood vessels, causing the relief of migraine in selective patients.

Indications

- Treatment of acute migraines with or without aura in adults

Contraindications and cautions

- Contraindicated with hypersensitivity to any component of eletriptan, allergy to other triptans, ischemic heart disease, cerebrovascular syndrome, peripheral vascular disease, uncontrolled hypertension, hemiplegic or basilar migraine, severe hepatic impairment, within 24 hr of using any other triptan- or ergotamine-containing medication.
- Use cautiously with pregnancy, lactation, hepatic impairment.

Available forms

Tablets—20, 40 mg

Dosages

Adults

Individualize dosage; 20–40 mg PO. If the headache improves but then returns, a second dose may be given after waiting at least 2 hr. Maximum daily dose, 80 mg.

Pediatric patients

Safety and efficacy not established.

Pharmacokinetics

Route	*Onset*	*Peak*
Oral	Rapid	1.5–2 hr

Metabolism: Hepatic; $T_{1/2}$: 4 hr
Distribution: May cross placenta; enters breast milk
Excretion: Urine, nonrenal processes

Adverse effects

- **CNS:** *Hypertonia, hypesthesia, vertigo,* abnormal dreams, anxiety
- **CV: Palpitations,** hypertension, tachycardia, angina, **MI**
- **GI:** Nausea, anorexia, constipation, esophagitis, flatulence
- **Respiratory:** *Pharyngitis,* dyspnea, asthma, URI, rhinitis
- **Other:** Fever, chills, *sweating,* bone pain

Interactions

✱ **Drug-drug** • Risk of prolonged vasospastic reactions if combined with ergot-containing drugs; do not use within 24 hr of each other • Risk of greatly elevated serum levels of CYP3A4 inhibitors—ketoconazole, itraconazole, nefazodone, clarithromycin, ritonavir, nelfinavir—and of eletriptan if combined; do not use within 72 hr of each other • Risk of combined effects if used within 24 hr of other triptans; do not use within 24 hr of each other • Risk of serotonin syndrome if combined with other serotonergic drugs, such as SSRIs

E

■ Nursing considerations

Assessment

- **History:** Hypersensitivity to any component of eletriptan, allergy to other triptans, presence of ischemic heart disease, cerebrovascular syndrome, peripheral vascular disease, uncontrolled hypertension, hemiplegic or basilar migraine, severe hepatic impairment, use within 24 hr of any other triptan- or ergotamine-containing medication, pregnancy, lactation, hepatic impairment
- **Physical:** T, orientation, reflexes, peripheral sensation; P, BP; R, adventitious sounds; abdominal examination; LFTs

Interventions

- Administer to relieve acute migraine, not as a prophylactic measure; supervise first dose of drug.
- Ensure that the patient has not taken an ergot-containing compound or other triptan within 24 hr.
- Do not administer more than two doses in a 24-hr period.
- Establish safety measures if CNS or visual disturbances occur.
- Control environment (eg, lighting, temperature) as appropriate to help relieve migraine.

⊗ ***Warning*** Monitor BP of patients with possible coronary artery disease; discontinue at any sign of angina, prolonged high BP, tachycardia, chest discomfort.

Teaching points

- Take drug exactly as prescribed, at the onset of headache or aura. Do not take this drug to prevent a migraine; it is used only to treat migraines that are occurring. If the headache persists after you take this drug, you may repeat the dose 2 hours later.

- Do not take more than two doses in 24-hour period. Do not take any other migraine medication while you are taking this drug. If your headache is not relieved, consult your health care provider.
- Maintain your usual procedures during a migraine—eg, control lighting, noise.
- Contact your health care provider immediately if you experience chest pain or pressure that is severe or does not go away.
- This drug interacts with many other drugs; consult with your health care provider if you are taking any other medications or if you add any drugs to your drug regimen.
- This drug should not be taken during pregnancy; if you suspect that you are pregnant, contact your health care provider and refrain from using drug.
- You may experience these side effects: Dizziness, drowsiness (avoid driving and using dangerous machinery while taking this drug); numbness, tingling, feelings of tightness or pressure.
- Report chest pain, numbness, chills.

eltrombopag

See Appendix W, *Less commonly used drugs*.

emtricitabine

*(em tra **cye'** tah ben)*

Emtriva

PREGNANCY CATEGORY B

Drug classes

Anti-HIV drug
Antiviral
Reverse transcriptase inhibitor

Therapeutic actions

HIV-1 reverse transcriptase inhibitor; competes with a natural substrate and is incorporated into the viral DNA, leading to chain termination.

Indications

- In combination with other antiretroviral drugs for the treatment of HIV-1 infection in adults and children
- **NEW INDICATION:** Off-label use: As monotherapy or in combination with clevudine for treatment of hepatitis B

Contraindications and cautions

- Contraindicated with allergy to any components of the product; lactation (HIV-infected mothers are discouraged from breastfeeding); concurrent use of lamivudine, *Atripla*, *Truvada*.
- Use cautiously with pregnancy; hepatic impairment; signs of lactic acidosis, risk factors for lactic acidosis including female gender and obesity; infection with hepatitis B virus; impaired renal function.

Available forms

Capsules—200 mg; oral solution—10 mg/mL

Dosages

Adults

200 mg daily PO, with or without food or 240 mg (24 mL) oral solution/day PO.

Pediatric patients 3 mo–17 yr

6 mg/kg/day PO to a maximum 240 mg (24 mL) oral solution; children weighing more than 33 kg and able to swallow a capsule may take one 200-mg capsule/day PO.

Pediatric patients up to 3 mo

3 mg/kg oral solution PO once daily

Patients with renal impairment

For dialysis patients, 200 mg PO every 96 hr. For renally impaired patients, use these dosages:

CrCl (mL/min)	*Capsule dosage (mg)*	*Oral solution dosage (mg)*
50 or more	200 daily	240 daily
30–49	200 every 48 hr	120 daily
15–29	200 every 72 hr	80 daily
Less than 15	200 every 96 hr	60 daily

Pharmacokinetics

Route	*Onset*	*Peak*
Oral	Rapid	1–2 hr

Metabolism: Hepatic; $T_{1/2}$: 10 hr

Distribution: May cross placenta; may enter breast milk
Excretion: Feces, urine

Adverse effects

- **CNS:** *Headache, asthenia,* depression, *insomnia, dizziness,* peripheral neurological symptoms, neuritis, paresthesias, *abnormal dreams*
- **GI:** *Nausea, diarrhea, abdominal pain,* vomiting, dyspepsia, **severe hepatomegaly with steatosis, sometimes fatal;** *elevated liver enzymes and bilirubin*
- **Metabolic: Lactic acidosis, sometimes severe,** hyperglycemia
- **Respiratory:** *Cough, rhinitis*
- **Other:** *Rash,* arthralgia, myalgia, fat redistribution

■ Nursing considerations

Assessment

- **History:** Allergy to any components of the product, lactation, pregnancy, hepatic impairment, signs of lactic acidosis, obesity, renal impairment, hepatitis B infection
- **Physical:** T; orientation, reflexes; R, adventitious sounds; abdominal examination, LFTs, renal function tests

Interventions

- Ensure that HIV antibody testing has been done before initiating therapy to reduce risk of emergence of HIV resistance.
- Ensure that patient is taking this drug in combination with other antiretroviral drugs.
- Monitor patients regularly to evaluate liver and renal function.

⊗ ***Black box warning*** Use caution if patient has or is suspected of having hepatitis B; serious resurgence of the disease can occur.

- Administer this drug without regard to food.

⊗ ***Black box warning*** Withdraw drug and monitor patient if patient develops signs of lactic acidosis or hepatotoxicity, including hepatomegaly and steatosis.

- Encourage women of childbearing age to use barrier contraceptives while taking this drug because the effects of the drug on the fetus are not known.
- Advise women who are breast-feeding to find another method of feeding the baby; HIV-infected woman are advised not to breast-feed.
- Advise patient that this drug does not cure the disease and there is still a risk of transmitting the disease to others.

Teaching points

- Take this drug once a day with or without food and in combination with your other antiviral drugs.
- Take the drug every day; if you miss a dose, take it as soon as you remember and then take the next dose at the usual time the next day. Do not double any doses.
- This drug does not cure your HIV infection and you will still be able to pass it to others; using condoms is advised. Women of childbearing age are encouraged not to become pregnant while taking this drug; barrier contraceptives are recommended.
- This drug may enter breast milk; if you are nursing a baby, you should find another method of feeding the baby.
- With some antiviral drugs, there is a redistribution of body fat—a "buffalo hump" appears and fat is distributed around the trunk and lost in the limbs; the long-term effects of this redistribution are not known.
- You may experience these side effects: Nausea, diarrhea, abdominal pain, headache (try to maintain your intake of nutrition and fluid as much as possible; eat frequent small meals and take the drug with food).
- Report severe weakness, muscle pain, trouble breathing, dizziness, cold feelings in your arms or legs, palpitations, yellowing of the eyes or skin, darkened urine or light-colored stools.

▽ enalapril maleate

*(e **nal'** a pril)*

Vasotec

enalaprilat

Vasotec I.V.

PREGNANCY CATEGORY D

Drug classes

ACE inhibitor
Antihypertensive

Therapeutic actions

Renin, synthesized by the kidneys, is released into the circulation where it acts on a plasma precursor to produce angiotensin I, which is converted by ACE to angiotensin II, a potent vasoconstrictor that also causes release of aldosterone from the adrenals; both of these actions increase BP. Enalapril blocks the conversion of angiotensin I to angiotensin II, decreasing BP, decreasing aldosterone secretion, slightly increasing serum K^+ levels, and causing Na^+ and fluid loss; increased prostaglandin synthesis also may be involved in the antihypertensive action. In patients with heart failure, peripheral resistance, afterload, preload, and heart size are decreased.

Indications

Oral

- Treatment of hypertension alone or in combination with other antihypertensives, especially thiazide-type diuretics
- Treatment of acute and chronic heart failure
- Treatment of asymptomatic left ventricular dysfunction (LVD)

Parenteral

- Treatment of hypertension when oral therapy is not possible

Contraindications and cautions

- Contraindicated with pregnancy, allergy to enalapril.
- Use cautiously with impaired renal function; salt or volume depletion (hypotension may occur); lactation.

Available forms

Tablets—2.5, 5, 10, 20 mg; injection—1.25 mg/mL

Dosages

Adults

Oral

- *Hypertension:*
  Patients not taking diuretics: Initial dose is 5 mg/day PO. Adjust dosage based on patient response. Usual range is 10–40 mg/day as a single dose or in two divided doses.
  Patients taking diuretics: Discontinue diuretic for 2–3 days if possible. If it is not possible to discontinue diuretic, give initial dose of 2.5 mg, and monitor for excessive hypotension for at least 2 hr.
  Converting to oral therapy from IV therapy: 5 mg daily with subsequent doses based on patient response.
- *Heart failure:* 2.5 mg PO daily or bid in conjunction with diuretics and digitalis. Maintenance dose is 2.5–20 mg/day given in two divided doses. Maximum daily dose is 40 mg.
- *Asymptomatic LVD:* 2.5 mg PO bid; target maintenance dose 20 mg/day in two divided doses.

Parenteral

Give IV only. 1.25 mg every 6 hr given IV over 5 min. A response is usually seen within 15 min, but peak effects may not occur for 4 hr.

- *Hypertension:*
  Converting to IV therapy from oral therapy: 1.25 mg every 6 hr; monitor patient response.
  Patients taking diuretics: 0.625 mg IV over 5 min. If adequate response is not seen after 1 hr, repeat the 0.625-mg dose. Give additional doses of 1.25 mg every 6 hr.

Pediatric patients 2 mo–16 yr

Oral

- *Hypertension:* Initial dose is 0.08 mg/kg PO once daily; maximum dose is 5 mg.

Geriatric patients and patients with renal impairment and heart failure

Oral

Excretion is reduced in renal failure; use smaller initial dose, and adjust upward to a maximum of 40 mg/day PO. For patients on dialysis, use 2.5 mg on dialysis days.

CrCl (mL/min)	*Serum Creatinine*	*Initial Dose*
More than 80	Not applicable	5 mg/day
80 or less–more than 30	Less than 3 mg/dL	5 mg/day
Less than 30	More than 3 mg/dL	2.5 mg/day

IV

If creatinine clearance is less than 30 mL/min, the initial dose is 0.625 mg, which may be repeated after 1 hr. Additional doses of 1.25 mg every 6 hr may be given with careful patient monitoring.

Pharmacokinetics

Route	*Onset*	*Peak*	*Duration*
Oral	60 min	4–6 hr	24 hr
IV	15 min	1–4 hr	6 hr

Metabolism: $T_{1/2}$: 11 hr
Distribution: Crosses placenta; enters breast milk
Excretion: Urine

IV FACTS

Preparation: Enalaprilat can be given as supplied or mixed with up to 50 mL of 5% dextrose injection, 0.9% sodium chloride injection, 0.9% sodium chloride injection in 5% dextrose, 5% dextrose in lactated Ringer's, *Isolyte E.* Stable at room temperature for 24 hr.
Infusion: Give by slow IV infusion over at least 5 min.

Adverse effects

- **CNS:** *Headache, dizziness, fatigue,* insomnia, paresthesias
- **CV:** Syncope, chest pain, palpitations, hypotension in salt- or volume-depleted patients
- **GI:** Gastric irritation, *nausea,* vomiting, *diarrhea,* abdominal pain, dyspepsia, elevated liver enzymes
- **GU:** Proteinuria, renal insufficiency, renal failure, polyuria, oliguria, urinary frequency, impotence
- **Hematologic:** *Decreased Hct and Hgb*
- **Other:** *Cough,* muscle cramps, hyperhidrosis

Interactions

✷ **Drug-drug** • Decreased hypotensive effect if taken concurrently with indomethacin, rifampin, NSAIDs

■ Nursing considerations

Assessment

- **History:** Allergy to enalapril, impaired renal function, salt or volume depletion, lactation, pregnancy
- **Physical:** Skin color, lesions, turgor; T; orientation, reflexes, affect, peripheral sensation; P, BP, peripheral perfusion; mucous membranes, bowel sounds, liver evaluation; urinalysis, LFTs, renal function tests, CBC, and differential

Interventions

⊗ ***Warning*** Alert surgeon, and mark the patient's chart with notice that enalapril is being taken; the angiotensin II formation subsequent to compensatory renin release during surgery will be blocked; hypotension may be reversed with volume expansion.

⊗ ***Black box warning*** Be aware that use of this drug in second and third trimesters can cause serious injury or death to the fetus; advise contraceptive use.

- Monitor patients on diuretic therapy for excessive hypotension after the first few doses of enalapril.
- Monitor patient closely in any situation that may lead to a drop in BP secondary to reduced fluid volume (excessive perspiration and dehydration, vomiting, diarrhea) because excessive hypotension may occur.
- Arrange for reduced dosage in patients with impaired renal function.

⊗ ***Warning*** Monitor patient carefully because peak effect may not be seen for 4 hr. Do not administer second dose until BP has been checked.

Teaching points

- Do not stop taking the medication without consulting your health care provider.
- Be careful in any situation that may lead to a drop in blood pressure (diarrhea, sweating, vomiting, dehydration).
- Avoid over-the-counter medications, especially cough, cold, and allergy medications that may interact with this drug.
- You may experience these side effects: GI upset, loss of appetite, change in taste perception (will pass with time); mouth sores (frequent mouth care may help); rash; fast heart rate; dizziness, light-headedness (usually passes in a few days; change position slowly, limit activities to those not requiring alertness and precision).
- Use of contraception is advised while taking this drug; fetal abnormalities or death may occur.
- Report mouth sores; sore throat, fever, chills; swelling of the hands, feet; irregular heartbeat, chest pains; swelling of the face, eyes, lips, tongue, difficulty breathing.

E

enfuvirtide

*(en foo **veer'** tide)*

Fuzeon

PREGNANCY CATEGORY B

Drug classes

Anti-HIV drug
Fusion inhibitor

Therapeutic actions

Prevents the entry of the HIV-1 virus into cells by inhibiting the fusion of the virus membrane with the viral and cellular membrane.

Indications

- In combination with other antiretrovirals for the treatment of HIV-1 infection in treatment-experienced patients with evidence of HIV-1 replication despite ongoing antiretroviral therapy

Contraindications and cautions

- Contraindicated with hypersensitivity to any component of enfuvirtide, lactation.
- Use cautiously with history of lung disease, pregnancy.

Available forms

Powder for injection—90 mg/mL

Dosages

Adults

90 mg bid by subcutaneous injection into the upper arm, anterior thigh, or abdomen.

Pediatric patients 6–16 yr

2 mg/kg bid by subcutaneous injection, up to a maximum of 90 mg/dose into the upper arm, anterior thigh, or abdomen.

Pharmacokinetics

Route	*Onset*	*Peak*
Subcut.	Slow	4–8 hr

Metabolism: Hepatic; $T_{1/2}$: 3.2–4.4 hr
Distribution: May cross placenta; may enter breast milk
Excretion: Tissue recycling of amino acids, not excreted

Adverse effects

- **CNS:** Dizziness, insomnia, depression, anxiety, peripheral neuropathy
- **GI:** Nausea, diarrhea, constipation, pancreatitis, abdominal pain, taste perversion, increased appetite
- **Respiratory: Pneumonia,** cough
- **Other:** Injection site reactions—pain, discomfort, redness, nodules; hypersensitivity reactions, fatigue, rash

■ Nursing considerations

Assessment

- **History:** Allergy to any components of the product, lactation, pregnancy, lung disease
- **Physical:** T; orientation, reflexes; R, adventitious sounds; skin evaluation

Interventions

- Make sure that the patient is taking this drug in combination with other antiretrovirals.
- Monitor patients regularly to evaluate lung function and viral load.
- Administer this drug by subcutaneous injection only; rotate sites regularly.
- Encourage women of childbearing age to use barrier contraceptives while taking this drug because the effects of the drug on the fetus are not known.
- Advise women who are breast-feeding to find another method of feeding the baby; HIV-infected women are advised not to breast-feed.
- Advise patient that this drug does not cure the disease and there is still a risk of transmitting the disease to others.

Teaching points

- Administer this drug by subcutaneous injection; you and a significant other should learn the proper method for preparing and administering the drug and for properly disposing of the syringes and needles.
- Administer the drug every day; if you miss a dose, contact your health care provider immediately.

- Rotate injection sites among the upper arm, abdomen, and anterior thigh; keep a record of the sites.
- Keep any reconstituted drug in the refrigerator; use within 24 hours.
- Bring refrigerated solution to room temperature before injecting; discard any unused portions.
- Continue taking your other antiviral drugs; the drugs are designed to be taken in combination.
- This drug does not cure the HIV infection and you will still be able to pass it to others; using condoms is advised. Women of childbearing age are discouraged from becoming pregnant while taking this drug; using barrier contraceptives is recommended.
- Select another method of feeding the baby if you are nursing a baby.
- Local reactions at the site of the injection occur commonly. Review the proper administration technique regularly, and rotate injection sites. If you experience severe pain, redness, or hardness at the site, consult your health care provider.
- You may experience these side effects: Nausea, diarrhea, abdominal pain, headache; (try to maintain your intake of nutrition and fluid as much as possible; eat frequent small meals); dizziness, lack of sleep (avoid driving and operating dangerous machinery if this occurs).
- Report chills, fever, any sign of infection, difficulty breathing or signs of respiratory infection, cough with fever, rapid breathing, shortness of breath.

DANGEROUS DRUG

▽enoxaparin

*(en **ocks'** a par in)*

Lovenox

PREGNANCY CATEGORY B

Drug classes
Antithrombotic
Low–molecular-weight heparin

Therapeutic actions
Low–molecular-weight heparin that inhibits thrombus and clot formation by blocking factor Xa, factor IIa, preventing the formation of clots.

Indications
- Prevention of DVT, which may lead to pulmonary embolism following hip replacement, knee replacement surgery, abdominal surgery
- Prevention of ischemic complications of unstable angina and non–Q-wave MI
- Treatment of DVT, pulmonary embolus with warfarin
- Prevention of DVT in medical patients who are at risk for thromboembolic complications due to severely restricted mobility during acute illnesses
- Treatment of acute ST-segment elevation MI, managed medically or with subsequent percutaneous coronary intervention

Contraindications and cautions
- Contraindicated with hypersensitivity to enoxaparin, heparin, pork products; severe thrombocytopenia; uncontrolled bleeding.
- Use cautiously with pregnancy or lactation, history of GI bleed, spinal tap, spinal/epidural anesthesia.

Available forms
Injection—30 mg/0.3 mL; 40 mg/0.4 mL; 60 mg/0.6 mL; 80 mg/0.8 mL; 100 mg/1 mL; 120 mg/0.8 mL; 150 mg/mL; 300 mg/3 mL

Dosages
Adults
- *DVT prophylaxis after hip or knee replacement surgery:* 30 mg subcutaneously bid with initial dose 12–24 hr after surgery. Continue throughout the postoperative period for 7–10 days; then 40 mg daily subcutaneously for up to 3 wk may be used.
- *Patients undergoing abdominal surgery:* 40 mg/day subcutaneously begun within 2 hr preoperatively and continued for 7–10 days.
- *Outpatient DVT treatment:* 1 mg/kg subcutaneously every 12 hr.
- *Inpatient DVT treatment:* 1.5 mg/kg subcutaneously once daily or 1 mg/kg every 12 hr.
- *Unstable angina and non–Q-wave MI:* 1 mg/kg subcutaneously every 12 hr for 2–8 days.

- *Prevention of DVT in high-risk medical patients:* 40 mg/day subcutaneously for 6–11 days; has been used up to 14 days.
- *Treatment of MI:*
  Younger than 75 yr: 30-mg IV bolus plus 1 mg/kg subcutaneous dose followed by 1 mg/kg subcutaneously every 12 hr with aspirin. (Maximum, 100 mg for first two doses only.)
  75 yr and older: 0.75 mg/kg subcutaneously every 12 hr. (Maximum, 75 mg for first two doses only.)

Pediatric patients

Safety and efficacy not established.

Patients with renal impairment (creatinine clearance less than 30 mL/min)

- *DVT prophylaxis:* 30 mg/day subcutaneously.
- *DVT treatment:* 1 mg/kg subcutaneously once daily.
- *MI treatment:* For patient younger than 75 yr, 30-mg IV bolus; then 1 mg/kg subcutaneously followed by 1 mg/kg/day subcutaneously. For patient 75 yr or older, 1 mg/kg/day subcutaneously.

Pharmacokinetics

Route	*Onset*	*Peak*	*Duration*
Subcut.	20–60 min	3–5 hr	12 hr

Metabolism: $T_{1/2}$: 4.5 hr
Distribution: May cross placenta; may enter breast milk
Excretion: Urine

Adverse effects

- **Hematologic: Hemorrhage;** *bruising;* thrombocytopenia; elevated AST, ALT levels; hyperkalemia
- **Hypersensitivity:** Chills, fever, urticaria, asthma
- **Other:** Fever; pain; local irritation, hematoma, erythema at site of injection, epidural or spinal hematoma with spinal tap, spinal/epidural anesthesia

Interactions

✱ **Drug-drug** • Increased bleeding tendencies with oral anticoagulants, salicylates, NSAIDs, penicillins, cephalosporins • Risk of severe bleeding if combined with heparin
✱ **Drug-lab test** • Increased AST, ALT levels
✱ **Drug-alternative therapy** • Increased risk of bleeding if combined with chamomile, garlic, ginger, ginkgo, and ginseng therapy, high-dose vitamin E

■ Nursing considerations

Assessment

- **History:** Recent surgery or injury; sensitivity to heparin, pork products, enoxaparin; lactation; history of GI bleed; pregnancy
- **Physical:** Peripheral perfusion, R, stool guaiac test, PTT or other tests of blood coagulation, platelet count, renal function tests

Interventions

- Give drug as soon as possible after hip surgery, within 12 hr of knee surgery, and within 2 hr preoperatively for abdominal surgery.

⊗ ***Black box warning*** Be aware of increased risk of spinal hematoma and neurologic damage if used with spinal/epidural anesthesia; if must be used, monitor patient closely.

- Give deep subcutaneous injections; do not give enoxaparin by IM injection.
- Administer by deep subcutaneous injection; patient should be lying down. Alternate between the left and right anterolateral and posterolateral abdominal wall. Introduce the whole length of the needle into a skinfold held between the thumb and forefinger; hold the skinfold throughout the injection.
- Apply pressure to all injection sites after needle is withdrawn; inspect injection sites for signs of hematoma; do not massage injection sites.
- Do not mix with other injections or infusions.
- Store at room temperature; fluid should be clear, colorless to pale yellow.
- Provide for safety measures (electric razor, soft toothbrush) to prevent injury to patient who is at risk for bleeding.
- Check patient for signs of bleeding; monitor blood tests.
- Alert all health care providers that patient is taking enoxaparin.

- Discontinue and initiate appropriate therapy if thromboembolic episode occurs despite enoxaparin therapy.

⊗ ***Warning*** Have protamine sulfate (enoxaparin antidote) readily available in case of overdose.

- Treat overdose as follows: Protamine sulfate (1% solution). Each mg of protamine neutralizes 1 mg enoxaparin. Give very slowly IV over 10 min.

Teaching points

- Have periodic blood tests to monitor your response to this drug.
- You and a significant other may need to learn to give the drug by subcutaneous injection and how to properly dispose of needles and syringes. Rotate injection sites.
- Avoid injury while you are taking this drug: Use an electric razor; avoid activities that might lead to injury.
- Report nosebleed, bleeding of the gums, unusual bruising, black or tarry stools, cloudy or dark urine, abdominal or lower back pain, severe headache.

▽ entacapone

*(en tah **kap'** own)*

Comtan

PREGNANCY CATEGORY C

Drug class

Antiparkinsonian

Therapeutic actions

Selectively and reversibly inhibits COMT, an enzyme that eliminates biologically active catecholamines, including dopa, dopamine, norepinephrine, epinephrine; when given with levodopa, entacapone's inhibition of COMT is believed to increase the plasma concentrations and duration of action of levodopa.

Indications

- Adjunct with levodopa and carbidopa in the treatment of the signs and symptoms of idiopathic Parkinson's disease in patients who are experiencing "wearing off" of drug effects

Contraindications and cautions

- Contraindicated with hypersensitivity to drug or its component.
- Use cautiously with hypertension, hypotension, hepatic or renal impairment, pregnancy, lactation.

Available forms

Tablets—200 mg

Dosages

Adults

200 mg PO taken concomitantly with the dose of levodopa–carbidopa, a maximum of eight times/day.

Pediatric patients

Safety and efficacy not established.

Pharmacokinetics

Route	*Onset*	*Peak*
Oral	Varies	1 hr

Metabolism: Hepatic; $T_{1/2}$: 0.4–0.7 hr, then 2.4 hr

Distribution: May cross placenta; may enter breast milk

Excretion: Feces, urine

Adverse effects

- **CNS:** *Disorientation, confusion,* memory loss, **hallucinations,** psychoses, agitation, nervousness, delusions, delirium, paranoia, euphoria, excitement, *light-headedness, dizziness,* depression, drowsiness, weakness, giddiness, paresthesias, heaviness of the limbs, numbness of fingers, *dyskinesias, hyperkinesia*
- **CV:** *Hypotension, orthostatic hypotension*
- **Dermatologic:** Rash, urticaria, other dermatoses
- **GI:** *Nausea, vomiting,* epigastric distress, flatulence, diarrhea
- **Respiratory:** URIs, dyspnea, sinus congestion, **rhabdomyolysis**
- **Other:** *Fever,* urine discoloration

Interactions

✱ **Drug-drug** • Increased toxicity and serum levels if combined with MAOIs; avoid this combination • Possible decreased excretion if combined with probenecid, cholestyramine, erythromycin, rifampin, ampicillin, or chloramphenicol; if one of these combinations is used, monitor patient closely • Risk of increased heart rate, arrhythmias, excessive BP changes if combined with norepinephrine, dopamine, dobutamine, methyldopa, isoetharine, isoproterenol, methyldopa, apomorphine, or epinephrine; administer with extreme caution and monitor patient closely

■ Nursing considerations

Assessment

- **History:** Hypersensitivity to drug or its components, hypertension, hypotension, hepatic or renal impairment, pregnancy, lactation
- **Physical:** Body weight; body T; skin color, lesions; orientation, affect, reflexes, bilateral grip strength, visual examination; P, BP, orthostatic BP, auscultation; bowel sounds, normal output, liver evaluation; urinary output, voiding pattern, LFTs, renal function tests

Interventions

⊗ ***Warning*** Administer only in conjunction with levodopa and carbidopa. Monitor patient response, customary levodopa dosage may need to be decreased.

- Provide sugarless lozenges or ice chips to suck if dry mouth is a problem.
- Give with meals if GI upset occurs; give before meals to patients bothered by dry mouth; give after meals if drooling is a problem or if drug causes nausea.
- Advise patient to use barrier contraceptives, serious birth defects can occur while using this drug; advise nursing mothers to use another means of feeding the baby because drug can enter breast milk and adversely affect the infant.
- Establish safety precautions if CNS, vision changes, hallucinations, or hypotension occurs (use side rails, accompany patient when ambulating).
- Provide additional comfort measures appropriate to patient with parkinsonism.

Teaching points

- Take this drug exactly as prescribed. Always take with your levodopa and carbidopa.
- Use barrier contraceptives while taking this drug; serious birth defects can occur. Do not nurse while on this drug; the drug enters breast milk and can adversely affect the baby.
- You may experience these side effects: Drowsiness, dizziness, confusion, blurred vision (avoid driving a car or engaging in activities that require alertness and visual acuity; if these occur, rise slowly when changing positions to help decrease dizziness); nausea (eat frequent small meals); dry mouth (suck sugarless lozenges or ice chips); hallucinations (this is a side effect of the drug; use care and have someone stay with you if this occurs); constipation (maintain adequate fluid intake and exercise regularly; if this does not help, consult your health care provider); reddish brown discoloration of urine (a drug effect).
- Report constipation, rapid or pounding heartbeat, confusion, eye pain, hallucinations, rash.

▽entecavir

*(en **tek'** ah veer)*

Baraclude

PREGNANCY CATEGORY C

Drug classes

Antiviral
Nucleoside analogue

Therapeutic actions

Blocks activities of reverse transcriptases preventing the formation of viral DNA and leading to decreased viral load associated with hepatitis B.

Indications

- Treatment of chronic hepatitis B infection in adults with evidence of active viral replication and either evidence of persistent elevations in serum aminotransferases or histologically active disease

Contraindications and cautions

- Contraindicated with known hypersensitivity to entecavir or any of its components, lactation, co-infection with HIV in patients not receiving highly active antiretroviral therapy.

- Use cautiously with pregnancy, renal impairment, liver transplant, concurrent use of drugs that alter renal function.

Available forms

Tablets—0.5, 1 mg; oral solution—0.05 mg/mL

Dosages

Adults and children 16 yr and older with no previous nucleoside treatment

0.5 mg/day PO on an empty stomach at least 2 hr after a meal or 2 hr before the next meal.

Adults and children 16 yr and older with a history of viremia also receiving lamivudine or with known resistance mutations

1 mg/day PO on an empty stomach at least 2 hr after a meal or 2 hr before the next meal.

Pediatric patients younger than 16 yr

Safety and efficacy not established.

Patients with renal impairment

Creatinine clearance of 50 mL/min or more, 0.5 mg/day PO (1 mg/day PO with lamivudine resistance); creatinine clearance of 30–less than 50 mL/min, 0.25 mg/day PO or 0.5 mg PO every 48 hr (0.5 mg/day PO or 1 mg every 48 hr with lamivudine resistance); creatinine clearance of 10–less than 30 mL/min, 0.15 mg/day PO or 0.5 mg PO every 72 hr (0.3 mg/day PO or 1 mg every 72 hr with lamivudine resistance); creatinine clearance less than 10 mL/min, 0.05 mg/day PO or 0.5 mg PO every 7 days (0.1 mg/day PO or 1 mg every 7 days with lamivudine resistance); in hemodialysis, 0.05 mg/day PO or 0.5 mg PO every 7 days (0.1 mg/day PO or 1 mg PO every 7 days with lamivudine resistance).

Pharmacokinetics

Route	*Onset*	*Peak*
Oral	Rapid	0.5–1.5 hr

Metabolism: $T_{1/2}$: 128–149 hr
Distribution: May cross placenta; may pass into breast milk
Excretion: Urine, unchanged

Adverse effects

- **CNS:** *Dizziness, headache, fatigue,* somnolence, insomnia
- **GI:** *Nausea,* vomiting, diarrhea, dyspepsia, lactic acidosis and severe hepatomegaly with steatosis
- **Other:** Acute exacerbations of hepatitis B (with discontinuation of therapy)

Interactions

✱ **Drug-drug** • Risk of decreased excretion and toxic effects if combined with drugs that alter renal function; monitor patient carefully and adjust dosages as needed

■ Nursing considerations

Assessment

- **History:** Allergy to any components of the product, lactation, pregnancy; renal impairment; signs of lactic acidosis
- **Physical:** T; orientation, reflexes; abdominal examination, LFTs, renal function tests

Interventions

- Assess renal function before beginning therapy; adjust dosage as appropriate.
- Maintain other measures used to help patient deal with chronic hepatitis B.
- Monitor patient regularly to evaluate effects of drug on the body.
- Administer this drug on an empty stomach, at least 2 hr after a meal or 2 hr before the next meal.

⊗ ***Black box warning*** Withdraw drug and monitor patient if patient develops signs of lactic acidosis or hepatotoxicity, including hepatomegaly and steatosis.

⊗ ***Black box warning*** Do not use in patients co-infected with HIV unless patient is receiving highly active antiretroviral therapy because of high risk of HIV resistance. HIV testing should be offered to all patients before starting entecavir therapy. Acute exacerbations of hepatitis B can also occur.

- Effects of the drug on a fetus are not known. Advise women of childbearing age to use barrier contraceptives while on this drug.
- Advise women who are nursing to find another method of feeding the baby; potential effects on the baby are not known.
- Advise patient that this drug does not cure the disease and there is still a risk of transmitting the disease to others.
- Monitor for worsening of hepatitis if drug is withdrawn.

E

Teaching points

- This drug is not a cure for hepatitis B. It may decrease the number of viruses in your body and may improve the condition of your liver.

⊗ ***Warning*** You should still take precautions to prevent the spread of hepatitis B; do not share any personal items that may have blood or body fluids on them; use condoms if having intercourse.

- Always take *Baraclude* on an empty stomach at least 2 hours after a meal and at least 2 hours before the next meal.
- If you are using the oral solution, use the measuring spoon provided to measure out your dose. Swallow the medicine directly from the measuring spoon. Rinse the spoon with water and allow to air dry after each use. Store the solution at room temperature.
- If you forget a dose of the drug, take that dose as soon as you remember, then take your next dose at the usual time. Do not take two doses at the same time.
- Do not run out of *Baraclude*. If you are running low, contact your health care provider; if you stop taking this drug, your hepatitis symptoms could get worse and become very serious.
- You will need to have regular health care, including blood tests, to monitor the effects of this drug on your body.
- It is not known how this drug could affect a nursing baby. If you are nursing a baby, another method of feeding the baby should be selected.
- It is not known how this drug could affect a fetus. If you are pregnant or decide to become pregnant while on this drug, consult your health care provider.
- You may experience the following side effects: Headache (consult your health care provider, medication may be available to help); dizziness (avoid driving a car or operating hazardous equipment if this occurs); nausea (frequent small meals may help).
- Report unusual muscle pain, trouble breathing, stomach pain with nausea and vomiting, feeling cold, lightheadedness, fast or irregular heartbeat, dark urine, yellowing of the eyes or skin, light-colored stools.

DANGEROUS DRUG

▽ephedrine sulfate

(e fed' rin)

PREGNANCY CATEGORY C

Drug classes

Bronchodilator
Sympathomimetic
Vasopressor

Therapeutic actions

Peripheral effects are mediated by receptors in target organs and are due in part to the release of norepinephrine from nerve terminals. Effects mediated by these receptors include vasoconstriction (increased BP, decreased nasal congestion alpha receptors), cardiac stimulation ($beta_1$), and bronchodilation ($beta_2$). Longer acting but less potent than epinephrine; also has CNS stimulant properties.

Indications

Parenteral

- Treatment of hypotensive states, especially those associated with spinal anesthesia; Stokes-Adams syndrome with complete heart block; CNS stimulant in narcolepsy and depressive states; acute bronchospasm; myasthenia gravis
- Pressor drug in hypotensive states following sympathectomy, overdosage with ganglionic-blocking drugs, antiadrenergic drugs, or other drugs used for lowering BP
- Relief of acute bronchospasm (epinephrine is the preferred drug)

Oral

- Treatment of allergic disorders, such as bronchial asthma, and temporary relief of wheezing, shortness of breath, and tightness of the chest

Contraindications and cautions

- Contraindicated with allergy to ephedrine, angle-closure glaucoma, anesthesia with cyclopropane or halothane, thyrotoxicosis, diabetes, hypertension, CV disorders, women in labor whose BP is lower than 130/80 mm Hg.

- Use cautiously with angina, arrhythmias, prostatic hypertrophy, unstable vasomotor syndrome, lactation.

Available forms

Capsules—25 mg; injection—50 mg/mL

Dosages

May be given PO, IM, slow IV, or subcutaneously.

Adults

Parenteral

- *Hypotensive episodes, allergic disorders:* 25–50 mg IM (fast absorption), subcutaneously (slower absorption), or 5–25 mg IV given slowly; may be repeated in 5–10 min.

Oral

- *Acute asthma:* Administer the smallest effective dose (12.5–25 mg PO every 4 hr).

Pediatric patients

Parenteral

0.5 mg/kg or 16.7 mg/m^2 IM or subcutaneously every 4–6 hr.

Oral

Not recommended for children younger than 12 yr.

Geriatric patients

More likely to experience adverse reactions; use with caution.

Pharmacokinetics

Route	Onset	Duration
Oral	30–40 min	3–5 hr
IM	10–20 min	1 hr
IV	Instant	1 hr

Metabolism: Hepatic; $T_{1/2}$: 3–6 hr
Distribution: May cross placenta; enters breast milk
Excretion: Urine

IV FACTS

Preparation: Administer as provided; no preparation required.
Infusion: Administer directly into vein or tubing of running IV; administer slowly, each 10 mg over at least 1 min.

Adverse effects

- **CNS:** *Fear, anxiety, tenseness, restlessness, headache, light-headedness, dizziness,* drowsiness, tremor, insomnia, hallucinations, psychological disturbances, **seizures,** CNS depression, weakness, blurred vision, ocular irritation, tearing, photophobia, symptoms of paranoid schizophrenia
- **CV:** Arrhythmias, **hypertension resulting in intracranial hemorrhage, CV collapse with hypotension, palpitations, tachycardia, precordial pain in patients with ischemic heart disease**
- **GI:** *Nausea,* vomiting, anorexia
- **GU:** Constriction of renal blood vessels and *decreased urine formation* (initial parenteral administration), *dysuria, vesical sphincter spasm* resulting in difficult and painful urination, urinary retention in males with prostatism
- **Other:** *Pallor,* respiratory difficulty, orofacial dystonia, sweating

Interactions

✱ **Drug-drug** • Severe hypertension with MAOIs, TCAs, furazolidone • Additive effects and increased risk of toxicity with urinary alkalinizers • Decreased vasopressor response with reserpine, methyldopa, urinary acidifiers • Decreased hypotensive action of guanethidine with ephedrine

✱ **Drug-alternative therapy** • Coadministration with ephedra, ma huang, guarana, and caffeine leads to additive effects and may lead to overstimulation, increased BP, CVA, and death

■ Nursing considerations

Assessment

- **History:** Allergy to ephedrine; angle-closure glaucoma; anesthesia with cyclopropane or halothane; thyrotoxicosis, diabetes, hypertension, CV disorders; prostatic hypertrophy, unstable vasomotor syndrome; lactation
- **Physical:** Skin color, T; orientation, reflexes, peripheral sensation, vision; P, BP, auscultation, peripheral perfusion; R, adventitious sounds; urinary output pattern, bladder percussion, prostate palpation

Interventions

- Protect solution from light; give only if clear; discard any unused portion.
- Monitor urine output with parenteral administration; initially renal blood vessels

may be constricted and urine formation decreased.

- Avoid prolonged use of systemic ephedrine (a syndrome resembling an anxiety effect may occur); temporary cessation of the drug usually reverses this syndrome.
- Monitor CV effects carefully; patients with hypertension may experience changes in BP because of the additional vasoconstriction. If a nasal decongestant is needed, give pseudoephedrine.

Teaching points

- Do not exceed recommended dose.
- Avoid over-the-counter medications. Many of them contain the same or similar drugs and serious overdosage can occur.
- You may experience these side effects: Dizziness, weakness, restlessness, tremor, lightheadedness, (avoid driving or operating dangerous equipment); urinary retention (empty your bladder before taking drug).
- Report nervousness, palpitations, sleeplessness, sweating.

DANGEROUS DRUG

epinephrine (adrenaline)

*(ep i **nef'** rin)*

epinephrine bitartrate

Aerosol: Primatene Mist

epinephrine borate

Ophthalmic solution: Epinal

epinephrine hydrochloride

Insect-sting emergencies: EpiPen Auto-Injector (delivers 0.3 mg IM adult dose), EpiPen Jr. Auto-Injector (delivers 0.15 mg IM for children)

OTC solutions for nebulization: AsthmaNefrin, microNefrin, Nephron, S_2

PREGNANCY CATEGORY C

Drug classes

Alpha-adrenergic agonist
Antiasthmatic
$Beta_1$- and $beta_2$-adrenergic agonist
Bronchodilator
Cardiac stimulant
Mydriatic
Nasal decongestant
Sympathomimetic
Vasopressor

Therapeutic actions

Naturally occurring neurotransmitter, the effects of which are mediated by alpha or beta receptors in target organs. Effects on alpha receptors include vasoconstriction, contraction of dilator muscles of iris. Effects on beta receptors include positive chronotropic and inotropic effects on the heart ($beta_1$ receptors); bronchodilation, vasodilation, and uterine relaxation ($beta_2$ receptors); decreased production of aqueous humor.

Indications

- IV: In ventricular standstill after all other measures have failed to restore circulation, given by trained personnel by intracardiac puncture and intramyocardial injection; treatment and prophylaxis of cardiac arrest and attacks of transitory AV heart block with syncopal seizures (Stokes-Adams syndrome); syncope due to carotid sinus syndrome; acute hypersensitivity (anaphylactoid) reactions, serum sickness, urticaria, angioneurotic edema; in acute asthmatic attacks to relieve bronchospasm not controlled by inhalation or subcutaneous injection; relaxation of uterine musculature; additive to local anesthetic solutions for injection to prolong their duration of action and limit systemic absorption
- Injection: Relief from respiratory distress of bronchial asthma.
- Aerosols and solutions for nebulization: Temporary relief from acute attacks of bronchial asthma, COPD
- Topical nasal solution: Temporary relief from nasal and nasopharyngeal mucosal congestion due to a cold, sinusitis, hay fever, or other upper respiratory allergies; adjunctive therapy in middle ear infections by decreasing congestion around eustachian ostia

- 0.1% ophthalmic solution: Conjunctivitis, during eye surgery to control bleeding, to produce mydriasis

Contraindications and cautions

- Contraindicated with allergy or hypersensitivity to epinephrine or components of preparation (many of the inhalant and ophthalmic products contain sulfites: Sodium bisulfite, sodium or potassium metabisulfite; check label before using any of these products in a sulfite-sensitive patient); narrow-angle glaucoma; shock other than anaphylactic shock; hypovolemia; general anesthesia with halogenated hydrocarbons or cyclopropane; organic brain damage, cerebral arteriosclerosis; cardiac dilation and coronary insufficiency; tachyarrhythmias; ischemic heart disease; hypertension; renal impairment (drug may initially decrease renal blood flow); COPD patients who have developed degenerative heart disease; diabetes mellitus; hyperthyroidism; lactation. Ophthalmic preparations are contraindicated for those wearing contact lenses (drug may discolor the contact lens), aphakic patients (maculopathy with decreased visual acuity may occur).
- Use cautiously with prostatic hypertrophy (may cause bladder sphincter spasm, difficult and painful urination), history of seizure disorders, psychoneurotic individuals, labor and delivery (may delay second stage of labor; can accelerate fetal heart beat; may cause fetal and maternal hypoglycemia), children (syncope has occurred when epinephrine has been given to asthmatic children). Use EpiPen Auto-Injector cautiously with hyperthyroidism, CAD, hypertension, diabetes, elderly patients, pregnancy, and patients weighing less than 30 kg.

Available forms

Solution for inhalation—1:100, 1:1,000, 1.125%, 1%; aerosol—0.35 mg, 0.5%, 0.22 mg; injection—1, 5 mg/mL; solution for injection—1:1,000, 1:2,000, 1:10,000, 1:100,000; suspension for injection—1:200; ophthalmic solution—0.1%

Dosages

Adults

Epinephrine injection

- *Hypersensitivity or bronchospasm:* 0.1–0.25 mg (1–2.5 mL of 1:10,000 solution) injected slowly.
- *Cardiac arrest:* 0.5–1 mg (5–10 mL of 1:10,000 solution) IV during resuscitation, 0.5 mg every 5 min. Intracardiac injection into left ventricular chamber, 0.3–0.5 mg (3–5 mL of 1:10,000 solution).

Intraspinal

0.2–0.4 mL added to anesthetic spinal fluid mixture. Concentrations of 1:100,000–1:20,000 are usually used.

1:1,000 solution

- *Respiratory distress:* 0.2–1 mL of 1:1,000 solution subcutaneously or IM.

1:200 suspension (for subcutaneous administration only)

- *Respiratory distress:* 0.1–0.3 mL (0.5–1.5 mg) subcutaneously.

Inhalation (aerosol)

Begin treatment at first symptoms of bronchospasm. Individualize dosage. Wait 1–5 min between inhalations to avoid overdose.

Inhalation (OTC)

4 yr and older: 1 inhalation, wait 1 min, then may use once more. Do not repeat for at least 3 hr.

Inhalation (nebulization)

Place not more than 10 drops into the nebulizer reservoir. Place nebulizer nozzle into partially opened mouth. Patient inhales deeply while bulb is squeezed one to three times (not more than every 3 hr).

Topical nasal solution

Apply locally as drops or spray or with a sterile swab, as required.

Pediatric patients

Epinephrine injection

- *1:1,000 solution, children:* 0.01 mg/kg or 0.3 mL/m^2 (0.01 mg/kg or 0.3 mg/m^2) subcutaneously; repeat every 4 hr if needed. Do not exceed 0.5 mL (0.5 mg) in a single dose. For infants, use 0.05 mg subcutaneously as initial dose, repeat every 20–30 min as needed. For neonates, use 0.01 mg/kg subcutaneously.
- *1:200 suspension, infants and children (1 mo–1 yr):* 0.005 mL/kg (0.025 mg/kg) subcutaneously.

E

- *Children 30 kg or less:* 0.15 mg or 0.01 mg/kg by autoinjector.
- *Hypersensitivity or bronchospasm:* For neonates, use 0.01 mg/kg IV. For infants, use 0.05 mg IV as initial dose and repeat every 20–30 min as needed with 1:10,000 solution.

Topical nasal solution

Apply locally as drops or spray or with a sterile swab, as required.

Geriatric patients or patients with renal failure

Use with caution.

Pharmacokinetics

Route	*Onset*	*Peak*	*Duration*
Subcut.	5–10 min	20 min	20–30 min
IM	5–10 min	20 min	20–30 min
IV	Instant	20 min	20–30 min
Inhalation	3–5 min	20 min	1–3 hr
Eye	Less than 1 hr	4–8 hr	24 hr

Metabolism: Neural
Distribution: Crosses placenta; enters breast milk
Excretion: Unknown

IV FACTS

Preparation: 0.5 mL dose may be diluted to 10 mL with sodium chloride injection for direct injection; prepare infusion by mixing 1 mg in 250 mL D_5W (4 mcg/mL).

Infusion: Administer by direct IV injection or into the tubing of a running IV, each 1 mg over 1 min, or run infusion at 1–4 mcg/min (15–60 mL/hr).

Adverse effects

Systemic administration

- **CNS:** *Fear, anxiety, tenseness, restlessness, headache, light-headedness, dizziness,* drowsiness, tremor, insomnia, hallucinations, psychological disturbances, seizures, CNS depression, weakness, blurred vision, ocular irritation, tearing, photophobia, symptoms of paranoid schizophrenia
- **CV:** Arrhythmias, **hypertension resulting in intracranial hemorrhage, CV collapse with hypotension, palpitations, tachycardia, precordial pain in patients with ischemic heart disease**
- **GI:** *Nausea,* vomiting, anorexia
- **GU:** Constriction of renal blood vessels and *decreased urine formation* (initial parenteral administration), *dysuria, vesical sphincter spasm* resulting in difficult and painful urination, urinary retention in males with prostatism
- **Other:** *Pallor,* respiratory difficulty, orofacial dystonia, sweating

Local injection

- **Local:** Necrosis at sites of repeat injections (due to intense vasoconstriction)

Nasal solution

- **Local:** Rebound congestion, local burning and stinging

Ophthalmic solutions

- **CNS:** *Headache, brow ache, blurred vision,* photophobia, difficulty with night vision, pigmentary (adrenochrome) deposits in the cornea, conjunctiva, or lids with prolonged use
- **Local:** *Transitory stinging on initial instillation,* eye pain or ache, conjunctival hyperemia

Interactions

✱ **Drug-drug** • Increased sympathomimetic effects with TCAs (eg, imipramine) • Excessive hypertension with propranolol, beta-blockers, furazolidone • Decreased cardiostimulating and bronchodilating effects with beta-adrenergic blockers (eg, propranolol) • Decreased vasopressor effects with chlorpromazine, phenothiazines • Decreased antihypertensive effect of methyldopa

■ Nursing considerations

Assessment

- **History:** Allergy or hypersensitivity to epinephrine or components of drug preparation; narrow-angle glaucoma; shock other than anaphylactic shock; hypovolemia; general anesthesia with halogenated hydrocarbons or cyclopropane; organic brain damage, cerebral arteriosclerosis; cardiac dilation and coronary insufficiency; tachyarrhythmias; ischemic heart disease; hypertension;

renal impairment; COPD; diabetes mellitus; hyperthyroidism; prostatic hypertrophy; history of seizure disorders; psychoneuroses; labor and delivery; lactation; contact lens use, aphakic patients (ophthalmic preparations)
- **Physical:** Weight; skin color, T, turgor; orientation, reflexes, IOP; P, BP; R, adventitious sounds; prostate palpation, normal urine output; urinalysis, renal function tests, blood and urine glucose, serum electrolytes, thyroid function tests, ECG

Interventions

⊗ ***Warning*** Use extreme caution when calculating and preparing doses; epinephrine is a very potent drug; small errors in dosage can cause serious adverse effects. Double-check pediatric dosage.
- Use minimal doses for minimal periods of time; "epinephrine-fastness" (a form of drug tolerance) can occur with prolonged use.
- Protect drug solutions from light, extreme heat, and freezing; do not use pink or brown solutions. Drug solutions should be clear and colorless (does not apply to suspension for injection).
- Shake the suspension for injection well before withdrawing the dose.
- Rotate subcutaneous injection sites to prevent necrosis; monitor injection sites frequently.

⊗ ***Warning*** Keep a rapidly acting alpha-adrenergic blocker (phentolamine) or a vasodilator (a nitrate) readily available in case of excessive hypertensive reaction.

⊗ ***Warning*** Have an alpha-adrenergic blocker or facilities for intermittent positive pressure breathing readily available in case pulmonary edema occurs.

⊗ ***Warning*** Keep a beta-adrenergic blocker (propranolol; a cardioselective beta-adrenergic blocker, such as atenolol, should be used in patients with respiratory distress) readily available in case cardiac arrhythmias occur.
- Do not exceed recommended dosage of inhalation products; administer pressurized inhalation drug forms during second half of inspiration, because the airways are open wider and the aerosol distribution is more extensive. If a second inhalation is needed, administer at peak effect of previous dose, 3–5 min.

Teaching points

- Do not exceed recommended dosage; adverse effects or loss of effectiveness may result. Read the instructions that come with respiratory inhalant products, and consult your health care provider or pharmacist if you have any questions.
- You may experience these side effects: Dizziness, drowsiness, fatigue, apprehension (use caution if driving or performing tasks that require alertness); anxiety, emotional changes; nausea, vomiting, change in taste (eat frequent small meals); fast heart rate. Nasal solution may cause burning or stinging when first used (transient).
- Report chest pain, dizziness, insomnia, weakness, tremor or irregular heart beat (respiratory inhalant), difficulty breathing, productive cough, failure to respond to usual dosage (respiratory inhalant).

epirubicin hydrochloride

See Appendix W, *Less commonly used drugs*.

eplerenone

*(ep **ler'** eh nown)*

Inspra

PREGNANCY CATEGORY B

Drug classes

Aldosterone receptor blocker
Antihypertensive

Therapeutic actions

Binds to aldosterone receptors, blocking the binding of aldosterone, leading to increased loss of sodium and water and lowering of BP.

Indications

- Treatment of hypertension, alone or in combination with other antihypertensive drugs
- Heart failure, post-MI, improvement in the survival of patients with left ventricular dysfunction after a heart attack
- Unlabeled uses: Alone or with ACE inhibitors to reduce left ventricular hypertrophy;

adjunct in diabetic hypertensives with microalbuminuria

Contraindications and cautions

- Contraindicated with allergy to eplerenone, hyperkalemia (exceeding 5.5 mEq/L), type 2 diabetes with microalbuminuria, severe renal impairment (creatinine clearance less than 50 mL/min or serum creatinine level higher than 2 mg/dL in males or 1.8 mg/dL in females), lactation.
- Use cautiously with hepatic impairment, pregnancy, concurrent treatment with potassium supplements, potassium-sparing diuretics, CYP450 and CYP3A4 inhibitors (eg, ketoconazole).

Available forms

Tablets—25, 50 mg

Dosages

Adults

- *Hypertension:* Initially, 50 mg/day PO as a single daily dose; if necessary, may be increased to 50 mg PO bid after a minimum of a 4-wk trial period. Maximum, 100 mg/day.
- *Heart failure post-MI:* Start with 25 mg/day PO titrate to 50 mg/day over 4 wk.
- *Heart failure:* If serum K^+ is lower than 5, increase dose; if 5–5.4, no adjustment necessary; if 5.5–5.9, decrease dose; if 6 or higher, withhold dose.

Pediatric patients

Safety and efficacy not established.

Pharmacokinetics

Route	*Onset*	*Peak*
Oral	Slow	1.5 hr

Metabolism: Hepatic; $T_{1/2}$: 4-6 hr
Distribution: May cross placenta; may enter breast milk
Excretion: Feces, urine

Adverse effects

CNS: Headache, dizziness, fatigue
CV: Angina, **MI**
GI: Diarrhea, abdominal pain
GU: Abnormal vaginal bleeding, albuminuria, changes in sexual function
Metabolic: Hypercholesterolemia, **hyperkalemia**
Respiratory: Cough
Other: Gynecomastia and breast pain in men, flulike symptoms

Interactions

✱ **Drug-drug** ⊗ ***Warning*** Risk of serious toxic effects if combined with strong inhibitors of the CYP450 3A4 system (ketoconazole, itraconazole, erythromycin, verapamil, saquinavir, fluconazole); if any of these drugs are being used, initiate treatment with 25 mg eplerenone and monitor patient closely.
• Increased risk of hyperkalemia if combined with ACE inhibitors and ARBs; monitor patient closely • Possible risk of lithium toxicity if combined with lithium; monitor serum lithium levels closely if this combination is necessary • Possible risk of decreased antihypertensive effect if combined with NSAIDs; monitor BP carefully • Risk of hyperkalemia also with potassium supplements, potassium-sparing diuretics such as spironolactone, amiloride, triamterene; avoid concomitant use

■ Nursing considerations

Assessment

- **History:** Allergy to eplerenone, hyperkalemia, type 2 diabetes mellitus, severe renal impairment, lactation, hepatic impairment, pregnancy, concurrent treatment with potassium supplements, CYP450 or CYP3A4 inhibitors
- **Physical:** Orientation, reflexes; BP; R; urinary output; LFTs, renal function tests, serum potassium levels, serum cholesterol

Interventions

- Arrange for pretreatment and periodic evaluation of serum potassium and renal function.
- Establish baseline patient weight to monitor drug effect.
- Administer once a day, in the morning, so increased urination will not interrupt sleep.
- Avoid giving patient any foods rich in potassium (see Appendix D, *Important Dietary*

Guidelines for Patient Teaching, for a complete list).
- Establish appropriate safety precautions if patient experiences adverse CNS effects.
- Suggest another method of feeding the baby if the drug is needed in a lactating woman.

Teaching points
- Take this drug early in the morning so any increase in urination will not affect sleep.
- Weigh yourself on a regular basis, at the same time of day and in the same clothes, and record this weight on your calendar.
- This drug may interact with many other medications. Alert any health care provider caring for you that you are taking this drug.
- This drug should not be taken during pregnancy or when nursing a baby; using barrier contraceptives is suggested.
- You will need periodic blood tests to evaluate the effect of this drug on your serum potassium level and cholesterol level.
- Avoid foods that are high in potassium (fruits, *Sanka* coffee).
- You may experience these side effects: Dizziness (use caution and avoid driving a car or performing other tasks that require alertness if you experience dizziness); enlargement or pain of the breasts (it may help to know that this is a drug effect and will pass when drug therapy is ended).
- Report weight change of more than 3 pounds in 1 day, severe dizziness, trembling, numbness, muscle weakness or cramps, palpitations.

▽epoetin alfa (EPO, erythropoietin)

*(e poe **e'** tin)*

Epogen, Eprex (CAN), Procrit

PREGNANCY CATEGORY C

Drug class
Recombinant human erythropoietin

Therapeutic actions
A natural glycoprotein produced in the kidneys, which stimulates red blood cell production in the bone marrow.

Indications
- Treatment of anemia associated with chronic renal failure, including patients older than 1 mo on dialysis
- Treatment of anemia related to therapy with azidothymidine (AZT) in HIV-infected patients
- Treatment of anemia related to chemotherapy in cancer patients
- Reduction of allogenic blood transfusions in surgical patients
- Unlabeled uses: Pruritus associated with renal failure; myelodysplastic syndromes; chronic inflammation associated with rheumatoid arthritis

Contraindications and cautions
- Contraindicated with uncontrolled hypertension; hypersensitivity to mammalian cell-derived products or to albumin human; contains benzyl alcohol, which can be fatal in premature infants.
- Use cautiously with pregnancy, lactation, sickle cell anemia, myelodysplastic syndromes, porphyria, hypercoagulable disorders.

Available forms
Injection—2,000, 3,000, 4,000, 10,000, 20,000, 40,000 units/mL

Dosages
Monitor patient closely; target Hgb 10–12 g/dL.

Adults
- *Anemia of chronic renal failure:* Starting dose, 50–100 units/kg three times weekly IV for dialysis patients and IV or subcutaneously for nondialysis patients. Reduce dose if Hgb increases more than 1 g/dL in any 2-wk period. Reduce dose by 25% if Hgb is 12 g/dL. Increase dose if Hgb does not increase by 1 g/dL after 4 wk of therapy or if Hgb is less than 10 g/dL. For maintenance dose, individualized based on Hgb—generally, 75–100 units/kg three times weekly. If on dialysis, median dose is 75 units/kg three times weekly. Target Hgb range is 10–12 g/dL.
- *Treatment of anemia in HIV-infected patients on AZT therapy:* For patients receiving AZT dose of 4,200 mg/wk or less with serum erythropoietin levels of 500 milliunits/mL or less, use 100 units/kg IV or subcutaneously

E

three times/wk for 8 wk; when desired response is achieved, titrate dose to maintain Hgb with lowest possible dose.

- *Treatment of anemia in cancer patients on chemotherapy (*Procrit *only):* 150 units/kg subcutaneously three times/wk or 40,000 units subcutaneously weekly; after 8 wk, can be increased to 300 units/kg or 60,000 units subcutaneously weekly.
- *Reduction of allogenic blood transfusions in surgery:* 300 units/kg/day subcutaneously for 10 days before surgery, on day of surgery, and 4 days after surgery. Or, 600 units/kg/day subcutaneously 21, 14, and 7 days before surgery and on day of surgery. Make sure that Hgb is higher than 10 g/dL and lower than 13 g/dL.
- *Chronic renal failure:* IV administration should be used instead of subcutaneous injection. Dosage should start slowly and be increased based on Hgb levels; check Hgb levels weekly until stable, then monthly.

Pediatric patients 1 mo–16 yr

- *Chronic renal failure:* 50 units/kg IV or subcutaneously 3 times/wk.
- *Anemia of prematurity:* 25–100 units/kg/dose 3 times/wk.
- *Cancer:* 600 units/kg/wk IV. Maximum dose, 60,000 units in children 5 yr and older.

Pharmacokinetics

Route	*Onset*	*Peak*	*Duration*
Subcut.	7–14 days	5–24 hr	24 hr

Metabolism: Serum; $T_{1/2}$: 4–13 hr
Distribution: Crosses placenta; enters breast milk
Excretion: Urine

IV FACTS

Preparation: As provided; no additional preparation. Enter vial only once; do not shake vial. Discard any unused solution. Refrigerate.
Infusion: Administer by direct IV injection or into tubing of running IV.
Incompatibilities: Do not mix with any other drug solution.

Adverse effects

- **CNS:** *Headache, arthralgias, fatigue, asthenia, dizziness,* **seizure, CVA,** TIA
- **CV:** *Hypertension, edema, chest pain*
- **GI:** *Nausea, vomiting, diarrhea*
- **Other:** Clotting of access line, **development of anti-erythropoietin antibodies with subsequent pure red cell aplasia and extreme anemia**

■ Nursing considerations

Assessment

- **History:** Uncontrolled hypertension, hypersensitivity to mammalian cell-derived products or to albumin human, lactation
- **Physical:** Reflexes, affect; BP, P; urinary output, renal function tests; CBC, Hct, iron levels, electrolytes

Interventions

⊗ ***Black box warning*** Risk of death and serious CV events is increased if Hgb target is higher than 12 g/dL. Use lowest levels of drug needed to increase Hgb to lowest level needed to avoid transfusion.

⊗ ***Black box warning*** Incidence of DVT is higher in patients who are receiving erythropoietin-stimulating agents preoperatively to reduce need for transfusion; consider antithrombotic prophylaxis if used for this purpose.

⊗ ***Black box warning*** Patients with cancer are at risk for more rapid tumor progression, shortened survival, and death when Hgb level target is more than 12 g/dL. Risk of death is increased in cancer patients not receiving radiation or chemotherapy.

- Confirm chronic, renal nature of anemia; not intended as a treatment of severe anemia or substitute for emergency transfusion.
- Patients with chronic renal failure on hemodialysis should receive the drug IV, not by subcutaneous injection, to decrease the risk of developing anti-erythropoietin antibodies.
- Gently mix; do not shake, shaking may denature the glycoprotein. Use only one dose per vial; do not reenter the vial. Discard unused portions.
- Do not give with any other drug solution.

- Administer dose three times per week. If administered independent of dialysis, administer into venous access line. If patient is not on dialysis, administer IV or subcutaneously.
- Monitor access lines for signs of clotting.
- Arrange for Hgb reading before administration of each dose to determine dosage. If patient fails to respond within 8 wk of therapy, evaluate patient for other etiologies of the problem.
- Monitor patient for sudden loss of response and severe anemia with low reticulocyte count; withhold drug and check patient for anti-erythropoietin antibodies. If antibodies are present, discontinue drug permanently and do not switch to any other erythropoietic agent; cross-sensitivity can occur.
- Monitor Hgb levels; target range is 10–12 g/dL; do not exceed 12 g/dL.
- Evaluate iron stores before and periodically during therapy. Supplemental iron may need to be ordered.
- Institute seizure precautions.

Teaching points

- Drug must be given three times per week and can only be given IV, subcutaneously, or into a dialysis access line. Prepare a schedule of administration dates.
- Keep appointments for blood tests needed to determine the effects of the drug on your blood count and to determine dosage.
- Maintain all of the usual activities and restrictions that apply to your chronic renal failure. If this becomes difficult, consult your health care provider.
- You may experience these side effects: Dizziness, headache, seizures (avoid driving or performing hazardous tasks); fatigue, joint pain (may be medicated); nausea, vomiting, diarrhea (proper nutrition is important).
- Report difficulty breathing, numbness or tingling, chest pain, seizures, severe headache.

▽epoprostenol sodium (prostacyclin, PGX, PGI_2)

See Appendix W, *Less commonly used drugs*.

▽eprosartan mesylate

*(ep row **sar'** tan)*

Teveten

PREGNANCY CATEGORY C (FIRST TRIMESTER)

PREGNANCY CATEGORY D (SECOND AND THIRD TRIMESTERS)

Drug classes

Antihypertensive
ARB

Therapeutic actions

Selectively blocks the binding of angiotensin II to specific tissue receptors found in the vascular smooth muscle and adrenal gland; this action blocks the vasoconstriction effect of the renin–angiotensin system as well as the release of aldosterone leading to decreased BP.

Indications

- Treatment of hypertension, alone or in combination with other antihypertensive drugs, particularly diuretics and calcium channel blockers
- Unlabeled use: Heart failure, left ventricular hypertrophy, diabetic nephropathy

Contraindications and cautions

- Contraindicated with hypersensitivity to any ARB, pregnancy (use during the second or third trimester can cause injury or even death to the fetus), lactation.
- Use cautiously with renal impairment, hypovolemia, hyperkalemia.

Available forms

Tablets—600 mg

Dosages

Adults

Usual starting dose is 600 mg PO daily. Can be administered in divided doses bid with a total daily dose of 400–800 mg/day being effective. Patients with moderate and severe renal impairment, maximum dose is 600 mg/day. If used as part of combination therapy, eprosartan should be added to established dose of other antihypertensive, starting at the lowest dose and increasing dosage based on patient response.

Pediatric patients

Safety and efficacy not established.

Pharmacokinetics

Route	Onset	Peak
Oral	Rapid	1–2 hr

Metabolism: Hepatic; $T_{1/2}$: 5–9 hr
Distribution: Crosses placenta; may enter breast milk
Excretion: Feces, urine

Adverse effects

- **CNS:** Headache, dizziness, syncope, muscle weakness, *fatigue, depression*
- **CV:** Hypotension
- **Dermatologic:** Rash, inflammation, urticaria, pruritus, alopecia, dry skin
- **GI:** Diarrhea, *abdominal pain,* nausea, constipation
- **Renal:** Hyperkalemia, increased BUN
- **Respiratory:** *URI symptoms,* cough, sinus disorders
- **Other:** Cancer (in preclinical studies), UTIs, **angioedema**

Interactions

✱ **Drug-drug** • Use caution when combining with other drugs that may elevate serum potassium concentrations—potassium-sparing diuretics, potassium supplements, or potassium-containing salt substitutes

■ Nursing considerations

Assessment

- **History:** Hypersensitivity to any ARB, pregnancy, lactation, renal impairment, hypovolemia, hyperkalemia
- **Physical:** Skin lesions, turgor; T; reflexes, affect; BP; R, respiratory auscultation; renal function tests

Interventions

- Administer without regard to meals.

⊠ ***Black box warning*** Ensure that patient is not pregnant before beginning therapy, suggest the use of barrier birth control while using eprosartan; fetal injury and deaths have been reported.

- Find an alternate method of feeding the infant if given to a nursing mother. Depression of the renin–angiotensin system in infants is potentially very dangerous.

⊗ ***Warning*** Alert surgeon and mark the patient's chart with notice that eprosartan is being taken. The blockage of the renin–angiotensin system following surgery can produce problems. Hypotension may be reversed with volume expansion.

- If BP control does reach desired levels, diuretics or other antihypertensives may be added to the drug regimen. Monitor patient's BP carefully.
- Monitor patient closely in any situation that may lead to a decrease in BP secondary to reduction in fluid volume—excessive perspiration, dehydration, vomiting, diarrhea—excessive hypotension can occur.

Teaching points

- Take drug without regard to meals. Do not stop taking this drug without consulting your health care provider.
- Use a barrier method of birth control while taking this drug; if you become pregnant or desire to become pregnant, consult your health care provider.
- You may experience these side effects: Dizziness (avoid driving a car or performing hazardous tasks); nausea, abdominal pain (proper nutrition is important, consult with your dietitian to maintain nutrition); symptoms of upper respiratory tract or urinary tract infection, cough (do not self-medicate, consult your health care provider if this becomes uncomfortable).
- Report fever, chills, dizziness, pregnancy, prolonged episodes of severe nausea, vomiting, and diarrhea.

DANGEROUS DRUG

▽ eptifibatide

(ep tiff ***ib'*** *ah tide)*

Integrilin

PREGNANCY CATEGORY B

Drug classes
Antiplatelet drug
Glycoprotein IIb/IIIa receptor agonist

Therapeutic actions
Inhibits platelet aggregation by binding to the glycoprotein IIb/IIIa receptor on the platelet, which prevents the binding of fibrinogen and other adhesive ligands to the platelet.

Indications
- Treatment of acute coronary syndrome
- Prevention of cardiac ischemic complications in patients undergoing elective, emergency, or urgent percutaneous coronary intervention

Contraindications and cautions
- Contraindicated with allergy to eptifibatide, bleeding diathesis, hemorrhagic CVA, active, abnormal bleeding or CVA within 30 days, uncontrolled or severe hypertension, major surgery within 6 wk, dialysis, severe renal impairment, low platelet count.
- Use cautiously in the elderly; with pregnancy, lactation, renal insufficiency.

Available forms
Injection—0.75, 2 mg/mL

Dosages
Adults
- *Acute coronary syndrome:* 180 mcg/kg IV (maximum of 22.6 mg) over 1–2 min as soon as possible after diagnosis, then 2 mcg/kg/min (maximum 15 mg/hr) by continuous IV infusion for up to 72 hr. If patient is to undergo percutaneous coronary intervention, continue for 18–24 hr after the procedure, up to 96 hr of therapy. Reduce infusion dose to 1 mcg/kg/min if serum creatinine is greater than 2 mg/dl.
- *Percutaneous coronary intervention:* 180 mcg/kg IV as a bolus immediately before the procedure, then 2 mcg/kg/min by continuous IV infusion for 18–24 hr. May give a second bolus of 180 mcg/kg 10 min after the first bolus is given.

Pediatric patients
Not recommended.

Pharmacokinetics

Route	*Onset*	*Peak*	*Duration*
IV	15 min	45 min	2–4 hr

Metabolism: Tissue; $T_{1/2}$: 1.5–2.5 hr
Distribution: May cross placenta; may enter breast milk
Excretion: Urine

IV FACTS
Preparation: Withdraw bolus from 10-mL vial. No preparation needed for continuous infusion. Spike the 100-mL vial with a vented infusion set. Protect from light.
Infusion: Infuse bolus quickly; infuse as continuous infusion using guidelines under Dosages section.
Compatibilities: May be given with alteplase, atropine, dobutamine, heparin, lidocaine, meperidine, metoprolol, morphine, nitroglycerin, verapamil.
Incompatibility: Do not mix with furosemide.

Adverse effects
- **CNS:** *Headache, dizziness,* weakness, syncope, flushing
- **Dermatologic:** *Rash,* pruritus
- **GI:** Nausea, GI distress, constipation, diarrhea
- **Hematologic:** Thrombocytopenia
- **Other:** *Bleeding, hypotension*

Interactions
✱ **Drug-drug** • Use caution when combining with other drugs that affect blood clotting—thrombolytics, anticoagulants, ticlopidine, dipyridamole, clopidogrel, NSAIDs; increased risk of bleeding or hemorrhage

■ Nursing considerations
Assessment
- **History:** Allergy to eptifibatide; bleeding diathesis; hemorrhagic CVA; active, abnormal bleeding or CVA within 30 days; uncontrolled or severe hypertension; major surgery within 6 wk; dialysis; severe renal impairment; low platelet count; pregnancy, lactation
- **Physical:** Skin color, temperature, lesions; orientation, reflexes, affect; P, BP, orthostatic BP, baseline ECG, peripheral perfusion;

respiratory rate, adventitious sounds, aPTT, PT, active clotting time

Interventions

- Use eptifibatide in conjunction with heparin and aspirin.

⊗ ***Warning*** As much as possible, avoid arterial and venous puncture, IM injection, catheterization, and intubation in patient using this drug to minimize blood loss.

- Avoid the use of noncompressible IV access sites to prevent excessive, uncontrollable bleeding.
- Arrange for baseline and periodic tests of CBC, PT, aPTT, and active clotting time. Maintain aPTT of 50–70 sec and active bleeding time of 300–350 sec.
- Properly care for femoral access site to minimize bleeding. Document aPTT lower than 45 sec or activated clotting time lower than 150 sec, and stop heparin for 3–4 hr before pulling sheath.
- Provide comfort measures and arrange for analgesics if headache occurs.

Teaching points

- This drug is given to minimize blood clotting and cardiac damage. It must be given IV.
- You will be monitored closely and periodic blood tests will be done to monitor the effects of this drug on your body.
- You may experience these side effects: Dizziness, light-headedness, bleeding.
- Report light-headedness, palpitations, pain at IV site, bleeding.

ergonovine maleate

*(er goe **noe'** veen)*

Ergotrate

PREGNANCY CATEGORY UNKNOWN

Drug class

Oxytocic

Therapeutic actions

Increases the strength, duration, and frequency of uterine contractions, and decreases postpartum uterine bleeding by direct effects at neuroreceptor sites.

Indications

- Prevention and treatment of postpartum and postabortal hemorrhage due to uterine atony
- Unlabeled use: Oxytocin challenge test, to diagnose coronary artery spasm in patients with variant angina

Contraindications and cautions

- Contraindicated with allergy to ergonovine, induction of labor, threatened spontaneous abortion, history of CVA.
- Use cautiously with hypertension, heart disease, venoatrial shunts, mitral-valve stenosis, obliterative vascular disease, sepsis, hepatic or renal impairment, lactation.

Available forms

Tablets—0.2 mg

Dosages

Adults

1–2 tablets (0.2–0.4 mg) PO every 6–12 hr until the danger of uterine atony has passed (usually 48 hr).

Pharmacokinetics

Route	*Onset*	*Duration*
Oral	6–15 min	90–180 min

Metabolism: Hepatic; $T_{1/2}$: 0.5–2 hr
Distribution: Crosses placenta; enters breast milk
Excretion: Feces, urine

Adverse effects

- **CNS:** *Dizziness, headache,* ringing in the ears
- **CV:** Elevation of BP—more common with ergonovine than other oxytocics
- **GI:** *Nausea, vomiting,* diarrhea
- **Hypersensitivity:** Allergic response, including shock
- **Other:** Ergotism—nausea, BP changes, weak pulse, dyspnea, chest pain, numbness

and coldness of the extremities, confusion, excitement, delirium, hallucinations, seizures, coma

■ Nursing considerations

Assessment

- **History:** Allergy to ergonovine, induction of labor, threatened spontaneous abortion, hypertension, heart disease, venoatrial shunts, peripheral vascular disease, sepsis, hepatic or renal impairment, lactation
- **Physical:** Uterine tone; orientation, reflexes, affect; P, BP, edema; R, adventitious sounds; CBC, LFTs, renal function tests

Interventions

- Initial therapy postpartum is usually with a parenteral drug, then switch to oral drug to minimize late postpartum bleeding.
- Monitor postpartum women for BP changes and amount and character of vaginal bleeding.
- Arrange for discontinuation of drug if signs of ergotism occur.
- Avoid prolonged use of the drug.

Teaching points

- Usually part of an immediate medical situation. Teaching about the complication of delivery or abortion should include drug. The patient needs to know the name of the drug and what she can expect once it is administered.
- You may experience these side effects: Nausea, vomiting, dizziness, headache, ringing in the ears.
- Report difficulty breathing, headache, numb or cold extremities, severe abdominal cramping.

ergotamine tartrate

See Appendix W, *Less commonly used drugs*.

erlotinib

See Appendix W, *Less commonly used drugs*.

ertapenem

(er tah ***pen'*** *em)*

Invanz

PREGNANCY CATEGORY B

Drug classes

Antibiotic
Methyl-carbapenem

Therapeutic actions

Bactericidal: Inhibits synthesis of susceptible bacterial cell wall causing cell death.

Indications

- Community-acquired pneumonia caused by *Streptococcus pneumoniae* (penicillin-susceptible strains only), *Haemophilus influenzae* (beta-lactamase–negative strains only), *Moraxella catarrhalis*
- Skin and skin structure infections including diabetic foot infections without osteomyelitis caused by *Staphylococcus aureus* (methicillin-susceptible strains only), *Streptococcus pyogenes, Escherichia coli, Streptococcus agalactiae, Klebsiella pneumoniae, Proteus mirabilis, Bacteroides fragilis, Porphyromonas asaccharolytica, Prevotella bivia, Peptostreptococcus* species
- Complicated GU infections, including pyelonephritis caused by *E. coli* or *K. pneumoniae.*
- Complicated intra-abdominal infections due to *E. coli, Clostridium clostridiiforme, Eubacterium lentum, Peptostreptococcus* species, *B. fragilis, Bacteroides distasonis, Bacteroides ovatus, Bacteroides thetaiotaomicron, Bacteroides uniformis*
- Acute pelvic infections, including postpartum endomyometritis, septic abortion, postsurgical gynecologic infections due to *S. agalactiae, E. coli, B. fragilis, P. asaccharolytica, Peptostreptococcus* species, *P. bivia*
- Prophylaxis of surgical-site infection after elective colorectal surgery in adults

Contraindications and cautions

- Contraindicated with allergies to any component of the drug and to beta lactam

antibiotics; allergy to amide-type local anesthetics (IM use); allergy to penicillins, cephalosporins, other allergens.
- Use cautiously with pregnancy; lactation, seizure disorder.

Available forms
Vials for reconstitution—1 g/vial

Dosages
Adults and children 13 yr and older
1 g IM or IV each day; length of treatment varies with infection—intra-abdominal, 5–14 days; urinary tract, 10–14 days; skin and skin structure, 7–14 days; community-acquired pneumonia, 10–14 days; acute pelvic infections, 3–10 days.
Prophylaxis: 1 g IV 1 hr before surgical incision.
Pediatric patients 3 mo to 12 yr
15 mg/kg IV or IM bid for 3–14 days; do not exceed 1 g/day.
Patients with renal impairment
For creatinine clearance of 30 mL/min or less, use 500 mg IV or IM daily.

Pharmacokinetics

Route	*Onset*	*Peak*
IV	Rapid	30 min
IM	10 min	2 hr

Metabolism: $T_{1/2}$: 4 hr
Distribution: Crosses the placenta; enters breast milk
Excretion: Urine, unchanged

IV FACTS
Preparation: Reconstitute 1-g vial with 10 mL of water for injection, 0.9% sodium chloride injection or bacteriostatic water for injection; do not dilute with diluents containing dextrose. Shake well to dissolve and transfer to 50 mL of 0.9% sodium chloride injection; use within 6 hr of reconstitution, or store refrigerated for up to 24 hr, but use within 4 hr of removal from refrigeration; inspect solution for particulate matter.
Infusion: Infuse over 30 min.
Incompatibilities: Do not mix in solution or in the same line as any other medications or any solution containing dextrose.

Adverse effects
- **CNS:** *Headache,* dizziness, asthenia, fatigue, insomnia, altered mental status, anxiety, **seizures**
- **CV:** Heart failure, arrhythmias, edema, swelling, hypotension, hypertension, chest pain
- **GI:** *Nausea,* vomiting, *diarrhea,* abdominal pain, constipation, dyspepsia, **pseudomembranous colitis,** liver toxicity, GERD
- **GU:** Vaginitis
- **Hypersensitivity:** *Ranging from rash* to *fever* to **anaphylaxis;** serum sickness reaction
- **Local:** *Pain, phlebitis,* thrombophlebitis, inflammation at IV site
- **Respiratory:** Pharyngitis, rales, respiratory distress, cough, dyspnea, rhonchi
- **Other:** Fever, rash, vaginitis

■ Nursing considerations

CLINICAL ALERT!
Name confusion has occurred between *Avinza* (extended-release morphine) and *Invanz* (ertapenem); use extreme caution.

Assessment
- **History:** Allergies to any component of the drug and to beta-lactam antibiotics; allergy to amide-type local anesthetics (IM use), penicillins, cephalosporins, other allergens; pregnancy, lactation, seizures
- **Physical:** T, skin status, swelling, orientation, reflexes, R, adventitious sounds, P, BP, peripheral perfusion, culture of affected area, sensitivity tests

Interventions
- Culture infected area and arrange for sensitivity tests before beginning drug therapy and during therapy if expected response is not seen.
- Prepare IM solution as follows: Reconstitute 1-g vials with 3.2 mL of 1% lidocaine injection without epinephrine; shake to form

solution; immediately withdraw contents for injection.
- Administer IM injections deeply into large muscle mass within 1 hr of reconstitution.

⊗ **Warning** Have emergency and life-support equipment readily available in case of severe hypersensitivity reaction.
- Discontinue drug if hypersensitivity reaction occurs.
- Monitor injection site for adverse reactions.
- Ensure ready access to bathroom facilities and provide frequent small meals if GI complications occur.
- Arrange for treatment of superinfections if they occur.

Teaching points
- You may experience these side effects: Nausea, diarrhea, dizziness, headache (consult your health care provider if any of these are severe).
- Report severe diarrhea, difficulty breathing, unusual tiredness or fatigue, pain at injection site.

erythromycin
*(er ith roe **mye'** sin)*

erythromycin base
Oral, ophthalmic ointment, topical dermatologic solution for acne, topical dermatologic ointment: Akne-mycin, A/T/S, Apo-Erythro (CAN), Apo-Erythro E-C (CAN), Erybid (CAN), EryDerm, Ery-Tab, Erythromycin Film-tabs, Ilotycin, PCE Dispertab

erythromycin estolate (CAN)
Novo-Rythro Estolate (CAN)

erythromycin ethylsuccinate
Oral: Apo-Erythro ES (CAN), E.E.S. 200, E.E.S. 400, E.E.S. Granules, EryPed, EryPed 200, EryPed 400, EryPed Drops, Novo-Rhythro Ethylsuccinate (CAN)

erythromycin gluceptate

erythromycin lactobionate
Erythrocin I.V. (CAN), Erythrocin Lactobionate

erythromycin stearate
Apo-Erythro-S (CAN)

PREGNANCY CATEGORY B

Drug class
Macrolide antibiotic

Therapeutic actions
Bacteriostatic or bactericidal in susceptible bacteria; binds to cell membrane, causing change in protein function, leading to cell death.

Indications
Systemic administration
- Acute infections caused by sensitive strains of *Streptococcus pneumoniae, Mycoplasma pneumoniae, Listeria monocytogenes, Legionella pneumophila*
- URIs, lower respiratory tract infections, skin and soft-tissue infections caused by group A beta-hemolytic streptococci when oral treatment is preferred to injectable benzathine penicillin
- PID caused by *Neisseria gonorrhoeae* in patients allergic to penicillin
- In conjunction with sulfonamides in URIs caused by *Haemophilus influenzae*
- As an adjunct to antitoxin in infections caused by *Corynebacterium diphtheriae* and *Corynebacterium minutissimum*
- Prophylaxis against alpha-hemolytic streptococcal endocarditis before dental or other procedures in patients allergic to penicillin who have valvular heart disease
- Oral erythromycin: Treatment of intestinal amebiasis caused by *Entamoeba histolytica;* infections in the newborn and in pregnancy that are caused by *Chlamydia trachomatis* and in adult chlamydial infections when tetracycline cannot be used; primary syphilis (*Treponema pallidum*) in penicillin-allergic patients; eliminating

Bordetella pertussis organisms from the nasopharynx of infected individuals and as prophylaxis in exposed and susceptible individuals
- Unlabeled uses: Erythromycin base is used with neomycin before colorectal surgery to reduce wound infection; treatment of severe diarrhea associated with *Campylobacter* enteritis or enterocolitis; treatment of genital, inguinal, or anorectal lymphogranuloma venereum infection; treatment of *Haemophilus ducreyi* (chancroid)

Ophthalmic ointment
- Treatment of superficial ocular infections caused by susceptible strains of microorganisms; prophylaxis of ophthalmia neonatorum caused by *N. gonorrhoeae* or *C. trachomatis*

Topical dermatologic solutions for acne
- Treatment of acne vulgaris

Topical dermatologic
- Granules used with flexible hydroactive dressings for dermal ulcers, pressure ulcers, leg ulcers, superficial wounds, and postoperative wounds
- Treatment of skin infections caused by sensitive microorganisms

Contraindications and cautions

Systemic administration
- Contraindicated with allergy to erythromycin.
- Use cautiously with hepatic impairment, lactation (secreted and may be concentrated in breast milk; may modify bowel flora of nursing infant and interfere with fever workups).

Ophthalmic ointment
- Contraindicated with allergy to erythromycin; viral, fungal, mycobacterial infections of the eye.

Available forms

Base: Tablets—250, 333, 500 mg; DR tablets—500 mg; DR capsules—250 mg; ophthalmic ointment—5 mg/g. Estolate: Tablets—500 mg; capsules—250 mg; suspension—125, 250 mg/5 mL. Stearate tablets—250, 500 mg ethylsuccinate: Ethylsuccinate tablets—200, 400 mg; suspension—200, 400 mg/5 mL, 100 mg/2–5 mL; powder for suspension—200 mg/5 mL; granules for suspension—400 mg/5 mL; topical solution—1.5%, 2%; topical gel, ointment—2%. Lactobionate injection—500, 1,000 mg.

Dosages

Systemic administration

Oral preparations of the different erythromycin salts differ in pharmacokinetics: 400 mg erythromycin ethylsuccinate produces the same free erythromycin serum levels as 250 mg of erythromycin base, stearate, or estolate.

Adults

15–20 mg/kg/day in continuous IV infusion or up to 4 g/day in divided doses every 6 hr; 250 mg (400 mg of ethylsuccinate) every 6 hr PO or 500 mg every 12 hr PO or 333 mg every 8 hr PO, up to 4 g/day, depending on the severity of the infection.
- *Streptococcal infections:* 250 mg every 6 hr or 500 mg every 12 hr (for group A beta-hemolytic streptococcal infections, continue therapy for at least 10 days).
- *Legionnaires disease:* 1–4 g/day PO or IV in divided doses for 10–21 days (ethylsuccinate 1.6 g/day; optimal doses not established).
- *Dysenteric amebiasis:* 250 mg (400 mg of ethylsuccinate) PO every 6 hr or 333 mg every 8 hr for 10–14 days.
- *Acute PID* (N. gonorrhoeae)*:* 500 mg of lactobionate or gluceptate IV every 6 hr for 3 days and then 500 mg stearate or base PO every 6 hr or 333 mg every 8 hr for 7 days.
- *Chlamydial infections:* Urogenital infections during pregnancy: 500 mg PO qid or 666 mg every 8 hr for at least 7 days, one-half this dose every 8 hr for at least 14 days if intolerant to first regimen. Urethritis in males: 800 mg of ethylsuccinate PO tid for 7 days.
- *Primary syphilis:* 30–40 g (48–64 g of ethylsuccinate) in divided doses over 10–15 days.
- *CDC recommendations for STDs:* 500 mg PO qid for 7–30 days, depending on the infection.

Pediatric patients

30–50 mg/kg/day PO in divided doses. Specific dosage determined by severity of infection, age, and weight.

- *Dysenteric amebiasis:* 30–50 mg/kg/day in divided doses for 10–14 days.
- *Pertussis:* 40–50 mg/kg/day PO daily in divided doses for 14 days.
- *Chlamydial infections:* 50 mg/kg/day PO in divided doses, for at least 2 (conjunctivitis of newborn) or 3 (pneumonia of infancy) wk.

Ophthalmic ointment

Adults and pediatric patients

One-half–inch ribbon instilled into conjunctival sac of affected eye two to six times per day, depending on severity of infection.

Topical

Adults and pediatric patients

- *Dermatologic solution for acne:* Apply to affected areas morning and evening.
- *Topical dermatologic:* Flexible hydroactive dressings and granules applied and kept in place for 1–7 days.

Pharmacokinetics

Route	*Onset*	*Peak*
Oral	1–2 hr	1–4 hr
IV	Rapid	1 hr

Metabolism: Hepatic; $T_{1/2}$: 1.5–2 hr
Distribution: Crosses placenta; enters breast milk
Excretion: Bile, urine

IV FACTS

Preparation: Reconstitute powder for IV infusion only with sterile water for injection without preservatives—10 mL for 250- and 500-mg vials, 20 mL for 1-g vials. Prepare intermittent infusion as follows: Dilute 250–500 mg in 100–250 mL of 0.9% sodium chloride injection or 5% dextrose in water. Prepare for continuous infusion by adding reconstituted drug to 0.9% sodium chloride injection, lactated Ringer's injection, or D_5W that will make a solution of 1 g/L.

Infusion: *Intermittent infusion:* Administer over 20–60 min qid; infuse slowly to avoid vein irritation. Administer continuous infusion within 4 hr, or buffer the solution to neutrality if administration is prolonged.

Incompatibilities: *Gluceptate*—do not add to aminophylline, pentobarbital, secobarbital, tetracycline. *Lactobionate*—do not mix with heparin, metoclopramide, tetracycline.

Y-site incompatibilities: Avoid chloramphenicol, heparin, phenobarbital, phenytoin.

Adverse effects

Systemic administration

- **CNS:** Reversible hearing loss, confusion, uncontrollable emotions, abnormal thinking
- **CV: Ventricular arrhythmias** (with IV)
- **GI:** *Abdominal cramping, anorexia, diarrhea, vomiting,* **pseudomembranous colitis,** hepatotoxicity
- **Hypersensitivity:** Allergic reactions ranging from rash to **anaphylaxis**
- **Other:** *Superinfections*

Ophthalmic ointment

- **Dermatologic:** Edema, urticaria, dermatitis, angioneurotic edema
- **Local:** *Irritation, burning, itching* at site of application

Topical dermatologic preparations

- **Local:** *Superinfections,* particularly with long-term use

Interactions

Systemic administration

✱ **Drug-drug** • Increased serum levels of digoxin • Increased effects of oral anticoagulants, theophylline, carbamazepine, ergot derivatives, disopyramide, calcium blockers, HMG-CoA reductase inhibitors, midazolam, proton pump inhibitors, quinidine • Increased therapeutic and toxic effects of corticosteroids • Increased levels of cyclosporine and risk of renal toxicity

✱ **Drug-food** • Decreased metabolism and increased risk of toxic effects if taken with grapefruit juice; avoid this combination

✱ **Drug-lab test** • Interferes with fluorometric determination of urinary catecholamines • Decreased urinary estriol levels due to inhibition of hydrolysis of steroids in the gut

Topical dermatologic solution for acne

✱ **Drug-drug** • Increased irritant effects with peeling, desquamating, or abrasive agents

E

■ Nursing considerations

Assessment

- **History:** Allergy to erythromycin, hepatic impairment, lactation; viral, fungal, mycobacterial infections of the eye (ophthalmologic), pregnancy
- **Physical:** Site of infection; skin color, lesions; orientation, affect, hearing tests; R, adventitious sounds; GI output, bowel sounds, liver evaluation; culture and sensitivity tests of infection, urinalysis, LFTs

Interventions

Systemic administration

- Culture site of infection before therapy.
- Administer oral erythromycin base or stearate on an empty stomach, 1 hr before or 2–3 hr after meals, with a full glass of water (oral erythromycin estolate, ethylsuccinate, and certain enteric-coated tablets [review the manufacturer's instructions] may be given without regard to meals).
- Administer around the clock to maximize effect; adjust schedule to minimize sleep disruption.
- Monitor liver function in patients on prolonged therapy.
- Give some preparations with meals, as directed, or substitute one of these preparations, if GI upset occurs with oral therapy.

Topical dermatologic solution for acne

- Wash affected area, rinse well, and dry before application.

Ophthalmic and topical dermatologic preparation

- Use topical products only when needed. Sensitization produced by the topical use of an antibiotic may preclude its later systemic use in serious infections. Topical antibiotic preparations not normally used systemically are best.
- Culture site before beginning therapy.
- Cover the affected area with a sterile bandage if needed (topical).

Teaching points

Systemic administration

- Take oral drug on an empty stomach, 1 hour before or 2–3 hours after meals, with a full glass of water; some forms may be taken without regard to meals. Do not drink grapefruit juice while on this drug. The drug should be taken around the clock; schedule to minimize sleep disruption. Finish the full course of the drug therapy.
- You may experience these side effects: Stomach cramping, discomfort (take the drug with meals, if appropriate); uncontrollable emotions, crying, laughing, abnormal thinking (reversible).
- Report severe or watery diarrhea, severe nausea or vomiting, dark urine, yellowing of the skin or eyes, loss of hearing, rash or itching.

Ophthalmic ointment

- Pull the lower eyelid down gently and squeeze a one-half–inch ribbon of the ointment into the sac, avoid touching the eye or lid. A mirror may be helpful. Gently close the eye, and roll the eyeball in all directions.
- Drug may cause temporary blurring of vision, stinging, or itching.
- Report stinging or itching that becomes pronounced.

Topical dermatologic solution for acne

- Wash and rinse area, and pat it dry before applying solution.
- Use fingertips or an applicator to apply; wash hands thoroughly after application.

▽escitalopram oxalate

*(ess si **tal'** oh pram)*

Lexapro

PREGNANCY CATEGORY C

Drug classes

Antidepressant
SSRI

Therapeutic actions

Potentiates serotonergic activity in the CNS by inhibiting reuptake of serotonin resulting in antidepressant effect with little effect on norepinephrine or dopamine; an isomer of citalopram.

Indications

- Treatment of major depressive disorder
- Maintenance treatment for patients with major depressive disorder
- Treatment of generalized anxiety disorder
- **NEW INDICATION:** Maintenance treatment for major depresssive disorder in patients 12–17 yr
- Unlabeled use: Panic disorder

Contraindications and cautions

- Contraindicated with MAOI, pimozide use; with allergy to drug or to citalopram or any component of the drug.
- Use cautiously in the elderly and with renal or hepatic impairment, illnesses of metabolism or hemodynamic response, pregnancy, lactation, suicidal patients, patients with mania or seizure disorders.

Available forms

Tablets—5, 10, 20 mg; oral solution—1 mg/5 mL

Dosages

Adults

- *Major depressive disorder:* Initially, 10 mg/day PO as a single daily dose; if needed, may be increased to 20 mg/day after a minimum of 1-wk trial period. For maintenance, 10–20 mg/day PO; reassess periodically.
- *Generalized anxiety disorder:* 10 mg/day PO; may be increased to 20 mg/day after 1 wk if needed. Treatment beyond 8 wk not tested.

Pediatric patients 12–17 yr

- *Major depressive disorder:* 10 mg/day PO as a single dose. Maximum dose, 20 mg/day.

Geriatric patients or adults with hepatic impairment

10 mg/day PO as a single dose; do not increase dose.

Pharmacokinetics

Route	Onset	Peak
Oral	Slow	3.5–6.5 hr

Metabolism: Hepatic; $T_{1/2}$: 27–32 hr
Distribution: Crosses placenta; enters breast milk
Excretion: Urine

Adverse effects

- **CNS:** *Somnolence, dizziness,* insomnia, fatigue, complex sleep disorders, serotonin syndrome (with abrupt discontinuation)
- **Dermatologic:** Sweating
- **GI:** *Nausea,* dry mouth, constipation, diarrhea, indigestion, abdominal pain, decreased appetite
- **GU:** *Ejaculatory disorders,* impotence, anorgasmia in females, decreased libido
- **Respiratory:** Rhinitis, sinusitis, flulike symptoms
- **Other: Anaphylaxis, angioedema,** serotonin syndrome

Interactions

✱ **Drug-drug** • Risk of serious toxic effects if combined with citalopram; do not use these drugs concomitantly • Increased escitalopram levels and toxicity if taken with MAOIs; ensure that patient has been off the MAOI for at least 14 days before administering escitalopram • Risk of serotonin syndrome—a syndrome characterized by increased BP, T, severe anxiety, agitation, rigidity, and can occur when multiple serotonin elevating drugs are used. Monitor patient carefully • Possible severe adverse effects if combined with other centrally acting CNS drugs including alcohol; use caution • Possible decreased effects of escitalopram if combined with carbamazepine, lithium; monitor patient closely

✱ **Drug-alternative therapy** • Increased risk of severe reaction if combined with St. John's wort; avoid this combination

■ Nursing considerations

CLINICAL ALERT!
There is potential for name confusion between escitalopram and citalopram and between *Lexapro* (escitalopram) and *Loxitane* (loxapine); use caution.

Assessment

- **History:** MAOI use; allergy to drug, citalopram, or any component of the drug; renal or hepatic impairment; older age; pregnancy; lactation; suicidal tendencies; metabolic illnesses or problems with hemodynamic response; alcoholism

- **Physical:** Orientation, reflexes; P, BP, perfusion; R, bowel sounds, normal output; urinary output; liver evaluation; LFTs, renal function tests

Interventions

⊗ ***Black box warning*** Monitor patient for risk of suicidality, especially when starting or altering dosage; children, adolescents, and young adults are at increased risk.

- Give once a day, in the morning or in the evening; may be taken with food if desired.
- Encourage patient to continue use for 4–6 wk, as directed, to ensure adequate levels to affect depression.

⊗ ***Warning*** Limit amount of drug given in prescription to potentially suicidal patients.

⊗ ***Warning*** If discontinuing drug after long-term use, taper dosage gradually to avoid withdrawal syndrome.

⊗ ***Warning*** Use during third trimester of pregnancy has led to prolonged hospitalization, need for respiratory support, and tube feedings for the baby.

- Advise any depressed patients to avoid the use of alcohol while being treated with antidepressive drugs.
- Establish appropriate safety precautions if patient experiences adverse CNS effects.
- Institute appropriate therapy for patient suffering from depression.

Teaching points

- Take this drug exactly as directed, and as long as directed; it may take several weeks to realize the benefits of the drug. The drug may be taken with food if desired.
- Do not stop taking this medication without consulting your health care provider.
- Avoid the use of alcohol while you are taking this drug.
- This drug should not be taken during pregnancy or when nursing a baby; using barrier contraceptives is suggested.
- You may experience these side effects: Drowsiness, dizziness, tremor (use caution and avoid driving a car or performing other tasks that require alertness if you experience daytime drowsiness); GI upset (frequent small meals, frequent mouth care may help); alterations in sexual function (this is a drug effect and will pass when drug therapy is ended); allergic reaction; swelling; complex sleep disorders.
- Report severe nausea, vomiting; blurred vision; excessive sweating, suicidal ideation, sexual dysfunction, insomnia.

DANGEROUS DRUG

esmolol hydrochloride

(ess' moe lol)

Brevibloc

PREGNANCY CATEGORY C

Drug classes

Antiarrhythmic

$Beta_1$-selective adrenergic blocker

Therapeutic actions

Blocks beta-adrenergic receptors in the heart and juxtaglomerular apparatus, reducing the influence of the sympathetic nervous system on these tissues; decreasing the excitability of the heart, cardiac output, and release of renin; and lowering BP and heart rate. At low doses, acts relatively selectively at the $beta_1$-adrenergic receptors of the heart; has very rapid onset and short duration.

Indications

- Supraventricular tachycardia, when rapid but short-term control of ventricular rate is desirable (atrial fibrillation, flutter, perioperative or postoperative situations)
- Noncompensatory tachycardia when heart rate requires specific intervention
- Intraoperative and postoperative tachycardia and hypertension when intervention is needed

Contraindications and cautions

- Contraindicated with decompensated heart failure, cardiogenic shock, second- or third-degree heart block (in the absence of a pacemaker), bradycardia.

- Use cautiously with bronchospastic disease, pregnancy, lactation.

Available forms

Injection—10 mg/mL, 250 mg/mL

Dosages

Adults

Individualize dosage by titration (loading dose followed by a maintenance dose). Initial loading dose of 500 mcg/kg/min IV for 1 min followed by a maintenance dose of 50 mcg/kg/min for 4 min. If adequate response is not observed in 5 min, repeat loading dose and follow with maintenance infusion of 100 mcg/kg/min. Repeat titration as necessary, increasing rate of maintenance dose in increments of 50 mcg/kg/min. As desired heart rate or safe end point is approached, omit loading infusion and decrease incremental dose in maintenance infusion to 25 mcg/kg/min (or less), or increase interval between titration steps from 5 to 10 min. Usual range is 50–200 mcg/kg/min. Infusions for up to 24 hr have been used; up to 48 hr may be well tolerated. Dosage should be individualized based on patient response; do not exceed 300 mcg/kg/min.

Pediatric patients

Safety and efficacy not established.

Pharmacokinetics

Route	*Onset*	*Peak*	*Duration*
IV	< 5 min	10–20 min	10–30 min

Metabolism: RBC esterases; $T_{1/2}$: 9 min
Distribution: Crosses placenta; may enter breast milk
Excretion: Urine

IV FACTS

Preparation: Dilute drug before infusing as follows: Add the contents of 2 ampules of esmolol (2.5 g) to a compatible diluent: 5% dextrose injection, 5% dextrose in Ringer's injection; 5% dextrose and 0.9% or 0.45% sodium chloride injection; lactated Ringer's injection; 0.9% or 0.45% sodium chloride injection after removing 20 mL from a 500 mL bottle, to make a drug solution with a concentration of 10 mg/mL. Diluted solution is stable for 24 hr at room temperature.
Infusion: Rate of infusion is determined by patient response; see Dosages section above.
Incompatibilities: Do not mix in solution with diazepam, furosemide, thiopental, or sodium bicarbonate.

Adverse effects

- **CNS:** *Light-headedness,* speech disorder, *midscapular pain, weakness, rigors,* somnolence, confusion
- **CV:** *Hypotension,* pallor, bradycardia
- **GI:** Taste perversion
- **GU:** Urine retention
- **Local:** *Inflammation,* induration, edema, erythema, burning at the site of infusion
- **Other:** Fever, rhonchi, flushing

Interactions

✱ **Drug-drug** • Increased therapeutic and toxic effects with verapamil • Impaired antihypertensive effects with ibuprofen, indomethacin, piroxicam

■ Nursing considerations

Assessment

- **History:** Cardiac, cerebrovascular disease; bronchospastic disease; pregnancy, lactation
- **Physical:** P, BP, ECG; orientation, reflexes; R, adventitious sounds; urinary output

Interventions

- Ensure that drug is not used in chronic settings when transfer to another drug is anticipated.
- Do not give undiluted drug.

⊗ ***Warning*** Do not mix with sodium bicarbonate, diazepam, furosemide, or thiopental.

- Monitor BP, HR, and ECG closely.

Teaching points

- This drug is reserved for emergency use; incorporate information about this drug into an overall teaching plan.

E

esomeprazole magnesium (perprazole, S-omeprazole)

*(ess oh **me'** pray zol)*

Nexium DNC, Nexium IV

PREGNANCY CATEGORY B

Drug classes

Antisecretory drug
Proton pump inhibitor

Therapeutic actions

Gastric acid-pump inhibitor: Suppresses gastric acid secretion by specific inhibition of the hydrogen–potassium ATPase enzyme system at the secretory surface of the gastric parietal cells; blocks the final step of acid production; is broken down less in the first pass through the liver than the parent compound omeprazole, allowing for increased serum levels.

Indications

- GERD—treatment of heartburn and other related symptoms
- Erosive esophagitis—short-term (4–8 wk) treatment for healing and symptom relief; also used for maintenance therapy following healing of erosive esophagitis
- Short-term treatment of GERD with a history of erosive esophagitis by IV route for up to 10 days, when oral therapy is not possible
- As part of combination therapy for the treatment of duodenal ulcer associated with *Helicobacter pylori*
- Reduction in occurrence of gastric ulcers associated with continuous NSAID use in patients at risk (60 yr and older, history of gastric ulcers) for developing gastric ulcers
- Treatment of pathological hypersecretory conditions, including Zollinger-Ellison syndrome
- Unlabeled uses: Non-GERD dyspepsia, Barrett esophagus, stress ulcer prophylaxis

Contraindications and cautions

- Contraindicated with hypersensitivity to omeprazole, esomeprazole, or other proton pump inhibitor.
- Use cautiously with hepatic impairment, pregnancy, lactation.

Available forms

DR capsules DNC—20, 40 mg; DR powder for suspension—20 mg, 40 mg; injection—20, 40 mg/vial

Dosages

Adults

- *Healing of erosive esophagitis:* 20–40 mg PO daily for 4–8 wk. An additional 4–8 wk course of therapy can be considered for patients who have not healed.
- *Maintenance of healing of erosive esophagitis:* 20 mg PO daily.
- *Symptomatic GERD:* 20 mg daily for 4 wk. An additional 4-wk course of therapy can be considered if symptoms have not resolved.
- *Short-term treatment of GERD when oral therapy is not possible:* 20–40 mg IV by injection over at least 3 min or IV infusion over 10–30 min.
- *Duodenal ulcer:* 40 mg/day PO for 10 days with 1,000 mg PO bid amoxicillin and 500 mg PO bid clarithromycin.
- *Reduction of risk of gastric ulcers with NSAID use:* 20–40 mg PO daily for 6 mo.

Pediatric patients (12–17 yr)

- *Short-term treatment of GERD:* 20–40 mg/day PO for up to 8 wk.

Pediatric patients (1–11 yr)

- *Treatment of GERD:* 10 mg/day PO for up to 8 wk.
- *Healing of erosive esophagitis:*
  Weight less than 20 kg: 10 mg/day PO for up to 8 wk.
  Weight of 20 kg or more: 10–20 mg/day PO for up to 8 wk.

Patients with hepatic impairment

Do not exceed 20 mg/day in patients with severe hepatic impairment.

Pharmacokinetics

Route	*Onset*	*Peak*	*Duration*
Oral	1–2 hr	1.5 hr	17 hr

Metabolism: Hepatic; $T_{1/2}$: 1–1.5 hr
Distribution: May cross placenta; may enter breast milk
Excretion: Bile, urine

IV FACTS

Preparation: Reconstitute with 5 mL of 0.9% sodium chloride injection; withdraw 5 mL of reconstituted solution. May be further diluted with 0.9% sodium chloride, lactated Ringer's, or 5% dextrose to a volume of 50 mL for infusion. Do not use if particulate matter is seen in solution, or solution is discolored. May be stored at room temperature for up to 12 hr.
Injection: Inject 5 mL directly or into line of running IV over no less than 3 min.
Infusion: Infuse dilute solution (50 mL) over 10–30 min.
Incompatibilities: Do not mix with other medications; flush tubing before and after each dose with 0.9% sodium chloride, lactated Ringer's, 5% dextrose.

Adverse effects

- **CNS:** *Headache, dizziness,* asthenia, vertigo, insomnia, apathy, anxiety, paresthesias, dream abnormalities
- **Dermatologic:** Rash, inflammation, urticaria, pruritus, alopecia, dry skin
- **GI:** *Diarrhea, abdominal pain, nausea, vomiting,* constipation, dry mouth, tongue atrophy, flatulence
- **Respiratory:** *URI symptoms, sinusitis,* cough, epistaxis

Interactions

✱ **Drug-drug** • Increased serum levels and potential increase in toxicity of benzodiazepines when taken concurrently • May interfere with absorption of drugs dependent upon presence of acidic environment (eg, ketoconazole, iron salts, digoxin) • Decreased levels of atazanavir if combined.

■ Nursing considerations

CLINICAL ALERT!
Potential for name confusion exists between esomeprazole and omeprazole; use caution. Name confusion has been reported between *Nexium* (esomeprazole) and *Nexavar* (sorafenib); use caution.

Assessment

- **History:** Hypersensitivity to any proton pump inhibitor; hepatic impairment; pregnancy, lactation
- **Physical:** Skin lesions; T; reflexes, affect; urinary output, abdominal examination; respiratory auscultation, LFTs

Interventions

⊗ ***Warning*** Arrange for further evaluation of patient after 4 wk of therapy for gastroesophageal reflux disorders. Symptomatic improvement does not rule out gastric cancer.

- If administering antacids, they may be administered concomitantly with esomeprazole.
- Administer IV for maximum of 10 days; switch to oral form as soon as possible.
- Prepare suspension by emptying packet into 15 mL water. Stir, let thicken 2–3 min, stir, and administer within 30 min. Rinse container with water and have patient drink.
- Ensure that the patient swallows capsule whole; do not crush, or chew; patients having difficulty swallowing may open capsule and sprinkle in applesauce or disperse in tap water, orange or apple juice, or yogurt; do not crush or chew pellets.
- To administer through a nasogastric (NG) tube, capsules can be opened and granules emptied into a syringe and delivered through the tube. For suspension form, add 15 mL of water to syringe, add packet, shake syringe, let thicken for 2–3 min, shake syringe, and inject through NG tube. Use within 30 min of preparation.
- Obtain baseline liver function tests and monitor periodically during therapy.
- Maintain supportive treatment as appropriate for underlying problem.
- Provide additional comfort measures to alleviate discomfort from GI effects and headache.

- Establish safety precautions if dizziness or other CNS effects occur (use side rails, accompany patient).

Teaching points

- Take the drug at least 1 hour before meals. Swallow the capsules whole; do not chew or crush. If you cannot swallow the capsule, it can be opened and sprinkled in applesauce or mixed in tap water, orange or apple juice, or yogurt; do not crush or chew the pellets. If using suspension, add 1 tablespoon water to packet, stir, let stand for 2–3 minutes to set, stir again, and drink within 30 minutes of preparing. Then rinse container with water and immediately drink remaining granules. This drug will need to be taken for 4–8 weeks, at which time your condition will be reevaluated.
- Arrange to have regular medical follow-up visits while you are using this drug.
- Maintain all of the usual activities and restrictions that apply to your condition. If this becomes difficult, consult your health care provider.
- You may experience these side effects: Dizziness (avoid driving a car or performing hazardous tasks); headaches (consult your health care provider if these become bothersome; medications may be available to help); nausea, vomiting, diarrhea (proper nutrition is important; consult with your dietitian to maintain nutrition; ensure ready access to bathroom); symptoms of upper respiratory tract infection, cough (it may help to know that this is a drug effect; do not self-medicate; consult your health care provider if this becomes uncomfortable).
- Report severe headache, worsening of symptoms, fever, chills, darkening of the skin, changes in color of urine or stool.

estazolam

*(es **taz'** e lam)*

ProSom

PREGNANCY CATEGORY X

CONTROLLED SUBSTANCE C-IV

Drug classes

Benzodiazepine
Sedative-hypnotic

Therapeutic actions

Exact mechanisms of action not understood; acts mainly at subcortical levels of the CNS, leaving the cortex relatively unaffected; potentiates the effects of GABA, an inhibitory neurotransmitter.

Indications

- Insomnia characterized by difficulty in falling asleep, frequent nocturnal awakenings, or early morning awakening
- Recurring insomnia or poor sleeping habits
- Acute or chronic medical situations requiring restful sleep

Contraindications and cautions

- Contraindicated with hypersensitivity to benzodiazepines, psychoses, acute narrow-angle glaucoma, shock, coma, acute alcoholic intoxication with depression of vital signs, pregnancy (increased risk of congenital malformations, neonatal withdrawal syndrome), labor and delivery ("floppy infant" syndrome reported), lactation (secreted in breast milk; chronic administration of diazepam, another benzodiazepine, to nursing mothers has caused infants to become lethargic and lose weight).
- Use cautiously with impaired liver or renal function, debilitation, depression, suicidal tendencies, history of substance abuse.

Available forms

Tablets—1, 2 mg

Dosages

Individualize dosage.

Adults

1 mg PO before bedtime; up to 2 mg may be needed.

Pediatric patients

Not for use in patients younger than 18 yr.

Geriatric patients or patients with debilitating disease

1 mg PO if healthy; start with 0.5 mg in debilitated patients.

Pharmacokinetics

Route	*Onset*	*Peak*
Oral	45–60 min	2 hr

Metabolism: Hepatic; $T_{1/2}$: 10–24 hr
Distribution: Crosses placenta; may enter breast milk
Excretion: Feces, urine

Adverse effects

- **CNS:** *Transient, mild drowsiness initially; sedation, depression, lethargy, apathy, fatigue, light-headedness, disorientation, restlessness, asthenia,* crying, delirium, headache, slurred speech, dysarthria, stupor, rigidity, tremor, dystonia, vertigo, euphoria, nervousness, difficulty in concentration, vivid dreams, psychomotor retardation, extrapyramidal symptoms, *mild paradoxical excitatory reactions during first 2 wk of treatment* (especially in psychiatric patients, aggressive children, and with high dosage), visual and auditory disturbances, diplopia, nystagmus, depressed hearing, nasal congestion, complex sleep disorders
- **CV:** *Bradycardia, tachycardia,* **CV collapse,** hypertension and hypotension, palpitations, edema
- **Dependence:** *Drug dependence with withdrawal syndrome* when drug is discontinued (more common with abrupt discontinuation of higher dosage used for longer than 4 mo)
- **Dermatologic:** Urticaria, pruritus, skin rash, dermatitis
- **GI:** *Constipation, diarrhea, dyspepsia,* dry mouth, salivation, nausea, anorexia, vomiting, difficulty in swallowing, gastric disorders, elevations of blood enzymes: LDH, alkaline phosphatase, AST, ALT; hepatic impairment, jaundice
- **GU:** *Incontinence, urinary retention, changes in libido,* menstrual irregularities
- **Hematologic:** Decreased Hct, blood dyscrasias
- **Other:** Hiccups, fever, diaphoresis, paresthesias, muscular disturbances, gynecomastia, **anaphylaxis, angioedema**

Interactions

✱ **Drug-drug** • Increased CNS depression when taken with alcohol, phenothiazines, opioids, barbiturates • Decreased sedative effects of estazolam if taken concurrently with theophylline, aminophylline, rifampin, and TCAs

■ Nursing considerations

Assessment

- **History:** Hypersensitivity to benzodiazepines; psychoses; acute narrow-angle glaucoma; shock; coma; acute alcoholic intoxication; pregnancy; labor; lactation; impaired liver or renal function, debilitation, depression, suicidal tendencies
- **Physical:** Skin color, lesions; T, orientation, reflexes, affect, ophthalmologic examination; P, BP; R, adventitious sounds; liver evaluation, abdominal examination, bowel sounds, normal output; CBC, LFTs, renal function tests

Interventions

- Arrange to monitor liver and renal function and CBC during long-term therapy.

⊗ ***Warning*** Taper dosage gradually after long-term therapy, especially in epileptic patients.

Teaching points

- Take drug exactly as prescribed; do not stop taking this drug without consulting your health care provider.
- Avoid alcohol, sleep-inducing, or over-the-counter drugs while taking this drug.
- Be aware that this drug provides symptomatic relief and is not a cure for insomnia. It may be habit-forming; it works best if used on an "as needed" basis and not every night.
- You may experience these side effects: Transient drowsiness, dizziness (avoid driving or engaging in dangerous activities); complex sleep disorders; allergic reaction; swelling; GI upset (take the drug with water); depression, dreams, emotional upset, crying; sleep may be disturbed for several nights after discontinuing the drug.
- Report severe dizziness, weakness, drowsiness that persists, rash or skin lesions, palpitations, swelling of the extremities, visual changes, difficulty voiding.

E

estradiol
(ess tra dye' ole)

estradiol
Oral: Estrace, Gynodiol
Transdermal system: Alora, Climara, Estraderm, Menostar, Vivelle, Vivelle Dot
Topical vaginal cream: Estrace
Vaginal ring: Estring
Topical emulsion: Estrasorb
Gel: Estrogel, Divigel
Topical spray: Evamist

estradiol acetate
Tablets: Femtrace
Vaginal ring: Femring

estradiol cypionate
Injection in oil: Depo-Estradiol

estradiol hemihydrate
Vaginal tablet: Vagifem

estradiol valerate
Injection in oil: Delestrogen

PREGNANCY CATEGORY X

Drug classes
Estrogen
Hormone

Therapeutic actions
Estradiol is the most potent endogenous female sex hormone. Estrogens are important in the development of the female reproductive system and secondary sex characteristics; affect the release of pituitary gonadotropins; cause capillary dilatation, fluid retention, protein anabolism and thin cervical mucus; conserve calcium and phosphorus and encourage bone formation; inhibit ovulation and prevent postpartum breast discomfort. They are responsible for proliferation of the endometrium; absence or decline of estrogen produces signs and symptoms of menopause on the uterus, vagina, breasts, cervix; relief in androgen-dependent prostatic carcinoma is attributable to competition with androgens for receptor sites, decreasing influence of the androgens.

Indications
- *Femtrace, Estrasorb,* estradiol cypionate, estradiol valerate: Vasomotor symptoms
- Estradiol acetate tablets (*Femtrace*), estradiol gel 0.1% (*Divigel*), estradiol spray (*Evamist*): Treatment of moderate to severe vasomotor symptoms associated with menopause
- *Vagifem, Estrace, Estring:* Vaginal atrophy
- *Femring,* tablets, transdermal (except *Menostar*), *Estrogel:* Vasomotor symptoms amd vaginal atrophy
- Estradiol oral, transdermal, estradiol valerate: Prevention of postmenopausal osteoporosis
- Estradiol oral, transdermal, estradiol cypionate, valerate: Treatment of female hypogonadism, female castration, primary ovarian failure
- Estradiol oral, estradiol valerate: Palliation of inoperable prostatic cancer
- Estradiol oral: Palliation of inoperable, progressing breast cancer

Contraindications and cautions
- Contraindicated with allergy to estrogens, allergy to tartrazine (in 2-mg oral tablets), breast cancer (with exceptions), estrogen-dependent neoplasm, undiagnosed abnormal genital bleeding, active or past history of thrombophlebitis or thromboembolic disorders, pregnancy (potential serious fetal defects; women of childbearing age should be advised of risks and birth control measures suggested), history of breast cancer.
- Use cautiously with metabolic bone disease, renal or hepatic insufficiency, heart failure, lactation.

Available forms
Transdermal—release rates of 0.014, 0.025, 0.0375, 0.05, 0.06, 0.075, 0.1 mg/24 hr; tablets—0.5, 1, 1.5, 2 mg; *Femtrace*—0.45, 0.9, 1.8 mg; injection—5, 10, 20, 40 mg/mL; vaginal cream—0.1 mg/g; vaginal ring—2 mg; *Femring*—0.05 mg/day, 0.1 mg/day; vaginal tablet—25 mcg; topical emulsion—

2.5 mg/g; gel—0.06%, 0.1%; topical spray—1.53 mg

Dosages

Adults

- *Moderate to severe vasomotor symptoms, atrophic vaginitis, kraurosis vulvae associated with menopause:* 1–2 mg/day PO. Adjust dose to control symptoms. For gel, 0.25 g of 0.1% gel applied to right or left upper thigh on alternating days; may be increased to 0.5 or 1 g/day to control symptoms. For topical spray (*Evamist*), 1 spray once daily to forearm; may be increased to 2–3 sprays daily. Cyclic therapy (3 wk on/1 wk off) is recommended, especially in women who have not had a hysterectomy. 1–5 mg estradiol cypionate in oil IM every 3–4 wk. 10–20 mg estradiol valerate in oil IM, every 4 wk. The 0.014- to 0.05-mg system is applied to the skin weekly or twice weekly. If oral estrogens have been used, start transdermal system 1 wk after withdrawal of oral form. Given on a cyclic schedule (3 wk on/1 wk off). Attempt to taper or discontinue medication every 3–6 mo.
- *Female hypogonadism, female castration, primary ovarian failure:* 1–2 mg/day PO. Adjust dose to control symptoms. Cyclic therapy (3 wk on/1 wk off) is recommended. 1.5–2 mg estradiol cypionate in oil IM at monthly intervals. 10–20 mg estradiol valerate in oil IM every 4 wk. The 0.05-mg system is applied to skin twice weekly as above.

Vaginal

- *Vaginal cream:* 2–4 g intravaginally daily for 1–2 wk, then reduce to one-half dosage for similar period followed by maintenance doses of 1 g one to three times/wk thereafter. Discontinue or taper at 3- to 6-mo intervals.
- *Vaginal ring:* Insert one ring high into vagina. Replace every 90 days.
- *Vaginal tablet:* 1 tablet inserted vaginally daily for 2 wk; then twice weekly.

Oral

- *Prostatic cancer (inoperable):* 1–2 mg PO tid. Administer long-term. 30 mg or more estradiol valerate in oil IM every 1–2 wk.
- *Breast cancer (inoperable, progressing):* 10 mg tid PO for at least 3 mo.
- *Prevention of postpartum breast engorgement:* 10–25 mg estradiol valerate in oil IM as a single injection at the end of the first stage of labor.
- *Osteoporosis prevention:* 0.5 mg/day PO given cyclically—23 days on, 5 days rest—starting as soon after menopause as possible.

Topical emulsion

Relief of menopausal symptoms: Apply lotion to legs, thighs, or calves once daily. Apply gel to one arm once daily.

Pediatric patients

Not recommended due to effect on growth of the long bones.

Pharmacokinetics

Route	Onset	Peak
Oral	Slow	Days

Metabolism: Hepatic; $T_{1/2}$: Not known
Distribution: Crosses placenta; enters breast milk
Excretion: Urine

Adverse effects

- **CNS:** Steepening of the corneal curvature with a resultant change in visual acuity and intolerance to contact lenses, *headache,* migraine, dizziness, mental depression, chorea, **seizures**
- **CV:** Increased BP, thromboembolic and thrombotic disease
- **Dermatologic:** *Photosensitivity, peripheral edema, chloasma,* erythema nodosum or multiforme, hemorrhagic eruption, loss of scalp hair, hirsutism, urticaria, dermatitis
- **GI:** Gallbladder disease (in postmenopausal women), **hepatic adenoma,** *nausea, vomiting, abdominal cramps, bloating,* **cholestatic jaundice, colitis, acute pancreatitis**
- **GU:** Increased risk of postmenopausal endometrial cancer, *breakthrough bleeding, change in menstrual flow, dysmenorrhea, premenstrual-like syndrome,* amenorrhea, vaginal candidiasis, cystitis-like syndrome, endometrial cystic hyperplasia
- **Hematologic:** Hypercalcemia, decreased glucose tolerance
- **Local:** *Pain at injection site,* sterile abscess, postinjection flare

- **Other:** Weight changes, reduced carbohydrate tolerance, aggravation of porphyria, edema, changes in libido, breast tenderness

Topical vaginal cream

Systemic absorption may cause uterine bleeding in menopausal women and may cause serious bleeding of remaining endometrial foci in sterilized women with endometriosis

Interactions

✱ **Drug-drug** • Increased therapeutic and toxic effects of corticosteroids • Decreased serum levels of estradiol with drugs that enhance hepatic metabolism of the drug—barbiturates, phenytoin, rifampin, carbamazepine

✱ **Drug-lab test** • Increased prothrombin and factors VII, VIII, IX, and X; thyroid-binding globulin with increased PBI, T_4, increased uptake of free T_3 resin (free T_4 is unaltered), serum triglycerides and phospholipid concentration • Decreased antithrombin III, pregnanediol excretion, response to metyrapone test, serum folate concentration • Impaired glucose tolerance

■ Nursing considerations

Assessment

- **History:** Allergy to estrogens, tartrazine; breast cancer, estrogen-dependent neoplasm; undiagnosed abnormal genital bleeding; active or previous thrombophlebitis or thromboembolic disorders; pregnancy; lactation; metabolic bone disease; renal insufficiency; heart failure
- **Physical:** Skin color, lesions, edema; breast examination; injection site; orientation, affect, reflexes; P, auscultation, BP, peripheral perfusion; R, adventitious sounds; bowel sounds, liver evaluation, abdominal examination; pelvic examination; serum calcium, phosphorus; LFTs, renal function tests; Papanicolaou (PAP) test, glucose tolerance test

Interventions

⊗ ***Black box warning*** Arrange for pretreatment and periodic (at least annual) history and physical, which should include BP, breasts, abdomen, pelvic organs, and a Pap test; may increase risk of endometrial cancer.

⊗ ***Black box warning*** Do not use to prevent CV events or dementia; may increase risk, including thrombophlebitis, pulmonary embolism, CVA, MI.

⊗ ***Black box warning*** Caution patient of the risks of estrogen use, the need to prevent pregnancy during treatment, for frequent medical follow-up, and for periodic rests from drug treatment.

- Administer cyclically for short-term only when treating postmenopausal conditions because of the risk of endometrial neoplasm; taper to the lowest effective dose, and provide a drug-free week each month.
- Apply transdermal system to a clean, dry area of skin on the trunk of the body, preferably the abdomen; do not apply to breasts; rotate the site at least 1 wk between applications; avoid the waistline because clothing may rub the system off; apply immediately after opening and compress for about 10 sec to attach.
- Apply topical gel to upper thighs, alternating right and left daily. Do not apply to irritated skin, and do not wash site for at least 1 hr.
- Apply topical spray to forearm. Let dry for at least 30 min.
- Insert vaginal ring as deeply as possible into upper one-third of vagina. Ring will remain in place for 3 months. Then, remove and evaluate need for continued therapy. If a ring falls out during 3 mo, rinse with warm water and reinsert.

⊗ ***Warning*** Arrange for the concomitant use of progestin therapy during long-term estrogen therapy in women with a uterus; this will mimic normal physiologic cycling and allow for a cyclic uterine bleeding that may decrease the risk of endometrial cancer. Women without a uterus do not need progestin.

- Administer parenteral preparations by deep IM injection only. Monitor injection sites and rotate with each injection to decrease development of abscesses.

Teaching points

- Use this drug in cycles or short term; prepare a calendar of drug days, rest days, and drug-free periods.

- Apply transdermal system and vaginal cream properly; insert vaginal tablet as high into the vagina as is comfortable.
- Apply gel to upper thighs, alternating right and left daily. Do not apply to irritated skin, and do not wash site for at least 1 hour.
- Apply one spray to forearm each day. Let dry for at least 30 minutes.
- Insert vaginal ring high in vagina; it should remain in place for 3 months. If it falls out before that time, rinse with warm water and reinsert.
- Potentially serious side effects include cancers, blood clots, and liver problems; it is very important to have periodic medical examinations throughout therapy.
- This drug cannot be given to pregnant women because of serious toxic effects to the baby; use of contraceptives is advised.
- You may experience these side effects: Nausea, vomiting, bloating; headache, dizziness, mental depression (use caution if driving or performing tasks that require alertness); sensitivity to sunlight (use a sunscreen and wear protective clothing); rash, loss of scalp hair, darkening of the skin on the face; changes in menstrual patterns.
- Report pain in the groin or calves of the legs, chest pain or sudden shortness of breath, abnormal vaginal bleeding, lumps in the breast, sudden severe headache, dizziness or fainting, changes in vision or speech, weakness or numbness in the arm or leg, severe abdominal pain, yellowing of the skin or eyes, severe mental depression, pain at injection site.

estrogens, conjugated

(ess' troe jenz)

Oral, topical vaginal cream: C.E.S. (CAN), Premarin

Parenteral: Premarin Intravenous

Synthetic: Cenestin, Enjuvia

PREGNANCY CATEGORY X

Drug classes

Estrogen
Hormone

Therapeutic actions

Estrogens are endogenous female sex hormones important in the development of the female reproductive system and secondary sex characteristics. They affect the release of pituitary gonadotropins; cause capillary dilatation, fluid retention, protein anabolism, and thin cervical mucus; conserve calcium and phosphorus; encourage bone formation; inhibit ovulation and prevent postpartum breast discomfort. They are responsible for the proliferation of the endometrium; absence or decline of estrogen produces signs and symptoms of menopause on the uterus, vagina, breasts, cervix. Their efficacy as palliation in male patients with androgen-dependent prostatic carcinoma is attributable to their competition with androgens for receptor sites, thus decreasing the influence of androgens.

Indications

Oral

- Palliation of moderate to severe vasomotor symptoms, atrophic vaginitis, or kraurosis vulvae associated with menopause
- Treatment of female hypogonadism; female castration; primary ovarian failure
- Osteoporosis: To retard progression
- Palliation of inoperable prostatic cancer
- Palliation of metastatic breast cancer
- *Cenestin:* Treatment of moderate to severe vasomotor symptoms associated with menopause

Parenteral

- Treatment of uterine bleeding due to hormonal imbalance in the absence of organic pathology

Vaginal cream

- Treatment of atrophic vaginitis and kraurosis vulvae associated with menopause

Contraindications and cautions

- Contraindicated with allergy to estrogens, breast cancer (with exceptions), estrogen-dependent neoplasm, undiagnosed abnormal genital bleeding, active or past thrombophlebitis or thromboembolic disorders from previous estrogen use, pregnancy (serious fetal defects; women of childbearing age should be advised of risks and birth control measures suggested).

E

- Use cautiously with metabolic bone disease, renal or hepatic insufficiency, heart failure, lactation.

Available forms

Tablets—0.3, 0.45, 0.625, 0.9, 1.25 mg; injection—25 mg; vaginal cream—0.625 mg/g

Dosages

Oral drug should be given cyclically (3 wk on/1 wk off) except in selected cases of carcinoma and prevention of postpartum breast engorgement.

Adults

- *Moderate to severe vasomotor symptoms associated with menopause:* 0.3–0.625 mg/day PO.
- *Atrophic vaginitis, kraurosis vulvae associated with menopause:* 0.5–2 g vaginal cream daily intravaginally or topically, depending on severity of condition. Taper or discontinue at 3- to 6-mo intervals. Or, 0.3 mg/day PO continually.
- *Female hypogonadism:* 0.3–0.625 mg/day PO for 3 wk followed by 1 wk of rest. Adjust dose depending on severity of symptoms and responsiveness of endometrium.
- *Female castration, primary ovarian failure:* 1.25 mg/day PO. Adjust dosage by patient response to lowest effective dose.
- *Prostatic cancer (inoperable):* 1.25–2.5 mg tid PO. Judge effectiveness by phosphatase determinations and by symptomatic improvement.
- *Osteoporosis:* Start with lowest dose, 0.3 mg/day PO given continuously or cyclically (25 days on/5 days off). Adjust dosage based on individual response.
- *Breast cancer (inoperable, progressing):* 10 mg tid PO for at least 3 mo.
- *Abnormal uterine bleeding due to hormonal imbalance:* 25 mg IV or IM. Repeat in 6–12 hr as needed. IV route provides a more rapid response.

Pediatric patients

Not recommended due to effect on growth of the long bones.

Pharmacokinetics

Route	*Onset*	*Peak*
Oral	Slow	Days
IV	Gradual	Hours

Metabolism: Hepatic; $T_{1/2}$: Unknown
Distribution: Crosses placenta; enters breast milk
Excretion: Urine

IV FACTS

Preparation: Reconstitute with provided diluent; add to normal saline, dextrose, and invert sugar solutions. Refrigerate unreconstituted parenteral solution; use reconstituted solution within a few hours. Refrigerated reconstituted solution is stable for 60 days; do not use solution if darkened or precipitates have formed.
Infusion: Inject slowly over 2–5 min.
Incompatibilities: Do not mix with protein hydrolysate, ascorbic acid, or any solution with an acid pH.

Adverse effects

- **CNS:** Steepening of the corneal curvature with a resultant change in visual acuity and intolerance to contact lenses, *headache,* migraine, dizziness, mental depression, chorea, **seizures**
- **CV:** Increased BP, thromboembolic and thrombotic disease
- **Dermatologic:** *Photosensitivity, peripheral edema, chloasma,* erythema nodosum or multiforme, hemorrhagic eruption, loss of scalp hair, hirsutism, urticaria, dermatitis
- **GI:** Gallbladder disease (in postmenopausal women), **hepatic adenoma,** *nausea, vomiting, abdominal cramps, bloating,* **cholestatic jaundice,** *colitis,* **acute pancreatitis**
- **GU:** Increased risk of endometrial cancer in postmenopausal women, *breakthrough bleeding, change in menstrual flow, dysmenorrhea, premenstrual-like syndrome,* amenorrhea, vaginal candidiasis, cystitis-like syndrome, endometrial cystic hyperplasia

- **Hematologic:** Hypercalcemia, decreased glucose tolerance
- **Local:** *Pain at injection site,* sterile abscess, postinjection flare
- **Other:** Weight changes, reduced carbohydrate tolerance, aggravation of porphyria, edema, changes in libido, breast tenderness

Topical vaginal cream

Systemic absorption may cause uterine bleeding in menopausal women and serious bleeding of remaining endometrial foci in sterilized women with endometriosis

Interactions

✱ Drug-drug • Increased therapeutic and toxic effects of corticosteroids • Decreased serum levels of estrogen with drugs that enhance hepatic metabolism of the drug: Barbiturates, phenytoin, rifampin, carbamazepine

✱ Drug-lab test • Increased prothrombin and factors VII, VIII, IX, and X; thyroid-binding globulin with increased PBI, T_4, increased uptake of free T_3 resin (free T_4 is unaltered), serum triglycerides and phospholipid concentration • Decreased antithrombin III, pregnanediol excretion, response to metyrapone test, serum folate concentration • Impaired glucose tolerance

■ Nursing considerations

Assessment

- **History:** Allergy to estrogens; breast cancer, estrogen-dependent neoplasm; undiagnosed abnormal genital bleeding; active or previous thrombophlebitis or thromboembolic disorders; pregnancy; lactation; metabolic bone disease; renal insufficiency; heart failure
- **Physical:** Skin color, lesions, edema; breast examination; injection site; orientation, affect, reflexes; P, auscultation, BP, peripheral perfusion; R, adventitious sounds; bowel sounds, liver evaluation, abdominal examination; pelvic examination; serum calcium, phosphorus; LFTs, renal function tests; Papanicolaou (Pap) test; glucose tolerance test

Interventions

⊗ ***Black box warning*** Arrange for pretreatment and periodic (at least annual) history and physical, which should include BP, breasts, abdomen, pelvic organs, and a Pap test; increased risk of endometrial cancer.

⊗ ***Black box warning*** Do not use to prevent CV events or dementia; may increase risk, including thrombophlebitis, pulmonary embolism, CVA, MI.

⊗ ***Black box warning*** Caution patient of the risks involved with estrogen use, the need to prevent pregnancy during treatment, for frequent medical follow-up, and periodic rests from drug treatment.

⊗ ***Warning*** Give cyclically for short term only when treating postmenopausal conditions because of the risk of endometrial neoplasm; taper to the lowest effective dose, and provide a drug-free week each month.

- Refrigerate unreconstituted parenteral solution; use reconstituted solution within a few hours.
- Refrigerated reconstituted solution is stable for 60 days; do not use solution if darkened or precipitates have formed.

⊗ ***Warning*** Arrange for the concomitant use of progestin therapy during long-term estrogen therapy in women with a uterus; this will mimic normal physiologic cycling and allow for cyclic uterine bleeding, which may decrease the risk of endometrial cancer. Women without a uterus do not need progestin.

Teaching points

- Use this drug cyclically or short term; prepare a calendar of drug days, rest days, and drug-free periods.
- Use vaginal cream properly.
- Potentially serious side effects can occur: Cancers, blood clots, liver problems; it is very important that you have periodic medical examinations throughout therapy.
- This drug cannot be given to pregnant women because of serious toxic effects to the baby; use of contraceptives is advised.
- You may experience these side effects: Nausea, vomiting, bloating; headache, dizziness, mental depression (use caution if driving or performing tasks that require alertness); sensitivity to sunlight (use a sunscreen and wear protective clothing); rash, loss of scalp hair, darkening of the skin on the face; changes in menstrual patterns.
- Report pain in the groin or calves of the legs, chest pain or sudden shortness of breath,

abnormal vaginal bleeding, lumps in the breast, sudden severe headache, dizziness or fainting, changes in vision or speech, weakness or numbness in the arm or leg, severe abdominal pain, yellowing of the skin or eyes, severe mental depression, pain at injection site.

estrogens, esterified

(ess' troe jenz)

Menest

PREGNANCY CATEGORY X

Drug classes

Estrogen
Hormone

Therapeutic actions

Estrogens are endogenous hormones important in the development of the female reproductive system and secondary sex characteristics. They cause capillary dilatation, fluid retention, protein anabolism, and thin cervical mucus; conserve calcium and phosphorus and encourage bone formation; inhibit ovulation and prevent postpartum breast discomfort. They are responsible for the proliferation of the endometrium; absence or decline of estrogen produces signs and symptoms of menopause on the uterus, vagina, breasts, cervix. Palliation with androgen-dependent prostatic carcinoma is attributable to competition for androgen receptor sites, decreasing the influence of androgens.

Indications

- Palliation of moderate to severe vasomotor symptoms, atrophic vaginitis, or kraurosis vulvae associated with menopause
- Treatment of female hypogonadism; female castration; primary ovarian failure
- Palliation of inoperable prostatic cancer
- Palliation of inoperable, metastatic breast cancer in men, postmenopausal women

Contraindications and cautions

- Contraindicated with allergy to estrogens, breast cancer (with exceptions), estrogen-dependent neoplasm, undiagnosed abnormal genital bleeding, active or past thrombophlebitis or thromboembolic disorders from previous estrogen use, pregnancy (serious fetal defects; women of childbearing age should be advised of the risks and birth control measures suggested).
- Use cautiously with metabolic bone disease, renal or hepatic insufficiency, heart failure, lactation.

Available forms

Tablets—0.3, 0.625, 1.25, 2.5 mg

Dosages

Administer PO only.

Adults

- *Moderate to severe vasomotor symptoms, atrophic vaginitis, kraurosis vulvae associated with menopause:* 0.3–1.25 mg/day PO for atrophic vaginitis and kraurosis vulvae. 1.25 mg/day PO for vasomotor symptoms. Adjust to lowest effective dose. Cyclic therapy (3 wk of daily estrogen followed by 1 wk of rest from drug therapy) is recommended. If patient has not menstruated in 2 mo, start at any time. If patient is still menstruating, start therapy on day 5 of bleeding.
- *Female hypogonadism:* 2.5–7.5 mg/day PO in divided doses for 20 days on/10 days off. If bleeding does not occur by the end of that period, repeat the same dosage schedule. If bleeding does occur before the end of the 10-day rest, begin a 20-day estrogen-progestin cyclic regimen with progestin given orally during the last 5 days of estrogen therapy. If bleeding occurs before this cycle is finished, restart course on day 5 of bleeding.
- *Female castration, primary ovarian failure:* 1.25 mg/day PO. Adjust dosage by patient response to lowest effective dose.
- *Prostatic cancer (inoperable):* 1.25–2.5 mg tid PO. In long-term therapy, judge effectiveness by symptomatic response and serum phosphatase determinations.
- *Breast cancer (inoperable, progressing):* 10 mg tid PO for at least 3 mo in selected men and postmenopausal women.

Pediatric patients

Not recommended due to effect on growth of the long bones.

Pharmacokinetics

Route	Onset	Peak
Oral	Slow	Days

Metabolism: Hepatic; $T_{1/2}$: Unknown
Distribution: Crosses placenta; enters breast milk
Excretion: Urine

Adverse effects

- **CNS:** Steepening of the corneal curvature with a resultant change in visual acuity and intolerance to contact lenses, *headache,* migraine, dizziness, mental depression, chorea, **seizures**
- **CV:** Increased BP, thromboembolic and thrombotic disease (with high doses in certain groups of susceptible women and in men receiving estrogens for prostatic cancer)
- **Dermatologic:** *Photosensitivity, peripheral edema, chloasma,* erythema nodosum or multiforme, hemorrhagic eruption, loss of scalp hair, hirsutism, urticaria, dermatitis
- **GI:** Gallbladder disease (in postmenopausal women), **hepatic adenoma** (rarely occurs, but may rupture and cause death), *nausea, vomiting, abdominal cramps, bloating,* cholestatic jaundice, colitis, acute pancreatitis
- **GU:** Increased risk of endometrial cancer in postmenopausal women, *breakthrough bleeding, change in menstrual flow, dysmenorrhea, premenstrual-like syndrome,* amenorrhea, vaginal candidiasis, cystitis-like syndrome, endometrial cystic hyperplasia
- **Hematologic:** Hypercalcemia (in breast cancer patients with bone metastases), decreased glucose tolerance
- **Other:** Weight changes, reduced carbohydrate tolerance, aggravation of porphyria, edema, changes in libido, breast tenderness

Interactions

✱ **Drug-drug** • Increased therapeutic and toxic effects of corticosteroids • Decreased serum levels of estrogen if taken with drugs that enhance hepatic metabolism of the drug: Barbiturates, phenytoin, rifampin, carbamazepine
✱ **Drug-lab test** • Increased prothrombin and factors VII, VIII, IX, and X; thyroid-binding globulin with increased PBI, T_4 increased uptake of free T_3 resin (free T_4 is unaltered), serum triglycerides and phospholipid concentration • Decreased antithrombin III, pregnanediol excretion, response to metyrapone test, serum folate concentration • Impaired glucose tolerance

■ Nursing considerations

Assessment

- **History:** Allergy to estrogens; breast cancer, estrogen-dependent neoplasm; undiagnosed abnormal genital bleeding; thrombophlebitis or thromboembolic disorders; pregnancy; lactation; metabolic bone disease; renal insufficiency; heart failure
- **Physical:** Skin color, lesions, edema; breast examination; injection site; orientation, affect, reflexes; P, auscultation, BP, peripheral perfusion; R, adventitious sounds; bowel sounds, liver evaluation, abdominal examination; pelvic examination; serum calcium, phosphorus; LFTs, renal function tests; Papanicolaou (Pap) test; glucose tolerance test

Interventions

⊗ ***Black box warning*** Arrange for pretreatment and periodic (at least annual) history and physical examination, which should include BP, breasts, abdomen, pelvic organs, and a Pap test; increased risk of endometrial cancer.

⊗ ***Black box warning*** Do not use to prevent CV events or dementia; may increase risk, including thrombophlebitis, pulmonary embolism, CVA, MI.

⊗ ***Black box warning*** Caution patient of the risks involved with estrogen use; the need to prevent pregnancy during treatment, for frequent medical follow-up, and for periodic rests from drug treatment.

⊗ ***Black box warning*** Give cyclically for short term only when treating postmenopausal conditions because of the risk of endometrial neoplasm; taper to the lowest effective dose, and provide a drug-free week each month.

⊗ ***Warning*** Arrange for progestin therapy during long-term estrogen therapy in postmenopausal women with a uterus; this will mimic normal physiologic cycling and allow for cyclic uterine bleeding, which may decrease the risk of endometrial cancer. Women without a uterus do not need progestin.

Teaching points

- Use this drug in cycles or short term; prepare a calendar of drug days, rest days, and drug-free periods (as appropriate).
- Potentially serious side effects can occur, including cancers, blood clots, liver problems; it is very important that you have periodic medical examinations throughout therapy.
- This drug cannot be given to pregnant women because of serious toxic effects to the baby; use of contraceptives is advised.
- You may experience these side effects: Nausea, vomiting, bloating; headache, dizziness, mental depression (use caution if driving or performing tasks that require alertness); sensitivity to sunlight (use a sunscreen and wear protective clothing); rash, loss of scalp hair, darkening of the skin on the face; changes in menstrual patterns.
- Report pain in the groin or calves of the legs, chest pain or sudden shortness of breath, abnormal vaginal bleeding, lumps in the breast, sudden severe headache, dizziness or fainting, changes in vision or speech, weakness or numbness in the arm or leg, severe abdominal pain, yellowing of the skin or eyes, severe mental depression.

▽ estropipate (piperazine estrone sulfate)

(ess' troe ***pi'*** *pate)*

Ogen

PREGNANCY CATEGORY X

Drug classes

Estrogen
Hormone

Therapeutic actions

Estrogens are endogenous female sex hormones important in the development of the female reproductive system and secondary sex characteristics. They cause capillary dilatation, fluid retention, protein anabolism, and thin cervical mucus; conserve calcium and phosphorus and encourage bone formation; inhibit ovulation and prevent postpartum breast discomfort. They are responsible for the proliferation of the endometrium; absence or decline of estrogen produces signs and symptoms of menopause on the uterus, vagina, breasts, cervix. Palliation with androgen-dependent prostatic carcinoma is attributable to competition with androgens for receptor sites, decreasing the influence of androgens.

Indications

- Palliation of moderate to severe vasomotor symptoms, atrophic vaginitis, or kraurosis vulvae associated with menopause
- Treatment of female hypogonadism, female castration, primary ovarian failure
- Prevention of osteoporosis

Contraindications and cautions

- Contraindicated with allergy to estrogens, breast cancer (with exceptions), estrogen-dependent neoplasm, undiagnosed abnormal genital bleeding, active or past thrombophlebitis or thromboembolic disorders from previous estrogen use, pregnancy (serious fetal defects; advise women of childbearing age of the potential risks and suggest birth control measures).
- Use cautiously with metabolic bone disease, renal or hepatic insufficiency, heart failure, lactation.

Available forms

Tablets—0.625, 1.25, 2.5, 5 mg

Dosages

Adults

- *Moderate to severe vasomotor symptoms, atrophic vaginitis, kraurosis vulvae associated with menopause:* 0.75–6 mg/day PO given cyclically (3 wk on and 1 wk off). Use lowest possible dose.
- *Female hypogonadism, female castration, primary ovarian failure:* 1.5–9 mg/day PO for the first 3 wk, followed by a rest period

of 8–10 days. Repeat if bleeding does not occur at end of rest period.

- *Prevention of osteoporosis:* 0.75 mg daily PO for 25 days of a 31-day cycle per month.

Pediatric patients

Not recommended due to effect on growth of the long bones.

Pharmacokinetics

Route	*Onset*	*Peak*
Oral	Slow	Days

Metabolism: Hepatic; $T_{1/2}$: Unknown
Distribution: Crosses placenta; enters breast milk
Excretion: Urine

Adverse effects

- **CNS:** Steepening of the corneal curvature with a resultant change in visual acuity and intolerance to contact lenses, *headache,* migraine, dizziness, mental depression, chorea, **seizures**
- **CV:** Increased BP, thromboembolic and thrombotic disease
- **Dermatologic:** *Photosensitivity, peripheral edema, chloasma,* erythema nodosum or multiforme, hemorrhagic eruption, loss of scalp hair, hirsutism, urticaria, dermatitis
- **GI:** Gallbladder disease (in postmenopausal women), **hepatic adenoma,** *nausea, vomiting, abdominal cramps, bloating,* **cholestatic jaundice,** *colitis,* acute pancreatitis
- **GU:** Increased risk of endometrial cancer in postmenopausal women, *breakthrough bleeding, change in menstrual flow, dysmenorrhea, premenstrual-like syndrome,* amenorrhea, vaginal candidiasis, cystitis-like syndrome, endometrial cystic hyperplasia
- **Hematologic:** Hypercalcemia, decreased glucose tolerance
- **Other:** Weight changes, reduced carbohydrate tolerance, aggravation of porphyria, edema, changes in libido, breast tenderness

Interactions

✱ **Drug-drug** • Increased therapeutic and toxic effects of corticosteroids • Decreased serum levels of estrogens if taken with drugs that enhance hepatic metabolism of the drug: barbiturates, phenytoin, rifampin, carbamazepine

✱ **Drug-lab test** • Increased prothrombin and factors VII, VIII, IX, and X; thyroid-binding globulin with increased PBI, T_4, increased uptake of free T_3 resin (free T_4 is unaltered), serum triglycerides and phospholipid concentration • Decreased antithrombin III, pregnanediol excretion, response to metyrapone test, serum folate concentration • Impaired glucose tolerance

■ Nursing considerations

Assessment

- **History:** Allergy to estrogens; breast cancer, estrogen-dependent neoplasm; undiagnosed abnormal genital bleeding; thrombophlebitis or thromboembolic disorders; pregnancy; lactation; metabolic bone disease; renal insufficiency; heart failure
- **Physical:** Skin color, lesions, edema; breast examination; injection site; orientation, affect, reflexes; P, auscultation, BP, peripheral perfusion; R, adventitious sounds; bowel sounds, liver evaluation, abdominal examination; pelvic examination; serum calcium, phosphorus; LFTs, renal function tests; Papanicolaou (Pap) test; glucose tolerance test

Interventions

⊠ ***Black box warning*** Arrange for pretreatment and periodic (at least annual) history and physical examination, which should include BP, breasts, abdomen, pelvic organs, and a Pap test; increased risk of endometrial cancer.

⊠ ***Black box warning*** Do not use to prevent CV events or dementia; may increase risk, including thrombophlebitis, pulmonary embolism, CVA, MI.

⊠ ***Black box warning*** Caution patient of the risks involved with estrogen use, the need to prevent pregnancy during treatment, for frequent medical follow-up, and for periodic rests from drug treatment.

⊠ ***Black box warning*** Give cyclically for short term only when treating postmenopausal conditions because of the risk of endometrial neoplasm. Taper to the lowest effective dose and provide a drug-free week each month.

⊗ ***Warning*** Arrange for the concomitant use of progestin therapy during long-term estrogen therapy in postmenopausal women with a uterus; this will mimic normal physiologic cycling and allow for a cyclic uterine bleeding, which may decrease the risk of endometrial cancer. Women without a uterus do not need progestin.

Teaching points

- Prepare a calendar of drug days, rest days, and drug-free periods.
- This drug cannot be given to pregnant women because of serious toxic effects to the baby; use of contraceptives is advised.
- Potentially serious side effects can occur, including cancers, blood clots, and liver problems; it is very important that you have periodic medical examinations throughout therapy.
- You may experience these side effects: Nausea, vomiting, bloating; headache, dizziness, mental depression (use caution driving or performing tasks that require alertness); sensitivity to sunlight (use a sunscreen and wear protective clothing); rash, loss of scalp hair, darkening of the skin on the face; changes in menstrual patterns.
- Report pain in the groin or calves of the legs, chest pain or sudden shortness of breath, abnormal vaginal bleeding, lumps in the breast, sudden severe headache, dizziness or fainting, changes in vision or speech, weakness or numbness in the arm or leg, severe abdominal pain, yellowing of the skin or eyes, severe mental depression.

eszopiclone

(ess zop' ah klone)

Lunesta DNC

PREGNANCY CATEGORY C

CONTROLLED SUBSTANCE SCHEDULE IV

Drug classes

Nonbenzodiazepine hypnotic
Sedative-hypnotic

Therapeutic actions

Exact mechanism of action is not known. It is thought to interact with GABA receptors at binding domains near benzodiazepine receptor sites, leading to sedation.

Indications

- Treatment of insomnia

Contraindications and cautions

- No known contraindications.
- Use cautiously with geriatric or debilitated patients, diseases or conditions that could affect metabolism or hemodynamics, signs or symptoms of depression, pregnancy, or lactation; history of substance abuse (may be habit-forming).

Available forms

Tablets DNC—1, 2, 3 mg

Dosage

Adult

Initial dose—2 mg PO taken immediately before bedtime. Dosage may be increased to 3 mg PO immediately before bedtime if clinically needed. The tablet should be swallowed whole, not cut or crushed.

Pediatric patients

Safety and efficacy not established.

Geriatric patients

Initial dose—1 mg PO taken immediately before bedtime if the primary complaint is falling asleep. If the primary complaint is difficulty staying asleep, 2 mg PO immediately before bedtime may be used.

Patients with severe hepatic impairment

1 mg PO immediately before bedtime. Use caution and monitor the patient closely.

Patients concurrently using CYP3A4 inhibitors

1 mg PO immediately before bedtime. May be increased to 2 mg with caution.

Pharmacokinetics

Route	*Onset*	*Peak*
Oral	Rapid	1 hr

Metabolism: Hepatic ; $T_{1/2}$: 6 hr

Distribution: May cross placenta; may pass into breast milk
Excretion: Urine

Adverse effects

- **CNS:** *Dizziness, somnolence, nervousness,* anxiety, depression, hallucinations, *headache,* complex sleep disorders, abnormal thinking
- **GI:** Unpleasant taste, dry mouth, dyspepsia, nausea, vomiting
- **GU:** Dysmenorrhea, gynecomastia
- **Respiratory:** Respiratory infection
- **Other:** Viral infection, rash, **anaphylaxis, angioedema**

Interactions

✱ **Drug-drug** • Risk of additional effects on psychomotor performance if combined with ethanol • Increased serum levels and risk of adverse effects if combined with potent CYP3A4 inhibitors (ketoconazole, itraconazole, clarithromycin, nefazodone, ritonavir, nelfinavir) • Risk of decreased serum levels and effectiveness if combined with rifampin

■ Nursing considerations

Assessment

- **History:** Lactation, pregnancy, depression, underlying medical conditions that could affect metabolism or hemodynamics
- **Physical:** Orientation, reflexes, affect; R, adventitious sounds; abdominal examination

Interventions

- Ensure that the patient swallows the tablet whole; do not cut, crush or allow patient to chew tablet.
- Administer drug only if patient is in bed and able to stay in bed for up to 8 hr; changes in cognition and motor function can be a safety issue.
- Monitor patients using drug for suicidal thoughts.
- Do not administer this drug after a fatty or large meal, absorption can be affected.
- Effects of the drug on a fetus are not known. Advise women of childbearing age to use barrier contraceptives while on this drug.
- It is not known if this drug would affect a nursing baby. Advise nursing women to use another method of feeding the baby.

Teaching points

- Take this drug exactly as prescribed. Do not use it longer than advised by your health care provider.
- Swallow the tablet whole, do not break or crush the tablet.
- Do not share this drug with anyone else. Store the drug in its original container and keep it out of the reach of children.
- Do not take this drug unless you are about to get into bed and are able to get 8 or more hours of sleep before you need to be alert again.
- Do not take this drug with or immediately after a high-fat or heavy meal, which could interfere with the absorption and effectiveness of the drug.
- Do not combine this drug with other sleep-inducing drugs, including over-the-counter products.
- It is not known how this drug would affect a pregnancy. If you think you are pregnant or would like to become pregnant, consult your health care provider.
- This drug should not be taken while nursing a baby. If you are nursing a baby, another method of feeding the baby should be used while you are using this drug.
- Do not drink alcohol while you are using this drug.
- You may experience sleeping problems the first night or two after stopping any sleep medicine, including *Lunesta*.
- You may experience these side effects: Changes in thinking, alertness (do not drive a car, operate potentially dangerous equipment, or make important legal decisions the day after you take this drug); complex sleep disorders; allergic reaction; swelling; headache (consult your health care provider for potential pain medications if this occurs); unpleasant taste, nausea (frequent mouth care, frequent small meals may help).
- Report depression, thoughts of suicide or disturbing thoughts, rash, severe headache, changes in behavior.

E

etanercept

(ee tan er' sept)

Enbrel

PREGNANCY CATEGORY B

Drug classes

Antiarthritic
Disease-modifying antirheumatic drug

Therapeutic actions

Genetically engineered tumor necrosis factor receptors from Chinese hamster ovary cells; keep inflammatory response to autoimmune disease in check by reacting with and deactivating free-floating tumor necrosis factor released by active leukocytes.

Indications

- Reduction of the signs and symptoms, inducing major clinical response, inhibiting the progression of structural damage, and improving physical function in patients with moderately to severely active rheumatoid arthritis; to delay the structural damage associated with rheumatoid arthritis; or may be used in combination with methotrexate when patients do not respond to methotrexate alone
- Reduction of signs and symptoms of moderately to severely active polyarticular juvenile idiopathic arthritis in patients 2 yr and older
- Reduction of signs and symptoms and to improve function in patients with psoriatic arthritis; may be used alone or in combination with methotrexate
- Treatment of ankylosing spondylitis
- Treatment of adult patients with chronic moderate to severe plaque psoriasis who are candidates for systemic therapy or phototherapy

NEW INDICATION: Unlabeled uses: Heart failure, Crohn's disease

Contraindications and cautions

- Contraindicated with allergy to etanercept or Chinese hamster products, lactation, pregnancy, cancer, severe infection including sepsis, CNS demyelinating disorders, myelosuppression.
- Use cautiously with renal or hepatic disorders, any infection, heart failure, latex allergy.

Available forms

Powder for injection—25 mg; prefilled single-use syringe—25, 50 mg/mL; single-use prefilled auto-injector—50 mg.

Dosages

Adults

- *Plaque psoriasis:* 50 mg/dose subcutaneously twice weekly 3 or 4 days apart for 3 mo; then maintenance dose of 50 mg/wk subcutaneously.
- *Ankylosing spondylitis, rheumatoid arthritis, psoriatic arthritis:* 50 mg/wk subcutaneously.

Pediatric patients 2–17 yr

0.8 mg/kg subcutaneously once weekly. Maximum dose, 50 mg/wk. 50-mg auto-injector may be used in patients weighing more than 63 kg. 25-mg prefilled syringe may be used for patients weighing 31–62 kg.

Pediatric patients younger than 2 yr

Safety and efficacy not established.

Pharmacokinetics

Route	*Onset*	*Peak*
Subcut.	Slow	72 hr

Metabolism: Tissue; $T_{1/2}$: 115 hr
Distribution: Crosses placenta; may enter breast milk
Excretion: Tissues

Adverse effects

- **CNS: CNS demyelinating disorders (MS, myelitis, optic neuritis),** dizziness, headache
- **CV:** hypotension, DVT, MI, heart failure
- **GI:** Abdominal pain, dyspepsia
- **Hematologic: Pancytopenia**
- **Respiratory:** *URIs,* congestion, rhinitis, cough, pharyngitis
- **Other:** *Irritation at injection site;* **increased risk of infections, cancers;** ANA development; autoimmune diseases, rash

■ Nursing considerations

Assessment

- **History:** Allergy to etanercept or Chinese hamster ovary products; pregnancy, lactation; serious infections; cancer; CNS demyelinating disorders, myelosuppression
- **Physical:** Skin lesions, color; R, adventitious sounds; injection site evaluation; range-of-motion to monitor drug effectiveness; CNS—neurologic evaluation, reflexes; CBC

Interventions

⊗ ***Warning*** Obtain a baseline and periodic CBC; discontinue drug at signs of severe bone marrow suppression.

⊗ ***Warning*** Obtain baseline values of neurologic function; discontinue drug at any sign of CNS demyelinating disorders.

- Advise patient that this drug does not cure the disease and appropriate therapies for rheumatoid arthritis should be used.
- Reconstitute for injection by slowly injecting 1 mL sterile bacteriostatic water provided with powder into the vial; swirl gently, do not shake; avoid foaming; liquid should be clear and free of particulate matter; use within 6 hr of reconstitution. Do not mix with any other medications.
- Rotate injection sites between abdomen, thigh, and upper arm. Maintain a chart to ensure that sites are rotated regularly.
- Teach patient and a significant other how to reconstitute and administer subcutaneous injections; observe the process periodically.

⊗ ***Black box warning*** Monitor patient for any sign of infection; discontinue drug if infection occurs; risk of serious infections, including TB, or death exists.

⊗ ***Black box warning*** There is an increased risk of lymphoma and other cancers in children taking this drug for juvenile rheumatoid arthritis, Crohn's disease, or other inflammatory conditions.

- Evaluate drug effectiveness periodically; 1–2 wk may be required before any change is noted; if no response has occurred within 3 mo, discontinue drug.
- Do not administer drug with any vaccinations; allow at least 2–3 wk between starting this drug and a vaccination.
- Stop drug if patient develops lupus-like symptoms.
- Protect patient from exposure to infections and ensure routine physical examinations and monitoring for potential cancers and autoimmune diseases.

Teaching points

- Take this drug exactly as prescribed. Note that this drug does not cure rheumatoid arthritis and appropriate therapies to deal with the disease should be followed. You and a significant other should learn how to prepare the drug and to administer subcutaneous injections. Prepare a chart of injection sites to ensure that sites are rotated on a regular basis. Consult your health care provider about proper disposal of needles and syringes.
- Arrange for frequent, regular medical follow-up visits, including blood tests to follow the effects of the drug on your body.
- You may experience these side effects: Signs and symptoms of upper respiratory infections, cough, sore throat (consult your health care provider for potential treatment if this becomes severe); headache (analgesics may be available to help); increased susceptibility to infections (avoid crowded areas and people who might have infections; use strict handwashing and good hygiene).
- Report fever, chills, lethargy; rash, difficulty breathing; swelling; worsening of arthritis; severe diarrhea; numbness, tingling; bruising, bleeding.

▽ethacrynic acid

See Appendix W, *Less commonly used drugs*.

▽ethambutol hydrochloride

*(e **tham'** byoo tole)*

Etibi (CAN), Myambutol

PREGNANCY CATEGORY C

Drug class

Antituberculotic (second line)

Therapeutic actions

Inhibits the synthesis of metabolites in growing mycobacterium cells, impairing cell metabolism, arresting cell multiplication, and causing cell death.

Indications

- Treatment of pulmonary TB in conjunction with at least one other antituberculotic

Contraindications and cautions

- Contraindicated with allergy to ethambutol; optic neuritis.
- Use cautiously with impaired renal function, lactation, pregnancy (use other antituberculotics), visual problems (cataracts, diabetic retinopathy).

Available forms

Tablets—100, 400 mg

Dosages

Ethambutol is not administered alone; use in conjunction with other antituberculotics.

Adults

- *Initial treatment:* 15 mg/kg/day PO as a single daily oral dose. Continue therapy until bacteriologic conversion has become permanent and maximal clinical improvement has occurred.
- *Retreatment:* 25 mg/kg/day as a single daily oral dose. After 60 days, reduce dose to 15 mg/kg/day as a single daily dose.

Pediatric patients

Not recommended for patients younger than 13 yr.

Pharmacokinetics

Route	*Onset*	*Peak*	*Duration*
Oral	Rapid	2–4 hr	20–24 hr

Metabolism: Hepatic; $T_{1/2}$: 3.3 hr
Distribution: Crosses placenta; enters breast milk
Excretion: Feces, urine

Adverse effects

- **CNS:** *Optic neuritis* (loss of visual acuity, changes in color perception), *fever, malaise, headache,* dizziness, mental confusion, disorientation, hallucinations, peripheral neuritis
- **GI:** *Anorexia, nausea, vomiting,* GI upset, abdominal pain, transient liver impairment
- **Hypersensitivity:** Allergic reactions—dermatitis, pruritus, anaphylactoid reaction
- **Other: Toxic epidermal necrolysis, thrombocytopenia,** joint pain, acute gout

Interactions

✱ **Drug-drug** • Decreased absorption with aluminum salts

■ Nursing considerations

Assessment

- **History:** Allergy to ethambutol, optic neuritis, impaired renal function, pregnancy, lactation
- **Physical:** Skin color, lesions; T, orientation, reflexes, ophthalmologic examination; liver evaluation, bowel sounds; CBC, LFTs, renal function tests

Interventions

- Administer with food if GI upset occurs.
- Administer in a single daily dose; must be used in combination with other antituberculotics.
- Arrange for follow-up of LFTs, renal function tests, CBC, ophthalmologic examinations.

Teaching points

- Take drug in a single daily dose; it may be taken with meals if GI upset occurs.
- Take this drug regularly; avoid missing doses. Do not discontinue this drug without first consulting your health care provider.
- Avoid using aluminum-containing antacids within at least 4 hours of taking drug.
- Arrange to have periodic medical checkups, which will include an eye examination and blood tests.
- You may experience these side effects: Nausea, vomiting, epigastric distress; skin rashes or lesions; visual changes, disorientation, confusion, drowsiness, dizziness (use caution if driving or operating dangerous machinery; use precautions to avoid injury).

- Report changes in vision (blurring, altered color perception), rash.

ethionamide

*(e thye on **am'** ide)*

Trecator

PREGNANCY CATEGORY C

Drug class

Antituberculotic (third line)

Therapeutic actions

Bacteriostatic against *Mycobacterium tuberculosis;* mechanism of action is not known.

Indications

- TB—any form that is not responsive to first-line antituberculotics—in conjunction with other antituberculotics

Contraindications and cautions

- Contraindicated with allergy to ethionamide, pregnancy.
- Use cautiously with hepatic impairment, diabetes mellitus, lactation.

Available forms

Tablets—250 mg

Dosages

Adults

Always use with at least one other antituberculotic. 15–20 mg/kg/day PO up to a maximum 1 g/day; dosage may be divided if GI upset is intolerable. Concomitant use of pyridoxine is recommended to prevent or minimize the symptoms of peripheral neuritis. Alternative dosing: 250 mg/day PO; gradually titrate to optimal dose.

Pediatric patients

10–20 mg/kg/day PO in two or three divided doses after meals (not to exceed 1 g/day) or 15 mg/kg/24 hr as a single daily dose.

Pharmacokinetics

Route	*Peak*	*Duration*
Oral	3 hr	9 hr

Metabolism: Hepatic; $T_{1/2}$: 2 hr

Distribution: Crosses placenta; may enter breast milk

Excretion: Urine

Adverse effects

- **CNS:** *Depression, drowsiness, asthenia,* seizures, peripheral neuritis, neuropathy, olfactory disturbances, blurred vision, diplopia, optic neuritis, dizziness, headache, restlessness, tremors, psychosis
- **CV:** Orthostatic hypotension
- **Dermatologic:** Rash, acne, alopecia, thrombocytopenia, pellagra-like syndrome
- **GI:** *Anorexia, nausea, vomiting, diarrhea, metallic taste,* stomatitis, hepatitis
- **Other:** Gynecomastia, impotence, menorrhagia, difficulty managing diabetes mellitus

■ Nursing considerations

Assessment

- **History:** Allergy to ethionamide; hepatic impairment, diabetes mellitus; pregnancy, lactation
- **Physical:** Skin color, lesions; orientation, reflexes, ophthalmologic examination, affect; BP, orthostatic BP; liver evaluation; LFTs, blood and urine glucose

Interventions

- Arrange for culture and sensitivity tests before use.
- Give only with other antituberculotics.

⊗ ***Warning*** Arrange for follow-up of LFTs before and every 2–4 wk during therapy.

- Monitor diabetic patients carefully.
- Caution patient to avoid pregnancy.

Teaching points

- Take drug once a day; take with food if GI upset occurs. Dose may be divided if GI upset is severe.
- Take this drug regularly; avoid missing doses. Do not discontinue this drug without first consulting your health care provider.
- Do not use this drug during pregnancy; serious fetal abnormalities have been reported. Use of barrier contraceptives is advised.
- Arrange to have regular, periodic medical checkups, including blood tests.
- You may experience these side effects: Loss of appetite, nausea, vomiting, metallic taste in mouth, increased salivation (take the drug

with food, frequent mouth care, frequent small meals may help), diarrhea; drowsiness, depression, dizziness, blurred vision (use caution operating a car or dangerous machinery; change position slowly; avoid injury); impotence, menstrual difficulties.
- Report unusual bleeding or bruising, severe GI upset, severe changes in vision.

ethosuximide

*(eth oh **sux'** i mide)*

Zarontin

PREGNANCY CATEGORY C

Drug classes

Antiepileptic
Succinimide

Therapeutic actions

Suppresses the EEG pattern associated with lapses of consciousness in absence (petit mal) seizures; reduces frequency of attacks; mechanism of action not understood, but may act in inhibitory neuronal systems.

Indications

- Control of absence (petit mal) seizures; may be given in combination with other antiepileptics especially when other forms of epilepsy coexist with absence seizures

Contraindications and cautions

- Contraindicated with hypersensitivity to succinimides, lactation.
- Use cautiously with hepatic, renal abnormalities; pregnancy, blood dyscrasias, intermittent porphyria.

Available forms

Capsules—250 mg; syrup—250 mg/5 mL

Dosages

Adults and pediatric patients 6 yr and older

Initial dose is 500 mg/day PO. Increase by small increments to maintenance level. One method is to increase the daily dose by 250 mg every 4–7 days until control is achieved with minimal side effects. Give dosage of more than 1.5 g/day in divided doses only under strict supervision (compatible with other antiepileptics when other forms of epilepsy coexist with absence seizures).

Pediatric patients 3–6 yr

Initial dose is 250 mg/day PO. Increase as described for adults above. The optimal dose for most children is 20 mg/kg/day in one dose or two divided doses.

Pharmacokinetics

Route	*Peak*
Oral	3–7 hr

Metabolism: Hepatic; $T_{1/2}$: 30 hr in children, 60 hr in adults
Distribution: Crosses placenta; enters breast milk
Excretion: Bile, urine

Adverse effects

- **CNS:** *Drowsiness, ataxia, dizziness, irritability, nervousness, headache, blurred vision,* myopia, photophobia, hiccups, euphoria, dreamlike state, lethargy, hyperactivity, fatigue, insomnia, increased frequency of **grand mal seizures** may occur when used alone in some patients with mixed types of epilepsy, confusion, instability, mental slowness, depression, hypochondriacal behavior, sleep disturbances, night terrors, aggressiveness, inability to concentrate
- **Dermatologic: Stevens-Johnson syndrome,** *pruritus, urticaria,* pruritic erythematous rashes, skin eruptions, erythema multiforme, systemic lupus erythematosus, alopecia, hirsutism
- **GI:** *Nausea, vomiting, vague gastric upset, epigastric and abdominal pain, cramps, anorexia, diarrhea, constipation, weight loss,* swelling of tongue, gum hypertrophy
- **Hematologic: Eosinophilia, granulocytopenia, leukopenia, agranulocytosis, aplastic anemia, monocytosis, pancytopenia**
- **Other:** Vaginal bleeding, periorbital edema, hyperemia, muscle weakness, abnormal LFTs, renal function tests

Interactions

✱ **Drug-drug** • Decreased serum levels of primidone • Risk of increased effects if combined with other CNS depressants including alcohol

■ Nursing considerations

Assessment

- **History:** Hypersensitivity to succinimides; hepatic, renal abnormalities; lactation, pregnancy
- **Physical:** Skin color, lesions; orientation, affect, reflexes, bilateral grip strength, vision examination; bowel sounds, normal output, liver evaluation; LFTs, renal function tests, urinalysis, CBC with differential, EEG

Interventions

⊗ ***Warning*** Reduce dosage, discontinue, or substitute other antiepileptic gradually; abrupt discontinuation may precipitate absence (petit mal) status.

- Monitor CBC and differential before and frequently during therapy.

⊗ ***Warning*** Discontinue drug if rash, depression of blood count, or unusual depression, aggressiveness, or behavioral alterations occur.

- Arrange counseling for women of childbearing age who need long-term maintenance therapy with antiepileptics and who wish to become pregnant.

⊗ ***Warning*** Evaluate for therapeutic serum levels (40–100 mcg/mL).

Teaching points

- Take this drug exactly as prescribed. Do not discontinue this drug abruptly or change dosage.
- Avoid alcohol, sleep-inducing, or over-the-counter drugs while you are using this drug.
- Arrange for frequent checkups to monitor this drug; keep all appointments for checkups.
- Wear a medical ID at all times so that any emergency medical personnel will know that you have epilepsy and are taking antiepileptic medication.
- You may experience these side effects: Drowsiness, dizziness, confusion, blurred vision (avoid driving or performing tasks requiring alertness or visual acuity); GI upset (take the drug with food or milk and eat frequent small meals).
- Report rash, joint pain, unexplained fever, sore throat, unusual bleeding or bruising, drowsiness, dizziness, blurred vision, pregnancy.

▽ethotoin

(eth' i toe in)

Peganone

PREGNANCY CATEGORY D

Drug classes

Antiepileptic
Hydantoin

Therapeutic actions

Has antiepileptic activity without causing general CNS depression; stabilizes neuronal membranes and prevents hyperexcitability caused by excessive stimulation; limits the spread of seizure activity from an active focus.

Indications

- Control of grand mal (tonic-clonic) and complex partial (psychomotor) seizures; may be combined with other antiepileptics

Contraindications and cautions

- Contraindicated with hypersensitivity to hydantoins, pregnancy, lactation, hepatic abnormalities, hematologic disorders.
- Use cautiously with acute intermittent porphyria; hypotension, severe myocardial insufficiency; diabetes mellitus, hyperglycemia.

Available forms

Tablets—250 mg

Dosages

Administer in four–six divided doses daily. Take after eating; space as evenly as possible.

Adults

Initial dose should be 1 g/day PO. Increase gradually over several days; usual maintenance dose is 2–3 g/day PO in four–six divided doses; less than 2 g/day is ineffective in most adults. If replacing another drug, reduce the dose of the other drug gradually as ethotoin dose is increased.

Pediatric patients

Initial dose should not exceed 750 mg/day PO in four–six divided doses; maintenance doses range from 500 mg/day to 1 g/day PO.

Pharmacokinetics

Route	*Onset*	*Peak*
Oral	Rapid	1–3 hr

Metabolism: Hepatic; $T_{1/2}$: 3–9 hr
Distribution: Crosses placenta; enters breast milk
Excretion: Urine

Adverse effects

- **CNS:** *Nystagmus, ataxia, dysarthria, slurred speech, mental confusion, dizziness, drowsiness, insomnia, transient nervousness, motor twitchings, fatigue, irritability, depression, numbness, tremor, headache,* photophobia, diplopia, conjunctivitis
- **Dermatologic:** Scarlatiniform, morbilliform, maculopapular, urticarial and nonspecific rashes; also serious and sometimes fatal dermatologic reactions: Bullous, exfoliative, or purpuric dermatitis, lupus erythematosus, and **Stevens-Johnson syndrome; toxic epidermal necrolysis,** hirsutism, alopecia, coarsening of the facial features, enlargement of the lips, Peyronie's disease
- **GI:** *Nausea,* vomiting, diarrhea, constipation, *gingival hyperplasia,* toxic hepatitis, **liver damage,** hypersensitivity reactions with hepatic involvement, including hepatocellular degeneration and **hepatocellular necrosis**
- **GU:** Nephrosis
- **Hematologic: Thrombocytopenia, leukopenia, granulocytopenia, agranulocytosis, pancytopenia; macrocytosis and megaloblastic anemia that usually respond to folic acid therapy; eosinophilia, monocytosis, leukocytosis, simple anemia, hemolytic anemia, aplastic anemia, hyperglycemia**
- **Respiratory: Pulmonary fibrosis,** acute pneumonitis
- **Other:** Lymph node hyperplasia, sometimes progressing to **frank malignant lymphoma,** monoclonal gammopathy and **multiple myeloma** (prolonged therapy), polyarthropathy, osteomalacia, weight gain, chest pain, periarteritis nodosa

Interactions

✱ **Drug-drug** • Increased pharmacologic effects with chloramphenicol, cimetidine, disulfiram, isoniazid, phenacemide, phenylbutazone, sulfonamides, trimethoprim • Complex interactions and effects when hydantoins and valproic acid are given together: Toxicity with apparently normal serum ethotoin levels; decreased plasma levels of valproic acid given with hydantoins; breakthrough seizures when the two drugs are given together • Decreased pharmacologic effects with antineoplastics, diazoxide, folic acid, rifampin, theophyllines • Increased pharmacologic effects and toxicity with primidone, oxyphenbutazone, fluconazole, amiodarone • Increased hepatotoxicity with acetaminophen • Decreased pharmacologic effects of these drugs: Corticosteroids, cyclosporine, disopyramide, doxycycline, estrogens, levodopa, methadone, metyrapone, mexiletine, hormonal contraceptives, carbamazepine

✱ **Drug-lab test** • Interference with the metyrapone and the 1-mg dexamethasone tests; avoid the use of hydantoins for at least 7 days prior to metyrapone testing

■ Nursing considerations

Assessment

- **History:** Hypersensitivity to hydantoins; hepatic abnormalities; hematologic disorders; acute intermittent porphyria; hypotension, severe myocardial insufficiency; diabetes mellitus, hyperglycemia; pregnancy; lactation
- **Physical:** T; skin color, lesions; lymph node palpation; orientation, affect, reflexes, vision examination; P, BP; R, adventitious sounds; bowel sounds, normal output, liver evaluation; periodontal examination; LFTs, urinalysis, CBC and differential, blood

proteins, blood and urine glucose, EEG, ECG

Interventions

- Give after food to enhance absorption and reduce GI upset; give in four–six divided doses as evenly spaced as possible.
- Administer with other antiepileptics to regulate seizures.

⊗ ***Warning*** Reduce dosage, discontinue, or substitute other antiepileptic gradually; abrupt discontinuation may precipitate status epilepticus.

⊗ ***Warning*** Discontinue drug if rash, depression of blood count, enlarged lymph nodes, hypersensitivity reaction, signs of liver damage, or Peyronie's disease (induration of the corpora cavernosa of the penis) occurs. Institute another antiepileptic promptly.

- Monitor hepatic function periodically during long-term therapy; monitor blood counts, urinalysis monthly.
- Monitor urine sugar of patients with diabetes mellitus regularly. Adjustment of dosage of hypoglycemic drug may be needed because antiepileptic may inhibit insulin release and induce hyperglycemia.

⊗ ***Warning*** Arrange to have lymph node enlargement occurring during therapy evaluated carefully. Lymphadenopathy, which simulates Hodgkin's disease, has occurred. Lymph node hyperplasia may progress to lymphoma.

- Monitor blood proteins to detect early malfunction of the immune system (multiple myeloma).
- Arrange dental consultation for patients on long-term therapy; proper oral hygiene can prevent development of gum hyperplasia.
- Arrange counseling for women of childbearing age who need long-term maintenance therapy with antiepileptics and who wish to become pregnant.

⊗ ***Warning*** Evaluate for therapeutic serum levels (15–50 mcg/mL).

Teaching points

- Take this drug exactly as prescribed, after food to enhance absorption and reduce GI upset. Space doses as evenly apart as possible throughout the day.
- Do not discontinue this drug abruptly or change dosage.
- Maintain good oral hygiene—regular brushing and flossing—to prevent gum disease while you are taking this drug.
- Arrange frequent dental checkups to prevent serious gum disease.
- Arrange for frequent checkups to monitor your response to this drug; keep all appointments for checkups.

⊗ ***Warning*** Monitor your blood sugar regularly, and report any abnormality if you are a diabetic.

⊗ ***Warning*** Use some form of contraception, other than birth control pills, while you are on this drug. This drug is not recommended for use during pregnancy. If you wish to become pregnant, discuss with your health care provider.

- Wear or carry a medical alert tag at all times so that any emergency medical personnel will know that you have epilepsy and are taking antiepileptic medication.
- You may experience these side effects: Drowsiness, dizziness, confusion, blurred vision (avoid driving or performing tasks requiring alertness or visual acuity); GI upset (take the drug with food and eat frequent small meals).
- Report rash, severe nausea or vomiting, drowsiness, slurred speech, impaired coordination, swollen glands, bleeding, swollen or tender gums, yellowish discoloration of the skin or eyes, joint pain, unexplained fever, sore throat, unusual bleeding or bruising, persistent headache, malaise, any indication of an infection or bleeding tendency, abnormal erection, pregnancy.

▽ etidronate disodium

*(e **tid'** ro nate)*

CO Etidronate (CAN), Didronel, Gen-Etidronate (CAN)

PREGNANCY CATEGORY C

Drug classes

Bisphosphonate
Calcium regulator

Therapeutic actions
Slows normal and abnormal bone resorption; reduces bone formation and bone turnover.

Indications
- Treatment of Paget's disease of bone
- Treatment of heterotopic ossification
- Unlabeled uses: Prevention and treatment of corticosteroid-induced osteoporosis, prevention of osteoporosis with spinal cord injury

Contraindications and cautions
- Contraindicated with allergy to bisphosphonates, hypocalcemia, pregnancy, lactation, severe renal impairment, clinically overt osteomalacia.
- Use cautiously with renal impairment, upper GI disease.

Available forms
Tablets—200, 400 mg

Dosages
Adults
- *Paget's disease:* 5–10 mg/kg/day PO for up to 6 mo; or 11–20 mg/kg/day PO for up to 3 mo. Doses above 10 mg/kg/day should be reserved for when lower doses are ineffective or when there is an urgent need to suppress rapid bone turnover or reduce elevated cardiac output. If retreatment is needed, wait at least 90 days between treatment regimens.
- *Heterotopic ossification:* 20 mg/kg/day PO for 2 wk followed by 10 mg/kg/day PO for 10 wk (following spinal cord injury); 20 mg/kg/day PO for 1 mo preoperatively if due to total hip replacement, then 20 mg/kg/day PO for 3 mo postoperatively.

Pediatric patients
Safety and efficacy not established.

Patients with renal impairment
Use caution and monitor patient frequently.

Pharmacokinetics

Route	*Onset*	*Duration*
Oral	Slow	90 days

Metabolism: Not metabolized; $T_{1/2}$: 1–6 hr
Distribution: Crosses placenta; may enter breast milk
Excretion: Urine

Adverse effects
- **CNS:** *Headache*
- **GI:** *Nausea, diarrhea,* altered taste, metallic taste
- **Hematologic:** Elevated BUN, serum creatinine
- **Skeletal:** *Increased or recurrent bone pain,* focal osteomalacia

Interactions
✱ **Drug-drug** • Increased risk of GI distress with aspirin • Decreased absorption with antacids, calcium, iron, multivalent cations; separate dosing by at least 2 hr
✱ **Drug-food** • Significantly decreased absorption and serum levels if taken with any food; administer on an empty stomach 2 hr before meals

■ Nursing considerations
Assessment
- **History:** Allergy to bisphosphonates, renal failure, upper GI disease, lactation, pregnancy
- **Physical:** Muscle tone, bone pain; bowel sounds; urinalysis, serum calcium, serum alkaline phosphatase, serum phosphate, renal function tests

Interventions
- Administer with a full glass of water, 2 hr before meals.
- Monitor serum calcium levels before, during, and after therapy.

⊗ ***Warning*** Ensure 3-mo rest period after treatment for Paget's disease if retreatment is required, 7 days between treatments for hypercalcemia of malignancy.

- Ensure adequate vitamin and calcium intake.
- Provide comfort measures if bone pain returns.

Teaching points
- Take this drug with a full glass of water 2 hours before meals.

- Periodic blood tests may be required to monitor your calcium levels.
- You may experience these side effects: Nausea, diarrhea, bone pain, headache (analgesics may be available to help).
- Report twitching, muscle spasms, dark-colored urine, severe diarrhea.

etodolac
(ee toe ***doe'*** *lak)*

PREGNANCY CATEGORY C

Drug classes
Analgesic (nonopioid)
NSAID

Therapeutic actions
Inhibits prostaglandin synthesis by inhibiting the enzyme, cyclo-oxygenase.

Indications
- Acute or long-term use in the management of signs and symptoms of osteoarthritis, rheumatoid arthritis, and juvenile rheumatoid arthritis
- Management of pain

Contraindications and cautions
- Contraindicated with significant renal impairment, pregnancy, lactation, hypersensitivity to aspirin, etodolac, or other NSAIDs.
- Use cautiously with impaired hearing; allergies; hepatic, hypertension, and GI conditions.

Available forms
Capsules—200, 300 mg; tablets—400, 500 mg; ER capsules—400, 500, 600 mg

Dosages
Adults
- *Osteoarthritis, rheumatoid arthritis:* Initially, 600–1,000 mg/day PO in divided doses; maintenance ranges, 600–1,200 mg/day in divided doses. Do not exceed 1,200 mg/day. Patients less than 60 kg: Do not exceed 20 mg/kg. ER: 400–1,000 mg/day PO; adjust based on patient response. Do not exceed 1,200 mg/day.
- *Analgesia, acute pain:* 200–400 mg every 6–8 hr PO. Do not exceed 1,200 mg/day.

Patients 6–16 yr
- *Juvenile rheumatoid arthritis:* The daily dose (given as single dose) should be based upon body weight as follows:
  20–30 kg: 400 mg/day PO.
  31–45 kg: 600 mg/day PO.
  46–60 kg: 800 mg/day PO.
  More than 60 kg: 1,000 mg/day PO.

Pharmacokinetics

Route	Onset	Peak
Oral	Varies	1–2 hr
Oral (ER)	Slow	6–7 hr

Metabolism: Hepatic; $T_{1/2}$: 7.3 hr, 8.3 hr (ER)
Distribution: Crosses placenta; enters breast milk
Excretion: Feces, urine

Adverse effects
- **CNS:** *Dizziness,* somnolence, insomnia, fatigue, tiredness, tinnitus, blurred vision
- **Dermatologic:** Rash, pruritus, sweating, dry mucous membranes, stomatitis
- **GI:** *Nausea, dyspepsia, GI pain, diarrhea,* vomiting, *constipation,* flatulence, **bleeding ulcers,** elevated liver enzymes, **hepatic failure**
- **GU:** Dysuria, **renal impairment or insufficiency**
- **Hematologic:** Bleeding, platelet inhibition with higher doses
- **Other:** Peripheral edema, **anaphylactoid reactions** to fatal anaphylactic shock

Interactions
✱ **Drug-drug** • Increased risk of bleeding if combined with anticoagulants, antiplatelet drugs • Possible decreased effectiveness of antihypertensives if taken with etodolac

■ Nursing considerations
Assessment
- **History:** Renal impairment, impaired hearing, allergy to aspirin or NSAIDs, hepatic, CV, and GI conditions, lactation, pregnancy
- **Physical:** Skin color and lesions; orientation, reflexes, ophthalmologic and audiometric evaluation, peripheral sensation; P, edema; R, adventitious sounds; liver

evaluation; CBC, clotting times, LFTs, renal function tests; serum electrolytes, stool guaiac

Interventions

⊗ ***Black box warning*** Be aware that patient may be at increased risk for CV events and GI bleeding; monitor accordingly.

- Give with food or after meals if GI upset occurs.
- Arrange for periodic ophthalmologic examination during long-term therapy.

⊗ ***Warning*** Institute emergency procedures if overdose occurs (gastric lavage, induction of emesis, supportive therapy).

Teaching points

- Take with food or meals if GI upset occurs.
- Take only the prescribed dosage.
- You may experience dizziness or drowsiness (avoid driving or the use of dangerous machinery while on this drug).
- Report sore throat, fever, rash, itching, weight gain, swelling in ankles or fingers; changes in vision; black, tarry stools; bleeding.

DANGEROUS DRUG

etoposide (VP-16)

*(e toe **poe'** side)*

Etopophos, Toposar, VePesid

PREGNANCY CATEGORY D

Drug classes

Antineoplastic
Mitotic inhibitor

Therapeutic actions

G2-specific cell toxic: Lyses cells entering mitosis; inhibits cells from entering prophase; inhibits DNA synthesis, leading to cell death.

Indications

- Refractory testicular tumors as part of combination therapy
- Treatment of small-cell lung carcinoma as part of combination therapy
- Unlabeled uses: Bladder cancer, lymphomas, leukemias, Ewing's sarcoma, Kaposi's sarcoma, brain tumors, gestational trophoblastic tumors, ovarian germ-cell tumors, rhabdomyosarcomas, Wilms' tumors, bone marrow transplants

Contraindications and cautions

- Contraindicated with allergy to etoposide, teniposide, *Cremophor EL;* pregnancy, lactation.
- Use cautiously with bone marrow suppression.

Available forms

Capsules—50 mg; injection—20 mg/mL; powder for injection—100 mg

Dosages

Modify dosage based on myelosuppression.

Adults

Parenteral

- *Testicular cancer:* 50–100 mg/m^2 per day IV on days 1 to 5 or 100 mg/ m^2 per day IV on days 1, 3, and 5, every 3–4 wk in combination with other chemotherapeutics.
- *Small-cell lung cancer:* 35 mg/m^2 per day IV for 4 days to 50 mg/ m^2 per day for 5 days; repeat every 3–4 wk after recovery from toxicity.

Oral

Small-cell lung cancer: Two times the IV dose rounded to the nearest 50 mg.

Pediatric patients

Safety and efficacy not established.

Patients with renal impairment

If creatinine clearance is less than 50 mL/min, reduce dosage and monitor patient closely.

Pharmacokinetics

Route	*Onset*	*Peak*	*Duration*
Oral	30–60 min	60–90 min	20–30 hr
IV	30 min	60 min	20–30 hr

Metabolism: Hepatic; $T_{1/2}$: 4–11 hr
Distribution: Crosses placenta; enters breast milk
Excretion: Bile, urine

IV FACTS

Preparation: Dilute with 5% dextrose injection or 0.9% sodium chloride injection to give a concentration of 0.2 or 0.4 mg/mL. Unopened vials are stable at room temperature for 2 yr; diluted solutions are stable at room temperature for 2 (0.4 mg/mL) or 4 (0.2 mg/mL) days.

Infusion: Administer slowly over 30–60 min. Etoposide phosphate solutions may be administered over 5–20 min. Do not give by rapid IV push.

Adverse effects

- **CNS:** *Somnolence, fatigue,* peripheral neuropathy
- **CV:** Hypotension (after rapid IV administration)
- **Dermatologic:** *Alopecia*
- **GI:** *Nausea, vomiting, anorexia, diarrhea,* stomatitis, aftertaste, liver toxicity
- **Hematologic:** *Myelotoxicity*
- **Hypersensitivity:** Chills, fever, tachycardia, **anaphylactic-like reaction, bronchospasm,** dyspnea
- **Other:** Carcinogenesis

■ Nursing considerations

Assessment

- **History:** Allergy to etoposide, teniposide, *Cremophor EL;* bone marrow suppression; pregnancy; lactation
- **Physical:** T; weight; hair; orientation, reflexes; BP, P; mucous membranes, abdominal examination; CBC

Interventions

- Do not administer IM or subcutaneously; severe local reaction and tissue necrosis occur.

⊗ ***Warning*** Avoid skin contact with this drug; use rubber gloves; if contact occurs, immediately wash with soap and water.

- Monitor BP during administration; if hypotension occurs, discontinue dose and consult with physician. Fluids and other supportive therapy may be needed.

⊠ ***Black box warning*** Obtain platelet count, Hgb, Hct, WBC count, differential before starting therapy and prior to each dose. If severe response occurs, discontinue therapy and consult with physician; severe myelosuppression is possible.

⊠ ***Black box warning*** Monitor patient for severe hypersensitivity reaction with any dose; arrange supportive care.

- Arrange for an antiemetic for severe nausea and vomiting.
- Arrange for wig or other suitable head covering before alopecia occurs. Teach patient the importance of covering the head at extremes of temperature.

Teaching points

- Keep a calendar for specific treatment days and additional courses of therapy.
- Avoid pregnancy while using this drug; you should use barrier contraceptives.
- Have regular blood tests to monitor the drug's effects.
- Avoid exposures to other people with infections, especially during periods of low blood counts.
- You may experience these side effects: Loss of appetite, nausea, vomiting, mouth sores (frequent mouth care, frequent small meals may help; try to maintain good nutrition; a dietitian may be able to help, and an antiemetic may be ordered); loss of hair (arrange for a wig or other suitable head covering before the hair loss occurs; it is important to keep the head covered at extremes of temperature).
- Report severe GI upset, diarrhea, vomiting, unusual bleeding or bruising, fever, chills, sore throat, difficulty breathing.

▽ etravirine

(eh tra vye' rin)

Intelence (DNC)

PREGNANCY CATEGORY B

Drug classes

Antiviral

Nonnucleoside reverse transcriptase inhibitor

Therapeutic actions

Binds directly to reverse transcriptase and blocks both RNA and DNA dependent polymerase activity leading to inability for viral replication, a decrease in viral load and subsequent increase, increases number of healthy $CD4^+$ cells; does not inhibit human DNA polymerase.

Indications

- In combination with other antiretroviral drugs, for treatment of HIV-1 infection in treatment-experienced adults who have evidence of viral replication and HIV-1 strains resistant to nonnucleotide reverse transcriptase inhibitors and other antiretroviral drugs

Contraindications and cautions

- No known contraindications.
- Women are advised not to nurse a baby while taking drug. Use cautiously with pregnancy.

Available forms

Tablets (DNC)—100 mg

Dosages

Adults

200 mg PO bid following a meal.

Pediatric patients

Safety and efficacy not established.

Pharmacokinetics

Route	Onset	Peak
Oral	Slow	2.5–4 hr

Metabolism: Hepatic: $T_{1/2}$: 21–61 hr
Distribution: May cross placenta, may enter breast milk
Excretion: Feces and urine

Adverse effects

- **CNS:** Headache, peripheral neuropathy, vertigo, blurred vision, insomnia, anxiety, paresthesias
- **CV:** Hypertension
- **Dermatologic: Stevens-Johnson syndrome, epidermal necrolysis,** *rash*
- **GI:** *Diarrhea,* nausea, abdominal pain, vomiting, dry mouth, flatulence
- **Other:** Fatigue; altered fat distribution, immune reconstitution syndrome; **severe hypersensitivity reactions**

Interactions

✱ **Drug-drug** • Risk of decreased serum levels and loss of effectiveness if used with efavirenz, nevirapine rifampin, rifapentine, rifabutin; avoid these combinations • Risk of increased serum levels and risk of toxic effects if used with delavirdine; avoid this combination • Risk of significant alteration in serum level of protease inhibitors (atazanavir, fosamprenavir, nelfinavir, indinavir) if combined; also use low dose ritonavir if this combination is used • Possible loss of therapeutic effect if combined with 600 mg bid ritonavir; avoid this combination • Risk of significant changes in therapeutic effect if combined with tipranavir and ritonavir; fosamprenavir and ritonavir; atazanavir and ritonavir; avoid these combinations • Risk of decreased effectiveness of antiarrhythmics; monitor patient closely if this combination is needed • Risk of increased bleeding tendencies with warfarin: if this combination is used; monitor patient closely and adjust dosage of warfarin as needed • Risk of significant decrease in effectiveness if combined with carbamazepine, phenobarbital, phenytoin; avoid these combinations • Risk of serum level concentration of azole antifungals if combined; monitor patient carefully and adjust antifungal dosage as appropriate • Risk of decreased effectiveness of clarithromycin if combined; suggest use of an alternate antibiotic

✱ **Drug-alternative therapy** • Risk of decreased serum levels and loss of effectiveness if combined with St. John's wort; avoid this combination

■ Nursing considerations

Assessment

- **History:** Hypersensitivity to any component of the drug, pregnancy, lactation, previous or current anti-HIV regimen
- **Physical:** T; skin color, lesions; orientation, affect; BP; abdominal examination

Interventions

- Give this drug with other antiretrovirals.

⊗ ***Warning*** Discontinue drug at first sign of severe skin or hypersensitivity reaction; fatalities have been reported.

- Review antiviral therapy and adjust dosage as needed to take into account effects on liver enzymes and numerous drug-drug interactions.

- Have patient swallow tablets whole with liquid, following a meal. Do not administer on an empty stomach. If patient is unable to swallow tablets, put them in a glass of water and stir, when water appears milky have the patient drink the whole glass and rinse several times and drink the rinse each time to get the full dose.
- Encourage nursing mothers to find a different method of feeding the baby while on this drug.

Teaching points

- Take this drug twice a day following a meal; never take on an empty stomach. Swallow the tablets whole; do not cut, crush, or chew the tablets.
- If you cannot swallow the tablets, you can place them in a glass of water, stir well, and when the water looks milky, drink immediately. Fill the glass with water several times and completely swallow each time to get any residue to make sure that you receive the entire dose.
- Always take this drug with other anti-HIV drugs that have been prescribed for you.
- Do not use St. John's wort while taking this drug; antiviral activity could be lost.
- If you miss a dose within 6 hours of the time you usually take it, take the dose following a meal, as soon as possible. Then take your next dose at the regular time. If you miss a dose by more than 6 hours, wait and take the next regularly scheduled dose. Do not double up doses and do not take more than the prescribed amount each day.
- Do not stop taking this drug; if you are running low, talk to your health care provider about a refill; the drug could stop working if stopped for even a short period.
- This drug does not cure HIV or AIDS; opportunistic infections may occur and regular medical care should be sought to deal with the disease.
- This drug does not reduce the risk of transmission of HIV to others by sexual contact or blood contamination; use appropriate precautions.
- It is not known if this drug could affect a fetus. If you wish to become pregnant, discuss this with your health care provider. If you become pregnant while taking this drug, consult your health care provider about enrolling in the *Antiretroviral Pregnancy Registry*.
- It is not known how this drug could affect a nursing baby. Because of the potential for passing the virus on to an infant, women with HIV infection are advised not to breastfeed; another method of feeding the baby should be used while you are taking this drug.
- Your health care provider will monitor $CD4^+$ levels regularly while you are taking this drug.
- You may experience these side effects: Headache, fever, rash (medication may be available to relieve these symptoms); dizziness (do not drive a car or operate dangerous machinery until you know how this drug will affect you); changes in fat distribution (decreased fat in the face, legs and arms; increased fat on the back, neck, chest).
- Report rash of any kind, any signs of infection (fever, swelling, redness), inability to eat, any changes in your prescribed medications, severe diarrhea.

everolimus

See Appendix W, *Less commonly used drugs*.

exemestane

See Appendix W, *Less commonly used drugs*.

exenatide

*(ex **enn'** ah tyde)*

Byetta

PREGNANCY CATEGORY C

Drug classes

Antidiabetic
Incretin mimetic drug

Therapeutic actions

An incretin that mimics the enhancement of glucose-dependent insulin secretion by pancreatic beta cells, depresses inappropriately elevated glucagon secretion, and slows gastric emptying, leading to lower blood glucose levels. Also associated with appetite suppression and weight loss.

Indications

- Adjunctive therapy to improve glycemic control in patients with type 2 diabetes who are taking metformin, a thiazolidinedione, a sulfonylurea, or a combination of metformin and a sulfonylurea or metformin and a thiazolidinedione but have not achieved glycemic control
- **NEW INDICATION:** Monotherapy, with diet and exercise, for treatment of adults with type 2 diabetes

Contraindications and cautions

- Contraindicated with hypersensitivity to exenatide or any of its components, end stage renal disease, severe GI disease, type 1 diabetes, diabetic ketoacidosis, lactation, history of pancreatitis.
- Use cautiously with pregnancy.

Available forms

Solution for injection, solution in a prefilled pen—5, 10 mcg/dose

Dosage

Adult

5 mcg by subcutaneous injection bid at any time within 60 min before the morning and evening meals or the two main meals of the day, approximately 6 hr apart. May be increased to 10 mcg bid after 1 month of therapy, if needed. Given in combination with oral antidiabetic drugs.

Pharmacokinetics

Route	*Onset*	*Peak*	*Duration*
Subcut.	Rapid	2 hr	8–10 hr

Metabolism: $T_{1/2}$: 2.4 hr
Distribution: Crosses placenta; may pass into breast milk
Excretion: Urine, unchanged

Adverse effects

- **CNS:** Headache, feeling jittery, dizziness
- **GI:** *Nausea,* vomiting, dyspepsia, diarrhea, **pancreatitis**
- **Other: Hypoglycemia,** injection site reaction, **hemorrhagic** or **necrotizing pancreatitis**

Interactions

✱ **Drug-drug** • Slowed gastric emptying and reduced absorption of some oral drugs; use with caution with oral drugs that require rapid absorption; space oral contraceptives and antibiotics at least 1 hr before administering exenatide

■ Nursing considerations

Assessment

- **History:** Hypersensitivity to exenatide or any of its components; end-stage renal disease, severe GI disease; type 1 diabetes, diabetic ketoacidosis; pancreatitis; lactation, pregnancy
- **Physical:** Orientation, reflexes, affect; abdominal examination; injection site; blood glucose levels

Interventions

- Inject subcutaneously within 60 min before the morning and evening meals or the two main meals of the day.
- Maintain other antidiabetic drugs, diet, and exercise regimen for control of diabetes.
- Monitor serum glucose levels and glycosylated Hgb levels to evaluate effectiveness of drug on controlling glucose levels.
- Monitor for pancreatitis. Stop drug and do not restart if signs of pancreatitis develop.
- Arrange for thorough diabetic teaching program to include disease, dietary control, exercise, signs and symptoms of hypoglycemia and hyperglycemia, avoidance of infection, and hygiene.

Teaching points

- Take drug subcutaneously. Use sterile technique. Dispose of the syringes appropriately.
- If you are using the prefilled pen, review your manual before each use. Be advised that the needles for the pen need to be purchased separately.
- Do not use solution that appears cloudy.
- Inject it into a site on your thigh, abdomen, or upper arm; rotate injection sites periodically.
- Store unopened vials in the refrigerator. Opened bottles may be kept at room temperature.

- Throw away any out-of-date bottles. Discard the pen after 30 days, even if solution remains in the pen.
- Inject this drug within 1 hour of your morning and evening meals or your two main meals of the day; do not use if you are not going to be eating. If you forget a dose, do not inject after you have eaten.
- Alcohol consumption can change your blood glucose levels and may alter your response to this drug.
- Do not take this drug if you are not able to eat or if you plan to skip a meal or if your blood sugar is too low.
- Do not change the dosage of this drug without consulting with your health care provider.
- It is not known how this drug would affect a pregnancy. If you think you are pregnant or would like to become pregnant, consult your health care provider.
- It is not known how this drug could affect a nursing baby. If you are nursing a baby, consult your health care provider.
- You will need to regularly monitor your blood glucose levels. Your health care provider may change the dose of exenatide or your other antidiabetic drugs, based on your blood glucose response.
- It is important that you follow the diet and exercise guidelines related to your disease.
- Review the signs and symptoms of hypoglycemia. Be prepared to treat hypoglycemia with fast-acting sugar or glucagon.
- Do not drive a car or operate potentially dangerous machinery until you are aware of how exenatide will affect your blood sugar. Low blood sugar can cause dizziness and changes in thinking.
- You may experience these side effects: Injection site reactions (proper injection and rotation of injection sites should help; if bothersome, consult your health care provider); hypoglycemia (use fast acting sugars or glucagons if this occurs; proper use and eating of meals should prevent this effect); nausea (this usually passes after a few days).
- Report continued nausea; hypoglycemic reactions; redness, pain or swelling at injection sites; stomach pain; vomiting.

▽ezetimibe

(ee zet' ah mibe)

Zetia

PREGNANCY CATEGORY C

Drug classes

Cholesterol absorption inhibitor
Cholesterol-lowering drug

Therapeutic actions

Localizes in the brush border of the small intestine and inhibits the absorption of cholesterol from the small intestine; this leads to a decrease delivery of dietary cholesterol to the liver, which will then increase the clearance of cholesterol from the blood and lead to a decrease in serum cholesterol.

Indications

- As an adjunct to diet and exercise to lower the cholesterol, LDL, and Apo-B levels in patients with primary hypercholesterolemia as monotherapy or in combination with HMG-CoA reductase inhibitors (statins)
- In combination with fenofibrate as adjunct to diet to reduce elevated total cholesterol, LDL cholesterol, apolipoprotein B, and non-HDL cholesterol levels in patients with mixed hyperlipidemia
- In combination with atorvastatin or simvastatin for the treatment of homozygous familial hypercholesterolemia as adjuncts to other lipid-lowering treatments
- As adjunctive therapy to diet for the treatment of homozygous sitosterolemia to reduce elevated sitosterol and campesterol levels
- As an adjunct to diet for the reduction of elevated total cholesterol, LDL, and apolipoprotein B as monotherapy in patients with primary hypercholesterolemia

Contraindications and cautions

- Contraindicated with allergy to any component of the drug. If given in combination with an HMG-CoA reductase inhibitor, contraindicated with pregnancy, lactation, active liver disease, or unexplained persistent increases in serum transaminase alkaline phosphorus levels.

- In monotherapy, use cautiously in the elderly and with hepatic impairment, pregnancy, lactation.

Available forms
Tablets—10 mg

Dosages
Adults and children 10 yr and older
10 mg/day PO taken without regard to food; may be taken at the same time as an HMG-CoA reductase inhibitor or fenofibrate; if combined with a bile acid sequestrant, should be taken at least 2 hr before or 4 hr after the bile acid sequestrant.

Pediatric patients younger than 10 yr
Safety and efficacy not established.

Pharmacokinetics

Route	*Onset*	*Peak*
Oral	Moderate	4–12 hr

Metabolism: Small intestine and hepatic; $T_{1/2}$: 22 hr
Distribution: May cross placenta; may enter breast milk
Excretion: Feces, urine

Adverse effects
- **CNS:** Headache, dizziness, fatigue
- **GI:** Abdominal pain, diarrhea
- **Respiratory:** Pharyngitis, sinusitis, *URI, cough*
- **Other:** Back pain, myalgia, arthralgia, viral infection

Interactions
✱ **Drug-drug** • Decreased serum levels and decreased effectiveness of ezetimibe if combined with cholestyramine; monitor patient closely and space ezetimibe dosing at least 2 hr before or 4 hr or more after the other drug • Increased serum levels of ezetimibe if combined with fenofibrate or gemfibrozil • Risk of cholethiasis if combined with fibrates • Risk of increased levels and toxicity of ezetimibe and cyclosporine if combined with cyclosporine; if this combination is used monitor patient very carefully.

■ Nursing considerations
Assessment
- **History:** Allergy to any component of the drug; pregnancy, hepatic impairment, lactation, evidence of diet and exercise program
- **Physical:** Skin lesions, color, T; orientation, affect; liver evaluation, bowel sounds; lipid studies, LFTs

Interventions
- Monitor serum cholesterol, LDLs, triglycerides before starting treatment and periodically during treatment.
- Determine that the patient has been on a low-cholesterol diet and exercise program for at least 2 wk before starting ezetimibe.
- If used as part of combination therapy; give drug at the same time as HMG-CoA reductase inhibitors or fenofibrate and at least 2 hr before or 4 hr or more after bile acid sequestrants.
- Encourage the use of barrier contraceptives if used with an HMG-CoA reductase inhibitor.
- Help mother to find another method of feeding her baby if this drug is needed for a nursing woman; it is not known if the drug enters breast milk.
- Consult with dietitian regarding low-cholesterol diets and provide information about exercise programs.
- Arrange for regular follow-up during long-term therapy.

Teaching points
- Take drug once each day at a time that is easy for you to remember. Do not take more than one tablet per day.
- Continue to take any other lipid-lowering drugs that have been prescribed for you. If you are also taking a bile acid sequestrant, take this drug at least 2 hours before or at least 4 hours after the bile acid sequestrant.
- Continue to follow your low-fat diet and participate in an exercise program.
- If you are nursing a baby, you should find another method of feeding the baby.
- Plan to return for periodic blood tests, including tests of liver function and cholesterol levels, to evaluate the effectiveness of this drug.

- You may experience these side effects: Abdominal pain, diarrhea (these usually pass with time, notify your health care provider if this becomes a problem); dizziness, (avoid driving and operating dangerous machinery until you know how this drug affects you); headache (analgesics may help).
- Report unusual muscle pain, weakness, or tenderness; severe diarrhea; respiratory infections.

▽factor IX concentrates

AlphaNine SD, Bebulin VH, BeneFix, Mononine, Profilnine SD

PREGNANCY CATEGORY C

Drug class

Antihemophilic

Therapeutic actions

Human factor IX complex consists of plasma fractions involved in the intrinsic pathway of blood coagulation; causes an increase in blood levels of clotting factors II, VII, VIII, IX, and X.

Indications

- Factor IX deficiency (hemophilia B, Christmas disease) to prevent or control bleeding

Contraindications and cautions

- Contraindicated with factor VII deficiencies; liver disease with signs of intravascular coagulation or fibrinolysis; do not use if hypersensitive to mouse or hamster protein (*Mononine* or *BeneFix*).
- Use cautiously with pregnancy, lactation.

Available forms

Injection—varies with brand, see label

Dosages

For factor IX deficiency, dosage depends on severity of deficiency and severity of bleeding; follow treatment carefully with factor IX level assays. Dosage should be calculated based on body weight and plasma factor IX levels and will vary for each preparation and intended use. See manufacturers' details.

Adults

- *BeneFix, Bebulin VH:* Administer IV daily–bid: minor hemorrhage—for 1–2 days; moderate hemorrhage—for 2–7 days; major hemorrhage—for 7–10 days.
- *Others:* 1 international unit/kg × body weight (kg) × desired increase (% of normal).
- *BeneFix:* 1.3 units/kg × body weight (kg) × desired increase (% of normal).

Adults and pediatric patients

- *Reversal of coumadin effect:* 15 units/kg IV is suggested.
- *Prophylaxis of factor IX deficiency:* 20–30 units/kg IV once or twice a week may prevent spontaneous bleeding in hemophilia B patients. Individualize dose. Increase dose if patient is exposed to trauma or surgery.

Pharmacokinetics

Route	Onset	Duration
IV	Immediate	1–2 days

Metabolism: Plasma; $T_{1/2}$: 24–32 hr
Distribution: Crosses placenta; enters breast milk
Excretion: Unknown

IV FACTS

Preparation: Prepare using diluents and needles supplied with product. Refrigerate.
Infusion: ⊗ ***Warning*** Infuse slowly. 100 units/min and 2–3 mL/min have been suggested. Do not exceed 3 mL/min, and stop or slow the infusion at any sign of headache; pulse, or BP changes.

Adverse effects

- **CNS:** *Headache,* flushing, chills, tingling, somnolence, lethargy
- **GI:** *Nausea,* vomiting, **hepatitis** (risk associated with use of blood products)
- **Hematologic:** *Thrombosis,* DIC, **AIDS** (risk associated with use of blood products; risk is lower with preparations treated with solvent detergents)
- **Other:** Chills, fever; BP changes, urticaria, *Creutzfeldt-Jakob disease*

■ Nursing considerations

Assessment

- **History:** Factor VII, factor IX deficiencies; liver disease with signs of intravascular coagulation or fibrinolysis; pregnancy; lactation
- **Physical:** Skin color, lesions; T; orientation, reflexes, affect; P, BP, peripheral perfusion; clotting factor levels, LFTs

Interventions

- Administer by IV route only.

⊗ ***Warning*** Decrease rate of infusion if headache, flushing, fever, chills, tingling, or urticaria occur; in some patients, the drug will need to be discontinued.

- Monitor patient's clinical response and factors II, VII, IX, and X levels regularly, and regulate dosage based on response.
- Monitor patient for any sign of thrombosis; use comfort and preventive measures when possible (eg, exercise, support stockings, ambulation, positioning).

Teaching points

- Dosage varies widely.
- Safety precautions are taken to ensure that this blood product is pure and the risk of AIDS and hepatitis is minimal.
- Wear or carry a medical ID to alert emergency medical personnel that you require this treatment.
- Report headache, rash, chills, calf pain, swelling, unusual bleeding, or bruising.

▽ famciclovir sodium

(fam sye' kloe vir)

Famvir

PREGNANCY CATEGORY B

Drug class

Antiviral

Therapeutic actions

Antiviral activity; inhibits viral DNA replication in acute herpes zoster.

Indications

- Management of acute herpes zoster (shingles)
- Treatment or suppression of recurrent episodes of genital herpes
- Treatment of recurrent herpes labialis (cold sores) in immunocompetent patients
- Treatment of recurrent orolabial or genital herpes simplex infections in HIV-infected patients
- Unlabeled use: Initial management of herpes genitalis

Contraindications and cautions

- Contraindicated with hypersensitivity to famciclovir or penciclovir, lactation.
- Use cautiously with pregnancy, impaired renal function.

Available forms

Tablets—125, 250, 500 mg

Dosages

Adults

- *Herpes zoster:* 500 mg every 8 hr PO for 7 days.
- *Genital herpes, first episode in immunecompetent patients:* 230 mg tid for 7–10 days.
- *Treatment of recurrent genital herpes:* 125 mg PO bid for 5 days or 1,000 mg PO bid for 1 day.
- *Chronic suppression of recurrent genital herpes:* 250 mg PO bid for up to 1 yr.
- *Recurrent orolabial or genital herpes simplex infection in HIV-infected patients:* 500 mg every 12 hr PO for 7 days.
- *Recurrent herpes labialis:* 1,500 mg PO as a single dose.

Pediatric patients

Safety and efficacy not established.

Patients with renal impairment

- *Herpes zoster:* Treat for 7 days as indicated below.

CrCl (mL/min)	*Dose*
60 or more	500 mg every 8 hr
40–59	500 mg every 12 hr
20–39	500 mg every 24 hr
Less than 20	250 mg every 24 hr
Dialysis	250 mg as a single dose after dialysis

- *Recurrent labialis:* Give a single dose as indicated below.

CrCl (mL/min)	*Dose*
60 or more	1,500 mg
40–59	750 mg
20–39	500 mg
Less than 20	250 mg
Dialysis	250 mg after dialysis

- *Treatment of recurrent genital herpes as single-day dosing:* Give drug as indicated below.

CrCl (mL/min)	*Dose*
60 and over	1,000 mg every 12 hr
40–59	500 mg every 12 hr
20–39	500 mg single dose
Less than 20	250 mg single dose

- *Treatment of recurrent genital herpes:* Treat for 5 days as indicated below.

CrCl (mL/min)	*Dose*
40 or more	125 mg every 12 hr
20–39	125 mg every 24 hr
Less than 20	125 mg every 24 hr
Dialysis	125 mg after dialysis

- *Suppression of recurrent genital herpes:*

CrCl (mL/min)	*Dose*
40 or more	250 mg every 12 hr
20–39	125 mg every 12 hr
Less than 20	125 mg every 24 hr
Dialysis	125 mg after dialysis

- *Recurrent orolabial or genital herpes simplex infection in HIV-infected patients:*

CrCl (mL/min)	*Dose*
40 or more	500 mg every 12 hr
20–39	500 mg every 24 hr
Less than 20	250 mg every 24 hr
Dialysis	250 mg after dialysis

Pharmacokinetics

Route	*Onset*	*Peak*
Oral	Varies	30–60 min

Metabolism: $T_{1/2}$: 2 hr
Distribution: Crosses placenta; may enter breast milk
Excretion: Feces, urine

Adverse effects

- **CNS:** Dreams, ataxia, coma, confusion, dizziness, *headache*
- **CV:** Arrhythmia, hypertension, hypotension
- **Dermatologic:** *Rash,* alopecia, pruritus, urticaria
- **GI:** Abnormal liver function tests, nausea, vomiting, anorexia, *diarrhea,* abdominal pain
- **Hematologic: Granulocytopenia, thrombocytopenia,** anemia
- **Other:** *Fever,* chills, **cancer,** sterility

Interactions

✱ **Drug-drug** • Increased serum concentration of famciclovir if taken with cimetidine • Increased digoxin levels if taken together

■ Nursing considerations

Assessment

- **History:** Hypersensitivity to famciclovir or penciclovir, cytopenia; impaired renal function; lactation, pregnancy
- **Physical:** Skin color, lesions; orientation; BP, P, auscultation, perfusion, edema; R, adventitious sounds; urinary output; CBC, Hct, BUN, creatinine clearance, LFTs

Interventions

- Decrease dosage in patients with impaired renal function.

⊗ ***Warning*** Arrange for CBC before and every 2 days during therapy and at least weekly thereafter. Consult with physician to reduce dosage if WBC or platelet counts fall.

Teaching points

- Take drug for 1, 5, or 7 full days as prescribed.
- Famciclovir does not cure genital herpes; use precautions to prevent transmission.
- You may experience these side effects: Decreased blood count leading to susceptibility to infection (blood tests may be needed; avoid crowds and exposure to disease), headache (analgesics may be ordered), diarrhea.
- Report bruising, bleeding, worsening of condition, fever, infection.

F

famotidine

(fa moe' ti deen)

Apo-Famotidine (CAN), Apo-Famotidine Injectable (CAN), Gen-Famotidine (CAN), Nu-Famotidine (CAN), Pepcid, Pepcid AC, Pepcid AC Maximum Strength, Pepcid RPD

PREGNANCY CATEGORY B

Drug class

Histamine-2 (H_2) receptor antagonist

Therapeutic actions

Competitively blocks the action of histamine at the H_2 receptors of the parietal cells of the stomach; inhibits basal gastric acid secretion and chemically induced gastric acid secretion.

Indications

- Short-term treatment and maintenance of duodenal ulcer
- Short-term treatment of benign gastric ulcer
- Treatment of pathologic hypersecretory conditions (eg, Zollinger-Ellison syndrome)
- Short-term treatment of GERD, esophagitis due to GERD
- OTC: Relief of symptoms of heartburn, acid indigestion, sour stomach
- Unlabeled uses: Part of combination therapy for *Helicobacter pylori,* perioperative suppression of gastric acid secretion, prevention of stress ulcers, prevention of aspiration pneumonitis, treatment of certain types of urticaria

Contraindications and cautions

- Contraindicated with allergy to famotidine; renal failure; lactation.
- Use cautiously with pregnancy, renal or hepatic impairment.

Available forms

Tablets—10, 20, 40 mg; chewable tablets—10 mg; orally disintegrating tablets—20, 40 mg; gelcaps—10 mg; powder for oral suspension—40 mg/5 mL; injection—10 mg/mL; injection, premixed—20 mg/50 mL in 0.9% sodium chloride

Dosages

Adults

- *Acute treatment of active duodenal ulcer:* 40 mg PO or IV at bedtime *or* 20 mg bid PO or IV. Therapy at full dosage should generally be discontinued after 6–8 wk. May be used with antacids for pain relief.
- *Maintenance therapy for duodenal ulcer:* 20 mg PO at bedtime.
- *Benign gastric ulcer:* 40 mg PO daily at bedtime.
- *Hypersecretory syndrome:* 20 mg every 6 hr PO initially. Doses up to 160 mg every 6 hr have been administered. 20 mg IV every 12 hr in patients unable to take oral drugs.
- *GERD:* 20 mg bid PO for up to 6 wk. For patients with esophagitis, the dose is 20–40 mg bid PO for up to 12 wk.
- *Heartburn, acid indigestion:* 10–20 mg PO for relief; 10–20 mg PO, 15–60 min before eating for prevention. Do not exceed 20 mg/24 hr.

Pediatric patients 1–12 yr

- *Peptic ulcer:* 0.5 mg/kg/day PO at bedtime or divided in two doses up to 40 mg/day; 0.25 mg/kg every 12 hr IV up to 40 mg/day if unable to take orally or for pathological hypersecretory conditions.
- *GERD with or without esophagitis:* 1 mg/kg/day PO divided in two doses up to 40 mg bid.

Infants

- *Younger than 3 mo:* 5 mg/kg/dose oral suspension once daily for up to 8 wk.
- *3 mo–1 yr:* 0.5 mg /kg PO bid for up to 8 wk.

Renal impairment

Reduce dosage to 20 mg PO at bedtime or 40 mg PO every 36–48 hr.

Pharmacokinetics

Route	Onset	Peak	Duration
Oral	Slow	1–3 hr	6–12 hr
IV	Less than 1 hr	0.5–3 hr	8–15 hr

Metabolism: Hepatic; $T_{1/2}$: 2.5–3.5 hr
Distribution: Crosses placenta; enters breast milk
Excretion: Urine

IV FACTS

Preparation: For direct injection, dilute 2 mL (solution contains 10 mg/mL) with 0.9% sodium chloride injection, water for injection, 5% or 10% dextrose injection, lactated Ringer's injection, or 5% sodium bicarbonate injection to a total volume of 5–10 mL. For infusion, 2 mL diluted with 100 mL 5% dextrose solution or other IVs. Stable for 48 hr at room temperature, 14 days if refrigerated.

Infusion: Inject directly slowly, over not less than 2 min. Infuse over 15–30 min; continuous infusion: 40 mg/24 hr.

Adverse effects

- **CNS:** *Headache,* malaise, *dizziness,* somnolence, insomnia
- **Dermatologic:** Rash
- **GI:** *Diarrhea, constipation,* anorexia, abdominal pain
- **Other:** Muscle cramp, increase in total bilirubin, sexual impotence

■ Nursing considerations

Assessment

- **History:** Allergy to famotidine; renal failure; lactation, pregnancy, hepatic impairment
- **Physical:** Skin lesions; liver evaluation, abdominal examination, normal output; renal function tests, serum bilirubin

Interventions

- If using one dose a day, administer drug at bedtime.
- Decrease doses with renal failure.
- Arrange for administration of concurrent antacid therapy to relieve pain.
- Reserve IV use for hospitalized patients not able to take oral medications; switch to oral medication as soon as possible.

Teaching points

- Take this drug at bedtime (or in the morning and at bedtime). Therapy may continue for 4–6 weeks or longer. Place rapidly disintegrating tablet on tongue and swallow with or without water.
- If needed, take antacid exactly as prescribed, being careful of the times of administration.
- Have regular medical follow-up while on this drug to evaluate your response.
- Take over-the-counter drug 1 hour before eating to prevent indigestion. Do not take more than two per day.
- You may experience these side effects: Constipation or diarrhea; loss of libido or impotence (reversible); headache (adjust lights, temperature, noise levels).
- Report sore throat, fever, unusual bruising or bleeding, severe headache, muscle or joint pain.

F

▽fat emulsion, intravenous

Intralipid 20%, 30%; Liposyn II 10%, 20%; Liposyn III 10%, 20%, 30%

PREGNANCY CATEGORY C

Drug classes

Caloric drug
Nutritional drug

Therapeutic actions

A preparation from soybean or safflower oil that provides neutral triglycerides, mostly unsaturated fatty acids; these are used as a source of energy, causing an increase in heat production, decrease in respiratory quotient, and increase in oxygen consumption.

Indications

- Source of calories and essential fatty acids for patients requiring parenteral nutrition for extended periods
- Essential fatty acid deficiency

Contraindications and cautions

- Contraindicated with disturbance of normal fat metabolism (hyperlipemia, lipoid nephrosis, acute pancreatitis), allergy to eggs.
- Use cautiously with severe liver damage, pulmonary disease, anemia, blood coagulation disorders, pregnancy, jaundiced or premature infants.

Available forms

Injection—10% (100, 200, 500 mL), 20% (50, 100, 250, 500 mL); 30% (500 mL)

Dosages

Adults

- *Parenteral nutrition:* Should not constitute more than 60% of total calorie intake. *10%:* Infuse IV at 1 mL/min for the first 15–30 min; may be increased to 2 mL/min. Infuse only 500 mL the first day, and increase the following day. Do not exceed 2.5 g/kg/day. *20%:* Infuse at 0.5 mL/min for the first 15–30 min; infuse only 250 mL *Liposyn II* or 500 mL *Intralipid* the first day, and increase the following day. Do not exceed 3 g/kg/day. *30%:* Infuse at 1 mL/min (0.1 g fat/min) for first 15–30 min; do not exceed 2.5 g/kg/day.
- *Fatty acid deficiency:* Supply 8%–10% of the caloric intake by IV fat emulsion.

Pediatric patients

- *Parenteral nutrition:* Should not constitute more than 60% of total calorie intake. *10%:* Initial IV infusion rate is 0.1 mL/min for the first 10–15 min. *20%:* Initial infusion rate is 0.05 mL/min for the first 10–15 min. If no untoward reactions occur, increase rate to 1 g/kg in 4 hr. Do not exceed 3 g/kg/day. *30%:* Initial infusion, 0.1 mL/min (0.01 g fat/min) for first 10–15 min; do not exceed 3 g/kg/day.

Pharmacokinetics

Route	Onset
IV	Rapid

Metabolism: Hepatic and tissue; $T_{1/2}$: Varies
Distribution: Crosses placenta; may enter breast milk
Excretion: Unknown

IV FACTS

Preparation: ⊗ ***Warning*** Supplied in single-dose containers; do not store partially used bottles; do not resterilize for later use; do not use with filters; do not use any bottle in which there appears to be separation from the emulsion.

Infusion: Infusion rate is 1 mL/min for 10% solution, monitor for 15–30 min; if no adverse reaction occurs, may be increased to 2 mL/min; 0.5 mL/min for 20% solution; 1 mL/min for 30%; may be increased if no adverse reactions. May be infused simultaneously with amino acid-dextrose mixtures by means of Y-connector located near the infusion site using separate flow rate; keep the lipid solution higher than the amino acid-dextrose line.

Incompatibilities: Do not mix or inject at Y site with amikacin, tetracycline. Monitor electrolyte and acid content; fat emulsion separates in acid solution.

Adverse effects

- **CNS:** *Headache,* flushing, fever, sweating, sleepiness, pressure over the eyes, dizziness
- **GI:** *Nausea,* vomiting
- **Hematologic:** *Thrombophlebitis,* **sepsis,** hyperlipidemia, hypercoagulability, **thrombocytopenia, leukopenia,** elevated liver enzymes
- **Other:** Irritation at infusion site, brown pigmentation in RES (IV fat pigment), cyanosis, infection

■ Nursing considerations

Assessment

- **History:** Disturbance of normal fat metabolism, allergy to eggs, severe liver damage, pulmonary disease, anemia, blood coagulation disorders, pregnancy, jaundiced or premature infants
- **Physical:** Skin color, lesions; T; orientation; P, BP, peripheral perfusion; CBC, plasma lipid profile (especially triglycerides), clotting factor levels, LFTs

Interventions

⊠ ***Black box warning*** Administer to preterm infants only if benefit clearly outweighs risk; deaths have occurred.

- Administer by IV route only.

⊗ ***Warning*** Inspect admixture for "breaking or oiling out" of the emulsion—seen as yellow streaking or accumulation of yellow droplets—or for the formation of any particulates; discard any admixture if these occur.

⊗ ***Warning*** Monitor patient carefully for fluid or fat overloading during infusion: Diluted serum electrolytes, overhydration, pulmonary edema, elevated jugular venous pressure, metabolic acidosis, impaired pulmonary diffusion capacity. Discontinue the infusion; reevaluate patient before restarting infusion at a lower rate.

- Monitor patient's clinical response, serum lipid profile (obtain triglycerides every week), weight gain, improved nitrogen balance.
- Monitor patient for thrombosis or sepsis; use comfort and preventive measures (such as exercise, support stockings, ambulation, positioning).

Teaching points

- Report pain at infusion site, difficulty breathing, chest pain, calf pain, excessive sweating.

febuxostat

*(feb **bux'** oh stat)*

Uloric

PREGNANCY CATEGORY C

Drug classes

Antigout drug
Xanthine oxidase inhibitor

Therapeutic actions

Blocks xanthine oxidase, an important enzyme in the process of uric acid formation; not thought to affect other enzymes involved in purine or pyrimidine synthesis.

Indications

- Long-term management of hyperuricemia in patients with gout

Contraindications and cautions

- Contraindicated with hypersensitivity to components of drug, concurrent treatment with azathioprine, mercaptopurine, or theophyllines.
- Use cautiously with severe renal or hepatic impairment, history of heart attack or stroke, pregnancy, lactation.

Available forms

Tablets—40, 80 mg

Dosages

Adults

Initially, 40 mg/day PO; if serum uric acid level is not less than 6 mg/dL in 2 weeks, dosage may be increased to 80 mg/day PO.

Pediatric patients

Safety and efficacy not established.

Patients with renal or hepatic impairment

No dosage change required with mild to moderate impairment; use caution with severe impairment (Child-Pugh Class C).

Pharmacokinetics

Route	*Onset*	*Peak*
Oral	Rapid	1–1.5 hr

Metabolism: Hepatic; $T_{1/2}$: 5–8 hr
Distribution: May cross placenta; may enter breast milk
Excretion: Urine, feces

Adverse effects

- **CNS:** Dizziness
- **CV:** Thromboembolic events, MI, stroke
- **GI:** Nausea, liver function abnormalities
- **Other:** Arthralgia, rash, gout flares

Interactions

✱ **Drug-drug** • Risk of decreased metabolism and increased serum levels of azathioprine, mercaptopurine, theophyllines when given with these drugs, causing toxicity; avoid these combinations; concurrent use is contraindicated

■ Nursing considerations

Assessment

- **History:** Hypersensitivity to components of drug, liver or renal dysfunction, heart attack or stroke, pregnancy, lactation
- **Physical:** Orientation, affect; skin—color, lesions; abdominal exam; serum uric acid level, liver and renal function tests, baseline ECG

Interventions

- Administer without regard to food. May be taken with antacids.
- Obtain baseline and periodic serum uric acid levels.

- Arrange for other medication if gout flare occurs.
- Monitor for signs and symptoms of heart attack or stroke; patient may be at increased risk.

Teaching points

- Take this drug once a day, with or without food. You may take this drug with antacids.
- Store this drug at room temperature, protected from light.
- If you miss a dose, take the next dose as soon as you remember.
- You may experience a flare-up of your gout symptoms when you start taking this drug. Do not stop taking the drug; contact your health care provider, who may give you other medications to handle the flare-up.
- You will be asked to have periodic blood tests to evaluate the effects of this drug on your body.
- It is not known how this drug affects a fetus. If you become pregnant while taking this drug, consult your health care provider.
- It is not known how this drug affects a nursing baby. Discuss the risks and benefits with your health care provider if you are nursing a baby.
- You may experience these side effects: Dizziness (do not drive a car or engage in activities that require alertness if these effects occur); nausea, joint pain, rash (these may lessen over time; consult your health care provider if they become too uncomfortable).
- Report chest pain, difficulty breathing, numbness or tingling, changes in the color of urine or stool, yellowing of the eyes or skin.

▽ felodipine

(fell oh' di peen)

Renedil (CAN) DNC

PREGNANCY CATEGORY C

Drug classes

Antihypertensive
Calcium channel blocker

Therapeutic actions

Inhibits the movement of calcium ions across the membranes of cardiac and vascular smooth muscle cells; greater selectivity for vascular smooth muscle as compared to cardiac muscle; leads to arterial and coronary artery vasodilation and decreased peripheral vascular resistance.

Indications

- Essential hypertension, alone or in combination with other antihypertensives

Contraindications and cautions

- Contraindicated with allergy to felodipine or other calcium channel blockers, sick sinus syndrome, heart block (second or third degree), lactation.
- Use cautiously with pregnancy, impaired hepatic function.

Available forms

ER tablets DNC—2.5, 5, 10 mg

Dosages

Adults

Initially, 5 mg PO daily; dosage may be gradually increased over at least 14 days. Usual dose is 2.5–10 mg PO daily. Doses greater than 10 mg PO daily are associated with an increased risk of peripheral edema.

Pediatric patients

Safety and efficacy not established.

Geriatric patients or patients with hepatic impairment

Monitor carefully; begin with 2.5 mg daily, and do not exceed 10 mg daily PO.

Pharmacokinetics

Route	Onset	Peak
Oral	2–5 hr	2.5–5 hr

Metabolism: Hepatic; $T_{1/2}$: 11–16 hr
Distribution: Crosses placenta; may enter breast milk
Excretion: Urine

Adverse effects

- **CNS:** *Dizziness, light-headedness, headache,* asthenia, *fatigue, lethargy*
- **CV:** *Peripheral edema,* arrhythmias

- **Dermatologic:** *Flushing,* rash
- **GI:** *Nausea,* abdominal discomfort, reflux, constipation

Interactions

✱ **Drug-drug** • Decreased serum levels with barbiturates, hydantoins, carbamazepine • Increased serum levels and toxicity with erythromycin, cimetidine, ranitidine, antifungals
✱ **Drug-food** • Decreased metabolism and increased risk of toxic effects if taken with grapefruit juice; avoid this combination

■ Nursing considerations

Assessment

- **History:** Allergy to felodipine, impaired hepatic function, sick sinus syndrome, heart block, lactation, pregnancy
- **Physical:** Skin lesions, color, edema; P, BP, baseline ECG, peripheral perfusion, auscultation, R, adventitious sounds; liver evaluation, GI normal output; LFTs, urinalysis

Interventions

- Have patient swallow tablet whole; do not chew or crush.
- Monitor patient carefully (BP, cardiac rhythm and output) while drug is being adjusted to therapeutic dose.
- Monitor cardiac rhythm regularly during stabilization of dosage and periodically during long-term therapy.
- Administer drug without regard to meals.

Teaching points

- Take this drug with meals if upset stomach occurs; swallow tablet whole, do not cut, crush, or chew. Do not drink grapefruit juice while using this drug.
- You may experience these side effects: Nausea, vomiting (eat frequent small meals); headache (adjust lighting, noise, and temperature; medication may be ordered if severe).
- Report irregular heart beat, shortness of breath, swelling of the hands or feet, pronounced dizziness, constipation.

▽ fenofibrate

*(fee no **fye'** brate)*

Antara, Apo-Fenofibrate (CAN), Fenoglide, Gen-Fenofibrate (CAN), Lipofen, Lofibra, PMS-Fenofibrate (CAN), ratio-Fenofibrate MC (CAN), TriCor, Triglide

PREGNANCY CATEGORY C

Drug class

Antihyperlipidemic

Therapeutic actions

Inhibits triglyceride synthesis in the liver resulting in a reduction in VLDL released into circulation; may also stimulate the breakdown of triglyceride-rich lipoproteins.

Indications

- Adjunct to diet in treating adults with primary hypercholesterolemia or mixed dyslipidemia
- Adjunct to diet for treatment of adults with hypertriglyceridemia
- Unlabeled use: Hyperuricemia

Contraindications and cautions

- Contraindicated with allergy to fenofibrate, hepatic or severe renal impairment, primary biliary cirrhosis, gall bladder disease, pregnancy.
- Use cautiously with lactation and in the elderly.

Available forms

Tablets—48, 50, 54, 145, 160 mg; capsules—43, 50, 67, 100, 130, 134, 150, 200 mg

Dosages

Adults

- *Hypertriglyceridemia:* Initially, 48–145 mg (*TriCor*) or 67–200 mg (*Lofibra*) with a meal or 50–160 mg/day (*Triglide*) daily PO or 43–130 mg/day PO (*Antara*), or 50–150 mg/day PO (*Lipofen*).
- *Primary hypercholesterolemia or mixed dyslipidemia:* 145 mg/day PO (*TriCor*) or 200 mg/day (*Lofibra*) with a meal or

160 mg/day (*Triglide*) or 130 mg/day PO (*Antara*), or 150 mg/day PO (*Lipofen*).

Pediatric patients

Safety and efficacy not established.

Geriatric patients

Initial dose, 48 mg/day PO (*TriCor*), 67 mg/day (*Lofibra*) with a meal or 50 mg/day (*Triglide*) or 43 mg/day PO (*Antara*), or 50 mg/day PO (*Lipofen*); adjust slowly with close monitoring.

Patients with renal impairment

Initiate therapy with 48 mg/day PO (*TriCor*), 67 mg/day (*Lofibra*) with a meal or 50 mg/day (*Triglide*) or 43 mg/day PO (*Antara*), or 50 mg/day PO (*Lipofen*); monitor renal function tests for 4–8 wk before increasing.

Pharmacokinetics

Route	*Onset*	*Peak*	*Duration*
Oral	Varies	6–8 hr	Wks

Metabolism: Hepatic; $T_{1/2}$: 20 hr

Distribution: Crosses placenta; enters breast milk

Excretion: Urine

Adverse effects

- **CV:** Angina, arrhythmias, swelling, phlebitis, thrombophlebitis
- **Dermatologic:** *Rash,* alopecia, dry skin, dry and brittle hair, pruritus, urticaria
- **GI:** *Nausea,* vomiting, diarrhea, dyspepsia, flatulence, bloating, stomatitis, gastritis, **pancreatitis,** peptic ulcer, GI hemorrhage
- **GU:** *Impotence, decreased libido,* dysuria, hematuria, proteinuria, decreased urine output
- **Hematologic:** Leukopenia, anemia, eosinophilia, increased AST and ALT, increased CPK
- **Other:** *Myalgia, flulike symptoms,* arthralgia, weight gain, polyphagia, increased perspiration, systemic lupus erythematosus, blurred vision, gynecomastia

Interactions

✱ **Drug-drug** • Increased bleeding tendencies if oral anticoagulants are given with fenofibrate; reduce dosage of anticoagulant • Possible rhabdomyolysis, acute renal failure if given with any statins; avoid this combination • Decreased absorption and effectiveness if given with bile acid sequestrants; administer at least 1 hr before or 4–6 hr after these drugs • Increased risk of renal toxicity if combined with immunosuppressants or other nephrotoxic drugs; use caution and monitor patient carefully

■ Nursing considerations

Assessment

- **History:** Allergy to fenofibrate, hepatic impairment, primary biliary cirrhosis, gall bladder disease, pregnancy, renal impairment, lactation
- **Physical:** Skin lesions, color, T, P, BP, auscultation, baseline ECG, peripheral perfusion, edema; bowel sounds, normal urine output, liver evaluation; lipid studies, CBC, LFTs, renal function tests, urinalysis

Interventions

- Differentiate between brand names used; dosage varies.
- Administer drug with meals (*Lofibra, Lipofen*).
- Monitor patient carefully.
- Ensure that patient continues strict dietary restrictions and exercise program.
- Arrange for regular follow-up, including blood tests for lipids, liver function, and CBC during long-term therapy.
- Give frequent skin care to deal with rashes and dryness.
- Monitor patient for muscle weakness, aches, especially if patient takes *TriCor* in combination with other cholesterol-lowering drugs.

Teaching points

- Take the drug with meals (*Lofibra, Lipofen*).
- Continue to follow strict dietary regimen and exercise program.
- Arrange to have regular follow-up visits to your health care provider, which will include blood tests.
- You may experience these side effects: Diarrhea, loss of appetite (ensure ready access to the bathroom if this occurs; frequent small meals may help).
- Report chest pain, shortness of breath, palpitations, myalgia, malaise, excessive fatigue, fever.

fenofibric acid
(feen oh fye' brick)

Trilipix DNC

PREGNANCY CATEGORY C

Drug class
Antihyperlipidemic

Therapeutic actions
Activates peroxisome proliferator activated receptor alpha, leading to an increase in lipolysis and elimination of triglyceride-rich particles from the plasma by activating lipoprotein lipase and reducing the production of lipase inhibitors. The decrease in triglycerides results in the production of large, buoyant LDL particles, which have a greater affinity for cholesterol receptors and are broken down rapidly; HDL levels are also increased.

Indications
- In combination with a statin to reduce triglycerides and increase HDL in patients with mixed dyslipidemia and CAD or at high risk for CAD who could achieve LDL goals
- As monotherapy to reduce triglycerides in patients with severe hypertriglyceridemia
- As monotherapy to reduced elevated LDL, total cholesterol, triglycerides and ApoB and to increase HDL in patients with primary hyperlipidemia or mixed dyslipidemia

Contraindications and cautions
- Contraindicated with hypersensitivity to components of drug or to fenofibrate, severe renal impairment, dialysis, active liver disease, gallbladder disease, lactation.
- Use cautiously with mild to moderate renal disease, history of liver dysfunction, pregnancy.

Available forms
DR capsules DNC—45, 135 mg

Dosages
Adults

Mixed dyslipidemia: 135 mg/day PO.
Hypertriglyceridemia: 45–135 mg/day PO.

Pediatric patients

Safety and efficacy not established.

Patients with renal impairment

45 mg/day PO.

Pharmacokinetics

Route	Onset	Peak
Oral	Slow	4–5 hr

Metabolism: Hepatic; $T_{1/2}$: 20 hr
Distribution: May cross placenta; enters breast milk
Excretion: Urine

Adverse effects
- **CNS:** Headache
- **GI:** Nausea, constipation, *abdominal pain,* pancreatitis, cirrhosis
- **Respiratory:** *URI*
- **Other:** Fatigue, myalgia, **rhabdomyolysis,** increased liver enzymes, renal toxicity, fever

Interactions
✱ **Drug-drug** • Increased risk of bleeding if combined with oral anticoagulants; monitor closely and adjust dosage of anticoagulant as needed • Risk of decreased effectiveness if taken with a bile acid sequestrant; fenofibric acid should be taken 1 hour before or 4 to 6 hours after these drugs • Possible increased risk of nephrotoxicity if combined with cyclosporine; monitor patient very closely; use of another lipid-lowering agent should be considered

■ Nursing considerations
Assessment
- **History:** Hypersensitivity to components of drug, fenofibrate; renal or liver dysfunction, gallbladder disease; pregnancy, lactation
- **Physical:** Orientation, affect; abdominal exam; respiratory auscultation; liver and renal function tests

Interventions
- Encourage patient to continue diet and exercise as prescribed.
- Administer without regard to food.
- Check patient's complete drug list and consider timing of drugs that might be affected by GI effects of this drug. If patient is also

F

taking a statin, the drugs can be taken at the same time.
- Do not cut, crush, or allow patient to chew capsule. Capsule should be swallowed whole.
- Advise patient who is nursing to select another method of feeding the baby.
- Arrange for regular monitoring of lipid profile and liver function.

Teaching points
- Take this drug once a day, with or without food.
- Continue the low-fat diet and exercise program you have been following.
- Do not cut, crush, or chew capsule. You should swallow the capsule whole. If you are also taking a statin, they may be taken at the same time.
- If you miss a dose, take the next dose as soon as you remember. If you remember you forgot a dose at about the same time you are scheduled for your next dose, just take the next dose. Do not double the doses. Do not take more than one dose a day.
- It is not known how this drug affects a fetus. If you become pregnant while taking this drug, consult your health care provider.
- It is not known how this drug affects a nursing baby. Because of the potential for serious adverse effects in an infant, you should use another method of feeding the baby while you are taking this drug.
- You may experience these side effects: Headache (consult your health care provider about potential treatment if it becomes uncomfortable); constipation, abdominal pain (these may lessen over time; consult your health care provide if they become too uncomfortable).
- You will need periodic blood tests to monitor the effects of this drug on your body.
- Report marked muscle weakness or pain, fever, abdominal pain accompanied by nausea and vomiting.

▽fenoprofen calcium
*(fen oh **proe'** fen)*

Nalfon

PREGNANCY CATEGORY B
(FIRST AND SECOND TRIMESTERS)

PREGNANCY CATEGORY D
(THIRD TRIMESTER)

Drug classes
Analgesic (nonopioid)
NSAID
Propionic acid derivative

Therapeutic actions
Analgesic, anti-inflammatory, and antipyretic activities largely related to inhibition of prostaglandin synthesis by inhibiting cyclooxygenase; exact mechanisms of action are not known.

Indications
- Acute and long-term treatment of rheumatoid arthritis and osteoarthritis
- Relief of mild to moderate pain
- Unlabeled uses: Treatment of juvenile rheumatoid arthritis; symptomatic treatment of sunburn, migraine headache

Contraindications and cautions
- Contraindicated with significant renal impairment, pregnancy, lactation, hypersensitivity to aspirin, fenoprofen, or other NSAIDs.
- Use cautiously with impaired hearing; hepatic, hypertension, and GI conditions.

Available forms
Capsules—200, 300, 400 mg; tablets—600 mg

Dosages
Do not exceed 3,200 mg/day.

Adults
- *Rheumatoid arthritis or osteoarthritis:* 300–600 mg PO tid or qid. Treatment for 2–3 wk may be required to see improvement.
- *Mild to moderate pain:* 200 mg every 4–6 hr PO, as needed.

Pediatric patients
Safety and efficacy not established.

Pharmacokinetics

Route	*Onset*	*Peak*
Oral	15–30 min	1–2 hr

Metabolism: Hepatic; $T_{1/2}$: 2–3 hr
Distribution: Crosses placenta; enters breast milk
Excretion: Urine

Adverse effects
NSAIDs
- **CNS:** *Headache, dizziness, somnolence, insomnia,* fatigue, tiredness, tinnitus, ophthalmologic effects
- **Dermatologic:** *Rash,* pruritus, sweating, dry mucous membranes, stomatitis
- **GI:** *Nausea, dyspepsia, GI pain,* diarrhea, vomiting, constipation, flatulence, **ulcer, GI bleed**
- **GU:** Dysuria, **renal impairment** (fenoprofen is one of the most nephrotoxic NSAIDs)
- **Hematologic:** Bleeding, platelet inhibition with higher doses, **neutropenia, eosinophilia, leukopenia, pancytopenia, thrombocytopenia, agranulocytosis, granulocytopenia, aplastic anemia,** decreased Hgb or Hct, **bone marrow depression,** menorrhagia
- **Respiratory:** Dyspnea, hemoptysis, pharyngitis, **bronchospasm,** rhinitis
- **Other:** Peripheral edema, **anaphylactoid reactions to fatal anaphylactic shock**

Interactions
✱ **Drug-drug** • Increased risk of bleeding with anticoagulants, antiplatelet drugs • Decreased effect when used with phenobarbital

■ Nursing considerations
Assessment
- **History:** Renal impairment, impaired hearing, allergy to aspirin or NSAIDs, hepatic, CV, and GI conditions, lactation, pregnancy
- **Physical:** Skin color and lesions; orientation, reflexes, ophthalmologic and audiometric evaluation, peripheral sensation; P, edema; R, adventitious sounds; liver evaluation; CBC, clotting times, LFTs, renal function tests; serum electrolytes, stool guaiac

Interventions
⊗ ***Black box warning*** Be aware that patient may be at increased risk for CV events, GI bleeding; monitor patient accordingly.
- Administer drug with food or after meals if GI upset occurs.
- Arrange for periodic ophthalmologic examination during long-term therapy.

⊗ ***Warning*** If overdose occurs, institute emergency procedures—gastric lavage, induction of emesis, supportive therapy.

Teaching points
- Take drug with food or meals if GI upset occurs.
- Take only the prescribed dosage.
- Do not take this drug during pregnancy; using contraceptives is advised.
- Dizziness or drowsiness can occur (avoid driving or using dangerous machinery).
- Report sore throat, fever, rash, itching, weight gain, swelling in ankles or fingers; changes in vision; black, tarry stools, bleeding.

DANGEROUS DRUG

▽ fentanyl
(fen' ta nil)

Actiq; Duragesic 12, 25, 50, 75, 100; Fentora, Ionsys, Onsolis, Sublimaze

PREGNANCY CATEGORY C

CONTROLLED SUBSTANCE C-II

Drug class
Opioid agonist analgesic

Therapeutic actions
Acts at specific opioid receptors, causing analgesia, respiratory depression, physical depression, euphoria.

Indications
- Analgesic action of short duration during anesthesia and immediate postoperative period
- Analgesic supplement in general or regional anesthesia
- Administration with a neuroleptic as an anesthetic premedication, for induction of anesthesia, and as an adjunct in maintenance of general and regional anesthesia

F

- For use as an anesthetic drug with oxygen in selected high-risk patients
- Transdermal system: Management of chronic pain in patients requiring continuous opioid analgesia over an extended period of time who cannot be managed by other means and who are already receiving opioid therapy
- *Actiq, Fentora, Onsolis:* Treatment of breakthrough pain in cancer patients being treated with and tolerant to opioids for underlying cancer pain

Contraindications and cautions

- Contraindicated with hypersensitivity to opioids, diarrhea caused by poisoning, acute bronchial asthma, upper airway obstruction, pregnancy.
- Use cautiously with bradycardia, history of seizures, lactation, renal impairment; history of drug addiction.

Available forms

Lozenge on a stick (*Actiq*)—200, 400, 600, 800, 1,200, 1,600 mcg; transdermal—12.5, 25, 50, 75, 100 mcg/hr; injection—50 mcg/mL; buccal tablets—100, 200, 400, 600, 800 mcg; buccal soluble film—200, 400, 600, 800, 1,200 mcg; ionic delivery system—40 mcg/10 min

Dosages

Individualize dosage; monitor vital signs.

Adults

Parenteral

- *Premedication:* 50–100 mcg IM 30–60 min before surgery.
- *Adjunct to general anesthesia:* Initial dosage is 2–20 mcg/kg. Maintenance dose, 2–50 mcg IV or IM; 25–100 mcg IV or IM when changes in vital signs indicate surgical stress or lightening of analgesia.
- *With oxygen for anesthesia:* Total high dose is 20–50 mcg/kg IV.
- *Adjunct to regional anesthesia:* 50–100 mcg IM or slowly IV over 1–2 min.
- *Postoperatively:* 50–100 mcg IM for the control of pain, tachypnea, or emergence delirium; repeat in 1–2 hr if needed.

Transdermal

Initiate therapy with 25 mcg/hr system; adjust dose as needed and tolerated. Apply to nonirritated and nonirradiated skin on a flat surface of the upper torso; may require replacement in 72 hr if pain has not subsided; do not use torn or damaged systems, serious overdose can occur.

Lozenges

- *Actiq:* Place unit in mouth between cheek and lower gum. Start with initial dose of 200 mcg. Until appropriate dose is reached, an additional dose can be used to treat an episode of breakthrough pain. Redosing may start 15 min after the previous lozenge has been completed. No more than two lozenges should be used for each breakthrough pain episode. Can consider increasing dose if requiring more than one lozenge for treatment of several consecutive breakthrough pain episodes. If more than four lozenges are needed daily, increase the dosage of long-acting opioid. *Actiq* should be sucked slowly over 15 min.
- *Buccal tablets:* Initially, 100-mcg tablet between cheek and gum for 14–25 min; may be repeated in 30 min if needed. Adjust slowly to control pain.
- *Buccal soluble film:* Remove film and place inside cheek; will dissolve within 5–30 min. Available only through FOCUS program.

Ionic delivery system

Apply to chest or upper, outer arm. With each activation, 40 mcg delivered over 10 min. Each system contains 80 doses. May use up to 3 units sequentially, if needed.

Pediatric patients 2–12 yr

Transdermal system

Children 2 yr and older initiating therapy on 25 mcg/hr system should be opioid tolerant and receiving at least 60 mg oral morphine equivalents/day.

Parenteral

2–3 mcg/kg IV as vital signs indicate.

Pharmacokinetics

Route	Onset	Duration
IV	1–2 min	0.5–1 hr
IM	7–8 min	1–2 hr
Transdermal	Gradual	72 hr
Transmucosal	15 min	1 hr

Metabolism: Liver; $T_{1/2}$: 1.5–6 hr
Distribution: Crosses placenta; may enter breast milk
Excretion: Unknown

IV FACTS

Preparation: May be used undiluted or diluted with 250 mL of D_5W. Protect vials from light.
Infusion: Administer slowly by direct injection, each milliliter over at least 1 min, or into running IV tubing.
Incompatibilities: Do not mix with methohexital, pentobarbital, thiopental.

Adverse effects

- **CNS:** *Sedation, clamminess, sweating, headache, vertigo, floating feeling, dizziness, lethargy, confusion, light-headedness,* nervousness, unusual dreams, agitation, euphoria, hallucinations, delirium, insomnia, anxiety, fear, disorientation, impaired mental and physical performance, mood changes, coma, weakness, headache, tremor, seizures
- **CV:** Palpitation, increase or decrease in BP, circulatory depression, **cardiac arrest, shock,** tachycardia, bradycardia, arrhythmia, palpitations
- **Dermatologic:** Rash, hives, pruritus, flushing, warmth, sensitivity to cold
- **EENT:** Diplopia, blurred vision
- **GI:** *Nausea, vomiting,* dry mouth, anorexia, *constipation,* biliary tract spasm
- **GU:** Ureteral spasm, spasm of vesical sphincters, urinary retention or hesitancy, oliguria, antidiuretic effect, reduced libido or potency
- **Local:** Phlebitis following IV injection, pain at injection site; tissue irritation and induration (subcutaneous injection)
- **Respiratory:** Slow, shallow respiration, **apnea,** suppression of cough reflex, laryngospasm, bronchospasm
- **Other:** Physical tolerance and dependence, psychological dependence; local skin irritation with transdermal system

Interactions

✱ **Drug-drug** • Potentiation of effects when given with other CNS acting drugs or barbiturate anesthetics; decrease dose of fentanyl when co-administering • Potentiation of effects may occur when given with macrolide antibiotics, ketoconazole, itraconazole, and protease inhibitors • Do not administer an MAOI within 14 days of fentanyl (increased CNS effects) • Increased risk of adverse effects and toxicity if combined with alcohol

✱ **Drug-food** • Decreased metabolism and risk of toxic effects if taken with grapefruit juice; avoid this combination

✱ **Drug-lab test** • Elevated biliary tract pressure may cause increases in plasma amylase, lipase; determinations of these levels may be unreliable for 24 hr after administration of opioids

■ Nursing considerations

CLINICAL ALERT!
Name confusion has occurred between fentanyl and sufentanil; use extreme caution.

Assessment

- **History:** Hypersensitivity to fentanyl or opioids, physical dependence on an opioid analgesic, pregnancy, labor, lactation, COPD, respiratory depression, anoxia, increased intracranial pressure, acute MI, ventricular failure, coronary insufficiency, hypertension, biliary tract surgery, renal or hepatic impairment
- **Physical:** Orientation, reflexes, bilateral grip strength, affect; pupil size, vision; P, auscultation, BP; R, adventitious sounds; bowel sounds, normal output; LFTs, renal function tests

Interventions

- Administer to women who are nursing a baby 4–6 hr before the next scheduled feeding to minimize the amount in milk.

⊗ ***Black box warning*** Keep opioid antagonist and facilities for assisted or controlled respiration readily available during parenteral administration; ensure appropriate use of drug because it is potentially dangerous. Respiratory depression and death can occur.

- Prepare site for transdermal form by clipping (not shaving) hair at site; do not use soap, oils, lotions, alcohol; let skin dry completely before application. Apply immediately after removal from the sealed package;

firmly press the transdermal system in place with the palm of the hand for 10–20 sec, making sure the contact is complete. Must be worn continually for 72 hr. Do not use any system that has been torn or damaged. Remove old patch before applying a new one.
- Note that the patch doesn't work quickly. It may take up to 12 hr to get the full therapeutic effect. Breakthrough medications may need to be used.
- Do not use *Actiq* in patients who never received opioids before; should be used only in opioid tolerant patients.
- Use caution with *Actiq* form to keep this drug out of the reach of children (it looks like a lollipop) and follow the distribution restrictions in place with this drug very carefully
- Use *Ionsys* only for hospitalized adults. Apply to intact, nonirritated skin on chest or upper arm. Patient presses button twice, firmly. System will deliver dose over 10 min. Up to 3 units may be used sequentially, if needed.
- Buccal soluble film is only available through FOCUS limited-access program. Dispose of unused films by removing from foil pack and flushing down toilet.

Teaching points
- Do not drink grapefruit juice while using this drug. If using the patch, do not use any patch that has been torn or damaged. Remove old patch before applying a new one. If using buccal soluble film, remove from the foil pack and place inside your cheek; it will dissolve within 5 to 30 minutes. Dispose of unused films by removing them from the foil pack, depositing them in the toilet and then flushing the toilet.
- You may experience these side effects: Dizziness, sedation, drowsiness, impaired visual acuity (ask for assistance if you need to move); nausea, loss of appetite (lie quietly, eat frequent small meals); constipation (a laxative may help).
- Report severe nausea, vomiting, palpitations, shortness of breath, or difficulty breathing.

ferrous salts
(fair' us)

ferrous fumarate
Femiron, Ferro-Sequels, Hemocyte, Ircon, Nephro-Fer, Palafer (CAN)

ferrous gluconate
Apo-Ferrous Gluconate (CAN), Fergon

ferrous sulfate
Apo-Ferrous Sulfate (CAN), Feosol, Fer-gen-sol, Fer-In-Sol

ferrous sulfate exsiccated
Feosol, Feratab, Ferodan (CAN), Slow Fe

PREGNANCY CATEGORY A

Drug class
Iron preparation

Therapeutic actions
Elevates the serum iron concentration, and is then converted to Hgb or trapped in the reticuloendothelial cells for storage and eventual conversion to a usable form of iron.

Indications
- Prevention and treatment of iron deficiency anemias
- Dietary supplement for iron
- Unlabeled use: Supplemental use during epoetin therapy to ensure proper hematologic response to epoetin

Contraindications and cautions
- Contraindicated with allergy to any ingredient; sulfite allergy; hemochromatosis, hemosiderosis, hemolytic anemias.
- Use cautiously with normal iron balance; peptic ulcer, regional enteritis, ulcerative colitis.

Available forms

Tablets—sulfate, 324, 325 mg; sulfate exsiccated, 200, 300 mg; gluconate, 240, 325 mg; fumarate, 63, 200, 324, 325, 350 mg; timed-release capsules—sulfate exsiccated, 160 mg; timed-release tablets—sulfate exsiccated, 160 mg; syrup—fumarate (*Ferro-Sequels*), 150 mg; sulfate, 90 mg/5 mL; elixir—sulfate, 220 mg/5 mL; drops—sulfate, 75 mg/0.6 mL, 125 mg/mL; fumarate, 45 mg/0.6 mL; tablet, chewable—fumarate, 100 mg; suspension—fumarate, 100 mg/5 mL

Dosages

Adults

- *Daily requirements:* Men, 8–11 mg/day PO; women, 8–18 mg/day PO; pregnant and lactating women, 9–27 mg/day PO.
- *Replacement in deficiency states:* 150–300 mg/day (6 mg/kg/day) PO for approximately 6–10 mo may be required.

Pediatric patients

- *Daily requirement:* 7–11 mg/day PO.
- *Replacement:* 3–6 mg/kg/day PO.

Pharmacokinetics

Route	*Onset*	*Peak*	*Duration*
Oral	4 days	7–10 days	2–4 mo

Metabolism: Recycled for use; $T_{1/2}$: Not known
Distribution: Crosses placenta; enters breast milk
Excretion: Unknown

Adverse effects

- **CNS:** CNS toxicity, acidosis, **coma and death with overdose**
- **GI:** *GI upset, anorexia, nausea, vomiting, constipation,* diarrhea, dark stools, temporary staining of the teeth (liquid preparations)

Interactions

✱ **Drug-drug** • Decreased anti-infective response to ciprofloxacin, norfloxacin, ofloxacin; separate doses by at least 2 hr • Decreased absorption with antacids, cimetidine • Decreased effects of levodopa if taken with iron • Increased serum iron levels with chloramphenicol • Decreased absorption of levothyroxine; separate doses by at least 2 hr

✱ **Drug-food** • Decreased absorption with antacids, eggs or milk, coffee and tea; avoid concurrent administration of any of these

■ Nursing considerations

Assessment

- **History:** Allergy to any ingredient, sulfite; hemochromatosis, hemosiderosis, hemolytic anemias; normal iron balance; peptic ulcer, regional enteritis, ulcerative colitis
- **Physical:** Skin lesions, color; gums, teeth (color); bowel sounds; CBC, Hgb, Hct, serum ferritin and iron levels

Interventions

- Confirm that patient does have iron deficiency anemia before treatment.
- Give drug with meals (avoiding milk, eggs, coffee, and tea) if GI discomfort is severe; slowly increase to build up tolerance.
- Administer liquid preparations in water or juice to mask the taste and prevent staining of teeth; have the patient drink solution with a straw.
- Warn patient that stool may be dark or green.
- Arrange for periodic monitoring of Hct and Hgb levels.

⊗ ***Black box warning*** Warn patient to keep drug out of children's reach; leading cause of fatal poisoning in children younger than 6 yr.

Teaching points

- Take drug on an empty stomach with water. Take after meals if GI upset is severe (avoid milk, eggs, coffee, and tea).
- Take liquid preparations diluted in water or juice, and sip them through a straw to prevent staining of the teeth.
- Treatment may not be necessary if cause of anemia can be corrected. It may be needed for several months to reverse anemia.
- Have periodic blood tests during therapy to determine the appropriate dosage.
- Do not take this preparation with antacids or tetracyclines. If these drugs are needed, they will be prescribed.
- You may experience these side effects: GI upset, nausea, vomiting (take drug with meals); diarrhea or constipation; dark or green stools.

F

- Keep this drug out of the reach of children.
- Report severe GI upset, lethargy, rapid respirations, constipation.

ferumoxytol

See Appendix W, *Less commonly used drugs.*

fesoterodine fumarate

(fess oh ***tear'*** *oh deen)*

Toviaz (DNC)

PREGNANCY CATEGORY C

Drug class

Antimuscarinic

Therapeutic actions

Competitively blocks muscarinic receptor sites: Bladder contraction is mediated by muscarinic receptors; blocking these receptors decreases bladder contraction and signs and symptoms of bladder overactivity.

Indications

- Treatment of overactive bladder with symptoms of urinary incontinence, urgency, and frequency in adults

Contraindications and cautions

- Contraindicated with known hypersensitivity to any component of the drug; urinary retention; gastric retention; uncontrolled narrow-angle glaucoma.
- Use cautiously with bladder outlet obstruction, decreased GI motility, controlled narrow-angle glaucoma, reduced hepatic function, myasthenia gravis, impaired renal function, pregnancy, lactation.

Available forms

ER tablets (DNC)—4, 8 mg

Dosages

Adults

4 mg/day PO; may be increased to a maximum of 8 mg/day if needed and tolerated.

Pediatric patients

Safety and efficacy not established.

Patients with renal impairment

No dosage adjustment needed in mild to moderate renal impairment. Limit dose to 4 mg/day PO in severe renal impairment.

Patients with hepatic impairment

Not recommended for patients with severe hepatic impairment.

Pharmacokinetics

Route	*Onset*	*Peak*
Oral	Rapid	5 hr

Metabolism: Hepatic; $T_{1/2}$: 7 hr

Distribution: May cross placenta; may enter breast milk

Excretion: Urine

Adverse effects

- **CNS:** Dry eyes, insomnia, drowsiness, blurred vision
- **CV:** Tachycardia
- **GI:** *Dry mouth, constipation*, dyspepsia, nausea, abdominal pain
- **GU:** Dysuria, urinary retention, UTI
- **Respiratory:** URI, cough, dry throat
- **Other:** Back pain, rash, decreased sweating

Interactions

✱ **Drug-drug** • Risk of increased serum levels and toxicity if given with any potent CYP3A4 inhibitor (ketoconazole, itraconazole, clarithromycin); dosage of fesoterodine should not exceed 4 mg/day and patient should be monitored closely

✱ **Drug-food** • Increased risk of drowsiness if combined with alcohol; advise patient to avoid this combination

■ Nursing considerations

Assessment

History: Hypersensitivity to any component of the drug, urinary retention, gastric retention, narrow-angle glaucoma, bladder outlet obstruction, decreased GI motility, reduced hepatic function, myasthenia gravis, impaired renal function, pregnancy, lactation

Physical: IOP reading; orientation; skin color and lesions; R, adventitious sounds; P; bowel sounds; urinary output, prostate palpation, LFT, renal function tests

Interventions

- Monitor IOP before and periodically during treatment if patient has glaucoma.
- Administer tablet with water. Ensure that tablet is swallowed whole, not cut, crushed, or chewed.
- Provide frequent mouth hygiene and sugarless lozenges if dry mouth is a problem.
- Provide frequent small meals if GI upset is a problem.
- Arrange for safety precautions if visual changes are a problem.
- Monitor bowel function and institute a bowel program if constipation becomes an issue.
- Monitor patient in hot environments; decreased ability to sweat can lead to heat prostration.

Teaching points

- Take this drug with water once a day as prescribed. Swallow the tablet whole; do not cut, crush, or chew it.
- You may experience these side effects: Dry mouth (sucking sugarless lozenges, frequent mouth care may help), constipation (ensure adequate fluid intake and fiber in the diet, consult your health care provider if this becomes a serious problem), dry eyes (this effect may pass with time; consult with your health care provider for possible treatment if this becomes severe), blurred vision (avoid driving or operating dangerous machinery until you know how this drug will affect you), difficulty emptying the bladder (it may help to empty your bladder before taking each dose of the drug), decreased ability to sweat (use caution in hot environments, make sure you have plenty of fluids and take precautions to avoid overheating).
- Be aware that alcohol may increase the sedation effects of this drug. Avoid drinking alcohol while on this drug.
- Report tremors, restlessness, thoughts of suicide, increased depression, inability to stay alert, sudden behavioral changes.

▽fexofenadine hydrochloride

(fecks oh ***fen'*** *a deen)*

Allegra, Allegra ODT

PREGNANCY CATEGORY C

Drug class

Antihistamine (nonsedating type)

Therapeutic actions

Competitively blocks the effects of histamine at peripheral H_1-receptor sites; has no anticholinergic (atropine-like) or sedating effects.

Indications

- Symptomatic relief of symptoms associated with seasonal allergic rhinitis in adults and children 2 yr and older
- Chronic idiopathic urticaria in adults and children 6 mo and older

Contraindications and cautions

- Contraindicated with allergy to any antihistamines, pregnancy, lactation.
- Use cautiously with hepatic or renal impairment, in geriatric patients.

Available forms

Tablets—30, 60, 180 mg; suspension—6 mg/mL; orally disintegrating tablets—30 mg

Dosages

Adults and patients 12 yr and older

- *Allergic rhinitis:* 60 mg PO bid or 180 mg once daily.
- *Chronic idiopathic urticaria:* 60 mg PO bid or 180 mg PO once daily.

Pediatric patients 6–11 yr

- *Allergic rhinitis and chronic idiopathic urticaria:* 30 mg orally disintegrating tablet PO bid.

Pediatric patients 2–11 yr

- *Allergic rhinitis and chronic idiopathic urticaria:* 30 mg PO bid.

Pediatric patients 6 mo–2 yr

- *Chronic idiopathic urticaria:* 15 mg (2.5 mL) PO bid.

F

Geriatric patients or patients with renal impairment
For geriatric patients or adults with renal impairment, use 60 mg PO daily. For children 2–11 yr with renal impairment, use 30 mg PO daily. For children 6 mo–2 yr with renal impairment, use 15 mg/day PO.

Pharmacokinetics

Route	*Onset*	*Peak*
Oral	Rapid	2.6 hr

Metabolism: Hepatic; $T_{1/2}$: 14.4 hr
Distribution: Crosses placenta; may enter breast milk
Excretion: Feces, urine

Adverse effects

- **CNS:** Fatigue, drowsiness
- **GI:** Nausea, dyspepsia
- **Other:** Dysmenorrhea, flulike symptoms

Interactions

✱ **Drug-drug** • Increased levels and possible toxicity with ketoconazole, itraconazole, erythromycin; fexofenadine dose may need to be decreased • Decreased effects when taken with antacids

■ Nursing considerations
Assessment

- **History:** Allergy to any antihistamines, renal impairment, pregnancy, lactation
- **Physical:** Mucous membranes, oropharynx, R, adventitious sounds; skin color, lesions; orientation, affect; renal function tests

Interventions

- Arrange for use of humidifier if thickening of secretions, nasal dryness become bothersome; encourage adequate intake of fluids.
- Provide supportive care for flulike symptoms.

Teaching points

- Avoid excessive dosage; take as prescribed.
- Do not take at the same time as antacids.
- Place orally disintegrating tablet on tongue; let disintegrate and then swallow with or without water.
- To maximize effects, take this medication in the morning before exposure to allergens.
- You may experience these side effects: Dizziness, sedation, drowsiness (use caution if driving or performing tasks that require alertness); thickening of bronchial secretions, dryness of nasal mucosa (use of a humidifier may help); menstrual irregularities; flulike symptoms (medication may be helpful).
- Report difficulty breathing, severe nausea, fever.

▽ fibrinogen concentrate, human

See Appendix W, *Less commonly used drugs.*

▽ filgrastim (granulocyte colony-stimulating factor, G-CSF)

*(fill **grass'** stim)*

Neupogen

PREGNANCY CATEGORY C

Drug class

Colony-stimulating factor

Therapeutic actions

Human granulocyte colony-stimulating factor produced by recombinant DNA technology; increases the production of neutrophils within the bone marrow with little effect on the production of other hematopoietic cells.

Indications

- To decrease the incidence of infection in patients with nonmyeloid malignancies receiving myelosuppressive anticancer drugs associated with a significant incidence of severe neutropenia with fever
- To reduce the time to neutrophil recovery and duration of fever, following induction or consolidation chemotherapy treatment of acute myeloid leukemia

- To reduce the duration of neutropenia following bone marrow transplant
- Treatment of severe chronic neutropenia
- Mobilization of hematopoietic progenitor cells into the blood for leukapheresis collection
- Orphan drug uses: Treatment of myelodysplastic syndrome, aplastic anemia, graft failure after bone marrow transplant, hairy cell leukemia, AIDs–drug-induced neutropenias.

Contraindications and cautions

- Contraindicated with hypersensitivity to *Escherichia coli* products.
- Use cautiously with lactation, pregnancy.

Available forms

Injection—300 mcg/mL, 480 mcg/1.6 mL single-dose vials; prefilled syringes—300 mcg/0.5 mL, 480 mcg/0.8 mL

Dosages

Adults

Starting dose is 5 mcg/kg/day subcutaneously or IV as a single daily injection. May be increased in increments of 5 mcg/kg for each chemotherapy cycle; 4–8 mcg/kg/day is usually effective.

- *Bone marrow transplant:* 10 mcg/kg/day IV or continuous subcutaneous infusion.
- *Severe chronic neutropenia:* 6 mcg/kg subcutaneously bid (congenital neutropenia); 5 mcg/kg/day subcutaneously as single injection (idiopathic or cyclic neutropenia).
- *Mobilization for harvesting:* 10 mcg/kg/day subcutaneously at least 4 days before first leukapheresis; continue to last leukapheresis.

Pediatric patients

Safety and efficacy not established.

Pharmacokinetics

Route	*Peak*	*Duration*
Subcut.	8 hr	4 days
IV	2 hr	4 days

Metabolism: Unknown; $T_{1/2}$: 210–231 min
Distribution: Crosses placenta; may enter breast milk
Excretion: Unknown

IV FACTS

Preparation: No special preparation required. Refrigerate; avoid shaking. Before injection, allow to warm to room temperature. Discard vial after one use, and do not reenter vial; discard any vial that has been at room temperature longer than 24 hr.
Infusion: Inject directly IV slowly over 15–30 min, or inject slowly into tubing of running IV over 4–24 hr.
Incompatibilities: Do not mix in solutions other than D_5W. Incompatible with numerous drugs in solution; check manufacturer's details before any combination.

Adverse effects

- **CNS:** Headache, fever, generalized weakness, fatigue
- **Dermatologic:** *Alopecia,* rash, mucositis
- **GI:** *Nausea, vomiting,* stomatitis, anorexia, *diarrhea,* constipation
- **Other:** *Bone pain,* generalized pain, sore throat, cough

■ Nursing considerations

Assessment

- **History:** Hypersensitivity to *E. coli* products, pregnancy, lactation
- **Physical:** Skin color, lesions, hair; T; abdominal examination, status of mucous membranes; CBC with differential, platelets

Interventions

- Obtain CBC and platelet count before and twice weekly during therapy; doses may be increased after chemotherapy cycles according to the duration and severity of bone marrow suppression.

⊗ ***Warning*** Do not give within 24 hr before and after chemotherapy.

- Give daily for up to 2 wk until the neutrophil count is 10,000/mm^3; discontinue therapy if this number is exceeded.
- Store in refrigerator; allow to warm to room temperature before use; if vial is at room temperature for longer than 24 hr, discard. Use each vial for one dose; do not reenter the vial. Discard any unused drug.
- Do not shake vial before use. If subcutaneous dose exceeds 1 mL, consider using two sites.

F

Teaching points

- Store drug in refrigerator; do not shake vial. Each vial can be used only once; do not reuse syringes or needles (proper container for disposal will be provided). Another person should be instructed in the proper administration technique. Use sterile technique.
- Avoid exposure to infection while you are receiving this drug (avoid crowds and people known to have infections).
- Keep appointments for frequent blood tests to evaluate effects of drug on your blood count.
- You may experience these side effects: Bone pain (analgesia may be ordered), nausea and vomiting (eat frequent small meals), loss of hair (it is very important to cover head in extreme temperatures).
- Report fever, chills, severe bone pain, sore throat, weakness, pain or swelling at injection site.

▽ finasteride

(fin as' teh ride)

Propecia, Proscar

PREGNANCY CATEGORY X

Drug class

Androgen hormone inhibitor

Therapeutic actions

Inhibits the intracellular enzyme that converts testosterone into a potent androgen (DHT); does not affect androgen receptors in the body; the prostate gland depends on DHT for its development and maintenance.

Indications

- *Proscar:* Treatment of symptomatic BPH; most effective with long-term use; reduces the need for prostate surgery and reduces the risk of urinary retention; with doxazosin, to reduce the risk of progression of BPH symptoms
- *Propecia:* Prevention of male pattern baldness (androgenetic alopecia) in patients with family history or early signs of loss
- Unlabeled uses: Adjuvant monotherapy following radical prostatectomy; prevention of the progression of first-stage prostate cancer; hirsutism; male chronic pelvic pain syndrome

Contraindications and cautions

- Contraindicated with allergy to finasteride or any component of the product, pregnancy, lactation.
- Use cautiously with hepatic impairment.

Available forms

Tablets—1 mg (*Propecia*), 5 mg (*Proscar*)

Dosages

Adults

- *BPH:* 5 mg daily PO with or without meals; may take 6–12 mo for response (*Proscar*).
- *Male pattern baldness:* 1 mg/day PO (*Propecia*).

Pediatric patients

Safety and efficacy not established.

Geriatric patients or patients with renal insufficiency

No dosage adjustment is needed.

Pharmacokinetics

Route	*Onset*	*Peak*	*Duration*
Oral	Rapid	8 hr	24 hr

Metabolism: Hepatic; $T_{1/2}$: 6 hr
Distribution: Crosses placenta; may enter breast milk (not used in women)
Excretion: Feces, urine

Adverse effects

- **GI:** Abdominal upset
- **GU:** *Impotence, decreased libido,* decreased volume of ejaculation
- **Other:** Gynecomastia

Interactions

✱ **Drug-lab test** • Decreased PSA levels when measured; false decrease does not mean patient is free of risk of prostate cancer

■ Nursing considerations

Assessment

- **History:** Allergy to finasteride or any component, hepatic impairment, pregnancy, lactation
- **Physical:** Liver evaluation, abdominal examination; renal function tests, normal urine output, prostate examination

Interventions

- Confirm that problem is BPH, and other disorders (prostate cancer, infection, strictures, hypotonic bladder) have been ruled out.
- Administer without regard to meals; protect container from light.
- Arrange for regular follow-up, including prostate examination, PSA levels, and evaluation of urine flow.
- Monitor urine flow and output; increase in urine flow may not occur in all situations.

⊗ ***Warning*** Do not allow pregnant women to handle crushed or broken tablets because of risk of inadvertent absorption, adversely affecting the fetus.

- Alert patient that libido may be decreased as well as the volume of ejaculate; usually reversible when the drug is stopped.

Teaching points

- Take this drug once a day without regard to meals; protect from light.
- Have regular medical follow-up to evaluate your response. Your health care provider will monitor your liver and kidney function as well as prostate-specific antigen levels.
- This drug has serious adverse effects on unborn babies. Do not allow a pregnant woman to handle the tablet if it is crushed or broken.
- You may experience these side effects: Loss of libido, impotence, decreased amount of ejaculate (usually reversible when the drug is stopped); breast enlargement, tenderness.
- Report inability to void, groin pain, sore throat, fever, weakness.

▽ flavoxate hydrochloride

(fla vox' ate)

Urispas

PREGNANCY CATEGORY B

Drug classes

Parasympathetic blocker
Urinary antispasmodic

Therapeutic actions

Counteracts smooth muscle spasm of the urinary tract by relaxing the detrusor and other muscles through action at the parasympathetic receptors; has local anesthetic and analgesic properties.

Indications

- Symptomatic relief of dysuria, urgency, nocturia, suprapubic pain, frequency and incontinence due to cystitis, prostatitis, urethritis, urethrocystitis, urethrotrigonitis

Contraindications and cautions

- Contraindicated with allergy to flavoxate, pyloric or duodenal obstruction, obstructive intestinal lesions or ileus, achalasia, GI hemorrhage, obstructive uropathies of the lower urinary tract.
- Use cautiously with glaucoma, pregnancy, lactation.

Available forms

Tablets—100 mg

Dosages

Adults and patients 12 yr and older

100–200 mg PO tid or qid. Reduce dose when symptoms improve. Use up to 1,200 mg/day in severe urinary urgency following pelvic radiotherapy.

Pediatric patients younger than 12 yr

Safety and efficacy not established.

Pharmacokinetics

Route	*Onset*	*Duration*
Oral	Slow	6 hr

Metabolism: $T_{1/2}$: 2–3 hr
Distribution: May cross placenta
Excretion: Feces, urine

Adverse effects

- **CNS:** *Nervousness, vertigo, headache, drowsiness,* mental confusion, hyperpyrexia, *blurred vision,* increased ocular tension, disturbance in accommodation
- **CV:** Tachycardia, palpitations
- **Dermatologic:** Urticaria, dermatoses
- **GI:** *Nausea, vomiting, dry mouth*
- **GU:** Dysuria
- **Hematologic: Eosinophilia, leukopenia**

Interactions

✱ **Drug-drug** • Risk of toxic effects if combined with anticholinergic drugs • Loss of effectiveness of cholinergic drugs such as Alzheimer's disease drugs if combined

■ Nursing considerations

Assessment

- **History:** Allergy to flavoxate, pyloric or duodenal obstruction, obstructive intestinal lesions or ileus, achalasia, GI hemorrhage, obstructive uropathies of the lower urinary tract, glaucoma, pregnancy, lactation
- **Physical:** Skin color, lesions; T; orientation, affect, reflexes, ophthalmic examination, ocular pressure measurement; P; bowel sounds, oral mucous membranes; CBC, stool guaiac

Interventions

- Arrange for definitive treatment of UTIs causing the symptoms being managed by flavoxate.
- Arrange for ophthalmic examination before and during therapy.

Teaching points

- Take drug three or four times a day.
- This drug is meant to relieve the symptoms you are experiencing; other medications will be used to treat the cause.
- You may experience these side effects: Dry mouth, GI upset (suck on sugarless lozenges and use frequent mouth care); drowsiness, blurred vision (avoid driving or performing tasks requiring alertness).
- Report blurred vision, fever, rash, nausea, vomiting.

▽ flecainide acetate

*(fle **ka'** nide)*

Tambocor

PREGNANCY CATEGORY C

Drug class

Antiarrhythmic

Therapeutic actions

Type 1c antiarrhythmic: Acts selectively to depress fast sodium channels, decreasing the height and rate of rise of cardiac action potentials and slowing conduction in all parts of the heart.

Indications

- Prevention and treatment of life-threatening ventricular arrhythmias, such as sustained ventricular tachycardia (not recommended for less severe ventricular arrhythmias)
- Prevention of paroxysmal atrial fibrillation or flutter (PAF) associated with symptoms and paroxysmal supraventricular tachycardias (PSVT), including atrioventricular nodal and atrioventricular reentrant tachycardia; other supraventricular tachycardias of unspecified mechanism with disabling symptoms in patients without structural heart disease

Contraindications and cautions

- Contraindicated with allergy to flecainide; heart failure; cardiogenic shock; cardiac conduction abnormalities (heart blocks of any kind, unless an artificial pacemaker is present to maintain heartbeat); MI; sick sinus syndrome; lactation, pregnancy.
- Use cautiously with endocardial pacemaker (permanent or temporary—stimulus parameters may need to be increased); heart failure; hepatic or renal disease; potassium imbalance.

Available forms

Tablets—50, 100, 150 mg

Dosages

Evaluation with close monitoring of cardiac response necessary for determining the correct dosage.

Adults

- *PSVT and PAF:* Starting dose of 50 mg every 12 hr PO; may be increased in increments of 50 mg bid every 4 days until efficacy is achieved; maximum dose is 300 mg/day.
- *Sustained ventricular tachycardia:* 100 mg every 12 hr PO. Increase in 50-mg increments twice a day every fourth day until efficacy is achieved. Maximum dose is 400 mg/day.
- *Heart failure:* Initial dose of no more than 100 mg every 12 hr PO. May increase in 50-mg increments bid every fourth day to a maximum of 200 mg/day; higher doses associated with increased heart failure.
- *Transfer to flecainide:* Allow at least 2–4 plasma half-lives to elapse after other antiarrhythmic drugs discontinued before starting flecainide. Consider hospitalization because withdrawal of a previous antiarrhythmic is likely to produce life-threatening arrhythmias.

Pediatric patients

Safety and efficacy in patients younger than 18 yr have not been established.

Patients with renal impairment

Initial dose, 100 mg daily PO or 50 mg every 12 hr. Wait about 4 days to reach a steady state, then increase dose cautiously.

Geriatric patients

Elimination may be slower. Usual dose should be used in patients up to 80 yr.

Pharmacokinetics

Route	*Onset*	*Peak*	*Duration*
Oral	30–60 min	3 hr	24 hr

Metabolism: Hepatic; $T_{1/2}$: 20 hr
Distribution: Crosses placenta; may enter breast milk
Excretion: Feces, urine

Adverse effects

- **CNS:** *Dizziness, fatigue, drowsiness, visual changes, headache*, tinnitus, paresthesias
- **CV:** *Cardiac arrhythmias*, heart failure, slowed cardiac conduction, *palpitations, chest pain*
- **GI:** *Nausea, vomiting, abdominal pain, constipation*, diarrhea
- **GU:** Polyuria, urinary retention, decreased libido
- **Other:** *Dyspnea,* sweating, hot flashes, night sweats, **leukopenia**

Interactions

✱ **Drug-drug** ⊗ ***Warning*** Risk of marked drop in cardiac output if combined with disopyramide or verapamil; avoid these combinations if possible.
• Risk of increased flecainide levels if combined with amiodarone, cimetidine, propranolol

■ Nursing considerations

Assessment

- **History:** Allergy to flecainide, heart failure, MI, cardiogenic shock, cardiac conduction abnormalities, sick sinus syndrome, endocardial pacemaker, hepatic or renal disease, potassium imbalance, lactation, pregnancy
- **Physical:** Weight; orientation, reflexes, vision; P, BP, auscultation, ECG, edema, R, adventitious sounds; bowel sounds, liver evaluation; urinalysis, CBC, serum electrolytes, LFTs, renal function tests

Interventions

⊗ ***Black box warning*** In patients with recent MI or chronic atrial fibrillation, treatment increases risk of nonfatal cardiac arrest and death.

- Monitor patient response carefully, especially when beginning therapy.
- Reduce dosage in patients with renal disease or hepatic failure.
- Check serum K^+ levels before giving.

⊗ ***Black box warning*** Monitor cardiac rhythm carefully; risk of potentially fatal proarrhythmias.

⊗ ***Warning*** Evaluate for therapeutic serum levels of 0.2–1 mcg/mL.

⊗ ***Warning*** Keep life support equipment, including pacemaker, readily available in case serious CVS, CNS effects occur—also keep dopamine, dobutamine, isoproterenol, or other positive inotropics nearby.

Teaching points

- You will need frequent monitoring of cardiac rhythm.
- Do not stop taking this drug for any reason without checking with your health care provider. Drug is taken at 12-hour intervals; work out a schedule so you take the drug as prescribed without waking up at night.
- Return for regular follow-up visits to check your heart rhythm and have a blood test to check your blood levels of this drug.
- You may experience these side effects: Drowsiness, dizziness, numbness, visual disturbances (avoid driving or using dangerous machinery); nausea, vomiting (frequent small meals may help); diarrhea, polyuria; sweating, night sweats, hot flashes, loss of libido (reversible after stopping the drug); palpitations.
- Report swelling of ankles or fingers, palpitations, fainting, chest pain.

▽ floxuridine

See Appendix W, *Less commonly used drugs.*

▽ fluconazole

(floo ***kon'*** *a zole)*

Apo-Fluconazole (CAN), Diflucan, Gen-Fluconazole (CAN), PMS-Fluconazole (CAN)

PREGNANCY CATEGORY C

Drug class

Antifungal

Therapeutic actions

Binds to sterols in the fungal cell membrane, changing membrane permeability; fungicidal or fungistatic depending on concentration and organism.

Indications

- Treatment of oropharyngeal, esophageal, vaginal, and systemic candidiasis, UTI and peritonitis caused by *Candida*
- Treatment of cryptococcal meningitis
- Prophylaxis of candidiasis in bone marrow transplants

Contraindications and cautions

- Contraindicated with hypersensitivity to fluconazole, lactation.
- Use cautiously with renal or hepatic impairment.

Available forms

Tablets—50, 100, 150, 200 mg; powder for oral suspension—10, 40 mg/mL; injection—2 mg/mL

Dosages

Individualize dosage; same for oral or IV routes because of rapid and almost complete absorption.

Adults

- *Oropharyngeal candidiasis:* 200 mg PO or IV on the first day, followed by 100 mg daily. Continue treatment for at least 2 wk to decrease likelihood of relapse.
- *Esophageal candidiasis:* 200 mg PO or IV on the first day, followed by 100 mg daily. Dosage up to 400 mg/day may be used in severe cases. Treat for a minimum of 3 wk; at least 2 wk after resolution.
- *Vaginal candidiasis:* 150 mg PO as a single dose.
- *Systemic candidiasis:* 400 mg PO or IV daily.
- *Candida UTI and peritonitis:* 50–200 mg/day PO.
- *Cryptococcal meningitis:* 400 mg PO or IV on the first day, followed by 200 mg daily. 400 mg daily may be needed. Continue treatment for 10–12 wk after cultures of CSF become negative.
- *Suppression of cryptococcal meningitis in AIDS patients:* 200 mg daily PO or IV.
- *Prevention of candidiasis in bone marrow transplants:* 400 mg PO daily for several days before onset of neutropenia and for 7 days after neutrophil count rises above 1,000 cells/mm^3.

Pediatric patients

Maximum daily dosage for children is 600 mg/day.

- *Oropharyngeal candidiasis:* 6 mg/kg PO or IV on the first day, followed by 3 mg/kg once daily for at least 2 wk.
- *Esophageal candidiasis:* 6 mg/kg PO or IV on the first day, followed by 3 mg/kg once daily. Treat for a minimum of 3 wk; at least 2 wk after resolution.
- *Systemic* Candida *infections:* Daily doses of 6–12 mg/kg/day PO or IV.
- *Cryptococcal meningitis:* 12 mg/kg PO or IV on the first day, followed by 6 mg/kg once daily. Continue treatment for 10–12 wk after cultures of CSF become negative.
- *Suppression of cryptococcal meningitis in children with AIDS:* 6 mg/kg daily PO or IV.

Patients with renal impairment

Initial dose of 50–400 mg PO or IV. If creatinine clearance is greater than 50 mL/min, use 100% of recommended dose; for creatinine clearance less than or equal to 50 mL/min, use 50% of recommended dose; for patients on hemodialysis, use one full dose after each dialysis.

Pharmacokinetics

Route	*Onset*	*Peak*	*Duration*
Oral	Slow	1–2 hr	2–4 days
IV	Rapid	1 hr	2–4 days

Metabolism: Hepatic; $T_{1/2}$: 30 hr
Distribution: Crosses placenta; may enter breast milk
Excretion: Urine

IV FACTS

Preparation: Do not remove overwrap until ready for use. Inner bag maintains sterility of product. Do not use plastic containers in series connections. Tear overwrap down side at slit, and remove solution container. Some opacity of plastic may occur; check for minute leaks, squeezing bag firmly. Discard solution if any leaks are found.
Infusion: Infuse at a maximum rate of 200 mg/hr given as a continuous infusion.
Incompatibilities: Do not add any supplementary medications.

Adverse effects

- **CNS:** *Headache*
- **GI:** *Nausea, vomiting, diarrhea, abdominal pain,* AST/ALT elevations
- **Other:** Rash

Interactions

✱ **Drug-drug** • Increased serum levels and therefore therapeutic and toxic effects of cyclosporine, phenytoin, benzodiazepines, oral hypoglycemics, warfarin anticoagulants, zidovudine • Decreased serum levels with rifampin, cimetidine

■ Nursing considerations

Assessment

- **History:** Hypersensitivity to fluconazole and other azoles, renal impairment, lactation, pregnancy
- **Physical:** Skin color, lesions; T; injection site; orientation, reflexes, affect; bowel sounds; LFTs, renal function tests; CBC and differential; culture of area involved

Interventions

- Culture infection before therapy; begin treatment before lab results are returned.
- Decrease dosage in cases of renal failure.
- Infuse IV only; not intended for IM or subcutaneous use.
- Do not add supplement medication to fluconazole.
- Administer through sterile equipment at a maximum rate of 200 mg/hr given as a continuous infusion.

⊗ ***Warning*** Monitor renal function tests weekly, discontinue or decrease dosage of drug at any sign of increased renal toxicity. Monitor liver function tests monthly during therapy.

Teaching points

- Drug may be given orally or IV as needed. The drug will need to be taken for the full course and may need to be taken long term.
- Use hygiene measures to prevent reinfection or spread of infection.
- Arrange for frequent follow-up while you are taking this drug. Be sure to keep all appointments, including those for blood tests.
- You may experience these side effects: Nausea, vomiting, diarrhea (frequent small meals may help); headache (analgesics may be ordered).
- Report rash, changes in stool or urine color, difficulty breathing, increased tears or salivation.

flucytosine (5-FC, 5-fluorocytosine)

(floo sye' toe seen)

Ancobon

PREGNANCY CATEGORY C

Drug class
Antifungal

Therapeutic actions
Affects cell membranes of susceptible fungi to cause fungus death; exact mechanism of action is not understood.

Indications
- Treatment of serious infections caused by susceptible strains of *Candida, Cryptococcus*

Contraindications and cautions
- Contraindicated with allergy to flucytosine, pregnancy, lactation.
- Use cautiously with renal impairment (drug accumulation and toxicity may occur), hepatic impairment, bone marrow depression.

Available forms
Capsules—250, 500 mg

Dosages
Adults

50–150 mg/kg/day PO at 6-hr intervals.

Pediatric patients

Safety and efficacy not established.

Patients with renal impairment

Adjust dosing interval based on creatinine clearance: maintain blood levels below 100 mcg/mL.

CrCl (mg/mL)	*Dosing Interval*
20–40	Every 12 hr
10–20	Every 24 hr
Less than 10	Every 24–48 hr

Pharmacokinetics

Route	*Onset*	*Peak*	*Duration*
Oral	Varies	2 hr	10–12 hr

Metabolism: Not significantly metabolized; $T_{1/2}$: 2–5 hr
Distribution: Crosses placenta; may enter breast milk
Excretion: Urine

Adverse effects
- **CNS:** Confusion, hallucinations, headache, sedation, vertigo
- **CV: Cardiac arrest,** chest pain
- **Dermatologic:** *Rash*
- **GI:** *Nausea, vomiting, diarrhea*
- **Hematologic:** *Anemia,* **leukopenia, thrombopenia,** elevation of liver enzymes, BUN, creatinine
- **Respiratory: Respiratory arrest,** shortness of breath

■ Nursing considerations
Assessment
- **History:** Allergy to flucytosine, renal impairment, bone marrow depression, lactation, pregnancy
- **Physical:** Skin color, lesions; orientation, reflexes, affect; bowel sounds, liver evaluation; LFTs, renal function tests; CBC and differential; serum flucytosine levels (in patients with renal impairment)

Interventions
- Administer capsules a few at a time over a 15-min period to decrease the GI upset and diarrhea.
- Monitor LFTs, renal function tests and hematologic function periodically throughout treatment.

⊗ ***Black box warning*** Monitor serum flucytosine levels in patients with renal impairment (levels higher than 100 mcg/mL associated with toxicity).

Teaching points
- Take the capsules a few at a time over a 15-minute period to decrease GI upset.
- You may experience these side effects: Nausea, vomiting, diarrhea (take capsules a few at a time over 15 minutes); sedation, dizziness, confusion (avoid driving or performing tasks that require alertness).

- Report rash, severe nausea, vomiting, diarrhea, fever, sore throat, unusual bleeding or bruising.

DANGEROUS DRUG

fludarabine phosphate

*(floo **dar'** a been)*

Fludara

PREGNANCY CATEGORY D

Drug classes

Antimetabolite
Antineoplastic

Therapeutic actions

Inhibits DNA polymerase alpha, ribonucleotide reductase and DNA primase, which inhibits DNA synthesis and prevents cell replication.

Indications

- Chronic lymphocytic leukemia (CLL); unresponsive B-cell CLL or no progress during treatment with at least one standard regimen that contains an alkylating drug
- Unlabeled uses: Non-Hodgkin's lymphoma, relapsing and secondary AML, acute lymphoblastic anemia

Contraindications and cautions

- Contraindicated with allergy to fludarabine or any component, lactation, pregnancy, severe bone marrow depression.
- Use cautiously with renal impairment.

Available forms

Powder for reconstitution—50 mg; injection—25 mg/mL

Dosages

Adults

25 mg/m^2 IV over 30 min for 5 consecutive days. Begin each 5-day course every 28 days. Recommendation is to use three additional cycles after a maximal response is achieved, then to discontinue drug.

Patients with renal impairment

Creatinine clearance of 30–70 mL/mm, reduce dosage by 20%; creatinine clearance of less than 30 mL/mm, do not administer.

Pharmacokinetics

Route	*Onset*	*Peak*
IV	Rapid	1–2 hr

Metabolism: Hepatic; $T_{1/2}$: 10 hr
Distribution: Crosses placenta; enters breast milk
Excretion: Urine

IV FACTS

Preparation: Reconstitute with 2 mL of sterile water for injection; the solid cake should dissolve in less than 15 sec; each mL of resulting solution will contain 25 mg fludarabine; may be further diluted in 100 or 125 mL of 5% dextrose injection or 0.9% sodium chloride; use within 8 hr of reconstitution; discard after that time. Store unreconstituted drug in refrigerator.
Infusion: Infuse slowly over no less than 30 min.

Adverse effects

- **CNS:** *Weakness, paresthesia, headache, visual disturbance,* hearing loss, sleep disorder, depression, **CNS toxicity**
- **CV:** *Edema,* angina
- **Dermatologic:** *Rash, pruritus,* seborrhea
- **GI:** *Diarrhea, anorexia, nausea, vomiting, stomatitis,* esophagopharyngitis, GI bleeding, mucositis
- **GU:** Dysuria, urinary infection, hematuria, **renal failure**
- **Hematologic:** *Bone marrow toxicity,* **autoimmune hemolytic anemia**
- **Respiratory:** *Cough, pneumonia, dyspnea, sinusitis,* URI, epistaxis, bronchitis, hypoxia
- **Other:** *Fever, chills, fatigue, infection, pain, malaise,* diaphoresis, hemorrhage, myalgia, arthralgia, osteoporosis, **tumor lysis syndrome**

F

■ Nursing considerations

Assessment

- **History:** Allergy to fludarabine or any component, lactation, pregnancy, severe bone marrow depression, renal impairment
- **Physical:** Weight; T; skin lesions, color, edema; hair; vision, speech, orientation, reflexes, sensation; R, adventitious sounds; mucous membranes, liver evaluation, abdominal examination; CBC, differential; Hgb, Hct, uric acid, LFTs, renal function tests; urinalysis, chest X-ray

Interventions

- Evaluate hematologic status before therapy and before each dose.

⊗ ***Black box warning*** Discontinue therapy if any sign of toxicity occurs (CNS complaints, stomatitis, esophagopharyngitis, rapidly falling WBC count, intractable vomiting, diarrhea, GI ulceration and bleeding, thrombocytopenia, hemorrhage); serious to life-threatening infections have occurred. Consult physician.

- Caution patient to avoid pregnancy while taking this drug.

Teaching points

- Prepare a calendar of treatment days.
- Use birth control while taking this drug; may cause birth defects or miscarriages.
- Have frequent, regular medical follow-up visits, including blood tests.
- You may experience these side effects: Nausea, vomiting, loss of appetite (medication; eat frequent small meals; maintain your nutrition while you are taking this drug); headache, fatigue, malaise, weakness, lethargy (avoid driving or operating dangerous machinery); mouth sores (practice frequent mouth care); diarrhea; increased susceptibility to infection (avoid crowds, exposure to infection; report any sign of infection—fever, fatigue).
- Report black, tarry stools; fever; chills; sore throat; unusual bleeding or bruising; chest pain; mouth sores; changes in vision; dizziness.

▽ fludrocortisone acetate

See Appendix W, *Less commonly used drugs.*

▽ flumazenil

*(floo **maz'** eh nill)*

Anexate (CAN), Romazicon

PREGNANCY CATEGORY C

Drug classes

Antidote
Benzodiazepine receptor antagonist

Therapeutic actions

Antagonizes the actions of benzodiazepines on the CNS and inhibits activity at GABA-benzodiazepine receptor sites.

Indications

- Complete or partial reversal of the sedative effects of benzodiazepines when general anesthesia has been induced or maintained with them, and when sedation has been produced for diagnostic and therapeutic procedures
- Management of benzodiazepine overdose

Contraindications and cautions

- Contraindicated with hypersensitivity to flumazenil or benzodiazepines; patients who have been given benzodiazepines to control potentially life-threatening conditions; patients showing signs of serious cyclic antidepressant overdose.
- Use cautiously with history of seizures, hepatic impairment, panic disorders, head injury, history of drug or alcohol dependence, pregnancy, lactation.

Available forms

Injection—0.1 mg/mL

Dosages

Use smallest effective dose possible.

Adults

- *Reversal of conscious sedation or in general anesthesia:* Give initial dose of 0.2 mg (2 mL) IV over 15 sec then wait 45 sec; if ineffectual, repeat dose at 60-sec intervals. Maximum cumulative dose of 1 mg (10 mL).
- *Management of suspected benzodiazepine overdose:* Give initial dose of 0.2 mg IV over 30 sec; repeat with 0.3 mg IV every 30 sec, up to a maximum cumulative dose of 3 mg.

Pediatric patients younger than 1 yr
Safety and efficacy not established.

Pediatric patients older than 1 yr

- *Reversal of conscious sedation with benzodiazepines:* 0.01 mg/kg (up to 0.2 mg) IV over 15 sec; if ineffectual after 45 sec, repeat dose at 60-sec intervals. Maximum cumulative dose, 0.05 mg/kg or 1 mg, whichever is lowest.

Pharmacokinetics

Route	Onset	Peak	Duration
IV	1–2 min	6–10 min	72 hr

Metabolism: Hepatic; $T_{1/2}$: 54 min
Distribution: Crosses placenta; may enter breast milk
Excretion: Unknown

IV FACTS

Preparation: Can be drawn into syringe with D_5W, lactated Ringer's, and normal saline solutions. Discard within 24 hr if mixed in solution. Do not remove from vial until ready for use.
Infusion: Infuse slowly over 15 sec for general anesthesia, over 30 sec for overdose. To reduce pain of injection, administer through a freely running IV infusion in a large vein.
Compatibilities: Stable with aminophylline, dobutamine, cimetidine, famotidine, ranitidine, heparin, lidocaine, procainamide.

Adverse effects

- **CNS:** *Dizziness, vertigo,* agitation, nervousness, dry mouth, tremor, palpitations, emotional lability, confusion, crying, vision changes, seizures
- **CV:** Vasodilation, flushing, arrhythmias, chest pain
- **GI:** *Nausea, vomiting,* hiccups
- **Other:** *Pain at injection site, increased sweating*

Interactions

✱ **Drug-food** • Ingestion of food during IV infusion decreases serum levels and effectiveness

■ Nursing considerations

Assessment

- **History:** Hypersensitivity to flumazenil or benzodiazepines; use of benzodiazepines for control of potentially life-threatening conditions; signs of serious cyclic antidepressant overdose, history of seizures, hepatic impairment, panic disorders, head injury, history of drug or alcohol dependence, pregnancy, lactation
- **Physical:** Skin color, lesions; T; orientation, reflexes, affect; P, BP, peripheral perfusion; serum drug levels

Interventions

- Administer by IV route only.

⊗ ***Warning*** Have emergency equipment ready, secure airway during administration.

⊗ ***Black box warning*** Drug may increase the risk of seizures, especially in patients on long-term benzodiazepine therapy and patients with serious cyclic antidepressant overdose; take appropriate precautions.

- Monitor clinical response carefully to determine effects of drug and need for repeated doses.
- Inject into running IV in a large vein to decrease pain of injection.
- Provide patient with written information after use; amnesia may be long-term, and teaching may not be remembered, including safety measures.

Teaching points

- Do not use any alcohol or over-the-counter drugs for 18–24 hours after use of this drug.
- Drug may cause changes in vision, dizziness, changes in alertness (avoid driving or operating hazardous machinery for at least 18–24 hours after drug use).
- Report difficulty breathing, pain at IV site, changes in vision, severe headache.

F

flunisolide

*(floo **niss'** oh lide)*

AeroBid, AeroBid-M, Aerospan HFA, Apo-Flunisolide (CAN), Nasarel, ratio-Flunisolide (CAN)

PREGNANCY CATEGORY C

Drug classes

Corticosteroid
Glucocorticoid
Hormone

Therapeutic actions

Anti-inflammatory effect; local administration into lower respiratory tract or nasal passages maximizes beneficial effects while decreasing possible adverse effects from systemic absorption.

Indications

- Intranasal: Relief and management of nasal symptoms of seasonal or perennial allergic rhinitis
- Inhalation: Maintenance treatment of asthma

Contraindications and cautions

- Contraindicated with systemic fungal infections, untreated local nasal infections, epistaxis, nasal trauma, septal ulcers, recent nasal surgery.
- Use cautiously with pregnancy, lactation, status asthmaticus.

Available forms

Intranasal solution, spray—25 mcg/actuation; inhalation—80 mcg/actuation, 250 mcg/actuation

Dosages

Intranasal

Each actuation of the inhaler delivers 25 mcg.

Adults

Initial dosage, two sprays (50 mcg) in each nostril bid (total dose 200 mcg/day); may be increased to two sprays in each nostril tid (total dose 300 mcg/day). Maximum daily dose, eight sprays in each nostril (400 mcg/day).

Pediatric patients 6–14 yr

Initial dosage, one spray in each nostril tid or two sprays in each nostril bid (total dose 150–200 mcg/day). Maximum daily dose, four sprays in each nostril (200 mcg/day). For maintenance dosage, reduce to smallest effective dose. Discontinue therapy after 3 wk if no significant symptomatic improvement.

Pediatric patients younger than 6 yr

Not recommended.

Inhalation

Each actuation of the inhaler delivers either 80 or 250 mcg.

Adults

Two inhalations by mouth bid. Maximum *AeroBid* dosage 2 mg/day; maximum *Aerospan* dosage 640 mcg.

Pediatric patients

- *AeroBid:* For 6–15 yr, dosage same as for adults. Maximum dosage 1 mg/day.
- *Aerospan:* For 12 yr and older, dosage same as for adults. For 6–11 yr, one inhalation bid. Maximum, 160 mcg bid. For younger than 6 yr, not recommended.

Pharmacokinetics

Route	*Onset*	*Peak*	*Duration*
Intranasal	Slow	10–30 min	4–6 hr
Inhalation	Fast	Unknown	Unknown

Metabolism: Hepatic; $T_{1/2}$: 1–2 hr
Distribution: Crosses placenta; enters breast milk
Excretion: Feces, urine

Adverse effects

- **CNS:** *Headache*
- **Dermatologic:** Urticaria
- **Endocrine:** HPA suppression, Cushing's syndrome with overdosage
- **GI:** Nausea
- **Local:** *Nasal irritation, fungal infection*
- **Respiratory:** *Epistaxis, rebound congestion,* perforation of the nasal septum, anosmia

■ Nursing considerations

Assessment

- **History:** Systemic fungal infections, untreated local nasal infections, epistaxis, nasal trauma, septal ulcers, recent nasal surgery, lactation
- **Physical:** Weight, T; BP, P, auscultation, R, adventitious sounds, examination of nares

Interventions

- Do not use during an acute asthmatic attack or to manage status asthmaticus.

⊗ ***Warning*** Taper systemic steroids carefully during transfer to inhalational steroids; deaths from adrenal insufficiency have occurred.

- Use decongestant nose drops to facilitate penetration if edema or excessive secretions are present.

Teaching points

- Do not use this drug more often than prescribed. Do not use this drug during an acute asthmatic attack.
- Do not stop using this drug without consulting your health care provider.
- Use decongestant nose drops first if nasal passages are blocked when using intranasal form.
- After using the inhaler, rinse your mouth with water or mouthwash to prevent oral candidiasis.
- You may experience these side effects: Local irritation (make sure you are using your device correctly), headache.
- Report sore mouth, sore throat.

DANGEROUS DRUG

▽fluorouracil (5-fluorouracil, 5-FU)

*(flure oh **yoor'** a sill)*

Adrucil, Carac, Efudex, Fluoroplex

PREGNANCY CATEGORY D

Drug classes

Antimetabolite
Antineoplastic

Therapeutic actions

Inhibits thymidylate synthetase, leading to inhibition of DNA synthesis and cell death.

Indications

- Parenteral: Palliative management of carcinoma of the colon, rectum, breast, stomach, pancreas in selected patients considered incurable by surgery or other means
- Topical treatment of multiple actinic or solar keratoses
- Topical treatment of superficial basal cell carcinoma
- Orphan drug uses: In combination with interferon alfa 2-a recombinant for esophageal and advanced colorectal carcinoma; with leucovorin for colon or rectum metastatic adenocarcinoma
- Unlabeled use: Topical treatment of condylomata acuminata

Contraindications and cautions

- Contraindicated with allergy to 5-FU; poor nutritional status; serious infections; lactation.
- Use cautiously with hematopoietic depression secondary to radiation or chemotherapy; impaired liver function; pregnancy.

Available forms

Injection—50 mg/mL; cream—0.5%, 1%, 5%; topical solution—2%, 5%

Dosages

IV

Adults

Initial dosage, 12 mg/kg IV daily for 4 successive days; do not exceed 800 mg/day. If no toxicity occurs, give 6 mg/kg on the days 6, 8, 10, and 12, with no drug therapy on days 5, 7, 9, and 11. Discontinue therapy at end of day 12, even if no toxicity.

Poor-risk or undernourished patients

6 mg/kg/day IV for 3 days. If no toxicity develops, give 3 mg/kg on the days 5, 7, and 9. No drug is given on days 4, 6, and 8. Do not exceed 400 mg/day.

Patients with hepatic failure

If serum bilirubin exceeds 5 mg/dL, do not administer 5-FU. For maintenance therapy, continue therapy on appropriate schedules:

- *For patients without toxicity:* Repeat dosage every 30 days after the last day of the previous treatment.

- *For patients with toxicity:* Give 10–15 mg/kg/wk as a single dose after signs of toxicity subside. Do not exceed 1 g/wk. Adjust dosage based on patient response; therapy may be prolonged (12–60 mo).

Topical

Adults

- *Actinic or solar keratoses:* Apply bid to cover lesions. Usually, 0.5% and 1% preparations are used on head, neck, and chest while 2% and 5% preparations are used on hands. Continue until inflammatory response reaches erosion, necrosis, and ulceration stage, then discontinue. Usual course of therapy is 2–4 wk. Complete healing may not be evident for 1–2 mo after cessation of therapy.
- *Superficial basal cell carcinoma:* Apply 5% strength bid in an amount sufficient to cover the lesions. Continue treatment for at least 3–6 wk. Treatment may be required for 10–12 wk.

Pharmacokinetics

Route	Onset	Peak	Duration
IV	Immediate	1–2 hr	6 hr

Metabolism: Hepatic; $T_{1/2}$: 18–20 min
Distribution: Crosses placenta; enters breast milk
Excretion: Lungs, urine

IV FACTS

Preparation: Store vials at room temperature; solution may discolor during storage with no adverse effects. Protect ampule from light. Precipitate may form during storage, heat to 60° C, and shake vigorously to dissolve. Cool to body temperature before administration. No dilution is required.
Infusion: Infuse slowly over 24 hr; inject into tubing of running IV to avoid pain on injection; direct injection over 1–3 min.
Incompatibilities: Do not mix with IV additives or other chemotherapeutic drugs.
Y-site incompatibility: Do not inject with droperidol.

Adverse effects

Parenteral

- **CNS:** *Lethargy, malaise, weakness,* euphoria, acute cerebellar syndrome, photophobia, lacrimation, decreased vision, nystagmus, diplopia
- **CV:** Myocardial ischemia, angina
- **Dermatologic:** *Alopecia, dermatitis, maculopapular rash, photosensitivity,* nail changes including nail loss, dry skin, fissures
- **GI:** *Diarrhea, anorexia, nausea, vomiting, cramps, enteritis, duodenal ulcer, duodenitis, gastritis, glossitis, stomatitis,* pharyngitis, esophagopharyngitis
- **Hematologic: Leukopenia, thrombocytopenia,** elevations in alkaline phosphatase, serum transaminase, serum bilirubin, lactate dehydrogenase
- **Other:** Fever, epistaxis

Topical

- **Hematologic:** Leukocytosis, **thrombocytopenia, toxic granulation,** eosinophilia
- **Local:** *Local pain, pruritus, hyperpigmentation, irritation, inflammation and burning at the site of application,* allergic contact dermatitis, scarring, soreness, tenderness, suppuration, scaling and swelling

Interactions

✱ **Drug-lab test** • 5-HIAA urinary excretion may increase • Plasma albumin may decrease due to protein malabsorption

■ Nursing considerations

Assessment

- **History:** Allergy to 5-FU, poor nutritional status, serious infections, hematopoietic depression, impaired liver function, pregnancy, lactation
- **Physical:** Weight; T; skin lesions, color; hair; vision, speech, orientation, reflexes, sensation; R, adventitious sounds; mucous membranes, liver evaluation, abdominal examination; CBC, differential; LFTs, renal function tests; urinalysis, chest X-ray

Interventions

- Evaluate hematologic status before beginning therapy and before each dose.

⊗ ***Black box warning*** Discontinue drug therapy at any sign of toxicity (stomatitis, esophagopharyngitis, rapidly falling WBC count, intractable vomiting, diarrhea, GI ulceration and bleeding, thrombocytopenia, hemorrhage); serious to life-threatening reactions have occurred. Consult physician.

- Arrange for biopsies of skin lesions to rule out frank neoplasm before beginning topical therapy and in all patients who do not respond to topical therapy.

⊗ ***Warning*** Thoroughly wash hands immediately after application of topical preparations. Use caution in applying near the nose, eyes, and mouth.

- Avoid occlusive dressings with topical application; the incidence of inflammatory reactions in adjacent skin areas is increased with these dressings. Use porous gauze dressings for cosmetic reasons.

Teaching points

- Prepare a calendar of treatment days. If using the topical application, wash hands thoroughly after application. Do not use occlusive dressings; a porous gauze dressing may be used for cosmetic reasons.
- Have frequent, regular medical follow-up visits, including frequent blood tests to evaluate drug effects.
- You may experience these side effects: Nausea, vomiting, loss of appetite (request medication; frequent small meals may help; maintain nutrition); decreased vision, tearing, double vision, malaise, weakness, lethargy (reversible; avoid driving or operating dangerous machinery); mouth sores (practice frequent mouth care); diarrhea; loss of hair (obtain a wig or other head covering; keep the head covered in extremes of temperature); rash, sensitivity of skin and eyes to sun and ultraviolet light (avoid exposure to the sun; use a sunscreen and protective clothing. With topical application, ultraviolet light will increase the severity of the local reaction); birth defects or miscarriages (use birth control); unsightly local reaction to topical application (transient; use a porous gauze dressing to cover areas); pain, burning, stinging, swelling at local application.
- Report black, tarry stools; fever; chills; sore throat; unusual bleeding or bruising; chest pain; mouth sores; severe pain; tenderness; scaling at site of local application.

▽fluoxetine hydrochloride

(floo ***ox'*** *e teen)*

Apo-Fluoxetine (CAN), Co-Fluoxetine (CAN), Gen-Fluoxetine (CAN), Novo-Fluoxetine (CAN), PMS-Fluoxetine (CAN), Prozac, Prozac Pulvules, Prozac Weekly, ratio-Fluoxetine (CAN), Sarafem

PREGNANCY CATEGORY C

Drug classes

Antidepressant
SSRI

Therapeutic actions

Acts as an antidepressant by inhibiting CNS neuronal uptake of serotonin; blocks uptake of serotonin with little effect on norepinephrine; little affinity for muscarinic, histaminergic, and $alpha_1$-adrenergic receptors.

Indications

- Treatment of depression; most effective in patients with major depressive disorder
- Treatment of OCD
- Treatment of bulimia
- Treatment of PMDD (*Sarafem*)
- Treatment of panic disorder with or without agoraphobia
- Unlabeled use: Raynaud's phenomenon, borderline personality disorder

Contraindications and cautions

- Contraindicated with hypersensitivity to fluoxetine, pregnancy.
- Use cautiously with impaired hepatic or renal function, diabetes mellitus, lactation, seizures; history of suicide attempts.

Available forms

Tablets—10, 15, 20 mg; capsules—10, 20, 40 mg; liquid—20 mg/5 mL; DR capsules—90 mg

F

Dosages

Adults

- *Antidepressant:* The full antidepressant effect may not be seen for up to 4–6 wk. Initially, 20 mg/day PO in the morning. If no clinical improvement is seen, increase dose after several weeks. Administer doses larger than 20 mg/day on a bid schedule or once a day in the morning. Do not exceed 80 mg/day. Once stabilized, may switch to 90-mg DR capsules once a week.
- *OCD:* Initially, 20 mg/day PO. If no clinical improvement is seen, increase the dose after several weeks. Usual dosage range is 20–60 mg/day PO; may require up to 5 wk for effectiveness. Do not exceed 80 mg/day.
- *Bulimia:* 60 mg/day PO in the morning.
- *PMDD (Sarafem):* 20 mg/day PO or 20 mg/day PO starting 14 days before the anticipated beginning of menses and continuing through the first full day of menses, then no drug until 14 days before next menses; do not exceed 80 mg/day.
- *Panic disorder (Prozac):* 10 mg/day PO for the first week; increase to 20 mg/day if needed. Maximum dose, 60 mg/day.

Pediatric patients 8–18 yr

- *Major depressive disorder:* 10 mg/day PO; may be increased to 20 mg/day after 1 wk or after several weeks for low-weight children.

Adolescents and higher-weight children

- *OCD:* Initially, 10 mg/day PO. After 2 wk increase to 20 mg/day. Suggested range, 20–60 mg/day PO.

Adolescents and lower-weight children

- *OCD:* Initially, 10 mg/day PO. Range, 20–30 mg/day.

Pediatric patients

Safety and efficacy not established.

Geriatric patients or patients with hepatic impairment

Give a lower or less frequent dose. Monitor response to guide dosage.

Pharmacokinetics

Route	*Onset*	*Peak*
Oral	Slow	6–8 hr

Metabolism: Hepatic; $T_{1/2}$: 9 days
Distribution: Crosses placenta; enters breast milk
Excretion: Feces, urine

Adverse effects

- **CNS:** *Headache, nervousness, insomnia, drowsiness, anxiety, tremor, dizziness, light-headedness,* agitation, sedation, abnormal gait, **seizures**
- **CV:** Hot flashes, palpitations
- **Dermatologic:** *Sweating, rash, pruritus,* acne, alopecia, contact dermatitis
- **GI:** *Nausea, vomiting, diarrhea, dry mouth, anorexia, dyspepsia, constipation, taste changes*, flatulence, gastroenteritis, dysphagia, gingivitis
- **GU:** *Painful menstruation, sexual dysfunction, frequency,* cystitis, impotence, urgency, vaginitis
- **Respiratory:** *URIs, pharyngitis,* cough, dyspnea, bronchitis, rhinitis
- **Other:** *weight changes, asthenia, fever*

Interactions

✱ Drug-drug ⊗ *Warning* Possible fatal reactions with MAOIs; do not administer together; 2-wk washout period needed.
• Increased therapeutic and toxic effects of TCAs • Do not use with thioridazine (increased levels of thioridazine) • Decreased effectiveness if taken while smoking • Increased toxicity of lithium; avoid this combination • Additive CNS effects if combined with benzodiazepines, alcohol; avoid these combinations • Avoid administration with other serotonergic drugs; may lead to serotonin syndrome

✱ Drug-alternative therapy • Increased risk of severe reaction if combined with St. John's wort therapy

■ Nursing considerations

CLINICAL ALERT!
Name confusion has occurred between *Sarafem* (fluoxetine) and *Serophene* (clomiphene); use caution.

Assessment

- **History:** Hypersensitivity to fluoxetine, impaired hepatic or renal function, diabetes mellitus, lactation, pregnancy, seizures
- **Physical:** Weight, T; skin rash, lesions; reflexes, affect; bowel sounds, liver evaluation; P, peripheral perfusion; urinary output, LFTs, renal function tests

Interventions

- Arrange for lower or less frequent doses in elderly patients and patients with hepatic impairment.

⊗ ***Black box warning*** Establish suicide precautions for severely depressed patients. Limit quantity of capsules dispensed; high risk of suicidality in children, adolescents, and young adults.

- Administer drug in the morning.
- Monitor patient for response to therapy for up to 4 wk before increasing dose.
- Switch to once a week therapy by starting weekly dose 7 days after last 20 mg/day dose. If response is not satisfactory, reconsider daily dosing.

⊗ ***Warning*** If discontinuing drug, dosage should be tapered gradually to avoid withdrawal syndrome.

Teaching points

- It may take up to 4 weeks before the full effect occurs. Take in the morning. If you feel sleepy or tired, you may take it at night. If you are taking the once-weekly capsule, mark calendar with reminders of drug day.
- Do not stop taking this drug without consulting your health care provider.
- Do not take this drug during pregnancy. If you think that you are pregnant or wish to become pregnant, consult your health care provider.
- Keep this drug, and all medications, out of the reach of children.
- You may experience these side effects: Dizziness, drowsiness, nervousness, insomnia (avoid driving or performing hazardous tasks); nausea, vomiting, weight loss (eat small frequent meals; monitor your weight loss); sexual dysfunction; flulike symptoms.
- Report rash, mania, seizures, severe weight loss, thoughts of suicide.

▽fluphenazine

*(floo **fen'** a zeen)*

fluphenazine decanoate

Injection: Modecate Concentrate (CAN)

fluphenazine hydrochloride

Oral tablets, concentrate, elixir, injection: Apo-Fluphenazine (CAN)

PREGNANCY CATEGORY C

Drug classes

Antipsychotic
Dopaminergic blocker
Phenothiazine

Therapeutic actions

Mechanism not fully understood: Antipsychotic drugs block postsynaptic dopamine receptors in the brain, depress the RAS, including the parts of the brain involved with wakefulness and emesis; anticholinergic, antihistaminic (H_1), and alpha-adrenergic blocking activity also may contribute to some of its therapeutic (and adverse) actions.

Indications

- Management of manifestations of psychotic disorders; the longer acting parenteral dosage forms, fluphenazine enanthate and fluphenazine decanoate, indicated for management of patients (chronic schizophrenics) who require prolonged parenteral therapy
- Fluphenazine decanoate: Management of behavioral complications in patients with mental retardation

Contraindications and cautions

- Contraindicated with hypersensitivity to fluphenazine, other phenothiazines, tartrazine, or aspirin; coma or severe CNS depression; bone marrow depression; blood dyscrasia; circulatory collapse; subcortical brain damage; Parkinson's disease; liver damage; cerebral arteriosclerosis; coronary disease; severe hypotension or hypertension; pregnancy.

- Use cautiously with respiratory disorders ("silent pneumonia"); glaucoma, prostatic hypertrophy (anticholinergic effects may exacerbate glaucoma and urinary retention); epilepsy or history of epilepsy (drug lowers seizure threshold); breast cancer (elevations in prolactin may stimulate a prolactin-dependent tumor); thyrotoxicosis; peptic ulcer, decreased renal function; myelography within previous 24 hr or myelography scheduled within 48 hr; exposure to heat or phosphorous insecticides; pregnancy; lactation; children younger than 12 yr, especially those with chickenpox, CNS infections (children are especially susceptible to dystonias that may confound the diagnosis of Reye's syndrome).

Available forms

Tablets—1, 2.5, 5, 10 mg; injection—25 mg/mL (decanoate); 2.5 mg/mL (hydrochloride); oral elixir—2.5 mg/5 mL; solution (concentrate)—5 mg/mL

Dosages

Full clinical effects may require 6 wk–6 mo of therapy. Patients who have never taken phenothiazines, poor-risk patients (those with disorders that predispose to undue reactions) should be treated initially with this shorter acting dosage form and then switched to the longer acting parenteral forms, fluphenazine enanthate or decanoate.

The duration of action of the esterified forms of fluphenazine is markedly longer than those of fluphenazine hydrochloride; the duration of action of fluphenazine enanthate is estimated to be 1–3 wk; the duration of action of fluphenazine decanoate is estimated to be 4 wk. No precise formula is available for the conversion of fluphenazine hydrochloride dosage to fluphenazine decanoate dosage, but one study suggests that 20 mg of fluphenazine hydrochloride daily was equivalent to 25 mg decanoate every 3 wk.

Adults

fluphenazine hydrochloride

Individualize dosage; begin with low dosage, and gradually increase.

Oral

2.5–10 mg/day in divided doses every 6–8 hr; usual maintenance dose is 1–5 mg/day, often as a single dose. Oral concentrate solution should be diluted in 60 mL of a suitable diluent that does not contain caffeine, tannic acid (eg, tea), or pectinates (eg, apple juice). Give daily doses greater than 20 mg with caution. When symptoms are controlled, gradually reduce dosage.

IM

Average starting dose is 1.25 mg (range 2.5–10 mg), divided and given every 6–8 hr; parenteral dose is one-third to one-half the oral dose. Give daily doses greater than 10 mg with caution.

fluphenazine decanoate

IM or subcutaneous: Initial dose, 12.5–25 mg IM or subcutaneously; determine subsequent doses and dosage interval based on patient response. If doses above 50 mg are needed, increase cautiously in 12.5-mg increments. Dose should not exceed 100 mg.

Pediatric patients

Generally not recommended for children younger than 12 yr.

Geriatric patients

Oral

Initial oral dose is 1–2.5 mg/day.

Pharmacokinetics

Route	*Onset*	*Peak*	*Duration*
Oral	1 hr	2 hr	6–8 hr
IM (HCl)	1 hr	1–2 hr	6–8 hr
IM (decanoate)	24–72 hr	Unknown	1–6 wk

Metabolism: Hepatic; $T_{1/2}$: 4.5–15.3 hr (fluphenazine hydrochloride), 6.8–9.6 days (fluphenazine decanoate)

Distribution: Crosses placenta; enters breast milk

Excretion: Urine, unchanged

Adverse effects

- **Autonomic:** Dry mouth, salivation, nasal congestion, nausea, vomiting, anorexia, fever, pallor, flushed facies, sweating, constipation, paralytic ileus, urinary retention, incontinence, polyuria, enuresis, priapism, ejaculation inhibition, male impotence

- **CNS:** *Drowsiness,* insomnia, vertigo, headache, weakness, tremor, ataxia, slurring, cerebral edema, **seizures,** exacerbation of psychotic symptoms, extrapyramidal syndromes *(pseudoparkinsonism); dystonias; akathisia,* tardive dyskinesias, potentially irreversible, **neuroleptic malignant syndrome,** hyperthermias, **autonomic disturbances** (rare, but 20% fatal)
- **CV:** Hypotension, orthostatic hypotension, hypertension, tachycardia, bradycardia, **cardiac arrest,** heart failure, cardiomegaly, **refractory arrhythmias,** pulmonary edema
- **Endocrine:** Lactation, breast engorgement in females, galactorrhea; SIADH; amenorrhea, menstrual irregularities; gynecomastia in males; changes in libido; hyperglycemia or **hypoglycemia;** glycosuria; hyponatremia; pituitary tumor with hyperprolactinemia; inhibition of ovulation, infertility, pseudopregnancy; reduced urinary levels of gonadotropins, estrogens, progestins
- **Hematologic: Eosinophilia, leukopenia,** leukocytosis, anemia; **aplastic anemia; hemolytic anemia; thrombocytopenic or nonthrombocytopenic purpura; pancytopenia**
- **Hypersensitivity:** Urticaria, angioneurotic edema, **laryngeal edema,** photosensitivity, eczema, asthma, **anaphylactoid reactions,** exfoliative dermatitis
- **Respiratory: Bronchospasm, laryngospasm,** dyspnea; suppression of cough reflex and potential for aspiration **(sudden death related to asphyxia or cardiac arrest has been reported)**

Interactions

✱ **Drug-drug** • Additive CNS depression with alcohol, barbiturates, or other sedatives • Additive anticholinergic effects and possibly decreased antipsychotic efficacy with anticholinergic drugs • Increased likelihood of seizures with metrizamide (contrast agent used in myelography)

✱ **Drug-lab test** • False-positive pregnancy tests (less likely if serum test is used)

■ Nursing considerations

Assessment

- **History:** Coma or severe CNS depression; bone marrow depression; blood dyscrasia; circulatory collapse; subcortical brain damage; Parkinson's disease; liver damage; cerebral arteriosclerosis; coronary disease; severe hypotension or hypertension; respiratory disorders; glaucoma, prostatic hypertrophy; epilepsy; breast cancer; thyrotoxicosis; peptic ulcer, decreased renal function; myelography within previous 24 hr or myelography scheduled within 48 hr; exposure to heat or phosphorous insecticides; age younger than 12 yr; chickenpox; CNS infections; pregnancy
- **Physical:** Weight, T; reflexes, orientation, IOP; P, BP, orthostatic BP; R, adventitious sounds; bowel sounds and normal output, liver evaluation; urinary output, prostate size; CBC, urinalysis, thyroid, LFTs, renal function tests

Interventions

- Oral concentrate solution should be diluted in 60 mL of a suitable diluent that does not contain caffeine, tannic acid (eg, tea), or pectinates (eg, apple juice).
- Arrange for discontinuation of drug if serum creatinine or BUN become abnormal or if WBC count is depressed.
- Monitor elderly patients for dehydration; institute remedial measures promptly. Sedation and decreased sensation of thirst related to CNS effects can lead to severe dehydration.
- Consult physician regarding appropriate warning of patient or patient's guardian about tardive dyskinesias.
- Consult physician about dosage reduction, use of anticholinergic antiparkinsonian drugs (controversial) if extrapyramidal effects occur.

Teaching points

- Take drug exactly as prescribed.
- Avoid driving or engaging in other dangerous activities if drowsiness, weakness, tremor, extrapyramidal symptoms, or vision changes occur.
- Avoid prolonged exposure to sun; use a sunscreen or cover skin if exposure is unavoidable.

F

- Maintain fluid intake, and use precautions against heatstroke in hot weather.
- Report sore throat, fever, unusual bleeding or bruising, rash, weakness, tremors, impaired vision, dark urine (pink or reddish brown urine is expected), pale stools, yellowing of skin or eyes.

flurazepam hydrochloride

(flur az' e pam)

Apo-Flurazepam (CAN)

PREGNANCY CATEGORY X

CONTROLLED SUBSTANCE C-IV

Drug classes
Benzodiazepine
Sedative-hypnotic

Therapeutic actions
Exact mechanisms not understood; acts mainly at subcortical levels of the CNS, leaving the cortex relatively unaffected; potentiates the effects of GABA, an inhibitory neurotransmitter.

Indications
- Insomnia characterized by difficulty in falling asleep, frequent nocturnal awakenings, or early morning awakening
- Recurring insomnia or poor sleeping habits
- Acute or chronic medical situations requiring restful sleep

Contraindications and cautions
- Contraindicated with hypersensitivity to benzodiazepines, psychoses, acute narrow-angle glaucoma, shock, coma, acute alcoholic intoxication with depression of vital signs, pregnancy (risk of congenital malformations, neonatal withdrawal syndrome), labor and delivery ("floppy infant" syndrome), lactation (infants become lethargic and lose weight).
- Use cautiously in the elderly or with impaired liver or renal function, debilitation, depression, suicidal tendencies.

Available forms
Capsules—15, 30 mg

Dosages
Individualize dosage.

Adults

30 mg PO at bedtime; 15 mg may suffice.

Pediatric patients

Not for use in patients younger than 15 yr.

Geriatric patients or patients with debilitating disease

Initially, 15 mg PO; adjust as needed.

Pharmacokinetics

Route	*Onset*	*Peak*
Oral	Fast	30–60 min

Metabolism: Hepatic; $T_{1/2}$: 47–100 hr
Distribution: Crosses placenta; enters breast milk
Excretion: Urine

Adverse effects
- **CNS:** *Transient, mild drowsiness initially; sedation, depression, lethargy, apathy, fatigue, lightheadedness, disorientation, restlessness, asthenia*, crying, delirium, headache, slurred speech, dysarthria, stupor, rigidity, tremor, dystonia, vertigo, euphoria, nervousness, difficulty in concentration, vivid dreams, psychomotor retardation, extrapyramidal symptoms; *mild paradoxical excitatory reactions during first 2 wk of treatment* (psychiatric patients, aggressive children, with high dosage), visual and auditory disturbances, diplopia, nystagmus, depressed hearing, nasal congestion, complex sleep disorders
- **CV:** *Bradycardia, tachycardia,* **CV collapse,** hypertension and hypotension, palpitations, edema
- **Dependence:** *Drug dependence with withdrawal syndrome* when drug is discontinued (common with abrupt cessation of high dosage used more than 4 mo)
- **Dermatologic:** Urticaria, pruritus, rash, dermatitis
- **GI:** *Constipation, diarrhea, dyspepsia,* dry mouth, salivation, nausea, anorexia, vomiting, difficulty in swallowing, gastric disorders, elevations of blood enzymes: LDH,

alkaline phosphatase, AST, ALT, hepatic impairment, jaundice
- **GU:** *Incontinence, urine retention, changes in libido*, menstrual irregularities
- **Hematologic:** Decreased Hct, blood dyscrasias
- **Other: Anaphylaxis, angioedema,** hiccups, fever, diaphoresis, paresthesias, muscular disturbances, gynecomastia

Interactions

✷ **Drug-drug** • Increased CNS depression with alcohol, phenothiazines, opioids, barbiturates, TCAs • Increased pharmacologic effects of flurazepam with cimetidine, disulfiram, hormonal contraceptives, SSRIs • Decreased sedative effects of flurazepam with theophylline, aminophylline, rifampin

■ Nursing considerations

Assessment

- **History:** Hypersensitivity to benzodiazepines; psychoses; acute narrow-angle glaucoma; shock; coma; acute alcoholic intoxication; pregnancy; labor; lactation; impaired liver or renal function, debilitation, depression, suicidal tendencies
- **Physical:** Skin color, lesions; T; orientation, reflexes, affect, ophthalmologic examination; P, BP; R, adventitious sounds; liver evaluation, abdominal examination, bowel sounds, normal output; CBC, LFTs, renal function tests

Interventions

- Monitor liver and renal function and CBC during long-term therapy.

⊗ ***Warning*** Taper dosage gradually after long-term therapy, especially in epileptic patients.
- Do not administer to pregnant women.

Teaching points

- Take drug exactly as prescribed.
- In long-term therapy, do not stop taking without consulting your health care provider.
- Avoid pregnancy while taking this drug; using barrier contraceptives is advised.
- You may experience these side effects: Drowsiness, dizziness (may lessen; avoid driving or engaging in other dangerous activities); GI upset (take with water); depression, dreams, emotional upset, crying; nocturnal sleep disturbance (may be prolonged after drug cessation).
- Report severe dizziness, weakness, drowsiness that persists, rash or skin lesions, palpitations, swelling of the extremities, visual changes, difficulty voiding.

▽ flurbiprofen

*(flure **bi'** proe fen)*

Ophthalmic solution: Ocufen
Oral: Ansaid, Apo-Flurbiprofen (CAN)

PREGNANCY CATEGORY B (ORAL), C (OPHTHALMIC)

Drug classes

Analgesic (nonopioid)
Anti-inflammatory
NSAID

Therapeutic actions

Analgesic, anti-inflammatory, and antipyretic activities largely related to inhibition of cyclooxygenase and prostaglandin synthesis; exact mechanisms of action are not known.

Indications

- Oral: Acute or long-term treatment of the signs and symptoms of rheumatoid arthritis and osteoarthritis
- Ophthalmic solution: Inhibition of intraoperative miosis
- Unlabeled uses of ophthalmic solution: Topical treatment of cystoid macular edema, inflammation after cataract surgery and uveitis syndromes

Contraindications and cautions

- Contraindicated with allergy to aspirin, flurbiprofen, or other NSAIDs, significant renal impairment, pregnancy, lactation.
- Use cautiously with impaired hearing, allergies, hepatic, CV, and GI conditions.

Available forms

Tablets—50, 100 mg; ophthalmic solution—0.03%

F

Dosages

Adults

Oral

Initial recommended daily dose of 200–300 mg PO, give in divided doses bid, tid, or qid. Largest recommended single dose is 100 mg. Doses above 300 mg/day PO are not recommended. Taper to lowest possible dose.

Ophthalmic solution

Instill 1 drop approximately every 30 min, beginning 2 hr before surgery (total of 4 drops).

Pediatric patients

Safety and efficacy not established.

Pharmacokinetics

Route	Onset	Peak
Oral	30–60 min	90 min

Metabolism: Hepatic; $T_{1/2}$: 5.7 hr
Distribution: Crosses placenta; enters breast milk
Excretion: Urine

Adverse effects

Oral

- **CNS:** *Headache, dizziness, somnolence, insomnia,* fatigue, tiredness, dizziness, tinnitus, ophthalmologic effects
- **CV:** Hypertension, heart failure
- **Dermatologic:** Rash, pruritus, sweating, dry mucous membranes, stomatitis
- **GI:** *Nausea, dyspepsia, GI pain,* diarrhea, vomiting, *constipation,* flatulence, **ulcer**
- **GU:** Dysuria, **renal impairment**
- **Hematologic: Bleeding,** platelet inhibition with higher doses, **neutropenia, eosinophilia, leukopenia, pancytopenia, thrombocytopenia, agranulocytosis, granulocytopenia, aplastic anemia,** decreased Hgb or Hct, **bone marrow depression,** menorrhagia
- **Respiratory:** Dyspnea, hemoptysis, pharyngitis, **bronchospasm,** rhinitis
- **Other:** Peripheral edema, **fatal anaphylactic shock**

Ophthalmic solution

- **Local:** *Transient stinging and burning on instillation, ocular irritation*

■ Nursing considerations

Assessment

- **History:** Renal impairment; impaired hearing; allergies; hepatic, CV, and GI conditions; lactation, pregnancy
- **Physical:** Skin color and lesions; orientation, reflexes, ophthalmologic and audiometric evaluation, peripheral sensation; P, edema; R, adventitious sounds; liver evaluation; CBC, clotting times, LFTs, renal function tests; serum electrolytes, stool guaiac

Interventions

⊗ ***Black box warning*** Be aware that patient may be at increased risk for CV event, GI bleeding; monitor accordingly.

- Administer drug with food or after meals if GI upset occurs.
- Assess patient receiving ophthalmic solutions for systemic effects because absorption does occur.
- Arrange for periodic ophthalmologic examinations during long-term therapy.

⊗ ***Warning*** If overdose occurs, institute emergency procedures—gastric lavage, induction of emesis, supportive therapy.

Teaching points

- Take drug with food or meals if GI upset occurs; take only the prescribed dosage.
- Avoid use during pregnancy, serious adverse effects could occur. Using barrier contraceptives is advised.
- Dizziness or drowsiness can occur (avoid driving or using dangerous machinery).
- Report sore throat, fever, rash, itching, weight gain, swelling in ankles or fingers, changes in vision, black or tarry stools, bleeding.

DANGEROUS DRUG

flutamide

(floo' ta mide)

Euflex (CAN), Novo-Flutamide (CAN)

PREGNANCY CATEGORY D

Drug classes

Antiandrogen
Antineoplastic

Therapeutic actions
Exerts potent antiandrogenic activity by inhibiting androgen uptake or by inhibiting nuclear binding of androgen in target tissues.

Indications
- Treatment of locally advanced and metastatic prostatic carcinoma in combination with LH-RH agonistic analogues (leuprolide acetate, goserelin)
- Unlabeled use: Treatment of hirsutism in women (250 mg/day)

Contraindications and cautions
- Contraindicated with hypersensitivity to flutamide or any component of the preparation, severe hepatic impairment, pregnancy, lactation.
- Use cautiously with smoking, G6PD deficiencies.

Available forms
Capsules—125 mg; tablets—250 mg (CAN)

Dosages
Adults
- *Locally advanced or metastatic prostatic cancer:* 250 mg PO tid. Treatment should begin at same as initiation of therapy with LH-RH analogue.

Pediatric patients
Safety and efficacy not established.

Pharmacokinetics

Route	*Onset*	*Peak*	*Duration*
Oral	Varies	2 hr	72 hr

Metabolism: Hepatic; $T_{1/2}$: 6 hr
Distribution: Crosses placenta; enters breast milk
Excretion: Urine

Adverse effects
- **CNS:** Drowsiness, confusion, depression, anxiety, nervousness
- **Dermatologic:** *Rash,* photosensitivity
- **Endocrine:** *Gynecomastia, hot flashes*
- **GI:** *Nausea, vomiting, diarrhea, GI disturbances,* jaundice, **hepatitis, hepatic necrosis,** elevated AST, ALT
- **GU:** *Impotence, loss of libido*
- **Hematologic:** *Anemia, leukopenia,* thrombocytopenia
- **Other:** Carcinogenesis, mutagenesis

■ Nursing considerations
Assessment
- **History:** Hypersensitivity to flutamide or any component of the preparation, hepatic impairment, smoking, G6PD deficiencies, pregnancy, lactation
- **Physical:** Skin color, lesions; reflexes, affect; urinary output; bowel sounds, liver evaluation; CBC, Hct, electrolytes, LFTs, PSA

Interventions
- Give flutamide with other drugs used for medical castration (LH-RH analogue).

⊗ ***Black box warning*** Arrange for periodic monitoring of liver function tests during long-term therapy; severe hepatic toxicity can occur.

Teaching points
- Take this drug with other drugs to treat your problem. Do not interrupt dosing or stop taking these medications without consulting your health care provider.
- Periodic blood tests will be needed to monitor the drug effects. Keep appointments for these tests.
- You may experience these side effects: Dizziness, drowsiness (avoid driving or performing hazardous tasks); nausea, vomiting, diarrhea (maintain nutrition, consult dietitian); impotence, loss of libido (reversible); sensitivity to light (use sunscreen or protective clothing).
- Report change in stool or urine color, yellow skin, difficulty breathing, malaise.

▽ fluvastatin sodium
*(flue va **sta'** tin)*

Lescol, Lescol XL (DNC)

PREGNANCY CATEGORY X

Drug classes
Antihyperlipidemic
Statin

Therapeutic actions
Inhibits the enzyme HMG-CoA that catalyzes the first step in the cholesterol synthesis pathway, resulting in a decrease in serum cholesterol, serum LDL (associated with increased risk of CAD), and either an increase or no change in serum HDL (associated with decreased risk of CAD).

Indications
- Adjunct to diet in the treatment of elevated total cholesterol and LDL cholesterol with primary hypercholesterolemia and mixed dyslipidemia (types IIa and IIb) where response to dietary restriction of saturated fat and cholesterol and other nonpharmacologic measures has not been adequate
- To slow progression of coronary atheroscleroses in patients with CAD, along with diet and exercise
- Reduction of the risk of undergoing coronary revascularization procedures in patients with CAD
- Treatment of heterozygous familial hypercholesterolemia in children 10–16 yr

Contraindications and cautions
- Contraindicated with allergy to fluvastatin, allergy to fungal byproducts, pregnancy, lactation.
- Use cautiously with impaired hepatic function, cataracts, myopathy.

Available forms
Capsules—20, 40 mg; extended-release tablets DNC—80 mg

Dosages
Adults
Initial dosage, 40 mg/day PO administered in the evening. Maintenance doses, 20–80 mg/day PO; give 80 mg/day as two 40-mg doses, or use 80-mg ER form.

Pediatric patients 10–16 yr
Initial dose, 20 mg/day PO. Adjust every 6 wk to a maximum dose of 40 mg bid or 80 mg of ER form PO once a day.

Pharmacokinetics

Route	*Onset*	*Peak*
Oral	Slow	4–6 wk

Metabolism: Hepatic; $T_{1/2}$: 3–7 hr
Distribution: Crosses placenta; enters breast milk
Excretion: Bile, feces

Adverse effects
- **CNS:** *Headache, blurred vision,* dizziness, insomnia, fatigue, muscle cramps, cataracts
- **GI:** *Flatulence, abdominal pain, cramps, constipation, nausea*, dyspepsia, heartburn
- **Hematologic:** Elevations of CPK, alkaline phosphatase, and transaminases
- **Other: Rhabdomyolysis**

Interactions
✱ Drug-drug ⊗ ***Warning*** Possible severe myopathy or rhabdomyolysis if taken with cyclosporine, erythromycin, gemfibrozil, niacin, other statins.
- Increased levels of phenytoin

✱ Drug-food • Decreased metabolism and increased risk of toxic effects if taken with grapefruit juice; avoid this combination

■ Nursing considerations
Assessment
- **History:** Allergy to fluvastatin, fungal byproducts; impaired hepatic function; cataracts (use caution); pregnancy; lactation
- **Physical:** Orientation, affect, ophthalmologic examination; liver evaluation; lipid studies, LFTs, muscle pain, CPK

Interventions
- Give in the evening; highest rates of cholesterol synthesis are between midnight and 5 AM. Doses of 80 mg/day of immediate-release product should be taken as two 40-mg doses.
- Before administering, ensure that patient is not pregnant and understands need to avoid pregnancy.
- Do not cut or crush ER tablets; ensure that patient swallows tablets whole.
- Arrange for regular follow-up during long-term therapy, including liver function tests.
- Arrange for periodic ophthalmologic examination to check for cataract development.

Teaching points

- Take drug in the evening. Do not drink grapefruit juice while taking this drug. Do not cut, crush, or chew tablets.
- Institute dietary changes, and maintain a low-cholesterol diet while taking this drug.
- This drug cannot be taken during pregnancy; using barrier contraceptives is advised.
- Arrange to have periodic ophthalmic examinations while you are taking this drug.
- You may experience these side effects: Nausea (eat frequent small meals); headache, muscle and joint aches and pains (may lessen).
- Report severe GI upset, changes in vision, unusual bleeding or bruising, dark urine or light-colored stools, muscle pain, fever.

fluvoxamine maleate

(floo vox' a meen)

Apo-Fluvoxamine (CAN),
CO Fluvoxamine (CAN),
Luvox CR DNC,
PMS-Fluvoxamine (CAN),
ratio-Fluvoxamine (CAN)

PREGNANCY CATEGORY C

Drug classes

Antidepressant
SSRI

Therapeutic actions

Selectively inhibits CNS neuronal uptake of serotonin; blocks uptake of serotonin with weak effect on norepinephrine; little affinity for muscarinic, histaminergic, and alpha$_1$-adrenergic receptors.

Indications

- Treatment of OCD
- Treatment of social anxiety disorder (CR capsules)
- Unlabeled uses: Treatment of depression, bulimia nervosa, panic disorder

Contraindications and cautions

- Contraindicated with hypersensitivity to fluvoxamine, lactation.
- Use cautiously with impaired hepatic or renal function, suicidal tendencies, seizures, mania, ECT therapy, CV disease, labor and delivery, pregnancy.

Available forms

Tablets—25, 50, 100 mg; CR capsules DNC—100, 150 mg

Dosages

Adults

Initially, 50 mg PO at bedtime. Increase in 50-mg increments at 4–7 day intervals. Usual range, 100–300 mg/day. Divide doses over 100 mg/day; give larger dose at bedtime. If symptoms do not improve within 10–12 wk, form of treatment should be reconsidered. CR capsules: 100–300 mg/day PO.

Pediatric patients 8–17 yr

Initially, 25 mg PO at bedtime. Increase dose by 25 mg/day every 4–7 days to achieve desired effect. Divide doses over 50 mg/day and give larger dose at bedtime. Maximum dose for children up to age 11 yr is 200 mg/day.

Geriatric patients or patients with hepatic impairment

Give a reduced dose (25 mg PO at bedtime), adjust more slowly.

Pharmacokinetics

Route	*Onset*	*Peak*
Oral	3–10 wk	2–8 hr

Metabolism: Hepatic; $T_{1/2}$: 15–20 hr
Distribution: Crosses placenta; enters breast milk
Excretion: Urine

Adverse effects

- **CNS:** *Headache, nervousness, insomnia, drowsiness, anxiety, tremor, dizziness, light-headedness,* agitation, *sedation,* abnormal gait, **seizures**
- **Dermatologic:** *Sweating, rash, pruritus,* acne, alopecia, contact dermatitis
- **GI:** *Nausea, vomiting, diarrhea, dry mouth, anorexia, dyspepsia, constipation, taste changes,* flatulence, gastroenteritis, dysphagia, gingivitis
- **GU:** *Sexual dysfunction, frequency,* cystitis, impotence, urgency, vaginitis
- **Respiratory:** *URIs, pharyngitis,* cough, dyspnea, bronchitis, rhinitis

F

Interactions

✱ **Drug-drug** • Do not administer with MAOIs (during or within 14 days) • Increased effects of triazolam, alprazolam, warfarin, carbamazepine, methadone, beta blockers, statins, diltiazem, TCAs, theophylline, clozapine; reduced dosages of these drugs will be needed • Decreased effects due to increased metabolism in cigarette smokers • Increased risk of serotonin syndrome if combined with other serotonergic drugs

✱ **Drug-alternative therapy** • Increased risk of severe reaction if combined with St. John's wort therapy

■ Nursing considerations

Assessment

- **History:** Hypersensitivity to fluvoxamine; lactation; impaired hepatic function; suicidal tendencies; seizures; mania; CV disease; labor and delivery; pregnancy
- **Physical:** Weight; T; skin rash, lesions; reflexes; affect; bowel sounds; liver evaluation; P, peripheral perfusion; LFTs, renal function tests

Interventions

- Give lower or less frequent doses in elderly patients and with hepatic or renal impairment.

⊗ ***Black box warning*** Establish suicide precautions for severely depressed patients, children, adolescents, and young adults. Limit quantity of tablets dispensed. Risk of suicidal ideation and behavior is increased.

- Administer drug at bedtime. If dose exceeds 100 mg, divide dose and administer the largest dose at bedtime.
- Ensure that patient does not cut, crush, or chew CR capsules.
- Monitor patient for therapeutic response for up to 4–7 days before increasing dose.
- Monitor patient for serotonin hypertension syndrome, elevated fever, severe anxiety, rigidity.

⊗ ***Warning*** When discontinuing the drug, taper dose by 50 mg/day every 5–7 days.

Teaching points

- Take this drug at bedtime; if a large dose is needed, the dose may be divided but take the largest dose at bedtime. Do not cut, crush, or chew controlled-release capsules.
- Do not stop taking this drug abruptly; it should be discontinued slowly.
- You may experience these side effects: Dizziness, drowsiness, nervousness, insomnia (avoid driving or performing hazardous tasks), nausea, vomiting, weight loss (eat frequent small meals), sexual dysfunction (reversible).
- Report rash, mania, seizures, severe weight loss, suicidal thoughts.

▽ folic acid (folate)

(foe' lik)

Folvite

PREGNANCY CATEGORY A

Drug classes

Folic acid
Vitamin supplement

Therapeutic actions

Required for nucleoprotein synthesis and maintenance of normal erythropoiesis.

Indications

- Treatment of megaloblastic anemias due to sprue, nutritional deficiency, pregnancy, infancy, and childhood

Contraindications and cautions

- Contraindicated with allergy to folic acid preparations; pernicious, aplastic, normocytic anemias.
- Use cautiously during lactation.

Available forms

Tablets—0.4, 0.8, 1 mg; injection—5 mg/mL

Dosages

Administer orally unless patient has severe intestinal malabsorption.

Adults

- *Therapeutic dose:* Up to 1 mg/day PO, IM, IV, or subcutaneously. Larger doses may be needed in severe cases.

- *Maintenance dose:* 0.4 mg/day.
- *Pregnancy and lactation:* 0.8 mg/day.

Pediatric patients

- *Maintenance dose:*
  Infants: 0.1 mg/day.
  Younger than 4 yr: Up to 0.3 mg/day.
  Older than 4 yr: 0.4 mg/day.

Pharmacokinetics

Route	*Onset*	*Peak*
Oral, IM, Subcut., IV	Varies	30–60 min

Metabolism: Hepatic; $T_{1/2}$: Unknown
Distribution: Crosses placenta; enters breast milk
Excretion: Urine

IV FACTS

Preparation: Solution is yellow to yellow-orange; may be added to hyperalimentation solution or dextrose solutions.
Infusion: Infuse at rate of 5 mg/min by direct IV injection; may be diluted in hyperalimentation for continuous infusion.

Adverse effects

- **Hypersensitivity:** Allergic reactions
- **Local:** *Pain and discomfort at injection site*

Interactions

✷ **Drug-drug** • Decrease in serum phenytoin and increase in seizure activity with folic acid preparations • Decreased absorption with sulfasalazine, aminosalicylic acid

■ Nursing considerations

CLINICAL ALERT!
Name confusion has occurred between folinic acid (leucovorin) and folic acid; use extreme caution.

Assessment

- **History:** Allergy to folic acid preparations; pernicious, aplastic, normocytic anemias; lactation
- **Physical:** Skin lesions, color; R, adventitious sounds; CBC, Hgb, Hct, serum folate levels, serum vitamin B_{12} levels, Schilling test

Interventions

- Administer orally if at all possible. With severe GI malabsorption or very severe disease, give IM, IV, or subcutaneously.
- Test using Schilling test and serum vitamin B_{12} levels to rule out pernicious anemia. Therapy may mask signs of pernicious anemia while the neurologic deterioration continues.

⊗ ***Warning*** Use caution when giving the parenteral preparations to premature infants. These preparations contain benzyl alcohol and may produce a fatal gasping syndrome in premature infants.

⊗ ***Warning*** Monitor patient for hypersensitivity reactions, especially if drug previously taken. Keep supportive equipment and emergency drugs readily available in case of serious allergic response.

Teaching points

- When the cause of megaloblastic anemia is treated or passes (infancy, pregnancy), there may be no need for folic acid because it normally exists in sufficient quantities in the diet.
- Report rash, difficulty breathing, pain or discomfort at injection site.

F

follitropin alfa

See Appendix W, *Less commonly used drugs.*

follitropin beta

See Appendix W, *Less commonly used drugs.*

fomepizole

See Appendix W, *Less commonly used drugs.*

DANGEROUS DRUG

fondaparinux

*(fon dah **pear'** ah nucks)*

Arixtra

PREGNANCY CATEGORY B

Drug classes

Antithrombotic
Factor Xa inhibitor

Therapeutic actions

Blocks naturally occurring factor Xa, leading to an alteration in the clot formation process; decreasing the risk of clot and thrombus formation.

Indications

- Prevention of venous thromboembolic events (including DVT and pulmonary emboli) in patient undergoing surgery for hip fracture, hip replacement, knee replacement or undergoing abdominal surgery
- Extended prophylaxis of DVT, which may lead to pulmonary embolism in patients undergoing hip fracture surgery
- Treatment of acute DVT in conjunction with warfarin
- Treatment of acute pulmonary embolism when administered in conjunction with warfarin when initial therapy is administered in the hospital

Contraindications and cautions

- Contraindicated with hypersensitivity to fondaparinux, severe renal impairment, adults weighing less than 50 kg, active major bleeding, bacterial endocarditis, thrombocytopenia.
- Use cautiously with pregnancy or lactation, mild to moderate renal impairment, adults older than 65 yr, bleeding disorders, history of heparin-induced thrombocytopenia, uncontrolled arterial hypertension, GI ulcers, diabetic retinopathy, spinal puncture, neuroaxial anesthesia.

Available forms

Prefilled syringes—2.5 mg/0.5 mL, 5 mg/0.4 mL, 7.5 mg/0.6 mL, 10 mg/0.8 mL

Dosages

Adults

2.5 mg/day subcutaneously starting 6–8 hr following surgical closure and continuing for 5–9 days. An additional 24 days may be added after the initial course for patients undergoing hip fracture surgery.

- *Treatment of DVT, acute pulmonary embolism in conjunction with warfarin:*

  Weight less than 50 kg: 5 mg/day subcutaneously for 5–9 days.

  Weight 50–100 kg: 7.5 mg/day subcutaneously for 5–9 days.

  Weight more than 100 kg: 10 mg/day subcutaneously for 5–9 days.

Warfarin therapy should begin within 72 hr.

Pediatric patients

Safety and efficacy not established.

Geriatric patients or patients with renal impairment

Contraindicated with severe renal impairment. Use caution with moderate renal impairment and with elderly patients. Monitor patient closely and discontinue drug if renal impairment increases or severe bleeding occurs.

Pharmacokinetics

Route	*Onset*	*Peak*
Subcut.	Rapid	3 hr

Metabolism: $T_{1/2}$: 17–21 hr
Distribution: May cross placenta; may enter breast milk
Excretion: Urine, unchanged

Adverse effects

- **CNS:** Insomnia, dizziness, confusion, headache
- **CV:** Edema, hypotension
- **GI:** *Nausea,* constipation, diarrhea, vomiting, dyspepsia
- **GU:** UTI, urinary retention
- **Hematologic: Hemorrhage;** *bruising;* thrombocytopenia; *anemia*
- **Hypersensitivity:** Chills, fever, urticaria, asthma
- **Metabolic:** Elevated AST, ALT levels; hypokalemia
- **Renal:** Impaired renal functions
- **Other:** *Fever;* pain; local irritation, hematoma, erythema at site of injection, rash

Interactions

✱ **Drug-drug** • Increased bleeding tendencies with oral anticoagulants, salicylates, penicillins, cephalosporins, NSAIDs

✱ **Drug-alternative therapy** • Increased bleeding with high dose of vitamin E, garlic, ginkgo

■ Nursing considerations

Assessment

- **History:** Recent surgery or injury; sensitivity to fondaparinux; renal impairment; pregnancy, lactation; recent bleeding, thrombocytopenia, bacterial endocarditis, spinal puncture
- **Physical:** Weight, peripheral perfusion, R, stool guaiac test, PTT or other tests of blood coagulation, platelet count, CBC, renal function tests

Interventions

- Arrange to give drug 6–8 hr following surgical closure; continue for 5–9 days. An additional 24-day course may be added for patients undergoing hip fracture surgery.

⊗ ***Black box warning*** Carefully monitor patients receiving spinal/epidural anesthesia; risk of spinal hematoma and neurologic damage.

- Give deep subcutaneous injections; do not give by IM injection.
- To administer by deep subcutaneous injection, patient should be lying down, and alternate administration between the left and right anterolateral and left and right posterolateral abdominal wall. Introduce the whole length of the needle into a skinfold held between the thumb and forefinger; hold the skinfold throughout the injection.
- Apply pressure to all injection sites after needle is withdrawn; inspect injection sites for signs of hematoma.
- Do not massage injection sites.
- Do not mix with other injections or infusions.
- Store at room temperature; fluid should be clear, colorless to pale yellow.
- Provide for safety measures (electric razor, soft toothbrush) to prevent injury to patient who is at risk for bleeding.
- Check patient for signs of bleeding; monitor blood tests.

Teaching points

- This drug must be given by subcutaneous injection; it is not taken orally. You and a significant other will be instructed in how to administer the drug if you are being discharged with it. Arrange for proper disposal of syringes and needles.
- Arrange for periodic blood tests that will be needed to monitor your response to this drug.
- Be careful to avoid injury while taking this drug: Use an electric razor; avoid activities that might lead to injury.
- Report nose bleed, bleeding of the gums, unusual bruising, black or tarry stools, cloudy or dark urine, abdominal or lower back pain, severe headache.

F

▽formoterol fumarate

*(for **moh'** te rol)*

Foradil Aerolizer, Perforomist

PREGNANCY CATEGORY C

Drug classes

Antiasthmatic
Beta$_2$ agonist

Therapeutic actions

Long-acting agonist that binds to beta$_2$ receptors in the lungs causing bronchodilation; may also inhibit the release of inflammatory mediators in the lung, blocking swelling and inflammation.

Indications

- Long-term maintenance treatment of asthma in adults and children 5 yr and older
- Prevention of exercise-induced bronchospasm in adults and children 12 yr and older when used on an occasional, as-needed basis
- Long-term maintenance treatment of bronchoconstriction in patients with COPD

Contraindications and cautions

- Contraindicated with hypersensitivity to adrenergics, amines, or to formoterol, acute asthma attack, acute airway obstruction.
- Use cautiously in the elderly and with pregnancy, lactation.

Available forms

Inhalation powder in capsules—12 mcg; inhalation solution—20 mcg/2 mL

Dosages

Adults

- *Maintenance treatment of COPD:* Oral inhalation of contents of 1 capsule (12 mcg) using *Aerolizer Inhaler* every 12 hr; do not exceed a total daily dose of 24 mcg. Or, one 20-mcg/2 mL vial by oral inhalation using a jet nebulizer connected to an air compressor twice daily, morning and evening; do not exceed 40 mcg/day.

Adults and pediatric patients 12 yr and older

- *Prevention of exercise-induced bronchospasm:* Oral inhalation of contents of one capsule (12 mcg) using the *Aerolizer Inhaler* 15 min before exercise. Use on an occasional, as-needed basis.

Adults and pediatric patients 5 yr and older

- *Maintenance treatment of asthma:* Oral inhalation of contents of 1 capsule (12 mcg) using the *Aerolizer Inhaler* every 12 hr. Do not exceed 1 capsule every 12 hr.

Pharmacokinetics

Route	Onset	Peak	Duration
Inhalation	1–3 min	1–3 hr	8–20 hr

Metabolism: Hepatic; $T_{1/2}$: 10–14 hr
Distribution: Crosses placenta; may enter breast milk
Excretion: Feces, urine

Adverse effects

- **CNS:** Tremor, dizziness, insomnia, dysphonia, *headache, nervousness*
- **CV:** Hypertension, tachycardia, chest pain
- **GI:** Nausea, dyspepsia, abdominal pain, *irritation of the throat and mouth*
- **Respiratory:** Bronchitis, respiratory infection, dyspnea, tonsillitis
- **Other:** *Viral infection* (most likely in children)

Interactions

✱ **Drug-drug** • Beta blockers and formoterol may inhibit each other's effects; avoid use together • Risk of prolonged QTc interval if combined with other drugs that prolong QTc interval; use with extreme caution

■ Nursing considerations

CLINICAL ALERT!
Name confusion has occurred between *Foradil* (formoterol) and *Toradol* (ketorolac); use extreme caution.

Assessment

- **History:** Hypersensitivity to adrenergics, amines, or formoterol, acute asthma attack, acute airway obstruction, pregnancy, lactation
- **Physical:** R, adventitious sounds, P, BP, ECG, orientation, reflexes

Interventions

⊗ ***Black box warning*** Long-acting beta-agonists may increase risk of asthma-related deaths; use only if clearly warranted.

- Instruct patient in the proper use of *Aerolizer Inhaler.* Ensure that patient does not swallow the capsule.
- Monitor use of inhaler. Patient should not wash the inhaler but should keep it dry; it should not be used for delivering any other medication. If a bronchodilator is needed between doses, consult with health care provider. Do not use more often than every 12 hr.
- Use a jet nebulizer connected to an air compressor for oral inhalation.
- Encourage patient who experiences exercise-induced asthma to use drug 15 min before activity, and to reserve this drug for occasional, as-needed use.
- Ensure that patient continues with appropriate use of corticosteroids or other drugs used to block bronchospasm, as appropriate.
- Arrange for periodic evaluation of respiratory condition during therapy.
- Arrange for analgesics as appropriate for headache.
- Establish safety precautions if tremor becomes a problem.

Teaching points

- This medication should not be used to relieve acute symptoms. For that purpose, use a short-acting $beta_2$-agonist.
- Use the *Aerolizer Inhaler* as instructed. This is the only inhaler that can be used with this drug.

- Use only twice a day. Do not wash the inhaler; keep it dry at all times. Do not use this inhaler to deliver any other drugs. Check the "use by" date on your drug and discard any capsules that have expired.
- For oral inhalation formulation, use a jet nebulizer connected to an air compressor.
- If drug is to be used periodically for exercise-induced asthma, use 15 minutes before activity.
- Arrange for periodic evaluation of your respiratory problem while using this drug; continue to use any other therapies that have been prescribed to control your asthma.
- You may experience these side effects: Headache (appropriate analgesics may be ordered); tremors (use care in performing dangerous tasks if this occurs); fast heartbeat, palpitations (monitor activity if this occurs, rest frequently).
- Report severe headache, irregular heartbeat, worsening of asthma, difficulty breathing.

▽fosamprenavir calcium

*(foss am **pren'** ah ver)*

Lexiva

PREGNANCY CATEGORY C

Drug classes
Antiviral
Protease inhibitor

Therapeutic actions
Antiviral activity; inhibits HIV protease activity, leading to the formation of immature, noninfectious virus particles.

Indications
- Treatment of HIV infection in adults in combination with other antiretrovirals (the use of fosamprenavir with ritonavir is not recommended for protease inhibitor-experienced patients)

Contraindications and cautions
- Contraindicated with allergy to any component of the drug or to amprenavir; concurrent use of drugs dependent on the CYP3A4 system for clearance, lactation; if used with ritonavir, use of flecainide and propafenone is contraindicated.
- Use cautiously with pregnancy, hepatic impairment, diabetes mellitus, lipid abnormalities, hemophilia, sulfonamide allergy.

Available forms
Tablets—700 mg; suspension—50 mg/mL

Dosages
Adults

1,400 mg PO bid.

- *With ritonavir:* 1,400 mg/day PO plus ritonavir 100 mg/day PO, 1,400 mg/day PO plus ritonavir 200 mg/day PO, or 700 mg PO bid with ritonavir 100 mg PO bid.
- *Protease-experienced patients:* 700 mg PO bid with ritonavir 100 mg PO bid.
- *In combination with ritonavir and efavirenz:* An additional 100 mg/day of ritonavir (300 mg/day total) is recommended.

Pediatric patients

- *Therapy-naïve children 2–5 yr:* 30 mg/kg oral suspension PO bid; do not exceed 1,400 mg bid.
- *Therapy-naïve children 6 yr and older:* 30 mg/kg oral suspension PO bid; do not exceed 1,400 mg bid. Or, 18 mg/kg oral suspension PO with ritonavir 3 mg/kg PO bid; do not exceed 700 mg fosamprenavir plus 100 mg ritonavir bid.
- *Therapy-experienced children 2–5 yr:* Safety and efficacy not established.
- *Therapy-experienced children 6 yr and older:* 18 mg/kg oral suspension with 3 mg/kg ritonavir PO bid; do not to exceed 700 mg fosamprenavir with 100 mg ritonavir bid.

Patients with hepatic impairment

- *Child Pugh score 5–6:* 700 mg PO bid without ritonavir (therapy-naïve patients) or 700 mg PO bid plus 100 mg/day ritonavir (therapy-naïve or protease-inhibitor–experienced patients).
- *Child Pugh score 7–9:* 700 mg PO bid without ritonavir (therapy naïve) or 450 mg PO bid with 100 mg/day ritonavir PO.
- *Child Pugh score 10–15:* 350 mg PO bid without ritonavir (therapy naïve) or 300 mg PO bid with ritonavir 100 mg/day PO.

Pharmacokinetics

Route	Onset	Peak
Oral	Varies	1.5–4 hr

Metabolism: Hepatic; $T_{1/2}$: 7.7 hr
Distribution: Crosses placenta; may enter breast milk
Excretion: Feces, urine

Adverse effects

- **CNS:** Headache, oral paresthesias, depression, mood disorders
- **Dermatologic:** Rash, **Stevens-Johnson syndrome,** pruritus
- **GI:** Nausea, vomiting, diarrhea, anorexia, abdominal pain, elevated liver enzymes
- **Hematologic:** Hyperglycemia, hypercholesterolemia, hypertriglyceridemia, neutropenia
- **Other:** Fatigue, redistribution of body fat (buffalo hump, thinning of arms and legs)

Interactions

✱ **Drug-drug** ⊗ ***Warning*** Potentially large increases in the serum concentration of flecainide, piroxicam, propafenone, rifabutin, simvastatin, lovastatin, midazolam, triazolam, dihydroergotamine, ergotamine, ergonovine, methylergonovine, pimozide, when taken with fosamprenavir. Potential for serious arrhythmias, seizure, rhabdomyolysis and fatal reactions. Do not administer fosamprenavir with any of these drugs.
• Potentially large increases in the serum concentration of the following: Antiarrhythmics—amiodarone, lidocaine, quinidine—monitor patient closely and adjust antiarrhythmic dosage as needed; antifungals—ketoconazole, itraconazole—reduced dosage of antifungals may be needed; rifabutin—reduce dosage to half recommended dose and monitor for neutropenia weekly; calcium channel blockers—diltiazem, felodipine, nifedipine, nicardipine, nimodipine, verapamil, amlodipine, nisoldipine, isradipine—increases calcium channel blocker concentrations; monitor patient very closely and use caution; atorvastatin—suggest use of a different HMG-CoA inhibitor; immunosuppressants—cyclosporine, tacrolimus—monitor serum concentration carefully and consider need for dosage reduction; sildenafil, vardenafil—reduce dosage and monitor patient carefully for adverse effects; TCAs—amitriptyline, imipramine—monitor serum concentrations closely and consider need for dosage reduction • Risk of decreased antiviral effectiveness when used with saquinavir, carbamazepine, phenobarbital, phenytoin, rifampin, delavirdine, efavirenz, nevirapine, lopinavir and ritonavir—check that appropriate dosage changes have been made; if any of these drugs are used together; monitor patient for progression of disease, adverse effects • Risk of decreased effectiveness of hormonal contraceptives; advise patient to use barrier contraceptives
✱ **Drug-alternative therapy** • Loss of virologic response if combined with St. John's wort; avoid this combination

■ Nursing considerations

Assessment

- **History:** Allergy to any component of the drug or to amprenavir; concurrent use of drugs dependent on the CYP3A4 system for clearance, lactation, pregnancy, hepatic impairment, diabetes mellitus, lipid abnormalities, hemophilia, sulfonamide allergy
- **Physical:** Orientation, affect, reflexes; bowel sounds; skin color, perfusion; LFTs, CBC, serum triglycerides and cholesterol

Interventions

⊗ ***Warning*** Do not administer with any of the drugs listed as contraindications. Check all other drugs in drug regimen for potential interaction and arrange for appropriate monitoring or dosage adjustment as needed.

- Use cautiously with any history of sulfonamide allergy; cross-reactivity may occur.
- Administer this drug with other antiretrovirals.
- Administer tablets without regard to food. Adults should take suspension without food; children should take suspension with food.
- Redose oral suspension if vomiting occurs within 30 min of dose.
- Monitor liver function and blood glucose levels before and periodically during therapy.
- Monitor patient for skin rash; arrange to discontinue drug if severe skin reaction occurs.

Teaching points

- Take this drug without regard to meals. Adults should take suspension without food; children should take suspension with food.
- Take the full course of therapy as prescribed; do not take double doses if one is missed; if you forget to take a dose for more than 4 hours, wait and take the next dose at the regular time; if you miss a dose by less than 4 hours, take your missed dose right away and your next dose at the regular time.
- Shake suspension vigorously before each use. Drug may be stored in refrigerator or at room temperature.
- Do not change dosage without consulting your health care provider. Take this drug with other antivirals as prescribed.
- This drug does not cure HIV infection; long-term effects are not yet known. Continue to take precautions as the risk of transmission is not reduced by this drug.
- Do not take other prescription or over-the-counter drugs without consulting your health care provider. This drug interacts with many other drugs; serious problems can occur.
- Consider using barrier contraceptives while taking this drug; hormonal contraceptives may not be effective.
- Use caution if taking sildenafil (*Viagra*), tadalafil (*Cialis*), or vardenafil (*Levitra*). There is an increased risk of adverse effects; consult your health care provider if adverse effects occur.
- Some diabetic patients may have changes in blood glucose while taking this drug; check your blood sugar often and consult your health care provider if control becomes a problem.
- Do not use St. John's wort while you are using this drug; consult your health care provider before using any herbal therapies.
- You may experience these side effects: Nausea, vomiting, diarrhea, abdominal pain (eat frequent small meals); headache, numbness and tingling (use caution if driving or operating dangerous machinery); redistribution of body fat with thinning of arms and legs, development of a buffalo hump (it may help to know that this is a drug effect).
- Report severe diarrhea, severe nausea, rash, changes in the color of urine or stool; increased thirst or urination.

▽fosfomycin tromethamine

*(foss foe **my'** sin troh **meth'** ah meen)*

Monurol

PREGNANCY CATEGORY B

Drug classes

Antibacterial
Urinary tract anti-infective

Therapeutic actions

Bactericidal; interferes with bacterial cell wall synthesis, blocks adherence of bacteria to uroepithelial cells.

Indications

- Uncomplicated UTIs in women caused by susceptible strains of *Escherichia coli* and *Enterococcus faecalis;* not indicated for the treatment of pyelonephritis or perinephric abscess

Contraindications and cautions

- Contraindicated with allergy to fosfomycin.
- Use cautiously with pregnancy, lactation.

Available forms

Granule packet—3 g

Dosages

Adults

1 packet dissolved in water PO.

Pediatric patients younger than 12 yr

Not recommended.

Pharmacokinetics

Route	*Onset*	*Peak*
Oral	Rapid	2–4 hr

Metabolism: Hepatic; $T_{1/2}$: 5.7 hr
Distribution: Crosses placenta; may enter breast milk
Excretion: Feces, urine

Adverse effects

- **CNS:** *Headache, dizziness,* back pain, asthenia

F

- **GI:** *Nausea,* abdominal cramps, dyspepsia, diarrhea
- **GU:** Vaginitis, dysmenorrhea
- **Other:** Rhinitis, rash

Interactions

✱ **Drug-drug** • Lowered serum concentration and urinary tract excretion with metoclopramide

■ Nursing considerations

Assessment

- **History:** Allergy to fosfomycin, pregnancy, lactation
- **Physical:** Skin color, lesions; orientation, reflexes; urine for analysis

Interventions

- Arrange for culture and sensitivity tests.
- Administer drug with food if GI upset occurs.

⊗ ***Warning*** Do not administer dry; mix a single dose packet in 90–120 mL of water and stir to dissolve; do not use hot water. Administer immediately.

- Monitor clinical response; if no improvement is seen or a relapse occurs, send urine for repeat culture and sensitivity tests.
- Encourage patient to observe other measures (avoid bubble baths, alkaline ash foods, sexual intercourse; drink lots of fluids) to decrease risk of UTI.

Teaching points

- This drug is meant to be a one-dose treatment for urinary tract infection; improvement should be seen in 2–3 days. If no improvement occurs, consult your health care provider.
- Take drug with food if GI upset occurs. Do not take in the dry form; mix a single dose packet in 90–120 milliliters of water and stir to dissolve; do not use hot water. Drink immediately after mixing.
- You may experience these side effects: Nausea, abdominal pain (eat frequent small meals; take the drug with meals); dizziness (observe caution if driving or using dangerous equipment).
- Report rash, visual changes, severe GI problems, weakness, tremors, worsening of urinary tract symptoms.

▽fosinopril sodium

*(foh **sin'** oh pril)*

Monopril

PREGNANCY CATEGORY C (FIRST TRIMESTER)

PREGNANCY CATEGORY D (SECOND AND THIRD TRIMESTERS)

Drug classes

ACE inhibitor
Antihypertensive

Therapeutic actions

Renin, synthesized by the kidneys, is released into the circulation where it acts on a plasma precursor to produce angiotensin I, which is converted by ACE to angiotensin II, a potent vasoconstrictor that also causes release of aldosterone from the adrenals; fosinopril blocks the conversion of angiotensin I to angiotensin II, leading to decreased BP, decreased aldosterone secretion, an increase in serum potassium levels, and sodium and fluid loss; increased prostaglandin synthesis may be involved in the antihypertensive action.

Indications

- Treatment of hypertension, alone or in combination with thiazide-type diuretics
- Management of heart failure as adjunctive therapy

Contraindications and cautions

- Contraindicated with allergy to fosinopril or other ACE inhibitors; pregnancy.
- Use cautiously with impaired renal or hepatic function, hyperkalemia, salt or volume depletion, lactation.

Available forms

Tablets—10, 20, 40 mg

Dosages

Adults

- *Hypertension:* Initial dose, 10 mg PO daily. Maintenance dose, 20–40 mg/day PO as a single dose or two divided doses. In patients receiving diuretic therapy, begin fosinopril therapy with 10 mg. Do not exceed maximum dose of 80 mg.

- *Heart failure:* Initially, 10 mg/day PO; observe for 2 hr for hypotension. If patient has moderate to severe renal failure, 5 mg/day PO.

Pediatric patients

Safety and efficacy not established.

Pharmacokinetics

Route	*Onset*	*Peak*	*Duration*
Oral	1 hr	3 hr	24 hr

Metabolism: Hepatic; $T_{1/2}$: 12 hr
Distribution: Crosses placenta; enters breast milk
Excretion: Feces, urine

Adverse effects

- **CV:** Angina pectoris, orthostatic hypotension in salt- or volume-depleted patients, palpitations
- **Dermatologic:** Rash, pruritus, diaphoresis, flushing
- **GI:** *Nausea,* abdominal pain, vomiting, diarrhea
- **Respiratory:** *Cough,* asthma, bronchitis, dyspnea, sinusitis
- **Other: Angioedema,** asthenia, myalgia, arthralgia, hyperkalemia

Interactions

✱ **Drug-drug** • Decreased effectiveness if combined with indomethacin or other NSAIDs • Risk of lithium toxicity if combined with ACE inhibitors • Risk of increased potassium levels if taken with potassium-sparing diuretics • Decreased absorption when given with antacids; separate by at least 2 hr

■ Nursing considerations

CLINICAL ALERT!
Name confusion has occurred between fosinopril and lisinopril; use caution.

Assessment

- **History:** Allergy to fosinopril and other ACE inhibitors, impaired renal or hepatic function, hyperkalemia, salt or volume depletion, lactation, pregnancy
- **Physical:** Skin color, lesions, turgor; T; P, BP, peripheral perfusion; mucous membranes, bowel sounds, liver evaluation; urinalysis, LFTs, renal function tests, CBC, and differential

Interventions

⊗ ***Warning*** Alert surgeon and mark the patient's chart with notice that fosinopril is being taken; the angiotensin II formation subsequent to compensatory renin release during surgery will be blocked; hypotension may be reversed with volume expansion.

⊠ ***Black box warning*** Suggest use of a contraceptive. Pregnancy should be avoided; fetal damage can occur.

- Arrange to switch to a different drug if pregnancy occurs; suggest use of barrier contraceptives.
- Monitor patient closely for a drop in BP secondary to reduction in fluid volume (excessive perspiration and dehydration, vomiting, diarrhea); excessive hypotension may occur.

Teaching points

- Do not stop taking the medication without consulting your health care provider.
- Avoid pregnancy while taking this drug; using barrier contraceptives is advised.
- Be careful with any conditions that may lead to a drop in blood pressure (such as diarrhea, sweating, vomiting, dehydration); if light-headedness or dizziness occurs, consult your health care provider.
- You may experience these side effects: GI upset, loss of appetite (these may be transient); lightheadedness (transient; change position slowly and limit activities to those that do not require alertness and precision); dry cough (not harmful).
- Report mouth sores; sore throat, fever, chills; swelling of the hands, feet; irregular heartbeat, chest pains; swelling of the face, eyes, lips, tongue, difficulty breathing, persistent cough.

F

fosphenytoin sodium

*(faws **fen'** i toe in)*

Cerebyx

PREGNANCY CATEGORY D

Drug classes

Antiepileptic
Hydantoin

Therapeutic actions

A prodrug that is converted to phenytoin; has antiepileptic activity without causing general CNS depression; stabilizes neuronal membranes and prevents hyperexcitability caused by excessive stimulation; limits the spread of seizure activity from an active focus.

Indications

- Short-term control of general convulsive status epilepticus
- Prevention and treatment of seizures occurring during or following neurosurgery
- **NEW INDICATION:** Short-term substitute for oral phenytoin

Contraindications and cautions

- Contraindicated with hypersensitivity to hydantoins, sinus bradycardia, sinoatrial block, second- or third-degree AV heart block, Stokes-Adams syndrome, pregnancy (data suggest an association between use of antiepileptic drugs by women with epilepsy and an elevated incidence of birth defects in children born to these women; however, do not discontinue antiepileptic therapy in pregnant women who are receiving therapy to prevent major seizures—this is likely to precipitate status epilepticus, with attendant hypoxia and risk to both mother and unborn child), lactation.
- Use cautiously with hypotension, severe myocardial insufficiency, porphyria, hepatic dysfunction.

Available forms

Injection—150-mg (100 mg phenytoin equivalents [PE]), 750-mg (500 mg PE) vial

Dosages

Dosage is given as PEs to facilitate transfer from phenytoin.

Adults

- *Status epilepticus:* Loading dose of 15–20 mg PE/kg administered at 100–150 mg PE/min IV.
- *Neurosurgery (prophylaxis):* Loading dose of 10–20 mg PE/kg IM or IV; maintenance dose of 4–6 mg PE/kg/day.
- *Substitution for oral phenytoin theraphy:* Substitute IM or IV at the same total daily dose as phenytoin, for short-term use only.

Pediatric patients

Not recommended.

Patients with renal or hepatic impairment

Use caution and monitor for early signs of toxicity—changes in the metabolism of the drug may result in increased risk of adverse effects.

Pharmacokinetics

Route	*Onset*	*Peak*
IV	Rapid	End of infusion

Metabolism: Hepatic; $T_{1/2}$: 15 min
Distribution: Crosses placenta; enters breast milk
Excretion: Urine

IV FACTS

Preparation: Dilute in 5% dextrose or 0.9% saline solution to a concentration of 1.5–25 mg PE/mL. Refrigerate; stable at room temperature for less than 48 hr.
Infusion: Infuse for status epilepticus at rate of 100–150 mg PE/min; never administer at a rate that exceeds 150 mg PE/min.

Adverse effects

- **CNS:** *Nystagmus, ataxia, dizziness, somnolence,* drowsiness, insomnia, transient nervousness, motor twitchings, fatigue, irritability, depression, numbness, tremor, headache, photophobia, diplopia, asthenia, back pain, suicidal ideation
- **CV:** *Hypotension,* vasodilation, tachycardia
- **Dermatologic:** *Pruritus*

- **GI:** *Nausea,* vomiting, dry mouth, taste perversion
- **Other:** Lymph node hyperplasia, sometimes progressing to frank malignant lymphoma, monoclonal gammopathy and multiple myeloma (prolonged therapy), polyarthropathy, osteomalacia, weight gain, chest pain, periarteritis nodosa

Interactions

No specific drug interactions have been reported, but since fosphenytoin is a metabolite of phenytoin, documented interactions with that drug should be considered.

✱ **Drug-drug** • Increased pharmacologic effects of hydantoins with chloramphenicol, cimetidine, disulfiram, phenacemide, phenylbutazone, sulfonamides, trimethoprim; reduced fosphenytoin dose may be needed • Complex interactions and effects when phenytoin and valproic acid are given together; phenytoin toxicity with apparently normal serum phenytoin levels; decreased plasma levels of valproic acid given with phenytoin; breakthrough seizures when the two drugs are given together • Increased pharmacologic effects and toxicity when primidone, oxyphenbutazone, amiodarone, chloramphenicol, fluconazole, isoniazid are given with hydantoins • Decreased pharmacologic effects of the following with hydantoins: Corticosteroids, cyclosporine, dicumarol, disopyramide, doxycycline, estrogens, furosemide, levodopa, methadone, metyrapone, mexiletine, hormonal contraceptives, quinidine, atracurium, pancuronium, tubocurarine, vecuronium, carbamazepine, diazoxide

✱ **Drug-lab test** • Interference with metyrapone and 1-mg dexamethasone tests for at least 7 days

■ Nursing considerations

CLINICAL ALERT!

Name confusion has occurred between *Cerebyx* (fosphenytoin), *Celebrex* (celecoxib), *Celexa* (citalopram), and *Xanax* (alprazolam); use caution.

Assessment

- **History:** Hypersensitivity to hydantoins; sinus bradycardia, sinoatrial block, second- or third-degree AV heart block, Stokes-Adams syndrome, pregnancy, lactation, hepatic failure, severe myocardial insufficiency, porphyria
- **Physical:** T; skin color, lesions; orientation, affect, reflexes, vision examination; P, BP; bowel sounds, normal output, liver evaluation; LFTs, CBC and differential, EEG and ECG

Interventions

- Continue supportive measures, including use of an IV benzodiazepine, until drug becomes effective against seizures.
- Possible increased risk of suicidal ideation; monitor patient accordingly.

⊗ ***Warning*** Administer IV slowly to prevent severe hypotension; margin of safety between full therapeutic and toxic doses is small. Continually monitor cardiac rhythm and check BP frequently and regularly during IV infusion and for 10–20 min after infusion.

- Monitor infusion site carefully—drug solutions are very alkaline and irritating.
- This drug is recommended for short-term use only (up to 5 days); switch to oral phenytoin as soon as possible.

⊗ ***Black box warning*** Suggest use of a contraceptive. Pregnancy should be avoided; fetal damage can occur.

Teaching points

- This drug can only be given IV and will be stopped as soon as you are able to take an oral drug.
- Use of a contraceptive is advised; drug should not be used during pregnancy.
- You may experience these side effects: Drowsiness, dizziness, GI upset.
- Report rash, severe nausea or vomiting, drowsiness, slurred speech, impaired coordination (ataxia), sore throat, unusual bleeding or bruising, persistent headache, malaise, pain at injection site, thoughts of suicide.

▽fospropofol disodium

*(foss **prob'** poh fall)*

Lusedra

PREGNANCY CATEGORY B

Drug class

Sedative-hypnotic

Therapeutic actions

Thought to increase sensitivity to GABA, leading to inhibition of neurotransmission and CNS depression.

Indications

- Monitored anesthesia care sedation in adults undergoing diagnostic and therapeutic procedures

Contraindications and cautions

- Contraindicated in hypersensitivity to components of drug.
- Use cautiously in elderly patients; severe systemic diseases, dehydration, decreased myocardial function or reduced vascular tone; pregnancy, lactation.

Available forms

Single-use vial—35 mg/mL

Dosages

Adults

6.5 mg/kg IV bolus followed by 1.6 mg/kg IV to maintain desired sedation. Bolus should not exceed 16.5 mL and IV infusion should not exceed 4 mL.

Pediatric patients

Safety and efficacy not established.

Geriatric patients and patients with severe systemic disease

75% of the standard dose is recommended.

IV FACTS

Preparation: Drug is ready to use and does not require further reconstitution. May be given with 5% dextrose, 5% dextrose with 0.2% or 0.45 % sodium chloride injection; 0.9% sodium chloride injection; lactated Ringer's solution; lactated Ringer's with 5% dextrose; 0.45% sodium chloride injection; 5% dextrose, 0.45% sodium chloride, and 20 mEq potassium chloride, USP. Does not need to be protected from light or infused through a filter. Solution should be clear, with no particulate matter. Discard vial after withdrawing drug.

Infusion: Administer through a freely flowing IV using a compatible solution. Flush line with normal saline before and after administering drug.

Incompatibilities: Do not mix with other drugs or solutions; physically incompatible with midazolam, meperidine.

Pharmacokinetics

Route	*Onset*	*Peak*
IV	Rapid	4–13 min

Metabolism: Hepatic; $T_{1/2}$: 0.8–0.9 hr

Distribution: May cross placenta; enters breast milk

Excretion: Urine

Adverse effects

- **CNS:** Headache, *paresthesia* (burning, tingling) *in perianal region,* **loss of responsiveness**
- **CV:** Hypotension
- **GI:** Nausea, vomiting
- **Respiratory: Hypoxemia, respiratory depression**
- **Other:** *Perianal pruritus*

Interactions

✱ **Drug-drug** • Risk of increased cardiac or respiratory depression if combined with other sedative-hypnotics (benzodiazepines, opioid analgesics)

■ Nursing considerations

Assessment

- **History:** Systemic diseases, pregnancy, lactation
- **Physical:** Orientation, affect; R, adventitious sounds; BP, ECG, state of hydration, skin lesions

Interventions

- Drug should only be administered by persons trained in administration of anesthesia who can continually monitor patient and are not involved in the diagnostic procedure or treatment being performed.
- Patient will require oxygen administration and continuous monitoring of pulse oximetry, ECG, and frequent blood pressure checks.
- Patients weighing more than 90 kg should be dosed as if they weigh 90 kg; patients less

than 60 kg should be dosed as if they weigh 60 kg.
- Emergency equipment should be readily available.
- Patient should be escorted after the procedure; driving is not advised.
- Alert patient that perianal burning, stinging, and tingling are common after injection of the drug and that these symptoms will pass and no treatment is required.

Teaching points

- You will be very relaxed and unaware during the procedure; you will require an escort at discharge because no driving is permitted immediately after the use of this drug.
- You may experience perianal burning, stinging, tingling, and rash, which are common effects when the drug is given. These symptoms are usually mild, last only a short time, and do not require treatment.

▽ frovatriptan succinate

*(frow vah **trip'** tan)*

Frova

PREGNANCY CATEGORY C

Drug classes

Antimigraine drug
Serotonin selective agonist
Triptan

Therapeutic actions

Binds to serotonin receptors to cause vascular constrictive effects on cranial blood vessels, causing the relief of migraine in selective patients.

Indications

- Treatment of acute migraines with or without aura in adults

Contraindications and cautions

- Contraindicated with allergy to frovatriptan, active CAD, ischemic heart disease, Prinzmetal's angina, peripheral or cerebral vascular syndromes, uncontrolled hypertension, hemiplegic or basilar migraine, use of an ergot compound or other triptan within 24 hr.
- Use cautiously with hepatic or renal impairment, risk factors for CAD, lactation, pregnancy.

Available forms

Tablets—2.5 mg

Dosages

Adults

2.5 mg PO as a single dose at first sign of migraine; if headache returns, may be repeated after 2 hr. Do not use more than 3 doses/24 hr. Safety of treating more than four headaches/30 days has not been established.

Pediatric patients

Safety and efficacy not established for patients younger than 18 yr.

Pharmacokinetics

Route	*Onset*	*Peak*
Oral	Varies	2–4 hr

Metabolism: Hepatic; $T_{1/2}$: 26 hr
Distribution: Crosses placenta; may enter breast milk
Excretion: Feces, urine

Adverse effects

- **CNS:** Dizziness, headache, anxiety, malaise, fatigue, weakness, myalgia, somnolence, paresthesia (tingling, burning, prickling, itching sensation), loss of sensation, abnormal vision, tinnitus
- **CV:** Palpitations, tightness or pressure in chest, flushing, **MI, cerebrovascular events, ventricular arrhythmias**
- **GI:** Vomiting, diarrhea, abdominal pain, dry mouth, dyspepsia, nausea
- **Musculoskeletal:** Skeletal pain
- **Other:** Warm or hot sensations, cold sensation, pain, increased sweating, rhinitis

Interactions

✱ Drug-drug ⊗ ***Warning*** Increased risk of weakness, hyperreflexia, CNS effects if combined with an SSRI (fluoxetine, fluvoxamine, paroxetine, sertraline); if combined with these drugs, appropriate safety precautions should be observed and patient monitored closely.

- Prolonged vasoactive reactions when taken concurrently with ergot-containing drugs or other triptans; space these drugs at least 24 hr apart

■ Nursing considerations

Assessment

- **History:** Allergy to frovatriptan, active coronary artery disease, Prinzmetal's angina, pregnancy, lactation, peripheral or cerebral vascular syndromes, uncontrolled hypertension, hemiplegic or basilar migraine, use of an ergot compound or other triptan within 24 hr, risk factors for CAD
- **Physical:** Skin color and lesions, orientation, reflexes, peripheral sensation, P, BP, LFTs, ECG

Interventions

- Ensure that the patient has been diagnosed with migraine headaches.
- Administer to relieve acute migraine, not as a prophylactic measure.
- Ensure that the patient has not taken an ergot-containing compound or other triptan within 24 hr.
- Do not administer more than three doses in a 24-hr period; space them at least 2 hr apart.
- Establish safety measures if CNS or visual disturbances occur.
- Provide environmental (lighting, temperature) control as appropriate to help relieve migraine.

⊗ ***Warning*** Monitor BP of patients with possible CAD; discontinue at any sign of angina, prolonged high BP, tachycardia, chest pain.

Teaching points

- Take drug exactly as prescribed, at the onset of headache or aura. Do not take this drug to prevent a migraine; it is only used to treat migraines that are occurring. If the headache persists after you take this drug, you may repeat the dose after 2 hours have passed.
- Do not take more than three doses in a 24-hour period. Do not take any other migraine medication while you are taking this drug. If the headache is not relieved, call your health care provider.
- This drug should not be taken during pregnancy; if you suspect that you are pregnant, contact your health care provider and refrain from using the drug.
- Maintain any procedures you usually use during a migraine (such as controlling lighting and noise).
- Contact your health care provider immediately if you experience chest pain or pressure that is severe or does not go away.
- You may experience these side effects: Dizziness, drowsiness (avoid driving or the use of dangerous machinery while taking this drug); numbness, tingling, feelings of tightness or pressure.
- Report feelings of heat, flushing, tiredness, feelings of sickness, swelling of lips or eyelids.

DANGEROUS DRUG

▽fulvestrant

(full ves' trant)

Faslodex

PREGNANCY CATEGORY D

Drug classes

Antineoplastic
Estrogen receptor antagonist

Therapeutic actions

Binds to estrogen receptors, has anti-estrogen effects; and inhibits growth of estrogen receptor–positive breast cancer cell lines.

Indications

- Treatment of hormone receptor-positive breast cancer in postmenopausal women with disease progression following anti-estrogen therapy

Contraindications and cautions

- Contraindicated with allergy to any component of the drug, pregnancy.
- Use cautiously with bleeding disorders, thrombocytopenia, hepatic impairment, lactation.

Available forms

Injection—50 mg/mL

Dosages

Adults

250 mg IM each month in the buttock as a single 5-mL injection or two concomitant 2.5-mL injections.

Pharmacokinetics

Route	*Onset*	*Peak*
IM	Slow	7 days

Metabolism: Hepatic; $T_{1/2}$: 40 days
Distribution: Crosses placenta; may enter breast milk
Excretion: Feces

Adverse effects

- **CNS:** Depression, light-headedness, dizziness, *headache,* hallucinations, vertigo, insomnia, paresthesia, anxiety, *asthenia*
- **CV:** Chest pain, *vasodilation*
- **Dermatologic:** *Hot flashes,* skin rash
- **GI:** *Nausea, vomiting,* food distaste, constipation, *diarrhea,* anorexia, *abdominal pain*
- **GU:** UTI, *pelvic pain*
- **Respiratory:** *Dyspnea, increased cough*
- **Other:** Peripheral edema, fever, pharyngitis, injection site reactions, pain, flulike symptoms, *increased sweat, anemia, back pain, bone pain, arthritis*

Interactions

✱ **Drug-drug** • Increased risk of bleeding if taken with oral anticoagulants

■ Nursing considerations

Assessment

- **History:** Allergy to any component of the drug; pregnancy, lactation; hepatic impairment, bleeding disorders, thrombocytopenia
- **Physical:** Skin color, lesions, turgor; pelvic examination; orientation, affect, reflex; BP, peripheral pulses, edema; LFTs

Interventions

- Ensure that the patient is not pregnant before administering drug.
- Counsel patient about the need to use contraceptives to avoid pregnancy while taking this drug. Inform patient that serious fetal harm could occur.
- Suggest an alternate method of feeding the baby if this drug is prescribed for a nursing mother.
- Mark a calendar for dates for monthly injections; periodically monitor injection sites if patient is self-administering drug.
- Provide comfort measures to help patient deal with drug effects: Hot flashes (environmental temperature control); headache, depression (monitoring light and noise); vaginal bleeding (hygiene measures); nausea, food distaste (eat frequent small meals).

Teaching points

- You and a significant other should learn the proper technique for administering an intramuscular injection; proper disposal of needles and syringes is important and should be reviewed.
- Mark your calendar with the date of your injection. If you are not able to self-administer the injection, mark your calendar with the dates to return to your health care provider for injections.
- This drug can cause serious fetal harm and must not be taken during pregnancy. Use contraceptives while you are taking this drug. If you become pregnant or decide that you would like to become pregnant, consult your health care provider immediately.
- You may experience these side effects: Hot flashes (staying in cool environment may help); nausea, vomiting (eat frequent small meals); weight gain; dizziness, headache, light-headedness (use caution if driving or performing tasks that require alertness if these occur).
- Report marked weakness, sleepiness, mental confusion, changes in color of urine or stool, pregnancy.

▽ furosemide

(fur oh' se mide)

Apo-Furosemide (CAN), Furosemide Special (CAN), Lasix

PREGNANCY CATEGORY C

Drug class

Loop diuretic

Therapeutic actions

Inhibits reabsorption of sodium and chloride from the proximal and distal tubules and ascending limb of the loop of Henle, leading to a sodium-rich diuresis.

Indications

- Oral, IV: Edema associated with heart failure, cirrhosis, renal disease
- IV: Acute pulmonary edema
- Oral: Hypertension

Contraindications and cautions

- Contraindicated with allergy to furosemide, sulfonamides; allergy to tartrazine (in oral solution); anuria, severe renal failure; hepatic coma; pregnancy; lactation.
- Use cautiously with SLE, gout, diabetes mellitus.

Available forms

Tablets—20, 40, 80 mg; oral solution—10 mg/mL, 40 mg/5 mL; injection—10 mg/mL

Dosages

Adults

- *Edema:* Initially, 20–80 mg/day PO as a single dose. If needed, a second dose may be given in 6–8 hr. If response is unsatisfactory, dose may be increased in 20- to 40-mg increments at 6- to 8-hr intervals. Up to 600 mg/day may be given. Intermittent dosage schedule (2–4 consecutive days/wk) is preferred for maintenance, *or* 20–40 mg IM or IV (slow IV injection over 1–2 min). May increase dose in increments of 20 mg in 2 hr. High-dose therapy should be given as infusion at rate not exceeding 4 mg/min.
- *Acute pulmonary edema:* 40 mg IV over 1–2 min. May be increased to 80 mg IV given over 1–2 min if response is unsatisfactory after 1 hr.
- *Hypertension:* 40 mg bid PO. If needed, additional antihypertensives may be added.

Pediatric patients

Premature infants, **do not exceed 1 mg/kg/day.** Stimulates prostaglandin E_2 synthesis and may increase incidence of patent ductus arteriosus and complicate RDS.

- *Edema:* Initially, 2 mg/kg/day PO. If needed, increase by 1–2 mg/kg in 6–8 hr. **Do not exceed 6 mg/kg.** Adjust maintenance dose to lowest effective level.
- *Pulmonary edema:* 1 mg/kg IV or IM. May increase by 1 mg/kg in 2 hr until the desired effect is seen. **Do not exceed 6 mg/kg.**

Patients with renal impairment

Up to 4 g/day has been tolerated. IV bolus injection should not exceed 1 g/day given over 30 min.

Pharmacokinetics

Route	*Onset*	*Peak*	*Duration*
Oral	60 min	60–120 min	6–8 hr
IV, IM	5 min	30 min	2 hr

Metabolism: Hepatic; $T_{1/2}$: 30–60 min
Distribution: Crosses placenta; enters breast milk
Excretion: Feces, urine

IV FACTS

Preparation: Store at room temperature; exposure to light may slightly discolor solution.
Infusion: Inject directly or into tubing of actively running IV; inject slowly over 1–2 min.
Incompatibilities: Do not mix with acidic solutions. Isotonic saline, lactated Ringer's injection, and 5% dextrose injection may be used after pH has been adjusted (if necessary); precipitates form with gentamicin, milrinone in 5% dextrose, 0.9% sodium chloride.

Adverse effects

- **CNS:** *Dizziness, vertigo, paresthesias, xanthopsia, weakness,* headache, drowsiness, fatigue, blurred vision, tinnitus, irreversible hearing loss
- **CV:** *Orthostatic hypotension,* volume depletion, cardiac arrhythmias, *thrombophlebitis*
- **Dermatologic:** *Photosensitivity, rash, pruritus, urticaria,* purpura, exfoliative dermatitis, erythema multiforme

- **GI:** *Nausea, anorexia, vomiting, oral and gastric irritation, constipation*, diarrhea, acute pancreatitis, jaundice
- **GU:** Polyuria, nocturia, glycosuria, *urinary bladder spasm*
- **Hematologic:** *Leukopenia, anemia, thrombocytopenia,* fluid and electrolyte imbalances, hyperglycemia, hyperuricemia
- **Other:** *Muscle cramps and muscle spasms*

Interactions

✱ **Drug-drug** • Increased risk of cardiac arrhythmias with cardiac glycosides (due to electrolyte imbalance) • Increased risk of ototoxicity with aminoglycoside antibiotics, cisplatin • Decreased absorption of furosemide with phenytoin • Decreased natriuretic and antihypertensive effects with indomethacin, ibuprofen, other NSAIDs • Decreased GI absorption with charcoal • May reduce effect of insulin or oral antidiabetics because blood glucose levels can become elevated

■ Nursing considerations

CLINICAL ALERT!

Name confusion has occurred between furosemide and torsemide; use extreme caution.

Assessment

- **History:** Allergy to furosemide, sulfonamides, tartrazine; electrolyte depletion anuria, severe renal failure; hepatic coma; SLE; gout; diabetes mellitus; lactation, pregnancy
- **Physical:** Skin color, lesions, edema; orientation, reflexes, hearing; pulses, baseline ECG, BP, orthostatic BP, perfusion; R, pattern, adventitious sounds; liver evaluation, bowel sounds; urinary output patterns; CBC, serum electrolytes (including calcium), blood sugar, LFTs, renal function tests, uric acid, urinalysis, weight

Interventions

⊗ ***Black box warning*** Profound diuresis with water and electrolyte depletion can occur; careful medical supervision is required.

- Administer with food or milk to prevent GI upset.
- Reduce dosage if given with other antihypertensives; readjust dosage gradually as BP responds.
- Give early in the day so that increased urination will not disturb sleep.
- Avoid IV use if oral use is at all possible.

⊗ ***Warning*** Do not mix parenteral solution with highly acidic solutions with pH below 3.5.

- Do not expose to light, which may discolor tablets or solution; do not use discolored drug or solutions.
- Discard diluted solution after 24 hr.
- Refrigerate oral solution.
- Measure and record weight to monitor fluid changes.
- Arrange to monitor serum electrolytes, hydration, liver and renal function.
- Arrange for potassium-rich diet or supplemental potassium as needed.

Teaching points

- Record intermittent therapy on a calendar or dated envelopes. When possible, take the drug early so increased urination will not disturb sleep. Take with food or meals to prevent GI upset.
- Weigh yourself on a regular basis, at the same time and in the same clothing, and record the weight on your calendar.
- Blood glucose levels may become temporarily elevated in patients with diabetes after starting this drug.
- You may experience these side effects: Increased volume and frequency of urination; dizziness, feeling faint on arising, drowsiness (avoid rapid position changes; hazardous activities, like driving; and consumption of alcohol); sensitivity to sunlight (use sunglasses, wear protective clothing, or use a sunscreen); increased thirst (suck on sugarless lozenges; use frequent mouth care); loss of body potassium (a potassium-rich diet or potassium supplement will be needed).
- Report loss or gain of more than 1.5 kg in 1 day, swelling in your ankles or fingers, unusual bleeding or bruising, dizziness, trembling, numbness, fatigue, muscle weakness or cramps.

gabapentin
*(gab ah **pen'** tin)*

Apo-Gabapentin (CAN), CO Gabapentin (CAN), Gen-Gabapentin (CAN), Neurontin, Novo-Gabapentin (CAN), PMS Gabapentin (CAN), ratio-Gabapentin (CAN)

PREGNANCY CATEGORY C

Drug class
Antiepileptic

Therapeutic actions
Mechanism of action not understood; antiepileptic activity may be related to its ability to inhibit polysynaptic responses and block posttetanic potentiation.

Indications
- Adjunctive therapy in the treatment of partial seizures with and without secondary generalization in adults and children 3–12 yr with epilepsy
- Orphan drug use: Treatment of amyotrophic lateral sclerosis
- Management of postherpetic neuralgia or pain in the area affected by herpes zoster after the disease has been treated
- Unlabeled uses: Hot flashes, neuropathic pain

Contraindications and cautions
- Contraindicated with hypersensitivity to gabapentin.
- Use cautiously with pregnancy, lactation.

Available forms
Capsules—100, 300, 400 mg; tablets—100, 300, 400, 600, 800 mg; oral solution—250 mg/5 mL

Dosages
Adults
- *Epilepsy:* Starting dose is 300 mg PO tid, then titrated up as needed. *Maintenance:* 900–1,800 mg/day PO in divided doses tid PO; maximum interval between doses should not exceed 12 hr. Up to 2,400–3,600 mg/day has been used.
- *Postherpetic neuralgia:* Initial dose of 300 mg/day PO; 300 mg bid PO on day 2; 300 mg tid PO on day 3.

Pediatric patients 3–12 yr

Initially, 10–15 mg/kg/day PO in three divided doses; adjust upward over about 3 days to 25–35 mg/kg daily in three divided doses in children 5 yr and older, and up to 40 mg/kg/day in three divided doses in children 3–4 yr.

Geriatric patients or patients with renal impairment

CrCl (mL/min)	*Dosage (mg/day)*
More than 60	900–3,600 in three divided doses
More than 30–59	400–1,400 in two divided doses
More than 15–29	200–700 in one dose
Less than 15	100–300 in one dose

Postdialysis supplemental dosing, 125–350 mg PO following each 4 hr of dialysis.

Pharmacokinetics

Route	*Onset*	*Duration*
Oral	Varies	6–8 hr

Metabolism: Hepatic; $T_{1/2}$: 5–7 hr
Distribution: Crosses placenta; enters breast milk
Excretion: Urine, unchanged

Adverse effects
- **CNS:** *Dizziness, insomnia,* nervousness, fatigue, *somnolence, ataxia,* diplopia, tremor
- **Dermatologic:** Pruritus, abrasion
- **GI:** Dyspepsia, vomiting, nausea, constipation, dry mouth, diarrhea
- **Respiratory:** Rhinitis, pharyngitis
- **Other:** Weight gain, facial edema, cancer, impotence, suicidal ideation

Interactions
✱ **Drug-drug** • Decreased serum levels with antacids

✱ **Drug-lab test** • False-positives may occur with *Ames N-Multistix SG* dipstick test for protein in the urine

■ Nursing considerations
Assessment
- **History:** Hypersensitivity to gabapentin; lactation, pregnancy
- **Physical:** Weight; T; skin color, lesions; orientation, affect, reflexes; P; R, adventitious sounds; bowel sounds, normal output

Interventions
- Give drug with food to prevent GI upset.
- Be aware that patient may be at increased risk for suicidality; monitor accordingly.
- Arrange for consultation with support groups for people with epilepsy.

⊗ ***Warning*** If overdose occurs, hemodialysis may be an option.

Teaching points
- Take this drug exactly as prescribed; do not discontinue abruptly or change dosage, except on the advice of your health care provider.
- Wear a medical alert ID at all times so that any emergency medical personnel will know that you have epilepsy and are taking antiepileptic medication.
- You may experience these side effects: Dizziness, blurred vision (avoid driving or performing other tasks requiring alertness or visual acuity); GI upset (take drug with food or milk, eat frequent small meals); headache, nervousness, insomnia; fatigue (periodic rest periods may help).
- Report severe headache, sleepwalking, rash, severe vomiting, chills, fever, difficulty breathing, thoughts of suicide.

▽ galantamine hydrobromide
*(gah **lan'** tah meen)*

Razadyne, Razadyne ER DNC

PREGNANCY CATEGORY B

Drug classes
Alzheimer's disease drug
Cholinesterase inhibitor

Therapeutic actions
Centrally acting, selective, long-acting, reversible cholinesterase inhibitor; causes elevated acetylcholine levels in the cortex, which is thought to slow the neuronal degradation that occurs in Alzheimer's disease.

Indications
- Treatment of mild to moderate dementia of the Alzheimer's type
- Unlabeled use: Vascular dementia

Contraindications and cautions
- Contraindicated with allergy to galantamine, severe hepatic impairment, severe renal impairment.
- Use cautiously with moderate renal or hepatic impairment, GI bleeding, seizures, asthma, COPD, pregnancy, lactation, and CV conditions.

Available forms
Tablets—4, 8, 12 mg; oral solution with dosing syringe—4 mg/mL; ER capsules DNC—8, 16, 24 mg

Dosages
Adults
Initially, 4 mg PO bid. If well tolerated after 4 wk, increase to 8 mg PO bid. If well tolerated after 4 more wk, increase to 12 mg PO bid. Range: 16–32 mg/day in two divided doses; ER capsules—initial dose, 8 mg/day PO; titrate to 16–24 mg/day PO.

Pediatric patients
Safety and efficacy not established.

Patients with hepatic or renal impairment
Do not exceed 16 mg/day. Contraindicated if creatinine clearance less than 9 mL/min or if Child-Pugh score is 10–15.

Pharmacokinetics

Route	*Onset*	*Peak*	*Duration*
Oral	Varies	1 hr	8 hr

Metabolism: Hepatic; $T_{1/2}$: 7 hr
Distribution: Crosses placenta; may enter breast milk
Excretion: Urine

Adverse effects
- **CNS:** *Insomnia,* tremor, *dizziness,* fatigue, sedation, somnolence, tremor, headache
- **CV:** Bradycardia, syncope

- **GI:** *Nausea, vomiting, diarrhea, dyspepsia, anorexia, abdominal pain,* weight loss
- **GU:** UTI, hematuria

Interactions

✱ **Drug-drug** • Increased galantamine concentration with drugs that are potent inhibitors of CYP2D6 or CYP3A4 • Increased effects and risk of galantamine toxicity if combined with cimetidine, ketoconazole, paroxetine, erythromycin, succinylcholine, or bethanechol; if any of these combinations are used, monitor patient closely and adjust dosage as needed

■ Nursing considerations

CLINICAL ALERT!
Because of name confusion, the manufacturer has changed the drug name *Reminyl* to *Razadyne.*

Assessment

- **History:** Allergy to galantamine, pregnancy, lactation, impaired renal or hepatic function, GI bleeding, seizures, asthma, COPD, CV conditions
- **Physical:** Orientation, affect, reflexes, BP, P, abdominal examination, LFTs, renal function tests

Interventions

- Establish baseline functional profile to allow evaluation of drug effectiveness.
- Ensure at least 4 wk at each dosage level to establish effectiveness and tolerance of adverse effects.
- Administer with food in the morning and evening to decrease GI discomfort.
- Mix solution with water, fruit juice, or soda to improve compliance.
- Ensure that patient swallows ER capsules whole; do not cut, crush, or allow patient to chew capsule. Capsule can be opened and contents sprinkled over soft food.
- Monitor patient for weight loss, diarrhea, and arrhythmias before use and periodically with prolonged use.
- Provide frequent small meals if GI upset is severe; antiemetics may be used if necessary.
- Provide patient safety measures if CNS effects occur.

⊗ **Warning** Notify surgeon that patient takes galantamine; exaggerated muscle relaxation may occur if succinylcholine-type drugs are used.

Teaching points

- Take drug exactly as prescribed, with food, in the morning and evening to decrease GI upset.
- Switch to oral solution if swallowing becomes difficult; mix with water, fruit juice, or soda to improve taste.
- Swallow capsules whole; do not cut, crush, or chew. Contents can be sprinkled over soft food if swallowing is difficult.
- This drug does not cure the disease but is thought to slow the degeneration associated with the disease.
- Dosage changes may be needed to achieve the best effects. If the drug is stopped for more than a few days, consult your health care provider; it should be restarted at the original, lower dose.
- You may experience these side effects: Nausea, vomiting (eat frequent small meals); insomnia, fatigue, confusion (use caution if driving or performing tasks that require alertness).
- Report severe nausea, vomiting, changes in stool or urine color, diarrhea, changes in neurologic functioning, palpitations.

▽ galsulfase

See Appendix W, *Less commonly used drugs.*

▽ ganciclovir sodium (DHPG)

(gan sye' kloe vir)

Cytovene (DNC), Vitrasert

PREGNANCY CATEGORY C

Drug class

Antiviral

Therapeutic actions

Antiviral activity; inhibits viral DNA replication in cytomegalovirus (CMV).

Indications

- IV and implant: Treatment of CMV retinitis in immunocompromised patients, including patients with AIDS
- IV: Prevention of CMV disease in transplant recipients at risk for CMV disease
- Oral: Alternative to IV for maintenance treatment of CMV retinitis
- Oral: Prevention of CMV disease in individuals with advanced HIV infection at risk of developing CMV disease
- Unlabeled use: Treatment of other CMV infections in immunocompromised patients

Contraindications and cautions

- Contraindicated with hypersensitivity to ganciclovir or acyclovir, lactation.
- Use cautiously with cytopenia, history of cytopenic reactions, impaired renal function, pregnancy.

Available forms

Capsules DNG—250, 500 mg; powder for injection—500 mg/vial; ocular implant—4.5 mg

Dosages

Adults

- *CMV retinitis:* Initial dose, 5 mg/kg given IV at a constant rate over 1 hr, every 12 hr for 14–21 days. For maintenance, 5 mg/kg given by IV infusion over 1 hr once daily, 7 days/wk *or* 6 mg/kg once daily, 5 days/wk; or 1,000 mg PO tid with food or 500 mg PO 6 times per day every 3 hr with food while awake. Implant surgically placed in affected eye every 5–8 mo.
- *Prevention of CMV disease in transplant recipients:* 5 mg/kg IV over 1 hr every 12 hr for 7–14 days; then 5 mg/kg/day once daily for 7 days/wk, *or* 6 mg/kg/day once daily for 5 days/wk. Prophylactic oral dose is 1,000 mg tid with food. Duration depends on duration and degree of immunosuppression.
- *Prevention of CMV disease with advanced AIDS:* 1,000 mg PO tid with food.

Pediatric patients

Safety and efficacy not established. Use only if benefit outweighs potential carcinogenesis and reproductive toxicity.

Patients with renal impairment

Initial IV dose

CrCl (mL/min)	*Dose IV (mg/kg)*	*Dosing Intervals*
70 or more	5 mg/kg	12 hr
50–69	2.5	12 hr
25–49	2.5	24 hr
10–24	1.25	24 hr
< 10	1.25	Three times/wk following hemodialysis

Maintenance

CrCl (mL/min)	*Dose IV (mg/kg)*	*Dosing Intervals*
70 or more	5 mg/kg	24 hr
50–69	2.5	24 hr
25–49	1.25	24 hr
10–24	0.625	24 hr
< 10	0.625	Three times/wk following hemodialysis

Oral dose

CrCl (mL/min)	*Dose PO (mg)*
70 or more	1,000 mg tid or 500 mg every 3 hr six times/day
50–69	1,500 daily or 500 tid
25–49	1,000 daily or 500 bid
10–24	500 daily
< 10	500 three times/wk following dialysis

Pharmacokinetics

Route	*Onset*	*Peak*
IV	Slow	1 hr
Oral	Slow	2–4 hr

Metabolism: Hepatic; $T_{1/2}$: 2–4 hr (IV), 4.8 hr (PO)

Distribution: Crosses placenta; may enter breast milk

Excretion: Feces, urine

IV FACTS

Preparation: Reconstitute vial by injecting 10 mL of sterile water for injection into vial; do not use bacteriostatic water for injection; shake vial to dissolve the drug. Discard vial if any particulate matter or discoloration is seen. Reconstituted solution in the vial is stable at

room temperature for 12 hr. Do not refrigerate reconstituted solution. Drug is stable for 14 days after mixing with 0.9% normal saline.
Infusion: Infuse slowly over 1 hr.
Compatibilities: Compatible with 0.9% sodium chloride, 5% dextrose, Ringer's injection, and lactated Ringer's injection.
Y-site incompatibilities: Do not combine with foscarnet, ondansetron.

Adverse effects

- **CNS:** Dreams, ataxia, coma, confusion, dizziness, headache
- **CV:** Arrhythmia, hypertension, hypotension
- **Dermatologic:** *Rash,* alopecia, pruritus, urticaria
- **GI:** *Abnormal liver function tests,* nausea, vomiting, anorexia, diarrhea, abdominal pain
- **Hematologic:** *Granulocytopenia, thrombocytopenia, anemia,* neutropenia
- **Local:** *Pain, inflammation at injection site,* phlebitis
- **Other:** *Fever,* chills, **cancer,** sterility

Interactions

✱ **Drug-drug** ⊗ ***Warning*** Use with extreme caution with cytotoxic drugs because the accumulation effect could cause severe bone marrow depression and other GI and dermatologic problems.
• Increased effects if taken with probenecid • Increased risk of seizures with imipenem-cilastatin • Extreme drowsiness and risk of bone marrow depression with zidovudine

■ Nursing considerations

Assessment

- **History:** Hypersensitivity to ganciclovir or acyclovir; cytopenia; impaired renal function; lactation, pregnancy
- **Physical:** Skin color, lesions; orientation; BP, P, auscultation, perfusion, edema; R, adventitious sounds; urinary output; CBC, Hct, BUN, creatinine clearance, LFTs

Interventions

- Give by IV infusion only. Do not give IM or subcutaneously; drug is very irritating to tissues.
- Do not exceed the recommended dosage, frequency, or infusion rates.
- Monitor infusion carefully; infuse at concentrations no greater than 10 mg/mL.
- Decrease dosage in patients with impaired renal function.
- Give oral doses with food.

⊠ ***Black box warning*** Obtain CBC before therapy, every 2 days during daily dosing, and at least weekly thereafter. Consult with physician and arrange for reduced dosage if WBC or platelet counts fall.

⊗ ***Warning*** Consult with pharmacy for proper disposal of unused solution. Precautions are required for disposal of nucleoside analogues.

⊗ ***Warning*** Avoid direct contact with skin or mucous membranes.

⊗ ***Warning*** Do not open or crush capsules.

- Provide patient with a calendar of drug days, and arrange convenient times for the IV infusion in outpatients.
- Advise patients having surgical implant of ganciclovir that procedure will need to be repeated every 5–8 mo.
- Arrange for periodic ophthalmic examinations. Drug is not a cure for the disease, and deterioration may occur.
- Advise patients that ganciclovir can decrease sperm production and cause birth defects in fetuses. Advise the patient to use contraception during ganciclovir therapy. Men receiving ganciclovir therapy should use barrier contraception during and for at least 90 days after ganciclovir therapy.
- Advise patient that ganciclovir has caused cancer in animals and that risk is possible in humans.

Teaching points

- Appointments will be made for you if you are an outpatient on IV therapy. Long-term therapy is frequently needed. Take the oral drug with food; do not open, crush, cut, or chew capsules. Surgical implant of drug will need to be repeated every 5–8 months.
- Frequent blood tests will be necessary to determine drug effects on your blood count and to adjust drug dosage. Keep appointments for these tests.
- Arrange for periodic ophthalmic examinations during therapy to evaluate progress of the disease. This drug is not a cure for your retinitis.

- If you also are receiving zidovudine, the two drugs cannot be given at the same time; severe adverse effects may occur.
- You may experience these side effects: Rash, fever, pain at injection site; decreased blood count leading to susceptibility to infection (frequent blood tests will be needed; avoid crowds and exposure to disease); birth defects and decreased sperm production (drug must not be taken during pregnancy; if pregnant or intending to become pregnant, consult your health care provider; use some form of contraception during therapy; male patients should use barrier contraception during therapy and for at least 90 days after therapy).
- Report bruising, bleeding, pain at injection site, fever, infection.

ganirelix acetate

See Appendix W, *Less commonly used drugs.*

gefitinib

See Appendix W, *Less commonly used drugs.*

DANGEROUS DRUG

gemcitabine hydrochloride

(jem site' ah ben)

Gemzar

PREGNANCY CATEGORY D

Drug classes

Antimetabolite
Antineoplastic
Pyrimidine analogue

Therapeutic actions

Cytotoxic: A nucleoside analogue that is cell cycle S–specific; causes cell death by disrupting and inhibiting DNA synthesis.

Indications

- First-line treatment of locally advanced or metastatic adenocarcinoma of pancreas; indicated for patients who have previously received 5-FU
- In combination with cisplatin as the first-line treatment of inoperable, locally advanced or metastatic non–small-cell lung cancer
- First-line therapy for metastatic breast cancer after failure of other adjuvant chemotherapy with an anthracycline, with paclitaxel
- In combination with carboplatin for the treatment of advanced ovarian cancer that has relapsed at least 6 mo after completion of a platinum-based therapy
- Unlabeled uses: Treatment of biliary cancer, bladder cancer, relapsed or refractory testicular cancer, squamous cell carcinoma of the head and neck

Contraindications and cautions

- Contraindicated with hypersensitivity to gemcitabine.
- Use cautiously with bone marrow suppression, renal or hepatic impairment, pregnancy, lactation.

Available forms

Powder for injection—200 mg/1 g

Dosages

Adults

- *Pancreatic cancer:* 1,000 mg/m^2 IV over 30 min given once weekly for up to 7 wk or until bone marrow suppression requires withholding treatment; subsequent cycles of once weekly for 3 out of 4 consecutive weeks can be given after 1-wk rest from treatment. For a patient who has completed the 7-wk course of initial therapy, the dose may be increased by 25% provided there is no significant hematologic toxicity.
- *Non–small-cell lung cancer:* 1,000 mg/m^2 IV over 30 min, days 1, 8, and 15 of each 28-day cycle with 100 mg/m^2 cisplatin on day 1 after gemcitabine infusion, *or* 1,250 mg/m^2 IV over 30 min, days 1 and 8 of each 21-day cycle with 100 mg/m^2 cisplatin on day 1 after gemcitabine infusion.
- *Metastatic breast cancer:* 1,250 mg/m^2 IV given over 30 min on days 1 and 8 of each 21-day cycle; with 175 mg/m^2 paclitaxel IV as a 3-hr infusion given before gemcitabine on day 1 of the cycle. Adjust dosage based on total granulocyte and

G

platelet counts taken on day 8 of the cycle for that dose.

- *Advanced ovarian cancer:* 1,000 mg/m^2 IV given over 30 min on days 1 and 8 of each 21-day cycle. Carboplatin is given on day 1 after gemcitabine.

Pediatric patients

Safety and efficacy not established.

Pharmacokinetics

Route	*Onset*	*Peak*
IV	Rapid	30 min

Metabolism: Hepatic; $T_{1/2}$: 42–70 min; half-life is linearly dependent on infusion time
Distribution: Crosses placenta; may enter breast milk
Excretion: Bile, urine

IV FACTS

Preparation: Use 0.9% sodium chloride injection as diluent for reconstitution of powder, 5 mL of 0.9% sodium chloride injection added to the 200-mg vial or 25 mL added to the 1-g vial. This will yield a concentration of 38 mg/mL; higher concentrations may lead to inadequate dissolution of powder. Resultant drug can be injected as reconstituted or further diluted in 0.9% sodium chloride injection. Stable for 24 hr at room temperature after reconstitution.
Infusion: Infuse slowly over 30 min; do not allow prolonged infusion; toxicity increases with length of infusion.

Adverse effects

- **CNS:** Somnolence, paresthesias
- **GI:** *Nausea, vomiting,* diarrhea, constipation, mucositis, GI bleeding, stomatitis, hepatic impairment
- **Hematologic: Bone marrow depression,** *infections*
- **Hepatic:** Elevated ALT
- **Pulmonary:** Dyspnea, **interstitial pneumonitis**
- **Renal:** Hematuria, proteinuria, elevated BUN and creatinine
- **Other:** *Fever, alopecia, pain, rash, edema, flulike symptoms*

■ Nursing considerations

Assessment

- **History:** Hypersensitivity to gemcitabine; bone marrow depression; renal or hepatic impairment; pregnancy, lactation
- **Physical:** T; skin color, lesions; R, adventitious sounds; abdominal examination, mucous membranes; LFTs, renal function tests, CBC with differential, urinalysis

Interventions

⊗ ***Warning*** Infuse over 30 min; longer infusions (more than 60 min) cause increased half-life and severe toxicity.

⊗ ***Warning*** Follow CBC, LFTs, and renal function tests carefully before and frequently during therapy; dosage adjustment may be needed if myelosuppression becomes severe or hepatic or renal impairment occurs.

- Protect patient from exposure to infection; monitor occurrence of infection at any site and arrange for appropriate treatment.
- Provide medication, frequent small meals for severe nausea and vomiting; monitor nutritional status.

Teaching points

- This drug must be given IV over 30 minutes once a week or as protocol dosing. Mark calendar with days to return for treatment. Regular blood tests will be needed to evaluate the effects of treatment.
- You may experience these side effects: Nausea and vomiting (may be severe; antiemetics may be helpful; eat frequent small meals); increased susceptibility to infection (avoid crowds and situations that may expose you to diseases); loss of hair (arrange for a wig or other head covering; keep the head covered at extremes of temperature).
- Report severe nausea and vomiting, fever, chills, sore throat, unusual bleeding or bruising, changes in color of urine or stool.

▽gemfibrozil

(jem fi' broe zil)

Apo-Gemfibrozil (CAN), Gen-Gemfibrozil (CAN), Lopid, PMS-Gemfibrozil (CAN)

PREGNANCY CATEGORY C

Drug class

Antihyperlipidemic

Therapeutic actions

Inhibits peripheral lipolysis and decreases the hepatic excretion of free fatty acids; this reduces hepatic triglyceride production; inhibits synthesis of VLDL carrier apolipoprotein; decreases VLDL production; increases HDL concentration.

Indications

- As adjunct to diet and exercise for hypertriglyceridemia in adult patients with very high elevations of triglyceride levels (type IV and V hyperlipidemia) at risk of pancreatitis unresponsive to diet therapy
- As adjunct to diet and exercise in reduction of coronary heart disease risk in patients who have not responded to diet, exercise, and other drugs and have low HDL levels in addition to high LDL and triglyceride levels

Contraindications and cautions

- Contraindicated with allergy to gemfibrozil, hepatic or renal impairment, primary biliary cirrhosis, gallbladder disease.
- Use cautiously with pregnancy, lactation, cholelithiasis, and renal impairment.

Available forms

Tablets—600 mg

Dosages

Adults

⊗ ***Warning*** 1,200 mg/day PO in two divided doses, 30 min before morning and evening meals. Caution: Use only if strongly indicated and lipid studies show a definite response; hepatic tumorigenicity occurs in laboratory animals.

Pediatric patients

Safety and efficacy not established.

Patients with renal or hepatic impairment

Contraindicated with hepatic impairment or severe renal impairment. Use caution with mild to moderate renal impairment.

Pharmacokinetics

Route	Onset	Peak
Oral	Varies	1–2 hr

Metabolism: Hepatic; $T_{1/2}$: 90 min
Distribution: Crosses placenta; enters breast milk
Excretion: Feces, urine

Adverse effects

- **CNS:** *Headache, dizziness, blurred vision,* vertigo, insomnia, paresthesia, tinnitus, *fatigue,* malaise, syncope
- **Dermatologic:** *Eczema, rash,* dermatitis, pruritus, urticaria
- **GI:** *Abdominal pain, epigastric pain, diarrhea, nausea, vomiting,* flatulence, dry mouth, constipation, anorexia, *dyspepsia,* cholelithiasis, elevated ALT and AST
- **GU:** Impairment of fertility
- **Hematologic:** Anemia, **eosinophilia, leukopenia,** hypokalemia, liver function changes, hyperglycemia
- **Other:** Painful extremities, back pain, arthralgia, muscle cramps, myalgia, swollen joints, myopathy

Interactions

✱ **Drug-drug** • Risk of rhabdomyolysis from 3 wk to several mo after therapy when combined with HMG-CoA reductase inhibitors (eg, lovastatin, simvastatin) • Risk of increased bleeding when combined with anticoagulants; monitor patient closely • Risk of hypoglycemia if combined with sulfonylureas and repaglinide; monitor closely

■ Nursing considerations

Assessment

- **History:** Allergy to gemfibrozil, hepatic or renal impairment, primary biliary cirrhosis, gallbladder disease, pregnancy, lactation
- **Physical:** Skin lesions, color, T; gait, range of motion; orientation, affect, reflexes; bowel sounds, normal output, liver evaluation;

G

lipid studies, CBC, LFTs, renal function tests, blood glucose

Interventions

- Administer drug with meals or milk if GI upset occurs.
- Ensure that patient continues diet and exercise programs.
- Arrange for regular follow-up visits, including blood tests for lipids, liver function, CBC, and blood glucose during long-term therapy.

Teaching points

- Take the drug with meals or with milk if GI upset occurs; changes in diet will be needed.
- Continue to follow diet and exercise recommendations for your high lipid levels.
- Have regular follow-up visits to your health care provider for blood tests to evaluate drug effectiveness.
- You may experience these side effects: Diarrhea, loss of appetite, flatulence (eat frequent small meals); muscular aches and pains, bone and joint discomfort; dizziness, faintness, blurred vision (use caution if driving or operating dangerous equipment).
- Report severe stomach pain with nausea and vomiting, fever and chills or sore throat, severe headache, vision changes.

▽ gemifloxacin mesylate

*(jem ah **flox'** a sin)*

Factive DNC

PREGNANCY CATEGORY C

Drug classes

Antibiotic
Fluoroquinolone

Therapeutic actions

Bactericidal; interferes with DNA replication, repair, transcription, and recombination in susceptible gram-negative and gram-positive bacteria, preventing cell reproduction and leading to cell death.

Indications

- Treatment of acute bacterial exacerbation of chronic bronchitis caused by *Streptococcus pneumoniae, Haemophilus influenzae, H. parainfluenzae, Moraxella catarrhalis*
- Treatment of community-acquired pneumonia caused by *S. pneumoniae* (including multi-drug–resistant strains), *H. influenzae, Moraxella catarrhalis, Mycoplasma pneumonia, Chlamydia pneumoniae, Klebsiella pneumoniae*

Contraindications and cautions

- Contraindicated with history of sensitivity to gemifloxacin or any fluoroquinolone antibiotic; history of prolonged QTc interval; uncorrected hypokalemia or hypomagnesemia; use of quinidine, procainamide, amiodarone, or sotalol antiarrhythmics.
- Use cautiously with epilepsy or predisposition to seizures; pregnancy; lactation.

Available forms

Tablets DNC—320 mg

Dosages

Adults

- *Acute bacterial exacerbation of chronic bronchitis:* 320 mg/day PO for 5 days.
- *Community-acquired pneumonia:* 320 mg/day PO for 7 days for known or suspected *S. pneumoniae, H. influenzae, M. pneumoniae,* or *C. pneumoniae* and 7 days for known or suspected multi-drug–resistant *S. pneumoniae, K. pneumoniae,* or *M. catarrhalis.*

Pediatric patients

Safety and efficacy not established.

Patients with renal impairment

For creatinine clearance greater than 40 mL/min, use usual dose; for creatinine clearance of 40 mL/min or less, use 160 mg/day PO.

Pharmacokinetics

Route	*Onset*	*Peak*
Oral	Rapid	0.5–2 hr

Metabolism: Hepatic; $T_{1/2}$: 4–12 hr
Distribution: May cross the placenta; may enter breast milk

Excretion: Feces, urine

Adverse effects

- **CNS:** Headache, dizziness, anorexia, tremor, vertigo, nervousness, insomnia
- **CV:** Increased QTc interval
- **GI:** Diarrhea, **ulcerative colitis,** nausea, abdominal pain, vomiting, taste perversion, gastroenteritis, dry mouth, dyspepsia, flatulence, elevated ALT
- **GU:** Fungal infection, genital moniliasis, vaginitis
- **Respiratory:** Pharyngitis, pneumonia
- **Other:** Rash, fatigue, back pain, eczema, urticaria, myalgia, photosensitivity, ruptured tendons

Interactions

✱ **Drug-drug** • Decreased absorption and serum levels if taken with calcium, sucalfrate, iron, didanosine, aluminum- or potassium-containing antacids; take these drugs 3 hr before or 2 hr after taking gemifloxacin • Increased risk of prolonged QT interval if combined with quinidine, procainamide, amiodarone or sotalol, erythromycin, antipsychotics, antidepressants; avoid these combinations

■ Nursing considerations

Assessment

- **History:** Allergy to fluoroquinolones; prolonged QT interval, uncorrected hypokalemia or hypomagnesemia; use of quinidine, procainamide, amiodarone, or sotalol antiarrhythmics; epilepsy or predisposition to seizures, pregnancy, lactation
- **Physical:** Skin color, lesions; T; orientation, reflexes, affect; R, adventitious sounds; mucous membranes, bowel sounds; LFTs, renal function tests, ECG, serum electrolytes

Interventions

⊠ ***Black box warning*** There is a risk of tendinitis and tendon rupture with drug administration. Risk increases in patients older than 60 yr, with concurrent corticosteroid use, and with kidney, heart, or lung transplant. Monitor these patients accordingly.

- Arrange for culture and sensitivity tests before beginning therapy.
- Continue therapy as indicated for condition being treated.
- Ensure that the tablet is swallowed whole, not cut, crushed, or chewed.

⊗ ***Warning*** Administer drug 3 hr before or at least 2 hr after antacids, iron, multivitamins, didanosine, or sucralfate.

⊗ ***Warning*** Discontinue drug at any sign of hypersensitivity (rash, photophobia) or with severe diarrhea.

- Discontinue drug and monitor ECG if palpitations or dizziness occurs.
- Monitor clinical response; if no improvement or a relapse occurs, repeat culture and sensitivity tests.

Teaching points

- Take drug once a day, at the same time each day, for the period prescribed, even if you are feeling much better. Swallow the tablet whole; do not cut, crush, or chew the tablet.
- If antacids, iron, multivitamins, sucralfate, or didanosine are being taken, you should take gemifloxacin 3 hours before or at least 2 hours after these drugs.
- Do not save tablets to self-treat other infections because this drug is very specific for the infection you have now.
- Drink plenty of fluids while you are taking this drug.
- Find another method of feeding your baby if you are nursing; the effects of this drug on the baby are not known.
- Stop the drug and notify your health care provider immediately if you experience acute pain or tenderness in a muscle or tendon; if you develop severe or bloody diarrhea or a severe rash.
- You may experience these side effects: Nausea, vomiting, abdominal pain (eat frequent small meals); diarrhea or constipation (consult your health care provider if this occurs); drowsiness, blurring of vision, dizziness (use caution if driving or using dangerous equipment); sensitivity to the sun (avoid exposure or use a sunscreen).
- Report palpitations, severe diarrhea, rash, fainting spells.

▽ gemtuzumab ozogamicin

See Appendix W, *Less commonly used drugs.*

gentamicin sulfate

*(jen ta **mye'** sin)*

Parenteral, intrathecal: Alcomicin (CAN), Pediatric Gentamicin Sulfate

Topical dermatologic cream, ointment: Garamycin

Ophthalmic: Garamycin, Gentacidin, Gentak, Genoptic, Genoptic S.O.P., Gentamicin impregnated

Implantable beads: Septopal

Gentamicin liposome injection: Maitec

PREGNANCY CATEGORY D

PREGNANCY CATEGORY C (OPHTHALMIC)

Drug class

Aminoglycoside

Therapeutic actions

Bactericidal: Inhibits protein synthesis in susceptible strains of gram-negative bacteria; appears to disrupt functional integrity of bacterial cell membrane, causing cell death.

Indications

Parenteral

- Serious infections caused by susceptible strains of *Pseudomonas aeruginosa, Proteus* species, *Escherichia coli, Klebsiella-Enterobacter-Serratia* species, *Citrobacter, Staphylococcus* species
- Serious infections when causative organisms are not known (often in conjunction with a penicillin or cephalosporin)
- Unlabeled use: With clindamycin as alternative regimen in PID

Intrathecal

- Gram-negative infections
- Serious CNS infections, such as meningitis, ventriculitis, infections caused by susceptible *Pseudomonas* species

Ophthalmic preparations

- Treatment of superficial ocular infections due to strains of microorganisms susceptible to gentamicin

Topical dermatologic preparation

- Infection prophylaxis in minor skin abrasions and treatment of superficial infections of the skin due to susceptible organisms amenable to local treatment

Gentamicin-impregnated PMAA beads on surgical wire

- Orphan drug use: Treatment of chronic osteomyelitis of posttraumatic, postoperative, or hematogenous origin

Gentamicin liposome injection

- Orphan drug use: Treatment of disseminated *Myobacterium avium-intracellulare* infection

Contraindications and cautions

- Contraindicated with allergy to any aminoglycosides.
- Use cautiously with renal or hepatic disease; sulfite sensitivity; preexisting hearing loss; active infection with herpes, vaccinia, varicella, fungal infections, mycobacterial infections (ophthalmic preparations); myasthenia gravis; parkinsonism; infant botulism; burn patients; lactation, pregnancy.

Available forms

Injection—10, 40 mg/mL; injection in 0.9% sodium chloride—0.8, 0.9, 1, 1.2, 1.4, 1.6 mg/mL; ophthalmic solution—3 mg/mL; ophthalmic ointment—3 mg/g; topical ointment—0.1%; topical cream—0.1%; ointment—1 mg; cream—1 mg; beads—2.8, 7.5 mg

Dosages

Dosage should be based on estimated lean body mass.

Parenteral

Adults

3 mg/kg/day in three equal doses every 8 hr IM or IV. Up to 5 mg/kg/day in three to four equal doses in severe infections, usually for 7–10 days. For IV use, a loading dose of 1–2 mg/kg may be infused over 30–60 min.

- *PID:* 2 mg/kg IV followed by 1.5 mg/kg tid plus clindamycin 600 mg IV qid. Continue for at least 4 days and at least 48 hr after patient improves, then continue clindamycin 450 mg orally qid for 10–14 days total therapy.

- *Surgical prophylaxis regimens:* Several complex, multidrug prophylaxis regimens are available for preoperative use; consult manufacturer's instructions.

Pediatric patients

2–2.5 mg/kg every 8 hr IM or IV.
Infants and neonates: 2.5 mg/kg every 8 hr.
Premature or full-term neonates: 2.5 mg/kg every 12 hr.

Geriatric patients or patients with renal failure

Reduce dosage or extend dosage intervals, and carefully monitor serum drug levels and renal function tests.

Ophthalmic solution

Adults and pediatric patients

1–2 drops into affected eye or eyes every 4 hr; use up to 2 drops hourly in severe infections.

Ophthalmic ointment

Adults and pediatric patients

Apply about ½″ to affected eye bid–tid.

Dermatologic preparations

Adults and pediatric patients

Apply tid–qid. Cover with sterile bandage if needed.

Pharmacokinetics

Route	*Onset*	*Peak*
IM, IV	Rapid	30–90 min

Metabolism: Hepatic; $T_{1/2}$: 2–3 hr
Distribution: Crosses placenta; enters breast milk
Excretion: Urine

IV FACTS

Preparation: Dilute single dose in 50–200 mL of sterile isotonic saline or D_5W. Do not mix in solution with any other drugs.
Infusion: Infuse over 30–120 min.
Incompatibilities: Do not mix in solution with any other drugs.

Adverse effects

- **CNS:** Ototoxicity—*tinnitus, dizziness,* vertigo, deafness (partially reversible to irreversible), vestibular paralysis, confusion, disorientation, depression, lethargy, nystagmus, visual disturbances, headache, *numbness, tingling,* tremor, paresthesias, muscle twitching, **seizures,** muscular weakness, **neuromuscular blockade**
- **CV:** Palpitations, hypotension, hypertension
- **GI:** Hepatic toxicity, *nausea, vomiting, anorexia,* weight loss, stomatitis, increased salivation
- **GU: Nephrotoxicity**
- **Hematologic:** *Leukemoid reaction,* **agranulocytosis, granulocytosis, leukopenia,** leukocytosis, **thrombocytopenia, eosinophelia, pancytopenia,** anemia, hemolytic anemia, increased or decreased reticulocyte count, electrolyte disturbances
- **Hypersensitivity:** *Purpura, rash,* urticaria, exfoliative dermatitis, itching
- **Local:** *Pain, irritation, arachnoiditis at IM injection sites*
- **Other:** Fever, **apnea,** splenomegaly, joint pain, *superinfections*

Ophthalmic preparations

- **Local:** *Transient irritation, burning, stinging, itching,* angioneurotic edema, urticaria, vesicular and maculopapular dermatitis, bacterial and fungal corneal ulcers

Topical dermatologic preparations

- **Local:** *Photosensitization,* superinfections

Interactions

✱ **Drug-drug** • Increased ototoxic, nephrotoxic, neurotoxic effects with other aminoglycosides, potent diuretics, cephalosporins, vancomycin, methoxyflurane, enflurane • Increased neuromuscular blockade and muscular paralysis with anesthetics, nondepolarizing neuromuscular blocking drugs, succinylcholine, citrate-anticoagulated blood • Potential inactivation of both drugs if mixed with beta-lactam–type antibiotics (space doses with concomitant therapy) • Increased bactericidal effect with penicillins, cephalosporins (to treat some gram-negative organisms and enterococci), carbenicillin, ticarcillin (to treat *Pseudomonas* infections)

■ Nursing considerations

Assessment

- **History:** Allergy to any aminoglycosides; renal or hepatic disease; preexisting hearing loss; active infection with herpes, vaccinia, varicella, fungal infections, mycobacterial infections (ophthalmic preparations);

G

myasthenia gravis; parkinsonism; infant botulism; lactation, pregnancy

- **Physical:** Site of infection; skin color, lesions; orientation, reflexes, eighth cranial nerve function; P, BP; R, adventitious sounds; bowel sounds, liver evaluation; urinalysis, BUN, serum creatinine, serum electrolytes, LFTs, CBC

Interventions

- Monitor serum concentrations when feasible to avoid potentially toxic levels. Peak levels should not exceed 12 mcg/mL (6–8 mcg/mL is usually adequate for most infections). Trough levels should not exceed 2 mcg/mL.
- Give by IM route if at all possible; give by deep IM injection.
- Culture infected area before therapy.
- Use 2 mg/mL intrathecal preparation without preservatives, for intrathecal use.
- Avoid long-term therapies because of increased risk of toxicities. Reduction in dose may be clinically indicated.
- Patients with edema or ascites may have lower peak concentrations due to expanded extracellular fluid volume.
- Cleanse area before application of dermatologic preparations.
- Ensure adequate hydration of patient before and during therapy.

⊗ ***Black box warning*** Monitor hearing with long-term therapy; ototoxicity can occur.

⊗ ***Black box warning*** Monitor renal function tests, CBC, and serum drug levels during long-term therapy. Consult with prescriber to adjust dosage as needed.

Teaching points

- Apply ophthalmic preparations by tilting head back; place medications into conjunctival sac and close eye; apply light pressure on lacrimal sac for 1 minute.
- Cleanse area before applying dermatologic preparations; area may be covered if necessary.
- You may experience these side effects: Ringing in the ears, headache, dizziness (reversible; use safety measures if severe); nausea, vomiting, loss of appetite (eat frequent small meals, perform frequent mouth care); burning, blurring of vision with ophthalmic preparations (avoid driving or performing dangerous activities if visual effects occur); photosensitization with dermatologic preparations (wear sunscreen and protective clothing).
- Report pain at injection site, severe headache, dizziness, loss of hearing, changes in urine pattern, difficulty breathing, rash or skin lesions; itching or irritation (ophthalmic preparations); worsening of the condition, rash, irritation (dermatologic preparation).

▽ glatiramer acetate

See Appendix W, *Less commonly used drugs.*

DANGEROUS DRUG

▽ glimepiride

*(glye **meh'** per ide)*

Amaryl, CO-Glimepiride (CAN), ratio-Glimepiride (CAN)

PREGNANCY CATEGORY C

Drug classes

Antidiabetic
Sulfonylurea (second generation)

Therapeutic actions

Stimulates insulin release from functioning beta cells in the pancreas; may improve binding between insulin and insulin receptors or increase the number of insulin receptors; thought to be more potent in effect than first-generation sulfonylureas.

Indications

- As an adjunct to diet to lower blood glucose in patients with type 2 diabetes mellitus whose hypoglycemia cannot be controlled by diet and exercise alone
- In combination with metformin or insulin to better control glucose as an adjunct to diet and exercise in patients with type 2 diabetes mellitus

Contraindications and cautions

- Contraindicated with allergy to sulfonylureas; diabetes complicated by fever, severe infections, severe trauma, major surgery, ketosis, acidosis, coma (insulin is indicated in these conditions);

type 1 or juvenile diabetes, serious hepatic or renal impairment, uremia, thyroid or endocrine impairment, glycosuria, hyperglycemia associated with primary renal disease; labor and delivery—if glimepiride is used during pregnancy, discontinue drug at least 1 mo before delivery; lactation, safety not established.
- Use cautiously with pregnancy.

Available forms
Tablets—1, 2, 4 mg

Dosages
Dose conservatively in elderly patients, debilitated or malnourished patients, and patients with renal or hepatic impairment.

Adults
Usual starting dose is 1–2 mg PO once daily with breakfast or first meal of the day; usual maintenance dose is 1–4 mg PO once daily, depending on patient response and glucose levels. Do not exceed 8 mg/day.
- *Combination with insulin therapy:* 8 mg PO daily with first meal of the day with low-dose insulin.
- *Transfer from other hypoglycemics:* No transition period is necessary.

Pediatric patients
Safety and efficacy not established.

Patients with renal or hepatic impairment; elderly, debilitated, malnourished patients; adrenal or pituitary insufficiency
Usual starting dose is 1 mg PO once daily; adjust dose carefully, lower maintenance doses may be sufficient to control blood sugar.

Pharmacokinetics

Route	Onset	Peak
Oral	1 hr	2–3 hr

Metabolism: Hepatic; $T_{1/2}$: 5.5–7 hr
Distribution: Crosses placenta; enters breast milk
Excretion: Bile, urine

Adverse effects
- **CNS:** Drowsiness, asthenia, nervousness, tremor, insomnia, blurred vision
- **CV: Increased risk of CV mortality** (possible)
- **Endocrine:** *Hypoglycemia,* SIADH
- **GI:** *Anorexia, nausea,* vomiting, *epigastric discomfort, heartburn, diarrhea*
- **Hematologic: Leukopenia, thrombocytopenia,** anemia
- **Hypersensitivity:** *Allergic skin reactions,* eczema, pruritus, erythema, urticaria, photosensitivity, fever, **eosinophilia,** jaundice
- **Other:** Diuresis, tinnitus, fatigue, weight gain, hyponatremia

Interactions
✱ **Drug-drug** • Increased risk of hypoglycemia with androgens, anticoagulants, azole antifungals, beta blockers, chloramphenicol, clofibrate, fenfluramine, fluconazole, gemfibrozil, histamine-2 blockers, magnesium salts, MAOIs, methyldopa, oxyphenbutazone, phenylbutazone, probenecid, salicylates, sulfinpyrazone, sulfonamides, TCAs, urinary acidifiers • Decreased effectiveness of both glimepiride and diazoxide if taken concurrently • Increased risk of hyperglycemia with rifampin, thiazides • Risk of hypoglycemia and hyperglycemia with ethanol; "disulfiram reaction" has also been reported • Possible decreased hypoglycemic effect with calcium channel blockers, cholestyramine, corticosteroids, diazoxide, estrogens, hydantoins, hormonal contraceptives, isoniazid, nicotinic acid, phenothiazines, rifampin, sympathomimetics, thiazide diuretics, thyroid drugs, urinary alkalinizers
✱ **Drug-alternative therapy** • Increased risk of hypoglycemia if taken with juniper berries, ginseng, garlic, fenugreek, coriander, dandelion root, celery

■ Nursing considerations
Assessment
- **History:** Allergy to sulfonylureas; diabetes complicated by fever, severe infections, severe trauma, major surgery, ketosis, acidosis, coma (insulin is indicated in these conditions); type 1 or juvenile diabetes, serious hepatic or renal impairment, uremia, thyroid or endocrine impairment, glycosuria, hyperglycemia associated with primary renal disease; pregnancy
- **Physical:** Skin color, lesions; T; orientation, reflexes, peripheral sensation; R, adventitious sounds; liver evaluation, bowel sounds; urinalysis, BUN, serum creatinine, LFTs, blood glucose, CBC

Interventions

- Monitor urine or serum glucose levels frequently to determine effectiveness of drug and dosage being used.

⊗ ***Warning*** Transfer to insulin therapy during periods of high stress (eg, infections, surgery, trauma).

- Use IV glucose if severe hypoglycemia occurs as a result of overdose.
- Arrange for consultation with dietitian to establish weight-loss program and dietary control.
- Arrange for thorough diabetic teaching program, including disease, dietary control, exercise, signs and symptoms of hypoglycemia and hyperglycemia, avoidance of infection, hygiene.

Teaching points

- Take this drug once a day with breakfast or the first main meal of the day.
- Do not discontinue this drug without consulting your health care provider.
- Continue with diet and exercise program for diabetes control.
- Monitor urine or blood for glucose and ketones as prescribed.
- Do not use this drug if you are pregnant.
- Avoid alcohol while taking this drug.
- Report fever, sore throat, unusual bleeding or bruising, rash, dark urine, light-colored stools, hypoglycemic or hyperglycemic reactions.

DANGEROUS DRUG

glipizide

(glip' i zide)

Glucotrol, Glucotrol XL (DNC)

PREGNANCY CATEGORY C

Drug classes

Antidiabetic
Sulfonylurea (second generation)

Therapeutic actions

Stimulates insulin release from functioning beta cells in the pancreas; may improve binding between insulin and insulin receptors or increase the number of insulin receptors; more potent in effect than first-generation sulfonylureas.

Indications

- Adjunct to diet and exercise to lower blood glucose with type 2 diabetes mellitus

Contraindications and cautions

- Contraindicated with allergy to sulfonylureas, diabetes with ketoacidosis, sole therapy of type 1 diabetes or diabetes complicated by pregnancy; diabetes complicated by fever, severe infections, severe trauma, major surgery, ketosis, acidosis, coma (insulin is indicated); type 1 diabetes, serious hepatic impairment, serious renal impairment.
- Use cautiously with uremia, thyroid or endocrine impairment, glycosuria, hyperglycemia associated with primary renal disease; labor and delivery (if glipizide is used during pregnancy, discontinue drug at least 1 mo before delivery); lactation; pregnancy.

Available forms

Tablets—5, 10 mg; ER tablets (DNC)—2.5, 5, 10 mg

Dosages

Dose conservatively in elderly patients, debilitated or malnourished patients, and patients with renal or hepatic impairment.

Give approximately 30 min before breakfast to achieve greatest reduction in postprandial hyperglycemia.

Adults

- *Initial therapy:* 5 mg PO before breakfast. Adjust dosage in increments of 2.5–5 mg as determined by blood glucose response. At least several days should elapse between adjustments. Maximum once-daily dose should not exceed 15 mg; above 15 mg, divide dose, and administer before meals. Do not exceed 40 mg/day. ER tablets: 5 mg/day. Adjust dosage in 5-mg increments every 3 mo; maximum dose—20 mg/day.
- *Maintenance therapy:* Total daily doses above 15 mg PO should be divided; total daily doses above 30 mg are given in divided doses bid.
- *ER form:* 5 mg/day with breakfast, may be increased to 10 mg/day after 3 mo if indicated.

Pediatric patients
Safety and efficacy not established.

Geriatric patients
Geriatric patients tend to be more sensitive to the drug. Start with initial dose of 2.5 mg/day PO. Monitor for 24 hr and gradually increase dose after several days as needed.

Pharmacokinetics

Route	*Onset*	*Peak*	*Duration*
Oral	1–1.5 hr	1–3 hr	10–24 hr
Oral (ER)	2–3 hr	6–12 hr	24 hr

Metabolism: Hepatic; $T_{1/2}$: 2–4 hr
Distribution: Crosses placenta; enters breast milk
Excretion: Bile, urine

Adverse effects
- **CNS:** Drowsiness, asthenia, nervousness, tremor, insomnia, tinnitus, fatigue, headache
- **CV: Increased risk of CV mortality,** syncope, blurred vision
- **Endocrine:** *Hypoglycemia,* SIADH
- **GI:** *Anorexia, nausea,* vomiting, *epigastric discomfort, heartburn, diarrhea,* flatulence
- **Hematologic: Leukopenia, thrombocytopenia,** anemia
- **Hypersensitivity:** *Allergic skin reactions,* eczema, pruritus, erythema, urticaria, photosensitivity, fever, eosinophilia, jaundice
- **Other:** Weight gain, arthralgia, leg cramps, hyponatremia

Interactions
✱ **Drug-drug** • Increased risk of hypoglycemia with sulfonamides, chloramphenicol, oxyphenbutazone, phenylbutazone, salicylates, clofibrate, beta blockers • Decreased effectiveness of glipizide and diazoxide if taken concurrently • Increased risk of hyperglycemia with rifampin, thiazides • Risk of hypoglycemia and hyperglycemia with ethanol; "disulfiram reaction" also has been reported
✱ **Drug-alternative therapy** • Increased risk of hypoglycemia if taken with juniper berries, ginseng, garlic, fenugreek, coriander, dandelion root, celery, karela

■ Nursing considerations
Assessment
- **History:** Allergy to sulfonylureas; diabetes mellitus with complications; type 1 diabetes mellitus, serious hepatic or renal impairment, uremia, thyroid or endocrine impairment, glycosuria, hyperglycemia associated with primary renal disease; pregnancy
- **Physical:** Skin color, lesions; T; orientation, reflexes, peripheral sensation; R, adventitious sounds; liver evaluation, bowel sounds; urinalysis, BUN, serum creatinine, LFTs, blood glucose, CBC

G

Interventions
- Give drug 30 min before breakfast; if severe GI upset occurs or more than 15 mg/day is required, dose may be divided and given before meals.
- Ensure that patient swallows ER tablets whole; do not allow patient to cut, crush, or chew them.
- Monitor urine or serum glucose levels frequently to determine drug effectiveness and dosage.

⊗ ***Warning*** Transfer to insulin therapy during periods of high stress (eg, infections, surgery, trauma).

⊗ ***Warning*** Use IV glucose if severe hypoglycemia occurs as a result of overdose.

Teaching points
- Take this drug 30 minutes before breakfast for best results.
- Do not discontinue this drug without consulting your health care provider.
- Monitor urine or blood for glucose and ketones.
- If taking ER tablets, swallow them whole; do not crush, chew, or divide tablets. The empty tablet may appear in your stool.
- Continue the prescribed diet and exercise regimen.
- Do not use this drug during pregnancy; consult your health care provider.
- Avoid alcohol while using this drug.
- Report fever, sore throat, unusual bleeding or bruising, rash, dark urine, light-colored stools, hypoglycemic or hyperglycemic reactions.

glucagon (rDNA origin)

(gloo' ka gon)

GlucaGen, GlucaGen Diagnostic Kit, GlucaGen HypoKit, Glucagon Emergency Kit

PREGNANCY CATEGORY B

Drug classes

Diagnostic agent
Glucose-elevating drug
Hormone

Therapeutic actions

Accelerates the breakdown of glycogen to glucose (glycogenolysis) in the liver, causing an increase in blood glucose level; relaxes smooth muscle of the GI tract and increases the force of contraction of the heart.

Indications

- Hypoglycemia: Counteracts severe hypoglycemic reactions in diabetic patients treated with insulin
- Diagnostic aid in the radiologic examination of the stomach, duodenum, small bowel, or colon when a hypotonic state is advantageous
- Unlabeled use: Treatment of beta blocker and calcium channel blocker overdose and in cardiac emergencies

Contraindications and cautions

- Contraindicated with hypersensitivity, pheochromocytoma, insulinoma.
- Use cautiously with pregnancy, lactation, insulinoma.

Available forms

Powder for injection—1 mg

Dosages

Adults and pediatric patients weighing more than 20 kg

- *Hypoglycemia:* 0.5–1.0 mg IV, IM, or subcutaneously. Response is usually seen in 5–20 min. If response is delayed, dose may be repeated one to two times. Use IV if possible.
- *Diagnostic aid:* Suggested dose, route, and timing of dose vary with the segment of GI tract to be examined and duration of effect needed. Carefully check manufacturer's literature before use.

Pediatric patients weighing less than 20 kg

0.5 mg IM, IV, or subcutaneously, or a dose equivalent to 20–30 mcg/kg.

Pharmacokinetics

Route	*Onset*	*Peak*	*Duration*
IV	1 min	15 min	9–20 min
IM	8–10 min	20–30 min	19–32 min

Metabolism: Hepatic; $T_{1/2}$: 3–10 min
Distribution: Crosses placenta; enters breast milk
Excretion: Bile, urine

IV FACTS

Preparation: Reconstitute with vial provided. Use immediately; refrigerated solution stable for 48 hr. If doses higher than 2 mg, reconstitute with sterile water for injection and use immediately.
Infusion: Inject directly into the IV tubing of an IV drip infusion, each 1 mg over 1 min.
Incompatibilities: Compatible with dextrose solutions, but precipitates may form in solutions of sodium chloride, potassium chloride, or calcium chloride.

Adverse effects

- **CV:** Hypotension, hypertension, tachycardia
- **GI:** *Nausea, vomiting*
- **Hematologic:** Hypokalemia in overdose
- **Hypersensitivity:** Urticaria, **respiratory distress,** hypotension

Interactions

✱ **Drug-drug** • Increased anticoagulant effect and risk of bleeding with oral anticoagulants

■ Nursing considerations

Assessment

- **History:** Insulinoma, pheochromocytoma, lactation, pregnancy

- **Physical:** Skin color, lesions, T; orientation, reflexes; P, BP, peripheral perfusion; R; liver evaluation, bowel sounds; blood and urine glucose, serum potassium

Interventions

⊗ ***Warning*** Arouse hypoglycemic patient as soon as possible after drug injection, and provide supplemental carbohydrates to restore liver glycogen and prevent secondary hypoglycemia.

- Arrange for evaluation of insulin dosage in cases of hypoglycemia as a result of insulin overdosage; insulin dosage may need to be adjusted.

Teaching points

- You and significant others should learn to administer the drug subcutaneously in case of hypoglycemia, and know when to notify your health care provider.

DANGEROUS DRUG

glyburide

(glye' byoor ide)

Apo-Glyburide (CAN), DiaBeta, Gen-Glybe (CAN), Glibenclamide, Glynase PresTab, Novo-Glyburide (CAN), PMS-Glyburide (CAN), ratio-Glyburide (CAN)

PREGNANCY CATEGORY B (GLYNASE)

PREGNANCY CATEGORY C (DIABETA)

Drug classes

Antidiabetic
Sulfonylurea

Therapeutic actions

Stimulates insulin release from functioning beta cells in the pancreas; may improve binding between insulin and insulin receptors or increase the number of insulin receptors; more potent in effect than first-generation sulfonylureas.

Indications

- Adjunct to diet to lower blood glucose with type 2 diabetes mellitus

Contraindications and cautions

- Contraindicated with allergy to sulfonylureas; diabetes mellitus with ketoacidosis, sole therapy of type 1 diabetes mellitus or diabetes mellitus complicated by pregnancy, serious hepatic or renal impairment, uremia; diabetes mellitus complicated by fever, severe infections, severe trauma, major surgery, ketosis, acidosis, coma (insulin is contraindicated).
- Use cautiously with pregnancy, lactation, thyroid or endocrine impairment, glycosuria, hyperglycemia associated with primary renal disease; labor and delivery (if glyburide is used during pregnancy, discontinue drug at least 1 mo before delivery).

Available forms

Tablets—1.25, 2.5, 5 mg; micronized tablets—1.5, 3, 4.5, 6 mg

Dosages

Adults

- *Initial therapy:* 2.5–5 mg PO with breakfast (*DiaBeta*); 1.5–3 mg/day PO (*Glynase*).
- *Maintenance therapy:* 1.25–20 mg/day PO given as a single dose or in divided doses. Increase in increments of no more than 2.5 mg (1.5 mg micronized) at weekly intervals based on patient's blood glucose response (*DiaBeta*); 0.75–12 mg/day PO (*Glynase*).

Patients sensitive to hypoglycemic drugs

Start with 1.25 mg daily (nonmicronized) or 0.75 mg daily (micronized).

Pediatric patients

Safety and efficacy not established.

Geriatric patients

Geriatric patients tend to be more sensitive to the drug; start with initial dose of 1.25 mg/day PO (*DiaBeta*); 0.75 mg/day PO (*Glynase*). Monitor for 24 hr, and gradually increase dose after at least 1 wk as needed.

Pharmacokinetics

Route	Onset	Peak	Duration
Oral			
Micronized	1 hr	2–3 hr	12–24 hr
Nonmicronized	2–4 hr	4 hr	12–24 hr

Metabolism: Hepatic; $T_{1/2}$: 4 hr
Distribution: Crosses placenta; enters breast milk
Excretion: Bile, urine

Adverse effects

- **CNS:** Drowsiness, tinnitus, fatigue, asthenia, nervousness, tremor, insomnia
- **CV: Increased risk of CV mortality**
- **Endocrine: Hypoglycemia**
- **GI:** *Anorexia, nausea,* vomiting, *epigastric discomfort, heartburn,* diarrhea, weight gain
- **Hematologic: Leukopenia, thrombocytopenia,** anemia
- **Hypersensitivity:** *Allergic skin reactions,* eczema, pruritus, erythema, urticaria, photosensitivity, fever, eosinophilia, jaundice
- **Other:** Blurred vision

Interactions

✱ **Drug-drug** • Increased risk of hypoglycemia with sulfonamides, chloramphenicol, oxyphenbutazone, phenylbutazone, salicylates, clofibrate • Decreased effectiveness of glyburide and diazoxide if taken concurrently • Increased risk of hyperglycemia with rifampin, thiazides • Risk of hypoglycemia and hyperglycemia with ethanol; "disulfiram reaction" has been reported

✱ **Drug-alternative therapy** • Increased risk of hypoglycemia if taken with juniper berries, ginseng, garlic, fenugreek, coriander, dandelion root, celery, karela

■ Nursing considerations

CLINICAL ALERT!
Name confusion has occurred between *DiaBeta* (glyburide) and *Zebeta* (bisoprolol); use caution.

Assessment

- **History:** Allergy to sulfonylureas; diabetes with complications; type 1 diabetes, serious hepatic or renal impairment, uremia, thyroid or endocrine impairment, glycosuria, hyperglycemia associated with primary renal disease, pregnancy
- **Physical:** Skin color, lesions; T; orientation, reflexes, peripheral sensation; R, adventitious sounds; liver evaluation, bowel sounds; urinalysis, BUN, serum creatinine, LFTs, blood glucose, CBC

Interventions

- Give drug before breakfast. If severe GI upset occurs, dose may be divided and given before meals.
- Monitor urine or serum glucose levels frequently to determine drug effectiveness and dosage.
- Monitor dosage carefully if switching to or from *Glynase.*

⊗ ***Warning*** Transfer to insulin therapy during periods of high stress (eg, infections, surgery, trauma).

⊗ ***Warning*** Use IV glucose if severe hypoglycemia occurs as a result of overdose.

Teaching points

- Do not discontinue this medication without consulting your health care provider.
- Monitor urine or blood for glucose and ketones; continue diet and exercise regimen for your diabetes.
- Do not use this drug during pregnancy; consult your health care provider.
- Avoid alcohol while using this drug.
- Report fever, sore throat, unusual bleeding or bruising, rash, dark urine, light-colored stools, hypoglycemic or hyperglycemic reactions.

▽ glycerin (glycerol)

(gli' ser in)

Colace Suppositories, Fleet Babylax, Osmoglyn, Sani-Supp

PREGNANCY CATEGORY C

Drug classes

Hyperosmolar laxative
Ophthalmic hyperosmolar preparation
Osmotic diuretic

Therapeutic actions

Elevates the osmolarity of the glomerular filtrate, thereby hindering the reabsorption of water and leading to a loss of water, sodium, and chloride; creates an osmotic gradient in the eye between plasma and ocular fluids, thereby reducing IOP; causes the local absorption of sodium and water in the stool, leading to a more liquid stool and local intestinal movement.

Indications

- *Osmoglyn:* For glaucoma, to interrupt acute attacks, or when a temporary drop in IOP is required
- *Osmoglyn:* Before ocular surgery performed under local anesthetic when a reduction in IOP is indicated
- Temporary relief of constipation
- Before rectal or bowel surgeries
- IV, unlabeled use (with proper preparation): To lower intracranial pressure or IOP

Contraindications and cautions

- Contraindicated with hypersensitivity to glycerin; symptoms of appendicitis, nausea, vomiting, fecal impaction, undiagnosed abdominal pain, intestinal obstruction; contraindicated as an osmotic diuretic with established anuria, severe dehydration, frank or impending acute pulmonary edema, severe cardiac decompensation.
- Use cautiously in the elderly; with hypervolemia, heart failure, confused mental states, severe dehydration, senility, diabetes, lactation, pregnancy.

Available forms

Oral solution—50% (0.6 mg/mL); liquid—4 mL/applicator; suppositories

Dosages

Adults

Oral

- *Reduction of IOP:* 2–3 mL of glycerin per kg of body weight (approximately 4–6 oz) given PO only, 1 hr–90 min before surgery (*Osmoglyn*).

Rectal

- *Laxative:* Insert one suppository high in rectum and retain 15–30 min; for rectal liquid, insert stem with tip pointing toward navel; squeeze unit until nearly all liquid is expelled, then remove.

Pediatric patients 2–6 yr

1 unit or as directed by physician.

Pediatric patients younger than 2 yr

Consult physician.

Pharmacokinetics

Route	*Onset*	*Peak*	*Duration*
Oral (*Osmoglyn*)	Varies	1 hr	5 hr

Metabolism: Hepatic; $T_{1/2}$: 2–3 hr
Distribution: Crosses placenta; may enter breast milk
Excretion: Urine

Adverse effects

- **CNS:** *Confusion, headache, syncope,* disorientation
- **CV:** Cardiac arrhythmias
- **Endocrine: Hyperosmolar nonketotic coma**
- **GI:** *Nausea, vomiting, diarrhea*
- **Other:** Severe dehydration, weight gain with continued use, local irritation ophthalmically, local irritation (suppository)

■ Nursing considerations

Assessment

- **History:** Hypersensitivity to glycerin, hypervolemia, heart failure, confused mental states, severe dehydration, elderly, senility, diabetes, lactation, pregnancy
- **Physical:** Skin color, edema; orientation, reflexes, muscle strength, pupillary reflexes; P, BP, perfusion; R, pattern, adventitious sounds; urinary output patterns; serum electrolytes, urinalysis

Interventions

- Give *Osmoglyn* orally only; it is not for injection.
- Give laxative as follows: Insert one suppository high in rectum, and have patient retain 15–30 min; for rectal liquid, insert stem with tip pointing toward navel; squeeze unit until nearly all liquid is expelled, then remove.
- Place a child on left side with knees bent and arms resting comfortably. Or use knee-chest position: Have child kneel and then lower

head and chest until left side of face is resting on the surface with left arm folded comfortably.
- May give local anesthetic before ophthalmic use because of local irritation that may occur.
- Monitor urinary output carefully.
- Monitor BP regularly.

Teaching points

- Take laxative as follows: Insert one suppository high in the rectum and retain for 15 minutes; for rectal liquid, insert stem with tip pointing toward navel; squeeze unit until nearly all liquid is expelled, then remove the unit. Some liquid will be left in the unit.
- You may experience these side effects: Increased urination, GI upset (eat frequent small meals), dry mouth (suck sugarless lozenges), headache, blurred vision (use caution when moving around; ask for assistance).
- Report severe headache, chest pain, confusion, rapid respirations, violent diarrhea.

▽ glycopyrrolate

*(glye koe **pye'** roe late)*

Robinul, Robinul Forte

PREGNANCY CATEGORY B

Drug classes

Anticholinergic (quaternary)
Antimuscarinic
Antispasmodic
Parasympatholytic

Therapeutic actions

Competitively blocks the effects of acetylcholine at receptors that mediate the effects of parasympathetic postganglionic impulses; depresses salivary and bronchial secretions; dilates the bronchi; inhibits vagal influences on the heart; relaxes the GI and GU tracts; inhibits gastric acid secretion.

Indications

- Oral: Adjunctive therapy in the treatment of peptic ulcer
- Parenteral: Reduction of salivary, tracheobronchial, and pharyngeal secretions preoperatively; reduction of the volume and free acidity of gastric secretions; and blocking of cardiac vagal inhibitory reflexes during induction of anesthesia and intubation; may be used intraoperatively to counteract drug-induced or vagal traction reflexes with the associated arrhythmias
- Parenteral: Protection against the peripheral muscarinic effects (eg, bradycardia, excessive secretions) of cholinergics (neostigmine, pyridostigmine) that are used to reverse the neuromuscular blockade produced by nondepolarizing neuromuscular junction blockers

Contraindications and cautions

- Contraindicated with glaucoma; adhesions between iris and lens; stenosing peptic ulcer; pyloroduodenal obstruction; paralytic ileus; intestinal atony; severe ulcerative colitis; toxic megacolon; symptomatic prostatic hypertrophy; bladder neck obstruction; bronchial asthma; COPD; cardiac arrhythmias; tachycardia; myocardial ischemia; lactation; impaired metabolic, liver, or kidney function; myasthenia gravis.
- Use cautiously in the elderly and with Down syndrome, brain damage, spasticity, hypertension, hyperthyroidism, pregnancy.

Available forms

Tablets—1, 2, mg; injection—0.2 mg/mL

Dosages

Adults

Oral

1 mg tid or 2 mg bid–tid. For maintenance, 1 mg bid. Maximum daily dose is 8 mg PO.

Parenteral

- *Peptic ulcer:* 0.1–0.2 mg IM or IV tid–qid.
- *Preanesthetic medication:* 0.004 mg/kg IM 30–60 min before anesthesia.
- *Intraoperative:* 0.1 mg IV; repeat as needed at 2- to 3-min intervals.
- *Reversal of neuromuscular blockade:* With neostigmine, pyridostigmine: 0.2 mg for each 1 mg neostigmine or 5 mg pyridostigmine; administer IV simultaneously.

Pediatric patients
Not recommended for children younger than 12 yr for peptic ulcer.

Parenteral
- *Preanesthetic medication:*
  Younger than 2 yr: 0.004 mg/kg IM 30 min to 1 hr before anesthesia.
  Younger than 12 yr: 0.002–0.004 mg/kg IM.
- *Intraoperative:* 0.004 mg/kg IV, not to exceed 0.1 mg in a single dose. May be repeated at 2- to 3-min intervals.
- *Reversal of neuromuscular blockade:* 0.2 mg for each 1 mg neostigmine or 5 mg pyridostigmine. Give IV simultaneously.

Pharmacokinetics

Route	*Onset*	*Peak*	*Duration*
Oral	60 min	60 min	8–12 hr
IM, Subcut.	15–30 min	30–45 min	2–7 hr
IV	1 min	End of infusion	Unknown

Metabolism: Hepatic; $T_{1/2}$: 2.5 hr
Distribution: Crosses placenta; enters breast milk
Excretion: Urine

IV FACTS
Preparation: No additional preparation required.
Infusion: Administer slowly into tubing of a running IV, each 0.2 mg over 1–2 min.
Incompatibilities: Do not combine with methylprednisolone; sodium succinate. May be incompatible with drugs that have more alkaline pH (greater than 6); eg, barbiturates, diazepam, lactated Ringer's solution.

Adverse effects
- **CNS:** Headache, flushing, nervousness, drowsiness, fever, mental confusion
- **CV:** Palpitations, tachycardia
- **GI:** *Dry mouth, altered taste perception, nausea, vomiting, dysphagia,* heartburn, constipation, bloated feeling, paralytic ileus, gastroesophageal reflux
- **GU:** *Urinary hesitancy and retention,* impotence
- **Local:** *Irritation at site of IM injection*
- **Ophthalmic:** *Blurred vision,* mydriasis, cycloplegia, photophobia, increased IOP
- **Other:** Decreased sweating and predisposition to heat prostration, suppression of lactation, nasal congestion

Interactions
✱ **Drug-drug** • Decreased antipsychotic effectiveness of haloperidol with anticholinergic drugs • Increased anticholinergic side effects (dry mouth, constipation, urinary retention) with amantadine and TCAs • Decreased antipsychotic effects and increased anticholinergic effects with phenothiazines

■ Nursing considerations
Assessment
- **History:** Glaucoma; adhesions between iris and lens, stenosing peptic ulcer, pyloroduodenal obstruction, paralytic ileus, intestinal atony, severe ulcerative colitis, toxic megacolon, symptomatic prostatic hypertrophy, bladder neck obstruction, COPD, cardiac arrhythmias, myocardial ischemia, impaired metabolic, liver or kidney function, myasthenia gravis; lactation; Down syndrome, brain damage, spasticity, hypertension, hyperthyroidism, pregnancy
- **Physical:** Bowel sounds, normal output; normal urinary output, prostate palpation; R, adventitious sounds; P, BP; IOP, vision; bilateral grip strength, reflexes; hepatic palpation, LFTs, renal function tests; skin color, lesions, texture

Interventions
- Ensure adequate hydration; provide environmental control (temperature) to prevent hyperpyrexia.
- Check pediatric dosage carefully; may be in mg/lb or mg/kg.
- Have patient void before each dose if urinary retention is a problem.

Teaching points
- Take this drug exactly as prescribed.
- Avoid hot environments (you will be heat-intolerant; dangerous reactions may occur).
- You may experience these side effects: Constipation (ensure adequate fluid intake, proper diet); dry mouth (suck sugarless lozenges, use frequent mouth care; this effect may lessen); blurred vision, sensitivity to light (reversible; avoid tasks that require acute

vision; wear sunglasses in bright light); impotence (reversible); difficulty in urination (empty bladder immediately before taking each dose).
- Report rash, flushing, eye pain, difficulty breathing, tremors, loss of coordination, irregular heartbeat, palpitations, headache, abdominal distention, hallucinations, severe or persistent dry mouth, difficulty swallowing, difficulty urinating, severe constipation, sensitivity to light.

gold sodium thiomalate

See Appendix W, *Less commonly used drugs.*

golimumab

*(goh **lim'** yoo mab)*

Simponi

PREGNANCY CATEGORY B

Drug classes
Antiarthritic
Monoclonal antibody
Tumor necrosis factor inhibitor

Therapeutic actions
Tumor necrosis factor antibody that binds to tumor necrosis factor, blocking an important mediator in the inflammatory response seen in chronic inflammatory diseases, such as rheumatoid arthritis, psoriatic arthritis, and ankylosing spondylitis.

Indications
- Treatment of moderately to severely active rheumatoid arthritis in adults in combination with methotrexate
- Treatment of active psoriatic arthritis in adults, as monotherapy or in combination with methotrexate
- Treatment of ankylosing spondylitis in adults

Contraindications and cautions
- Contraindicated with hypersensitivity to components of drug, active infection, active tuberculosis, lactation.
- Use cautiously with heart failure, history of exposure to fungal infections, hepatitis B, malignancies, demyelinating disorders such as multiple sclerosis, pregnancy.

Available forms
Single-use prefilled syringe—50 mg/0.5 mL; single-use autoinjector—50 mg/0.5 mL

Dosages
Adults
50 mg by subcutaneous injection once a month.
Pediatric patients
Safety and efficacy not established.

Pharmacokinetics

Route	*Onset*	*Peak*
Subcut.	Slow	2–6 days

Metabolism: Hepatic; $T_{1/2}$: 2 wk
Distribution: May cross placenta; may enter breast milk
Excretion: Tissues

Adverse effects
- **CNS:** Dizziness, **increased risk of demyelinating disorders**
- **CV:** Hypertension, heart failure
- **Respiratory:** *URI, nasopharyngitis,* bronchitis, sinusitis, rhinitis
- **Other:** Fever, injection-site reaction, **risk of infection,** psoriasis

Interactions
✱ **Drug-drug** • Increased risk of potentially serious infection if combined with anakinra, abatacept, rituximab, other TNF blockers (infliximab, adalimumab, etanercept, certolizumab); avoid this combination • Risk of infection if live vaccines are given while patient is taking this drug; avoid this combination

■ Nursing considerations
Assessment
- **History:** Tuberculosis, malignancy, heart failure, multiple sclerosis, travel exposure to invasive fungal infections, hepatitis B, pregnancy, lactation
- **Physical:** T, orientation; R, adventitious sounds; BP

Interventions

⊗ ***Black box warning*** Potentially serious infections are possible with drug administration, including TB, sepsis, invasive fungal infections. Discontinue drug if patient develops infection or sepsis. Perform TB test before beginning therapy. If TB is present, start TB treatment and monitor patient carefully throughout therapy.

⊗ ***Black box warning*** There is increased risk of lymphoma and other cancers in children and adolescents being treated with golimumab.

- Store syringes in refrigerator. Allow prefilled syringe or autoinjector to sit at room temperature for 30 min before giving subcutaneous injection. Solution should be clear and free of particles. Discard unused solution.
- Rotate injection sites; do no inject into areas that are bruised, red, or hard. Monitor sites for infection.
- Monitor patient with history of hepatitis B for possible reactivation; if reactivation occurs, stop golimumab and begin antiviral therapy.
- Monitor patient for possible demyelinating disorders.
- Do not administer live vaccines to patient taking this drug.
- Monitor patient for signs and symptoms of infection and discontinue drug if infection occurs.
- Protect patient from exposure to infections and ensure regular physical exams and monitoring for infections or cancer development.

Teaching points

- You will need to have a TB test before beginning therapy with this drug.
- Take this drug exactly as prescribed, once a month by subcutaneous injection. Mark your calendar with the injection dates. This drug does not cure your rheumatic disease, and you may be taking other drugs to help with the signs and symptoms.
- You and a significant other should learn how to administer subcutaneous injections. Store the syringes in the refrigerator. Let the syringe sit at room temperature for 30 minutes before injecting drug. Make sure the solution is clear and free of particles. Discard any leftover solution. Consult your health care provider about the proper disposal of needles and syringes.
- Arrange for periodic medical follow-up to evaluate the effects of the drug on your body.
- This drug may appear in breast milk and cause adverse effects in a nursing baby; if you are nursing a baby, you should use another method of feeding the baby.
- You should not receive live vaccines while you are taking this drug.
- You may experience these side effects: dizziness (avoid driving or operating hazardous machinery if this occurs); upper respiratory infection, runny nose (consult your health care provider for potential treatments if this becomes uncomfortable); increased susceptibility to infections (avoid people who might have infections and crowded areas; use strict hand-washing technique and good hygiene).
- Report fever, rash, chills, lethargy, swelling, numbness, tingling, worsening of arthritis symptoms, difficulty breathing.

G

▽gonadorelin hydrochloride

See Appendix W, *Less commonly used drugs*.

DANGEROUS DRUG

▽goserelin acetate

(goe' se rel in)

Zoladex, Zoladex LA (CAN)

PREGNANCY CATEGORY X

PREGNANCY CATEGORY D (IN BREAST CANCER)

Drug classes

Antineoplastic
Hormone

Therapeutic actions

An analogue of LH-RH or gonadotropin-releasing hormone; potent inhibitor of pituitary gonadotropin secretion; initial administration causes an increase in FSH and LH and resultant increase in testosterone levels;

with long-term administration, these hormone levels fall to levels normally seen with surgical castration within 2–4 wk, as pituitary is inhibited. In women this leads to a decrease in serum estradiol levels and therefore a reduction in ovarian size and function, uterus and mammary gland size, and a repression of sex hormone–responsive tumors.

Indications

- Palliative treatment of advanced prostatic cancer when orchiectomy or estrogen administration is not indicated or is unacceptable
- Stage B_2–C prostatic cancer with flutamide for locally confined T2b–T4 carcinoma
- Management of endometriosis, including pain relief and reduction of endometriotic lesions
- Palliative treatment of advanced breast cancer in premenopausal and perimenopausal women
- Endometrial thinning drug before endometrial ablation

Contraindications and cautions

- Contraindicated with pregnancy, lactation, hypersensitivity to LH-RH or any component, undiagnosed vaginal bleeding.
- Use cautiously with hypercalcemia, high lipid levels.

Available forms

Implant—3.6, 10.8 mg

Dosages

Adults

3.6 mg subcutaneously every 28 days or 10.8 mg every 3 mo into the upper abdominal wall.

- *Prostatic or breast carcinoma:* Long-term use of 3.6 mg.
- *Endometriosis:* Continue therapy with 3.6 mg for 6 mo.
- *Endometrial thinning:* One to two 3.6-mg subcutaneous depots 4 wk apart; surgery should be done 4 wk after first dose—within 2–4 wk after second depot if two are used.
- *Stage B_2–C prostatic cancer:* Start therapy 8 wk before initiating radiation therapy and continue during radiation therapy. Treatment regimen is one 3.6 mg depot 8 wk before radiation followed by one 10.8-mg depot 28 days later. Or, four injections of 3.6-mg depot at 28-day intervals, two depots preceding and two during radiotherapy.

Pediatric patients

Safety and efficacy not established.

Pharmacokinetics

Route	*Onset*	*Peak*
Subcut.	Slow (men) 8–22 days (women)	12–15 days (men) 8–22 days (women)

Metabolism: Hepatic; $T_{1/2}$: 4.2 hr (men), 2.3 hr (women)
Distribution: Crosses placenta; may enter breast milk
Excretion: Urine

Adverse effects

- **CNS:** Insomnia, dizziness, lethargy, anxiety, depression, headache, emotional lability
- **CV:** Heart failure, edema, hypertension, arrhythmia, chest pain, vasodilation, hypotension
- **GI:** Nausea, anorexia
- **GU:** *Hot flashes, sexual dysfunction, dysmenorrhea, decreased erections, lower urinary tract symptoms, vaginitis,* gynecomastia
- **Other:** Rash, sweating, cancer, pain, breast atrophy, peripheral edema

■ Nursing considerations

Assessment

- **History:** Pregnancy, lactation
- **Physical:** Skin T, lesions; reflexes, affect; BP, P; urinary output; pregnancy test if appropriate, calcium levels, lipid levels

Interventions

⊗ ***Warning*** Ensure that patient is not pregnant before use; advise patient to use barrier contraceptives.

- Use syringe provided. Discard if package is damaged. Remove sterile syringe immediately before use. Use a local anesthetic before injection to decrease pain and discomfort.

- Administer using aseptic technique under the supervision of a physician familiar with the implant technique.
- Bandage area after injection of implant.
- Repeat injection in 28 days; keep as close to this schedule as possible.

Teaching points

- This drug will be implanted into your upper abdomen every 28 days or 3 months as appropriate. It is important to keep to this schedule. Mark a calendar of injection dates.
- Do not take this drug if you are pregnant; if you think you are pregnant or wish to become pregnant, consult your health care provider.
- You may experience these side effects: Hot flashes (keep environment cool); sexual dysfunction—regression of sex organs, impaired fertility, decreased erections; pain at injection site (a local anesthetic will be used; if discomfort is severe, analgesics may be ordered).
- Report chest pain, increased signs and symptoms of your cancer, difficulty breathing, dizziness, severe pain at injection site.

▽ granisetron hydrochloride

(gran iz' e tron)

Kytril, Sancuso

PREGNANCY CATEGORY B

Drug classes

Antiemetic
5-HT_3 receptor antagonist

Therapeutic actions

Selectively binds to serotonin (5-HT_3) receptors in the CTZ, blocking the nausea and vomiting caused by the release of serotonin by mucosal cells during chemotherapy, which stimulates the CTZ and causes nausea and vomiting.

Indications

- Prevention and treatment of nausea and vomiting associated with emetogenic chemotherapy and radiation
- Prevention and treatment of postoperative nausea and vomiting (injection)
- **NEW INDICATION:** Unlabeled use: Postanesthetic shivering

Contraindications and cautions

- Contraindicated with history of hypersensitivity, concurrent use of apomorphine.
- Use cautiously with colitis, hepatic or renal impairment, pregnancy, lactation.

Available forms

Tablets—1 mg; injection—0.1, 1 mg/mL; oral solution—1 mg/5 mL; transdermal system—3.1 mg/24 hr

Dosages

Adults and patients 2 yr and older

IV

- *Chemotherapy-induced nausea and vomiting:* 10 mcg/kg IV over 5 min starting within 30 min of chemotherapy; only on days of chemotherapy.
- *Postoperative nausea and vomiting:* 1 mg IV over 30 seconds before induction or reversal of anesthesia.

Oral

1 mg PO bid or 2 mg/day as 1 dose, beginning up to 1 hr before chemotherapy and second dose 12 hr after chemotherapy; only on days of chemotherapy.

- *Radiation therapy:* 2 mg once daily taken 1 hr before radiation.

Transdermal

Apply 1 patch to clean, dry skin on the upper, outer arm 24–48 hr before chemotherapy. Keep patch in place a minimum of 24 hr after completion of chemotherapy and then remove it. Patch may be left in place for up to 7 days.

Pediatric patients younger than 18 yr

Safety and efficacy of transdermal use not established.

Pediatric patients younger than 2 yr

Oral and IV use not recommended.

Pharmacokinetics

Route	Onset	Peak
IV	Rapid	30–45 min
Oral	Moderate	60–90 min

Metabolism: Hepatic; $T_{1/2}$: 5 hr (IV), 6.2 hr (oral)
Distribution: Crosses placenta; enters breast milk, protein-bound
Excretion: Urine

IV FACTS

Preparation: Dilute in 0.9% sodium chloride or 5% dextrose to a total volume of 20–50 mL; stable up to 24 hr refrigerated; protect from light.
Infusion: Inject slowly over 5 min.
Incompatibilities: Do not mix in solution with other drugs.

Adverse effects

- **CNS:** *Headache,* asthenia, somnolence, dizziness, insomnia
- **CV:** Hypertension, angina
- **GI:** Diarrhea or constipation, nausea, abdominal pain, vomiting, decreased appetite, dyspepsia
- **Other:** Fever, chills, shivering, increased AST and ALT, alopecia

■ Nursing considerations

Assessment

- **History:** Allergy to granisetron, pregnancy, lactation, liver or renal impairment, colitis
- **Physical:** Orientation, reflexes, affect; BP; bowel sounds; T

Interventions

- Provide mouth care and sugarless lozenges to suck to help alleviate nausea.
- Give drug only on days of chemotherapy, or before radiation therapy, or before surgery or reversal of anesthesia.

Teaching points

- This drug may be given IV, orally, or as a transdermal patch when you are receiving your chemotherapy; it will help decrease nausea and vomiting.
- If using the transdermal patch, apply one patch to clean, dry skin on the upper, outer arm 24–48 hr before chemotherapy. Keep patch in place a minimum of 24 hr after completion of chemotherapy and then remove it. Patch may be left in place for up to 7 days.
- You may experience these side effects: Lack of sleep, drowsiness (use caution if driving or performing tasks that require alertness); diarrhea or constipation; headache (ask for medication).
- Report severe headache, fever, numbness or tingling, severe diarrhea or constipation.

▽ guaifenesin (glyceryl guaiacolale)

*(gwye **fen'** e sin)*

Allfen; Altarussin; Diabetic Tussin; Guiatuss; Ganidin NR; Liquibid; Mucinex (DNC); Naldecon Senior Ex; Organidin NR; Robitussin; Scot-Tussin Expectorant; Siltussin SA

PREGNANCY CATEGORY C

Drug class

Expectorant

Therapeutic actions

Enhances the output of respiratory tract fluid by reducing adhesiveness and surface tension, facilitating the removal of viscous mucus.

Indications

- Symptomatic relief of respiratory conditions characterized by dry, nonproductive cough and when there is mucus in the respiratory tract

Contraindications and cautions

- Contraindicated with allergy to guaifenesin.
- Use cautiously with pregnancy, lactation, and persistent coughs.

Available forms

Syrup—100 mg/5 mL; liquid—100, 200 mg/5 mL; capsules—200 mg; tablets—100, 200, 400 mg; ER tablets (DNC)—600, 1,200 mg; granules—50, 100 mg per packet

Dosages

Adults and patients older than 12 yr

200–400 mg PO every 4 hr; do not exceed 2.4 g/day. For 600-mg ER tablets, 1–2 tablets every 12 hr; do not exceed 2.4 g/day.

Pediatric patients 6–12 yr

100–200 mg PO every 4 hr. Do not exceed 1.2 g/day or 600 mg (ER) PO every 12 hr.

Pediatric patients 2–6 yr

50–100 mg PO every 4 hr. Do not exceed 600 mg/day.

Pharmacokinetics

Route	*Onset*	*Duration*
Oral	30 min	4–6 hr

Metabolism: Not known; $T_{1/2}$: 1 hr
Distribution: Not known
Excretion: Urine

Adverse effects

- **CNS:** Headache, dizziness
- **Dermatologic:** Rash, urticaria
- **GI:** *Nausea, vomiting,* GI discomfort

Interactions

✱ **Drug-lab test** • Color interference and false results of 5-HIAA and VMA urinary determinations

■ Nursing considerations

CLINICAL ALERT!
Name confusion has been reported between *Mucinex* (guaifenesin) and *Mucomyst* (acetylcysteine); use caution.

Assessment

- **History:** Allergy to guaifenesin; persistent cough due to smoking, asthma, or emphysema; very productive cough; pregnancy
- **Physical:** Skin lesions, color; T; orientation, affect; R, adventitious sounds

Interventions

⊗ ***Warning*** Monitor reaction to drug; persistent cough for longer than 1 wk, fever, rash, or persistent headache may indicate a more serious condition.

Teaching points

- Some extended-release formulations may be cut in half but cannot be crushed or chewed. *Mucinex* cannot be crushed, chewed, or cut.
- Do not take for longer than 1 week; if fever, rash, or headache occur, consult your health care provider.
- You may experience these side effects: Nausea, vomiting (eat frequent small meals); dizziness, headache (avoid driving or operating dangerous machinery).
- Report fever, rash, severe vomiting, persistent cough.

▽ guanabenz acetate

(gwahn' a benz)

Wytensin

PREGNANCY CATEGORY C

Drug classes

Antihypertensive
Sympatholytic (centrally acting)

Therapeutic actions

Stimulates CNS $alpha_2$-adrenergic receptors, reduces sympathetic nerve impulses from the vasomotor center to the heart and blood vessels, decreases peripheral vascular resistance, and lowers systemic BP.

Indications

- Management of hypertension, alone or in combination with a thiazide diuretic

Contraindications and cautions

- Contraindicated with hypersensitivity to guanabenz.
- Use cautiously with severe coronary insufficiency, recent MI, CV disease, severe renal or hepatic failure, pregnancy, lactation.

Available forms

Tablets—4, 8 mg

Dosages

Adults

Individualize dosage. Initial dose of 4 mg PO bid, alone or with a thiazide diuretic; increase in increments of 4–8 mg/day every 1–2 wk. Maximum dose, 32 mg bid, but doses this high are rarely needed.

Pediatric patients

Safety and efficacy not established for children younger than 12 yr.

Pharmacokinetics

Route	*Onset*	*Peak*	*Duration*
Oral	45–60 min	2–5 hr	6–12 hr

Metabolism: Unknown; $T_{1/2}$: 6 hr
Distribution: Crosses placenta; enters breast milk
Excretion: Feces, urine

Adverse effects

- **CNS:** *Sedation, weakness, dizziness, headache,* drowsiness
- **CV:** Chest pain, edema, **arrhythmias**
- **Dermatologic:** Rash, pruritus
- **GI:** *Dry mouth*

Interactions

✱ **Drug-drug** • Additive sedative effects seen with CNS depressants

■ Nursing considerations

Assessment

- **History:** Hypersensitivity to guanabenz; severe coronary insufficiency, cerebrovascular disease, severe renal or hepatic failure; lactation, pregnancy
- **Physical:** Orientation, affect, reflexes; P, BP, orthostatic BP, perfusion, auscultation; LFTs, renal function tests, ECG

Interventions

- Store tightly sealed, protected from light.

⊗ ***Warning*** Do not discontinue drug abruptly; discontinue therapy by reducing the dosage gradually over 2–4 days to avoid rebound hypertension, increased blood and urinary catecholamines, anxiety, nervousness, and other subjective effects.

- Assess compliance with drug regimen in a nonthreatening, supportive manner.

Teaching points

- Take this drug exactly as prescribed; do not miss doses. Do not discontinue unless instructed to do so by your health care provider. Do not discontinue abruptly. Store tightly sealed, protected from light.
- You may experience these side effects: Drowsiness, dizziness, light-headedness, headache, weakness (transient; use caution while driving or performing other tasks that require alertness or physical dexterity).
- Report persistent or severe drowsiness, dry mouth.

▽ guanfacine hydrochloride

(gwahn' fa seen)

Intuniv (DNC), Tenex

PREGNANCY CATEGORY B

Drug classes

Antihypertensive
Sympatholytic (centrally acting)

Therapeutic actions

Stimulates central (CNS) alpha_2-adrenergic receptors, reduces sympathetic nerve impulses from the vasomotor center to the heart and blood vessels, decreases peripheral vascular resistance, and lowers systemic BP.

Indications

- Management of hypertension, alone or with a thiazide diuretic
- **NEW INDICATION:** Treatment of ADHD in patients 6–17 yr (ER tablets)
- Unlabeled use: Amelioration of symptoms in heroin withdrawal; reduced frequency of migraine headaches and reduced nausea and vomiting

Contraindications and cautions

- Contraindicated with hypersensitivity to guanfacine, labor and delivery, lactation.
- Use cautiously with severe coronary insufficiency, recent MI, CV disease, chronic renal or hepatic failure, pregnancy.

Available forms

Tablets—1, 2 mg; ER tablets DNC—1, 2, 3, 4 mg

Dosages

Adults

Recommended dose is 1 mg/day PO given at bedtime to minimize somnolence. If 1 mg/day does not give a satisfactory result after 3–4 wk of therapy, doses of 2 mg and then 3 mg may be given, although most of the drug's effect is seen at 1 mg. If BP rises toward the end of the dosing interval, divided dosage should be used. Higher daily doses (rarely up to 4 mg/day in divided doses) have been used, but adverse reactions increase with doses larger than 3 mg/ day, and there is no evidence of increased efficacy. Taper ER form when discontinuing; decrease by no more than 1 mg every 3–7 days.

Pediatric patients 6–17 yr

1 mg/day PO (ER tablet); increase by 1 mg/day/week to maximum of 4 mg/day. Withdraw gradually.

Pharmacokinetics

Route	*Onset*	*Peak*	*Duration*
Oral	2 hr	1–4 hr	24 hr

Metabolism: Hepatic; $T_{1/2}$: 10–30 hr
Distribution: Crosses placenta; enters breast milk
Excretion: Urine

Adverse effects

- **CNS:** *Sedation, weakness, dizziness,* headache, insomnia, amnesia, confusion, depression, conjunctivitis, iritis, vision disturbance, malaise, paresthesia, paresis, taste perversion, tinnitus, hypokinesia, somnolence
- **CV:** Bradycardia, palpitations, substernal pain, hypotension
- **Dermatologic:** Dermatitis, pruritus, purpura, sweating
- **GI:** *Dry mouth, constipation,* abdominal pain, diarrhea, dyspepsia, dysphagia, nausea
- **GU:** *Impotence,* libido decrease, testicular disorder, urinary incontinence
- **Other:** Rhinitis, leg cramps, taste alterations, fatigue

■ Nursing considerations

Assessment

- **History:** Hypersensitivity to guanfacine; severe coronary insufficiency, cerebrovascular disease; chronic renal or hepatic failure; pregnancy; lactation
- **Physical:** Skin color, lesions; orientation, affect, reflexes; ophthalmologic examination; P, BP, orthostatic BP, perfusion, auscultation; R, adventitious sounds; bowel sounds, normal output; normal urinary output, voiding pattern; LFTs, renal function tests, ECG

G

Interventions

⊗ ***Warning*** Do not discontinue drug abruptly; discontinue therapy by reducing the dosage gradually over 2–4 days to avoid rebound hypertension (much less likely than with clonidine; BP usually returns to pretreatment levels in 2–4 days without ill effects).

- Assess compliance with drug regimen in a nonthreatening, supportive manner.
- Ensure that patient does not cut, crush, or chew ER tablets.

Teaching points

- Take this drug exactly as prescribed; it is important that you do not miss doses. Swallow ER tablets whole with water, milk, or other liquid. Do not cut, crush, or chew tablets. Do not discontinue the drug unless instructed to do so by your health care provider. Do not discontinue drug abruptly.
- You may experience these side effects: Drowsiness, dizziness, light-headedness, headache, weakness (transient; observe caution while driving or performing other tasks that require alertness or physical dexterity); dry mouth (suck sugarless lozenges or ice chips); GI upset (eat frequent small meals); dizziness, light-headedness when you change position (get up slowly; use caution when climbing stairs); impotence, other sexual dysfunction, decreased libido; palpitations.
- Report urinary incontinence, changes in vision, rash.

haloperidol
*(ha loe **per'** i dole)*

haloperidol
Apo-Haloperidol (CAN), Haldol, Haloperidol LA (CAN), Novo-Peridol (CAN)

haloperidol decanoate
Haldol Decanoate, Haldol Decanoate 50, Haldol Decanoate 100

PREGNANCY CATEGORY C

Drug classes
Antipsychotic
Dopaminergic blocker

Therapeutic actions
Mechanism not fully understood; antipsychotics block postsynaptic dopamine receptors in the brain, depress the RAS, including those parts of the brain involved with wakefulness and emesis; chemically resembles the phenothiazines.

Indications
- Management of manifestations of psychotic disorders
- Control of tics and vocalizations in Tourette syndrome in adults and children
- Behavioral problems in children with combative, explosive hyperexcitability that cannot be attributed to immediate provocation
- Short-term treatment of hyperactive children with excessive motor activity, mood lability
- Haloperidol decanoate: Prolonged parenteral therapy of chronic schizophrenia
- Unlabeled uses: Control of nausea and vomiting, control of acute psychiatric situations (IV use), treatment of intractable hiccoughs, agitation, hyperkinesia, infantile autism

Contraindications and cautions
- Contraindicated with hypersensitivity to typical antipsychotics, coma or severe CNS depression, bone marrow depression, blood dyscrasia, circulatory collapse, subcortical brain damage, Parkinson's disease, liver damage, cerebral arteriosclerosis, coronary disease, severe hypotension or hypertension.
- Use cautiously with pregnancy; lactation; respiratory disorders ("silent pneumonia"); glaucoma, prostatic hypertrophy (anticholinergic effects may exacerbate glaucoma and urinary retention); epilepsy or history of epilepsy (drug lowers seizure threshold); tardive dyskinesia; NMS; breast cancer (elevations in prolactin may stimulate a prolactin-dependent tumor); thyrotoxicosis; peptic ulcer; decreased renal function; myelography within previous 24 hr or scheduled within 48 hr; exposure to heat or phosphorous insecticides; children younger than 12 yr, especially those with chickenpox, CNS infections (children are especially susceptible to dystonias that may confound the diagnosis of Reye's syndrome); allergy to aspirin if giving the 1-, 2-, 5-, and 10-mg tablets (these tablets contain tartrazine).

Available forms
Tablets—0.5, 1, 2, 5, 10, 20 mg; oral concentrate—2 mg/mL; injection—50, 100 mg/mL as decanoate, 5 mg/mL as lactate

Dosages
Full clinical effects may require 6 wk–6 mo of therapy. Children, debilitated and geriatric patients, and patients with a history of adverse reactions to neuroleptic drugs may require lower dosage.

Adults
Oral

Initial dosage range, 0.5–2 mg bid–tid PO with moderate symptoms; 3–5 mg bid–tid PO for more resistant patients. Daily dosages up to 100 mg/day (or more) have been used, but safety of prolonged use has not been demonstrated. For maintenance, reduce dosage to lowest effective level.
- *Tourette syndrome:* 0.5–1.5 mg tid as starting dose; up to 10 mg/day may be needed.

IM

2–5 mg (up to 10–30 mg) every 60 min or every 4–8 hr IM as necessary for prompt control of acutely agitated patients with severe symptoms. Switch to oral dosage as soon as feasible, using total IM dosage in previous 24 hr as a guide to total daily oral dosage.

IM, haloperidol decanoate injection

Maintenance, 10–15 times the daily oral dose in elderly patients stabilized on 10 mg/day or less; 20 times the daily oral dose in patients stabilized on high doses and tolerant to oral haloperidol. Do not exceed 3 mL per injection site; repeat at 4-wk intervals. Initial dose should not exceed 100 mg. If more than 100 mg is needed, divide into two doses of 100 mg on day 1 and give rest of dose 3–7 days later.

Pediatric patients 3–12 yr or 15–40 kg

Initial dose, 0.5 mg/day (25–50 mcg/kg/day) PO; may increase in increments of 0.5 mg every 5–7 days as needed. Total daily dose may be divided and given bid–tid.

- *Psychiatric disorders:* 0.05–0.15 kg/day PO given bid–tid. Severely disturbed psychotic children may require higher dosage.
- *Nonpsychotic and Tourette syndromes, behavioral disorders, hyperactivity:* 0.05–0.075 mg/kg/day PO given bid–tid. In severely disturbed nonpsychotic children, short-term administration may suffice. There is little evidence of improved effects at doses greater than 6 mg/day.

Geriatric patients

Use lower doses (0.5–2.0 mg bid–tid), and increase dosage more gradually than in younger patients.

Pharmacokinetics

Route	*Onset*	*Peak*
Oral	Varies	3–5 hr
IM	Rapid	20 min
IM, decanoate	Slow	6 days

Metabolism: Hepatic; $T_{1/2}$: 21–24 hr, 3 wk for decanoate

Distribution: Crosses placenta; enters breast milk

Excretion: Bile, urine

Adverse effects

Not all effects have been reported with haloperidol; however, because haloperidol has certain pharmacologic similarities to the phenothiazine class of antipsychotic drugs, all adverse effects associated with phenothiazine therapy should be kept in mind when haloperidol is used.

- **Autonomic:** Dry mouth, salivation, nasal congestion, nausea, vomiting, anorexia, fever, pallor, facial flushing, sweating, constipation, paralytic ileus, urinary retention, incontinence, polyuria, enuresis, priapism, ejaculation inhibition
- **CNS:** *Drowsiness,* insomnia, vertigo, headache, weakness, tremor, ataxia, slurring, cerebral edema, seizures, exacerbation of psychotic symptoms, extrapyramidal syndromes—*pseudoparkinsonism; dystonias; akathisia,* tardive dyskinesias, potentially irreversible (no known treatment), **NMS**—extrapyramidal symptoms, hyperthermia, autonomic disturbances
- **CV:** Hypotension, orthostatic hypotension, hypertension, tachycardia, bradycardia, **cardiac arrest,** cardiomegaly, **refractory arrhythmias,** pulmonary edema
- **Endocrine:** Lactation, breast engorgement in females, galactorrhea; SIADH; amenorrhea, menstrual irregularities; gynecomastia in males; changes in libido; hyperglycemia or hypoglycemia; glycosuria; hyponatremia; pituitary tumor with hyperprolactinemia; inhibition of ovulation, infertility, pseudopregnancy
- **Hematologic:** Eosinophilia, leukopenia, leukocytosis, anemia; aplastic anemia; hemolytic anemia; thrombocytopenic or nonthrombocytopenic purpura; pancytopenia
- **Hypersensitivity:** Jaundice, urticaria, angioneurotic edema, laryngeal edema, photosensitivity, eczema, asthma, **anaphylactoid reactions,** exfoliative dermatitis
- **Respiratory:** Bronchospasm, laryngospasm, dyspnea; **suppression of cough reflex and potential for aspiration**

Interactions

✱ **Drug-drug** • Additive anticholinergic effects and possibly decreased antipsychotic efficacy with anticholinergic drugs • Increased risk of toxic side effects with lithium • Decreased effectiveness with carbamazepine

✱ **Drug-lab test** • False-positive pregnancy tests (less likely if serum test is used) • Increase in PBI, not attributable to an increase in thyroxine

H

✱ **Drug-alternative therapy** • With ginkgo biloba, increased drug effectiveness and decreased extrapyramidal effects of haloperidol

■ Nursing considerations

Assessment

- **History:** Severe CNS depression; bone marrow depression; blood dyscrasia; circulatory collapse; subcortical brain damage; Parkinson's disease; liver damage; cerebral arteriosclerosis; coronary disease; severe hypotension or hypertension; respiratory disorders; glaucoma, prostatic hypertrophy; epilepsy or history of epilepsy; breast cancer; thyrotoxicosis; peptic ulcer, decreased renal function; myelography within previous 24 hr or scheduled within 48 hr; exposure to heat or phosphorus insecticides; children younger than 12 yr, especially those with chickenpox, CNS infections; allergy to aspirin, pregnancy, lactation
- **Physical:** Weight, T; reflexes, orientation, IOP; P, BP, orthostatic BP; R, adventitious sounds; bowel sounds and normal output, liver evaluation; urinary output, prostate size, CBC, urinalysis, thyroid, LFTs, renal function tests

Interventions

- Do not give children IM injections.
- Do not use haloperidol decanoate for IV injections.

⊗ ***Warning*** Gradually withdraw drug when patient has been on maintenance therapy to avoid withdrawal-emergent dyskinesias.

⊗ ***Warning*** Discontinue drug if serum creatinine or BUN become abnormal or if WBC count is depressed.

⊗ ***Warning*** Monitor elderly patients for dehydration; institute remedial measures promptly; sedation and decreased thirst related to CNS effects can lead to severe dehydration.

- Consult physician regarding appropriate warning of patient or patient's guardian about tardive dyskinesias.
- Consult physician about reducing dosage and using anticholinergic antiparkinsonians (controversial) if extrapyramidal effects occur.

Teaching points

- Take this drug exactly as prescribed.
- Avoid driving or engaging in other dangerous activities if dizziness or drowsiness or vision changes occur.
- Avoid prolonged exposure to sun, or use a sunscreen or covering garments.
- Maintain fluid intake, and use precautions against heatstroke in hot weather.
- You may experience these side effects: dry mouth (sucking sugarless lozenges may help); urinary retention (empty your bladder before taking the drug), constipation (medication may be available to help).
- Report sore throat, fever, unusual bleeding or bruising, rash, weakness, tremors, impaired vision, dark-colored urine (pink or reddish brown urine is to be expected), pale stools, yellowing of the skin or eyes.

DANGEROUS DRUG

▽ heparin

(hep' ah rin)

heparin sodium and 0.9% sodium chloride

heparin sodium and 0.45% sodium chloride

heparin sodium injection

Hepalean (CAN), Heparin LEO (CAN)

heparin sodium lock flush solution

Hepalean-Lok (CAN), Hepflush-10, Hep-Lock, Hep-Lock U/P

PREGNANCY CATEGORY C

Drug class

Anticoagulant

Therapeutic actions

Heparin inactivates factor Xa, therefore inhibiting thrombus and clot formation by blocking the conversion of prothrombin to thrombin and fibrinogen to fibrin, the final steps in the clotting process. Heparin also inhibits the activation of factor XIII and thrombin-induced activation of factors V and VIII

Indications

- Prevention and treatment of venous thrombosis, pulmonary embolism, and peripheral arterial embolism
- Treatment of atrial fibrillation with embolization
- Diagnosis and treatment of DIC
- Prevention of clotting in blood samples and heparin lock sets and during dialysis procedures
- Unlabeled uses: Adjunct in therapy of coronary occlusion with acute MI, prevention of left ventricular thrombi and CVA post-MI, prevention of cerebral thrombosis in the evolving CVA

Contraindications and cautions

- Contraindicated with hypersensitivity to heparin; severe thrombocytopenia; uncontrolled bleeding; any patient who cannot be monitored regularly with blood coagulation tests; labor and immediate postpartum period.
- Use cautiously with pregnancy; women older than 60 yr who are at high risk for hemorrhaging, dysbetalipoproteinemia; recent surgery or injury.

Available forms

Injection—1,000, 2,000, 2,500, 5,000, 7,500, 10,000, 12,500, 20,000, 40,000 units/mL; also single-dose and unit-dose forms; lock flush solution—10, 100 units/mL

Dosages

Adjust dosage according to coagulation tests. Dosage is adequate when WBCT = 2.5–3 times control—or aPTT = 1.5–2 times control value. The following are guidelines to dosage:

Adults

Subcutaneous (deep subcutaneous injection)

- *For general anticoagulation:* IV loading dose of 5,000 units and then 10,000–20,000 units subcutaneously followed by 8,000–10,000 units every 8 hr or 15,000–20,000 units every 12 hr.
- *Prophylaxis of postoperative thromboembolism:* 5,000 units by deep subcutaneous injection 2 hr before surgery and every 8–12 hr thereafter for 7 days or until patient is fully ambulatory.

IV

- *Intermittent IV:* Initial dose of 10,000 units and then 5,000–10,000 units every 4–6 hr.
- *Continuous IV infusion:* Loading dose of 5,000 units and then 20,000–40,000 units/day.
- *Surgery of heart and blood vessels for patients undergoing total body perfusion:* Not less than 150 units/kg; guideline often used is 300 units/kg for procedures less than 60 min, 400 units/kg for longer procedures.
- *Clot prevention in blood samples:* 70–150 units/10–20 mL of whole blood.
- *Heparin lock and extracorporal dialysis:* See manufacturer's instructions.

Pediatric patients

Initial IV bolus of 50 units/kg and then 100 units/kg IV every 4 hr, or 20,000 units/m^2 per 24 hr by continuous IV infusion.

Pharmacokinetics

Route	*Onset*	*Peak*	*Duration*
IV	Immediate	Minutes	2–6 hr
Subcut.	20–60 min	2–4 hr	8–12 hr

Metabolism: $T_{1/2}$: 30–180 min
Distribution: Does not cross placenta, does not enter breast milk; broken down in liver
Excretion: Urine

IV FACTS

Continuous infusion: Can be mixed in normal saline, D_5W, Ringer's; mix well; invert bottle numerous times to ensure adequate mixing. Monitor patient closely; infusion pump is recommended.

Single dose: Direct, undiluted IV injection of up to 5,000 units (adult) or 50 units/kg (pediatric), given over 60 seconds.

Monitoring: Blood should be drawn for coagulation testing 30 min before each intermittent IV dose or every 4–6 hr if patient is on continuous infusion pump.

Incompatibilities: Heparin should not be mixed in solution with any other drug unless specifically ordered; direct incompatibilities in solution and at Y-site seen with amikacin,

H

codeine, chlorpromazine, cytarabine, diazepam, dobutamine, doxorubicin, droperidol, ergotamine, erythromycin, gentamicin, haloperidol, hydrocortisone, kanamycin, levorphanol, meperidine, methadone, methicillin, methotrimeprazine, morphine, netilmicin, pentazocine, phenytoin, polymyxin B, promethazine, streptomycin, tetracycline, tobramycin, vancomycin.

Adverse effects

- **Dermatologic:** Loss of hair
- **Hematologic: Hemorrhage;** *bruising;* thrombocytopenia; elevated AST, ALT levels, hyperkalemia
- **Hypersensitivity:** Chills, fever, urticaria, asthma
- **Other:** Osteoporosis, suppression of renal function (long-term, high-dose therapy), **white clot syndrome**

Interactions

✷ **Drug-drug** • Increased bleeding tendencies with oral anticoagulants, salicylates, penicillins, cephalosporins, low–molecular-weight heparins, platelet inhibitors • Decreased anticoagulation effects if taken concurrently with nitroglycerin

✷ **Drug-lab test** • Increased AST, ALT levels • Increased thyroid function tests • Altered blood gas analyses, especially levels of carbon dioxide, bicarbonate concentration, and base excess

✷ **Drug-alternative therapy** • Increased risk of bleeding if combined with chamomile, garlic, ginger, ginkgo, and ginseng therapy; high-dose vitamin E

■ Nursing considerations

Assessment

- **History:** Recent surgery or injury; sensitivity to heparin; hyperlipidemia; pregnancy
- **Physical:** Peripheral perfusion, R, stool guaiac test, PTT or other tests of blood coagulation, platelet count, renal function tests

Interventions

- Adjust dose according to coagulation test results performed just before injection (30 min before each intermittent dose or every 4–6 hr if continuous IV dose). Therapeutic range aPTT: 1.5–2.5 times control.
- Always check compatibilities with other IV solutions.
- Use heparin lock needle to avoid repeated injections.
- Give deep subcutaneous injections; do not give heparin by IM injection.
- Do not give IM injections to patients on heparin therapy (heparin predisposes to hematoma formation).

⊗ ***Warning*** Apply pressure to all injection sites after needle is withdrawn; inspect injection sites for signs of hematoma; do not massage injection sites.

- Mix well when adding heparin to IV infusion.
- Do not add heparin to infusion lines of other drugs, and do not piggyback other drugs into heparin line. If this must be done, ensure drug compatibility.
- Provide for safety measures (electric razor, soft toothbrush) to prevent injury from bleeding.
- Check for signs of bleeding; monitor blood tests.
- Alert all health care providers of heparin use.

⊗ ***Warning*** Have protamine sulfate (heparin antidote) readily available in case of overdose. Each mg of protamine neutralizes 100 USP heparin units. Give very slowly IV over 10 min, not to exceed 50 mg. Establish dose based on blood coagulation studies.

Teaching points

- This drug must be given by a parenteral route (cannot be taken orally).
- Frequent blood tests are needed to determine whether blood clotting time is within the correct range.
- Be careful to avoid injury: Use an electric razor, avoid contact sports, and avoid other activities that might lead to injury.
- You may experience loss of hair.
- Report nose bleed, bleeding of the gums, unusual bruising, black or tarry stools, cloudy or dark urine, abdominal or lower back pain, severe headache.

hetastarch (hydroxyethyl starch, HES)

(het' a starch)

Hespan, Voluven

PREGNANCY CATEGORY C

Drug class

Plasma expander

Therapeutic actions

Complex mixture of various sized molecules with colloidal properties that approximate those of human albumin and raise human plasma volume when administered IV; increases the erythrocyte sedimentation rate and improves the efficiency of granulocyte collection by centrifugal means.

Indications

- Adjunctive therapy for plasma volume expansion in shock due to hemorrhage, burns, surgery, sepsis, trauma
- Adjunctive therapy in leukapheresis to improve harvesting and increase the yield of granulocytes

Contraindications and cautions

- Contraindicated with allergy to hetastarch, severe bleeding disorders, severe cardiac failure, renal failure with anuria or oliguria.
- Use cautiously with hepatic impairment, pregnancy, lactation.

Available forms

Injection—6 g/100 mL in 500 mL IV infusion bottle

Dosages

Adults

- *Plasma volume expansion:* 500–1,000 mL IV. Do not usually exceed 1,500 mL/day. In acute hemorrhagic shock, rates approaching 20 mL/kg/hr are often needed (*Hespan*); up to 50 mL/kg/day *Voluven* injection.
- *Leukapheresis (Hespan):* 250–700 mL hetastarch infused at a constant fixed ratio of 1:8 to 1:13 to venous whole blood. Safety of up to two procedures per week and a total of seven to ten procedures using hetastarch have been established.

Pediatric patients

Safety and efficacy not established.

Pharmacokinetics

Route	Onset	Peak	Duration
IV	Immediate	24 hr	24–36 hr

Metabolism: Renal; $T_{1/2}$: 17 days, then 48 days

Distribution: Crosses placenta; enters breast milk

Excretion: Urine

IV FACTS

Preparation: Use as prepared by manufacturer; store at room temperature; do not use if turbid deep brown or if crystalline precipitate forms.

Infusion: Rate of infusion should be determined by patient response; start at approximately 20 mL/kg, reduce rate to lowest possible needed to maintain hemodynamics.

Incompatibilities: Do not mix in solution with any other drug and do not add at Y-site with any other drugs.

Adverse effects

- **CNS:** *Headache,* muscle pain
- **GI:** *Vomiting, submaxillary and parotid glandular enlargement*
- **Hematologic:** Prolongation of PT, PTT; **bleeding and increased clotting times**
- **Hypersensitivity:** Periorbital edema, urticaria, wheezing
- **Other:** *Mild temperature elevations, chills, itching, mild influenza-like symptoms,* peripheral edema of the lower extremities

■ Nursing considerations

Assessment

- **History:** Allergy to hetastarch, severe bleeding disorders, severe cardiac congestion, renal failure or anuria; hepatic impairment; pregnancy, lactation
- **Physical:** T; submaxillary and parotid gland evaluation; P, BP, adventitious sounds, peripheral and periorbital edema; R, adventitious sounds; liver evaluation; urinalysis,

LFTs, renal function tests, clotting times, PT, PTT, Hgb, Hct, CBC with differential

Interventions

- Administer by IV infusion only; monitor rates based on patient response.

⊗ ***Warning*** Keep life-support equipment readily available in cases of shock.

⊗ ***Warning*** Ensure that no other drugs are mixed with or added to hetastarch.

Teaching points

- This drug can only be given IV.
- Report difficulty breathing, headache, muscle pain, rash, unusual bleeding or bruising.

histrelin implant

See Appendix W, *Less commonly used drugs*.

hyaluronic acid derivatives

See Appendix W, *Less commonly used drugs*.

hyaluronidase

See Appendix W, *Less commonly used drugs*.

hydralazine hydrochloride

*(hye **dral'** a zeen)*

Apo-Hydralazine (CAN), Apresoline

PREGNANCY CATEGORY C

Drug classes

Antihypertensive
Vasodilator (peripheral)

Therapeutic actions

Acts directly on vascular smooth muscle to cause vasodilation, primarily arteriolar, decreasing peripheral resistance; maintains or increases renal and cerebral blood flow.

Indications

- Oral: Essential hypertension alone or in combination with other drugs
- Parenteral: Severe essential hypertension when drug cannot be given orally or when need to lower BP is urgent
- Unlabeled uses: Reducing afterload in the treatment of heart failure, severe aortic insufficiency, and after valve replacement (doses up to 800 mg tid)

Contraindications and cautions

- Contraindicated with hypersensitivity to hydralazine, tartrazine (in 100-mg tablets marketed as *Apresoline*); CAD, mitral valvular rheumatic heart disease (implicated in MI).
- Use cautiously with CVAs; increased intracranial pressure (drug-induced BP decrease increases risk of cerebral ischemia); severe hypertension with uremia; advanced renal damage; slow acetylators (higher plasma levels may be achieved; lower dosage may be adequate); lactation, pregnancy, pulmonary hypertension.

Available forms

Tablets—10, 25, 50, 100 mg; injection—20 mg/mL

Dosages

Adults

Oral

Initiate therapy with gradually increasing dosages. Start with 10 mg qid PO for the first 2–4 days; increase to 25 mg qid PO for the first week. Second and subsequent weeks: 50 mg qid. For maintenance, adjust to lowest effective dosage; twice daily dosage may be adequate. Some patients may require up to 300 mg/day. Incidence of toxic reactions, particularly the lupus-like syndrome, is high in patients receiving large doses.

Parenteral

- *Hypertension:* Patient should be hospitalized. Give IV or IM. Use parenteral therapy only when drug cannot be given orally. Usual dose is 20–40 mg, repeated as necessary. Monitor BP frequently; average maximal decrease occurs in 10–80 min. Transfer to oral form as soon as possible.

- *Eclampsia:* 5–10 mg every 20 min via IV bolus; if no response after 20 mg, try another drug.

Pediatric patients

Although safety and efficacy have not been established by controlled clinical trials, hydralazine has been used in children.

Oral

0.75 mg/kg/day PO, given in divided doses every 6–12 hr. Dosage may be gradually increased over the next 3–4 wk to a maximum of 7.5 mg/kg/day PO or 200 mg/day PO.

Parenteral

1.7–3.5 mg/kg divided into 4–6 doses.

Pharmacokinetics

Route	*Onset*	*Peak*	*Duration*
Oral	Rapid	1–2 hr	6–12 hr
IM, IV	Rapid	10–20 min	2–4 hr

Metabolism: Hepatic; $T_{1/2}$: 3–7 hr
Distribution: Crosses placenta; may enter breast milk
Excretion: Urine

IV FACTS

Preparation: No further preparation required, use as provided.
Infusion: Inject slowly over 1 min, directly into vein or into tubing of running IV; monitor BP response continually.
Incompatibilities: Do not mix with aminophylline, ampicillin, chlorothiazide, edetate, hydrocortisone, nitroglycerin, phenobarbital, verapamil.
Y-site incompatibilities: Do not mix with aminophylline, ampicillin, diazoxide, furosemide.

Adverse effects

- **CNS:** *Headache,* peripheral neuritis, dizziness, tremors; psychotic reactions characterized by depression, disorientation, or anxiety
- **CV:** *Palpitations, tachycardia, angina pectoris,* hypotension, paradoxical pressor response, orthostatic hypotension
- **GI:** *Anorexia, nausea, vomiting, diarrhea,* constipation, paralytic ileus
- **GU:** Difficult micturition, impotence
- **Hematologic:** Blood dyscrasias
- **Hypersensitivity:** Rash, urticaria, pruritus; fever, chills, arthralgia, eosinophilia; rarely, hepatitis, obstructive jaundice
- **Other:** Nasal congestion, flushing, edema, muscle cramps, lymphadenopathy, splenomegaly, dyspnea, lupus-like syndrome, possible carcinogenesis, lacrimation, conjunctivitis

Interactions

✱ **Drug-drug** • Increased pharmacologic effects of beta-adrenergic blockers and hydralazine when given concomitantly; dosage of beta blocker may need adjustment
✱ **Drug-food** • Increased bioavailability of oral hydralazine given with food

H

■ Nursing considerations

Assessment

- **History:** Hypersensitivity to hydralazine, tartrazine; heart disease; CVA; increased intracranial pressure; severe hypertension; advanced renal damage; slow acetylators; lactation, pregnancy
- **Physical:** Weight; T; skin color, lesions; lymph node palpation; orientation, affect, reflexes; examination of conjunctiva; P, BP, orthostatic BP, supine BP, perfusion, edema, auscultation; R, adventitious sounds, status of nasal mucous membranes; bowel sounds, normal output; voiding pattern, normal output; CBC with differential, lupus-like cell preparations, ANA determinations, renal function tests, urinalysis

Interventions

- Give oral drug with food to increase bioavailability (drug should be given in a consistent relationship to ingestion of food for consistent response to therapy).

⊗ ***Warning*** Use parenteral drug immediately after opening ampule. Use as quickly as possible after drawing through a needle into a syringe. Hydralazine changes color after contact with metal, and discolored solutions should be discarded.

⊗ ***Warning*** Withdraw drug gradually, especially from patients who have experienced marked BP reduction. Rapid withdrawal may cause a possible sudden increase in BP.

- Drug may cause a syndrome resembling SLE. Arrange for CBC, lupus erythematosus (LE) cell preparations, and ANA titers before and periodically during prolonged therapy, even in the asymptomatic patient. Discontinue if blood dyscrasias occur. Reevaluate therapy if ANA or LE tests are positive.

⊗ ***Warning*** Discontinue or reevaluate therapy if patient develops arthralgia, fever, chest pain, or continued malaise.

- Arrange for pyridoxine therapy if patient develops symptoms of peripheral neuritis.
- Monitor patient for orthostatic hypotension, which is most marked in the morning and in hot weather, and with alcohol or exercise.

Teaching points

- Take this drug exactly as prescribed. Take with food. Do not discontinue or reduce dosage without consulting your health care provider.
- You may experience these side effects: Dizziness, weakness (these are most likely when changing position, in the early morning, after exercise, in hot weather, and when you have consumed alcohol; some tolerance may occur; avoid driving or engaging in tasks that require alertness; change position slowly; use caution in climbing stairs; lie down for a while if dizziness persists); GI upset (eat frequent small meals); constipation; impotence; numbness, tingling (vitamin supplements may ameliorate symptoms); stuffy nose.
- Report persistent or severe constipation; unexplained fever or malaise, muscle or joint aching; chest pain; rash; numbness, tingling.

▽hydrochlorothiazide

*(hye droe klor oh **thye'** a zide)*

Apo-Hydro (CAN), Ezide, HydroDIURIL, Hydro-Par, Microzide Capsules

PREGNANCY CATEGORY B

Drug class

Thiazide diuretic

Therapeutic actions

Inhibits reabsorption of sodium and chloride in distal renal tubule, increasing the excretion of sodium, chloride, and water by the kidney.

Indications

- Adjunctive therapy in edema associated with heart failure, cirrhosis, corticosteroid, and estrogen therapy; renal impairment
- Hypertension as sole therapy or in combination with other antihypertensives
- Unlabeled uses: Calcium nephrolithiasis alone or with amiloride or allopurinol to prevent recurrences in hypercalciuric or normal calciuric patients; diabetes insipidus, especially nephrogenic diabetes insipidus; osteoporosis

Contraindications and cautions

- Contraindicated with allergy to thiazides, sulfonamides; fluid or electrolyte imbalance; renal disease (can lead to azotemia); liver disease (risk of hepatic coma); anuria.
- Use cautiously with gout (risk of attack); SLE; glucose tolerance abnormalities, diabetes mellitus; hyperparathyroidism; manic-depressive disorder (aggravated by hypercalcemia); pregnancy; lactation, elevated triglyceride levels.

Available forms

Tablets—12.5, 25, 50, 100 mg; capsules—12.5 mg

Dosages

Adults

- *Edema:* 25–100 mg daily PO until dry weight is attained. Then, 25–100 mg daily PO or intermittently, up to 200 mg/day.
- *Hypertension:* 12.5–50 mg PO.
- *Calcium nephrolithiasis:* 50 mg daily or bid PO.

Pediatric patients

General guidelines: 1–2 mg/kg/day PO in 1 or 2 doses.

Maximum dose:

2–12 yr: 37.5–100 mg/day in 2 doses.

6 mo–2 yr: 12.5–37.5 mg/day in 2 doses.

Younger than 6 mo: Up to 3 mg/kg/day in 2 doses.

Geriatric patients

Initiate with 12.5 mg/day; increase in 12.5-mg increments, monitoring patient closely.

Pharmacokinetics

Route	Onset	Peak	Duration
Oral	2 hr	4–6 hr	6–12 hr

Metabolism: Hepatic; $T_{1/2}$: 5.6–14.8 hr
Distribution: Crosses placenta; enters breast milk
Excretion: Urine

Adverse effects

- **CNS:** *Dizziness, vertigo,* paresthesias, weakness, headache, drowsiness, fatigue
- **CV:** Orthostatic hypotension, venous thrombosis, volume depletion, cardiac arrhythmias, chest pain
- **Dermatologic:** Photosensitivity, rash, purpura, exfoliative dermatitis, hives, alopecia
- **GI:** *Nausea, anorexia, vomiting, dry mouth,* diarrhea, constipation, jaundice, hepatitis, pancreatitis
- **GU:** *Polyuria, nocturia,* impotence, loss of libido, hyperuricemia
- **Hematologic:** Leukopenia, thrombocytopenia, agranulocytosis, aplastic anemia, neutropenia
- **Other:** Muscle cramps and muscle spasms, fever, gouty attacks, flushing, weight loss, rhinorrhea, electrolyte imbalances, hyperglycemia

Interactions

✱ **Drug-drug** • Altered electrolytes with loop diuretics, amphotericin B, corticosteroids • Increased neuromuscular blocking effects and respiratory depression with nondepolarizing muscle relaxants • Decreased absorption with cholestyramine, colestipol • Increased risk of cardiac glycoside toxicity if hypokalemia occurs • Increased risk of lithium toxicity • Decreased effectiveness of antidiabetic drugs

✱ **Drug-lab test** • Decreased PBI levels without clinical signs of thyroid disturbance

■ Nursing considerations

Assessment

- **History:** Allergy to thiazides, sulfonamides; fluid or electrolyte imbalance; renal or liver disease; gout; SLE; glucose tolerance abnormalities, diabetes mellitus; hyperparathyroidism; manic-depressive disorders; lactation, pregnancy
- **Physical:** Skin color, lesions, edema; orientation, reflexes, muscle strength; pulses, baseline ECG, BP, orthostatic BP, perfusion; R, pattern, adventitious sounds; liver evaluation, bowel sounds, urinary output patterns; CBC, serum electrolytes, blood glucose, LFTs, renal function tests, serum uric acid, urinalysis

Interventions

- Give with food or milk if GI upset occurs.
- Mark calendars or provide other reminders of drug for alternate day or 3–5 days/wk therapy.
- Reduce dosage of other antihypertensives by at least 50% if given with thiazides; readjust dosages gradually as BP responds.
- Administer early in the day so increased urination will not disturb sleep.
- Measure and record weights to monitor fluid changes.

Teaching points

- Record intermittent therapy on a calendar, or use prepared, dated envelopes. Take drug early so increased urination will not disturb sleep. Drug may be taken with food or meals if GI upset occurs.
- Weigh yourself on a regular basis, at the same time and in the same clothing: Record weight on your calendar.
- You may experience these side effects: Increased volume and frequency of urination; dizziness, feeling faint on arising, drowsiness (avoid rapid position changes; hazardous activities, like driving; alcohol); sensitivity to sunlight (use sunglasses, wear protective clothing, or use a sunscreen); decrease in sexual function; increased thirst (sucking on sugarless lozenges and frequent mouth care may help); gout attack (report any sudden joint pain).
- Report weight change of more than 3 pounds in 1 day, swelling in your ankles or fingers, unusual bleeding or bruising, dizziness, trembling, numbness, fatigue, muscle weakness or cramps.

hydrocortisone

*(hye droe **kor'** ti zone)*

hydrocortisone acetate

Dermatologic cream, ointment: Cortaid with Aloe, Cortef Cream (CAN), Cortef Feminine Itch, Corticaine, Cortoderm (CAN), Gynecort Female Creme, Lanacort-5, Lanacort-10, Maximum Strength Caldecort, Maximum Strength Cortaid, Tucks, U-Cort

hydrocortisone butyrate

Dermatologic ointment and cream: Locoid

hydrocortisone cypionate

Oral suspension: Cortef

hydrocortisone probutate

Pandel

hydrocortisone sodium succinate

IV, IM injection: A-Hydrocort, Solu-Cortef

hydrocortisone valerate

Dermatologic cream, ointment, lotion: Westcort

PREGNANCY CATEGORY C

Drug classes

Adrenocortical steroid
Corticosteroid (short-acting)
Glucocorticoid
Hormone

Therapeutic actions

Enters target cells and binds to cytoplasmic receptors; initiates many complex reactions that are responsible for its anti-inflammatory, immunosuppressive (glucocorticoid), and salt-retaining (mineralocorticoid) actions. Some actions may be undesirable, depending on drug use.

Indications

- Replacement therapy in adrenal cortical insufficiency
- Allergic states—severe or incapacitating allergic conditions
- Hypercalcemia associated with cancer
- Short-term inflammatory and allergic disorders, such as rheumatoid arthritis, collagen diseases (SLE), dermatologic diseases (pemphigus), status asthmaticus, and autoimmune disorders
- Hematologic disorders—thrombocytopenic purpura, erythroblastopenia
- Trichinosis with neurologic or myocardial involvement
- Ulcerative colitis, acute exacerbations of MS, and palliation in some leukemias and lymphomas
- Intra-articular or soft-tissue administration: Arthritis, psoriatic plaques
- Retention enema: For ulcerative colitis, proctitis
- Topical preparations: Minor skin irritation and rashes due to seborrheic dermatitis and psoriasis
- Dermatologic preparations: To relieve inflammatory and pruritic manifestations of dermatoses that are steroid responsive
- Anorectal cream, suppositories: To relieve discomfort of hemorrhoids and perianal itching or irritation

Ophthalmic

- Ophthalmic diseases: Acute and chronic severe allergic or inflammatory conditions including herpes zoster ophthalmicus, iritis, iridocyclitis, chorioretinitis, uveitis and choroiditis, optic neuritis, sympathetic ophthalmia, allergic conjunctivitis, keratitis, allergic corneal marginal ulcers, anterior segment inflammation

Contraindications and cautions

Systemic administration

- Contraindicated with allergy to any component of the drug, fungal infections, amebiasis, hepatitis B, vaccinia, or varicella, and antibiotic-resistant infections, immunosuppression.

- Use cautiously with kidney disease (risk for edema); liver disease, cirrhosis, hypothyroidism; ulcerative colitis with impending perforation; diverticulitis; recent GI surgery; active or latent peptic ulcer; inflammatory bowel disease (risks exacerbations or bowel perforation); hypertension, heart failure; thromboembolic tendencies, thrombophlebitis, osteoporosis, convulsive disorders, metastatic carcinoma, diabetes mellitus; TB; lactation.

Retention enemas, intrarectal foam

- Contraindicated with systemic fungal infections, recent intestinal surgery, extensive fistulas.
- Use cautiously with pregnancy.

Topical dermatologic administration

- Contraindicated with fungal, tubercular, herpes simplex skin infections; vaccinia, varicella; ear application when eardrum is perforated.
- Use cautiously with pregnancy, lactation.

Available forms

Tablets—5, 10, 20 mg; oral suspension—10 mg/5 mL, 25, 50 mg/mL; injection—25, 50 mg/mL, 100, 250, 500, 1,000 mg/vial; topical lotion—0.25%, 0.5%, 1%, 2%, 2.5%; topical liquid—1%; topical oil—1%; topical solution—1%; topical spray—1%; cream—0.2%, 0.5%, 1%, 2.5%; ointment—0.5%, 1%, 2.5%; topical gel—1%, 2%; stick, roll-on—1%; pump spray—1%

Dosages

Adults

Individualize dosage, based on severity and response. Give daily dose before 9 AM to minimize adrenal suppression. If long-term therapy is needed, alternate-day therapy should be considered. After long-term therapy, withdraw drug slowly to avoid adrenal insufficiency. For maintenance therapy, reduce initial dose in small increments at intervals until lowest clinically satisfactory dose is reached.

IM, IV (hydrocortisone sodium succinate)

100–500 mg initially and every 2, 4, or 6 hr, based on condition and response.

Pediatric patients

Individualize dosage based on severity and response rather than on formulae that correct adult doses for age or weight. Carefully observe growth and development in infants and children on prolonged therapy.

Oral (hydrocortisone cypionate)

20–240 mg/day in single or divided doses.

Adults and pediatric patients

IM, IV (hydrocortisone sodium succinate)

Reduce dose, based on condition and response, but give no less than 25 mg/day.

Retention enema (hydrocortisone)

100 mg nightly for 21 days.

Intrarectal foam (hydrocortisone acetate)

1 applicator daily or bid for 2 or 3 wk and every second day thereafter.

Topical dermatologic preparations

Apply sparingly to affected area bid–qid.

Pharmacokinetics

Route	*Onset*	*Peak*	*Duration*
Oral	1–2 hr	1–2 hr	1–1.5 days
IM	Rapid	4–8 hr	1–1.5 days
IV	Immediate	Unknown	1–1.5 days
Rectal	Slow	3–5 days	4–6 days

Metabolism: Hepatic; $T_{1/2}$: 80–120 min

Distribution: Crosses placenta; enters breast milk

Excretion: Urine

IV FACTS

Preparation: Give directly or dilute in normal saline or D_5W. Administer within 24 hr of diluting.

Infusion: Inject slowly, directly or dilute, and infuse hydrocortisone phosphate at a rate of 25 mg/min; hydrocortisone sodium succinate at rate of each 500 mg over 30 sec–10 min.

Incompatibilities: Do not mix or inject at Y-site with amobarbital, ampicillin, bleomycin, dimenhydrinate, doxapram, doxorubicin, ephedrine, ergotamine, heparin, hydralazine, metaraminol, methicillin, nafcillin, pentobarbital, phenobarbital, phenytoin, prochlorperazine, promethazine, secobarbital.

Adverse effects

Systemic

- **CNS:** *Vertigo, headache,* paresthesias, insomnia, seizures, psychosis
- **CV:** *Hypotension, shock,* hypertension and heart failure secondary to fluid retention, thromboembolism, thrombophlebitis, fat embolism, cardiac arrhythmias secondary to electrolyte disturbances
- **Dermatologic:** *Thin, fragile skin; petechiae; ecchymoses;* purpura; striae; subcutaneous fat atrophy
- **EENT:** Cataracts, glaucoma (long-term therapy), increased IOP
- **Endocrine:** *Amenorrhea, irregular menses,* growth retardation, decreased carbohydrate tolerance and diabetes mellitus, cushingoid state (long-term therapy), HPA suppression systemic with therapy longer than 5 days, Cushing's syndrome, hyperglycemia
- **GI:** *Peptic or esophageal ulcer, pancreatitis,* abdominal distention, nausea, vomiting, increased appetite and weight gain (long-term therapy)
- **Hematologic:** *Na^+ and fluid retention, hypokalemia,* hypocalcemia, increased blood sugar, increased serum cholesterol, decreased serum T_3 and T_4 levels
- **Hypersensitivity:** Anaphylactoid or hypersensitivity reactions
- **Musculoskeletal:** *Muscle weakness,* steroid myopathy and loss of muscle mass, osteoporosis, spontaneous fractures (long-term therapy)
- **Other:** *Immunosuppression, aggravation or masking of infections, impaired wound healing*

Adverse effects related to specific routes of administration

- **IM repository injections:** Atrophy at injection site
- **Intra-articular:** Osteonecrosis, tendon rupture, infection
- **Intralesional therapy, head and neck:** Blindness (rare)
- **Intraspinal:** Meningitis, adhesive arachnoiditis, conus medullaris syndrome
- **Intrathecal administration:** Arachnoiditis
- **Retention enema:** Local pain, burning; rectal bleeding; systemic absorption and adverse effects (see Systemic Adverse Effects)
- **Topical dermatologic ointments, creams, sprays:** Local burning, irritation, acneiform lesions, striae, skin atrophy

Interactions

✱ **Drug-drug** • Increased steroid blood levels with hormonal contraceptives, troleandomycin, ketoconazole, estrogen • Decreased steroid blood levels with phenytoin, phenobarbital, rifampin, cholestyramine • Decreased serum level of salicylates • Decreased effectiveness of anticholinesterases (ambenonium, edrophonium, neostigmine, pyridostigmine); ketoconazole, estrogen • Use cautiously with anticoagulants; monitor PT/INR

✱ **Drug-lab test** • False-negative nitroblue tetrazolium test for bacterial infection (with systemic absorption) • Suppression of skin test reactions • May decrease serum potassium levels, T_3, and T_4 levels

■ Nursing considerations

Assessment

- **History:** Infections; kidney disease; liver disease, hypothyroidism; ulcerative colitis with impending perforation; diverticulitis; recent GI surgery; active or latent peptic ulcer; inflammatory bowel disease; hypertension, heart failure; thromboembolic tendencies, thrombophlebitis, osteoporosis, seizure disorders, metastatic carcinoma, diabetes mellitus; lactation. ***Retention enemas, intrarectal foam:*** Systemic fungal infections; recent intestinal surgery, extensive fistulas. ***Topical dermatologic administration:*** Fungal, tubercular, herpes simplex skin infections; vaccinia, varicella; ear application when eardrum is perforated
- **Physical:** ***Systemic administration:*** Weight, T; reflexes, affect, bilateral grip strength, ophthalmologic examination; BP, P, auscultation, peripheral perfusion, discoloration, pain or prominence of superficial vessels; R, adventitious sounds, chest X-ray; upper GI X-ray (history or symptoms of peptic ulcer), liver palpation; CBC, serum electrolytes,

2-hr postprandial blood glucose, urinalysis, thyroid function tests, serum cholesterol. ***Topical, dermatologic preparations:*** Affected area, integrity of skin

Interventions

Systemic administration

⊗ **Warning** Give daily before 9 AM to mimic normal peak diurnal corticosteroid levels and minimize HPA suppression.

- Space multiple doses evenly throughout the day.
- Do not give IM injections if patient has thrombocytopenic purpura.
- Rotate sites of IM repository injections to avoid local atrophy.
- Use minimal doses for minimal duration to minimize adverse effects.
- Taper doses when discontinuing high-dose or long-term therapy.
- Arrange for increased dosage when patient is subject to unusual stress.
- Ensure that adequate amount of Ca^{2+} is taken if prolonged administration of steroids.
- Use alternate-day maintenance therapy with short-acting corticosteroids whenever possible.

⊗ **Warning** Do not give live virus vaccines with immunosuppressive doses of hydrocortisone.

- Provide antacids between meals to help avoid peptic ulcer.

Topical dermatologic administration

- Use caution with occlusive dressings; tight or plastic diapers over affected area can increase systemic absorption.
- Avoid prolonged use, especially near eyes, in genital and rectal areas, on face, and in skin creases.

Teaching points

Systemic administration

- Take this drug exactly as prescribed. Do not stop taking this drug without notifying your health care provider; slowly taper dosage to avoid problems.
- Dosage reductions may create adrenal insufficiency. Report any fatigue, muscle and joint pains, anorexia, nausea, vomiting, diarrhea, weight loss, weakness, dizziness, or low blood sugar (if you monitor blood sugar).
- Take with meals or snacks if GI upset occurs.
- Take single daily or alternate-day doses before 9 AM; mark calendar or use other measures as reminder of treatment days.
- Do not overuse joint after intra-articular injections, even if pain is gone.
- Frequent follow-up visits to your health care provider are needed to monitor drug response and adjust dosage.
- Wear a medical alert ID (if you are using long-term therapy) so that any emergency medical personnel will know that you are taking this drug.
- You may experience these side effects: Increase in appetite, weight gain (some of gain may be fluid retention; monitor intake); heartburn, indigestion (eat frequent small meals, use of antacids may help); increased susceptibility to infection (avoid crowds during peak cold or flu seasons, and avoid anyone with a known infection); poor wound healing (if injured or wounded, consult health care provider); muscle weakness, fatigue (frequent rest periods may help).
- Report unusual weight gain, swelling of lower extremities, muscle weakness, black or tarry stools, vomiting of blood, epigastric burning, puffing of face, menstrual irregularities, fever, prolonged sore throat, cold or other infection, worsening of symptoms.

Intra-articular, intralesional administration

- Do not overuse the injected joint even if the pain is gone. Adhere to rules of proper rest and exercise.

Topical dermatologic administration

- Apply sparingly, and rub in lightly.
- Avoid contacting your eye with the medication.
- Report burning, irritation, or infection of the site, worsening of the condition.
- Avoid prolonged use.

Anorectal preparations

- Maintain normal bowel function with proper diet, adequate fluid intake, and regular exercise.
- Use stool softeners or bulk laxatives if needed.
- Notify your health care provider if symptoms do not improve in 7 days or if bleeding, protrusion, or seepage occurs.

hydroflumethiazide

See Appendix W, *Less commonly used drugs*.

DANGEROUS DRUG

hydromorphone hydrochloride

(hye droe ***mor'*** *fone)*

Dilaudid, Dilaudid-HP, Hydromorph Contin (CAN), Hydromorph HP 10, 20, 50 (CAN), Hydromorph HP Forte (CAN), PMS-Hydromorphone (CAN)

PREGNANCY CATEGORY C

PREGNANCY CATEGORY D (LABOR AND DELIVERY)

CONTROLLED SUBSTANCE C-II

Drug class

Opioid agonist analgesic (phenanthrene)

Therapeutic actions

Acts as agonist at specific mu-opioid receptors in the CNS to produce analgesia, euphoria, sedation; the receptors mediating these effects are thought to be the same as those mediating the effects of endogenous opioids (enkephalins, endorphins).

Indications

- Relief of moderate to severe pain, acute and chronic pain

Contraindications and cautions

- Contraindicated with hypersensitivity to opioids, tartrazine (2- and 4-mg tablets, *Dilaudid*); physical dependence on an opioid analgesic (drug may precipitate withdrawal); severe or acute bronchial asthma, upper airway obstruction. Liquid and tablets contraindicated in labor and delivery and status asthmaticus.
- Use cautiously with pregnancy (readily crosses placenta; neonatal withdrawal if mother used drug during pregnancy); bronchial asthma, COPD, respiratory depression, anoxia, increased intracranial pressure, acute MI, ventricular failure, coronary insufficiency, hypertension, biliary tract disease, renal or hepatic impairment, lactation.

Available forms

Injection—1, 2, 4, 10 mg/mL; tablets—2, 4, 8 mg; suppositories—3 mg; powder for injection—250 mg/vial; oral solution—1 mg/mL; injection—1, 2, 4 mg/mL; injection concentrate—10 mg/mL

Dosages

Individualize to each patient.

Adults

Oral

Tablet, 2–4 mg every 4–6 hr; more than 4 mg may be needed for severe pain. Liquid, 2.5–10 mg every 3–6 hr.

Parenteral

1–2 mg IM, subcutaneously every 4–6 hr as needed. May be given by slow IV injection over 2–3 min if no other route is tolerated.

Rectal

3 mg every 6–8 hr.

Pediatric patients

Safety and efficacy not established. Contraindicated in premature infants.

Geriatric patients or patients with renal or hepatic impairment

Use caution; respiratory depression may occur in elderly, the very ill, those with respiratory problems. Reduced dosage may be necessary.

Pharmacokinetics

Route	Onset	Peak	Duration
Oral	Varies	30–60 min	4–5 hr
IM	15–30 min	30–60 min	4–5 hr

Metabolism: Hepatic; $T_{1/2}$: 2–3 hr; ER capsules, 18 hr

Distribution: Crosses placenta; enters breast milk

Excretion: Urine

IV FACTS

Preparations: Administer undiluted or diluted in normal saline or D_5W.

Infusion: Inject slowly, each 2 mg over 2–5 min, directly into vein or into tubing of running IV.

Adverse effects

- **CNS:** *Light-headedness, dizziness, sedation,* euphoria, dysphoria, delirium, insomnia, agitation, anxiety, fear, hallucinations, disorientation, drowsiness, lethargy, impaired mental and physical performance, coma, mood changes, weakness, headache, tremor, seizures, miosis, visual disturbances, suppression of cough reflex
- **CV:** Facial flushing, peripheral circulatory collapse, tachycardia, bradycardia, arrhythmia, palpitations, chest wall rigidity, hypertension, hypotension, orthostatic hypotension, syncope
- **Dermatologic:** Pruritus, urticaria, laryngospasm, bronchospasm, edema, diaphoresis
- **GI:** *Nausea, vomiting,* dry mouth, anorexia, *constipation,* biliary tract spasm; increased colonic motility in patients with chronic ulcerative colitis
- **GU:** Ureteral spasm, spasm of vesical sphincters, urinary retention or hesitancy, oliguria, antidiuretic effect, reduced libido or potency
- **Hypersensitivity:** Anaphylactoid reactions (IV administration)
- **Local:** Phlebitis following IV injection pain at injection site; tissue irritation and induration (subcutaneous injection)
- **Major hazards: Respiratory depression, apnea, circulatory depression, respiratory arrest, shock, cardiac arrest**
- **Other:** *Sweating,* physical tolerance and dependence, psychological dependence

Interactions

✱ **Drug-drug** • Potentiation of effects of hydromorphone with barbiturate anesthetics, alcohol; decrease dose of hydromorphone when coadministering • Opioid agonist/antagonists may reduce effects of hydromorphone; use caution

✱ **Drug-lab test** • Elevated biliary tract pressure (an effect of opioids) may cause increases in plasma amylase, lipase; determinations of these levels may be unreliable for 24 hr after administration of opioids

■ Nursing considerations

Assessment

- **History:** Hypersensitivity to opioids, tartrazine; physical dependence on an opioid analgesic; pregnancy; lactation; COPD, respiratory depression, anoxia, increased intracranial pressure, acute MI, ventricular failure, coronary insufficiency, hypertension, biliary tract surgery, renal or hepatic impairment
- **Physical:** Orientation, reflexes, bilateral grip strength, affect; pupil size, vision; P, auscultation, BP; R, adventitious sounds; bowel sounds, normal output; thyroid, LFTs, renal function tests

Interventions

⊠ ***Black box warning*** Monitor dosage and intended use; it varies with form. Serious effects can occur.

- Give to nursing women 4–6 hr before next scheduled feeding to minimize drug in milk.

⊗ ***Warning*** Ensure opioid antagonist and facilities for assisted or controlled respiration are readily available during parenteral administration.

⊗ ***Warning*** Use caution when injecting subcutaneously into chilled body areas or in patients with hypotension or in shock; impaired perfusion may delay absorption. With repeated doses, an excessive amount may be absorbed when circulation is restored.

- Refrigerate rectal suppositories.

Teaching points

- Learn how to administer rectal suppositories; refrigerate suppositories.
- Take drug exactly as prescribed.
- Avoid alcohol, antihistamines, sedatives, tranquilizers, and over-the-counter drugs.
- Do not take leftover medication; do not let anyone else take the prescription.
- You may experience these side effects: Nausea, loss of appetite (take drug with food, lie quietly, eat frequent small meals); constipation (laxative may help); dizziness, sedation, drowsiness, impaired vision (avoid tasks that require alertness, visual acuity).
- Report severe nausea, vomiting, constipation, shortness of breath or difficulty breathing.

hydroxocobalamin

See Appendix X, *Less commonly used drugs*.

hydroxyethyl starch in sodium choride

See Appendix X, *Less commonly used drugs*.

DANGEROUS DRUG

hydroxyurea

*(hye drox ee yoor **ee'** a)*

Droxia, Gen-Hydroxyurea (CAN), Hydrea

PREGNANCY CATEGORY D

Drug class

Antineoplastic

Therapeutic actions

Cytotoxic: Inhibits an enzyme that is crucial for DNA synthesis, but exact mechanism of action is not fully understood.

Indications

- Melanoma
- Resistant chronic myelocytic leukemia
- Recurrent, metastatic, or inoperable ovarian cancer
- Concomitant therapy with irradiation for primary squamous cell carcinoma of the head and neck, excluding the lip
- Polycythemia vera
- Cervical cancer and, in combination with radiation therapy, brain tumors, cervical tumors, and head and neck tumors
- To reduce the frequency of painful crises and to reduce the need for blood transfusions in adult patients with sickle cell anemia (*Droxia*)
- Unlabeled uses: Essential thrombocythemia, psoriasis, HIV treatment with didanosine

Contraindications and cautions

- Contraindicated in severe bone marrow suppression, allergy to hydroxyurea.
- Use cautiously in patients with impaired hepatic and renal functions, mild to moderate bone marrow suppression, pregnancy, lactation.

Available forms

Capsules—500 mg; *Droxia* capsules—200, 300, 400 mg

Dosages

Adults

⊗ ***Warning*** Base dosage on ideal or actual body weight, whichever is less. Interrupt therapy if WBC count falls below 2,500/mm^3 or platelet count below 100,000/mm^3. Recheck in 3 days and resume therapy when counts approach normal (*Hydrea*).

- *Solid tumors:* Intermittent therapy: 80 mg/kg PO as a single dose every third day. Continuous therapy: 20–30 mg/kg PO as a single daily dose.
- *Concomitant therapy with irradiation:* 80 mg/kg as a single daily dose every third day. Begin hydroxyurea 7 days before irradiation, and continue during and for a prolonged period after radiation therapy (*Hydrea*).
- *Resistant chronic myelocytic leukemia:* 20–30 mg/kg as a single daily dose (*Hydrea*).
- *Reduction of sickle cell anemia crises (Droxia):* 15 mg/kg/day PO as a single dose; may be increased by 5 mg/kg/day PO as a single dose; may be increased by 5 mg/kg/day every 12 wk until maximum tolerated dose or 35 mg/kg/day is reached. If blood levels become toxic, stop drug and resume at 2.5 mg/kg/day less than the dose that resulted in toxicity when blood levels return to normal. May increase every 12 wk in 2.5-mg/kg/day intervals if blood levels stay acceptable.

Patients with renal impairment

Consider need to decrease dosage, and monitor patient closely.

Pediatric patients

Dosage regimen not established.

Pharmacokinetics

Route	*Onset*	*Peak*	*Duration*
Oral	Varies	1–4 hr	18–20 hr

Metabolism: Hepatic; $T_{1/2}$: 3–4 hr
Distribution: Crosses placenta; enters breast milk
Excretion: Urine

Adverse effects

- **CNS:** *Headache, dizziness,* disorientation, hallucinations
- **Dermatologic:** Maculopapular rash, facial erythema
- **GI:** *Stomatitis, anorexia, nausea, vomiting,* diarrhea, constipation, elevated hepatic enzymes
- **GU:** Impaired renal tubular function
- **Hematologic:** *Bone marrow depression*
- **Local:** Mucositis at the site, especially in combination with irradiation
- **Other:** Fever, chills, malaise, **cancer,** pulmonary reactions

Interactions

✱ **Drug-drug** • Uricosuric agents may increase uric acid levels; adjust dose of uricosuric agent

✱ **Drug-lab test** • Serum uric acid, BUN, and creatinine levels may increase with hydroxyurea therapy • Drug causes self-limiting abnormalities in erythrocytes that resemble those of pernicious anemia but are not related to vitamin B_{12} or folate deficiency

■ Nursing considerations

Assessment

- **History:** Allergy to hydroxyurea, irradiation, leukopenia, impaired hepatic and renal function, lactation, pregnancy
- **Physical:** Weight; T; skin color, lesions; reflexes, orientation, affect; mucous membranes, abdominal examination; CBC, LFTs, renal function tests

Interventions

- Give in oral form only. Do not cut, crush, or allow patient to chew capsules. If patient is unable to swallow capsules, empty capsules into a glass of water, and give immediately (inert products may not dissolve).
- Encourage patient to drink 10–12 glasses of fluid each day.
- Check CBC before administration before therapy and every 2 wk.
- Caution patient to avoid pregnancy while using this drug; using barrier contraceptives is advised.

Teaching points

- Prepare a calendar for dates to return for diagnostic testing and treatment days. If you are unable to swallow the capsule, empty the capsule into a glass of water and take immediately (some of the material may not dissolve).
- This medication can cause serious adverse effects. Avoid handling it, store it safely away from children and pets, and dispose of it in a closed container.
- Avoid pregnancy while using this drug, fetal abnormalities have been reported; using barrier contraceptives is advised.
- Arrange for regular blood tests at least every 2 weeks to monitor the drug's effects.
- Drink at least 10–12 glasses of fluid each day while using this drug.
- You may experience these side effects: Loss of appetite, nausea, vomiting, mouth sores (frequent mouth care, frequent small meals may help; maintain good nutrition; an antiemetic may be ordered); constipation or diarrhea (a bowel program may be established); disorientation, dizziness, headache (take precautions to avoid injury); red face, rash (reversible).
- Report fever, chills, sore throat, unusual bleeding or bruising, severe nausea, vomiting, loss of appetite, sores in the mouth or on the lips, pregnancy (it is advisable to use birth control while on this drug).

▽ hydroxyzine

*(hye **drox'** i zeen)*

hydroxyzine hydrochloride

Oral preparations: Apo-Hydroxyzine (CAN), Vistaril

Parenteral preparations: Vistaril

hydroxyzine pamoate

Oral preparation: Vistaril

PREGNANCY CATEGORY C

Drug classes

Antiemetic
Antihistamine
Anxiolytic

Therapeutic actions

Mechanisms of action not understood; actions may be due to suppression of subcortical areas of the CNS; has clinically demonstrated antihistaminic, analgesic, antispasmodic, antiemetic, mild antisecretory, and bronchodilator activity.

Indications

- Symptomatic relief of anxiety and tension associated with psychoneurosis; adjunct in organic disease states in which anxiety is manifested; alcoholism and asthma; before dental procedures
- Management of pruritus due to allergic conditions, such as chronic urticaria, atopic and contact dermatosis, and in histamine-mediated pruritus
- Sedation when used as premedication and following general anesthesia
- Control of nausea and vomiting and as adjunct to analgesia preoperatively and postoperatively (parenteral) to allow decreased opioid dosage
- IM administration: Management of the acutely disturbed or hysterical patient; the acute or chronic alcoholic with anxiety withdrawal symptoms or delirium tremens; as preoperative and postoperative adjunct to permit reduction in opioid dosage, allay anxiety, and control emesis

Contraindications and cautions

- Contraindicated with allergy to hydroxyzine or cetirizine; pregnancy, lactation.
- Use cautiously with uncomplicated vomiting in children (may contribute to Reye's syndrome or unfavorably influence its outcome; extrapyramidal effects may obscure diagnosis of Reye's syndrome).

Available forms

Tablets—10, 25, 50 mg; syrup—10 mg/5 mL; capsules—25, 50, 100 mg; oral suspension—25 mg/5 mL; injection—25, 50 mg/mL

Dosages

Start patients on IM therapy when indicated; use oral therapy for maintenance. Adjust dosage to patient's response.

Adults

Oral

- *Symptomatic relief of anxiety:* 50–100 mg qid.
- *Management of pruritus:* 25 mg tid–qid.
- *Sedative (preoperative and postoperative):* 50–100 mg.

IM

- *Psychiatric and emotional emergencies:* 50–100 mg immediately and every 4–6 hr as needed.
- *Preoperative and postoperative sedation:* 50–100 mg.
- *Pruritus:* 25 mg tid–qid.

Pediatric patients

Oral

- *Anxiety, pruritus:*

Younger than 6 yr: 50 mg/day in divided doses.

Older than 6 yr: 50–100 mg/day in divided doses.

- *Sedative:* 0.6 mg/kg.

IM

- *Preoperative and postoperative sedation:* 0.6 mg/kg.

Pharmacokinetics

Route	Onset	Peak	Duration
Oral, IM	15–30 min	3 hr	4–6 hr

Metabolism: Hepatic; $T_{1/2}$: 3 hr

Distribution: Crosses placenta; may enter breast milk

Excretion: Urine

Adverse effects

- **CNS:** *Drowsiness,* involuntary motor activity, including tremor and seizures
- **GI:** *Dry mouth,* reflux, constipation
- **GU:** Urinary retention
- **Hypersensitivity:** Wheezing, dyspnea, chest tightness

Interactions

✱ **Drug-drug** • Potentiating action when used concomitantly with CNS depressants (opioids, barbiturates)

■ Nursing considerations

Assessment

- **History:** Allergy to hydroxyzine or cetirizine, uncomplicated vomiting in children, lactation, pregnancy
- **Physical:** Skin color, lesions, texture; orientation, reflexes, affect; R, adventitious sounds

Interventions

⊗ ***Warning*** Determine and treat underlying cause of vomiting. Drug may mask signs and symptoms of serious conditions, such as brain tumor, intestinal obstruction, or appendicitis.

⊗ ***Warning*** Do not administer parenteral solution subcutaneously, IV, or intra-arterially; tissue necrosis has occurred with subcutaneous and intra-arterial injection, and hemolysis with IV injection.

- Give IM injections deep into a large muscle: In adults, use upper outer quadrant of buttocks or midlateral thigh; in children, use midlateral thigh muscles; use deltoid area only if well developed.

Teaching points

- Take as prescribed. Avoid excessive dosage.
- You may experience these side effects: Dizziness, sedation, drowsiness (use caution if performing tasks that require alertness); avoid alcohol, sedatives, sleep aids (serious overdosage could result); dry mouth (mouth care, sucking sugarless lozenges may help).
- Report difficulty breathing, tremors, loss of coordination, sore muscles, or muscle spasm.

▽hylan B gel

See Appendix W, *Less commonly used drugs*.

▽hyoscyamine sulfate (L-hyoscyamine)

(high ah' ska meen)

Anaspaz, Cystospaz, ED-SPAZ, IB-Stat, Levbid DNC, Levsin, Levsin/SL, Levsinex Timecaps DNC, Mar-Spas, Neosol, NuLev, Symax Duotab, Symax Fastab, Symax-SL DNC, Symax-SR DNC

PREGNANCY CATEGORY C

Drug classes

Anticholinergic
Antimuscarinic
Antispasmodic
Belladonna alkaloid
Parasympatholytic

Therapeutic actions

Direct GI smooth muscle relaxant; competitively blocks the effects of acetylcholine at muscarinic cholinergic receptors that mediate the effects of parasympathetic postganglionic impulses, thus relaxing the GI tract. Also has antisecretory effects along the GI.

Indications

- Adjunctive therapy in IBS, peptic ulcer, spastic or functional GI disorders, cystitis, neurogenic bladder or bowel disorders, parkinsonism, biliary or renal colic
- Rhinitis and anticholinesterase poisoning
- **NEW INDICATION:** Reduction of rigidity and tremors and control of sialorrhea and hyperhidrosis associated with parkinsonism
- Partial heart block associated with vagal activity
- Preoperatively to decrease secretions
- Parenterally to improve radiological imaging tests

Contraindications and cautions

- Contraindicated with hypersensitivity to anticholinergic drugs, glaucoma, adhesions between iris and lens, stenosing peptic ulcer, pyloroduodenal obstruction, paralytic ileus, intestinal atony, severe ulcerative colitis, toxic megacolon, symptomatic prostatic hypertrophy, bladder neck obstruction, bronchial asthma, COPD, myocardial ischemia, myasthenia gravis, tachycardia, renal disease.
- Use cautiously with high environmental temperatures, fever, diarrhea, hyperthyroidism, CV disease, hypertension, heart failure, arrhythmias, renal disease, hiatal hernia, pregnancy, lactation.

Available forms

Tablets—0.125 mg, 0.15 mg; sublingual tablets—0.125 mg; ER tablets DNC—0.375 mg; ER capsules DNC—0.375 mg; orally disintegrating tablets—0.125 mg; oral spray—

0.125 mg/mL; elixir—0.125 mg/5 mL; solution—0.125 mg/mL; injection—0.5 mg/mL

Dosages

Adults

Oral or sublingual

0.125–0.25 mg 3–4 times per day.
Oral solution: 1–2 mL every 4 hr as needed; do not exceed 12 mL per day.
Oral spray: 1–2 sprays every 4 hr as needed; do not exceed 12 sprays per day.
Orally disintegrating tablets: ½–1 tablet 3–4 times per day 30 min–1 hr before meals and at bedtime.
Elixir: 1–2 teaspoons every 4 hr as needed; do not exceed 12 teaspoons per day.

ER

0.375–0.75 mg PO every 12 hr. May give 1 capsule every 8 hr if needed; do not exceed 4 capsules per day.

Parenteral

- *GI disorders:* 0.25–0.5 mg subcutaneously, IM, or IV 2–4 times per day as needed.
- *Preanesthetic:* 0.005 mg/kg IV or IM 30–60 min before induction.
- *Treatment of bradycardia:* 0.125 mg (0.25 mL) IV. Repeat as needed.
- *Reversal of neuromuscular blockade:* 0.2 mg IV, IM, or subcutaneously for every 1 mg neostigmine.

Pediatric patients

Regular and sublingual tablets, orally disintegrating tablets (except Mar-Spas*)*

12 yr and older: 1–2 tablets PO every 4 hr as needed; do not exceed 12 tablets in 24 hr.
2 yr to younger than 12 yr: ½–1 tablet PO every 4 hr as needed; do not exceed 6 tablets in 24 hr.

Mar-Spas *orally disintegrating tablets*

12 yr and older: ½–1 tablet PO tid–qid 30 min–1 hr before meals and at bedtime.
Younger than 12 yr: Not recommended.

Extended release and timed-release capsules

12 yr and older: 1–2 capsules PO every 12 hr; adjust to 1 capsule every 8 hr if needed. Do not exceed 4 capsules in 24 hr.

Oral solution

12 yr and older: 1–2 mL PO every 4 hr or as needed; do not exceed 12 mL in 24 hr.
2 yr to younger than 12 yr: 0.25–1 mL PO every 4 hr or as needed; do not exceed 6 mL in 24 hr.
Younger than 2 yr:

Weight (kg)	*Dose (drops)*	*Maximum drops/day*
3.4	4	24
5	5	30
7	6	36
10	8	48

Elixir

12 yr and older: 1–2 tsp PO every 4 hr or as needed; do not exceed 12 tsp in 24 hr.
2 yr to younger than 12 yr: Give dose based on weight every 4 hr as needed; do not exceed 6 tsp PO in 24 hr.

Weight (kg)	*Dose (tsp)*
10	0.25 (1.25 mL)
20	0.5 (2.5 mL)
40	0.75 (3.75 mL)
50	1 (5 mL)

Oral spray

12 yr and older: 1–2 sprays every 4 hr as needed.

Injectable

Older than 2 yr:
Preanesthetic: 5 mcg/kg IV 30–60 min before anesthesia.
Treatment of drug-induced bradycardia: 0.25 mL IV during surgery; repeat as needed.
Reversal of neuromuscular blockade: 0.2 mg IV for every 1 mg neostigmine.

Pharmacokinetics

Route	*Onset*	*Peak*	*Duration*
Oral tablets	20–30 min	30–60 min	4 hr
Sublingual	5–20 min	30–60 min	4hr
ER	20–30 min	40–90 min	12 hr
Parenteral	2–3 min	15–30 min	4 hr

Metabolism: Hepatic; $T_{1/2}$: 9–10 hr (injection, 3.5 hr)
Distribution: Crosses placenta; enters breast milk
Excretion: Urine

Adverse effects

- **CNS:** *Dizziness,* blurred vision, dilated pupils confusion, *drowsiness,* psychosis, headache
- **CV:** *Palpitations,* hypertension, chest pain, tachycardia
- **GI:** *Nausea, dry mouth,* taste loss, *constipation,* vomiting
- **GU:** *Urinary hesitancy,* impotence
- **Other:** *Decreased sweating, fever, anaphylaxis, urticaria,* heat prostration

Interactions

✱ **Drug-drug** • Additive effects with other anticholinergics, amantadine, haloperidol, phenothiazines, MAOIs, TCAs, or antihistamines; monitor patient closely and adjust dosages as needed • Decreased absorption if combined with antacids; space 2–4 hr apart

■ Nursing considerations

Assessment

- **History:** Glaucoma, adhesions between iris and lens, stenosing peptic ulcer, pyloroduodenal obstruction, paralytic ileus, intestinal atony, severe ulcerative colitis, toxic megacolon, symptomatic prostatic hypertrophy, bladder neck obstruction, bronchial asthma, COPD, myocardial ischemia, myasthenia gravis, fever, diarrhea, hyperthyroidism, CV disease, hypertension, heart failure, arrhythmias, renal disease, hiatal hernia, pregnancy, lactation
- **Physical:** Bowel sounds, normal output; normal urinary output, prostate palpation; R, adventitious sounds; P, BP; IOP, vision; bilateral grip strength, reflexes; liver palpation, LFTs, renal function tests; skin color, lesions, texture

Interventions

- Ensure adequate hydration; control environment (temperature) to prevent hyperpyrexia.
- Use caution in geriatric patients who may be more sensitive to anticholinergic effects.
- Encourage patient to void before each dose if urinary retention becomes a problem.
- Ensure ER forms are not cut, crushed, or chewed.
- Monitor lighting to minimize discomfort of photophobia.
- Establish safety precautions (side rails, assistance with ambulation, proper lighting) if visual effects occur.
- Provide sugarless lozenges, ice chips to suck (if permitted) if dry mouth occurs.
- Provide frequent small meals if GI upset is severe.

Teaching points

- Take drug exactly as prescribed; do not cut, crush, or chew ER tablets.
- Take 30–60 minutes before meals.
- Avoid hot environments while taking this drug (you will be heat-intolerant and dangerous reactions may occur).
- You may experience these side effects: Dry mouth (sugarless lozenges, frequent mouth care may help; this effect sometimes lessens over time); blurred vision, sensitivity to light (these effects will go away when you discontinue the drug; avoid tasks that require acute vision and wear sunglasses when in bright light); impotence (this effect will go away when you discontinue the drug; you may wish to discuss it with your health care provider); difficulty in urination (it may help to empty the bladder immediately before taking each dose).
- Report skin rash, flushing, eye pain, difficulty breathing, tremors, loss of coordination, irregular heartbeat, palpitations, headache, abdominal distention, hallucinations, difficulty swallowing, difficulty urinating.

I

▽ ibandronate sodium

*(eh **ban'** drow nate)*

Boniva DNC

PREGNANCY CATEGORY C

Drug classes

Bisphosphonate
Calcium regulator

Therapeutic actions

Inhibits osteoclast activity and reduces bone resorption and turnover, without inhibiting bone formation or mineralization.

Indications

- Treatment and prevention of osteoporosis in postmenopausal women
- Unlabed use: Treatment of metastatic bone disease in breast cancer

Contraindications and cautions

- Contraindicated with known allergy to any component of the tablet, uncorrected hypocalcemia, inability to stand or sit upright for at least 60 minutes (oral form).
- Use caution with known upper GI abnormalities, pregnancy, lactation.

Available forms

Prefilled syringe—1 mg/mL; tablets DNC—2.5, 150 mg

Dosages

Adults

One 2.5-mg tablet/day PO or one 150-mg tablet PO once per month on the same date each month or 3 mg IV, given over 15–30 sec, every 3 mo.

Pediatric patients

Safety and efficacy not established.

For patients with renal impairment

Not recommended with severe renal impairment (creatinine clearance less than 30 mL/min).

Pharmacokinetics

Route	*Onset*	*Peak*
Oral	Rapid	0.5–2 hr
IV	Rapid	Unknown

Metabolism: $T_{1/2}$: 37–157 hr
Distribution: May cross placenta; may pass into breast milk
Excretion: Urine, unchanged

Adverse effects

- **CNS:** *Headache,* dizziness, vertigo, nerve root lesion, asthenia, insomnia
- **CV:** Angina, *hypertension*
- **GI:** *Diarrhea, dyspepsia, abdominal pain,* constipation, vomiting, gastritis, tooth disorder, dysphagia, esophagitis, esophageal ulcers, gastric ulcers
- **Respiratory:** *URI, bronchitis, pneumonia,* pharyngitis
- **Other: Jaw osteonecrosis** (increased risk with cancer, chemotherapy, radiation therapy, preexisting dental disease), *back pain,* infection, *myalgia,* joint pain, hypercholesterolemia

Interactions

✱ **Drug-drug** • Decreased absorption of ibandronate if taken at the same time as multivalent cations (aluminum, iron, magnesium), antacids

✱ **Drug-food** • Milk or food; ibandronate should be taken on an empty stomach, first thing in the morning, 60 min before any food or other medications

■ Nursing considerations

Assessment

- **History:** Allergy to any component of the tablet, uncorrected hypocalcemia, inability to stand or sit upright for at least 60 min, upper GI abnormalities, pregnancy, lactation
- **Physical:** Orientation, reflexes; BP; respiratory evaluation; abdominal examination, serum calcium levels, renal function tests

Interventions

⊗ ***Warning*** Administer in the morning with a full glass of water at least 60 min before the first beverage, food, or medication of the day. Patient must stay upright for 60 min after taking the tablet to avoid potentially serious esophageal erosion.

- Monitor serum calcium levels before, during, and after therapy.
- Ensure adequate intake of vitamin D and calcium.
- Make calendar for patient using once-a-month or once every 3 mo dosing as a reminder to take drug.
- Provide comfort measures and possible analgesics for headache and pain.
- Encourage frequent small meals if GI effects are uncomfortable.

Teaching points

- Take this drug in the morning with a full glass of water, at least 60 minutes before any food, beverage, or other medications. You must stay upright for at least 60 minutes after taking the tablet to prevent potentially serious problems with your esophagus. If you are taking the once a month dose, be sure to mark your calendar as a reminder of when to take the drug. Swallow the tablet whole; do not suck on it or chew it. If taking once every 3 months IV, reschedule the missed dose as soon as possible. Subsequent injections should be rescheduled for once every 3 months from that month.

- If you miss a dose of the daily medication, do not take the dose later in the day. Return to your usual routine the next morning. Do not take more than 1 tablet each day. If you miss a dose of the monthly medication or if the next scheduled dose is more than 7 days away, take the 150-mg tablet the morning following the day that you remembered. Then return to taking the tablet every month on your original date. If your next scheduled dose is 1–7 days away, wait and take the tablet on the scheduled day, then every month on that same date as scheduled. Never take two 150-mg tablets in the same week.
- Take vitamin D and calcium to increase the effectiveness of this drug.
- You may need to have periodic bone density tests to evaluate the effects of this drug on your body.
- It is not known how this drug could affect a nursing baby. If you are nursing a baby, you should choose another method of feeding the baby.
- It is not known how this drug could affect a fetus. If you are pregnant or would like to become pregnant while on this drug, consult your health care provider.
- You may experience these side effects: Headache (consult with your health care provider; medication may be available to help); nausea, diarrhea (frequent small meals may help).
- Report pain or trouble swallowing, chest pain, very bad heartburn, or heartburn that does not get better.

ibritumomab

See Appendix W, *Less commonly used drugs*.

ibuprofen

*(eye **byoo'** proe fen)*

Advil, Advil Liqui-Gels, Advil Migraine, Advil Pediatric Drops, Apo-Ibuprofen (CAN), Apo-Ibuprofen Prescription (CAN), Caldolor, Children's Advil, Children's Motrin, Genpril, Ibutab, Infants' Motrin, Junior Strength Advil, Junior Strength Motrin, Menadol, Midol, Midol Maximum Strength Cramp Formula, Motrin, Motrin IB, Motrin Migraine Pain, PediaCare Fever, Pediatric Advil Drops

PREGNANCY CATEGORY B

PREGNANCY CATEGORY D (THIRD TRIMESTER)

Drug classes

Analgesic (nonopioid)
NSAID
Propionic acid derivative

Therapeutic actions

Anti-inflammatory, analgesic, and antipyretic activities largely related to inhibition of prostaglandin synthesis; exact mechanisms of action are not known. Inhibits both cyclooxygenase (COX) 1 and 2. Ibuprofen is slightly more selective for COX-1.

Indications

- Relief of signs and symptoms of rheumatoid arthritis and osteoarthritis
- Relief of mild to moderate pain
- Treatment of primary dysmenorrhea
- Prevention and treatment of migraine headache
- Fever reduction
- Unlabeled uses: Prevention of adverse reactions with DTP vaccine in patients at risk for seizures

Contraindications and cautions

- Contraindicated with allergy to ibuprofen, salicylates, or other NSAIDs (more common in patients with rhinitis, asthma, chronic urticaria, nasal polyps).

Black box warning Contraindicated for treatment of perioperative pain after coronary artery bypass graft.

- Use cautiously with CV dysfunction, hypertension, peptic ulceration, GI bleeding, pregnancy, lactation, impaired hepatic or renal function.

Available forms

Tablets—100, 200, 400, 600, 800 mg; chewable tablets—50, 100 mg; capsules—200 mg; suspension—100 mg/2.5 mL,100 mg/5 mL; oral drops—40 mg/mL; injection—400 mg/4 mL, 800 mg/8 mL

Dosages

Adults

Do not exceed 3,200 mg/day.

- *Mild to moderate pain:* 400 mg every 4–6 hr PO.
- *Migraine:* 400 mg PO at onset of headache.
- *Osteoarthritis or rheumatoid arthritis:* 1,200–3,200 mg/day PO (300 mg qid or 400, 600, 800 mg tid or qid; individualize dosage. Therapeutic response may occur in a few days, but often takes 2 wk).
- *Primary dysmenorrhea:* 400 mg every 4 hr PO.
- *IV use:* 400–800 mg IV over 30 min every 6 hr for pain; 400 mg IV over 30 min for fever, can be followed by 400 mg every 4–6 hr or 100–200 mg every 4 hr to control fever.
- *OTC use:* 200–400 mg every 4–6 hr PO while symptoms persist; do not exceed 1,200 mg/day. Do not take for more than 10 days for pain or 3 days for fever, unless so directed by health care provider.

Pediatric patients

Give dose every 6–8 hr according to weight (shown below) but no more than qid.

Weight (kg)	*Dose (mg)*
5–7	50
8–10	75
11–15	100
16–21	150
22–26	200
27–31	250
32–43	300

- *Juvenile arthritis:* 30–40 mg/kg/day PO in three to four divided doses; 20 mg/kg/day for milder disease.
- *Fever (6 mo–12 yr):* 5–10 mg/kg PO every 6–8 hr; do not exceed 40 mg/kg/day.

Oral drops

5–8 kg (12–17 lb) or age 6–11 months: 1.25 mL (50 mg)

9–11 kg (18–23 lb) or age 12–23 months: 1.875 mL (75 mg)

Pharmacokinetics

Route	*Onset*	*Peak*	*Duration*
Oral	30 min	1–2 hr	4–6 hr

Metabolism: Hepatic; $T_{1/2}$: 1.8–2.5 hr

Distribution: Crosses placenta; may enter breast milk

Excretion: Urine

IV FACTS

Preparation: Dilute to a concentration of 4 mg/mL or less using 0.9% sodium chloride, 5% dextrose, or lactated Ringer's. Solution should be particulate matter–free and not discolored. Diluted solution is stable for up to 24 hr at room temperature.

Infusion: Infuse over no less than 30 min.

Adverse effects

- **CNS:** *Headache, dizziness, somnolence, insomnia,* fatigue, tiredness, dizziness, tinnitus, ophthalmologic effects
- **CV:** Hypertension, palpitations, arrhythmia, heart failure
- **Dermatologic:** *Rash,* pruritus, sweating, dry mucous membranes, stomatitis
- **GI:** *Nausea, dyspepsia, GI pain,* diarrhea, vomiting, *constipation,* flatulence, **GI bleeding**
- **GU:** Dysuria, renal impairment, menorrhagia
- **Hematologic:** Bleeding, platelet inhibition with higher doses, neutropenia, eosinophilia, leukopenia, pancytopenia, thrombocytopenia, agranulocytosis, granulocytopenia, aplastic anemia, decreased Hgb or Hct, bone marrow depression
- **Respiratory:** Dyspnea, hemoptysis, pharyngitis, **bronchospasm,** rhinitis

- **Other:** Peripheral edema, **anaphylactoid reactions to anaphylactic shock**

Interactions

✱ **Drug-drug** • Increased toxic effects of lithium with ibuprofen • Decreased diuretic effect with loop diuretics—bumetanide, furosemide, ethacrynic acid • Potential decrease in antihypertensive effect of beta-adrenergic blocking drugs and ACE inhibitors • Increased risk of gastric ulceration with bisphosphonates • Increased risk of bleeding with anticoagulants

✱ **Drug-alternative therapy** • Increased risk of bleeding with concurrent use of ginkgo biloba

■ Nursing considerations

Assessment

- **History:** Allergy to ibuprofen, salicylates or other NSAIDs; CV dysfunction, hypertension; peptic ulceration, GI bleeding; impaired hepatic or renal function; pregnancy; lactation
- **Physical:** Skin color, lesions; T; orientation, reflexes, ophthalmologic evaluation, audiometric evaluation, peripheral sensation; P, BP, edema; R, adventitious sounds; liver evaluation, bowel sounds; CBC, clotting times, urinalysis, LFTs, renal function tests, serum electrolytes, stool guaiac

Interventions

⊗ ***Black box warning*** Be aware that patient may be at increased risk of CV event, GI bleeding; monitor accordingly.

- Ensure that patient is well hydrated if using IV form.
- Administer drug with food or after meals if GI upset occurs.
- Arrange for periodic ophthalmologic examination during long-term therapy.
- Discontinue drug if eye changes, symptoms of hepatic impairment, or renal impairment occur.

⊗ ***Warning*** Institute emergency procedures if overdose occurs: Gastric lavage, induction of emesis, and supportive therapy.

Teaching points

- Use drug only as suggested; avoid overdose. Take the drug with food or after meals if GI upset occurs. Do not exceed the prescribed dosage.
- Avoid over-the-counter drugs. Many of these drugs contain similar medication, and serious overdosage can occur.
- You may experience these side effects: Nausea, GI upset, dyspepsia (take drug with food); diarrhea or constipation; drowsiness, dizziness, vertigo, insomnia (use caution when driving or operating dangerous machinery).
- Report sore throat, fever, rash, itching, weight gain, swelling in ankles or fingers, changes in vision, black or tarry stools.

DANGEROUS DRUG

▽ibutilide fumarate

*(eye **byu'** ti lyed **foo'** mah rate)*

Corvert

PREGNANCY CATEGORY C

Drug class

Antiarrhythmic (predominantly class III)

Therapeutic actions

Prolongs cardiac action potential, increases atrial and ventricular refractoriness; produces mild slowing of sinus rate and AV conduction; delays repolarization by activating inward current rather than blocking outward current.

Indications

- Rapid conversion of atrial fibrillation or flutter of recent onset to sinus rhythm; most effective in arrhythmias of less than 90 days' duration

Contraindications and cautions

- Contraindicated with hypersensitivity to ibutilide; second- or third-degree AV heart block, prolonged QTc intervals.
- Use cautiously with ventricular arrhythmias, pregnancy, lactation, renal and hepatic impairment.

Available forms

Solution—0.1 mg/mL

Dosages

Adults weighing 60 kg or more

1 vial (1 mg) infused IV over 10 min; may be repeated after 10 min if arrhythmia is not terminated.

Adults weighing less than 60 kg

0.1 mL/kg (0.01 mg/kg) infused IV over 10 min; may be repeated after 10 min if arrhythmia is not terminated.

Pediatric patients

Not recommended.

Pharmacokinetics

Route	*Onset*	*Peak*
IV	Immediate	10 min

Metabolism: Hepatic; $T_{1/2}$: 6 hr
Distribution: Crosses placenta, may enter breast milk
Excretion: Feces, urine

IV FACTS

Preparation: May be diluted in 50 mL of diluent, 0.9% sodium chloride, or 5% dextrose injection; one 10-mL vial added to 50 mL of diluent yields a concentration of 0.017 mg/mL; may also be infused undiluted; diluted solution is stable for 24 hr at room temperature or for 48 hr refrigerated.
Infusion: Infuse slowly over 10 min.
Compatibilities: Compatible with 5% dextrose injection, 0.9% sodium chloride injection.
Incompatibilities: Do not mix in solution with any other drugs.

Adverse effects

- **CNS:** Headache, light-headedness, dizziness, tingling in arms, numbness
- **CV: Ventricular arrhythmias,** hypotension, hypertension, tachycardia
- **GI:** *Nausea*

Interactions

✱ **Drug drug** • Increased risk of serious to life-threatening arrhythmias with disopyramide, quinidine, procainamide, amiodarone, sotalol; do not give together • Increased risk of proarrhythmias with phenothiazines, TCAs, antihistamines • Use cautiously with digoxin because ibutilide may mask digoxin cardiotoxicity

■ Nursing considerations

Assessment

- **History:** Hypersensitivity to ibutilide; second- or third-degree AV heart block, time of onset of atrial arrhythmia; prolonged QTc intervals; pregnancy, lactation; ventricular arrhythmias
- **Physical:** Orientation; BP, P, auscultation, ECG; R, adventitious sounds

Interventions

- Determine time of onset of arrhythmia and potential benefit before beginning therapy. Conversion is more likely in patients with arrhythmias of short (fewer than 90 days') duration.

⊗ ***Warning*** Ensure that patient is adequately anticoagulated, generally for at least 2 wk, if atrial fibrillation lasts more than 2–3 days.

- Monitor ECG continually during and for at least 4 hr after administration. Be alert for possible arrhythmias, including PVCs, sinus tachycardia, sinus bradycardia, and varying degrees of block at time of conversion.

⊠ ***Black box warning*** Keep emergency equipment readily available during and for at least 4 hr after administration; can cause potentially life-threatening arrhythmias.

- Provide appointments for continued follow-up care, including ECG monitoring; tendency to revert to atrial arrhythmia after conversion increases with length of time patient was in abnormal rhythm.

Teaching points

- This drug can only be given by intravenous infusion. You will need electrocardiographic monitoring during and for 4 hours after administration.
- Arrange for follow-up medical evaluation, including electrocardiography, which is important to monitor the effect of the drug on your heart.
- You may experience these side effects: Rapid or irregular heartbeat (usually passes shortly), headache.

- Report chest pain, difficulty breathing, numbness, or tingling.

DANGEROUS DRUG

idarubicin hydrochloride

(eye da roo' bi sin)

Idamycin PFS

PREGNANCY CATEGORY D

Drug classes

Antibiotic (anthracycline)
Antineoplastic

Therapeutic actions

Cytotoxic: Binds to DNA and inhibits DNA synthesis in susceptible cells.

Indications

- In combination with other approved antileukemic drugs for the treatment of AML in adults
- Orphan drug uses: Acute nonlymphocytic leukemia and ALL in pediatric patients

Contraindications and cautions

- Contraindicated with allergy to idarubicin, other anthracycline antibiotics; myelosuppression; cardiac disease; pregnancy; lactation.
- Use cautiously with impaired hepatic or renal function.

Available forms

Injection—1 mg/mL

Dosages

Adults

- *Induction therapy in adults with AML:* 12 mg/m² daily for 3 days by slow IV injection (10–15 min) in combination with cytarabine. Cytarabine may be administered as 100 mg/m² daily given by continuous infusion for 7 days or as a 25-mg/m² IV bolus followed by 200 mg/m² daily for 5 days by continuous infusion. A second course may be administered when toxicity has subsided, if needed, at a 25% dose reduction.

Pediatric patients

Safety and efficacy not established.

Patients with renal or hepatic impairment

Reduce dosage by 25%. Do not administer if bilirubin level exceeds 5 mg/dL.

Pharmacokinetics

Route	*Onset*	*Peak*
IV	Rapid	Minutes

Metabolism: Hepatic; $T_{1/2}$: 22 hr
Distribution: Crosses placenta; enters breast milk
Excretion: Bile, urine

IV FACTS

Preparation: Use extreme caution when preparing drug. Using goggles and gloves is recommended as drug can cause severe skin reactions. If skin is accidentally exposed to idarubicin, wash with soap and water; use standard irrigation techniques if eyes are contaminated. Store solution in the refrigerator and protect from light.
Infusion: Administer slowly (over 10–15 min) into tubing of a freely running IV infusion of sodium chloride injection or 5% dextrose injection. Attach the tubing to a butterfly needle inserted into a large vein; avoid veins over joints or in extremities with poor perfusion.
Incompatibilities: ⊗ ***Warning*** Do not mix idarubicin with other drugs, especially heparin (a precipitate forms, and the IV solution must not be used) and any alkaline solution.

Adverse effects

- **CV: Cardiac toxicity,** heart failure, phlebosclerosis
- **Dermatologic:** *Complete but reversible alopecia,* hyperpigmentation of nailbeds and dermal creases, facial flushing
- **GI:** *Nausea, vomiting, mucositis,* anorexia, diarrhea, abdominal cramping
- **Hematologic: Myelosuppression,** hyperuricemia due to cell lysis
- **Hypersensitivity:** Fever, chills, urticaria, **anaphylaxis**
- **Local:** Severe local cellulitis, vesication and tissue necrosis if extravasation occurs

I

- **Other:** Carcinogenesis, infertility, infection, headache, infection

Nursing considerations
Assessment
- **History:** Allergy to idarubicin, other anthracycline antibiotics; myelosuppression; cardiac disease; impaired hepatic or renal function; pregnancy; lactation
- **Physical:** T; skin color, lesions; weight; hair; nailbeds; local injection site; cardiac auscultation, peripheral perfusion, pulses, ECG; R, adventitious sounds; liver evaluation, mucous membranes; CBC, LFTs, renal function tests, uric acid levels

Interventions
⊠ ***Black box warning*** Do not give IM or subcutaneously because severe local reaction and tissue necrosis occur. Give IV only.

⊠ ***Black box warning*** Be aware that patient is at risk for myocardial toxicity; monitor accordingly.

⊗ ***Warning*** Monitor injection site for extravasation; ask about burning or stinging. If extravasation occurs, discontinue infusion immediately, and restart in another vein. For local subcutaneous extravasation, local infiltration with corticosteroid may be ordered; flood area with normal saline, and apply cold compress to area. If ulceration begins, arrange consultation with plastic surgeon.

⊠ ***Black box warning*** Monitor the patient's response to therapy frequently at beginning of therapy: Serum uric acid level, CBC, cardiac output (listen for S_3), liver function tests, CBC changes may require a decrease in the dose; consult physician.

- Ensure adequate hydration to prevent hyperuricemia.
- Ensure that patient is not pregnant; explain the importance of avoiding pregnancy.

Teaching points
- Prepare a calendar for days to return for drug therapy. Drug can only be given IV.
- This drug should not be used during pregnancy; using barrier contraceptives is advised.
- Have regular medical follow-up care, including blood tests to monitor the drug's effects.
- You may experience these side effects: Rash, skin lesions, loss of hair, changes in nails (obtain a wig before hair loss occurs; skin care may help); loss of appetite, nausea, mouth sores (perform frequent mouth care, frequent small meals may help; maintain good nutrition; consult a dietitian; an antiemetic may be ordered); red urine (transient).
- Report difficulty breathing, sudden weight gain, swelling, burning or pain at injection site, unusual bleeding or bruising; chest pain.

idursulfase

See Appendix W, *Less commonly used drugs*.

DANGEROUS DRUG

ifosfamide

*(eye **foss'** fa mide)*

Ifex

PREGNANCY CATEGORY D

Drug classes
Alkylating drug
Antineoplastic
Nitrogen mustard

Therapeutic actions
Cytotoxic: Exact mechanism of action is not known, although metabolite of ifosfamide alkylates DNA, interferes with the replication of susceptible cells; immunosuppressive: Lymphocytes are especially sensitive to drug effects.

Indications
- In combination with other approved neoplastic drugs for third-line chemotherapy of germ cell testicular cancer; prophylactically with mesna to prevent hemorrhagic cystitis
- Orphan drug uses: Third-line chemotherapy in the treatment of bone sarcomas, soft-tissue sarcomas
- Unlabeled uses: Possible effectiveness in the treatment of lung, breast, ovarian, pancreatic and gastric cancer; sarcomas; acute leukemias; malignant lymphomas; bladder and cervical cancer

Contraindications and cautions

- Contraindicated with allergy to ifosfamide, hematopoietic depression, pregnancy, lactation.
- Use cautiously with impaired hepatic or renal function.

Available forms

Powder for injection—1, 3 g

Dosages

Adults

Administer IV at a dose of 1.2 g/m^2 per day for 5 consecutive days. Treatment is repeated every 3 wk or after recovery from hematologic toxicity. For prevention of bladder toxicity, give more than 2 L of fluid per day IV or PO. Also use mesna IV to prevent hemorrhagic cystitis.

Pediatric patients

Safety and efficacy not established.

Patients with renal impairment

Data not available on appropriate dosage. Reduced dosage is advisable; use caution.

Pharmacokinetics

Route	*Onset*
IV	Rapid

Metabolism: Hepatic; $T_{1/2}$: 15 hr
Distribution: Crosses placenta; enters breast milk
Excretion: Urine

IV FACTS

Preparation: Add sterile water for injection or bacteriostatic water for injection to the vial, and shake gently. Use 20 mL diluent with 1-g vial, giving a final concentration of 50 mg/mL, or use 60-mL diluent with 3-g vial, giving a final concentration of 50 mg/mL. Solutions may be further diluted to achieve concentrations of 0.6–20 mg/mL in 5% dextrose injection, 0.9% sodium chloride injection, lactated Ringer's injection, and sterile water for injection. Solution is stable for at least 1 wk at room temperature or 6 wk if refrigerated. Dilutions not prepared with bacteriostatic water for injection should be refrigerated and used within 6 hr.

Infusion: Administer as a slow IV infusion lasting a minimum of 30 min.

Adverse effects

- **CNS:** *Somnolence, confusion, hallucinations,* coma, depressive psychosis, dizziness, seizures
- **Dermatologic:** *Alopecia,* darkening of skin and fingernails
- **GI:** *Anorexia, nausea, vomiting,* diarrhea, stomatitis
- **GU:** *Hemorrhagic cystitis,* bladder fibrosis, *hematuria* to **potentially fatal hemorrhagic cystitis,** increased urine uric acid levels, gonadal suppression
- **Hematologic:** *Leukopenia,* thrombocytopenia, anemia (rare), increased serum uric acid levels
- **Other:** Immunosuppression, secondary neoplasia, hepatic impairment, infection

Interactions

✱ **Drug-food** • Decreased metabolism and risk of toxic effects if taken with grapefruit juice; avoid this combination

■ Nursing considerations

Assessment

- **History:** Allergy to ifosfamide, hematopoietic depression, impaired hepatic or renal function, pregnancy, lactation
- **Physical:** Reflexes, affect; skin lesions, hair; urinary output, renal function; LFTs, renal function tests, CBC, Hct

Interventions

⊗ ***Black box warning*** Arrange for blood tests to evaluate hematopoietic function before beginning therapy and weekly during therapy; serious hemorrhagic toxicities have occurred.

⊗ ***Black box warning*** Arrange for extensive hydration consisting of at least 2 L of oral or IV fluid per day to prevent bladder toxicity.

⊗ ***Black box warning*** Arrange to administer a protector, such as mesna, to prevent hemorrhagic cystitis.

- Counsel male patients not to father a child during or immediately after therapy; infant cardiac and limb abnormalities have occurred. Counsel female patients not to become pregnant while using this drug; severe birth defects have occurred.

Teaching points

- This drug can only be given IV.
- Have frequent blood tests to monitor your response to this drug. All appointments for follow-up care should be kept.
- Avoid grapefruit juice while using this drug.
- Men or women should use birth control while using drug and for a time afterwards; this drug can cause severe birth defects.
- You may experience these side effects: Nausea, vomiting, loss of appetite (take drug with food, eat frequent small meals); maintain your fluid intake and nutrition (drink at least 10–12 glasses of fluid each day); darkening of the skin and fingernails, loss of hair (obtain a wig or arrange for some other head covering before hair loss occurs; keep head covered in extreme temperatures).
- Report unusual bleeding or bruising, fever, chills, sore throat, cough, shortness of breath, blood in the urine, painful urination, unusual lumps or masses, flank, stomach or joint pain, sores in mouth or on lips, yellow discoloration of skin or eyes.

iloperidone

*(il oh **pair'** ih dohn)*

Fanapt

PREGNANCY CATEGORY C

Drug classes

Atypical antipsychotic
Benzisoxazole derivative

Therapeutic actions

Mechanism of action not fully understood; blocks dopamine and serotonin receptors in the brain, depresses the reticular activating system; suppresses many of the negative aspects of schizophrenia, including blunted affect, social withdrawal, lack of motivation, anger.

Indications

- Acute treatment of schizophrenia in adults. Consider first using drugs that do not prolong QT interval. Consider need to slowly titrate drug, prolonging time until therapeutic effect is seen; faster-acting drugs may be more appropriate.

Contraindications and cautions

- Contraindicated with hypersensitivity to components of drug, pregnancy, lactation.
- Use cautiously with prolonged QT interval, history of seizures, diabetes, suicidal ideation.

Available forms

Tablets—1, 2, 4, 6, 8 10, 12 mg

Dosages

Adults

Target dose: 12–24 mg/day PO. Titrate based on orthostatic hypotension tolerance—initially, 1 mg PO bid; then 2, 4, 6, 8, 10, and 12 mg PO bid on days 2, 3, 4, 5, 6, and 7, respectively.

Pediatric patients

Safety and efficacy not established.

Patients with hepatic impairment

Not recommended.

Pharmacokinetics

Route	Onset	Peak
Oral	Rapid	2–4 hr

Metabolism: Hepatic; $T_{1/2}$: 18–23 hr
Distribution: May cross placenta; may enter breast milk
Excretion: Urine, feces

Adverse effects

- **CNS:** *Dizziness, somnolence,* extrapyramidal disorders, tremor, lethargy, blurred vision, altered thinking
- **CV:** Orthostatic hypotension, hypotension, tachycardia, prolonged QT interval
- **GI:** *Nausea,* diarrhea, dry mouth, abdominal discomfort
- **GU:** Priapism, ejaculation failure
- **Respiratory:** URI, nasal pharyngitis
- **Other:** Fatigue, lethargy, bone marrow suppression, **neuroleptic malignant syndrome,** hyperglycemia, weight gain, gynecomastia, galactorrhea

Interactions

✱ **Drug-drug** • Increased risk of serious cardiac arrhythmias if taken with other drugs that prolong QT interval; avoid this combination. If combination must be used, monitor patient carefully • Possible increased serum levels and toxicity if combined with ketoconazole, fluoxetine, itraconazole, paroxetine; iloperidone dosage should be halved if these drug combinations are used • Risk of increased effectiveness of antihypertensives if used with iloperidone; monitor patient closely and adjust antihypertensive dosage as needed • Risk of increased CNS effects if combined with centrally acting drugs or alcohol; use caution if this combination is used

✱ **Drug-alternative therapy** • Possible increased toxicity if combined with St. John's wort

■ Nursing considerations

Assessment

- **History:** Hypersensitivity to components of drug; prolonged QT interval, history of seizures, diabetes, suicidal ideation, pregnancy, lactation
- **Physical:** Orientation, affect, reflexes; BP, P; abdominal exam; liver evaluation; ECG, LFTs, CBC

Interventions

⊠ ***Black box warning*** There is an increased risk of death if used in elderly patients with dementia-related psychosis. Do not use for these patients; not approved for this use.

- Obtain baseline ECG to rule out prolonged QT interval; monitor patient periodically throughout therapy.
- Titrate drug over first week to decrease effect of orthostatic hypotension.
- Monitor patient regularly for signs and symptoms of increased blood glucose level.
- Advise patient who is nursing to select another method of feeding the baby.
- Monitor patient for signs and symptoms of neuroleptic malignant syndrome (high temperature, muscle rigidity, altered mental status, high or low blood pressure, diaphoresis, tachycardia); discontinue drug and support patient if these occur. Carefully consider reintroduction of drug because recurrence is likely.
- Provide safety measures as needed if patient develops extrapyramidal effects or orthostatic hypotension.
- Because of the risk of suicidal ideation with treatment, limit amount of drug dispensed to the smallest effective amount to decrease chances of overdose.
- Continue other measures used to deal with schizophrenia.

Teaching points

- Take this drug once a day, exactly as prescribed. Carefully follow directions for increasing the dosage over the first week.
- If you miss a dose, take the next dose as soon as you remember. Do not take more than the prescribed amount each day.
- Avoid alcohol while taking this drug. Tell your health care provider about other drugs, over-the-counter drugs, or herbal therapies that you are using because serious drug interactions are possible.
- If you are diabetic, monitor your blood glucose level very carefully and adjust treatment as ordered.
- It is not known how this drug affects a fetus. If you become pregnant while taking this drug, consult your health care provider.
- It is not known how this drug affects a nursing baby. Because of the potential for serious adverse effects on an infant, you should use another method of feeding the baby while you are taking this drug.
- This drug may cause your blood pressure to fall when you stand up; this is called *orthostatic hypotension.* Use care when standing or changing positions. Orthostatic hypotension is most likely to occur when starting the drug and when changing dosage.
- You may experience these side effects: Dizziness, changes in motor performance and impaired thinking (do not drive a car or engage in activities that require alertness if these effects occur); nausea, dry mouth (small, frequent meals may help; sucking sugarless lozenges may also be helpful).
- Report fever accompanied by sweating, changes in mental status, muscle rigidity; heart palpitations, feeling faint, loss of consciousness, thoughts of suicide.

iloprost

See Appendix W, *Less commonly used drugs*.

DANGEROUS DRUG

imatinib mesylate

(eh mat' eh nib mess' ah late)

Gleevec (DNC)

PREGNANCY CATEGORY D

Drug classes

Antineoplastic
Protein tyrosine kinase inhibitor

Therapeutic actions

A protein tyrosine kinase inhibitor that selectively inhibits the Bcr-Abl tyrosine kinase created by the Philadelphia chromosome abnormality in CML; this inhibits proliferation and induces apoptosis in the Bcr-Abl positive cell lines as well as fresh leukemic cells, leading to an inhibition of tumor growth in CML patients in blast crisis.

Indications

- Treatment of patients with Philadelphia-chromosome–positive CML in blast crisis, accelerated phase or in chronic phase after failure with interferon-alfa therapy
- Treatment of patients with Kit (CD117) positive unresectable or metastatic malignant GI stromal tumors (GISTs)
- Treatment of adults with relapsed or refractory Philadelphia-chromosome–positive ALL
- Treatment of aggressive systemic mastocytosis (ASM)
- Treatment of adults with unresectable, recurrent, or metastatic dermatofibrosarcoma protuberans (DFSP)
- Treatment of adults with myelodysplastic/myeloproliferative diseases (MDS/MPD)
- Treatment of hypereosinophilic syndrome and chronic eosinophilic leukemia (HES/CEL) in adults
- Treatment of pediatric patients with Philadelphia chromosome positive CML in chronic phase, whose disease recurred after stem cell transplant or who are resistant to interferon alfa therapy

Contraindications and cautions

- Contraindicated with allergy to imatinib or any of its components, pregnancy, lactation.
- Use cautiously with hepatic or renal impairment; bone marrow suppression; cardiac disease, risk factors for heart failure.

Available forms

Tablets (DNC)—100, 400 mg

Dosages

Dosage should be adjusted based on bone marrow function and liver toxicity.

When used with CYP3A4 inducers, increase imatinib dosage by 50% and carefully monitor patient. For dosages of 800 mg or more, use 400 mg tablets to avoid increase in iron.

Adults

- *Chronic phase CML:* 400 mg/day PO as a once-a-day dose; increase to 600 mg/day may be considered if response is not satisfactory and patient can tolerate the drug.
- *Accelerated phase or blast crisis CML:* 600 mg/day PO as a single dose; increase to 400 mg PO bid may be considered if response is not satisfactory and patient can tolerate the drug.
- *ALL:* 600 mg/day PO.
- *ASM:* 400 mg/day PO.
- *DFSP:* 800 mg/day PO.
- *HES/CEL:* 400 mg/day PO.
- *MDS/MPD:* 400 mg/day PO.
- *GIST:* 400 or 800 mg/day PO.

Pediatric patients older than 2 yr

Newly diagnosed CML: 340 mg/m^2 PO; maximum dose 600 mg/day.
Chronic phase CML: 260 mg/m^2/day PO given as one dose, or divided and given morning and evening.

Patients with hepatic impairment

Severe impairment, decrease dosage by 25%.

Patients with renal impairment

For creatinine clearance of 20–39 mL/min, reduce starting dose by 50%; increase as tolerated. Doses of 400 mg not recommended. For creatinine clearance of 40–59 mL/min, doses of 600 mg not recommended.

Pharmacokinetics

Route	*Onset*	*Peak*
Oral	Slow	2–4 hr

Metabolism: Hepatic; $T_{1/2}$: 14–17 hr
Distribution: Crosses placenta; may enter breast milk; 95% protein-bound
Excretion: Feces, urine

Adverse effects

- **CNS:** Malaise, insomnia, *headache,* dizziness
- **CV: Severe heart failure, left ventricular dysfunction**
- **GI:** Abdominal pain, *vomiting, nausea, diarrhea,* dyspepsia, anorexia, constipation, hepatotoxicity, GI irritation
- **Hematologic:** *Neutropenia, thrombocytopenia*
- **Respiratory:** Pulmonary edema, pneumonia, URI, cough
- **Other:** Myalgia, fever, *rash, sudden weight gain, fluid retention,* night sweats, joint pain, muscle cramps, fatigue, hemorrhage, pruritus, rigors, hemorrhage

Interactions

✱ **Drug-drug** ⊗ ***Warning*** Increased serum levels of simvastatin, cyclosporine, or pimozide when combined with imatinib; avoid these combinations if possible.
• Risk of increased imatinib effects with ketoconazole, itraconazole, azithromycin, or clarithromycin; use caution if this combination is used • Risk of decreased imatinib effects if combined with dexamethasone, phenytoin, carbamazepine, rifampicin, or phenobarbital; use caution if this combination is required • Increased risk of bleeding with warfarin; if anticoagulation is needed, use of a heparin is recommended
✱ **Drug-food** • Increased risk of toxic effects with grapefruit juice; avoid this combination
✱ **Drug-alternative therapy** • Decreased effectiveness of imatinib if taken with St. John's wort; avoid this combination

■ Nursing considerations

Assessment

- **History:** Allergy to imatinib or any of its components, pregnancy, lactation, hepatic or renal impairment
- **Physical:** T, body weight, P, BP, R, adventitious sounds, CBC with differential, LFTs, Hgb, Hct, cardiac function

Interventions

- Administer once a day with a meal and a large glass of water. Pediatric patients may have the dose divided and given half in the morning and half in the evening.
- If patient cannot swallow tablets, they may be dispersed in a glass of water or apple juice and given immediately. Use 50 mL for 10-mg tablet and 200 mL for 400-mg tablet. Do not cut or crush tablet.
- Provide frequent small meals if GI upset occurs.
- Arrange for nutritional consult if nausea and vomiting are persistent.
- Provide analgesics if headache or muscle pain is a problem.
- Advise women of child-bearing age to use a barrier form of contraception while taking this drug.
- Increase imatinib dose by at least 50% when administering with a potent CYP3A4 inducer such as rifampin or phenytoin.

⊗ ***Warning*** Monitor CBC before and periodically during therapy; arrange for dosage adjustment as indicated if bone marrow suppression occurs.

⊗ ***Warning*** Monitor patient for fluid retention and edema; severe cases may require dosage reduction or discontinuation of drug.

- Arrange for appropriate consultation to help patient cope with the high cost of drug.

Teaching points

- This drug should be taken once a day as a single dose, with a meal and a large glass of water. Do not crush tablet. If tablet is crushed, avoid contact with skin and mucous membranes. If contact occurs, flush area immediately with water. Children may split the dose in two, taking half in the morning and half in the evening.
- This drug has been linked to serious fetal abnormalities; women of childbearing age who are taking this drug should use a barrier contraceptive.
- Avoid infection while taking this drug; avoid crowded areas or people with known infections.
- Do not use any alternative therapy, including St. John's wort, while you are in this treatment program; it may decrease the effectiveness of the drug.

I

- You will need regular blood tests to monitor the effects of this drug on your blood.
- You may experience these side effects: Nausea, vomiting (eat frequent small meals or suck on sugarless lozenges or chewing gum); headache, muscle cramps, pain (use of an analgesic may help; consult your health care provider); fluid retention and sudden weight gain (monitor daily weights and report sudden increases or difficulty breathing).
- Report fever, chills, unusual bleeding or bruising, difficulty breathing, yellowing of your skin or eyes, any signs of infection, sudden weight gain, severe swelling.

imipramine
*(im **ip'** ra meen)*

imipramine hydrochloride
Tofranil

imipramine pamoate
Tofranil-PM

PREGNANCY CATEGORY C

Drug class
TCA (tertiary amine)

Therapeutic actions
Mechanism of action unknown; the TCAs are structurally related to the phenothiazine antipsychotic drugs (eg, chlorpromazine), but unlike the phenothiazines, TCAs inhibit the presynaptic reuptake of the neurotransmitters norepinephrine and serotonin; anticholinergic at CNS and peripheral receptors; sedative; the relation of these effects to clinical efficacy is unknown.

Indications
- Relief of symptoms of depression (endogenous depression most responsive); sedative effects of tertiary amine TCAs may be helpful in patients whose depression is associated with anxiety and sleep disturbance
- Enuresis in children 6 yr and older
- Unlabeled use: Control of chronic pain (eg, intractable pain of cancer, peripheral neuropathies, postherpetic neuralgia, tic douloureux, central pain syndromes), migraine prophylaxis

Contraindications and cautions
- Contraindicated with hypersensitivity to any tricyclic drug or to tartrazine (in preparations marketed as *Tofranil, Tofranil-PM;* patients with aspirin allergy are commonly allergic to tartrazine); concomitant therapy with an MAOI; EST with coadministration of TCAs; recent MI; myelography within previous 24 hr or scheduled within 48 hr; pregnancy.
- Use cautiously with preexisting CV disorders; seizure disorders (TCAs lower the seizure threshold); hyperthyroidism; angle-closure glaucoma, increased IOP, urinary retention, ureteral or urethral spasm; impaired hepatic, renal function; psychiatric patients (schizophrenic or paranoid patients may exhibit a worsening of psychosis with TCA therapy; manic-depressive patients may shift to hypomanic or manic phase); elective surgery; lactation; history of suicide attempts; use with alcohol.

Available forms
Tablets (imipramine hydrochloride, imipramine pamoate)—10, 25, 50 mg; capsules (imipramine pamoate)—75, 100, 125, 150 mg

Dosages
Adults
- *Depression:* Hospitalized patients—Initially, 100–150 mg/day PO in divided doses. Gradually increase to 200 mg/day as required. If no response after 2 wk, increase to 250–300 mg/day. Total daily dosage may be given at bedtime. Outpatients—Initially, 75 mg/day PO, increasing to 150 mg/day. Dosages more than 200 mg/day not recommended. Total daily dosage may be given at bedtime. Maintenance dose is 50–150 mg/day.
- *Chronic pain:* 50–200 mg/day PO.

Adolescent and geriatric patients
- *Depression:* 30–40 mg/day PO; doses greater than 100 mg/day generally are not needed.

Pediatric patients 6 yr and older
Imipramine pamoate capsules should not be used in children because of potential for overdose. Capsules can be used in adults if daily dosage is 75 mg or higher.

- *Childhood enuresis:* Initially, 25 mg/day 1 hr before bedtime. If response is not satisfactory after 1 wk, increase to 50 mg nightly in children younger than 12 yr, 75 mg nightly in children older than 12 yr. Doses or more than 75 mg/day do not have greater efficacy but are more likely to increase side effects. Do not exceed 2.5 mg/kg per day. Early-night bedwetters may be more effectively treated with earlier and divided dosage (25 mg midafternoon, repeated at bedtime). Institute drug-free period after successful therapy, gradually tapering dosage.

Pharmacokinetics

Route	*Onset*	*Peak*
Oral	Varies	2–4 hr

Metabolism: Hepatic; $T_{1/2}$: 8–16 hr
Distribution: Crosses placenta; enters breast milk
Excretion: Urine

Adverse effects

Adult use

- **CNS:** *Sedation and anticholinergic effects,* dry mouth, blurred vision, disturbance of accommodation for near vision, mydriasis, increased IOP; *confusion, disturbed concentration,* hallucinations, disorientation, decreased memory, feelings of unreality, delusions, anxiety, nervousness, restlessness, agitation, panic, insomnia, nightmares, hypomania, mania, exacerbation of psychosis, drowsiness, weakness, fatigue, headache, numbness, tingling, paresthesias of extremities, incoordination, motor hyperactivity, akathisia, ataxia, tremors, peripheral neuropathy, extrapyramidal symptoms, *seizures,* dysarthria, tinnitus, altered EEG, suicidal ideation
- **CV:** *Orthostatic hypotension,* hypertension, syncope, tachycardia, palpitations, **MI,** arrhythmias, heart block, precipitation of heart failure, CVA
- **Endocrine:** Elevated or depressed blood sugar, elevated prolactin levels, inappropriate ADH secretion
- **GI:** *Dry mouth, constipation,* paralytic ileus, *nausea,* vomiting, anorexia, epigastric distress, diarrhea, flatulence, dysphagia, peculiar taste, increased salivation, stomatitis, glossitis, parotid swelling, abdominal cramps, black tongue, hepatitis
- **GU:** Urinary retention, delayed micturition, dilation of the urinary tract, gynecomastia, testicular swelling in men; breast enlargement, menstrual irregularity and galactorrhea in women; increased or decreased libido; impotence
- **Hematologic: Bone marrow depression,** including agranulocytosis; eosinophilia, purpura, thrombocytopenia, leukopenia
- **Hypersensitivity:** Rash, pruritus, vasculitis, petechiae, photosensitization, edema (generalized, facial, tongue), drug fever
- **Withdrawal:** Abrupt discontinuation of prolonged therapy—nausea, headache, vertigo, nightmares, malaise
- **Other:** Nasal congestion, excessive appetite, weight gain or loss; sweating (paradoxical effect in a drug with prominent anticholinergic effects), alopecia, lacrimation, hyperthermia, flushing, chills

Pediatric use for enuresis

- **CNS:** *Nervousness, sleep disorders, tiredness,* seizures, anxiety, emotional instability, syncope, collapse
- **CV:** ECG changes of unknown significance when given in doses of 5 mg/kg/day
- **GI:** Constipation, *mild GI disturbances*
- **Other:** Adverse reactions reported with adult use

Interactions

✱ **Drug-drug** • Increased TCA levels and pharmacologic (especially anticholinergic) effects with cimetidine, fluoxetine, or ranitidine • Increased serum levels and risk of bleeding with oral anticoagulants • Altered response, including arrhythmias and hypertension, with sympathomimetics • Risk of severe hypertension with clonidine • Hyperpyretic crises, severe seizures, hypertensive episodes, and deaths when MAOIs are given with TCAs • Decreased hypotensive activity of guanethidine with imipramine

Note: MAOIs and TCAs have been used successfully in some patients resistant to therapy with single drugs; however, the combination can cause serious and potentially fatal adverse effects.

✱ **Drug-alternative therapy** • Plasma imipramine levels may be reduced with St. John's wort

■ Nursing considerations

Assessment

- **History:** Hypersensitivity to any tricyclic drug or to tartrazine; concomitant therapy with an MAOI; EST with coadministration of TCAs; recent MI; myelography within previous 24 hr or scheduled within 48 hr; preexisting CV disorders; seizure disorders; hyperthyroidism; angle-closure glaucoma, increased IOP, urinary retention, ureteral or urethral spasm; impaired hepatic, renal function; psychiatric patients; elective surgery; pregnancy; lactation
- **Physical:** Weight; T; skin color, lesions; orientation, affect, reflexes, vision and hearing; P, BP, auscultation, orthostatic BP, perfusion; bowel sounds, normal output, liver evaluation; urine flow, normal output; usual sexual function, frequency of menses, breast and scrotal examination; LFTs, urinalysis, CBC, ECG

Interventions

- Obtain baseline ECG to monitor cardiac arrhythmias.

⊠ ***Black box warning*** Limit drug access for depressed and potentially suicidal patients; increased risk of suicidality especially in children, adolescents, and young adults; monitor patients accordingly.

- Give IM only when oral therapy is impossible. Do not give IV.
- Give major portion of dose at bedtime if drowsiness, severe anticholinergic effects occur (note that elderly may not tolerate single-daily-dose therapy).

⊗ ***Warning*** Reduce dosage if minor side effects develop; discontinue if serious side effects occur.

- Arrange for CBC if fever, sore throat, or other sign of infection develops during therapy.

Teaching points

- Take drug exactly as prescribed. Do not stop taking drug abruptly or without consulting your health care provider; clinical effects may take 4–6 weeks to be seen.
- Avoid prolonged exposure to sunlight or sunlamps; use a sunscreen or wear protective garments.
- Use of barrier contraceptives is recommended. If nursing, choose another method to feed the baby.
- You may experience these side effects: Headache, dizziness, drowsiness, weakness, blurred vision (reversible; safety measures may need to be taken if severe; avoid driving or performing tasks that require alertness); nausea, vomiting, constipation, loss of appetite (eat frequent small meals; frequent mouth care may help); dry mouth (sucking sugarless candies may help); disorientation, difficulty concentrating, emotional changes; changes in sexual function, impotence, changes in libido.
- Report dry mouth, difficulty in urination, excessive sedation, fever, chills, sore throat, palpitations, suicidal thoughts.

DANGEROUS DRUG

▽ inamrinone lactate

*(in **am'** ri none)*

PREGNANCY CATEGORY C

Drug classes

Cardiotonic
Inotropic

Therapeutic actions

Increases force of contraction of ventricles (positive inotropic effect); causes vasodilation by a direct relaxant effect on vascular smooth muscle.

Indications

- Heart failure: Short-term management of patients who have not responded to cardiac glycosides, diuretics, or vasodilators.

Contraindications and cautions

- Contraindicated with allergy to inamrinone or bisulfites.

- Use cautiously with severe aortic or pulmonic valvular disease, acute MI, decreased fluid volume, pregnancy, lactation.

Available forms
Injection—5 mg/mL

Dosages
Adults
- *Initial dose:* 0.75 mg/kg IV bolus, given over 2–3 min. A supplemental IV bolus of 0.75 mg/kg may be given after 30 min if needed.
- *Maintenance infusion:* 5–10 mcg/kg/min. Do not exceed a total of 10 mg/kg/day.

Pediatric patients
Not recommended.

Pharmacokinetics

Route	Onset	Peak	Duration
IV	Immediate	10 min	2 hr

Metabolism: Hepatic; $T_{1/2}$: 3.6–5.8 hr
Distribution: Crosses placenta; may enter breast milk
Excretion: Feces, urine

IV FACTS
Preparation: Give as supplied or dilute in normal or one-half normal saline solution to a concentration of 1–3 mg/mL. Use diluted solution within 24 hr. Protect ampules from exposure to light.
Infusion: Administer IV bolus slowly over 2–3 min. Maintenance infusion should not exceed 5–10 mcg/kg/min. Monitor doses; do not exceed a daily dose of 10 mg/kg.
Incompatibilities: Do not mix directly with dextrose-containing solutions; may be injected into a Y-connector or into tubing when a dextrose solution is running; precipitates can form.
Y-site incompatibilities: Do not mix with furosemide, sodium bicarbonate. Do not inject with furosemide.

Adverse effects
- **CV:** *Arrhythmias,* hypotension
- **GI:** Nausea, vomiting, abdominal pain, anorexia, hepatotoxicity
- **Hematologic:** *Thrombocytopenia*
- **Hypersensitivity:** Pericarditis, pleuritis, ascites, vasculitis
- **Other:** Fever, chest pain, burning at injection site

■ Nursing considerations

CLINICAL ALERT!
Name confusion had occurred between amiodarone when drug name was amrinone; although inamrinone is a new name, confusion may still occur.

Assessment
- **History:** Allergy to inamrinone or bisulfites, severe aortic or pulmonic valvular disease, acute MI, decreased fluid volume, lactation, pregnancy
- **Physical:** Weight, orientation, P, BP, cardiac auscultation, peripheral pulses, peripheral perfusion; R, adventitious sounds; bowel sounds, liver evaluation; urinary output; serum electrolyte levels, platelet count, liver enzymes

Interventions
- Protect drug vial from light.
- Monitor BP and pulse, and reduce dose if marked decreases occur.
- Monitor input and output and electrolyte levels; record daily weight.

⊗ ***Warning*** Monitor platelet counts if patient is on prolonged therapy. Consider reducing dosage if platelet levels fall to less than 150,000/mm^3.

Teaching points
- You will need to have your blood pressure and pulse monitored frequently.
- You may experience increased voiding while using this drug.
- Report pain at IV injection site, dizziness, weakness, fatigue, numbness or tingling.

indapamide
(in dap' a mide)

Apo-Indapamide (CAN),
Gen-Indapamide (CAN),
PMS-Indapamide (CAN)

PREGNANCY CATEGORY B

Drug class
Thiazide-like diuretic (indoline)

Therapeutic actions
Inhibits reabsorption of sodium and chloride in distal renal tubule, increasing excretion of sodium, chloride, and water by the kidney; may decrease peripheral resistance.

Indications
- Edema associated with heart failure
- Hypertension, as sole therapy or in combination with other antihypertensives
- Unlabeled use: Diabetes insipidus, especially nephrogenic diabetes insipidus

Contraindications and cautions
- Contraindicated with allergy to thiazides, sulfonamides; hepatic coma or precoma, anuria.
- Use cautiously with fluid or electrolyte imbalance; renal disease (risk of azotemia); liver disease (may precipitate hepatic coma); gout (risk of precipitation of attack); SLE; glucose tolerance abnormalities, diabetes mellitus; hyperparathyroidism; bipolar disorder (aggravated by hypercalcemia); pregnancy; lactation.

Available forms
Tablets—1.25, 2.5 mg

Dosages
Adults
- *Edema:* 2.5 mg/day PO as single dose in the morning. May be increased to 5 mg/day if response is not satisfactory after 1 wk.
- *Hypertension:* 1.25 mg/day PO. May be increased up to 2.5 mg/day if response is not satisfactory after 4 wk. May increase to a maximum of 5 mg/day or consider adding another antihypertensive. If combination antihypertensive therapy is needed, reduce the dosage of other drugs by 50%, then adjust according to patient's response.

Pediatric patients
Safety and efficacy not established.

Pharmacokinetics

Route	*Onset*	*Peak*	*Duration*
Oral	1–2 hr	2 hr	36 hr

Metabolism: Hepatic; $T_{1/2}$: 14 hr
Distribution: Crosses placenta; enters breast milk
Excretion: Urine

Adverse effects
- **CNS:** *Dizziness, vertigo,* paresthesias, weakness, headache, drowsiness, fatigue, anxiety, nervousness
- **CV:** Orthostatic hypotension, venous thrombosis, volume depletion, cardiac arrhythmias, chest pain
- **Dermatologic:** Photosensitivity, rash, purpura, exfoliative dermatitis, hives
- **GI:** *Nausea, anorexia, vomiting, dry mouth,* diarrhea, constipation, jaundice, hepatitis, pancreatitis, dyspepsia
- **GU:** *Polyuria, nocturia,* impotence, decreased libido
- **Hematologic:** Leukopenia, thrombocytopenia, agranulocytosis, aplastic anemia, neutropenia
- **Other:** Hypokalemia, muscle cramps and muscle spasms, fever, gouty attacks, flushing, weight loss, rhinorrhea, infection, pain, back pain

Interactions
✱ **Drug-drug** • Consider risk of interactions seen with all thiazides • Increased thiazide effects if taken with diazoxide • Decreased absorption with cholestyramine, colestipol • Increased risk of cardiac glycoside toxicity if hypokalemia occurs • Increased risk of lithium toxicity • Decreased effectiveness of antidiabetics

✱ **Drug-lab test** • Decreased PBI levels without clinical signs of thyroid disturbance

■ Nursing considerations

Assessment

- **History:** Allergy to thiazides, sulfonamides; fluid or electrolyte imbalance; renal or liver disease; gout; SLE; glucose tolerance abnormalities, diabetes mellitus; hyperparathyroidism; manic-depressive disorders; lactation, pregnancy
- **Physical:** Skin color, lesions, edema; orientation, reflexes, muscle strength; pulses, baseline ECG, BP, orthostatic BP, perfusion; R, pattern, adventitious sounds; liver evaluation, bowel sounds, urinary output patterns; CBC, serum electrolytes, blood glucose, LFTs, renal function tests, serum uric acid, urinalysis

Interventions

- Give with food or milk if GI upset occurs.
- Mark calendars or provide other reminders for outpatients on alternate-day or 3–5 days/wk therapy.
- Give early in the day so increased urination will not disturb sleep.
- Measure and record regular weight to monitor fluid changes.

Teaching points

- Record intermittent therapy on a calendar, or use prepared, dated envelopes. Take the drug early in the day so increased urination will not disturb sleep. The drug may be taken with food or meals if GI upset occurs.
- Weigh yourself on a regular basis, at the same time of the day and in the same clothing; record the weight on your calendar.
- You may experience these side effects: Increased volume and frequency of urination; dizziness, feeling faint on arising, drowsiness (avoid rapid position changes; hazardous activities, like driving a car; and alcohol, which can intensify these problems); sensitivity to sunlight (use sunglasses, wear protective clothing, or use a sunscreen); decrease in sexual function; increased thirst (sucking on sugarless lozenges, frequent mouth care may help).
- Report weight change of more than 3 pounds in 1 day, swelling in ankles or fingers, unusual bleeding or bruising, dizziness, trembling, numbness, fatigue, muscle weakness or cramps.

▽indinavir sulfate

*(in **din'** ah ver)*

Crixivan

PREGNANCY CATEGORY C

Drug classes

Antiretroviral
Antiviral
Protease inhibitor

Therapeutic actions

Antiviral activity; inhibits HIV protease activity, leading to production of immature, noninfective HIV particles.

Indications

- Treatment of HIV infection in adults; used in combination with other drugs

Contraindications and cautions

- Contraindicated with allergy to component of indinavir.
- Use cautiously with pregnancy, hepatic or renal impairment, lactation.

Available forms

Capsules—100, 200, 333, 400 mg

Dosages

Adults

800 mg PO every 8 hr. With delavirdine, 600 mg PO every 8 hr with delavirdine 400 mg tid; with didanosine, administer more than 1 hr apart on an empty stomach; with itraconazole, 600 mg PO every 8 hr with itraconazole 200 mg bid; with ketoconazole, 600 mg PO every 8 hr; with rifabutin, 1,000 mg (three 333-mg capsules) PO every 8 hr, reduce rifabutin by 50%.

Pediatric patients

Safety and efficacy not established in children younger than 12 yr.

Patients with hepatic impairment

600 mg PO every 8 hr with mild to moderate hepatic impairment.

Pharmacokinetics

Route	*Onset*	*Peak*
Oral	Rapid	0.8 hr

Metabolism: Hepatic; $T_{1/2}$: 3–4 hr

Distribution: Crosses placenta; enters breast milk; 60% bound to human plasma proteins
Excretion: Feces, urine

Adverse effects

- **CNS:** *Headache,* dizziness, insomnia, somnolence
- **CV:** Palpitations
- **Dermatologic:** Acne, dry skin, contact dermatitis, rash, body odor
- **GI:** *Nausea, vomiting, diarrhea,* anorexia, dry mouth, acid regurgitation, *hyperbilirubinemia,* abdominal pain, increased appetite
- **GU:** Dysuria, hematuria, nocturia, pyelonephritis, nephrolithiasis, urolithiasis
- **Respiratory:** Cough, dyspnea, sinusitis
- **Other:** Hypothermia, chills, back pain, flank pain, flulike symptoms, appetite increase, fever, back pain, fatigue, taste perversion

Interactions

✱ **Drug-drug** ⊗ ***Warning*** Potentially large increase in serum concentration of triazolam, midazolam, pimozide and ergot derivatives with indinavir; potential for serious arrhythmias, seizure, and fatal reactions; do not administer indinavir with any of these drugs.

• Azole antifungals, delavirdine, nelfinavir, ritonavir, interleukins may increase indinavir concentrations and cause toxicity • Decreased effectiveness with didanosine; give these two drugs 1 hr apart on empty stomach to decrease effects of interaction • Significant decrease in serum levels with nevirapine—avoid this combination; if combination is necessary, increase indinavir to 1,000 mg every 8 hr with nevirapine 200 mg bid; carefully monitor effectiveness of indinavir if starting or stopping nevirapine • Decreased indinavir concentrations with efavirenz, carbamazepine, phenobarbital, phenytoin, rifabutin, venlafaxine • Indinavir may cause increased concentrations of fentanyl, rifamycin, benzodiazepines, ritonavir, and sildenafil

✱ **Drug-food** • Absorption is decreased by presence of food and grapefruit juice; give on empty stomach with full glass of water

✱ **Drug-alternative therapy** • Decreased effectiveness if combined with St. John's wort

■ Nursing considerations

Assessment

- **History:** Allergy to indinavir, hepatic or renal impairment, pregnancy, lactation
- **Physical:** T; orientation, reflexes; BP, P, peripheral perfusion; R, adventitious sounds; bowel sounds; urinary output; skin color, perfusion; LFTs, renal function tests

Interventions

- Capsules should be protected from moisture; store in container provided and keep desiccant in bottle. Give drug every 8 hr around the clock.
- Give on an empty stomach, 1 hr before or 2 hr after meal with a full glass of water. If GI upset is severe, give with a light meal; avoid grapefruit juice and foods high in calories, fat, or protein.

⊗ ***Warning*** Carefully screen drug history to avoid potentially dangerous drug interactions.

- Monitor patient to maintain hydration; if nephrolithiasis occurs, therapy will need to be interrupted or stopped.

Teaching points

- Take this drug on an empty stomach, 1 hour before or 2 hours after a meal, with a full glass of water. If GI upset is severe, take with a light meal; avoid grapefruit juice and foods high in calories, fat, or protein.
- Store the capsules in the original container and leave the desiccant in the bottle. These capsules are very sensitive to moisture.
- Take the full course of therapy as prescribed; do not take double doses if one is missed; do not change dosage without consulting your health care provider. Take drug every 8 hours around the clock.
- Drink 1.5 liters or more of water per day to ensure adequate hydration.
- This drug does not cure HIV infection; long-term effects are not yet known; continue to take precautions as the risk of transmission is not reduced by this drug.
- Do not take any other prescription or over-the-counter drugs without consulting your health care provider; this drug interacts with many other drugs and serious problems can occur.

- You may experience these side effects: Nausea, vomiting, loss of appetite, diarrhea, abdominal pain, headache, dizziness, insomnia.
- Report severe diarrhea, severe nausea, personality changes, changes in color of urine or stool, flank pain, fever or chills.

indomethacin

(in mdoe eth' a sin)

indomethacin

Indocid P.D.A. (CAN), Indocin, Indocin-SR

indomethacin sodium trihydrate

Apo-Indomethacin (CAN), Indocin I.V.

PREGNANCY CATEGORY B

PREGNANCY CATEGORY D (THIRD TRIMESTER)

Drug class

NSAID

Therapeutic actions

Anti-inflammatory, analgesic, and antipyretic activities largely related to inhibition of prostaglandin synthesis; exact mechanisms of action are not known. Inhibits both cyclooxygenase (COX) 1 and 2. Indomethacin is mainly COX-1 selective.

Indications

- Oral, topical, suppositories: Relief of signs and symptoms of moderate to severe rheumatoid arthritis and moderate to severe osteoarthritis, moderate to severe ankylosing spondylitis, acute painful shoulder (bursitis, tendinitis), acute gouty arthritis (*not* SR form)
- Parenteral use: Closure of hemodynamically significant patent ductus arteriosus in premature infants weighing 500–1,750 g, if 48 hr of usual medical management is not effective
- Unlabeled uses for oral form: Pharmacologic closure of persistent patent ductus arteriosus in premature infants; juvenile rheumatoid arthritis; prevention of premature labor
- Unlabeled use of topical eye drops: Cystoid macular edema
- Unlabeled uses: To reduce incidence of patent ductus arteriosus in patients at risk for the condition.

Contraindications and cautions

Oral and rectal

- Contraindicated with allergy to indomethacin, salicylates, or other NSAIDs; history of proctitis or rectal bleeding (suppositories); pregnancy in the third trimester, lactation, labor; pain associated with coronary artery bypass graft surgery.
- Use cautiously with CV dysfunction, hypertension, peptic ulceration, GI bleeding, impaired renal or hepatic function, pregnancy.

IV

- Contraindicated with proven or suspected infection; bleeding, thrombocytopenia, coagulation defects; necrotizing enterocolitis; neonates with significant renal impairment, congenital heart disease when patency of ductus arteriosus is needed for blood flow.
- Use cautiously with renal impairment.

Available forms

Capsules—25, 50 mg; SR capsules—75 mg; oral suspension—25 mg/5 mL; suppositories—50 mg; powder for injection—1 mg

Dosages

Adults

- *Osteoarthritis or rheumatoid arthritis, ankylosing spondylitis:* 25 mg PO bid or tid. If tolerated, increase dose by 25- or 50-mg increments if needed up to total daily dose of 150–200 mg/day PO. SR dose may be used.
- *Acute painful shoulder:* 75–150 mg/day PO, in three or four divided doses. Discontinue drug after inflammation is controlled, usually 7–14 days. SR dose may be used.
- *Acute gouty arthritis:* 50 mg PO, tid until pain is tolerable, then rapidly decrease dose until no longer needed, usually within 3–5 days. Do not use SR dose. In those who have persistent night pain or morning stiffness, a total daily dose of 100 mg may be given at bedtime. Do not exceed 200 mg.

Pediatric patients

Safety and efficacy not established. When special circumstances warrant use in children older than 2 yr, initial dose is 2 mg/kg/day in divided doses PO. Do not exceed 4 mg/kg/day or 150–200 mg/day, whichever is less.

IV

Three IV doses given at 12- to 24-hr intervals.

Age	*1st Dose*	*2nd Dose*	*3rd Dose*
Younger than 48 hr	0.2 mg/kg	0.1 mg/kg	0.1 mg/kg
2–7 days	0.2 mg/kg	0.2 mg/kg	0.2 mg/kg
Older than 7 days	0.2 mg/kg	0.25 mg/kg	0.25 mg/kg

If marked anuria or oliguria occurs, do not give additional doses. If ductus reopens, repeat course of therapy at 12- to 24-hr intervals.

Pharmacokinetics

Route	*Onset*	*Peak*	*Duration*
Oral	30 min	1–2 hr	4–6 hr
IV	Immediate	Unknown	15–30 min

Metabolism: Hepatic; $T_{1/2}$: 4.5–6 hr
Distribution: Crosses placenta; enters breast milk
Excretion: Urine

IV FACTS

Preparation: Reconstitute solution with 1–2 mL of 0.9% sodium chloride injection or water for injection; diluents should be preservative free. If 1 mL of diluent is used, concentration is 0.1 mg/0.1 mL. If 2 mL of diluent is used, concentration is 0.05 mg/0.1 mL. Discard any unused portion of the solution; prepare fresh solution before each dose.
Infusion: Inject reconstituted solution IV over 5–10 sec; further dilution is not recommended.

Adverse effects

Oral, suppositories

- **CNS:** *Headache, dizziness, somnolence, insomnia,* fatigue, tiredness, dizziness, tinnitus, ophthalmologic effects
- **CV: Thrombotic events, MI, CVA**
- **Dermatologic:** *Rash,* pruritus, sweating, dry mucous membranes, stomatitis
- **GI:** *Nausea, dyspepsia, GI pain,* diarrhea, vomiting, *constipation,* flatulence, **GI bleed**
- **GU:** Dysuria, renal impairment
- **Hematologic: Bleeding ulcer,** platelet inhibition with higher doses, neutropenia, eosinophilia, leukopenia, pancytopenia, thrombocytopenia, agranulocytosis, granulocytopenia, aplastic anemia, decreased Hgb or Hct, bone marrow depression, menorrhagia
- **Respiratory:** Dyspnea, hemoptysis, pharyngitis, **bronchospasm,** rhinitis
- **Other:** Peripheral edema, **anaphylactoid reactions to anaphylactic shock**

IV preparation

- **GI: GI bleeding,** *vomiting,* abdominal distention, transient ileus
- **GU:** Renal impairment
- **Hematologic:** *Increased bleeding problems,* including intracranial bleed, **DIC,** hyponatremia, hyperkalemia, hypoglycemia, fluid retention
- **Respiratory:** *Apnea, exacerbation of pulmonary infection,* **pulmonary hemorrhage**
- **Other:** Retrolental fibroplasia, local irritation with extravasation

Interactions

✱ **Drug-drug** • Increased toxic effects of lithium • Decreased diuretic effect with loop diuretics: Bumetanide, furosemide, ethacrynic acid • Potential decrease in antihypertensive effect of beta-adrenergic blocking drugs, ACE inhibitors, and ARBs • Increased risk of gastric ulceration with bisphosphonates • Increased risk of bleeding with anticoagulants • Indomethacin may potentiate potassium-sparing properties of potassium-sparing diuretics

✱ **Drug-lab test** • False-negative results in dexamethasone suppression test

■ Nursing considerations

Assessment

- **History:** Oral and rectal preparations: Allergy to indomethacin, salicylates, or other NSAIDs; CV dysfunction, hypertension, recent history of coronary artery bypass surgery; peptic ulceration, GI bleeding; history of proctitis or rectal bleeding; impaired hepatic or renal function; pregnancy; labor and delivery. IV preparations: Proven or suspected infection; bleeding, thrombocytopenia, coagulation defects; necrotizing enterocolitis; renal impairment; local irritation if extravasation occurs

- **Physical:** Skin color, lesions; T; orientation, reflexes, ophthalmologic evaluation, audiometric evaluation, peripheral sensation; P, BP, edema; R, adventitious sounds; liver evaluation, bowel sounds; CBC, clotting times, urinalysis, LFTs, renal function tests, serum electrolytes, stool guaiac

Interventions

Oral and rectal preparations

⊠ ***Black box warning*** Be aware that patient may be at increased risk for CV events, GI bleeding; monitor accordingly. Adverse reactions are dose-related; use lowest effective dose.

- Do not give SR tablets for gouty arthritis.
- Give drug with food or after meals if GI upset occurs.
- Arrange for periodic ophthalmologic examination during long-term therapy.

⊗ ***Warning*** Discontinue drug if eye changes or symptoms of hepatic or renal impairment occur.

⊗ ***Warning*** For overdose, use emergency procedures—gastric lavage, induction of emesis, support.

⊗ ***Warning*** Test renal function between doses. If severe renal impairment is noted, do not give the next dose.

Teaching points

- Parents of infants receiving IV therapy for patent ductus arteriosus will need support and encouragement and an explanation of the drug's action; this is best incorporated into the teaching about the disease.
- Use the drug only as suggested; avoid overdose. Take with food or after meals if GI upset occurs. Do not exceed the prescribed dosage. Do not use with over-the-counter analgesics; serious toxicity can occur.
- You may experience these side effects: Nausea, GI upset, dyspepsia (take drug with food); diarrhea or constipation; drowsiness, dizziness, vertigo, insomnia (use caution if driving or operating dangerous machinery).
- Report sore throat, fever, rash, itching, weight gain, swelling in ankles or fingers, changes in vision, black tarry stools.

infliximab

See Appendix W, *Less commonly used drugs*.

insoluble Prussian blue

See Appendix W, *Less commonly used drugs*.

DANGEROUS DRUG

insulin

(in' su lin)

Insulin injection: Humulin R, Novolin Toronto (CAN), Novolin R, Novolin R PenFill

Insulin injection concentrate: Humulin R Regular U-500

Insulin lispro: Humalog

Isophane insulin suspension (NPH): Humulin N, Novolinge (CAN), Novolin NPH (CAN), Novolin N, Novolin N PenFill

Insulin aspart: NovoLog

Insulin detemir: Levemir

Insulin glargine: Lantus

Insulin glulisine: Apidra, Apidra SoloSTAR

Combination insulins: Humalog 75/25, Humulin 50/50, Humulin 70/30, Novolin 70/30, Novolin 70/30 PenFill, Novolinge 10/90, 20/80, 30/70, 40/60, 50/50 (CAN), NovoLog 50/50, NovoLog 70/30

PREGNANCY CATEGORY B

PREGNANCY CATEGORY C (INSULIN GLARGINE, INSULIN ASPART, INSULIN GLULISINE)

Drug classes

Antidiabetic
Hormone

Therapeutic actions

Insulin is a hormone secreted by beta cells of the pancreas that, by receptor-mediated effects, promotes the storage of the body's fuels, facilitating the transport of metabolites and ions (potassium) through cell membranes and stimulating the synthesis of glycogen from glucose, of fats from lipids, and proteins from amino acids.

Indications

- Treatment of type 1 diabetes mellitus
- Treatment of type 2 diabetes mellitus that cannot be controlled by diet or oral drugs
- Regular insulin injection: Treatment of severe ketoacidosis or diabetic coma
- Treatment of hyperkalemia with infusion of glucose to produce a shift of potassium into the cells
- Highly purified and human insulins promoted for short courses of therapy (surgery, intercurrent disease), newly diagnosed patients, patients with poor metabolic control, and patients with gestational diabetes
- Insulin injection concentrated: Treatment of diabetic patients with marked insulin resistance (requiring more than 200 units/day)
- Glargine (*Lantus*): Treatment of adult patients with type 2 diabetes mellitus who require basal insulin control of hyperglycemia
- Treatment of adults and children 6 yr and older who require basal insulin control
- Determir (*Levemir*): Treatment of adults with diabetes who require basal insulin for the control of hyperglycemia
- Aspart (*NovoLog*): To maintain glycemic control in children 4–18 yr using a continuous subcutaneous infusion pump

Contraindications and cautions

- Contraindicated with allergy to pork products (varies with preparations; human insulin not contraindicated with pork allergy); during episodes of hypoglycemia.
- Use cautiously with pregnancy (keep patients under close supervision; rigid control is desired; following delivery, requirements may drop for 24–72 hr, rising to normal levels during next 6 wk); lactation (monitor mother carefully; insulin requirements may decrease during lactation).

Available forms

Injection—100 units/mL, 500 units/mL (concentrated); prefilled cartridges and pens—100 units/mL

Dosages

Adults and pediatric patients

General guidelines, 0.5–1 unit/kg/day. The number and size of daily doses, times of administration, and type of insulin preparation are determined after close medical scrutiny of the patient's blood and urine glucose, diet, exercise, and intercurrent infections and other stresses. Usually given subcutaneously. Regular insulin and insulin glulisine may be given IV in diabetic coma or ketoacidosis. Insulin injection concentrated may be given subcutaneously or IM but do not administer IV.

Adults with type 2 diabetes mellitus requiring basal insulin control

10 units/day subcutaneously, given at the same time each day. Range, 2–100 units/day (*Lantus*) or 0.1–0.2 units/kg subcutaneously in the evening or 10 units once or twice a day (*Levemir*).

Pharmacokinetics

Type	*Onset*	*Peak*	*Duration*
Regular	30–60 min	2–3 hr	6–12 hr
NPH	1–1.5 hr	4–12 hr	24 hr
Lente	1–2.5 hr	7–15 hr	24 hr
Ultralente	4–8 hr	10–30 hr	> 36 hr
Lispro	< 15 min	30–90 min	2–5 hr
Aspart	10–20 min	1–3 hr	3–5 hr
Detemir	Slow	3–6 hr	6–11 hr
Glargine	60 min	None	24 hr
Glulisine	2–5 min	30–90 min	2 hr
Combination insulins	30–60 min, then 1–2 hr	2–4 hr, then 6–12 hr	6–8 hr, then 18–24 hr

Metabolism: Cellular; $T_{1/2}$: Varies with preparation
Distribution: Crosses placenta; does not enter breast milk
Excretion: Unknown

IV FACTS

Preparation: May be mixed with standard IV solutions; use of plastic tubing or bag will change the amount of insulin delivered.
Infusion: Use of a monitored delivery system is suggested. Rate should be determined by patient response and glucose levels.
Incompatibilities: Do not add to aminophylline, amobarbital, chlorothiazide, cytarabine, dobutamine, methylprednisolone, pentobarbital, phenobarbital, phenytoin, secobarbital, sodium bicarbonate, thiopental.

Adverse effects

- **Hypersensitivity:** Rash, **anaphylaxis or angioedema**
- **Local:** Allergy—local reactions at injection site—redness, swelling, itching; usually resolves in a few days to a few weeks; a change in type or species source of insulin may be tried; lipodystrophy; pruritus
- **Metabolic:** Hypoglycemia; ketoacidosis
- **Respiratory:** Decline in pulmonary function (inhaled insulin)

Interactions

✷ **Drug-drug** • Increased hypoglycemic effects of insulin with MAOIs, beta blockers, salicylates, or alcohol • Delayed recovery from hypoglycemic episodes and masked signs and symptoms of hypoglycemia if taken with beta-adrenergic blocking drugs • Decreased effectiveness of insulin with corticosteroids, diuretics, atypical antipsychotics

✷ **Drug-alternative therapy** • Increased risk of hypoglycemia if taken with juniper berries, ginseng, garlic, fenugreek, coriander, dandelion root, celery

■ Nursing considerations

Assessment

- **History:** Allergy to pork products; pregnancy; lactation
- **Physical:** Skin color, lesions; eyeball turgor; orientation, reflexes, peripheral sensation; P, BP; R, adventitious sounds; urinalysis, blood glucose

Interventions

- Ensure uniform dispersion of insulin suspensions by rolling the vial gently between hands; avoid vigorous shaking.
- Give maintenance doses subcutaneously, rotating injection sites regularly to decrease incidence of lipodystrophy; give regular insulin IV or IM in severe ketoacidosis or diabetic coma.
- Monitor patients receiving insulin IV carefully; plastic IV infusion sets have been reported to remove 20%–80% of the insulin; dosage delivered to the patient will vary.
- Do not give insulin injection concentrated IV; severe anaphylactic reactions can occur.
- Use caution when mixing two types of insulin; always draw the regular insulin into the syringe first; if mixing with insulin lispro, draw the lispro first; use mixtures of regular and NPH or regular and Lente insulins within 5–15 min of combining them; *Lantus* (insulin glargine) and *Levemir* (insulin detemir) cannot be mixed in solution with any other drug, including other insulins.

⊗ ***Warning*** Double-check, or have a colleague check, the dosage drawn up for pediatric patients, for patients receiving concentrated insulin injection, or patients receiving very small doses; even small errors in dosage can cause serious problems.

- Carefully monitor patients being switched from one type of insulin to another; dosage adjustments are often needed. Human insulins often require smaller doses than beef or pork insulin; monitor cautiously if patients are switched; lispro insulin is given 15 min before a meal. *Levemir* is given in the evening.
- Store insulin in a cool place away from direct sunlight. Refrigeration is preferred. Do not freeze insulin. Insulin prefilled in glass or plastic syringes is stable for 1 wk refrigerated; this is a safe way of ensuring proper dosage for patients with limited vision or who have problems with drawing up insulin.
- Monitor urine or serum glucose levels frequently to determine effectiveness of drug and dosage. Patients can learn to adjust insulin dosage on a sliding scale based on test results.
- Monitor insulin needs during times of trauma or severe stress; dosage adjustments may be needed.

⊗ ***Warning*** Keep life-support equipment and glucose readily available to deal with ketoacidosis or hypoglycemic reactions.

Teaching points

- Use the same type and brand of syringe; use the same type and brand of insulin to avoid dosage errors. Arrange for proper disposal of syringes.
- Do not change the order of mixing insulins. Rotate injection sites regularly (keep a chart of sites used) to prevent breakdown at injection sites.
- Dosage may vary with activities, stress, or diet. Monitor blood or urine glucose levels, and consult your health care provider if problems arise.
- Store drug in the refrigerator or in a cool place out of direct sunlight; do not freeze insulin.
- If refrigeration is not possible, drug is stable at controlled room temperature and out of direct sunlight for up to 1 month.
- Monitor your urine or blood levels for glucose and ketones as prescribed.
- Wear a medical alert tag stating that you have diabetes and are taking insulin so that emergency medical personnel will take proper care of you.
- Avoid alcohol; serious reactions can occur.
- Report fever, sore throat, vomiting, hypoglycemic or hyperglycemic reactions, rash.

DANGEROUS DRUG

▽interferon alfa-2b (IFN-a2, rIFN-a2, a-2-interferon)

*(in ter **feer'** on)*

Intron-A

PREGNANCY CATEGORY C

Drug classes

Antineoplastic
Immunomodulator
Interferon

Therapeutic actions

Inhibits growth of tumor cells; mechanism of action is not clearly understood; prevents the replication of tumor cells and enhances host immune response. Interferons are produced by human leukocytes in response to viral infections and other stimuli. Interferon alfa-2b is produced by recombinant DNA technology using *Escherichia coli.*

Indications

- Hairy cell leukemia in patients 18 yr and older
- Intralesional treatment of condylomata acuminata in patients 18 yr and older
- AIDS-related Kaposi's sarcoma in patients 18 yr and older
- Adjunct to surgical treatment of malignant melanoma in patients older than 18 yr who are free of disease, but at high risk of recurrence with 56 days of surgery
- Treatment of chronic hepatitis C in patients 18 yr and older
- Treatment of chronic hepatitis B in patients 1 yr and older
- Follicular lymphoma, as initial treatment of clinically aggressive follicular non-Hodgkin's lymphoma with other chemotherapy in patient 18 yr and older
- Orphan drug uses: CML, metastatic renal cell carcinoma, ovarian carcinoma, invasive carcinoma of cervix, primary malignant brain tumors, laryngeal papillomatosis, carcinoma in situ of urinary bladder, chronic delta hepatitis, acute hepatitis B

Contraindications and cautions

- Contraindicated with allergy to interferon-alfa or any components of the product, severe hepatic impairment.
- Use cautiously with cardiac disease, pulmonary disease, diabetes mellitus prone to ketoacidosis, coagulation disorders, bone marrow depression, pregnancy, neuropsychiatric disorders, autoimmune diseases, lactation.

Available forms

Powder for injection—10, 18, 50 million international units/vial; solution for injection—18, 25 million international units/vial; injection—3, 5, 10 million international units/dose (in multidose pens)

Dosages

Adults

- *Hairy cell leukemia:* 2 million international units/m^2 subcutaneously or IM three times/wk for up to 6 mo. Continue for several months, depending on clinical and hematologic response. Patient with platelet count less than 50,000/mm^3 should not receive IM injection.
- *Condylomata acuminata:* 1 million international units/lesion three times/wk for 3 wk intralesionally. Maximum response occurs 4–8 wk after initiation of therapy. Up to five lesions can be treated at one time. May repeat course at 12–16 wk.
- *Chronic hepatitis C:* 3 million international units subcutaneously or IM, three times/wk for 18–24 mo.
- *AIDS-related Kaposi's sarcoma:* 30 million international units/m^2 three times/wk subcutaneously or IM. Maintain dosage until disease progresses rapidly or severe intolerance occurs. Do not use the multidose pens or multidose vials due to inappropriate concentration.
- *Chronic hepatitis B:* 30–35 million international units/wk subcutaneously or IM either as 5 million international units daily or 10 million international units three times/wk for 16 wk.
- *Follicular lymphoma:* 5 million international units subcutaneously, three times/wk for 18 mo with other chemotherapy. Adjust dosage based on blood counts.
- *Malignant melanoma:* 20 million international units/m^2 IV on 5 consecutive days/wk for 4 wk; maintenance, 10 million international units/m^2 IV three times/wk for 48 wk.

Pediatric patients

- *Chronic hepatitis B:* 3 million international units/m^2 subcutaneously three times/wk for the first wk, then increase to 6 million international units/m^2 subcutaneously three times/wk for a total of 16–24 wk (maximum dose, 10 million international units, three times/wk). Adjust dosage based on blood counts.

Pharmacokinetics

Route	*Onset*	*Peak*
IM, Subcut.	Rapid	3–12 hr
IV	Rapid	End of infusion

Metabolism: Renal; $T_{1/2}$: 2–3 hr
Distribution: Crosses placenta; may enter breast milk
Excretion: Unknown

IV FACTS

Powder for injection is not indicated for pediatric patients because diluent contains benzyl alcohol.

Preparation: Inject diluent (bacteriostatic water for injection) into vial using chart provided by manufacturer; agitate gently, withdraw with sterile syringe, inject into 100 mL of normal saline.

Infusion: Administer each dose slowly over 20 min.

I

Adverse effects

- **CNS:** *Dizziness, confusion,* paresthesias, numbness, lethargy, decreased mental status, depression, visual disturbances, sleep disturbances, nervousness
- **CV:** Hypotension, edema, hypertension, chest pain, arrhythmias, palpitations
- **Dermatologic:** *Rash,* dryness or inflammation of the oropharynx, *dry skin, pruritus,* partial alopecia
- **GI:** *Anorexia, nausea,* diarrhea, vomiting, change in taste
- **GU:** Impaired fertility in women, transient impotence
- **Hematologic:** Leukopenia, neutropenia, thrombocytopenia, anemia, decreased Hgb; increased levels of AST, LDH, alkaline phosphatase, bilirubin, uric acid, serum creatinine, BUN, blood sugar, serum phosphorus, neutralizing antibodies; hypocalcemia
- **Other:** *Flulike symptoms,* weight loss, diaphoresis, arthralgia

■ Nursing considerations

Assessment

- **History:** Allergy to interferon-alfa or product components, cardiac or pulmonary disease, diabetes mellitus prone to ketoacidosis, coagulation disorders, bone marrow depression, pregnancy, lactation
- **Physical:** Weight; T; skin color, lesions; orientation, reflexes; P, BP, edema, ECG; liver evaluation; CBC, blood glucose, LFTs, renal function tests, urinalysis

Interventions

- Obtain laboratory tests (CBC, differential, granulocytes and hairy cells, bone marrow and hairy cells, LFTs) before therapy and monthly during therapy.
- Prepare solution as follows:

Vial Strength (Million International Units)	*Final Amount of Diluent (mL)*	*Concentration (Million International Units/mL)*
3	1	3
5	1	5
10	2	5
25	5	5
10	1	10
50	1	50

- Use bacteriostatic water for injection as diluent. Agitate gently. After reconstitution, stable for 1 mo if refrigerated.
- Administer IM or subcutaneously.

⊗ ***Black box warning*** Monitor for severe reactions, including hypersensitivity reactions and neuropsychiatric, autoimmune, ischemic, and infectious disorders; notify physician immediately; dosage reduction or discontinuation may be necessary; risk of serious to life-threatening reactions.

- Ensure that patient is well hydrated, especially during initiation of treatment.

Teaching points

- Prepare a calendar to check off as drug is given. You and a significant other should learn proper subcutaneous or IM injection technique for outpatient use. Do not change brands of interferon without consulting your health care provider. Arrange for proper disposal of syringes and needles.
- Arrange for regular blood tests to monitor the drug's effects.
- You may experience these side effects: Loss of appetite, nausea, vomiting (frequent mouth care, frequent small meals may help; maintain good nutrition; a dietitian may be able to help; an antiemetic also may be ordered); fatigue, confusion, dizziness, numbness, visual disturbances, depression (use special precautions to avoid injury; avoid driving or using dangerous machinery); flulike symptoms (take drug at bedtime; ensure rest periods for yourself; a medication may be ordered for fever).
- Report fever, chills, sore throat, unusual bleeding or bruising, chest pain, palpitations, dizziness, changes in mental status.

interferon alfacon-1

See Appendix W, *Less commonly used drugs*.

interferon alfa-n3

See Appendix W, *Less commonly used drugs*.

interferon beta-1a

*(in ter **feer'** on)*

Avonex, Rebif

PREGNANCY CATEGORY C

Drug classes

Immunomodulator
Interferon
MS drug

Therapeutic actions

Interferons are produced by human leukocytes in response to viral infections and other stimuli; interferon beta-1a blocks replication of viruses and stimulates the host immunoregulatory activities. It is produced by Chinese hamster ovary cells.

Indications

- MS—treatment of relapsing forms of MS to slow accumulation of physical disability and decrease frequency of clinical exacerbations

Contraindications and cautions

- Contraindicated with allergy to beta interferon, human albumin, or any components of product, lactation.
- Use cautiously with chronic progressive MS, suicidal tendencies or mental disorders, cardiac disease, seizures, pregnancy.

Available forms

Powder for injection—33 mcg (*Avonex*), prefilled syringe—30 mcg/0.5 mL (*Avonex*);

injection—8.8 mcg/0.2 mL, 22 mcg/0.5 mL, 44 mcg/0.5 mL (*Rebif*)

Dosages

Adults

30 mcg IM once per week (*Avonex*) 22 or 44 mcg subcutaneously 3 times per week (*Rebif*)—start with 8.8 mcg 3 times per week and titrate up over 5 wk to full dose of 22–44 mcg.

Pediatric patients

Safety and efficacy not established in patients younger than 18 yr.

Pharmacokinetics

Route	*Onset*	*Peak*	*Duration*
IM	12 hr	48 hr	4 days

Metabolism: Hepatic and renal; $T_{1/2}$: 10 hr
Distribution: Crosses placenta; may enter breast milk
Excretion: Urine

Adverse effects

- **CNS:** *Dizziness, confusion,* paresthesias, numbness, lethargy, decreased mental status, depression, visual disturbances, sleep disturbances, nervousness, asthenia
- **CV:** Hypotension, edema, hypertension, chest pain, arrhythmias, palpitations
- **Dermatologic:** *Photosensitivity,* rash, alopecia, sweating
- **GI:** *Anorexia, nausea,* diarrhea, vomiting, change in taste
- **GU:** Impairment of fertility in women, transient impotence
- **Hematologic:** Leukopenia, neutropenia, thrombocytopenia, anemia, decreased Hgb; increased levels of AST, LDH, alkaline phosphatase, bilirubin, uric acid, serum creatinine, BUN, blood sugar, serum phosphorus, neutralizing antibodies; hypocalcemia
- **Other:** *Flulike symptoms,* weight loss, diaphoresis, arthralgia, injection site reaction

■ Nursing considerations

Assessment

- **History:** Allergy to beta interferon or any component of product, mental disorders, suicidal tendencies, cardiac disease, seizures, depression, pregnancy, lactation
- **Physical:** Weight; T; skin color, lesions; orientation, reflexes; P, BP, edema, ECG; liver evaluation; CBC, blood glucose, LFTs, renal function tests, urinalysis

Interventions

- Arrange for laboratory tests—CBC, differential, granulocytes and hairy cells and bone marrow hairy cells, and liver function tests—before and monthly during therapy.
- Reconstitute with 1.1 mL of diluent and swirl gently to dissolve; use within 6 hr (*Avonex*).
- Ensure that patient is well hydrated, especially during initiation of treatment.
- Ensure regular follow-up and treatment of MS; this drug is not a cure.
- If flulike symptoms occur, arrange for supportive treatment—rest, acetaminophen for fever and headache, environmental control.
- Carefully monitor patients with any history of mental disorders or suicidal tendencies.
- Counsel female patients to use birth control while using this drug. Drug should not be used in pregnancy.

Teaching points

- *Avonex* needs to be taken weekly. If you or a significant other can give an IM injection: Store vial in refrigerator, reconstitute with 1.1 milliliters of diluent and swirl gently, use within 6 hours. Do not give in the same site each week.
- *Rebif* needs to be given three times per week subcutaneously, preferably at the same time of day and on the same days of the week. Store in refrigerator, reconstitute with solution provided, and discard any solution remaining in the syringe. Rotate injection sites.
- Keep a chart of injection sites to prevent overuse of one area. Arrange for proper disposal of needles and syringes.
- Have regular treatment and follow-up of MS; this drug is not a cure.
- You may experience these side effects: Loss of appetite, nausea, vomiting (use frequent mouth care; eat frequent small meals; maintain good nutrition if possible—dietitian may be able to help; antiemetics may be ordered); fatigue, confusion, dizziness, numbness, visual disturbances, depression (use caution to avoid injury; avoid driving or using dangerous machinery); impotence

(usually transient); sensitivity to sunlight (use a sunscreen, wear protective clothing if exposure to sun cannot be prevented).
- Report fever, chills, sore throat, unusual bleeding or bruising, chest pain, palpitations, dizziness, changes in mental status.

▽interferon beta-1b (rIFN-B)

(in ter ***feer'*** *on)*

Betaseron, Extava

PREGNANCY CATEGORY C

Drug classes
Immune modulator
Interferon
MS drug

Therapeutic actions
Interferons are produced by human leukocytes in response to viral infections and other stimuli; interferon beta-1b block replication of viruses and stimulate the host immunoregulatory activities. Interferon beta-1b is produced by recombinant DNA technology using *Escherichia coli.*

Indications
- Reduce the frequency of clinical exacerbations in relapsing, remitting MS

Contraindications and cautions
- Contraindicated with allergy to beta interferon, human albumin, or product components; lactation.
- Use cautiously with chronic progressive MS, suicidal tendencies, mental disorders, pregnancy.

Available forms
Powder for injection—0.3 mg

Dosages
Adults

0.25 mg subcutaneously every other day; discontinue use if disease is unremitting for more than 6 mo. Initially, 0.0625 mg subcutaneously every other day, weeks 1–2; then 0.125 mg subcutaneously every other day, weeks 3–4; 0.1875 mg subcutaneously every other day, weeks 5–6; target 0.25 mg subcutaneously every other day by week 7.

Pediatric patients

Safety and efficacy not established in patients younger than 18 yr.

Pharmacokinetics

Route	*Onset*	*Peak*
Subcut.	Slow	1–8 hr

Metabolism: Hepatic and renal; $T_{1/2}$: 8 min–4.3 hr
Distribution: Crosses placenta; may enter breast milk
Excretion: Urine

Adverse effects
- **CNS:** *Dizziness, confusion,* paresthesias, numbness, lethargy, decreased mental status, depression, visual disturbances, sleep disturbances, nervousness
- **CV:** Hypotension, edema, hypertension, chest pain, arrhythmias, palpitations
- **Dermatologic:** *Photosensitivity,* rash, alopecia, sweating
- **GI:** *Anorexia, nausea,* diarrhea, vomiting, change in taste, abdominal pain
- **GU:** Impairment of fertility in women, transient impotence, metrorrhagia
- **Hematologic:** Leukopenia, neutropenia, thrombocytopenia, anemia, decreased Hgb; increased levels of AST, LDH, alkaline phosphatase, bilirubin, uric acid, serum creatinine, BUN, blood sugar, serum phosphorus, neutralizing antibodies; hypocalcemia
- **Other:** *Flulike symptoms,* weight loss, diaphoresis, arthralgia, injection site reaction

■ Nursing considerations
Assessment
- **History:** Allergy to interferon beta or any components of the product, mental disorders, suicidal tendencies, pregnancy, lactation
- **Physical:** Weight; T; skin color, lesions; orientation, reflexes; P, BP, edema, ECG; liver evaluation; CBC, blood glucose, LFTs, renal function tests, urinalysis

Interventions

- Obtain laboratory tests (CBC, differential, granulocytes and hairy cells, bone marrow hairy cells, and liver function tests) before therapy and monthly during therapy.

⊗ ***Warning*** Monitor for severe reactions; notify physician immediately; you may need to reduce dosage or discontinue drug.

- Reconstitute by using a sterile syringe and needle to inject 1.2 mL supplied diluent into vial; gently swirl vial to dissolve drug completely; do not shake. Discard if any particulate matter or discoloration has occurred. After reconstitution, vial contains 0.25 mg/mL solution. Withdraw 1 mL of reconstituted solution with a sterile syringe fitted with a 27-gauge needle. Inject subcutaneously into arms, abdomen, hips, or thighs. Vial is for single use only. Discard any unused portions. Refrigerate. Use reconstituted solution within 3 hr.
- Ensure that patient is well hydrated, especially during initiation of treatment.
- Ensure regular follow-up and treatment of MS; this drug is not a cure.

⊗ ***Warning*** Carefully monitor patients with any mental disorders or suicidal tendencies.

- Counsel female patients to use birth control. Drug should not be used in pregnancy.

Teaching points

- Reconstitute by using a sterile syringe and needle to inject 1.2 milliliters supplied diluent into vial; gently swirl the vial to dissolve the drug completely; do not shake. Discard if any particulate matter or discoloration has occurred. After reconstitution, vial contains 0.25 mg/mL solution. Withdraw 1 milliliter of reconstituted solution with a sterile syringe fitted with a 27-gauge needle. Inject subcutaneously into arms, abdomen, hips, or thighs. Vial is for single use only. Discard any unused portions. Refrigerate. Use reconstituted solution within 3 hours.
- Keep a chart of injection sites to prevent overuse of one area. Arrange for proper disposal of needles and syringes.
- Have regular treatment and follow-up of MS; this drug is not a cure.
- Using barrier contraceptives is advised; the drug should not be used during pregnancy.
- You may experience these side effects: Loss of appetite, nausea, vomiting (frequent mouth care, frequent small meals may help; maintain good nutrition; a dietitian may be able to help; an antiemetic also may be ordered); fatigue, confusion, dizziness, numbness, visual disturbances, depression (use special precautions to avoid injury; avoid driving or using dangerous machinery); impotence (transient and reversible); sensitivity to the sun (use sunscreen and wear protective clothing if exposed to sun).
- Report fever, chills, sore throat, unusual bleeding or bruising, chest pain, palpitations, dizziness, changes in mental status, thoughts of suicide.

▽ interferon gamma-1b

(in ter feer' on)

Actimmune

PREGNANCY CATEGORY C

Drug classes

Immunomodulator
Interferon

Therapeutic actions

Interferons are produced by human leukocytes in response to viral infections and other stimuli; interferon gamma-1b block has potent phagocyte-activating effects; acts as an interleukin; produced by *Escherichia coli* bacteria.

Indications

- For reducing the frequency and severity of serious infections associated with chronic granulomatous disease
- For delaying time to disease progression in patients with severe, malignant osteopetrosis
- Orphan drug use: Renal cell carcinoma

Contraindications and cautions

- Contraindicated with allergy to interferon gamma, *E. coli,* or product components; lactation.
- Use cautiously with seizure disorders, compromised CNS function, cardiac disease, myelosuppression, pregnancy.

Available forms
Injection—100 mcg/0.5 mL (2 million international units)

Dosages
Adults
50 mcg/m^2 (1 million international units/m^2) subcutaneously three times/wk in patients who have a body surface area greater than 0.5 m^2; 1.5 mcg/kg per dose in patients who have a body surface area less than 0.5 m^2 subcutaneously three times/wk. Reduce dose by 50% or hold therapy for severe reactions.
Pediatric patients
Safety and efficacy not established in patients younger than 18 yr.

Pharmacokinetics

Route	*Onset*	*Peak*
Subcut.	Slow	7 hr

Metabolism: Hepatic and renal; $T_{1/2}$: 2.9–5.9 hr
Distribution: Crosses placenta; may enter breast milk
Excretion: Urine

Adverse effects
- **CNS:** *Dizziness, confusion,* paresthesias, headache, numbness, lethargy, decreased mental status, depression, visual disturbances, sleep disturbances, nervousness
- **CV:** Hypotension, edema, hypertension, chest pain, arrhythmias, palpitations
- **GI:** *Anorexia, nausea,* diarrhea, vomiting, change in taste, pancreatitis
- **Other:** *Flulike symptoms,* weight loss, diaphoresis, arthralgia, injection site reaction, fever, rash, chills, fatigue, myalgia

■ Nursing considerations
Assessment
- **History:** Allergy to interferon gamma, *E. coli,* or product components; pregnancy, lactation, seizure disorders, compromised CNS function, cardiac disease, myelosuppression
- **Physical:** Weight; T; skin color, lesions; orientation, reflexes; P, BP, edema, ECG; liver evaluation; CBC, blood glucose, LFTs, renal function tests, urinalysis

Interventions
- Obtain laboratory tests (CBC, differential, granulocytes and hairy cells, bone marrow and hairy cells, and liver function tests) before therapy and monthly during therapy.

⊗ ***Warning*** Monitor for severe reactions and notify physician immediately; dosage may need to be reduced or drug discontinued.

- Store in refrigerator; each vial is for one use only, discard after that time. Discard any vial that has been unrefrigerated for 12 hr.
- Give drug at bedtime if flulike symptoms become a problem.
- Advise women of childbearing age to use barrier contraceptives; drug should not be used during pregnancy.

Teaching points
- Store in refrigerator; each vial is for one use only; discard after that time. Discard vial that has been unrefrigerated for 12 hours. You and a significant other should learn the proper technique for subcutaneous injections. Product does not contain a preservative.
- Keep a chart of injection sites to prevent overuse of one area. Arrange for proper disposal of needles and syringes.
- Using barrier contraceptives is advised; this drug should not be used in pregnancy.
- You may experience these side effects: Loss of appetite, nausea, vomiting (frequent mouth care, frequent small meals may help; maintain good nutrition; a dietitian may be able to help; an antiemetic also may be ordered); fatigue, confusion, dizziness, numbness, visual disturbances, depression (use special precautions to avoid injury; avoid driving or using dangerous machinery); flulike symptoms (fever, chills, aches, pains; rest, take acetaminophen for fever and headache; take drug at bedtime).
- Report fever, chills, sore throat, unusual bleeding or bruising, chest pain, palpitations, dizziness, changes in mental status.

iodine thyroid products

(eye' oh dine)

Lugol's Solution, Strong Iodine Solution, Thyro-Block, ThyroShield

PREGNANCY CATEGORY D

Drug class
Thyroid suppressant

Therapeutic actions
Inhibits synthesis of the active thyroid hormones T_3 and T_4 and inhibits the release of these hormones into circulation.

Indications
- Hyperthyroidism: Adjunctive therapy with antithyroid drugs in preparation for thyroidectomy, treatment of thyrotoxic crisis, or neonatal thyrotoxicosis
- Thyroid blocking in a radiation emergency
- Unlabeled uses: Potassium iodide has been effective with Sweet's syndrome, treatment of lymphocutaneous sporotrichosis in combination with a potent topical steroid

Contraindications and cautions
- Contraindicated with allergy to iodides.
- Use cautiously with pulmonary edema, pulmonary TB (sodium iodide); pregnancy; lactation.

Available forms
Solution—5% iodine, 10% potassium iodide; tablets—130 mg potassium iodide; ThyroShield solution—65 mg/mL. *Note:* Potassium iodide tablets and drops are available only to state and federal agencies.

Dosages
Adults and pediatric patients older than 1 yr
- *RDA:* 150 mcg PO.
- *Preparation for thyroidectomy:* 2–6 drops strong iodine solution tid PO for 10 days before surgery.
- *Thyroid blocking in a radiation emergency used as directed by state or local health authorities:* 1 tablet (130 mg potassium iodide) PO or 6 drops (21 mg potassium iodide/drop) added to one-half glass of liquid per day for 10 days.
- *ThyroShield:* As directed by local public health authorities; don't give more than 1 dose per 24 hr.
  For adults and children older than 12 yr and weighing more than 68 kg: 2 mL per 24 hr.
  For pediatric patients 12–18 yr weighing less than 68 kg and patients 3–12 yr: 1 mL per 24 hr.
  For pediatric patients 1 mo-3 yr: 0.5 mL per 24 hr.
  For infants to 1 mo: 0.25 mL per 24 hr.

Pediatric patients younger than 1 yr
- *Thyroid blocking in a radiation emergency:* One-half of a crushed tablet or 3 drops in a small amount of liquid per day for 10 days.

Pharmacokinetics

Route	*Onset*	*Peak*	*Duration*
Oral	24 hr	10–15 days	6 wk

Metabolism: Hepatic; $T_{1/2}$: Unknown
Distribution: Crosses placenta; may enter breast milk
Excretion: Urine

Adverse effects
- **Dermatologic:** *Rash*
- **Endocrine:** Hypothyroidism, hyperthyroidism, goiter
- **GI:** *Swelling of the salivary glands, iodism* (metallic taste, burning mouth and throat, sore teeth and gums, head cold symptoms, stomach upset, diarrhea)
- **Hypersensitivity:** Allergic reactions—fever, joint pains, swelling of the face or body, shortness of breath

Interactions
✱ **Drug-drug** • Increased risk of hypothyroidism if taken concurrently with lithium

■ Nursing considerations
Assessment
- **History:** Allergy to iodides, pulmonary edema, pulmonary TB, lactation

- **Physical:** Skin color, lesions, edema; R, adventitious sounds; gums, mucous membranes; T_3 and T_4

Interventions

- Test skin for idiosyncrasy to iodine before giving parenteral doses.
- Dilute strong iodine solution with fruit juice or water to improve taste.
- Crush tablets for small children.

⊗ ***Warning*** Discontinue drug if symptoms of acute iodine toxicity occur: Vomiting, abdominal pain, diarrhea, or circulatory collapse.

Teaching points

- Drops may be diluted in fruit juice or water. Tablets may be crushed.
- Discontinue use and report fever, rash, swelling of the throat, metallic taste, sore teeth and gums, head cold symptoms, severe GI distress, enlargement of the thyroid gland.

▽iodoquinol (diiodohydroxyquinoline)

(eye oh doe ***kwin'*** *ole)*

Yodoxin

PREGNANCY CATEGORY C

Drug class

Amebicide

Therapeutic actions

Directly amebicidal by an unknown mechanism; is poorly absorbed in the GI tract and is able to exert its amebicidal action directly in the large intestine.

Indications

- Acute or chronic intestinal amebiasis

Contraindications and cautions

- Contraindicated with hepatic failure, allergy to iodine preparations or 8-hydroxyquinolines.
- Use cautiously with thyroid disease, pregnancy, lactation.

Available forms

Tablets—210, 650 mg; powder—25 g

Dosages

Adults

650 mg tid PO after meals for 20 days.

Pediatric patients

10–13.3 mg/kg/day PO, in 3 divided doses for 20 days. Maximum dose, 650 mg/dose. Do not exceed 1.95 g in 24 hr for 20 days.

Pharmacokinetics

Route	Onset
Oral	Slow

Very poorly absorbed; exerts effects locally in the intestine.

Excretion: Feces

Adverse effects

- **CNS:** Blurring of vision, weakness, fatigue, optic atrophy, peripheral neuropathy, vertigo, numbness, headache
- **Dermatologic:** *Rash, pruritus,* urticaria
- **GI:** *Nausea, vomiting, diarrhea,* anorexia, abdominal cramps, pruritus ani
- **Other:** Thyroid enlargement, fever, chills

Interactions

✱ **Drug-lab test** • Interferes with many tests of thyroid function; interference may last up to 6 mo after drug is discontinued

■ Nursing considerations

Assessment

- **History:** Hepatic failure, allergy to iodine preparations or 8-hydroxyquinolines, thyroid disease, lactation, pregnancy
- **Physical:** Skin rashes, lesions; check reflexes, ophthalmologic examination; BP, P, R; LFTs, thyroid function tests (PBI, T_3, and T_4)

Interventions

- Administer drug after meals.
- Administer for full course of therapy.
- Maintain patient's nutrition.

Teaching points

- Take drug after meals.

- You may experience these side effects: GI upset, nausea, vomiting, diarrhea (eat frequent small meals; frequent mouth care often helps).
- Report severe GI upset, rash, blurring of vision, unusual fatigue, fever.

ipratropium bromide

*(i pra **troe'** pee um)*

Apo-Ipravent (CAN), Atrovent, Atrovent HFA, Gen-Ipratropium (CAN), ratio-Ipratropium (CAN), ratio-Ipratropium UDV (CAN)

PREGNANCY CATEGORY B

Drug classes

Anticholinergic
Antimuscarinic
Bronchodilator
Parasympatholytic

Therapeutic actions

Anticholinergic, chemically related to atropine, which blocks vagally mediated reflexes by antagonizing the action of acetylcholine. Causes bronchodilation and inhibits secretion from serous and seromucous glands lining the nasal mucosa.

Indications

- Bronchodilator for maintenance treatment of bronchospasm associated with COPD (solution, aerosol), chronic bronchitis, and emphysema
- Nasal spray: Symptomatic relief of rhinorrhea associated with perennial rhinitis, common cold, seasonal allergic rhinitis

Contraindications and cautions

- Contraindicated with hypersensitivity to atropine or its derivatives, soybean or peanut allergies (aerosol).
- Use cautiously with narrow-angle glaucoma, prostatic hypertrophy, bladder neck obstruction, pregnancy, lactation.

Available forms

Aerosol—17, 18 mcg/actuation; solution for inhalation—0.02%; (500 mcg/vial); nasal spray—0.03% (21 mcg/spray), 0.06% (42 mcg/spray)

Dosages

Aerosol

Adults

The usual dosage is 2 inhalations qid. Patients may take additional inhalations as required. Do not exceed 12 inhalations/24 hr.

Solution for inhalation

Adults and pediatric patients 12 yr and older

500 mcg tid–qid via nebulizer, with doses 6–8 hr apart.

Nasal spray

Adults and pediatric patients 12 yr and older

2 sprays 0.06% per nostril tid–qid for relief with common cold.

Adults and pediatric patients 6 yr and older

2 sprays 0.03% per nostril bid–tid for rhinitis.

Adults and pediatric patients older than 5 yr

- *Rhinorrhea in seasonal allergic rhinitis:* 2 sprays 0.06% qid for 3 wk.

Pediatric patients 5–11 yr

2 sprays 0.06% per nostril tid for relief with common cold.

Pharmacokinetics

Route	*Onset*	*Peak*	*Duration*
Inhalation	15 min	1–2 hr	3–4 hr

Metabolism: Hepatic, $T_{1/2}$: 2 hr
Distribution: May cross placenta; may enter breast milk
Excretion: Unknown

Adverse effects

- **CNS:** *Nervousness, dizziness, headache,* fatigue, insomnia, *blurred vision*
- **GI:** *Nausea,* GI distress, *dry mouth*
- **Respiratory:** Dyspnea, bronchitis, bronchospasms, URI, *cough,* exacerbation of symptoms, hoarseness, pharyngitis
- **Other:** Back pain, chest pain, allergic-type reactions, palpitations, rash

■ Nursing considerations

Assessment

- **History:** Hypersensitivity to atropine, soybeans, peanuts (aerosol preparation); acute bronchospasm, narrow-angle glaucoma, prostatic hypertrophy, bladder neck obstruction, pregnancy, lactation

- **Physical:** Skin color, lesions, texture; T; orientation, reflexes, bilateral grip strength; affect; ophthalmic examination; P, BP; R, adventitious sounds; bowel sounds, normal output; normal urinary output, prostate palpation

Interventions

- Protect solution for inhalation from light. Store unused vials in foil pouch.
- Use nebulizer mouthpiece instead of face mask to avoid blurred vision or aggravation of narrow-angle glaucoma.
- Can mix with albuterol in nebulizer for up to 1 hr.
- Ensure adequate hydration; control environment (temperature) to prevent hyperpyrexia.
- Have patient void before taking medication to avoid urinary retention.
- Teach patient proper use of inhaler.

Teaching points

- Use this drug as an inhalation product. Review the proper use of inhalator; for nasal spray, initiation of pump requires 7 actuations; if not used for 24 hours, 2 actuations will be needed before use. If not used for more than 7 days, reprime pump with 7 sprays. Protect from light; do not freeze.
- For *Atrovent HFA,* use only the supplied HFA aerosol inhalation mouthpiece.
- You may experience these side effects: Dizziness, headache, blurred vision (avoid driving or performing hazardous tasks); nausea, vomiting, GI upset (proper nutrition is important; consult with a dietitian to maintain nutrition); cough.
- Report rash, eye pain, difficulty voiding, palpitations, vision changes.

irbesartan

(er bah sar' tan)

Avapro

PREGNANCY CATEGORY C (FIRST TRIMESTER)

PREGNANCY CATEGORY D (SECOND AND THIRD TRIMESTERS)

Drug classes

Antihypertensive
ARB

Therapeutic actions

Selectively blocks the binding of angiotensin II to specific tissue receptors found in the vascular smooth muscle and adrenal gland; this action blocks the vasoconstriction effect of the renin-angiotensin system as well as the release of aldosterone, leading to decreased BP.

Indications

- Treatment of hypertension as monotherapy or in combination with other antihypertensives
- Slowing of the progression of nephropathy in patients with hypertension and type 2 diabetes

Contraindications and cautions

- Contraindicated with hypersensitivity to irbesartan, pregnancy (use during the second or third trimester can cause injury or even death to the fetus).
- Use cautiously with hepatic or renal impairment, hypovolemia, volume or sodium depletion, lactation.

Available forms

Tablets—75, 150, 300 mg

Dosages

Adults

- *Diabetic nephropathy:* 300 mg/day PO as a single dose.
- *Hypertension:* 150 mg PO daily as one dose; adjust slowly to determine effective dose; maximum daily dose, 300 mg.

Pediatric patients 13–16 yr
150 mg/day PO; maximum dose, 300 mg.
Pediatric patients 6–12 yr
75 mg/day PO, titrate to a maximum of 150 mg/day.
Pediatric patients younger than 6 yr
Not recommended.
Volume- or salt-depleted patients
75 mg/day PO.

Pharmacokinetics

Route	*Onset*	*Peak*
Oral	Varies	1–3 hr

Metabolism: Hepatic; $T_{1/2}$: 11–15 hr
Distribution: Crosses placenta; enters breast milk
Excretion: Feces, urine

Adverse effects

- **CNS:** *Headache, dizziness,* syncope, muscle weakness, sleep disturbance
- **CV:** Hypotension, orthostatic hypotension, flushing
- **Dermatologic:** Rash, inflammation, urticaria, pruritus, alopecia, dry skin
- **GI:** *Diarrhea, abdominal pain, nausea,* constipation, dry mouth, dental pain, dyspepsia
- **Respiratory:** *URI symptoms, cough,* sinus disorders
- **Other:** Cancer in preclinical studies, back pain, fever, gout, *fatigue,* neutropenia, **angioedema**

Interactions

✷ **Drug-drug** • Use caution with drugs metabolized by CYP2C9; anticipated effects may be altered

■ Nursing considerations

Assessment

- **History:** Hypersensitivity to irbesartan, pregnancy, lactation, hepatic or renal impairment, hypovolemia
- **Physical:** Skin lesions, turgor; T; reflexes, affect; BP; R, respiratory auscultation; LFTs, renal function tests

Interventions

- Administer without regard to meals.

⊠ ***Black box warning*** Ensure that patient is not pregnant before beginning therapy; suggest using barrier birth control while using irbesartan; fetal injury and deaths have been reported.

- Find an alternative method of feeding the baby if giving drug to a nursing mother. Depression of the renin-angiotensin system in infants is potentially very dangerous.

⊗ ***Warning*** Alert surgeon and mark the patient's chart with notice that irbesartan is being taken. The blockage of the renin-angiotensin system following surgery can produce problems. Hypotension may be reversed with volume expansion.

- Monitor patient closely in any situation that may lead to a decrease in BP secondary to reduction in fluid volume (excessive perspiration, dehydration, vomiting, diarrhea); excessive hypotension can occur.

Teaching points

- Take this drug without regard to meals. Do not stop taking this drug without consulting your health care provider.
- Use a barrier method of birth control while using this drug; if you become pregnant or desire to become pregnant, consult your health care provider.
- You may experience these side effects: Dizziness (more likely to occur in any situation where you may be fluid depleted [extreme heat, exertion]; avoid driving or performing hazardous tasks); headache (medications may be available to help); nausea, vomiting, diarrhea (proper nutrition is important; consult a dietitian); symptoms of upper respiratory tract infection, cough (do not self-medicate; consult your health care provider if this becomes uncomfortable).
- Report fever, chills, dizziness, pregnancy.

DANGEROUS DRUG

▽ irinotecan hydrochloride

*(eh rin **oh'** te kan)*

Camptosar

PREGNANCY CATEGORY D

Drug classes

Antineoplastic
DNA topoisomerase inhibitor

Therapeutic actions

Cytotoxic: Causes death of cells during cell division by causing damage to the DNA strand during DNA synthesis; specific to cells using topoisomerase I, DNA, and irinotecan complexes.

Indications

- First-line therapy in combination with 5-FU and leucovorin for patients with metastatic colon or rectal carcinomas
- Treatment of patients with metastatic colon or rectal cancer whose disease has recurred or progressed following 5-FU therapy
- Unlabeled uses: Cervical cancer, lung cancer, gastric cancer, CNS tumor

Contraindications and cautions

- Contraindicated with allergy to irinotecan, lactation, pregnancy.
- Use cautiously with bone marrow depression, severe diarrhea.

Available forms

Injection—20 mg/mL

Dosages

Adults

Monitor patient for toxicity at each visit, and modify dose based on patient tolerance.

- *Single-drug use:* 125 mg/m² IV over 90 min once weekly for 4 wk, then a 2-wk rest; repeat 6-wk regimen or 350 mg/m² IV over 90 min once every 3 wk.
- *Combination drugs:* 125 mg/m² IV over 90 min, days 1, 8, 15, and 22 with leucovorin 20 mg/m² IV bolus days 1, 8, 15, and 22 and 5-FU, 500 mg/m² IV days 1, 8, 15, and 22. Restart cycle on day 43. *Or* 180 mg/m² IV over 90 min days 1, 15, and 29 with leucovorin—200 mg/m² IV over 2 hr days 1, 2, 15, 16, 29, and 30 and 5-FU—400 mg/m² as IV bolus days 1, 2, 15, 16, 29, and 30 followed by 5-FU 600 mg/m² IV infusion over 22 hr on days 1, 2, 15, 16, 29, and 30. Restart cycle on day 43.

Pediatric patients

Not recommended.

Pharmacokinetics

Route	*Onset*	*Peak*
IV	Immediate	1–2 hr

Metabolism: Hepatic; $T_{1/2}$: 6–12 hr
Distribution: Crosses placenta; may enter breast milk, binds to albumin
Excretion: Bile, urine

IV FACTS

Preparation: Dilute in 5% dextrose injection or 0.9% sodium chloride injection to final concentration of 0.12–2.8 mg/mL. Store diluted drug protected from light; use within 48 hr if refrigerated or within 24 hr if at room temperature (5% dextrose only). Store vials at room temperature, protected from light.
Infusion: Infuse total dose over 90 min.
Incompatibilities: Do not add any other drugs to solution.

Adverse effects

- **CNS:** Insomnia, dizziness, asthenia, confusion
- **Dermatologic:** *Alopecia,* sweating, flushing, rashes
- **GI:** *Nausea, vomiting, diarrhea,* constipation, stomatitis, flatulence, dyspepsia, abdominal pain, anorexia, mucositis
- **Hematologic: Neutropenia, leukopenia, anemia, thrombocytopenia**
- **Respiratory:** *Dyspnea,* cough, rhinitis
- **Other:** Fatigue, malaise, pain, infections, fever, cramping, weight loss, pain, infection

Interactions

✱ **Drug-drug** • Irinotecan used with other antineoplastics may cause excessive diarrhea, myelosuppression, and other associated adverse reactions • Increased risk of dehydration if patient is also on diuretics; withhold diuretics if patient has nausea and vomiting • Risk of severe toxicity with ketoconazole; combination is contraindicated

✱ **Drug-alternative therapy** • May decrease irinotecan plasma levels and efficacy if taken with St. John's wort; combination is contraindicated

■ Nursing considerations

Assessment

- **History:** Allergy to irinotecan, diarrhea, pregnancy, lactation, bone marrow depression
- **Physical:** T; skin lesions, color, turgor; orientation, affect, reflexes; R; abdominal examination, bowel sounds; CBC with differential

Interventions

⊠ ***Black box warning*** Obtain CBC before each infusion; do not give to patients with a baseline neutrophil count of less than 1,500 cells/mm^2; consult with physician for reduction in dose or withholding of drug if bone marrow depression becomes evident; severe bone marrow depression can occur.

⊗ ***Warning*** Ensure that patient is not pregnant before beginning therapy; advise the use of barrier contraceptives.

- Monitor infusion site; if extravasation occurs, flush with sterile water and apply ice.

⊠ ***Black box warning*** Monitor for diarrhea; assess hydration and arrange to decrease dose if 4–6 stools/day; omit a dose if 7–9 stools/day; if 10 or more stools/day, consult a physician. Early diarrhea may be prevented or ameliorated by atropine 0.25–1 mg IV or subcutaneously; treat late diarrhea lasting more than 24 hr with loperamide.

- Protect patient from any exposure to infection.
- Arrange for wig or other appropriate head covering when alopecia occurs.

Teaching points

- This drug can only be given by IV infusion, which will run over 90 minutes. Mark calendar with days to return for infusion. A blood test will be required before each dose.
- This drug cannot be used during pregnancy; using barrier contraceptives is suggested.
- You may experience these side effects: Increased susceptibility to infection (avoid crowded areas or people with known infections; report any injury); nausea, vomiting (eat frequent small meals; medication may be ordered); headache; loss of hair (arrange for a wig or other head covering; it is important to protect the head from extreme temperatures); diarrhea.
- Report pain at injection site, any injury or illness, fatigue, severe nausea or vomiting, increased, severe, or bloody diarrhea.

▽ iron dextran

DexFerrum, INFeD, Infufer (CAN)

PREGNANCY CATEGORY C

Drug class

Iron preparation

Therapeutic actions

Elevates the serum iron concentration and is then converted to Hgb or trapped in the reticuloendothelial cells for storage and eventual conversion to usable form of iron.

Indications

- Treatment of iron deficiency anemia only when oral administration of iron is unsatisfactory or impossible
- Unlabeled use: May be required for patients receiving epoetin therapy

Contraindications and cautions

- Contraindicated with allergy to iron dextran, anemias other than iron deficiency anemia, acute phase of infectious renal disease.
- Use cautiously with impaired hepatic function, rheumatoid arthritis, allergies, asthma, lactation, pregnancy.

Available forms

Injection—50 mg/mL

Dosages

Adults and pediatric patients

- *Iron deficiency anemia:* Administer a 0.5 mL IM or IV test dose before therapy. Base dosage on hematologic response with frequent Hgb determinations.

For patients weighing more than 15 kg: Use the following formula:
Dose (mL) = [0.0442 (desired Hgb − observed Hgb) × LBW] + (0.26 × LBW),

where Hgb = Hgb in g/dL and LBW = lean body weight.
Determine LBW as follows:
For males: LBW = 50 kg + 2.3 kg for each inch of patient's height over 5 ft.
For females: LBW = 45.5 kg + 2.3 kg for each inch of patient's height over 5 ft.
For children 5–15 kg and older than 4 mo: Use the following formula:
Dose (mL) = 0.0442 (desired Hgb – observed Hgb) × W + (0.26 × W), where W = actual weight in kg.

- *Iron replacement for blood loss:* Determine dosage by the following formula: Replacement iron (in mg) = blood loss (in mL) × Hct

IM

Inject only into the upper outer quadrant of the buttocks. Give test dose of 0.5 mL IM. If tolerated, do not exceed 0.5 mL (25 mg) for infants weighing less than 5 kg; 1 mL for those more than 5 to less than 10 kg; 2 mL for all others.

IV injection

Give a test dose of 0.5 mL over at least 5 min before beginning therapy. May give up to 2 mL per daily dose (100 mg). Give slowly at 50 mg/min or less, undiluted.

Pharmacokinetics

Route	*Onset*	*Peak*
IM	Slow	1–2 wk

Metabolism: $T_{1/2}$: 6 hr
Distribution: Crosses placenta; enters breast milk
Excretion: Blood loss

IV FACTS

Preparation: *Intermittent IV:* Calculate dose from formula. Give individual doses of 2 mL or less per day. Use single-dose ampules without preservatives. *IV infusion:* Dilute needed dose in 200–250 mL of normal saline.
Infusion: *Intermittent IV:* Give undiluted and slowly—1 mL or less/min. *IV infusion (not approved by the FDA):* Infuse over 1–2 hr after a test dose of 25 mL. Do not mix with other drugs or add to parenteral nutrition.

Adverse effects

- **CNS:** Headache, backache, dizziness, malaise, transitory paresthesias, seizures, numbness, syncope, unconsciousness
- **CV:** Hypotension, chest pain, shock, tachycardia, **cardiac arrest,** hypertension, arrhythmias
- **GI:** *Nausea, vomiting,* diarrhea, abdominal pain, altered taste
- **Hypersensitivity:** Hypersensitivity reactions, including **anaphylaxis;** dyspnea, urticaria, rash and itching, arthralgia and myalgia, fever, sweating, purpura
- **Local:** *Pain, inflammation and sterile abscesses at injection site, brown skin discoloration* (IM use); *lymphadenopathy, local phlebitis, peripheral vascular flushing* (IV administration)
- **Other:** *Arthritic reactivation,* fever, shivering, sweating, rash, pruritus, arthritis, iron overload, cyanosis

Interactions

✱ **Drug-drug** • Delayed response to iron dextran therapy in patients taking chloramphenicol
✱ **Drug-lab test** • Use caution when interpreting serum iron levels when done within 4 hr of iron dextran injection • Serum may be discolored to a brownish color following IV injection • Bone scans using Tc-99m diphosphonate may have abnormal areas following IM injection

■ Nursing considerations

Assessment

- **History:** Allergy to iron dextran, anemias other than iron deficiency anemia, impaired liver function, rheumatoid arthritis, allergies or asthma, lactation, pregnancy
- **Physical:** Skin lesions, color; T; injection site examination; range of motion, joints; R, adventitious sounds; liver evaluation; CBC, Hgb, Hct, serum ferritin assays, LFTs

Interventions

- Verify that patient has iron deficiency anemia before treatment.
- Arrange treatment of underlying cause of iron deficiency anemia.

- Give IM injections using the Z-track technique (displace skin laterally before injection) to avoid injection into the tissue and tissue staining. Use a large-gauge needle; if patient is standing, have patient support self on leg not receiving the injection. If patient is lying down, have the injection site uppermost.

⊗ ***Black box warning*** Monitor patient for hypersensitivity reactions; test dose is highly recommended. Keep epinephrine readily available in case severe hypersensitivity reaction occurs.

- Monitor serum ferritin levels periodically; these correlate well with iron stores. Do not give with oral iron preparations.
- Caution patients with rheumatoid arthritis that acute exacerbation of joint pain and swelling may occur; provide appropriate comfort measures.

Teaching points

- Treatment will end if anemia is corrected.
- Have periodic blood tests during therapy to assess drug response and determine appropriate dosage.
- Do not take oral iron products or vitamins with iron added while using this drug.
- You may experience these side effects: Pain at injection site, headache, joint and muscle aches, GI upset.
- Report difficulty breathing, pain at injection site, rash, itching.

▽iron sucrose

See Appendix W, *Less commonly used drugs*.

▽isocarboxazid

See Appendix W, *Less commonly used drugs*.

▽isoniazid (isonicotinic acid hydrazide, INH)

*(eye soe **nye'** a zid)*

Isotamine (CAN), Nydrazid

PREGNANCY CATEGORY C

Drug class

Antituberculotic

Therapeutic actions

Bactericidal: Interferes with lipid and nucleic acid biosynthesis in actively growing tubercle bacilli.

Indications

- TB, all forms in which organisms are susceptible
- Prophylaxis in specific patients who are tuberculin reactors or household members of recently diagnosed tuberculars or who are considered to be high risk (patients with HIV, IV drug users, recent converters [5 mm or more increase on skin test within 2 yr in patients younger than 35 yr or 15 mm or more increase in patients older than 35 yr] and children younger than 4 yr with 10 mm or more induration on purified protein derivative tuberculin skin test)
- Unlabeled use of 300–400 mg/day, increased over 2 wk to 20 mg/kg/day, for improvement of severe tremor in patients with MS

Contraindications and cautions

- Contraindicated with allergy to isoniazid, isoniazid-associated hepatic injury or other severe adverse reactions to isoniazid, acute hepatic disease.
- Use cautiously with renal impairment, lactation, pregnancy.

Available forms

Tablets—100, 300 mg; syrup—50 mg/5 mL; injection—100 mg/mL

Dosages

Adults

- *Treatment of active TB:* 5 mg/kg/day (up to 300 mg) PO in a single dose, with other effective drugs or 15 mg/kg (up to 900 mg) PO two or three times per week. "First-line treatment" is considered to be 300 mg INH plus 600 mg rifampin, each given in a single daily oral dose. Consult manufacturer's guidelines for other possible combinations.
- *Prophylaxis for TB:* 300 mg/day PO in a single dose.
- Concomitant administration of 10–50 mg/day of pyridoxine is recommended for those

who are malnourished or predisposed to neuropathy (alcoholics, diabetics).

Pediatric patients

- *Treatment of active TB:* 10–15 mg/kg/day (up to 300 mg) PO in a single dose, with other effective drugs or 20–40 mg/kg (up to 900 mg/day) two or three times per week.
- *Prophylaxis for TB:* 10 mg/kg/day (up to 300 mg) PO in a single dose.

Pharmacokinetics

Route	*Onset*	*Peak*	*Duration*
Oral	Varies	1–2 hr	24 hr

Metabolism: Hepatic; $T_{1/2}$: 1–4 hr
Distribution: Crosses placenta; enters breast milk
Excretion: Urine

Adverse effects

- **CNS:** *Peripheral neuropathy,* seizures, toxic encephalopathy, optic neuritis and atrophy, memory impairment, toxic psychosis
- **GI:** *Nausea, vomiting, epigastric distress,* bilirubinemia, bilirubinuria, *elevated AST,* ALT levels, jaundice, **hepatitis**
- **Hematologic:** Agranulocytosis, hemolytic or aplastic anemia, **thrombocytopenia,** eosinophilia, pyridoxine deficiency, pellagra, hyperglycemia, metabolic acidosis, hypocalcemia, hypophosphatemia due to altered vitamin D metabolism
- **Hypersensitivity:** Fever, skin eruptions, lymphadenopathy, vasculitis
- **Local:** *Local irritation at IM injection site*
- **Other:** Gynecomastia, rheumatic syndrome, SLE syndrome

Interactions

✱ **Drug-drug** • Increased incidence of isoniazid-related hepatitis with alcohol and possibly if taken in high doses with rifampin • Increased serum levels of phenytoin • Increased effectiveness and risk of toxicity of carbamazepine • Risk of high output renal failure in fast INH acetylators with enflurane • Increased risk of hepatotoxicity with acetaminophen, rifampin

✱ **Drug-food** • Risk of sympathetic-type reactions with tyramine-containing foods and exaggerated response (headache, palpitations, sweating, hypotension, flushing, diarrhea, itching) to histamine-containing food (fish [skipjack, tuna] sauerkraut juice, yeast extracts)

■ Nursing considerations

Assessment

- **History:** Allergy to isoniazid, isoniazid-associated adverse reactions; acute hepatic disease; renal impairment; lactation, pregnancy
- **Physical:** Skin color, lesions; T; orientation, reflexes, peripheral sensitivity, bilateral grip strength; ophthalmologic examination; R, adventitious sounds; liver evaluation; CBC, LFTs, renal function tests, blood glucose

Interventions

- Give on an empty stomach, 1 hr before or 2 hr after meals; may be given with food if GI upset occurs.
- Give in a single daily dose. Reserve parenteral dose for patients unable to take oral medications.
- Decrease foods containing tyramine or histamine in patient's diet.
- Consult with physician and arrange for daily pyridoxine in diabetic, alcoholic, or malnourished patients; also for patients who develop peripheral neuritis, and those with HIV.

⊗ ***Warning*** Discontinue drug, and consult with physician if signs of hypersensitivity occur.

☒ ***Black box warning*** Monitor liver enzymes monthly; risk of serious to fatal hepatitis.

Teaching points

- Take this drug in a single daily dose. Take drug on an empty stomach, 1 hour before or 2 hours after meals. If GI distress occurs, may be taken with food.
- Take this drug regularly; avoid missing doses; do not discontinue without first consulting your health care provider.
- Do not drink alcohol, or drink as little as possible. There is an increased risk of hepatitis if these two drugs are combined.
- Avoid foods containing tyramine; consult a dietitian to obtain a list of foods containing tyramine or histamine.

- Have periodic medical check-ups, including an eye examination and blood tests, to evaluate the drug effects.
- You may experience these side effects: Nausea, vomiting, epigastric distress (take drug with meals); skin rashes or lesions; numbness, tingling, loss of sensation (use caution to prevent injury or burns).
- Report weakness, fatigue, loss of appetite, nausea, vomiting, yellowing of skin or eyes, darkening of the urine, numbness or tingling in hands or feet.

DANGEROUS DRUG

isoproterenol
*(eye soe proe **ter'** e nole)*

isoproterenol hydrochloride
Isuprel

PREGNANCY CATEGORY C

Drug classes
Antiasthmatic
$Beta_1$- and $beta_2$-adrenergic agonist
Bronchodilator
Sympathomimetic
Vasopressor in shock

Therapeutic actions
Effects are mediated by $beta_1$- and $beta_2$-adrenergic receptors; acts on $beta_1$-receptors in the heart to produce positive chronotropic and positive inotropic effects and to increase automaticity; acts on $beta_2$-receptors in the bronchi to cause bronchodilation; acts on $beta_2$-receptors in smooth muscle in the walls of blood vessels in skeletal muscle and splanchnic beds to cause dilation (cardiac stimulation, vasodilation may be adverse effects when drug is used as bronchodilator).

Indications
- Management of bronchospasm during anesthesia; a vasopressor in shock
- Adjunct in the management of shock (hypoperfusion syndrome) and in the treatment of cardiac standstill or arrest; carotid sinus hypersensitivity; heart block; Stokes-Adams syndrome; heart failure; ventricular tachycardia and ventricular arrhythmias that require increased inotropic activity for therapy

Contraindications and cautions
- Contraindicated with hypersensitivity to isoproterenol; tachyarrhythmias, tachycardia caused by digoxin toxicity; acute angina; general anesthesia with halogenated hydrocarbons or cyclopropane (sensitize the myocardium to catecholamines); labor and delivery (may delay second stage of labor; can accelerate fetal heart beat; may cause hypoglycemia, hypokalemia, pulmonary edema in the mother, and hypoglycemia in the neonate).
- Use cautiously with unstable vasomotor system disorders, hypertension, coronary insufficiency, history of CVA, COPD patients with degenerative heart disease, diabetes mellitus, hyperthyroidism, history of seizure disorders, psychoneuroses, lactation, pregnancy.

Available forms
Injection—0.02 (1:50,000), 0.2 (1:5,000) mg/mL

Dosages
Adults
Injection
- *Bronchospasm during anesthesia:* 0.01–0.02 mg (0.5–1 mL of diluted solution) bolus IV; repeat when necessary.
- *Shock:* 0.5–5 mcg/min; infuse IV at a rate adjusted on the basis of HR, CVP, systemic BP, and urine flow.
- *Cardiac standstill and arrhythmias:* IV injection, 0.02–0.06 mg using diluted solution. IV infusion, 5 mcg/min using diluted solution.

Pediatric patients
There are no well-controlled studies in children. The American Heart Association recommends an infusion of 0.1 mcg/kg/min as an initial dose; range, 0.1–1 mcg/kg/min.
- *Bronchospasm during anesthesia (patients 7–19 yr):* 0.05–0.17 mcg/kg/min. Maximum dose, 1.3–2.7 mcg/kg/min. Postoperative cardiac patients will need a lower dose than patients with asthma.

Geriatric patients

Patients older than 60 yr are more likely to experience side effects; use with extreme caution.

Pharmacokinetics

Route	Onset	Duration
IV	Immediate	1–2 min

Metabolism: Tissue; $T_{1/2}$: Unknown
Distribution: Crosses placenta; enters breast milk
Excretion: Urine

IV FACTS

Preparation: Dilute the 1:5,000 solutions for IV injection or infusion with 5% dextrose or sodium chloride injection; a convenient dilution is 1 mg isoproterenol (5 mL) in 500 mL diluent (final concentration 1:500,000 or 2 mcg/mL).
Infusion: Dosage of 5 mcg/min is provided by infusing 2.5 mL/min; adjust dosage to keep heart rate less than 110 beats per min.
Incompatibilities: Do not combine with aminophylline, barbiturates, lidocaine, sodium bicarbonate.

Adverse effects

- **CNS:** *Restlessness, apprehension, anxiety, fear,* CNS stimulation, hyperkinesia, insomnia, tremor, drowsiness, irritability, weakness, vertigo, headache
- **CV:** *Cardiac arrhythmias, tachycardia, palpitations,* anginal pain, changes in BP, paradoxical precipitation of Stokes-Adams seizures during normal sinus rhythm or transient heart block
- **GI:** *Nausea, vomiting, heartburn,* unusual or bad taste, swelling of the parotid glands
- **Respiratory:** *Respiratory difficulties,* dyspnea, **pulmonary edema,** *coughing, bronchospasm, paradoxical airway resistance with repeated, excessive use*
- **Other:** *Sweating, pallor,* flushing, muscle cramps, blurred vision

Interactions

✱ **Drug-drug** • Increased peripheral vasoconstriction if given with ergot alkaloids; if this combination is used, monitor BP and perfusion carefully • Increased BP response may occur if combined with TCAs, halogenated hydrocarbon anesthetics, oxytocic drugs; monitor patient closely and adjust dosage as needed • Possible arrhythmias with epinephrine; do not administer together

■ Nursing considerations

Assessment

- **History:** Hypersensitivity to isoproterenol; tachyarrhythmias; general anesthesia with halogenated hydrocarbons or cyclopropane; unstable vasomotor system disorders; hypertension; CAD; history of CVA; COPD patients with degenerative heart disease; diabetes mellitus; hyperthyroidism; seizure disorders; psychoneurotic disorders; labor and delivery; lactation
- **Physical:** Weight; skin color, T, turgor; orientation, reflexes; P, BP; R, adventitious sounds; blood and urine glucose, serum electrolytes, thyroid function tests, ECG

Interventions

- Protect drug from light, and keep in original carton until use.
- Use minimal doses for minimum periods; drug tolerance can occur with prolonged use.

⊗ ***Warning*** Keep a beta-adrenergic blocker (a cardioselective beta-adrenergic blocker, such as atenolol, should be used in patients with respiratory distress) readily available in case cardiac arrhythmias occur.

Teaching points

- This drug is given IV.
- You may experience these side effects: Drowsiness, dizziness, inability to sleep (use caution); nausea, vomiting (eat frequent small meals); anxiety; rapid heart rate.
- Report chest pain, dizziness, insomnia, weakness, tremor or irregular heart beat.

isosorbide nitrates

(eye soe sor' bide)

isosorbide dinitrate

Apo-ISDN (CAN), Dilatrate SR (DNC), Isochron (DNC), Isordil Dinitrate, Isordil Titradose

isosorbide mononitrate

Imdur (DNC), ISMO, Monoket

PREGNANCY CATEGORY C

PREGNANCY CATEGORY B (IMDUR, MONOKET)

Drug classes

Antianginal
Nitrate
Vasodilator

Therapeutic actions

Relaxes vascular smooth muscle with a resultant decrease in venous return and decrease in arterial BP, which reduces left ventricular workload and decreases myocardial oxygen consumption.

Indications

- Dinitrate: Treatment and prevention of angina pectoris
- Mononitrate: Prevention of angina pectoris; treatment of angina pectoris (*Monoket*)
- Unlabeled use (dinitrate): Used with hydralazine in black patients with advanced heart failure; acute angle-closure glaucoma in emergent situations; achalasia
- Unlabeled use (mononitrate): Used with nadolol to prevent recurrent variceal bleeding

Contraindications and cautions

- Contraindicated with allergy to nitrates, severe anemia, head trauma, cerebral hemorrhage, hypertrophic cardiomyopathy, narrow-angle glaucoma, orthostatic hypotension.
- Use cautiously with pregnancy, lactation, acute MI, heart failure.

Available forms

Dinitrate: Tablets—5, 10, 20, 30, 40 mg; ER tablets (DNC)—40 mg; SR capsules (DNC)—40 mg; SL tablets—2.5, 5 mg

Mononitrate: Tablets —10, 20 mg; ER tablets (DNC)—30, 60, 120 mg

Dosages

Adults

To avoid tolerance to drug, take short-acting products bid or tid with last dose no later than 7 PM and ER or SR products once daily or bid at 8 AM and 2 PM. This creates a nitrate-free period.

Isosorbide dinitrate

- *Angina pectoris:* Starting dose, 2.5–5 mg sublingual or 5- to 20-mg oral tablets. For maintenance, 10–40 mg every 6 hr or tid oral tablets or capsules; SR or ER, initially 40 mg, then 40–80 mg PO every 8–12 hr.
- *Acute prophylaxis:* Initial dosage, 2.5–5 mg sublingually every 2–3 hr. Give 15 min before activity that may cause angina.

Isosorbide mononitrate

- *Prevention of angina:* 20 mg PO bid given 7 hr apart. In smaller patients, start with 5 mg (one-half of 10-mg tablet) but then increase to at least 10 mg by day 2 or 3 of therapy. Give first dose when waking and second dose 7 hr later. This creates a nitrate-free period and minimizes tolerance to drug. ER tablets—30–60 mg/day PO may be increased to 120 mg/day if needed.

Pediatric patients

Safety and efficacy not established.

Pharmacokinetics

Route	Onset	Duration
Oral	15–45 min	4–6 hr
Oral SR, ER	Up to 4 hr	6–8 hr
SL	2–5 min	1–2 hr

Metabolism: Hepatic; $T_{1/2}$: 5 min, then 2–5 hr

Distribution: May cross placenta; may enter breast milk

Excretion: Urine

Adverse effects

- **CNS:** *Headache, apprehension, restlessness, weakness,* vertigo, dizziness, faintness
- **CV:** *Tachycardia, retrosternal discomfort, palpitations, hypotension,* **syncope,** *collapse, orthostatic hypotension, angina, rebound hypertension,* atrial fibrillation

- **Dermatologic:** Rash, exfoliative dermatitis, cutaneous vasodilation with flushing
- **GI:** *Nausea,* vomiting, incontinence of feces, abdominal pain, diarrhea, ulcer
- **GU:** Dysuria, impotence, urinary frequency
- **Other:** Muscle twitching, pallor, perspiration, cold sweat, arthralgia, bronchitis, thrombocytopenia

Interactions

✱ **Drug-drug** • Increased systolic BP and decreased antianginal effect if taken concurrently with ergot alkaloids

✱ **Drug-lab test** • False report of decreased serum cholesterol if done by the Zlatkis-Zak color reaction

■ Nursing considerations

CLINICAL ALERT!
Name confusion has occurred between *Isordil* (isosorbide) and *Plendil* (felodipine); use caution.

Assessment

- **History:** Allergy to nitrates, severe anemia, GI hypermobility, head trauma, cerebral hemorrhage, hypertrophic cardiomyopathy, pregnancy, lactation
- **Physical:** Skin color, T, lesions; orientation, reflexes, affect; P, BP, orthostatic BP, baseline ECG, peripheral perfusion; R, adventitious sounds; liver evaluation, normal output; CBC, Hgb

Interventions

- Give sublingual preparations under the tongue or in the buccal pouch; discourage the patient from swallowing.
- Create a nitrate-free period to minimize tolerance.

⊗ ***Warning*** Give chewable tablets slowly, only 5 mg initially, because severe hypotension can occur; ensure that patient does not chew or crush SR or ER preparations.

- Give oral preparations on an empty stomach, 1 hr before or 2 hr after meals; take with meals if severe, uncontrolled headache occurs.

⊗ ***Warning*** Keep life-support equipment readily available if overdose occurs or cardiac condition worsens.

⊗ ***Warning*** Gradually reduce dose if anginal treatment is being terminated; rapid discontinuation can lead to problems of withdrawal.

Teaching points

- Place sublingual tablets under your tongue or in your cheek; do not chew, swallow, or crush the tablet. Take the isosorbide before chest pain begins, when activities or situation may precipitate an attack. Take oral isosorbide dinitrate on an empty stomach, 1 hour before or 2 hours after meals; do not chew or crush extended- or sustained-release preparations; do not take isosorbide mononitrate to relieve acute anginal episodes.
- You may experience these side effects: Dizziness, light-headedness (may be transient; use care to change positions slowly); headache (lie down in a cool environment, rest; over-the-counter preparations may not help; take drug with meals); flushing of the neck or face (reversible).
- Report blurred vision, persistent or severe headache, rash, more frequent or more severe angina attacks, fainting.

▽ isotretinoin (13-*cis*-retinoic acid, vitamin A metabolite)

*(eye so **tret'** i noyn)*

Amnesteem (DNC), Claravis (DNC), Sotret (DNC)

PREGNANCY CATEGORY X

Drug classes

Acne product
Retinoid (first generation)
Vitamin metabolite

Therapeutic actions

Decreases sebaceous gland size and inhibits sebaceous gland differentiation, resulting in a reduction in sebum secretion; inhibits follicular keratinization; exact mechanism of action is not known.

Indications

- Treatment of severe recalcitrant nodular acne unresponsive to conventional treatments
- Unlabeled uses: Treatment of cutaneous disorders of keratinization, cutaneous T-cell lymphoma and leukoplakia, psoriasis, rosacea, pityriasis rubra pilaris, keratoacanthomas

Contraindications and cautions

- Contraindicated with allergy to isotretinoin, parabens, or product component; pregnancy (has caused severe fetal malformations and spontaneous abortions); lactation.
- Use cautiously with history of severe depression, suicidal ideation, diabetes mellitus, pediatric patients with genetic predisposition to age-related osteoporosis, a history of childhood osteoporosis, osteomalacia, other diseases of bone metabolism.

Available forms

Capsules DNC—10, 20, 30, 40 mg; soft gel capsules DNC—10, 20, 30, 40 mg

Dosages

Adults and pediatric patients 12 yr and older

Individualize dosage based on side effects and disease response. Initial dose, 0.5–1 mg/kg/day PO; usual dosage range is 0.5–2 mg/kg/day divided into two doses for 15–20 wk. Maximum daily dose, 2 mg/kg. If a second course of therapy is needed, allow a rest period of at least 8 wk between courses. Must take with food or absorption of drug will decrease.

Pharmacokinetics

Route	*Onset*	*Peak*	*Duration*
Oral	Varies	2.9–3.2 hr	6–20 hr

Metabolism: Hepatic; $T_{1/2}$: 10–20 hr
Distribution: Crosses placenta; may enter breast milk
Excretion: Urine

Adverse effects

- **CNS:** *Lethargy, insomnia, fatigue, headache,* pseudotumor cerebri (papilledema, headache, nausea, vomiting, visual disturbances); depression, psychoses, **suicide,** aggressive or violent behavior
- **CV:** Palpitations, tachycardia, vascular thrombotic disease
- **Dermatologic:** *Skin fragility, dry skin, pruritus, rash,* thinning of hair, peeling of palms and soles, skin infections, photosensitivity, nail brittleness, petechiae
- **EENT:** *Cheilitis, eye irritation, conjunctivitis,* corneal opacities, epistaxis
- **GI:** *Nausea, vomiting, abdominal pain,* anorexia, inflammatory bowel disease, dry mouth, gum irritation
- **GU:** *White cells in the urine, proteinuria, hematuria*
- **Hematologic:** Elevated sedimentation rate, hypertriglyceridemia, abnormal liver function tests, increased fasting serum glucose
- **Musculoskeletal:** Skeletal hyperostosis, arthralgia, bone and joint pain and stiffness
- **Respiratory:** *Epistaxis, dry nose, bronchospasms*

Interactions

✸ **Drug-drug** • Increased toxicity when taken with vitamin A; avoid this combination • Risk of increased adverse effects if combined with systemic corticosteroids, phenytoin; use caution if these combinations are used • Risk of pseudotumor cerebri with concomitant tetracycline use

■ Nursing considerations

Assessment

- **History:** Allergy to isotretinoin, parabens, or product component; diabetes mellitus; pregnancy; lactation; history of depression
- **Physical:** Skin color, lesions, turgor, texture; joint range of motion; orientation, reflexes, affect, ophthalmologic examination; mucous membranes, bowel sounds; serum triglycerides, HDL, sedimentation rate, CBC and differential, urinalysis, pregnancy test

Interventions

⊗ ***Black box warning*** Ensure that patient reads and signs the consent form that comes with this drug. Place this form in the patient's permanent record.

⊗ ***Black box warning*** Ensure that patient is not pregnant before therapy; test for pregnancy within 2 wk of beginning therapy.

Advise patient to use two forms of contraception starting 1 mo before therapy, during treatment, and for 1 mo after treatment is discontinued. Patient must sign consent form acknowledging this information; form should be kept in patient's medical record. Pharmacists must register patients in iPLEDGE program before dispensing drug. Patient may obtain no more than a 30-day supply.

- Do not give a second course of therapy within 8 wk of first course.
- Give drug with meals; do not crush capsules.
- Do not give vitamin supplements that contain vitamin A.

⊗ ***Warning*** Discontinue drug if signs of papilledema occur; consult with a neurologist for further care.

⊗ ***Warning*** Discontinue drug at any indication of severe depression or psychoses. Patient must sign informed consent concerning risk of suicide; form should be kept in patient's medical record.

- Discontinue drug if visual disturbances occur; arrange for an ophthalmologic examination.

⊗ ***Warning*** Discontinue drug if abdominal pain, rectal bleeding, or severe diarrhea occurs; consult with physician.

- Monitor triglycerides during therapy; if elevation occurs, institute measures to lower serum triglycerides: Reduce weight, reduce dietary fat, exercise, increase intake of insoluble fiber, decrease alcohol consumption.
- Monitor diabetic patients with frequent blood glucose determinations.
- Do not allow blood donation from patients taking isotretinoin due to the teratogenic effects of the drug.

Teaching points

- Only 1 month's prescription can be given at a time. You will need to complete a consent form before this drug is prescribed.
- Take drug with meals; do not crush capsules.
- Transient flare-ups of acne may occur at beginning of therapy.
- There is a risk of injury in pediatric patients who participate in sports that involve repetitive impact; parents should monitor activity and alert coaches.
- Use two forms of contraception 1 month before treatment, during treatment, and for 1 month after treatment is discontinued. This drug has been associated with severe birth defects and miscarriages; it is contraindicated in pregnant women. If you think that you are pregnant, consult your health care provider immediately. You must sign a consent form stating your understanding of the need for contraception.
- Do not donate blood while using this drug because of its potential effects on the fetus of a blood recipient.
- Avoid vitamin supplements containing vitamin A; serious toxic effects may occur. Limit your consumption of alcohol. You also may need to limit your intake of fats and increase exercise to limit drug effects on blood triglyceride levels.
- Avoid wax expilation and skin resurfacing during and for 6 months after therapy; scarring could occur.
- You may experience these side effects: Dizziness, lethargy, headache, visual changes (avoid driving or performing tasks that require alertness); sensitivity to the sun (avoid sunlamps, exposure to the sun; use sunscreens, protective clothing); diarrhea, abdominal pain, loss of appetite (take drug with meals); dry mouth (suck sugarless lozenges); eye irritation and redness, inability to wear contact lenses; dry skin, itching, redness, nose bleeds.
- Report headache with nausea and vomiting, severe diarrhea or rectal bleeding, visual difficulties, depression, suicidal ideation, violent or aggressive behavior.

▽isradipine

*(eyes **rad'** i peen)*

DynaCirc, DynaCirc CR DNC

PREGNANCY CATEGORY C

Drug classes

Antihypertensive
Calcium channel blocker

Therapeutic actions
Inhibits the movement of calcium ions across the membranes of cardiac and arterial muscle cells; calcium is involved in the generation of the action potential in specialized automatic and conducting cells in the heart and in arterial smooth muscle and excitation-contraction coupling in cardiac muscle cells; inhibition of transmembrane calcium flow results in the depression of impulse formation in specialized cardiac pacemaker cells, slowing of the velocity of conduction of the cardiac impulse, the depression of myocardial contractility, and the dilation of coronary arteries and arterioles and peripheral arterioles. These effects lead to decreased cardiac work, cardiac energy consumption, and BP.

Indications
- Management of hypertension alone or in combination with thiazide-type diuretics

Contraindications and cautions
- Contraindicated with allergy to isradipine; sick sinus syndrome, except with ventricular pacemaker; heart block (second or third degree); IHSS; cardiogenic shock.
- Use cautiously in the elderly and with hypotension, impaired hepatic or renal function (repeated doses may accumulate), pregnancy, lactation, heart failure.

Available forms
Capsules—2.5, 5 mg; CR tablets DNC—5, 10 mg

Dosages
Adults
Initial dose of 2.5 mg PO bid. An antihypertensive effect is usually seen within 2–3 hr; maximal response may require 2–4 wk. Dosage may be increased in increments of 5 mg/day at 2- to 4-wk intervals. Maximum dose, 20 mg/day. CR: 5–10 mg PO daily as monotherapy or combined with thiazide diuretic.
Pediatric patients
Safety and efficacy are not established.
Geriatric patients and patients with hepatic or renal impairment
Starting dose is 5 mg/day PO for CR tablets; 2.5 mg PO bid for capsules.

Pharmacokinetics

Route	*Onset*	*Peak*
Oral	40 min	90 min
CR	NA	7–8 hr

Metabolism: Hepatic; $T_{1/2}$: 8 hr
Distribution: Crosses placenta; enters breast milk; 95% protein-bound
Excretion: Feces, urine

Adverse effects
- **CNS:** *Dizziness,* vertigo, emotional depression, sleepiness, *headache*
- **CV:** *Peripheral edema, hypotension,* arrhythmias, bradycardia, **AV heart block, angina, MI, CVA** (increased risk with isradipine than with other calcium channel blockers)
- **GI:** *Nausea,* constipation, abdominal discomfort, diarrhea
- **Other:** Muscle fatigue, diaphoresis, fatigue, rash

Interactions
✱ **Drug-drug** • Increased cardiac depression with beta-adrenergic blocking drugs • Increased serum levels of digoxin, carbamazepine, prazosin, and quinidine • Increased respiratory depression with atracurium, pancuronium, tubocurarine, and vecuronium • Decreased effects with calcium and rifampin • Increased isradipine levels with azole antifungals and H_2 antagonists • Risk of severe hypotension with fentanyl anesthesia; use caution

■ Nursing considerations
Assessment
- **History:** Allergy to isradipine; sick sinus syndrome, heart block; IHSS; cardiogenic shock, severe heart failure; hypotension; impaired hepatic or renal function; pregnancy; lactation
- **Physical:** Skin color, edema; orientation, reflexes; P, BP, baseline ECG, peripheral perfusion, auscultation; R, adventitious sounds; liver evaluation, normal output; LFTs, renal function tests, urinalysis

Interventions
- Consider increased risk of angina, MI, and CVA with use of this drug; select patients carefully.

⊗ ***Warning*** Monitor patient carefully (BP, cardiac rhythm, and output) while drug is being adjusted to therapeutic dose.

- Monitor BP very carefully with concurrent doses of other antihypertensive drugs.
- Monitor cardiac rhythm regularly during stabilization of dosage and periodically during long-term therapy.

⊗ ***Warning*** Monitor patients with renal or hepatic impairment carefully for drug accumulation and adverse reactions.

Teaching points

- Swallow controlled-release tablets whole. Do not crush, chew, or divide them. The empty shell is eliminated in the stool.
- You may experience these side effects: Nausea, vomiting (eat frequent small meals); headache (monitor lighting, noise, and temperature; medication may be ordered if severe); dizziness, sleepiness (avoid driving or operating dangerous equipment); emotional depression (should pass when the drug is stopped); constipation (measures may be taken to alleviate this problem).
- Report irregular heart beat, shortness of breath, swelling of the hands or feet, pronounced dizziness, constipation.

▽itraconazole

*(eye tra **kon'** a zole)*

Sporanox

PREGNANCY CATEGORY C

Drug class

Antifungal—triazole

Therapeutic actions

Binds to sterols in the fungal cell membrane, changing membrane permeability; fungicidal or fungistatic depending on concentration and organism.

Indications

- Parenteral and oral: Treatment of blastomycosis, histoplasmosis in immunocompromised and nonimmunocompromised patients
- Parenteral and oral: Treatment of aspergillosis in patients intolerant or refractory to amphotericin B
- Treatment of onychomycosis due to dermatophytes (capsules only)
- Parenteral and oral: Treatment of febrile neutropenic patients with suspected fungal infections
- Oral solution: Treatment of fungal, candidiasis infections of the esophagus or mouth
- Unlabeled uses: Treatment of superficial and systemic mycoses, fungal keratitis, cutaneous leishmaniasis; used as an alternative to fluconazole for HIV patients to prevent candiasis, cryptococcosis, and coccidiodomycosis

Contraindications and cautions

- Contraindicated with hypersensitivity to itraconazole or other azoles, lactation, heart failure, history of prolonged QTc interval.
- Use cautiously with hepatic or renal impairment, arrhythmias, pregnancy.

Available forms

Capsules—100 mg; oral solution—10 mg/mL

Dosages

Adults

- *Empiric febrile neutropenia:* 200 mg PO bid until clinically significant neutropenia resolves.
- *Candidiasis:* 200 mg/day PO (oral solution only) for 1–2 wk (oro-pharyngeal); 100 mg/day for a minimum of 3 wk (esophageal); 200 mg/day in AIDS patients and neutropenic patients.
- *Blastomycosis or chronic histoplasmosis:* 200 mg/day PO for a minimum of 3 mo, may increase to a maximum of 400 mg/day.
- *Other systemic mycoses:* 100–200 mg/day for 3–6 mo.
- *Dermatophytoses:* 100–200 mg/day to bid for 7–28 days, determined by specific infection.
- *Fingernail onychomycosis:* 200 mg bid PO for 1 wk, followed by 3-wk rest period; repeat.
- *Toenail onychomycosis:* 200 mg/day PO for 12 wk.
- *Aspergillosis:* 200–400 mg/day PO.

Oral solution
100–200 mg (10–20 mL), rinse and hold, swallow solution daily for 1–3 wk.

Pediatric patients
Safety and efficacy not established.

Patients with renal impairment
Do not give to patients if creatinine clearance less than 30 mL/min.

Pharmacokinetics

Route	*Onset*	*Peak*	*Duration*
Oral	Slow	4.6 hr	4–6 days

Metabolism: Hepatic; $T_{1/2}$: 21 hr, then 64 hr
Distribution: Crosses placenta; may enter breast milk, highly protein-bound
Excretion: Feces, urine

Adverse effects

- **CNS:** *Headache,* dizziness
- **CV: Heart failure**
- **GI:** *Nausea, vomiting, diarrhea, abdominal pain,* anorexia, hepatic function abnormality
- **Other:** *Rash, edema,* fever, malaise

Interactions

✱ Drug-drug ⊗ ***Black box warning*** Potential for serious CV events, including ventricular tachycardia and death, with lovastatin, simvastatin, triazolam, midazolam, pimozide, dofetilide, and quinidine; avoid these combinations.

• Increased serum levels and therefore therapeutic and toxic effects of cyclosporine, digoxin, oral hypoglycemics, warfarin anticoagulants, phenytoin, and buspirone • Decreased serum levels with histamine-2 antagonists, antacids, proton pump inhibitors, isoniazid, phenytoin, rifampin, carbamazepine, phenobarbital, and nevirapine • Increased plasma level of itraconazole with macrolide antibiotics and protease inhibitors • Potential for prolonged sedation if combined with benzodiazepines • Increased risk of rhabdomyolysis with lovastatin

✱ Drug-food • Risk of decreased effectiveness if combined with grapefruit juice, orange juice • Risk of increased effects if combined with cola beverages; avoid this combination

■ Nursing considerations

Assessment

- **History:** Hypersensitivity to itraconazole, hepatic impairment, lactation, heart failure, prolonged QTc interval, pregnancy
- **Physical:** Skin color, lesions; T; orientation, reflexes, affect; bowel sounds, BP, P, auscultation; LFTs; culture of area involved, ECG

Interventions

- Culture of infection before beginning therapy; begin treatment before laboratory results are returned.
- Screen medications to prevent serious drug interactions.
- Decrease dosage in cases of hepatic failure.

⊗ ***Black box warning*** Do not administer to patients with evidence of cardiac dysfunction or heart failure; risk of severe heart failure.

- Give oral capsules with meals to facilitate absorption.

⊗ ***Warning*** Monitor LFTs regularly in patients with a history of hepatic impairment; discontinue or decrease dosage at signs of increased liver toxicity.

- Discontinue drug at any sign of active liver disease—elevated enzymes, hepatitis; or signs of heart failure.

Teaching points

- Take the full course of drug therapy that has been prescribed. Therapy may need to be long term.
- Take capsules with food; take oral solution without food.
- Adopt hygiene measures to prevent reinfection or spread of infection.
- Have frequent follow-up visits while you are using this drug. Keep all appointments, which may include those for blood tests.
- Women of childbearing age should use contraceptives during therapy and for 1 month after therapy is stopped.
- You may experience these side effects: Nausea, vomiting, diarrhea (eat frequent small meals); headache (analgesics may be ordered); rash, itching (appropriate medication may help).
- Report unusual fatigue, anorexia, vomiting, jaundice, dark urine, pale stool, edema, difficulty breathing.

I

ivermectin

See Appendix W, *Less commonly used drugs.*

ixabepilone

See Appendix W, *Less commonly used drugs.*

kanamycin sulfate

(kan a ***mye'*** *sin)*

Kantrex

PREGNANCY CATEGORY D

Drug class

Aminoglycoside antibiotic

Therapeutic actions

Bactericidal: Inhibits protein synthesis in strains of gram-negative bacteria; functional integrity of cell membrane appears to be disrupted, causing cell death.

Indications

- Infections caused by susceptible strains of *Escherichia coli, Proteus, Enterobacter aerogenes, Klebsiella pneumoniae, Serratia marcescens, Acinetobacter*
- Treatment of severe infections due to susceptible strains of staphylococci in patients allergic to other antibiotics
- As part of a multidrug therapy for *Mycobacterium avium* complex (an infection in AIDS patients)

Contraindications and cautions

- Contraindicated with allergy to aminoglycosides; intestinal obstruction, pregnancy, lactation.
- Use cautiously with elderly or any patient with diminished hearing, decreased renal function, dehydration, neuromuscular disorders.

Available forms

Injection—500 mg, 1 g; pediatric injection—75 mg

Dosages

Adults and pediatric patients

Do not exceed 1.5 g/day.

IM

7.5 mg/kg every 12 hr or 15 mg/kg/day in equally divided doses every 6–8 hr. Usual duration is 7–10 days. Do not exceed 1.5 g per day. If no effect in 3–5 days, discontinue therapy.

IV

15 mg/kg/day divided into two or three equal doses, administered over 30–60 min.

Intraperitoneal

500 mg diluted in 20 mL sterile water instilled into the wound closure.

Aerosol

250 mg bid–qid, nebulized.

Geriatric patients or patients with renal failure

Reduce dosage, and carefully monitor serum drug levels and renal function tests. When not possible, reduce frequency of administration. Calculate dosing interval from the following: Dosage interval in hr = serum creatinine (mg/dL) × 9.

Pharmacokinetics

Route	*Onset*	*Peak*
IM, IV	Rapid	30–120 min

Metabolism: $T_{1/2}$: 2–3 hr
Distribution: Crosses placenta; enters breast milk
Excretion: Urine, feces

IV FACTS

Preparation: Do not mix with other antibacterial drugs; administer separately; dilute contents of 500-mg vial with 100–200 mL of normal saline or D_5W; dilute 1 g-vial with 200–400 mL of diluent; vials may darken during storage, does not affect potency.
Infusion: Administer dose slowly over 30–60 min (especially important in children).
Incompatibilities: Do not combine with amphotericin B, cephapirin, chlorpheniramine, colistimethate, heparin, methohexital, or other antibacterials.

Adverse effects

- **CNS:** *Ototoxicity–tinnitus, dizziness, vertigo, deafness* (partially reversible to irreversible), confusion, disorientation, depression, lethargy, nystagmus, visual disturbances, headache, fever, tremor, paresthesias, muscle twitching, seizures, muscular weakness, neuromuscular blockade, apnea
- **CV:** Palpitations, hypotension, hypertension
- **GI:** *Nausea, vomiting, anorexia, diarrhea,* weight loss, increased salivation, malabsorption syndrome
- **GU:** *Nephrotoxicity* (may be irreversible)
- **Hematologic:** Leukemoid reaction, agranulocytosis, granulocytosis, leukopenia, leukocytosis, thrombocytopenia, eosinophilia, anemia, hemolytic anemia, increased or decreased reticulocyte count
- **Hepatic:** Hepatic toxicity; hepatomegaly
- **Hypersensitivity:** Purpura, rash, urticaria, exfoliative dermatitis
- **Other:** *Superinfections, pain and irritation at IM injection sites*

Interactions

✱ **Drug-drug** • Increased ototoxic and nephrotoxic effects with potent diuretics and other ototoxic and nephrotoxic drugs (cephalosporins, penicillins) • Increased likelihood of neuromuscular blockade if given shortly after general anesthetics, depolarizing and nondepolarizing neuromuscular junction blockers, or succinylcholine • Decreased absorption and therapeutic levels of digoxin with kanamycin and methotrexate • Increased effect of warfarin with oral kanamycin due to decreased absorption of vitamin K

✱ **Drug-lab test** • Inactivation between aminoglycosides and beta-lactam antibiotics may result in false low-aminoglycoside readings

■ Nursing considerations

Assessment

- **History:** Allergy to aminoglycosides; intestinal obstruction, lactation, diminished hearing, decreased renal function, dehydration, neuromuscular disorders; pregnancy
- **Physical:** Site of infection, skin color, lesions; orientation, reflexes, eighth cranial nerve function; P, BP; R, bowel sounds; urinalysis, BUN, serum creatinine, serum electrolytes, LFTs, CBC

Interventions

- Arrange culture and sensitivity tests before beginning therapy.
- Therapeutic serum levels are peaks of 20–25 mcg/mL and troughs of less than 10 mcg/mL. Monitor with fourth dose, then weekly thereafter.

⊗ ***Black box warning*** Monitor length of treatment: Usual duration, 7–10 days. If clinical response does not occur within 3–5 days, stop therapy. Prolonged treatment risks increased toxicity. If drug is used longer than 10 days, monitor auditory and renal function daily.

- Give IM dosage by deep IM injection in upper outer quadrant of the gluteal muscle.
- Ensure that patient is well hydrated before and during therapy.

⊗ ***Black box warning*** Monitor patients receiving a total dose of more than 15 g, elderly patients, and those with preexisting tinnitus or vertigo for signs of eighth cranial nerve damage.

Teaching points

- You may experience these side effects: Ringing in the ears, headache, dizziness (reversible; use safety measures); nausea, vomiting, loss of appetite (eat frequent small meals; frequent mouth care may help).
- Report severe headache, dizziness, loss of hearing, severe diarrhea, increased urine output.

▽ketoconazole

*(kee toe **koe'** na zole)*

Apo-Ketoconazole (CAN), Extina, Kuric, Nizoral A-D, Xolegel

PREGNANCY CATEGORY C

Drug class

Antifungal (Imidazole)

Therapeutic actions

Impairs the synthesis of ergosterol, the main sterol of fungal cell membranes, allowing

K

increased permeability and leakage of cellular components and causing cell death.

Indications

- Treatment of systemic fungal infections: Candidiasis, chronic mucocutaneous candidiasis, oral thrush, candiduria, blastomycosis, coccidioidomycosis, histoplasmosis, chromomycosis, paracoccidioidomycosis
- Treatment of dermatophytosis (recalcitrant infections not responding to topical or griseofulvin therapy)
- Topical treatment of seborrheic dermatitis in patients older than 12 yr
- Cream: Tinea corporis (ringworm), tinea cruris (jock itch), and tinea pedis (athlete's foot)
- Shampoo: Reduction of scaling due to dandruff
- Orphan drug use: With cyclosporine to diminish cyclosporine-induced nephrotoxicity in organ transplant
- Unlabeled uses: Treatment of onychomycosis, pityriasis versicolor, vaginal candidiasis, tinea pedis, tinea corporis, tinea cruris, tinea capitis; CNS fungal infections at high doses (800–1,200 mg/day); advanced prostate cancer at doses of 400 mg every 8 hr; Cushing's syndrome (800–1,200 mg/day); refractory depression

Contraindications and cautions

- Contraindicated with allergy to ketoconazole; fungal meningitis; administration with terfenadine, astemizole, oral triazolam; pregnancy; lactation.
- Use cautiously with hepatic failure (increased risk of hepatocellular necrosis).

Available forms

Tablets—200 mg; shampoo—1% (OTC), 2%; topical gel—2%; cream—2%; topical foam—2%

Dosages

Adults

200 mg PO daily. Up to 400 mg/day in severe infections. Treatment period must be long enough to prevent recurrence, 1 wk–6 mo, depending on infecting organism and site.

Pediatric patients older than 2 yr

3.3–6.6 mg/kg/day PO as a single dose.

Pediatric patients younger than 2 yr

Safety and efficacy not established.

Shampoo

Moisten hair and scalp thoroughly with water; apply sufficient shampoo to produce a lather; leave on hair for 5 min. Shampoo twice a week for 4 wk with at least 3 days between shampooing.

Topical

Patients older than 12 yr

- *Tinea pedis:* Apply thin film of gel, foam, or cream once daily to affected areas for 2 wk; do not wash this area for 3 hr after applying. Wait 20 min before applying makeup or sunscreen. May require 6 wk of treatment.

Foam

- *Seborrheic dermatitis:* Apply foam bid for 4 wk.

Pharmacokinetics

Route	Onset	Peak
Oral	Varies	1–2 hr
Topical	Slow	Unknown

Metabolism: Hepatic; $T_{1/2}$: 8 hr
Distribution: Crosses placenta; enters breast milk
Excretion: Bile, urine

Adverse effects

- **CNS:** Headache, dizziness, somnolence, photophobia
- **GI:** Hepatotoxicity, *nausea, vomiting,* abdominal pain
- **GU:** Impotence, oligospermia (with very high doses)
- **Hematologic:** Thrombocytopenia, leukopenia, hemolytic anemia
- **Hypersensitivity:** Urticaria to **anaphylaxis**
- **Local:** Severe irritation, *pruritus, stinging* with topical application
- **Other:** *Pruritus,* fever, chills, gynecomastia

Interactions

✱ **Drug-drug** • Decreased blood levels of ketoconazole with rifampin • Increased blood levels of cyclosporine and risk of toxicity • Increased duration of adrenal suppression with corticosteroids • Decreased absorption if taken with antacids, histamine-2 blockers, proton pump inhibitors; space these at least 2 hr apart • Potent inhibitor of CYP3A4 enzyme system. Use with drugs metabolized via this system (eg, tacrolimus, warfarin) may lead to increased plasma levels and toxicity; use is contraindicated

■ Nursing considerations

Assessment

- **History:** Allergy to ketoconazole, fungal meningitis, hepatic failure, pregnancy, lactation
- **Physical:** Skin color, lesions; orientation, reflexes, affect; bowel sounds; LFTs; CBC and differential; culture of area involved

Interventions

- Culture fungus before therapy; begin treatment before return of laboratory results.

⊗ ***Warning*** Keep epinephrine readily available in case of severe anaphylaxis after first dose.

☒ ***Black box warning*** Risk of serious to fatal hepatic toxicity; monitor patient closely.

- Administer oral drug with food to decrease GI upset.
- Do not administer with antacids, H_2-blockers, proton pump inhibitors; ketoconazole requires an acidic environment for absorption; if antacids are required, administer at least 2 hr apart.
- Continue administration for long-term therapy until infection is eradicated: Candidiasis, 1–2 wk; other systemic mycoses, 6 mo; chronic mucocutaneous candidiasis, often requires maintenance therapy; tinea versicolor, 2 wk of topical application.
- Stop treatment, and consult physician about diagnosis if no improvement is seen within 2 wk of topical application.
- Administer shampoo as follows: Moisten hair and scalp thoroughly with water; apply sufficient shampoo to produce a lather; gently massage for 1 min; rinse hair with warm water; repeat, leaving on hair for 3 min.
- Arrange to monitor hepatic function tests before therapy and monthly or more frequently throughout treatment.

Teaching points

- Take the full course of drug therapy. Long-term use of the drug will be needed; beneficial effects may not be seen for several weeks.
- Take oral drug with meals to decrease GI upset.
- If using shampoo, moisten hair and scalp thoroughly with water; apply sufficient shampoo to produce a lather; leave on hair for 5 minutes. Shampoo twice a week for 4 weeks with at least 3 days between shampooing.
- Apply thin layer of gel, foam, or cream to affected area for 2 weeks. Wait 20 minutes before applying makeup or sunscreen to area, and do not wash area for 3 hours.
- Use appropriate hygiene measures to prevent reinfection or spread of infection.
- Do not take antacids, histamine-2 blockers, proton pump inhibitors with this drug; if they are needed, take this drug at least 2 hours after their administration.
- You may experience these side effects: Nausea, vomiting, diarrhea (take drug with food); sedation, dizziness, confusion (avoid driving or performing tasks that require alertness); stinging, irritation (local application).
- Report rash, severe nausea, vomiting, diarrhea, fever, sore throat, unusual bleeding or bruising, yellow skin or eyes, dark urine or pale stools, severe irritation (local application).

ketoprofen

*(kee toe **proe'** fen)*

PREGNANCY CATEGORY B (FIRST AND SECOND TRIMESTERS)

PREGNANCY CATEGORY D (THIRD TRIMESTER)

Drug classes

Nonopioid analgesic
NSAID

Therapeutic actions

Anti-inflammatory and analgesic activity; inhibits prostaglandin and leukotriene synthesis and has antibradykinin and lysosomal membrane-stabilizing actions.

K

Indications
- Acute and long-term treatment of rheumatoid arthritis and osteoarthritis
- Relief of mild to moderate pain
- Treatment of dysmenorrhea
- Reduction of fever (OTC indication)

Contraindications and cautions
- Contraindicated with significant renal impairment, pregnancy, lactation; allergy to ketoprofen, aspirin.
- Use cautiously with impaired hearing; allergies; hepatic, CV, and GI conditions.

Available forms
Capsules—50, 75 mg; ER capsules—100, 150, 200 mg

Dosages
Adults
Do not exceed 300 mg/day, or 200 mg/day ER.
- *Rheumatoid arthritis, osteoarthritis:* Starting dose, 75 mg tid or 50 mg qid PO. Maintenance dose, 150–300 mg PO in three or four divided doses. ER, 200 mg PO daily.
- *Mild to moderate pain, primary dysmenorrhea:* 25–50 mg PO every 6–8 hr as needed.

Pediatric patients
Safety and efficacy not established.

Geriatric patients or patients with hepatic or renal impairment
Reduce starting dose by one-half or one-third; maximum dose, 100 mg/day.

Pharmacokinetics

Route	*Onset*	*Peak*
Oral	30–60 min	0.5–2 hr
ER oral	30–60 min	6–7 hr

Metabolism: Hepatic; $T_{1/2}$: 2–4 hr, 5–6 hr for ER
Distribution: Crosses placenta; enters breast milk
Excretion: Urine

Adverse effects
- **CNS:** *Headache, dizziness,* somnolence, *insomnia,* fatigue, tiredness, tinnitus, ophthalmologic effects
- **Dermatologic:** *Rash,* pruritus, sweating, dry mucous membranes
- **GI:** *Nausea, dyspepsia, GI pain,* diarrhea, vomiting, *constipation,* flatulence, **gastric or duodenal ulcer**
- **GU:** Dysuria, **renal impairment**
- **Hematologic:** Bleeding, platelet inhibition with higher doses, neutropenia, eosinophilia, leukopenia, thrombocytopenia, agranulocytosis, aplastic anemia, menorrhagia
- **Respiratory:** Dyspnea, hemoptysis, pharyngitis, bronchospasm, rhinitis
- **Other:** Peripheral edema, **anaphylactoid reactions to anaphylactic shock**

Interactions
✱ **Drug-drug** • Increased risk of nephrotoxicity with other nephrotoxins (aminoglycosides, cyclosporine, diuretics) • Increased risk of bleeding with anticoagulants (warfarin) and aspirin

■ Nursing considerations
Assessment
- **History:** Renal impairment, impaired hearing, allergies, hepatic, CV, and GI conditions, lactation, pregnancy
- **Physical:** Skin color and lesions; orientation, reflexes, ophthalmologic and audiometric evaluation, peripheral sensation; P, BP, edema; R, adventitious sounds; liver evaluation; CBC, clotting times, LFTs, renal function tests; serum electrolytes, stool guaiac

Interventions
⊠ ***Black box warning*** Be aware that patient may be at increased risk for CV events, GI bleeding; monitor accordingly.
- Administer drug with food or after meals if GI upset occurs.
- Arrange for periodic ophthalmologic examination during long-term therapy.

⊗ ***Warning*** If overdose occurs, institute emergency procedures: Gastric lavage, induction of emesis, supportive therapy.

Teaching points
- Take drug with food or meals if GI upset occurs; take only the prescribed dosage.

- Use during pregnancy is not advised; if an analgesic is needed, consult your health care provider.
- Dizziness, drowsiness can occur (avoid driving or using dangerous machinery).
- For over-the-counter use: Do not take for more than 3 days for fever or for more than 10 days for pain. If symptoms persist, contact your health care provider.
- Report sore throat, fever, rash, itching, weight gain, swelling in ankles or fingers; changes in vision; black, tarry stools, easy bruising.

ketorolac tromethamine

*(**kee'** toe role ak)*

Acular LS, Acular PF

PREGNANCY CATEGORY C (FIRST AND SECOND TRIMESTERS)

PREGNANCY CATEGORY D (THIRD TRIMESTER)

Drug classes

Antipyretic
Nonopioid analgesic
NSAID

Therapeutic actions

Anti-inflammatory and analgesic activity; inhibits prostaglandins and leukotriene synthesis.

Indications

- Short-term management of pain (up to 5 days)
- Ophthalmic: Relief of ocular itching due to seasonal conjunctivitis and relief of postoperative inflammation after cataract surgery

Contraindications and cautions

- Contraindicated with significant renal impairment, during labor and delivery, lactation; patients wearing soft contact lenses (ophthalmic); aspirin allergy; concurrent use of NSAIDs; active peptic ulcer disease, recent GI bleed or perforation, history of peptic ulcer disease or GI bleeding; hypersensitivity to ketorolac; as prophylactic analgesic before major surgery; treatment of perioperative pain in CABG; suspected or confirmed cerebrovascular bleeding; hemorrhagic diathesis, incomplete hemostasis, high risk of bleeding; use with probenecid, pentoxyphylline.
- Use cautiously with impaired hearing; allergies; hepatic, CV and GI conditions.

Available forms

Ophthalmic solution—0.4%, 0.5%; tablets—10 mg; injection—15, 30 mg/mL

Dosages

For short-term use only (up to 5 days). Potent NSAID with many adverse effects.

Adults

Parenteral

- *Single-dose treatment:* 60 mg IM or 30 mg IV.
- *Multiple-dose treatment:* 30 mg IM or IV every 6 hr to a maximum 120 mg/day.

Oral

- *Transfer to oral:* 20 mg PO as a first dose for patients who received 60 mg IM or 30 mg IV as a single dose or 30-mg multiple dose, followed by 10 mg every 4–6 hr; do not exceed 40 mg/24 hr.

Ophthalmic

- *Itching from allergic conjunctivitis:* 1 drop qid.
- *Acular PF:* For cataract surgery, begin 1 drop qid 24 hr after and continue for 2 wk.
- *Acular LS:* 1 drop qid prn for burning and stinging for up to 4 days after surgery. For pain and photophobia, use for 3 days.

Pediatric patients 2–16 yr

Use one single-dose injection—1 mg/kg IM up to a maximum of 30 mg, or 0.5 mg/kg IV up to a maximum of 15 mg.

Geriatric patients 65 yr and older, patients with renal impairment, and patients weighing less than 50 kg

Parenteral

- *Single-dose treatment:* 30 mg IM or 15 mg IV.
- *Multiple-dose treatment:* 15 mg IM or IV every 6 hr to a maximum of 60 mg/day.

Oral

- *Transfer to oral:* 10 mg PO as first dose for patients who received 30 mg IM or 15 mg IV single dose or 15 mg IM or IV multiple dose, then 10 mg PO every 4–6 hr; do not exceed 40 mg/24 hr.

Pharmacokinetics

Route	Onset	Peak	Duration
Oral	Varies	30–60 min	6 hr
IM, IV	30 min	1–2 hr	6 hr

Metabolism: Hepatic; $T_{1/2}$: 2.4–8.6 hr
Distribution: Crosses placenta; enters breast milk
Excretion: Urine

IV FACTS

Preparation: No further preparation is required.
Infusion: Infuse slowly as a bolus over no less than 15 sec.
Incompatibilities: Do not mix with morphine, sulfate, meperidine, promethazine, or hydroxyzine; a precipitate will form. Protect injection from light.

Adverse effects

- **CNS:** *Headache, dizziness, somnolence, insomnia,* fatigue, tinnitus, ophthalmologic effects
- **Dermatologic:** *Rash,* pruritus, sweating, dry mucous membranes
- **GI:** *Nausea, dyspepsia, GI pain,* diarrhea, vomiting, *constipation,* flatulence, **gastric or duodenal ulcers**
- **GU:** Dysuria, **renal impairment**
- **Hematologic:** Bleeding, platelet inhibition with higher doses, neutropenia, eosinophilia, leukopenia, pancytopenia, thrombocytopenia, agranulocytosis, granulocytopenia, aplastic anemia, decreased Hgb or Hct, bone marrow depression, menorrhagia
- **Respiratory:** Dyspnea, hemoptysis, pharyngitis, bronchospasm, rhinitis
- **Other:** Peripheral edema; anaphylactoid reactions to anaphylactic shock; local burning, stinging (ophthalmic)

Interactions

✱ **Drug-drug** • Increased risk of nephrotoxicity with other nephrotoxins (aminoglycosides, cyclosporine) • Increased risk of bleeding with anticoagulants (warfarin), aspirin

■ Nursing considerations

Assessment

- **History:** Renal impairment; impaired hearing; allergies; hepatic, CV, and GI conditions; lactation, pregnancy
- **Physical:** Skin color and lesions; orientation, reflexes, ophthalmologic and audiometric evaluation, peripheral sensation; P, edema, BP; R, adventitious sounds; liver evaluation; CBC, clotting times, LFTs, renal function tests; serum electrolytes, stool guaiac

Interventions

⊗ ***Black box warning*** Be aware that patient may be at increased risk for CV events, GI bleeding, renal toxicity; monitor accordingly.

⊗ ***Black box warning*** Do not use during labor, delivery, or while nursing; serious adverse effects to the fetus or baby are possible.

⊗ ***Black box warning*** May increase risk of bleeding. Do not use with high risk of bleeding or prophylactically before surgery.

⊗ ***Black box warning*** There is increased risk of severe hypersensitivity with known hypersensitivity to aspirin, NSAIDs. Contraindicated for use with aspirin or NSAIDs because of risk of serious cumulative NSAID effects.

⊗ ***Warning*** Keep emergency equipment readily available at time of initial dose, in case of severe hypersensitivity reaction.

- Protect drug vials from light.
- Administer every 6 hr to maintain serum levels and control pain.

Teaching points

- Every effort will be made to administer the drug on time to control pain; dizziness, drowsiness can occur (avoid driving or using dangerous machinery); burning and stinging on application (ophthalmic).
- Do not use ophthalmic drops with contact lenses.
- Report sore throat, fever, rash, itching, weight gain, swelling in ankles or fingers; changes in vision; black, tarry stools, easy bruising.

DANGEROUS DRUG

labetalol hydrochloride

*(la **bet'** a lol)*

Normodyne, Trandate

PREGNANCY CATEGORY C

Drug classes

Alpha- and beta-adrenergic blocker
Antihypertensive

Therapeutic actions

Competitively blocks $alpha_1$- and $beta_1$- and $beta_2$-adrenergic receptors, and has some sympathomimetic activity at $beta_2$-receptors. Alpha- and beta-blocking actions contribute to the BP-lowering effect; beta blockade prevents the reflex tachycardia seen with most alpha-blocking drugs and decreases plasma renin activity.

Indications

- Hypertension, alone or with other oral drugs, especially diuretics
- Parenteral preparations: Severe hypertension
- Unlabeled uses: Control of BP in pheochromocytoma; clonidine withdrawal hypertension

Contraindications and cautions

- Contraindicated with sinus bradycardia, second- or third-degree heart block, cardiogenic shock, heart failure, asthma.
- Use cautiously with diabetes or hypoglycemia (can mask cardiac signs of hypoglycemia), nonallergic bronchospasm (oral drug—IV is absolutely contraindicated), pheochromocytoma (paradoxical increases in BP have occurred), hepatic impairment, pregnancy, lactation.

Available forms

Tablets—100, 200, 300 mg; injection—5 mg/mL

Dosages

Adults

Oral

Initial dose, 100 mg bid. After 2–3 days, using standing BP as indicator, adjust dosage in increments of 100 mg bid every 2–3 days. For maintenance, 200–400 mg bid. May need up to 2,400 mg/day; to improve tolerance, divide total daily dose and give tid.

Parenteral

- *Severe hypertension:* For repeated IV injection, 20 mg (0.25 mg/kg) slowly over 2 min. Individualize dosage using supine BP; additional doses of 40 or 80 mg can be given at 10-min intervals until desired BP is achieved or until a 300-mg dose has been injected. For continuous IV infusion, dilute ampule (see IV facts), infuse at a rate of up to 2 mg/min, adjust according to BP response up to 300 mg total dose. Transfer to oral therapy as soon as possible.

Pediatric patients

Safety and efficacy not established.

Geriatric patients

Generally require lower maintenance doses between 100 and 200 mg bid.

Pharmacokinetics

Route	Onset	Peak	Duration
Oral	Varies	1–2 hr	8–12 hr
IV	Immediate	5 min	5.5 hr

Metabolism: Hepatic; $T_{1/2}$: 6–8 hr
Distribution: Crosses placenta; enters breast milk
Excretion: Urine

IV FACTS

Preparation: Add 200 mg to 160 mL of a compatible IV fluid to make a 1 mg/mL solution; infuse at 2 mL/min, or add 200 mg (2 ampules) to 250 mg of IV fluid to make a 2 mg/3 mL solution, infuse at 3 mL/min. Compatible IV fluids include Ringer's, lactated Ringer's, 0.9% sodium chloride, 2.5% dextrose and 0.45% sodium chloride, 5% dextrose, 5% dextrose and Ringer's, 5% dextrose and 5% lactated Ringer's, and 5% dextrose and 0.2%, 0.33%, or 0.9% sodium chloride. Stable for 24 hr in these solutions at concentrations between 1.25 and 3.75 mg/mL.
Infusion: Administer infusion at 2–3 mL/min; inject slowly over 2 min.
Incompatibilities: Do not dilute drug in 5% sodium bicarbonate injection or other alkaline solutions, including furosemide.
Y-site incompatibilities: Do not give with nafcillin.

Adverse effects

- **CNS:** *Dizziness, vertigo, fatigue,* depression, paresthesias, sleep disturbances, hallucinations, disorientation, memory loss, slurred speech
- **CV:** Heart failure, cardiac arrhythmias, peripheral vascular insufficiency, claudication, CVA, pulmonary edema, hypotension
- **Dermatologic:** Rash, pruritus, sweating, dry skin
- **EENT:** Eye irritation, dry eyes, conjunctivitis, blurred vision
- **GI:** *Gastric pain, flatulence, constipation, diarrhea, nausea, vomiting,* anorexia, ischemic colitis, renal and mesenteric arterial thrombosis, retroperitoneal fibrosis, hepatomegaly, acute pancreatitis, taste alteration
- **GU:** *Impotence, decreased libido,* Peyronie's disease, dysuria, nocturia, polyuria, priapism, urinary retention
- **Respiratory: Bronchospasm,** *dyspnea, cough,* bronchial obstruction, nasal stuffiness, rhinitis, pharyngitis
- **Other:** *Decreased exercise tolerance,* development of antinuclear antibodies, hyperglycemia or hypoglycemia, elevated liver enzymes

Interactions

✱ **Drug-drug** • Risk of excessive hypotension with enflurane, halothane, or isoflurane • Potential for added antihypertensive effects with nitroglycerin • Additive AV block with calcium channel blockers

✱ **Drug-lab test** • Possible falsely elevated urinary catecholamines in lab tests using a trihydroxyindole reaction

■ Nursing considerations

Assessment

- **History:** Sinus bradycardia, second- or third-degree heart block, cardiogenic shock, heart failure, asthma, pregnancy, lactation, diabetes or hypoglycemia, nonallergic bronchospasm, pheochromocytoma
- **Physical:** Weight, skin condition, neurologic status, P, BP, ECG, respiratory status, renal and thyroid function, blood and urine glucose

Interventions

⊗ ***Warning*** Do not discontinue drug abruptly after long-term therapy. (Hypersensitivity to catecholamines may have developed, causing exacerbation of angina, MI and ventricular arrhythmias; taper drug gradually over 2 wk with monitoring.)

- Consult with physician about withdrawing the drug if the patient is to undergo surgery (withdrawal is controversial).
- Keep patient supine during parenteral therapy, and assist initial ambulation.
- Position to decrease effects of edema.
- Provide support and encouragement to deal with drug effects and disease.

Teaching points

- Take drug with meals.
- Do not stop taking drug unless instructed to do so by your health care provider.
- If you have diabetes, monitor your blood glucose carefully. This drug may mask usual symptoms of hypoglycemia.
- You may experience these side effects: Dizziness, light-headedness, loss of appetite, nightmares, depression, sexual impotence.
- Report difficulty breathing, night cough, swelling of extremities, slow pulse, confusion, depression, rash, fever, sore throat.

▽ lacosamide

*(lah **koss'** ah mide)*

Vimpat

PREGNANCY CATEGORY C

Drug class

Antiepileptic

Therapeutic actions

Mechanism of action not fully understood; inhibits voltage-sensitive sodium channels, resulting in stabilization of neuronal membranes and inhibition of repetitive neuronal firing.

Indications

- Adjunctive therapy for the treatment of partial-onset seizures in patients 17 yr and older; IV use is indicated for short-term treatment when oral administration is not feasible

Contraindications and cautions

- Contraindicated with hypersensitivity to components of drug, pregnancy, lactation.
- Use cautiously with cardiac conduction problems, MI, heart failure, drugs that prolong the PR interval, suicidal ideation, hepatic dysfunction, renal impairment.

Available forms

Tablets—50, 100, 150, 200 mg; single-use vial—200 mg/20 mL

Dosages

Adults

Initially, 50 mg PO bid; may be increased, if needed and tolerated, at weekly intervals by 100 mg/day given in two divided doses. Usual effective dosage is 200–400 mg/day PO. IV dosage is the same as oral dosage and may be used short-term if oral dosing is not feasible; transfer patient to oral form as soon as feasible.

Pediatric patients younger than 17 yr

Safety and efficacy not established.

Patients with renal impairment

Patients with severe renal impairment (CrCl ≤30 mL/min) should receive a maximum of 300 mg/day.

Patients with hepatic impairment

Increase dosage with caution. Maximum dosage is 300 mg/day with mild to moderate hepatic impairment; not recommended for use with severe hepatic impairment.

Pharmacokinetics

Route	*Onset*	*Peak*
Oral	Rapid	1–4 hr
IV	Rapid	End of infusion

Metabolism: Hepatic; $T_{1/2}$: 13 hr
Distribution: May cross placenta; may enter breast milk
Excretion: Urine

IV FACTS

Preparation: Solution may be given as provided or diluted in 0.9% sodium chloride injection, 5% dextrose injection, or lactated Ringer's injection. Solution should be clear; discard solution that is discolored or contains particulate matter. Discard unused portion. Stable for 24 hr at room temperature when diluted in appropriate solutions.
Infusion: Infuse slowly over 30–60 min.
Incompatibilities: Do not administer in the same line as other medications.

Adverse effects

- **CNS:** *Dizziness, ataxia, diplopia,* somnolence, tremor, *headache,* nystagmus, gait disorder, balance disorder, blurred vision, vertigo
- **CV:** Prolonged PR interval
- **GI:** *Nausea, vomiting,* diarrhea
- **Other:** Fatigue, pruritus

Interactions

✱ **Drug-drug** • Increased risk of prolonged PR interval if combined with other drugs known to prolong PR interval; monitor patient closely if such a combination is needed

■ Nursing considerations

Assessment

- **History:** Hypersensitivity to components of drug, cardiac conduction problems, MI, heart failure, use of drugs that prolong PR interval, suicidal ideation, hepatic dysfunction, renal impairment, pregnancy, lactation
- **Physical:** Orientation, affect, reflexes; BP, P, bowel sounds, LFTs, renal function tests, baseline ECG

Interventions

⊗ ***Warning*** There is an increased risk of suicidal ideation when used in children, adolescents, or young adults; monitor patient accordingly.

⊗ ***Warning*** Taper drug slowly when discontinuing; risk of seizures increases if drug is stopped abruptly.

- Be aware that dosage is the same for PO and IV routes. IV route should be reserved for short-term use when oral dosing is not feasible. Switch to oral route as soon as possible.
- Provide safety measures if CNS effects occur.

Teaching points

- Take this drug exactly as prescribed; be aware that the dosage may be slowly increased.

- Do not discontinue this drug abruptly. If the drug is discontinued, it will need to be slowly tapered to prevent seizures.
- You will need to have regular medical follow-up to monitor your response to this drug.
- It is not known how this drug affects a fetus; use of contraceptives is advised when you are taking this drug.
- If you are nursing a baby, you should use another method of feeding the baby while you are taking this drug because the drug could cause serious adverse effects in the baby.
- You may experience these side effects: Headache (medications may be available to help); nausea and vomiting (small, frequent meals may help; medication may be available to relieve these symptoms); dizziness, sleepiness, problems with vision and balance (avoid driving or performing tasks that require alertness or visual acuity until you know how this drug will affect you; take special precautions to avoids falls); thoughts of suicide, depression (be aware of changes in thoughts or thoughts of suicide; report changes to your health care provider immediately).
- Report thoughts of suicide, sudden changes in personality, excessive activity or thoughts of aggression, severe nausea or vomiting.

lactulose

(lak' tyoo lose)

Ammonia-reducing drug: Apo-Lactulose (CAN), Cephulac, Enulose

Laxative: Chronulac, Constilac, Constulose, Duphalac, Kristalose, PMS-Lactulose (CAN), ratio-Lactulose (CAN)

PREGNANCY CATEGORY B

Drug classes

Ammonia reduction drug
Laxative

Therapeutic actions

The drug passes unchanged into the colon where bacteria break it down to organic acids that increase the osmotic pressure in the colon and slightly acidify the colonic contents, resulting in an increase in stool water content, stool softening, laxative action. This also results in migration of blood ammonia into the colon contents with subsequent trapping and expulsion in the feces.

Indications

- Treatment of constipation
- Prevention and treatment of portal-systemic encephalopathy

Contraindications and cautions

- Contraindicated with allergy to lactulose, low-galactose diet.
- Use cautiously with diabetes, pregnancy, and lactation.

Available forms

Syrup, solution—10 g/15 mL

Dosages

Adults

Laxative

15–30 mL/day PO; may be increased to 60 mL/day as needed.

Oral

- *Portal-systemic encephalopathy:* 30–45 mL tid or qid. Adjust dosage every 1–2 days to produce two or three soft stools/day. 30–45 mL/hr may be used if needed. Return to standard dose as soon as possible.

Rectal

- *Portal-systemic encephalopathy:* 300 mL lactulose mixed with 700 mL water or physiologic saline as a retention enema, retained for 30–60 min. May be repeated every 4–6 hr. Start oral drug as soon as feasible and before stopping enemas.

Pediatric patients

Laxative

Safety and efficacy not established.

Oral

- *Portal-systemic encephalopathy:* Standards not clearly established. Initial dose of 2.5–10 mL/day in divided dose for small children or 40–90 mL/day for older children is suggested. Attempt to produce two or three soft stools daily.

Pharmacokinetics

Route	Onset	Peak	Duration
Oral	Varies	20 hr	24–48 hr

Very minimal systemic absorption

Adverse effects

- **GI:** *Transient flatulence, distention, intestinal cramps, belching,* diarrhea, nausea
- **Other:** Acid–base imbalances, electrolyte imbalance

■ Nursing considerations

Assessment

- **History:** Allergy to lactulose, low-galactose diet, diabetes, lactation, pregnancy
- **Physical:** Abdominal examination, bowel sounds, serum electrolytes, serum ammonia levels

Interventions

⊗ ***Warning*** Do not freeze laxative form. Extremely dark or cloudy syrup may be unsafe; do not use.

- Give laxative syrup orally with fruit juice, water, or milk to increase palatability.
- Administer retention enema using a rectal balloon catheter. Do not use cleansing enemas containing soapsuds or other alkaline drugs that counteract the effects of lactulose.
- Do not administer other laxatives while using lactulose.
- Monitor serum ammonia levels.
- Monitor with long-term therapy for potential electrolyte and acid–base imbalances.
- Carefully monitor blood glucose levels in diabetic patients.

Teaching points

- Do not use other laxatives. The drug may be mixed in water, juice, or milk to make it more tolerable.
- For laxative use, do not use continuously for longer than 1 week unless directed by your health care provider.
- Make sure you have ready access to bathroom; bowel movements will be increased to two or three per day.
- You may experience these side effects: Abdominal fullness, flatulence, belching.
- Report diarrhea, severe belching, abdominal fullness.

▽lamivudine (3TC)

(lam ah ***vew'*** *den)*

Epivir, Epivir-HBV

PREGNANCY CATEGORY C

Drug classes

Antiviral
Reverse transcriptase inhibitor

Therapeutic actions

Nucleoside analogue inhibitor of HIV reverse transcriptase via DNA viral chain termination and HBV polymerase.

Indications

- Treatment of HIV infection in combination with other antiretroviral drugs
- Treatment of chronic hepatitis B (*Epivir-HBV*) with active liver inflammation

Contraindications and cautions

- Contraindicated with life-threatening allergy to any component.
- Use cautiously with compromised bone marrow function, impaired renal function, hepatic impairment, obesity, pregnancy, lactation.

Available forms

Tablets—100 (*Epivir–HBV*); 150, 300 mg (*Epivir*); oral solution—5 mg/mL (*Epivir–HBV*), 10 mg/mL (*Epivir*)

Dosages

Adults

- *Hepatitis B:* 100 mg PO daily.

Adults and patients 16 yr and older

- *HIV infection:* 150 mg PO bid or 300 mg/day PO as a single dose in combination with other antiretroviral drugs.

Pediatric patients

- *HIV infection:*
  3 mo–16 yr: 4 mg/kg PO bid; up to a maximum of 150 mg bid.

or:
Patients weighing 14–21 kg: 75 mg (one-half tablet) PO bid.
Patients weighing more than 21 kg but less than 30 kg: 75 mg (one-half tablet) PO

L

in the morning and then 150 mg (1 tablet) PO in the evening.
Patients weighing 30 kg or more: 150 mg (1 tablet) PO bid.
- *Hepatitis B:*
2–17 yr: 3 mg/kg PO daily up to a maximum of 100 mg daily.

Patients with impaired renal function

- *HIV infection:*

CrCl (mL/min)	*Dosage (PO)*
50 or more	150 mg bid or 300 mg daily
30–49	150 mg daily
15–29	150 mg first dose, then 100 mg daily
5–14	150 mg first dose, then 50 mg daily
Less than 5	50 mg first dose, then 25 mg daily

- *Hepatitis B:*

CrCl (mL/min)	*Dosage (PO)*
50 or more	100 mg daily
30–49	100 mg first dose, then 50 mg daily
15–29	100 mg first dose, then 25 mg daily
5–14	35 mg first dose, then 15 mg daily
Less than 5	35 mg first dose, then 10 mg daily

Pharmacokinetics

Route	*Onset*	*Peak*
Oral	Slow	2–4 hr

Metabolism: Unknown; $T_{1/2}$: 5–7 hr
Distribution: Crosses placenta; enters breast milk
Excretion: Urine

Adverse effects

- **CNS:** *Headache,* insomnia, myalgia, *asthenia,* malaise, dizziness, paresthesias, somnolence
- **GI:** *Nausea, GI pain, diarrhea,* anorexia, vomiting, dyspepsia, **pancreatitis** (children), **hepatomegaly with lactic acidosis, steatosis**
- **Hematologic:** *Agranulocytosis*
- **Respiratory:** *Nasal signs and symptoms, cough*
- **Other:** Fever, rash, taste perversion

Interactions

✱ **Drug-drug** • Increased levels of lamivudine taken concurrently with trimethoprim-sulfamethoxazole • Lamivudine and zalcitabine inhibit the effects of each other; avoid concurrent use

■ Nursing considerations

Assessment

- **History:** Life-threatening allergy to any component, compromised bone marrow function, impaired renal function, pregnancy, lactation, hepatic impairment, obesity
- **Physical:** Skin rashes, lesions, texture; T; affect, reflexes, peripheral sensation; bowel sounds, liver evaluation; renal function tests, CBC and differential

Interventions

⊗ ***Black box warning*** Arrange to monitor hematologic indices and liver function every 2 wk during therapy; severe hepatomegaly with steatosis, lactic acidosis has occurred.

⊗ ***Black box warning*** Counsel and periodically test patients receiving *Epivir-HBV.* Severe, acute exacerbations of HBV have been reported in patients with both HIV and HBV infection who stop taking lamivudine.

- Monitor children for any sign of pancreatitis and discontinue immediately if it occurs.
- Monitor patient for signs of opportunistic infections that will need to be treated appropriately.
- Administer the drug concurrently with other antiretrovirals for HIV infection.
- Offer support and encouragement to the patient to deal with the diagnosis as well as the effects of drug therapy and the high expense of treatment.

Teaching points

- Take drug as prescribed; take concurrently with other drugs prescribed for HIV treatment.
- These drugs are not a cure for AIDS, AIDS-related complex, or hepatitis B; opportunistic infections may occur and regular medical care should be sought to deal with the disease.
- Arrange for frequent blood tests during the course of treatment; results of blood counts

may indicate a need to decrease dosage or discontinue the drug for a time.

- Lamivudine does not reduce the risk of transmission of HIV or hepatitis B to others by sexual contact or blood contamination—use appropriate precautions.
- Avoid pregnancy while using this drug; using barrier contraceptives is urged.
- You may experience these side effects: Nausea, loss of appetite, change in taste (eat frequent small meals); dizziness, loss of feeling (take appropriate precautions); headache, fever, muscle aches (an analgesic may help, consult your health care provider).
- Report extreme fatigue, lethargy, severe headache, severe nausea, vomiting, difficulty breathing, rash.

lamotrigine

(la mo' tri geen)

Apo-Lamotrigine (CAN), Gen-Lamotrigine (CAN), Lamictal, Lamictal Chewable Dispersible Tablets, Lamictal XR DNG, PMS-Lamotrigine (CAN), ratio-Lamotrigine (CAN)

PREGNANCY CATEGORY C

Drug class

Antiepileptic

Therapeutic actions

Mechanism not well understood; may inhibit voltage-sensitive sodium channels, stabilizing the neuronal membrane and modulating calcium-dependent presynaptic release of excitatory amino acids.

Indications

- Adjunctive therapy in the treatment of partial seizures in adults and children 2 yr and older with epilepsy
- **NEW INDICATION:** ER form—once daily adjunctive therapy for patients 13 yr and older with partial onset seizures
- Adjunctive therapy for the treatment of Lennox-Gastaut syndrome in infants, children, and adults; primary generalized tonic-clonic seizures in adults and children 2 yr and older
- Monotherapy in adults with partial seizures that have not been controlled by other therapies
- Conversion to monotherapy in adults with partial seizures receiving treatment with a single enzyme-inducing antiepileptic drug
- Long-term maintenance of bipolar 1 disorder, to delay the occurrence of acute mood episodes in patients on standard therapy
- Unlabeled uses: Absence seizures (children), temporal lobe seizures, migraine headache

Contraindications and cautions

- Contraindicated with allergy to drug, lactation.
- Use cautiously with impaired hepatic, renal, or cardiac function; patients younger than 16 yr, pregnancy.

Available forms

Tablets—25, 100, 150, 200 mg; chewable tablets—2, 5, 25 mg; orally disintegrating tablets—25, 50, 100, 200 mg; ER tablets DNG—25, 50, 100, 200 mg

Dosages

Adults

- *Epilepsy*

Patients taking enzyme-inducing antiepileptics (ie, carbamazepine, phenytoin, phenobarbital) and not valproic acid: 50 mg PO daily for 2 wk; then 100 mg PO daily in two divided doses for 2 wk; may increase by 100 mg/day every wk up to a maintenance dose of 300–500 mg/day in two divided doses. Patients older than 13 yr (ER tablets): wk 1–2, 50 mg/day PO; wk 3–4, 100 mg/day PO; wk 5, 200 mg/day PO; wk 6, 300 mg/day PO; wk 7, 400 mg/day PO. Range, 400–600 mg/day.

Patients taking enzyme-inducing antiepileptics (ie, carbamazepine, phenytoin, phenobarbital) and also valproic acid: 25 mg PO every other day for 2 wk; then 25 mg PO daily for 2 wk, then may increase by 25–50 mg every 1–2 wk up to a maintenance dose of 100–400 mg/day PO in two divided doses.

L

Conversion of patients to lamotrigine monotherapy: Titrate as above to a target dose of 500 mg/day in two divided doses, then attempt to decrease other antiepileptic by 20% weekly.

- *Bipolar I disorder*
  Patients taking valproic acid: 25 mg every other day for 2 wk; then 25 mg once daily for 2 wk. After 4 wk, dose may be doubled at weekly intervals to target of 100 mg/day.
  Patients taking enzyme-inducing antiepileptics but not valproic acid: 50 mg/day for 2 wk; then 100 mg daily in two divided doses for 2 wk. After 4 wk, dose may be increased in 100-mg increments at weekly intervals to target maintenance dosage of 400 mg/day in two divided doses.
  Patients taking neither enzyme-inducing antiepileptics nor valproic acid: 25 mg/day for 2 wk; then 50 mg daily for 2 wk. After 4 wk, dose may be doubled at weekly intervals to maintenance dosage of 200 mg/day.

Pediatric patients 2–12 yr

- *Patients taking non–enzyme-inducing antiepileptics with valproic acid*—0.15 mg/kg/day in one to two divided doses for 2 wk. Then 0.3 mg/kg/day in one to two divided doses, rounded down to nearest 5 mg for 2 wk. For maintenance, 1–5 mg/kg/day in one to two divided doses, to a maximum of 200 mg/day.
- *Single enzyme-inducing antiepileptic without valproic acid:* 0.6 mg/kg/day in two divided doses for 2 wk, then 1.2 mg/kg/day in two divided doses for 2 wk. For maintenance, 5–15 mg/kg/day in two divided doses, to a maximum of 400 mg/day.

Pediatric patients older than 12 yr

- *Patients taking valproic acid*—25 mg PO every other day for 2 wk, then 25 mg PO daily for 2 wk. For maintenance, 100–400 mg/day in one to two divided doses. *Without valproic acid:* 50 mg/day PO for 2 wk, then 100 mg/day in two divided doses for 2 wk. For maintenance, 300–500 mg/day in one to two divided doses, to a maximum of 500 mg/day.

Pharmacokinetics

Route	Onset	Peak
Oral	Rapid	2–5 hr

Metabolism: Hepatic; $T_{1/2}$: 25–33 hr
Distribution: Crosses placenta; may enter breast milk
Excretion: Urine

Adverse effects

- **CNS:** *Dizziness,* insomnia, headache, somnolence, *ataxia,* diplopia, blurred vision
- **Dermatologic: Stevens-Johnson syndrome, rash, toxic epidermal necrosis with multiorgan failure**
- **GI:** *Nausea,* vomiting, abdominal pain, constipation, diarrhea

Interactions

✱ **Drug-drug** • Decrease in lamotrigine levels of 40%–50% with enzyme-inducing antiepileptics—carbamazepine, phenytoin, phenobarbital, primidone • Decreased clearance of lamotrigine, requiring a lower dose, if taken with valproic acid

■ Nursing considerations

CLINICAL ALERT!
Name confusion has occurred between *Lamictal* (lamotrigine) and *Lamisil* (terbinafine); use extreme caution.

Assessment

- **History:** Lactation; impaired hepatic, renal or cardiac function; pregnancy
- **Physical:** Weight; T; skin color, lesions; orientation, affect, reflexes; P, BP, perfusion; bowel sounds, normal output; LFTs, renal function tests

Interventions

- Monitor renal and hepatic function before and periodically during therapy; if abnormal, reevaluate therapy.

⊗ ***Warning*** Monitor drug doses carefully when starting therapy and with each increase in dose; special care will be needed when changing the dose or frequency of any other antiepileptic.

☒ ***Black box warning*** Monitor patient for any sign of rash; discontinue lamotrigine immediately if rash appears and be prepared with appropriate life support if needed; potential for serious or life-threatening rash.

- Administer only whole dispersible tablets.
- Administer chewable, dispersible tablets with a small amount of water or fruit juice if chewed; to disperse, add tablet to 1 tsp water, wait 1 min, swirl and administer immediately.
- Taper drug slowly over a 2-wk period when discontinuing.

Teaching points

- Take this drug exactly as prescribed.
- Do not discontinue this drug abruptly or change dosage, except on the advice of your health care provider.
- Wear or carry a medical ID tag to alert emergency medical personnel that you are an epileptic taking antiepileptic medication.
- If rash occurs, notify your health care provider immediately.
- You may experience these side effects: Dizziness, drowsiness (avoid driving or performing tasks requiring alertness or visual acuity); GI upset (take drug with food or milk, eat frequent small meals); headache (medication can be ordered).
- Report yellowing of skin, abdominal pain, changes in color of urine or stools, fever, sore throat, mouth sores, unusual bleeding or bruising, rash.

▽lanreotide acetate

See Appendix W, *Less commonly used drugs.*

▽lansoprazole

*(lanz **ah'** pray zol)*

Prevacid ODC, Prevacid IV

PREGNANCY CATEGORY B

Drug classes

Antisecretory drug
Proton pump inhibitor

Therapeutic actions

Gastric acid-pump inhibitor: Suppresses gastric acid secretion by specific inhibition of the hydrogen–potassium ATPase enzyme system at the secretory surface of the gastric parietal cells; blocks the final step of acid production.

Indications

- Short-term treatment (up to 4 wk) of active duodenal ulcer
- Short-term treatment (up to 8 wk) of gastric ulcers
- Healing of NSAID-related gastric ulcer
- Risk reduction for NSAID-related gastric ulcer
- Short-term treatment (up to 8 wk) of GERD: Severe erosive esophagitis; poorly responsive symptomatic GERD
- Long-term treatment of pathological hypersecretory conditions (eg, Zollinger-Ellison syndrome, multiple adenomas, systemic mastocytosis)
- Maintenance therapy for healing of erosive esophagitis, duodenal ulcers
- Eradication of *Helicobacter pylori* infection in patients with active or recurrent duodenal ulcers in combination with clarithromycin and amoxicillin
- Short-term treatment (up to 7 days) of all grades of erosive esophagitis when patient is unable to take oral medication (IV)

L

Contraindications and cautions

- Contraindicated with hypersensitivity to lansoprazole or any of its components.
- Use cautiously with pregnancy, lactation.

Available forms

DR capsules ODC—15, 30 mg; orally disintegrating DR tablets—15, 30 mg; DR granules for oral suspension—15, 30 mg; powder for injection—30 mg/vial

Dosages

Adults

- *Active duodenal ulcer:* 15 mg PO daily before eating for 4 wk. For maintenance, 15 mg PO daily.
- *Gastric ulcer:* 30 mg/day PO for up to 8 wk.
- *Risk reduction of gastric ulcer with NSAIDS:* 15 mg/day PO for up to 12 wk.
- *Duodenal ulcers associated with* H. pylori: 30 mg lansoprazole, 500 mg clarithromycin, 1 g amoxicillin, all given PO bid for 10–14 days; or 30 mg lansoprazole and 1 g amoxicillin PO tid for 14 days.
- *GERD:* 15 mg/day PO for up to 8 wk.
- *Erosive esophagitis or poorly responsive GERD:* 30 mg PO daily before eating for up to 8 wk. An additional 8-wk course may be

helpful for patients who do not heal with 8-wk therapy.
- *Maintenance of healing of erosive esophagitis:* 15 mg/day PO.
- *Pathological hypersecretory conditions:* Individualize dosage. Initial dose is 60 mg PO daily. Doses up to 90 mg bid have been used. Administer daily doses of more than 120 mg in divided doses.
- *Short-term treatment of all grades of erosive esophagitis:* 30 mg/day IV, over 30 min for up to 7 days; switch to oral form as soon as possible for total of 8 wk treatment.

Pediatric patients 12–17 yr

Nonerosive GERD: 15 mg/day PO for up to 8 wk.

Erosive esophagitis: 30 mg/day PO for up to 8 wk.

Pediatric patients 1–11 yr

Give as oral suspension, or capsules may be opened and the granules sprinkled on soft food. Do not cut, crush, or chew granules.

Patients weighing 30 kg or less: 15 mg/day PO for up to 12 wk.

Patients weighing more than 30 kg: 30 mg/day PO for up to 12 wk.

Patients with hepatic impairment

Consider reducing dose and monitoring patient response.

Pharmacokinetics

Route	*Onset*	*Peak*
Oral	Varies	1.7 hr
IV	Rapid	End of transfusion

Metabolism: Hepatic; $T_{1/2}$: 2 hr, 1.3 hr (IV)
Distribution: Crosses placenta; may enter breast milk
Excretion: Bile

IV FACTS

Preparation: Reconstitute with 5 mL sterile water for injection (resulting solution 6 mg/mL); mix gently until powder is dissolved; reconstituted solution is stable for 1 hr before dilution. Dilute in 50 mL 0.9% sodium chloride injection, lactated Ringer's, or 5% dextrose injection. Stable for 24 hr (0.9% sodium chloride, lactated Ringer's) or 12 hr (5% dextrose).

Infusion: Use in-line filter provided with product. Infuse over 30 min; flush line with appropriate dilution fluid.
Incompatibilities: Do not administer with other drugs.

Adverse effects

- **CNS:** *Headache,* dizziness, asthenia, vertigo, insomnia, anxiety, paresthesias, dream abnormalities
- **Dermatologic:** Rash, inflammation, urticaria, pruritus, alopecia, dry skin, acne
- **GI:** *Diarrhea, abdominal pain, nausea, vomiting,* constipation, dry mouth
- **Respiratory:** *URI symptoms,* cough, epistaxis
- **Other:** Gastric cancer in preclinical studies, back pain, fever

Interactions

✱ **Drug-drug** • Decreased serum levels if taken concurrently with sucralfate • Decreased serum levels of ketoconazole, theophylline when taken with lansoprazole

■ Nursing considerations

Assessment

- **History:** Hypersensitivity to lansoprazole or any of its components; pregnancy; lactation
- **Physical:** Skin lesions; body T; reflexes, affect; urinary output, abdominal examination; respiratory auscultation

Interventions

- Administer before meals. Caution patient to swallow capsules whole, not to chew or crush. If patient has difficulty swallowing, open capsule and sprinkle granules on apple sauce, *Ensure,* yogurt, cottage cheese, or strained pears. For nasogastric tube, place 15- or 30-mg tablet in a syringe and draw 4 or 10 mL of water; shake gently for quick dispersal. After dispersal, inject through nasogastric tube into the stomach within 15 min. If using capsules with nasogastric tube, mix granules from capsule with 40 mL apple juice and inject through tube, flush tube with more apple juice; or granules for oral suspension can be added to 30 mL water, stir well, and have patient drink immediately.

Place orally disintegrating tablet on tongue; follow with water after it dissolves.

⊗ ***Warning*** Arrange for further evaluation of patient after 4 wk of therapy for acute gastroesophageal reflux disorders if symptomatic improvement does not rule out gastric cancer, which did occur in preclinical studies.

- Switch to oral drug from IV as soon as patient is able to take oral drugs. Use of IV drug for more than 7 days is not approved.

Teaching points

- Take the drug before meals. Swallow the capsules whole—do not chew, open, or crush. If you are unable to swallow capsule, open and sprinkle granules on applesauce, or use granules, which can be added to 30 milliliters water, stirred, and drunk immediately. If using orally disintegrating tablet, place on your tongue and allow to dissolve. Follow with a drink of water.
- Arrange to have regular medical follow-up care while you are taking this drug.
- You may experience these side effects: Dizziness (avoid driving a car or performing hazardous tasks); headache (medications may be available to help); nausea, vomiting, diarrhea (proper nutrition is important, consult with a dietitian to maintain nutrition); symptoms of upper respiratory tract infection, cough (reversible; do not self-medicate, consult your health care provider if this becomes uncomfortable).
- Report severe headache, worsening of symptoms, fever, chills.

lanthanum carbonate

See Appendix W, *Less commonly used drugs.*

lapatinib

See Appendix W, *Less commonly used drugs.*

laronidase

See Appendix W, *Less commonly used drugs.*

leflunomide

(leh flew' no mide)

Arava

PREGNANCY CATEGORY X

Drug classes

Antiarthritic
Pyrimidine synthesis inhibitor

Therapeutic actions

Reversibly inhibits the enzyme dihydroorotate dehydrogenase, which is active in the autoimmune process that leads to rheumatoid arthritis; blocking this enzyme relieves the signs and symptoms of inflammation and blocks the structural damage caused by the inflammatory response to the autoimmune process.

Indications

- Treatment of active rheumatoid arthritis; to relieve symptoms and slow progression
- Improvement in physical functioning in adults with active rheumatoid arthritis

Contraindications and cautions

- Contraindicated with allergy to leflunomide, lactation, pregnancy, childbearing age when not using a reliable method of contraception, significant hepatic impairment, hepatitis B or C, severe immune deficiency.
- Use cautiously with renal or hepatic disorders.

Available forms

Tablets—10, 20, 100 mg

Dosages

Adults

Loading dose, 100 mg PO daily for 3 days; maintenance dose, 20 mg PO daily. If not well tolerated or if ALT elevates to more than two times upper level of normal, may reduce to 10 mg PO daily. If elevation of ALT is between two and three times upper limit of normal, monitor closely if continued therapy is desired; if it is three times or greater than upper limit of normal, use of cholestyramine may decrease absorption; consider discontinuation.

Pediatric patients
Safety and efficacy not established.
Patients with hepatic impairment
Do not use with serious hepatic impairment. Decrease dosage and monitor patient closely with mild to moderate hepatic impairment.

Pharmacokinetics

Route	*Onset*	*Peak*
Oral	Varies	6–12 hr

Metabolism: Hepatic; $T_{1/2}$: 14–18 days
Distribution: Crosses placenta; enters breast milk
Excretion: Urine

Adverse effects

- **CNS:** *Headache,* drowsiness, blurred vision, fatigue, dizziness, paresthesias
- **Dermatologic:** *Erythematous rashes,* pruritus, urticaria, *transient alopecia*
- **GI:** Nausea, vomiting, *diarrhea,* **hepatic toxicity**
- **Other:** Serious birth defects, pancytopenia, agranulocytosis, thrombocytopenia

Interactions

✱ **Drug-drug** • Possible severe hepatic impairment if combined with other hepatotoxic drugs; use with caution • Decreased absorption and effectiveness if combined with charcoal, cholestyramine • Increased risk of toxicity if combined with rifampin; monitor patient closely if this combination is used

■ Nursing considerations

Assessment

- **History:** Allergy to leflunomide, childbearing age, pregnancy, lactation, hepatitis B or C, severe hepatic impairment
- **Physical:** Weight; skin lesions, color; hair; orientation, liver evaluation, abdominal examination; LFTs

Interventions

⊗ ***Warning*** Monitor LFTs before and periodically during therapy. Discontinue drug if hepatic impairment occurs.

- Advise patient that this drug does not cure the disease and appropriate therapies for rheumatoid arthritis should be used.
- Arrange for patient to obtain a wig or some other suitable head covering if alopecia occurs; ensure that head is covered at extreme temperatures; loss of hair is usually reversible.
- Provide appropriate skin care; arrange for treatment of skin lesions as needed.

⊗ ***Black box warning*** Advise women of childbearing age of the risks associated with becoming pregnant while using this drug. Arrange for counseling for appropriate contraceptive measures while this drug is being used. If patient decides to become pregnant, a withdrawal program to rid the body of leflunomide is recommended. Cholestyramine may be used to rapidly decrease serum levels if unplanned pregnancy occurs.

Teaching points

- Take this drug exactly as prescribed. Note that this drug does not cure rheumatoid arthritis, and appropriate therapies to deal with the disease should be followed.
- This drug may cause birth defects or miscarriages. It is advisable to use birth control while using this drug and for 8 weeks thereafter. Consult your health care provider if you decide to become pregnant; a withdrawal program is available.
- Arrange for frequent, regular medical follow-up care, including frequent blood tests to follow the effects of the drug on your body.
- You may experience these side effects: Nausea, vomiting, diarrhea (medication may be ordered to help; eat frequent small meals); dizziness, drowsiness (these are all effects of the drug; consult with your nurse or physician if these occur; dosage adjustment may be needed; avoid driving or operating dangerous machinery if these occur); loss of hair (you may wish to obtain a wig or other suitable head covering; it is important to keep the head covered at extremes of temperature); rash (avoid exposure to the sun, use a sunscreen and protective clothing if exposed to sun).
- Report black, tarry stools; fever, chills, sore throat; unusual bleeding or bruising; cough or shortness of breath; darkened or bloody

urine; abdominal, flank, or joint pain; yellow color to the skin or eyes; mouth sores.

lenalidomide

See Appendix W, *Less commonly used drugs.*

lepirudin

See Appendix W, *Less commonly used drugs.*

letrozole

(le' tro zol)

Femara

PREGNANCY CATEGORY D

Drug classes

Antiestrogen
Antineoplastic
Aromatase inhibitor

Therapeutic actions

Inhibits the conversion of androgens to estrogens by the aromatase enzyme system (in postmenopausal women, the aromatase system is the main source of estrogens); reduces estrogen levels in all tissues, including tumors.

Indications

- Treatment of advanced breast cancer in postmenopausal women as a first-line treatment and with disease progression following traditional antiestrogen therapy
- Adjuvant treatment of early, receptor-positive breast cancer in postmenopausal women
- Extended adjuvant treatment of breast cancer in postmenopausal women who have received 5 yr of tamoxifen therapy

Contraindications and cautions

- Contraindicated with allergy to letrozole, pregnancy.
- Use cautiously with hepatic impairment, lactation.

Available forms

Tablets—2.5 mg

Dosages

Adults

2.5 mg PO daily; continue until tumor progression is evident.

Patients with hepatic impairment

Reduce dose by 50% in patients with cirrhosis or severe hepatic impairment; give 2.5 mg every other day. No adjustment needed for mild to moderate impairment.

Pharmacokinetics

Route	*Onset*	*Peak*
Oral	Varies	2–6 wk

Metabolism: Hepatic; $T_{1/2}$: 2 days
Distribution: Crosses placenta; may enter breast milk
Excretion: Urine

Adverse effects

- **CNS:** Depression, *headache,* fatigue, somnolence, anxiety, vertigo, dizziness, insomnia
- **CV:** Thromboembolic events, CV events, cerebrovascular events
- **Dermatologic:** Alopecia, *hot flashes,* rash
- **GI:** *Nausea, GI upset,* elevated liver enzymes, diarrhea, vomiting, constipation, abdominal pain, dyspepsia
- **Respiratory:** Cough, dyspnea, chest wall pain
- **Other:** Peripheral edema; arthralgia, bone pain, back pain

■ Nursing considerations

Assessment

- **History:** Allergy to letrozole, hepatic impairment, pregnancy, lactation
- **Physical:** Skin lesions, color, turgor; orientation, affect, reflexes; peripheral pulses, edema; LFTs, estrogen receptor evaluation of tumor cells

Interventions

⊗ ***Warning*** Counsel patient about the need to use contraceptive measures to avoid pregnancy while taking this drug; inform patient that serious fetal harm could occur.

- Provide comfort measures to help patient deal with drug effects: Hot flashes (control environmental temperature); headache, depression (monitor light and noise); vaginal bleeding (hygiene measures).

- Discontinue drug at signs that tumor is progressing.

Teaching points

- This drug can cause serious fetal harm and must not be taken during pregnancy. Contraceptive measures should be used while you are taking this drug. If you become pregnant or decide that you would like to become pregnant, consult your health care provider immediately.
- You may experience these side effects: Hot flashes (stay in cool temperatures); nausea, GI upset (eat frequent small meals); headache, light-headedness (use caution if driving or performing tasks that require alertness).
- Report changes in color of urine or stool, increased fatigue, rash, fever, chills, severe depression.

leucovorin calcium (citrovorum factor, folinic acid)

*(loo koe **vor'** in)*

PREGNANCY CATEGORY C

Drug class

Folic acid derivative

Therapeutic actions

Active reduced form of folic acid; required for nucleoprotein synthesis and maintenance of normal hematopoiesis.

Indications

- "Leucovorin rescue"—after high-dose methotrexate therapy for various cancers
- Parenteral form: Treatment of megaloblastic anemias due to sprue, nutritional deficiency, pregnancy, and infancy when oral folic acid therapy is not feasible
- IV: With 5-FU for palliative treatment of metastatic colorectal cancer
- To decrease toxicity of methotrexate caused by decreased elimination or for inadvertent overdose of folic acid antagonists such as trimethoprim

Contraindications and cautions

- Contraindicated with allergy to leucovorin on previous exposure, pernicious anemia or other megaloblastic anemias in which vitamin B_{12} is deficient.
- Use cautiously with pregnancy, lactation.

Available forms

Tablets—5, 10, 15, 25 mg; injection—3 mg/mL, 10 mg/mL; powder for injection—50, 100, 200, 350, 500 mg/vial

Dosages

Adults

- *Rescue after methotrexate therapy:* Begin therapy within 24 hr of methotrexate dose. 10 mg/m^2 PO every 6 hr for 10 doses or until methotrexate level is less than 0.05 micromolar. If at 24 hr following methotrexate administration, serum creatinine is 100% greater than the pretreatment level, or based on methotrexate levels, increase the leucovorin dose to 150 mg IV every 3 hr until the serum methotrexate level is less than 1.0 micromolar; then 15 mg IV every 3 hr until methotrexate level is less than .05 micromolar.
- *Megaloblastic anemia:* Up to 1 mg/day IM may be used. Do not exceed 1 mg/day.
- *Metastatic colon cancer:* Give 200 mg/m^2 by slow IV injection over up to 3 min, followed by 5-FU 370 mg/m^2 IV *or* 20 mg/m^2 IV, followed by 5-FU 425 mg/m^2 IV. Repeat daily for 5 days; may be repeated at 4-wk intervals.

Pharmacokinetics

Route	*Onset*	*Peak*	*Duration*
Oral	30 min	2.4 hr	3–6 hr
IM	Rapid	52 min	3–6 hr
IV	Immediate	10 min	3–6 hr

Metabolism: Hepatic; $T_{1/2}$: 5.7 hr (oral), 6.2 hr (IV, IM)
Distribution: Crosses placenta; enters breast milk
Excretion: Urine

IV FACTS

Preparation: Prepare solution by diluting a 50-mg vial of powder with 5 mL bacteriostatic

water for injection that contains benzyl alcohol and use within 7 days, or reconstitute with water for injection, and use immediately. Protect from light.
Infusion: Infuse slowly over 3–5 min; not more than 160 mg/min.
Incompatibility: Do not mix with floxuridine or 5-FU.
Y-site incompatibility: Do not inject with droperidol.

Adverse effects

- **Hypersensitivity:** Allergic reactions
- **Local:** *Pain, discomfort at injection site*

Interactions

✱ **Drug-drug** • Leucovorin increases the efficacy and potential side effects of 5-FU; adjust dosage of 5-FU and monitor.

■ Nursing considerations

CLINICAL ALERT!
Name confusion has occurred between leucovorin and *Leukeran* (chlorambucil) and between folinic acid (leucovorin) and folic acid; use extreme caution.

Assessment

- **History:** Allergy to leucovorin on previous exposure, pernicious anemia or other megaloblastic anemias, lactation, pregnancy
- **Physical:** Skin lesions, color; R, adventitious sounds; CBC, Hgb, Hct, serum folate levels, serum methotrexate levels

Interventions

⊗ ***Warning*** Do not use benzyl alcohol solutions when giving leucovorin to premature infants; a fatal gasping syndrome has occurred.

- Begin leucovorin rescue within 24 hr of methotrexate administration. Arrange for fluid loading and urine alkalinization during this procedure to decrease methotrexate toxicity.
- Give drug orally unless intolerance to oral route develops due to nausea and vomiting from chemotherapy or clinical condition. Switch to oral drug when feasible. Doses more than 25 mg should be divided or given IV.

⊗ ***Warning*** Monitor patient for hypersensitivity reactions, especially if drug has been used previously. Keep supportive equipment and emergency drugs readily available in case of serious allergic response.

⊗ ***Warning*** Do not administer intrathecally; doing so can be fatal.

Teaching points

- Leucovorin "rescues" normal cells from the effects of methotrexate and allows them to survive.
- Leucovorin used to treat anemias or colorectal cancer must be given IV. Mark calendars with treatment days.
- Report rash, difficulty breathing, pain, or discomfort at injection site.

▽ leuprolide acetate

*(loo **proe'** lide)*

Eligard, Lupron, Lupron Depot, Lupron Depot-PED, Lupron Depot—3 Month, Lupron Depot—4 Month, Lupron for Pediatric Use

PREGNANCY CATEGORY X

Drug class

Gonadotropin-releasing hormone (GnRH) analogue

Therapeutic actions

An LH-RH agonist that occupies pituitary gonadotropin-releasing hormone receptors and desensitizes them; inhibits gonadotropin secretion when given continuously, leading to an initial increase, then profound decrease in LH and FSH levels.

Indications

- Advanced prostatic cancer—palliation, alternative to orchiectomy or estrogen therapy
- Depot only: Endometriosis
- Central precocious puberty
- Depot only: Uterine leiomyomata
- Unlabeled uses: Treatment of breast, ovarian, and endometrial cancer; infertility; prostatic hypertrophy

Contraindications and cautions

- Contraindicated with allergy to leuprolide, pregnancy, undiagnosed vaginal bleeding, lactation.

Available forms

Injection—5 mg/mL; *Depot*—3.75, 7.5 mg; *Depot-Ped*—7.5, 11.25, 15 mg; 3-mo *Depot*—11.25, 22.5, 45 mg; 4-mo *Depot*—30 mg, 72 mg; powder for injection—7.5 mg

Dosages

Adults

- *Advanced prostate cancer:* 1 mg/day subcutaneously; use only the syringes that come with the drug.
  Depot: 7.5 mg IM monthly (every 28–33 days). Do not use needles smaller than 22 gauge.
  3-mo depot: 22.5 mg IM or subcutaneously every 3 mo (84 days).
  4-mo depot: 30 mg IM or subcutaneously every 4 mo.
- *6-mo depot:* 45 mg subcutaneously every 6 mo.
- *Endometriosis:* 3.75 mg as a single monthly IM injection or 11.25 mg IM every 3 mo. Continue for 6 mo.
- *Uterine leiomyomata:* 3.75 mg as a single monthly injection for 3 mo *or* 11.25 mg IM once; give with concomitant iron treatment.

Pediatric patients

- *Central precocious puberty:* 50 mcg/kg/day subcutaneously; may be titrated up by 10 mcg/kg/day increments.
  Depot: 0.3 mg/kg IM monthly every 4 wk. Round to nearest depot size; minimum, 7.5 mg.

Pharmacokinetics

Route	*Onset*	*Peak*	*Duration*
IM depot	4 hr	Variable	1, 3, or 4 mo

Metabolism: Unknown; $T_{1/2}$: 3 hr (subcutaneous injection)
Distribution: Crosses placenta; may enter breast milk
Excretion: Unknown

Adverse effects

- **CNS:** *Dizziness, headache, pain,* paresthesia, blurred vision, lethargy, fatigue, insomnia, memory disorder
- **CV:** *Peripheral edema,* cardiac arrhythmias, thrombophlebitis, heart failure, **MI**
- **Dermatologic:** Rash, alopecia, itching, erythema
- **GI:** GI bleeding, *nausea, vomiting, anorexia,* sour taste, *constipation*
- **GU:** *Frequency, hematuria,* decrease in size of testes, increased BUN and creatinine, impotence, decreased libido, gynecomastia
- **Local:** Ecchymosis at injection site
- **Respiratory:** Difficulty breathing, pleural rub, worsening of pulmonary fibrosis
- **Other:** *Hot flashes, sweats,* bone pain

■ Nursing considerations

Assessment

- **History:** Allergy to leuprolide; pregnancy, lactation
- **Physical:** Skin lesions, color, turgor; testes; injection sites; orientation, affect, reflexes, peripheral sensation; peripheral pulses, edema, P; R, adventitious sounds; serum testosterone and serum PSA levels

Interventions

- Administer only with the syringes provided with the drug.
- Administer subcutaneously; monitor injection sites for bruising and rash; rotate injection sites to decrease local reaction.
- Give depot injection deep into muscle. Prepare a calendar of monthly (28–33 days every 3, 4, or 6 mo) return visits for new injection.
- Store below room temperature (25° C or 77° F); avoid freezing. Depot suspension is stable for 24 hr following reconstitution; product does not contain preservatives, so discard if not used properly.
- Arrange for periodic serum testosterone and PSA determinations.

⊗ ***Warning*** Consider stopping therapy for central precocious puberty before 11 yr in females, 12 yr in males. Monitor patient with GnRH stimulation test, sex steroids, and Tanner staging.

- Advise patient to use barrier contraceptives; serious fetal harm can occur.

- Teach patient and significant other the technique for subcutaneous injection, and observe administration before home administration of daily doses.

Teaching points

- Administer subcutaneously only, using the syringes that come with the drug; arrange to dispose of needles and syringes appropriately. If depot is used, drug may be given IM or subcutaneously; prepare calendar for return dates, stressing the importance of receiving each injection.
- Do not stop taking this drug without first consulting your health care provider.
- This drug cannot be taken during pregnancy; using barrier contraceptives is advised.
- You may experience these side effects: Bone pain, difficulty urinating (usually transient); hot flashes (stay in cool places); nausea, vomiting (eat frequent small meals); dizziness, headache, light-headedness (use caution when driving or performing tasks that require alertness); decreased libido, impotence.
- Report injection site pain, burning, itching, swelling, numbness, tingling, severe GI upset, pronounced hot flashes.

▽ levalbuterol

*(lev al **byoo'** ter ole)*

levalbuterol hydrochloride

Xopenex

levalbuterol tartrate

Xopenex HFA

PREGNANCY CATEGORY C

Drug classes

Antiasthmatic
Beta$_2$-selective adrenergic agonist
Bronchodilator
Sympathomimetic

Therapeutic actions

In low doses, acts relatively selectively at beta$_2$-adrenergic receptors to cause bronchodilation and vasodilation; at higher doses, beta$_2$-selectivity is lost and the drug also acts at beta$_1$ receptors to cause typical sympathomimetic cardiac effects.

Indications

- Treatment and prevention of bronchospasm in adults and children 4 yr and older, (tartrate) and 6 yr and older (hydrochloride) with reversible obstructive pulmonary disease

Contraindications and cautions

- Contraindicated with hypersensitivity to albuterol or levalbuterol; tachyarrhythmias, tachycardia caused by digoxin toxicity; general anesthesia with halogenated hydrocarbons or cyclopropane (these sensitize the myocardium to catecholamines); unstable vasomotor system disorders; hypertension; coronary insufficiency, coronary artery disease; history of CVA; COPD in patients who have developed degenerative heart disease.
- Use cautiously in psychoneurotic individuals and with hyperthyroidism; history of seizure disorders; pregnancy; lactation.

Available forms

Solution for inhalation—0.31 mg/3 mL, 0.63 mg/3 mL, 1.25 mg/3 mL; solution for inhalation concentrate—1.25 mg/0.5 mL; inhalation—45 mcg/actuation

Dosages

Levalbuterol hydrochloride

Adults and patients 12 yr and older

0.63 mg tid, every 6–8 hr by nebulization; if patient does not respond, the dose may be increased to up to 1.25 mg tid by nebulization.

Pediatric patients 6–11 yr

0.31 mg tid by nebulization; do not exceed 0.63 mg tid.

Pediatric patients younger than 6 yr

Safety and efficacy not established.

Levalbuterol tartrate

Adults and children 4 yr and older

Two inhalations (90 mcg) repeated every 4–6 hr; some patients may respond to 1 inhalation (45 mcg) every 4 hr.

Pharmacokinetics

Route	*Onset*	*Peak*	*Duration*
Inhalation	5 min	1 hr	6–8 hr

L

Metabolism: Hepatic; $T_{1/2}$: 4–6 hr
Distribution: Crosses placenta; enters breast milk
Excretion: Urine

Adverse effects

- **CNS:** *Apprehension, anxiety, fear, CNS stimulation,* hyperkinesia, insomnia, tremor, dizziness, irritability, weakness, vertigo, headache
- **CV:** Cardiac arrhythmias, tachycardia, palpitations, PVCs (rare), anginal pain (less likely with bronchodilator doses of this drug than with bronchodilator doses of a nonselective beta-agonist, eg, isoproterenol), increases or decreases in BP
- **Dermatologic:** Sweating, pallor, flushing
- **GI:** *Nausea,* vomiting, heartburn, unusual or bad taste
- **Respiratory:** Respiratory difficulties, pulmonary edema, coughing, URI, **bronchospasm**

Interactions

✱ **Drug-drug** • Risk of increased sympathomimetic effects when given with other sympathomimetics • Risk of increased toxicity, especially cardiac, when used in combination with theophylline, aminophylline • Possible decreased bronchodilating effects when given with beta-adrenergic blockers (eg, propranolol) • Risk of severe toxicity if combined with MAO inhibitors; use extreme caution

■ Nursing considerations

Assessment

- **History:** Hypersensitivity to levalbuterol or albuterol; tachyarrhythmias, tachycardia caused by digoxin toxicity; general anesthesia with halogenated hydrocarbons or cyclopropane; unstable vasomotor system disorders; hypertension; coronary artery disease; history of CVA; COPD in patients who have developed degenerative heart disease; diabetes mellitus; hyperthyroidism; history of seizure disorders; history of psychiatric illness; pregnancy, lactation
- **Physical:** Weight, skin color, T, turgor; orientation, reflexes, affect; P, BP; R, adventitious sounds; blood and urine glucose, serum electrolytes, thyroid function tests, ECG

Interventions

⊗ ***Warning*** Keep unopened drug in foil pouch until ready to use; protect from heat and light. Once foil pouch is open, use the vial within 2 wk, protected from light and heat. Once a vial is removed from foil pouch, use immediately. If not used, protect from light and use within 1 wk. Discard vial if solution is not colorless.

- Teach patient correct use of inhaler and maintenance of actuator (*Xopenex HFA*).
- Continue use to control recurrent bouts of bronchospasm; most effective with regular use.
- Do not exceed recommended dosage; administer inhalation drug forms during second half of inspiration, because the airways are open wider and the aerosol distribution is more extensive.

⊗ ***Warning*** Monitor patient response; if usual effective dosage regimen does not provide relief, this usually indicates a serious worsening of the asthma and indicates need for reassessment of drug regimen.

- Establish safety precautions if CNS changes occur.
- Reassure patients with acute respiratory distress; provide appropriate supportive measures.
- Monitor environmental temperature if patient has flushing or sweating.

Teaching points

- Do not exceed recommended dosage—adverse effects or loss of effectiveness may result; read the instructions for use that come with the product for proper administration of nebulized drug.
- Keep unopened drug in foil pouch until ready to use; protect from heat and light. Once foil pouch is open, use the vial within 2 weeks, protected from light and heat. Once a vial is removed from its foil pouch, use immediately. If not used, protect from light and use within 1 week. Discard the vial if the solution is not colorless.
- You may experience these side effects: Dizziness, fatigue, headache (use caution if driving or performing tasks that require alertness if these effects occur); nausea, vomiting, change in taste (eat frequent small meals;

consult your health care provider if this is prolonged); rapid heart rate, anxiety, sweating, flushing.
- If using a metered inhaler (*Xopenex HFA*), prime the inhaler before use; blow out all the air you can expel, place the actuator in your mouth and slowly breathe in while pressing down on the top of the metal canister. Hold your breath for 10 seconds. If you are prescribed two inhalations, wait 10 seconds and then repeat the process. Wash and air dry the actuator at least once a week. Discard the metal canister after 200 sprays, even if you think the canister is not empty.
- Report chest pain, dizziness, insomnia, weakness, tremors or irregular heartbeat, difficulty breathing, productive cough, failure to respond to usual dosage.

levetiracetam

(lev ah ty ray' ca tam)

Keppra, Keppra XR DNC

PREGNANCY CATEGORY C

Drug class
Antiepileptic

Therapeutic actions
Mechanism of action not well understood; antiepileptic activity may be related to its ability to inhibit polysynaptic responses and block posttetanic potentiation.

Indications
- Adjunctive therapy in the treatment of partial-onset seizures in adults and children 4 yr and older with epilepsy, when used with other epilepsy medication
- Adjunctive therapy in the treatment of myoclonic seizures in patients 12 yr and older
- Adjunctive therapy in treatment of primary generalized tonic-clonic seizures in adults and children 6 yr and older with idiopathic generalized epilepsy
- Unlabeled uses: Migraine, adjunctive therapy for bipolar disease, monotherapy for new-onset pediatric epilepsy.

Contraindications and cautions
- Contraindicated with hypersensitivity to levetiracetam.
- Use cautiously with lactation, pregnancy, renal impairment.

Available forms
Tablets—250, 500, 750, 1,000 mg; oral solution—100 mg/mL; injection—500 mg/5 mL; ER tablets DNC—500 mg

Dosages
Adults and children older than 16 yr
- *Partial-onset seizures:* 1,000 mg/day given as 500 mg PO or IV bid; may be increased in 1,000-mg/day increments every 2 wk; maximum dose, 3,000 mg/day. ER tablets: 1,000 mg/day PO; increase every 2 wk in 1,000 mg/day intervals to maximum dosage 3,000 mg/day.
- *Generalized tonic-clonic seizures:* Initially, 1,000 mg/day PO given as 500 mg bid; increase by 1,000 mg/day every 2 wk to recommended 3,000 mg/day.

Adults and children 12 yr and older
- *Myoclonic seizures:* 1,000 mg/day given as 500 mg PO bid; slowly increase to recommended maximum dose, 3,000 mg/day.

Pediatric patients 6–15 yr
- *Generalized tonic-clonic seizures:* Initially, 20 mg/kg/day PO in two divided doses of 10 mg/kg. Increase every 2 wk by 20-mg/kg increments to recommended dosage of 60 mg/kg/day given as 30 mg/kg bid.

Pediatric patients 4–16 yr
- *Partial-onset seizures:* 10 mg/kg PO bid (500–1,000 mg/day), may be increased every 2 wk in 20 mg/kg increments to 30 mg/kg bid (1,500–3,000 mg/day). To determine daily dose of oral solution: total dose (mL/day) = daily dose (mg/kg/day) × patient weight (kg) divided by 100 mg/mL.

Patients with renal impairment

CrCl (mL/min)	*Dosage (mg)*
More than 80	500–1,500 every 12 hr
50–80	500–1,000 every 12 hr
30–50	250–750 every 12 hr
Less than 30	250–500 every 12 hr

L

For patients on dialysis, use 500–1,000 mg every 24 hr.

Pharmacokinetics

Route	Onset	Peak
Oral	Rapid	1 hr

Metabolism: $T_{1/2}$: 6–8 hr
Distribution: Crosses placenta; may enter breast milk
Excretion: Urine, unchanged

IV FACTS

Preparation: Dilute desired dose in 100 mL of 0.9% sodium chloride, lactated Ringer's solution, or 5% dextrose solution.
Infusion: Infuse over 15 min.
Compatibilities: Compatible with lorazepam, diazepam, valproate sodium.

Adverse effects

- **CNS:** *Dizziness, headache,* vertigo, nervousness, fatigue, *somnolence, ataxia,* diplopia, suicidal ideation
- **Dermatologic:** Pruritus
- **GI:** Dyspepsia, vomiting, nausea, constipation, anorexia
- **Respiratory:** Rhinitis, pharyngitis
- **Other:** Weight gain, facial edema, impotence

■ Nursing considerations

CLINICAL ALERT!
Name confusion has occurred between *Keppra* (levetiracetam) and *Kaletra* (lopinavir and ritonavir); use extreme caution.

Assessment

- **History:** Hypersensitivity to levetiracetam; lactation, renal impairment, pregnancy
- **Physical:** Body weight; body T; skin color, lesions; orientation, affect, reflexes; P, R, adventitious sounds; bowel sounds, normal output, renal function tests

Interventions

- Reserve IV use for short-term, when oral administration is not feasible; revert to oral use as soon as patient is able.
- Give drug with food to prevent GI upset; use oral solution for children or adults with difficulty swallowing. Ensure that patient does not cut, crush, or chew ER tablets.
- If CNS, vision, or coordination changes occur, establish safety precautions (use side rails, accompany patient when ambulating).
- Advise using barrier contraceptives while this drug is being used.

⊗ ***Warning*** Do not stop drug abruptly. Risk of seizure precipitation; withdraw gradually.

- Offer support and encouragement for dealing with epilepsy and adverse drug effects; arrange for consultation with support groups for people with epilepsy as needed.

Teaching points

- Take this drug exactly as prescribed. Do not cut, crush, or chew ER tablets; swallow them whole.
- Do not discontinue this drug abruptly or change dosage, except on the advice of your health care provider.
- Do not take this drug if you are pregnant or plan to become pregnant, serious fetal effects can occur, using barrier contraceptives is recommended.
- Wear or carry a medical alert tag at all times so that any emergency medical personnel taking care of you will know that you have epilepsy and are taking an antiepileptic.
- You may experience these side effects: Dizziness, blurred vision (avoid driving a car or performing other tasks requiring alertness or visual acuity if this occurs); GI upset (taking the drug with food or milk and eating frequent small meals may help); headache, nervousness (if these become severe, consult your health care provider); fatigue (periodic rest periods may be helpful).
- Report severe headache, sleepwalking, rash, severe vomiting, chills, fever, difficulty breathing.

▽ levocetirizine dihydrochloride

*(lev oh seh **teer'** ih zeen)*

Xyzal

PREGNANCY CATEGORY B

Drug class
Antihistamine

Therapeutic actions
Potent histamine (H_1) receptor antagonist; inhibits histamine release and eosinophil chemotaxis during inflammation, reducing swelling and inflammatory response.

Indications
- Relief from symptoms of seasonal and perennial allergic rhinitis in adults and children 6 mo and older
- Treatment of uncomplicated skin effects in chronic idiopathic urticaria in patients 2 yr and older

Contraindications and cautions
- Contraindicated with hypersensitivity to levocetirizine, any of its components, or cetirizine; end-stage renal disease; renal impairment in children 6–11 yr; lactation.
- Use cautiously with pregnancy and with use of CNS depressants.

Available forms
Tablets—5 mg; oral solution—2.5 mg/5 mL

Dosages
Adults and children 12 yr and older

5 mg/day PO, taken in the evening.

Children 6–11 yr

2.5 mg/day PO taken in the evening.

Children 6 mo–5 yr

1.25 mg (½ tsp oral solution) PO once daily in the evening.

Patients with renal impairment

12 yr and older: If creatinine clearance is 50–80 mL/min, give 2.5 mg/day PO; if creatinine clearance is 30–50 mL/min, give 2.5 mg PO every other day; if creatinine clearance is 10–30 mL/min, give 2.5 mg PO twice weekly (once every 3–4 days); if creatinine clearance is less than 10 mL/min, drug is not recommended.

Pharmacokinetics

Route	*Onset*	*Peak*
Oral	Rapid	1 hr

Metabolism: $T_{1/2}$: 8 hr

Distribution: May cross placenta; enters breast milk

Excretion: Urine, unchanged

Adverse effects
- **CNS:** *Somnolence,* asthenia
- **GI:** Dry mouth
- **Respiratory:** *Nasopharyngitis,* cough, pharyngitis, epistaxis
- **Other:** *Fatigue,* fever

Interactions
✱ Drug-drug • Risk of increased CNS depression and altered mental alertness if combined with alcohol or other CNS depressing drugs; avoid this combination

■ Nursing considerations
Assessment
- **History:** Hypersensitivity to any component of the drug or to cetirizine, renal impairment, pregnancy, lactation, use of CNS depressants
- **Physical:** T; orientation, affect, reflexes; R, adventitious sounds; renal function tests

Interventions
- Administer once each day, in the evening.
- Alert patient to possible alterations in mental alertness while taking this drug.
- Encourage use of humidifiers and adequate intake of fluids to help prevent severe dryness of mucous membranes.
- Provide skin care for urticaria.

Teaching points
- Take this drug once each day, in the evening. Do not take more than the prescribed dose in any one day.
- It is not known how this drug could affect a nursing baby. If you are nursing a baby, another method of feeding the baby should be selected.
- It is not known how this drug could affect a fetus; if you are pregnant, consult your health care provider.
- Avoid the use of alcohol or any CNS depressants while you are using this drug; these could increase the effects on mental alertness.
- You may experience these side effects: Sleepiness, decreased mental alertness (avoid driving

a car, operating dangerous machinery, or engaging in tasks that require mental alertness while you are on this drug); cough, nosebleed, sore throat (use a humidifier, and make sure you drink plenty of fluids to help prevent severe drying of your mucous membranes).
- Report difficulty breathing, nosebleeds, and marked changes in mental functioning.

levodopa

*(lee voe **doe'** pa)*

PREGNANCY CATEGORY C

Drug class
Antiparkinsonian

Therapeutic actions
Biochemical precursor of the neurotransmitter dopamine, which is deficient in the basal ganglia of parkinsonism patients; unlike dopamine, levodopa penetrates the blood–brain barrier. It is transformed in the brain to dopamine; thus, levodopa is a form of replacement therapy. It is efficacious for 2–5 yr in relieving the symptoms of parkinsonism but not drug-induced extrapyramidal disorders.

Indications
- Treatment of parkinsonism (postencephalitic, arteriosclerotic, and idiopathic types) and symptomatic parkinsonism following injury to the nervous system by carbon monoxide or manganese intoxication
- Given with carbidopa (*Lodosyn;* fixed combinations, *Sinemet*), an enzyme inhibitor that decreases the activity of dopa decarboxylase in the periphery, thus reducing blood levels of levodopa and decreasing the intensity and incidence of many of the adverse effects of levodopa
- Unlabeled uses: Relief of herpes zoster (shingles) pain; restless leg syndrome

Contraindications and cautions
- Contraindicated with hypersensitivity to levodopa; allergy to tartrazine (an ingredient in *Dopar*); glaucoma, especially angle-closure glaucoma; lactation.
- Use cautiously in psychiatric patients, especially the depressed or psychotic; and with severe CV or pulmonary disease; occlusive cerebrovascular disease; history of MI with residual arrhythmias; bronchial asthma; renal, hepatic, endocrine disease; history of peptic ulcer; pregnancy.

Available forms
Available only in combination products

Dosages
Adults
Individualize dosage. Increase dosage gradually to minimize side effects; titrate dosage carefully to optimize benefits and minimize side effects. Initially, 0.5–1 g PO daily divided into two or more doses given with food. Increase gradually in increments not exceeding 0.75 g/day every 3–7 days as tolerated. Do not exceed 8 g/day, except for exceptional patients. A significant therapeutic response may not be obtained for 6 mo.
Pediatric patients
Safety for use in children younger than 12 yr not established.

Pharmacokinetics

Route	*Onset*	*Peak*
Oral	Varies	0.5–2 hr

Metabolism: Hepatic; $T_{1/2}$: 1–3 hr
Distribution: Crosses placenta; enters breast milk
Excretion: Urine

Adverse effects
- **CNS:** *Adventitious movement (eg, dystonic movements), ataxia, increased hand tremor, headache, dizziness, numbness, weakness and faintness,* bruxism, confusion, insomnia, nightmares, hallucinations and delusions, agitation and anxiety, malaise, fatigue, euphoria, mental changes (including paranoid ideation), psychotic episodes, depression with or without suicidal tendencies, dementia, bradykinesia ("on-off" phenomenon), muscle twitching and blepharospasm, diplopia, blurred vision, dilated pupils
- **CV:** Cardiac irregularities, palpitations, orthostatic hypotension

- **Dermatologic:** Flushing, hot flashes, increased sweating, rash
- **GI:** *Anorexia, nausea, vomiting, abdominal pain or distress, dry mouth, dysphagia, dysgeusia,* bitter taste, sialorrhea, trismus, burning sensation of the tongue, diarrhea, constipation, flatulence, weight change, upper GI hemorrhage in patients with history of peptic ulcer
- **GU:** Urinary retention, urinary incontinence
- **Hematologic:** Leukopenia, anemia, elevated BUN, AST, ALT, LDH, bilirubin, alkaline phosphatase, protein-bound iodine
- **Respiratory:** Bizarre breathing patterns

Interactions

✱ Drug-drug ⊗ ***Warning*** Increased therapeutic effects and possible hypertensive crisis with MAOIs; withdraw MAOIs at least 14 days before starting levodopa therapy
• Decreased efficacy with pyridoxine (vitamin B_6), phenytoin, papaverine, TCAs, benzodiazepines

✱ Drug-lab test • May interfere with urine tests for sugar or ketones • False Coombs' test results • False elevations of uric acid when using colorimetric method

■ Nursing considerations

Assessment

- **History:** Hypersensitivity to levodopa, tartrazine; glaucoma; history of melanoma; suspicious or undiagnosed skin lesions; severe CV or pulmonary disease; occlusive cerebrovascular disease; history of MI with residual arrhythmias; bronchial asthma; renal, hepatic, endocrine disease; history of peptic ulcer; psychiatric disorders; lactation, pregnancy
- **Physical:** Weight; T; skin color, lesions; orientation, affect, reflexes, bilateral grip strength, vision examination; P, BP, orthostatic BP, auscultation; R, depth, adventitious sounds; bowel sounds, normal output, liver evaluation; voiding pattern, normal output, prostate palpation; LFTs, renal function tests; CBC with differential

Interventions

⊗ ***Warning*** Arrange to decrease dosage if therapy is interrupted; observe for the development of suicidal tendencies.

- Give with meals if GI upset occurs.
- Ensure that patient voids before receiving dose if urinary retention is a problem.
- Monitor hepatic, renal, hematopoietic, and CV function.
- For patients who take multivitamins, provide a preparation without pyridoxine.

Teaching points

- Take this drug exactly as prescribed.
- Do not take multivitamin preparations with pyridoxine. These may prevent any therapeutic effect of levodopa. Notify your health care provider if you need vitamins.
- You may experience these side effects: Drowsiness, dizziness, confusion, blurred vision (avoid driving or engaging in activities that require alertness and visual acuity); nausea (take with meals, eat frequent small meals); dry mouth (suck sugarless lozenges or ice chips); painful or difficult urination (empty bladder before each dose); constipation (maintain adequate fluid intake and exercise regularly, request correctives); dark sweat or urine (not harmful); dizziness or faintness when you get up (change position slowly and use caution when climbing stairs).
- Report fainting, light-headedness, dizziness; uncontrollable movements of the face, eyelids, mouth, tongue, neck, arms, hands, or legs; mental changes; irregular heartbeat or palpitations; difficult urination; severe or persistent nausea or vomiting.

L

▽ levofloxacin

*(lee voe **flox'** a sin)*

Levaquin

PREGNANCY CATEGORY C

Drug classes

Antibiotic
Fluoroquinolone

Therapeutic actions

Bactericidal: Interferes with DNA by inhibiting DNA gyrase replication in susceptible gram-negative and gram-positive bacteria, preventing cell reproduction.

Indications

- Treatment of adults with community-acquired pneumonia, bacterial sinusitis caused by susceptible bacteria including multidrug resistant strains
- Treatment of acute exacerbation of chronic bronchitis caused by susceptible bacteria
- Treatment of complicated and uncomplicated skin and skin structure infections caused by susceptible bacteria
- Treatment of complicated and uncomplicated UTIs and acute pyelonephritis caused by susceptible bacteria
- Treatment of complicated UTIs caused by *Escherichia coli, Klebsiella pneumoniae,* or *Proteus mirabilis* and acute pyelonephritis caused by *E. coli*
- Treatment of chronic bacterial prostatitis caused by *E. coli, Enterococcus faecalis, Staphylococcus*
- Treatment of nosocomial pneumonia due to methicillin-sensitive *Staphylococcus aureus, Pseudomonas strains, Serratia, E. coli, Klebsiella, Haemophilus influenzae, Streptococcus pneumoniae*
- Treatment of postexposure inhalational anthrax
- Unlabeled uses: Traveler's diarrhea, epididymitis, gonococcal infection, pelvic inflamatory disease, urethritis

Contraindications and cautions

- Contraindicated with allergy to fluoroquinolones, lactation.
- Use cautiously with renal impairment, seizures, pregnancy.

Available forms

Tablets—250, 500, 750 mg; oral solution—25 mg/mL; injection—5 mg/mL; injection concentrate—25 mg/mL

Dosages

Adults

- *Community-acquired pneumonia:* 500 mg daily PO or IV for 7–14 days.
- *Sinusitis:* 500 mg daily PO or IV for 10–14 days or 750 mg/day PO or IV for 5 days.
- *Chronic bronchitis:* 500 mg daily PO or IV for 7 days.
- *Skin infection:* 500–750 mg daily PO or IV for 7–14 days.
- *UTIs:* 250 mg daily PO or IV for 3–10 days; complicated, 750 mg/day PO or IV for 5 days.
- *Pyelonephritis:* 250 mg daily PO or IV for 10 days or 750 mg PO or IV for 5 days.
- *Nosocomial pneumonia:* 750 mg daily PO or IV for 7–14 days.
- *Chronic prostatitis:* 500 mg/day PO for 28 days or 500 mg/day by slow IV infusion over 60 min for 28 days.
- *Postexposure anthrax:* 500 mg/day PO or IV for 60 days.

Pediatric patients

- *Inhalational anthrax:* 6 mo or older weighing more than 50 kg: 500 mg/day PO for 60 days; 6 mo or older weighing less than 50 kg: 8 mg/kg every 12 hr PO for 60 days. Do not exceed 250 mg/dose.

Patients with renal impairment

CrCl (mL/min)	*Dose*
50–80	No adjustment
20–49	500 mg initially, then 250 mg daily; or 750 mg then 750 mg every 48 hr
10–19	500 mg initially, then 250 mg every 48 hr; or 750 mg, then 500 mg every 48 hr

For patients on dialysis, 750 mg initially, then 500 mg every 48 hr; or 500 mg initially, then 250 mg every 48 hr.

Pharmacokinetics

Route	*Onset*	*Peak*	*Duration*
Oral	Varies	1–2 hr	3–5 hr
IV	Rapid	End of infusion	3–5 hr

Metabolism: Hepatic; $T_{1/2}$: 6–8 hr
Distribution: Crosses placenta; enters breast milk
Excretion: Urine

IV FACTS

Preparation: No further preparation is needed if using the premixed solution; dilute single-use vials in 50–100 mL D_5W.
Infusion: Administer slowly over at least 60–90 min. Do not administer IM or subcutaneously.

Compatibilities: Can be further diluted in 0.9% sodium chloride injection, 5% dextrose injection, 5% dextrose/0.9% sodium chloride, 5% dextrose in lactated Ringer's, *Plasma-Lyte 56* and *5% Dextrose* injection, 5% dextrose/0.45% sodium chloride, 0.15% potassium chloride, sodium lactate injection.

Adverse effects

- **CNS:** *Headache,* dizziness, *insomnia,* fatigue, somnolence, blurred vision
- **GI:** *Nausea,* vomiting, dry mouth, *diarrhea,* abdominal pain (occur less with this drug than with ofloxacin), constipation, flatulence, abnormal liver function
- **GU:** Abnormal renal function, acute renal failure, UTI, urine retention
- **Hematologic:** Elevated BUN, serum creatinine, and alkaline phosphatase; neutropenia, anemia
- **Other:** Fever, rash, photosensitivity, *muscle and joint tenderness,* increased serum glucose, tendinitis

Interactions

✱ **Drug-drug** • Decreased therapeutic effect with iron salts, sucralfate, antacids, zinc, magnesium (separate by at least 2 hr) • Increased risk of seizures with NSAIDs; avoid this combination • Risk of prolonged QT interval if combined with other drugs known to prolong QT interval; use caution

✱ **Drug-alternative therapy** • Increased risk of severe photosensitivity reactions if combined with St. John's wort therapy

■ Nursing considerations

Assessment

- **History:** Allergy to fluoroquinolones, renal impairment, seizures, lactation, pregnancy
- **Physical:** Skin color, lesions; T; orientation, reflexes, affect; mucous membranes, bowel sounds; LFTs, renal function tests; blood glucose (patients with diabetes)

Interventions

⊗ ***Black box warning*** There is a risk of tendinitis and tendon rupture with drug administration. Risk increase in patients older than 60 yr, with concurrent corticosteroids use, and with kidney, heart, or lung transplant.

- Arrange for culture and sensitivity tests before beginning therapy.
- Continue therapy as indicated for condition being treated.
- Administer oral drug without regard to meals with a glass of water; separate oral drug from other cation administration, including antacids, by at least 2 hr.
- Ensure that patient is well hydrated during course of therapy.

⊗ ***Warning*** Discontinue drug at any sign of hypersensitivity (rash, photophobia) or at complaint of tendon pain, inflammation, or rupture.

- Monitor clinical response; if no improvement is seen or a relapse occurs, repeat culture and sensitivity test.

Teaching points

- Take oral drug without regard to meals. If an antacid is needed, do not take it within 2 hours of levofloxacin dose.
- Drink plenty of fluids while you are using this drug.
- You may experience these side effects: Nausea, vomiting, abdominal pain (eat frequent small meals); diarrhea or constipation (consult your health care provider); drowsiness, blurred vision, dizziness (use caution if driving or operating dangerous equipment); sensitivity to sunlight (avoid exposure, use a sunscreen if needed).
- Report rash, visual changes, severe GI problems, weakness, tremors, muscle pain.

▽ levoleucovorin

See Appendix W, *Less commonly used drugs*.

DANGEROUS DRUG

▽ levorphanol tartrate

(lee vor' fa nole)

Levo-Dromoran

PREGNANCY CATEGORY C

CONTROLLED SUBSTANCE C-II

Drug class

Opioid agonist analgesic

Therapeutic actions

Acts as agonist at specific opioid receptors in the CNS to produce analgesia, euphoria, sedation; the receptors are thought to be the same as those mediating the effects of endogenous opioids (enkephalins, endorphins).

Indications

- Relief of moderate to severe acute and chronic pain
- Preoperative medication to allay apprehension, provide prolonged analgesia, reduce thiopental requirements, and shorten recovery time (*Levo-Dromoran*)

Contraindications and cautions

- Contraindicated with hypersensitivity to opioids, diarrhea caused by poisoning (before toxins are eliminated), pregnancy (neonatal withdrawal), labor or delivery (respiratory depression of neonate—premature infants are especially at risk; may prolong labor), bronchial asthma, acute alcoholism, increased intracranial pressure, respiratory depression, anoxia.
- Use cautiously with COPD, cor pulmonale, acute abdominal conditions, CV disease, supraventricular tachycardias, myxedema, seizure disorders, delirium tremens, cerebral arteriosclerosis, ulcerative colitis, kyphoscoliosis, Addison's disease, prostatic hypertrophy, urethral stricture, recent GI or GU surgery, toxic psychosis, and renal or hepatic impairment.

Available forms

Tablets—2 mg; injection—2 mg/mL

Dosages

Adults

Starting dose is 2 mg PO repeated every 6–8 hr (*Levo-Dromoran*) or 3–6 hr (levorphanol). Increase to 3 mg if necessary (*Levo-Dromoran*). Higher doses may be needed in opioid-tolerant patients or patients with severe pain. Usual dose 8–16 mg/day (levorphanol) or 6–12 mg/day (*Levo-Dromoran*).

IM or subcutaneous

1–2 mg; repeat in 6–8 hr as needed. Do not exceed 8 mg/day IM.

Geriatric patients or impaired adults

Use caution—respiratory depression may occur in the elderly, the very ill, and those with respiratory problems. Reduced dosage (by up to 50%) may be necessary.

Pharmacokinetics

Route	*Onset*	*Peak*	*Duration*
Oral	30–90 min	0.5–1 hr	6–8 hr

Metabolism: Hepatic; $T_{1/2}$: 12–16 hr
Distribution: Crosses placenta; enters breast milk
Excretion: Urine

Adverse effects

- **CNS:** *Light-headedness, dizziness, sedation,* euphoria, dysphoria, delirium, insomnia, agitation, anxiety, fear, hallucinations, disorientation, drowsiness, lethargy, impaired mental and physical performance, coma, mood changes, weakness, headache, tremor, seizures, miosis, visual disturbances, suppression of cough reflex
- **CV:** Facial flushing, peripheral circulatory collapse, tachycardia, bradycardia, arrhythmia, palpitations, chest wall rigidity, hypertension, hypotension, orthostatic hypotension, syncope
- **Dermatologic:** Pruritus, urticaria, edema, hemorrhagic urticaria (rare)
- **GI:** *Nausea, vomiting,* dry mouth, anorexia, *constipation,* biliary tract spasm; increased colonic motility in patients with chronic ulcerative colitis
- **GU:** Ureteral spasm, spasm of vesicle sphincters, urinary retention or hesitancy, oliguria, antidiuretic effect, reduced libido or potency
- **Respiratory: Bronchospasm, laryngospasm**
- **Major hazards:** Respiratory depression, apnea, circulatory depression, **respiratory arrest, shock, cardiac arrest**
- **Other:** *Sweating* (more common in ambulatory patients and those without severe pain), physical tolerance and dependence, psychological dependence

Interactions

✱ **Drug-drug** • Potentiation of effects of levorphanol when given with barbiturate anesthetics; decrease dose of levorphanol when coadministering • Increased risk of CNS effects with ethanol, barbiturates, antihistamines, and other sedating drugs

✱ **Drug-lab test** • Elevated biliary tract pressure may cause increases in plasma amylase and lipase; determinations of these levels may be unreliable for 24 hr after administration of opioids

■ Nursing considerations

Assessment

- **History:** Hypersensitivity to opioids, diarrhea caused by poisoning, labor or delivery, bronchial asthma, acute alcoholism, increased intracranial pressure, respiratory depression, cor pulmonale, acute abdominal conditions, CV disease, myxedema, seizure disorders, delirium tremens, cerebral arteriosclerosis, ulcerative colitis, fever, kyphoscoliosis, Addison's disease, prostatic hypertrophy, urethral stricture, recent GI or GU surgery, toxic psychosis, renal or hepatic impairment
- **Physical:** T; skin color, texture, lesions; orientation, reflexes, pupil size, bilateral grip strength, affect; P, auscultation, BP, orthostatic BP, perfusion; R, adventitious sounds; bowel sounds, normal output; frequency and pattern of voiding, normal output; ECG; EEG; thyroid, LFTs, renal function tests

Interventions

- Give to lactating women 4–6 hr before the next feeding to minimize the amount in milk.
- Reassure patient that most people who receive opiates for medical reasons do not develop psychological dependency.

Teaching points

- Take drug exactly as prescribed.
- Do not take leftover medication for other disorders, and do not let anyone else take your prescription.
- You may experience these side effects: Nausea, loss of appetite (take with food, lie quietly, eat frequent small meals); constipation (laxative may help); dizziness, sedation, drowsiness, impaired visual acuity (avoid driving, performing other tasks that require alertness or visual acuity).
- Report severe nausea, vomiting, constipation, shortness of breath, or difficulty breathing.

▽levothyroxine sodium (L-thyroxine, T_4)

(lee voe thye rox' een)

Levothroid, Levoxine, Levoxyl, Synthroid, Thyro-Tabs, Unithroid

PREGNANCY CATEGORY A

Drug class

Thyroid hormone

Therapeutic actions

Increases the metabolic rate of body tissues, thereby increasing oxygen consumption; respiration and HR; rate of fat, protein, and carbohydrate metabolism; and growth and maturation.

Indications

- Replacement therapy in hypothyroidism
- Pituitary TSH suppression in the treatment and prevention of euthyroid goiters and in the management of thyroid cancer
- Treatment of thyrotoxicosis in conjunction with antithyroid drugs and to prevent goitrogenesis, hypothyroidism, and thyrotoxicosis during pregnancy
- Treatment of myxedema coma

Contraindications and cautions

- Contraindicated with allergy to active or extraneous constituents of drug, untreated thyrotoxicosis, and acute MI uncomplicated by hypothyroidism.
- Use cautiously with Addison's disease (treat hypoadrenalism with corticosteroids before thyroid therapy), lactation, patients with coronary artery disease or angina.

Available forms

Tablets—25, 50, 75, 88, 100, 112, 125, 137, 150, 175, 200, 300 mcg; powder for injection—200, 500 mcg/vial; capsules—13, 25, 50, 75, 100, 125, 150 mcg

L

Dosages

50–100 mcg equals approximately 60 mg (1 grain) desiccated thyroid.

Adults

- *Hypothyroidism:* Initial dose, 50 mcg PO, with increasing increments of 25 mcg PO every 6–8 wk; maintenance up to 200 mcg/day. IV or IM injection can be substituted for the oral dosage form when oral ingestion is not possible. Usual IV dose is 50% of oral dose. Start at 25 mcg/day or less in patients with long-standing hypothyroidism or known cardiac disease. Usual replacement 1.7 mcg/kg per day.
- *Myxedema coma without severe heart disease:* 200–500 mcg IV as initial dose. An additional 100–300 mcg or more may be given the second day if necessary. Switch to PO once patient is able. Full effect not seen for 24 hr; dose based on improvement.
- *TSH suppression in thyroid cancer, nodules, and euthyroid goiters:* Doses should be individualized based on specific disease and patient. Larger amounts than used for normal suppression.
- *Thyroid suppression therapy:* 2.6 mcg/kg/day PO for 7–10 days.
- Older patients may require less than 1 mcg/kg/day. For most patients older than 50 yr or under age 50 with cardiac disease, an initial dose of 12.5 to 25 mcg/day with increases of 25 mcg/day every 6–8 wk.

Pediatric patients

- *Congenital hypothyroidism:* Infants require replacement therapy from birth.
  0–3 mo: 10–15 mcg/kg/day.
  3–6 mo: 8–10 mcg/kg/day.
  6–12 mo: 6–8 mcg/kg/day.
  1–5 yr: 5–6 mcg/kg/day.
  6–12 yr: 4–5 mcg/kg/day.
  Older than 12 yr: 2–3 mcg/kg/day.

Pharmacokinetics

Route	Onset	Peak
Oral	Slow	1–3 wk
IV	6–8 hr	24–48 hr

Metabolism: Hepatic; $T_{1/2}$: 6–7 days
Distribution: Crosses placenta; enters breast milk
Excretion: Urine

IV FACTS

Preparation: Add 5 mL 0.9% sodium chloride injection. Shake the vial to ensure complete mixing. Use immediately after reconstitution. Discard any unused portion.
Infusion: Inject directly, each 100 mcg over 1 min.
Incompatibilities: Do not mix with any other IV fluids.

Adverse effects

- **CNS:** Tremors, headache, nervousness, insomnia
- **CV:** Palpitations, tachycardia, angina, **cardiac arrest**
- **Dermatologic:** Allergic skin reactions, partial loss of hair in first few months of therapy in children
- **GI:** Diarrhea, nausea, vomiting, gagging, tablet stuck in throat, choking, esophageal atresia

Interactions

✱ **Drug-drug** • Decreased absorption of oral thyroid preparation with cholestyramine, colestipol, aluminum- and magnesium-containing antacids, iron, sucralfate • Increased risk of bleeding with warfarin—reduce dosage of anticoagulant when T_4 is begun • Decreased effectiveness of cardiac glycosides if taken with thyroid replacement • Decreased theophylline clearance when patient is in hypothyroid state; monitor levels and patient response as euthyroid state is achieved

■ Nursing considerations

Assessment

- **History:** Allergy to active or extraneous constituents of drug, thyrotoxicosis, acute MI uncomplicated by hypothyroidism, Addison's disease, lactation
- **Physical:** Skin lesions, color, T, texture; T; muscle tone, orientation, reflexes; P, auscultation, baseline ECG, BP; R, adventitious sounds; thyroid function tests

Interventions

⊗ ***Black box warning*** Do not use for weight loss; large doses may cause serious adverse effects.

- Monitor response carefully at start of therapy, and adjust dosage. Full therapeutic effect may not be seen for several days.
- Ensure that patient swallows tablet with a full glass of water.
- Do not change brands of T_4 products, due to possible bioequivalence problems.
- Do not add IV doses to other IV fluids.
- Use caution in patients with CV disease.
- Administer oral drug as a single daily dose before breakfast with a full glass of water.
- Arrange for regular, periodic blood tests of thyroid function.
- For children and other patients who cannot swallow tablets, crush and suspend in a small amount of water or formula, or sprinkle over soft food. Administer immediately.

⊗ ***Warning*** Most CV and CNS adverse effects indicate that the dose is too high. Check thyroid function tests and arrange to adjust dosage as necessary.

Teaching points

- Take as a single dose before breakfast with a full glass of water.
- This drug replaces an important hormone and will need to be taken for life. Do not discontinue drug without consulting your health care provider; serious problems can occur.
- Carry a medical ID tag to alert emergency medical personnel that you are use this drug.
- Arrange to have periodic blood tests and medical evaluations. Keep your scheduled appointments.
- Report headache, chest pain, palpitations, fever, weight loss, sleeplessness, nervousness, irritability, unusual sweating, intolerance to heat, diarrhea.

DANGEROUS DRUG

▽ lidocaine hydrochloride

(lye' doe kane)

lidocaine HCl in 5% dextrose

lidocaine HCl without preservatives

Antiarrhythmic preparations: Xylocaine HCl IV for Cardiac Arrhythmias

Local anesthetic preparations: Octocaine, Xylocaine HCl (injectable)

Topical for mucous membranes: Anestacon, Burn-O-Jel, DentiPatch, DermaFlex, Xylocaine, Zilactin-L

Topical Dermatologic: L-M-X4, Lidamantle, Numby Stuff, Regenecare, Solarcaine, Xylocaine

Transdermal: Lidoderm

PREGNANCY CATEGORY B

Drug classes

Antiarrhythmic
Local anesthetic

Therapeutic actions

Type 1b antiarrhythmic: Decreases diastolic depolarization, decreasing automaticity of ventricular cells; increases ventricular fibrillation threshold.

Local anesthetic: Blocks the generation and conduction of action potentials in sensory nerves by reducing sodium permeability, reducing height and rate of rise of the action potential, increasing excitation threshold, and slowing conduction velocity.

Indications

- As antiarrhythmic: Management of acute ventricular arrhythmias during cardiac surgery and MI (IV use). Use IM when IV administration is not possible or when ECG monitoring is not available and the danger of ventricular arrhythmias is great (single-dose IM use, for example, by paramedics in a mobile coronary care unit)
- As alternative to amiodarone to treat ventricular fibrillation or tachycardia with cardiac arrest
- As anesthetic: Infiltration anesthesia, peripheral and sympathetic nerve blocks, central nerve blocks, spinal and caudal anesthesia, retrobulbar and transtracheal injection; topical anesthetic for skin disorders and accessible mucous membranes

- As local analgesia for pain associated with postherpetic neuralgia

Contraindications and cautions

- Contraindicated with allergy to lidocaine or amide-type local anesthetics, heart failure, cardiogenic shock, second- or third-degree heart block (if no artificial pacemaker), Stokes-Adams syndrome, Wolff-Parkinson-White syndrome.
- Use cautiously with hepatic or renal disease, inflammation or sepsis in the region of injection (local anesthetic), labor and delivery (epidural anesthesia may prolong the second stage of labor; monitor for fetal and neonatal CV and CNS toxicity), and lactation.

Available forms

Direct injection—10, 20 mg/mL; IV injection (admixture)—5, 10, 15, 20, 40, 100 mg/mL; IV infusion—2, 4, 8 mg/mL; topical liquid—2.5%; topical ointment—5%; topical cream—0.5%, 3%, 4%; topical gel—0.5%, 2%, 2.5%, 4%, 5%; topical spray—0.5%, 10%; topical solution—2%, 4%; transdermal system—5%, topical lotion—3%

Dosages

Adults

IM

- *Arrhythmia:* Use only the 10% solution for IM injection. 300 mg in deltoid or thigh muscle. Switch to IV lidocaine or oral antiarrhythmic as soon as possible. Repeat dose in 60–90 min if necessary.

IV bolus

- *Arrhythmia:* Use only lidocaine injection labeled for IV use and without preservatives or catecholamines. Monitor ECG constantly. Give 50–100 mg at rate of 25–50 mg/min. Give second bolus dose after 5 min if needed. Do not exceed 200–300 mg in 1 hr.

IV, continuous infusion

- *Arrhythmia:* Give 1–4 mg/min (or 20–50 mcg/kg/min). Titrate the dose down as soon as the cardiac rhythm stabilizes. Use lower doses in patients with heart failure, liver disease, and in patients older than 70 yr.

Topical, intratissue, epidural

- *Local anesthesia:* Preparations containing preservatives should not be used for spinal or epidural anesthesia. Drug concentration and diluent should be appropriate to particular local anesthetic use: 5% solution with glucose is used for spinal anesthesia, 1.5% solution with dextrose for low spinal or "saddle block" anesthesia. Dosage varies with the area to be anesthetized and the reason for the anesthesia; use the lowest dose possible to achieve results.

Topical analgesia

- *Transdermal:* Apply up to 3 patches to area of pain for up to 12 hr within 24 hr.
- *Cream, ointment, gel, solution, spray:* Apply as directed 1–3 times per day.

Pediatric patients

IV

- *Arrhythmia:* Safety and efficacy have not been established. American Heart Association recommends bolus of 0.5–1 mg/kg IV, followed by 30 mcg/kg/min with caution.

Topical, intratissue, epidural

- *Local anesthesia:* See adult dosage discussion. Use lower concentrations.

Geriatric or debilitated patients, patients with liver disease or heart failure

Use lower concentrations in these patients.

Pharmacokinetics

Route	Onset	Peak	Duration
IM	5–10 min	5–15 min	2 hr
IV	Immediate	Immediate	10–20 min

Metabolism: Hepatic; $T_{1/2}$: 10 min, then 1.5–3 hr

Distribution: Crosses placenta; may enter breast milk

Excretion: Urine

IV FACTS

Preparation: Prepare solution for IV infusion as follows: 1–2 g lidocaine to 1 L D_5W = 0.1%–0.2% solution; 1–2 mg lidocaine/mL. Stable for 24 hr after dilution.

Infusion: IV bolus: Give 50–100 mg at rate of 25–50 mg/min. Continuous infusion: Give at a rate of 1–4 mL/min of a 1 mg/mL solution will provide 1–4 mg lidocaine/min. Use only preparations of lidocaine specifically labeled for IV infusion.

Adverse effects

Antiarrhythmic with systemic administration

- **CNS:** *Dizziness or light-headedness, fatigue, drowsiness,* unconsciousness, tremors, twitching, vision changes; may progress to **seizures**
- **CV:** *Cardiac arrhythmias,* **cardiac arrest,** vasodilation, *hypotension*
- **GI:** *Nausea,* vomiting
- **Hypersensitivity:** Rash, **anaphylactoid reactions**
- **Respiratory:** Respiratory depression, **Respiratory arrest**
- **Other:** Malignant hyperthermia, fever, local injection site reaction

Injectable local anesthetic for epidural or caudal anesthesia

- **CNS:** *Headache, backache,* septic meningitis, persistent sensory, motor, or autonomic deficit of lower spinal segments, sometimes with incomplete recovery
- **CV:** *Hypotension* due to sympathetic block
- **Dermatologic:** Urticaria, pruritus, erythema, edema
- **GU:** *Urinary retention, urinary or fecal incontinence*

Topical local anesthetic

- **Dermatologic:** Contact dermatitis, urticaria, cutaneous lesions
- **Hypersensitivity: Anaphylactoid reactions**
- **Local:** *Burning, stinging, tenderness, swelling, tissue irritation,* tissue sloughing and necrosis
- **Other:** Methemoglobinemia, **seizures** (children)

Interactions

✱ **Drug-drug** • Increased lidocaine levels with beta blockers (propranolol, metoprolol, nadolol, pindolol, atenolol), cimetidine • Prolonged neuromuscular blockade with succinylcholine

✱ **Drug-lab test** • Increased CPK if given IM

■ Nursing considerations

Assessment

- **History:** Allergy to lidocaine or amide-type local anesthetics, heart failure, cardiogenic shock, second- or third-degree heart block, Wolff-Parkinson-White syndrome, Stokes-Adams syndrome, hepatic or renal disease, inflammation or sepsis in region of injection, lactation, pregnancy
- **Physical:** T; skin color, rashes, lesions; orientation, speech, reflexes, sensation and movement (local anesthetic); P, BP, auscultation, continuous ECG monitoring during use as antiarrhythmic; edema; R, adventitious sounds; bowel sounds, liver evaluation; urine output; serum electrolytes, LFTs, renal function tests

Interventions

⊗ ***Warning*** Check drug concentration carefully; many concentrations are available.

- Reduce dosage with hepatic or renal failure.
- Continuously monitor response when used as antiarrhythmic or injected as local anesthetic.

⊗ ***Warning*** Keep life-support equipment and vasopressors readily available in case severe adverse reaction (CNS, CV, or respiratory) occurs when lidocaine is injected.

⊗ ***Warning*** Establish safety precautions if CNS changes occur; have IV diazepam or short-acting barbiturate (thiopental, thiamylal) readily available in case of seizures.

⊗ ***Warning*** Monitor for malignant hyperthermia (jaw muscle spasm, rigidity); have life-support equipment and IV dantrolene readily available.

- Titrate dose to minimum needed for cardiac stability, when using lidocaine as antiarrhythmic.
- Reduce dosage when treating arrhythmias in heart failure, digoxin toxicity with AV block, and geriatric patients.
- Monitor fluid load carefully; more concentrated solutions can be used to treat arrhythmias in patients on fluid restrictions.
- Have patients who have received lidocaine as a spinal anesthetic remain lying flat for 6–12 hr afterward, and ensure that they are adequately hydrated to minimize risk of headache.

⊗ ***Warning*** Large amounts of anesthetics used during cosmetic procedures may result in severe, life-threatening adverse effects. Amount used should be as small as possible and monitored by an experienced physician.

⊗ ***Warning*** Check lidocaine preparation carefully; epinephrine is added to solutions of lidocaine to retard the absorption of the local anesthetic from the injection site. Make sure that such solutions are used only to produce local anesthesia. These solutions should be injected cautiously in body areas supplied by end arteries and used cautiously in patients with peripheral vascular disease, hypertension, thyrotoxicosis, or diabetes.

- Use caution to prevent choking. Patient may have difficulty swallowing after using oral topical anesthetic. Do not give food or drink for 1 hr after use of oral anesthetic.
- Apply lidocaine ointments or creams to a gauze or bandage before applying to the skin.

⊗ ***Warning*** Monitor for safe and effective serum drug concentrations (antiarrhythmic use: 1–5 mcg/mL). Concentrations of 6 or more mcg/mL are usually toxic.

Teaching points

- Dosage is changed frequently in response to cardiac rhythm on monitor.
- Oral lidocaine can cause numbness of the tongue, cheeks, and throat. Do not eat or drink for 1 hour after using oral lidocaine to prevent biting the inside of your mouth or tongue and choking.
- You may experience these side effects: Drowsiness, dizziness, numbness, double vision; nausea, vomiting; stinging, burning, local irritation (local anesthetic).
- Report difficulty speaking, thick tongue, numbness, tingling, difficulty breathing, pain or numbness at IV site, swelling, or pain at site of local anesthetic use.

▽ lincomycin hydrochloride

See Appendix W, *Less commonly used drugs.*

▽ linezolid

*(lah **nez'** oh lid)*

Zyvox

PREGNANCY CATEGORY C

Drug class

Oxazolidinone antibiotic

Therapeutic actions

Bacteriostatic and bacteriocidal: Interferes with protein synthesis on the bacterial ribosome; effective in VRE, *Staphylococcus,* and methicillin-resistant *S. aureus* (MRSA) and penicillin-resistant *pneumococci* and *S. aureus;* is a reversible, nonselective MAOI.

Indications

- Treatment of infections due to vancomycin-resistant *Enterococcus faecium* (VREF)
- Treatment of nosocomial and community-acquired pneumonia due to *S. aureus* and penicillin-susceptible *Streptococcus pneumoniae*
- Treatment of skin and skin structure infections including those caused by MRSA
- Treatment of diabetic foot infections without osteomyelitis caused by gram-positive organisms including MRSA, *Streptococcus pyogenes,* or *Streptococcus agalactiae*

Contraindications and cautions

- Contraindicated with allergy to linezolid; lactation; phenylketonuria (oral suspension).
- Use cautiously with bone marrow suppression, hepatic impairment, hypertension, hyperthyroidism, pheochromocytoma, carcinoid syndrome, pregnancy.

Available forms

Tablets—600 mg; powder for oral suspension—100 mg/5 mL; injection—2 mg/mL

Dosages

No dosage adjustment is needed if switching between oral and IV forms.

Adults

- *VREF, MRSA, pneumonia, complicated skin and skin structure infections, including diabetic foot ulcers without osteomyelitis:* 600 mg IV or PO every 12 hr for 10–28 days, depending on infection.
- *Uncomplicated skin and skin structure infections:* 400–600 mg PO every 12 hr for 10–14 days.

Pediatric patients

- *VREF, CAP, nosocomial pneumonia, complicated skin, and skin structure infections: 11 yr or younger:* 10 mg/kg IV or PO every 8 hr.
- *Uncomplicated skin and skin structure infections:*
  Younger than 5 yr: 10 mg/kg PO every 8 hr.
  5–11 yr: 10 mg/kg PO every 12 hr.

Pharmacokinetics

Route	*Onset*	*Peak*
Oral	Rapid	1–2 hr
IV	Rapid	30 min

Metabolism: Hepatic; $T_{1/2}$: 5 hr
Distribution: Crosses placenta; enters breast milk
Excretion: Urine

IV FACTS

Preparation: Use premixed solution—available in 100, 200, and 300 mL forms; store at room temperature, protect from light, leave overwrap in place until ready to use; appears yellow.
Infusion: Infuse over 30–120 min, switch to oral form as soon as appropriate. May be infused into line using 5% dextrose injection, 0.9% sodium chloride, or lactated Ringer's.
Incompatibilities: ⊗ ***Warning*** Do not introduce additives into this solution; do not mix in solution or at Y-connection with any other drugs. If other drugs are being given through the same line, the line should be flushed before and after linezolid administration.

Adverse effects

- **CNS:** *Headache,* dizziness, *insomnia,* fatigue, somnolence, depression, nervousness
- **GI:** *Nausea,* vomiting, dry mouth, *diarrhea,* anorexia, gastritis, **pseudomembranous colitis**
- **Hematologic: Thrombocytopenia**
- **Other:** Fever, rash, sweating, photosensitivity, tendinitis

Interactions

✱ **Drug-drug** • Risk of hypertension and related adverse effects if combined with drugs containing pseudoephedrine, SSRIs, MAOIs; use caution and monitor patient carefully if any of these combinations are used • Increased risk of bleeding and thrombocytopenia if combined with antiplatelet drugs (aspirin, dipyridamole, NSAIDs); monitor platelet counts carefully

✱ **Drug-food** ⊗ ***Warning*** Risk of severe hypertension if combined with large amounts of food containing tyramine (see Appendix D, *Important dietary guidelines for patient teaching,* for tyramine food lists); patient should be cautioned to avoid eating large amounts of these foods.

■ Nursing considerations

CLINICAL ALERT!
Name confusion has occurred between *Zyvox* (linezolid) and *Zovirax* (acyclovir); use caution.

Assessment

- **History:** Allergy to linezolid; hepatic impairment, bone marrow depression, hypertension, phenylketonuria, hyperthyroidism, carcinoid syndrome, pheochromocytoma, pregnancy, lactation
- **Physical:** Culture site; skin color, lesions; T; orientation, reflexes, affect; P, BP; mucous membranes, bowel sounds; LFTs, CBC, and differential

Interventions

- Arrange for culture and sensitivity tests before beginning therapy.
- Reserve use of this drug for cases of well-documented bacteria-sensitive infections.
- Continue therapy as indicated for condition being treated.
- Monitor platelet counts regularly if drug is used for 2 wk or longer.
- Monitor BP before and periodically during therapy if patient is on antidepressants or drugs containing sympathomimetics.
- Advise patient to avoid foods high in tyramine to avoid risk of severe hypertension.
- Advise patient of high cost of drug and refer for financial support as needed.
- Monitor clinical response—if no improvement is seen or a relapse occurs, repeat culture and sensitivity tests.

Teaching points

- Take drug every 12 hours or every 8 hours as prescribed; take the full course of the drug; drug may be taken with or without food.
- Avoid foods high in tyramine (a list will be provided) while you are using this drug.
- You may experience these side effects: Nausea, vomiting, abdominal pain (eat frequent small meals; take the drug with food); diarrhea (consult your health care provider if this occurs).
- Report rash, severe GI problems, weakness, tremors, anxiety, increased bleeding.

▽ liothyronine sodium (T_3, triiodithyronine)

(lye' oh thye' roe neen)

Cytomel, Triostat

PREGNANCY CATEGORY A

Drug class

Thyroid hormone

Therapeutic actions

Increases the metabolic rate of body tissues, thereby increasing oxygen consumption; respiratory and HR; rate of fat, protein, and carbohydrate metabolism; and growth and maturation.

Indications

- Replacement therapy in hypothyroidism
- Pituitary TSH suppression in the treatment and prevention of euthyroid goiters and in the management of thyroid cancer
- Thyrotoxicosis in conjunction with antithyroid drugs and to prevent goitrogenesis, hypothyroidism, and thyrotoxicosis during pregnancy
- Synthetic hormone used with patients allergic to desiccated thyroid or thyroid extract derived from pork or beef
- Diagnostic use: T_3 suppression test to differentiate suspected hyperthyroidism from euthyroidism
- IV: Treatment of myxedema coma and precoma

Contraindications and cautions

- Contraindicated with allergy to active or extraneous constituents of drug, untreated thyrotoxicosis, and acute MI uncomplicated by hypothyroidism.
- Use cautiously with Addison's disease (treat hypoadrenalism with corticosteroids before thyroid therapy), lactation, patients with coronary artery disease or angina, pregnancy.

Available forms

Tablets—5, 25, 50 mcg; injection—10 mcg/mL

Dosages

15–37.5 mcg equals approximately 60 mg (1 grain) desiccated thyroid.

Adults

- *Hypothyroidism:* Initial dosage, 25 mcg/day PO. May be increased every 1–2 wk in increments of 12.5–25-mcg. For maintenance, 25–75 mcg/day.
- *Myxedema:* Initial dosage, 5 mcg/day PO. Increase in increments of 5–10 mcg every 1–2 wk. For maintenance, 50–100 mcg/day.
- *Myxedema coma and precoma:* 25–50 mcg IV every 4–12 hr; do not give IM or subcutaneously. In patients with cardiac disease, start at 10–20 mcg IV. Do not exceed 100 mcg/24 hr.
- *Simple goiter:* Initial dosage, 5 mcg/day PO. May be increased by increments of 5–10 mcg every 1–2 wk. For maintenance, 75 mcg/day.
- *T_3 suppression test:* 75–100 mcg/day PO for 7 days, then repeat iodine 131 (^{131}I) uptake test. ^{131}I uptake will be unaffected in the hyperthyroid patient but will be decreased by 50% or more in the euthyroid patient.

Pediatric patients

- *Congenital hypothyroidism:* Infants require replacement therapy from birth. Starting dose is 5 mcg/day PO with 5-mcg increments every 3–4 days until the desired dosage is reached. Usual maintenance dosage, 20 mcg/day PO up to age 1 yr; 50 mcg/day for age 1–3 yr. Use adult dosage after age 3 yr.

Geriatric patients
Start therapy with 5 mcg/day PO. Increase by only 5-mcg increments at 2-wk intervals, and monitor patient response.

Pharmacokinetics

Route	*Onset*	*Peak*	*Duration*
Oral	Varies	2–3 days	3–4 days
IV	Rapid	End of infusion	Unkown

Metabolism: Hepatic; $T_{1/2}$: 1–2 days
Distribution: Does not cross placenta; enters breast milk
Excretion: Urine

▼ IV FACTS

Preparation: No further preparation is needed; refrigerate vials before use; discard unused portions.
Infusion: Infuse slowly, each 10 mcg over 1 min. Switch to oral form as soon as possible.

Adverse effects

- **Dermatologic:** Allergic skin reactions, partial loss of hair in first few months of therapy in children
- **Endocrine:** Mainly symptoms of hyperthyroidism: *Palpitations, elevated pulse pressure, tachycardia, arrhythmias,* angina pectoris, **cardiac arrest;** tremors, *headache, nervousness, insomnia; nausea,* diarrhea, changes in appetite; weight loss, menstrual irregularities, sweating, heat intolerance, fever
- **Other:** Esophageal atresia

Interactions

✱ **Drug-drug** • Decreased absorption of oral thyroid preparation with cholestyramine • Increased risk of bleeding with warfarin—reduce dosage of anticoagulant when thyroid hormone is begun • Decreased effectiveness of cardiac glycosides with thyroid replacement • Decreased clearance of theophyllines if patient is in hypothyroid state; monitor response and adjust dosage as patient approaches euthyroid state

■ Nursing considerations

Assessment

- **History:** Allergy to active or extraneous constituents of drug, thyrotoxicosis, acute MI uncomplicated by hypothyroidism, Addison's disease, lactation, pregnancy
- **Physical:** Skin lesions, color, T, texture; T; muscle tone, orientation, reflexes; P, auscultation, baseline ECG, BP; R, adventitious sounds; thyroid function tests

Interventions

⊗ ***Black box warning*** Do not use for weight loss; large doses may cause serious adverse effects.

- Monitor patient response carefully at start of therapy; adjust dosage.
- Monitor exchange from one form of thyroid replacement to T_3. Discontinue the other medication, then begin this drug at a low dose with gradual increases based on the patient's response.

⊗ ***Warning*** Most CV and CNS adverse effects indicate a too high dose. Stop medication for several days and reinstitute at a lower dose.

- Administer as a single daily dose before breakfast with a full glass of water.
- Arrange for regular, periodic blood tests of thyroid function.
- Monitor cardiac response.

Teaching points

- Take as a single dose before breakfast with a full glass of water.
- This drug replaces an important hormone and will need to be taken for life. Do not discontinue drug for any reason without consulting your health care provider; serious problems can occur.
- Wear or carry a medical ID tag to alert emergency medical personnel that you are using this drug.
- Have periodic blood tests and medical evaluations.
- Nausea and diarrhea may occur (dividing the dose may help).
- Report headache, chest pain, palpitations, fever, weight loss, sleeplessness, nervousness, irritability, unusual sweating, intolerance to heat, diarrhea.

liotrix
(lye' oh trix)

Thyrolar

PREGNANCY CATEGORY A

Drug class
Thyroid hormone (contains synthetic T_3 and T_4 in a ratio of 1 to 4 by weight)

Therapeutic actions
Increases the metabolic rate of body tissues, thereby increasing oxygen consumption; respiratory and HR; rate of fat, protein, and carbohydrate metabolism; and growth and maturation.

Indications
- Replacement therapy in hypothyroidism
- Congenital hypothyroidism
- Pituitary TSH suppression in the treatment and prevention of euthyroid goiters and in the management of thyroid cancer
- Treatment of thyrotoxicosis in conjunction with antithyroid drugs and to prevent goitrogenesis, hypothyroidism, and thyrotoxicosis during pregnancy
- Diagnostic test for thyroid disease

Contraindications and cautions
- Contraindicated with allergy to active or extraneous constituents of drug, untreated thyrotoxicosis, and acute MI uncomplicated by hypothyroidism.
- Use cautiously with Addison's disease (hypoadrenalism; treat with corticosteroids before thyroid therapy), lactation, coronary artery disease, or angina, pregnancy.

Available forms
Tablets—¼, ½, 1, 2, 3 grains equivalent to 15, 30, 60, 120, 180 mg thyroid, respectively

Dosages
60 mg equals 65 mg (1 grain) desiccated thyroid; administered only PO.

Adults
- *Hypothyroidism:* Initial dosage, 30 mg/day PO. Increase gradually every 2–3 wk in 15-mg (thyroid equivalent) increments (2 wk in children). In patients with cardiac disease, start with 15 mg/day (thyroid equivalent).
- *Maintenance dose:* 60–120 mg/day PO (thyroid equivalent).
- *Thyroid cancer:* Use larger doses than required for replacement surgery.
- *Diagnostic test:* 1.56 mcg/kg/day PO for 7–10 days.

Pediatric patients older than 12 yr
More than 90 mg/day (thyroid equivalent PO).

Pediatric patients 6–12 yr
60–90 mg/day (thyroid equivalent PO).

Pediatric patients 1–5 yr
45–60 mg/day (thyroid equivalent PO).

Pediatric patients 6–12 mo
30–45 mg/day (thyroid equivalent PO).

Pediatric patients 0–6 mo
15–30 mg/day (thyroid equivalent PO).

Pharmacokinetics

Route	Onset	Peak	Duration
Oral	Varies	2–3 days	3 days

Metabolism: Hepatic; $T_{1/2}$: 1–6 days
Distribution: Does not cross placenta; enters breast milk
Excretion: Urine

Adverse effects
- **Dermatologic:** Allergic skin reactions, partial hair loss in first few months of therapy in children
- **Endocrine:** Mainly symptoms of hyperthyroidism: *Palpitations, elevated pulse pressure, tachycardia, arrhythmias,* angina pectoris, **cardiac arrest;** tremors, *headache, nervousness, insomnia; nausea,* diarrhea, changes in appetite; weight loss, menstrual irregularities, sweating, heat intolerance, fever
- **Other:** Esophageal atresia

Interactions
✱ **Drug-drug** • Decreased absorption of oral thyroid preparation with cholestyramine • Increased risk of bleeding with warfarin—reduce dosage of anticoagulant when T_4 is begun • Decreased effectiveness of cardiac glycosides if taken with thyroid replacement • Decreased clearance of theophyllines in hypothyroid state; monitor response and adjust dosage as patient approaches euthyroid state

✱ **Drug-lab test** • Androgens, corticosteroids, estrogens, oral contraceptives, iodine-containing preparations may alter thyroid tests

■ Nursing considerations

Assessment

- **History:** Allergy to active or extraneous constituents of drug, thyrotoxicosis, acute MI uncomplicated by hypothyroidism, Addison's disease, lactation, pregnancy
- **Physical:** Skin lesions, color, T, texture; T; muscle tone, orientation, reflexes; P, auscultation, baseline ECG, BP; R, adventitious sounds; thyroid function tests

Interventions

⊠ ***Black box warning*** Do not use for weight loss; large doses may cause serious adverse effects.

- Monitor response carefully at start of therapy, and adjust dosage.

⊗ ***Warning*** Most CV and CNS adverse effects indicate a dose that is too high. Stop drug for several days and reinstitute at a lower dose.

- Administer as a single daily dose before breakfast with a full glass of water.
- Carefully check dosage; dosing can be confusing when converting from grains to thyroid-equivalent dosages.
- Arrange for regular, periodic blood tests of thyroid function.
- Monitor cardiac response.

Teaching points

- Take as a single dose before breakfast with a full glass of water.
- This drug replaces an important hormone and will need to be taken for life. Do not discontinue without consulting your health care provider; serious problems can occur.
- If you are also diabetic, dosages of your diabetic medications may need to be changed.
- Wear a medical ID tag to alert emergency medical personnel that you take this drug.
- Have periodic blood tests and medical evaluations.
- Nausea and diarrhea may occur (divide the dose).
- Report headache, chest pain, palpitations, fever, weight loss, sleeplessness, nervousness, irritability, unusual sweating, intolerance to heat, diarrhea.

▽ lisdexamfetamine dimesylate

*(liss dex am **fet'** a meen)*

Vyvanse

PREGNANCY CATEGORY C

CONTROLLED SUBSTANCE C-II

Drug classes

Amphetamine
CNS stimulant

Therapeutic actions

Thought to block reuptake of norepinephrine and dopamine in the presynaptic neuron and increase release of these monamines into the extraneuronal space, stimulating CNS activity and leading to suppressed appetite, increased alertness, elevated mood, improved physical performance when fatigue and sleep deprivation have caused impairment; mode of action in attention deficit/hyperactivity disorder (ADHD) is not understood.

Indications

- Treatment of ADHD in patients 6 yr and older

Contraindications and cautions

- Contraindicated with hypersensitivity to any component of the drug, advanced arteriosclerosis, symptomatic CV disease, moderate to severe hypertension, hyperthyroidism, hypersensitivity or idiosyncratic reaction to sympathetic amines, glaucoma, agitated states, history of drug abuse, during or within 14 days following treatment with an MAOI, lactation.
- Use cautiously with history of seizures, preexisting psychosis or bipolar disorder, pregnancy.

Available forms

Capsules—20, 30, 40, 50, 60, 70 mg

Dosages

Adults and children 6 yr and older

30 mg/day PO in the morning; may increase at weekly intervals in increments of 10–20 mg/day to a maximum of 70 mg/day.

L

Pharmacokinetics

Route	Onset	Peak
Oral	Rapid	3.5 hr

Metabolism: Hepatic; $T_{1/2}$: 1 hr
Distribution: May cross placenta; enters breast milk
Excretion: Urine

Adverse effects

- **CNS:** *Headache,* dizziness, somnolence, *insomnia,* tics, *irritability,* aggression, mania, affect lability, seizures, visual disturbances
- **CV: Serious cardiac events, sudden death,** hypertension, tachycardia
- **GI:** *Abdominal pain, diarrhea,* nausea, *vomiting,* dry mouth, *decreased appetite*
- **Other:** Fever, *weight loss,* rash, drug dependence, slowed growth

Interactions

✱ **Drug-drug** • Risk of decreased effectiveness if combined with urine acidifying agents, methenamine • Risk of increased activity of TCAs and sympathomimetic agents and increased risk of CV events • Risk of toxic neurologic effects and potentially fatal malignant hyperpyrexia if combined with MAOIs; do not use for 14 days after stopping MAOI • Blocked effects if combined with chlorpromazine; do not use this combination (chlorpromazine may be used to treat amphetamine poisoning) • Decreased CNS stimulation if combined with haloperidol • Enhanced effects of meperidine, norepinephrine if combined with lisdexamfetamine • Risk of excessive CNS stimulation and fatal seizures if combined with propoxyphene overdose

✱ **Drug-lab test** • Significant elevation in plasma corticosteroid level, particularly in the evening

■ Nursing considerations

⊗ ***Black box warning*** High risk of abuse could lead to drug dependence; misuse of amphetamines has caused serious CV events and sudden death.

Assessment

- **History:** Hypersensitivity to any component of the drug, advanced arteriosclerosis, symptomatic CV disease, moderate to severe hypertension, hyperthyroidism, known hypersensitivity or idiosyncrasy to sympathetic amines, glaucoma, agitated states, history of drug abuse, during or within 14 days following treatment with an MAOI, lactation; history of seizures, preexisting psychosis or bipolar disorder, pregnancy
- **Physical:** Skin color, lesions; orientation, affect, reflexes; BP, P; height and weight

Interventions

- Ensure proper diagnosis before administering to children for behavioral syndromes; drug should not be used until other causes (learning disabilities, EEG abnormalities, neurologic deficits) are ruled out.
- Drug therapy should be part of a comprehensive program to help with the problem.
- Interrupt drug therapy periodically to determine if symptomatic response still validates drug therapy.
- Monitor growth of children on long-term therapy; failure to grow may indicate need to stop drug.
- Dispense the lowest feasible dose to minimize risk of overdosage; drug should be stored securely out of the reach of anyone who might abuse drug (drug is a controlled substance).
- If child cannot swallow capsules, empty the capsule contents into a glass of water and have the child drink it right away. Do not try to divide doses or save contents.
- Administer drug early in the day to help prevent insomnia.
- Provide small, frequent meals if GI upset is a problem.
- Monitor BP periodically.

Teaching points

- Store this drug at room temperature in a dry place (not in the bathroom or near the kitchen sink). It is a controlled substance with abuse potential; store it out of the reach of children.
- Give this drug once a day in the morning. If you or your child cannot swallow the capsule, open it, dissolve the entire contents in a glass of water, and drink or have the child drink it right away.
- You or your child will need to have periodic blood tests, blood pressure checks, and

height and weight checks to monitor the effects of this drug.
- This drug should be used as part of a comprehensive ADHD treatment program that includes behavior modification.
- The effectiveness of this drug may be changed by combining with certain other drugs, especially antidepressants such as MAOIs, antipsychotic drugs, blood pressure drugs, seizure drugs, and opioid pain relievers. Tell all of your child's health care providers that your child is taking this drug so that appropriate dosage adjustments and precautions can be taken.
- You or your child may experience the following side effects: Irritability, insomnia (monitor the child, especially at the start of drug therapy); dry mouth, loss of appetite, abdominal pain (sucking sugarless candies may help, but make sure to safeguard the child's nutrition); slowing of growth, weight loss (report any marked changes to your health care provider).
- Report aggression, vision changes, manic symptoms, marked weight loss, seizures.

▽ lisinopril

*(lyse **in'** oh pril)*

Prinivil, Zestril

PREGNANCY CATEGORY C (FIRST TRIMESTER)

PREGNANCY CATEGORY D (SECOND AND THIRD TRIMESTERS)

Drug classes

ACE inhibitor
Antihypertensive

Therapeutic actions

Renin, synthesized by the kidneys, is released into the circulation where it acts on a plasma precursor to produce angiotensin I, which is converted by ACE to angiotensin II, a potent vasoconstrictor that also causes release of aldosterone from the adrenals. Lisinopril blocks the conversion of angiotensin I to angiotensin II, leading to decreased BP, decreased aldosterone secretion, a small increase in serum potassium levels, and sodium and fluid loss.

Indications

- Treatment of hypertension alone or in combination with other antihypertensives
- Adjunctive therapy in heart failure for patients unresponsive to diuretics and digoxin alone
- Treatment of stable patients within 24 hr of acute MI to improve survival with standard treatments

Contraindications and cautions

- Contraindicated with allergy to lisinopril, other ACE inhibitors, history of angioedema.
- Use cautiously with impaired renal function, heart failure, salt or volume depletion, IHSS, pregnancy, lactation.

Available forms

Tablets—2.5, 5, 10, 20, 30, 40 mg

Dosages

Adults not taking diuretics

Initial dose, 10 mg/day PO. Adjust dosage based on response. Usual range is 20–40 mg/day as a single dose.

Adults taking diuretics

Discontinue diuretic for 2–3 days. If it is not possible to discontinue, give initial dose of 5 mg, and monitor for excessive hypotension.
- *Heart failure:* 5 mg PO daily with diuretics and digitalis. Effective range, 5–20 mg/day (*Prinivil*) and 5–40 mg/day (*Zestril*).
- *Acute MI:* Start within 24 hr of MI with 5 mg PO followed in 24 hr by 5 mg PO; 10 mg PO after 48 hr, then 10 mg PO daily for 6 wk.

Pediatric patients 6 yr and older

Usual starting dose is 0.07 mg/kg once daily up to 5 mg total.

Pediatric patients younger than 6 yr

Safety and efficacy not established; drug usually not recommended.

Geriatric patients and patients with renal impairment

Excretion is reduced in renal failure. Use smaller initial dose, and adjust upward to a maximum of 40 mg/day PO.

L

CrCl (mL/min)	*Initial Dose*
More than 30	10 mg/day
10–30	5 mg/day (2.5 mg for HF)
Less than 10	2.5 mg/day

For patients on dialysis, give 2.5 mg on day of dialysis.

Pharmacokinetics

Route	*Onset*	*Peak*	*Duration*
Oral	1 hr	7 hr	24 hr

Metabolism: Hepatic; $T_{1/2}$: 12 hr
Distribution: Crosses placenta; may enter breast milk
Excretion: Urine

Adverse effects

- **CNS:** *Headache, dizziness, insomnia, fatigue,* paresthesias
- **CV:** *Orthostatic hypotension,* tachycardia, angina pectoris, **MI,** Raynaud's syndrome, heart failure, severe hypotension in salt- or volume-depleted patients
- **GI:** *Gastric irritation, nausea, diarrhea,* peptic ulcers, dysgeusia, cholestatic jaundice, hepatocellular injury, anorexia, constipation
- **GU:** Proteinuria, renal insufficiency, renal failure, polyuria, oliguria, frequency
- **Hematologic:** Neutropenia, agranulocytosis, thrombocytopenia, hemolytic anemia, **pancytopenia,** hyperkalemia
- **Other:** *Angioedema* (particularly of the face, extremities, lips, tongue, larynx; death has been reported with **airway obstruction;** *cough,* muscle cramps, impotence, rash, pruritus

Interactions

✱ **Drug-drug** • Decreased antihypertensive effects and increased risk of renal damage if taken with NSAIDs • Exacerbation of cough if combined with capsaicin

■ Nursing considerations

CLINICAL ALERT!
Name confusion has occurred between lisinopril and fosinopril; use caution.

Assessment

- **History:** Allergy to lisinopril or other ACE inhibitors, impaired renal function, heart failure, salt or volume depletion, lactation, pregnancy
- **Physical:** Skin color, lesions, turgor; T; P, BP, peripheral perfusion; mucous membranes, bowel sounds, liver evaluation; urinalysis, LFTs, renal function tests, CBC and differential, potassium

Interventions

- Begin drug within 24 hr of acute MI; ensure that patient is also receiving standard treatment (eg, aspirin, beta-adrenergic blockers, thrombolytics).

⊗ ***Warning*** Keep epinephrine readily available in case of angioedema of the face or neck region; if breathing difficulty occurs, consult physician, and administer epinephrine.

⊗ ***Warning*** Alert surgeon, and mark the patient's chart with notice that lisinopril is being taken. The angiotensin II formation subsequent to compensatory renin release during surgery will be blocked. Hypotension may be reversed with volume expansion.

- Monitor patients on diuretic therapy for excessive hypotension following the first few doses of lisinopril.
- Monitor patients closely in any situation that may lead to a decrease in BP secondary to reduction in fluid volume (excessive perspiration and dehydration, vomiting, diarrhea) because excessive hypotension may occur.
- Arrange for reduced dosage in patients with impaired renal function.

⊗ ***Black box warning*** Suggest the use of contraceptives; if pregnancy should occur, discontinue drug as soon as possible; fetal injury or death may occur.

Teaching points

- Take this drug once a day. It may be taken with meals. Do not stop taking drug without consulting your health care provider.
- Be careful with any conditions that may lead to a drop in blood pressure (such as diarrhea, sweating, vomiting, dehydration). If lightheadedness or dizziness occurs, consult your health care provider.

- Do not take this during pregnancy; use of contraceptive measures is advised.
- You may experience these side effects: GI upset, loss of appetite, change in taste perception (may be transient; take with meals); rash; fast heart rate; dizziness, light-headedness (transient; change position slowly, and limit activities to those that do not require alertness and precision); headache, fatigue, sleeplessness.
- Report mouth sores; sore throat; fever; chills; swelling of the hands or feet; irregular heartbeat; chest pains; swelling of the face, eyes, lips, or tongue; and difficulty breathing.

lithium
(lith' ee um)

lithium carbonate
Apo-Lithium Carbonate (CAN), Carbolith (CAN), Duralith (CAN), Eskalith, Eskalith CR, Lithane (CAN), Lithobid, Lithonate, Lithotabs, PMS-Lithium Carbonate (CAN)

lithium citrate

PREGNANCY CATEGORY D

Drug class
Antimanic drug

Therapeutic actions
Mechanism is not known; alters sodium transport in nerve and muscle cells; inhibits release of norepinephrine and dopamine, but not serotonin, from stimulated neurons; slightly increases intraneuronal stores of catecholamines; decreases intraneuronal content of second messengers and may thereby selectively modulate the responsiveness of hyperactive neurons that might contribute to the manic state.

Indications
- Treatment of manic episodes of bipolar disorder; maintenance therapy to prevent or diminish frequency and intensity of subsequent manic episodes
- Unlabeled uses: Prophylaxis of cluster headache and cyclic migraine headache, treatment of SIADH, hypothyroidism (doses of 600–900 mg/day), borderline personality disorder, major depression

Contraindications and cautions
- Contraindicated with hypersensitivity to tartrazine; significant renal or CV disease; severe debilitation, dehydration; sodium depletion, patients on diuretics (lithium decreases sodium reabsorption, and hyponatremia increases lithium retention); use of ACE inhibitors; pregnancy; lactation.
- Use cautiously with protracted sweating and diarrhea; suicidal or impulsive patients; infection with fever.

Available forms
Capsules—150, 300, 600 mg; tablets—300 mg; SR tablets—300 mg; CR tablets—450 mg; syrup—300 mg/5 mL

Dosages
Individualize dosage according to serum levels and clinical response.

Adults
- *Acute mania:* 600 mg PO tid or 900 mg slow-release form PO bid to produce effective serum levels between 1 and 1.5 mEq/L. Serum levels should be determined twice per week in samples drawn immediately before a dose (at least 8–12 hr after previous dose).
- *Long-term use:* 300 mg PO tid–qid to produce a serum level of 0.6–1.2 mEq/L. Serum levels should be determined at least every 2 mo in samples drawn immediately before a dose (at least 8–12 hr after previous dose).
- *Conversion from conventional to slow-release dosage forms:* Give the same total daily dose divided into two or three doses.

Pediatric patients
Safety and efficacy for children younger than 12 yr not established.

Geriatric patients and patients with renal impairment
Reduced dosage may be needed. Elderly patients often respond to reduced dosage and may exhibit signs of toxicity at serum levels tolerated

by other patients. Plasma half-life is prolonged in renal impairment.

Pharmacokinetics

Route	Onset	Peak
Oral (tablets, capsules)	Unknown	0.5–3 hr
Oral (SR, CR tablets, capsules)	Unknown	4–12 hr

Metabolism: $T_{1/2}$: 24 hr
Distribution: Crosses placenta; enters breast milk
Excretion: Urine

Adverse effects

Reactions are related to serum lithium levels. (Toxic lithium levels are close to therapeutic levels: Therapeutic levels in acute mania range between 1 and 1.5 mEq/L; therapeutic levels for maintenance are 0.6–1.2 mEq/L.)

Less than 1.5 mEq/L

- **CNS:** *Lethargy, slurred speech, muscle weakness, fine hand tremor*
- **GI:** Nausea, vomiting, diarrhea, thirst
- **GU:** Polyuria

1.5–2 mEq/L (mild to moderate toxic reactions)

- **CNS:** Coarse hand tremor, mental confusion, hyperirritability of muscles, drowsiness, incoordination
- **CV:** ECG changes
- **GI:** Persistent GI upset, gastritis, salivary gland swelling, abdominal pain, excessive salivation, flatulence, indigestion

2–2.5 mEq/L (moderate to severe toxic reactions)

- **CNS:** Ataxia, giddiness, fasciculations, tinnitus, blurred vision, clonic movements, seizures, stupor, coma
- **CV:** Serious ECG changes, severe hypotension with **cardiac arrhythmias**
- **GU:** Large output of dilute urine
- **Respiratory:** Fatalities secondary to **pulmonary complications**

Greater than 2.5 mEq/L (life-threatening toxicity)

- **General:** Complex involvement of multiple organ systems, including seizures, arrhythmias, **CV collapse,** stupor, coma

Reactions unrelated to serum levels

- **CNS:** Headache, worsening of organic brain syndromes, fever, reversible short-term memory impairment, dyspraxia
- **CV:** ECG changes; hyperkalemia associated with ECG changes; syncope; tachycardia-bradycardia syndrome; rarely, arrhythmias, heart failure, diffuse myocarditis, **death**
- **Dermatologic:** Pruritus with or without rash; maculopapular, acneiform, and follicular eruptions; cutaneous ulcers; edema of ankles or wrists
- **Endocrine:** Diffuse nontoxic goiter; hypothyroidism; hypercalcemia associated with hyperparathyroidism; transient hyperglycemia; irreversible nephrogenic diabetes insipidus, which improves with diuretic therapy; impotence or sexual dysfunction
- **GI:** Dysgeusia (taste distortion), salty taste; swollen lips; dental caries
- **Other:** Weight gain (5–10 kg); chest tightness; swollen or painful joints, eye irritation, worsening of cataracts, disturbance of visual accommodation, leukocytosis

Interactions

✱ **Drug-drug** • Increased risk of toxicity with thiazide diuretics due to decreased renal clearance of lithium—reduced lithium dosage may be needed • Increased plasma lithium levels with indomethacin and some other NSAIDs (phenylbutazone, piroxicam, ibuprofen) and fluoxetine, methyldopa, and metronidazole • Increased CNS toxicity with carbamazepine • Encephalopathic syndrome (weakness, lethargy, fever, tremulousness, confusion, extrapyramidal symptoms, leukocytosis, elevated serum enzymes) with irreversible brain damage when taken with haloperidol • Greater risk of hypothyroidism with iodide salts • Decreased effectiveness due to increased excretion of lithium with urinary alkalinizers, including antacids, tromethamine • Risk of increased adverse effects with SSRIs

✱ **Drug-alternative therapy** • Increased effects and toxicity with juniper, dandelion

■ Nursing considerations

Assessment

- **History:** Hypersensitivity to tartrazine; significant renal or CV disease; severe debilitation, dehydration; sodium depletion, patients on diuretics; protracted sweating, diarrhea; suicidal or impulsive patients; infection with fever; pregnancy; lactation
- **Physical:** Weight and T; skin color, lesions; orientation, affect, reflexes; ophthalmic examination; P, BP, R, adventitious sounds; bowel sounds, normal output; normal fluid intake, normal output, voiding pattern; thyroid, renal glomerular and tubular function tests, urinalysis, CBC and differential, baseline ECG

Interventions

- Give with caution and frequent monitoring of serum lithium levels to patients with renal or CV disease, debilitation, or dehydration or life-threatening psychiatric disorders.
- Give drug with food or milk or after meals.

⊠ ***Black box warning*** Monitor clinical status closely, especially during initial stages of therapy; monitor for therapeutic serum levels of 0.6–1.2 mEq/L; toxicity is closely related to serum levels.

- Individuals vary in their response to this drug; some patients may exhibit toxic signs at serum lithium levels considered within the therapeutic range.
- Advise patient that this drug may cause serious fetal harm and cannot be used during pregnancy; urge use of barrier contraceptives.
- Decrease dosage after the acute manic episode is controlled; lithium tolerance is greater during the acute manic phase and decreases when manic symptoms subside.

⊗ ***Warning*** Ensure that patient maintains adequate intake of salt and adequate intake of fluid (2,500–3,000 mL/day).

Teaching points

- Take this drug exactly as prescribed, after meals or with food or milk. Swallow sustained- or controlled-release tablets whole; do not chew or crush.
- Eat a normal diet with normal salt intake; maintain adequate fluid intake (at least 2.5 quarts/day).
- Arrange for frequent checkups, including blood tests. Keep all appointments for checkups to get the most benefits with the least toxicity.
- Use contraception to avoid pregnancy. If you wish to become pregnant or believe that you have become pregnant, consult your health care provider.
- Discontinue drug and notify your health care provider if toxicity occurs—diarrhea, vomiting, ataxia, tremor, drowsiness, lack of coordination or muscular weakness.
- You may experience these side effects: Drowsiness, dizziness (avoid driving or performing tasks that require alertness); GI upset (eat frequent small meals); mild thirst, greater than usual urine volume, fine hand tremor (may persist throughout therapy; notify your heath care provider if severe).
- Report diarrhea or fever.

DANGEROUS DRUG

▽lomustine (CCNU)

*(loe **mus'** teen)*

CeeNU

PREGNANCY CATEGORY D

Drug classes

Alkylating drug, nitrosourea
Antineoplastic

Therapeutic actions

Cytotoxic: Exact mechanism of action not known, but it involves alkylation of DNA, thus inhibiting DNA, RNA, and protein synthesis; cell-cycle nonspecific.

Indications

- Treatment with other drugs for primary and metastatic brain tumors and secondary treatment of Hodgkin's disease in patients who relapse following primary therapy

Contraindications and cautions

- Contraindicated with allergy to lomustine, myelosuppression, pregnancy (teratogenic and embryotoxic in preclinical studies), and lactation.
- Use cautiously with impaired renal or hepatic function.

L

Available forms

Capsules—10, 40, 100 mg

Dosages

Adults and pediatric patients

130 mg/m² PO as a single dose every 6 wk. Adjustments must be made with bone marrow suppression; initially reduce the dose to 100 mg/m² PO every 6 wk; do not give a repeat dose until platelets exceed 100,000/mm² and leukocytes exceed 4,000/mm²; adjust dosage after initial dose based on hematologic response as follows:

Minimum (nadir) count after prior dose:

Leukocytes mm²	*Platelets mm²*	*Percentage of Prior Dose to Give*
More than 4,000	More than 100,000	100
3,000–3,999	75,000–99,999	100
2,000–2,999	25,000–74,999	70
Less than 2,000	Less than 25,000	50

Pharmacokinetics

Route	*Onset*	*Peak*	*Duration*
Oral	10 min	1.6 hr	48 hr

Metabolism: Hepatic; $T_{1/2}$: 16–72 hr
Distribution: Crosses placenta; enters breast milk
Excretion: Urine

Adverse effects

- **CNS:** Ataxia, lethargy
- **Dermatologic:** Alopecia
- **GI:** *Nausea, vomiting,* stomatitis, hepatotoxicity
- **GU:** Renal toxicity
- **Hematologic:** *Leukopenia; thrombocytopenia; anemia,* delayed for 4–6 wk; immunosuppression
- **Respiratory:** Pulmonary fibrosis
- **Other:** Secondary malignancies

■ Nursing considerations

Assessment

- **History:** Allergy to lomustine, radiation therapy, chemotherapy, hematopoietic depression, impaired renal or hepatic function, pregnancy, lactation
- **Physical:** T; weight; mucous membranes, liver evaluation; CBC, differential; urinalysis, LFTs, renal function tests

Interventions

⊠ ***Black box warning*** Arrange for blood tests to evaluate hematopoietic function before therapy and weekly for at least 6 wk thereafter; severe bone marrow suppression is possible.

⊗ ***Warning*** Do not give full dosage within 2–3 wk after a full course of radiation therapy or chemotherapy due to risk of severe bone marrow depression; reduced dosage may be needed.

- Advise patient that drug cannot be taken during pregnancy; suggest using barrier contraceptives.
- Reduce dosage in patients with depressed bone marrow function.
- Administer tablets on an empty stomach to decrease GI upset; antiemetics may be needed for nausea and vomiting.
- Monitor pulmonary function because of risk of pulmonary fibrosis.

Teaching points

- Take this drug on an empty stomach.
- Maintain your fluid intake and nutrition.
- Use birth control; this drug can cause severe birth defects.
- You may experience these side effects: Nausea, vomiting, loss of appetite (take on an empty stomach, an antiemetic may be ordered; frequent small meals may help), hair loss.
- Report unusual bleeding or bruising, fever, chills, sore throat, stomach or flank pain, sores on your mouth or lips, unusual tiredness, confusion, difficulty breathing.

loperamide hydrochloride

*(loe **per'** a mide)*

Prescription: Apo-Loperamide (CAN)

OTC: Diar-Aid Caplets, Imodium A-D, K-Pek II, Neo-Diaral, Pepto Diarrhea Control

PREGNANCY CATEGORY B

Drug class
Antidiarrheal

Therapeutic actions
Slows intestinal motility and affects water and electrolyte movement through the bowel by inhibiting peristalsis through direct effects on the circular and longitudinal muscles of the intestinal wall.

Indications
- Control and symptomatic relief of acute nonspecific diarrhea and chronic diarrhea associated with inflammatory bowel disease
- Reduction of volume of discharge from ileostomies
- OTC use: Control of diarrhea, including traveler's diarrhea

Contraindications and cautions
- Contraindicated with allergy to loperamide, patients who must avoid constipation, diarrhea associated with organisms that penetrate the intestinal mucosa (*Escherichia coli, Salmonella, Shigella, Clostridium difficile*).
- Use cautiously with hepatic impairment, acute ulcerative colitis, pregnancy, and lactation.

Available forms
Tablets—2 mg; capsules—2 mg; liquid—1 mg/5 mL; 1 mg/7.5 mL

Dosages
Adults
- *Acute diarrhea:* Initial dose of 4 mg PO followed by 2 mg after each unformed stool. Do not exceed 16 mg/day unless directed by a physician. Clinical improvement is usually seen within 48 hr.
- *Chronic diarrhea:* Initial dose of 4 mg PO followed by 2 mg after each unformed stool until diarrhea is controlled. Individualize dose based on patient response. Average daily maintenance dose is 4–8 mg. If no clinical improvement is seen with dosage of 16 mg/day for 10 days, further treatment will probably not be effective.
- *Traveler's diarrhea (OTC):* 4 mg PO after first loose stool, followed by 2 mg after each subsequent stool; do not exceed 16 mg/day.

Pediatric patients
Avoid use in children younger than 2 yr, and use extreme caution in younger children. Do not use OTC product with children.
- *Acute diarrhea:* First-day dosage schedule:

Age	Weight	Dose Form	Dosage
2–5 yr	13–20 kg	Liquid	1 mg tid
6–8 yr	20–30 kg	Liquid or capsule	2 mg bid
8–12 yr	More than 30 kg	Liquid or capsule	2 mg tid

  Subsequent doses: Administer 1 mg/10 kg PO only after a loose stool. Daily dosage should not exceed recommended first-day dosage.
- *Chronic diarrhea:* Dosage schedule has not been established.
- *Traveler's diarrhea (OTC):*
  Younger than 6 yr (21 kg and less): Consult with physician; not recommended.
  6–8 yr (22–26 kg): 2 mg PO after first loose stool, followed by 1 mg after each subsequent loose stool; do not exceed 4 mg/day for more than 2 days.
  9–11 yr (27–43 kg): 2 mg PO after first loose stool followed by 1 mg after each subsequent stool; do not exceed 6 mg/day for more than 2 days.

Pharmacokinetics

Route	Onset	Peak
Oral	Varies	1–6 hr

Metabolism: Hepatic; $T_{1/2}$: first phase, 6 hr; second phase, 1–2 days
Distribution: May cross placenta and enter breast milk
Excretion: Feces, urine

Adverse effects

- **CNS:** Tiredness, drowsiness, dizziness
- **GI: Toxic megacolon** (in patients with ulcerative colitis), *abdominal pain, distention or discomfort, constipation, dry mouth, nausea,* vomiting
- **Hematologic:** Myelosuppression
- **Hypersensitivity:** Rash
- **Respiratory:** Pulmonary infiltrates, pulmonary fibrosis

■ Nursing considerations

Assessment

- **History:** Allergy to loperamide, patients who must avoid constipation, diarrhea associated with organisms that penetrate the intestinal mucosa (*E. coli, Salmonella, Shigella*); hepatic impairment, acute ulcerative colitis, lactation
- **Physical:** Skin color, lesions; orientation, reflexes; abdominal examination, bowel sounds, liver evaluation; serum electrolytes (with extended use)

Interventions

- Monitor for response. If improvement is not seen within 48 hr, discontinue treatment and notify health care provider.
- Give drug after each unformed stool. Keep track of amount given to avoid exceeding the recommended daily dosage unless directed by a physician.

⊗ ***Warning*** Have the opioid antagonist naloxone readily available in case of overdose and CNS depression.

Teaching points

- Take drug as prescribed. Do not exceed prescribed dosage or recommended daily dosage.
- Drink clear fluids to prevent dehydration.
- You may experience these side effects: Abdominal fullness, nausea, vomiting; dry mouth (suck on sugarless lozenges); dizziness.
- Report abdominal pain or distention, fever, and diarrhea that does not stop after a few days.

▽ lopinavir (lopinavir and ritonavir)

(low ***pin'*** *ah ver)*

Kaletra DNC

PREGNANCY CATEGORY C

Drug classes

Antiviral

Protease inhibitor combination

Therapeutic actions

Lopinavir in this combination exhibits antiviral activity; inhibits HIV protease activity, leading to the decrease in production of HIV particles; ritonavir in this preparation inhibits metabolism of lopinavir, allowing for increased plasma levels of lopinavir.

Indications

- Treatment of HIV infection in combination with other antiretrovirals

Contraindications and cautions

- Contraindicated with allergy to lopinavir, ritonavir.
- Use cautiously with pregnancy, hepatic impairment, pancreatitis, lactation.

Available forms

Tablets DNC—100 mg lopinavir/25 mg ritonavir, 200 mg lopinavir/50 mg ritonavir; oral solution—400 mg lopinavir/100 mg ritonavir/5 mL

Dosages

Dose is based on lopinavir component of lopinavir/ritonavir solution (400 mg/100 mg/ 5 mL).

Once-daily lopinavir/ritonavir is not recommended for treatment-experienced patients.

Adults and pediatric patients older than 12 yr and weighing more than 40 kg

- *HIV infection, with other antiretrovirals in treatment-naive patients:* 800 mg lopinavir and 200 mg ritonavir (four tablets or 10 mL) PO once daily or divided evenly bid.
- *HIV infection, with other antiretrovirals in treatment-experienced patients:* 400 mg

lopinavir and 100 mg ritonavir (two tablets or 5 mL) PO bid.

- *Taken with efavirenz, nevirapine, fosamprenavir without ritonavir, or nelfinavir:* 600 mg lopinavir and 150 mg ritonavir (three tablets) PO bid for treatment-experienced patients. No dosage adjustment needed for treatment-naive patients.
- *Patients using oral solution and also taking efavirenz, nevirapine, amprenavir, or nelfinavir:* Dosage should be adjusted to 533 mg lopinavir and 133 mg ritonavir (6.5 mL) bid with food.

Pediatric patients

Tablets

Dosage is based on weight.

Weight (kg)	*Dosage*
7–less than 15	12 mg/kg PO bid
15–40	10 mg/kg PO bid
More than 40	400 mg PO bid

Solution

Dosage is based on weight.

Weight (kg)	*Dosage*
7–10	1.25 mL PO bid
More than 10–less than 15	1.75 mL PO bid
15–20	2.25 mL PO bid
More than 20–25	2.75 mL PO bid
More than 25–30	3.5 mL PO bid
More than 30–35	4 mL PO bid
More than 35–40	4.75 mL PO bid
More than 40	5 mL PO bid

Younger than 6 mo: Not recommended.

- *Taken with amprenavir, efavirenz, or nevirapine:*

Tablets: More than 45 kg: Use adult dose.
15–45 kg: 11 mg/kg PO bid.
7–15 kg: 13 mg/kg PO bid.

Solution

Dosage is based on weight.

Weight (kg)	*Dosage*
7–10	1.5 mL PO bid
More than 10–less than 15	2 mL PO bid
15–20	2.5 mL PO bid
More than 20–25	3.25 mL PO bid
More than 25–30	4 mL PO bid
More than 30–35	4.5 mL PO bid
More than 35–40	5 mL PO bid
More than 40–45	5.75 mL PO bid
More than 45	6.5 mL PO bid

Pharmacokinetics

Route	*Onset*	*Peak*
Oral	Varies	3–4 hr

Metabolism: Hepatic; $T_{1/2}$: 5–6 hr
Distribution: Crosses placenta; may enter breast milk
Excretion: Feces and urine

Adverse effects

- **CNS:** *Asthenia, peripheral and circumoral paresthesias,* anxiety, dreams, *headache,* dizziness, hallucinations, personality changes
- **CV:** DVTs, hypotension, syncope, tachycardia, chest pain
- **Dermatologic:** Rash, acne, alopecia, dry skin, exfoliative dermatitis
- **Endocrine:** *Increased triglycerides and cholesterol,* hyperglycemia, hyperuricemia, gynecomastia, hypothyroidism, hypogonadism
- **GI:** *Nausea, vomiting, diarrhea, anorexia, abdominal pain,* pancreatitis, *taste perversion,* dry mouth, hepatitis, hepatic impairment, dehydration
- **Hematologic:** Leukopenia, anemia
- **Other:** Hypothermia, chills, back pain, edema, cachexia

Interactions

✱ **Drug-drug** ⊗ ***Warning*** Potentially large increase in serum concentration of drugs metabolized by CYP450 3A4 (caused by ritonavir). Do not administer lopinavir with any of these drugs, including amiodarone, bepridil, bupropion, clozapine, encainide, flecainide, meperidine, piroxicam, propafenone, propoxy-phene, quinidine, and rifabutin. Potential for serious arrhythmias, seizures, and fatal reactions.

⊗ ***Warning*** Potentially large increases in serum concentration of these sedatives and hypnotics: Alprazolam, clonazepam, diazepam, estazolam, flurazepam, midazolam, triazolam, zolpidem. Extreme sedation and respiratory depression could occur. Do not administer lopinavir with any of these drugs.

• May increase level and adverse effects of phosphodiesterase 5 inhibitors (e.g., sildenafil, vardenafil, tadalafil) including hypotension and prolonged erection • May decrease effectiveness of hormonal contraceptives; using barrier contraceptives is advised

L

✱ **Drug-food** • Absorption of lopinavir oral solution is increased by the presence of food; taking the oral solution with food is strongly recommended

✱ **Drug-alternative therapy** • Potential for reduced effectiveness if combined with St. John's wort; avoid this combination

■ Nursing considerations

CLINICAL ALERT!

Name confusion has occurred between *Kaletra* (lopinavir/ritonavir) and *Keppra* (levetiracetam); use extreme caution.

Assessment

- **History:** Allergy to lopinavir, ritonavir, hepatic impairment, pancreatitis, pregnancy, lactation
- **Physical:** T; orientation, reflexes; BP, P, peripheral perfusion; R, adventitious sounds; bowel sounds; skin color, perfusion; LFTs, serum amylase levels, triglycerides, cholesterol, electrolytes

Interventions

- Solution should be stored in the refrigerator; may be left at room temperature but should be used within 60 days; protect from light and extreme heat. Oral solution contains 42% alcohol.
- Obtain baseline triglycerides, cholesterol levels, electrolytes, and glucose levels. Monitor periodically during therapy.

⊗ ***Warning*** Screen medication history before administration to avoid potentially serious drug interactions.

- Administer oral solution with meals or food to increase absorption. Tablets may be taken without regard to food; ensure that tablets are swallowed whole and are not cut, crushed, or chewed.
- Didanosine and lopinavir/ritonavir tablets may be administered simultaneously without food.
- Administer didanosine 1 hr before or 2 hr after lopinavir solution.

Teaching points

- Take the oral solution with meals or food; store the solution in the refrigerator. The taste of the solution may be improved if mixed with chocolate milk, *Ensure,* or *Advera* 1 hour before taking.
- Tablets must be swallowed whole and may be taken with or without food. Do not crush, chew, or divide tablets.
- Take the full course of therapy as prescribed; do not take a double dose if one is missed; do not change dosage without consulting your health care provider. Take this drug with your other HIV medications.
- This drug does not cure HIV infection; long-term effects are not yet known; continue to take precautions because the risk of transmission is not reduced by this drug.
- This drug may cause hormonal contraceptives to be ineffective; using barrier contraceptives is advised.
- Do not take any other drug, prescription or over-the-counter, or use any herbal therapies without consulting with your health care provider; this drug interacts with many other drugs and serious problems can occur.
- You may experience these side effects: Nausea, vomiting, loss of appetite, diarrhea, abdominal pain; headache, dizziness, numbness, and tingling.
- Report severe diarrhea, severe nausea, personality changes, changes in the color of urine or stool, fever or chills, severe abdominal pain.

▽ loratadine

*(lor **at'** a deen)*

Alavert, Alavert Childrens, Apo-Loratadine (CAN), Claritin, Claritin Hives Relief, Claritin Reditabs, Claritin 24-Hour Allergy, Dimetapp Children's ND Non-Drowsy Allergy, Triaminic Allerchews

PREGNANCY CATEGORY B

Drug class

Antihistamine (nonsedating type)

Therapeutic actions

Competitively blocks the effects of histamine at peripheral histamine-1 receptor sites; has anticholinergic (atropine-like) and antipruritic effects.

Indications

- Symptomatic relief of perennial and seasonal allergic rhinitis, vasomotor rhinitis, allergic conjunctivitis, and mild, uncomplicated urticaria and angioedema
- Treatment of rhinitis and chronic urticaria in children 2 yr and older

Contraindications and cautions

- Contraindicated with allergy to any antihistamines.
- Use cautiously with lactation, pregnancy.

Available forms

Tablets—10 mg; syrup—5 mg/5 mL; chewable tablets—5 mg; orally disintegrating tablets—5, 10 mg

Dosages

Place rapid dissolving tablets on tongue. Administer with or without water.

Adults and pediatric patients 6 yr and older

10 mg daily PO on an empty stomach.

Pediatric patients 2–5 yr

5 mg PO daily (syrup, chewable tablets).

Geriatric patients or patients with renal or hepatic impairment

10 mg PO every other day.

Pharmacokinetics

Route	*Onset*	*Peak*	*Duration*
Oral	1–3 hr	8–12 hr	24 hr

Metabolism: Hepatic; $T_{1/2}$: 8.4 hr
Distribution: Crosses placenta; enters breast milk
Excretion: Feces, urine

Adverse effects

- **CNS:** *Headache, nervousness, dizziness,* depression, drowsiness
- **CV:** Palpitations, edema
- **GI:** *Appetite increase,* nausea, diarrhea, abdominal pain
- **Respiratory: Bronchospasm,** pharyngitis
- **Other:** Fever, photosensitivity, rash, myalgia, arthralgia, angioedema, *weight gain,* dry mouth

Interactions

✱ **Drug-drug** • Additive CNS depressant effects with alcohol or other CNS depressants
✱ **Drug-lab test** • False skin testing procedures if done while patient is taking antihistamines

■ Nursing considerations

Assessment

- **History:** Allergy to any antihistamines; lactation, pregnancy
- **Physical:** Skin color, lesions, texture; orientation, reflexes, affect; vision examinations; R, adventitious sounds; prostate palpation; serum transaminase levels

Interventions

- Administer without regard to meals.

Teaching points

- If using rapid or orally disintegrating tablets, place on tongue; tablet will dissolve within seconds. Swallow with or without water.
- Avoid the use of alcohol; serious sedation could occur.
- You may experience these side effects: Dizziness, sedation, drowsiness (use caution if driving or performing tasks that require alertness); headache; thickening of bronchial secretions, dryness of nasal mucosa (use a humidifier).
- Report difficulty breathing, hallucinations, tremors, loss of coordination, irregular heartbeat.

▽ lorazepam

(lor a' ze pam)

Apo-Lorazepam (CAN), Ativan, Lorazepam Intensol, PMS-Lorazepam (CAN)

PREGNANCY CATEGORY D

CONTROLLED SUBSTANCE C-IV

Drug classes
Anxiolytic
Benzodiazepine
Sedative-hypnotic

Therapeutic actions
Exact mechanisms are not understood; acts mainly at subcortical levels of the CNS, binding to benzodiazepine receptors on postsynaptic GABA neurons in the CNS, leaving the cortex relatively unaffected. Main sites of action may be the limbic system and reticular formation; benzodiazepines potentiate the effects of GABA, an inhibitory neurotransmitter; anxiolytic effects occur at doses well below those needed to cause sedation and ataxia.

Indications
- Oral: Management of anxiety disorders or for short-term relief of symptoms of anxiety or anxiety associated with depression; insomnia due to anxiety or transient situational stress
- Parenteral: Preanesthetic medication in adults to produce sedation, relieve anxiety, and decrease recall of events related to surgery; treatment of status epilepticus

Contraindications and cautions
- Contraindicated with hypersensitivity to benzodiazepines, propylene glycol, polyethylene glycol or benzyl alcohol (parenteral lorazepam); psychoses; acute narrow-angle glaucoma; shock; coma; acute alcoholic intoxication with depression of vital signs; pregnancy (crosses placenta; risk of congenital malformations and neonatal withdrawal syndrome); labor and delivery ("floppy infant" syndrome); lactation.
- Use cautiously with impaired hepatic or renal function.

Available forms
Injection—2, 4 mg/mL; oral solution—2 mg/mL; tablets—0.5, 1, 2 mg

Dosages
Adults
Oral
Usual dose is 2–6 mg/day; range, 1–10 mg/day in divided doses with largest dose at bedtime.
- *Insomnia due to transient stress:* 2–4 mg given at bedtime.

IM
0.05 mg/kg up to a maximum of 4 mg administered at least 2 hr before operative procedure.

IV
Initial dose is 2 mg total or 0.044 mg/kg, whichever is smaller. Do not exceed this dose in patients older than 50 yr. Doses as high as 0.05 mg/kg up to a total of 4 mg may be given 15–20 min before the procedure to those benefited by a greater lack of recall.
- *Status epilepticus:* For patients older than 18 yr, 4 mg slowly at 2 mg/min. May give another 4 mg after 10–15 min if needed.

Pediatric patients
Drug should not be used in children younger than 12 yr.

Patients with renal or hepatic impairment
Initially, 1–2 mg/day in divided doses. Adjust as needed and tolerated.

Pharmacokinetics

Route	Onset	Peak	Duration
Oral	Intermediate	1 hr	12–24 hr
IM	15–30 min	60–90 min	12–24 hr
IV	1–5 min	10–15 min	12–24 hr

Metabolism: Hepatic; $T_{1/2}$: 10–20 hr
Distribution: Crosses placenta; enters breast milk
Excretion: Urine

IV FACTS
Preparation: Dilute lorazepam immediately before IV use. For direct IV injection or injection into IV line, dilute with an equal volume of compatible solution (sterile water for injection, sodium chloride injection, or 5% dextrose injection); do not use if solution is discolored or contains a precipitate. Protect from light.
Infusion: Direct inject slowly, or infuse at maximum rate of 2 mg/min.
Y-site incompatibilities: Do not mix with foscarnet, ondansetron, aztreonam, imipenem/cilastatin, omeprazole.

Adverse effects
- **CNS:** *Transient, mild drowsiness initially; sedation, depression, lethargy, apathy, fatigue, light-headedness, disorientation,*

anger, hostility, episodes of mania and hypomania, *restlessness, confusion,* crying, delirium, *headache,* slurred speech, dysarthria, stupor, rigidity, tremor, dystonia, vertigo, euphoria, nervousness, difficulty concentrating, vivid dreams, psychomotor retardation, extrapyramidal symptoms; *mild paradoxical excitatory reactions during first 2 wk of treatment,* anterograde amnesia
- **CV:** Bradycardia, tachycardia, **CV collapse,** hypertension and hypotension, palpitations, edema
- **Dermatologic:** Urticaria, pruritus, rash, dermatitis
- **EENT:** Visual and auditory disturbances, diplopia, nystagmus, depressed hearing, nasal congestion
- **GI:** Constipation, diarrhea, *dry mouth,* salivation, *nausea,* anorexia, vomiting, difficulty in swallowing, gastric disorders, hepatic impairment
- **GU:** Incontinence, urinary retention, libido changes, menstrual irregularities
- **Other:** Hiccups, fever, diaphoresis, paresthesias, muscular disturbances, gynecomastia; *drug dependence with withdrawal syndrome when drug is discontinued; more common with abrupt discontinuation of higher dosage used for longer than 4 mo*

Interactions

✱ **Drug-drug** • Increased CNS depression with alcohol and other sedating medications, such as barbiturates and opioids • Decreased effectiveness with theophyllines • Risk of toxicity if combined with probenecid, valproate; reduce lorazepam dose by 50%

✱ **Drug-alternative therapy** • Kava kava increases the sedative effects of benzodiazepines; coma has been reported with concurrent use

■ Nursing considerations

CLINICAL ALERT!

Name confusion has occurred between lorazepam and alprazolam; use caution.

Assessment

- **History:** Hypersensitivity to benzodiazepines, propylene glycol, polyethylene glycol or benzyl alcohol; psychoses; acute narrow-angle glaucoma; shock; coma; acute alcoholic intoxication with depression of vital signs; pregnancy; lactation; impaired liver or renal function, debilitation
- **Physical:** Skin color, lesions; T; orientation, reflexes, affect, ophthalmologic examination; P, BP; R, adventitious sounds; liver evaluation, abdominal examination, bowel sounds, normal output; CBC, LFTs, renal function tests

Interventions

- Sublingual administration has more rapid absorption than PO, and bioavailability compares to IM use.
- Do not administer intra-arterially; arteriospasm or gangrene may result.
- Give IM injections of undiluted drug deep into muscle mass, monitor injection sites.
- Do not use solutions that are discolored or contain a precipitate. Protect drug from light, and refrigerate oral solution.
- Oral solution may be mixed with water, juice, soda, applesauce, or pudding.

⊗ ***Warning*** Keep equipment to maintain a patent airway readily available when drug is given IV.

- Refrigerate injection and oral solution (36° F to 46° F). Can be stored at room temperature for 60 days.
- Reduce dose of opioid analgesics by at least half in patients who have received parenteral lorazepam.
- Keep patients who have received parenteral doses under close observation, preferably in bed, up to 3 hr. Do not permit ambulatory patients to drive following an injection.

⊗ ***Warning*** Taper dosage gradually after long-term therapy, especially in patients with epilepsy.

Teaching points

- Take drug exactly as prescribed; do not stop taking drug (in long-term therapy) without consulting your health care provider.
- You may experience these side effects: Drowsiness, dizziness (may be transient; avoid driving or engaging in dangerous activities); GI upset (take drug with food); nocturnal sleep disturbances for several nights after discontinuing the drug if used as a sedative and hypnotic; depression, dreams, emotional upset, crying.

- Report severe dizziness, weakness, drowsiness that persists, rash or skin lesions, palpitations, edema of the extremities; visual changes; difficulty voiding.

losartan potassium

*(low **sar'** tan)*

Cozaar

PREGNANCY CATEGORY C (FIRST TRIMESTER)

PREGNANCY CATEGORY D (SECOND AND THIRD TRIMESTERS)

Drug classes

Antihypertensive
ARB

Therapeutic actions

Selectively blocks the binding of angiotensin II to specific tissue receptors found in the vascular smooth muscle and adrenal gland; this action blocks the vasoconstriction effect of the renin-angiotensin system as well as the release of aldosterone leading to decreased BP.

Indications

- Treatment of hypertension, alone or in combination with other antihypertensives
- Treatment of diabetic nephropathy with an elevated serum creatinine and proteinuria in patients with type 2 (non–insulin-dependent) diabetes and a history of hypertension
- Reduction of the risk of CVA in patients with hypertension and left ventricular hypertrophy

Contraindications and cautions

- Contraindicated with hypersensitivity to losartan, pregnancy (use during the second or third trimester can cause injury or even death to the fetus), lactation.
- Use cautiously with hepatic or renal impairment, hypovolemia, history of angioedema.

Available forms

Tablets—25, 50, 100 mg

Dosages

Adults

- *Hypertension:* Starting dose of 50 mg PO daily. Patients on diuretics or hypovolemic patients may only require 25 mg daily. Dosage ranges from 25–100 mg daily PO given once or twice a day have been used.
- *Diabetic nephropathy:* 50 mg/day PO once daily; may be increased to 100 mg/day once daily based on BP response.
- *CVA reduction:* 50 mg/day PO with 12.5 mg/day hydrochlorothiazide. May be increased to 100 mg/day PO with 25 mg/day hydrochlorothiazide if needed.

Pediatric patients 6 yr and older

- *Hypertension:* 0.7 mg/kg once daily up to 50 mg/day total.

Pharmacokinetics

Route	*Onset*	*Peak*
Oral	Varies	1–3 hr

Metabolism: Hepatic; $T_{1/2}$: 2 hr, then 6–9 hr
Distribution: Crosses placenta; enters breast milk
Excretion: Feces, urine

Adverse effects

- **CNS:** Headache, *dizziness,* syncope, insomnia
- **CV:** Hypotension
- **Dermatologic:** Rash, urticaria, pruritus, alopecia, dry skin
- **GI:** *Diarrhea, abdominal pain, nausea,* constipation, dry mouth
- **Respiratory:** *URI symptoms, cough,* sinus disorders
- **Other:** Back pain, fever, gout, muscle weakness

Interactions

✱ **Drug-drug** • Decreased serum levels and effectiveness if taken concurrently with phenobarbital, indomethacin, and rifamycin • Losartan is converted to an active metabolite by CYP450 3A4, and 2C9 (fluconazole); drugs that inhibit 3A4 (ketoconazole, fluconazole) may increase antihypertensive effects of losartan

■ Nursing considerations

Assessment

- **History:** Hypersensitivity to losartan, pregnancy, lactation, hepatic or renal impairment, hypovolemia
- **Physical:** Skin lesions, turgor; T; reflexes, affect; BP; R, respiratory auscultation; LFTs, renal function tests

Interventions

- Administer without regard to meals.

⊠ ***Black box warning*** Ensure that patient is not pregnant before beginning therapy, suggest the use of barrier birth control while using losartan; fetal injury and deaths have been reported.

- Find an alternative method of feeding the baby if given to a nursing mother. Depression of the renin-angiotensin system in infants is potentially very dangerous.

⊗ ***Warning*** Alert surgeon and mark the patient's chart with notice that losartan is being taken. The blockage of the renin-angiotensin system following surgery can produce problems. Hypotension may be reversed with volume expansion.

- Monitor patient closely in any situation that may lead to a decrease in BP secondary to reduction in fluid volume—excessive perspiration, dehydration, vomiting, diarrhea—excessive hypotension can occur.

Teaching points

- Take drug without regard to meals. Do not stop taking this drug without consulting your health care provider.
- Use a barrier method of birth control while using this drug; if you become pregnant or desire to become pregnant, consult with your health care provider. If you are breast-feeding, you should find another method of feeding the baby.
- You may experience these side effects: Dizziness (avoid driving a car or performing hazardous tasks); headache (request medications); nausea, vomiting, diarrhea (proper nutrition is important, consult a dietitian to maintain nutrition); symptoms of upper respiratory tract infection, cough (do not self-medicate; consult your health care provider if uncomfortable).
- Report fever, chills, dizziness, pregnancy.

▽lovastatin (mevinolin)

*(loe va **sta'** tin)*

Altoprev (DNC), Apo-Lovastatin (CAN), Co-Lovastatin (CAN), Gen-Lovastatin (CAN), Mevacor, Nu-Lovastatin (CAN), PMS-Lovastatin (CAN), ratio-Lovastatin (CAN)

PREGNANCY CATEGORY X

Drug classes

Antihyperlipidemic
HMG-CoA reductase inhibitor

Therapeutic actions

Inhibits the enzyme that catalyzes the rate-limiting step in the cholesterol synthesis pathway, resulting in a decrease in serum cholesterol, serum LDLs (the lipids associated with the development of coronary artery disease), and either an increase or no change in serum HDLs (the lipids associated with decreased risk of CAD).

Indications

- Treatment of familial hypercholesterolemia
- Adjunctive treatment of type II hyperlipidemia (ER only)
- To slow the progression of atherosclerosis in patients with CAD
- Primary prevention of coronary heart disease in patients without symptomatic disease; average to moderately elevated total cholesterol and LDL cholesterol, and low HDLs
- Treatment of primary hypercholesterolemia with diet and exercise to decrease total and LDL cholesterol
- As adjunct to diet to reduce total cholesterol, LDLs, apolipoprotein B levels in adolescent boys and girls who are at least 1 yr postmenarche who have heterozygous familial hypercholesterolemia

Contraindications and cautions

- Contraindicated with allergy to lovastatin, active liver disease, unexplained persistent serum transaminase, pregnancy.
- Use cautiously with impaired hepatic function, cataracts, lactation.

L

Available forms

Tablets—10, 20, 40 mg; ER tablets (DNC)—10, 20, 40, 60 mg

Dosages

Adults

Initially, 20 mg/day PO given in the evening with meals. Maintenance range, 10–80 mg/day PO single or divided doses. Do not exceed 80 mg/day. For ER tablets, 10–60 mg/day as single dose PO, taken in the evening. Adjust at intervals of 4 wk or more. Maximum daily dose, 40 mg/day if taking amiodarone or verapamil. Patients receiving cyclosporine should start at 10 mg daily and not exceed 20 mg daily. May be combined with bile acid sequestrants. If combined with fibrates or niacin, do not exceed 20 mg daily.

Pediatric patients

- *Adolescent boys and postmenarchal girls, 10–17 yr:* 10–40 mg/day PO; may increase to a maximum of 40 mg/day.

Patients with renal impairment

For creatinine clearance less than 30 mL/min, use doses more than 20 mg/day with caution.

Pharmacokinetics

Route	Onset	Peak
Oral	2 wk	4–6 wk

Metabolism: Hepatic; $T_{1/2}$: 2–4 hr
Distribution: Crosses placenta; enters breast milk
Excretion: Bile, feces

Adverse effects

- **CNS:** *Headache,* blurred vision, dizziness, insomnia, fatigue, muscle cramps, cataracts
- **GI:** *Flatulence, abdominal pain, cramps, constipation, nausea,* dyspepsia, heartburn, elevations of alkaline phosphatase, transaminases
- **Other:** Myalgia, rhabdomyolysis, rash

Interactions

✱ **Drug-drug** ⊗ ***Warning*** Possibility of severe myopathy or rhabdomyolysis with cyclosporine, amiodarone, verapamil, or gemfibrozil or other HMG-CoA inhibitors, or niacin and azole antifungals; avoid these combinations.
• Increased serum levels and risk of myopathy if combined with drugs that inhibit CYP450 3A4 (e.g., itraconazole, ketoconazole); reduce lovastatin dose or interrupt treatment if these drugs are needed

✱ **Drug-food** • Decreased metabolism and increased risk of toxic effects if taken with grapefruit juice; avoid this combination

■ Nursing considerations

Assessment

- **History:** Allergy to lovastatin, impaired hepatic function, cataracts, pregnancy, lactation
- **Physical:** Orientation, affect, ophthalmologic examination; liver evaluation; lipid studies, LFTs

Interventions

- Give in the evening; highest rates of cholesterol synthesis are between midnight and 5 AM.
- Arrange for regular checkups.
- Advise patient that this drug cannot be taken during pregnancy; urge the use of barrier contraceptives.
- Arrange for periodic ophthalmologic examinations to check for cataract development, and liver function studies every 4–6 wk during first 15 mo and then periodically.
- Administer only when diet restricted in cholesterol and saturated fats fails to lower cholesterol and lipids adequately.
- Discontinue lovastatin if LFTs increase to three times the upper limit of normal.

Teaching points

- Take drug in the evening. Continue following a cholesterol-lowering diet while taking this medication. Avoid drinking grapefruit juice while taking this drug.
- Do not cut, crush, or chew extended-release tablets.
- Use a barrier contraceptive while you are taking this drug; if you think you are pregnant or wish to become pregnant, consult your health care provider.
- Have periodic ophthalmologic examinations.
- You may experience these side effects: Nausea (eat frequent small meals), headache, muscle and joint aches and pains (may lessen).
- Report severe GI upset, changes in vision, unusual bleeding or bruising, dark urine, or light-colored stools, severe muscle pain, soreness.

loxapine
(lox' a peen)

loxapine hydrochloride

loxapine succinate

Apo-Loxapine (CAN), Loxapac (CAN), Loxitane, PMS-Loxapine (CAN)

PREGNANCY CATEGORY C

Drug classes
Antipsychotic
Dopaminergic blocker

Therapeutic actions
Mechanism of action is not fully understood: Antipsychotic drugs block postsynaptic dopamine receptors in the brain, but this may not be necessary and sufficient for antipsychotic activity.

Indications
- Treatment of schizophrenia

Contraindications and cautions
- Contraindicated with coma or severe CNS depression; bone marrow depression; blood dyscrasia; circulatory collapse; subcortical brain damage; Parkinson's disease; liver disease; cerebral arteriosclerosis; coronary disease; severe hypotension or hypertension.
- Use cautiously with respiratory disorders ("silent pneumonia"); glaucoma, prostatic hypertrophy; epilepsy or history of epilepsy; breast cancer (elevations in prolactin may stimulate a prolactin-dependent tumor); thyrotoxicosis; peptic ulcer, decreased renal function; exposure to heat or phosphorus insecticides; pregnancy; and lactation.

Available forms
Capsules—5, 10, 25, 50 mg

Dosages
Adults
Oral

Individualize dosage, and administer in divided doses bid–qid, initially 10 mg bid. Severely disturbed patients may need up to 50 mg/day. Increase dosage fairly rapidly over the first 7–10 days until symptoms are controlled. Usual dosage range is 60–100 mg/day; dosage greater than 250 mg/day is not recommended. For maintenance, reduce to minimum effective dose. Usual range is 20–60 mg/day.

Pediatric patients
Not recommended for patients younger than 16 yr.

Geriatric patients
Use lower doses, and increase dosage more gradually than in younger patients.

Pharmacokinetics

Route	*Onset*	*Peak*	*Duration*
Oral	30 min	1.5–3 hr	12 hr

Metabolism: Hepatic; $T_{1/2}$: 1–14 hr
Distribution: Unknown
Excretion: Urine

Adverse effects
Adverse effects listed are those of antipsychotic drugs.

- **Autonomic:** Dry mouth, salivation, nasal congestion, nausea, vomiting, anorexia, fever, pallor, facial flushing, sweating, constipation, paralytic ileus, urinary retention, incontinence, polyuria, enuresis, priapism, ejaculation inhibition, male impotence
- **CNS:** *Drowsiness,* insomnia, vertigo, headache, weakness, tremor, ataxia, slurring, cerebral edema, seizures, exacerbation of psychotic symptoms, extrapyramidal syndromes—*pseudoparkinsonism; dystonias; akathisia,* tardive dyskinesias, potentially irreversible, **neuroleptic malignant syndrome**
- **CV:** Hypotension, orthostatic hypotension, hypertension, tachycardia, bradycardia, cardiac arrest, heart failure, cardiomegaly, **refractory arrhythmias,** pulmonary edema
- **Endocrine:** Lactation, breast engorgement, galactorrhea; SIADH; amenorrhea, menstrual irregularities; gynecomastia; changes in libido; hyperglycemia or hypoglycemia; glycosuria; hyponatremia; pituitary tumor with hyperprolactinemia; inhibition of ovulation, infertility, pseudopregnancy; reduced urinary levels of gonadotropins, estrogens, progestins

L

- **Hematologic:** Eosinophilia, leukopenia, leukocytosis, anemia; aplastic anemia; hemolytic anemia; thrombocytopenic or nonthrombocytopenic purpura; pancytopenia
- **Hypersensitivity:** Jaundice, urticaria, angioneurotic edema, laryngeal edema, photosensitivity, eczema, asthma, anaphylactoid reactions, exfoliative dermatitis
- **Respiratory: Bronchospasm, laryngospasm,** dyspnea; suppression of cough reflex and potential for aspiration

Interactions

✱ **Drug-drug** • Increased risk of CNS effects if combined with other CNS medications

■ Nursing considerations

CLINICAL ALERT!
Name confusion has been reported between *Loxitane* (loxapine) and *Lexapro* (escitalopram); use caution.

Assessment

- **History:** Coma or severe CNS depression; blood dyscrasia; circulatory collapse; subcortical brain damage; Parkinson's disease; liver damage; cerebral arteriosclerosis; coronary disease; severe hypotension or hypertension; respiratory disorders; glaucoma, prostatic hypertrophy; epilepsy; breast cancer; thyrotoxicosis; peptic ulcer, decreased renal function; myelography within previous 24 hr or myelography scheduled within 48 hr; exposure to heat or phosphorus insecticides; pregnancy, lactation
- **Physical:** Weight, T; reflexes, orientation, IOP; P, BP, orthostatic BP; R, adventitious sounds; bowel sounds and normal output, liver evaluation; urinary output, prostate size; CBC, urinalysis, thyroid, LFTs, renal function tests

Interventions

⊗ ***Black box warning*** There is increased risk of mortality when antipsychotics are used in elderly patients with dementia-related psychosis. Avoid this use; not approved for this use.

⊗ ***Warning*** Arrange for discontinuation if WBC count is depressed.

⊗ ***Warning*** Monitor elderly patients for dehydration; institute remedial measures promptly; sedation and decreased thirst sensation due to CNS effects can lead to severe dehydration.

- Consult physician about appropriate warning of patient or patient's guardian about tardive dyskinesias.
- Consult physician about dosage reduction and use of anticholinergic antiparkinsonian drugs (controversial) if extrapyramidal effects occur.

Teaching points

- Take drug exactly as prescribed.
- Avoid driving or engaging in dangerous activities if dizziness or vision changes occur.
- Avoid prolonged exposure to sun or use a sunscreen or covering garments.
- Maintain fluid intake, and use precautions against heatstroke in hot weather.
- Report sore throat, fever, unusual bleeding or bruising, rash, weakness, tremors, impaired vision, dark urine, pale stools, and yellowing of the skin or eyes.

▽ lutropin

See Appendix W, *Less commonly used drugs.*

▽ magaldrate (aluminum magnesium hydroxide) sulfate

(mag' al drate)

Iosopan, Riopan

PREGNANCY CATEGORY C

Drug class

Antacid

Therapeutic actions

Neutralizes or reduces gastric acidity, resulting in an increase in the pH of the stomach and duodenal bulb and inhibiting the proteolytic activity of pepsin; the combination of magnesium (causes diarrhea when administered alone) and aluminum (constipating when administered alone) salts usually minimizes adverse GI effects.

Indications

- Symptomatic relief of upset stomach associated with hyperacidity
- Hyperacidity associated with peptic ulcer, gastritis, peptic esophagitis, gastric hyperacidity, and hiatal hernia
- Treatment of hypomagnesemia, hypocalcemia, hyperphosphatemia

Contraindications and cautions

- Contraindicated with allergy to magnesium or aluminum products.
- Use cautiously with renal insufficiency, gastric outlet obstruction (aluminum salt may inhibit gastric emptying), pregnancy, lactation.

Available forms

Suspension—540 mg/5 mL; liquid—540 mg/5 mL

Dosages

Adults

540–1,080 mg (5–10 mL) PO between meals and at bedtime. Do not exceed 80 mL (16 teaspoonfuls) in 24 hr. Do not use maximum dosage for more than 2 wk.

Pharmacokinetics

Route	Onset	Peak
Oral	30 min	30–60 min

Generally no systemic absorption

Adverse effects

- **GI:** *Rebound hyperacidity,* diarrhea, constipation
- **Metabolic:** Decreased absorption of fluoride and accumulation of aluminum in serum, bone, CNS (aluminum may be neurotoxic, especially in patients with renal failure); *alkalosis;* hypermagnesemia and toxicity in patients with renal failure

Interactions

✱ **Drug-drug** ⊗ ***Warning*** Do not administer other oral drugs within 1–2 hr of antacid administration; change in gastric pH may interfere with absorption of oral drugs.
• Decreased pharmacologic effect of tetracyclines, penicillamine, nitrofurantoin, fluoroquinolones, ketoconazole • Decreased absorption and therapeutic effects of clindamycin and lincomycin

■ Nursing considerations

Assessment

- **History:** Allergy to magnesium or aluminum products, renal insufficiency, gastric outlet obstruction, pregnancy, lactation
- **Physical:** Bone and muscle strength; abdominal examination, bowel sounds; renal function tests, serum magnesium as appropriate

Interventions

- Do not administer other oral drugs within 1–2 hr of antacid administration.
- Give between meals and at bedtime.

⊗ ***Warning*** Monitor patients on long-term therapy for signs of aluminum accumulation: Bone pain, muscle weakness, malaise. Discontinue drug as needed.

Teaching points

- Take between meals and at bedtime.
- Do not take with any other oral medications; absorption of those medications can be inhibited. Take other oral medications at least 1–2 hours after aluminum salt.
- Report bone pain, muscle weakness, coffee-ground vomitus, black tarry stools, no relief from symptoms being treated.

M

▽ magnesium salts

*(mag **nee'** zee um)*

magnesia

magnesium citrate

Citro-Mag (CAN)

magnesium hydroxide

Milk of Magnesia, Phillips' Chewable

magnesium oxide

Mag-Ox 400, Maox 420, Uro-Mag

PREGNANCY CATEGORY C

PREGNANCY CATEGORY A (ANTACID)

PREGNANCY CATEGORY B (LAXATIVE)

Drug classes
Antacid
Laxative

Therapeutic actions
Antacid (magnesium hydroxide, magnesium oxide): Neutralizes or reduces gastric acidity, resulting in an increase in the pH of the stomach and duodenal bulb and inhibition of the proteolytic activity of pepsin. Laxative (magnesium citrate, magnesium hydroxide): Attracts and retains water in intestinal lumen and distends bowel; causes the duodenal secretion of cholecystokinin, which stimulates fluid secretion and intestinal motility.

Indications
- Symptomatic relief of upset stomach associated with hyperacidity
- Hyperacidity associated with peptic ulcer, gastritis, peptic esophagitis, gastric hyperacidity, and hiatal hernia
- Prophylaxis of GI bleeding, stress ulcers, aspiration pneumonia
- Short-term relief of constipation; evacuation of the colon for rectal and bowel examination

Contraindications and cautions
- Contraindicated with allergy to magnesium products.
- Use cautiously with renal insufficiency, pregnancy, lactation.

Available forms
Tablets—311 (chewable), 400, 420, 500 mg; capsules—140 mg; liquid—various

Dosages
Adults
Magnesium citrate
- *Laxative:* 300 mL or in divided doses with a full glass of water.

Magnesium hydroxide
- *Antacid:* 5–15 mL liquid or 622–1,244 mg tablets PO qid (adult and patients older than 12 yr).
- *Laxative:* 15–60 mL PO taken with liquid.

Magnesium oxide
- *Capsules:* 140 mg PO tid–qid.
- *Tablets:* 400–800 mg/day PO.

Pediatric patients
Magnesium citrate
- *Laxative:* 90–210 mL for ages 6–12 yr with full glass of water; 60 mL for ages 2–6 yr with full glass of water.

Magnesium hydroxide
- *Laxative:*
  Younger than 2 yr: Do not administer unless directed by a physician.
  2–5 yr: 5–15 mL PO.
  6–11 yr: 15–30 mL PO.

Pharmacokinetics
Route	Onset
Oral	20–60 min

Minimal systemic absorption
Excretion: Renal

Adverse effects
- **CNS:** Dizziness, fainting, sweating
- **GI:** *Diarrhea, nausea, perianal irritation*
- **Metabolic:** Hypermagnesemia and toxicity in patients with renal failure

Interactions
✱ **Drug-drug** ⊗ ***Warning*** Do not give other oral drugs within 1–2 hr of antacid administration; change in gastric pH may interfere with absorption.
- Decreased pharmacologic effect of tetracyclines, penicillamine, nitrofurantoin, fluoroquinolones, ketoconazole

■ Nursing considerations
Assessment
- **History:** Allergy to magnesium products; renal insufficiency
- **Physical:** Abdominal examination, bowel sounds; renal function tests, serum magnesium

Interventions
- Do not administer other oral drugs within 1–2 hr of antacid administration.
- Have patient chew antacid tablets thoroughly before swallowing; follow with a glass of water.
- Give antacid between meals and at bedtime.

Teaching points

- Take antacid between meals and at bedtime. If tablets are being used, chew thoroughly before swallowing, and then drink a glass of water.
- Do not use laxatives if you have abdominal pain, nausea, or vomiting.
- Refrigerate magnesium citrate solutions to keep them effective and improve their taste.
- Do not take with any other oral medications; absorption of those medications can be inhibited. Take other oral medications at least 1–2 hours after aluminum salt.
- Diarrhea may occur with antacid therapy.
- Do not use laxatives long-term. Prolonged or excessive use can lead to serious problems. You should increase your intake of water (to 6–8 glasses/day) and fiber, and exercise regularly.
- You may experience these side effects: Excessive bowel activity, cramping, diarrhea, nausea, dizziness (be careful not to fall).
- With antacid use, report diarrhea; coffee-ground vomitus; black, tarry stools; no relief from symptoms being treated. With laxative use, report rectal bleeding, muscle cramps or pain, weakness, dizziness (not related to abdominal cramps and bowel movement), unrelieved constipation.

DANGEROUS DRUG (IV)

▽magnesium sulfate (epsom salt)

(mag ***nee'*** *zee um)*

PREGNANCY CATEGORY A

PREGNANCY CATEGORY B (LAXATIVE)

Drug classes

Antiepileptic
Electrolyte
Laxative

Therapeutic actions

Cofactor of many enzyme systems involved in neurochemical transmission and muscular excitability; prevents or controls seizures by blocking neuromuscular transmission; attracts and retains water in the intestinal lumen and distends the bowel to promote mass movement and relieve constipation.

Indications

- Acute nephritis (children), to control hypertension
- IV: Hypomagnesemia, replacement therapy
- IV or IM: Preeclampsia or eclampsia
- PO: Short-term treatment of constipation
- PO: Evacuation of the colon for rectal and bowel examinations
- To correct or prevent hypomagnesemia in patients on parenteral nutrition
- Unlabeled uses: Inhibition of premature labor (parenteral), adjunct treatment of exacerbations of acute asthma; treatment torsades de pointes, atypical ventricular arrhythmias

Contraindications and cautions

- Contraindicated with allergy to magnesium products; heart block, myocardial damage; abdominal pain, nausea, vomiting, or other symptoms of appendicitis; acute surgical abdomen, fecal impaction, intestinal and biliary tract obstruction, hepatitis. Do not give during 2 hr preceding delivery because of risk of magnesium toxicity in the neonate.
- Use cautiously with renal insufficiency.

Available forms

Granules—40 mEq/5 g; injection—0.325, 0.65, 1, 4 mEq/mL

Dosages

Adults

- *Parenteral nutrition:* 8–24 mEq/day IV.
- *Mild magnesium deficiency:* 1 g IM or IV every 6 hr for 4 doses (32.5 mEq/24 hr).
- *Severe hypomagnesemia:* Up to 2 mEq/kg IM within 4 hr or 5 g (40 mEq)/1,000 mL D_5W or 0.9% normal saline IV infused over 3 hr.
- *Eclampsia, severe preeclampsia:* Total initial dose of 10–14 g. May infuse 4–5 g in 250 mL 5% dextrose injection or 0.9% sodium chloride while giving IM doses up to 10 g (5 g or 10 mL of undiluted 50% solution in each buttock). Or, may give initial IV dose of 4 g by diluting 50% solution to 10% or 20%; may inject diluted fluid (40 mL of 10% or 20 mL of 20% solution) IV over 3–4 min.

M

Then inject 4–5 g (8 to 10 mL of 50% solution) IM into alternate buttocks every 4 hr as needed depending on patellar reflex and respiratory function. Or, after initial IV dose, may give 1–2 g/hr by constant IV infusion. Continue until paroxysms stop. To control seizures, optimal serum magnesium level is 6 mg/100 mL. Do not exceed 30–40 g in 24 hr.

IM

- *Toxemia:* 4–5 g of a 50% solution every 4 hr as needed.

IV

1–4 g of a 10%–20% solution. Do not exceed 1.5 mL/min of a 10% solution. Or, 4–5 g in 250 mL of 5% dextrose. Do not exceed 3 mL/min.

- *Arrhythmias:* 3–4 g IV over several min; then 3–20 mg/min continuous infusion for 5–48 hr.
- *Acute MI:* 2 g IV over 5–15 min followed by 18 g IV over 24 hr.

PO

- *Laxative:* 10–30 g daily given as single dose or divided doses.

Pediatric patients

- *Laxative:*
  6–11 yr: 5–10 g daily in single dose or divided doses; 15–30 mL/day.
  2–5 yr: 2.5–5 g daily in single dose or divided doses; 5–15 mL/day.

IM

100 mg/kg (0.8 mEq/kg or 0.2 mL/kg of a 50% solution) IM every 4–6 hr as needed. Or, 20–40 mg/kg (0.16–0.32 mEq/kg or 0.1–0.2 mL/kg of a 20% solution).

IV

For severe symptoms, 100–200 mg/kg of a 1%–3% solution IV over 1 hr with half of dose given in first 15–20 min (seizure control).

Patients with renal impairment

- *Severe preeclampsia, eclampsia:* In severe impairment, maximum dosage is 20 g in 48 hr. Check serum magnesium level often.

Pharmacokinetics

Route	*Onset*	*Duration*
IV	Immediate	30 min
IM	60 min	3–4 hr
Oral	1–2 hr	3–4 hr

Metabolism: $T_{1/2}$: Unknown
Distribution: Crosses placenta, enters breast milk
Excretion: Urine

IV FACTS

Preparation: Dilute IV infusion to a concentration of 20% or less before IV administration; dilute 4–5 g in 250 mL D_5W or sodium chloride solution.
Infusion: Do not exceed 1.5 mL of a 10% solution per minute IV or 3 mL/min IV infusion.
Incompatibilities: Do not mix with other IV drugs.

Adverse effects

- **CNS:** *Weakness, dizziness,* fainting, sweating (PO)
- **CV:** Palpitations
- **GI:** *Excessive bowel activity, perianal irritation* (PO)
- **Metabolic:** *Magnesium intoxication* (flushing, sweating, hypotension, depressed reflexes, flaccid paralysis, hypothermia, circulatory collapse, cardiac and CNS depression—parenteral); hypocalcemia with tetany (secondary to treatment of eclampsia—parenteral)

Interactions

✱ **Drug-drug** • Potentiation of neuromuscular blockade produced by nondepolarizing neuromuscular relaxants (atracurium, pancuronium, vecuronium)

■ Nursing considerations

Assessment

- **History:** Allergy to magnesium products; renal insufficiency; heart block, myocardial damage; symptoms of appendicitis; acute surgical abdomen, fecal impaction, intestinal and biliary tract obstruction, hepatitis
- **Physical:** Skin color, texture; muscle tone; T; orientation, affect, reflexes, peripheral sensation; P, auscultation, BP, rhythm strip; abdominal examination, bowel sounds; renal function tests, serum magnesium and calcium, LFTs (oral use)

Interventions

- Reserve IV use in eclampsia for immediate life-threatening situations.
- Give IM route by deep IM injection of the undiluted (50%) solution for adults; dilute to a 20% solution for children.

⊗ ***Warning*** Monitor serum magnesium levels during parenteral therapy. Arrange to discontinue administration as soon as levels are within normal limits (1.5–3 mEq/L) and desired clinical response is obtained.

⊗ ***Warning*** Monitor knee-jerk reflex before repeated parenteral administration. If knee-jerk reflexes are suppressed, do not administer magnesium because respiratory center failure may occur.

- Give oral magnesium sulfate as a laxative only as a temporary measure. Arrange for dietary measures (fiber, fluids), exercise, and environmental control to return to normal bowel activity.
- Do not give oral magnesium sulfate with abdominal pain, nausea, or vomiting.
- Monitor bowel function; if diarrhea and cramping occur, discontinue oral drug.
- Maintain urine output at a level of 100 mL every 4 hr during parenteral administration.

Teaching points

- Use only as a temporary measure to relieve constipation. Do not take if abdominal pain, nausea, or vomiting occurs.
- You may experience diarrhea with oral use. If this occurs, discontinue drug and consult your health care provider.
- Report sweating, flushing, muscle tremors or twitching, inability to move extremities.

▽mannitol

(man' i tole)

Osmitrol

PREGNANCY CATEGORY B

Drug classes

Diagnostic agent
Osmotic diuretic
Urinary irrigant

Therapeutic actions

Elevates the osmolarity of the glomerular filtrate, thereby hindering the reabsorption of water and leading to a loss of water, sodium, chloride (used for diagnosis of glomerular filtration rate); creates an osmotic gradient in the eye between plasma and ocular fluids, thereby reducing IOP; creates an osmotic effect, leading to decreased swelling in post-transurethral prostatic resection.

Indications

- Prevention and treatment of the oliguric phase of renal failure
- Reduction of intracranial pressure and treatment of cerebral edema; of elevated IOP when the pressure cannot be lowered by other means
- Promotion of the urinary excretion of toxic substances
- Diagnostic use: Measurement of GFR
- Irrigant in transurethral prostatic resection or other transurethral procedures

Contraindications and cautions

- Contraindicated with anuria due to severe renal disease.
- Use cautiously with pulmonary congestion, active intracranial bleeding (except during craniotomy), dehydration, renal disease, heart failure, pregnancy, lactation.

Available forms

Injection—5%, 10%, 15%, 20%, 25%; solution—5 g/100 mL

Dosages

Adults

IV infusion only; individualize concentration and rate of administration. Dosage is 50–200 g/day. Adjust dosage to maintain urine flow of 30–50 mL/hr.

- *Prevention of oliguria:* 50–100 g IV as a 5%–25% solution.
- *Treatment of oliguria:* 50–100 g IV of a 15%–25% solution.
- *Reduction of intracranial pressure and cerebral edema:* 1.5–2 g/kg IV as a 15%–25% solution over 30–60 min. Evidence of reduced pressure should be seen in 15 min.

- *Reduction of IOP:* Infuse 1.5–2 g/kg IV as a 25% solution, 20% solution, or 15% solution over 30 min. If used preoperatively, use 60–90 min before surgery for maximal effect.
- *Adjunctive therapy to promote diuresis in intoxications:* Maximum of 200 g IV of mannitol with other fluids and electrolytes.
- *Measurement of glomerular filtration rate:* Dilute 100 mL of a 20% solution with 180 mL of sodium chloride injection. Infuse this 280 mL of 7.2% solution IV at a rate of 20 mL/min. Collect urine with a catheter for the specified time for measurement of mannitol excreted in mg/min. Draw blood at the start and at the end of the time for measurement of mannitol in mg/mL plasma.
- *Test dose of mannitol for patients with inadequate renal function:* 0.2 g/kg IV (about 50 mL of a 25% solution, 75 mL of a 20% solution) in 3–5 min to produce a urine flow of 30–50 mL/hr. If urine flow does not increase, repeat dose. If no response to second dose, reevaluate patient situation.
- *Urologic irrigation:* Use prepared 5 g/100 mL distilled water solution; irrigate as needed.

Pediatric patients

Dosage for children younger than 12 yr not established.

Pharmacokinetics

Route	*Onset*	*Peak*	*Duration*
IV	30–60 min	1 hr	6–8 hr
Irrigant	Rapid	Rapid	Short

Metabolism: $T_{1/2}$: 15–100 min
Distribution: Crosses placenta; may enter breast milk
Excretion: Urine

IV FACTS

Preparation: Mannitol may crystallize at low temperatures, especially solutions of more than 15%. If crystals are observed, warm solution to dissolve.

Infusion: Infuse at rates listed (above). Use an infusion set with a filter if concentrated mannitol is used.

Incompatibilities: Do not add to blood products.

Adverse effects

- **CNS:** *Dizziness,* headache, blurred vision, **seizures**
- **CV:** Hypotension, hypertension, edema, HF, thrombophlebitis, tachycardia, chest pain
- **Dermatologic:** Urticaria, skin necrosis with infiltration
- **GI:** *Nausea, anorexia, dry mouth, thirst*
- **GU:** *Diuresis,* urine retention
- **Hematologic:** Fluid and electrolyte imbalances, hyponatremia
- **Respiratory:** Pulmonary congestion, rhinitis

■ Nursing considerations

Assessment

- **History:** Pulmonary congestion, active intracranial bleeding, dehydration, renal disease, heart failure, pregnancy, lactation
- **Physical:** Skin color, lesions, edema, hydration; orientation, muscle strength, reflexes, pupils; pulses, BP, perfusion; R, pattern, adventitious sounds; urinary output patterns; serum electrolytes, urinalysis, renal function tests

Interventions

⊗ ***Warning*** Do not give electrolyte-free mannitol with blood. If blood must be given, add at least 20 mEq of sodium chloride to each liter of mannitol solution.

- Do not expose solutions to low temperatures; crystallization may occur. If crystals are seen, warm the bottle in a hot water bath, then cool to body temperature before administering.
- Make sure the infusion set contains a filter if giving concentrated mannitol.
- Monitor serum electrolytes periodically with prolonged therapy.

Teaching points

- You may experience these side effects: Increased urination; GI upset (eat frequent small meals); dry mouth (suck sugarless lozenges); headache, blurred vision (use caution when moving, ask for assistance).
- Report difficulty breathing, pain at the IV site, chest pain.

maprotiline hydrochloride

(ma ***proe'*** *ti leen)*

Novo-Maprotiline (CAN)

PREGNANCY CATEGORY B

Drug class

Antidepressant (tetracyclic)

Therapeutic actions

Mechanism of action unknown; appears to act similarly to TCAs; the TCAs act to inhibit the presynaptic reuptake of the neurotransmitters norepinephrine (primarily) and serotonin; anticholinergic at CNS and peripheral receptors; sedating; the relation of these effects to clinical efficacy is unknown.

Indications

- Treatment of depressive illness in patients with depressive neurosis (dysthymic disorder)
- Treatment of depression in patients with bipolar disorder (depressed type)
- Treatment of anxiety associated with depression

Contraindications and cautions

- Contraindicated with hypersensitivity to tricyclic drugs, concomitant therapy with an MAOI, recent MI, myelography within previous 24 hr or scheduled within 48 hr, known or suspected seizure disorder, pregnancy (limb reduction abnormalities reported), lactation.
- Use cautiously with EST; preexisting CV disorders (increased risk of serious CV toxicity); angle-closure glaucoma, increased IOP, urine retention, ureteral or urethral spasm; seizure disorders (lowers seizure threshold); hyperthyroidism (predisposes to CV toxicity, including cardiac arrhythmias); impaired hepatic, renal function; psychiatric disorders (schizophrenic or paranoid patients may worsen); manic-depression (may shift to hypomanic or manic phase); elective surgery (stop use as soon as possible before surgery).

Available forms

Tablets—25, 50, 75 mg

Dosages

Adults

- *Mild to moderate depression:* Initially, 75 mg/day PO in outpatients. Maintain initial dosage for 2 wk due to long drug half-life. Dosage may then be increased gradually in 25-mg increments. Most patients respond to 150 mg/day, but some may require up to 225 mg/day.
- *More severe depression:* Initially, 100–150 mg/day PO in hospitalized patients. If needed, gradually increase to 225 mg/day.
- *Maintenance:* Reduce dosage to lowest effective level, usually 75–150 mg/day PO.

Pediatric patients

Not recommended in patients younger than 18 yr.

Geriatric patients

Give lower doses to patients older than 60 yr; begin at 25 mg PO daily and gradually increase to 50–75 mg/day PO for maintenance.

Pharmacokinetics

Route	*Onset*	*Peak*	*Duration*
Oral	Slow	12 hr	2–4 wk

Metabolism: Hepatic; $T_{1/2}$: 51 hr

Distribution: Crosses placenta; enters breast milk

Excretion: Feces, urine

Adverse effects

- **CNS:** *Sedation and anticholinergic (atropine-like) effects; confusion* (especially in elderly), *disturbed concentration,* hallucinations, disorientation, decreased memory, feelings of unreality, delusions, anxiety, nervousness, restlessness, agitation, panic, insomnia, nightmares, hypomania, mania, exacerbation of psychosis, drowsiness, weakness, fatigue, headache, numbness, tingling, paresthesias of extremities, incoordination, motor hyperactivity, akathisia, ataxia, tremors, peripheral neuropathy, extrapyramidal symptoms, **seizures,** speech blockage, dysarthria, tinnitus, altered EEG, suicidal ideation
- **CV:** *Orthostatic hypotension,* hypertension, syncope, tachycardia, palpitations, **MI,** arrhythmias, heart block, precipitation of HF, CVA

M

- **Endocrine:** Elevated or depressed blood sugar, elevated prolactin levels, inappropriate ADH secretion
- **GI:** *Dry mouth, constipation,* paralytic ileus, *nausea,* vomiting, anorexia, epigastric distress, diarrhea, flatulence, dysphagia, peculiar taste, increased salivation, stomatitis, glossitis, parotid swelling, abdominal cramps, black tongue, hepatitis, jaundice (rare), elevated transaminases, altered alkaline phosphatase
- **GU:** Urine retention, delayed micturition, dilation of the urinary tract, gynecomastia, testicular swelling; breast enlargement, menstrual irregularity and galactorrhea; increased or decreased libido; impotence
- **Hematologic:** Bone marrow depression, eosinophilia, thrombocytopenia, leukopenia
- **Hypersensitivity:** Rash, pruritus, vasculitis, petechiae, photosensitization, edema
- **Withdrawal:** Symptoms with abrupt discontinuation of prolonged therapy: Nausea, headache, vertigo, nightmares, malaise
- **Other:** Nasal congestion, excessive appetite, weight gain or loss; sweating (paradoxical effect in a drug with prominent anticholinergic effects), alopecia, lacrimation, hyperthermia, flushing, chills

Interactions

✱ **Drug-drug** • Risk of seizures if taken with benzodiazepines (or if benzodiazepines are rapidly tapered during maprotiline therapy), phenothiazines • Additive atropine-like effects if combined with anticholinergics, sympathomimetics; monitor patient closely and adjust dosages as needed • Increased risk of cardiotoxicity if taken with thyroid medications; monitor patient closely

■ Nursing considerations

Assessment

- **History:** Hypersensitivity to any tricyclic drug; concomitant therapy with an MAOI; recent MI; myelography within previous 24 hr or scheduled within 48 hr; lactation; EST; preexisting CV disorders; angle-closure glaucoma, increased IOP, urine retention, ureteral or urethral spasm; seizure disorders; hyperthyroidism; impaired hepatic, renal function; psychiatric problems; bipolar disorder; elective surgery, pregnancy, lactation
- **Physical:** Weight; T; skin color, lesions; orientation, affect, reflexes, vision and hearing; P, BP, orthostatic BP, perfusion; bowel sounds, normal output, liver evaluation; urine flow, normal output; usual sexual function, frequency of menses, breast and scrotal examination; LFTs, urinalysis, CBC, ECG

Interventions

⊗ ***Warning*** Limit drug access to depressed and potentially suicidal patients.

⊠ ***Black box warning*** Monitor children, adolescents, and young adults for increased risk of suicidal thinking and behavior.

- Expect clinical response in 3 wk, although some have improved in 3–7 days.
- Give major portion of dose at bedtime if drowsiness or severe anticholinergic effects occur.
- Reduce dosage with minor side effects; discontinue drug if serious side effects occur.
- Arrange for CBC if patient develops fever, sore throat, or signs of infection.

Teaching points

- Take drug exactly as prescribed, and do not stop taking this drug without consulting your health care provider.
- Avoid pregnancy while taking this drug, fetal abnormalities have been reported; using barrier contraceptive is advised.
- Avoid alcohol, sleep-inducing drugs, and over-the-counter drugs.
- Avoid prolonged exposure to sunlight or sunlamps, use sunscreen or protective garments if exposure is unavoidable.
- You may experience these side effects: Headache, dizziness, drowsiness, weakness, blurred vision (reversible; use caution if severe, avoid driving or performing tasks that require alertness); nausea, vomiting, loss of appetite, dry mouth (frequent small meals, frequent mouth care, sucking sugarless candies may help); nightmares, inability to concentrate, confusion; changes in sexual function.
- Report dry mouth, difficulty in urination, excessive sedation, chest pain, thoughts of suicide.

maraviroc
(mar ah vye' rock)

Selzentry

PREGNANCY CATEGORY B

Drug classes
Antiviral
CCR5 co-receptor antagonist

Therapeutic actions
Selectively binds to the human chemokine receptor CCR5 on the cell membrane, preventing interaction of HIV-1 and CCR5 needed for HIV to enter the cell and multiply.

Indications
- Combination antiretroviral treatment of adults infected with detectable CCR5-tropic HIV-1 who have evidence of viral replication and HIV-1 strains resistant to multiple antiretroviral drugs

Contraindications and cautions
- Contraindicated with hypersensitivity to any component of the drug, lactation.
- Use cautiously with co-infection with hepatitis B, liver disease, increased risk of CV events, hypotension, pregnancy.

Available forms
Tablets—150, 300 mg

Dosages
Adults
When given with strong CYP3A inhibitors, protease inhibitors (except tipranavir/ritonavir), delavirdine, 150 mg PO bid. When given with tipranavir/ritonavir, nevirapine, enfuvirtide, nucleoside reverse transcriptase inhibitors, other drugs that are not strong CYP3A inhibitors, 300 mg PO bid. When given with efavirenz, rifampin, carbamazepine, phenobarbital, phenytoin, 600 mg PO bid.
Pediatric patients younger than 16 yr
Safety and efficacy not established.

Pharmacokinetics

Route	*Onset*	*Peak*
Oral	Slow	0.5–4 hr

Metabolism: Hepatic; $T_{1/2}$: 14–18 hr
Distribution: May cross placenta; enters breast milk
Excretion: Feces, urine

Adverse effects
- **CNS:** *Dizziness,* paresthesias, dysesthesias, peripheral neuropathies, sensory abnormalities, depression, sleep disturbances
- **GI:** *Abdominal pain,* constipation, dyspepsia, stomatitis, appetite disorder, **hepatotoxicity**
- **Respiratory:** *Cough,* URI, sinusitis, bronchitis, pneumonia
- **Other:** *Fever, musculoskeletal symptoms,* pruritus, dermatitis, infections

Interactions
✱ **Drug-drug** • Increased serum levels and toxicity when combined with CYP3A inhibitors (ketoconazole, lopinavir/ritonavir, ritonavir, saquinavir, atazanavir, delavirdine); adjust maraviroc dosage accordingly • Decreased serum levels and loss of effectiveness if combined with CYP3A inducers (nevirapine, rifampin, efavirenz); adjust maraviroc dose accordingly
✱ **Drug-alternative therapy** • Loss of effectiveness if taken with St. John's wort; avoid this combination

■ Nursing considerations
☒ ***Black box warning*** Risk of severe hepatotoxicity, possibly preceded by evidence of systemic allergic reaction (rash, eosinophilia, elevated IgE level); immediately evaluate and support patient with any sign of hepatitis or allergic reaction.

Assessment
- **History:** Hypersensitivity to any component of the drug, history of liver impairment, hepatitis B infection, risk factors for cardiovascular events, pregnancy, lactation
- **Physical:** T; orientation, affect; BP; R, lung sounds; abdominal exam; LFTs

Interventions

- Give this drug with other antiretroviral drugs.
- Review antiviral therapy and adjust dosage according to effects on liver enzyme systems.
- Ensure that patient swallows tablet whole; do not cut, crush, or allow patient to chew tablet.
- Monitor patient for any sign of allergic reaction or hepatitis; severe hepatoxicity could occur. Check CBC and IgE markers.
- Encourage nursing mothers to find a different method of feeding the baby while on this drug.
- Protect patient from exposure to infection, and encourage patient to avoid situations that increase risk of infection.

Teaching points

- Take this drug twice a day without regard to food. Swallow the tablets whole; do not cut, crush, or chew them.
- Always take this drug with other anti-HIV drugs that have been prescribed for you.
- Do not take St. John's wort while on this drug; antiviral activity could be lost.
- If you miss a dose, take it as soon as you remember and then take the regularly scheduled dose at the regular time. If it is less than 6 hours until the next scheduled dose, skip the missed dose and just take the next scheduled dose. Do not double doses. Do not take more than two doses on any one day.
- Do not stop taking this drug; it could lose effect if stopped for even a short period of time. If you are running low, talk to your health care provider about a refill.
- This drug does not cure HIV or AIDS; you may still develop opportunistic infections, and you should seek regular medical care to manage the disease.
- Maraviroc does not reduce the risk of transmitting HIV to others by sexual contact or blood contamination; use appropriate precautions.
- It is not known if this drug could affect a fetus. If you wish to become pregnant, discuss this with your health care provider. If you become pregnant while taking this drug, consult your health care provider about enrolling in the Antiretroviral Pregnancy Registry.
- It is not known how this drug could affect a nursing baby. Because of the risk of serious adverse effects on an infant, you should choose another method of feeding the baby while you are on this drug.
- Your health care provider will monitor your CD4 levels and your liver function regularly while you are on this drug.
- You may experience these side effects: Headache, fever, rash (medication may be available to relieve these symptoms); dizziness (do not drive a car or operate dangerous machinery until you know how this drug will affect you); increased risk of infection, cancer (have regular screenings, and consult your health care provider at the first sign of infection).
- Report rash, difficulty breathing, changes in the color of your stool or urine, fainting, yellowing of the eyes or skin, infections.

▽ mebendazole

*(me **ben'** da zole)*

Vermox

PREGNANCY CATEGORY C

Drug class

Anthelmintic

Therapeutic actions

Irreversibly blocks glucose uptake by susceptible helminths, depleting glycogen stores needed for survival and reproduction of the helminths, causing death.

Indications

- Treatment of *Trichuris trichiura* (whipworm), *Enterobius vermicularis* (pinworm), *Ascaris lumbricoides* (roundworm), *Ancylostoma duodenale* (common hookworm), *Necator americanus* (American hookworm)

Contraindications and cautions

- Contraindicated with allergy to mebendazole, pregnancy (embryotoxic and teratogenic; avoid use, especially during first trimester).
- Use cautiously with lactation.

Available forms
Chewable tablets—100 mg

Dosages
Adults and patients 2 yr and older
- *Trichuriasis, ascariasis, hookworm infections:* 1 tablet PO morning and evening on 3 consecutive days.
- *Enterobiasis:* 1 tablet PO once. If not cured 3 wk after treatment, a second treatment course is advised.

Pediatric patients younger than 2 yr
Safety and efficacy not established.

Pharmacokinetics

Route	Onset	Peak
Oral	Slow	2–4 hr

Metabolism: Hepatic; $T_{1/2}$: 2.5–9 hr
Distribution: Crosses placenta; may enter breast milk
Excretion: Feces

Adverse effects
- **GI:** *Transient abdominal pain, diarrhea*
- **Other:** Fever

■ Nursing considerations
Assessment
- **History:** Allergy to mebendazole, pregnancy, lactation
- **Physical:** T; bowel sounds, output

Interventions
- Culture for ova and parasites.
- Administer drug with food; tablets may be chewed, swallowed whole, or crushed and mixed with food.
- Arrange for second course of treatment if patient is not cured 3 weeks after treatment.
- Treat all family members for pinworm infestation.
- Disinfect toilet facilities after patient use (pinworms).
- Arrange for daily laundry of bed linens, towels, nightclothes, and undergarments (pinworms).

Teaching points
- Chew or swallow whole or crushed and mixed with food.
- Pinworms are easily transmitted; all family members should be treated for complete eradication.
- Use strict handwashing and hygiene measures. Launder undergarments, bed linens, and nightclothes daily. Disinfect toilet facilities daily and bathroom floors periodically (pinworms).
- You may experience these side effects: Nausea, abdominal pain, diarrhea (eat frequent small meals).
- Report fever, return of symptoms, severe diarrhea.

DANGEROUS DRUG

▽mechlorethamine hydrochloride (HN_2, nitrogen mustard)
*(me klor **eth'** a meen)*

Mustargen

PREGNANCY CATEGORY D

Drug classes
Alkylating drug
Antineoplastic
Nitrogen mustard

Therapeutic actions
Cytotoxic: Reacts chemically with DNA, RNA, other proteins to prevent replication and function of susceptible cells, causing cell death; cell-cycle nonspecific.

Indications
- IV use: Palliative treatment of bronchogenic carcinoma, Hodgkin's disease, lymphosarcoma, chronic myelogenous leukemia, chronic lymphocytic leukemia, mycosis fungoides, polycythemia vera
- Intrapleural, intraperitoneal, intrapericardial use: Palliative treatment of effusion secondary to metastatic carcinoma
- Unlabeled use: Topical treatment of cutaneous mycosis fungoides

Contraindications and cautions
- Contraindicated with allergy to mechlorethamine, active infection, pregnancy, lactation.

- Use cautiously with amyloidosis, hematopoietic depression, concomitant steroid therapy.

Available forms

Powder for injection—10 mg

Dosages

Individualize dosage based on hematologic profile and response.

Adults

IV

Usual dose, total of 0.4 mg/kg IV for each course of therapy as a single dose or in two to four divided doses of 0.1–0.2 mg/kg/day. Give at night in case sedation is required for side effects. Interval between courses of therapy is usually 3–6 wk.

Intracavitary

Dose and preparation vary greatly with cavity and disease treated. Consult manufacturer's label; usual dose 0.2–0.4 mg/kg.

Pharmacokinetics

Route	*Onset*	*Peak*	*Duration*
IV	Immediate	Seconds	Minutes

Metabolism: $T_{1/2}$: A few minutes
Distribution: Crosses placenta; may enter breast milk
Excretion: Urine

IV FACTS

Preparation: Reconstitute vial with 10 mL of sterile water for injection or sodium chloride injection; resultant solution contains 1 mg/mL of mechlorethamine hydrochloride. Prepare solution immediately before use; decomposes on standing.

Infusion: Inject into tubing of a flowing IV infusion slowly over 3–5 min.

Adverse effects

- **CNS:** *Weakness,* vertigo, tinnitus, diminished hearing
- **Dermatologic:** Maculopapular rash, alopecia, herpes zoster
- **GI:** *Nausea, vomiting, anorexia,* diarrhea, jaundice
- **GU:** *Impaired fertility*
- **Hematologic:** *Bone marrow depression,* immunosuppression, hyperuricemia
- **Local:** *Vesicant thrombosis, thrombophlebitis,* tissue necrosis if extravasation occurs

■ Nursing considerations

Assessment

- **History:** Allergy to mechlorethamine, active infection, amyloidosis, hematopoietic depression, concomitant steroid therapy, pregnancy, lactation
- **Physical:** T; weight; skin color, lesions; injection site; orientation, reflexes, hearing evaluation; CBC, differential, uric acid

Interventions

- Arrange for blood tests to evaluate hematopoietic function before and during therapy.

⊗ ***Black box warning*** Use caution when preparing drug for administration; use chemo-safe nonpermeable gloves for handling drug; drug is highly toxic and a vesicant. Avoid inhalation of dust or vapors and contact with skin or mucous membranes (especially the eyes). If eye contact occurs, immediately irrigate with copious amount of ophthalmic irrigating solution, and obtain an ophthalmologic consultation. If skin contact occurs, irrigate with copious amount of water for 15 min, followed by application of 2% sodium thiosulfate.

⊗ ***Warning*** Use caution when determining correct amount of drug for injection. The margin of safety is very small; double check dosage before administration.

⊗ ***Black box warning*** Monitor injection site for any sign of extravasation. Painful inflammation and induration or sloughing of skin may occur. If leakage is noted, promptly infiltrate with sterile isotonic sodium thiosulfate (1/6M), and apply an ice compress for 6–12 hr. Notify physician.

- Consult physician for premedication with antiemetics or sedatives to prevent severe nausea and vomiting. Giving at night may help alleviate the problem.
- Ensure that patient is well hydrated before treatment.
- Caution patient to avoid pregnancy while taking this drug; advise using barrier contraceptives.

- Monitor uric acid levels; ensure adequate fluid intake, and prepare for appropriate treatment if hyperuricemia occurs.

Teaching points

- This drug must be given IV or directly into a body cavity.
- Use birth control. This drug cannot be taken during pregnancy; serious fetal effects can occur. If you think you are pregnant or wish to become pregnant, consult your health care provider.
- You may experience these side effects: Nausea, vomiting, loss of appetite (use antiemetic or sedative at night; maintain fluid intake and nutrition); weakness, dizziness, ringing in the ears or loss of hearing (use special precautions to avoid injury); infertility, from irregular menses to complete amenorrhea; men may stop producing sperm (may be irreversible).
- Report pain, burning at IV site, severe GI distress, sore throat, rash, joint pain, fever.

▽ meclizine hydrochloride

(mek' li zeen)

Bonamine (CAN), Bonine

Oral prescription tablets:
Antivert, Antrizine, Dramamine Less Drowsy Formula, Meni-D

PREGNANCY CATEGORY B

Drug classes

Anticholinergic
Antiemetic
Antihistamine
Anti–motion-sickness drug

Therapeutic actions

Reduces sensitivity of the labyrinthine apparatus; probably acts at least partly by blocking cholinergic synapses in the vomiting center, which receives input from the CTZ and from peripheral nerve pathways; peripheral anticholinergic effects may contribute to efficacy.

Indications

- Prevention and treatment of nausea, vomiting, motion sickness
- Possibly effective for the management of vertigo associated with diseases affecting the vestibular system

Contraindications and cautions

- Contraindicated with allergy to meclizine or cyclizine; tartrazine sensitivity (more common in patients with aspirin hypersensitivity).
- Use cautiously with lactation, narrow-angle glaucoma, stenosing peptic ulcer, symptomatic prostatic hypertrophy, bronchial asthma, bladder neck obstruction, pyloroduodenal obstruction, cardiac arrhythmias, postoperative state (hypotensive effects may be confusing and dangerous), pregnancy.

Available forms

Tablets—12.5, 25, 50 mg; chewable tablets—25 mg; capsules—25 mg

Dosages

Adults

- *Motion sickness:* 25–50 mg PO 1 hr before travel. May repeat dose every 24 hr for the duration of the journey.
- *Vertigo:* 25–100 mg PO daily in divided doses.

Pediatric patients

Not recommended for children younger than 12 yr.

Geriatric patients

More likely to cause dizziness, sedation, syncope, toxic confusional states, and hypotension in elderly patients; use with caution.

Pharmacokinetics

Route	Onset	Peak	Duration
Oral	1 hr	1–2 hr	4–24 hr

Metabolism: $T_{1/2}$: 6 hr
Distribution: Crosses placenta; may enter breast milk
Excretion: Feces

Adverse effects

- **CNS:** *Drowsiness, confusion,* euphoria, nervousness, restlessness, insomnia and

excitement, seizures, vertigo, tinnitus, blurred vision, diplopia, auditory and visual hallucinations
- **CV:** Hypotension, palpitations, tachycardia
- **Dermatologic:** Urticaria, rash
- **GI:** *Dry mouth, anorexia, nausea,* vomiting, diarrhea or constipation
- **GU:** *Urinary frequency, difficult urination,* urine retention
- **Respiratory: Respiratory depression, death** (due to overdose, especially in young children), dry nose and throat

Interactions

✱ **Drug-drug** • Increased sedation with alcohol or other CNS depressants

■ Nursing considerations

Assessment

- **History:** Allergy to meclizine or cyclizine, pregnancy, narrow-angle glaucoma, stenosing peptic ulcer, symptomatic prostatic hypertrophy, bronchial asthma, bladder neck obstruction, pyloroduodenal obstruction, cardiac arrhythmias, postoperative patients, lactation, pregnancy
- **Physical:** Skin color, lesions, texture; orientation, reflexes, affect; ophthalmic examination; P, BP; R, adventitious sounds; bowel sounds, normal output, status of mucous membranes; prostate palpation, urinary output

Interventions

- Monitor I & O, and take appropriate measures with urine retention.

Teaching points

- Take as prescribed. Avoid excessive dosage. If you are using chewable tablets, chew them carefully before swallowing.
- Anti–motion-sickness drugs work best if used ahead of time for prevention.
- Avoid alcohol; serious sedation could occur.
- You may experience these side effects: Dizziness, sedation, drowsiness (use caution driving or performing tasks that require alertness); epigastric distress, diarrhea, or constipation (take with food); dry mouth (practice frequent mouth care, suck sugarless lozenges); dryness of nasal mucosa (try another motion-sickness or antivertigo remedy).
- Report difficulty breathing, hallucinations, tremors, loss of coordination, visual disturbances, irregular heartbeat.

DANGEROUS DRUG

medroxyprogesterone acetate

*(me **drox'** ee proe **jess'** te rone)*

Oral: Apo-Medroxyprogesterone (CAN), Gen-Medroxy (CAN), Provera

Parenteral: Depo-Provera, Depo-subQ Provera 104

PREGNANCY CATEGORY X

Drug classes

Antineoplastic
Contraceptive
Hormone
Progestin

Therapeutic actions

Progesterone derivative; endogenous progesterone transforms proliferative endometrium into secretory endometrium; inhibits the secretion of pituitary gonadotropins, which prevents follicular maturation and ovulation; inhibits spontaneous uterine contraction.

Indications

- Reduction of endometrial hyperplasia in postmenopausal women
- Oral: Treatment of secondary amenorrhea
- Oral: Abnormal uterine bleeding due to hormonal imbalance in the absence of organic pathology
- Parenteral: Adjunctive therapy and palliation of inoperable, recurrent, and metastatic endometrial carcinoma or renal carcinoma; long acting contraceptive (*Depo-Provera*)
- Subcutaneous depot: Long-acting contraceptive; management of endometriosis-associated pain (*Depo-subQ Provera 104*)
- Unlabeled use for depot form: Treatment of breast cancer

2011 Quick-access photoguide to pills and capsules

This photoguide presents over 350 tablets and capsules, representing the most commonly prescribed generic and trade drugs. These drugs, organized alphabetically by generic name, are shown in actual size and color with cross-references to drug information. Each product is labeled with its trade name and its strength.

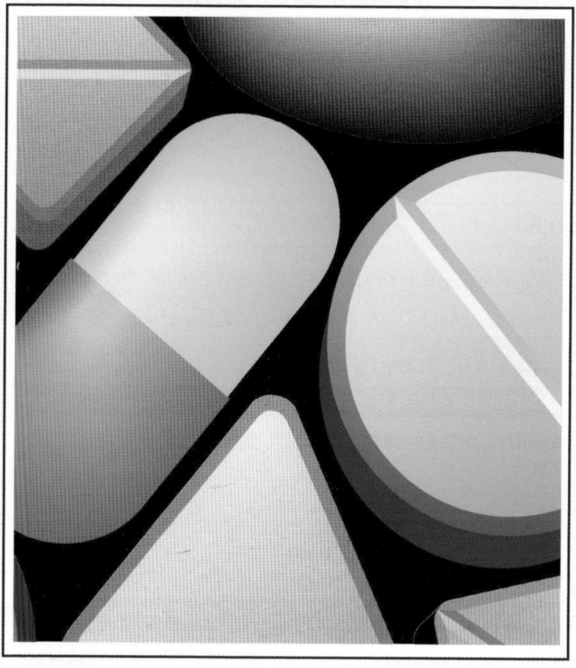

ACAMPROSATE CALCIUM

Campral
(page 67)

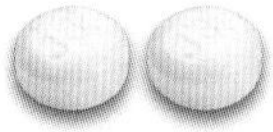

333 mg

ACETAMINOPHEN AND HYDROCODONE BITARTRATE

Lortab
(page 1305)

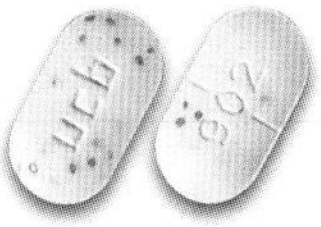

500 mg/5 mg

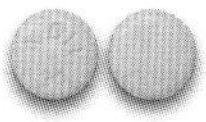

500 mg/7.5 mg

Vicodin
(page 1305)

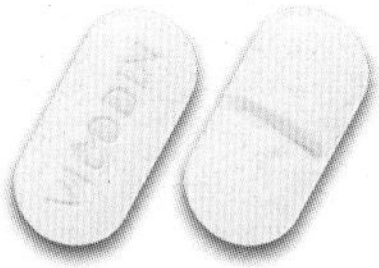

500 mg/5 mg

Vicodin ES
(page 1305)

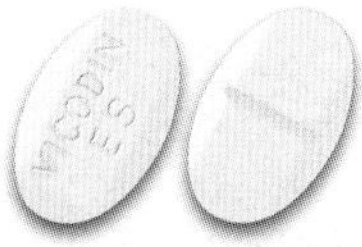

750 mg/7.5 mg

ACETAMINOPHEN WITH CODEINE

Tylenol with Codeine No. 3
(page 1304)

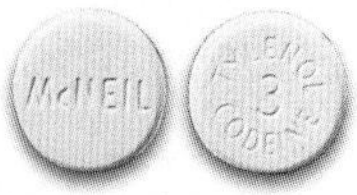

300 mg/30 mg

ALENDRONATE SODIUM

Fosamax
(page 85)

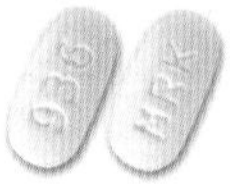

10 mg

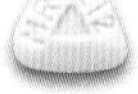

40 mg

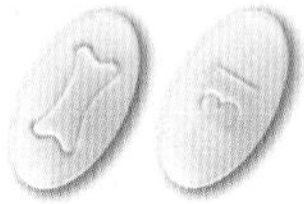

70 mg

ALFUZOSIN HYDROCHLORIDE

Uroxatral
(page 86)

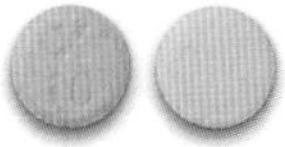

10 mg

ALPRAZOLAM

Xanax
(page 94)

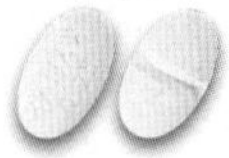

0.25 mg

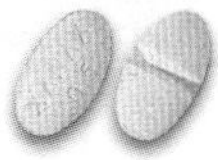

0.5 mg

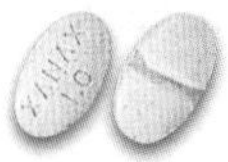

1 mg

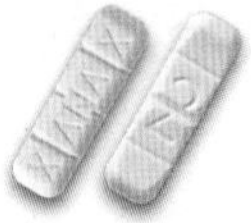

2 mg

AMLODIPINE BESYLATE

Norvasc
(page 119)

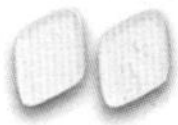

2.5 mg

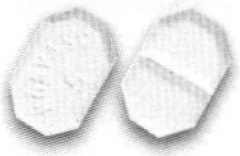

5 mg

ANASTROZOLE

Arimidex
(page 133)

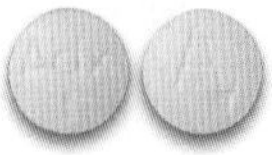

1 mg

ARIPIPRAZOLE

Abilify
(page 141)

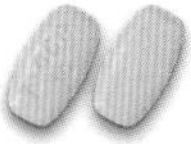
10 mg

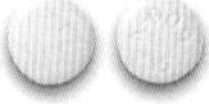
15 mg

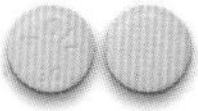
30 mg

ATAZANAVIR SULFATE

Reyataz
(page 151)

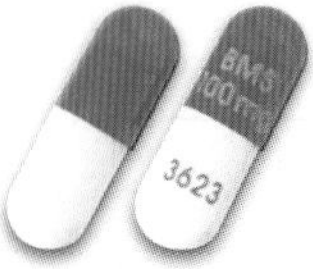

100 mg

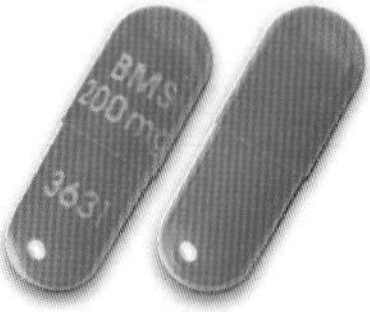

200 mg

ATENOLOL

Tenormin
(page 153)

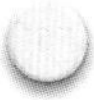
25 mg

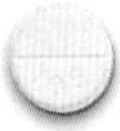
50 mg

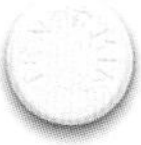
100 mg

ATOMOXETINE HYDROCHLORIDE

Strattera
(page 155)

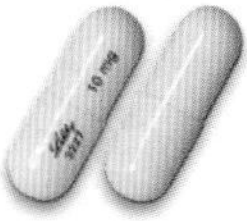
10 mg

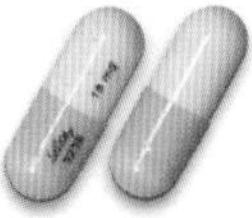
18 mg

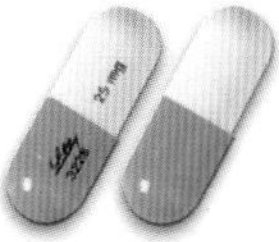
25 mg

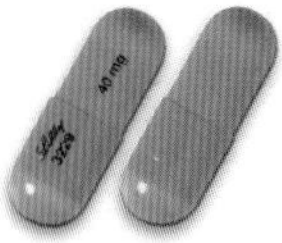
40 mg

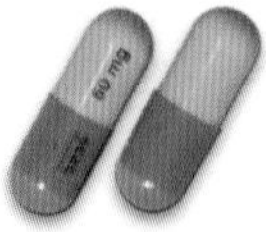
60 mg

ATORVASTATIN CALCIUM

Lipitor
(page 157)

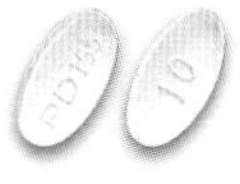
10 mg

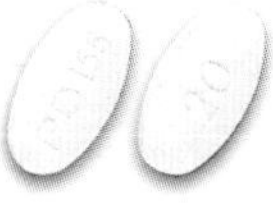
20 mg

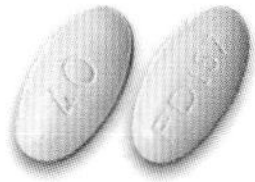
40 mg

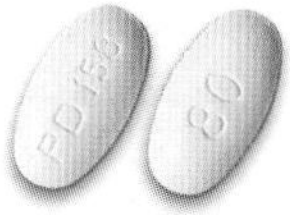
80 mg

AZITHROMYCIN

Zithromax
(page 164)

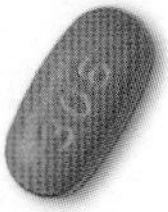
250 mg

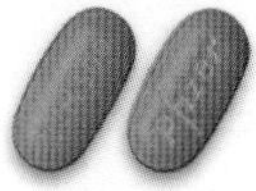
500 mg

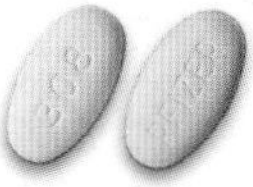
600 mg

BENAZEPRIL HYDROCHLORIDE

Lotensin
(page 173)

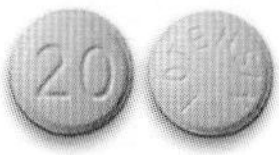
20 mg

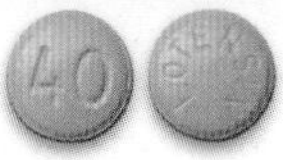
40 mg

BUMETANIDE

Bumex
(page 202)

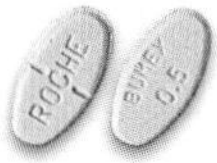
0.5 mg

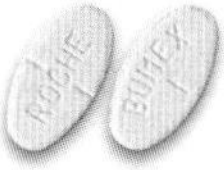
1 mg

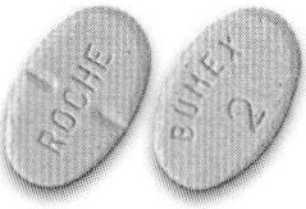
2 mg

BUSPIRONE HYDROCHLORIDE

BuSpar
(page 207)

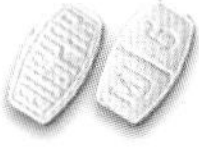
5 mg

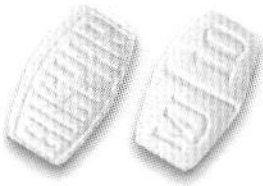
10 mg

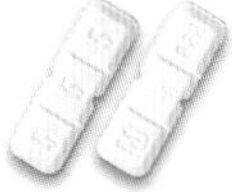
15 mg

CARBIDOPA AND LEVODOPA

Sinemet
(page 1323)

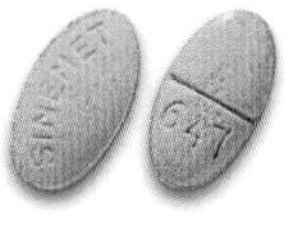

10 mg/100 mg

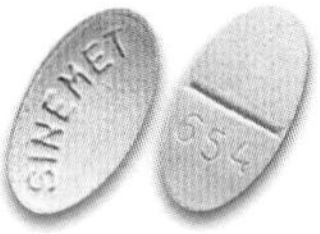

25 mg/250 mg

Sinemet CR
(page 1323)

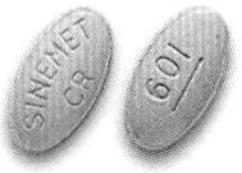

25 mg/100 mg

CARBIDOPA, LEVODOPA, AND ENTACAPONE

Stalevo
(page 1324)

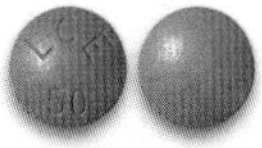

12.5 mg/50 mg/200 mg

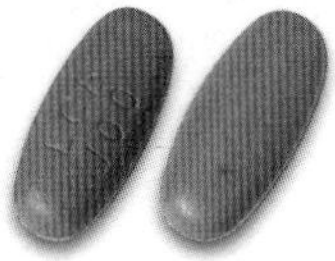

25 mg/100 mg/200 mg

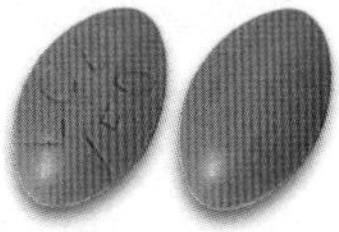

37.5 mg/150 mg/200 mg

CARISOPRODOL

Soma
(page 233)

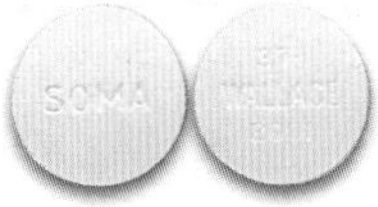

350 mg

CEFPROZIL

Cefzil
(page 252)

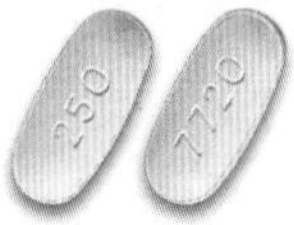

250 mg

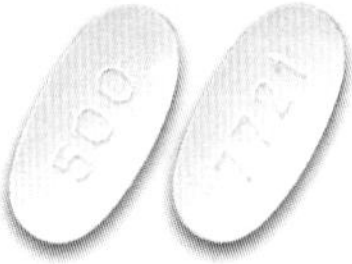

500 mg

CELECOXIB

Celebrex
(page 263)

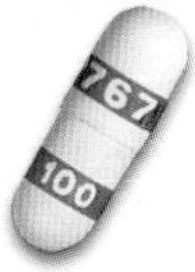

100 mg

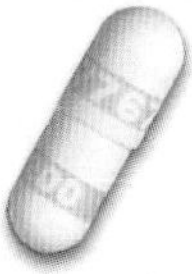

200 mg

CIPROFLOXACIN

Cipro
(page 292)

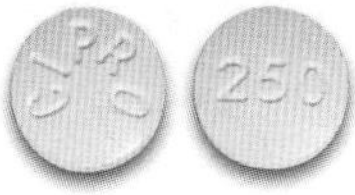

250 mg

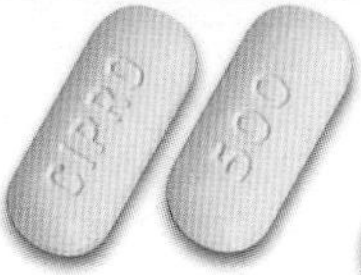

500 mg

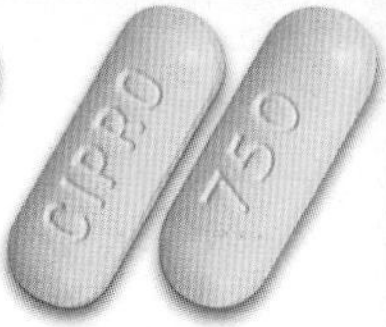

750 mg

CITALOPRAM HYDROBROMIDE

Celexa
(page 296)

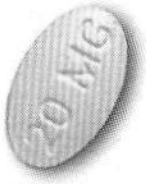

20 mg

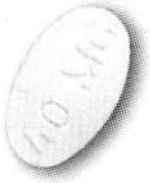

40 mg

CLARITHROMYCIN

Biaxin
(page 299)

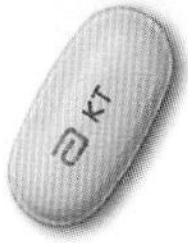

250 mg

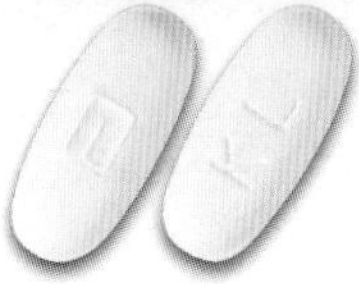

500 mg

Biaxin XL
(page 299)

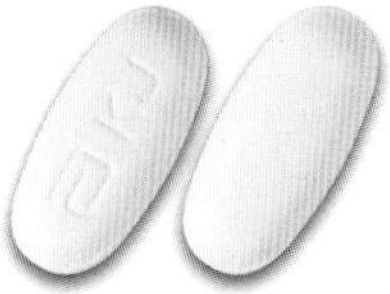

500 mg

CLONAZEPAM

Klonopin
(page 309)

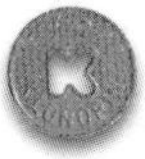
0.5 mg

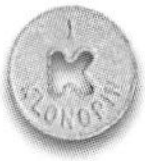
1 mg

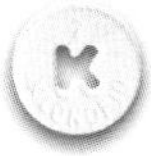
2 mg

DARIFENACIN HYDROBROMIDE

Enablex
(page 352)

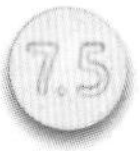

7.5 mg

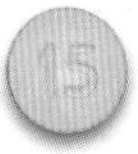

15 mg

DESLORATADINE

Clarinex
(page 359)

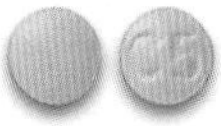

5 mg

DIAZEPAM

Valium
(page 378)

2 mg

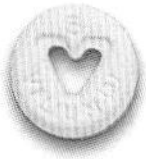
5 mg

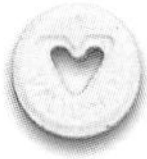
10 mg

DILTIAZEM HYDROCHLORIDE

Cardizem
(page 393)

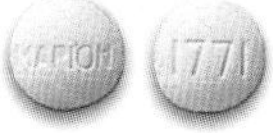
30 mg

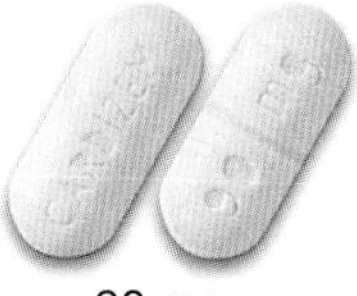
90 mg

Cardizem CD
(page 393)

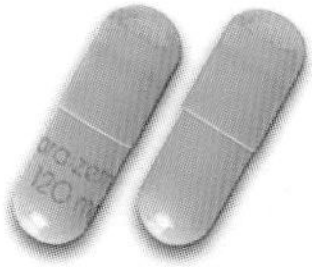
120 mg

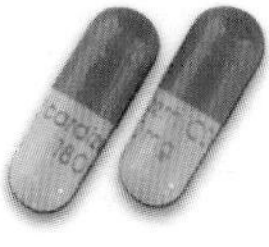
180 mg

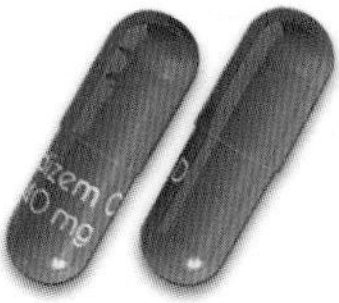
240 mg

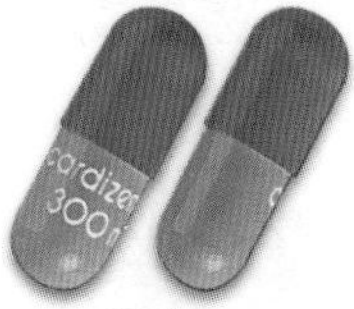
300 mg

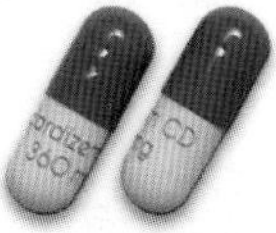
360 mg

Cardizem LA
(page 393)

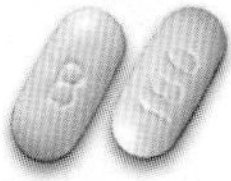
180 mg

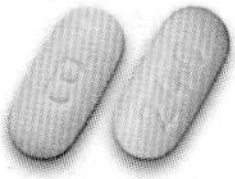
240 mg

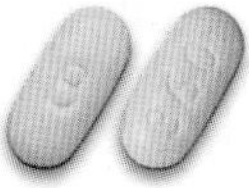
360 mg

DIVALPROEX SODIUM

Depakote
(page 1210)

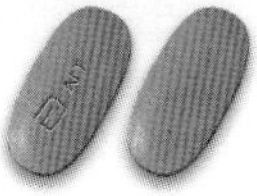
125 mg

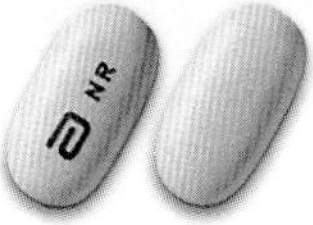

250 mg

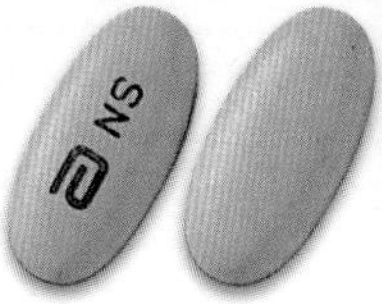

500 mg

Depakote Sprinkle
(page 1210)

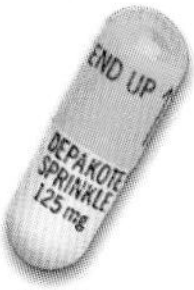

125 mg

DOXAZOSIN MESYLATE

Cardura
(page 415)

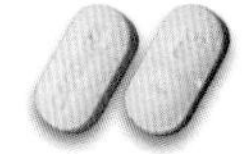

1 mg

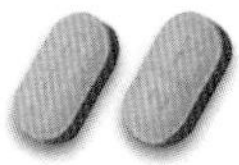

2 mg

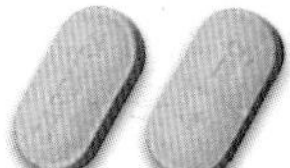

4 mg

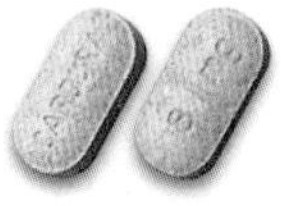

8 mg

DULOXETINE HYDROCHLORIDE

Cymbalta
(page 428)

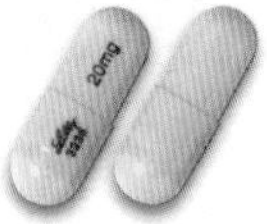

20 mg

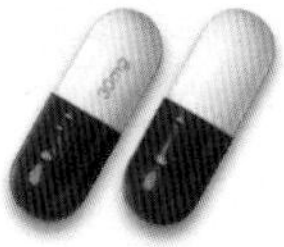

30 mg

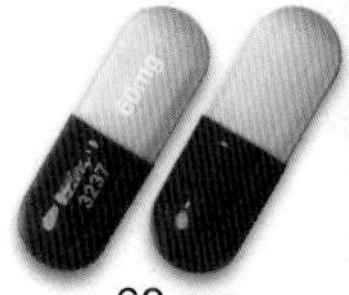

60 mg

ELETRIPTAN HYDROBROMIDE

Relpax
(page 438)

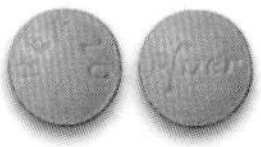

20 mg

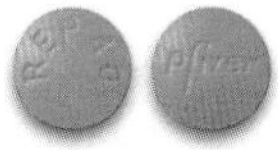

40 mg

ENALAPRIL MALEATE

Vasotec
(page 441)

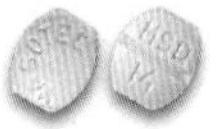

2.5 mg

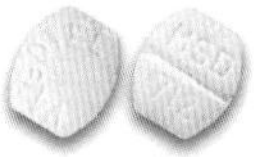

5 mg

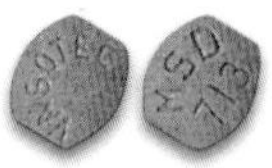

10 mg

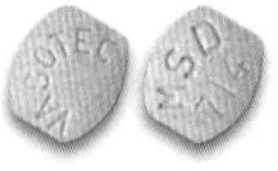

20 mg

ERYTHROMYCIN BASE

Ery-Tab
(page 465)

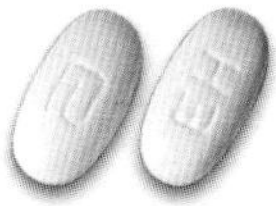

333 mg

ESCITALOPRAM OXALATE

Lexapro
(page 468)

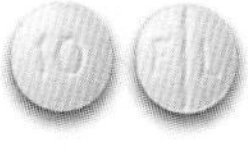

10 mg

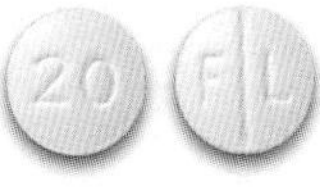

20 mg

ESTRADIOL

Estrace
(page 476)

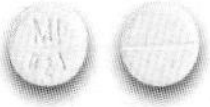

0.5 mg

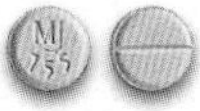

1 mg

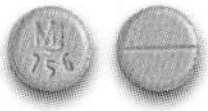

2 mg

ESTROGENS, CONJUGATED

Premarin
(page 479)

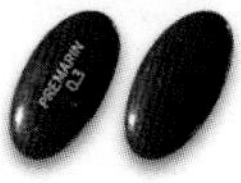

0.3 mg

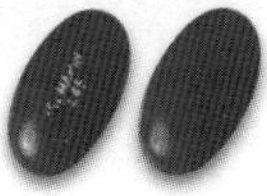

0.45 mg

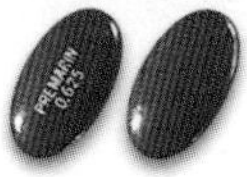

0.625 mg

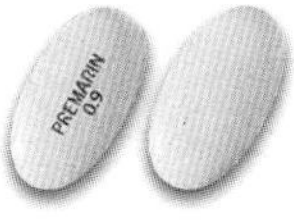

0.9 mg

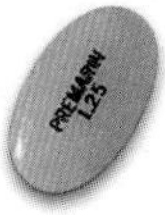

1.25 mg

ESZOPICLONE

Lunesta
(page 486)

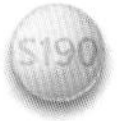
1 mg

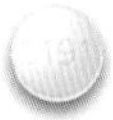
2 mg

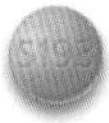
3 mg

EZETIMIBE

Zetia
(page 503)

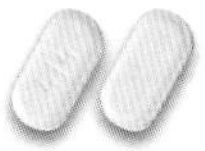
10 mg

FAMOTIDINE

Pepcid
(page 508)

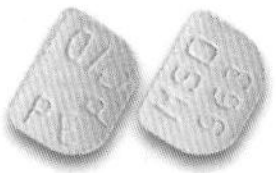
20 mg

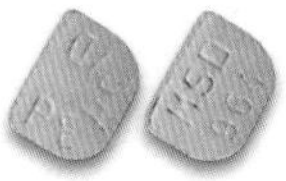
40 mg

FEXOFENADINE HYDROCHLORIDE

Allegra
(page 523)

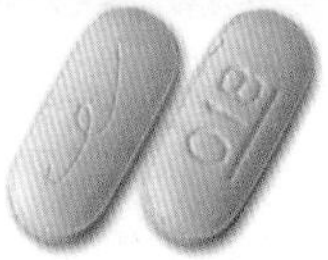
180 mg

FLUCONAZOLE

Diflucan
(page 530)

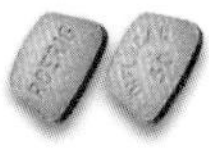
50 mg

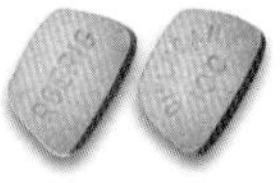
100 mg

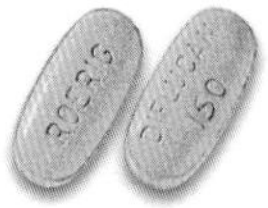
150 mg

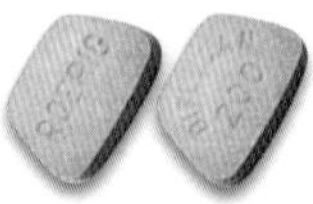
200 mg

FLUOXETINE HYDROCHLORIDE

Prozac
(page 539)

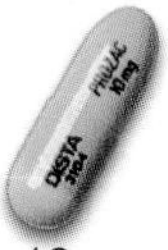

10 mg

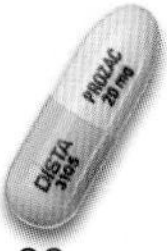

20 mg

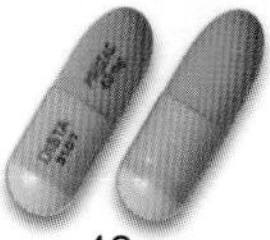

40 mg

Prozac Weekly
(page 539)

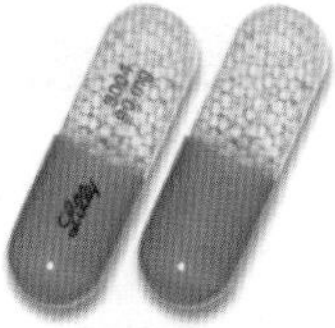

90 mg

Sarafem
(page 539)

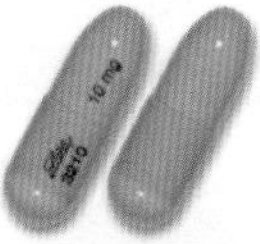

10 mg

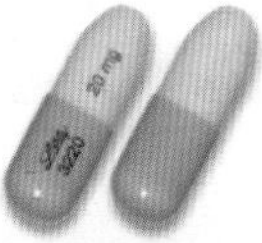

20 mg

FLUVASTATIN SODIUM

Lescol
(page 547)

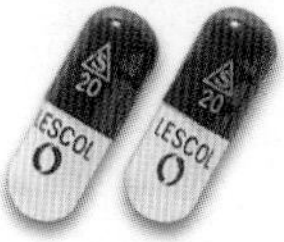

20 mg

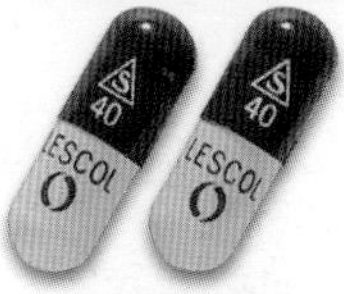

40 mg

FOSINOPRIL SODIUM

Monopril
(page 558)

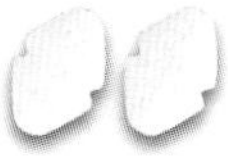

10 mg

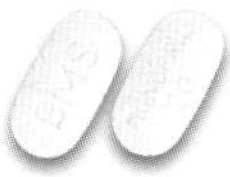

20 mg

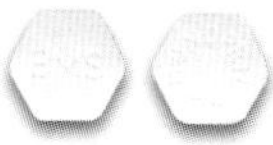

40 mg

FROVATRIPTAN SUCCINATE

Frova
(page 563)

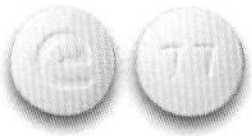

2.5 mg

FUROSEMIDE

Lasix
(page 565)

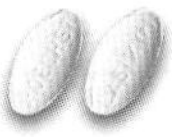

20 mg

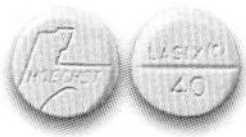

40 mg

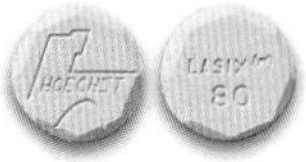

80 mg

GABAPENTIN

Neurontin
(page 568)

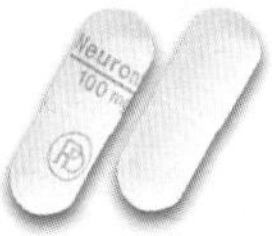

100 mg

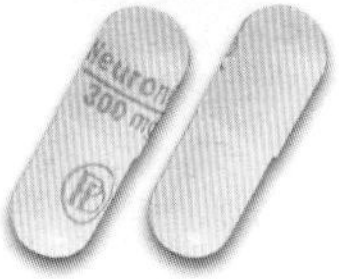

300 mg

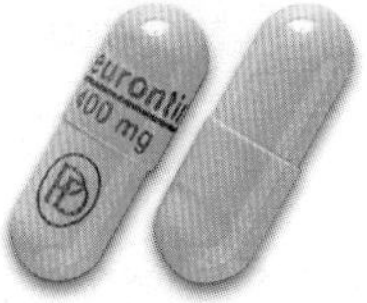

400 mg

GEMFIBROZIL

Lopid
(page 575)

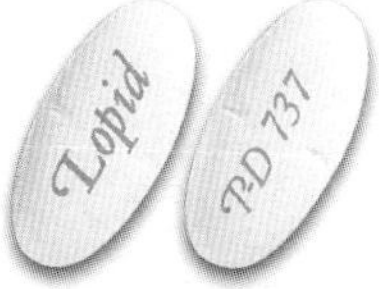

600 mg

GLIPIZIDE

Glucotrol
(page 582)

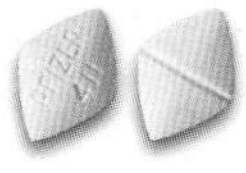

5 mg

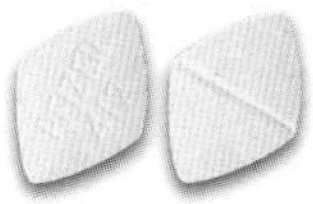

10 mg

Glucotrol XL
(page 582)

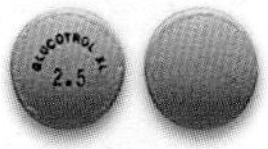

2.5 mg

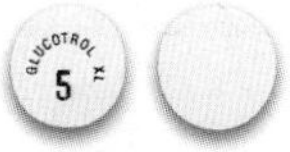

5 mg

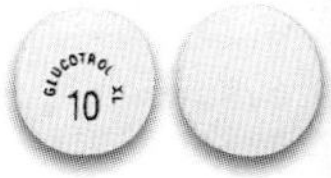

10 mg

GLYBURIDE

DiaBeta
(page 585)

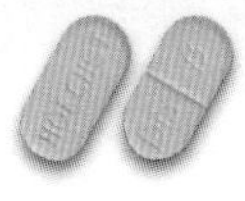

1.25 mg

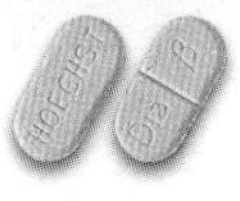

2.5 mg

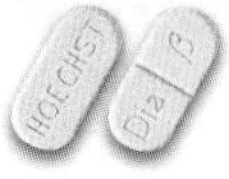

5 mg

INDINAVIR SULFATE

Crixivan
(page 637)

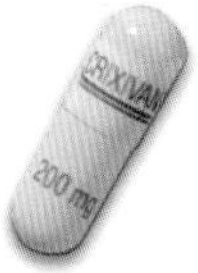

200 mg

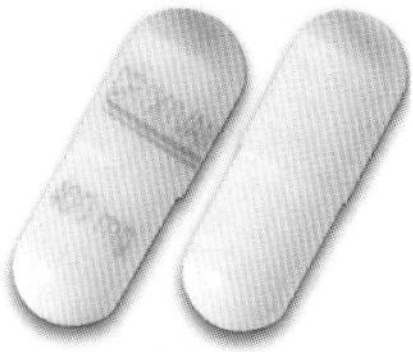

400 mg

LAMIVUDINE AND ZIDOVUDINE

Combivir
(page 1326, 1334)

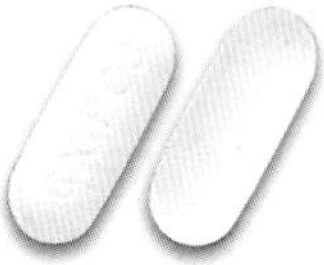

150 mg/300 mg

LANSOPRAZOLE

Prevacid
(page 685)

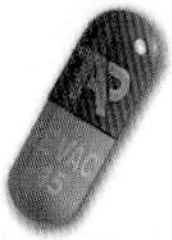

15 mg

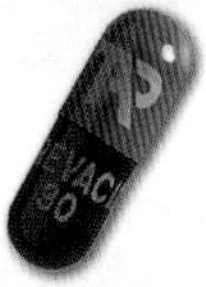

30 mg

LEVOFLOXACIN

Levaquin
(page 699)

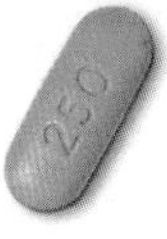

250 mg

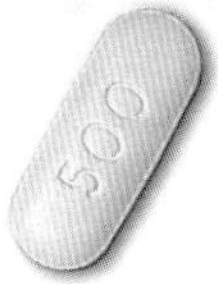

500 mg

LEVOTHYROXINE SODIUM

Levoxyl
(page 703)

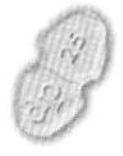
25 mcg

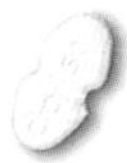
50 mcg

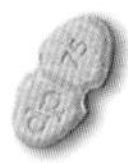
75 mcg

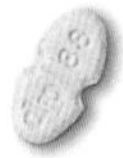
88 mcg

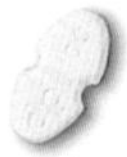
100 mcg

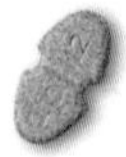
112 mcg

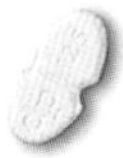
125 mcg

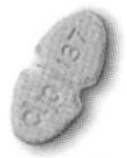
137 mcg

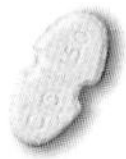
150 mcg

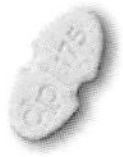
175 mcg

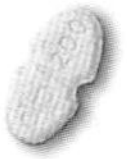
200 mcg

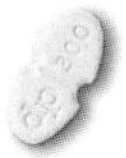
300 mcg

Synthroid
(page 703)

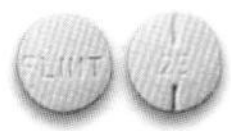
25 mcg

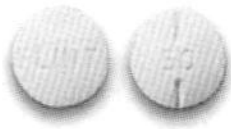
50 mcg

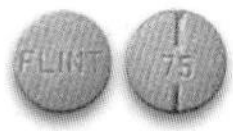
75 mcg

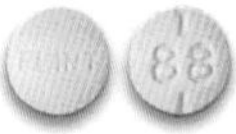
88 mcg

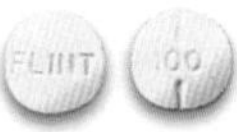
100 mcg

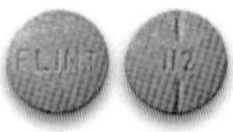
112 mcg

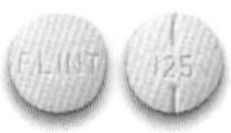
125 mcg

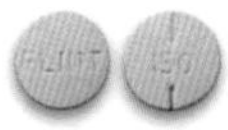
150 mcg

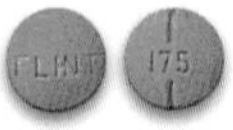
175 mcg

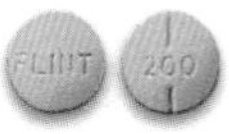
200 mcg

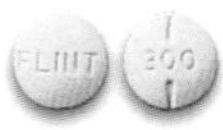
300 mcg

LISINOPRIL

Prinivil
(page 715)

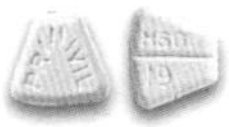

5 mg

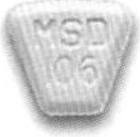

10 mg

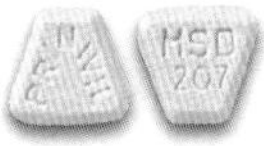

20 mg

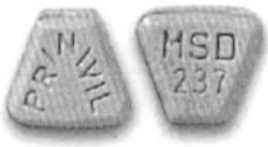

40 mg

Zestril
(page 715)

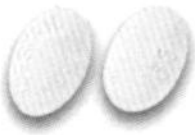

2.5 mg

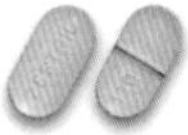

5 mg

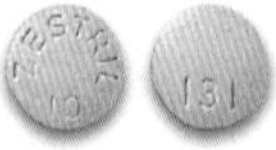

10 mg

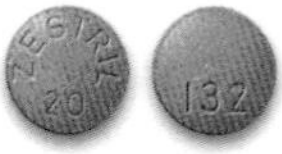

20 mg

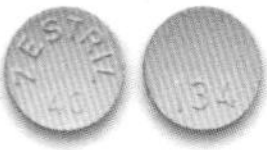

40 mg

LOPINAVIR AND RITONAVIR

Kaletra
(page 722)

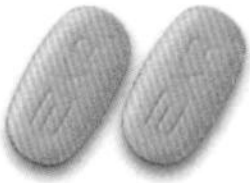

200 mg/50 mg

LOSARTAN POTASSIUM

Cozaar
(page 728)

25 mg 50 mg

LOVASTATIN

Mevacor
(page 729)

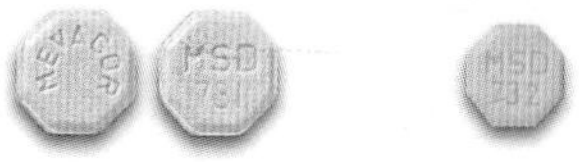

20 mg 40 mg

LUBIPROSTONE

Amitiza
(page 1300)

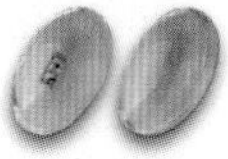

24 mcg

MEDROXYPROGESTERONE ACETATE

Provera
(page 746)

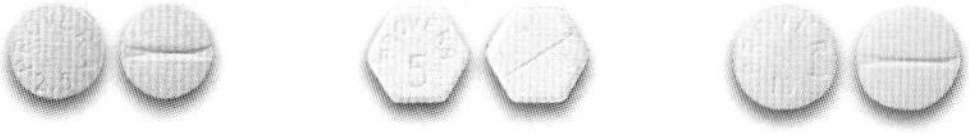

2.5 mg 5 mg 10 mg

MEPERIDINE HYDROCHLORIDE

Demerol
(page 756)

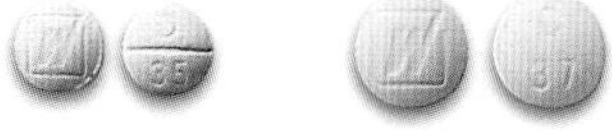

50 mg 100 mg

METFORMIN HYDROCHLORIDE

Glucophage
(page 767)

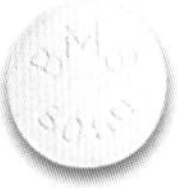

500 mg

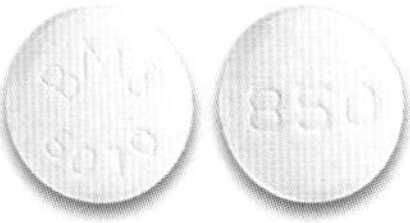

850 mg

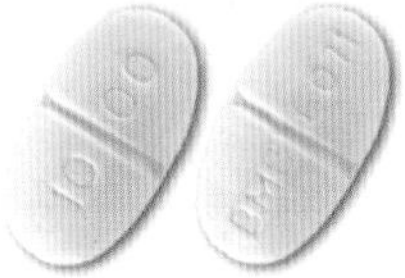

1,000 mg

Glucophage XR
(page 767)

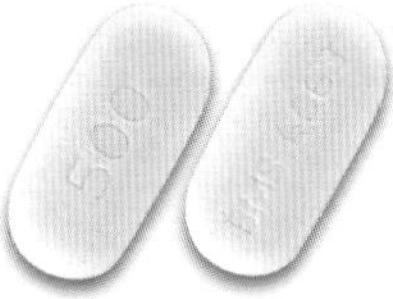

500 mg

METHYLPHENIDATE HYDROCHLORIDE

Concerta
(page 786)

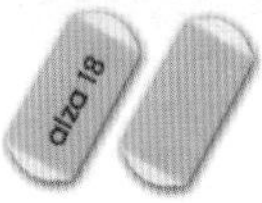

18 mg

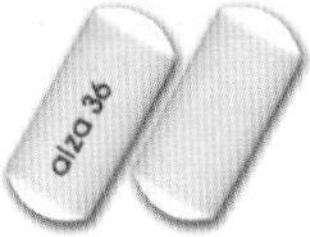

36 mg

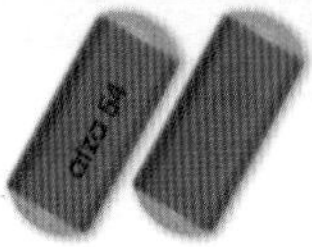

54 mg

Ritalin
(page 786)

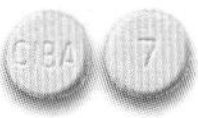

5 mg

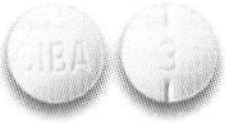

10 mg

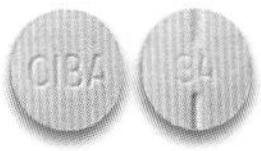

20 mg

Ritalin-SR
(page 786)

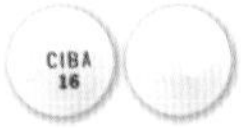

20 mg

METHYLPREDNISOLONE

Medrol
(page 788)

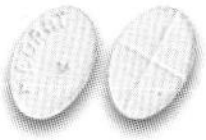
4 mg

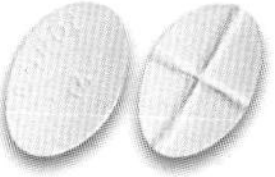
16 mg

METOPROLOL SUCCINATE

Toprol-XL
(page 794)

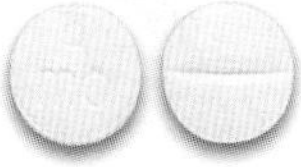
50 mg

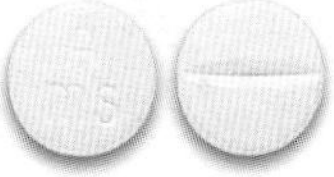
100 mg

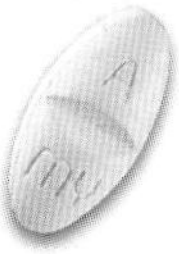
200 mg

MONTELUKAST SODIUM

Singulair
(page 825)

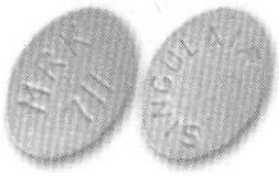
4 mg

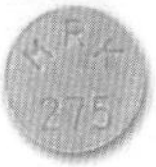

5 mg

10 mg

NAPROXEN

Naprosyn
(page 846)

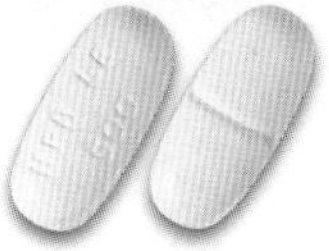
500 mg

NIFEDIPINE

Procardia XL
(page 867)

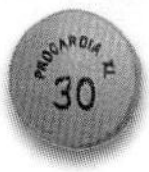

30 mg

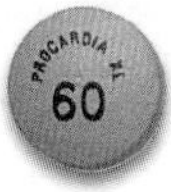

60 mg

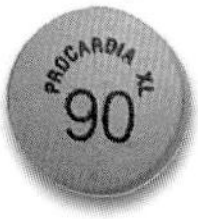

90 mg

NITROFURANTOIN

Macrobid
(page 869)

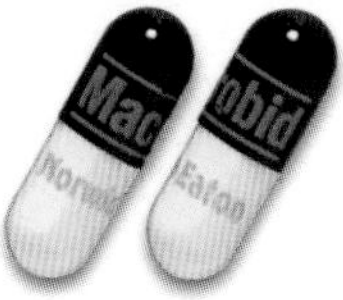

100 mg

NITROGLYCERIN

Nitrostat
(page 871)

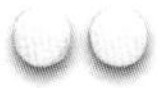

0.4 mg

NORTRIPTYLINE HYDROCHLORIDE

Pamelor
(page 883)

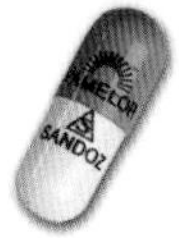

10 mg

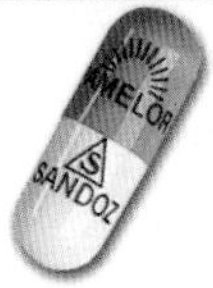

25 mg

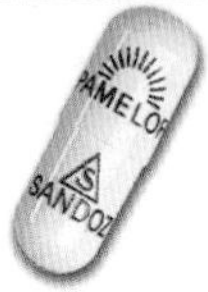

50 mg

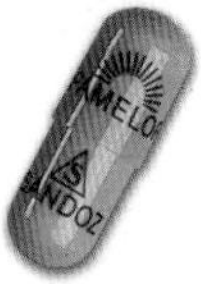

75 mg

OLMESARTAN MEDOXOMIL

Benicar
(page 891)

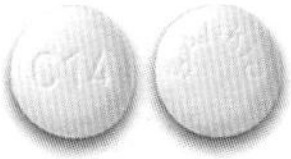

20 mg

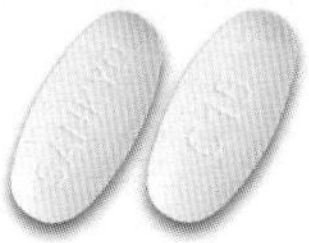

40 mg

OMEPRAZOLE

Prilosec
(page 894)

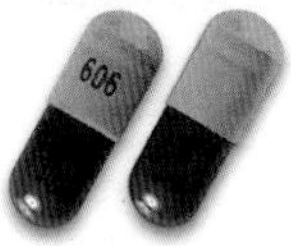

10 mg

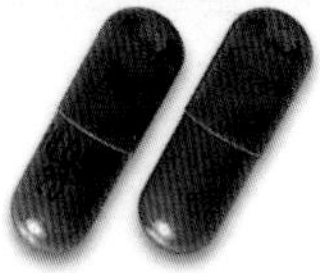

20 mg

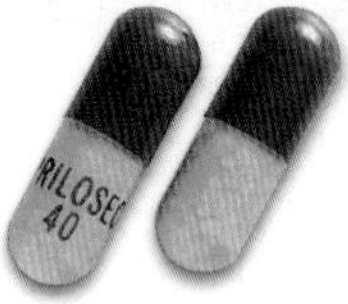

40 mg

OXYCODONE HYDROCHLORIDE

OxyContin
(page 913)

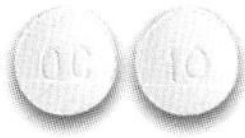

10 mg

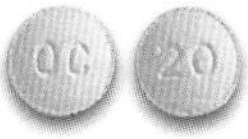

20 mg

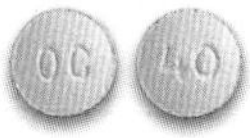

40 mg

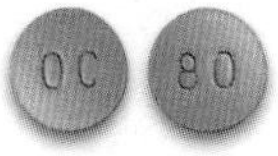

80 mg

PENTOXIFYLLINE

Trental
(page 948)

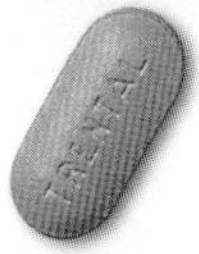

400 mg

PHENYTOIN SODIUM

Dilantin Kapseals
(page 962)

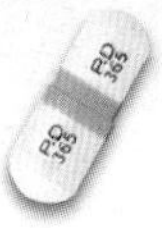

30 mg

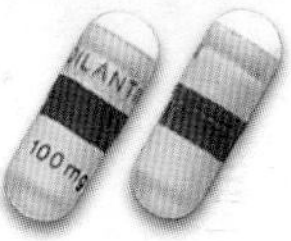

100 mg

PRAVASTATIN SODIUM

Pravachol
(page 987)

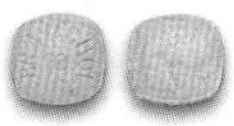

10 mg

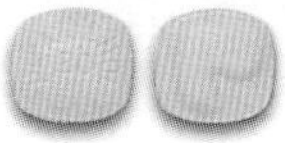

20 mg

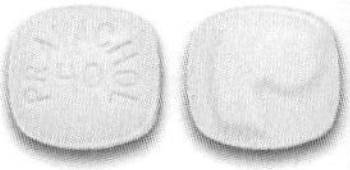

40 mg

PROPRANOLOL HYDROCHLORIDE

Inderal
(page 1012)

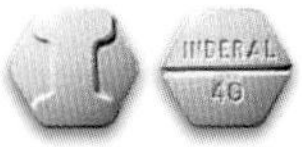

40 mg

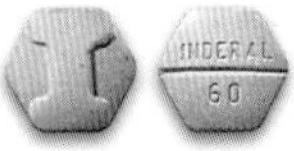

60 mg

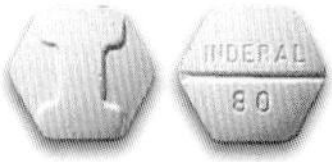

80 mg

Inderal LA
(page 1012)

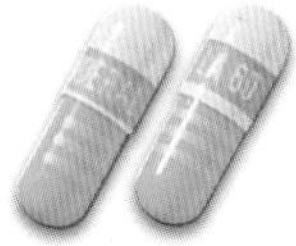

60 mg

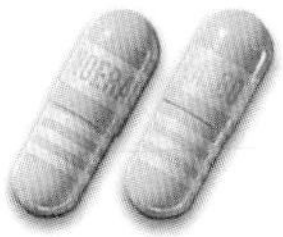

80 mg

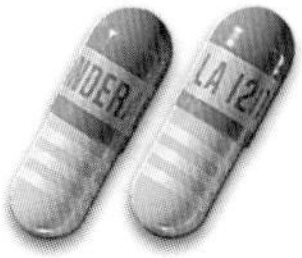

120 mg

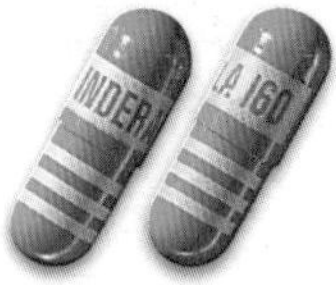

160 mg

QUINAPRIL HYDROCHLORIDE

Accupril
(page 1028)

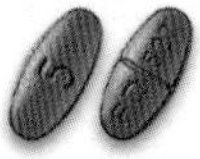

5 mg

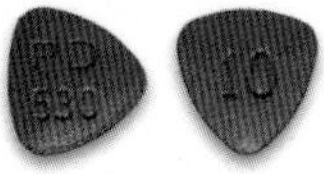

10 mg

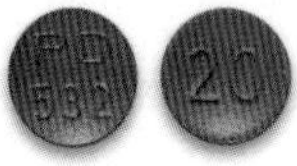

20 mg

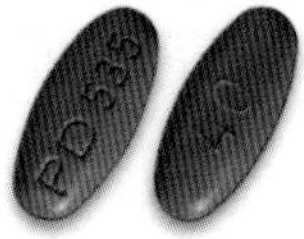

40 mg

RALOXIFENE HYDROCHLORIDE

Evista
(page 1032)

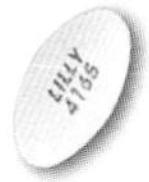

60 mg

RANITIDINE HYDROCHLORIDE

Zantac
(page 1038)

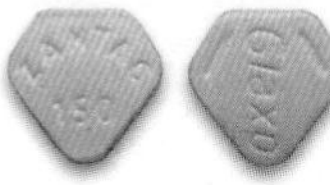

150 mg

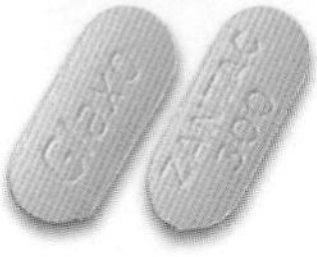

300 mg

RANOLAZINE

Ranexa
(page 1040)

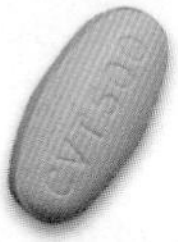

500 mg

RASAGILINE MESYLATE

Azilect
(page 1041)

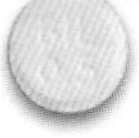

0.5 mg

1 mg

RISEDRONATE SODIUM

Actonel
(page 1052)

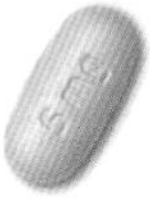

5 mg

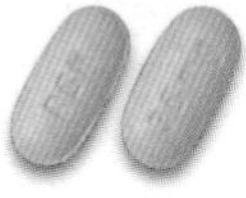

35 mg

RISPERIDONE

Risperdal
(page 1053)

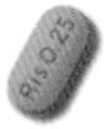

0.25 mg

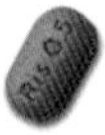

0.5 mg

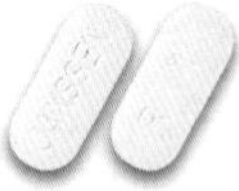

1 mg

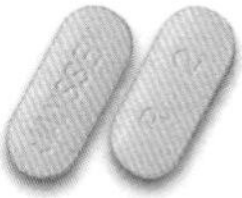

2 mg

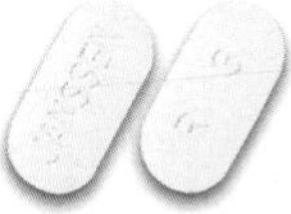

3 mg

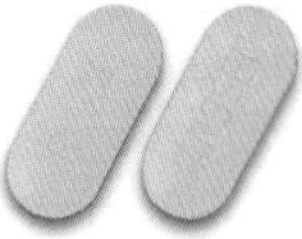

4 mg

ROSIGLITAZONE MALEATE

Avandia
(page 1061)

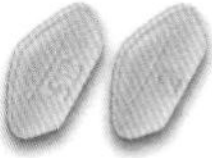

2 mg

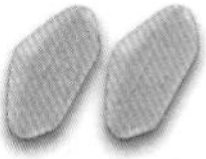

4 mg

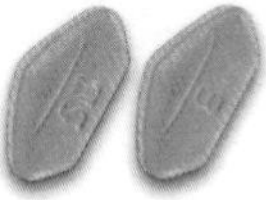

8 mg

ROSUVASTATIN CALCIUM

Crestor
(page 1062)

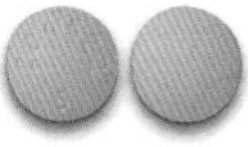

5 mg

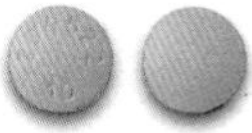

10 mg

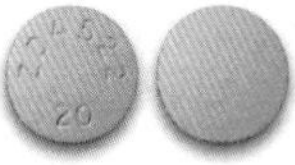

20 mg

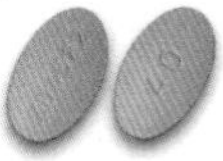

40 mg

SERTRALINE HYDROCHLORIDE

Zoloft
(page 1078)

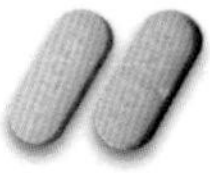
50 mg

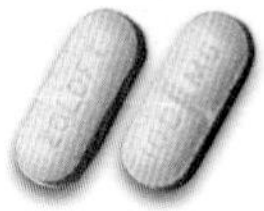
100 mg

SILDENAFIL CITRATE

Viagra
(page 1081)

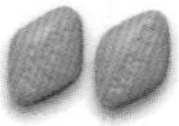
25 mg

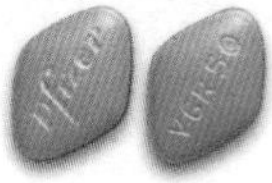

50 mg

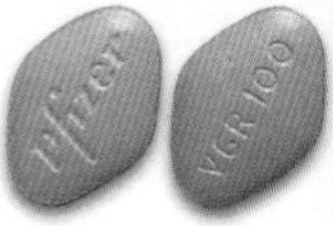

100 mg

SIMVASTATIN

Zocor
(page 1085)

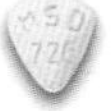
5 mg

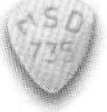
10 mg

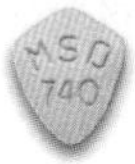

20 mg

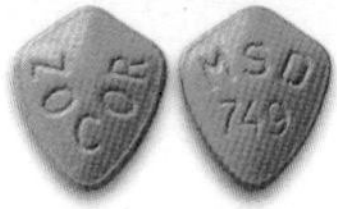

40 mg

SITAGLIPTIN PHOSPHATE

Januvia
(page 1087)

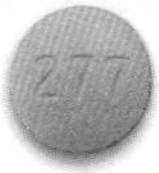

100 mg

SORAFENIB

Nexavar
(page 1420)

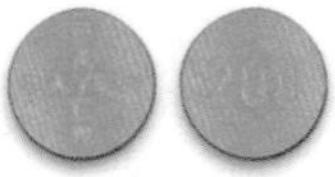

200 mg

SUCRALFATE

Carafate
(page 1105)

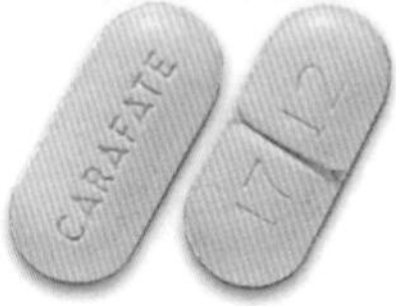

1 g

SULFAMETHOXAZOLE AND TRIMETHOPRIM

Bactrim DS
(page 1309)

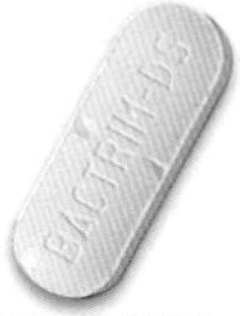

800 mg/160 mg

SUMATRIPTAN SUCCINATE

Imitrex
(page 1112)

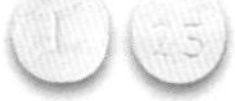

25 mg

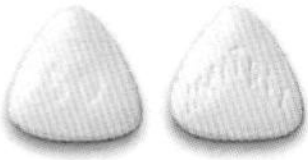

50 mg

SUNITINIB MALATE

Sutent
(page 1421)

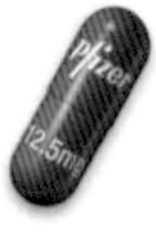

12.5 mg

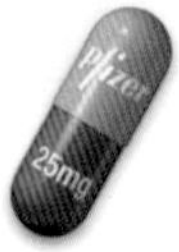

25 mg

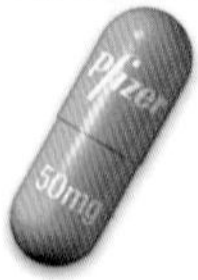

50 mg

TEMAZEPAM

Restoril
(page 1126)

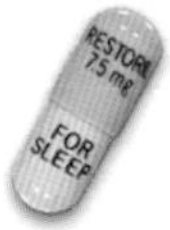

7.5 mg

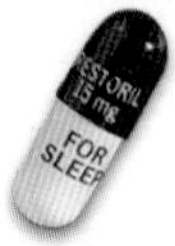

15 mg

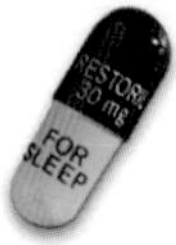

30 mg

TENOFOVIR DISOPROXIL FUMARATE

Viread
(page 1130)

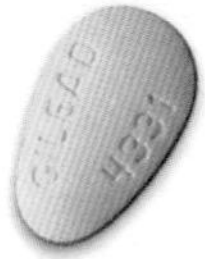

300 mg

TERAZOSIN HYDROCHLORIDE

Hytrin
(page 1131)

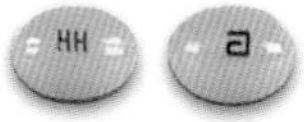

1 mg

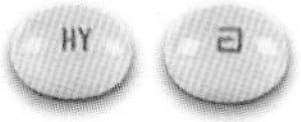

2 mg

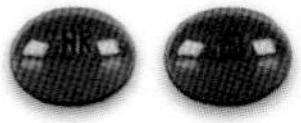
5 mg

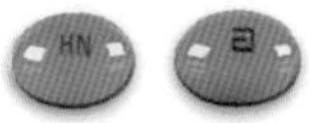

10 mg

TICLOPIDINE HYDROCHLORIDE

Ticlid
(page 1154)

250 mg

TOLTERODINE TARTRATE

Detrol
(page 1173)

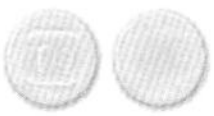
1 mg

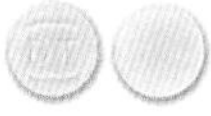
2 mg

TRAMADOL HYDROCHLORIDE AND ACETAMINOPHEN

Ultracet
(page 1307)

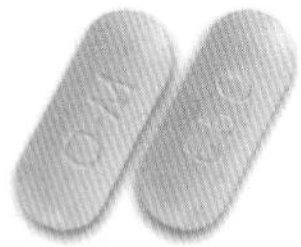

37.5 mg/325 mg

VALSARTAN

Diovan
(page 1213)

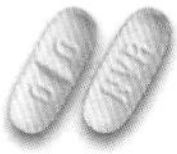

40 mg

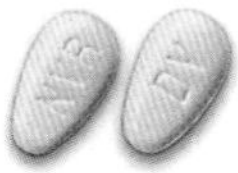

80 mg

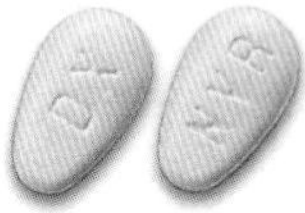

160 mg

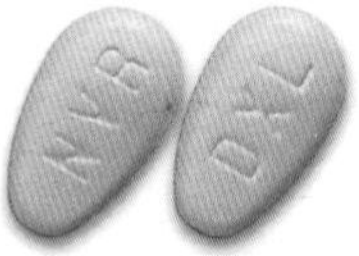

320 mg

VARDENAFIL HYDROCHLORIDE

Levitra
(page 1216)

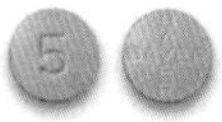

5 mg

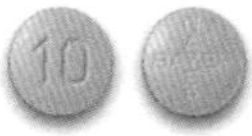

10 mg

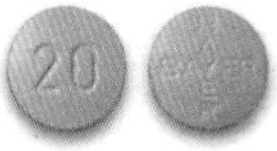

20 mg

VARENICLINE TARTRATE

Chantix
(page 1217)

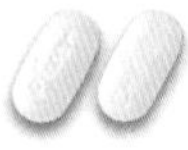

0.5 mg

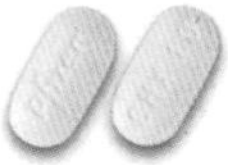

1 mg

VENLAFAXINE HYDROCHLORIDE

Effexor
(page 1219)

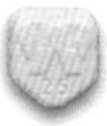

25 mg

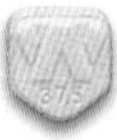

37.5 mg

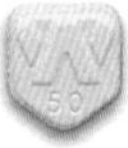

50 mg

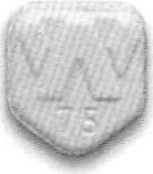

75 mg

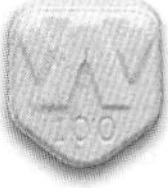

100 mg

Effexor XR
(page 1219)

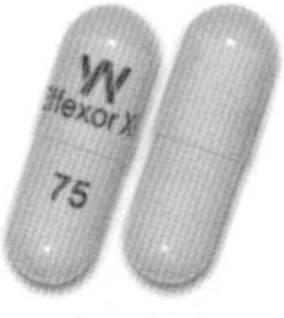

75 mg

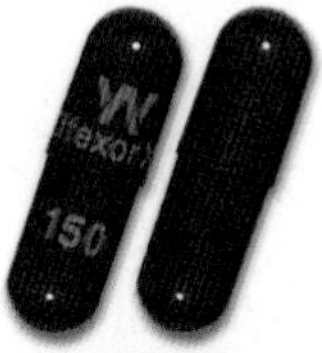

150 mg

VERAPAMIL HYDROCHLORIDE

Calan
(page 1220)

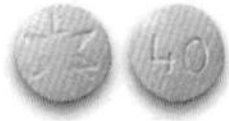

40 mg

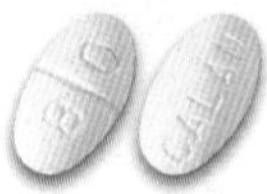

80 mg

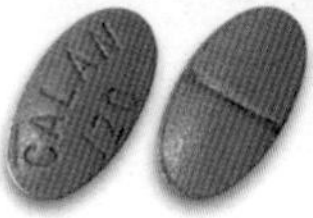

120 mg

Isoptin SR
(page 1220)

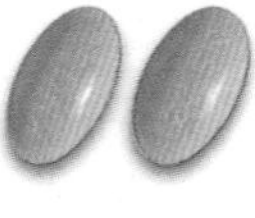

120 mg

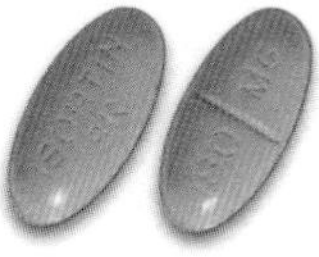

180 mg

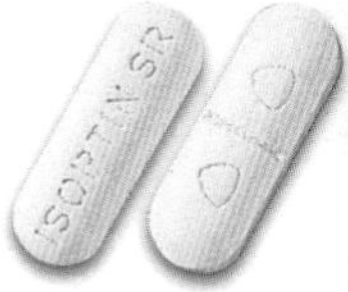

240 mg

Verelan
(page 1220)

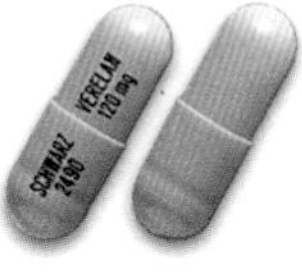

120 mg

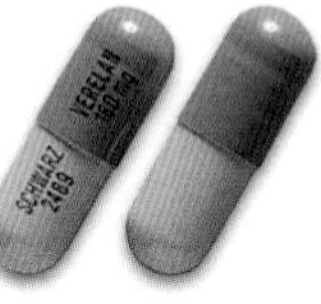

180 mg

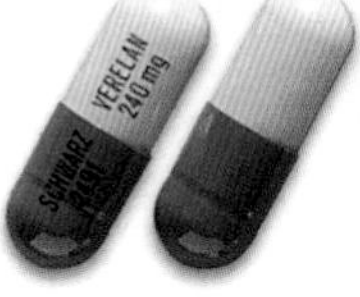

240 mg

WARFARIN SODIUM

Coumadin
(page 1230)

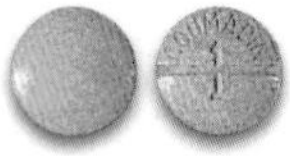

1 mg

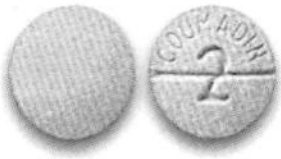

2 mg

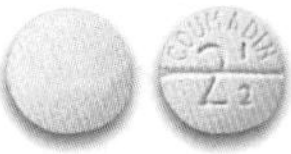

2.5 mg

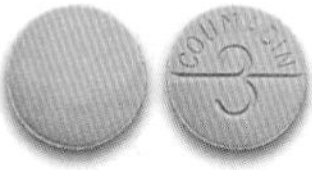

3 mg

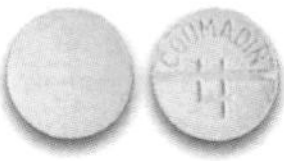

4 mg

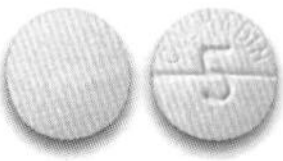

5 mg

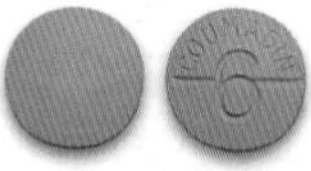

6 mg

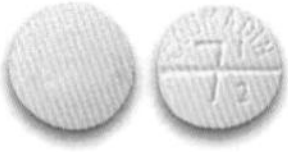

7.5 mg

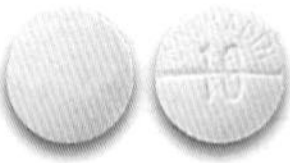

10 mg

ZIDOVUDINE

Retrovir
(page 1237)

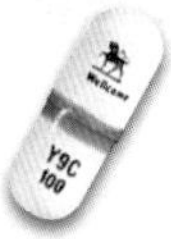

100 mg

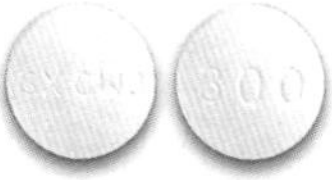

300 mg

ZOLPIDEM TARTRATE

Ambien
(page 1244)

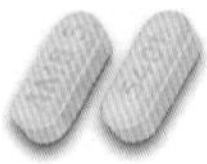

5 mg

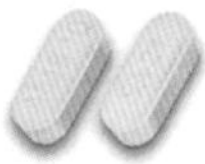

10 mg

Contraindications and cautions

- Contraindicated with allergy to progestins; thrombophlebitis, thromboembolic disorders, cerebral hemorrhage or history of these conditions; hepatic disease, carcinoma of the breast, ovaries, or endometrium, undiagnosed vaginal bleeding, missed abortion; pregnancy (fetal abnormalities, including masculinization of the female fetus have been reported); lactation.
- Use cautiously with epilepsy; migraine; asthma; cardiac or renal impairment.

Available forms

Tablets—2.5, 5, 10 mg; injection—150, 400 mg/mL; 104 mg/0.65 mL (Depo-subQ)

Dosages

Adults

- *Contraception monotherapy:* 150 mg IM every 3 mo. For *Depo-subQ Provera:* 104 mg subcutaneously into thigh or abdomen every 12–14 wk.
- *Secondary amenorrhea:* 5–10 mg/day PO for 5–10 days. A dose for inducing an optimum secretory transformation of an endometrium that has been primed with exogenous or endogenous estrogen is 10 mg/day for 10 days. Start therapy at any time; withdrawal bleeding usually occurs 3–7 days after therapy ends.
- *Abnormal uterine bleeding:* 5–10 mg/day PO for 5–10 days, beginning on the 16th or 21st day of the menstrual cycle. To produce an optimum secretory transformation of an endometrium that has been primed with estrogen, give 10 mg/day PO for 10 days, beginning on the 16th day of the cycle. Withdrawal bleeding usually occurs 3–7 days after discontinuing therapy. If bleeding is controlled, administer two subsequent cycles.
- *Endometrial or renal carcinoma:* 400–1,000 mg/wk IM. If improvement occurs within a few weeks or months and the disease appears stabilized, it may be possible to maintain improvement with as little as 400 mg/mo IM.
- *Reduction of endometrial hyperplasia:* 5–10 mg/day PO for 12–14 consecutive days/mo. Start on 1st or 16th day of cycle.
- *Management of endometriosis-associated pain:* 104 mg subcutaneously (*Depo-subQ Provera*) into anterior thigh or abdomen every 12–14 wk; do not use for longer than 2 yr.

Pharmacokinetics

Route	*Onset*	*Peak*
Oral	Slow	Unknown
IM	Weeks	Months

Metabolism: Hepatic; $T_{1/2}$: 50 days (IM)
Distribution: Crosses placenta; enters breast milk
Excretion: Unknown

Adverse effects

- **CNS:** Sudden, partial, or complete loss of vision; proptosis, diplopia, migraine, precipitation of acute intermittent porphyria, mental depression, pyrexia, insomnia, somnolence, nervousness, fatigue
- **CV:** Thrombophlebitis, cerebrovascular disorders, retinal thrombosis, pulmonary embolism, thromboembolic and thrombotic disease, increased BP
- **Dermatologic:** *Rash with or without pruritus, acne,* melasma or chloasma, alopecia, hirsutism, photosensitivity, pruritus, urticaria
- **GI:** Cholestatic jaundice, nausea
- **GU:** *Breakthrough bleeding, spotting, change in menstrual flow, amenorrhea,* changes in cervical erosion and cervical secretions, breast tenderness and secretion
- **Other:** *Fluid retention, edema, increase or decrease in weight,* decreased glucose tolerance; bone loss

Interactions

✱ **Drug-lab test** • Inaccurate tests of hepatic and endocrine function

■ Nursing considerations

Assessment

- **History:** Allergy to progestins; thrombophlebitis; thromboembolic disorders; cerebral hemorrhage; hepatic disease; carcinoma of the breast, ovaries, or endometrium; undiagnosed vaginal bleeding; missed abortion; epilepsy; migraine; asthma; cardiac dysfunction; renal impairment; pregnancy; lactation
- **Physical:** Skin color, lesions, turgor; hair; breasts; pelvic examination; orientation,

affect; ophthalmologic examination; P, auscultation, peripheral perfusion, edema; R, adventitious sounds; liver evaluation; LFTs, renal function tests, glucose tolerance, Papanicolaou (Pap) test

Interventions

- Arrange for pretreatment and periodic (at least annual) history and physical, which should include BP, breasts, abdomen, pelvic organs, and a Pap test.

⊗ ***Black box warning*** Before therapy begins, ensure that patient is not pregnant and caution patient to prevent pregnancy and to have frequent medical follow-up visits.

⊗ ***Warning*** Discontinue medication and consult physician if sudden, partial, or complete loss of vision occurs; if papilledema or retinal vascular lesions are present, discontinue drug.

⊗ ***Warning*** Discontinue medication and consult physician at the first sign of thromboembolic disease (leg pain, swelling, peripheral perfusion changes, shortness of breath).

Teaching points

- If you are taking the oral form of this drug, mark days you should take the medication on a calendar.
- If using the subcutaneous depot form of this drug, mark your calendar for days you should receive new injections.
- This drug should not be taken during pregnancy due to risk of serious fetal abnormalities. If drug is used for indications other than contraception, using barrier contraceptives is suggested.
- You may experience these side effects: Sensitivity to light (avoid exposure to the sun; use sunscreen and protective clothing); dizziness, sleeplessness, depression (use caution driving or performing tasks that require alertness); skin rash, color changes, loss of hair; fever; nausea.
- Report pain or swelling and warmth in the calves, acute chest pain or shortness of breath, sudden severe headache or vomiting, dizziness or fainting, visual disturbances, numbness or tingling in the arm or leg.

▽ mefenamic acid

*(me fe **nam'** ik)*

Apo-Mefenamic (CAN), Ponstel

PREGNANCY CATEGORY C

Drug class

NSAID

Therapeutic actions

Anti-inflammatory, analgesic, and antipyretic activities related to inhibition of prostaglandin synthesis; exact mechanisms of action are not known.

Indications

- Relief of moderate pain when therapy will not exceed 1 wk
- Treatment of primary dysmenorrhea

Contraindications and cautions

- Contraindicated with hypersensitivity to mefenamic acid, aspirin allergy, and as treatment of perioperative pain with coronary artery bypass grafting.
- Use cautiously with asthma, renal or hepatic impairment, peptic ulcer disease, GI bleeding, hypertension, heart failure, pregnancy, lactation.

Available forms

Capsules—250 mg

Dosages

Adults and patients older than 14 yr

- *Acute pain:* Initially, 500 mg PO followed by 250 mg every 6 hr as needed. Do not exceed 1 wk of therapy.
- *Primary dysmenorrhea:* Initially, 500 mg PO then 250 mg every 6 hr starting with the onset of bleeding. Can be initiated at start of menses and should not be necessary for longer than 2–3 days.

Pediatric patients

Safety and efficacy for patients younger than 14 yr not established.

Pharmacokinetics

Route	Onset	Peak	Duration
Oral	Varies	2–4 hr	6 hr

Metabolism: Hepatic; $T_{1/2}$: 2–4 hr
Distribution: Crosses placenta; enters breast milk
Excretion: Feces, urine

Adverse effects
- **CNS:** *Headache, dizziness,* somnolence, *insomnia,* fatigue, tiredness, dizziness, tinnitus, ophthalmic effects
- **Dermatologic:** *Rash,* pruritus, sweating, dry mucous membranes, stomatitis
- **GI:** *Nausea, dyspepsia, GI pain, diarrhea,* vomiting, *constipation,* flatulence, ulcers, GI bleed
- **GU:** Dysuria, **renal impairment**
- **Hematologic:** Bleeding, platelet inhibition with higher doses, neutropenia, eosinophilia, leukopenia, pancytopenia, thrombocytopenia, agranulocytosis, granulocytopenia, aplastic anemia, decreased Hgb or Hct, bone marrow depression, menorrhagia
- **Respiratory:** Dyspnea, hemoptysis, pharyngitis, bronchospasm, rhinitis
- **Other:** Peripheral edema, **anaphylactoid reactions** to **anaphylactic shock**

Interactions
✱ **Drug-drug** • Increased risk of GI bleeds with ASA, anticoagulants, other NSAIDs
✱ **Drug-lab test** • False-positive reaction for urinary bile using the Diazo tablet test

■ Nursing considerations
Assessment
- **History:** Allergies; renal, hepatic, CV, GI conditions; pregnancy; lactation
- **Physical:** Skin color and lesions; orientation, reflexes, ophthalmologic and audiometric evaluation, peripheral sensation; P, edema; R, adventitious sounds; liver evaluation; CBC, clotting times, LFTs, renal function tests; serum electrolytes, stool guaiac

Interventions
⊗ ***Black box warning*** Be aware that patient may be at increased risk for CV events, GI bleeding; monitor accordingly.
- Give with milk or food to decrease GI upset.
- Arrange for periodic ophthalmologic examinations during long-term therapy.

⊗ ***Warning*** If overdose occurs, institute emergency procedures—supportive therapy and induced emesis, activated charcoal, and/or an osmotic cathartic.

Teaching points
- Take drug with food; take only the prescribed dosage; do not take the drug longer than 1 week.
- Discontinue drug and consult your health care provider if rash, diarrhea, or digestive problems occur.
- Dizziness or drowsiness can occur (avoid driving and using dangerous machinery).
- Report sore throat, fever, rash, itching, weight gain, swelling in ankles or fingers; changes in vision; black, tarry stools; severe diarrhea, right upper abdominal pain, flulike symptoms.

DANGEROUS DRUG

(as antineoplastic)

megestrol acetate
(me jess' trole)

Apo-Megestrol (CAN), Megace, Megace ES, Megace OS (CAN)

PREGNANCY CATEGORY X (ORAL SUSPENSION)

PREGNANCY CATEGORY D (TABLETS)

Drug classes
Antineoplastic
Hormone
Progestin

Therapeutic actions
Inhibits secretion of pituitary gonadotropins with resulting decrease in estrogen secretion; exerts cytotoxic effects on tumor cells.

Indications
- Tablets: Palliation of advanced carcinoma of the breast or endometrium and as an adjunct to surgery or radiation

- Suspension: Appetite stimulant in HIV-related cachexia, anorexia or unexplained weight loss
- Unlabeled uses: Appetite stimulant for cachexia in advanced cancer; treatment for hot flashes

Contraindications and cautions

- Contraindicated with allergy to progestins; thrombophlebitis, thromboembolic disorders, cerebral hemorrhage or history of these conditions; hepatic disease, undiagnosed vaginal bleeding, missed abortion; pregnancy (masculinization of female fetus); lactation.
- Use cautiously with epilepsy, migraine, asthma, cardiac dysfunction, renal impairment.

Available forms

Tablets—20, 40 mg; suspension—40 mg/mL; extra strength suspension—125 mg/mL

Dosages

Adults

- *Breast cancer:* 160 mg/day PO (40 mg qid).
- *Endometrial cancer:* 40–320 mg/day PO in divided doses.
- *Cachexia with HIV:* Initially, 800 mg/day; normal range, 400–800 mg/day (suspension only) or 625 mg/day ES suspension.

Pharmacokinetics

Route	Onset	Peak
Oral	Slow	Weeks

Metabolism: Hepatic; $T_{1/2}$: 13–105 hr (tablets)
Distribution: Crosses placenta; enters breast milk
Excretion: Urine, feces

Adverse effects

- **CNS:** Paresthesia, confusion, seizures, depression, neuropathy, hypesthesia, abnormal thinking
- **CV:** Thrombophlebitis, cerebrovascular disorders, retinal thrombosis, **pulmonary embolism,** thromboembolic and thrombotic disease, increased BP
- **Dermatologic:** *Rash with or without pruritus, acne,* melasma or chloasma, alopecia, hirsutism, photosensitivity, pruritus, urticaria
- **GI:** Cholestatic jaundice, nausea
- **GU:** *Breakthrough bleeding, spotting, change in menstrual flow, amenorrhea,* changes in cervical erosion and cervical secretions, breast tenderness and secretion
- **Other:** *Fluid retention, edema, increase in weight,* decreased glucose tolerance

Interactions

✱ **Drug-lab test** • Inaccurate tests of hepatic and endocrine function

■ Nursing considerations

Assessment

- **History:** Allergy to progestins; thrombophlebitis, thromboembolic disorders, cerebral hemorrhage; hepatic disease; carcinoma of the breast or genital organs, undiagnosed vaginal bleeding, missed abortion; epilepsy, migraine, asthma, cardiac dysfunction, renal impairment; pregnancy; lactation
- **Physical:** Skin color, lesions, turgor; hair; breasts; pelvic examination; orientation, affect; ophthalmologic examination; P, auscultation, peripheral perfusion, edema; R, adventitious sounds; liver evaluation; LFTs, renal function tests, glucose tolerance, Papanicolaou test

Interventions

⊗ ***Warning*** Discontinue drug and consult physician at signs of thromboembolic disease—leg pain, swelling, peripheral perfusion changes, shortness of breath.

⊠ ***Black box warning*** Caution patient to avoid using drug during pregnancy because of risks to the fetus; advise using barrier contraceptives.

- Shake suspension well before use; store in a tightly closed bottle in a cool place.

Teaching points

- If the suspension form is ordered, store in a cool place in a tightly closed bottle; shake well before each use. Take care to differentiate long-acting from regular suspension.
- This drug causes serious fetal abnormalities or fetal death; avoid pregnancy. Use of barrier contraceptives is advised.
- You may experience these side effects: Sensitivity to light (avoid exposure to the sun;

use sunscreen and protective clothing); dizziness, sleeplessness, depression (use caution if driving or performing tasks that require alertness); skin rash, color changes, loss of hair; fever; nausea.
- Report pain or swelling and warmth in the calves, acute chest pain or shortness of breath, sudden severe headache or vomiting, dizziness or fainting, numbness or tingling in the arm or leg.

meloxicam
(mel ox' i kam)

Apo-Meloxicam (CAN), CO Meloxicam (CAN), Gen-Meloxicam (CAN), Mobic, Novo-Meloxicam (CAN), PMS-Meloxicam (CAN), ratio-Meloxicam (CAN)

PREGNANCY CATEGORY C (FIRST AND SECOND TRIMESTERS)

PREGNANCY CATEGORY D (THIRD TRIMESTER)

Drug class
NSAID (oxicam derivative)

Therapeutic actions
Anti-inflammatory, analgesic, and antipyretic activities related to inhibition of the enzyme cyclooxygenase (COX), which is required for the synthesis of prostaglandins and thromboxanes. Somewhat more selective for COX-2 sites (found in the brain, kidney, ovary, uterus, cartilage, bone, and at sites of inflammation) than for COX-1 sites, which are found throughout the tissues and are related to protection of the GI mucosa.

Indications
- Relief from the signs and symptoms of osteoarthritis and rheumatoid arthritis
- Relief from the signs and symptoms of pauciarticular or polyarticular course juvenile rheumatoid arthritis in patients 2 yr or older
- Unlabeled uses: Treatment of ankylosing spondylitis, acute shoulder pain

Contraindications and cautions
- Contraindicated with allergy to aspirin or meloxicam; for perioperative pain after coronary artery bypass surgery.
- Use cautiously with allergies; renal, hepatic, CV, GI conditions; bleeding disorders; pregnancy; lactation.

Available forms
Tablets—7.5, 15 mg; oral suspension—7.5 mg/5 mL

Dosages
Adults
Starting dose, 7.5 mg PO daily. Maximum dosage, 15 mg PO daily.
Pediatric patients
0.125 mg/kg PO once daily up to a maximum dose of 7.5 mg, using oral suspension.

Pharmacokinetics

Route	Onset	Peak
Oral	1 hr	5–6 hr

Metabolism: Hepatic; $T_{1/2}$: 15–20 hr
Distribution: Crosses placenta; enters breast milk
Excretion: Feces, urine

Adverse effects
- **CNS:** *Headache, dizziness,* somnolence, *insomnia,* fatigue, tiredness, tinnitus, ophthalmologic effects
- **Dermatologic:** *Rash,* pruritus, sweating, dry mucous membranes, stomatitis
- **GI:** *Nausea, dyspepsia, GI pain, diarrhea,* vomiting, constipation, flatulence
- **GU:** Dysuria, renal impairment
- **Hematologic:** Bleeding, platelet inhibition (with higher doses), neutropenia, eosinophilia, leukopenia, pancytopenia, thrombocytopenia, agranulocytosis, granulocytopenia, aplastic anemia, decreased Hgb or Hct, bone marrow depression, menorrhagia
- **Respiratory:** Dyspnea, hemoptysis, pharyngitis, bronchospasm, rhinitis

M

- **Other:** Peripheral edema, anaphylactoid reactions to **anaphylactic shock**

Interactions

✱ **Drug-drug** • Increased serum lithium levels and risk of toxicity if taken concurrently; monitor patient carefully • Possible increased risk of renal failure if combined with ACE inhibitors, diuretics • Increased risk of GI bleeding if combined with aspirin, anticoagulants, oral corticosteroids

■ Nursing considerations

Assessment

- **History:** Allergies; renal, hepatic, CV, and GI bleeding; history of ulcers; pregnancy; lactation; bleeding disorders
- **Physical:** Skin color and lesions; orientation, reflexes, peripheral sensation; P, edema; R, adventitious sounds; liver evaluation; CBC, clotting times, LFTs, renal function tests; serum electrolytes, stool guaiac

Interventions

⊗ ***Black box warning*** Be aware that patient may be at increased risk for CV events, GI bleeding; monitor accordingly.

- Administer drug with food or milk if GI upset occurs.
- Establish safety measures if CNS disturbances occur.
- Monitor patient on prolonged therapy for signs of GI bleeding or hepatic toxicity.

⊗ ***Warning*** If overdose occurs, institute emergency procedures—gastric lavage followed by activated charcoal, supportive therapy.

- Provide further comfort measures to reduce pain (positioning, environmental control), and to reduce inflammation (warmth, positioning, rest).

Teaching points

- Take drug with food if GI upset occurs.
- Take only the prescribed dosage.
- You may experience these side effects: Dizziness, drowsiness (avoid driving or using dangerous machinery while taking this drug).
- Report sore throat, fever, rash, itching, weight gain, swelling in ankles or fingers, changes in vision, black, tarry stools.

DANGEROUS DRUG

melphalan (L-Pam, L-Phenylalanine Mustard, L-Sarcolysin)

(mel' fa lan)

Alkeran

PREGNANCY CATEGORY D

Drug classes

Alkylating drug
Antineoplastic
Nitrogen mustard

Therapeutic actions

Cytotoxic: Alkylates cellular DNA, thus interfering with the replication of susceptible cells, causing cell death; cell-cycle nonspecific.

Indications

- Treatment of multiple myeloma, nonresectable epithelial ovarian carcinoma; use IV only when oral therapy is not possible
- Unlabeled uses: Breast cancer, testicular cancer, bone marrow transplantation

Contraindications and cautions

- Contraindicated with allergy to melphalan, lactation.
- Use cautiously with radiation therapy, chemotherapy, pregnancy (potentially mutagenic and teratogenic; avoid use in the first trimester).

Available forms

Tablets—2 mg; powder for injection—50 mg

Dosages

Individualize dosage based on hematologic profile and response.

Adults

Oral

- *Multiple myeloma:* 6 mg/day PO. After 2–3 wk, stop drug for up to 4 wk, and monitor blood counts. When blood counts are rising, institute maintenance dose of 2 mg/day PO. Response may occur gradually over many months (many alternative regimens, some including prednisone, are used).

- *Epithelial ovarian carcinoma:* 0.2 mg/kg/day PO for 5 days as a single course. Repeat courses every 4–6 wk, depending on hematologic response.

IV

- *Multiple myeloma:* 16 mg/m^2 administered as a single infusion over 15–20 min; administered at 2-wk intervals for 4 doses, then at 4-wk intervals.

Pediatric patients

Safety and efficacy not established.

Patients with renal impairment

Consider reducing initial oral dosage in patients with moderate to severe impairment; reduce IV dosage by 50% in patients with BUN of 30 mg/dL or more.

Pharmacokinetics

Route	*Onset*	*Peak*
Oral	Varies	2 hr
IV	Rapid	1 hr

Metabolism: $T_{1/2}$: 90 min (oral)
Distribution: Crosses placenta; enters breast milk
Excretion: Urine

IV FACTS

Preparation: Reconstitute with 10 mL of supplied diluent, and shake vigorously until a clear solution is obtained; this provides 5 mg/mL solution. Immediately dilute in 0.9% sodium chloride injection to a dilution of less than 0.45 mg/mL. Complete infusion within 60 min of reconstitution. Protect from light. Dispense in glass containers. Do not refrigerate reconstituted solution.
Infusion: Administer dilute product over a minimum of 15 min; complete within 60 min of reconstitution.

Adverse effects

- **Dermatologic:** Maculopapular rash, urticaria, *alopecia*
- **GI:** *Nausea, vomiting,* oral ulceration, diarrhea
- **Hematologic: Bone marrow depression,** hyperuricemia
- **Respiratory:** Bronchopulmonary dysplasia, **pulmonary fibrosis**
- **Other:** *Amenorrhea,* cancer, acute leukemia, **anaphylaxis**

Interactions

✱ **Drug-lab test** • Increased urinary 5-HIAA levels due to tumor cell destruction

■ Nursing considerations

Assessment

- **History:** Allergy to melphalan or chlorambucil, radiation therapy, chemotherapy, pregnancy, lactation
- **Physical:** T; weight; skin color, lesions; R, adventitious sounds; liver evaluation; CBC, differential, Hgb, renal function tests

Interventions

⊗ ***Black box warning*** Arrange for blood tests to evaluate hematopoietic function before therapy and weekly during therapy; severe bone marrow suppression may occur.

⊗ ***Warning*** Do not give full dosage until 4 wk after a full course of radiation therapy or chemotherapy due to risk of severe bone marrow depression.

- Consider dosage reductions in patients with impaired renal function.
- Ensure that patient is well hydrated before treatment.

⊗ ***Black box warning*** Caution patient to avoid pregnancy while taking this drug; drug is considered to be mutagenic.

- Divide single daily dose if nausea and vomiting occur.

Teaching points

- Take drug once a day. If nausea and vomiting occur, consult with your health care provider about dividing the dose.
- Refrigerate tablets in glass bottle.
- This drug causes severe birth defects; use of barrier contraceptives is advised.
- You may experience these side effects: Nausea, vomiting, loss of appetite (divided dose, frequent small meals may help; maintain fluid intake and nutrition; drink at least 10–12 glasses of fluid each day); skin rash, loss of hair (obtain a wig if hair loss occurs; head should be covered at extremes of temperature).
- Report unusual bleeding or bruising, fever, chills, sore throat, cough, shortness of breath,

black tarry stools, flank or stomach pain, joint pain.

memantine hydrochloride

*(meh **man'** teen)*

Namenda

PREGNANCY CATEGORY B

Drug classes

Alzheimer's disease drug
N-methyl-*D*-aspartate (NMDA) receptor antagonist

Therapeutic actions

Exerts a low to moderate affinity for NMDA receptor sites with no effects on GABA, dopamine, histamine, glycine, or adrenergic receptor sites; persistent activation of the CNS NMDA receptors by the excitatory amino acid glutamate has been suggested to contribute to the symptomatology of Alzheimer's disease.

Indications

- Treatment of moderate to severe dementia of the Alzheimer's type
- Unlabeled uses: Treatment of vascular dementia, treatment of ADHD

Contraindications and cautions

- Contraindicated with allergy to memantine or any component of the drug.
- Use cautiously with pregnancy, lactation, renal impairment.

Available forms

Tablets—5, 10 mg; oral solution—2 mg/mL

Dosages

Adults

Initially, 5 mg/day PO, increase at weekly intervals to 5 mg bid (10 mg/day), 15 mg/day (5 mg and 10 mg doses) with a target dose of 20 mg/day (10 mg bid). Use solution-dosing device if solution is used.

Pediatric patients

Safety and efficacy not established.

Patients with renal impairment

Consider dosage reduction and closely monitor the patient; avoid use with severe renal impairment.

Pharmacokinetics

Route	Onset	Peak
Oral	Varies	3–7 hr

Metabolism: Hepatic metabolism; $T_{1/2}$: 60–80 hr
Distribution: May cross placenta; may enter breast milk
Excretion: Urine

Adverse effects

- **CNS:** Fatigue, *headache, dizziness, confusion,* somnolence, hallucinations, agitation, insomnia, anxiety
- **CV:** Hypertension, peripheral edema
- **GI:** Vomiting, diarrhea, *constipation*
- **GU:** UTI, urinary incontinence
- **Respiratory:** Cough, dyspnea, URI, bronchitis
- **Other:** Pain, back pain, arthralgia

Interactions

✱ **Drug-drug** • Increased effects and risk of toxicity of memantine if taken with drugs that alkalinize the urine, including carbonic anhydrase inhibitors, sodium bicarbonate; monitor patient closely and make dosage adjustments as needed • Potential for increased effects and toxicity if combined with amantadine, ketamine, or dextromethorphan; use caution if this combination is used

■ Nursing considerations

Assessment

History: Allergy to memantine or component of the drug, pregnancy, lactation, renal impairment
Physical: Orientation, affect, reflexes; BP; R, adventitious sounds, assessment of normal function

Interventions

- Establish baseline functional profile to follow evaluation of drug effectiveness.

- Administer without regard to food; may take with food if GI upset is a problem; switch to oral solution if swallowing is difficult.
- Provide patient safety measures if CNS effects occur.
- Establish bowel program if constipation becomes an issue.

Teaching points

- Take drug exactly as prescribed; take with food to decrease GI upset; learn to use the solution-dosing device rather than spoon to determine exact dose of solution.
- This drug does not cure the disease; it is not thought to prevent or slow the degeneration associated with the disease.
- Dosage changes will be needed and will be made on a weekly basis until the target dosage is reached.
- You may experience these side effects: Headache (an analgesic may be available); dizziness, fatigue, confusion (use caution if driving or performing tasks that require alertness); constipation (consult your health care provider for an appropriate bowel program).
- Report severe nausea, vomiting, severe headache, swelling of the legs, respiratory problems, lack of improvement in day-to-day functioning.

▽ menotropins

*(men oh **troe'** pins)*

Menopur, Repronex

PREGNANCY CATEGORY X

Drug classes

Fertility drug
Hormone

Therapeutic actions

A purified preparation of human gonadotropins; in women, produces ovarian follicular growth; when followed by administration HCG, produces ovulation; used with HCG for at least 3 mo to induce spermatogenesis in men with primary or secondary pituitary hypofunction who have previously achieved adequate masculinization with HCG administration.

Indications

- Women: Given with HCG sequentially to induce ovulation and pregnancy in anovulatory infertile patients without primary ovarian failure; used with HCG to stimulate multiple follicles for in vitro fertilization programs
- Unlabeled use: Treatment of male infertility caused by hypogonotropic hypogonadism

Contraindications and cautions

- Contraindicated with known sensitivity to menotropins; high gonadotropin levels, indicating primary ovarian failure; overt thyroid or adrenal dysfunction; abnormal bleeding of undetermined origin; ovarian cysts or enlargement not due to polycystic ovary syndrome; intracranial lesion, such as pituitary tumor; pregnancy (women); normal gonadotropin levels, indicating pituitary function; elevated gonadotropin levels, indicating primary testicular failure; infertility disorders other than hypogonadotropin hypogonadism (men).
- Use cautiously with lactation.

Available forms

Powder or pellet for injection—75 international units FSH/75 international units LH; 150 international units FSH/150 international units LH

Dosages

Women

To achieve ovulation, HCG must be given following menotropins when clinical assessment indicates sufficient follicular maturation as indicated by urinary excretion of estrogens.

Menopur, Repronex

225 units IM; then 75–150 units/day by subcutaneous injection up to a maximum of 450 units/day for no longer than 12 days (*Repronex*) or 20 days (*Menopur*). Base actual dose on follicular development.

Repronex

Patients who have received gonadotropin-releasing hormone agonists or pituitary suppression: Initially, 150 international units subcutaneously or IM daily for first 5 days; adjust dosage as needed after 2 or more days. Do not adjust by more than 150 international units per adjustment and do not exceed maximum daily dose of 450 international units. Do not use longer than 12 days. If patient response is adequate, give HCG 5,000–10,000 units 1 day following last dose of menotropins.

Pharmacokinetics

Route	Onset	Peak	Duration
IM	Slow	Weeks	Months

Metabolism: $T_{1/2}$: 11–13 hr (*Menopur*), 53–59 hr (*Repronex*)
Distribution: Crosses placenta
Excretion: Urine

Adverse effects

Women

- **CNS:** Dizziness
- **CV:** Arterial thromboembolism, tachycardia
- **GI:** Nausea, vomiting, abdominal pain, bloating
- **GU:** *Ovarian enlargement,* hyperstimulation syndrome, hemoperitoneum
- **Hypersensitivity:** Hypersensitivity reactions
- **Other:** *Febrile reactions;* birth defects in resulting pregnancies, *multiple pregnancies*

■ Nursing considerations

Assessment

- **History:** Sensitivity to menotropins; high gonadotropin levels; overt thyroid or adrenal dysfunction, abnormal bleeding of undetermined origin, ovarian cysts or enlargement not due to polycystic ovary syndrome, intracranial lesion, pregnancy, lactation (women); normal gonadotropin levels; elevated gonadotropin levels; infertility disorders other than hypogonadotropin hypogonadism (men)
- **Physical:** Abdominal examination, pelvic examination; testicular examination; serum gonadotropin levels; 24 hr urinary estrogens and estriol excretion (women); T; masculinization, serum testosterone levels (men)

Interventions

- Dissolve contents of 1–6 vials in 1–2 mL of sterile saline. Administer subcutaneously immediately. *Repronex* may also be given IM. Discard any unused portion.
- Store ampules at room temperature or in refrigerator; do not freeze.
- Monitor women for any sign of ovarian enlargement at least every other day during treatment and for 2 wk after treatment.

⊗ ***Warning*** Discontinue drug at any sign of ovarian overstimulation, and arrange to have patient admitted to the hospital for observation and supportive measures. Do not attempt to remove ascitic fluid because of the risk of injury to the ovaries. Have the patient refrain from intercourse if ovarian enlargement occurs.

- Provide women with calendar of treatment days and explanations about what signs of estrogen and progesterone activity to watch for. Caution patient that 24-hr urine collections will be needed periodically, that HCG also must be given to induce ovulation, and that daily intercourse should begin 1 day prior to HCG administration and until ovulation occurs.
- Alert patient to risks and hazards of multiple births.

Teaching points

- Prepare a calendar showing the treatment schedule; drug can only be given intramuscularly and must be used with human chorionic gonadotropin (HCG) to achieve the desired effects. If you are administering the drug yourself, dispose of needles and syringes properly.
- Know that there is a risk of multiple pregnancy when using this drug.
- Have intercourse daily beginning on the day prior to HCG therapy until ovulation occurs.
- Report pain at injection site, severe abdominal or lower back pain, fever, fluid in the abdomen.

DANGEROUS DRUG

▽ meperidine hydrochloride (pethidine)

(me ***per'*** *i deen)*

Demerol

PREGNANCY CATEGORY B

PREGNANCY CATEGORY D (PROLONGED USE)

CONTROLLED SUBSTANCE C-II

Drug class
Opioid agonist analgesic

Therapeutic actions
Acts as agonist at specific opioid receptors in the CNS to produce analgesia, euphoria, sedation; the receptors mediating these effects are thought to be the same as those mediating the effects of endogenous opioids (enkephalins, endorphins).

Indications
- Oral, parenteral: Relief of moderate to severe acute pain
- Parenteral: Preoperative medication, support of anesthesia, and obstetric analgesia

Contraindications and cautions
- Contraindicated with hypersensitivity to opioids, diarrhea caused by poisoning (before toxins are eliminated), bronchial asthma, COPD, cor pulmonale, respiratory depression, anoxia, kyphoscoliosis, acute alcoholism, increased intracranial pressure, pregnancy, seizure disorder, renal impairment. Contraindicated in premature infants.
- Use cautiously with acute abdominal conditions, CV disease, supraventricular tachycardias, myxedema, delirium tremens, cerebral arteriosclerosis, ulcerative colitis, fever, Addison's disease, prostatic hypertrophy, urethral stricture, recent GI or GU surgery, toxic psychosis, labor or delivery (opioids given to the mother can cause respiratory depression of neonate; premature infants are especially at risk), renal or hepatic impairment, lactation.

Available forms
Tablets—50, 100 mg; syrup—50 mg/5 mL; injection—10, 25, 50, 75, 100 mg/mL; oral solution—50 mg/5 mL

Dosages
Adults
- *Relief of pain:* Individualize dosage; 50–150 mg IM, subcutaneously, or PO every 3–4 hr as needed. Diluted solution may be given by slow IV injection. IM route is preferred for repeated injections.
- *Preoperative medication:* 50–100 mg IM or subcutaneously, 30–90 min before beginning anesthesia.
- *Support of anesthesia:* Dilute to 10 mg/mL, and give repeated doses by slow IV injection, or dilute to 1 mg/mL and infuse continuously. Individualize dosage.
- *Obstetric analgesia:* When contractions become regular, 50–100 mg IM or subcutaneously; repeat every 1–3 hr.

Pediatric patients
Contraindicated in premature infants.
- *Relief of pain:* 1.1–1.75 mg/kg IM, subcutaneously, or PO up to adult dose every 3–4 hr as needed.
- *Preoperative medication:* 1.1–2.2 mg/kg IM or subcutaneously, up to adult dose, 30–90 min before beginning anesthesia.

Geriatric or debilitated patients
Use caution; respiratory depression may occur in elderly, the very ill, and those with respiratory problems. Reduced dosage may be needed.

Pharmacokinetics

Route	*Onset*	*Peak*	*Duration*
Oral	15 min	60–90 min	2–4 hr
IM, Subcut.	10–15 min	3–50 min	2–4 hr
IV	Immediate	5–7 min	2–4 hr

Metabolism: Hepatic; $T_{1/2}$: 3–4 hr
Distribution: Crosses placenta; enters breast milk
Excretion: Urine

IV FACTS
Preparation: Dilute parenteral solution prior to IV injection using 5% dextrose and lactated Ringer's; dextrose-saline combinations; 2.5%, 5%, or 10% dextrose in water, Ringer's, or lactated Ringer's; 0.45% or 0.9% sodium chloride; 1/6M sodium lactate.
Infusion: Administer by slow IV injection over 4–5 min or by continuous infusion when diluted to 1 mg/mL.
Incompatibilities: ⊗ ***Warning*** Do not mix meperidine solutions with solutions of barbiturates, aminophylline, heparin, morphine sulfate, methicillin, phenytoin, sodium bicarbonate, iodide, sulfadiazine, sulfisoxazole.
Y-site incompatibilities: Do not give with other drugs.

M

Adverse effects

- **CNS:** *Light-headedness, dizziness, sedation,* euphoria, dysphoria, delirium, insomnia, agitation, anxiety, fear, hallucinations, disorientation, drowsiness, lethargy, impaired mental and physical performance, coma, mood changes, weakness, headache, tremor, seizures, miosis, visual disturbances, suppression of cough reflex
- **CV:** Facial flushing, peripheral circulatory collapse, tachycardia, bradycardia, arrhythmia, palpitations, chest wall rigidity, hypertension, hypotension, orthostatic hypotension, syncope
- **Dermatologic:** Pruritus, urticaria, laryngospasm, bronchospasm, edema
- **GI:** *Nausea, vomiting,* dry mouth, anorexia, *constipation,* biliary tract spasm, increased colonic motility in patients with chronic ulcerative colitis
- **GU:** Ureteral spasm, spasm of vesical sphincters, urine retention or hesitancy, oliguria, antidiuretic effect, reduced libido or potency
- **Local:** Tissue irritation and induration (subcutaneous injection)
- **Major hazards: Respiratory depression, apnea, circulatory depression, respiratory arrest, shock, cardiac arrest**
- **Other:** *Sweating,* physical tolerance and dependence, psychological dependence

Interactions

✱ **Drug-drug** ⊗ ***Warning*** Severe and sometimes fatal reactions (resembling opioid overdose; characterized by seizures, hypertension, hyperpyrexia) when given to patients receiving or who have recently received MAOIs; do not give meperidine to patients on MAOIs • Potentiation of effects with barbiturate anesthetics; decrease dose of meperidine when coadministering • Increased likelihood of respiratory depression, hypotension, profound sedation, or coma with phenothiazines

✱ **Drug-lab test** • Elevated biliary tract pressure may cause increases in plasma amylase, lipase; determinations of these levels may be unreliable for 24 hr after administration of opioids

■ Nursing considerations

Assessment

- **History:** Hypersensitivity to opioids, diarrhea caused by poisoning, bronchial asthma, COPD, cor pulmonale, respiratory depression, anoxia, kyphoscoliosis, acute alcoholism, increased intracranial pressure, acute abdominal conditions, CV disease, supraventricular tachycardias, myxedema, seizure disorders, delirium tremens, cerebral arteriosclerosis, ulcerative colitis, fever, Addison's disease, prostatic hypertrophy, urethral stricture, recent GI or GU surgery, toxic psychosis, renal or hepatic impairment, pregnancy, lactation
- **Physical:** T; skin color, texture, lesions; orientation, reflexes, bilateral grip strength, affect, pupil size; P, auscultation, BP, orthostatic BP, perfusion; R, adventitious sounds; bowel sounds, normal output; frequency and pattern of voiding, normal output; ECG; EEG; LFTs, renal and thyroid function tests

Interventions

- Administer to lactating women 4–6 hr before the next feeding to minimize the amount in milk.

⊗ ***Warning*** Keep opioid antagonist and facilities for assisted or controlled respiration readily available during parenteral administration.

⊗ ***Warning*** Use caution when injecting subcutaneously into chilled areas of the body or in patients with hypotension or in shock; impaired perfusion may delay absorption; with repeated doses, an excessive amount may be absorbed when circulation is restored.

- Reduce dosage of meperidine by 25%–50% in patients receiving phenothiazines or other tranquilizers.
- Give each dose of the oral syrup in half glass of water. If taken undiluted, it may exert a slight local anesthetic effect on mucous membranes.
- Reassure patient that addiction is unlikely; most patients who receive opiates for medical reasons do not develop dependence syndromes.

⊗ ***Warning*** Use meperidine with extreme caution in patients with renal impairment or those requiring repeated dosing due to accumulation of normeperidine, a toxic metabolite that may cause seizures.

Teaching points
- Take drug exactly as prescribed.
- Avoid alcohol, antihistamines, sedatives, tranquilizers, and over-the-counter drugs.
- Do not take leftover medication for other disorders, and do not let anyone else take this prescription.
- You may experience these side effects: Nausea, loss of appetite (take with food and lie quietly, eat frequent small meals); constipation (request a laxative); dizziness, sedation, drowsiness, impaired visual acuity (avoid driving, performing other tasks that require alertness or visual acuity).
- Report severe nausea, vomiting, constipation, shortness of breath, or difficulty breathing.

meprobamate
*(me proe **ba'** mate)*

Miltown

PREGNANCY CATEGORY D

CONTROLLED SUBSTANCE C-IV

Drug class
Anxiolytic

Therapeutic actions
Has effects at many sites in the CNS, including the thalamus and limbic system; inhibits multineuronal spinal reflexes; is mildly tranquilizing; has some antiepileptic and central skeletal muscle relaxing properties.

Indications
- Management of anxiety disorders for the short-term relief of the symptoms of anxiety (anxiety or tension associated with the stress of everyday life usually does not require treatment with anxiolytic drugs); effectiveness for longer than 4 mo not established.

Contraindications and cautions
- Contraindicated with hypersensitivity to meprobamate or to related drugs, such as carisoprodol; acute intermittent porphyria; hepatic or renal impairment; pregnancy; lactation.
- Use cautiously with epilepsy (drug may precipitate seizures).

Available forms
Tablets—200, 400 mg

Dosages
Adults
1,200–1,600 mg/day PO in three or four divided doses. Do not exceed 2,400 mg/day.
Pediatric patients 6–12 yr
100–200 mg PO bid–tid.
Pediatric patients younger than 6 yr
Safety and efficacy not established.
Geriatric patients
Use lowest effective dose to avoid oversedation.

Pharmacokinetics

Route	*Onset*	*Peak*
Oral	Varies	1–3 hr

Metabolism: Hepatic; $T_{1/2}$: 6–14 hr
Distribution: Crosses placenta; enters breast milk
Excretion: Urine

Adverse effects
- **CNS:** *Drowsiness, ataxia, dizziness, headache, slurred speech, vertigo, weakness, impairment of visual accommodation,* euphoria, overstimulation, paradoxical excitement, paresthesias
- **CV:** *Palpitations, tachycardia,* various arrhythmias, syncope, **hypotensive crisis**
- **GI:** *Nausea, vomiting, diarrhea*
- **Hematologic:** Agranulocytosis, aplastic anemia; thrombocytopenic purpura; exacerbation of porphyric symptoms
- **Hypersensitivity:** Allergic or idiosyncratic reactions (usually seen between first and fourth doses in patients without previous drug exposure): *Itchy, urticarial or erythematous maculopapular rash;* leukopenia, acute nonthrombocytopenic purpura, petechiae, ecchymoses, eosinophilia, peripheral edema, adenopathy, fever, fixed drug eruption; hyperpyrexia, chills, angioneurotic edema, bronchospasm, oliguria, anuria, anaphylaxis, erythema multiforme, exfoliative dermatitis, stomatitis, proctitis; **Stevens-Johnson syndrome,** bullous dermatitis
- **Other:** Physical, psychological dependence; withdrawal reaction

Interactions

✱ **Drug-drug** • Additive CNS depression with alcohol, opioids, barbiturates, and other CNS depressants

■ Nursing considerations

Assessment

- **History:** Hypersensitivity to meprobamate or to related drugs; acute intermittent porphyria; hepatic or renal impairment; epilepsy; pregnancy; lactation
- **Physical:** T; skin color, lesions; orientation, affect, reflexes, vision examination; P, BP; R, adventitious sounds; bowel sounds, normal output, liver evaluation; LFTs, renal function tests, CBC and differential, EEG and ECG

Interventions

- Supervise dose and amount for patients who are addiction prone or alcoholic.

⊗ ***Warning*** Dispense least amount of drug feasible to patients who are depressed or suicidal.

- Withdraw gradually over 2 wk if patient has been maintained on high doses for weeks or months.
- Withdraw drug if allergic or idiosyncratic reactions occur.
- Caution patient about the need to avoid pregnancy while taking this drug.

⊗ ***Warning*** Keep epinephrine, antihistamines, corticosteroids, and life-support equipment readily available in case allergic or idiosyncratic reaction occurs.

Teaching points

- Take this drug exactly as prescribed. This drug may not be effective after several months of therapy; continue to see your health care provider.
- Avoid alcohol, sleep-inducing, or over-the-counter drugs; these could cause dangerous effects.
- Use barrier method of birth control while taking this drug; do not take this drug during pregnancy. Consult your health care provider immediately if you decide to become pregnant or find that you are pregnant.
- You may experience these side effects: Drowsiness, dizziness, light-headedness, blurred vision (avoid driving or performing other tasks requiring alertness or visual acuity); GI upset (eat frequent small meals).
- Report rash, sore throat, fever, easy bruising, bleeding, thoughts of suicide.

DANGEROUS DRUG

▽ mercaptopurine (6-mercaptopurine, 6-MP)

*(mer kap toe **pyoor'** een)*

Purinethol

PREGNANCY CATEGORY D

Drug classes

Antimetabolite
Antineoplastic

Therapeutic actions

Tumor-inhibiting properties, probably due to interference with purine nucleotide synthesis and hence with RNA and DNA synthesis, leading to cell death; cell-cycle specific.

Indications

- Remission induction, remission consolidation, and maintenance therapy of acute leukemia (lymphocytic, myelogenous)

Contraindications and cautions

- Contraindicated with allergy to mercaptopurine, prior resistance to mercaptopurine (cross-resistance with thioguanine is frequent), hematopoietic depression, pregnancy, lactation.
- Use cautiously with impaired renal function (slower elimination and greater accumulation; reduce dosage).

Available forms

Tablets—50 mg

Dosages

Adults and pediatric patients

- *Induction therapy:* Usual initial dose is 2.5 mg/kg/day PO (about 100–200 mg in adults, 50 mg in the average 5-yr-old child). Continue daily for several weeks. After 4 wk, if no clinical improvement or toxicity, increase to 5 mg/kg/day.

- *Maintenance therapy after complete hematologic remission:* 1.5–2.5 mg/kg/day PO as a single daily dose. Often effective in children with ALL, especially in combination with methotrexate.

Patients with renal impairment

Reduce dosage and monitor patient closely.

Pharmacokinetics

Route	*Onset*	*Peak*
Oral	Varies	2 hr

Metabolism: Hepatic; $T_{1/2}$: 47 min (adults)
Distribution: Crosses placenta; may enter breast milk
Excretion: Urine

Adverse effects

- **GI:** Hepatotoxicity; oral lesions (resembling thrush); nausea; vomiting; anorexia, pancreatitis
- **Hematologic:** *Bone marrow depression, immunosuppression, hyperuricemia* as consequence of antineoplastic effect and cell lysis
- **Other:** Drug fever, **cancer,** chromosomal aberrations, rash, hyperpigmentation

Interactions

✱ **Drug-drug** • Increased risk of severe toxicity with allopurinol; reduce mercaptopurine to one-third to one-fourth the usual dose

■ Nursing considerations

CLINICAL ALERT!

Name confusion has occurred between *Purinethol* (mercaptopurine) and propylthiouracil; use extreme caution.

Assessment

- **History:** Allergy to mercaptopurine; prior resistance to mercaptopurine; hematopoietic depression; impaired renal function; pregnancy; lactation
- **Physical:** T; mucous membranes, liver evaluation, abdominal examination; CBC, differential, Hgb, platelet counts; LFTs, renal function tests; urinalysis; serum uric acid

Interventions

- Evaluate hematopoietic status before and frequently during therapy.
- Round dose to nearest 25 mg (tablets are scored).
- Ensure that patient is well hydrated before and during therapy to minimize adverse effects of hyperuricemia.
- Caution patient about the risk of serious fetal harm while taking this drug; advise patient to use barrier contraceptives.
- Administer as a single daily dose.

Teaching points

- Drink adequate fluids; drink at least 8–10 glasses of fluid each day.
- Have frequent, regular medical follow-up visits, including blood tests to follow the drug effects.
- You may experience these side effects: Mouth sores (practice frequent mouth care); miscarriages (use barrier contraceptives); nausea, vomiting.
- Report fever, chills, sore throat, unusual bleeding or bruising, yellow discoloration of the skin or eyes, abdominal pain, flank pain, joint pain, fever, weakness, diarrhea.

▽ meropenem

*(mare oh **pen' ehm**)*

Merrem IV

PREGNANCY CATEGORY B

Drug class

Antibiotic (carbapenem)

Therapeutic actions

Bactericidal: Inhibits synthesis of bacterial cell wall and causes cell death in susceptible cells.

Indications

- Susceptible intra-abdominal infections caused by viridans group streptococci, *Escherichia coli, Klebsiella pneumoniae,*

Pseudomonas aeruginosa, Bacteroides fragilis, Bacteroides thetaiotaomicron, and *Peptostreptococcus*

- Bacterial meningitis caused by *Streptococcus pneumoniae, Haemophilus influenzae, Neisseria meningitidis* in pediatric patients 3 mo and older
- Treatment of complicated skin and skin structure infections due to *Staphylococcus aureus* (beta-lactamase and non–beta-lactamase–producing methicillin-susceptible isolates only), *Streptococcus pyogenes, Streptococcus agalactiae,* viridans group streptococci, *Enterococcus faecalis* (excluding vancomycin-resistant isolates), *Pseudomonas aeruginosa, E. coli, Proteus mirabilis, Bacteroides fragilis, Peptostreptococcus* species
- Unlabeled uses: Community-acquired pneumonia, therapy for patients with febrile neutropenia

Contraindications and cautions

- Contraindicated with allergy to cephalosporins, penicillins, beta-lactams; lactation.
- Use cautiously with CNS disorders, seizures, renal or hepatic impairment, pregnancy.

Available forms

Powder for injection—500 mg, 1 g

Dosages

Adults

- *Meningitis, intra-abdominal infections:* 1 g IV every 8 hr.
- *Skin and skin structure infections:* 500 mg IV every 8 hr.

Pediatric patients 3 mo and older

- *Intra-abdominal infections:* If less than 50 kg, 20 mg/kg IV every 8 hr. If more than 50 kg, 1 g IV every 8 hr.
- *Meningitis:* If less than 50 kg, 40 mg/kg IV every 8 hr; if more than 50 kg, 2 g IV every 8 hr.
- *Skin and skin structure infections:* If less than 50 kg,10 mg/kg IV every 8 hr; if more than 50 kg, 500 mg IV every 8 hr.

Pediatric patients younger than 3 mo

Not recommended.

Patients with impaired renal function

CrCl (mL/min)	*Dose (meningitis, intra-abdominal infections)*	*Dose (skin, skin structure infections)*
26–50	1 g IV every 12 hr	500 mg IV every 12 hr
10–25	500 mg IV every 12 hr	250 mg IV every 12 hr
Less than 10	500 mg IV every 24 hr	250 mg IV every 24 hr

Pharmacokinetics

Route	*Onset*	*Peak*	*Duration*
IV	Immediate	5 min	10–12 min

Metabolism: $T_{1/2}$: 1 hr
Distribution: Unknown whether crosses placenta; may enter breast milk
Excretion: Urine, unchanged

IV FACTS

Preparation: Dilute in 0.9% sodium chloride injection; 5% or 10% dextrose injection; dextrose in sodium chloride, potassium chloride, sodium bicarbonate, Normosol-M, Ringer's lactate; 2.5% mannitol injection; Ringer's injection; Ringer's lactate injection; sodium lactate injection 1/6N; sodium bicarbonate. Store at room temperature or 39° F (4° C); stability in each solution varies—consult manufacturer's instructions if not used immediately.
Infusion: Infuse over 15–30 min or give by direct IV injection over 3–5 min.
Incompatibilities: Do not mix in solution with other drugs.

Adverse effects

- **CNS:** *Headache,* dizziness, lethargy, paresthesias, **seizures,** insomnia
- **GI:** *Nausea, vomiting, diarrhea, anorexia, abdominal pain, flatulence,* **pseudomembranous colitis,** liver toxicity
- **Other:** *Superinfections,* abscess (redness, tenderness, heat, tissue sloughing), inflammation at injection site, *phlebitis, rash,* urticaria, pruritus

Interactions

✱ **Drug-drug** • Possible toxic levels if combined with probenecid; avoid this combination

■ Nursing considerations

Assessment

- **History:** Allergy to cephalosporins, penicillins, beta lactams; renal failure; CNS disorders, seizures, renal or hepatic impairment; pregnancy, lactation
- **Physical:** Orientation, affect; skin color, lesions; culture site of infection; R, adventitious sounds; bowel sounds, abdominal examination; LFTs, renal function tests

Interventions

- Culture infected area and arrange for sensitivity tests before beginning therapy.
- Monitor for superinfections and arrange treatment as appropriate.

⊗ ***Warning*** Discontinue drug at any sign of colitis and arrange for appropriate supportive treatment.

Teaching points

- This drug can only be given IV.
- You may experience these side effects: Stomach upset, loss of appetite, nausea (take drug with food); diarrhea (stay near bathroom); headache, dizziness.
- Report severe diarrhea, difficulty breathing, unusual tiredness, pain at injection site.

▽mesalamine (5-aminosalicylic acid, 5-ASA)

*(me **sal'** a meen)*

Apriso, Asacol DNC, CANASA, Lialda DNC, Mesasal (CAN), Pentasa DNC, Rowasa, Salofalk (CAN)

PREGNANCY CATEGORY B

Drug class

Anti-inflammatory

Therapeutic actions

Mechanism of action is unknown; thought to be a direct, local anti-inflammatory effect in the colon where mesalamine blocks cyclooxygenase and inhibits prostaglandin production in the colon.

Indications

- Oral: Remission and treatment, and induction of remission with one daily dose, of active mild to moderate ulcerative colitis
- Suppository: Treatment of active, distal, mild to moderate ulcerative colitis, ulcerative proctitis, or proctosigmoiditis

Contraindications and cautions

- Contraindicated with hypersensitivity to mesalamine, salicylates, any component of the formulation.
- Use cautiously with renal impairment, pregnancy, lactation.

Available forms

DR tablets DNC—400 mg, 1.2 g; CR capsules DNC—250, 500 mg; ER capsules DNC—375 mg; suppositories—1 g; rectal suspension—4 g/60 mL

Dosages

Adults

Rectal

- *Suspension enema:* 60 mL units in one rectal instillation (4 g) once a day, preferably at bedtime, and retained for approximately 8 hr. Usual course of therapy is 3–6 wk. Effects may be seen within 3–21 days.
- *Rectal suppository:* 1 g (1 suppository) bid. Retain suppository for 1–3 hr or longer. Usual course is 3–6 wk.

Oral

- *DR tablets:* 2–4 1.2 g tablets PO once daily with food for total dose of 2.4–4.8 g. Treatment beyond 8 wk has not been studied (*Lialda*).
- *ER capsules:* 1.5 g/day PO (4 capsules) in the morning (*Apriso*).
- *CR capsules:* 1 g PO qid for a total daily dose of 4 g for up to 8 wk (*Pentasa*).
- *DR tablets:* 1.6 g/day PO in divided doses (*Asacol*).

Pediatric patients

Safety and efficacy not established.

M

Pharmacokinetics

Route	Onset	Peak
Oral	Varies	3–6 hr
Rectal	Slow	3–6 hr

Metabolism: $T_{1/2}$: 5–10 hr
Distribution: Crosses placenta; may enter breast milk
Excretion: Feces

Adverse effects

- **CNS:** *Headache, fatigue, malaise,* dizziness, asthenia, insomnia
- **GI:** *Abdominal pain, cramps, discomfort; gas; flatulence; nausea;* diarrhea, bloating, hemorrhoids, rectal pain, constipation
- **GU:** Urinary urgency, dysmenorrhea
- **Other:** *Flulike symptoms, fever, cold,* rash, back pain, hair loss, peripheral edema, pruritus

■ Nursing considerations

Assessment

- **History:** Hypersensitivity to mesalamine, salicylates, any component of the formulation; renal impairment; lactation, pregnancy
- **Physical:** T, hair status; reflexes, affect; abdominal examination, rectal examination; urinary output; renal function tests

Interventions

- Administer enemas as follows: Shake bottle well to ensure suspension is homogeneous. Remove protective applicator sheath; hold bottle at the neck to ensure that none of the dose is lost. Have patient lie on the left side (to facilitate migration of drug into the sigmoid colon) with the lower leg extended and the upper leg flexed forward. Knee-chest position can be used if more acceptable to the patient. Gently insert the application tip into the rectum pointing toward the umbilicus; steadily squeeze the bottle to discharge the medication. Patient must retain medication for approximately 8 hr.
- Administer rectal suppository as follows: Remove the foil wrapper; avoid excessive handling (suppository will melt at body temperature); insert completely into the rectum with pointed end first; have patient retain for 1–3 hr or longer.
- Caution patient not to chew tablet or capsule; swallow whole. Notify physician if intact tablets are found in the stool.
- Monitor patients with renal impairment for possible side effects.

Teaching points

- This drug may be given as a suspension enema, so the medication must be retained for approximately 8 hours; it is best given at bedtime to facilitate the retention; the effects of the drug are usually seen within 3–21 days, but a full course of therapy is about 6 weeks. (Review administration with patient and significant other.)
- Administer rectal suppository as follows: Remove the foil wrapper; avoid excessive handling (suppository will melt at body temperature); insert completely into the rectum with pointed end first; retain for 3 hours or longer; staining of clothing may occur, using a protective pad is suggested.
- Do not chew oral tablets or capsules; swallow whole. If intact tablets are seen in the stool, notify your health care provider.
- You may experience these side effects: Abdominal cramping, discomfort, pain, gas (relax; maintain the position used for insertion to relieve pressure on the abdomen); headache, fatigue, fever, flulike symptoms (request medication); hair loss (usually mild and transient).
- Report difficulty breathing, rash, severe abdominal pain, fever, headache.

▽ mesna

See Appendix X, *Less commonly used drugs.*

▽ metaproterenol sulfate

*(met a proe **ter'** e nole)*

PREGNANCY CATEGORY C

Drug classes

Antiasthmatic
$Beta_2$-selective adrenergic agonist
Bronchodilator
Sympathomimetic

Therapeutic actions

In low doses, acts relatively selectively at $beta_2$-adrenergic receptors to cause bronchodilation; at higher doses, $beta_2$ selectivity is lost and the drug also acts at $beta_1$ receptors to cause typical sympathomimetic cardiac effects.

Indications

- Prophylaxis and treatment of bronchial asthma and reversible bronchospasm that may occur with bronchitis and emphysema

Contraindications and cautions

- Contraindicated with hypersensitivity to metaproterenol; tachyarrhythmias, tachycardia caused by digitalis intoxication.
- Use cautiously with unstable vasomotor system disorders; hypertension; CAD; history of CVA; COPD in patients who have developed degenerative heart disease; hyperthyroidism; history of seizure disorders; psychoneurotic individuals; pregnancy; labor and delivery (may inhibit labor; parenteral use of $beta_2$-adrenergic agonists can accelerate fetal heartbeat, cause hypoglycemia, hypokalemia, and pulmonary edema in the mother and hypoglycemia in the neonate); lactation.

Available forms

Tablets—10, 20 mg; syrup—10 mg/5 mL

Dosages

Adults and children 12 yr and older

Oral

20 mg PO tid–qid.

Pediatric patients

Oral

Younger than 6 yr: Not recommended.

6–9 yr or weight less than 27 kg: 10 mg PO tid–qid.

Older than 9 yr or weight more than 27 kg: 20 mg PO tid–qid.

Geriatric patients

Patients older than 60 yr are more likely to develop side effects; use extreme caution.

Pharmacokinetics

Route	*Onset*	*Peak*	*Duration*
Oral	1 hr	2–3 hr	3–6 hr

Metabolism: Liver and tissue; $T_{1/2}$: Unknown
Excretion: Feces

Adverse effects

- **CNS:** *Restlessness, apprehension, anxiety, fear, CNS stimulation,* hyperkinesia, insomnia, tremor, drowsiness, irritability, weakness, vertigo, headache
- **CV:** Cardiac arrhythmias, *tachycardia,* palpitations, PVCs (rare), anginal pain—less likely with bronchodilator doses of this drug than with bronchodilator doses of a nonselective beta-agonist (isoproterenol), changes in BP
- **GI:** *Nausea, vomiting, heartburn,* unusual or bad taste in mouth
- **Respiratory:** Respiratory difficulties, pulmonary edema, coughing, **bronchospasm,** paradoxical airway resistance with repeated, excessive use of inhalation preparations
- **Other:** *Sweating, pallor, flushing*

■ Nursing considerations

Assessment

- **History:** Hypersensitivity to metaproterenol; tachyarrhythmias; unstable vasomotor system disorders; hypertension; CAD; CVA; COPD patients who have developed degenerative heart disease; hyperthyroidism; seizure disorders; psychoneuroses; pregnancy; labor; lactation
- **Physical:** Weight; skin color, T, turgor; orientation, reflexes; P, BP; R, adventitious sounds; blood and urine glucose, serum electrolytes, thyroid function tests, ECG

Interventions

- Use minimal doses for minimal periods–drug tolerance can occur with prolonged use.
- Switch to syrup if swallowing is difficult.

⊗ ***Warning*** Keep a beta-adrenergic blocker (a cardioselective beta-blocker such as atenolol should be used in patients with respiratory distress) readily available in case cardiac arrhythmias occur.

- Do not exceed recommended dosage.

Teaching points

- If taking tablets, protect from moisture.
- Do not exceed recommended dosage; adverse effects or loss of effectiveness may result.

M

Read product instructions and ask your health care provider or pharmacist if you have any questions.

- You may experience these side effects: Nausea, vomiting, change in taste (eat small frequent meals); dizziness, drowsiness, fatigue, weakness (use caution if driving or performing tasks that require alertness); irritability, apprehension, sweating, flushing.
- Report chest pain, dizziness, insomnia, weakness, tremor or irregular heartbeat, difficulty breathing, productive cough, failure to respond to usual dosage.

metaxalone

*(me **tax'** ah lone)*

Skelaxin

PREGNANCY CATEGORY C

Drug class

Skeletal muscle relaxant (centrally acting)

Therapeutic actions

Precise mechanism of action not known, but may be due to general CNS depression; does not directly relax tense skeletal muscles or directly affect the motor endplate or motor nerves.

Indications

- Adjunct to rest, physical therapy, and other measures for the relief of discomfort associated with acute, painful musculoskeletal disorders

Contraindications and cautions

- Contraindicated with hypersensitivity to metaxalone; tendency for hemolytic or other anemias; severe renal or hepatic impairment, lactation.
- Use cautiously with mild hepatic impairment, pregnancy.

Available forms

Tablets—800 mg

Dosages

Adults and patients 12 yr and older

800 mg PO tid–qid.

Pediatric patients younger than 12 yr

Not recommended.

Pharmacokinetics

Route	*Onset*	*Peak*	*Duration*
Oral	60 min	3 hr	4–6 hr

Metabolism: Hepatic; $T_{1/2}$: 2–4 hr
Distribution: Crosses placenta; may enter breast milk
Excretion: Urine

Adverse effects

- **CNS:** *Light-headedness, dizziness, drowsiness,* headache, fever, blurred vision
- **Dermatologic:** Urticaria, pruritus, rash
- **GI:** *Nausea,* vomiting, GI upset, hepatic impairment
- **Other: Hemolytic anemia, leukopenia**

Interactions

✱ **Drug-drug** • Increased risk of sedation with other CNS depressants and alcohol
✱ **Drug-lab test** • False-positive Benedict's test; use of a more specific glucose test is advised

■ Nursing considerations

Assessment

- **History:** Hypersensitivity to metaxalone; tendency for hemolytic or other anemias; severe renal or hepatic impairment; lactation, pregnancy
- **Physical:** T; skin color, lesions; orientation, affect, vision examination, reflexes; bowel sounds, normal output; CBC, LFTs, renal function tests

Interventions

- Establish safety precautions if dizziness, drowsiness, or blurred vision occurs (use side rails, accompany patient when ambulating).
- Arrange for analgesics if headache occurs (and possibly as adjunct for relief of discomfort of muscle spasm).
- Provide positioning, massage, and warm soaks as appropriate for relief of pain of muscle spasm.

- Provide support and encouragement to deal with discomfort of underlying condition and drug effects.

Teaching points

- Take this drug exactly as prescribed. Do not take a higher dosage than that prescribed.
- Continue the use of rest, physical therapy, and other measures to relieve the discomfort.
- Avoid the use of alcohol, sleep-inducing, or over-the-counter drugs while you are taking this drug. These could cause dangerous effects. If you feel that you need one of these preparations, consult your health care provider.
- You may experience these side effects: Drowsiness, dizziness (avoid driving a car or engaging in activities that require alertness if these occur); nausea (take drug with food and eat frequent small meals).
- Report rash, itching, yellow discoloration of the skin or eyes.

DANGEROUS DRUG

metformin hydrochloride

(met fore' min)

Apo-Metformin (CAN), CO Metformin Coated (CAN), Fortamet, Gen-Metformin (CAN), Glucophage, Glucophage XR (DNC), Glumetza (DNC), Metformin HCl ER (DNC), Nu-Metformin (CAN), PMS-Metformin (CAN), ratio-Metformin (CAN), Riomet

PREGNANCY CATEGORY B

Drug class

Antidiabetic

Therapeutic actions

Exact mechanism is not understood; possibly increases peripheral utilization of glucose, decreases hepatic glucose production, and alters intestinal absorption of glucose.

Indications

- Adjunct to diet to lower blood glucose with type 2 diabetes mellitus in patients 10 yr and older; ER in patients 17 yr and older; 18 yr and older for *Glumetza*
- As part of combination therapy with a sulfonylurea or insulin when either drug alone cannot control glucose levels in patients with type 2 diabetes mellitus
- Unlabeled uses: Treatment of anovulation in women with polycystic ovary syndrome; treatment of antipsychotic drug-induced weight gain

Contraindications and cautions

- Contraindicated with allergy to metformin; heart failure; diabetes complicated by fever, severe infections, severe trauma, major surgery, ketosis, acidosis, coma (use insulin); type 1 diabetes, serious hepatic impairment, serious renal impairment, uremia, thyroid or endocrine impairment, glycosuria, hyperglycemia associated with primary renal disease; labor and delivery (if metformin is used during pregnancy, discontinue drug at least 1 mo before delivery); lactation (safety not established).
- Use cautiously with the elderly.

Available forms

Tablets—500, 850, 1,000 mg; ER tablets (DNC)—500, 750, 1,000 mg; oral solution—500 mg/5 mL

Dosages

Adults

500 mg bid or 850 mg once daily PO. May increase 500 mg/wk or 850 mg/2 wk to maximum of 2,550 mg/day in divided doses. Dosage should be adjusted based on response and blood glucose level. ER tablet: Initially, 500 mg/day PO with evening meal; may be increased by 500 mg/wk to a maximum of 2,550 mg once daily.

Pediatric patients 10–16 yr

500 mg bid with meals. May increase 500 mg/wk to maximum of 2,000 mg/day in divided doses. ER tablet is not recommended.

Geriatric patients and patients with renal impairment

Smaller doses may be necessary; monitor closely and adjust slowly.

Pharmacokinetics

Route	*Peak*	*Duration*
Oral	2–2.5 hr	10–16 hr

M

Metabolism: $T_{1/2}$: 6.2 and 17.6 hr
Distribution: Crosses placenta; enters breast milk
Excretion: Urine

Adverse effects

- **Endocrine:** Hypoglycemia, **lactic acidosis**
- **GI:** *Anorexia, nausea,* vomiting, *epigastric discomfort, heartburn, diarrhea,* flatulence
- **Hypersensitivity:** *Allergic skin reactions,* eczema, pruritus, erythema, urticaria

Interactions

✱ **Drug-drug** • Increased risk of hypoglycemia with sulfonylureas, cimetidine, furosemide, cationic drugs such as digoxin, amiloride, vancomycin • Increased risk of lactic acidosis with ethanol • Increased risk of acute renal failure and lactic acidosis with iodinated contrast material used in radiologic studies; stop metformin at or before time of procedure and hold for 48 hr afterward

✱ **Drug-alternative therapy** • Increased risk of hypoglycemia if taken with juniper berries, ginseng, garlic, fenugreek, coriander, dandelion root, celery

■ Nursing considerations

Assessment

- **History:** Allergy to metformin; diabetes complicated by fever, severe infections, severe trauma, major surgery, ketosis, acidosis, coma; type 1 diabetes, serious hepatic or renal impairment, uremia, thyroid or endocrine impairment, glycosuria, hyperglycemia associated with primary renal disease; HF; pregnancy, lactation
- **Physical:** Skin color, lesions; T, orientation, reflexes, peripheral sensation; R, adventitious sounds; liver evaluation, bowel sounds; urinalysis, BUN, serum creatinine, LFTs, blood glucose, CBC

Interventions

⊗ ***Black box warning*** Risk of severe lactic acidosis; monitor patient, and treat any suspicion of lactic acidosis.

- Monitor urine or serum glucose levels frequently to determine effectiveness of drug and dosage.

⊗ ***Warning*** Arrange for transfer to insulin therapy during periods of high stress (infections, surgery, trauma).

⊗ ***Warning*** Use IV glucose if severe hypoglycemia occurs as a result of overdose.

Teaching points

- Do not discontinue this medication without consulting your health care provider.
- Monitor blood for glucose and ketones as prescribed.
- Swallow extended-release tablets whole; do not cut, crush, or chew.
- Do not use this drug during pregnancy; if you become pregnant, consult your health care provider for appropriate therapy.
- Avoid using alcohol while taking this drug.
- Report fever, sore throat, unusual bleeding or bruising, rash, dark urine, light-colored stools, hypoglycemic or hyperglycemic reactions.

DANGEROUS DRUG

▽ methadone hydrochloride

(meth' a done)

Dolophine, Methadone HCl Diskets, Methadone HCl Intensol, Methadose

PREGNANCY CATEGORY C

CONTROLLED SUBSTANCE C-II

Drug class

Opioid agonist analgesic

Therapeutic actions

Acts as agonist at specific opioid receptors in the CNS to produce analgesia, euphoria, sedation; the receptors mediating these effects are thought to be the same as those mediating the effects of endogenous opioids (enkephalins, endorphins); when used in approved methadone maintenance programs, can substitute for heroin, other illicit opioids in patients who want to terminate a drug use.

Indications

- Relief of severe pain not responsive to nonopioid analgesics

- Detoxification and temporary maintenance treatment of opioid addiction (ineffective for relief of general anxiety)

Contraindications and cautions

- Contraindicated with hypersensitivity to opioids, diarrhea caused by poisoning (before toxins are eliminated), bronchial asthma, COPD, cor pulmonale, respiratory depression, anoxia, kyphoscoliosis, acute alcoholism, increased intracranial pressure.
- Use cautiously with acute abdominal conditions, CV disease, supraventricular tachycardias, myxedema, seizure disorders, delirium tremens, cerebral arteriosclerosis, ulcerative colitis, fever, Addison's disease, prostatic hypertrophy, urethral stricture, recent GI or GU surgery, toxic psychosis, pregnancy before labor (crosses placenta; neonatal withdrawal observed in infants born to drug-using mothers; safety in pregnancy before labor not established), labor or delivery (administration of opioids to mother can cause respiratory depression of neonate—risk greatest for premature neonates), renal or hepatic impairment, lactation.

Available forms

Tablets—5, 10 mg; oral solution—5 mg/5 mL, 10 mg/5 mL; oral concentrate—10 mg/mL; injection—10 mg/mL; dispersible tablets—40 mg

Dosages

Oral methadone is approximately one-half as potent as parenteral methadone.

Adults

- *Relief of pain:* 2.5–10 mg IM, subcutaneously, or PO every 3–4 hr as necessary. IM route is preferred to subcutaneous for repeated doses (subcutaneous use may cause local irritation). Individualize dosage; patients with excessively severe pain and those who have become tolerant to the analgesic effect of opioids may need higher dosage.
- *Detoxification:* Initially 20–30 mg PO or parenteral; PO preferred. Increase dose to suppress withdrawal signs. 40 mg/day in single or divided doses is usually an adequate stabilizing dose for those physically dependent on high doses. Continue stabilizing doses for 2–3 days, then gradually decrease dosage every day or every 2 days. A daily reduction of 20% of the total dose may be tolerated. Provide sufficient dosage to keep withdrawal symptoms at tolerable level. Treatment should not exceed 21 days and may not be repeated earlier than 4 wk after completion of previous course. Detoxification treatment continued longer than 21 days becomes maintenance treatment, which may be undertaken only by approved programs (addicts hospitalized for other medical conditions may receive methadone maintenance treatment).
- *Maintenance treatment:* For patients who are heavy heroin users up until hospital admission, initial dose of 20 mg 4–8 hr after heroin is stopped or 40 mg in a single dose PO. For patients with little or no opioid tolerance, half this dose may suffice. Dosage should suppress withdrawal symptoms but not produce acute opioid effects of sedation, respiratory depression. Give additional 10-mg doses if needed to suppress withdrawal syndrome. Adjust dosage, up to 120 mg/day.

Pediatric patients

Not recommended for relief of pain in children due to insufficient documentation.

Geriatric patients or impaired adults

Use caution. Respiratory depression may occur in the elderly, the very ill, and those with respiratory problems. Reduced dosage may be necessary.

Pharmacokinetics

Route	Onset	Peak	Duration
Oral	30–60 min	1.5–2 hr	4–12 hr
IM	10–20 min	1–2 hr	4–8 hr
Subcut.	10–20 min	1–2 hr	4–8 hr

Metabolism: Hepatic; $T_{1/2}$: 25 hr
Distribution: Crosses placenta; enters breast milk
Excretion: Bile, feces, urine

Adverse effects

- **CNS:** *Light-headedness, dizziness, sedation,* euphoria, dysphoria, delirium, insomnia, agitation, anxiety, fear, hallucinations, disorientation, drowsiness, lethargy, impaired

M

mental and physical performance, coma, mood changes, weakness, headache, tremor, seizures, miosis, visual disturbances, suppression of cough reflex
- **CV:** Facial flushing, peripheral circulatory collapse, arrhythmia, palpitations, chest wall rigidity, hypertension, hypotension, orthostatic hypotension, syncope, prolonged QT interval
- **Dermatologic:** Pruritus, urticaria, laryngospasm, bronchospasm, edema, hemorrhagic urticaria (rare)
- **GI:** *Nausea, vomiting,* dry mouth, anorexia, constipation, biliary tract spasm; increased colonic motility in patients with chronic ulcerative colitis
- **GU:** Ureteral spasm, spasm of vesical sphincters, urine retention or hesitancy, oliguria, antidiuretic effect, reduced libido or potency
- **Local:** Tissue irritation and induration (subcutaneous injection)
- **Major hazards: Respiratory depression, apnea, circulatory depression, respiratory arrest, shock, cardiac arrest**
- **Other:** Sweating (more common in ambulatory patients and those without severe pain), physical tolerance and dependence, psychological dependence

Interactions

✱ **Drug-drug** • Potentiation of effects of methadone with barbiturate anesthetics—decrease dose of methadone when coadministering • Decreased effectiveness of methadone with hydantoins, rifampin, urinary acidifiers (ammonium chloride, potassium acid phosphate, sodium acid phosphate) • Numerous interactions with HIV antiretrovirals, especially protease inhibitors

✱ **Drug-lab test** • Elevated biliary tract pressure (opioid effect) may cause increases in plasma amylase, lipase; determinations of these levels may be unreliable for 24 hr after administration of opioids

■ Nursing considerations

Assessment

- **History:** Hypersensitivity to opioids, diarrhea caused by poisoning, bronchial asthma, COPD, cor pulmonale, respiratory depression, kyphoscoliosis, acute alcoholism, increased intracranial pressure; acute abdominal conditions, CV disease, supraventricular tachycardias, myxedema, seizure disorders, delirium tremens, cerebral arteriosclerosis, ulcerative colitis, fever, Addison's disease, prostatic hypertrophy, urethral stricture, recent GI or GU surgery, toxic psychosis; pregnancy; labor; lactation
- **Physical:** T; skin color, texture, lesions; orientation, reflexes, bilateral grip strength, affect, pupil size; pulse, auscultation, BP, orthostatic BP, perfusion; R, adventitious sounds; bowel sounds, normal output; frequency and pattern of voiding; ECG; EEG; LFTs, renal and thyroid function tests

Interventions

⊠ ***Black box warning*** Use for opioid addiction should be part of an approved program. Deaths have been reported during initiation of treatment for opioid dependence. Use care to determine all drugs patient is using, and keep emergency services on standby.

⊠ ***Black box warning*** Monitor patient for QT interval prolongation, especially at higher doses.

- Give to lactating women 4–6 hr before the next feeding to minimize the amount in milk.

⊗ ***Warning*** Keep opioid antagonist and equipment for assisted or controlled respiration readily available during parenteral administration.

⊗ ***Warning*** Use caution when injecting subcutaneously into chilled body areas or in patients with hypotension or in shock—impaired perfusion may delay absorption; with repeated doses, an excessive amount may be absorbed when circulation is restored.

Teaching points

- Take drug exactly as prescribed.
- Avoid alcohol—serious adverse effects may occur.
- Do not take leftover medication for other disorders; do not let anyone else take the prescription.
- Avoid pregnancy while taking this drug; using barrier contraceptives is advised.
- You may experience these side effects: Nausea, loss of appetite (take with food, lie

quietly, eat frequent small meals); constipation (laxative may help); dizziness, sedation, drowsiness, impaired visual acuity (avoid driving, performing other tasks that require alertness or visual acuity).
- Report severe nausea, vomiting, constipation, shortness of breath, or difficulty breathing.

methazolamide

See Appendix W, *Less commonly used drugs.*

methenamine
(meth en' a meen)

methenamine
Dehydral (CAN)

methenamine hippurate
Hiprex, Urex

PREGNANCY CATEGORY C

Drug classes
Antibacterial
Urinary tract anti-infective

Therapeutic actions
Hydrolyzed in acid urine to ammonia and formaldehyde, which is bactericidal; the hippurate and mandelate salts help to maintain an acid urine.

Indications
- Suppression or elimination of bacteriuria associated with pyelonephritis, cystitis, chronic UTIs, residual urine (accompanying some neurologic disorders), and in anatomic abnormalities of the urinary tract

Contraindications and cautions
- Contraindicated with allergy to methenamine, tartrazine (in methenamine hippurate marketed as *Hiprex*), aspirin (associated with tartrazine allergy), lactation.
- Use cautiously with hepatic or renal impairment, gout (causes urate crystals to precipitate in urine), pregnancy, severe dehydration.

Available forms
Tablets—1 g

Dosages
Adults

Methenamine
1 g qid PO after meals and at bedtime.

Methenamine hippurate
1 g bid PO.

Pediatric patients

Methenamine
Younger than 6 yr: 50 mg/kg/day PO divided into three doses.
6–12 yr: 500 mg qid PO.

Methenamine hippurate
6–12 yr: 0.5–1 g bid PO.
Older than 12 yr: 1 g bid PO.

Pharmacokinetics

Route	*Onset*	*Peak*
Oral	Rapid	30–90 min
Oral (hippurate)	Rapid	2 hr

Metabolism: Hepatic; $T_{1/2}$: 3–6 hr
Distribution: Crosses placenta; enters breast milk
Excretion: Urine

Adverse effects
- **Dermatologic:** Pruritus, urticaria, erythematous eruptions, rash
- **GI:** Nausea, abdominal cramps, vomiting, diarrhea, anorexia, stomatitis
- **GU:** *Bladder irritation, dysuria,* proteinuria, hematuria, frequency, urgency, crystalluria
- **Other:** Headache, dyspnea, generalized edema, elevated serum transaminase (with hippurate salt)

Interactions
✱ **Drug-lab test** • False increase in 17-hydroxycorticosteroids, catecholamines • False decrease in 5-HIAA • Inaccurate measurement of urine estriol levels by acid hydrolysis procedures during pregnancy

■ Nursing considerations
Assessment
- **History:** Allergy to methenamine, tartrazine, aspirin; renal or hepatic impairment; dehydration; gout; pregnancy, lactation

M

- **Physical:** Skin color, lesions; hydration; ear lobes—tophi; joints; liver evaluation; urinalysis, LFTs; serum uric acid

Interventions

- Arrange for culture and sensitivity tests before and during therapy.
- Administer drug with food to prevent GI upset; give drug around-the-clock for best effects.
- Ensure patient avoids foods and medications that alkalinize the urine.
- Ensure adequate hydration for patient.
- Monitor clinical response; if no improvement is seen or a relapse occurs, repeat urine culture and sensitivity tests.
- Monitor LFTs with methenamine hippurate.

Teaching points

- Take drug with food. Complete the full course of therapy to resolve the infection.
- Take this drug at regular intervals around-the-clock; develop a schedule with the help of your health care provider.
- Avoid alkalinizing foods: Citrus fruits, milk products; or alkalinizing medications (sodium bicarbonate).
- Review other medications with your health care provider.
- Drink plenty of fluids.
- You may experience these side effects: Nausea, vomiting, abdominal pain (eat frequent small meals); diarrhea; painful urination, frequency, blood in urine (drink plenty of fluids).
- Report rash, painful urination, severe GI upset.

methimazole

*(meth **im'** a zole)*

Northyx, Tapazole

PREGNANCY CATEGORY D

Drug class

Antithyroid drug

Therapeutic actions

Inhibits the synthesis of thyroid hormones.

Indications

- Treatment of hyperthyroidism

Contraindications and cautions

- Contraindicated with allergy to antithyroid products, pregnancy (use only if absolutely necessary and when mother has been informed about potential harm to the fetus; if an antithyroid drug is required, propylthiouracil is the drug of choice), lactation.
- Use cautiously with bone marrow depression.

Available forms

Tablets—5, 10, 15, 20 mg

Dosages

Adults

Initial dose, 15–60 mg/day PO in three equal doses every 8 hr. Maintenance dose, 5–15 mg/day PO.

Pediatric patients

Initially, give 0.4 mg/kg/day PO, followed by maintenance dose of approximately one-half the initial dose; actual dose is determined by the patient's response. Alternatively, give initial dose of 0.5–0.7 mg/kg/day or 15–20 mg/m^2/day PO in three divided doses, followed by maintenance dose of one-third to two-thirds of initial dose, starting when patient becomes euthyroid. Maximum dose is 30 mg/24 hr.

Pharmacokinetics

Route	Onset	Peak	Duration
Oral	30–40 min	60 min	2–4 hr

Metabolism: $T_{1/2}$: 6–13 hr
Distribution: Crosses placenta; enters breast milk
Excretion: Urine

Adverse effects

- **CNS:** *Paresthesias, neuritis,* vertigo, drowsiness, neuropathies, depression, headache
- **Dermatologic:** *Rash,* urticaria, pruritus, skin pigmentation, exfoliative dermatitis, lupuslike syndrome, loss of hair
- **GI:** Nausea, vomiting, epigastric distress, loss of taste, sialadenopathy, jaundice, hepatitis
- **GU:** Nephritis

- **Hematologic:** *Agranulocytosis, granulocytopenia, thrombocytopenia, hypoprothrombinemia, bleeding,* vasculitis, periarteritis
- **Other:** Arthralgia, myalgia, edema, lymphadenopathy, drug fever

Interactions

✱ **Drug-drug** • Increased theophylline clearance and decreased effectiveness if given to hyperthyroid patients; clearance will change as patient approaches euthyroid state • Altered effects of oral anticoagulants with methimazole • Increased therapeutic effects and toxicity of cardiac glycosides, metoprolol, propranolol when hyperthyroid patients become euthyroid

■ Nursing considerations

Assessment

- **History:** Allergy to antithyroid products; pregnancy, lactation
- **Physical:** Skin color, lesions, pigmentation; orientation, reflexes, affect; liver evaluation; CBC, differential, PT, LFTs, renal function tests

Interventions

- Give drug in three equally divided doses at 8-hr intervals; try to schedule to allow patient to sleep at his or her regular time.
- Obtain regular, periodic blood tests to monitor bone marrow depression and bleeding tendencies.
- Advise medical and surgical personnel that patient is taking this drug, which increases the risk of bleeding problems.
- Ensure patient is not pregnant before giving this drug; advise patient to use barrier contraceptives.

Teaching points

- Take this drug around-the-clock at 8-hour intervals. Establish a schedule, with the aid of your health care provider, which fits your routine.
- This drug will need to be taken for a prolonged period to achieve the desired effects.
- Using barrier contraceptives is advised while taking this drug; serious fetal abnormalities may occur.
- If you are nursing a baby, another method of feeding the baby should be used.
- You may experience these side effects: Dizziness, weakness, vertigo, drowsiness (use caution driving or operating dangerous machinery); nausea, vomiting, loss of appetite (eat frequent small meals); rash, itching.
- Report fever, sore throat, unusual bleeding or bruising, headache, general malaise.

▽ methocarbamol

*(meth oh **kar'** ba mole)*

Robaxin, Robaxin-750

PREGNANCY CATEGORY C

Drug class

Skeletal muscle relaxant (centrally acting)

Therapeutic actions

Precise mechanism of action not known but may be due to general CNS depression; does not directly relax tense skeletal muscles or directly affect the motor end plate or motor nerves.

Indications

- Relief of discomfort associated with acute, painful musculoskeletal conditions, as an adjunct to rest, physical therapy, and other measures
- Control of neuromuscular manifestations of tetanus

Contraindications and cautions

- Contraindicated with hypersensitivity to methocarbamol; known or suspected renal pathology (parenteral methocarbamol is contraindicated because of polyethylene glycol 300 in vehicle).
- Use cautiously in patients with epilepsy, pregnancy, lactation.

Available forms

Tablets—500, 750 mg; injection—100 mg/mL

Dosages

Adults

Oral

Initially, 1.5 g qid PO. For the first 48–72 hr, 6 g/day or up to 8 g/day is recommended. For maintenance, 1 g qid or 750 mg every 4 hr PO or 1.5 g tid for total dosage of 4–4.5 g/day.

M

- *Tetanus:* Up to 24 g/day may be needed.

Parenteral

1 g IM or IV; 2–3 g may be needed in severe cases. Do not exceed 3 g for longer than 3 days except when treating tetanus.

Pediatric patients

Oral

Not recommended.

Parenteral

- *Tetanus:* 15 mg/kg IV, repeated every 6 hr as needed.

Pharmacokinetics

Route	*Onset*	*Peak*
Oral	30 min	2 hr
IM/IV	Unknown	Unknown

Metabolism: Hepatic; $T_{1/2}$: 1–2 hr
Distribution: Crosses placenta; may enter breast milk
Excretion: Feces, urine

IV FACTS

Preparation: Administer undiluted, as provided.
Infusion: Administer at maximum rate of 3 mL/min. May dilute 1 vial in no more than 250 mL sodium chloride injection or 5% dextrose solution. For tetanus, inject 1–2 g directly into IV tubing; add 1–2 g to infusion bottle for total dose of 3 g or less. May repeat every 6 hr.

Adverse effects

- **CNS:** *Light-headedness, dizziness, drowsiness,* headache, fever, blurred vision
- **CV:** Bradycardia, flushing, hypotension, syncope
- **Dermatologic:** *Urticaria,* pruritus, rash
- **GI:** *Nausea,* vomiting, dyspepsia
- **Other:** Conjunctivitis with nasal congestion

Interactions

✱ **Drug-lab test** • May cause interference with color reactions in tests for 5-HIAA and vanillylmandelic acid

■ Nursing considerations

Assessment

- **History:** Hypersensitivity to methocarbamol; known or suspected renal pathology, epilepsy (use caution with parenteral administration), pregnancy, lactation
- **Physical:** T; skin color, lesions; nasal mucous membranes, conjunctival examination; orientation, affect, vision examination, reflexes; P, BP; bowel sounds, normal output; urinalysis, renal function tests

Interventions

- Do not exceed 3 g total dosage for longer than 3 days except when treating tetanus.
- Have patient remain recumbent during and for at least 15 min after IV injection.
- For IM use, do not inject more than 5 mL into each gluteal region; repeat at 8-hr intervals.
- Switch from parenteral to oral route as soon as possible.
- Ensure patient is not pregnant before use; use in pregnancy only if benefits clearly outweigh risk to the fetus.
- Patient's urine may darken on standing.

Teaching points

- Take this drug exactly as prescribed. Do not take a higher dosage than prescribed, and do not take it longer than prescribed.
- Avoid alcohol, sleep-inducing, or over-the-counter drugs; these could cause dangerous effects.
- Your urine may darken to a brown, black, or green color on standing.
- You may experience these side effects: Drowsiness, dizziness, blurred vision (avoid driving or engaging in activities that require alertness); nausea (take with food, eat frequent small meals).
- Report rash, itching, fever, or nasal congestion.

DANGEROUS DRUG

▽ methotrexate (amethopterin, MTX)

*(meth oh **trex'** ate)*

ratio-Methotrexate (CAN), Rheumatrex, Rheumatrex Dose Pack, Trexall

PREGNANCY CATEGORY X

Drug classes
Antimetabolite
Antineoplastic
Antipsoriatic
Antirheumatic

Therapeutic actions
Inhibits dihydrofolic acid reductase, leading to inhibition of DNA synthesis and inhibition of cellular replication; selectively affects the most rapidly dividing cells (neoplastic and psoriatic cells).

Indications
- Treatment of gestational choriocarcinoma, chorioadenoma destruens, hydatidiform mole
- Treatment and prophylaxis of meningeal leukemia, mycosis fungoides
- Symptomatic control of severe, recalcitrant, disabling psoriasis
- Management of severe, active, classical, or definite rheumatoid arthritis
- Management of polyarticular course juvenile rheumatoid arthritis
- High-dose regimen followed by leucovorin rescue for adjuvant therapy of nonmetastatic osteosarcoma (orphan drug designation)
- Unlabeled uses: To reduce corticosteroid requirements in patients with severe corticosteroid-dependent asthma; as a maintenance regimen for Wegener's agranulomatosis, dermatomyositis, relapsing-remitting MS, myositis, ulcerative colitis, refractory Crohn's disease, uveitis, SLE, psoriatic arthritis

Contraindications and cautions
- Contraindicated with pregnancy, lactation, alcoholism, chronic liver disease, immune deficiencies, blood dyscrasias, hypersensitivity to methotrexate.
- Use cautiously with renal disease, infection, peptic ulcer, ulcerative colitis, debility.

Available forms
Tablets—2.5, 5, 7.5, 10, 15 mg; powder for injection—20 mg, 1 g per vial; injection—25 mg/mL

Dosages
Adults
- *Choriocarcinoma and other trophoblastic diseases:* 15–30 mg PO or IM daily for a 5-day course. Repeat courses three to five times with rest periods of 1 wk or longer between courses until toxic symptoms subside. Continue one to two courses of methotrexate after chorionic gonadotropin hormone levels are normal.
- *Leukemia:* Induction: 3.3 mg/m^2 of methotrexate PO or IM with 60 mg/m^2 of prednisone daily for 4–6 wk. Maintenance: 30 mg/m^2 methotrexate PO or IM twice weekly or 2.5 mg/kg IV every 14 days. If relapse occurs, return to induction doses.
- *Meningeal leukemia:* Give methotrexate intrathecally in cases of lymphocytic leukemia as prophylaxis. 12 mg/m^2 intrathecally at intervals of 2–5 days and repeat until cell count of CSF is normal.
- *Lymphomas:* Burkitt's tumor, stages I and II: 10–25 mg/day PO for 4–8 days. In stage III, combine with other neoplastic drugs. All usually require several courses of therapy with 7- to 10-day rest periods between doses.
- *Mycosis fungoides:* 2.5–10 mg/day PO for weeks or months or 50 mg IM once weekly or 25 mg IM twice weekly. Alternatively, in early stage, 5–50 mg PO or IM once weekly, or 15–37.5 mg PO or IM twice weekly; can also give IV with combination chemotherapy regimens in advanced disease.
- *Osteosarcoma:* Starting dose is 12 g/m^2 or up to 15 g/m^2 IV to give a peak serum concentration of 1,000 micromol. Must be used as part of a cytotoxic regimen with leucovorin rescue.
- *Severe psoriasis:* 10–25 mg/wk PO, IM, or IV as a single weekly dose. Do not exceed 30 mg/wk. Or 2.5 mg PO at 12-hr intervals for three doses each wk. Do not exceed 30 mg/wk. After optimal clinical response is achieved, reduce dosage to lowest possible with longest rest periods and consider return to conventional, topical therapy.
- *Severe rheumatoid arthritis:* Starting dose: Single doses of 7.5 mg/wk PO or divided dosage of 2.5 mg PO at 12-hr intervals for three doses given as a course once weekly. Dosage may be gradually increased, based on response. Do not exceed 20 mg/wk. Therapeutic response usually begins within 3–6 wk, and improvement may continue for another 12 wk. Improvement may

M

be maintained for up to 2 yr with continued therapy.

Pediatric patients

- *Meningeal leukemia:*
  Younger than 1 yr: 6 mg intrathecally every 2–5 days.
  1–2 yr: 8 mg intrathecally every 2–5 days.
  2–3 yr: 10 mg intrathecally every 2–5 days.
  3 yr or older: 12 mg intrathecally every 2–5 days.
- *Polyarticular course juvenile rheumatoid arthritis (2–16 yr):* Initially, 10 mg/m² PO weekly. Dosage may be increased based on patient response. Maximum 20 mg/m²/wk. Therapeutic response usually begins in 3–6 wk.

Pharmacokinetics

Route	*Onset*	*Peak*
Oral	Varies	1–2 hr
IM, IV	Rapid	0.5–1 hr

Metabolism: $T_{1/2}$: 3–15 hr
Distribution: Crosses placenta; enters breast milk
Excretion: Urine

IV FACTS

Preparation: Reconstitute 20-mg vials with an appropriate sterile preservative-free medium, 5% dextrose solution, or sodium chloride injection to a concentration no greater than 25 mg/mL; reconstitute 1-g vial with 19.4 mL to a concentration of 50 mg/mL.
Infusion: Administer diluted drug by direct IV injection at a rate of not more than 10 mg/min. ⊗ ***Warning*** Do not give formulations with benzyl alcohol or preservatives intrathecally or for high-dose therapy.
Incompatibilities: Do not combine with bleomycin, prednisolone.
Y-site incompatibility: Do not give with droperidol.

Adverse effects

- **CNS:** Headache, drowsiness, blurred vision, aphasia, hemiparesis, paresis, seizures, *fatigue, malaise, dizziness*
- **Dermatologic:** *Erythematous rashes,* pruritus, urticaria, photosensitivity, depigmentation, *alopecia,* ecchymosis, telangiectasia, acne, furunculosis
- **GI:** *Ulcerative stomatitis,* gingivitis, pharyngitis, anorexia, *nausea,* vomiting, diarrhea, hematemesis, melena, GI ulceration and bleeding, enteritis, **hepatic toxicity**
- **GU:** Renal failure, *effects on fertility* (defective oogenesis, defective spermatogenesis, transient oligospermia, menstrual dysfunction, infertility, abortion, fetal defects)
- **Hematologic: Severe bone marrow depression,** *increased susceptibility to infection*
- **Hypersensitivity: Anaphylaxis, sudden death**
- **Respiratory: Interstitial pneumonitis,** chronic interstitial obstructive pulmonary disease
- **Other:** *Chills and fever,* metabolic changes (diabetes, osteoporosis), cancer

Interactions

✷ **Drug-drug** ⊗ ***Warning*** Potentially serious to fatal reactions when given with NSAIDs; use extreme caution if this combination is used.
⊗ ***Warning*** Risk of toxicity if combined with alcohol; avoid this combination.
• Increased risk of toxicity with salicylates, phenytoin, probenecid, sulfonamides • Decreased serum levels and therapeutic effects of digoxin • May decrease theophylline clearance

■ Nursing considerations

Assessment

- **History:** Allergy to methotrexate, hematopoietic depression, severe hepatic or renal disease, infection, peptic ulcer, ulcerative colitis, debility, psoriasis, pregnancy, lactation
- **Physical:** Weight; T; skin lesions, color; hair; vision, speech, orientation, reflexes, sensation; R, adventitious sounds; mucous membranes, liver evaluation, abdominal examination; CBC, differential; LFTS, renal function tests; urinalysis, blood and urine glucose, glucose tolerance test, chest X-ray

Interventions

⊗ ***Black box warning*** Arrange for tests to evaluate CBC, urinalysis, renal and liver function tests, and chest X-ray before therapy, during therapy, and for several weeks after therapy; severe toxicity could occur.

⊗ **Black box warning** Ensure that patient is not pregnant before administering this drug; counsel patient about the severe risks of fetal abnormalities associated with this drug.

⊗ **Warning** Reduce dosage or discontinue if renal failure occurs.

- Reconstitute powder for intrathecal use with preservative-free sterile sodium chloride injection; intended for one dose only; discard remainder. The solution for injection contains benzyl alcohol and should not be given intrathecally.

⊗ **Warning** Arrange to have leucovorin or levoleucovorin readily available as antidote for methotrexate overdose or when large doses are used. In general, doses of leucovorin (calcium leucovorin or levoleucovorin) should be equal or higher than doses of methotrexate and should be given within the first hour. Up to 75 mg IV within 12 hr, followed by 12 mg IM every 6 hr for four doses. For average doses of methotrexate that cause adverse effects, give 6–12 mg leucovorin IM, every 6 hr for four doses or 10 mg/m^2 PO followed by 10 mg/m^2 every 6 hr for 72 hr.

- Arrange for an antiemetic if nausea and vomiting are severe.
- Arrange for adequate hydration during therapy to reduce the risk of hyperuricemia.
- Do not administer any other medications containing alcohol.

Teaching points

- Prepare a calendar of treatment days.
- This drug may cause birth defects or miscarriages. Use birth control while taking this drug and for 3 months thereafter. Men using this drug should also use barrier contraceptives.
- Avoid alcohol and NSAIDs; serious side effects may occur.
- Arrange for frequent, regular medical follow-up visits, including blood tests to follow the drug's effects.
- You may experience these side effects: Nausea, vomiting (request medication; eat frequent small meals); numbness, tingling, dizziness, drowsiness, blurred vision, difficulty speaking (drug effects; seek dosage adjustment; avoid driving or operating dangerous machinery); mouth sores (frequent mouth care is needed); infertility; loss of hair (obtain a wig or other suitable head covering; keep the head covered at extremes of temperature); rash, sensitivity to sun and ultraviolet light (avoid sun; use a sunscreen and protective clothing).
- Report black, tarry stools; fever; chills; sore throat; unusual bleeding or bruising; cough or shortness of breath; darkened or bloody urine; abdominal, flank, or joint pain; yellow color to the skin or eyes; mouth sores.

▽ methoxsalen

See Appendix W, *Less commonly used drugs.*

▽ methoxy polyethylene glycol–epoetin beta

*(meth **oks'** ee polly **eth'** ah leen gleye' kol eh poe **eh'** tin **bay'** tah)*

Mircera

PREGNANCY CATEGORY C

M

Drug class

Erythropoiesis stimulator

Therapeutic actions

An erythropoietin receptor activator with a longer half-life than natural erythropoietin; stimulates RBC production in bone marrow in the same manner as natural erythropoietin, a hormone released into bloodstream in response to renal hypoxia.

Indications

- Management of anemia associated with chronic renal failure (not chemotherapy) in adults, including those receiving and not receiving dialysis

Contraindications and cautions

- Contraindicated with known hypersensitivity to any component of this drug or drugs in this class; uncontrolled hypertension; anemia caused by cancer chemotherapy.
- Use cautiously with hypertension, history of seizures, pregnancy, lactation.

Available forms
Single-use vials—50, 100, 200, 300, 400, 600, 1,000 mcg/mL; prefilled syringes—50, 75, 100, 150, 200, 250 mcg/0.3 mL; 400, 600, 800 mcg/0.6 mL

Dosages
Adults
Initially, 0.6 mcg/kg once every 2 wk by subcutaneous or IV injection; dosage should be adjusted to keep hemoglobin at 10–12 g/dL. Once hemoglobin has been maintained, drug may be given once monthly using twice the dose given every 2 wk.
Patients being treated with other erythropoiesis stimulators
See table below.

Pharmacokinetics

Route	*Onset*	*Peak*
IV	Slow	48 hr
Subcut.	Slow	72 hr

Metabolism: $T_{1/2}$: 134 +/- 65 hr (IV); 139 +/- 67 hr (subcutaneous)
Distribution: May cross placenta; may enter breast milk
Excretion: Urine

IV FACTS
Preparation: Administer as provided; no additional preparation is required. Enter vial only once, and discard used solution. Refrigerate vial. Do not shake vial. Inspect for discoloration or particulate matter before use.
Injection: Administer by direct IV injection or into the tubing of a running IV.
Incompatibilities: Do not mix with or add to solutions containing any other drugs.

Adverse effects
- **CNS:** *Headache, fatigue,* asthenia, dizziness, **seizures**
- **CV:** *Hypertension,* hypotension, **serious CV events, thromboembolic events, septic shock**
- **GI:** *Diarrhea,* vomiting, constipation
- **Respiratory:** *Nasopharyngitis, URI*
- **Other: Increased mortality and tumor progression in patient with cancer, pure red cell aplasia with anti-erythropoietin antibodies,** injection site reactions

■ Nursing considerations
Assessment
- **History:** Hypersensitivity to methoxy polyethylene glycol—epoetin beta or any drugs of this class, hypertension, history of seizures, pregnancy, lactation
- **Physical:** Reflexes, affect, BP, P, R, adventitious sounds, urinary output, renal function tests, CBC, Hct, hemoglobin, electrolytes

Interventions
⊗ ***Black box warning*** There is increased risk of death and serious CV and thromboembolic events when patients receiving erythropoiesis stimulating agents have a target Hgb level exceeding 12 g/dL; target dosage to maintain Hgb level between 10 and 12 g/dL.
⊗ ***Black box warning*** There is increased risk of death and tumor progression if this drug is used for anemia secondary to cancer chemotherapy. It is not indicated for this use.
- Store vials in the refrigerator or at room temperature for up to 7 days; prefilled syringes may be kept at room temperature for up to 30 days, protected from light.
- Do not shake vials or syringes. Inspect solution. Do not use if color changes or particulate matter appears.
- Rotate sites, if giving subcutaneous injections, to prevent injection site irritation.

Weekly epoetin alfa dose (units)	*Weekly darbepoetin alfa dose (mcg)*	*Monthly methoxy polyethylene glycol–epoetin beta dose (mcg)*	*Every-2-wk methoxy polyethylene glycol–epoetin beta dose (mcg)*
Less than 8,000	Less than 40	120	60
8,000–16,000	40–80	200	100
More than 16,000	More than 80	360	180

- Target dose to achieve a Hgb level between 10 and 12 g/dL. If patient does not respond to drug within 4 wk, evaluate cause of anemia.
- Evaluate iron stores before and periodically during therapy; supplemental iron may be needed.
- Monitor patient for sudden loss of response and severe anemia with low reticulocyte count; withhold drug and check patient for anti-erythropoietin antibodies. If antibodies are present, discontinue drug permanently and do not switch to another erythropoiesis stimulating agent; cross sensitivity can occur.
- Establish safety precautions (e.g., side rails, environmental control, lighting) if CNS effects occur.
- Maintain seizure precautions during administration.
- Provide additional comfort measures as necessary to alleviate discomfort from GI effects, headache.
- Offer support and encouragement to deal with chronic disease and need for prolonged therapy and testing.

Teaching points

- This drug is given once every 2 weeks by IV or subcutaneous injection. Mark your calendar for treatment days. After your response to the drug has stabilized, you may receive the drug once monthly.
- You and a significant other should learn to prepare and administer the drug by subcutaneous injection. Rotate injection sites to prevent irritation. Dispose of syringes and needles in an appropriate disposal box.
- Store vials in the refrigerator, protected from light; if using prefilled syringes, they may be kept at room temperature, protected from light, for up to 30 days.
- Do not shake the vial or syringe; inspect the solution to make sure it has not changed color and that it contains no particles in the solution.
- If you miss a dose, administer it as soon as you remember and then return to the usual dose schedule. If you miss two doses, contact your health care provider.
- Your health care provider will follow your body's response to this drug carefully with regular blood tests. Your hemoglobin should be 10–12 g/dL.
- It is not known how this drug could affect a fetus; if you are pregnant or decide to become pregnant while on this drug, consult your health care provider.
- It is not known how this drug could affect a nursing baby. If you are nursing a baby, discuss this with your health care provider.
- You may experience these side effects: Headache (consult your health care provider because medication may be available to help); nausea (frequent small meals may help); diarrhea (if this becomes severe, contact your health care provider immediately); irritation and inflammation at the injection site.
- Report trouble breathing, chest pain, sudden confusion or trouble speaking, trouble seeing, trouble walking, sudden severe headache, sudden numbness or weakness, loss of consciousness.

▽ methscopolamine bromide

*(meth skoe **pol'** a meen)*

Pamine, Pamine Forte

PREGNANCY CATEGORY C

Drug classes

Anticholinergic
Antimuscarinic
Antispasmodic
Parasympatholytic

Therapeutic actions

Competitively blocks the effects of acetylcholine at muscarinic cholinergic receptors that mediate the effects of parasympathetic postganglionic impulses, relaxing the GI tract and inhibiting gastric acid secretion.

Indications

- Adjunctive therapy in the treatment of peptic ulcer

Contraindications and cautions

- Contraindicated with known hypersensitivity to the drug; glaucoma; adhesions between

M

iris and lens; stenosing peptic ulcer, pyloroduodenal obstruction, paralytic ileus, intestinal atony, severe ulcerative colitis, toxic megacolon, symptomatic prostatic hypertrophy, bladder neck obstruction; bronchial asthma, COPD; cardiac arrhythmias, myocardial ischemia; sensitivity to anticholinergic drugs, bromides, tartrazine (tartrazine sensitivity is more common with allergy to aspirin); impaired metabolic, liver, or renal function; myasthenia gravis.
- Use cautiously with hypertension, hyperthyroidism, pregnancy, lactation.

Available forms
Tablets—2.5, 5 mg

Dosages
Adults
2.5 mg PO 30 min before meals and 2.5–5 mg PO at bedtime.

Pediatric patients
Safety and efficacy not established.

Pharmacokinetics

Route	*Onset*	*Duration*
Oral	1 hr	4–6 hr

Metabolism: Hepatic; $T_{1/2}$: 2–3 hr
Distribution: Crosses placenta; may enter breast milk
Excretion: Bile, urine

Adverse effects
- **CNS:** *Blurred vision,* mydriasis, cycloplegia, photophobia, increased IOP
- **CV:** Palpitations, tachycardia
- **GI:** *Dry mouth, altered taste perception, nausea, vomiting, dysphagia,* heartburn, constipation, bloated feeling, paralytic ileus, gastroesophageal reflux
- **GU:** *Urinary hesitancy and retention;* impotence
- **Other:** Decreased sweating and predisposition to heat prostration, suppression of lactation, nasal congestion, xerostomia

Interactions
✱ **Drug-drug** • Decreased antipsychotic effectiveness of haloperidol with anticholinergic drugs

■ Nursing considerations
Assessment
- **History:** Hypersensitivity to methscopolamine; glaucoma, adhesions between iris and lens; stenosing peptic ulcer, pyloroduodenal obstruction, paralytic ileus, intestinal atony, severe ulcerative colitis, toxic megacolon, symptomatic prostatic hypertrophy, bladder neck obstruction; bronchial asthma, COPD; cardiac arrhythmias, myocardial ischemia; sensitivity to anticholinergic drugs, bromides, tartrazine, impaired metabolic, liver, or renal function; myasthenia gravis; hypertension; hyperthyroidism; pregnancy; lactation
- **Physical:** Bowel sounds, normal output; urinary output, prostate palpation; R; adventitious sounds; P, BP; IOP, vision; bilateral grip strength, reflexes; liver palpation, LFTs, renal function tests; skin color, lesions, texture

Interventions
- Ensure adequate hydration; control environment (temperature) to prevent hyperpyrexia.
- Encourage patient to void before each dose of medication if urine retention becomes a problem.

Teaching points
- Take drug exactly as prescribed.
- Avoid hot environments (you will be heat intolerant, and dangerous reactions may occur).
- You may experience these side effects: Constipation (ensure adequate fluid intake, proper diet); dry mouth (suck sugarless lozenges, use frequent mouth care); blurred vision, sensitivity to light (avoid tasks that require acute vision; wear sunglasses when in bright light); impotence (reversible); difficulty with urination (empty bladder immediately before taking dose).
- Report rash, flushing, eye pain, difficulty breathing, tremors, loss of coordination, irregular heartbeat, palpitations, headache, abdominal distention, hallucinations, severe or persistent dry mouth, difficulty swallowing, difficulty in urination, severe constipation, sensitivity to light.

methsuximide

See Appendix X, *Less commonly used drugs.*

methyclothiazide

*(meth i kloe **thye'** a zide)*

Enduron

PREGNANCY CATEGORY B

Drug class

Thiazide diuretic

Therapeutic actions

Inhibits reabsorption of sodium and chloride in distal renal tubule, thereby increasing excretion of sodium, chloride, and water by the kidney.

Indications

- Adjunctive therapy in edema associated with heart failure, cirrhosis, corticosteroid and estrogen therapy, renal impairment
- Hypertension, as sole therapy or in combination with other antihypertensives

Contraindications and cautions

- Contraindicated with hypersensitivity to thiazides.
- Use cautiously with fluid or electrolyte imbalances, renal or liver disease, gout, SLE, glucose tolerance abnormalities, hyperparathyroidism.

Available forms

Tablets—2.5, 5 mg

Dosages

Adults

- *Edema:* 2.5–10 mg daily PO. Maximum single dose is 10 mg.
- *Hypertension:* 2.5–5 mg daily PO. If BP is not controlled by 5 mg daily within 8–12 wk, another antihypertensive may be needed.

Pharmacokinetics

Route	Onset	Peak	Duration
Oral	2 hr	6 hr	24 hr

Metabolism: $T_{1/2}$: Unknown

Distribution: Crosses placenta; enters breast milk

Excretion: Urine

Adverse effects

- **CNS:** *Dizziness, vertigo,* paresthesias, weakness, headache, drowsiness, fatigue
- **CV:** Orthostatic hypotension, volume depletion
- **Dermatologic:** Photosensitivity, rash, purpura, hives
- **GI:** *Nausea, anorexia, vomiting, dry mouth,* diarrhea, constipation, jaundice
- **GU:** *Polyuria, nocturia*
- **Hematologic:** Leukopenia, thrombocytopenia, agranulocytosis, aplastic anemia, neutropenia
- **Other:** Muscle cramp, hyperglycemia, hyperuricemia, electrolyte imbalance

Interactions

✱ **Drug-drug** • Risk of hyperglycemia with diazoxide • Decreased absorption with cholestyramine, colestipol • Increased risk of digoxin toxicity if hypokalemia occurs • Increased risk of lithium toxicity when taken with thiazides • Increased fasting blood glucose leading to need to adjust dosage of antidiabetics

✱ **Drug-lab test** • Decreased PBI levels without clinical signs of thyroid disturbances

■ Nursing considerations

Assessment

- **History:** Fluid or electrolyte imbalances, renal or liver disease, gout, SLE, glucose tolerance abnormalities, hyperparathyroidism, bipolar disorders, pregnancy, lactation
- **Physical:** Skin color and lesions; orientation, reflexes, muscle strength; pulses, BP, orthostatic BP, perfusion, edema, baseline ECG; R, adventitious sounds; liver evaluation, bowel sounds; CBC, serum electrolytes, blood glucose, LFTs, renal function tests, serum uric acid, urinalysis

Interventions

- Give with food or milk if GI upset occurs.
- Administer early in the day so increased urination will not disturb sleep.
- Measure and record regular body weights to monitor fluid changes.

Teaching points

- Take drug early in the day so sleep will not be disturbed by increased urination.
- Weigh yourself daily, and record weight on a calendar.
- Protect skin from exposure to sun or bright lights (sensitivity may occur).
- Increased urination will occur.
- Use caution if you feel dizzy, drowsy, or faint.
- Report rapid weight change, swelling in ankles or fingers, unusual bleeding or bruising, muscle cramps.

▽methyldopa

(meth ill doe' pa)

methyldopa

Apo-Methyldopa (CAN)

methyldopate hydrochloride

PREGNANCY CATEGORY B (ORAL)

PREGNANCY CATEGORY C (IV)

Drug classes

Antihypertensive

Sympatholytic (centrally acting)

Therapeutic actions

Mechanism of action not conclusively demonstrated; probably due to drug's metabolism, which lowers arterial BP by stimulating CNS $alpha_2$-adrenergic receptors, which in turn decreases sympathetic outflow from the CNS.

Indications

- Hypertension
- IV methyldopate: Acute hypertensive crisis; not drug of choice because of slow onset of action
- Unlabeled use: Hypertension of pregnancy

Contraindications and cautions

- Contraindicated with hypersensitivity to methyldopa, active hepatic disease, previous methyldopa therapy associated with liver disorders.
- Use cautiously with previous liver disease, renal failure, dialysis, bilateral cerebrovascular disease, pregnancy, lactation.

Available forms

Tablets—250, 500 mg; injection—50 mg/mL

Dosages

Adults

Oral therapy (methyldopa)

- *Initial therapy:* 250 mg bid–tid in the first 48 hr. Adjust dosage at minimum intervals of at least 2 days until response is adequate. Increase dosage in the evening to minimize sedation. For maintenance, 500 mg–2 g/day in two to four doses. Usually given in two doses; some patients may be controlled with a single dose at bedtime.
- *Concomitant therapy:* With antihypertensives other than thiazides, limit initial dosage to 500 mg/day in divided doses. When added to a thiazide, dosage of thiazide need not be changed.

IV therapy (methyldopate)

250–500 mg every 6 hr as required (maximum 1 g every 6 hr). Switch to oral therapy as soon as control is attained; use the dosage schedule used for parenteral therapy.

Pediatric patients

Oral therapy (methyldopa)

Individualize dosage; initial dosage is based on 10 mg/kg/day in two to four doses. Maximum dosage is 65 mg/kg/day or 3 g/day, whichever is less.

IV therapy (methyldopate)

20–40 mg/kg/day in divided doses every 6 hr. Maximum dosage is 65 mg/kg or 3 g/day, whichever is less.

Geriatric patients and patients with impaired renal function

Reduce dosage. Drug is largely excreted by the kidneys.

Pharmacokinetics

Route	Onset	Peak	Duration
Oral	Varies	2–4 hr	12–24 hr
IV	4–6 hr	4–6 hr	10–16 hr

Metabolism: Hepatic; $T_{1/2}$: 1.8 hr
Distribution: Crosses placenta; enters breast milk
Excretion: Urine

IV FACTS

Preparation: Add the dose to 100 mL of 5% dextrose, or give in D_5W in a concentration of 10 mg/mL.
Infusion: Administer over 30–60 min.
Incompatibilities: Do not combine with barbiturates or sulfonamides.

Adverse effects

- **CNS:** *Sedation, headache, asthenia, weakness* (usually early and transient), dizziness, light-headedness, symptoms of cerebrovascular insufficiency, paresthesias, parkinsonism, Bell's palsy, decreased mental acuity, involuntary choreoathetotic movements, psychic disturbances
- **CV:** *Bradycardia,* prolonged carotid sinus hypersensitivity, aggravation of angina pectoris, paradoxical pressor response, pericarditis, **myocarditis,** orthostatic hypotension, edema
- **Dermatologic:** Rash seen as eczema or lichenoid eruption, toxic epidermal necrolysis fever, lupuslike syndrome
- **Endocrine:** Breast enlargement, gynecomastia, lactation, hyperprolactinemia, amenorrhea, galactorrhea, impotence, failure to ejaculate, decreased libido
- **GI:** *Nausea, vomiting, distention, constipation,* flatus, diarrhea, colitis, dry mouth, sore or black tongue, pancreatitis, sialadenitis, abnormal liver function tests, jaundice, hepatitis, **hepatic necrosis**
- **Hematologic:** Positive Coombs' test, hemolytic anemia, bone marrow depression, leukopenia, granulocytopenia, thrombocytopenia, positive tests for antinuclear antibody, lupuslike syndrome, and rheumatoid factor
- **Other:** Nasal stuffiness, mild arthralgia, myalgia, septic shock–like syndrome

Interactions

✱ **Drug-drug** • Potentiation of the pressor effects of sympathomimetic amines • Increased hypotension with levodopa • Risk of hypotension during surgery with central anesthetics; monitor patient carefully

✱ **Drug-lab test** • Methyldopa may interfere with tests for urinary uric acid, serum creatinine, AST, urinary catecholamines

■ Nursing considerations

Assessment

- **History:** Hypersensitivity to methyldopa; hepatic disease; previous methyldopa therapy associated with liver disorders; renal failure; dialysis; bilateral cerebrovascular disease; lactation, pregnancy
- **Physical:** Weight; T; skin color, lesions; mucous membrane color, lesions; orientation, affect, reflexes; P, BP, orthostatic BP, perfusion, edema, auscultation; bowel sounds, normal output, liver evaluation; breast examination; LFTs, renal function tests, urinalysis, CBC and differential, direct Coombs' test

Interventions

- Administer IV slowly over 30–60 min; monitor injection site.

⊗ ***Warning*** Monitor hepatic function, especially in the first 6–12 wk of therapy or if unexplained fever appears. Discontinue drug if fever, abnormalities in liver function tests, or jaundice occurs. Ensure that methyldopa is not reinstituted in such patients.

⊗ ***Warning*** Monitor blood counts periodically to detect hemolytic anemia; a direct Coombs' test before therapy and 6 and 12 mo later may be helpful. Discontinue drug if Coombs'-positive hemolytic anemia occurs. If hemolytic anemia is related to methyldopa, ensure that drug is not reinstituted.

⊗ ***Warning*** Discontinue therapy if involuntary choreoathetotic movements occur.

⊗ ***Warning*** Discontinue if edema progresses or signs of HF occur.

- Add a thiazide to drug regimen or increase dosage if methyldopa tolerance occurs (second and third month of therapy).

⊗ ***Warning*** Monitor BP carefully when discontinuing methyldopa; drug has short duration of action, and hypertension usually returns within 48 hr.

Teaching points

- Take this drug exactly as prescribed; it is important that you not miss doses.

M

- You may experience these side effects: Drowsiness, dizziness, light-headedness, headache, weakness (often transient; avoid driving or engaging in tasks that require alertness); GI upset (eat frequent small meals); dreams, nightmares, memory impairment (reversible); dizziness, light-headedness when you get up (get up slowly; use caution when climbing stairs); urine that darkens on standing (expected effect); impotence, failure of ejaculation, decreased libido; breast enlargement, sore breasts.
- Report unexplained, prolonged general tiredness; yellowing of the skin or eyes; fever; bruising; rash.

▽ methylene blue
(meth' i leen)

Methblue 65, Urolene Blue

PREGNANCY CATEGORY C

Drug classes
Antidote
Diagnostic agent
Urinary tract anti-infective

Therapeutic actions
Oxidation-reduction agent that converts the ferrous iron of reduced Hgb to the ferric form, producing methemoglobin; weak germicide in lower doses; tissue staining.

Indications
- Treatment of cyanide poisoning and drug-induced methemoglobinemia
- May be useful in the management of patients with oxalate urinary tract calculi
- GU antiseptic for cystitis and urethritis
- Unlabeled uses: Delineation of body structures and fistulas through dye effect; neonatal glutaricacidura II unresponsive to riboflavin

Contraindications and cautions
- Contraindicated with allergy to methylene blue, renal insufficiency, intraspinal injections.
- Use cautiously with G6PD deficiency; anemias; CV deficiencies; pregnancy, lactation.

Available forms
Tablets—65 mg; injection—10 mg/mL

Dosages
Adults
Oral

65–130 mg tid with a full glass of water.

IV

1–2 mg/kg (0.1–0.2 mL/kg) injected over several minutes.

Pharmacokinetics

Route	*Onset*	*Peak*
Oral	Varies	Unknown
IV	Immediate	End of infusion

Metabolism: Tissue; $T_{1/2}$: Unknown
Excretion: Bile, feces, urine

IV FACTS
Preparation: No preparation required.
Infusion: Inject directly IV or into tubing of actively running IV; inject slowly over several minutes.

Adverse effects
- **CNS:** Dizziness, headache, mental confusion, sweating
- **CV:** Precordial pain
- **GI:** *Nausea,* vomiting, diarrhea, abdominal pain, *blue-green stool*
- **GU:** *Discolored urine* (blue-green); bladder irritation
- **Other:** Necrotic abscess (subcutaneous injection); fetal anemia and distress (amniotic injection); neural damage, paralysis (intrathecal injection); *skin stained blue*

■ Nursing considerations
Assessment
- **History:** Allergy to methylene blue, renal insufficiency, presence of G6PD deficiency; anemias; CV deficiencies; pregnancy, lactation
- **Physical:** Skin color, lesions; urinary output, bladder palpation; abdominal examination, normal output; CBC with differential

Interventions

- Give oral drug after meals with a full glass of water.
- Give IV slowly over several minutes; avoid exceeding recommended dosage.

⊗ ***Warning*** Use care to avoid subcutaneous injection; monitor intrathecal sites used for diagnostic injection for necrosis and damage.

- Contact with skin will dye the skin blue; stain may be removed by hypochlorite solution.
- Monitor CBC for signs of marked anemia.

Teaching points

- Take drug after meals with a full glass of water.
- Avoid bubble baths, excessive ingestion of citrus juice, and sexual contacts if bladder infection or urethritis is being treated.
- You may experience these side effects: Urine or stool discolored blue-green; abdominal pain, nausea, vomiting (eat frequent small meals).
- Report difficulty breathing, severe nausea or vomiting, fatigue.

▽ methylergonovine maleate

*(meth ill er goe **noe'** veen)*

Methergine

PREGNANCY CATEGORY C

Drug class

Oxytocic

Therapeutic actions

A partial agonist or antagonist at alpha receptors; as a result, it increases the strength, duration, and frequency of uterine contractions.

Indications

- Routine management after delivery of the placenta
- Treatment of postpartum atony and hemorrhage; subinvolution of the uterus
- Uterine stimulation during the second stage of labor following the delivery of the anterior shoulder, under strict medical supervision

Contraindications and cautions

- Contraindicated with allergy to methylergonovine, hypertension, toxemia, lactation, pregnancy.
- Use cautiously with sepsis, obliterative vascular disease, hepatic or renal impairment.

Available forms

Tablets—0.2 mg; injection—0.2 mg/mL

Dosages

Adults

IM

0.2 mg after delivery of the placenta, after delivery of the anterior shoulder, or during puerperium. May be repeated every 2–4 hr.

IV

Same dosage as IM; infuse slowly over at least 60 sec. Monitor BP very carefully as severe hypertensive reaction can occur; reserve this route for emergency situations.

Oral

0.2 mg PO tid or qid daily in the puerperium for up to 1 wk.

Pharmacokinetics

Route	*Onset*	*Peak*	*Duration*
Oral	5–10 min	30–60 min	3 hr
IM	2–5 min	30 min	3 hr
IV	Immediate	2–3 min	1–3 hr

Metabolism: Hepatic; $T_{1/2}$: 1.5–12.7 hr
Distribution: Crosses placenta; enters breast milk
Excretion: Feces

IV FACTS

Preparation: No additional preparation required.
Infusion: Inject directly IV or into tubing of running IV; inject very slowly, over no less than 60 sec; rapid infusion can result in sudden hypertension or cerebral events.

Adverse effects

- **CNS:** *Dizziness, headache,* tinnitus, diaphoresis
- **CV:** *Hypertension,* palpitations, chest pain, dyspnea
- **GI:** *Nausea,* vomiting

M

Interactions

✱ **Drug-drug** • Risk of severe hypertension, vasoconstriction, MI if combined with vasoconstrictors, ergot alkaloids; use extreme caution • Avoid use with potent CYP3A4 inhibitors

■ Nursing considerations

Assessment

- **History:** Allergy to methylergonovine, hypertension, toxemia, sepsis, obliterative vascular disease, hepatic or renal impairment, lactation, pregnancy
- **Physical:** Uterine tone, vaginal bleeding; orientation, reflexes, affect; P, BP, edema; CBC, LFTs, renal function tests; fetal monitoring when used during labor

Interventions

- Administer by IM injection or orally unless emergency requires IV use. Complications are more frequent with IV use.
- Monitor postpartum women for BP changes and amount and character of vaginal bleeding.
- Discontinue if signs of toxicity occur.
- Avoid prolonged use of the drug.

Teaching points

- This drug should not be needed for longer than 1 week.
- The patient receiving a parenteral oxytocic is usually receiving it as part of an immediate medical situation, and the drug teaching should be incorporated into the teaching about delivery. The patient needs to know the name of the drug and what she can expect after it is administered.
- You may experience these side effects: Nausea, vomiting, dizziness, headache, ringing in the ears (short-term use may make it tolerable).
- Report difficulty breathing, headache, numb or cold extremities, severe abdominal cramping.

▽ methylnaltrexone bromide

See Appendix W, *Less commonly used drugs.*

▽ methylphenidate hydrochloride

*(meth ill **fen'** i date)*

Apo-Methylphenidate (CAN), Apo-Methylphenidate SR (CAN), Biphentin (CAN), Concerta DNC, Daytrana, Metadate CD DNC, Metadate ER DNC, Methylin, Methylin ER DNC, PMS-Methylphenidate (CAN), Ritalin, Ritalin LA DNC, Ritalin-SR DNC

PREGNANCY CATEGORY C

CONTROLLED SUBSTANCE C-II

Drug class

CNS stimulant

Therapeutic actions

Mild cortical stimulant with CNS actions similar to those of the amphetamines; efficacy in hyperkinetic syndrome, attention-deficit disorders in children appear paradoxical and are not understood.

Indications

- Narcolepsy (*Ritalin, Ritalin SR, Metadate ER, Methylin*)
- Attention-deficit disorders, hyperkinetic syndrome, minimal brain dysfunction in children or adults with a behavioral syndrome characterized by the following symptoms: Moderate to severe distractibility, short attention span, hyperactivity, emotional lability, and impulsivity, not secondary to environmental factors or psychiatric disorders
- Unlabeled use: Treatment of depression in the elderly, cancer and CVA patients; alleviation of neurobehavioral symptoms after traumatic brain injury; improvement in pain control and sedation in patients receiving opiates

Contraindications and cautions

- Contraindicated with hypersensitivity to methylphenidate; marked anxiety, tension, and agitation; glaucoma; motor tics, family history or diagnosis of Tourette syndrome; severe depression of endogenous or exogenous origin; normal fatigue states; concurrent use or use within 2 wk of MAOI.

- Use cautiously with seizure disorders; hypertension; drug dependence, alcoholism; emotional instability, psychosis; seizures; lactation, pregnancy; short gut syndrome, peritonitis, esophageal motility disorders (*Concerta*).

Available forms
Tablets—5, 10, 20 mg; chewable tablets—2.5, 5, 10 mg; SR tablets DNC—20 mg; ER tablets DNC—10, 18, 20, 27, 36, 54 mg; ER capsules DNC—20, 30 mg (*Metadate CD* DNC); and 10, 20, 30, 40, 50, 60 mg (*Ritalin LA* DNC); transdermal patch—1.1, 1.6, 2.2, 3.3 mg/hr; solution—1, 2 mg/mL

Dosages
Adults
Individualize dosage. Give orally in divided doses bid or tid, preferably 30–45 min before meals; dosage ranges from 10–60 mg/day PO. If insomnia is a problem, drug should be taken before 6 PM. Timed-release tablets have a duration of 8 hr and may be used when timing and dosage are adjusted to the 8-hr daily regimen. ER forms: 18 mg PO daily in the morning; may be increased by 18 mg/day at 1-wk intervals to a maximum of 54 mg/day (*Concerta*); 10- to 20-mg/day increments to a maximum 60 mg/day (*Metadate CD, Ritalin LA*).

Pediatric patients 13–17 yr
Initially, 18 mg/day PO taken in the morning without regard to food; titrate to a maximum 72 mg/day PO. Do not exceed 2 mg/kg/day. Tablets must be swallowed whole and should not be cut, crushed, or chewed (*Concerta*). Or, 10–30 mg/day by transdermal patch; apply patch 2 hr before effect needed and remove after 9 hr.

Pediatric patients 6–12 yr
Start with small oral doses (5 mg PO before breakfast and lunch with gradual increments of 5–10 mg weekly). Daily dosage of more than 60 mg not recommended. Discontinue use after 1 mo if no improvement. Discontinue periodically to assess condition; usually discontinued after puberty. ER forms: Use adult dosage. Or, 10–30 mg/day by transdermal patch; apply patch 2 hr before effect needed and remove after 9 hr.

Pediatric patients younger than 6 yr
Not recommended.

Pharmacokinetics

Route	Onset	Peak	Duration
Oral	Varies	1–3 hr	3–6 hr
Oral (ER)	Varies	5–8 hr	3–12 hr
Transdermal	2 hr	3 hr	Up to 3 hr after removal

Metabolism: Hepatic; $T_{1/2}$: 1–3 hr (6.8 hr ER; 3–4 hr transdermal)
Distribution: Crosses placenta; may enter breast milk
Excretion: Urine

Adverse effects
- **CNS:** *Nervousness, insomnia,* dizziness, headache, dyskinesia, chorea, drowsiness, tics, Tourette's syndrome, toxic psychosis, blurred vision, accommodation difficulties
- **CV:** *Increased or decreased pulse and BP; tachycardia,* angina, cardiac arrhythmias, palpitations
- **Dermatologic:** Rash, urticaria, fever, exfoliative dermatitis, erythema multiforme with necrotizing vasculitis and thrombocytopenic purpura, loss of scalp hair
- **GI:** *Anorexia, nausea, abdominal pain,* weight loss
- **Hematologic:** Leukopenia, anemia
- **Other:** Tolerance, psychological dependence, abnormal behavior with abuse, arthralgia

Interactions
✱ **Drug-drug** • Increased effects and toxicity of methylphenidate with MAOIs • Increased serum levels of phenytoin, TCAs, oral anticoagulants, SSRIs with methylphenidate; monitor for toxicity

✱ **Drug-lab test** • Methylphenidate may increase the urinary excretion of epinephrine

■ Nursing considerations
Assessment
- **History:** Hypersensitivity to methylphenidate; marked anxiety, tension, and agitation; glaucoma; motor tics, Tourette syndrome; severe depression; normal fatigue state;

seizure disorders; hypertension; drug dependence, alcoholism, emotional instability; pregnancy, lactation
- **Physical:** Weight; T; skin color, lesions; orientation, affect, ophthalmologic examination (tonometry); P, BP, auscultation; R, adventitious sounds; bowel sounds, normal output; CBC with differential, platelet count, baseline ECG

Interventions

⊗ ***Black box warning*** Be aware that drug has potential for abuse; use caution with emotionally unstable patients.

- Ensure proper diagnosis before administering to children for behavioral syndromes; drug should not be used until other causes or concomitants of abnormal behavior (learning disability, EEG abnormalities, neurologic deficits) are ruled out.
- Ensure that patient does not have underlying cardiac problems before beginning therapy; serious cardiac effects have been reported.
- Apply transdermal patch to clean, dry area of the hip approximately 2 hr before effect needed. Remove after 9 hr. Alternate hips.
- Interrupt drug dosage periodically in children to determine if symptoms warrant continued drug therapy.
- Monitor growth of children on long-term methylphenidate therapy.
- Ensure that all timed-release tablets and capsules are swallowed whole, not chewed or crushed.
- Dispense the smallest feasible dose to minimize risk of overdose.
- Give before 6 PM to prevent insomnia.
- Monitor CBC and platelet counts periodically in patients on long-term therapy.
- Monitor BP frequently early in treatment.

Teaching points

- Take this drug exactly as prescribed. Timed-release tablets and capsules must be swallowed whole, not chewed or crushed. *Metadate CD* capsules may be opened and entire contents sprinkled on soft food—do not chew or crush granules. Transdermal patch should be applied to clean, dry area of the hip. Remove after 9 hours. Alternate hips.
- Chewable tablets must be taken with at least 8 ounces of water to reduce the risk of choking.
- Take drug before 6 PM to avoid nighttime sleep disturbance.
- Avoid alcohol and over-the-counter drugs, including nose drops, cold remedies; some over-the-counter drugs could cause dangerous effects.
- You may experience these side effects: Nervousness, restlessness, dizziness, insomnia, impaired thinking (may lessen over time; avoid driving or engaging in activities that require alertness); headache; loss of appetite; dry mouth.
- Avoid heating pads, electric blankets if wearing the transdermal patch; heat will alter drug's effects.
- Keep drug in secure place; do not share with others; upon removing the transdermal patch, fold patch so adhesive sides stick together and discard in a container with a lid.
- Report nervousness, insomnia, palpitations, vomiting, rash, fever.

▽methylprednisolone

*(meth ill pred **niss'** oh lone)*

methylprednisolone

Oral: Medrol

methylprednisolone acetate

IM injection: depMedalone, Depo-Medrol

methylprednisolone sodium succinate

IV, IM injection: A-Methapred, Solu-Medrol

PREGNANCY CATEGORY C

Drug classes

Corticosteroid
Glucocorticoid
Hormone

Therapeutic actions

Enters target cells and binds to intracellular corticosteroid receptors, initiating many complex reactions that are responsible for its anti-inflammatory and immunosuppressive effects.

Indications

- Short-term management of various inflammatory and allergic disorders, such as rheumatoid arthritis, collagen diseases (eg, SLE), dermatologic diseases (eg, pemphigus), status asthmaticus, and autoimmune disorders (eg, MS)
- Hematologic disorders: Thrombocytopenia purpura, erythroblastopenia
- Ulcerative colitis, acute exacerbations of MS, and palliation in some leukemias and lymphomas
- Trichinosis with neurologic or myocardial involvement
- Prevention of nausea and vomiting associated with chemotherapy
- Unlabeled use: Septic shock, RDS, acute spinal cord injury

Contraindications and cautions

- Contraindicated with infections, especially TB, fungal infections, amebiasis, vaccinia and varicella, and antibiotic-resistant infections; lactation.
- Administration of live vaccines is contraindicated in patients receiving immunosuppressive doses.
- Use cautiously with kidney or liver disease, hypothyroidism, ulcerative colitis with impending perforation, diverticulitis, active or latent peptic ulcer, inflammatory bowel disease, heart failure, hypertension, thromboembolic disorders, osteoporosis, seizure disorders, diabetes mellitus, pregnancy.

Available forms

Tablets—2, 4, 8, 16, 24, 32 mg; powder for injection—40, 125, 500 mg/vial; 1, 2 g/vial; suspension for injection—20, 40, 80 mg/mL

Dosages

Adults

Individualize dosage, depending on severity and response. Give daily dose before 9 AM to minimize adrenal suppression. For maintenance, reduce initial dose in small increments at intervals until the lowest satisfactory clinical dose is reached. If long-term therapy is needed, consider alternate-day therapy with a short-acting corticosteroid. After long-term therapy, withdraw drug slowly to prevent adrenal insufficiency.

Oral

4–48 mg/day. For alternate-day therapy, give twice the usual dose every other morning.

IV, IM

10–40 mg IV administered over 30 min. Give subsequent doses IV or IM.

⊗ ***Warning*** Rapid IV administration of large doses (more than 0.5–1 g in less than 10–120 min) has caused serious cardiac complications.

Methylprednisolone acetate

- *Rheumatoid arthritis, maintenance:* 40–120 mg IM weekly.
- *Adrenogenital syndrome:* 40 mg IM every 2 wk.
- *Dermatologic lesions:* 40–120 mg IM weekly for 1–4 wk.
- *Asthma and allergic rhinitis:* 80–120 mg IM.
- *Intralesional:* 20–60 mg.
- *Intra-articular dose depends on site of injection:* 4–10 mg (small); 10–40 mg (medium); 20–80 mg (large joints).

Pediatric patients

Individualize dosage on the basis of severity and response rather than by formulae of correct doses for age or weight. Carefully observe growth and development in infants and children on prolonged therapy. Minimum dose of methylprednisolone is 0.5 mg/kg per 24 hr.

- *High-dose therapy:* 30 mg/kg IV infused over 10–30 min; may repeat every 4–6 hr but not longer than 72 hr.

Pharmacokinetics

Route	*Onset*	*Peak*	*Duration*
Oral	Varies	1–2 hr	1.2–1.5 days
IV	Rapid	Rapid	Unknown
IM	8–12 hr	Unknown	4–8 days

Metabolism: Hepatic; $T_{1/2}$: 78–188 min
Distribution: Crosses placenta; enters breast milk
Excretion: Urine

M

IV FACTS

Preparation: No additional preparation is required.

Infusion: Inject directly into vein or into tubing of running IV; administer slowly, over at least 30 min, to reduce cardiac effects. Acetate form should not be given IV.

Incompatibilities: Do not combine with allopurinol, calcium gluconate, ciprofloxacin, docetaxel, etoposide, filgrastim, gemcitabine, glycopyrrolate, insulin, nafcillin, ondansetron, paclitaxel, penicillin G sodium, propofol, sargramostim, tetracycline, vinorelbine.

Adverse effects

Effects depend on dose, route, and duration of therapy.

- **CNS:** *Vertigo, headache,* paresthesias, insomnia, seizures, psychosis, cataracts, increased IOP, glaucoma
- **CV:** Hypotension, **shock,** hypertension and heart failure secondary to fluid retention, thromboembolism, thrombophlebitis, fat embolism, cardiac arrhythmias
- **Electrolyte imbalance:** *Na^+ and fluid retention,* hypokalemia, hypocalcemia
- **Endocrine:** Amenorrhea, irregular menses, growth retardation, decreased carbohydrate tolerance, diabetes mellitus, cushingoid state (long-term effect), increased blood sugar, increased serum cholesterol, decreased T_3 and T_4 levels, HPA suppression with systemic therapy longer than 5 days
- **GI:** Peptic or esophageal ulcer, pancreatitis, abdominal distention, nausea, vomiting, *increased appetite, weight gain*
- **Hypersensitivity:** Anaphylactoid reactions
- **Musculoskeletal:** Muscle weakness, steroid myopathy, loss of muscle mass, osteoporosis, spontaneous fractures
- **Other:** *Immunosuppression; aggravation or masking of infections; impaired wound healing;* thin, fragile skin; petechiae, ecchymoses, purpura, striae; subcutaneous fat atrophy

Interactions

✱ **Drug-drug** • Increased therapeutic and toxic effects with erythromycin, azole antifungals, troleandomycin • Risk of severe deterioration of muscle strength when given to myasthenia gravis patients who are receiving ambenonium, edrophonium, neostigmine, pyridostigmine • Decreased steroid blood levels with barbiturates, phenytoin, rifampin • Decreased effectiveness of salicylates

✱ **Drug-lab test** • False-negative nitroblue-tetrazolium test for bacterial infection • Suppression of skin test reactions

■ Nursing considerations

Assessment

- **History:** Infections; recent vaccinations; kidney or liver disease, hypothyroidism, ulcerative colitis, diverticulitis, active or latent peptic ulcer, inflammatory bowel disease, heart failure, hypertension, thromboembolic disorders, osteoporosis, seizure disorders, diabetes mellitus; pregnancy; lactation
- **Physical:** Weight, T, reflexes and grip strength, affect and orientation, P, BP, peripheral perfusion prominence of superficial veins, R and adventitious sounds, serum electrolytes, blood glucose

Interventions

- Use caution with the 24-mg tablets marketed as *Medrol;* these contain tartrazine, which may cause allergic reactions, especially in people who are allergic to aspirin.
- Give daily dose before 9 AM to mimic normal peak corticosteroid blood levels.
- Monitor glucose levels with prolonged therapy; dietary adjustments may be needed.
- Increase dosage when patient is subject to stress.

⊗ ***Warning*** Taper doses when discontinuing high-dose or long-term therapy to allow adrenal recovery.

⊗ ***Warning*** Do not give live-virus vaccines with immunosuppressive doses of corticosteroids.

⊗ ***Warning*** Some injectable products contain benzyl alcohol. Do not administer them to neonates or inject intrathecally.

Teaching points

- Do not stop taking the oral drug without consulting your health care provider.
- Avoid exposure to infections.

- Report unusual weight gain, swelling of the extremities, muscle weakness, black or tarry stools, fever, prolonged sore throat, colds or other infections, worsening of disorder.

metoclopramide

*(met oh kloe **pra'** mide)*

Apo-Metoclop (CAN), Maxolon, Metozolv ODT, Nu-Metoclopramide (CAN), Octamide PFS, Reglan

PREGNANCY CATEGORY B

Drug classes

Antiemetic
Dopaminergic blocker
GI stimulant

Therapeutic actions

Stimulates motility of upper GI tract without stimulating gastric, biliary, or pancreatic secretions; appears to sensitize tissues to action of acetylcholine; relaxes pyloric sphincter, which, when combined with effects on motility, accelerates gastric emptying and intestinal transit; little effect on gallbladder or colon motility; increases lower esophageal sphincter pressure; has sedative properties; induces release of prolactin.

Indications

- Relief of symptoms of acute and recurrent diabetic gastroparesis
- Short-term therapy (4–12 wk) for adults with symptomatic gastroesophageal reflux who fail to respond to conventional therapy
- Parenteral: Prevention of nausea and vomiting associated with emetogenic cancer chemotherapy
- Prophylaxis of postoperative nausea and vomiting when nasogastric suction is undesirable
- Single-dose parenteral use: Facilitation of small-bowel intubation when tube does not pass the pylorus with conventional maneuvers
- Single-dose parenteral use: Stimulation of gastric emptying and intestinal transit of barium when delayed emptying interferes with radiologic examination of the stomach or small intestine
- Unlabeled uses: Improvement of lactation (doses of 30–45 mg/day); treatment of nausea and vomiting of a variety of etiologies: Emesis during pregnancy and labor, gastric ulcer, anorexia nervosa

Contraindications and cautions

- Contraindicated with allergy to metoclopramide; GI hemorrhage, mechanical obstruction or perforation; pheochromocytoma (may cause hypertensive crisis); epilepsy.
- Use cautiously with previously detected breast cancer (one-third of such tumors are prolactin dependent); lactation, pregnancy; fluid overload; renal impairment.

Available forms

Tablets—5, 10 mg; oral solution (syrup)—1 mg/mL; injection—5 mg/mL; orally disintegrating tablets—5, 10 mg

Dosages

Adults

- *Relief of symptoms of gastroparesis:* 10 mg PO 30 min before each meal and at bedtime for 2–8 wk. If symptoms are severe, initiate therapy with 10 mg IM or IV administration for up to 10 days until symptoms subside.
- *Symptomatic gastroesophageal reflux:* 10–15 mg PO up to four times/day 30 min before meals and at bedtime. If symptoms occur only at certain times or in relation to specific stimuli, single doses of 20 mg may be preferable; guide therapy by endoscopic results. Do not use longer than 12 wk.
- *Prevention of postoperative nausea and vomiting:* 10–20 mg IM at the end of surgery.
- *Prevention of chemotherapy-induced emesis:* Dilute and give by IV infusion over at least 15 min. Give first dose 30 min before chemotherapy; repeat every 2 hr for two doses, then every 3 hr for three doses. The initial two doses should be 2 mg/kg for highly emetogenic drugs (cisplatin, dacarbazine); 1 mg/kg may suffice for other chemotherapeutic drugs. If extrapyramidal symptoms occur, administer 50 mg of diphenhydramine IM.
- *Facilitation of small bowel intubation, gastric emptying:* 10 mg (2 mL) by direct IV injection over 1–2 min.

M

Pediatric patients

- *Facilitation of intubation, gastric emptying:*
  Younger than 6 yr: 0.1 mg/kg by direct IV injection over 1–2 min.
  6–14 yr: 2.5–5 mg by direct IV injection over 1–2 min.

Pharmacokinetics

Route	*Onset*	*Peak*	*Duration*
Oral	30–60 min	60–90 min	1–2 hr
IM	10–15 min	60–90 min	1–2 hr
IV	1–3 min	60–90 min	1–2 hr

Metabolism: Hepatic; $T_{1/2}$: 5–6 hr
Distribution: Crosses placenta; enters breast milk
Excretion: Urine

IV FACTS

Preparation: Dilute dose in 50 mL of a parenteral solution (D_5W, sodium chloride injection, dextrose 5% in 0.45% sodium chloride, Ringer's injection, or lactated Ringer's injection). May be stored for up to 48 hr if protected from light or up to 24 hr under normal light.
Infusion: Give direct IV doses slowly (over 1–2 min); give infusions over at least 15 min.
Incompatibilities: Do not mix with solutions containing chloramphenicol, sodium bicarbonate, cisplatin, erythromycin.
Y-site incompatibilities: Do not give with allopurinol, furosemide, cefepime.

Adverse effects

- **CNS:** *Restlessness, drowsiness, fatigue, lassitude,* insomnia, *extrapyramidal reactions,* parkinsonism-like reactions, akathisia, dystonia, myoclonus, dizziness, anxiety
- **CV:** Transient hypertension
- **GI:** *Nausea, diarrhea*

Interactions

✱ **Drug-drug** • Decreased absorption of digoxin from the stomach • Increased toxic and immunosuppressive effects of cyclosporine • Increased neuromuscular blocking effects with succinylcholine

■ Nursing considerations

Assessment

- **History:** Allergy to metoclopramide, GI hemorrhage, mechanical obstruction or perforation, depression, pheochromocytoma, epilepsy, lactation, previously detected breast cancer
- **Physical:** Orientation, reflexes, affect; P, BP; bowel sounds, normal output; EEG

Interventions

⊗ ***Black box warning*** Long-term treatment has been associated with permanent tardive dyskinesia; the risk increases with patients older than 60 yr, especially women. Use the smallest dose possible; do not exceed 3-mo therapy.

- Monitor BP carefully during IV administration.
- Monitor for extrapyramidal reactions, and consult physician if they occur.
- Monitor patients with diabetes, arrange for alteration in insulin dose or timing if diabetic control is compromised by alterations in timing of food absorption.

⊗ ***Warning*** Keep diphenhydramine injection readily available in case extrapyramidal reactions occur (50 mg IM).

⊗ ***Warning*** Have phentolamine readily available in case of hypertensive crisis (most likely to occur with undiagnosed pheochromocytoma).

Teaching points

- Take this drug exactly as prescribed.
- Do not use alcohol, sleep remedies, or sedatives; serious sedation could occur.
- You may experience these side effects: Drowsiness, dizziness (do not drive or perform other tasks that require alertness); restlessness, anxiety, depression, headache, insomnia (reversible); nausea, diarrhea.
- Report involuntary movement of the face, eyes, or limbs, severe depression, severe diarrhea.

metolazone

*(me **tole'** a zone)*

Zaroxolyn

PREGNANCY CATEGORY B

Drug class
Thiazide-like diuretic

Therapeutic actions
Inhibits reabsorption of sodium and chloride in distal renal tubule, increasing excretion of sodium, chloride, and water by the kidney.

Indications
- Treatment of salt and water retention, including edema of HF and renal disease, nephrotic syndrome, and diminished renal function
- Hypertension, as monotherapy or in combination with other antihypertensives
- Unlabeled uses: Osteoporosis, diabetes insipidus

Contraindications and cautions
- Contraindicated with hypersensitivity to thiazides, hepatic coma, fluid or electrolyte imbalances, renal or liver disease, sulfonamide derivatives.
- Use cautiously with gout, SLE, glucose tolerance abnormalities, hyperparathyroidism, bipolar disorder, lactation, pregnancy.

Available forms
Tablets: 2.5, 5, 10 mg

Dosages
Adults
- *Hypertension:* 2.5–5 mg daily PO.
- *Edema of renal disease:* 5–20 mg daily PO.
- *Edema of heart failure:* 5–20 mg daily PO.

Pediatric patients
Not recommended.

Pharmacokinetics

Route	Onset	Peak	Duration
Oral	1 hr	8 hr	12–24 hr

Metabolism: Hepatic; $T_{1/2}$: 8–14 hr
Distribution: Crosses placenta; may enter breast milk
Excretion: Urine

Adverse effects
- **CNS:** *Dizziness, vertigo,* paresthesias, weakness, *headache,* drowsiness, *fatigue*
- **CV:** Orthostatic hypotension, venous thrombosis, volume depletion, cardiac arrhythmias, chest pain
- **Dermatologic:** Photosensitivity, rash, purpura, exfoliative dermatitis
- **GI:** *Nausea, anorexia, vomiting, dry mouth, diarrhea, constipation,* jaundice, hepatitis, pancreatitis
- **GU:** *Polyuria, nocturia, impotence,* decreased libido
- **Hematologic:** Leukopenia, thrombocytopenia, neutropenia, agranulocytosis, aplastic anemia, fluid and electrolyte imbalances
- **Other:** Muscle cramps and muscle spasms, fever, hives, gouty attacks, flushing

Interactions
✱ Drug-drug • Increased thiazide effects and chance of acute hyperglycemia with diazoxide • Decreased absorption with cholestyramine, colestipol • Increased risk of cardiac glycoside toxicity if hypokalemia occurs • Increased risk of lithium toxicity • Increased dosage of antidiabetics may be needed • Increased risk of severe hypokalemia with dofetilide; combination is contraindicated
✱ Drug-lab test • Decreased PBI levels without clinical signs of thyroid disturbances

M

■ Nursing considerations
Assessment
- **History:** Fluid or electrolyte imbalances, renal or liver disease, gout, SLE, glucose tolerance abnormalities, hyperparathyroidism, bipolar disorder, hepatic coma or precoma, lactation, pregnancy
- **Physical:** Skin color and lesions; orientation, reflexes, muscle strength; pulses, BP, orthostatic BP, perfusion, edema, baseline ECG; R, adventitious sounds; liver evaluation, bowel sounds; CBC, serum electrolytes, blood glucose, LFTs, renal function tests, serum uric acid, urinalysis

Interventions
⊠ ***Black box warning*** Do not interchange *Zaroxolyn* with other formulations; they are not therapeutically equivalent.
⊗ ***Warning*** Withdraw drug 2–3 days before elective surgery; for emergency surgery, reduce dosage of preanesthetic or anesthetic.
- Give with food or milk if GI upset occurs.
- Measure and record body weight to monitor fluid changes.

Teaching points

- Take drug early in the day so sleep will not be disturbed by increased urination.
- Weigh yourself daily and record weights.
- Protect skin from the sun and bright lights.
- You may experience these side effects: Increased urination; dizziness, drowsiness, feeling faint (use caution; avoid driving or operating dangerous machinery); headache.
- Report rapid weight change, swelling in ankles or fingers, unusual bleeding or bruising, muscle cramps.

DANGEROUS DRUG

metoprolol

(me toe' proe lole)

metoprolol

Apo-Metoprolol SR (CAN) DNC, Gen-Metoprolol (CAN), Lopressor, Novo-Metoprol (CAN), Nu-Metop (CAN)

metoprolol succinate

Toprol-XL DNC

metoprolol tartrate

Apo-Metoprolol (CAN), Lopressor Injection, PMS-Metoprolol-L (CAN)

PREGNANCY CATEGORY C

Drug classes

Antihypertensive
Beta$_1$-selective adrenergic blocker

Therapeutic actions

Competitively blocks beta-adrenergic receptors in the heart and juxtaglomerular apparatus, decreasing the influence of the sympathetic nervous system on these tissues and the excitability of the heart, decreasing cardiac output and the release of renin, and lowering BP; acts in the CNS to reduce sympathetic outflow and vasoconstrictor tone.

Indications

- Hypertension, alone or with other drugs, especially diuretics
- Immediate-release tablets and injection: Prevention of reinfarction in MI patients who are hemodynamically stable or within 3–10 days of the acute MI
- Long-term treatment of angina pectoris
- *Toprol-XL* only: Treatment of stable, symptomatic heart failure of ischemic, hypertensive, or cardiomyopathic origin

Contraindications and cautions

- Contraindicated with sinus bradycardia (HR less than 45 beats/min), second- or third-degree heart block (PR interval more than 0.24 sec), cardiogenic shock, HF, second and third trimesters of pregnancy.
- Use cautiously with diabetes or thyrotoxicosis; asthma or COPD; pregnancy.

Available forms

Tablets—25, 50, 100 mg; ER tablets DNC—25, 50, 100, 200 mg; injection—1 mg/mL

Dosages

Adults

- *Hypertension:* Initially, 100 mg/day PO in single or divided doses; gradually increase dosage at weekly intervals. Usual maintenance dose is 100–450 mg/day.
- *Angina pectoris:* Initially, 100 mg/day PO in two divided doses; may be increased gradually, effective range, 100–400 mg/day.
- *MI, early treatment:* Three IV bolus doses of 5 mg each at 2-min intervals with careful monitoring. If these are tolerated, give 50 mg PO 15 min after the last IV dose and every 6 hr for 48 hr. Thereafter, give a maintenance dose of 100 mg PO bid. Reduce initial PO doses to 25 mg, or discontinue in patients who do not tolerate the IV doses.
- *MI, late treatment:* 50–100 mg PO bid as soon as possible after infarct, continuing for at least 3 mo and possibly for 1–3 yr.

ER tablets

- *Hypertension:* 25–100 mg/day PO as one dose; may increase at weekly intervals to a maximum of 400 mg/day.
- *Angina:* 100 mg/day PO as one dose.
- *HF:* 12.5–25 mg/day *Toprol-XL* for 2 wk; may then be increased by 25 mg every 2 wk to a maximum of 200 mg.

Pediatric patients
Safety and efficacy not established.

Pharmacokinetics

Route	Onset	Peak	Duration
Oral	15 min	90 min	Varies
IV	Immediate	60–90 min	15–19 hr

Metabolism: Hepatic; $T_{1/2}$: 3–4 hr
Distribution: Crosses placenta; enters breast milk
Excretion: Urine

IV FACTS

Preparation: No additional preparation is required.
Infusion: Inject directly into vein or into tubing of running IV over 1 min. Inject as a bolus; monitor carefully; wait 2 min between doses; do not give if bradycardia is less than 45 beats/min, heart block, systolic pressure less than 100 mm Hg.
Incompatibilities: Do not mix with amino acids, amphotericin B complex, aztreonam, dopamine.

Adverse effects

- **Allergic:** Pharyngitis, erythematous rash, fever, sore throat, **laryngospasm**
- **CNS:** Dizziness, vertigo, tinnitus, fatigue, emotional depression, paresthesias, sleep disturbances, hallucinations, disorientation, memory loss, slurred speech
- **CV:** *Heart failure, cardiac arrhythmias,* peripheral vascular insufficiency, claudication, CVA, pulmonary edema, hypotension
- **Dermatologic:** Rash, pruritus, sweating, dry skin, worsening of psoriasis
- **EENT:** Eye irritation, dry eyes, conjunctivitis, blurred vision
- **GI:** *Gastric pain, flatulence, constipation, diarrhea, nausea, vomiting,* anorexia, ischemic colitis, renal and mesenteric arterial thrombosis, retroperitoneal fibrosis, hepatomegaly, acute pancreatitis
- **GU:** *Impotence, decreased libido,* dysuria, Peyronie's disease, nocturia, frequent urination
- **Musculoskeletal:** Joint pain, arthralgia, muscle cramp
- **Respiratory: Bronchospasm,** dyspnea, cough, bronchial obstruction, nasal stuffiness, rhinitis, pharyngitis
- **Other:** *Decreased exercise tolerance, development of ANA,* hyperglycemia or hypoglycemia, elevated serum transaminase, alkaline phosphatase

Interactions

✷ **Drug-drug** • Increased effects of metoprolol with verapamil, cimetidine, methimazole, propylthiouracil • Increased effects of both drugs if metoprolol is taken with hydralazine • Increased serum levels and toxicity of IV lidocaine, if given concurrently • Increased risk of orthostatic hypotension with prazosin • Decreased antihypertensive effects if taken with NSAIDs, clonidine, rifampin • Decreased therapeutic effects with barbiturates • Hypertension followed by severe bradycardia if given concurrently with epinephrine
✷ **Drug-lab test** • Possible false results with glucose or insulin tolerance tests (oral)

■ Nursing considerations

Assessment

- **History:** Sinus bradycardia (HR less than 45 beats/min), second- or third-degree heart block (PR interval greater than 0.24 sec), cardiogenic shock, heart failure, systolic BP less than 100 mm Hg; diabetes or thyrotoxicosis; asthma or COPD; lactation, pregnancy
- **Physical:** Weight, skin condition, neurologic status, P, BP, ECG, respiratory status, renal and thyroid function tests, blood and urine glucose

Interventions

⊗ ***Warning*** Do not discontinue drug abruptly after long-term therapy (hypersensitivity to catecholamines may have developed, causing exacerbation of angina, MI, and ventricular arrhythmias). Taper drug gradually over 2 wk with monitoring.

- Ensure that patient swallows the ER tablets whole; do not cut, crush, or chew. *Toprol XL* tablets may be divided at the score; divided tablets should be swallowed whole, not crushed or chewed.
- Consult physician about withdrawing drug if patient is to undergo surgery (controversial).

- Give oral drug with food to facilitate absorption.
- Provide continual cardiac monitoring for patients receiving IV metoprolol.

Teaching points

- Do not stop taking this drug unless instructed to do so by your health care provider.
- Swallow the extended-release tablets whole; do not cut, crush, or chew. If using *Toprol XL,* you can divide the tablets at the score; divided tablets must be swallowed whole, not crushed or chewed.
- You may experience these side effects: Dizziness, drowsiness, light-headedness, blurred vision (avoid driving or dangerous activities); nausea, loss of appetite (eat frequent small meals); nightmares, depression (discuss change of medication); sexual impotence.
- Report difficulty breathing, night cough, swelling of extremities, slow pulse, confusion, depression, rash, fever, sore throat.

▽metronidazole

(me troe ***ni'*** *da zole)*

Apo-Metronidazole (CAN), Flagyl, Flagyl 375, Flagyl ER, Flagyl IV, MetroGel, MetroGel-Vaginal, NidaGel (CAN), Noritate, Protostat, Vandazole

PREGNANCY CATEGORY B

Drug classes

Amebicide
Antibacterial
Antibiotic
Antiprotozoal

Therapeutic actions

Bactericidal: Inhibits DNA synthesis in specific (obligate) anaerobes, causing cell death; antiprotozoal-trichomonacidal, amebicidal: Biochemical mechanism of action is not known.

Indications

- Acute infection with susceptible anaerobic bacteria
- Acute intestinal amebiasis
- Amebic liver abscess
- Trichomoniasis (acute and partners of patients with acute infection)
- Bacterial vaginosis
- Preoperative, intraoperative, postoperative prophylaxis for patients undergoing colorectal surgery
- Topical application: Treatment of inflammatory papules, pustules, and erythema of rosacea
- Unlabeled uses: Prophylaxis for patients undergoing gynecologic, abdominal surgery; hepatic encephalopathy; Crohn's disease; antibiotic-associated pseudomembranous colitis; treatment of *Gardnerella vaginalis,* giardiasis (use recommended by the CDC); infected decubitus ulcers; perioral dermatitis

Contraindications and cautions

- Contraindicated with hypersensitivity to metronidazole; pregnancy (do not use for trichomoniasis in first trimester).
- Use cautiously with CNS diseases, hepatic disease, candidiasis (moniliasis), blood dyscrasias, lactation.

Available forms

Tablets—250, 500 mg; ER tablets—750 mg; capsules—375 mg; powder for injection—500 mg; injection—500 mg/100 mL; lotion, cream, gel—0.75%; cream, gel—1%; vaginal gel—0.75%

Dosages

Adults

Oral

- *Amebiasis:* 750 mg PO tid for 5–10 days. (In amebic dysentery, combine with iodoquinol 650 mg PO tid for 20 days.)
- *Antibiotic-associated pseudomembranous colitis:* 1–2 g/day PO in 3–4 divided doses for 7–10 days.
- *Gardnerella vaginalis:* 500 mg PO bid for 7 days.
- *Giardiasis:* 250 mg PO tid for 7 days.
- *Trichomoniasis:* 2 g PO in 1 day (1-day treatment) *or* 250 mg PO tid for 7 days.

- *Bacterial vaginosis:*
  Nonpregnant women: 500 mg PO bid for 7 days or a single 2-g dose followed by 750 mg PO daily for 7 days.
  Pregnant women: 500 mg PO bid or 250 mg PO tid for 7 days; avoid treatment in the first trimester.

IV

- *Anaerobic bacterial infection:* 15 mg/kg IV infused over 1 hr; then 7.5 mg/kg infused over 1 hr every 6 hr for 7–10 days, not to exceed 4 g/day.
- *Prophylaxis:* 15 mg/kg infused IV over 30–60 min and completed about 1 hr before surgery. Then 7.5 mg/kg infused over 30–60 min at 6- to 12-hr intervals after initial dose during the day of surgery only.

***Topical* (MetroGel)**

- *Treatment of inflammatory papules, pustules, and erythema of rosacea:* Apply and rub in a thin film twice daily, morning and evening, to entire affected areas after washing; results should be seen within 3 wk; treatment through 9 wk has been effective.

***Vaginal* (MetroGel-Vaginal)**

- *Nonpregnant women:* 1 applicatorful intravaginally one to two times/day for 5 days.

Pediatric patients

- *Anaerobic bacterial infection:* Not recommended.
- *Amebiasis:* 35–50 mg/kg/day PO in three divided doses for 10 days.

Pharmacokinetics

Route	Onset	Peak
Oral	Varies	1–2 hr
IV	Rapid	1–2 hr

Metabolism: Hepatic; $T_{1/2}$: 6–8 hr
Distribution: Crosses placenta; enters breast milk
Excretion: Feces, urine

IV FACTS

Preparation: Reconstitute by adding 4.4 mL of sterile water for injection, bacteriostatic water for injection, 0.9% sodium chloride injection, or bacteriostatic 0.9% sodium chloride injection to the vial and mix thoroughly. Resultant volume is 5 mL with a concentration of 100 mg/mL. Solution should be clear to pale yellow to yellow-green; do not use if cloudy or contains precipitates; use within 24 hr; protect from light. Add reconstituted solution to glass or plastic container containing 0.9% sodium chloride injection, 5% dextrose injection or lactated Ringer's to a final concentration of 8 mg/mL or less before administering; discontinue other solutions while running metronidazole.

Infusion: Before administration, add 5 mEq sodium bicarbonate injection for each 500 mg used (if not using premixed bags); mix thoroughly. Do not refrigerate neutralized solution. Do not administer solution that has not been neutralized. Infuse over 1 hr.

Adverse effects

- **CNS:** *Headache, dizziness, ataxia,* vertigo, incoordination, insomnia, seizures, peripheral neuropathy, fatigue
- **GI:** *Unpleasant metallic taste, anorexia, nausea, vomiting, diarrhea,* GI upset, cramps
- **GU:** Dysuria, incontinence, *darkening of the urine*
- **Local:** Thrombophlebitis (IV); *redness, burning, dryness, and skin irritation* (topical)
- **Other:** Severe, disulfiram-like interaction with alcohol, candidiasis (superinfection)

Interactions

✱ Drug-drug • Decreased effectiveness with barbiturates • Disulfiram-like reaction (flushing, tachycardia, nausea, vomiting) with alcohol • Psychosis if taken with disulfiram • Increased bleeding tendencies with oral anticoagulants

✱ Drug-lab test • False-low (or zero) values in AST, ALT, LDH, triglycerides, hexokinase glucose tests

■ Nursing considerations

Assessment

- **History:** CNS or hepatic disease, candidiasis (moniliasis), blood dyscrasias, pregnancy, lactation
- **Physical:** Reflexes, affect; skin lesions, color (with topical application); abdominal examination, liver palpation; urinalysis, CBC, LFTs

M

Interventions

⊗ ***Black box warning*** Avoid use unless needed. Metronidazole may be carcinogenic.

- Administer oral doses with food.
- Apply topically (*MetroGel*) after cleansing the area. Advise patient that cosmetics may be used over the area after application.
- Reduce dosage in hepatic disease.

Teaching points

- Take full course of drug therapy; take the drug with food if GI upset occurs.
- Do not drink alcohol (beverages or preparations containing alcohol, cough syrups) for 24–72 hr of drug use; severe reactions may occur.
- Your urine may be a darker color than usual; this is expected.
- Refrain from sexual intercourse during treatment for trichomoniasis, unless partner wears a condom.
- Apply the topical preparation by cleansing the area and then rubbing a thin film into the affected area. Avoid contact with the eyes. Cosmetics may be applied to the area after medication is dry.
- You may experience these side effects: Dry mouth with strange metallic taste (frequent mouth care, sucking sugarless candies may help); nausea, vomiting, diarrhea (eat frequent small meals).
- Report severe GI upset, dizziness, unusual fatigue or weakness, fever, chills.

▽ metyrosine

See Appendix W, *Less commonly used drugs.*

DANGEROUS DRUG

▽ mexiletine hydrochloride

*(mex **ill'** i teen)*

Mexitil, Novo-Mexiletine (CAN)

PREGNANCY CATEGORY C

Drug class

Antiarrhythmic

Therapeutic actions

Type I antiarrhythmic: Decreases automaticity of ventricular cells by membrane stabilization.

Indications

- Treatment of documented life-threatening ventricular arrhythmias (use with lesser arrhythmias is not recommended)
- Unlabeled uses: Prophylactic use to decrease arrhythmias in acute phase of acute MI (mortality may not be affected); reduction of pain, dysesthesia, and paresthesia associated with diabetic neuropathy

Contraindications and cautions

- Contraindicated with allergy to mexiletine, cardiogenic shock, hypotension, second- or third-degree heart block (without artificial pacemaker), lactation.
- Use cautiously with hepatic disease, seizure disorders, hypotension, severe HF, pregnancy.

Available forms

Capsules—150, 200, 250 mg

Dosages

Adults

200 mg every 8 hr PO. Increase in 50- to 100-mg increments every 2–3 days until desired antiarrhythmic effect is obtained. Maximum dose, 1,200 mg/day PO. Rapid control, 400 mg loading dose, then 200 mg every 8 hr PO.

- *Transferring from other antiarrhythmics: Lidocaine:* Stop the lidocaine with the first dose of mexiletine; leave IV line open until adequate arrhythmia suppression is ensured. *Quinidine sulfate:* Initial dose of 200 mg 6–12 hr PO after the last dose of quinidine. *Procainamide:* Initial dose of 200 mg 3–6 hr PO after the last dose of procainamide. *Disopyramide:* 200 mg 6–12 hr PO after the last dose of disopyramide.

Pediatric patients

Safety and efficacy not established.

Pharmacokinetics

Route	Onset	Peak
Oral	0.5–2 hr	2–3 hr

Metabolism: Hepatic; $T_{1/2}$: 10–12 hr
Distribution: Crosses placenta; enters breast milk
Excretion: Urine

Adverse effects

- **CNS:** *Dizziness, light-headedness, headache,* fatigue, drowsiness, *tremors, coordination difficulties, visual disturbances,* numbness, nervousness, *sleep difficulties*
- **CV:** *Cardiac arrhythmias, chest pain*
- **GI:** *Nausea, vomiting, heartburn,* abdominal pain, diarrhea, liver injury
- **Hematologic:** Positive ANA, thrombocytopenia, leukopenia
- **Respiratory:** *Dyspnea*
- **Other:** *Rash*

Interactions

✱ **Drug-drug** • Decreased mexiletine levels with hydantoins and rifampin • Increased theophylline levels and toxicity with mexiletine • Increased mexiletine levels with propafenone

■ Nursing considerations

Assessment

- **History:** Allergy to mexiletine, HF, cardiogenic shock, hypotension, second- or third-degree heart block, hepatic disease, seizure disorders, lactation, pregnancy
- **Physical:** Weight; orientation, reflexes; P, BP, auscultation, ECG, edema; R, adventitious sounds; bowel sounds, liver evaluation; urinalysis, urine pH, CBC, electrolytes, LFTs, renal function tests

Interventions

⊠ ***Black box warning*** Reserve use for life-threatening arrhythmias; may have serious proarrhythmic effects.

- Monitor patient response carefully, especially when beginning therapy.
- Reduce dosage with hepatic failure.

⊗ ***Warning*** Monitor for safe and effective serum levels (0.5–2 mcg/mL).

Teaching points

- Take with food to reduce GI problems.
- Frequent monitoring of cardiac rhythm is needed.
- Do not stop taking this drug without consulting your health care provider.
- Return for regular follow-up visits to check your heart rhythm and to have blood tests.
- Do not change your diet. Maintain acidity level in urine. Discuss dietary change with your health care provider.
- You may experience these side effects: Drowsiness, dizziness, numbness, visual disturbances (avoid driving or working with dangerous machinery); nausea, vomiting, heartburn (eat frequent small meals); diarrhea; headache; sleep disturbances.
- Report fever, chills, sore throat, excessive GI discomfort, chest pain, excessive tremors, numbness, lack of coordination, headache, sleep disturbances.

▽ micafungin sodium

(mick ah ***fun'*** *gin)*

Mycamine

PREGNANCY CATEGORY C

Drug classes

Antifungal
Echinocandin

Therapeutic actions

Inhibits the synthesis of components needed for the production of fungal cell walls, leading to cell death.

Indications

- Treatment of patients with esophageal candidiasis
- Prevention of *Candida* infections in patients undergoing hematopoietic stem cell transplantation
- Treatment of candidemia, acute disseminated candidiasis, *Candida* peritonitis and absesses

Contraindications and cautions

- Contraindicated with known hypersensitivity to micafungin.
- Use cautiously with liver impairment, renal impairment, pregnancy, lactation.

Available forms

Powder for injection—50 mg

Dosages

Adults

- *Treatment of esophageal candidiasis:* 150 mg/day by IV infusion over 1 hr for 10–30 days.
- *Prophylaxis of* Candida *infection:* 50 mg/day by IV infusion over 1 hr for about 19 days.
- *Treatment of* Candida *infections:* 100 mg/day IV infused over 1 hr for 10–47 days based on infection being treated.

Pharmacokinetics

Route	*Onset*	*Peak*
IV	Rapid	End of infusion

Metabolism: $T_{1/2}$: 14–17 hr
Distribution: May cross placenta; may pass into breast milk
Excretion: Feces, urine

IV FACTS

Preparation: Reconstitute with 5 mL 0.9% sodium chloride without bacteriostatic agent to yield 10 mg/mL using sterile technique. Swirl to mix; do not shake vigorously. Solution should be clear with no particulate matter. Protect reconstituted solution from light. Further dilute in 100 mL 0.9% sodium chloride injection. Discard any unused solution. Store diluted solution at room temperature for up to 24 hr; diluted solution protected from light, is stable for 24 hr.
Infusion: Infuse over 1 hr; flush the tubing of any running IV with 0.9% sodium chloride injection before infusing micafungin.
Incompatibilites: Do not mix in solution with any other drug; has been shown to form precipitates with many commonly used drugs.

Adverse effects

- **CNS:** Delirium, *headache,* dizziness, somnolence
- **CV:** Arrhythmias, changes in BP, cyanosis
- **GI:** Nausea, abdominal pain, vomiting, elevated liver enzymes
- **Hematologic:** Leukopenia, neutropenia, thrombocytopenia, anemia, lymphopenia, **hemolytic anemia**
- **Other: Potentially serious hypersensitivity reaction,** rash, *phlebitis*

Interactions

✱ **Drug-drug** • Concentrations of sirolimus and nifedipine may increase when used with micafungin; monitor for toxicity

■ Nursing considerations

Assessment

- **History:** Hypersensitivity to micafungin, hepatic impairment, renal impairment, pregnancy, lactation
- **Physical:** Orientation, reflexes; abdominal examination; skin color, lesions; LFTs, renal function tests, CBC with differential

Interventions

- Establish baseline liver function, renal function, and CBC before beginning therapy.
- Use sterile technique in preparing solution for IV infusion, there are no bacteriostatic agents in the preparation.
- Monitor injection site for any sign of reaction or the development of phlebitis.
- Maintain life support equipment on hand when beginning therapy, potentially serious hypersensitivity reactions have been reported.
- Advise the use of contraceptives during therapy.
- If the patient is nursing during therapy, suggest another method of feeding the baby.
- Provide comfort measures and possible analgesics for headache and pain.
- Encourage frequent small meals if GI effects are uncomfortable.

Teaching points

- You will receive *Mycamine* as a 1-hour IV infusion each day. If you are being treated for an infection, this will last 10–47 days depending on your response. If prevention of the infection is the goal of therapy, treatment will last for about 19 days.
- If you experience shortness of breath or difficulty breathing, consult your health care provider immediately.
- It is not known how this drug could affect a nursing baby. If you are nursing a baby, another method of feeding the baby should be selected.
- It is not known how this drug could affect a fetus, if you are pregnant or decide to become pregnant while on this drug, consult

your health care provider. Use of contraceptive measures is advised.

- You will need to have periodic blood tests to evaluate the effects of this drug on your body.
- You may experience these side effects: Headache (consult your health care provider, medication may be available to help); nausea, diarrhea (eating frequent small meals may help); dizziness (do not drive a car or operate hazardous machinery if this occurs).
- Report redness, pain or swelling at the IV site; changes in the color of urine or stool, rash, yellowing of the skin or eyes, difficulty breathing, increased bleeding or bruising.

miconazole nitrate

*(mi **kon'** a zole)*

Topical: Breeze Mist Antifungal, Fungoid Tincture, Lotrimin AF, Micatin, Neosporin AF, Tetterine, Ting, Triple Paste AF, Zeasorb-AF

Vaginal suppositories, topical: Femizol-M, Micozole (CAN), Monistat 1, Monistat 1 Combination Pack (CAN), Monistat 1 Vaginal Ovule, Monistat 3, Monistat 3 Vaginal Ovule (CAN), Monistat 7, Monistat Dual Pak, M-Zole 3, M-Zole 7 Dual Pack

PREGNANCY CATEGORY B

Drug class

Antifungal

Therapeutic actions

Fungicidal: Alters fungal cell membrane permeability, causing cell death; also may alter fungal cell DNA and RNA metabolism or cause accumulation of toxic peroxides intracellularly.

Indications

- Vaginal suppositories: Local treatment of vulvovaginal candidiasis (moniliasis)
- Topical administration: Tinea pedis, tinea cruris, tinea corporis caused by *Trichophyton rubrum, Trichophyton mentagrophytes, Epidermophyton floccosum;* cutaneous candidiasis (moniliasis), tinea versicolor

Contraindications and cautions

- Contraindicated with allergy to miconazole or components used in preparation.
- Use cautiously with pregnancy, lactation.

Available forms

Vaginal suppositories—100, 200, 1,200 mg; topical cream—2%; vaginal cream—2%; topical powder—2%; topical spray—1%, 2%; topical ointment—2%; spray powder or liquid—2%; solution–2%

Dosages

Adults

Vaginal suppositories

- *Monistat 3:* Insert 1 suppository intravaginally once daily at bedtime for 3 days. *Monistat 7:* One applicator cream or 1 suppository in the vagina daily at bedtime for 7 days. Repeat course if needed. Alternatively, one 1,200-mg suppository at bedtime for 1 dose.

Topical

- *Cream and lotion:* Cover affected areas bid, morning and evening. Powder: Spray or sprinkle powder liberally over affected area in the morning and evening.

Pediatric patients

Topical

2 yr and older: Use adult dosage.
Younger than 2 yr: Not recommended.

Pharmacokinetics

Route	Onset	Peak
Topical	Rapid	Unknown
Vaginal	Unknown	Unknown

Metabolism: Hepatic; $T_{1/2}$: 21–24 hr
Distribution: Crosses placenta; may enter breast milk
Excretion: Feces, urine

Adverse effects

Vaginal suppositories

- **Local:** *Irritation,* sensitization or vulvovaginal burning, pelvic cramps
- **Other:** Rash, headache

Topical application

- **Local:** *Irritation, burning, maceration,* allergic contact dermatitis

■ Nursing considerations

Assessment

- **History:** Allergy to miconazole or components used in preparation; lactation, pregnancy
- **Physical:** Skin color, lesions, area around lesions; T; orientation, affect; culture of area involved

Interventions

- Culture fungus involved before therapy.
- Insert vaginal suppositories high into the vagina; have patient remain recumbent for 10–15 min after insertion; provide sanitary napkin to protect clothing from stains.
- Monitor response; if none is noted, arrange for further cultures to determine causative organism.
- Apply lotion to intertriginous areas if topical application is required; if cream is used, apply sparingly to avoid maceration of the area.
- Ensure patient receives the full course of therapy to eradicate the fungus and to prevent recurrence.

⊗ ***Warning*** Discontinue topical or vaginal administration if rash or sensitivity occurs.

Teaching points

- Take the full course of drug therapy even if symptoms improve. Continue during menstrual period even if vaginal route is being used. Long-term use will be needed; beneficial effects may not be seen for several weeks.
- Insert vaginal suppositories high into the vagina.
- Use hygiene measures to prevent reinfection or spread of infection.
- This drug is for the fungus being treated; do not self-medicate other problems with this drug.
- Refrain from sexual intercourse, or advise partner to use a condom to avoid reinfection; with vaginal form of drug, use a sanitary napkin to prevent staining of clothing.
- You may experience these side effects: Irritation, burning, stinging.
- Report local irritation, burning (topical application); rash, irritation, pelvic pain (vaginal use).

DANGEROUS DRUG

▽ midazolam hydrochloride

*(mid **ay'** zoh lam)*

Apo-Midazolam (CAN)

PREGNANCY CATEGORY D

CONTROLLED SUBSTANCE C-IV

Drug classes

Benzodiazepine (short-acting)
CNS depressant

Therapeutic actions

Exact mechanisms of action not understood; acts mainly at the limbic system and reticular formation; potentiates the effects of GABA, an inhibitory neurotransmitter; anxiolytic and amnesia effects occur at doses below those needed to cause sedation, ataxia; has little effect on cortical function.

Indications

- IV or IM: Sedation, anxiolysis, and amnesia prior to diagnostic, therapeutic, or endoscopic procedures or surgery
- Induction of general anesthesia
- Continuous sedation of intubated and mechanically ventilated patients as a component of anesthesia or during treatment in the critical care setting
- Unlabeled uses: Treatment of epileptic seizure or refractory status epilepticus

Contraindications and cautions

- Contraindicated with hypersensitivity to benzodiazepines, allergy to cherries (syrup), psychoses, acute narrow-angle glaucoma, shock, coma, acute alcoholic intoxication, pregnancy (cleft lip or palate, inguinal hernia, cardiac defects, microcephaly, pyloric stenosis have been reported when used in first trimester; neonatal withdrawal syndrome reported in infants) and in neonates.

- Use cautiously in elderly or debilitated patients; in patients being treated for open-angle glaucoma; with impaired liver or renal function, lactation.

Available forms

Injection—5 mg/mL, 1 mg/mL, syrup—2 mg/mL

Dosages

⊗ ***Black box warning*** Midazolam should only be administered by a person trained in general anesthesia and with equipment for maintaining airway and resuscitation on hand; respiratory depression and respiratory arrest can occur. Administer IV with continuous monitoring of respiratory and CV function. Individualize dosage; use lower dosage in the elderly and debilitated patients. Adjust dosage according to use of other premedication.

⊗ ***Warning*** Rapid injection should be avoided in neonates, especially when given with fentanyl.

⊗ ***Warning*** Midazolam syrup has been associated with respiratory depression and arrest, especially when given with opioids.

Adults

- *Preoperative sedation, anxiety, amnesia:* *Younger than 60 yr:* 70–80 mcg/kg IM 1 hr before surgery (usual dose, 5 mg).
  Older than 60 yr or debilitated: 20–50 mcg/kg IM 1 hr before surgery (usual dose, 1–3 mg).
- *Conscious sedation for short procedures:* *Younger than 60 yr:* 1–2.5 mg IV initially, maintenance dose of 25% of initial dose.
  Older than 60 yr: 1–1.5 mg IV initially, maintenance dose of 25% initial dose.
- *Induction of anesthesia:*
  Younger than 55 yr: 300–350 mcg/kg IV (up to a total of 600 mcg/kg).
  Older than 55 yr: 150–300 mcg/kg IV as initial dose.
  Debilitated adults: 150–250 mcg/kg IV as initial dose.
- *Sedation in critical care areas:* 10–50 mcg/kg (0.5–4 mg usual dose) as a loading dose; may repeat every 10–15 min until desired effect is seen; continuous infusion of 20–100 mcg/kg/hr to sustain effect.

Pediatric patients

- *Preoperative sedation, anxiety, amnesia:* *6 mo–16 yr:* 0.1–0.15 mg/kg IM; do not exceed 10 mg/dose.
- *Conscious sedation for short procedures:* *Older than 12 yr:* 1–2.5 mg IV initially, maintenance dose of 25% of initial dose.
- *Conscious sedation for short procedures prior to anesthesia:*
  6–12 yr: 25–50 mcg/kg IV initially. Up to 400 mcg/kg may be used; do not exceed 10 mg/dose.
  6 mo–5 yr: 50–100 mcg/kg IV. Do not exceed 6 mg total dose.
- *Sedation in critical care areas for intubated patients only:* 50–200 mcg/kg IV as a loading dose, then continuous infusion of 60–120 mcg/kg/hr.
  Neonates older than 32 wk gestation: 60 mcg/kg/hr IV.
  Neonates younger than 32 wk gestation: 30 mcg/kg/hr IV.

IV FACTS

Preparation: Do not mix with other solutions; do not mix in plastic bags or tubing; may be used undiluted or diluted in D_5W, 0.9% normal saline, or lactated Ringer's.

Infusion: Inject slowly into large vein over 2 min, monitoring patient response.

Y-site incompatibilities: Albumin, ampicillin, ceftazidime, cefuroxime, clonidine, dexamethasone, foscarnet, furosemide, hydrocortisone, methotrexate, nafcillin, omeprazole, sodium bicarbonate.

Pharmacokinetics

Route	*Onset*	*Peak*	*Duration*
IM	15 min	30 min	2–6 hr
IV	3–5 min	Less than 30 min	2–6 hr

Metabolism: Hepatic metabolism; $T_{1/2}$: 1.8–6.8 hr

Distribution: Crosses placenta; enters breast milk

Excretion: Urine

Adverse effects

- **CNS:** Transient and mild drowsiness (initially), sedation, depression, lethargy, apathy, fatigue, light-headedness, disorientation,

M

restlessness, confusion, crying, delirium, headache, slurred speech, dysarthria, stupor, rigidity, tremor, dystonia, vertigo, euphoria, nervousness, difficulty in concentration, vivid dreams, psychomotor retardation, extrapyramidal symptoms, mild paradoxical excitatory reactions (during first 2 wk of treatment), visual and auditory disturbances, diplopia, nystagmus, depressed hearing, nasal congestion

- **CV:** Bradycardia, tachycardia, CV collapse, hypertension, hypotension, palpitations, edema
- **Dependence:** Drug dependence with withdrawal syndrome when drug is discontinued (more common with abrupt discontinuation of higher dosage used for longer than 4 mo)
- **Dermatologic:** Urticaria, pruritus, skin rash, dermatitis
- **GI:** Constipation, diarrhea, dry mouth, salivation, nausea, anorexia, vomiting, difficulty in swallowing, gastric disorders, elevations of blood enzymes: LDH, alkaline phosphatase, AST, ALT, hepatic impairment, jaundice
- **GU:** Incontinence, urine retention, changes in libido, menstrual irregularities
- **Hematologic:** Decreased Hct, blood dyscrasias
- **Other:** Phlebitis and thrombosis at IV injection sites, hiccups, fever, diaphoresis, paresthesias, muscular disturbances, gynecomastia; pain, burning, and redness after IM injection

Interactions

✱ **Drug-drug** • Risk of increased CNS depression if combined with alcohol, antihistamines, opioids, other sedatives; protease inhibitors, decrease midazolam dose by up to 50% if any of these combinations are used • Decreased effectiveness if given with carbamazepine, phenytoin, rifampin, rifabutin, phenobarbital; monitor patient's response carefully

✱ **Drug-food** • Decreased metabolism and increased effects of midazolam with grapefruit juice; avoid this combination

■ Nursing considerations

Assessment

- **History:** Hypersensitivity to benzodiazepines; psychoses, acute narrow-angle glaucoma, shock, coma, acute alcoholic intoxication with depression of vital signs; elderly or debilitated; impaired liver or renal function; pregnancy, lactation
- **Physical:** Weight; skin color, lesions; orientation, affect, reflexes, sensory nerve function, ophthalmologic examination; P, BP; R, adventitious sounds; bowel sounds, normal output, liver evaluation; normal output; LFTs, renal function tests, CBC

Interventions

⊗ *Warning* Do not administer intra-arterially, which may produce arteriospasm or gangrene.

- Do not use small veins (dorsum of hand or wrist) for IV injection.
- Administer IM injections deep into muscle.
- Monitor IV injection site for extravasation.
- Arrange to reduce dosage of midazolam if patient is also being given opioid analgesics; reduce dosage by at least 50% and monitor patient closely.
- Monitor level of consciousness before, during, and for at least 2–6 hr after administration of midazolam.
- Carefully monitor P, BP, and respirations carefully during administration.

⊗ *Warning* Keep resuscitative facilities readily available; have flumazenil available as antidote if overdose should occur.

- Keep patients in bed for 3 hr; do not permit ambulatory patients to operate a vehicle following an injection.
- Arrange to monitor liver and renal function and CBC at intervals during long-term therapy.
- Establish safety precautions if CNS changes occur (use side rails, accompany ambulating patient).
- Provide comfort measures and reassurance for patients receiving diazepam for tetanus.
- Arrange to taper dosage gradually after long-term therapy.
- Provide patient with written information regarding recovery and follow-up care. Midazolam is a potent amnesiac and memory may be altered.

Teaching points

- This drug will help you to relax and will make you go to sleep; this drug is a potent

amnesiac and you will not remember what has happened to you.
- Avoid using alcohol or sleep-inducing or over-the-counter drugs before receiving this drug. If you feel that you need one of these preparations, consult your health care provider.
- You may experience these side effects: Drowsiness, dizziness (these may become less pronounced after a few days; avoid driving a car or engaging in other dangerous activities if these occur); GI upset; dreams, difficulty concentrating, fatigue, nervousness, crying (it may help to know that these are effects of the drug; consult your health care provider if these become bothersome).
- Report severe dizziness, weakness, drowsiness that persists, rash or skin lesions, visual or hearing disturbances, difficulty voiding.

▽ midodrine hydrochloride

(mid' oh dryn)

ProAmatine

PREGNANCY CATEGORY C

Drug classes
Alpha agonist
Antihypotensive

Therapeutic actions
Activates alpha receptors in the arteriolar and venous vasculature, producing an increase in vascular tone and elevation of BP.

Indications
- Treatment of symptomatic orthostatic hypotension in patients whose lives are considerably impaired by the disorder and who do not respond to other therapy
- Unlabeled use: Management of urinary incontinence at doses of 2.5–5 mg bid–tid

Contraindications and cautions
- Contraindicated with severe CAD, acute renal disease, urine retention, pheochromocytoma, thyrotoxicosis, persistent or excessive supine hypertension.
- Use cautiously with renal or hepatic impairment, lactation, pregnancy, visual problems. May cause severe hypertension.

Available forms
Tablets—2.5, 5, 10 mg

Dosages
Adults

10 mg PO tid during daytime hours when upright.

Pediatric patients

Safety and efficacy not established.

Patients with renal impairment

Starting dose of 2.5 mg PO tid.

Pharmacokinetics

Route	*Onset*	*Peak*
Oral	Rapid	30 min

Metabolism: Hepatic and tissue; $T_{1/2}$: 25 min
Distribution: Crosses placenta; may enter breast milk
Excretion: Urine

Adverse effects
- **CNS:** Headache, *paresthesias, pain,* dizziness, vertigo, visual field changes
- **CV:** *Supine hypertension, bradycardia*
- **Dermatologic:** *Piloerection, pruritus,* rash
- **Other:** *Dysuria, chills*

Interactions
✱ **Drug-drug** • Increased effects and toxicity of cardiac glycosides, beta blockers, alpha-adrenergic agents, steroids (fludrocortisone) with midodrine; monitor patient carefully and adjust dosage as needed

■ Nursing considerations
Assessment
- **History:** Severe CAD, acute renal disease, urine retention, pheochromocytoma, thyrotoxicosis, persistent or excessive supine hypertension, renal or hepatic impairment, lactation, pregnancy, visual problems
- **Physical:** T; orientation, visual field checks; skin color, lesions, T; BP—sitting, standing, supine, P; LFTs, renal function tests

M

Interventions

- Establish baseline hepatic and renal function and evaluate periodically during therapy.

⊠ ***Black box warning*** Monitor BP carefully, especially if used with any drug that causes vasoconstriction, because drug can cause marked increase in blood pressure. Give only to patients who are ambulatory—do not give to bedridden patients or before bed.

⊗ ***Warning*** Monitor HR when beginning therapy. Bradycardia is common as therapy begins; persistent bradycardia should be evaluated and drug discontinued.

⊗ ***Warning*** Monitor patients with known visual problems or who are taking fludrocortisone for any change in visual fields. Discontinue drug and consult physician if changes occur.

- Encourage patient to take drug after voiding if urine retention is a problem.

Teaching points

- Take this drug during the day when you will be up and around. Do not take it before going to bed or lying down.
- Empty your bladder before taking this drug if urine retention has been a problem.
- Return for regular medical evaluation of your blood pressure and response to this drug.
- You may experience these side effects: Numbness or tingling in the extremities (avoid injury); slow heart rate; rash, goose bumps.
- Report changes in vision, pounding in the head when lying down, very slow heart rate, difficulty urinating.

▽ mifepristone (RU-486)

*(miff eh **prist' own**)*

Mifeprex

PREGNANCY CATEGORY X

Drug class

Abortifacient

Therapeutic actions

Acts as an antagonist of progesterone sites in the endometrium, allowing prostaglandins to stimulate uterine contractions, causing implanted trophoblast to separate from the placental wall; may also decrease placental viability and accelerate degenerative changes resulting in sloughing of the endometrium.

Indications

- Termination of pregnancy through 49 days gestational age; most effective when combined with a prostaglandin
- Unlabeled uses: Postcoital contraception, endometriosis, unresectable meningioma, fetal death, or nonviable early pregnancy

Contraindications and cautions

- Contraindicated with allergy to prostaglandin preparations; acute PID; active cardiac, hepatic, pulmonary, renal disease; undiagnosed adrenal mass; hemorrhagic disorder, anticoagulation; ectopic pregnancy; and in patients with an IUD in place.
- Use cautiously with history of asthma; anemia, jaundice, diabetes, epilepsy, scarred uterus, cervicitis, infected endocervical lesions, acute vaginitis.

Available forms

Tablets—200 mg

Dosages

Adults

Day 1: 600 mg (3 tablets) PO taken as a single dose. Day 3: If termination of pregnancy cannot be confirmed, 400 mcg (2 tablets) misoprostol (*Cytotec*). Day 14: Evaluation for termination of pregnancy; if unsuccessful, surgical intervention is suggested at this time.

Pharmacokinetics

Route	*Onset*	*Peak*
Oral	Rapid	1–3 hr

Metabolism: Tissue; $T_{1/2}$: 18 hr
Distribution: Crosses placenta; may enter breast milk
Excretion: Feces, urine

Adverse effects

- **CNS:** *Headache,* dizziness
- **GI:** *Vomiting, diarrhea, nausea, abdominal pain*

- **GU:** Heavy uterine bleeding, endometritis, uterine or vaginal pain
- **Other: Potentially serious to fatal infection**

■ Nursing considerations

CLINICAL ALERT!
Name confusion has occurred between mifepristone and misoprostol and between *Mifeprex* and *Mirapex* (pramipexole); use extreme caution.

Assessment

- **History:** Allergy to prostaglandin preparations; acute PID; active cardiac, hepatic, pulmonary, renal disease; history of asthma; hypotension; hypertension; CV, adrenal, renal, or hepatic disease; anemia; jaundice; diabetes; epilepsy; scarred uterus; cervicitis, infected endocervical lesions, acute vaginitis
- **Physical:** T; BP, P, auscultation; bowel sounds, liver evaluation; vaginal discharge, pelvic examination, uterine tone; LFTs, renal function tests, WBC count, urinalysis, CBC

Interventions

⊗ ***Black box warning*** Serious or fatal infection may develop after abortion. Monitor patient for sustained fever, prolonged heavy bleeding, severe abdominal pain. Urge patient to seek emergency medical help if these occur.

- Provide appropriate referrals and counseling for abortion.
- Alert patient that menses usually begins within 5 days of treatment and lasts for 1–2 wk.
- Arrange to follow drug within 48 hr with a prostaglandin (*Cytotec*) as appropriate.

⊗ ***Warning*** Ensure that abortion is complete or that other measures are used to complete the abortion if drug effects are not sufficient.

- Prepare for dilatation and curettage if heavy bleeding does not resolve.
- Provide analgesic and antiemetic as needed to increase comfort.
- Ensure patient follow-up; serious to fatal infections have been reported.

Teaching points

Teaching about mifepristone should be incorporated into the total teaching plan for the patient undergoing an abortion; specific information that should be included follows:

- Menses begins within 5 days of treatment and will last 1–2 weeks.
- You may experience these side effects: Nausea, vomiting, diarrhea (medication may be ordered); uterine or vaginal pain, headache (an analgesic may be ordered).
- Be aware that another pregnancy could occur before normal menses begin; start contraception as soon as termination of pregnancy is confirmed and sexual intercourse is resumed.
- Report immediately sustained fever, severe abdominal pain, prolonged heavy bleeding, dizziness on arising, or persistent malaise.

DANGEROUS DRUG

▽ miglitol

(mig' lab tall)

Glyset

PREGNANCY CATEGORY B

Drug classes

Alpha-glucosidase inhibitor
Antidiabetic

Therapeutic actions

An alpha-glucosidase inhibitor that delays the digestion of ingested carbohydrates, leading to a smaller increase in blood glucose following meals and a decrease in glycosylated Hgb; does not enhance insulin secretion and so its effects are additive to those of the sulfonylureas in controlling blood glucose.

Indications

- Adjunct to diet to lower blood glucose in patients with type 2 diabetes mellitus whose hyperglycemia cannot be managed by diet alone
- Combination therapy with a sulfonylurea to enhance glycemic control in those patients with type 2 diabetes who do not receive adequate control with diet and either drug

Contraindications and cautions

- Contraindicated with hypersensitivity to the drug; diabetic ketoacidosis; cirrhosis;

M

inflammatory bowel disease; intestinal obstruction or predisposition to intestinal obstruction; colon ulceration; type 1 diabetes; conditions that would deteriorate with increased gas in the bowel.
- Use cautiously with renal impairment, pregnancy, lactation.

Available forms

Tablets—25, 50, 100 mg

Dosages

Adults

- *Monotherapy:* Initial dose, 25 mg PO tid at the first bite of each meal; may start at 25 mg PO daily if severe GI effects are seen. For maintenance, 50 mg PO tid at first bite of each meal. Maximum dose, 100 mg PO tid.
- *Combination with a sulfonylurea:* Blood glucose may be much lower; monitor closely and adjust dosages of each drug accordingly.

Pediatric patients

Safety and efficacy not established.

Pharmacokinetics

Route	*Onset*	*Peak*
Oral	Rapid	2–3 hr

Metabolism: Not metabolized; $T_{1/2}$: 2 hr
Distribution: Very little
Excretion: Urine

Adverse effects

- **Dermatologic:** Rash
- **Endocrine:** *Hypoglycemia* (taken in combination with other antidiabetic drugs)
- **GI:** Abdominal pain, flatulence, diarrhea, anorexia, nausea, vomiting

Interactions

✱ **Drug-drug** • Decreased bioavailability and effectiveness of propranolol, ranitidine • Miglitol is less effective if taken with digestive enzymes or charcoal; avoid combining
✱ **Drug-alternative therapy** • Increased risk of hypoglycemia if taken with juniper berries, ginseng, garlic, fenugreek, coriander, dandelion root, celery

■ Nursing considerations

Assessment

- **History:** Hypersensitivity to the drug; diabetic ketoacidosis; cirrhosis; inflammatory bowel disease; intestinal obstruction or predisposition to intestinal obstruction; type 1 diabetes; conditions that would deteriorate with increased gas in the bowel; renal impairment; pregnancy; lactation
- **Physical:** Skin color, lesions; T; orientation, reflexes, peripheral sensation; R, adventitious sounds; liver evaluation, bowel sounds; urinalysis, BUN, blood glucose, renal function tests

Interventions

- Give drug tid with the first bite of each meal.
- Monitor urine or serum glucose levels often to determine effectiveness of drug and dosage.
- Tell patient abdominal pain and flatulence are likely.
- Arrange for consult with dietitian to establish weight loss program and dietary control as appropriate. Plan thorough diabetic teaching program to include disease, dietary control, exercise, signs and symptoms of hypoglycemia and hyperglycemia, avoidance of infection, and hygiene.

Teaching points

- Do not discontinue this medication without consulting your health care provider.
- Take this drug three times a day with the first bite of each meal.
- Monitor blood for glucose and ketones as prescribed.
- Continue diet and exercise program established for control of diabetes.
- You may experience these side effects: Abdominal pain, flatulence, bloating.
- Report fever, sore throat, unusual bleeding or bruising, severe abdominal pain.

▽ miglustat

See Appendix W, *Less commonly used drugs.*

▽ milnacipran

See Appendix W, *Less commonly used drugs.*

DANGEROUS DRUG

milrinone lactate

(mill' ri none)

Primacor

Pregnancy Category C

Drug class

Inotropic

Therapeutic actions

Increases force of contraction of ventricles (positive inotropic effect); causes vasodilation by a direct relaxant effect on vascular smooth muscle.

Indications

- Heart failure: Short-term IV management of patients with acute decompensated heart failure

Contraindications and cautions

- Contraindicated with allergy to milrinone or bisulfites; severe aortic or pulmonic valvular disease.
- Use cautiously in the elderly, and with pregnancy, lactation.

Available forms

Injection—1 mg/mL

Dosages

Adults

Loading dose, 50 mcg/kg IV bolus, given over 10 min. Maintenance infusion, 0.375–0.75 mcg/kg/min. Do not exceed a total of 1.13 mg/kg/day.

Pediatric patients

Not recommended.

Geriatric patients or patients with renal impairment

Do not exceed 1.13 mg/kg/day. For patients with renal impairment, refer to this table:

CrCl (mL/min)	*Infusion Rate (mcg/kg/min)*
5	0.2
10	0.23
20	0.28
30	0.33
40	0.38
50	0.43

Pharmacokinetics

Route	*Onset*	*Peak*	*Duration*
IV	Immediate	5–15 min	8 hr

Metabolism: Hepatic; $T_{1/2}$: 2.3–2.5 hr

Distribution: Crosses placenta; may enter breast milk

Excretion: Urine

IV FACTS

Preparation: Add diluent of 0.45% or 0.9% sodium chloride injection, USP or 5% dextrose injection, USP. Add 180 mL per 20-mg vial to prepare solution of 100 mcg/mL; 113 mL per 20-mg vial to prepare a solution of 150 mcg/mL; add 80 mL diluent to 20-mg vial to prepare solution of 200 mcg/mL. Or, premixed infusion may be used without further dilution.

Infusion: Administer while carefully monitoring patient's hemodynamic and clinical response; see manufacturer's insert for detailed guidelines.

Incompatibility: Do not mix directly with other drugs. Furosemide should not be administered through same IV line because precipitate may form.

Adverse effects

- **CNS:** Headache
- **CV:** *Ventricular arrhythmias,* hypotension, supraventricular arrhythmias, chest pain, angina, **death**
- **Hematologic:** Thrombocytopenia, hypokalemia

Interactions

*** Drug-drug** • Precipitate formation in solution if given in the same IV line with furosemide; avoid this combination

■ Nursing considerations

Assessment

- **History:** Allergy to milrinone or bisulfites, severe aortic or pulmonic valvular disease, lactation, pregnancy
- **Physical:** Weight, orientation, P, BP, cardiac auscultation, peripheral pulses and perfusion, R, adventitious sounds, serum electrolyte levels, platelet count, ECG, renal function tests

M

Interventions

- Monitor cardiac rhythm continually.
- Monitor BP and P and reduce dose if marked decreases occur.
- Monitor I & O and electrolyte levels.

Teaching points

- You will need frequent monitoring of your blood pressure, pulse, and heart activity during therapy.
- You may experience increased voiding; appropriate bathroom arrangements will be made.
- Report pain at IV injection site, numbness or tingling, shortness of breath, chest pain.

minocycline hydrochloride

*(mi noe **sye'** kleen)*

Apo-Minocycline (CAN), Arestin, Cleervue-M, Dynacin, Gen-Minocycline (CAN), Minocin, Myrac, ratio-Minocycline (CAN), Solodyn

PREGNANCY CATEGORY D

Drug classes

Antibiotic
Tetracycline

Therapeutic actions

Bacteriostatic: Inhibits protein synthesis of susceptible bacteria, causing cell death.

Indications

- Infections caused by rickettsiae; *Mycoplasma pneumoniae*; agents of psittacosis, ornithosis, lymphogranuloma venereum and granuloma inguinale; *Borrelia recurrentis; Haemophilus ducreyi; Pasteurella pestis; Pasteurella tularensis; Bartonella bacilliformis; Bacteroides; Vibrio comma; Vibrio fetus; Brucella; Escherichia coli; Enterobacter aerogenes; Shigella; Acinetobacter calcoaceticus; Haemophilus influenzae; Klebsiella; Diplococcus pneumoniae; Staphylococcus aureus*
- When penicillin is contraindicated, infections caused by *Neisseria gonorrhoeae, Treponema pallidum, Treponema pertenue, Listeria monocytogenes, Clostridium, Bacillus anthracis*
- As an adjunct to amebicides in acute intestinal amebiasis
- Oral tetracyclines are indicated for treatment of severe acne, uncomplicated urethral, endocervical, or rectal infections in adults caused by *Chlamydia trachomatis*

NEW INDICATION: Treatment of inflammatory lesions of nonnodule, moderate to severe acne vulgaris in patients 12 yr and older (ER tablets)

- Oral minocycline is indicated in treatment of asymptomatic carriers of *N. meningitidis* (not useful for treating the infection); infections caused by *Mycobacterium marinum;* uncomplicated urethral, endocervical, or rectal infections caused by *Ureaplasma urealyticum;* uncomplicated gonococcal urethritis in men due to *N. gonorrhoeae*
- *Arestin:* Adjunct to scaling and root planing to reduce pocket depth in patients with adult periodontitis
- Unlabeled use: Alternative to sulfonamides in the treatment of nocardiosis; treatment of early rheumatoid arthritis, gallbladder infection caused by *Escherichia coli*

Contraindications and cautions

- Contraindicated with allergy to tetracyclines.
- Use cautiously with renal or hepatic impairment, pregnancy, lactation, asthma.

Available forms

Capsules—50, 75, 100 mg; pellet-filled capsules—50, 100 mg; oral suspension—50 mg/5 mL; tablets—50, 75, 100 mg; sustained release microsphere—1 mg; ER tablets—45, 90, 115, 135 mg; injection—100 mg/vial

Dosages

Adults

200 mg initially, followed by 100 mg every 12 hr PO. May be given as 100–200 mg initially and then 50 mg qid PO.

- *Syphilis:* Usual PO dose for 10–15 days.

- *Urethral, endocervical, rectal infections:* 100 mg bid PO for 7 days.
- *Gonococcal urethritis in men:* 100 mg bid PO for 5 days.
- *Gonorrhea:* 200 mg PO followed by 100 mg every 12 hr for 4 days; get post-therapy cultures within 2–3 days.
- *Meningococcal carrier state:* 100 mg every 12 hr PO for 5 days.
- *Adult periodontitis:* Unit dose cartridge discharged in subgingival area.
- *Moderate to severe acne vulgaris (12 yr and older)*: 1 mg/kg/day PO for upto 12 wk (ER tablets).

IV

200 mg followed by 100 mg every 12 hr. Do not exceed 400 mg/day. Switch to oral form as soon as possible.

Pediatric patients older than 8 yr

4 mg/kg PO followed by 2 mg/kg every 12 hr PO.

ER tablets

Once daily based on patient weight:
45–59 kg: 45 mg.
60–90 kg: 90 mg.
91–136 kg: 135 mg.

IV

4 mg/kg followed by 2 mg/kg every 12 hr. Switch to oral form as soon as possible.

Geriatric patients or patients with renal failure

Decrease recommended dosage; increase dosing interval with renal impairment. Do not exceed 200 mg *Minocin* in 24 hr in patients with renal impairment.

Pharmacokinetics

Route	*Onset*	*Peak*
Oral	Rapid	2–3 hr

Metabolism: Hepatic; $T_{1/2}$: 11–24 hr
Distribution: Crosses placenta; enters breast milk
Excretion: Feces, urine

IV FACTS

Preparation: Reconstitute with 5 mL sterile water for injection and immediately dilute with 500–1,000 mL sodium chloride injection, dextrose, dextrose and sodium chloride injection, Ringer's injection, or lactated Ringer's. Administer immediately. Stable 24 hr at room temperature. Discard unused portion.
Infusion: Avoid rapid administration.
Incompatibilities: Do not mix in solution with other drugs, calcium, or whole blood.

Adverse effects

- **Dental:** *Discoloring and inadequate calcification of primary teeth of fetus if used by pregnant women; discoloring and inadequate calcification of permanent teeth if used during period of dental development*
- **Dermatologic:** *Phototoxic reactions, rash,* exfoliative dermatitis (more frequent and severe with this tetracycline than with others)
- **GI:** Fatty liver, **liver failure,** *anorexia, nausea, vomiting, diarrhea, glossitis,* dysphagia, enterocolitis, esophageal ulcer, dyspepsia
- **Hematologic:** Hemolytic anemia, thrombocytopenia, neutropenia, eosinophilia, leukocytosis, leukopenia
- **Local:** Local irritation at injection site
- **Other:** Superinfections, nephrogenic diabetes insipidus syndrome

M

Interactions

✱ **Drug-drug** • Decreased absorption of minocycline with antacids, iron, alkali • Increased digoxin toxicity • Increased nephrotoxicity with methoxyflurane • Decreased activity of penicillin
✱ **Drug-food** • Decreased absorption of minocycline if taken with food, dairy products

■ Nursing considerations

Assessment

- **History:** Allergy to tetracyclines, renal or hepatic impairment, pregnancy, lactation
- **Physical:** Skin status, orientation and reflexes, R and adventitious sounds, GI function and liver evaluation, urinalysis and BUN, LFTs, renal function tests; culture of infected area

Interventions

- Administer oral medication without regard to food or meals; if GI upset occurs, give with meals.
- Reserve IV use for situations in which oral use is not possible. Switch from IV to oral route as soon as possible.

Teaching points

- Take drug throughout the day for best results.
- Take with meals if GI upset occurs.
- *Arestin:* After treatment, avoid eating hard, crunchy, or sticky foods for 1 week and postpone brushing for 12 hours.
- You may experience these side effects: Sensitivity to sunlight (wear protective clothing, use sunscreen); diarrhea, nausea (take with meals; eat frequent small meals).
- Report rash, itching; difficulty breathing; dark urine or light-colored stools; severe cramps, watery diarrhea.

▽minoxidil

(mi nox' i dill)

Topical: Rogaine, Rogaine Extra Strength

PREGNANCY CATEGORY C

Drug classes

Antihypertensive
Vasodilator

Therapeutic actions

Acts directly on vascular smooth muscle to cause vasodilation, reducing elevated systolic and diastolic BP; does not interfere with CV reflexes; does not usually cause orthostatic hypotension but does cause reflex tachycardia and renin release, leading to sodium and water retention; mechanism in stimulating hair growth is not known, possibly related to arterial dilation.

Indications

- Severe hypertension that is symptomatic or associated with target organ damage and is not manageable with maximum therapeutic doses of a diuretic plus two other antihypertensive drugs; use in milder hypertension not recommended
- Topical use (when compounded as a 1%–5% lotion or 1% ointment): Alopecia areata and male pattern alopecia

Contraindications and cautions

- Contraindicated with hypersensitivity to minoxidil or any component of the topical preparation (topical); pheochromocytoma (may stimulate release of catecholamines from tumor); acute MI; dissecting aortic aneurysm; lactation.
- Use cautiously with malignant hypertension, HF (use diuretic), angina pectoris (use a beta-blocker), pregnancy.

Available forms

Tablets—2.5, 10 mg; topical 2%, 5%

Dosages

Adults and patients 12 yr and older

Oral

- *Monotherapy:* Initial dosage is 5 mg/day PO as a single dose. Daily dosage can be increased to 10, 20, then 40 mg in single or divided doses. Effective range is usually 10–40 mg/day PO. Maximum dosage is 100 mg/day. If supine diastolic BP has been reduced less than 30 mm Hg, administer the drug only once a day. If reduced more than 30 mm Hg, divide the daily dose into two equal parts. Dosage adjustment should normally be at least at 3-day intervals; in emergencies, every 6 hr with careful monitoring is possible.
- *Concomitant therapy with diuretics:* Use minoxidil with a diuretic in patients relying on renal function for maintaining salt and water balance; the following diuretic dosages have been used when starting minoxidil therapy: Hydrochlorothiazide, 50 mg bid; chlorthalidone, 50–100 mg daily; furosemide, 40 mg bid. If excessive salt and water retention result in weight gain more than 5 lb, change diuretic therapy to furosemide; if patient already takes furosemide, increase dosage.
- *Concomitant therapy with beta-adrenergic blockers or other sympatholytics:* The following dosages are recommended when starting minoxidil therapy: Propranolol, 80–160 mg/day; other beta blockers, dosage equivalent to the above; methyldopa 250–750 mg bid (start methyldopa at least 24 hr before minoxidil); clonidine, 0.1–0.2 mg bid.

Topical

Apply 1 mL to the total affected areas of the scalp twice daily. The total daily dosage should not exceed 2 mL. Twice daily application for longer than 4 mo may be required before evidence of hair regrowth is observed. Once hair growth is realized, twice daily application is necessary for continued and additional hair regrowth. Balding process reported to return to untreated state 3–4 mo after cessation of the drug.

Pediatric patients younger than 12 yr

Experience is limited, particularly in infants; use recommendations as a guide; careful adjustment is necessary. Initial dosage is 0.2 mg/kg/day PO as a single dose. May increase by 50%–100% increments until optimum BP control is achieved. Effective range is usually 0.25–1 mg/kg/day; maximum dose is 50 mg daily. Experience in children is limited; monitor carefully.

Geriatric patients or patients with impaired renal function

Smaller doses may be required; closely supervise to prevent cardiac failure or exacerbation of renal failure.

Pharmacokinetics

Route	*Onset*	*Peak*	*Duration*
Oral	30 min	2–3 hr	75 hr

Metabolism: Hepatic; $T_{1/2}$: 4.2 hr
Distribution: Crosses placenta; enters breast milk
Excretion: Urine

Adverse effects

- **CNS:** Fatigue, headache
- **CV:** Tachycardia (unless given with beta-adrenergic blocker or other sympatholytic drug), pericardial effusion and tamponade; *changes in direction and magnitude of T-waves;* cardiac necrotic lesions (reported in patients with known ischemic heart disease, but risk of minoxidil-associated cardiac damage cannot be excluded)
- **Dermatologic:** *Temporary edema, hypertrichosis* (elongation, thickening, and enhanced pigmentation of fine body hair occurring within 3–6 wk of starting therapy; usually first noticed on temples, between eyebrows and extending to other parts of face, back, arms, legs, scalp); rashes including bullous eruptions; **Stevens-Johnson syndrome;** darkening of the skin
- **GI:** Nausea, vomiting
- **Hematologic:** Initial decrease in Hct, Hgb, RBC count
- **Local:** *Irritant dermatitis, allergic contact dermatitis, eczema, pruritus, dry skin or scalp, flaking, alopecia* (topical use)
- **Respiratory:** *Bronchitis, upper respiratory infection, sinusitis* (topical use)

■ Nursing considerations

Assessment

- **History:** Hypersensitivity to minoxidil or any component of the topical preparation; pheochromocytoma; acute MI, dissecting aortic aneurysm; malignant hypertension; heart failure; angina pectoris; lactation, pregnancy
- **Physical:** Skin color, lesions, hair, scalp; P, BP, orthostatic BP, supine BP, perfusion, edema, auscultation; bowel sounds, normal output; CBC with differential, renal function tests, urinalysis, ECG

Interventions

- Apply topical preparation to affected area; if you use your fingers, wash hands thoroughly afterward.
- Do not apply other topical drugs, including topical corticosteroids, retinoids, and petrolatum or agents known to enhance cutaneous drug absorption.
- Do not apply topical preparation to open lesions or breaks in the skin, which could increase risk of systemic absorption.

⊗ ***Warning*** Arrange to withdraw oral drug gradually, especially from children; rapid withdrawal may cause a sudden increase in BP (rebound hypertension has been reported in children, even with gradual withdrawal; use caution and monitor BP closely when withdrawing from children).

⊗ ***Black box warning*** Arrange for echocardiographic evaluation of possible pericardial effusion if using oral drug; more vigorous diuretic therapy, dialysis, other treatment (including minoxidil withdrawal) may be required.

Teaching points

Oral

- Take this drug exactly as prescribed. Take all other medications that have been prescribed. Do not discontinue any drug or reduce the

M

dosage without consulting your health care provider.

- You may experience these side effects: Enhanced growth and darkening of fine body and face hair (do not discontinue medication without consulting your health care provider); GI upset (eat frequent small meals).
- Report increased heart rate of 20 beats or more per minute over normal (your normal heart rate is ___ beats per minute); rapid weight gain of more than 5 pounds; unusual swelling of the extremities, face, or abdomen; difficulty breathing, especially when lying down; new or aggravated symptoms of angina (chest, arm, or shoulder pain); severe indigestion; dizziness, light-headedness, or fainting.

Topical

- Apply the prescribed amount to the affected area twice a day. If using your fingers, wash hands thoroughly after application. It may take 4 months or longer for any noticeable hair regrowth to appear. Response to this drug is very individual. If no response is seen within 4 months, consult your health care provider about efficacy of continued use.
- Do not apply more frequent or larger applications. This will not speed up or increase hair growth but may increase side effects.
- If one or two daily applications are missed, restart twice-daily applications, and return to usual schedule. Do not attempt to make up missed applications.
- Do not apply any other topical medication to the area while you are using this drug.
- Do not apply to any sunburned, broken skin or open lesions; this increases the risk of systemic effects. Do not apply to any part of the body other than the scalp.
- Twice-daily use of the drug will be needed to retain or continue the hair regrowth.

▽ mirtazapine

*(mer **tab'** zah peen)*

Gen-Mirtazapine (CAN), Novo-Mirtazapine OD (CAN), Remeron, Remeron SolTab, Sandoz-Mirtazapine (CAN)

PREGNANCY CATEGORY C

Drug class

Antidepressant (tetracyclic)

Therapeutic actions

Mechanism of action unknown; appears to act similarly to TCAs, which inhibit the presynaptic reuptake of the neurotransmitters norepinephrine and serotonin; anticholinergic at CNS and peripheral receptors; sedating; relation of these effects to clinical efficacy is unknown.

Indications

- Treatment of major depressive disorder
- **NEW INDICATION:** Unlabeled uses: Chronic urticaria, hot flashes, drug-induced hyperhidrosis, pruritus

Contraindications and cautions

- Contraindicated with hypersensitivity to any tricyclic or tetracyclic drug; concomitant therapy with an MAOI; pregnancy (limb reduction abnormalities reported); lactation.
- Use cautiously with ECT; preexisting CV disorders (eg, severe coronary heart disease, progressive HF, angina pectoris, paroxysmal tachycardia [possible increased risk of serious CVS toxicity with TCAs]); angle-closure glaucoma, increased IOP; urine retention, ureteral or urethral spasm; seizure disorders (TCAs lower the seizure threshold); hyperthyroidism (predisposes to CVS toxicity, including cardiac arrhythmias); impaired hepatic, renal function; psychiatric patients (schizophrenic or paranoid patients may exhibit a worsening of psychosis with TCAs); bipolar disorder (may shift to hypomanic or manic phase); elective surgery (TCAs should be discontinued as long as possible before surgery).

Available forms

Tablets—7.5, 15, 30, 45 mg; orally disintegrating tablet—15, 30, 45 mg

Dosages

Adults

Initial dose, 15 mg PO daily, as a single dose in evening. May be increased up to 45 mg/day as needed. Change dose only at intervals greater than 1–2 wk. Continue treatment for up to 6 mo for acute episodes.

- *Switching from MAOI:* Allow at least 14 days between discontinuation of MAOI and beginning of mirtazapine therapy. Allow 14 days after stopping mirtazapine before starting MAOI.

Pediatric patients
Not recommended in patients younger than 18 yr.

Geriatric patients and patients with renal or hepatic impairment
Give lower doses to patients older than 60 yr.

Pharmacokinetics

Route	*Onset*	*Peak*	*Duration*
Oral	Slow	2–4 hr	2–4 wk

Metabolism: Hepatic; $T_{1/2}$: 20–40 hr
Distribution: Crosses placenta; enters breast milk
Excretion: Feces, urine

Adverse effects

- **CNS:** *Sedation and anticholinergic (atropine-like) effects, confusion* (especially in elderly), *disturbed concentration,* hallucinations, disorientation, decreased memory, feelings of unreality, delusions, anxiety, nervousness, restlessness, agitation, panic, insomnia, nightmares, hypomania, mania, exacerbation of psychosis, drowsiness, weakness, fatigue, headache, numbness, agitation (less likely with this drug than with other antidepressants)
- **CV:** Orthostatic hypotension, hypertension, syncope, tachycardia, palpitations, **MI,** arrhythmias, **heart block,** precipitation of heart failure, CVA
- **Endocrine:** Elevated or depressed blood sugar; elevated prolactin levels; inappropriate ADH secretion
- **GI:** *Dry mouth, constipation,* paralytic ileus, *nausea* (less likely with this drug than with other antidepressants), *increased appetite, weight gain,* vomiting, anorexia, epigastric distress, diarrhea, flatulence, dysphagia, peculiar taste, increased salivation, stomatitis, glossitis, parotid swelling, abdominal cramps, black tongue, liver enzyme elevations
- **GU:** Urine retention, delayed micturition, dilation of urinary tract, gynecomastia, testicular swelling in men; breast enlargement, menstrual irregularity, galactorrhea in women; increased or decreased libido; impotence
- **Hematologic: Agranulocytosis,** *neutropenia*
- **Hypersensitivity:** Rash, pruritus, vasculitis, petechiae, photosensitization, edema

Interactions

✱ **Drug-drug** ⊗ ***Warning*** Risk of serious, sometimes fatal reactions if combined with MAOIs; do not use this combination or within 14 days of MAOI therapy.

■ Nursing considerations

Assessment

- **History:** Hypersensitivity to any antidepressant; concomitant therapy with MAOI; recent MI; myelography within previous 24 hr or scheduled within 48 hr; lactation; ECT; preexisting CV disorders; angle-closure glaucoma, increased IOP; urine retention, ureteral or urethral spasm; seizure disorders; hyperthyroidism; impaired hepatic, renal function; psychiatric problems; bipolar disorder; elective surgery; pregnancy, lactation
- **Physical:** Body weight; T; skin color, lesions; orientation, affect, reflexes, vision and hearing; P, BP, orthostatic BP, perfusion; bowel sounds, normal output, liver evaluation; urine flow, normal output; usual sexual function, frequency of menses, breast and scrotal examination; LFTs, urinalysis, CBC, renal function tests; ECG

Interventions

⊠ ***Black box warning*** Ensure that depressed and potentially suicidal patients have access only to limited quantities of the drug; increased risk of suicidality in children, adolescents, and young adults. Monitor accordingly.

- Administer orally disintegrating tablets to patients who have difficulty swallowing: Open blister pack and have patient place tablet on tongue. Do not split tablet.
- Expect clinical response in 3–7 days up to 3 wk (latter is more usual).

M

- Arrange for CBC if patient develops fever, sore throat, or other sign of infection during therapy.
- Establish safety precautions if CNS changes occur (raise side rails, accompany patient when ambulating).

Teaching points

- Take this drug exactly as prescribed; do not stop taking the drug abruptly or without consulting your health care provider.
- Place orally disintegrating tablet on tongue; it can be swallowed without water. Open blister pack with dry hands and use tablet immediately; do not cut or break tablet.
- Avoid using alcohol, other sleep-inducing drugs, or over-the-counter drugs while using this drug.
- Avoid prolonged exposure to sunlight or sunlamps; use a sunscreen or protective garments if long exposure to sunlight is unavoidable.
- You may experience these side effects: Headache, dizziness, drowsiness, weakness, blurred vision (reversible; avoid driving or performing tasks that require alertness); nausea, vomiting, loss of appetite, dry mouth (eat frequent small meals; use frequent mouth care, suck on sugarless candies); nightmares, inability to concentrate, confusion; changes in sexual function.
- Report fever, flulike symptoms, any infection, dry mouth, difficulty urinating, excessive sedation, suicidal thoughts.

▽ misoprostol

*(mye soe **prost'** ole)*

Apo-Misoprostol (CAN), Cytotec

PREGNANCY CATEGORY X

Drug class

Prostaglandin

Therapeutic actions

A synthetic prostaglandin E_1 analogue; inhibits gastric acid secretion and increases bicarbonate and mucus production, protecting the lining of the stomach.

Indications

- Prevention of NSAID (including aspirin)-induced gastric ulcers in patients at high risk of complications from a gastric ulcer (the elderly; patients with concomitant debilitating disease, history of ulcers)
- With mifepristone as an abortifacient (see mifepristone)
- Unlabeled use: Appears effective in treating but not preventing duodenal ulcers in patients unresponsive to histamine-2 antagonists; cervical ripening and labor induction; postpartum hemorrhage; chronic idiopathic constipation

Contraindications and cautions

- Contraindicated with history of allergy to prostaglandins; pregnancy (abortifacient; advise women of childbearing age in written and oral form of use, have a negative serum pregnancy test within 2 wk prior to therapy, provide contraceptives, and begin therapy on the second or third day of the next normal menstrual period); lactation.
- Use cautiously in the elderly, and with renal impairment, duodenal ulcers.

Available forms

Tablets—100, 200 mcg

Dosages

Adults

200 mcg four times daily PO with food. If this dose cannot be tolerated, 100 mcg can be used. Take misoprostol for the duration of the NSAID therapy. Take the last dose of the day at bedtime.

Pediatric patients

Safety and efficacy in patients younger than 18 yr not established.

Geriatric patients or patients with renal impairment

Dosage adjustment is usually not needed, but dosage can be reduced if 200-mcg PO dose cannot be tolerated.

Pharmacokinetics

Route	*Onset*	*Peak*
Oral	Rapid	12–15 min

Metabolism: Hepatic; $T_{1/2}$: 20–40 min
Distribution: Crosses placenta; may enter breast milk
Excretion: Urine

Adverse effects

- **GI:** *Nausea, diarrhea, abdominal pain, flatulence,* vomiting, dyspepsia, constipation
- **GU:** *Miscarriage,* excessive bleeding, *spotting, cramping,* hypermenorrhea, menstrual disorders, dysmenorrhea
- **Other:** Headache

■ Nursing considerations

CLINICAL ALERT!
Name confusion has occurred between misoprostol and mifepristone; use extreme caution.

Assessment

- **History:** Allergy to prostaglandins; pregnancy, lactation; renal impairment, duodenal ulcer
- **Physical:** Abdominal examination, normal bowel function, urinary output

Interventions

- Give to patients at high risk for developing NSAID-induced gastric ulcers; give for the full term of the NSAID use.

⊗ ***Black box warning*** Arrange for serum pregnancy test for any woman of childbearing age; women must have a negative test within 2 wk of beginning therapy; drug can act as an abortifacient.

- Arrange for oral and written explanation of the risks to pregnancy; appropriate contraceptive measures must be taken; begin therapy on the second or third day of a normal menstrual period.

Teaching points

- Take this drug four times a day, with meals and at bedtime. Continue to take your NSAID while taking this drug. Take the drug exactly as prescribed. Do not give this drug to anyone else.
- This drug can cause miscarriage and is often associated with dangerous bleeding. Do not take if pregnant; do not become pregnant while taking this medication. If pregnancy occurs, discontinue drug, and consult your health care provider immediately.
- You may experience these side effects: Abdominal pain, nausea, diarrhea, flatulence (take with meals); menstrual cramping, abnormal menstrual periods, spotting, even in postmenopausal women (request analgesics); headache.
- Report severe diarrhea, spotting or menstrual pain, severe menstrual bleeding, pregnancy.

DANGEROUS DRUG

▽mitomycin (mitomycin-C, MTC)

(mye toe ***mye'*** *sin)*

PREGNANCY CATEGORY D

Drug classes

Antibiotic
Antineoplastic

Therapeutic actions

Cytotoxic: Inhibits DNA synthesis and cellular RNA and protein synthesis in susceptible cells, causing cell death.

Indications

- Disseminated adenocarcinoma of the stomach or pancreas; part of combination therapy or as palliative measure when other modalities fail
- Unlabeled use: Intravesical route—superficial bladder cancer; opthalmic route—may be useful adjunct to surgery in primary or recurrent pterygia; other unlabeled uses include colorectal cancer, breast cancer, squamous cell carcinoma of the head, neck, lungs, and cervix

Contraindications and cautions

- Contraindicated with allergy to mitomycin; thrombocytopenia, coagulation disorders, or increase in bleeding tendencies; severe impaired renal function (creatinine level above 1.7 mg/dL); myelosuppression; pregnancy; lactation.
- Use cautiously with renal impairment.

Available forms

Powder for injection—5-, 20-, 40-mg vials

Dosages

Adults

After hematologic recovery from previous chemotherapy, use the following schedule at 6- to 8-wk intervals: 15 mg/m² IV as a single dose. Reevaluate patient for hematologic response between courses of therapy; adjust dosage accordingly:

Leukocytes (mm³)	*Platelets (mm³)*	*% of Prior Dose to Be Given*
More than 4,000	More than 100,000	100
3,000–3,999	75,000–99,999	100
2,000–2,999	25,000–74,999	70
Less than 2,000	Less than 25,000	50

Do not repeat dosage until leukocyte count has returned to 4,000/mm³ and platelet count to 100,000/mm³.

Pharmacokinetics

Route	*Onset*	*Peak*
IV	Slow	Unknown

Metabolism: Hepatic; $T_{1/2}$: 17 min
Distribution: Crosses placenta; may enter breast milk
Excretion: Urine

IV FACTS

Preparation: Reconstitute 5- to 20-mg vial with 10 or 40 mL of sterile water for injection, respectively; reconstitute 40-mg vial with 80 mL sterile water. Shake vial to improve dissolution. If product does not dissolve immediately, allow to stand at room temperature until solution is obtained. This solution is stable for 14 days if refrigerated, 7 days at room temperature; further dilution in various IV fluids reduces stability—check manufacturer's insert.
Infusion: Infuse slowly over 5–10 min; monitor injection site to avoid local reaction.
Incompatibility: Do not mix with bleomycin.

Adverse effects

- **CNS:** Headache, blurred vision, confusion, drowsiness, syncope, fatigue
- **GI:** *Anorexia, nausea, vomiting,* diarrhea, hematemesis, stomatitis
- **GU:** Renal toxicity, **hemolytic uremic syndrome**
- **Hematologic: Bone marrow toxicity,** microangiopathic hemolytic anemia (a syndrome of anemia, thrombocytopenia, renal failure, hypertension)
- **Respiratory: Pulmonary toxicity, acute respiratory distress syndrome**
- **Other:** *Fever,* cancer in preclinical studies, *cellulitis at injection site, alopecia*

■ Nursing considerations

Assessment

- **History:** Allergy to mitomycin; thrombocytopenia, coagulation disorders or increase in bleeding tendencies; impaired renal function; myelosuppression; pregnancy; lactation
- **Physical:** T; skin color, lesions; weight; hair; local injection site; orientation, reflexes; R, adventitious sounds; mucous membranes; CBC, clotting tests, renal function tests

Interventions

- Do not give IM or subcutaneously due to severe local reaction and tissue necrosis.

⊗ ***Warning*** Monitor injection site for extravasation: If patient reports burning or stinging, discontinue infusion immediately and restart in another vein.

⊗ ***Black box warning*** Monitor patient response frequently at beginning of therapy (CBC, renal function tests, pulmonary examination) because of the risk of bone marrow suppression and hemolytic uremic syndrome with renal failure. Adverse effects may require a decreased dose or discontinuation of drug; consult with physician.

Teaching points

- Prepare a calendar with return dates for drug therapy; this drug can only be given IV.
- Take precautions to avoid pregnancy while using this drug; using barrier contraceptives is advised.
- Have regular medical follow-up visits, including blood tests to monitor drug's effects.
- You may experience these side effects: Rash, skin lesions, loss of hair (obtain a wig; skin care may help); loss of appetite, nausea, mouth sores (frequent mouth care,

eat frequent small meals; maintain good nutrition; consult a dietitian; request an antiemetic); drowsiness, dizziness, syncope, headache (use caution driving or operating dangerous machinery; take special precautions to prevent injuries).
- Report difficulty breathing, sudden weight gain, swelling, burning or pain at injection site, unusual bleeding or bruising.

mitotane

See Appendix W, *Less commonly used drugs.*

DANGEROUS DRUG

mitoxantrone hydrochloride

(mye toe ***zan'*** *trone)*

Novantrone

PREGNANCY CATEGORY D

Drug classes

Antineoplastic
MS drug

Therapeutic actions

Cytotoxic; cell-cycle nonspecific, appears to be DNA reactive, causing the death of both proliferating and nonproliferating cells.

Indications

- As part of combination therapy in the treatment of acute nonlymphocytic leukemia in adults, including myelogenous, promyelocytic, monocytic, and erythroid acute leukemias
- Treatment of pain in patients with advanced prostatic cancer, in combination with steroids
- Treatment of chronic progressive, progressive relapsing, or worsening relapsing-remitting MS
- Unlabeled uses: Treatment of breast cancer, refractory lymphomas, autologous bone marrow transplantation

Contraindications and cautions

- Contraindicated with hypersensitivity to mitoxantrone, pregnancy.
- Use cautiously with bone marrow suppression, HF, lactation.

Available forms

Injection—2 mg/mL

Dosages

Adults

- *Combination therapy:* For induction, 12 mg/m^2 IV per day on days 1–3, with 100 mg/m^2 of cytosine arabinoside for 7 days given as a continuous infusion on days 1–7. If remission does not occur, a second series can be used, with mitoxantrone given for 2 days and cytosine arabinoside for 5 days.
- *Consolidation therapy:* Mitoxantrone 12 mg/m^2 IV for days 1 and 2, and cytosine arabinoside 100 mg/m^2 given as a continuous 24-hr infusion on days 1–5; given 6 wk after induction therapy if needed. Severe myelosuppression may occur.
- *Hormone-refractory prostate cancer:* 12–14 mg/m^2 as short IV infusion every 21 days.
- *MS:* 12 mg/m^2 IV over 5–15 min every 3 mo; do not exceed cumulative lifetime dose of 140 mg/m^2.

Pediatric patients

Safety and efficacy not established.

Pharmacokinetics

Route	Onset	Duration
IV	Rapid	2–3 days

Metabolism: Hepatic; $T_{1/2}$: 5.8 days
Distribution: Crosses placenta; may enter breast milk
Excretion: Bile, urine

IV FACTS

Preparation: Dilute solution to at least 50 mL in either 0.9% sodium chloride or D_5W; may be further diluted in D_5W, normal saline, or dextrose 5% in normal saline if needed. Inject this solution into tubing of a freely running IV of 0.9% sodium chloride injection or 5% dextrose injection over period of at least 3 min. Use immediately after dilution and discard any leftover solution immediately. Wear gloves and goggles and avoid any contact with skin or mucous membranes.

M

Infusion: Inject slowly over at least 3 min.
Incompatibilities: Do not mix in solution with heparin; a precipitate may form. Do not mix in solution with any other drug; studies are not yet available regarding the safety of such mixtures.

Adverse effects

- **CNS:** Headache, seizures
- **CV: Heart failure,** potentially fatal; arrhythmias; chest pain
- **GI:** *Nausea, vomiting, diarrhea,* abdominal pain, mucositis, GI bleeding, jaundice
- **Hematologic: Bone marrow depression,** *infections of all kinds, hyperuricemia*
- **Respiratory:** *Cough,* dyspnea
- **Other:** *Fever, alopecia, cancer in laboratory animals*

■ Nursing considerations

Assessment

- **History:** Hypersensitivity to mitoxantrone, bone marrow depression, HF, pregnancy, lactation
- **Physical:** Neurologic status, T; P, BP, auscultation, peripheral perfusion; R, adventitious sounds; abdominal examination, mucous membranes; LFTs, CBC with differential

Interventions

⊗ ***Black box warning*** Follow CBC and LFTs carefully before and frequently during therapy; dose adjustment may be needed if myelosuppression becomes severe.

- Monitor patient for hyperuricemia, which frequently occurs as a result of rapid tumor lysis; monitor serum uric acid levels and arrange for appropriate treatment as needed.

⊗ ***Warning*** Handle drug with great care; the use of gloves, gowns, and goggles is recommended; if drug comes in contact with skin, wash immediately with warm water; clean spills with calcium hypochlorite solution.

⊗ ***Black box warning*** Monitor IV site for signs of extravasation; if extravasation occurs, stop administration and restart at another site immediately.

⊗ ***Black box warning*** Left ventricular ejection fraction (LVEF) should be evaluated before each dose when treating MS. Yearly evaluations should be done after finishing treatment to detect late cardiac toxic effects; decreased LVEF and frank HF can occur.

⊗ ***Black box warning*** Monitor BP, P, cardiac output regularly during administration; supportive care for heart failure should be started at the first sign of failure.

- Protect patient from exposure to infection; monitor occurrence of infection at any site and arrange for appropriate treatment.

Teaching points

- This drug will need to be given IV for 3 days in conjunction with cytosine therapy; mark calendar with days of treatment. Regular blood tests will be needed to evaluate the effects of this treatment (antineoplastic).
- This drug will be given IV every 3 months when being used to treat MS.
- Using barrier contraceptives is advised; fetal harm may occur if you are pregnant while taking this drug.
- You may experience these side effects: Nausea, vomiting (may be severe; antiemetics may be helpful; eat frequent small meals); increased susceptibility to infection (avoid crowds and exposure to disease); loss of hair (obtain a wig; it is important to keep your head covered in extremes of temperature); blue-green color of the urine (may last for 24 hours after treatment is finished; the whites of the eyes may also be tinted blue for a time; this finding is expected and will pass).
- Report severe nausea and vomiting; fever, chills, sore throat; unusual bleeding or bruising; fluid retention or swelling; severe joint pain.

▽modafinil

(moe ***daff'*** *in ill)*

Alertec (CAN), Provigil

PREGNANCY CATEGORY C

CONTROLLED SUBSTANCE C-IV

Drug classes

CNS stimulant
Narcolepsy drug

Therapeutic actions

A CNS stimulant that helps to improve vigilance and decrease excessive daytime sleepiness associated with narcolepsy and other sleep disorders; may act through dopaminergic mechanisms; exact mechanism of action is not known. Not associated with the cardiac and other systemic stimulatory effects of amphetamines.

Indications

- Treatment of narcolepsy with excessive daytime sleepiness
- Improvement in wakefulness in patients with shift-work sleep disorder (SWSD)
- Improvement in wakefulness in patients with obstructive sleep apnea/hypopnea syndrome (OSAHS)
- Unlabeled use: Treatment of fatigue associated with MS

Contraindications and cautions

- Contraindicated with hypersensitivity to modafinil, left ventricular hypertrophy, ischemic ECG changes, mitral valve prolapse.
- Use cautiously with impaired renal or hepatic function, epilepsy, emotional instability, psychosis, depression, mania, pregnancy, lactation.

Available forms

Tablets—100, 200 mg

Dosages

Adults

- *Narcolepsy, OSAHS:* 200 mg PO daily given as a single dose. Up to 400 mg/day as a single dose may be used.
- *SWSD:* 200 mg/day taken 1 hr before start of shift.

Pediatric patients

Safety and efficacy not established.

Geriatric patients or patients with hepatic impairment

In elderly patients, elimination may be reduced; monitor response and consider use of lower dose. With severe hepatic impairment, reduce dosage to 50%.

Pharmacokinetics

Route	*Onset*	*Peak*
Oral	Gradual	2–3 hr

Metabolism: Hepatic; $T_{1/2}$: 15 hr
Distribution: Crosses placenta; may enter breast milk
Excretion: Urine

Adverse effects

- **CNS:** *Insomnia, headache, nervousness, anxiety,* fatigue
- **Dermatologic:** Rashes, **Stevens-Johnson syndrome**
- **GI:** Dry mouth, choking, nausea, diarrhea, anorexia

Interactions

✱ **Drug-drug** • Increased plasma levels of triazolam when used concurrently; triazolam dosage may need reduction • Possible decreased effectiveness of hormonal contraceptives; suggest the use of barrier contraceptives • Risk of increased levels and effects of warfarin, phenytoin, and TCAs; monitor patient and decrease dosage as appropriate

M

■ Nursing considerations

Assessment

- **History:** Hypersensitivity to modafinil, left ventricular hypertrophy, mitral valve prolapse, ischemic ECG changes, epilepsy, pregnancy, lactation, drug dependence, emotional instability
- **Physical:** Body weight; T; skin color, lesions; orientation, affect, reflexes; P, BP, auscultation; R, adventitious sounds; bowel sounds, normal output; LFTs, renal function tests, baseline ECG

Interventions

- Ensure proper diagnosis before administering to rule out underlying medical problems.

⊗ ***Warning*** Arrange to dispense the least feasible amount of drug at any one time to minimize risk of overdose.

- Administer drug once a day in the morning.
- Arrange to monitor liver function tests periodically in patients on long-term therapy.
- Establish safety precautions if CNS changes occur (use side rails, accompany patient when ambulating).

Teaching points

- Take this drug exactly as prescribed; if taking to improve wakefulness with shift work, take 1 hour before the start of your shift.
- Avoid pregnancy while using this drug; using barrier contraceptives is advised.
- You may experience these side effects: Insomnia, nervousness, restlessness, dizziness, impaired thinking (these effects may become less pronounced after a few days; avoid driving a car or engaging in activities that require alertness if these effects occur, notify your health care provider if they are pronounced or bothersome), headache.
- Report insomnia, abnormal body movements, rash, severe diarrhea, pale-colored stools, yellowing of the skin or eyes.

moexipril

(mo ex' ah pril)

Univasc

PREGNANCY CATEGORY C (FIRST TRIMESTER)

PREGNANCY CATEGORY D (SECOND AND THIRD TRIMESTERS)

Drug classes

ACE inhibitor
Antihypertensive

Therapeutic actions

Renin, synthesized by the kidneys, is released into the circulation where it acts on a plasma precursor to produce angiotensin I, which is converted by ACE to angiotensin II, a potent vasoconstrictor that also causes release of aldosterone from the adrenals. Both of these actions increase BP; moexipril blocks the conversion of angiotensin I to angiotensin II, leading to decreased BP, decreased aldosterone secretion, a small increase in serum potassium levels, and sodium and fluid loss; increased prostaglandin synthesis may also be involved in the antihypertensive action.

Indications

- Treatment of hypertension, alone or in combination with other antihypertensives such as thiazide-type diuretics

Contraindications and cautions

- Contraindicated with allergy to ACE inhibitors, impaired renal function, HF, salt or volume depletion, history of ACE inhibitor-induced angioedema, lactation, pregnancy.
- Use cautiously with hepatic impairment and in elderly patients.

Available forms

Tablets—7.5, 15 mg

Dosages

Adults

- *Patients not receiving diuretics:* Initially, 7.5 mg PO daily, given 1 hr before a meal; for maintenance, 7.5–30 mg PO daily or in one to two divided doses 1 hr before meals.
- *Patients receiving diuretics:* Discontinue diuretic for 2 or 3 days before beginning moexipril; follow dosage listed above, if BP is not controlled, diuretic therapy may be added. If diuretic cannot be stopped, start moexipril therapy with 3.75 mg and monitor for symptomatic hypotension.

Pediatric patients

Safety and efficacy not established.

Geriatric patients and patients with renal impairment

Excretion is reduced in renal failure; use with caution. If creatinine clearance 40 mL/min or less, start with 3.75 mg PO daily, adjust up to a maximum of 15 mg/day.

Pharmacokinetics

Route	Onset	Peak	Duration
Oral	1 hr	3–4 hr	24 hr

Metabolism: $T_{1/2}$: 2–9 hr
Distribution: Crosses placenta; enters breast milk
Excretion: Urine

Adverse effects

- **CV:** *Tachycardia,* angina pectoris, **MI,** hypotension in salt- or volume-depleted patients
- **GI:** *Gastric irritation, aphthous ulcers, peptic ulcers, diarrhea, dysgeusia,* cholestatic jaundice, hepatocellular injury, anorexia, constipation
- **GU:** *Proteinuria,* renal insufficiency, renal failure, polyuria, oliguria, urinary frequency
- **Hematologic:** Neutropenia, agranulocytosis, thrombocytopenia, hemolytic anemia, **pancytopenia**
- **Skin:** *Rash, pruritus, flushing,* scalded mouth sensation, exfoliative dermatitis, photosensitivity, alopecia
- **Other:** *Cough,* malaise, dry mouth, lymphadenopathy, *flulike symptoms, dizziness,* angioedema

Interactions

✱ **Drug-drug** • Increased risk of hyperkalemia with potassium supplements, potassium-sparing diuretics, salt substitutes • Risk of excessive hypotension with diuretics • Risk of abnormal response with lithium

✱ **Drug-lab test** • False-positive test for urine acetone

■ Nursing considerations

Assessment

- **History:** Allergy to ACE inhibitors, impaired renal or hepatic function, HF, salt or volume depletion, pregnancy, lactation
- **Physical:** Skin color, lesions, turgor; T; P, BP, peripheral perfusion; mucous membranes, bowel sounds, liver evaluation; urinalysis, LFTs, renal function tests, CBC and differential

Interventions

⊗ ***Warning*** Alert the surgeon and mark patient's chart with notice that moexipril is being taken; the angiotensin II formation subsequent to compensatory renin release during surgery will be blocked; hypotension may be reversed with volume expansion.

⊠ ***Black box warning*** Do not administer during pregnancy; drug may cause serious fetal injury or death.

- Monitor patient closely for a fall in BP secondary to reduction in fluid volume from excessive perspiration and dehydration, vomiting, or diarrhea; excessive hypotension may occur. Monitor potassium levels carefully in patients receiving potassium supplements, using potassium-sparing diuretics or salt substitutes.
- Reduce dosage in patients with impaired renal function.
- Monitor for excessive hypotension with any diuretic therapy.

Teaching points

- Do not stop taking this drug without consulting your health care provider. Take tablet 1 hr before meals.
- This drug is associated with fetal defects; using barrier contraceptives is advised to prevent pregnancy.
- Be careful in any situation that may lead to a drop in blood pressure (diarrhea, sweating, vomiting, dehydration); if light-headedness or dizziness occurs, consult your health care provider.
- You may experience these side effects: GI upset, diarrhea, loss of appetite, change in taste perception; mouth sores (frequent mouth care may help); rash; fast heart rate; dizziness, light-headedness (transient; change position slowly and limit activities to those that do not require alertness and precision).
- Report mouth sores; sore throat, fever, chills; swelling of the hands or feet; irregular heartbeat, chest pains; swelling of the face, eyes, lips, tongue; difficulty breathing; leg cramps.

▽ molindone hydrochloride

*(moe **lin'** done)*

Moban

PREGNANCY CATEGORY C

Drug classes

Antipsychotic
Dopaminergic blocker

Therapeutic actions

Mechanism of action not fully understood. Antipsychotic drugs block postsynaptic dopamine receptors in the brain, but this may not be necessary and sufficient for antipsychotic activity;

clinically resembles the piperazine phenothiazines (fluphenazine).

Indications

- Management of schizophrenia

Contraindications and cautions

- Contraindicated with coma or severe CNS depression, bone marrow depression, blood dyscrasia, circulatory collapse, subcortical brain damage, Parkinson's disease, liver damage, cerebral arteriosclerosis, coronary disease, severe hypotension or hypertension.
- Use cautiously with respiratory disorders ("silent pneumonia"), glaucoma, prostatic hypertrophy, epilepsy or history of epilepsy (drug lowers seizure threshold), breast cancer (elevations in prolactin may stimulate a prolactin-dependent tumor), thyrotoxicosis, peptic ulcer, decreased renal function, exposure to heat or phosphorous insecticides, pregnancy, lactation and in children younger than 12 yr, especially those with chickenpox, CNS infections (children are especially susceptible to dystonias that may confound the diagnosis of Reye's syndrome).

Available forms

Tablets—5, 10, 25, 50 mg

Dosages

Adults

Initially, 50–75 mg/day PO increased to 100 mg/day in three or four divided doses. Individualize dosage; severe symptoms may require up to 225 mg/day. For maintenance of mild symptoms, 5–15 mg PO tid–qid; for maintenance of moderate symptoms, 10–25 mg PO tid–qid; for maintenance of severe symptoms, 225 mg/day.

Pediatric patients

Not recommended for children younger than 12 yr.

Geriatric patients

Use lower doses and increase dosage more gradually than in younger patients.

Pharmacokinetics

Route	*Onset*	*Peak*	*Duration*
Oral	Varies	90 min	24–36 hr

Metabolism: Hepatic; $T_{1/2}$: 1.5 hr
Distribution: Crosses placenta; enters breast milk
Excretion: Feces, urine

Adverse effects

- **Autonomic:** Dry mouth, salivation, nasal congestion, nausea, vomiting, anorexia, fever, pallor, flushed facies, sweating, constipation, paralytic ileus, urine retention, incontinence, polyuria, enuresis, priapism, ejaculation inhibition, male impotence
- **CNS:** *Drowsiness,* insomnia, vertigo, headache, weakness, tremor, ataxia, slurring, cerebral edema, seizures, exacerbation of psychotic symptoms, extrapyramidal syndromes (*pseudoparkinsonism, dystonias, akathisia,* tardive dyskinesias, potentially irreversible [no known treatment]), **NMS** (extrapyramidal symptoms, hyperthermia, autonomic disturbances [rare, but 20% fatal])
- **CV:** Hypotension, orthostatic hypotension, hypertension, tachycardia, bradycardia, cardiac arrest, HF, cardiomegaly, **refractory arrhythmias,** pulmonary edema
- **Endocrine:** Lactation, breast engorgement, galactorrhea; SIADH; amenorrhea, menstrual irregularities; gynecomastia; changes in libido; hyperglycemia or hypoglycemia; glycosuria; hyponatremia; pituitary tumor with hyperprolactinemia; inhibition of ovulation; infertility, pseudopregnancy; reduced urinary levels of gonadotropins, estrogens, progestins
- **Hematologic:** Eosinophilia, leukopenia, leukocytosis, anemia; aplastic anemia; hemolytic anemia; thrombocytopenic or nonthrombocytopenic purpura
- **Hypersensitivity:** Jaundice, urticaria, angioneurotic edema, laryngeal edema, eczema, asthma, anaphylactoid reactions, exfoliative dermatitis
- **Respiratory: Bronchospasm, laryngospasm,** dyspnea; suppression of cough reflex and potential for aspiration (sudden death related to **asphyxia** or **cardiac arrest**)

Interactions

✱ **Drug-drug** • Decreased absorption of oral phenytoin, tetracycline

✱ **Drug-lab test** • False-positive pregnancy tests (less likely if serum test is used) • Increase in PBI, not attributable to an increase in thyroxine

■ Nursing considerations
Assessment
- **History:** Coma or severe CNS depression, bone marrow depression, circulatory collapse, subcortical brain damage, Parkinson's disease, liver damage, cerebral arteriosclerosis, coronary disease, severe hypotension or hypertension, respiratory disorders, glaucoma, prostatic hypertrophy, epilepsy, breast cancer, thyrotoxicosis, peptic ulcer, decreased renal function, exposure to heat or phosphorous insecticides, pregnancy, lactation, age younger than 12 yr
- **Physical:** Weight, T; reflexes, orientation, IOP; P, BP, orthostatic BP; R, adventitious sounds; bowel sounds and normal output, liver evaluation; urinary output, prostate size; CBC, urinalysis, LFTs, renal and thyroid function tests

Interventions
⊠ ***Black box warning*** Risk of death is increased if drug is used to treat elderly patients with dementia-related psychosis. Drug is not approved for this use.

⊗ ***Warning*** Discontinue drug if serum creatinine or BUN become abnormal or if WBC count is depressed.
- Monitor elderly patients for dehydration, and institute remedial measures promptly; sedation and decreased sensation of thirst related to CNS effects can lead to severe dehydration.
- Consult physician regarding appropriate warning of patient or patient's guardian about tardive dyskinesias.
- Consult physician about dosage reduction, use of anticholinergic antiparkinsonian drugs (controversial) if extrapyramidal effects occur.

Teaching points
- Take drug exactly as prescribed.
- Avoid driving or engaging in other dangerous activities if central nervous system or vision changes occur.
- Maintain fluid intake, and use precautions against heatstroke in hot weather.
- Report sore throat, fever, unusual bleeding or bruising, rash, weakness, tremors, impaired vision, dark urine (pink or reddish brown urine is to be expected), pale stools, yellowing of the skin or eyes.

▽ montelukast sodium
*(mon tell **oo'** kast)*

Singulair

PREGNANCY CATEGORY B

Drug classes
Antasthmatic
Leukotriene receptor antagonist

Therapeutic actions
Selectively and competitively blocks the receptor that inhibits leukotriene formation, thus blocking many of the signs and symptoms of asthma—neutrophil and eosinophil migration, neutrophil and monocyte aggregation, leukocyte adhesion, increased capillary permeability, and smooth muscle contraction. These actions contribute to inflammation, edema, mucus secretion, and bronchoconstriction associated with the signs and symptoms of asthma.

Indications
- Prophylaxis and chronic treatment of asthma in adults and children 12 mo and older
- Relief of symptoms of seasonal allergic rhinitis in adults and children 2 yr and older
- Relief of symptoms of perennial allergic rhinitis in adults and children 6 mo and older
- Prevention of exercise-induced bronchoconstriction in patients 15 yr and older
- Unlabeled uses: Chronic urticaria, atopic dermatitis

Contraindications and cautions
- Contraindicated with hypersensitivity to montelukast or any of its components; acute asthma attacks; status asthmaticus.
- Use cautiously with pregnancy and lactation.

M

Available forms

Tablets—10 mg; chewable tablets—4, 5 mg; granules—4 mg/packet

Dosages

Adults and patients 15 yr and older

One 10-mg tablet PO daily, taken in the evening. For exercise-induced bronchoconstriction, dose taken 2 hr before exercise and not repeated for at least 24 hr.

Pediatric patients

6 mo–23 mo (perennial allergic rhinitis): 1 packet (4 mg) PO per day.
12–23 mo (asthma only): 4-mg granules PO daily, taken in the evening.
2–5 yr: One 4-mg chewable tablet PO daily, taken in the evening.
6–14 yr: One 5-mg chewable tablet PO daily, taken in the evening.

Pharmacokinetics

Route	*Onset*	*Peak*
Oral	Rapid	2–4 hr

Metabolism: Hepatic; $T_{1/2}$: 2.7–5.5 hr
Distribution: Crosses placenta and enters breast milk
Excretion: Feces, urine

Adverse effects

- **CNS:** Headache, dizziness, fatigue, neuropsychiatric events
- **GI:** Nausea, diarrhea, abdominal pain, dental pain, liver impairment
- **Respiratory:** Influenza, cold, nasal congestion
- **Other:** Generalized pain, fever, rash, fatigue

Interactions

✱ **Drug-drug** • Decreased effects and bioavailability if taken with phenobarbital; monitor patient and adjust dosage as needed

■ Nursing considerations

Assessment

- **History:** Hypersensitivity to montelukast or any of its components, acute asthma attacks, status asthmaticus, pregnancy, lactation
- **Physical:** T; orientation, reflexes; R, adventitious sounds; GI evaluation

Interventions

- Administer in the evening without regard to food.
- Ensure that drug is taken continually for optimal effect.
- Do not administer for acute asthma attack or acute bronchospasm.
- Be aware of the risk of neuropsychiatric events, including behavior and mood changes; monitor patient accordingly.
- Avoid the use of aspirin or NSAIDs in patients with known sensitivities while they are using this drug.

⊗ ***Warning*** Ensure that patient has a readily available rescue medication for acute asthma attacks or situations when a short-acting inhaled drug is needed.

Teaching points

- Take this drug regularly as prescribed; do not stop taking this drug during symptom-free periods; do not stop taking this drug without consulting your health care provider. Continue taking any other drugs for treating your asthma that have been prescribed for you. Notify your health care provider if your asthma becomes worse.
- Do not take this drug for an acute asthma attack or acute bronchospasm; this drug is not a bronchodilator, and routine emergency procedures should be followed during acute attacks.
- If taking this drug to prevent exercise-induced bronchoconstriction, take it at least 2 hours before exercising, and do not take another dose for at least 24 hours.
- Avoid using aspirin or NSAIDs if you have a known sensitivity to these drugs. Montelukast will not prevent reactions.
- You may experience these side effects: Dizziness (use caution when driving or performing activities that require alertness); nausea, vomiting (eat frequent small meals, take drug with food); headache (analgesics may be available).
- Report fever, acute asthma attacks, flulike symptoms, lethargy, changes in behavior or mood.

DANGEROUS DRUG

morphine sulfate

(mor' feen)

Timed-release: Avinza DNC, Kadian DNC, MS Contin DNC, Oramorph SR DNC, ratio-Morphine SR (CAN) DNC

Oral solution: MSIR, Roxanol, Roxanol T

Rectal suppositories: RMS

Injection: Astramorph PF, Duramorph, Morphine HP Injection (CAN), MOS Sulfate (CAN), PMS Morphine (CAN)

Preservative-free concentrate for microinfusion devices for intraspinal use: Infumorph, Morphine LP Injection (CAN), Morphine LP Epidural (CAN)

Liposome injection: DepoDur

PREGNANCY CATEGORY C

CONTROLLED SUBSTANCE C-II

Drug class

Opioid agonist analgesic

Therapeutic actions

Principal opium alkaloid; acts as agonist at specific opioid receptors in the CNS to produce analgesia, euphoria, sedation; the receptors mediating these effects are thought to be the same as those mediating the effects of endogenous opioids (enkephalins, endorphins).

Indications

- Relief of moderate to severe acute and chronic pain
- Preoperative medication to sedate and allay apprehension, facilitate induction of anesthesia, and reduce anesthetic dosage
- Analgesic adjunct during anesthesia
- Component of most preparations that are oral alcoholic solutions used for chronic severe pain, especially in terminal cancer patients
- Intraspinal use with microinfusion devices for the relief of intractable pain
- Treatment of pain following major surgery, ER liposome injection for single-dose administration by epidural route at the lumbar level
- Unlabeled use: Relief of pain associated with MI

Contraindications and cautions

- Contraindicated with hypersensitivity to opioids; during labor or delivery of a premature infant (may cross immature blood–brain barrier more readily); after biliary tract surgery or surgical anastomosis; with pregnancy, labor (respiratory depression in neonate; may prolong labor).
- Use cautiously with head injury and increased intracranial pressure; acute asthma, COPD, cor pulmonale, preexisting respiratory depression, hypoxia, hypercapnia (may decrease respiratory drive and increase airway resistance); lactation (wait 4–6 hr after administration to nurse the baby); acute abdominal conditions; CV disease, supraventricular tachycardias; myxedema, seizure disorders, acute alcoholism, delirium tremens; cerebral arteriosclerosis; ulcerative colitis; fever; kyphoscoliosis; Addison's disease; prostatic hypertrophy, urethral stricture, recent GI or GU surgery, toxic psychosis, renal or hepatic impairment.

Available forms

Injection—0.5, 1, 2, 4, 5, 8, 10, 15, 25, 50 mg/mL; tablets—15, 30 mg; CR tablets DNC —15, 30, 60, 100, 200 mg; ER tablets DNC— 15, 30, 60, 100, 200 mg; soluble tablets—10, 15, 30 mg; oral solution—10, 20, 100 mg/5 mL; concentrated oral solution—20 mg/mL, 100 mg/5 mL; suppositories—5, 10, 20, 30 mg; SR capsules DNC—20, 30, 50, 60, 100 mg; ER capsules DNC: 10, 20, 30, 50, 60, 80, 90, 100, 120 mg; liposome injection—10 mg/mL

Dosages

Adults

Oral

One-third to one-sixth as effective as parenteral administration because of first-pass metabolism; 10–30 mg every 4 hr PO. CR, ER, and SR: 30 mg every 8–12 hr PO or as directed by physician; *Kadian:* 20–100 mg PO daily–24-hr release system; *MS Contin:* 200 mg PO every 12 hr; *Avinza:* 30 mg PO daily; if opioid naive, increase by 30 mg (or lower) increments every 4 days.

IM or subcutaneous

10 mg (range, 5–20 mg) every 4 hr or as directed by physician.

IV

2–10 mg/70 kg of body weight in 4–5 mL water for injection administered over 4–5 min, or as directed by physician. Continuous IV infusion: 0.1–1 mg/mL in D_5W by controlled infusion device.

Rectal

10–30 mg every 4 hr or as directed by physician.

Epidural

Initial injection of 5 mg in the lumbar region may provide pain relief for up to 24 hr. If adequate pain relief is not achieved within 1 hr, incremental doses of 1–2 mg may be given at intervals sufficient to assess effectiveness, up to 10 mg/24 hr. For continuous infusion, initial dose of 2–4 mg/24 hr is recommended. Further doses of 1–2 mg may be given if pain relief is not achieved initially.

Liposome injection

10–15 mg by lumbar epidural injection using a catheter or needle prior to major surgery or after clamping the umbilical cord during cesarean section.

Intrathecal

Dosage is usually one-tenth that of epidural dosage; a single injection of 0.2–1 mg may provide satisfactory pain relief for up to 24 hr. Do not inject more than 2 mL of the 5-mg/10 mL ampule or more than 1 mL of the 10-mg/10 mL ampule. Use only in the lumbar area. Repeated intrathecal injections are not recommended; use other routes if pain recurs. For epidural or intrathecal dosing, use preservative-free morphine preparations only.

Pediatric patients

Do not use in premature infants.

IM, subcutaneous, or IV

0.1–0.2 mg/kg (up to 15 mg per dose) every 4 hr or as directed by physician.

Geriatric patients or impaired adults

Use caution. Respiratory depression may occur in the elderly, the very ill, those with respiratory problems. Reduced dosage may be needed.

Epidural

Use extreme caution; injection of less than 5 mg in the lumbar region may provide adequate pain relief for up to 24 hr.

Intrathecal

Use lower dosages than recommended above for adults.

Pharmacokinetics

Route	*Onset*	*Peak*	*Duration*
Oral	Varies	60 min	5–7 hr
Rectal	Rapid	20–60 min	5–7 hr
Subcut.	Rapid	50–90 min	5–7 hr
IM	Rapid	30–60 min	5–6 hr
IV	Immediate	20 min	5–6 hr

Metabolism: Hepatic; $T_{1/2}$: 1.5–2 hr

Distribution: Crosses placenta; enters breast milk

Excretion: Bile, urine

IV FACTS

Preparation: No further preparation needed for direct injection; dilute for infusion to a concentration of 0.1–1 mg/mL in D_5W.

Infusion: Inject slowly directly IV or into tubing of running IV, each 15 mg over 4–5 min; monitor by controlled infusion device to maintain pain control.

Incompatibilities: Do not mix with aminophylline, amobarbital, chlorothiazide, heparin, meperidine, phenobarbital, phenytoin, sodium bicarbonate, sodium iodide, thiopental.

Y-site incompatibilities: Do not give with minocycline, tetracycline.

Adverse effects

- **CNS:** *Light-headedness, dizziness, sedation,* euphoria, dysphoria, delirium, insomnia, agitation, anxiety, fear, hallucinations, disorientation, drowsiness, lethargy, impaired mental and physical performance, coma, mood changes, weakness, headache, tremor, seizures, miosis, visual disturbances, suppression of cough reflex
- **CV:** Facial flushing, peripheral circulatory collapse, tachycardia, bradycardia, arrhythmia, palpitations, chest wall rigidity,

hypertension, hypotension, orthostatic hypotension, syncope

- **Dermatologic:** Pruritus, urticaria, **laryngospasm, bronchospasm,** edema
- **GI:** *Nausea, vomiting,* dry mouth, anorexia, constipation, biliary tract spasm; increased colonic motility in patients with chronic ulcerative colitis
- **GU:** Ureteral spasm, spasm of vesical sphincters, urine retention or hesitancy, oliguria, antidiuretic effect, reduced libido or potency
- **Local:** Tissue irritation and induration (subcutaneous injection)
- **Major hazards: Respiratory depression, apnea, circulatory depression, respiratory arrest, shock, cardiac arrest**
- **Other:** *Sweating,* physical tolerance and dependence, psychological dependence

Interactions

✷ **Drug-drug** • Increased likelihood of respiratory depression, hypotension, profound sedation or coma in patients receiving barbiturate general anesthetics • Risk of toxicity if combined with alcohol (ER forms especially likely)

✷ **Drug-lab test** • Elevated biliary tract pressure (an effect of opioids) may cause increases in plasma amylase, lipase; determinations of these levels may be unreliable for 24 hr

■ Nursing considerations

Assessment

- **History:** Hypersensitivity to opioids; diarrhea caused by poisoning; labor or delivery of a premature infant; biliary tract surgery or surgical anastomosis; head injury and increased intracranial pressure; acute asthma, COPD, cor pulmonale, preexisting respiratory depression; acute abdominal conditions; CV disease, supraventricular tachycardias, myxedema, seizure disorders, acute alcoholism, delirium tremens; cerebral arteriosclerosis; ulcerative colitis; fever; kyphoscoliosis; Addison's disease; prostatic hypertrophy, urethral stricture, recent GI or GU surgery, toxic psychosis, renal or hepatic impairment; pregnancy; lactation
- **Physical:** T; skin color, texture, lesions; orientation, reflexes, bilateral grip strength, affect; P, auscultation, BP, orthostatic BP, perfusion; R, adventitious sounds; bowel sounds, normal output; urinary frequency, voiding pattern, normal output; ECG; EEG; LFTs, renal and thyroid function tests

Interventions

⊠ ***Black box warning*** Caution patient not to chew or crush CR, ER, or SR preparations and ensure appropriate use of these forms.

⊠ ***Black box warning*** Make sure patient is observed for at least 24 hr in a fully equipped and staffed environment if morphine is given by epidural or intrathecal route because of risk of serious adverse effects.

⊗ ***Warning*** Dilute and administer slowly IV to minimize likelihood of adverse effects.

- Tell patient to lie down during IV administration.

⊗ ***Warning*** Keep opioid antagonist and facilities for assisted or controlled respiration readily available during IV administration.

⊗ ***Warning*** Use caution when injecting IM or subcutaneously into chilled areas or in patients with hypotension or in shock; impaired perfusion may delay absorption; with repeated doses, an excessive amount may be absorbed when circulation is restored.

- Reassure patients that they are unlikely to become addicted; most patients who receive opiates for medical reasons do not develop dependence syndromes.

⊠ ***Black box warning*** Liposome preparation is for lumbar epidural injection only; it should not be given intrathecally, IV, or IM.

Teaching points

- Take this drug exactly as prescribed. Avoid alcohol, antihistamines, sedatives, tranquilizers, and over-the-counter drugs.
- Swallow controlled-release, extended-release, or sustained-release preparations (*MS Contin, Oramorph SR*) whole; do not cut, crush, or chew.
- Do not take leftover medication for other disorders, and do not let anyone else take your prescription.
- You may experience these side effects: Nausea, loss of appetite (take with food, lie quietly); constipation (use laxative); dizziness, sedation, drowsiness, impaired visual acuity (avoid driving or performing tasks that require alertness and visual acuity).

M

- Report severe nausea, vomiting, constipation, shortness of breath or difficulty breathing, rash.

moxifloxacin hydrochloride

*(mocks ee **flox'** a sin)*

Avelox, Avelox IV, Vigamox

PREGNANCY CATEGORY C

Drug classes

Antibiotic
Fluoroquinolone

Therapeutic actions

Bactericidal; interferes with DNA replication, repair, transcription, and recombination in susceptible gram-negative and gram-positive bacteria, preventing cell reproduction and leading to cell death.

Indications

- Treatment of adults with community-acquired pneumonia caused by susceptible strains of *Streptococcus pneumoniae* (including multidrug resistant strains), *Haemophilus influenzae, Mycoplasma pneumoniae, Chlamydia pneumoniae, Moraxella catarrhalis, Staphylococcus aureus, Klebsiella pneumoniae*
- Treatment of bacterial sinusitis caused by *S. pneumoniae, H. influenzae, M. catarrhalis*
- Treatment of acute bacterial exacerbation of chronic bronchitis caused by *S. pneumoniae, H. influenzae, H. parainfluenzae, K. pneumoniae, S. aureus, M. catarrhalis*
- Treatment of uncomplicated skin and skin structure infections caused by *S. aureus* or *Streptococcus pyogenes*
- Treatment of complicated skin and skin structure infections and complicated intra-abdominal infections caused by methicillin–susceptible *S. aureus, E. coli, K. pneumoniae, Enterobacter cloacae*

Contraindications and cautions

- Contraindicated with allergy to fluoroquinolones, prolonged QT interval, hypokalemia, pregnancy, lactation.
- Use cautiously with hepatic impairment, seizures.

Available forms

Tablets—400 mg; injection—400 mg in 250 mL

Dosages

Adults

- *Pneumonia:* 400 mg PO or IV daily for 7–14 days.
- *Sinusitis:* 400 mg PO or IV daily for 10 days.
- *Acute exacerbation of chronic bronchitis:* 400 mg PO or IV daily for 5 days.
- *Uncomplicated skin and skin structure infections:* 400 mg PO daily for 7 days.
- *Complicated skin and skin structure infections:* 400 mg PO or IV daily for 7–21 days.
- *Complicated intra-abdominal infections:* 400 mg PO or IV for 5–14 days.

Pediatric patients

Not recommended in patients younger than 18 yr.

Pharmacokinetics

Route	Onset	Peak
Oral	Varies	1–3 hr
IV	Rapid	Minutes

Metabolism: Hepatic; $T_{1/2}$: 12–13.5 hr
Distribution: Crosses placenta; enters breast milk
Excretion: Feces, urine

IV FACTS

Preparation: Supplied in premixed 250-mL bags; do not refrigerate; single use only, discard any excess.
Infusion: Infuse over 60 min by direct infusion or into Y-site of running IV.
Compatibilities: Compatible with 0.9% sodium chloride injection, 1M sodium chloride injection, 5% or 10% dextrose injection, sterile water for injection, lactated Ringer's for injection.

Adverse effects

- **CNS:** *Headache,* dizziness, *insomnia,* fatigue, somnolence, depression, nervousness, anxiety, paresthesia
- **CV:** Palpitations, tachycardia, hypertension, hypotension, **prolonged QT interval**
- **GI:** *Nausea,* vomiting, dry mouth, *diarrhea,* anorexia, gastritis, stomatitis
- **Hematologic:** Altered PT, thrombocytopenia, eosinophilia
- **Respiratory:** Asthma, cough, dyspnea, pharyngitis, rhinitis
- **Other:** Fever, rash, sweating, photosensitivity, tendonitis, tendon rupture

Interactions

✱ **Drug-drug** ⊗ ***Warning*** Risk of severe cardiac arrhythmias if combined with any other drug known to prolong the QTc interval (quinidine, procainamide, amiodarone, sotalol, phenothiazines); avoid these combinations.

• Decreased absorption and therapeutic effectiveness of moxifloxacin if taken with sucralfate, metal medications (antacids), multivitamins, didanosine chewable; moxifloxacin should be taken 4 hr before or at least 8 hr after any of these drugs • Increased risk of seizures if fluoroquinolones are combined with NSAIDs; monitor patient closely

■ Nursing considerations

Assessment

- **History:** Allergy to fluoroquinolones, prolonged QTc interval, hypokalemia, hepatic impairment, seizures, lactation, pregnancy
- **Physical:** Skin color, lesions; T; orientation, reflexes, affect; R, adventitious sounds; P, BP; mucous membranes, bowel sounds; LFTs, ECG, CBC

Interventions

- Arrange for culture and sensitivity tests before beginning therapy.
- Continue therapy as indicated for condition being treated.
- Administer oral drug 4 hr before or at least 8 hr after antacids or other anion-containing drugs.
- Do not change dosage when switching from IV to oral dose.

⊗ ***Warning*** Discontinue drug at any sign of hypersensitivity (rash, photophobia) or with severe diarrhea.

⊠ ***Black box warning*** Risk of tendonitis and tendon rupture increases, especially in patients older than age 60 yr, patients taking corticosteroids, and those who have received a kidney, heart, or lung transplant.

⊗ ***Warning*** Discontinue drug and monitor ECG if palpitations or dizziness occurs.

- Monitor clinical response; if no improvement is seen or a relapse occurs, repeat culture and sensitivity tests.

Teaching points

- Take oral drug once a day for the period prescribed. If antacids are being taken, take drug 4 hours before or at least 8 hours after the antacid.
- You may experience these side effects: Nausea, vomiting, abdominal pain (eat frequent small meals); diarrhea or constipation (consult your health care provider); drowsiness, blurring of vision, dizziness (observe caution if driving or using dangerous equipment); sensitivity to the sun (avoid exposure, use a sunscreen).
- Report rash, visual changes, severe GI problems, weakness, tremors, palpitations, sensitivity to light, pain or inflammation in tendons.

▽ muromonab-CD3

(mew ***ro'*** *mon ab)*

Orthoclone OKT3

PREGNANCY CATEGORY C

Drug classes

Immunosuppressant
Monoclonal antibody

Therapeutic actions

A murine monoclonal antibody to the antigen of human T cells; functions as an immunosuppressant by blocking T cells.

Indications

- Acute allograft rejection in renal transplant patients

M

- Treatment of steroid-resistant acute allograft rejection in cardiac and hepatic transplant patients

Contraindications and cautions

- Contraindicated with allergy to muromonab or any murine product, fluid overload as evidenced by chest X-ray, or more than 3% weight gain in 1 wk.
- Use cautiously with fever (use antipyretics to decrease fever before therapy); previous administration of muromonab-CD3 (antibodies frequently develop, risks serious reactions on repeat administration); pregnancy.

Available forms

Injection—5 mg/5 mL

Dosages

Give only as an IV bolus in less than 1 min. Do not infuse or give by any other route.

Adults

5 mg/day for 10–14 days. Begin treatment once acute renal rejection is diagnosed. It is strongly recommended that methylprednisolone sodium succinate 8 mg/kg IV be given 1–4 hr prior to muromonab-CD3.

Pediatric patients weighing 30 kg or less

Initially, 2.5 mg/day IV for 10–14 days.

Pediatric patients weighing more than 30 kg

5 mg/day IV for 10–14 days. May increase 2.5 mg/day increments if needed.

Pharmacokinetics

Route	Onset	Peak	Duration
IV	Minutes	2–7 days	7 days

Metabolism: Tissue; $T_{1/2}$: 47–100 hr
Distribution: Crosses placenta
Excretion: Unknown

IV FACTS

Preparation: Draw solution into a syringe through a low protein-binding 0.2- or 0.22-mcm filter. Discard filter and attach needle for IV bolus injection. Solution may develop fine translucent particles that do not affect its potency. Refrigerate solution; do not freeze or shake. Use immediately; discard unused portions.
Infusion: Administer as an IV bolus over less than 1 min. Do not give as an IV infusion or with other drug solutions. Flush line with saline before and after IV injection.
Incompatibilities: Do not mix with any other drug solution; do not infuse simultaneously with any other drug. If sequential infusions are required, flush line with saline before and after administering muromonab.

Adverse effects

- **CNS:** Malaise, *tremors,* coma, seizures, headache
- **GI:** *Vomiting, nausea, diarrhea*
- **Respiratory: Acute pulmonary edema,** *dyspnea, chest pain,* wheezing
- **Other:** Lymphomas, *increased susceptibility to infection, fever, chills,* **cytokine-release syndrome** ("flu" to shock)

Interactions

✱ **Drug-drug** • Reduce dosage of other immunosuppressive drugs; severe immunosuppression can lead to increased susceptibility to infection and increased risk of lymphomas; other immunosuppressives can be restarted about 3 days prior to cessation of muromonab • Risk of encephalopathy and CNS effects with indomethacin

■ Nursing considerations

Assessment

- **History:** Allergy to muromonab or any murine product; fluid overload; fever; previous administration of muromonab-CD3; pregnancy; lactation
- **Physical:** T, weight; P, BP; R, adventitious sounds; chest X-ray, CBC

Interventions

- Obtain chest X-ray within 24 hr of therapy to ensure chest is clear.
- Arrange for antipyretics (acetaminophen) if patient is febrile before therapy.
- Monitor WBC levels and circulating T cells periodically during therapy.

⊗ ***Black box warning*** Monitor patient very closely after first dose; acetaminophen

PRN should be ordered to cover febrile reactions; cooling blanket may be needed in severe cases. Equipment for intubation and respiratory support should be readily available for severe pulmonary reactions; anaphylactoid reactions may occur with any dose.

Teaching points

- There is often a severe reaction to the first dose, including high fever and chills, difficulty breathing, and chest congestion (you will be closely watched, and comfort measures will be given).
- Avoid infection; people may wear masks and rubber gloves when caring for you; visitors may be limited.
- Report chest pain, difficulty breathing, nausea, chills.

▽ mycophenolate

*(my coe **fen'** oh late)*

mycophenolate mofetil

IV injection: CellCept

mycophenolate sodium

Oral: Myfortic

PREGNANCY CATEGORY D

Drug class

Immunosuppressant

Therapeutic actions

Immunosuppressant: Inhibits T-lymphocyte activation; exact mechanism of action unknown, but binds to intracellular protein, which may prevent the generation of nuclear factor of activated T cells, and suppresses the immune activation and response of T cells; inhibits proliferative responses of T and B cells.

Indications

- Prophylaxis of organ rejection in patients receiving allogeneic renal, hepatic, and heart transplants; intended to be used concomitantly with corticosteroids and cyclosporine; *Myfortic* used for renal transplants only
- Unlabeled uses: Refractory uveitis as 2 g/day alone or in combination therapy; second-line agent for Churg-Strauss syndrome; combined with prednisolone for diffuse proliferative lupus nephritis

Contraindications and cautions

- Contraindicated with allergy to mycophenolate, pregnancy, lactation.
- Use cautiously with impaired renal function.

Available forms

Capsules—250 mg; tablets—500 mg; DR tablets—180, 360 mg (*Myfortic*); powder for oral suspension—200 mg/mL; powder for injection—500 mg/vial

Dosages

Adults

- *Renal transplantation:* 1 g bid PO or IV (administered over at least 2 hr) starting within 24 hr of transplant; 720 mg PO bid on an empty stomach (*Myfortic*).
- *Cardiac transplantation:* 1.5 g PO bid or IV (IV over at least 2 hr).
- *Hepatic transplantation:* 1 g IV bid or 1.5 g PO bid (over at least 2 hr).

Pediatric patients

- *Renal transplantation:* 600 mg/m^2 oral suspension PO bid (up to a maximum daily dose of 2 g/10 mL oral suspension); 400 mg/m^2 PO bid to a maximum 720 mg bid (*Myfortic*).

Geriatric patients

Maximum recommended dose is 720 mg PO bid (DR tablets).

Patients with severe renal impairment

Avoid doses of more than 1 g bid. Monitor patient carefully for adverse response.

Pharmacokinetics

Route	*Onset*	*Peak*
Oral	Varies	45–60 min

Metabolism: Hepatic; $T_{1/2}$: 17.9 hr
Distribution: Crosses placenta; enters breast milk
Excretion: Urine

IV FACTS

Preparation: Reconstitute and dilute to 6 mg/mL with 5% dextrose injection. Reconstitute each 500-mg vial with 14 mL 5% dextrose injection. Gently shake. Solution should be slightly yellow without precipitates. For a 1-g dose, dilute contents of two reconstituted vials into 140 mL of D_5W; for a 1.5-g dose, dilute contents of three reconstituted vials into 210 mL of D_5W. Use caution to avoid contact with solution. If contact occurs, wash with soap and water.

Infusion: Infuse over at least 2 hr. Begin within 24 hr of transplant and continue for 14 days or less.

Incompatibilities: Do not mix with any other drugs or infusion admixtures.

Adverse effects

- **CNS:** *Tremor, headache, insomnia,* paresthesias
- **CV:** Chest pain, *hypertension,* peripheral edema
- **GI: Hepatotoxicity,** *constipation, diarrhea, nausea, vomiting,* anorexia
- **GU:** *Renal impairment,* nephrotoxicity, *UTI,* oliguria
- **Hematologic:** Leukopenia, *anemia,* hyperkalemia, hypokalemia, hyperglycemia, red blood cell aplasia
- **Other:** Abdominal pain, fever, asthenia, back pain, ascites, neoplasms, *infection*

Interactions

✱ **Drug-drug** • Decreased levels and effectiveness with cholestyramine, antacids • Decreased levels and effectiveness of theophylline, phenytoin

■ Nursing considerations

Assessment

- **History:** Allergy to mycophenolate; pregnancy, lactation; renal function
- **Physical:** T; skin color, lesions; BP, peripheral perfusion; liver evaluation, bowel sounds, gum evaluation; LFTs, renal function tests, CBC

Interventions

⊗ ***Warning*** Monitor renal and liver function before and periodically during therapy; marked decreases in function may require dosage change or discontinuation of therapy.

- Use caution; do not confuse *Myfortic* and *CellCept*.
- Prepare oral suspension by tapping closed bottle several times, adding 47 mL water to bottle, and shaking closed bottle for 1 min. Add another 47 mL water; shake for 1 min.

⊗ ***Black box warning*** Protect patient from exposure to infections and maintain sterile technique for invasive procedures; risk for serious to life-threatening infection exists.

⊗ ***Black box warning*** Monitor patient for possible lymphoma development related to drug action.

- Risk of pure red blood cell aplasia; monitor patient accordingly.

Teaching points

- Avoid infection while using this drug; avoid crowds or people with infections. Notify your health care provider immediately if you injure yourself.
- Avoid sun exposure; use sunscreen if you cannot avoid exposure.
- Have periodic blood tests to monitor your response to the drug and its effects.
- Do not discontinue this drug without consulting your health care provider.
- This drug should not be taken during pregnancy. If you think you are pregnant or you want to become pregnant, consult your health care provider.
- You may experience these side effects: Nausea, vomiting (take drug with food); diarrhea; headache (request analgesics).
- Report unusual bleeding or bruising, fever, sore throat, mouth sores, tiredness.

nabilone

(nah' bah lone)

Cesamet

PREGNANCY CATEGORY C

CONTROLLED SUBSTANCE C-II

Drug classes

Antiemetic
Cannabinoid

Therapeutic actions

A synthetic cannabinoid that interacts with the cannabinoid receptor systems in the CNS, causing an antiemetic effect as well as effects on mental state, dry mouth, and hypotension.

Indications

Treatment of nausea and vomiting associated with chemotherapy in patients who have had inadequate response to conventional antiemetic therapies

Contraindications and cautions

- Contraindicated with hypersensitivity to any component of the drug.
- Use cautiously with pregnancy, lactation; current or previous psychiatric disorder; current therapy with sedatives, hypnotics, or psychoactive drugs; history of substance abuse, hypertension, heart disease.

Available forms

Capsules—1 mg

Dosages

Adults

1–2 mg PO bid. Initial dose given 1–3 hr before chemotherapy begins. Maximum recommended dose, 6 mg/day PO, divided and given tid. May be given daily during each chemotherapy cycle and for 48 hr after last dose in cycle, if needed. Patient should be under close supervision because of risk of altered mental state.

Pediatric patients younger than 18 yr

Safety and efficacy not established.

Pharmacokinetics

Route	*Onset*	*Peak*
Oral	Rapid	2 hr

Metabolism: Hepatic; $T_{1/2}$: 2–35 hr (active metabolites)
Distribution: May cross placenta; may enter breast milk
Excretion: Feces

Adverse effects

- **CNS:** *Drowsiness, vertigo, euphoria, ataxia,* headache, *difficulty concentrating,* sleep disturbance, disorientation, depersonalization, vision disturbances
- **CV:** Orthostatic hypotension, hypotension, tachycardia, palpitations, hypertension, arrhythmia
- **Dependence:** Risk of psychological dependence
- **GI:** *Dry mouth,* nausea, anorexia, increased appetite, diarrhea, constipation
- **Other:** Fatigue, malaise

Interactions

✱ Drug-drug • Risk of additive hypertension, tachycardia, cardiac toxicity if combined with amphetamines, cocaine, sympathomimetics; use caution • Risk of tachycardia, drowsiness if combined with atropine, scopolamine, antihistamines, anticholinergics; use caution • Risk of tachycardia, hypertension, drowsiness if combined with amitriptyline, amoxapine, desipramine, TCAs; use caution • Risk of additive CNS depression if combined with barbiturates, benzodiazepines, ethanol, lithium, opioids, buspirone, antihistamines, muscle relaxants, other CNS depressants; use caution

■ Nursing considerations

Assessment

- **History:** Allergy to any component of the drug; pregnancy, lactation; current or previous psychiatric disorders; concurrent therapy with sedatives, hypnotics, or psychoactive drugs; history of substance abuse, hypertension, heart disease
- **Physical:** Orientation, affect, reflexes; BP, standing BP, P; abdominal examination

Interventions

- Limit prescriptions to the minimum amount needed for a single chemotherapy cycle because of abuse potential.
- Warn patient about drug's profound effects on mental state and abuse potential before starting therapy. Patient should receive full information about potential drug effects; they can persist 48–72 hr after stopping drug.
- Warn patient about potential effects on mood and behavior to prevent panic if these occur.
- Patient should be supervised by a responsible adult while taking this drug; monitor patient during first round of chemotherapy to determine effects and their duration to establish guidelines for supervision. Super-

vision should begin again whenever dosage changes.
- Provide safety measures if dizziness and lightheadedness occur.

⊗ ***Warning*** Discontinue drug if psychotic reaction occurs; observe patient closely until evaluated and counseled. Patient should participate in decision about further use of drug, perhaps at a lower dosage.

Teaching points

- This drug is called a cannabinoid. It works in the brain much like marijuana. It has many of the associated mental changes and dependency issues that occur with marijuana.
- Take this drug exactly as prescribed. Take the first dose of the cycle 1–3 hours before chemotherapy starts. Take the drug every day during the chemotherapy cycle; you may need the drug for 1–2 days after the cycle to maintain relief of nausea and vomiting.
- If you miss a dose of the daily medication, take the dose as soon as you remember; then return to your usual routine. Do not double the dose.
- Be aware that the effects of this drug may continue 2–3 days after you stop taking it.
- It is not known how this drug could affect a nursing baby. If you are nursing, consult your health care provider.
- It is not known how this drug could affect a fetus. If you are pregnant or you decide to become pregnant while taking this drug, consult your health care provider.
- This drug interacts with many other drugs, and the interaction could cause serious side effects. Tell any health care provider who is taking care of you that you are taking this drug.
- Do not drink alcohol while taking this drug.
- You may experience these side effects: Dizziness, drowsiness, anxiety, disorientation, dry mouth. Do not drive a car or operate dangerous machinery while taking this drug, and avoid making any important decisions. For dry mouth, practice frequent mouth care; sucking sugarless lozenges may help.
- Report chest pain, rapid heartbeat, depression, feelings of panic, hallucinations.

▽nabumetone

*(nah **byoo'** meh tone)*

Apo-Nabumetone (CAN), Gen-Nabumetone (CAN)

PREGNANCY CATEGORY C (FIRST AND SECOND TRIMESTERS)

PREGNANCY CATEGORY D (THIRD TRIMESTER)

Drug classes

Analgesic (nonopioid)
NSAID

Therapeutic actions

Analgesic, anti-inflammatory, and antipyretic activities largely related to inhibition of prostaglandin synthesis; exact mechanisms of action are not known.

Indications

- Acute and long-term treatment of signs and symptoms of rheumatoid arthritis and osteoarthritis

Contraindications and cautions

- Contraindicated with significant renal impairment, allergy to NSAIDs, pregnancy, lactation.
- Use cautiously with hepatic, CV, and GI conditions.

Available forms

Tablets—500, 750 mg

Dosages

Adults

1,000 mg PO as a single dose with or without food. 1,500–2,000 mg/day have been used. May be given in divided doses.

Pediatric patients

Safety and efficacy not established.

Patients with renal impairment

Maximum starting dose should not exceed 750 mg daily for moderate insufficiency, 500 mg for severe insufficiency.

Pharmacokinetics

Route	Onset	Peak
Oral	30 min	30–60 min

Metabolism: Hepatic; $T_{1/2}$: 22.5–30 hr
Distribution: Crosses placenta; enters breast milk
Excretion: Urine

Adverse effects

- **CNS:** *Headache, dizziness, somnolence, insomnia,* fatigue, tiredness, dizziness, tinnitus, ophthalmic effects
- **Dermatologic:** *Rash,* pruritus, sweating, dry mucous membranes, stomatitis
- **GI:** *Nausea, dyspepsia, GI pain,* diarrhea, vomiting, *constipation,* flatulence
- **GU:** Dysuria, **renal impairment**
- **Hematologic:** Bleeding, platelet inhibition with higher doses, neutropenia, eosinophilia, leukopenia, pancytopenia, thrombocytopenia, agranulocytosis, granulocytopenia, aplastic anemia, decreased Hgb or Hct, bone marrow depression, menorrhagia
- **Respiratory:** Dyspnea, hemoptysis, pharyngitis, **bronchospasm,** rhinitis
- **Other:** Peripheral edema, anaphylactoid reactions to **fatal anaphylactic shock**

Interactions

✱ **Drug-drug** • Increased risk of bleeding if combined with warfarin, aspirin

■ Nursing considerations

Assessment

- **History:** Renal impairment; impaired hearing; allergies; hepatic, CV, and GI conditions; lactation; pregnancy
- **Physical:** Skin color and lesions; orientation, reflexes, ophthalmic and audiometric evaluation, peripheral sensation; P, edema; R, adventitious sounds; liver evaluation; CBC, clotting times, LFTs, renal function tests; serum electrolytes, stool guaiac

Interventions

⊗ ***Black box warning*** Be aware that patient may be at increased risk for CV events or GI bleeding; monitor accordingly.

- Administer drug with food or after meals if GI upset occurs.
- Arrange for periodic ophthalmologic examinations during long-term therapy.

⊗ ***Warning*** If overdose occurs, institute emergency procedures—gastric lavage, induction of emesis, supportive therapy.

Teaching points

- Take drug with food or meals if GI upset occurs; take only the prescribed dosage.
- Dizziness, drowsiness can occur (avoid driving or using dangerous machinery).
- Report sore throat, fever, rash, itching, weight gain, swelling in ankles or fingers; changes in vision; black, tarry stools.

▽ nadolol

(nay doe' lol)

Corgard

PREGNANCY CATEGORY C

Drug classes

Antianginal
Antihypertensive
Beta-adrenergic blocker (nonselective)

Therapeutic actions

Competitively blocks beta-adrenergic receptors in the heart and juxtaglomerular apparatus, decreasing the influence of the sympathetic nervous system on these tissues and decreasing the excitability of the heart, cardiac output, oxygen consumption, renin release, and BP.

Indications

- Hypertension alone or with other drugs, especially diuretics
- Long-term management of angina pectoris
- Unlabeled uses: Treatment of ventricular arrhythmias, migraines, lithium-induced tremors, essential tremors

Contraindications and cautions

- Contraindicated with sinus bradycardia (HR less than 45 beats/min), second- or third-degree heart block (PR interval greater than 0.24 sec), cardiogenic shock, HF, asthma, COPD, lactation.

- Use cautiously with diabetes or thyrotoxicosis, pregnancy.

Available forms

Tablets—20, 40, 80, 120, 160 mg

Dosages

Adults

- *Hypertension:* Initially, 40 mg PO daily; gradually increase dosage in 40- to 80-mg increments until optimum response is achieved. Usual maintenance dose is 40–80 mg/day; up to 320 mg daily may be needed. To discontinue, reduce dosage gradually over a 1- to 2-wk period.
- *Angina:* Initially, 40 mg PO daily; gradually increase dosage in 40- to 80-mg increments at 3- to 7-day intervals until optimum response is achieved or heart rate markedly decreases. Usual maintenance dose is 40–80 mg daily; up to 240 mg/day may be needed. Safety and efficacy of larger doses not established. To discontinue, reduce dosage gradually over 1- to 2-wk period.

Pediatric patients

Safety and efficacy not established.

Geriatric patients or patients with renal failure

CrCl (mL/min)	*Dosage Intervals (hr)*
More than 50	24
31–50	24–36
10–30	24–48
Less than 10	40–60

Pharmacokinetics

Route	*Onset*	*Peak*	*Duration*
Oral	Varies	3–4 hr	17–24 hr

Metabolism: $T_{1/2}$: 20–24 hr
Distribution: Crosses placenta; enters breast milk
Excretion: Urine

Adverse effects

- **Allergic reactions:** Pharyngitis, erythematous rash, fever, sore throat, **laryngospasm,** respiratory distress
- **CNS:** Dizziness, vertigo, tinnitus, fatigue, emotional depression, paresthesias, sleep disturbances, hallucinations, disorientation, memory loss, slurred speech
- **CV:** *Heart failure, cardiac arrhythmias,* peripheral vascular insufficiency, claudication, CVA, **pulmonary edema,** hypotension
- **Dermatologic:** Rash, pruritus, sweating, dry skin
- **EENT:** Eye irritation, dry eyes, conjunctivitis, blurred vision
- **GI:** *Gastric pain, flatulence, constipation, diarrhea, nausea, vomiting,* anorexia, ischemic colitis, renal and mesenteric arterial thrombosis, retroperitoneal fibrosis, hepatomegaly, acute pancreatitis
- **GU:** *Impotence, decreased libido,* Peyronie's disease, dysuria, nocturia, urinary frequency
- **Musculoskeletal:** Joint pain, arthralgia, muscle cramp
- **Respiratory:** Bronchospasm, dyspnea, cough, bronchial obstruction, nasal stuffiness, rhinitis, pharyngitis (less likely than with propranolol)
- **Other:** *Decreased exercise tolerance, development of antinuclear antibodies,* hyperglycemia or hypoglycemia, elevated serum transaminase

Interactions

✱ **Drug-drug** • Increased effects with verapamil • Increased serum levels and toxicity of IV lidocaine, theophylline • Increased risk of orthostatic hypotension with prazosin • Increased risk of peripheral ischemia with ergotamine, dihydroergotamine • Decreased antihypertensive effects with NSAIDs, clonidine • Hypertension followed by severe bradycardia with epinephrine

✱ **Drug-lab test** • Possible false results with glucose or insulin tolerance tests

■ Nursing considerations

Assessment

- **History:** Sinus bradycardia, second- or third-degree heart block, cardiogenic shock, heart failure; asthma, COPD; diabetes or thyrotoxicosis; pregnancy; lactation
- **Physical:** Weight, skin condition, neurologic status, P, BP, ECG, respiratory status, renal and thyroid function tests, blood and urine glucose

Interventions

⊗ ***Warning*** Do not discontinue drug abruptly after long-term therapy (hypersensitivity to catecholamines may have developed, causing exacerbation of angina, MI, and ventricular arrhythmias). Taper drug gradually over 2 wk with monitoring.

- Consult with physician about withdrawing drug if patient is to undergo surgery (controversial).

Teaching points

- Do not stop taking unless instructed to do so by your health care provider; drug must be stopped gradually to prevent serious adverse effects.
- Avoid driving or dangerous activities if dizziness, disorientation occur.
- Report difficulty breathing, night cough, swelling of extremities, slow pulse, confusion, depression, rash, fever, sore throat.

▽nafarelin acetate

(naf' a re lin)

Synarel

PREGNANCY CATEGORY X

Drug class

Gonadotropin-releasing hormone (GnRH)

Therapeutic actions

A potent agonistic analogue of GnRH, which is released from the hypothalamus to stimulate LH and FSH release from the pituitary; these hormones are responsible for regulating reproductive status. Repeated dosing abolishes the stimulatory effect on the pituitary gland, leading to decreased secretion of gonadal steroids by about 4 wk; consequently, tissues and functions that depend on gonadal steroids for their maintenance become quiescent.

Indications

- Treatment of endometriosis, including pain relief and reduction of endometriotic lesions
- Treatment of central precocious puberty in children of both sexes

Contraindications and cautions

- Contraindicated with known sensitivity to GnRH, GnRH-agonist analogues, excipients in the product; undiagnosed abnormal vaginal bleeding; pregnancy; lactation (potential androgenic effects on the fetus).
- Use cautiously with rhinitis.

Available forms

Nasal solution—2 mg/mL (200 mcg/spray)

Dosages

Adults

- *Endometriosis:* 400 mcg/day. One spray (200 mcg) into one nostril in the morning and 1 spray into the other nostril in the evening. Start treatment between days 2 and 4 of the menstrual cycle. 800-mcg dose may be administered as 1 spray into each nostril in the morning (a total of 2 sprays) and again in the evening for patients with persistent regular menstruation after 2 months of treatment. Treatment for 6 mo is recommended. Retreatment is not recommended because safety has not been established.

Pediatric patients

- *Central precocious puberty:* 1,600 mcg/day. Two sprays (400 mcg) in each nostril in the morning and 2 sprays in each nostril in the evening; may be increased to 1,800 mcg/day. If 1,800 mcg are needed, give 3 sprays into alternating nostrils three times/day. Continue until resumption of puberty is desired.

Pharmacokinetics

Route	*Onset*	*Peak*
Nasal	Rapid	4 wk

Metabolism: $T_{1/2}$: 2–4 hr
Distribution: Crosses placenta; may enter breast milk
Excretion: Urine

Adverse effects

- **CNS:** Dizziness, headache, sleep disorders, fatigue
- **Endocrine:** *Androgenic effects* (acne, edema, mild hirsutism, decrease in breast size, deepening of the voice, oily skin or hair, weight gain, clitoral hypertrophy or testicular atrophy), *hypoestrogenic effects* (flushing,

N

sweating, vaginitis, nervousness, emotional lability)
- **GI:** Hepatic impairment
- **GU:** Fluid retention, vaginal dryness, ovarian cysts
- **Local:** *Nasal irritation*
- **Other:** Rash, pruritus; with prolonged therapy, bone density loss has been noted

■ Nursing considerations
Assessment
- **History:** Sensitivity to GnRH, GnRH-agonist analogues, excipients in the product; undiagnosed abnormal genital bleeding; pregnancy; lactation; rhinitis
- **Physical:** Weight; hair distribution pattern; skin color, texture, lesions; breast examination; nasal mucosa; orientation, affect, reflexes; P, auscultation, BP, peripheral edema; liver evaluation; bone density studies in long-term therapy

Interventions
- Ensure that patient is not pregnant before therapy; begin therapy for endometriosis during menstrual period, days 2–4; advise the use of barrier contraceptives.
- Store drug upright; protect from exposure to light.
- Arrange for bone age and growth velocity studies before therapy and periodically thereafter if retreatment is suggested because of return of endometriosis.
- Ensure patient has enough of the drug to prevent interruption of therapy.
- Caution patient that androgenic effects may not be reversible when the drug is withdrawn.
- Monitor nasal mucosa for signs of erosion during course of therapy.
- If a topical decongestant needs to be used, wait at least 2 hr after dosing with nafarelin.

Teaching points
- Use this drug without interruption; be sure that you have enough on hand to prevent interruption. Store the drug upright. Protect the bottle from exposure to light. Clear nasal passages by gently blowing your nose before administering drug.
- Regular menstruation should cease within 4–6 weeks of therapy. Breakthrough bleeding or ovulation may still occur.
- Consult with your health care provider if you need a topical nasal decongestant; a decongestant should be used at least 2 hours after nafarelin use.
- This drug is contraindicated during pregnancy; use a nonhormonal form of birth control during therapy. If you become pregnant, discontinue the drug and consult your health care provider immediately.
- You may experience these side effects: Masculinizing effects (acne, hair growth, deepening of voice, oily skin or hair; may not be reversible); low estrogen effects (flushing, sweating, vaginal irritation, nervousness); nasal irritation.
- Report abnormal growth of facial hair, deepening of the voice, unusual bleeding or bruising, fever, chills, sore throat, vaginal itching or irritation, nasal irritation or burning.

DANGEROUS DRUG

▽ nalbuphine hydrochloride

(nal' byoo feen)

Nubain

PREGNANCY CATEGORY B

PREGNANCY CATEGORY D (PROLONGED USE OR WITH HIGH DOSES AT TERM)

Drug class
Opioid agonist-antagonist analgesic

Therapeutic actions
Nalbuphine acts as an agonist at specific opioid receptors in the CNS to produce analgesia and sedation but also acts to cause hallucinations and is an antagonist at mu receptors.

Indications
- Relief of moderate to severe pain
- Preoperative analgesia, as a supplement to surgical anesthesia, and for obstetric analgesia during labor and delivery

- Unlabeled use: Prevention and treatment of intrathecal morphine–induced pruritus after cesarean section

Contraindications and cautions

- Contraindicated with hypersensitivity to nalbuphine, sulfites.
- Use cautiously with emotionally unstable patients or those with a history of opioid abuse, pregnancy prior to labor (neonatal withdrawal may occur if mothers used drug during pregnancy), labor or delivery (use with caution during delivery of premature infants, who are especially sensitive to respiratory depressant effects of opioids), bronchial asthma, COPD, respiratory depression, anoxia, increased intracranial pressure, acute MI when nausea and vomiting are present, biliary tract surgery (may cause spasm of the sphincter of Oddi), lactation.

Available forms

Injection—1.5 mg/mL, 10 mg/mL, 20 mg/mL

Dosages

Adults

Usual dose is 10 mg for a 70-kg person IM, IV, or subcutaneously every 3–6 hr as needed. Individualize dosage. In nontolerant patients, the recommended single maximum dose is 20 mg, with a maximum total daily dose of 160 mg. Patients dependent on opioids may experience withdrawal symptoms with administration of nalbuphine; control by small increments of morphine by slow IV administration until relief occurs. If the previous opioid was morphine, meperidine, codeine, or another opioid with similar duration of activity, administer one-fourth the anticipated nalbuphine dose initially, and observe for signs of withdrawal. If no untoward symptoms occur, progressively increase doses until analgesia is obtained.

- *Supplement to anesthesia:* Induction—0.3–3 mg/kg IV over 10–15 min; maintenance—0.25–0.5 mg/kg IV.

Pediatric patients younger than 18 yr

Not recommended.

Patients with renal or hepatic impairment

Reduce dosage.

Pharmacokinetics

Route	Onset	Peak	Duration
IV	2–3 min	15–20 min	3–6 hr
Subcut., IM	Less than 15 min	30–60 min	3–6 hr

Metabolism: Hepatic; $T_{1/2}$: 5 hr
Distribution: Crosses placenta; enters breast milk
Excretion: Urine

IV FACTS

Preparation: No additional preparation is required.
Infusion: Administer by direct injection or into the tubing of a running IV.
Y-site incompatibilities: Do not give with nafcillin, ketorolac.

Adverse effects

- **CNS:** *Sedation, clamminess, sweating, headache,* nervousness, restlessness, depression, crying, confusion, faintness, hostility, unusual dreams, hallucinations, euphoria, dysphoria, unreality, *dizziness, vertigo,* floating feeling, feeling of heaviness, numbness, tingling, flushing, warmth, blurred vision
- **CV:** Hypotension, hypertension, bradycardia, tachycardia
- **Dermatologic:** Pruritus, burning, urticaria
- **GI:** Nausea, vomiting, cramps, dyspepsia, bitter taste, *dry mouth*
- **GU:** Urinary urgency
- **Respiratory:** Respiratory depression, dyspnea, asthma

Interactions

✱ **Drug-drug** • Potentiation of effects with barbiturate anesthetics or other CNS depressants

■ Nursing considerations

Assessment

- **History:** Hypersensitivity to nalbuphine, sulfites; lactation; emotional instability or history of opioid abuse; pregnancy; bronchial asthma, COPD, respiratory depression; anoxia; increased intracranial pressure; MI; biliary tract surgery

N

- **Physical:** Orientation, reflexes, bilateral grip strength, affect; pupil size, vision; pulse, auscultation, BP; R, adventitious sounds; bowel sounds, normal output; urine output; LFTs, renal function tests

Interventions

⊗ ***Warning*** Taper dosage when discontinuing after prolonged use to avoid withdrawal symptoms.

⊗ ***Warning*** Keep opioid antagonist and facilities for assisted or controlled respiration available in case of respiratory depression.

- Reassure patient about addiction liability; most patients who receive opiates for medical reasons do not develop dependence syndromes.

Teaching points

- You may experience these side effects: Dizziness, sedation, drowsiness, impaired visual acuity (avoid driving, performing tasks that require alertness), nausea, loss of appetite (lying quietly, eating frequent small meals may help).
- Report severe nausea, vomiting, palpitations, shortness of breath, or difficulty breathing.

nalidixic acid

(nal i ***dix'*** *ik)*

NegGram

PREGNANCY CATEGORY C

Drug classes

Antibacterial
Urinary tract anti-infective

Therapeutic actions

Bactericidal; interferes with DNA and RNA synthesis in susceptible gram-negative bacteria, causing cell death.

Indications

- UTIs caused by susceptible gram-negative bacteria, including *Proteus* strains, *Klebsiella* species, *Enterobacter* species, *Escherichia coli*

Contraindications and cautions

- Contraindicated with allergy to nalidixic acid, epilepsy, porphyria, concomitant therapy with melphalan, alkylating agents.
- Use cautiously with G6PD deficiency, renal or hepatic impairment, cerebral arteriosclerosis, pregnancy, lactation.

Available forms

Tablets—500 mg

Dosages

Adults and children 12 yr and older

Initial therapy, 1 g PO qid for 1–2 wk. For prolonged therapy, total dose may be reduced to 2 g/day.

Pediatric patients 3 mo–younger than 12 yr

Exact dosage is based on weight; total daily dose for initial therapy, 55 mg/kg/day PO divided into 4 equal doses. For prolonged therapy, may be reduced to 33 mg/kg/day.

Pediatric patients younger than 3 mo

Not recommended.

Pharmacokinetics

Route	*Onset*	*Peak*
Oral	Varies	1–2 hr

Metabolism: Hepatic; $T_{1/2}$: 1–2.5 hr
Distribution: Crosses placenta; enters breast milk
Excretion: Urine

Adverse effects

- **CNS:** *Drowsiness, weakness, headache, dizziness, vertigo,* visual disturbances
- **Dermatologic:** Photosensitivity reactions
- **GI:** *Abdominal pain, nausea, vomiting, diarrhea*
- **Hematologic:** Thrombocytopenia, leukopenia, hemolytic anemia
- **Hypersensitivity:** Rash, pruritus, urticaria, angioedema, eosinophilia, arthralgia
- **Other:** Achilles tendon rupture

Interactions

✱ **Drug-drug** • Increased risk of bleeding if given with oral anticoagulants • Increased risk of serious GI toxicity with melphalan or other alkylating agents; combination is contraindicated

✱ **Drug-lab test** • False-positive urinary glucose results when using Benedict's reagent, Fehling's reagent, *Clinitest* tablets • False elevations of urinary 17-keto and ketogenic steroids when assay uses m-dinitrobenzene

■ Nursing considerations

Assessment

- **History:** Allergy to nalidixic acid, seizures, epilepsy, G6PD deficiency, renal or hepatic impairment, cerebral arteriosclerosis, pregnancy, lactation
- **Physical:** Skin color, lesions; joints; orientation, reflexes; CBC, LFTs, renal function tests

Interventions

- Arrange for culture and sensitivity tests.
- Give with food if GI upset occurs.
- Obtain periodic blood counts, renal and liver function tests during prolonged therapy.
- Encourage patient to implement nondrug measures to help fight UTIs—avoid bubble baths, void after intercourse, avoid alkaline ash foods, use proper hygiene, increase fluid intake.
- Monitor clinical response; if no improvement is seen or a relapse occurs, send urine for repeat culture and sensitivity tests.

Teaching points

- Take drug with food. Complete the full course of therapy to ensure resolution of the infection.
- You may experience these side effects: Nausea, vomiting, abdominal pain (eat frequent small meals); diarrhea; sensitivity to sunlight (wear protective clothing, and use sunscreen); drowsiness, blurring of vision, dizziness (observe caution if driving or using dangerous equipment).
- Use measures to help decrease urinary tract infections—avoid bubble baths, void after intercourse, avoid citrus juices, increase fluid intake; wipe from front to back.
- Report severe rash, visual changes, weakness, tremors, severe headaches, seizures, changes in behavior.

▽ naloxone hydrochloride

*(nal **ox'** one)*

Narcan

PREGNANCY CATEGORY C

Drug classes

Diagnostic agent
Opioid antagonist

Therapeutic actions

Pure opioid antagonist; reverses the effects of opioids, including respiratory depression, sedation, hypotension; can reverse the psychotomimetic and dysphoric effects of opioid agonist-antagonists, such as pentazocine.

Indications

- Complete or partial reversal of opioid depression, including respiratory depression induced by opioids, including natural and synthetic narcotics, propoxyphene, methadone, nalbuphine, butorphanol, pentazocine
- Diagnosis of suspected acute opioid overdose
- Unlabeled uses: Improvement of circulation in refractory shock, reversal of alcoholic coma, dementia of Alzheimer's or schizophrenic type

Contraindications and cautions

- Contraindicated with allergy to opioid antagonists.
- Use cautiously with opioid addiction, CV disorders, pregnancy, lactation.

Available forms

Injection—0.02 mg/mL, 0.4 mg/mL

Dosages

IV administration is recommended in emergencies when rapid onset of action is required.

Adults

- *Opioid overdose:* Initial dose of 0.4–2 mg, IV. Additional doses may be repeated at 2- to 3-min intervals. If no response after 10 mg, question the diagnosis. IM or subcutaneous routes may be used if IV route is unavailable.
- *Postoperative opioid depression:* Titrate dose to patient's response. Initial dose of

0.1–0.2 mg IV at 2- to 3-min intervals until desired degree of reversal. Repeat doses may be needed within 1- to 2-hr intervals, depending on amount and type of opioid. Supplemental IM doses produce a longer-lasting effect.

Pediatric patients

- *Opioid overdose:* Initial dose is 0.01 mg/kg IV. Subsequent dose of 0.1 mg/kg may be administered if needed. May be given IM or subcutaneously in divided doses.
- *Postoperative opioid depression:* For the initial reversal of respiratory depression, inject in increments of 0.005–0.01 mg IV at 2- to 3-min intervals to the desired degree of reversal.

Pharmacokinetics

Route	*Onset*	*Duration*
IV	2 min	4–6 hr
IM, Subcut.	3–5 min	4–6 hr

Metabolism: Hepatic; $T_{1/2}$: 30–81 min
Distribution: Crosses placenta; may enter breast milk
Excretion: Urine

IV FACTS

Preparation: Dilute in normal saline or 5% dextrose solutions for IV infusions. The addition of 2 mg in 500 mL of solution provides a concentration of 0.004 mg/mL; titrate rate by response. Use diluted mixture within 24 hr. After that time, discard any remaining solution.
Infusion: Inject directly, or titrate rate of infusion based on response.
Incompatibilities: Do not mix naloxone with preparations containing bisulfite, metabisulfite, high–molecular-weight anions, alkaline pH solutions.

Adverse effects

- **Acute opioid abstinence syndrome:** *Nausea, vomiting, sweating, tachycardia, increased BP, tremulousness*
- **CNS:** Reversal of analgesia and excitement (postoperative use)
- **CV:** *Hypotension, hypertension,* ventricular tachycardia and **fibrillation, pulmonary edema** (postoperative use)

■ Nursing considerations

Assessment

- **History:** Allergy to opioid antagonists; opioid addiction; CV disorders; lactation
- **Physical:** Sweating; reflexes, pupil size; P, BP; R, adventitious sounds

Interventions

- Monitor patient continuously after use of naloxone; repeat doses may be needed, depending on duration of opioid and time of last dose.

⊗ ***Warning*** Maintain open airway and provide artificial ventilation, cardiac massage, vasopressor drugs if needed to counteract acute opioid overdose.

Teaching points

- Report sweating, feelings of tremulousness.

naltrexone hydrochloride

(nal trex' one)

ReVia, Vivitrol

PREGNANCY CATEGORY C

Drug class

Opioid antagonist

Therapeutic actions

Pure opiate antagonist; markedly attenuates or completely, reversibly blocks the subjective effects of IV opioids, including those with mixed opioid agonist-antagonist properties.

Indications

- Adjunct to treatment of alcohol or opioid dependence as part of a comprehensive treatment program
- Unlabeled uses: Treatment of postconcussional syndrome unresponsive to other treatments; eating disorders

Contraindications and cautions

- Contraindicated with allergy to opioid antagonists, acute hepatitis, liver failure.
- Use cautiously with opioid addiction (may produce withdrawal symptoms; do not

administer unless patient has been opioid-free for 7–10 days); opioid withdrawal; lactation; depression, suicidal tendencies; pregnancy.

Available forms

Tablets—25, 50, 100 mg; injection—380 mg/vial

Dosages

⊗ ***Warning*** Give naloxone challenge before use except in patients already showing clinical signs of opioid withdrawal.

Adults

IV challenge

Draw 2 ampules of naloxone, 2 mL (0.8 mg) into a syringe. Inject 0.5 mL (0.2 mg). Leave needle in vein, and observe for 30 sec. If no signs of withdrawal occur, inject remaining 1.5 mL (0.6 mg), and observe for 20 min for signs and symptoms of withdrawal (stuffiness or running nose, tearing, yawning, sweating, tremor, vomiting, piloerection, feeling of temperature change, joint or bone and muscle pain, abdominal cramps, skin crawling).

Subcutaneous challenge

Administer 2 mL (0.8 mg) naloxone, and observe for signs and symptoms of withdrawal for 20 min. If any of the signs and symptoms of withdrawal occur or if there is any doubt that the patient is opioid free, do not administer naltrexone. Confirmatory rechallenge can be done within 24 hr. Inject 4 mL IV, and observe for signs and symptoms of withdrawal. Repeat until no signs and symptoms are seen and patient is no longer at risk.

Naltrexone

- *Alcoholism:* 50 mg/day PO or 380 mg IM into upper outer quadrant of gluteal muscle once every 4 wk (*Vivitrol*). Alternate buttock with each administration.
- *Opioid dependence:* Initial dose of 25 mg PO. Observe for 1 hr; if no signs or symptoms are seen, complete dose with 25 mg. Usual maintenance dose is 50 mg/24 hr PO. Flexible dosing schedule can be used with 100 mg every other day or 150 mg every third day.

Pediatric patients

Safety has not been established in patients younger than 18 yr.

Pharmacokinetics

Route	*Onset*	*Peak*	*Duration*
Oral	15–30 min	60 min	24–72 hr

Metabolism: Hepatic; $T_{1/2}$: 3.9–12.9 hr
Distribution: Crosses placenta; enters breast milk
Excretion: Urine

Adverse effects

- **CNS:** *Difficulty sleeping, anxiety, nervousness, headache, low energy,* increased energy, irritability, dizziness, blurred vision, burning, light sensitivity
- **CV:** Phlebitis, edema, increased BP, nonspecific ECG changes
- **Dermatologic:** *Rash,* oily skin, pruritus, acne
- **GI: Hepatocellular injury,** *abdominal pain or cramps, nausea, vomiting,* loss of appetite, diarrhea, constipation
- **GU:** *Delayed ejaculation, decreased potency,* increased frequency of or discomfort with voiding
- **Respiratory:** Nasal congestion, rhinorrhea, sneezing, sore throat, excess mucus or phlegm, sinus trouble, epistaxis, injection site reaction
- **Other:** *Chills, increased thirst,* increased appetite, weight change, yawning, swollen glands, *joint and muscle pain,* injection site reaction

Interactions

✱ **Drug-drug** • Decreased effectiveness of opioid analgesics or other opioid-containing preparations

■ Nursing considerations

Assessment

- **History:** Allergy to opioid antagonists; opioid addiction; opioid withdrawal; acute hepatitis, liver failure; lactation; depression, suicidal tendencies; pregnancy
- **Physical:** Sweating; skin lesions, color; reflexes, affect, orientation, muscle strength; P, BP, edema, baseline ECG; R, adventitious sounds; liver evaluation; urine screen for opioids, LFTs

Interventions

⊗ ***Warning*** Do not use until patient has been opioid free for 7–10 days; check urine opioid levels.

⊗ ***Warning*** Do not administer until patient has passed a naloxone challenge.

- Administer IM injection in the gluteal region, alternating buttocks.
- Initiate treatment slowly, and monitor until patient has been given naltrexone in the full daily dose with no signs and symptoms of withdrawal.

⊗ ***Black box warning*** Obtain periodic liver function tests during therapy; discontinue therapy at sign of increasing hepatic impairment (risk of hepatocellular injury).

- Do not use opioid drugs for analgesia, cough, and cold; do not use opioid antidiarrheal preparations; patient will not respond; use a nonopioid preparation.
- Ensure that patient is actively participating in a comprehensive treatment program.

Teaching points

- This drug will help facilitate abstinence from alcohol or opioids.
- This drug blocks the effects of opioids and other opiates.
- Wear or carry a medical ID tag to alert emergency medical personnel that you are taking this drug.
- Small doses of heroin or other opiate drugs will not have an effect. Self-administration of large doses of heroin or other opioids can overcome the blockade effect but may cause death, serious injury, or coma.
- You may experience these side effects: Drowsiness, dizziness, blurred vision, anxiety (avoid driving or operating dangerous machinery); diarrhea, nausea, vomiting (take drug with food to decrease these effects); decreased sexual function.
- Report unusual bleeding or bruising; dark, tarry stools; yellowing of eyes or skin; running nose; tearing; sweating; chills; joint or muscle pain.

▽naproxen

*(na **prox'** en)*

naproxen

Apo-Naproxen (CAN), Apo-Naproxen EC (CAN), Apo-Naproxen SR (CAN), EC-Naprosyn, Gen-Naproxen EC (CAN), Naprelan DNC, Naprosyn, Novo-Naprox (CAN), Novo-Naprox-EC (CAN)

naproxen sodium

Aleve, Anaprox, Anaprox DS DNC, Apo-Napro-Na (CAN), Apo-Napro-Na DS (CAN) DNC, Midol Extended Relief, Novo Naprox Sodium (CAN), Novo Naprox Sodium DS (CAN) DNC, Novo Naprox SR (CAN)

PREGNANCY CATEGORY C

Drug classes

Analgesic (nonopioid)
NSAID

Therapeutic actions

Analgesic, anti-inflammatory, and antipyretic activities largely related to inhibition of prostaglandin synthesis; exact mechanisms of action are not known.

Indications

- Mild to moderate pain
- Treatment of primary dysmenorrhea, rheumatoid arthritis, osteoarthritis, ankylosing spondylitis, tendinitis, bursitis, acute gout
- OTC use: Temporary relief of minor aches and pains associated with the common cold, headache, toothache, muscular aches, backache, minor pain of arthritis, pain of menstrual cramps, reduction of fever
- Treatment of juvenile arthritis (*Naproxen*)

Contraindications and cautions

- Contraindicated with allergy to naproxen, salicylates, other NSAIDs; pregnancy; lactation.
- Use cautiously with asthma, chronic urticaria, CV dysfunction, hypertension, GI bleeding, peptic ulcer, impaired hepatic or renal function.

Available forms

Tablets—200, 250, 375, 500 mg; 220, 275, 500 mg (as naproxen sodium); DR tablets—375, 500 mg; CR tablets—375, 500 mg; suspension—125 mg/5 mL

Dosages

Do not exceed 1,250 mg/day (1,375 mg/day naproxen sodium).

Adults

- *Rheumatoid arthritis or osteoarthritis, ankylosing spondylitis:*

***DR* (EC-Naprosyn)** DNC
375–500 mg PO bid.
***CR* (Naprelan)** DNC
750–1,000 mg PO daily as a single dose.
Naproxen sodium
275–550 mg bid PO. May increase to 1.65 g/day for a limited period.
Naproxen tablets
250–500 mg PO bid.
Naproxen suspension
250 mg (10 mL), 375 mg (15 mL), 500 mg (20 mL) PO bid.

- *Acute gout:*

***CR* (Naprelan)** DNC
1,000–1,500 mg PO daily as a single dose.
Naproxen sodium
825 mg PO followed by 275 mg every 8 hr until attack subsides.
Naproxen
750 mg PO, followed by 250 mg every 8 hr until attack subsides.

- *Mild to moderate pain:*

***CR* (Naprelan)** DNC
1,000 mg PO daily as a single dose.
Naproxen sodium
550 mg PO followed by 275 mg every 6–8 hr.
Naproxen
500 mg followed by 500 mg every 12 hr or 250 mg every 6–8 hr.
OTC
200 mg PO every 8–12 hr with a full glass of liquid while symptoms persist. Do not exceed 600 mg in 24 hr.

Pediatric patients

- *Juvenile arthritis:*

Naproxen
10 mg/kg/day PO given in two divided doses.
Naproxen sodium
Safety and efficacy not established.
OTC
Do not give to children younger than 12 yr unless under advice of physician.

Geriatric patients

Do not give more than 200 mg every 12 hr PO.

Pharmacokinetics

Drug	*Onset*	*Peak*	*Duration*
Naproxen	1 hr	2–4 hr	7 hr or less
Naproxen sodium	1 hr	1–2 hr	7 hr or less

Metabolism: Hepatic; $T_{1/2}$: 12–15 hr
Distribution: Crosses placenta; enters breast milk
Excretion: Urine

Adverse effects

- **CNS:** *Headache, dizziness, somnolence, insomnia,* fatigue, tiredness, dizziness, tinnitus, ophthalmic effects
- **Dermatologic:** *Rash,* pruritus, sweating, dry mucous membranes, stomatitis
- **GI:** *Nausea, dyspepsia, GI pain,* diarrhea, vomiting, *constipation,* flatulence
- **GU:** Dysuria, renal impairment, including renal failure, interstitial nephritis, hematuria
- **Hematologic:** Bleeding, platelet inhibition with higher doses, neutropenia, eosinophilia, leukopenia, pancytopenia, thrombocytopenia, agranulocytosis, granulocytopenia, aplastic anemia, decreased Hgb or Hct, menorrhagia
- **Respiratory:** Dyspnea, hemoptysis, pharyngitis, **bronchospasm,** rhinitis
- **Other:** Peripheral edema, **anaphylactoid reactions** to **anaphylactic shock**

Interactions

✱ **Drug-drug** • Increased serum lithium levels and risk of toxicity with naproxen
✱ **Drug-lab test** • Falsely increased values for urinary 17-ketogenic steroids; discontinue naproxen therapy for 72 hr before adrenal function tests • Inaccurate measurement of urinary 5-HIAA

■ Nursing considerations

Assessment

- **History:** Allergy to naproxen, salicylates, other NSAIDs; asthma, chronic urticaria, CV dysfunction; hypertension; GI bleeding;

N

peptic ulcer; impaired hepatic or renal function; pregnancy; lactation
- **Physical:** Skin color and lesions; orientation, reflexes, ophthalmologic and audiometric evaluation, peripheral sensation; P, BP, edema; R, adventitious sounds; liver evaluation; CBC, clotting times, LFTs, renal function tests; serum electrolytes; stool guaiac

Interventions

⊠ ***Black box warning*** Be aware that patient may be at increased risk for CV events, GI bleeding; monitor accordingly.
- Give with food or after meals if GI upset occurs. Do not cut, crush, or allow patient to chew DR or CR forms.
- Arrange for periodic ophthalmologic examination during long-term therapy.

⊗ ***Warning*** If overdose occurs, institute emergency procedures—gastric lavage, induction of emesis, supportive therapy.

Teaching points

- Take drug with food or meals if GI upset occurs; take only the prescribed dosage. Do not cut, crush, or chew extended-release forms.
- Dizziness, drowsiness can occur (avoid driving or using dangerous machinery).
- Report sore throat; fever; rash; itching; weight gain; swelling in ankles or fingers; changes in vision; black, tarry stools.

▽ naratriptan

*(nar ah **trip'** tan)*

Amerge

PREGNANCY CATEGORY C

Drug classes

Antimigraine drug (triptan)
Serotonin selective agonist

Therapeutic actions

Binds to serotonin receptors to cause vascular constrictive effects on cranial blood vessels, causing the relief of migraine in selective patients; migraine is believed to be caused by vasodilation of cranial blood vessels in these patients.

Indications

- Treatment of acute migraine attacks with or without aura

Contraindications and cautions

- Contraindicated with allergy to any triptan, active CAD, uncontrolled hypertension, cerebrovascular disease or peripheral vascular syndromes, severe renal or hepatic impairment.
- Use cautiously in the elderly; with lactation, pregnancy.

Available forms

Tablets—1, 2.5 mg

Dosages

Adults

Single dose of 1 mg PO or 2.5 mg PO; may be repeated in 4 hr if needed. Do not exceed 5 mg/24 hr.

Pediatric patients

Safety and efficacy not established.

Patients with renal or hepatic impairment

Contraindicated in severe renal impairment (creatinine clearance less than 15 mL/min) or severe hepatic impairment (Child-Pugh grade C). In mild or moderate renal or hepatic impairment, start with lowest dose and do not exceed 2.5 mg/24 hr.

Pharmacokinetics

Route	*Onset*	*Peak*
Oral	Slow	2–3 hr

Metabolism: Hepatic; $T_{1/2}$: 6 hr
Distribution: Crosses placenta; enters breast milk
Excretion: Urine

Adverse effects

- **CNS:** *Dizziness,* headache, anxiety, fatigue, drowsiness, paresthesias, corneal defects
- **CV:** BP alterations, tightness or pressure in chest
- **Other:** *Neck, throat, or jaw discomfort;* generalized pain, nausea

Interactions

✱ Drug-drug • Prolonged vasoactive reactions when taken concurrently with ergot-containing drugs; avoid this combination • Increased blood levels and prolonged effects if combined with hormonal contraceptives; monitor patient and adjust dosage as appropriate

■ Nursing considerations

Assessment

- **History:** Allergy to any triptan, active CAD, uncontrolled hypertension, severe renal or hepatic impairment, pregnancy, lactation
- **Physical:** Orientation, reflexes, peripheral sensation; P, BP; LFTs, renal function tests

Interventions

- Administer to relieve acute migraine, not as a prophylactic measure; administer with food.
- Establish safety measures if CNS or visual disturbances occur.
- Provide appropriate analgesics as needed for pain related to therapy.
- Recommend the use of barrier contraceptives to women of childbearing age; serious birth defects could occur.
- Control environment (lighting, temperature) as appropriate to help relieve migraine.

⊗ ***Warning*** Monitor BP of patients with possible coronary artery disease; discontinue naratriptan at any sign of angina or prolonged high BP.

Teaching points

- Take drug to relieve migraine; do not use as a means of prevention. Take drug with food.
- Dosage may be repeated in 4 hours if headache returns or has not been relieved. Do not take more than 5 milligrams in one 24-hour period.
- This drug should not be taken during pregnancy; if you suspect that you are pregnant, stop taking the drug, and contact your health care provider.
- Continue to do anything that usually helps you during a migraine—adjust lighting, control noise, and so forth.

⊗ ***Warning*** Contact your health care provider immediately if you experience chest pain or pressure that is severe or does not go away.

- You may experience these side effects: Dizziness, drowsiness (avoid driving or using dangerous machinery while taking this drug); numbness, tingling, feelings of tightness or pressure.
- Report severe pain or discomfort, visual changes, palpitations, unrelieved headache.

▽natalizumab

*(nah tah **liz'** yoo mab)*

Tysabri

PREGNANCY CATEGORY C

Drug classes

Monoclonal antibody
MS drug

Therapeutic actions

Monoclonal antibody specific for the alpha-4 subunit on the surface of all leukocytes except neutrophils. Binding with this subunit inhibits adhesion of leukocytes to their counter-receptors, including those on vascular endothelium. Preventing leukocyte adhesion inhibits migration of leukocytes into inflamed tissue and may inhibit recruitment and inflammatory activity of activated immune cells. The exact mechanism of action in MS (thought to be an autoimmune disorder) is not known, but natalizumab may prevent migration of leukocytes into the brain and reduce plaque formation.

Indications

Monotherapy for patients with relapsing MS to delay physical disability and decrease the frequency of exacerbations; reserved for patients who have had inadequate response to or cannot tolerate other MS therapies

- Treatment of Crohn's disease in patients who have not responded to other therapies.

Contraindications and cautions

- Contraindicated with allergy to any component of the preparation, progressive multifocal leukoencephalopathy (PML) or history of it, lactation.
- Use caution with immune supression, pregnancy.

N

Available forms
Single-use vials—300 mg/15 mL

Dosages
Adults
300 mg by IV infusion over 1 hr every 4 wk.
Pediatric patients
Safety and efficacy not established.

Pharmacokinetics

Route	*Onset*	*Peak*
IV	Slow	7–8 days

Metabolism: Tissue; $T_{1/2}$: 11–15 days
Distribution: May cross placenta; may enter breast milk
Excretion: Tissue

IV FACTS
Preparation: Withdraw 15 mL of natalizumab from vial using a sterile syringe and needle. Inject drug into 100 mL 0.9% sodium chloride injection. Gently invert to mix completely. Do not shake. Inspect solution; it should be clear and free of particulates. Use immediately, or refrigerate and use within 8 hr. Do not freeze. If refrigerated, warm to room temperature before infusion.
Infusion: Infuse over approximately 1 hr. After infusion, flush with 0.9% sodium chloride solution. Observe patient during and for 1 hr after infusion to detect hypersensitivity reactions.
Incompatibilities: Do not mix with any other drug.

Adverse effects
- **CNS:** *Headache, depression,* dizziness, suicidal ideation, tremor, rigors, **PML**
- **GI:** *Gastroenteritis, abdominal discomfort, diarrhea,* abnormal liver function, tooth infections
- **GU:** Irregular menses, dysmenorrhea, amenorrhea, urinary urgency, urinary frequency, UTI
- **Hematologic:** *Increased levels of circulating lymphocytes, monocytes, eosinophils, basophils, nucleated RBCs*
- **Respiratory:** *Lower respiratory tract infections,* tonsillitis
- **Skin:** *Rash,* pruritus, dermatitis
- **Other:** *Infection, fatigue, arthralgia,* **anaphylactic reactions,** infusion reaction (headache, dizziness, fatigue, urticaria, pruritus, rigors, hypersensitivity reactions), weight changes

Interactions
✱ **Drug-drug** • Increased risk of infection if combined with corticosteroids or other immune suppressants; avoid this combination

■ Nursing considerations
Assessment
- **History:** Allergy to any component of the preparation; pregnancy, lactation; immune suppression, PML
- **Physical:** T; skin color, lesions; orientation, reflexes; R, adventitious sounds

Interventions
⊗ ***Black box warning*** Be aware that drug increases the risk of PML, which can be fatal. Natalizumab is available only through the TOUCH prescribing program; patients should be monitored closely for signs of PML, and drug should be stopped immediately if they occur. Drug is available only to prescribers and patients who have entered the TOUCH program and understand risks of the drug and need to monitor closely.
- Withhold drug at any sign of PML (change in eyesight, thought disturbances, loss of balance or strength); an MRI will be ordered to evaluate the patient.
- Make sure patient is not immune suppressed or taking immunosuppressants.
- Refrigerate vials. Product contains no preservatives; do not use after expiration date. Protect from light. Do not freeze.
- Monitor patient during infusion and for 1 hr afterward for hypersensitivity reaction (headache, dizziness, urticaria, pruritus, rigors). Discontinue drug immediately at first sign of hypersensitivity reaction. Provide supportive care if reaction occurs after infusion.
- Do not administer drug to patient who has had a hypersensitivity reaction to it.
- Urge women of childbearing age to use barrier contraceptive; effects of this drug on a fetus are not known.

- If woman is lactating, suggest another method of feeding the baby during therapy.

Teaching points

- You must enroll in the TOUCH Prescribing Program before you can receive this drug; the program includes careful monitoring and education about the risk of a serious, viral, brain lesion from using this drug.
- This drug is given by IV infusion every 4 weeks. The infusion will take about 1 hour, and you will need to be monitored for another hour. Keep a calendar to remind you of the dates for each infusion.
- This drug should not be taken during pregnancy or when nursing a baby unless absolutely necessary; use a barrier contraceptive, effects of the drug on a fetus or nursing baby are not known.
- This drug increases your risk of infection. Contact your health care provider if fever or other signs of infection occur.
- You may experience these side effects: Headache (medication may be available to help); respiratory infection, urinary tract infection (avoid crowded areas and people with infections, and wash your hands often); upset stomach, GI discomfort (small, frequent meals may help).
- Report fever, hives, rash, depression, any sign of infection; changes in thinking, balance, strength, or eyesight that last for several days.

DANGEROUS DRUG

▽ nateglinide

(nah teg' lah nyde)

Starlix

PREGNANCY CATEGORY C

Drug classes

Antidiabetic
Meglitinide

Therapeutic actions

Closes potassium channels in the beta cells of the pancreas, which causes the opening of calcium channels and a resultant increase in insulin release; highly selective for pancreatic potassium channels with little effect on the vasculature. Glucose-lowering abilities depend on the existence of functioning beta cells in the pancreas.

Indications

- Adjunct to diet and exercise to lower blood glucose in patients with type 2 diabetes mellitus whose hyperglycemia cannot be managed by diet and exercise alone
- Combination therapy with metformin or a thiazolidinedione for glycemic control in those patients with type 2 diabetes who do not receive adequate control with diet and either drug

Contraindications and cautions

- Contraindicated with hypersensitivity to the drug, diabetic ketoacidosis, type 1 diabetes, pregnancy, lactation.
- Use cautiously with hepatic impairment.

Available forms

Tablets—60, 120 mg

Dosages

Adults

120 mg PO tid taken 1–30 min before meals; 60 mg PO tid may be tried if patient is near HbA_{1c} goal.

Pediatric patients

Safety and efficacy not established.

Pharmacokinetics

Route	*Onset*	*Peak*	*Duration*
Oral	Rapid	1 hr	4 hr

Metabolism: Hepatic; $T_{1/2}$: 1.5 hr
Distribution: Crosses placenta; may enter breast milk
Excretion: Feces, urine

Adverse effects

- **CNS:** *Headache,* paresthesias, dizziness
- **Endocrine:** Hypoglycemia (low risk)
- **GI:** Nausea, diarrhea, constipation, vomiting, dyspepsia
- **Respiratory:** *URI,* sinusitis, rhinitis, bronchitis

Interactions

✱ **Drug-drug** • Increased risk of hypoglycemia if taken with salicylates, NSAIDs, beta-blockers, MAOIs; monitor patient closely

N

■ Nursing considerations

Assessment

- **History:** Hypersensitivity to the drug, diabetic ketoacidosis, type 1 diabetes, renal or hepatic impairment, pregnancy, lactation
- **Physical:** Skin color, lesions; T; orientation, reflexes, peripheral sensation; R, adventitious sounds; liver evaluation, bowel sounds; blood glucose, LFTs, renal function tests

Interventions

- Administer drug three times a day 1–30 min before meals; if a patient skips or adds a meal, the dosage should be skipped or added appropriately.
- Monitor urine or serum glucose levels and HbA_{1c} levels frequently to determine effectiveness of drug and dosage being used.
- Arrange for consult with dietitian to establish weight loss program and dietary control as appropriate.
- Arrange for thorough diabetic teaching program to include disease, dietary control, exercise, signs and symptoms of hypoglycemia and hyperglycemia, avoidance of infection, and hygiene.

Teaching points

- Do not discontinue this medication without consulting your health care provider.
- Take this drug 1–30 minutes before meals (three times a day); if you skip a meal, skip the dosage; if you add a meal, take your dosage before that meal also.
- Monitor urine or blood for glucose and ketones as prescribed.
- Return for regular follow-up visits to monitor your response to the drug and possible need for dosage adjustment.
- Continue diet and exercise program established for control of diabetes.
- Know the signs and symptoms of hypoglycemia and hyperglycemia and appropriate treatment as indicated; report the incidence of either to your health care provider.
- You may experience these side effects: Headache, increased upper respiratory infections, nausea.
- Report fever, sore throat, unusual bleeding or bruising; severe abdominal pain.

▽nebivolol

*(nah **bev'** ah loll)*

Bystolic

PREGNANCY CATEGORY C

Drug classes

Antihypertensive
Beta-adrenergic blocker

Therapeutic actions

Decreases heart rate and contractility, suppresses renin release, and vasodilates and decreases peripheral vascular resistance, all leading to decreased blood pressure and decreased cardiac output and oxygen consumption.

Indications

- Treatment of hypertension, as monotherapy or with other antihypertensives

Contraindications and cautions

- Contraindicated with hypersensitivity to any component of the drug, severe bradycardia, heart block, cardiogenic shock, decompensated HF, sick sinus syndrome (unless a pacemaker is in place), severe hepatic impairment (Child-Pugh greater than grade B), lactation.
- Use cautiously with bronchospastic diseases, surgery, diabetes, hypoglycemia, thyroid dysfunction, renal impairment, hepatic impairment, history of anaphylactic reactions, pheochromocytoma, pregnancy.

Available forms

Tablets—2.5, 5, 10, 20 mg

Dosages

Adults

Starting dose: 5 mg/day PO; may be increased at 2-wk intervals to a maximum of 40 mg/day PO based on patient response.

Pediatric patients

Safety and efficacy not established.

Patients with severe renal impairment

If creatinine clearance is less than 30 mL/min, starting dose 2.5 mg/day PO; titrate slowly and monitor patient closely.

Patients with hepatic impairment
In moderate impairment, starting dose of 2.5 mg/day PO; titrate slowly and monitor patient closely. In severe impairment, drug not recommended.

Pharmacokinetics

Route	Onset	Peak
Oral	Rapid	1.5–4 hr

Metabolism: Hepatic; $T_{1/2}$: Not reported
Distribution: May cross placenta; may enter breast milk
Excretion: Urine, feces

Adverse effects

- **CNS:** *Headache,* dizziness, insomnia
- **CV:** Chest pain, bradycardia, arrhythmias, peripheral edema, hypotension
- **GI:** Nausea, diarrhea
- **Respiratory:** Dyspnea
- **Other:** Fatigue

Interactions

✱ **Drug-drug** • Risk of decreased HR and impaired conduction if combined with calcium antagonists (particularly verapamil, diltiazem), antiarrhythmics, cardiac glycosides; monitor patient closely because dosage adjustments may be needed • Risk of severe suppression of sympathetic activity if combined with other beta blockers, catecholamine-depleting drugs; avoid this combination or, if it must be used, monitor patient closely • Risk of unexpected BP response if combined with CYP2D6 inhibitors or inducers (quinidine, propafenone, fluoxetine, paroxetine); monitor patient response very closely and adjust dosage as needed • Risk of serious side effects when discontinuing combined use of clonidine and nebivolol; taper nebivolol and discontinue for several days before gradually tapering clonidine

■ Nursing considerations

Assessment

- **History:** Hypersensitivity to any component of drug, sinus bradycardia, heart block, HF, cardiogenic shock, renal impairment, liver impairment, diabetes, bronchospastic disorders, thyroid dysfunction, pregnancy, lactation, anaphylactic reactions
- **Physical:** Orientation, affect, reflexes; P, BP, heart sounds, peripheral perfusion; R, adventitious sounds; ECG, renal function tests, LFTs, thyroid levels, blood glucose

Interventions

⊗ ***Warning*** Do not stop this drug abruptly after long-term therapy; hypersensitivity to catecholamines can exacerbate angina, MI, ventricular arrhythmia. Taper drug gradually over 2 wk while monitoring patient.

- Consult surgeon about withdrawing drug if patient is to have surgery (withdrawal is controversial).
- Establish safety precautions if CNS changes occur (dizziness, altered thought process).

Teaching points

- This drug may be used with other antihypertensives; follow your drug regimen carefully.
- Take this drug once a day, with or without food. Try to take it at about the same time each day.
- If you miss a dose, take the next dose as soon as you remember. Do not make up or double doses; do not take more than one dose each day.
- Do not run out of tablets, and do not stop taking this drug suddenly. If it is decided that you need to stop this drug, the dose will be tapered slowly over 1 to 2 weeks to prevent possible side effects.
- If you have diabetes, be aware that this drug may block the signs or symptoms of hypoglycemia and hyperglycemia. You will need to monitor yourself carefully while taking this drug.
- Do not drive or operate dangerous machinery until you know how this drug affects you; it may cause dizziness and loss of alertness.
- It is not known how this drug could affect an unborn fetus. You should use contraception while you are taking this drug. If you become pregnant while taking this drug, consult your health care provider.
- It is not known how this drug could affect a nursing baby. Because of the risk of serious side effects in an infant, you should choose another method of feeding the baby while taking this drug.

- You may experience these side effects: Dizziness, insomnia (do not drive a car or engage in activities that require alertness if these effects occur); headache (consult your health care provider about medication to relieve headache).
- Report difficulty breathing, increasing shortness of breath, swelling in the ankles or legs, sudden weight gain, or a very slow heart rate.

nefazodone

See Appendix W, *Less commonly used drugs.*

nelarabine

See Appendix W, *Less commonly used drugs.*

nelfinavir mesylate

*(nell **fin'** a veer)*

Viracept

PREGNANCY CATEGORY B

Drug classes

Antiviral
Protease inhibitor

Therapeutic actions

Inhibitor of the HIV-1 protease; prevents viral cleavage resulting in the production of immature, noninfectious virus. Though no controlled trials of the effectiveness of nelfinavir exist, studies may indicate effectiveness in combination with nucleoside analogues.

Indications

- Treatment of HIV infection when antiretroviral therapy is warranted in combination with nucleoside analogues or other antiretroviral drugs
- Unlabeled use: Postexposure prophylaxis following exposure to HIV

Contraindications and cautions

- Contraindicated with life-threatening allergy to any component, concurrent use of drugs dependent on CYP3A for clearance (amiodarone, quinidine, ergot derivatives, pimozide, midazolam, triazolam, lovastatin, simvastatin).
- Use cautiously with renal and hepatic impairment, hemophilia, pregnancy, lactation.

Available forms

Tablets—250, 625 mg; powder—50 mg/g

Dosages

Adults and patients older than 13 yr

750 mg PO tid or 1,250 mg PO bid in combination with other antiretroviral drugs.

Pediatric patients 2–13 yr

45–55 mg/kg PO bid or 25–35 mg/kg PO tid.

Pediatric patients younger than 2 yr

Not recommended.

Pharmacokinetics

Route	*Onset*	*Peak*
Oral	Slow	2–4 hr

Metabolism: Hepatic; $T_{1/2}$: 3.5–5 hr
Distribution: May cross placenta; may enter breast milk
Excretion: Feces

Adverse effects

- **CNS:** Anxiety, depression, insomnia, myalgia, dizziness, paresthesias, **seizures,** suicide ideation
- **Dermatologic:** Dermatitis, folliculitis, fungal dermatitis, rash, sweating, urticaria
- **GI:** *Diarrhea, nausea, GI pain,* anorexia, vomiting, dyspepsia, liver enzyme elevations
- **Respiratory:** Dyspnea, pharyngitis, rhinitis, sinusitis
- **Other:** Eye disorders, sexual dysfunction

Interactions

✱ **Drug-drug** ⊗ ***Warning*** Risk of severe toxic effects and life-threatening arrhythmias with rifampin, triazolam, midazolam, amiodarone, quinidine, ergot derivatives, pimozide, lovastatin, simvastatin; avoid these combinations • Decreased effectiveness with rifabutin, phenobarbital, phenytoin, dexamethasone, carbamazepine • Possible loss of effectiveness of hormonal contraceptives with nelfinavir; recommend using barrier contraceptives

✷ Drug-food • Decreased metabolism and risk of toxic effects if combined with grapefruit juice; avoid this combination

✷ Drug-alternative therapy • Decreased effectiveness of nelfinavir if combined with St. John's wort

■ Nursing considerations

CLINICAL ALERT!

Name confusion has occurred between *Viracept* (nelfinavir) and *Viramune* (nevirapine); use caution.

Assessment

- **History:** Life-threatening allergy to any component; impaired hepatic or renal function; pregnancy, lactation; hemophilia; concurrent drug, herbal therapy use
- **Physical:** T; affect, reflexes, peripheral sensation; R, adventitious sounds; bowel sounds, liver evaluation; LFTs, renal function tests

Interventions

- Administer with meals or a light snack; powder may be mixed with a small amount of nonacidic food or beverage; use within 6 hr of mixing.
- Monitor patient for signs of opportunistic infections that will need to be treated appropriately.
- Arrange for loperamide to control diarrhea if it occurs.
- Recommend that patient use barrier contraceptives while using this drug.

Teaching points

- Take drug exactly as prescribed; take missed doses as soon as possible and return to normal schedule; do not take double doses.
- Take with meals or a light snack; do not drink grapefruit juice while using this drug.
- Powder may be mixed with water, milk, baby formula, soy milk, ice cream, pudding, or liquid dietary supplements; use within 6 hours of mixing; take in combination with nucleoside analogues.
- These drugs are not a cure for AIDS or AIDS-related complex; opportunistic infections may occur and regular medical care should be sought to deal with the disease.
- The long-term effects of this drug are not yet known.
- This drug combination does not reduce the risk of transmission of HIV to others by sexual contact or blood contamination; use appropriate precautions.
- Use barrier contraceptives; this drug may block the effectiveness of hormonal contraceptives.
- Avoid St. Johns wort while taking this drug.
- You may experience these side effects: Nausea, loss of appetite, diarrhea (eat frequent small meals; medication is available to control diarrhea); dizziness, loss of feeling (take appropriate precautions).
- Report extreme fatigue, lethargy, severe headache, severe nausea, vomiting, difficulty breathing, rash, changes in color of urine or stool.

▽neomycin sulfate

(nee o mye' sin)

Mycifradin, Neo-fradin, Neo-Tabs

PREGNANCY CATEGORY D

Drug class

Aminoglycoside

Therapeutic actions

Bactericidal: Inhibits protein synthesis in susceptible strains of bacteria; functional integrity of bacterial cell membrane appears to be disrupted, causing cell death. Due to poor PO absorption, oral neomycin is used to suppress GI bacterial flora.

Indications

- Preoperative suppression of GI bacterial flora
- Adjunct treatment in hepatic coma to reduce ammonia-forming bacteria in the GI tract

Contraindications and cautions

- Contraindicated with allergy to aminoglycosides, intestinal obstruction, pregnancy, lactation.
- Use cautiously in the elderly or with any patient with diminished hearing, decreased renal function, dehydration, neuromuscular

disorders (myasthenia gravis, parkinsonism, infant botulism).

Available forms

Tablets—500 mg; oral solution—125 mg/ 5 mL

Dosages

Adults

- *Preoperative preparation for elective colorectal surgery:* See manufacturer's recommendations for a complex 3-day regimen that includes oral erythromycin, bisacodyl, magnesium sulfate, enemas, and dietary restrictions.
- *Hepatic coma:* 4–12 g/day in divided doses for 5–6 days, as adjunct to protein-free diet and supportive therapy, including transfusions, as needed.

Pediatric patients

- *Hepatic coma:* 50–100 mg/kg/day in divided doses for 5–6 days, as adjunct to protein-free diet and supportive therapy including transfusions, as needed.

Geriatric patients or patients with renal failure

Reduce dosage and carefully monitor serum drug levels and renal function tests throughout treatment. If this is not possible, reduce frequency of administration.

Pharmacokinetics

Route	Onset	Peak
Oral	Varies	1–4 hr

Metabolism: $T_{1/2}$: 3 hr
Distribution: Crosses placenta; enters breast milk
Excretion: Feces, urine

Adverse effects

Although limited absorption occurs across the intact GI mucosa, the risk of absorption from ulcerated area requires consideration of all side effects with oral and parenteral therapy.

- **CNS:** Ototoxicity—*tinnitus, dizziness,* vertigo, deafness (partially reversible to irreversible), vestibular paralysis, confusion, disorientation, depression, lethargy, nystagmus, visual disturbances, headache, *numbness, tingling,* tremor, paresthesias, muscle twitching, **seizures**
- **CV:** Palpitations, hypotension, hypertension
- **GI:** Hepatic toxicity, *nausea, vomiting, anorexia,* weight loss, stomatitis, increased salivation
- **GU: Nephrotoxicity**
- **Hematologic:** *Leukemoid reaction,* agranulocytosis, granulocytosis, leukopenia, leukocytosis, thrombocytopenia, eosinophilia, pancytopenia, anemia, hemolytic anemia, increased or decreased reticulocyte count, electrolyte disturbances
- **Hypersensitivity:** Hypersensitivity reactions—*purpura, rash,* urticaria, exfoliative dermatitis, itching
- **Local:** *Pain, irritation*
- **Other:** Fever, apnea, splenomegaly, joint pain, *superinfection*

Interactions

✷ **Drug-drug** • Increased ototoxic, nephrotoxic, neurotoxic effects with other aminoglycosides, potent diuretics • Increased neuromuscular blockade and muscular paralysis with anesthetics, nondepolarizing neuromuscular blocking drugs, succinylcholine, citrate-anticoagulated blood • Potential inactivation of both drugs if mixed with beta-lactam–type antibiotics • Increased bactericidal effect with penicillins, cephalosporins, carbenicillin, ticarcillin • Decreased absorption and therapeutic effects of digoxin

✷ **Drug-lab test** • Falsely low serum aminoglycoside levels with penicillin or cephalosporin therapy; these antibiotics can inactivate aminoglycosides after the blood sample is drawn

■ Nursing considerations

Assessment

- **History:** Allergy to aminoglycosides; intestinal obstruction, diminished hearing, decreased renal function, dehydration, neuromuscular disorders; pregnancy, lactation
- **Physical:** Renal function, eighth cranial nerve function, state of hydration, CBC, skin color and lesions, orientation and affect, reflexes, bilateral grip strength, body weight, bowel sounds

Interventions
- Ensure that the patient is well hydrated.

Teaching points
- Report hearing changes, dizziness, severe diarrhea.

neostigmine
(nee oh ***stig'*** *meen)*
neostigmine bromide

neostigmine methylsulfate
Prostigmin

PREGNANCY CATEGORY C

Drug classes
Antidote
Antimyasthenic
Cholinesterase inhibitor
Parasympathomimetic
Urinary tract drug

Therapeutic actions
Increases the concentration of acetylcholine at the sites of cholinergic transmission, and prolongs and exaggerates the effects of acetylcholine by reversibly inhibiting the enzyme acetylcholinesterase, causing parasympathomimetic effects and facilitating transmission at the skeletal neuromuscular junction; also has direct cholinomimetic activity on skeletal muscle; may have direct cholinomimetic activity on neurons in autonomic ganglia and the CNS.

Indications
- Prevention and treatment of postoperative distention and urinary retention
- Symptomatic control of myasthenia gravis
- Diagnosis of myasthenia gravis (edrophonium preferred)
- Antidote for nondepolarizing neuromuscular junction blockers (tubocurarine or pancuronium) after surgery

Contraindications and cautions
- Contraindicated with hypersensitivity to anticholinesterases; adverse reactions to bromides (neostigmine bromide); intestinal or urogenital tract obstruction, peritonitis; pregnancy (may stimulate uterus and induce premature labor); lactation.
- Use cautiously with asthma, peptic ulcer, bradycardia, cardiac arrhythmias, recent coronary occlusion, vagotonia, hyperthyroidism, epilepsy.

Available forms
Injection—1:1,000 (1 mg/mL), 1:2,000 (0.5 mg/mL), 1:4,000 (0.25 mg/mL); tablets—15 mg

Dosages
Adults
- *Prevention of postoperative distention and urinary retention:* 1 mL of the 1:4,000 solution (0.25 mg) neostigmine methylsulfate subcutaneously or IM as soon as possible after operation. Repeat every 4–6 hr for 2–3 days.
- *Treatment of postoperative distention:* 1 mL of the 1:2,000 solution (0.5 mg) neostigmine methylsulfate subcutaneously or IM, as required.
- *Treatment of urinary retention:* 1 mL of the 1:2,000 solution (0.5 mg) neostigmine methylsulfate subcutaneously or IM. If urination does not occur within 1 hr, catheterize the patient. After the bladder is emptied, continue 0.5-mg injections every 3 hr for at least five injections.
- *Symptomatic control of myasthenia gravis:* 1 mL of the 1:2,000 solution (0.5 mg) subcutaneously or IM. Individualize subsequent doses. Should be used with atropine to counteract adverse muscarinic effects. Tablets—15–375 mg/day PO; average daily dose is 150 mg.
- *Diagnosis of myasthenia gravis:* 0.022 mg/kg IM.
- *Antidote for nondepolarizing neuromuscular blockers:* Give atropine sulfate 0.6–1.2 mg IV several min before slow IV injection of neostigmine 0.5–2 mg. Repeat as required. Total dose should usually not exceed 5 mg.

Pediatric patients
- *Prevention, treatment of postoperative distention and urinary retention:* Safety and efficacy not established.
- *Symptomatic control of myasthenia gravis:* 0.01–0.04 mg/kg per dose IM, IV, or

subcutaneously every 2–3 hr as needed. Tablets—2 mg/kg/day PO every 3–4 hr as needed.
- *Diagnosis of myasthenia gravis:* 0.04 mg/kg IM.
- *As antidote for nondepolarizing neuromuscular blocker:* Give 0.008–0.025 mg/kg atropine sulfate IV several min before slow IV injection of neostigmine 0.025–0.08 mg/kg.

Pharmacokinetics

Route	*Onset*	*Peak*	*Duration*
Subcut., IM	20–30 min	20–30 min	2.5–4 hr
IV	10–30 min	20–30 min	2.5–4 hr
Oral	20–30 min	20–30 min	2–4 hr

Metabolism: Hepatic; $T_{1/2}$: 47–60 min
Distribution: May cross placenta or enter breast milk
Excretion: Urine

IV FACTS

Preparation: No further preparation is required.
Infusion: Inject slowly directly into vein or into tubing of running IV, each 0.5 mg over 1 min.

Adverse effects

- **CNS:** Seizures, dysarthria, dysphonia, drowsiness, dizziness, headache, loss of consciousness
- **CV:** *Cardiac arrhythmias,* **cardiac arrest,** decreased cardiac output leading to hypotension, syncope
- **Dermatologic:** Diaphoresis, flushing, rash, urticaria, anaphylaxis
- **EENT:** *Lacrimation, miosis,* spasm of accommodation, diplopia, conjunctival hyperemia
- **GI:** *Salivation, dysphagia, nausea, vomiting, increased peristalsis, abdominal cramps,* flatulence, diarrhea
- **GU:** *Urinary frequency and incontinence,* urinary urgency
- **Local:** Thrombophlebitis after IV use
- **Peripheral:** Skeletal muscle weakness, fasciculations, muscle cramps, arthralgia
- **Respiratory:** *Increased pharyngeal and tracheobronchial secretions,* **laryngospasm, bronchospasm,** bronchiolar constriction, dyspnea, respiratory muscle paralysis, central respiratory paralysis

Interactions

✱ **Drug-drug** • Prolonged neuromuscular blockade of succinylcholine • Decreased effects and possible muscular depression with corticosteroids • Increased neuromuscular blocking effect due to aminoglycoside antibiotics

■ Nursing considerations

Assessment

- **History:** Hypersensitivity to anticholinesterases; adverse reactions to bromides; intestinal or urogenital tract obstruction, peritonitis; asthma, peptic ulcer, cardiac arrhythmias, recent coronary occlusion, vagotonia, hyperthyroidism, epilepsy; lactation, pregnancy
- **Physical:** Skin color, texture, lesions; reflexes, bilateral grip strength; P, auscultation, BP; R, adventitious sounds; salivation, bowel sounds, normal output; frequency, voiding pattern, normal output; EEG, thyroid tests

Interventions

- Administer IV slowly.
- Overdose with anticholinesterase drugs can cause muscle weakness (cholinergic crisis) that is difficult to differentiate from myasthenic weakness. The administration of atropine may mask the parasympathetic effects of anticholinesterase overdose and further confound the diagnosis.

⊗ ***Warning*** Keep atropine sulfate readily available as an antidote and antagonist in case of cholinergic crisis or hypersensitivity reaction.

⊗ ***Warning*** Discontinue drug, and consult physician if excessive salivation, emesis, frequent urination, or diarrhea occurs.

- Decrease dosage if excessive sweating or nausea occurs.

Teaching points

- Take this drug exactly as prescribed; patient and a significant other should receive extensive teaching about the effects of the drug, the signs and symptoms of myasthenia

gravis, the fact that muscle weakness may be related both to drug overdose and to exacerbation of the disease, and that it is important to report muscle weakness promptly to your health care provider so that proper evaluation can be made.
- You may experience these side effects: Blurred vision, difficulty with far vision, difficulty with dark adaptation (use caution while driving, especially at night, or performing hazardous tasks in reduced light); increased urinary frequency, abdominal cramps; sweating (avoid hot or excessively humid environments).
- Report muscle weakness, nausea, vomiting, diarrhea, severe abdominal pain, excessive sweating, excessive salivation, frequent urination, urinary urgency, irregular heartbeat, difficulty breathing.

▽nesiritide (hBNP)

See Appendix W, *Less commonly used drugs.*

▽nevirapine

(neh veer' ah pine)

Viramune

PREGNANCY CATEGORY C

Drug classes
Antiviral
Nonnucleoside reverse transcriptase inhibitor

Therapeutic actions
Antiretroviral activity; binds directly to HIV-1 reverse transcriptase and blocks the replication of HIV by changing the structure of the HIV enzyme.

Indications
- Treatment of HIV-1 infection in combination with other antiretroviral drugs

Contraindications and cautions
- Contraindicated with allergy to nevirapine; lactation.
- Use cautiously with renal or hepatic impairment, rash, pregnancy.

Available forms
Tablets—200 mg; oral suspension—50 mg/5 mL

Dosages
Adults
200 mg PO daily for 14 days; if no rash appears, then 200 mg PO bid with other antivirals. Daily dose should not exceed 400 mg/day.
Pediatric patients 8 yr and older
4 mg/kg PO daily for 14 days, then 4 mg/kg PO bid. Daily dose should not exceed 400 mg/day.
Pediatric patients 2 mo–8 yr
4 mg/kg PO daily for 14 days, then 7 mg/kg PO bid. Daily dose should not exceed 400 mg/day.

Pharmacokinetics

Route	*Onset*	*Peak*
Oral	Rapid	4 hr

Metabolism: Hepatic; $T_{1/2}$: 45 hr, then 25–30 hr
Distribution: Crosses placenta; enters breast milk
Excretion: Urine

Adverse effects
- **CNS:** *Headache*
- **Dermatologic: Stevens-Johnson syndrome, rash, toxic epidermal necrolysis**
- **GI:** *Nausea, vomiting, diarrhea,* dry mouth, **hepatic impairment including hepatitis, hepatic necrosis**
- **Other:** Infection, chills, fever

Interactions
✱ **Drug-drug** • Avoid concurrent use with protease inhibitors, hormonal contraceptives (metabolism is increased and effectiveness decreased) • Decreased ketoconazole, itraconazole, clarithromycin, rifampin levels and effects; avoid this combination
✱ **Drug-alternative therapy** • Decreased effectiveness if combined with St. John's wort

■ Nursing considerations

CLINICAL ALERT!
Name confusion has occurred between *Viramune* (nevirapine) and *Viracept* (nelfinavir); use caution.

Assessment

- **History:** Allergy to nevirapine, renal or hepatic impairment, pregnancy, lactation, rash
- **Physical:** T; orientation, reflexes; peripheral perfusion; urinary output; skin color, perfusion, hydration; LFTs, renal function tests

Interventions

- Administer in combination with nucleoside analogues.

⊗ ***Black box warning*** Monitor renal and hepatic function tests before and during treatment. Discontinue drug at any sign of hepatic impairment; severe to life-threatening hepatotoxicity is possible.

⊗ ***Black box warning*** Do not administer if severe rash occurs, especially accompanied by fever, blistering, lesion, swelling, general malaise; discontinue if rash recurs on rechallenge; severe to life-threatening reactions are possible.

- Shake suspension gently before use. Rinse oral dosing cup and administer rinse to patient.

Teaching points

- Take this drug exactly as prescribed; do not take double doses if you miss a dose. Take your other HIV drugs as prescribed.
- If you are using the suspension form, shake gently before use. Dosing syringe is recommended to ensure the correct dose.
- Use some method of barrier birth control (not hormonal contraceptives) while using this medication. Severe birth defects can occur, and this drug causes loss of effectiveness of hormonal contraceptives.
- This drug does not cure HIV infection. Follow routine preventive measures and continue any other medication that has been prescribed.
- You may experience these side effects: Nausea, vomiting, loss of appetite, diarrhea, headache, fever.
- Report rash, any lesions or blistering, changes in color of stool or urine, fever, muscle or joint pain.

▽niacin

(nye' ah sin)

Niacor, Niaspan, Slo-Niacin

PREGNANCY CATEGORY C

Drug classes

Antihyperlipidemic
Vitamin

Therapeutic actions

May partially inhibit the release of free fatty acids from adipose tissue and increase lipoprotein activity, which could increase the rate of triglyceride removal from plasma; these actions reduce the total LDL and triglycerides and increase HDL. Niacin also decreases serum levels of apo B and lipoprotein A.

Indications

- Adjunct to diet for treatment of adults with very high serum triglyceride levels (types IV and V hyperlipidemia) who present a risk of pancreatitis and who do not respond adequately to dietary control
- Adjunct for treatment of adults with hypercholesterolemia
- Treatment of pellagra, niacin deficiency

Contraindications and cautions

- Contraindicated with hepatic impairment, active peptic ulcer disease, arterial bleeding, lactation.
- Use cautiously with history of jaundice, hepatobiliary disease, peptic ulcer, high alcohol consumption, renal impairment, unstable angina, gout, recent surgery, pregnancy.

Available forms

ER tablets DNC—500, 750, 1,000 mg; tablets—50, 100, 250, 500 mg; OTC CR tablets DNC—250, 500, 750 mg; OTC CR capsules DNC—250, 400 mg; OTC SR capsules DNC—125, 500 mg

Dosages

Adults and pediatric patients older than 16 yr

Dyslipidemia: Initially, 100 mg PO tid, increased to 1,000 mg PO tid (immediate-release form); 500 mg/day PO at bedtime for 4 wk, then 1,000 mg/day PO at bedtime (extended-release form), maximum dosage is 2,000 mg/day; 1,000–2,000 mg/day PO (sustained-release form).

CAD, post MI: 500 mg/day PO at bedtime, titrated at 4-wk intervals to maximum of 1,000–2,000 mg/day.

Pellagra: 50–100 mg PO tid to maximum of 500 mg/day.

Pediatric patients 16 yr and younger

Dyslipidemia: 100–250 mg/day PO in three divided doses with meals; may be increased at 2- to 3-wk intervals to maximum of 10 mg/kg/day (immediate-release form).

Pellagra: 50–100 mg PO tid.

Pharmacokinetics

Route	*Onset*	*Peak*
Oral	Rapid	45 min

Metabolism: Hepatic; $T_{1/2}$: Unknown
Distribution: Crosses placenta, enters breast milk
Excretion: Urine

Adverse effects

- **CNS:** *Headache,* anxiety
- **CV:** Arrhythmias, hypotension
- **Dermatologic:** *Flushing,* acanthosis nigricans, dry skin, *rash*
- **GI:** *GI upset,* peptic ulcer, abnormal liver function tests, *diarrhea, nausea, vomiting*
- **Hematologic:** Hyperuricemia
- **Other:** Glucose intolerance

Interactions

✱ **Drug-drug** • Increased risk of rhabdomyolysis with HMG-CoA inhibitors • Increased effectiveness of antihypertensives, vasoactive drugs • Increased risk of bleeding with anticoagulants; monitor PT and platelet counts and adjust dosage accordingly • Decreased absorption with bile acid sequestrants; separate doses by at least 4–6 hr

■ Nursing considerations

Assessment

- **History:** Hepatic impairment, active peptic ulcer disease, arterial bleeding, lactation, hepatobiliary disease, peptic ulcer, high alcohol consumption, renal impairment, unstable angina, gout, recent surgery, pregnancy
- **Physical:** Skin lesions, color, T; orientation, affect, reflexes; P, auscultation, baseline ECG, BP; liver evaluation; lipid studies, LFTs

Interventions

- Administer drug at bedtime to minimize effects of flushing.
- When flushing is persistent, recommend 325 mg aspirin taken 30 min before each scheduled dose of niacin.

⊗ ***Warning*** Do not substitute ER products for immediate-release products at equivalent doses. Severe hepatic toxicity has occurred.

- Avoid ingestion of hot liquids or alcohol around the time of niacin administration to minimize flushing.
- Consult with a dietitian regarding a low-cholesterol diet.
- Arrange for regular follow-up during long-term therapy.

Teaching points

- Take drug at bedtime. The dose will change each week until the desired response is achieved. Do not cut, crush, or chew extended-release forms.
- Take your bile acid sequestrant (if appropriate) 4–6 hours apart from niacin; avoid alcohol while using this medication.
- Maintain your diet and exercise program for lowering lipid level.
- You may experience these side effects: Nausea, heartburn, loss of appetite (eat frequent small meals); headache (may lessen over time; if bothersome, consult your health care provider); rash, flushing (take drug at bedtime). You may take an aspirin or nonsteroidal anti-inflammatory drug 30 minutes before each dose to reduce GI distress and flushing.
- Report unusual bleeding or bruising, palpitations, fainting, rash, fever.

N

▽ nicardipine hydrochloride

*(nye **kar'** de peen)*

Cardene, Cardene IV, Cardene SR

PREGNANCY CATEGORY C

Drug classes
Antianginal
Antihypertensive
Calcium channel blocker

Therapeutic actions
Inhibits the movement of calcium ions across the membranes of cardiac and arterial muscle cells; calcium is involved in the generation of the action potential in specialized automatic and conducting cells in the heart, in arterial smooth muscle, and in excitation-contraction coupling in cardiac muscle cells. Inhibition of calcium flow results in the depression of impulse formation in specialized cardiac pacemaker cells, in slowing of the velocity of conduction of the cardiac impulse, in the depression of myocardial contractility, and in the dilation of coronary arteries and arterioles and peripheral arterioles; these effects lead to decreased cardiac work, decreased cardiac energy consumption, and increased delivery of oxygen to myocardial cells.

Indications
- Immediate-release only: Chronic stable (effort-related) angina. Use alone or with beta blockers
- Immediate-release and SR: Management of essential hypertension alone or with other antihypertensives
- IV: Short-term treatment of hypertension when oral use is not feasible

Contraindications and cautions
- Contraindicated with allergy to nicardipine, pregnancy, lactation.
- Use cautiously with impaired hepatic or renal function, sick sinus syndrome, heart block (second- or third-degree), HF.

Available forms
Capsules—20, 30 mg; SR capsules—30, 45, 60 mg; injection—2.5 mg/mL; premixed bags—20 mg/200 mL, 40 mg/200 mL

Dosages
Adults
Oral
- *Angina:* Immediate-release only—individualize dosage. Usual initial dose is 20 mg tid PO. Range, 20–40 mg tid PO. Allow at least 3 days before increasing dosage to ensure steady-state plasma levels.
- *Hypertension:* Immediate-release—initial dose, 20 mg tid PO. Range, 20–40 mg tid. The maximum BP-lowering effect occurs in 1–2 hr. Adjust dosage based on BP response, allow at least 3 days before increasing dosage. SR—initial dose is 30 mg bid PO. Range, 30–60 mg bid.

IV
- *Hypertension:* For gradual reduction, begin infusion at 5 mg/hr. Increase by 2.5 mg/hr every 15 min to maximum of 15 mg/hr. For rapid reduction, begin infusion at 5 mg/hr. Increase by 2.5 mg/hr every 5 min to maximum of 15 mg/hr. Once BP is controlled, reduce to 3 mg/hr.

Pediatric patients
Safety and efficacy not established.

Patients with renal or hepatic impairment
For patients with renal impairment, adjust dosage beginning with 20 mg tid PO (immediate-release) or 30 mg bid PO (SR). For patients with hepatic impairment, starting dose 20 mg bid PO (immediate-release) with individual adjustment.

Pharmacokinetics

Route	*Onset*	*Peak*
Oral	20 min	0.5–2 hr

Metabolism: Hepatic; $T_{1/2}$: 2–4 hr
Distribution: Crosses placenta; enters breast milk
Excretion: Urine

IV FACTS
Preparation: Dilute each ampule with 240 mL of solution to a concentration of 0.1 mg/mL; store at room temperature; protect from light; stable for 24 hr.
Infusion: Slow IV infusion; begin with 5 mg/hr. Increase by 2.5 mg/hr every 5 min (rapid control) or 15 min (slow control) to maximum of 15 mg/hr. When BP is controlled, use maintenance rate of 3 mg/hr (rapid control).
Compatibilities: Compatible with dextrose 5% injection, dextrose 5% and sodium chloride

0.45% or 0.9% injection; dextrose 5% with potassium; 0.45% or 0.9% sodium chloride.
Incompatibilities: Do not mix with 5% sodium bicarbonate or lactated Ringer's.

Adverse effects
- **CNS:** *Dizziness, light-headedness, headache, asthenia,* fatigue
- **CV:** *Peripheral edema, angina,* hypotension, arrhythmias, *bradycardia, AV block,* asystole
- **Dermatologic:** *Flushing,* rash
- **GI:** *Nausea,* hepatic injury

Interactions
✱ **Drug-drug** • Increased serum levels and toxicity of cyclosporine

■ Nursing considerations
Assessment
- **History:** Allergy to nicardipine, impaired hepatic or renal function, sick sinus syndrome, heart block (second- or third-degree), pregnancy, lactation
- **Physical:** Skin lesions, color, edema; P, BP, baseline ECG, peripheral perfusion, auscultation; R, adventitious sounds; liver evaluation, normal GI output; LFTs, renal function tests, urinalysis

Interventions
- Monitor the patient carefully (BP, cardiac rhythm, and output) while drug is being titrated to therapeutic dose; dosage may be increased more rapidly in hospitalized patients under close supervision.

⊗ ***Warning*** Monitor BP very carefully with concurrent doses of nitrates.

- Monitor cardiac rhythm regularly during stabilization of dosage and long-term therapy.
- Provide small frequent meals if GI upset occurs.

Teaching points
- Take exactly as prescribed; do not exceed the prescribed daily dose.
- You may experience these side effects: Nausea, vomiting (eat frequent small meals); headache (monitor lighting, noise, and temperature; request medication if severe).
- Report irregular heart beat, shortness of breath, swelling of the hands or feet, pronounced dizziness, constipation.

▽nicotine
(nik' oh teen)

Nicoderm CQ, Nicotrol, Nicotrol Inhaler, Nicotrol NS

PREGNANCY CATEGORY D

Drug class
Smoking deterrent

Therapeutic actions
Nicotine acts at nicotinic receptors in the peripheral and CNS; produces behavioral stimulation and depression, cardiac acceleration, peripheral vasoconstriction, and elevated BP.

Indications
- Temporary aid to the cigarette smoker seeking to give up smoking while in a behavioral modification program under medical supervision
- Unlabeled use: Improvement of symptoms of Tourette syndrome

Contraindications and cautions
- Contraindicated with allergy to nicotine, arrhythmias, angina pectoris, pregnancy, lactation, and during the post-MI period. Inhaler is contraindicated with asthma, COPD.
- Use cautiously with hyperthyroidism, pheochromocytoma, type 2 diabetes (releases catecholamines from the adrenal medulla), hypertension, peptic ulcer disease.

Available forms
Transdermal system—7, 14, 21 mg/day; 5, 10, 15 mg/16 hr (*Nicotrol*); nasal spray— 0.5 mg/actuation (10 mg/mL); inhaler—4 mg/actuation

Dosages
Adults
Topical
Apply system, 5–21 mg, once every 24 hr. Dosage is based on response and stage of withdrawal.

Nicoderm: 21 mg/day for first 6 wk; 14 mg/day for next 2 wk; 7 mg/day for next 2 wk. *Nicotrol:* 15 mg/day for first 6 wk; 10 mg/day for next 2 wk; 5 mg/day for last 2 wk.

Nasal spray

1 spray in each nostril as needed, one to two doses each hour, up to five doses/hr and 40 doses/day.

Nasal inhaler

1 spray in each nostril, one to two doses/hr to a maximum five doses/hr or 40 doses/day. Dosage is individualized; in studies, best results were achieved by continuous, frequent puffing over 20 min. Do not use longer than 6 mo. Patients are treated for 12 wk, then weaned off the daily dose over next 6–12 wk.

Pediatric patients

Safety and efficacy in children and adolescents who smoke have not been established.

Pharmacokinetics

Route	*Onset*	*Peak*	*Duration*
Dermal	1–2 hr	4–6 min	4–24 hr
Nasal	Rapid	15 min	NA

Metabolism: Hepatic; $T_{1/2}$: 1–4 hr
Distribution: Crosses placenta; enters breast milk
Excretion: Urine

Adverse effects

- **CNS:** *Headache, insomnia,* abnormal dreams, dizziness, light-headedness, sweating
- **GI:** Diarrhea, constipation, nausea, dyspepsia, abdominal pain, dry mouth
- **Local:** *Erythema, burning, pruritus* at site of patch; local edema
- **Respiratory:** Cough, pharyngitis, sinusitis
- **Other:** Backache, chest pain, asthenia, dysmenorrhea, flulike symptoms

Interactions

✱ **Drug-drug** • Increased circulating levels of cortisol, catecholamines with nicotine use; smoking dosage of adrenergic agonists, adrenergic blockers may need to be adjusted according to nicotine, smoking status of patient • Smoking increases metabolism and lowers blood levels of caffeine, theophylline, imipramine, pentazocine; decreases effects of furosemide, propranolol • Cessation of smoking may decrease metabolism of propoxyphene

■ Nursing considerations

Assessment

- **History:** Allergy to nicotine; nonsmoker; post-MI, arrhythmias, angina pectoris; hyperthyroidism, pheochromocytoma, type 2 diabetes; hypertension, peptic ulcer disease; pregnancy; lactation
- **Physical:** Orientation, affect; P, auscultation, BP; oral mucous membranes, abdominal examination; thyroid function tests

Interventions

- Protect systems from heat; slight discoloration of system is not significant.
- Apply system to nonhairy, clean, dry skin site on upper body or upper outer arm; use only when the pouch is intact; use immediately after removal from pouch; use each system only once. Remove old system before applying a new system.
- Wash hands thoroughly after application; do not touch eyes.
- Wrap used system in foil pouch of newly applied system; fold over and dispose of immediately to prevent access by pets or children.
- Apply new system after 24 hr; do not reuse same site for at least 1 wk. *Nicotrol:* Apply a new system each day after waking, and remove at bedtime.

⊗ ***Warning*** Handle nasal spray carefully; if it comes in contact with skin, flush immediately; dispose of bottle with cap in place.

- Ensure that patient has stopped smoking; if the patient is unable to stop smoking within the first 4 wk of therapy, drug therapy should be stopped.
- Encourage patients who have been unsuccessful at any dose to take a "therapy holiday" before trying again; counseling should explore factors contributing to their failure and other means of success.

Teaching points

- Protect systems from heat; slight discoloration of system is not significant.
- Apply system to nonhairy, clean, dry skin site on upper body or upper outer arm; use only

when the pouch is intact; use immediately after removal from pouch; use each system only once. Remove old system before applying a new system.
- Wash hands thoroughly after application; do not touch eyes. Wrap used system in foil pouch of newly applied system; fold over and dispose of immediately to prevent access by pets or children.
- Apply new system after 24 hours; do not reuse same site for at least 1 week. *Nicotrol:* Apply a new system each day after waking, and remove at bedtime.
- Tilt head back to administer spray; do not sniff, swallow, or inhale while spray is administered. If spray comes in contact with skin, flush immediately; discard bottle with cap in place.
- Store reusable mouthpiece for inhaler in plastic case; wash with soap and water. Throw inhaler cartridge away out of reach of children and pets.
- Abstain from smoking.
- You may experience these side effects: Dizziness, headache, light-headedness (use caution driving or performing tasks that require alertness); nausea, vomiting, constipation or diarrhea (frequent small meals, regular mouth care may help); skin redness, swelling at application site (good skin care, switching sites daily may help).
- Report nausea and vomiting, diarrhea, cold sweat, chest pain, palpitations, burning or swelling at application site.

▽nicotine polacrilex (nicotine resin complex)

(nik' oh teen)

Commit, Nicorette, Nicorette DS, Nicotine Gum

PREGNANCY CATEGORY C

Drug class
Smoking deterrent

Therapeutic actions
Acts as an agonist at nicotinic receptors in the peripheral and CNS; produces behavioral stimulation and depression, cardiac acceleration, peripheral vasoconstriction, and elevated BP.

Indications
- Temporary aid to the cigarette smoker seeking to give up smoking while in a behavioral modification program under medical supervision

Contraindications and cautions
- Contraindicated with allergy to nicotine or resin used, arrhythmias, angina pectoris, active TMJ disease, pregnancy, lactation, and during the post-MI period.
- Use cautiously with hyperthyroidism, pheochromocytoma, type 2 diabetes (releases catecholamines from the adrenal medulla), hypertension, peptic ulcer disease.

Available forms
Chewing gum—2 or 4 mg/square; lozenge—2, 4 mg

Dosages
Adults

Chewing gum

If patient smokes less than 25 cigarettes/day, start with 2 mg; if more than 25 cigarettes/day, start with 4 mg. Have patient chew one piece of gum whenever the urge to smoke occurs. Have the patient chew each piece slowly until it tingles, then place it between the cheek and gums; when tingle is gone, have patient chew gum again and repeat the process. Gum usually lasts for about 30 min to promote even, slow, buccal absorption of nicotine. Patients often require 10 pieces daily during the first month. Do not exceed 24 pieces daily. Therapy may be effective for up to 3 mo; 4–6 mo for complete cessation has been used. Should not be used for longer than 4 mo.

Lozenge

Start with 2 mg if patient first smokes more than 30 min after waking up; 4 mg if patient starts smoking within 30 min of waking. Patient must place lozenge in mouth, let dissolve over 20–30 min, and avoid eating or drinking anything other than water for 15 min before use. In week 1–6, use 1 lozenge every 1–2 hr; in week 7–9, use 1 lozenge every 2–4 hr; in week 10–12, use 1 lozenge every 4–8 hr. Do not exceed 5 lozenges in 6 hr or 20 daily.

N

Pediatric patients
Safety and efficacy in children and adolescents who smoke have not been established.

Pharmacokinetics

Route	*Onset*	*Peak*
Oral	Slow	15–30 min

Metabolism: Hepatic; $T_{1/2}$: 30–120 min
Distribution: Crosses placenta; enters breast milk
Excretion: Urine

Adverse effects
- **CNS:** Dizziness, light-headedness
- **GI:** *Mouth or throat soreness; hiccups, nausea, vomiting,* nonspecific GI distress, excessive salivation
- **Local:** Mechanical effects of chewing gum—traumatic injury to oral mucosa or teeth, *jaw ache,* eructation secondary to air swallowing

Interactions
✱ **Drug-drug** • Increased circulating levels of cortisol, catecholamines with nicotine use, smoking—dosage of adrenergic agonists, adrenergic blockers may need to be adjusted according to nicotine, smoking status of patient • Smoking increases metabolism and lowers blood levels of caffeine, theophylline, imipramine, pentazocine; decreases effects of furosemide, propranolol • Cessation of smoking may decrease metabolism of propoxyphene

■ Nursing considerations
Assessment
- **History:** Allergy to nicotine or resin used; nonsmoker; post-MI period; arrhythmias; angina pectoris; active TMJ disease; hyperthyroidism, pheochromocytoma, type 2 diabetes; hypertension, peptic ulcer disease; pregnancy; lactation
- **Physical:** Jaw strength, symmetry; orientation, affect; P, auscultation, BP; oral mucous membranes, abdominal examination; thyroid function tests

Interventions
- Review mechanics of chewing gum with patient; patient must chew the gum slowly and intermittently to promote even, slow absorption of nicotine; discard chewed gum in wrapper to prevent access by children or pets.
- Have patient place lozenge in mouth and allow to dissolve in mouth over 20–30 min; do not allow patient to eat or drink for 15 min before use.
- Arrange to withdraw or taper use of gum or lozenges in abstainers at 3 mo; effectiveness after that time has not been established, and patients may be using gum as substitute source for nicotine dependence.

Teaching points
- Chew one piece of gum every time you have the desire to smoke. Chew each piece slowly until it tingles. Then place the gum between the cheek and gums. When the tingle is gone, chew again and repeat the process. Do not chew more than 24 pieces of gum each day. Discard chewed gum in wrapper to prevent access by children or pets.
- Place lozenge in mouth and allow to dissolve over 20–30 minutes; do not eat or drink for 15 minutes before use. Do not use more than 5 lozenges in 6 hours or 20 in 1 day. If you remove a lozenge, wrap it up carefully to prevent access by children or pets.
- Do not consume liquids within 15 minutes before or while chewing gum or using lozenge; they may interfere with nicotine absorption.
- Abstain from smoking.
- Do not offer to nonsmokers; serious reactions can occur if used by nonsmokers.
- You may experience these side effects: Dizziness, headache, light-headedness (use caution driving or performing tasks that require alertness); nausea, vomiting, increased burping; jaw muscle ache (modify chewing technique).
- Report nausea and vomiting, increased salivation, diarrhea, cold sweat, headache, disturbances in hearing or vision, chest pain, palpitations.

nifedipine

(nye fed' i peen)

Adalat CC, Adalat XL (CAN), Afeditab CR ONC, Apo-Nifed (CAN), Apo-Nifed AP (CAN), Nifediac CC, Nifedical XL, Procardia, Procardia XL

PREGNANCY CATEGORY C

Drug classes

Antianginal
Antihypertensive
Calcium channel blocker

Therapeutic actions

Inhibits the movement of calcium ions across the membranes of cardiac and arterial muscle cells; inhibition of transmembrane calcium flow results in the depression of impulse formation in specialized cardiac pacemaker cells, in slowing of the velocity of conduction of the cardiac impulse, in the depression of myocardial contractility, and in the dilation of coronary arteries and arterioles and peripheral arterioles; these effects lead to decreased cardiac work, decreased cardiac energy consumption, and increased delivery of oxygen to myocardial cells.

Indications

- Angina pectoris due to coronary artery spasm (Prinzmetal's variant angina)
- Chronic stable angina (effort-associated angina)
- ER preparation only: Treatment of hypertension
- Orphan drug use: Treatment of interstitial cystitis
- Unlabeled uses: Anal fissures, ureteral stones, topical use to improve wound healing

Contraindications and cautions

- Contraindicated with allergy to nifedipine.
- Use cautiously with lactation, pregnancy, HF, aortic stenosis.

Available forms

ER tablets ONC—30, 60, 90 mg; capsules—10, 20 mg

Dosages

Adults

Initial dose, 10 mg tid PO. Maintenance range, 10–20 mg tid. Higher doses (20–30 mg tid–qid) may be required, depending on patient response. Adjust over 7–14 days. More than 180 mg/day is not recommended.

ER ONC

30–60 mg PO once daily. Adjust over 7–14 days. Usual maximum dose is 90–120 mg/day.

Pharmacokinetics

Route	*Onset*	*Peak*
Oral	20 min	30 min
ER	20 min	2.5–6 hr

Metabolism: Hepatic; $T_{1/2}$: 2–5 hr
Distribution: Crosses placenta; enters breast milk
Excretion: Feces, urine

Adverse effects

- **CNS:** *Dizziness, light-headedness, headache, asthenia, fatigue, nervousness,* sleep disturbances, blurred vision, *weakness, tremor, mood changes*
- **CV:** *Peripheral edema, angina,* hypotension, arrhythmias, *AV block,* asystole
- **Dermatologic:** *Flushing, rash,* dermatitis, pruritus, urticaria
- **GI:** *Nausea, diarrhea, constipation,* cramps, flatulence, hepatic injury
- **Other:** *Nasal congestion, cough,* fever, chills, shortness of breath, muscle cramps, joint stiffness, sexual difficulties

Interactions

✱ **Drug-drug** • Increased effects with cimetidine

✱ **Drug-food** • Risk of increased toxic effects; avoid use with grapefruit juice

■ Nursing considerations

Assessment

- **History:** Allergy to nifedipine, pregnancy, lactation
- **Physical:** Skin lesions, color, edema; orientation, reflexes; P, BP, baseline ECG, peripheral perfusion, auscultation; R, adventitious sounds; liver evaluation, normal GI output; LFTs

N

Interventions

⊗ ***Warning*** Monitor patient carefully (BP, cardiac rhythm, and output) while drug is being adjusted to therapeutic dose; the dosage may be increased more rapidly in hospitalized patients under close supervision. Do not exceed 30 mg/dose increases.

- Ensure that patients do not chew or divide ER tablets.
- Taper dosage of beta blockers before nifedipine therapy.
- Protect drug from light and moisture.

Teaching points

- Do not chew, cut, or crush extended-release tablets. Swallow whole.
- Avoid grapefruit juice while taking this drug; it can cause increased toxicity.
- You may experience these side effects: Nausea, vomiting (eat frequent small meals); dizziness, light-headedness, vertigo (avoid driving and operating dangerous machinery; take special precautions to avoid falling); muscle cramps, joint stiffness, sweating, sexual difficulties (reversible).
- Report irregular heartbeat, shortness of breath, swelling of the hands or feet, pronounced dizziness, constipation.

nilotinib

See Appendix W, *Less commonly used drugs.*

nimodipine

See Appendix W, *Less commonly used drugs.*

nisoldipine

(nye sole' di peen)

Sular DNC

PREGNANCY CATEGORY C

Drug classes

Antihypertensive
Calcium channel blocker

Therapeutic actions

Inhibits the movement of calcium ions across the membranes of cardiac and arterial muscle cells; inhibits transmembrane calcium flow, which results in the depression of impulse formation in specialized cardiac pacemaker cells, slowing of the velocity of conduction of the cardiac impulse, depression of myocardial contractility, and dilation of coronary arteries and arterioles and peripheral arterioles; these effects in turn lead to decreased cardiac work, decreased cardiac energy consumption.

Indications

- Essential hypertension, alone or in combination with other antihypertensives

Contraindications and cautions

- Contraindicated with allergy to nisoldipine, impaired hepatic function, sick sinus syndrome, HF, heart block (second- or third-degree).
- Use cautiously with MI or severe CAD (increased severity of disease has occurred), lactation, pregnancy.

Available forms

ER tablets DNC—8.5, 17, 25.5, 34 mg

Dosages

Adults

Initial dose of 17 mg PO daily; increase in weekly increments of 8.5 mg/wk until BP is controlled. Usual maintenance dose is 17–34 mg PO daily. Maximum dose, 34 mg/day.

Pediatric patients

Safety and efficacy not established.

Geriatric patients or patients with hepatic impairment

Monitor BP very carefully. Reduced starting doses (no more than 8.5 mg) and reduced maintenance doses are recommended.

Pharmacokinetics

Route	*Onset*	*Peak*	*Duration*
Oral	Slow	6–12 hr	24 hr

Metabolism: Hepatic; $T_{1/2}$: 7–12 hr
Distribution: Crosses placenta; may enter breast milk
Excretion: Urine

Adverse effects
- **CNS:** *Dizziness, light-headedness, headache, asthenia, fatigue,* lethargy
- **CV:** *Peripheral edema,* arrhythmias, **MI, increased angina**
- **Dermatologic:** *Flushing, rash*
- **GI:** *Nausea,* abdominal discomfort

Interactions
✱ **Drug-drug** • Possible increased serum levels and toxicity of cyclosporine • Possible increased serum levels and toxicity with cimetidine • Increased risk of toxic cardiac effects with quinidine
✱ **Drug-food** • Decreased metabolism and increased risk of toxic effects if combined with grapefruit juice; avoid this combination • Excessive drug concentration if taken with a high-fat meal; avoid this combination

■ Nursing considerations
Assessment
- **History:** Allergy to nisoldipine, impaired hepatic function, sick sinus syndrome, heart block (second- or third-degree), lactation, HF, CAD, pregnancy
- **Physical:** Skin lesions, color, edema; P, BP; baseline ECG, peripheral perfusion, auscultation, R, adventitious sounds; liver evaluation, GI normal output; LFTs, renal function tests, urinalysis

Interventions
⊗ ***Warning*** Monitor patient carefully (BP, cardiac rhythm and output) while drug is being adjusted to therapeutic dose; dosage may be increased more rapidly in hospitalized patients under close supervision.
- Monitor BP very carefully if patient is on concurrent doses of nitrates or other antihypertensives.
- Monitor cardiac rhythm regularly during stabilization of dosage and periodically during long-term therapy.
- Administer drug without regard to meals. Do not cut, crush, or allow patient to chew tablets.

Teaching points
- Take this drug with meals if upset stomach occurs; do not take with high-fat meals or grapefruit juice. Do not drink grapefruit juice while using this drug.
- Swallow tablet whole; do not chew, cut, or crush.
- You may experience these side effects: Nausea, vomiting (eat frequent small meals); headache (monitor lighting, noise, and temperature; request medication if severe).
- Report irregular heart beat, shortness of breath, swelling of the hands or feet, pronounced dizziness, constipation, chest pain.

▽ nitazoxanide
See Appendix W, *Less commonly used drugs.*

▽ nitrofurantoin
*(nye troe fyoor **an'** toyn)*

nitrofurantoin
Apo-Nitrofurantoin (CAN), Furadantin, Novo-Furantoin (CAN)

nitrofurantoin macrocrystals
Macrobid, Macrodantin

PREGNANCY CATEGORY B

Drug classes
Antibacterial
Urinary tract anti-infective

Therapeutic actions
Bacteriostatic in low concentrations, possibly by interfering with bacterial carbohydrate metabolism; bactericidal in high concentrations, possibly by disrupting bacterial cell wall formation, causing cell death.

Indications
- Treatment of UTIs, including acute cystitis, caused by susceptible strains of *Escherichia coli, Staphylococcus aureus, Klebsiella, Enterobacter, Proteus*
- Prophylaxis or long-term suppression of UTIs

Contraindications and cautions
- Contraindicated with allergy to nitrofurantoin, renal impairment, pregnancy, lactation.

N

- Use cautiously in patients with G6PD deficiency, anemia, diabetes.

Available forms

Capsules—25, 50, 100 mg; dual-release capsules—100 mg; oral suspension—25 mg/5 mL

Dosages

Adults

50–100 mg PO qid for 10–14 days or 100 mg bid for 7 days (*Macrobid*). Do not exceed 400 mg/day.

- *Long-term suppressive therapy:* 50–100 mg PO at bedtime.

Pediatric patients

5–7 mg/kg/day in four divided doses PO. Not recommended in children younger than 1 mo.

- *Long-term suppressive therapy:* As low as 1 mg/kg/day PO in one to two doses.

Pharmacokinetics

Route	*Onset*	*Peak*
Oral	Rapid	30 min

Metabolism: Hepatic; $T_{1/2}$: 20–60 min
Distribution: Crosses placenta; enters breast milk
Excretion: Urine

Adverse effects

- **CNS:** Peripheral neuropathy, headache, dizziness, nystagmus, drowsiness, vertigo
- **Dermatologic:** Exfoliative dermatitis, **Stevens-Johnson syndrome,** alopecia, pruritus, urticaria, angioedema
- **GI:** *Nausea, abdominal cramps, vomiting, diarrhea, anorexia,* parotitis, pancreatitis, **hepatotoxicity**
- **Hematologic:** Hemolytic anemia in G6PD deficiency; granulocytopenia, agranulocytosis, leukopenia, thrombocytopenia, eosinophilia, megaloblastic anemia
- **Respiratory: Pulmonary hypersensitivity**
- **Other:** Superinfections of the GU tract; hypotension; muscular aches; *brown-rust urine*

Interactions

✱ **Drug-drug** • Delayed or decreased absorption with magnesium trisilicate, magaldrate

✱ **Drug-lab test** • False elevations of urine glucose, bilirubin, alkaline phosphatase, BUN, urinary creatinine • False-positive urine glucose when using Benedict's or Fehling's reagent

■ Nursing considerations

Assessment

- **History:** Allergy to nitrofurantoin, renal impairment, G6PD deficiency, anemia, diabetes, pregnancy, lactation
- **Physical:** Skin color, lesions; orientation, reflexes; R, adventitious sounds; liver evaluation; CBC; LFTs, renal function tests; serum electrolytes; blood, urine glucose, urinalysis

Interventions

- Arrange for culture and sensitivity tests before and during therapy.
- Give with food or milk to prevent GI upset.
- Continue drug for at least 3 days after a sterile urine specimen is obtained.
- Monitor clinical response; if no improvement is seen or a relapse occurs, send urine for repeat culture and sensitivity.

⊗ ***Warning*** Monitor pulmonary function carefully; reactions can occur within hours or weeks of nitrofurantoin therapy.

- Arrange for periodic CBC and liver function tests during long-term therapy.

Teaching points

- Take drug with food or milk. Complete the full course of drug therapy to ensure a resolution of the infection. Take this drug at regular intervals around-the-clock; consult your nurse or pharmacist to set up a convenient schedule.
- You may experience these side effects: Nausea, vomiting, abdominal pain (eat frequent small meals); diarrhea; drowsiness, blurring of vision, dizziness (observe caution driving or using dangerous equipment); brown or yellow-rust urine (expected effect).
- Report fever, chills, cough, chest pain, difficulty breathing, rash, numbness or tingling of the fingers or toes.

nitroglycerin
*(nye troe **gli'** ser in)*

Intravenous: generic
Spray: Nitrolingual Pumpspray
Sublingual: Gen-Nitroglycerin (CAN), NitroQuick, Nitrostat
Sustained-release: Nitro-Time DNC
Topical: Nitro-Bid
Transdermal: Minitran, Nitrek, Nitro-Dur, Transderm-Nitro
Translingual: Nitrolingual

PREGNANCY CATEGORY C

Drug classes
Antianginal
Nitrate

Therapeutic actions
Relaxes vascular smooth muscle with a resultant decrease in venous return and decrease in arterial BP, which reduces left ventricular workload and decreases myocardial oxygen consumption.

Indications
- Sublingual, translingual preparations: Acute angina
- Oral SR, sublingual, topical, transdermal, translingual preparations: Prophylaxis of angina
- IV: Angina unresponsive to recommended doses of organic nitrates or beta blockers
- IV: Perioperative hypertension
- IV: HF associated with acute MI
- IV: To produce controlled hypotension during surgery
- Unlabeled uses: Reduction of cardiac workload in acute MI and in HF (sublingual, topical); adjunctive treatment of Raynaud's disease (topical)

Contraindications and cautions
- Contraindicated with allergy to nitrates, severe anemia, early MI, head trauma, cerebral hemorrhage, hypertrophic cardiomyopathy, pregnancy, lactation.
- Use cautiously with hepatic or renal disease, hypotension or hypovolemia, increased intracranial pressure, constrictive pericarditis, pericardial tamponade, low ventricular filling pressure or low PCWP.

Available forms
Injection for solution (requires dilution)—5 mg/mL; injection (premixed)—100, 200, 400 mcg/mL; sublingual tablets—0.3, 0.4, 0.6 mg; ER buccal tablets—2.3 mg; translingual spray—0.4 mg/spray; oral SR capsules—2.5, 6.5, 9 mg; transdermal—0.1, 0.2, 0.3, 0.4, 0.6, 0.8 mg/hr; topical ointment—2%

Dosages
Adults
IV
Initial dose, 5 mcg/min delivered through an infusion pump. Increase by 5-mcg/min increments every 3–5 min as needed. If no response at 20 mcg/min, increase increments to 10–20 mcg/min. Once a partial BP response is obtained, reduce dose and lengthen dosage intervals; continually monitor response and titrate carefully.

Sublingual
- *Acute attack:* Dissolve one tablet under tongue or in buccal pouch at first sign of anginal attack; repeat every 5 min until relief is obtained. Do not take more than three tablets/15 min. If pain continues or increases, patient should call physician or go to hospital.
- *Prophylaxis:* Use 5–10 min before activities that might precipitate an attack.

Buccal
Place tablet between the lip and gum and allow it to dissolve over 3–5 min. Do not chew or swallow the tablet. Initial dose is 1 mg every 5 hr while awake. Maintenance dose is 2 mg tid.

SR (oral) DNC
Initial dose, 2.5–9 mg every 12 hr. Increase to every 8 hr as needed and tolerated. Doses as high as 26 mg given qid have been used.

Topical
Initial dose, one-half inch every 8 hr. Increase by one-half inch to achieve desired results. Usual dose is 1–2 inches every 8 hr; up to 4–5 inches every 4 hr have been used. 1 inch = 15 mg nitroglycerin.

Transdermal
Apply one patch each day. Adjust to higher doses by using patches that deliver more drug or

N

by applying more than one patch. Apply patch to arm; remove at bedtime.

Translingual

Spray preparation delivers 0.4 mg/metered dose. At onset of attack, spray one to two metered doses into oral mucosa; no more than three doses/15 min should be used. If pain persists, seek medical attention. May be used prophylactically 5–10 min before activity that might precipitate an attack.

Pediatric patients

Safety and efficacy not established.

Pharmacokinetics

Route	*Onset*	*Duration*
IV	1–2 min	3–5 min
Sublingual	1–3 min	30–60 min
Translingual spray	2 min	30–60 min
Oral, SR	20–45 min	8–12 hr
Topical ointment	30–60 min	4–8 hr
Transdermal	30–60 min	24 hr

Metabolism: Hepatic; $T_{1/2}$: 1–4 min
Distribution: Crosses placenta; enters breast milk
Excretion: Urine

IV FACTS

Preparation: Dilute in 5% dextrose injection or 0.9% sodium chloride injection. Do not mix with other drugs; check the manufacturer's instructions carefully because products vary considerably in concentration and volume per vial. Use only with glass IV bottles and the administration sets provided. Protect from light and extremes of temperature.
Infusion: Do not give by IV push; regulate rate based on patient response and BP.
Incompatibilities: Do not mix in solution with other drugs.

Adverse effects

- **CNS:** Headache, apprehension, restlessness, weakness, vertigo, dizziness, faintness
- **CV:** Tachycardia, retrosternal discomfort, palpitations, **hypotension,** syncope, collapse, orthostatic hypotension, angina
- **Dermatologic:** Rash, exfoliative dermatitis, cutaneous vasodilation with flushing, pallor, perspiration, cold sweat, contact dermatitis—transdermal preparations, topical allergic reactions—topical nitroglycerin ointment
- **GI:** Nausea, vomiting, incontinence of urine and feces, abdominal pain
- **Local:** Local burning sensation at the point of dissolution (sublingual)
- **Other:** Ethanol intoxication with high-dose IV use (alcohol in diluent)

Interactions

✱ **Drug-drug** • Increased risk of hypertension and decreased antianginal effect with ergot alkaloids • Decreased pharmacologic effects of heparin • Risk of severe hypotension and adverse CV events with sildenafil, tadalafil, vardenafil; avoid this combination

✱ **Drug-lab test** • False report of decreased serum cholesterol if done by the Zlatkis-Zak color reaction

■ Nursing considerations

CLINICAL ALERT!

Name confusion has occurred between *NitroBid* (nitroglycerin) and *Nicotrol* (nicotine); between nitroglycerin and nitroprusside; use caution.

Assessment

- **History:** Allergy to nitrates, severe anemia, early MI, head trauma, cerebral hemorrhage, hypertrophic cardiomyopathy, hepatic or renal disease, xerostania, hypotension or hypovolemia, increased intracranial pressure, constrictive pericarditis, pericardial tamponade, low ventricular filling pressure or low PCWP, pregnancy, lactation
- **Physical:** Skin color, T, lesions; orientation, reflexes, affect; P, BP, orthostatic BP, baseline ECG, peripheral perfusion; R, adventitious sounds; liver evaluation, normal output; LFTs, renal function tests (IV); CBC, Hgb

Interventions

- Give sublingual preparations under the tongue or in the buccal pouch. Encourage patient not to swallow. Ask patient if the tablet "fizzles" or burns. Always check the expiration date on the bottle; store at room temperature, protected from light. Discard unused drug 6 mo after bottle is opened (conventional tablets); stabilized tablets (*Nitrostat*) are less subject to loss of potency.

- Give SR preparations with water; warn the patient not to chew the tablets or capsules; do not crush these preparations.
- Administer topical ointment by applying the ointment over a 6″ × 6″ area in a thin, uniform layer using the applicator. Cover area with plastic wrap held in place by adhesive tape. Rotate sites of application to decrease the chance of inflammation and sensitization; close tube tightly when finished.
- Administer transdermal systems to skin site free of hair and not subject to much movement. Shave areas that have a lot of hair. Do not apply to distal extremities. Change sites slightly to decrease the chance of local irritation and sensitization. Remove transdermal system before attempting defibrillation or cardioversion. Remove old system before applying a new one.
- Administer the translingual spray directly onto the oral mucosa; preparation is not to be inhaled or swallowed.

⊗ ***Warning*** Arrange to withdraw drug gradually; 4–6 wk is the recommended withdrawal period for the transdermal preparations.

Teaching points

- For sublingual tablets, place tablet under your tongue or in your cheek; do not chew or swallow the tablet; the tablet should burn or "fizzle" under the tongue. Take the nitroglycerin before chest pain begins, when you anticipate that your activities or situation may precipitate an attack. Sit or lie down before taking nitroglycerin. You may repeat your dose every 5 minutes for a total of three tablets. If the pain is still not relieved, contact emergency medical services. Do not buy large quantities; this drug does not store well. Keep the drug in a dark, dry place, in a dark-colored glass bottle with a tight lid; do not combine with other drugs.
- For buccal tablets, place tablet between your lip and gum and allow it to dissolve over 3–5 minutes. Do not chew or swallow the tablet.
- Do not chew or crush the timed-release preparations; take on an empty stomach.
- Spread a thin layer of topical ointment on the skin using the applicator. Do not rub or massage the area. Cover with plastic wrap held in place with adhesive tape. Wash your hands after application. Keep the tube tightly closed. Rotate the sites frequently to prevent local irritation.
- To use transdermal systems, you may need to shave an area for application. Apply to a slightly different area each day. Remove the old system before you apply a new one. Use care if changing brands; each system has a different concentration. Remove the old system before applying a new system.
- Spray translingual spray directly onto oral mucous membranes; do not inhale or swallow. Use 5–10 minutes before activities that you anticipate will precipitate an attack.
- You may experience these side effects: Dizziness, light-headedness (may be transient; change positions slowly); headache (lie down in a cool environment and rest; over-the-counter preparations may not help); flushing of the neck or face (transient).
- Report blurred vision, persistent or severe headache, rash, more frequent or more severe angina attacks, fainting.

N

▽nitroprusside sodium

(nye troe ***pruss'*** *ide)*

Nipride (CAN), Nitropress

PREGNANCY CATEGORY C

Drug classes

Antihypertensive
Vasodilator

Therapeutic actions

Acts directly on vascular smooth muscle to cause vasodilation (arterial and venous) and reduce BP. Mechanism involves interference with calcium influx and intracellular activation of calcium. CV reflexes are not inhibited and reflex tachycardia, increased renin release occur.

Indications

- Hypertensive crises for immediate reduction of BP

- Production of controlled hypotension during anesthesia to reduce bleeding in surgical procedures
- Acute HF
- Unlabeled uses: Acute MI, with dopamine; left ventricular failure, with oxygen, morphine, loop diuretic

Contraindications and cautions

- Contraindicated with treatment of compensatory hypertension; to produce controlled hypotension during surgery with known inadequate cerebral circulation; emergency use in moribund patients; acute HF with peripheral vascular disease.
- Use cautiously with hepatic, renal insufficiency (drug decomposes to cyanide, which is metabolized by the liver and kidneys to thiocyanate ion); hypothyroidism (thiocyanate inhibits the uptake and binding of iodine); pregnancy; lactation.

Available forms

Powder for injection—50 mg/vial

Dosages

Administer only by continuous IV infusion with sterile D_5W.

Adults and pediatric patients

In patients not receiving antihypertensive medication, the average dose is 3 mcg/kg/min (range 0.5–10 mcg/kg/min). At this rate, diastolic BP is usually lowered by 30%–40% below pretreatment diastolic levels. Use smaller doses in patients on antihypertensive medication. Do not exceed infusion rate of 10 mcg/kg/min. If this rate of infusion does not reduce BP within 10 min, discontinue administration.

Geriatric patients or patients with renal impairment

Use with caution and in initial low dosage. The elderly may be more sensitive to the hypotensive effects.

Pharmacokinetics

Route	*Onset*	*Duration*
IV	1–2 min	1–10 min

Metabolism: Hepatic; $T_{1/2}$: 2 min

Distribution: Crosses placenta; may enter breast milk

Excretion: Urine

IV FACTS

Preparation: Dissolve contents of 50-mg vial in 2–3 mL of D_5W. Dilute the prepared stock solution in 250–1,000 mL of D_5W, and promptly wrap container in aluminum foil or other opaque material to protect from light; the administration set tubing does not need to be covered. Observe solution for color changes. Freshly prepared solution has a faint brown tint; discard it if highly colored (blue, green, or dark red). If properly protected from light, reconstituted solution is stable for 24 hr. Do not use the infusion fluid for administration of any other drugs. Do not infuse undiluted solution.

Infusion: Infuse slowly to reduce likelihood of adverse effects; use an infusion pump, microdrip regulator, or similar device to allow precise control of flow rate; carefully monitor BP and regulate dose based on response.

Incompatibilities: Do not mix in solution with any other drugs.

Adverse effects

- **CNS:** *Apprehension, headache, restlessness, muscle twitching,* dizziness
- **CV:** *Retrosternal pressure, palpitations, hypotension,* bradycardia, tachycardia, ECG changes
- **Cyanide toxicity:** Increasing tolerance to drug and metabolic acidosis are early signs, followed by dyspnea, headache, vomiting, dizziness, ataxia, loss of consciousness, imperceptible pulse, absent reflexes, widely dilated pupils, pink skin color, distant heart sounds, shallow breathing (seen in overdose)
- **Dermatologic:** *Diaphoresis,* flushing
- **Endocrine:** Hypothyroidism
- **GI:** *Nausea, vomiting, abdominal pain*
- **Hematologic:** Methemoglobinemia, antiplatelet effects
- **Local:** Irritation at injection site

■ Nursing considerations

Assessment

- **History:** Hepatic or renal insufficiency, hypothyroidism, pregnancy, lactation

- **Physical:** Reflexes, affect, orientation, pupil size; BP, P, orthostatic BP, supine BP, perfusion, edema, auscultation; R, adventitious sounds; LFTs, renal and thyroid function tests, blood acid–base balance

Interventions
- Monitor injection site carefully to prevent extravasation.

⊠ ***Black box warning*** Do not let BP drop too rapidly; do not lower systolic BP below 60 mm Hg. Monitor BP closely.

⊗ ***Warning*** Provide amyl nitrate inhalation, materials to make 3% sodium nitrite solution, sodium thiosulfate on standby in case of overdose of nitroprusside and depletion of the patient's body stores of sulfur occur, leading to cyanide toxicity.

⊠ ***Black box warning*** Monitor blood acid-base balance (metabolic acidosis is early sign of cyanide toxicity), serum thiocyanate levels daily during prolonged therapy, especially in patients with renal impairment.

Teaching points
- Anticipate frequent monitoring of blood pressure, blood tests, checks of IV dosage and rate.
- Report pain at injection site, chest pain.

▽ nizatidine
(nigh za' ti deen)

Apo-Nizatidine (CAN), Axid, Axid AR, Axid Pulvules, Gen-Nizatidine (CAN), PMS-Nizatidine (CAN)

PREGNANCY CATEGORY B

Drug class
Histamine-2 (H_2) antagonist

Therapeutic actions
Inhibits the action of histamine at the H_2 receptors of the parietal cells of the stomach, inhibiting basal gastric acid secretion and gastric acid secretion that is stimulated by food, caffeine, insulin, histamine, cholinergic agonists, gastrin, and pentagastrin. Total pepsin output also is reduced.

Indications
- Short-term and maintenance treatment of duodenal ulcer
- Short-term treatment of benign gastric ulcer
- GERD
- OTC: Prevention of heartburn, acid indigestion, and sour stomach brought on by eating
- Unlabeled uses: Prevention of olanzapine-related weight gain; prevention of NSAID-related ulcers

Contraindications and cautions
- Contraindicated with allergy to nizatidine, lactation.
- Use cautiously with impaired renal or hepatic function, pregnancy.

Available forms
Capsules—150, 300 mg; OTC tablets—75 mg; oral solution—15 mg/mL

Dosages
Adults
- *Active duodenal ulcer:* 300 mg PO daily at bedtime. 150 mg PO bid may be used. Most ulcers heal in 4 wk.
- *Maintenance of healed duodenal ulcer:* 150 mg PO daily at bedtime.
- *GERD:* 150 mg PO bid.
- *Benign gastric ulcer:* 150 mg PO bid or 300 mg daily at bedtime.
- *Prevention of heartburn, acid indigestion:* 75 mg PO 30–60 min before food or beverages that cause the problem, taken with water.

Pediatric patients
Safety and efficacy not established.

Geriatric patients or patients with renal impairment
For creatinine clearance 20–50 mL/min, use 150 mg/day PO for active ulcer; 150 mg every other day for maintenance. For creatinine clearance less than 20 mL/min, use 150 mg PO every other day for active ulcer; 150 mg PO every 3 days for maintenance.

Pharmacokinetics

Route	*Onset*	*Peak*
Oral	Varies	0.5–3 hr

Metabolism: Hepatic; $T_{1/2}$: 1–2 hr

Distribution: Crosses placenta; enters breast milk
Excretion: Urine

Adverse effects

- **CNS:** *Dizziness, somnolence, headache, confusion, hallucinations,* peripheral neuropathy; symptoms of brainstem dysfunction (dysarthria, ataxia, diplopia)
- **CV:** Cardiac arrhythmias, **cardiac arrest**
- **GI:** *Diarrhea,* hepatitis, pancreatitis, hepatic fibrosis
- **Hematologic:** Neutropenia, agranulocytosis, increases in plasma creatinine, serum transaminase
- **Other:** *Impotence,* gynecomastia, rash, arthralgia, myalgia

Interactions

✱ **Drug-drug** • Increased serum salicylate levels with aspirin
✱ **Drug-lab test** • False-positive tests for urobilinogen

■ Nursing considerations

Assessment

- **History:** Allergy to nizatidine, impaired renal or hepatic function, pregnancy, lactation
- **Physical:** Skin lesions; orientation, affect; P, baseline ECG; liver evaluation, abdominal examination, normal output; CBC, LFTs, renal function tests

Interventions

- Administer drug at bedtime.
- Decrease doses in renal and hepatic impairment.
- Switch to oral solution if swallowing is difficult.
- Arrange for regular follow-up, including blood tests to evaluate effects.

Teaching points

- Use oral solution if prescribed; may be stored at room temperature.
- Take over-the-counter drug 30–60 minutes before the food or beverage that causes the problem; take with water.
- Take drug at bedtime. Therapy may continue for 4–6 weeks or longer.
- Take antacids exactly as prescribed, being careful of the times of administration. Do not take over-the-counter drugs, and avoid alcohol. Many over-the-counter drugs contain ingredients that might interfere with this drug's effectiveness.
- Tell all health care providers, including dentists, that you are taking this drug. Dosage and timing of all your medications must be coordinated. If anything about the drugs that you are taking changes, consult your health care providers.
- Have regular medical follow-up visits to evaluate drug response.
- Report sore throat, fever, unusual bruising or bleeding, tarry stools, confusion, hallucinations, dizziness, muscle or joint pain.

DANGEROUS DRUG

▽ norepinephrine bitartrate (levarterenol)

*(nor ep i **nef'** rin)*

Levophed

PREGNANCY CATEGORY C

Drug classes

Alpha-adrenergic agonist
$Beta_1$-adrenergic agonist
Cardiac stimulant
Sympathomimetic
Vasopressor

Therapeutic actions

Vasopressor and cardiac stimulant; effects are mediated by $alpha_1$- or $beta_1$-adrenergic receptors in target organs; potent vasoconstrictor (alpha effect) acting in arterial and venous beds; potent positive inotropic agent ($beta_1$ effect), increasing the force of myocardial contraction and increasing coronary blood flow.

Indications

- Restoration of BP in controlling certain acute hypotensive states (pheochromocytomectomy, sympathectomy, poliomyelitis, spinal anesthesia, MI, septicemia, blood transfusion, and drug reactions)

• Adjunct in the treatment of cardiac arrest and profound hypotension

Contraindications and cautions

• Contraindicated with hypovolemia (not a substitute for restoration of fluids, plasma, electrolytes, and should not be used when there are blood volume deficits except as an emergency measure to maintain coronary and cerebral perfusion until blood volume replacement can be effected; if administered continuously to maintain BP when there is hypovolemia, perfusion of vital organs may be severely compromised and tissue hypoxia may result); general anesthesia with halogenated hydrocarbons or cyclopropane; profound hypoxia or hypercarbia; mesenteric or peripheral vascular thrombosis (risk of extending the infarct).
• Use cautiously with pregnancy, lactation.

Available forms

Injection—1 mg/mL (as base)

Dosages

Individualize infusion rate based on response.

Adults

• *Restoration of BP in acute hypotensive states:* Add 4 mL of the solution (1 mg/mL) to 1,000 mL of 5% dextrose solution for a concentration of 4 mcg base/mL. Initially, give 8–12 mcg base per min. Adjust dose gradually to maintain desired BP (usually 80–100 mm Hg systolic). Average maintenance dose is 2–4 mcg base/min. Occasionally enormous daily doses are needed (68 mg base/day). Continue the infusion until adequate BP and tissue perfusion are maintained without therapy. Treatment may be required up to 6 days (vascular collapse due to acute MI). Reduce infusion gradually.
• *Adjunct in cardiac arrest:* Administer IV during cardiac resuscitation to restore and maintain BP after effective heartbeat and ventilation established. Dosages are similar to those used in acute hypotensive states.

Pediatric patients

Safety and efficacy not established.

Pharmacokinetics

Route	*Onset*	*Duration*
IV	Rapid	1–2 min

Metabolism: Neural; $T_{1/2}$: Unknown
Distribution: Crosses placenta
Excretion: Urine

IV FACTS

Preparation: Dilute drug in 5% dextrose solution in distilled water or 5% dextrose in saline solution; these dextrose solutions protect against oxidation. Do not administer in saline solution alone.
Infusion: Infusion rate is determined by response with constant BP monitoring; check manufacturer's insert for detailed guidelines.
Incompatibilities: Do not mix with blood products, aminophylline, amobarbital, lidocaine, pentobarbital, phenobarbital, phenytoin, secobarbital, sodium bicarbonate, thiopental.

Adverse effects

• **CNS:** *Headache*
• **CV:** *Bradycardia,* hypertension

Interactions

✱ **Drug-drug** • Increased hypertensive effects with TCAs (imipramine), reserpine, methyldopa • Decreased vasopressor effects with phenothiazines

■ Nursing considerations

Assessment

• **History:** Hypovolemia, general anesthesia with halogenated hydrocarbons or cyclopropane, profound hypoxia or hypercarbia, mesenteric or peripheral vascular thrombosis, lactation, pregnancy
• **Physical:** Weight; skin color, T, turgor; P, BP; R, adventitious sounds; urine output; serum electrolytes, ECG

Interventions

• Give whole blood or plasma separately, if indicated.
• Administer IV infusions into a large vein, preferably the antecubital fossa, to prevent extravasation.

N

- Do not infuse into femoral vein in elderly patients or those suffering from occlusive vascular disease (atherosclerosis, arteriosclerosis, diabetic endarteritis, Buerger's disease); occlusive vascular disease is more likely to occur in lower extremity.
- Avoid catheter tie-in technique, if possible, because stasis around tubing may lead to high local concentrations of drug.
- Monitor BP every 2 min from the start of infusion until desired BP is achieved, then monitor every 5 min if infusion is continued.
- Monitor infusion site for extravasation.

⊗ ***Black box warning*** Provide phentolamine on standby in case extravasation occurs (5–10 mg phentolamine in 10–15 mL saline should be used to infiltrate the affected area).

⊗ ***Warning*** Do not use drug solutions that are pink or brown; drug solutions should be clear and colorless.

Teaching points

Because norepinephrine is used only in acute emergency situations, patient teaching will depend on patient's awareness and will relate mainly to patient's status and to monitoring being done, rather than specifically to therapy with norepinephrine.

▽norethindrone acetate

(nor eth ***in'*** *drone)*

Aygestin

PREGNANCY CATEGORY X

Drug classes

Hormone
Progestin

Therapeutic actions

Progesterone derivative. Progesterone transforms proliferative endometrium into secretory endometrium; inhibits the secretion of pituitary gonadotropins, which prevents follicular maturation and ovulation; and inhibits spontaneous uterine contraction. Progestins have varying profiles of estrogenic, antiestrogenic, anabolic, and androgenic activity.

Indications

- Treatment of amenorrhea, abnormal uterine bleeding due to hormonal imbalance
- Treatment of endometriosis
- Base: Component of some hormonal contraceptive preparations

Contraindications and cautions

- Contraindicated with allergy to progestins; thrombophlebitis, thromboembolic disorders, cerebral hemorrhage or history of these conditions; hepatic disease; carcinoma of the breast or genital organs; undiagnosed vaginal bleeding; missed abortion; pregnancy; lactation.
- Use cautiously with epilepsy, migraine, asthma, cardiac dysfunction, or renal impairment.

Available forms

Tablets—5 mg

Dosages

Administer orally only.

Adults

- *Amenorrhea; abnormal uterine bleeding:* 2.5–10 mg PO for 5–10 days during second half of theoretical menstrual cycle.
- *Endometriosis:* 5 mg/day PO for 2 wk. Increase in increments of 2.5 mg/day every 2 wk until 15 mg/day is reached. May be maintained for 6–9 mo or until breakthrough bleeding demands temporary termination.

Pharmacokinetics

Route	*Onset*
Oral	Varies

Metabolism: Hepatic; $T_{1/2}$: Unknown
Distribution: Crosses placenta; enters breast milk
Excretion: Feces, urine

Adverse effects

- **CNS:** Sudden, partial, or complete loss of vision; proptosis; diplopia; migraine; precipitation of acute intermittent porphyria;

mental depression; pyrexia; insomnia; somnolence

- **CV:** Thrombophlebitis, cerebrovascular disorders, retinal thrombosis, **pulmonary embolism,** thromboembolic and thrombotic disease, increased BP
- **Dermatologic:** *Rash with or without pruritus, acne,* melasma or chloasma, alopecia, hirsutism, photosensitivity
- **GI:** Cholestatic jaundice, nausea
- **GU:** *Breakthrough bleeding, spotting, change in menstrual flow, amenorrhea,* changes in cervical erosion and cervical secretions, breast tenderness and secretion
- **Other:** Decreased glucose tolerance, *fluid retention, edema, increase in weight*

Interactions

✱ **Drug-lab test** • Inaccurate tests of hepatic and endocrine function

■ Nursing considerations

Assessment

- **History:** Allergy to progestins; thrombophlebitis, thromboembolic disorders, cerebral hemorrhage; hepatic disease; carcinoma of the breast or genital organs; undiagnosed vaginal bleeding; missed abortion; pregnancy; lactation; epilepsy, migraine; asthma; cardiac dysfunction, or renal impairment
- **Physical:** Skin color, lesions, turgor; hair; breasts; pelvic examination; orientation, affect; ophthalmologic examination; P, auscultation, peripheral perfusion, edema; R, adventitious sounds; liver evaluation; LFTs, renal function tests, glucose tolerance, Papanicolaou (Pap) test

Interventions

- Arrange for pretreatment and periodic (at least annual) history and physical, including BP, breasts, abdomen, pelvic organs, and a Pap test.
- Warn patient prior to therapy to prevent pregnancy and to obtain frequent medical follow-up care.

⊗ ***Warning*** Use caution when administering drug to ensure preparation ordered is the one being used; norethindrone acetate is approximately twice as potent as norethindrone.

⊗ ***Warning*** Discontinue medication and consult physician if sudden, partial, or complete loss of vision occurs; if papilledema or retinal vascular lesions are present, discontinue drug.

⊗ ***Warning*** Discontinue medication and consult physician at sign of thromboembolic disease—leg pain, swelling, peripheral perfusion changes, shortness of breath.

Teaching points

- Take drugs in accordance with a marked calendar.
- Avoid pregnancy; serious fetal abnormalities or fetal death could occur.
- You may experience these side effects: Sensitivity to light (avoid exposure to the sun; use sunscreen and protective clothing); dizziness, sleeplessness, depression (use caution driving or performing tasks that require alertness); skin rash, color changes, loss of hair; fever; nausea.
- Report pain or swelling and warmth in the calves, acute chest pain or shortness of breath, sudden severe headache or vomiting, dizziness or fainting, numbness or tingling in the arm or leg.

N

▽ norfloxacin

(nor ***flox'*** *a sin)*

Apo-Norflox (CAN), CO-Norfloxacin (CAN), Noroxin

PREGNANCY CATEGORY C

Drug classes

Antibiotic
Fluoroquinolone
Urinary tract anti-infective

Therapeutic actions

Bactericidal; interferes with DNA replication in susceptible gram-negative bacteria, leading to cell death.

Indications

- For the treatment of adults with UTIs caused by susceptible bacteria, including *Escherichia coli, Proteus mirabilis, Klebsiella pneumoniae, Enterobacter cloacae,*

Proteus vulgaris, Providencia rettgeri, Morganella morganii, Proteus aeruginosa, Citrobacter freundii, Staphylococcus aureus, S. epidermidis, group D streptococci
- Uncomplicated urethral and cervical gonorrhea caused by *Neisseria gonorrhoeae*
- Prostatitis caused by *E. coli*

Contraindications and cautions

- Contraindicated with allergy to norfloxacin, nalidixic acid, or cinoxacin; lactation; history of tendonitis or tendon rupture.
- Use cautiously in patients with renal impairment, seizures, pregnancy.

Available forms

Tablets—400 mg

Dosages

Adults

- *Uncomplicated UTIs:* 400 mg every 12 hr PO for 7–10 days. Maximum dose, 800 mg/day.
- *Uncomplicated cystitis due to* E. coli, K. pneumonia, *or* P. mirabilis: 400 mg every 12 hr PO for 3 days.
- *Complicated UTI:* 400 mg PO every 12 hr for 10–21 days.
- *Uncomplicated gonorrhea:* 800 mg PO as a single dose.
- *Prostatitis:* 400 mg every 12 hr PO for 28 days.

Pediatric patients

Not recommended; produced lesions of joint cartilage in immature experimental animals.

Geriatric patients or patients with impaired renal function

For creatinine clearance of 30 mL/min or less use 400 mg/day, PO for 7–10 days.

Pharmacokinetics

Route	*Onset*	*Peak*
Oral	Varies	2–3 hr

Metabolism: Hepatic; $T_{1/2}$: 3–4.5 hr
Distribution: Crosses placenta; enters breast milk
Excretion: Urine

Adverse effects

- **CNS:** *Headache,* dizziness, insomnia, fatigue, somnolence, depression, blurred vision
- **GI:** *Nausea,* vomiting, dry mouth, diarrhea, abdominal pain, dyspepsia, flatulence, constipation, heartburn
- **Hematologic:** Elevated BUN, AST, ALT, serum creatinine and alkaline phosphatase; decreased WBC count, neutrophil count, Hct
- **Other:** Fever, rash, photosensitivity

Interactions

✱ **Drug-drug** • Decreased therapeutic effect with iron salts, sucralfate • Decreased absorption with antacids • Increased serum levels and toxic effects of theophyllines, cyclosporine • Increased risk of QT prolongation with other drugs that prolong QT interval
✱ **Drug-alternative therapy** • Increased risk of severe photosensitivity reactions if combined with St. John's wort therapy

■ Nursing considerations

Assessment

- **History:** Allergy to norfloxacin, nalidixic acid, or cinoxacin; renal impairment; seizures; pregnancy; lactation
- **Physical:** Skin color, lesions; T; orientation, reflexes, affect; mucous membranes, bowel sounds; LFTs, renal function tests

Interventions

⊠ ***Black box warning*** Risk of tendonitis and tendon rupture is increased, especially in patients older than 60 yr; patients who have undergone kidney, heart, or lung transplant; and those taking corticosteroids.
- Arrange for culture and sensitivity tests before therapy.
- Administer drug 1 hr before or 2 hr after meals or ingestion of milk or dairy products. Give with a glass of water.
- Ensure that patient is well hydrated.
- Administer antacids, multivitamins, and other products containing iron or zinc at least 2 hr after dosing.
- Monitor clinical response; if no improvement is seen or a relapse occurs, send urine for repeat culture and sensitivity.

Teaching points

- Take drug on an empty stomach, 1 hour before or 2 hours after meals, milk, or dairy

products. If an antacid is needed, do not take it within 2 hours of the norfloxacin dose.
- Drink plenty of fluids.
- You may experience these side effects: Nausea, vomiting, abdominal pain (eat frequent small meals); diarrhea or constipation; drowsiness, blurring of vision, dizziness (observe caution driving or using dangerous equipment).
- Report rash, visual changes, severe GI problems, weakness, tremors, tendon pain, severe diarrhea.

▽norgestrel

(nor jess' trel)

PREGNANCY CATEGORY X

Drug classes

Hormonal contraceptive
Hormone
Progestin

Therapeutic actions

Progestational agent; the endogenous female progestin, progesterone, transforms proliferative endometrium into secretory endometrium; inhibits the secretion of pituitary gonadotropins, which prevents follicular maturation and ovulation; and inhibits spontaneous uterine contractions. The primary mechanism by which norgestrel prevents conception is not known, but progestin-only hormonal contraceptives alter the cervical mucus, exert a progestational effect on the endometrium that interferes with implantation, and in some patients, suppress ovulation.

Indications

- Prevention of pregnancy using hormonal contraceptives; somewhat less efficacious (3 pregnancies per 100 woman years) than the combined estrogen/progestin hormonal contraceptives (about 1 pregnancy per 100 woman years, depending on formulation)

Contraindications and cautions

- Contraindicated with allergy to progestins, tartrazine; thrombophlebitis, thromboembolic disorders, cerebral hemorrhage, or history of these conditions; CAD; hepatic disease; carcinoma of the breast or genital organs, undiagnosed vaginal bleeding, missed abortion; as a diagnostic test for pregnancy; pregnancy (fetal abnormalities—masculinization of the female fetus, congenital heart defects, and limb reduction defects); lactation.
- Use cautiously with epilepsy, migraine, asthma, cardiac dysfunction, or renal impairment.

Available forms

Tablets—0.075 mg

Dosages

Adults

Administer daily, starting on the first day of menstruation. Take one tablet, PO, at the same time each day, every day of the year. Missed dose: one tablet—take as soon as remembered, then take the next tablet at regular time; two consecutive tablets—take one of the missed tablets, discard the other, and take daily tablet at usual time; three consecutive tablets—discontinue immediately and use additional form of birth control until menses or pregnancy is ruled out.

Pharmacokinetics

Route	Onset
Oral	Varies

Metabolism: Hepatic; $T_{1/2}$: Unknown
Distribution: Crosses placenta; enters breast milk
Excretion: Urine

Adverse effects

- **CNS:** Neuro-ocular lesions, mental depression, migraine, *changes in corneal curvature,* contact lens intolerance
- **CV:** *Thrombophlebitis, thrombosis,* **pulmonary embolism,** coronary thrombosis, **MI,** cerebral thrombosis, Raynaud's disease, arterial thromboembolism, renal artery thrombosis, **cerebral hemorrhage,** hypertension
- **Dermatologic:** Rash with or without pruritus, acne, melasma
- **GI:** Gallbladder disease, liver tumors, hepatic lesions, *nausea, vomiting,* abdominal cramps, bloating, cholestatic jaundice

N

- **GU:** *Breakthrough bleeding, spotting, change in menstrual flow, amenorrhea,* changes in cervical erosion and cervical secretions, endocervical hyperplasia, vaginal candidiasis
- **Other:** *Breast tenderness and secretion, enlargement;* fluid retention, edema, increase or decrease in weight

Interactions

✱ **Drug-drug** • Decreased effectiveness of hormonal contraceptives with barbiturates, hydantoins, carbamazepine, rifampin, griseofulvin, penicillins, tetracyclines; use alternate form of birth control if these drugs are needed
✱ **Drug-alternative therapy** • Decreased effectiveness if taken with St. John's wort

■ Nursing considerations

Assessment

- **History:** Allergy to progestins, tartrazine; thrombophlebitis, thromboembolic disorders, cerebral hemorrhage; CAD; hepatic disease; carcinoma of the breast or genital organs, undiagnosed vaginal bleeding, missed abortion; epilepsy, migraine, asthma, cardiac dysfunction, or renal impairment; pregnancy; lactation
- **Physical:** Skin color, lesions, turgor; hair; breasts; pelvic examination; orientation, affect; ophthalmologic examination; P, auscultation, peripheral perfusion, edema; R, adventitious sounds; liver evaluation; LFTs, renal function tests, glucose tolerance, Papanicolaou (Pap) test, pregnancy test

Interventions

- Arrange for pretreatment and periodic (at least annual) history and physical, including BP, breasts, abdomen, pelvic organs, and a Pap test.
- Start no earlier than 4 wk postpartum for postpartum use.

⊗ ***Warning*** Discontinue medication and consult physician if sudden, partial, or complete loss of vision occurs; if papilledema or retinal vascular lesions are present on examination, discontinue.

⊗ ***Warning*** Discontinue drug and consult physician at any sign of thromboembolic disease—leg pain, swelling, peripheral perfusion changes, shortness of breath.

Teaching points

- Take exactly as prescribed at intervals not exceeding 24 hours. Take at bedtime or with a meal to establish a routine; medication must be taken daily for prevention of pregnancy; if you miss one tablet, take as soon as remembered, then take the next tablet at regular time. If you miss two consecutive tablets, take one of the missed tablets, discard the other, and take daily tablet at usual time. If you miss three consecutive tablets, discontinue immediately, and use another method of birth control until your cycle starts again. It is a good idea to use an additional method of birth control if any tablets are missed.
- Discontinue drug and consult your health care provider if you decide to become pregnant. It may be suggested that you use a nonhormonal form of birth control for a few months before becoming pregnant.
- Do not take this drug during pregnancy; serious fetal abnormalities have been reported. If you think that you are pregnant, consult your health care provider immediately.
- Tell all health care providers, including dentists, that you take this drug. If other medications are prescribed, they may decrease the effectiveness of hormonal contraceptives and an additional method of birth control may be needed.
- You may experience these side effects: Sensitivity to light (avoid exposure to the sun; use sunscreen and protective clothing); dizziness, sleeplessness, depression (use caution driving or performing tasks that require alertness); rash, skin color changes, loss of hair; fever; nausea; breakthrough bleeding or spotting (transient); intolerance to contact lenses due to corneal changes.
- Report pain or swelling and warmth in the calves, acute chest pain or shortness of breath, sudden severe headache or vomiting, dizziness or fainting, visual disturbances, numbness or tingling in the arm or leg, breakthrough bleeding or spotting that lasts into the second month of therapy.

nortriptyline hydrochloride

*(nor **trip'** ti leen)*

Apo-Nortriptyline (CAN), Aventyl, Gen-Nortriptyline (CAN), Pamelor, ratio-Nortriptyline (CAN)

PREGNANCY CATEGORY D

Drug class

TCA (secondary amine)

Therapeutic actions

Mechanism of action unknown; the TCAs are structurally related to the phenothiazine antipsychotic drugs (eg, chlorpromazine), but inhibit the presynaptic reuptake of the neurotransmitters norepinephrine and serotonin; anticholinergic at CNS and peripheral receptors; sedating; the relationship of these effects to clinical efficacy is unknown.

Indications

- Relief of symptoms of depression (endogenous depression most responsive)
- Unlabeled uses: Treatment of panic disorders (25–75 mg/day), premenstrual depression (50–125 mg/day), dermatologic disorders (75 mg/day), chronic pain, headache prophylaxis

Contraindications and cautions

- Contraindicated with hypersensitivity to any tricyclic drug, concomitant therapy with an MAOI, recent MI, myelography within previous 24 hr or scheduled within 48 hr, pregnancy (limb reduction abnormalities), lactation.
- Use cautiously with EST (increased hazard with TCAs); preexisting CV disorders (possibly increased risk of serious CVS toxicity); angle-closure glaucoma, increased IOP; urinary retention, ureteral or urethral spasm (anticholinergic effects may exacerbate these conditions); seizure disorders; hyperthyroidism (predisposes to CVS toxicity, including cardiac arrhythmias); impaired hepatic, renal function; psychiatric patients (schizophrenic or paranoid patients may exhibit a worsening of psychosis); bipolar disorder (may shift to hypomanic or manic phase); elective surgery (discontinued as long as possible before surgery).

Available forms

Capsules—10, 25, 50, 75 mg; solution—10 mg/5 mL

Dosages

Adults

25 mg tid–qid PO. Begin with low dosage and gradually increase as required and tolerated. Doses of more than 150 mg/day are not recommended.

Pediatric patients 12 yr and older

30–50 mg/day PO in divided doses.

Pediatric patients younger than 12 yr

Not recommended.

Geriatric patients

30–50 mg/day PO in divided doses.

Pharmacokinetics

Route	*Onset*	*Peak*	*Duration*
Oral	Varies	2–4 hr	2–4 wk

Metabolism: Hepatic; $T_{1/2}$: 18–28 hr
Distribution: Crosses placenta; enters breast milk
Excretion: Urine

Adverse effects

- **CNS:** *Sedation and anticholinergic (atropine-like) effects* (dry mouth, blurred vision, disturbance of accommodation for near vision, mydriasis, increased IOP), *confusion* (especially in elderly), *disturbed concentration,* hallucinations, disorientation, decreased memory, feelings of unreality, delusions, anxiety, nervousness, restlessness, agitation, panic, insomnia, nightmares, hypomania, mania, exacerbation of psychosis, drowsiness, weakness, fatigue, headache, numbness, tingling, paresthesias of extremities, incoordination, motor hyperactivity, akathisia, ataxia, tremors, peripheral neuropathy, extrapyramidal symptoms, **seizures,** speech blockage, dysarthria
- **CV:** *Orthostatic hypotension,* hypertension, syncope, tachycardia, palpitations, MI, arrhythmias, heart block, precipitation of heart failure, CVA

- **Endocrine:** Elevated or depressed blood sugar; elevated prolactin levels; inappropriate ADH secretion
- **GI:** *Dry mouth, constipation,* paralytic ileus, *nausea,* vomiting, anorexia, epigastric distress, diarrhea, flatulence, dysphagia, peculiar taste, increased salivation, stomatitis, glossitis, parotid swelling, abdominal cramps, black tongue, hepatitis; elevated transaminase, altered alkaline phosphatase
- **GU:** Urinary retention, delayed micturition, dilation of the urinary tract, gynecomastia, testicular swelling; breast enlargement, menstrual irregularity and galactorrhea; increased or decreased libido; impotence
- **Hematologic:** Bone marrow depression, including agranulocytosis; eosinophilia; purpura; thrombocytopenia; leukopenia
- **Hypersensitivity:** Rash, pruritus, vasculitis, petechiae, photosensitization, edema (generalized, facial, tongue), drug fever
- **Withdrawal:** Symptoms with abrupt discontinuation of prolonged therapy: Nausea, headache, vertigo, nightmares, malaise
- **Other:** Nasal congestion, excessive appetite, weight gain or loss; sweating, alopecia, lacrimation, hyperthermia, flushing, chills

Interactions

✱ **Drug-drug** • Increased TCA levels and pharmacologic (especially anticholinergic) effects with cimetidine, fluoxetine • Altered response, including arrhythmias and hypertension with sympathomimetics • Risk of severe hypertension with clonidine • Hyperpyretic crises, severe seizures, hypertensive episodes, and deaths when MAOIs are given with TCAs *Note:* MAOIs and TCAs have been used successfully in some patients resistant to therapy with single agents; however, case reports indicate that the combination can cause serious and potentially fatal adverse effects.

■ Nursing considerations

Assessment

- **History:** Hypersensitivity to any tricyclic drug; concomitant therapy with an MAOI; recent MI; myelography within previous 24 hr or scheduled within 48 hr; pregnancy; lactation; EST; preexisting CV disorders; angle-closure glaucoma, increased IOP; urinary retention, ureteral or urethral spasm; seizure disorders; hyperthyroidism; impaired hepatic, renal function; psychiatric disorders; bipolar disorder; elective surgery
- **Physical:** Weight; T; skin color, lesions; orientation, affect, reflexes, vision and hearing; P, BP, orthostatic BP, perfusion; bowel sounds, normal output, liver evaluation; urine flow, normal output; usual sexual function, frequency of menses, breast and scrotal examination; LFTs, urinalysis, CBC, ECG

Interventions

⊗ ***Black box warning*** Limit access to drug by depressed and potentially suicidal patients; risk of suicidality in children and adolescents and young adults. Monitor accordingly.

- When doses larger than 100 mg/day are given, plasma levels of nortriptyline should be monitored and maintained in the range of 50–150 ng/mL.
- Give major portion of dose at bedtime if drowsiness or severe anticholinergic effects occur.
- Reduce dosage if minor side effects develop; discontinue if serious side effects occur.
- Arrange for CBC if patient develops fever, sore throat, or other sign of infection.

Teaching points

- Take drug exactly as prescribed; do not stop taking this drug abruptly or without consulting your health care provider.
- Avoid alcohol, other sleep-inducing, or over-the-counter drugs.
- Avoid prolonged exposure to sunlight or sunlamps; use a sunscreen or protective garments if possible.
- You may experience these side effects: Headache, dizziness, drowsiness, weakness, blurred vision (reversible; use safety measures if severe; avoid driving or performing tasks that require alertness); nausea, vomiting, loss of appetite, dry mouth (eat frequent small meals, perform frequent mouth care, suck sugarless candy); nightmares, inability to concentrate, confusion; changes in sexual function.
- Report dry mouth, difficulty in urination, excessive sedation, thoughts of suicide.

nystatin

(nye stat' in)

Oral, oral troche: Candistatin (CAN), Mycostatin, Nilstat, ratio-Nystatin (CAN)

Vaginal preparations: Mycostatin

Topical application: Mycostatin, Nilstat

PREGNANCY CATEGORY C

Drug class

Antifungal

Therapeutic actions

Fungicidal and fungistatic: Binds to sterols in the cell membrane of the fungus with a resultant change in membrane permeability, allowing leakage of intracellular components and causing cell death.

Indications

- Oral: Treatment of oropharyngeal candidiasis
- Troche: Treatment of oral candidiasis
- Vaginal: Local treatment of vaginal candidiasis (moniliasis)
- Topical applications: Treatment of cutaneous or mucocutaneous mycotic infections caused by *Candida albicans* and other *Candida* species

Contraindications and cautions

- Contraindicated with allergy to nystatin or components used in preparation.
- Use cautiously with pregnancy, lactation.

Available forms

Tablets—500,000 units; suspension—100,000 units/mL; vaginal tablets—100,000 units; troche—200,000 units; topical cream, ointment, powder—100,000 units/g

Dosages

Adults

Vaginal preparations

1 tablet (100,000 units) or 1 applicator of cream (100,000 units) daily–bid for 2 wk.

Topical

- *Vaginal preparations:* Apply to affected area two to three times daily until healing is complete.
- *Topical foot powder:* For fungal infections of the feet, dust powder on feet and in shoes and socks.

Adults and pediatric patients except infants

Oral

- *Tablets:* 500,000–1,000,000 units tid. Continue for at least 48 hr after clinical cure.
- *Troche:* Dissolve 1–2 tablets in mouth four to five times/day for up to 14 days.
- *Suspension:* 400,000–600,000 units four times/day for 14 days and for at least 48 hr after symptoms subside.

Pharmacokinetics

No general systemic absorption

Excretion: Feces, unchanged (oral use)

Adverse effects

Oral

- **GI:** *Nausea, vomiting, diarrhea, GI distress*

Vaginal

- **Local:** *Irritation, vulvovaginal burning*

Topical

- **Local:** *Local irritation*

■ Nursing considerations

Assessment

- **History:** Allergy to nystatin or components used in preparation, pregnancy, lactation
- **Physical:** Skin color, lesions, area around lesions; bowel sounds; culture of area involved

Interventions

- Culture fungus before therapy.
- Have patient retain oral suspension in mouth as long as possible before swallowing. Paint suspension on each side of the mouth. Continue local treatment for at least 48 hr after clinical improvement is noted.
- Prepare nystatin in the form of frozen flavored popsicles to improve oral retention of the drug for local application.
- Administer nystatin troche orally for the treatment of oral candidiasis; have patient dissolve 1–2 tablets in mouth.

- Insert vaginal suppositories high into the vagina. Have patient remain recumbent for 10–15 min after insertion. Provide sanitary napkin to protect clothing from stains.
- Clean affected area before topical application, unless otherwise indicated.
- Monitor response to drug therapy. If no response is noted, arrange for further cultures to determine causative organism.
- Ensure that patient receives the full course of therapy to eradicate the fungus and to prevent recurrence.
- Discontinue topical or vaginal administration if rash or sensitivity occurs.

Teaching points

- Take the full course of drug therapy even if symptoms improve. Continue during menstrual period if vaginal route is being used. Long-term use of the drug may be needed; beneficial effects may not be seen for several weeks. Vaginal suppositories should be inserted high into the vagina.
- Use appropriate hygiene measures to prevent reinfection or spread of infection.
- This drug is for the fungus being treated; do not self-medicate other problems.
- Refrain from sexual intercourse or advise partner to use a condom to avoid reinfection; use a sanitary napkin to prevent staining of clothing with vaginal use.
- You may experience these side effects: Nausea, vomiting, diarrhea (oral use); irritation, burning, stinging (local use).
- Report worsening of condition; local irritation, burning (topical application); rash, irritation, pelvic pain (vaginal use); nausea, GI distress (oral administration).

octreotide acetate

(ok tree' oh tide)

Sandostatin, Sandostatin LAR Depot

PREGNANCY CATEGORY B

Drug classes

Antidiarrheal
Hormone

Therapeutic actions

Mimics the natural hormone somatostatin; suppresses secretion of serotonin, gastrin, vasoactive intestinal peptide, insulin, glucagon, secretin, motilin, and pancreatic polypeptide; also suppresses growth hormone and decreases splanchnic blood flow.

Indications

- Symptomatic treatment of patients with metastatic carcinoid tumors to suppress or inhibit the associated severe diarrhea and flushing episodes
- Treatment of the profuse watery diarrhea associated with vasoactive intestinal polypeptide tumors (VIPomas)
- Reduction of growth hormone blood levels in patients with acromegaly not responsive to other treatment
- Unlabeled uses: GI fistula, variceal bleeding, diarrheal states, pancreatic fistulas, IBS, dumping syndrome

Contraindications and cautions

- Contraindicated with hypersensitivity to octreotide or any of its components.
- Use cautiously with renal impairment, thyroid disease, diabetes mellitus, pregnancy, lactation.

Available forms

Injection—0.05, 0.1, 0.2, 0.5, 1 mg/mL; depot injection—10, 20, 30 mg/5 mL

Dosages

Adults

Subcutaneous injection is the route of choice. Initial dose is 50 mcg subcutaneously two to three times daily; the number of injections is increased based on response, usually bid–tid. IV bolus injections have been used in emergency situations—not recommended. Depot injection: Do not administer IV or subcutaneously; inject intragluteally at 4-wk intervals. Patients should be stabilized on subcutaneous octreotide for at least 2 wk before switching to long-acting depot.

- *Carcinoid tumors:* First 2 wk of therapy: 100–600 mcg/day subcutaneously in two to four divided doses (mean daily dosage, 300 mcg).

- *VIPomas:* 200–300 mcg subcutaneously in two to four divided doses during initial 2 wk of therapy to control symptoms. Range, 150–750 mcg subcutaneously; doses above 450 mcg are usually not required. Depot injection: 20 mg IM every 4 wk.
- *Acromegaly:* 50 mcg tid subcutaneously, adjusted up to 100–500 mcg tid. Withdraw for 4 wk once yearly. Depot injection: 20 mg IM intragluteally once every 4 wk; after 2–3 mo, reevaluate patient to adjust dosage as needed.

Pediatric patients

Safety and efficacy for depot injection not established.

- *GI tumors:* 1–10 mcg/kg/day subcutaneously.

Geriatric patients or patients with renal impairment

Half-life may be prolonged; adjust dosage.

Pharmacokinetics

Route	*Onset*	*Peak*
Subcut.	Rapid	15 min

Metabolism: Hepatic; $T_{1/2}$: 1.5 hr
Distribution: May cross placenta; may enter breast milk
Excretion: Urine

Adverse effects

- **CNS:** Anxiety, *headache, dizziness, lightheadedness,* fatigue, seizures, depression, drowsiness, vertigo, hyperesthesia, irritability, forgetfulness, malaise, nervousness, visual disturbances
- **CV:** Shortness of breath, hypertension, thrombophlebitis, ischemia, heart failure, palpitations, *bradycardia*
- **Dermatologic:** *Flushing,* edema, hair loss, thinning of skin, skin flaking, bruising, pruritus, rash
- **Endocrine:** *Hyperglycemia, hypoglycemia,* galactorrhea, clinical hypothyroidism
- **GI:** *Nausea, vomiting, diarrhea, abdominal pain, loose stools,* fat malabsorption, constipation, flatulence, hepatitis, rectal spasm, GI bleeding, heartburn, cholelithiasis, dry mouth, burning mouth
- **Local:** *Injection site pain*
- **Musculoskeletal:** Asthenia, weakness, leg cramps, muscle pain, joint pain, backache
- **Respiratory:** Rhinorrhea

■ Nursing considerations

Assessment

- **History:** Hypersensitivity to octreotide or any of its components; renal impairment; thyroid disease, diabetes mellitus; lactation
- **Physical:** Skin lesions, hair; reflexes, affect; BP, P, orthostatic BP; abdominal examination, liver evaluation, mucous membranes; renal and thyroid function tests, blood glucose, electrolytes

Interventions

- Administer by subcutaneous injection; avoid multiple injections in the same site within short periods.
- Administer depot injection by deep IM intragluteal injection; avoid deltoid injections. Administer LAR depot immediately after mixing.

⊗ ***Warning*** Monitor patients with renal function impairment closely; reduced dosage may be necessary.

- Store ampules in the refrigerator; may be at room temperature on day of use. Do not use if particulates or discoloration are observed.
- Monitor patient closely for endocrine reactions—blood glucose alterations, thyroid hormone changes, growth hormone level.
- Arrange for baseline and periodic gallbladder ultrasound to detect cholelithiasis.
- Monitor blood glucose, especially at start of therapy, to detect hypoglycemia or hyperglycemia. Patients with diabetes will require close monitoring.
- Arrange to withdraw the drug for 4 wk (8 wk for depot injection) once yearly when treating acromegaly.

Teaching points

- This drug must be injected. You and a significant other can be instructed in the procedure of subcutaneous injections. Review technique and process periodically. Do not use the same site for repeated injections; rotate injection sites. Dispose of needles and syringes properly. Dosage will be adjusted based on your response. Depot injection must be given IM once every 4 weeks.

- Arrange for periodic medical examinations, including blood tests and gallbladder tests.
- You may experience these side effects: Headache, dizziness, light-headedness, fatigue (avoid driving or performing tasks that require alertness); nausea, diarrhea, abdominal pain (eat frequent small meals; maintain nutrition); flushing, dry skin, flaking of skin (skin care may prevent breakdown); pain at the injection site.
- Report sweating, dizziness, severe abdominal pain, fatigue, fever, chills, infection, or severe pain at injection sites.

ofatumumab

See Appendix W, *Less commonly used drugs.*

ofloxacin

*(oh **flox'** a sin)*

Floxin, Floxin Otic, Ocuflox

PREGNANCY CATEGORY C

Drug classes

Antibiotic
Fluoroquinolone

Therapeutic actions

Bactericidal; interferes with DNA replication in susceptible gram-positive and gram-negative bacteria, preventing cell reproduction.

Indications

- Lower respiratory tract infections caused by *Haemophilus influenzae, Streptococcus pneumoniae*
- Acute, uncomplicated urethral and cervical gonorrhea due to *Neisseria gonorrhoeae*, nongonococcal urethritis, and cervicitis due to *Chlamydia trachomatis*, mixed infections due to both
- Uncomplicated skin and soft tissue infections due to *Staphylococcus aureus, Streptococcus pyogenes, Proteus mirabilis*
- Uncomplicated UTIs caused by *Citrobacter diversus, Enterobacter aerogenes, Escherichia coli, Klebsiella pneumoniae, Pseudomonas aeruginosa,* and *P. mirabilis* caused by *C. trachomatis* and *N. gonorrhoeae*
- Complicated UTIs caused by *C. diversus, E. coli, K. pneumoniae, P. aeruginosa, P. mirabilis*
- Oral: Primary treatment of PID; complicated UTIs due to susceptible bacteria, including *E. coli, K. pneumoniae, P. mirabilis, C. diversus,* or *P. aeruginosa*
- Prostatitis due to *E. coli*
- Ophthalmic solution: Treatment of ocular infections caused by susceptible organisms
- Orphan drug use: Treatment of bacterial corneal ulcers
- Otic: Otitis externa (patients 6 mo and older), chronic suppurative otitis media (patients 12 yr and older), acute otitis media (patients 1 yr and older); once daily treatment of swimmer's ear (otitis externa) caused by *E. coli, P. aeruginosa, S. aureus* (adults and children 6 mo and older)

Contraindications and cautions

- Contraindicated with allergy to fluoroquinolones, lactation.
- Use cautiously with renal impairment, seizures, pregnancy.

Available forms

Ophthalmic solution—3 mg/mL (0.3%); tablets—200, 300, 400 mg; otic solution—0.3%

Dosages

Adults

- *Uncomplicated UTIs:* 200 mg every 12 hr PO for 3–7 days.
- *Complicated UTIs:* 200 mg bid PO for 10 days.
- *Lower respiratory tract infections:* 400 mg every 12 hr PO for 10 days.
- *Mild to moderate skin infections:* 400 mg every 12 hr PO for 10 days.
- *Prostatitis:* 300 mg every 12 hr PO for 6 wk.
- *Acute, uncomplicated gonorrhea:* 400 mg PO as a single dose.
- *Cervicitis, urethritis:* 300 mg every 12 hr PO for 7 days.
- *Ocular infections:* 1–2 drops per eye as indicated.
- *Otic infections:* 10 drops in affected ear tid for 10–14 days.

- *Swimmer's ear:* 10 drops (1.5 mg) in affected ear, once daily for 7 days.
- *Chronic suppurative otitis media:* 10 drops in affected ear bid for 14 days.

Pediatric patients younger than 18 yr

Systemic

Not recommended; produced lesions of joint cartilage in immature experimental animals.

Otic

1 yr–younger than 12 yr:

- *Swimmer's ear, acute otitis media with tympanostomy tubes:* 5 drops in affected ear bid for 10 days.

12 yr and older:

- *Swimmer's ear:* 10 drops in affected ear bid for 10 days.
- *Chronic otitis media:* 10 drops in affected ear bid for 14 days.

6 mo–13 yr:

- *Swimmer's ear:* 5 drops (0.75 mg) in affected ear once daily for 7 days.

Geriatric patients or patients with impaired renal function

For creatinine clearance 20–50 mL/min, use a 24-hr interval; for creatinine clearance less than 20 mL/min, use a 24-hr interval and half the recommended dose.

Pharmacokinetics

Route	*Onset*	*Peak*	*Duration*
Oral	Varies	1–2 hr	9 hr

Metabolism: Hepatic; $T_{1/2}$: 5–10 hr
Distribution: Crosses placenta; enters breast milk
Excretion: Bile, urine

Adverse effects

- **CNS:** *Headache,* dizziness, *insomnia,* fatigue, somnolence, depression, blurred vision
- **GI:** *Nausea,* vomiting, dry mouth, *diarrhea,* abdominal pain
- **Hematologic:** Elevated BUN, AST, ALT, serum creatinine and alkaline phosphatase; decreased WBC count, neutrophil count, Hct
- **Other:** Fever, rash, *photosensitivity;* ocular burning

Interactions

✱ **Drug-drug** • Decreased therapeutic effect with iron salts, zinc, sucralfate • Decreased absorption with antacids

✱ **Drug-alternative therapy** • Increased risk of severe photosensitivity reactions if combined with St. John's wort

■ Nursing considerations

Assessment

- **History:** Allergy to fluoroquinolones, renal impairment, seizures, lactation, pregnancy
- **Physical:** Skin color, lesions; T; orientation, reflexes, affect; mucous membranes, bowel sounds; LFTs, renal function tests

Interventions

⊗ ***Black box warning*** Fluoroquinolones are associated with increased risk of tendinitis and tendon rupture; risk is higher in patients older than 60 yr, women, and patients with kidney, heart, or lung transplants.

- Arrange for culture and sensitivity tests before beginning therapy.
- Continue therapy for 2 days after the signs of infection have disappeared.
- Administer oral drug 1 hr before or 2 hr after meals with a glass of water.
- Ensure that patient is well hydrated.
- Administer antacids at least 2 hr before or after dosing.
- Monitor clinical response; if no improvement is seen or a relapse occurs, repeat culture and sensitivity tests.

Teaching points

- Take oral drug on an empty stomach, 1 hour before or 2 hours after meals. If an antacid is needed, do not take it within 2 hours of ofloxacin dose.
- Use eye or ear drops as instructed; keep tip away from surfaces; wash hands before administering.
- Drink plenty of fluids.
- Avoid prolonged exposure to sunlight.
- You may experience these side effects: Nausea, vomiting, abdominal pain (eat frequent small meals); diarrhea or constipation; drowsiness, blurring of vision, dizziness (use caution if driving or using dangerous equipment).

- Report rash, visual changes, severe GI problems, weakness, tremors, tendon pain.

olanzapine

*(oh **lan'** za peen)*

Zyprexa, Zyprexa IntraMuscular, Zyprexa Zydis

PREGNANCY CATEGORY C

Drug classes

Antipsychotic
Dopaminergic blocker

Therapeutic actions

Mechanism of action not fully understood; blocks dopamine receptors in the brain, depresses the RAS; blocks serotonin receptor sites; anticholinergic, antihistaminic (H_1), and alpha-adrenergic blocking activity may contribute to some of its therapeutic (and adverse) actions; produces fewer extrapyramidal effects than most antipsychotics.

Indications

- Treatment of schizophrenia
- Treatment of acute mixed or manic episodes associated with bipolar 1 disorder and maintenance of bipolar 1 disorder as monotherapy, or combined with lithium or valproate
- Treatment of agitation associated with schizophrenia and bipolar 1 mania (injection)

Contraindications and cautions

- Contraindicated with allergy to olanzapine, myeloproliferative disorders, severe CNS depression, comatose states, lactation.
- Use cautiously in elderly or debilitated patients or with CV or cerebrovascular disease, dehydration, seizure disorders, Alzheimer's disease, prostate enlargement, narrow-angle glaucoma, history of paralytic ileus or breast cancer, pregnancy, phenylketonuria (if using orally disintegrating tablets, contain phenylalanine).

Available forms

Tablets—2.5, 5, 7.5, 10, 15, 20 mg; orally disintegrating tablets—5, 10, 15, 20 mg; powder for injection—10 mg

Dosages

Adults

- *Schizophrenia:* Initially, 5–10 mg PO daily, increase to 10 mg PO daily within several days; may be increased by 5 mg/day at 1-wk intervals to achieve desired effect. Do not exceed 20 mg/day.
- *Bipolar mania:* 10–15 mg/day PO; adjust at 5-mg intervals as needed, not less than every 24 hr. Maximum dose, 20 mg/day. For maintenance, 5–20 mg/day PO. The initial dose is 10 mg of olanzapine when combined with lithium or valproate.
- *Agitation:* 10 mg IM; range 5–10 mg IM; dose may be repeated in 2 hr if needed; safety of giving more than 30 mg/24 hr not established.

Pediatric patients

Safety and efficacy not established in patients younger than 18 yr.

Geriatric patients

5 mg IM.

Debilitated patients

Start with initial dose of 5 mg; 2.5 mg IM.

Pharmacokinetics

Route	*Onset*	*Peak*	*Duration*
Oral	Varies	6 hr	Weeks
IM	Rapid	15–45 min	Weeks

Metabolism: Hepatic; $T_{1/2}$: 30 hr
Distribution: Crosses placenta; enters breast milk
Excretion: Feces, urine

Adverse effects

- **CNS:** *Somnolence, dizziness,* nervousness, headache, akathisia, personality disorders, tardive dyskinesia, **neuroleptic malignant syndrome**
- **CV:** *Orthostatic hypotension,* peripheral edema, tachycardia
- **GI:** *Constipation,* abdominal pain
- **Respiratory:** Cough, pharyngitis
- **Other:** *Fever,* weight gain, joint pain, development of diabetes mellitus, increased lipid levels

Interactions

✱ **Drug-drug** • Increased risk of orthostatic hypotension with antihypertensives, alcohol, benzodiazepines; avoid use of alcohol and use caution with antihypertensives • Increased risk of seizures with anticholinergics, CNS drugs • May decrease effectiveness of levodopa, dopamine agonists • Decreased effectiveness with rifampin, omeprazole, carbamazepine, smoking • Increased risk of toxicity with fluvoxamine

■ Nursing considerations

CLINICAL ALERT!

Name confusion has occurred between *Zyprexa* (olanzapine) and *Zyrtec* (cetirizine); use caution.

Assessment

- **History:** Allergy to olanzapine, myeloproliferative disorders, severe CNS depression, comatose states, history of seizure disorders, lactation, CV or cerebrovascular disease, dehydration, Alzheimer's disease, prostate enlargement, narrow-angle glaucoma, history of paralytic ileus or breast cancer, elderly or debilitated, pregnancy
- **Physical:** T, weight; reflexes, orientation, IOP, ophthalmologic examination; P, BP, orthostatic BP, ECG; R, adventitious sounds; bowel sounds, normal output, liver evaluation; prostate palpation, normal urine output; CBC, urinalysis, LFTs, renal function tests

Interventions

- Do not dispense more than 1-wk supply at a time.
- Peel back foil on blister pack of disintegrating tablets; do not push through foil; use dry hands to remove tablet and place in mouth.
- Prepare solution for IM injection using 2.1 mL sterile water for injection. Resulting solution contains 5 mg/mL. Solution should be clear yellow. Use within 1 hr of reconstitution. Discard any unused portion.
- Monitor for the many possible drug interactions before beginning therapy.

⊗ ***Black box warning*** Risk of death is increased when drug is used to treat elderly patients with dementia-related psychosis; drug is not approved for this use.

- Encourage patient to void before taking the drug to help decrease anticholinergic effects of urinary retention.
- Monitor for elevations of temperature and differentiate between infection and neuroleptic malignant syndrome.
- Monitor for orthostatic hypotension and provide appropriate safety measures as needed.
- Monitor patient regularly for signs and symptoms of diabetes mellitus; monitor lipid and triglyceride levels.

Teaching points

- Take this drug exactly as prescribed; do not change dose without consulting your health care provider.
- Peel back foil on blister pack of disintegrating tablets; do not push through foil; use dry hands to remove tablet, place entire tablet in mouth.
- This drug cannot be taken during pregnancy. If you think you are pregnant or wish to become pregnant, contact your health care provider.
- You may experience these side effects: Drowsiness, dizziness, sedation, seizures (avoid driving, operating machinery, or performing tasks that require concentration); dizziness, faintness on arising (change positions slowly, use caution); increased salivation (if bothersome, contact your health care provider); constipation (consult your health care provider for appropriate relief measures); fast heart rate (rest and take your time if this occurs).
- Report lethargy, weakness, fever, sore throat, malaise, mouth ulcers, and flulike symptoms.

▽ olmesartan medoxomil

(ol ma sar' tan)

Benicar

PREGNANCY CATEGORY C (FIRST TRIMESTER)

PREGNANCY CATEGORY D (SECOND AND THIRD TRIMESTERS)

Drug classes
Angiotensin II receptor antagonist
Antihypertensive

Therapeutic actions
Selectively blocks the binding of angiotensin II to specific tissue receptors found in the vascular smooth muscle and adrenal gland; this action blocks the vasoconstricting effect of the renin-angiotensin system as well as the release of aldosterone leading to decreased BP; may prevent the vessel remodeling associated with the development of atherosclerosis.

Indications
- Treatment of hypertension, alone or in combination with other antihypertensives

Contraindications and cautions
- Contraindicated with hypersensitivity to any component of the drug, pregnancy (use during the second or third trimester can cause injury or death to the fetus), lactation.
- Use cautiously with renal impairment, hypovolemia, salt depletion.

Available forms
Tablets—5, 20, 40 mg

Dosages
Adults
20 mg/day PO as a once-daily dose; may titrate to 40 mg/day if needed after 2 wk.
Pediatric patients
Safety and efficacy not established.

Pharmacokinetics

Route	*Onset*	*Peak*
Oral	Varies	1–2 hr

Metabolism: Hydrolyzed in GI tract; $T_{1/2}$: 13 hr
Distribution: Crosses placenta; enters breast milk
Excretion: Feces, urine

Adverse effects
- **CNS:** *Headache,* dizziness, syncope, muscle weakness
- **CV:** Hypotension, tachycardia
- **Dermatologic:** Rash, inflammation, urticaria, pruritus, alopecia, dry skin
- **GI:** *Diarrhea, abdominal pain, nausea,* constipation, dry mouth, dental pain
- **Hematologic:** Increased CPK, hyperglycemia, hypertriglyceridemia
- **Respiratory:** *URI symptoms, bronchitis, cough,* sinusitis, rhinitis, pharyngitis
- **Other:** *Back pain, flulike symptoms,* fatigue, hematuria, arthritis, **angioedema**

■ Nursing considerations
Assessment
- **History:** Hypersensitivity to any component of the drug, pregnancy, lactation, hepatic or renal impairment, hypovolemia, salt depletion
- **Physical:** Skin lesions, turgor; body T; reflexes, affect; BP; R, respiratory auscultation; LFTs, renal function tests, serum electrolytes

Interventions
- Administer without regard to meals.

⊗ ***Black box warning*** Ensure that patient is not pregnant before beginning therapy. Suggest the use of barrier birth control while using olmesartan; fetal injury and deaths have been reported.
- Find an alternate method of feeding the infant if given to a nursing mother. Depression of the renin-angiotensin system in infants is potentially very dangerous.

⊗ ***Warning*** Alert the surgeon and mark the patient's chart with notice that olmesartan is being taken. The blockage of the renin-angiotensin system following surgery can produce problems. Hypotension may be reversed with volume expansion.
- Monitor patient closely in any situation that may lead to a decrease in BP secondary to reduction in fluid volume—excessive perspiration, dehydration, vomiting, diarrhea; excessive hypotension can occur.

Teaching points
- Take drug without regard to meals. Do not stop taking this drug without consulting your health care provider.
- Use a barrier method of birth control while using this drug; if you become pregnant or

desire to become pregnant, consult your health care provider.
- Take special precautions to maintain your fluid intake and provide safety precautions in any situation that might cause a loss of fluid volume—excessive perspiration, dehydration, vomiting, diarrhea; excessive hypotension can occur.
- You may experience these side effects: Dizziness (avoid driving a car or performing hazardous tasks); headache (medications may be available to help); nausea, vomiting, diarrhea (proper nutrition is important, consult a dietitian to maintain nutrition); symptoms of upper respiratory tract, cough (do not self-medicate, consult your health care provider if this becomes uncomfortable).
- Report fever, chills, dizziness, pregnancy, swelling.

▽ olsalazine sodium

See Appendix W, *Less commonly used drugs.*

▽ omalizumab

See Appendix W, *Less commonly used drugs.*

▽ omega-3-acid ethyl esters

(oh may gah-three-ass' id)

Lovaza

PREGNANCY CATEGORY C

Drug classes
Lipid-lowering drug
Omega-3 fatty acid

Therapeutic actions
Inhibits liver enzyme systems leading to a decrease in the synthesis of triglycerides in the liver, lowering serum triglyceride levels.

Indications
- As an adjunct to diet to reduce very high (greater than 500 mg/dL) triglyceride levels in adult patients

Contraindications and cautions
- Contraindicated with known allergy to any component of the capsule.
- Use caution with known sensitivity to fish products, pregnancy, lactation.

Available forms
Capsules—1 g

Dosages
Adults
4 g/day PO taken as a single dose (4 capsules) or divided into two doses—2 capsules PO bid.
Pediatric patients
Safety and efficacy not established.

Pharmacokinetics

Route	*Onset*	*Peak*
Oral	Rapid	Unknown

Metabolism: $T_{1/2}$: Unknown
Distribution: May cross placenta; may pass into breast milk
Excretion: Tissues

Adverse effects
- **CV:** Angina
- **GI:** Taste perversion, dyspepsia, *eructation*
- **Other:** Pain, back pain, rash, flulike symptoms, *infection*

Interactions
✱ **Drug-drug** • Potential risk for increased bleeding if combined with anticoagulants; monitor patient closely and adjust anticoagulant dosage if needed

■ Nursing considerations

CLINICAL ALERT!
Name confusion has occurred between *Omacor* (the former trade name of omega-3-acid ethyl esters) and *Amicar* (amino caproic acid). Although the name of omega-3-acid esters has been changed to *Lovaza,* confusion may still occur; use caution.

Assessment
- **History:** Allergy to any component of the tablet, sensitivity to fish products, pregnancy, lactation

O

- **Physical:** T; abdominal examination; skin color, lesions; triglyceride levels

Interventions

- Reserve use for patients with very high triglyceride levels; obtain baseline level and periodically monitor levels.
- Assess patient for any potential underlying causes for elevated triglycerides.
- Ensure that patient continues diet and exercise program to control lipids.
- Suggest the use of contraceptive measures; it is not known if this drug could affect a fetus.
- Suggest another method of feeding the baby if a woman is nursing; it is not known if this drug crosses into breast milk.
- Encourage frequent small meals if GI effects are uncomfortable.

Teaching points

- Take this drug in one dose of four capsules, or you can take two doses of two capsules each. You can take this drug with meals.
- If you miss a dose of the daily medication, take it as soon as you remember and then return to your normal schedule. Do not make up doses. Do not take more than four capsules in one day.
- You should continue your dietary and exercise program to control your lipid levels.
- You may be asked to have periodic blood tests to evaluate the effects of this drug on your body.
- It is not known how this drug could affect a nursing baby. If you are nursing a baby, another method of feeding the baby should be selected.
- It is not known how this drug could affect a fetus, if you are pregnant or decide to become pregnant while on this drug, consult your health care provider; use of contraceptive measures is advised while you are on this drug.
- You may experience these side effects: Taste changes, GI upset, frequent burping (this may stop after you have used the drug for awhile; frequent small meals may help); rash, fever, flulike symptoms (consult your health care provider; analgesics may be available to help).
- Report chest pain, severe headache, swelling, difficulty breathing.

▽omeprazole

(oh me' pray zol)

Losec (CAN) DNC, Prilosec DNC, Prilosec OTC DNC, Zegerid (with sodium bicarbonate) DNC

PREGNANCY CATEGORY C

Drug classes

Antisecretory drug
Proton pump inhibitor

Therapeutic actions

Gastric acid-pump inhibitor: Suppresses gastric acid secretion by specific inhibition of the hydrogen-potassium ATPase enzyme system at the secretory surface of the gastric parietal cells; blocks the final step of acid production.

Indications

- Short-term treatment of active duodenal ulcer
- Treatment of heartburn or symptoms of GERD
- Short-term treatment of active benign gastric ulcer
- GERD, severe erosive esophagitis, poorly responsive symptomatic GERD
- Long-term therapy: Treatment of pathologic hypersecretory conditions (Zollinger-Ellison's syndrome, multiple adenomas, systemic mastocytosis)
- Eradication of *Helicobacter pylori* with amoxicillin or metronidazole and clarithromycin
- *Prilosec OTC:* Treatment of frequent heartburn (2 or more days per week)
- *Zegerid* oral suspension: Reduction of risk of upper GI bleeding in critically ill patients; includes sodium bicarbonate
- Unlabeled use: Posterior laryngitis

Contraindications and cautions

- Contraindicated with hypersensitivity to omeprazole or its components.
- Use cautiously with pregnancy, lactation.

Available forms

DR capsules DNC—10, 20, 40 mg; DR tablets DNC—20 mg (OTC); powder for oral suspension—20, 40 mg/packet (*Zegerid*); capsules DNC—20, 40 mg (*Zegerid*)

Dosages

Adults

- *Active duodenal ulcer:* 20 mg PO daily for 2–8 wk. Should not be used for maintenance therapy.
- *Active gastric ulcer:* 40 mg PO daily for 4–8 wk.
- *Severe erosive esophagitis or poorly responsive GERD:* 20 mg PO daily for 4–8 wk. Do not use as maintenance therapy. An additional 4–8 wk course can be considered if needed.
- *Pathologic hypersecretory conditions:* Individualize dosage. Initial dose is 60 mg PO daily. Doses up to 120 mg tid have been used. Administer daily amounts greater than 80 mg in divided doses.
- *Frequent heartburn (2 or more days per week):* 20 mg (*Prilosec OTC* tablet) PO once daily before eating in the morning for 14 days. May repeat the 14-day course every 4 mo.
- *Upper GI bleeding in critically ill patients:* 40 mg PO followed by 40 mg PO in 6–8 hr on day 1; then 40 mg/day for up to 14 days (*Zegerid*).

Pediatric patients 2 yr and older

- *GERD or other acid-related disorder:* 10 mg if patient weighs less than 20 kg; 20 mg if 20 kg or more.

Pediatric patients younger than 2 yr

Safety and efficacy not established.

Pharmacokinetics

Route	Onset	Peak
Oral	Varies	0.5–3.5 hr

Metabolism: Hepatic; $T_{1/2}$: 0.5–1 hr
Distribution: Crosses placenta; may enter breast milk
Excretion: Bile, urine

Adverse effects

- **CNS:** *Headache, dizziness,* asthenia, vertigo, insomnia, apathy, anxiety, paresthesias, dream abnormalities
- **Dermatologic:** Rash, inflammation, urticaria, pruritus, alopecia, dry skin
- **GI:** *Diarrhea, abdominal pain, nausea, vomiting,* constipation, dry mouth, tongue atrophy
- **Respiratory:** *URI symptoms,* cough, epistaxis
- **Other:** Cancer in preclinical studies, back pain, fever

Interactions

✷ **Drug-drug** ⊗ ***Warning*** Increased serum levels and potential increase in toxicity of benzodiazepines, phenytoin, warfarin; if these combinations are used, monitor patient closely.

- Decreased absorption with sucralfate; give these drugs at least 30 min apart

■ Nursing considerations

Assessment

- **History:** Hypersensitivity to omeprazole or any of its components, pregnancy, lactation
- **Physical:** Skin lesions; T; reflexes, affect; urinary output, abdominal examination; respiratory auscultation

Interventions

- Administer before meals. Caution patient to swallow capsules whole—not to open, chew, or crush them. If using oral suspension, empty packet into a small cup containing 2 tbsp of water. Stir and have patient drink immediately; fill cup with water and have patient drink this water. Do not use any other diluent.

⊗ ***Warning*** Arrange for further evaluation of patient after 8 wk of therapy for GERD; not intended for maintenance therapy. Symptomatic improvement does not rule out gastric cancer, which did occur in preclinical studies.

- Administer antacids with, if needed.
- If patient cannot swallow *Prilosec* capsules, contents of capsule may be added to or sprinkled on 1 tablespoon applesauce. Mix capsule contents into applesauce and have patient swallow immediately without chewing pellets. Follow with a glass of water.
- *Zegerid* capsules should not be opened and contents should not be sprinkled on applesauce. Use suspension if swallowing is difficult.

Teaching points

- Take the drug before meals. Swallow the capsules whole; do not chew, open, or crush them. If using the oral suspension, empty packet into a small cup containing 2 tablespoons of water. Stir and drink immediately; fill cup with water and drink the water. Do not use any other liquid or food to dissolve the packet. This drug will need to be taken for up to 8 weeks (short-term therapy) or for a prolonged period (more than 5 years in some cases).
- If you take *Prilosec* capsules and cannot swallow them whole, capsule contents may be added to or sprinkled on 1 tablespoon of applesauce. Mix with applesauce, swallow immediately without chewing pellets, and follow with a glass of water. *Zegerid* capsules should not be opened or added to food.
- Have regular medical follow-up visits.
- You may experience these side effects: Dizziness (avoid driving or performing hazardous tasks); headache (request medications); nausea, vomiting, diarrhea (maintain proper nutrition); symptoms of URI, cough (do not self-medicate; consult your health care provider if uncomfortable).
- Report severe headache, worsening of symptoms, fever, chills, severe diarrhea.

▽ondansetron hydrochloride

*(on **dan'** sah tron)*

Zofran, Zofran ODT

PREGNANCY CATEGORY B

Drug class

Antiemetic

Therapeutic actions

Blocks specific receptor sites (5-HT_3), which are associated with nausea and vomiting in the chemoreceptor trigger zone, centrally and at specific sites peripherally. It is not known whether its antiemetic actions are from actions at the central, peripheral, or combined sites.

Indications

- Parenteral and oral: Prevention of nausea and vomiting associated with emetogenic cancer chemotherapy in patients older than 6 mo
- Prevention of postoperative nausea and vomiting—to prevent further episodes or, when postoperative nausea and vomiting must be avoided (oral), prophylactically (parenteral) in patients older than 1 mo
- Prevention of nausea and vomiting associated with radiotherapy
- Unlabeled uses: Treatment of nausea and vomiting associated with acetaminophen poisoning, prostacyclin therapy

Contraindications and cautions

- Contraindicated with allergy to ondansetron.
- Use cautiously with pregnancy, lactation, hepatic impairment.

Available forms

Tablets—4, 8, 24 mg; orally disintegrating tablets—4, 8 mg; oral solution—4 mg/5 mL; injection—2 mg/mL, 32 mg/50 mL

Dosages

Adults

Parenteral

- *Prevention of chemotherapy-induced nausea and vomiting:* Three 0.15 mg/kg doses IV: First dose is given over 15 min, beginning 30 min before chemotherapy; subsequent doses are given at 4 and 8 hr, or a single 32-mg dose is infused over 15 min beginning 30 min before the start of the chemotherapy.

Oral

- *Prevention of nausea and vomiting associated with cancer chemotherapy:* 8 mg PO 30 min prior to chemotherapy, then 8 mg 8 hr later; give 8 mg every 12 hr for 1–2 days after completion of chemotherapy. For highly emetogenic chemotherapy, give 24 mg PO 30 min before starting chemotherapy.
- *Prevention of nausea and vomiting associated with radiotherapy:* 8 mg PO tid. For total-body radiotherapy, administer 1–2 hr before radiation each day. For single high-dose radiotherapy to abdomen, give 1–2 hr before radiotherapy, then every 8 hr

for 1–2 days after completion of therapy. For daily fractionated radiotherapy to abdomen, give 1–2 hr before therapy, then every 8 hr for each day therapy is given.

Parenteral or oral

- *Prevention of postoperative nausea and vomiting:* 4 mg undiluted IV, preferably over 2–5 min, or as a single IM dose immediately before induction of anesthesia or 16 mg PO 1 hr before anesthesia.

Pediatric patients

- *Prevention of chemotherapy-induced nausea and vomiting:*

Parenteral

6 mo–18 yr: Three doses of 0.15 mg/kg IV over 15 min given 30 min before the start of the chemotherapy, then 4 and 8 hr later.

Oral

12 yr and older: Same as adult.

4–11 yr: 4 mg PO 30 min prior to chemotherapy, 4 mg at 4 and 8 hr, then 4 mg PO tid for 1–2 days after completion of chemotherapy.

Younger than 4 yr: Safety and efficacy not established.

- *Prevention of postoperative nausea and vomiting:*

1 mo–12 yr: 0.1 mg/kg IV if patient weighs less than 40 kg or a single dose of 4 mg IV if more than 40 kg, preferably given 2–5 min before or following induction of anesthesia. Infuse over at least 30 sec.

Patients with hepatic impairment

Maximum daily dose of 8 mg IV or PO.

Pharmacokinetics

Route	*Onset*	*Peak*
Oral	30–60 min	1.7–2.2 hr
IV	Immediate	Immediate

Metabolism: Hepatic; $T_{1/2}$: 3.5–6 hr

Distribution: Crosses placenta; may enter breast milk

Excretion: Urine

▼ IV FACTS

Preparation: Dilute in 50 mL of 5% dextrose injection or 0.9% sodium chloride injection; stable for 48 hr at room temperature after dilution.

Infusion: Infuse slowly over 15 min diluted or 2–5 min undiluted.

Compatibilities: May be diluted with 0.9% sodium chloride injection, 5% dextrose injection, 5% dextrose and 0.9% sodium chloride injection; 5% dextrose and 0.45% sodium chloride injection; 3% sodium chloride injection.

Incompatibilities: Do not mix with alkaline solutions.

Adverse effects

- **CNS:** *Headache, dizziness,* drowsiness, shivers, malaise, fatigue, weakness, *myalgia*
- **CV:** Chest pain, hypotension
- **Dermatologic:** Pruritus
- **GI:** Abdominal pain, constipation, liver impairment, *diarrhea*
- **GU:** Urinary retention
- **Local:** Pain at injection site

Interactions

✱ **Drug-food** • Increased extent of absorption if taken orally with food

■ Nursing considerations

Assessment

- **History:** Allergy to ondansetron, pregnancy, lactation, nausea and vomiting
- **Physical:** Skin color and texture; orientation, reflexes, bilateral grip strength, affect; P, BP; abdominal examination; urinary output

Interventions

- Ensure that the timing of drug doses corresponds to that of the chemotherapy or radiation.
- Administer oral drug for 1–2 days following completion of chemotherapy or radiation.
- For *Zofran ODT,* peel foil backing of one blister and remove tablet gently. Do not push tablet through the foil backing. Immediately place tablet on tongue , where it will dissolve in seconds, and have patient swallow it with saliva.

Teaching points

- Take oral drug for 1–2 days following chemotherapy or radiation therapy to maximize prevention of nausea and vomiting. Take the drug every 8 hours around-the-clock for best results.

- For *Zofran ODT,* peel foil backing of one blister and remove tablet gently. Do not push tablet through the foil backing. Immediately place tablet on tongue, where it will dissolve in seconds, and swallow with saliva.
- You may experience these side effects: Weakness, dizziness (change position slowly to avoid injury); dizziness, drowsiness (do not drive or perform tasks that require alertness).
- Report continued nausea and vomiting, pain at injection site, chest pain, palpitations.

DANGEROUS DRUG

opium preparations

(oh' pee um)

Camphorated tincture: Paregoric
Deodorized tincture: Opium Tincture, Deodorized

PREGNANCY CATEGORY C

CONTROLLED SUBSTANCE C-III (PAREGORIC)

CONTROLLED SUBSTANCE C-II (OPIUM TINCTURE, DEODORIZED)

Drug classes

Antidiarrheal
Opioid agonist analgesic

Therapeutic actions

Activity is primarily due to morphine content; acts as agonist at specific opioid receptors in the CNS to produce analgesia, euphoria, sedation; the receptors mediating these effects are thought to be the same as those mediating the effects of endogenous opioids (enkephalins, endorphins); inhibits peristalsis and diarrhea by producing spasm of GI tract smooth muscle.

Indications

- Antidiarrheal
- Unlabeled uses: Neonatal abstinence syndrome, management of short-bowel syndrome

Contraindications and cautions

- Contraindicated with hypersensitivity to opioids, diarrhea caused by poisoning (before toxins are eliminated), pregnancy, labor or delivery (opioids given to mother can cause respiratory depression of neonate; premature infants are at special risk; may prolong labor), bronchial asthma, COPD, cor pulmonale, respiratory depression, anoxia, kyphoscoliosis, acute alcoholism, increased intracranial pressure, lactation.
- Use cautiously with acute abdominal conditions, CV disease, supraventricular tachycardias, myxedema, seizure disorders, delirium tremens, cerebral arteriosclerosis, ulcerative colitis, fever, Addison's disease, prostatic hypertrophy, urethral stricture, recent GI or GU surgery, toxic psychosis, renal or hepatic impairment.

Available forms

Liquid—2 mg morphine equivalent/5 mL (*Paregoric*); 10 mg/mL (*Opium Tincture, Deodorized*)

Dosages

⊗ ***Warning*** Caution: *Opium Tincture, Deodorized,* contains 25 times more morphine than *Paregoric.* Do not confuse dosage; severe toxicity can occur.

Adults

Paregoric

5–10 mL PO daily–qid (5 mL is equivalent to 2 mg morphine).

Opium Tincture, Deodorized

0.6 mL qid. Maximum, 6 mL/day.

Pediatric patients

Contraindicated in premature infants.

Paregoric

0.25–0.5 mL/kg PO daily–qid.

Geriatric patients or impaired adults

⊗ ***Warning*** Use caution; respiratory depression may occur in the elderly, the very ill, those with respiratory problems. Reduced dosage may be necessary.

Pharmacokinetics

Route	*Onset*	*Peak*	*Duration*
Oral	Varies	0.5–1 hr	3–7 hr

Metabolism: Hepatic; $T_{1/2}$: 1.5–2 hr

Distribution: Crosses placenta; enters breast milk
Excretion: Urine

Adverse effects

- **CNS:** *Light-headedness, dizziness, sedation,* euphoria, dysphoria, delirium, insomnia, agitation, anxiety, fear, hallucinations, disorientation, drowsiness, lethargy, impaired mental and physical performance, coma, mood changes, weakness, headache, tremor, seizures, miosis, visual disturbances
- **CV:** Facial flushing, peripheral circulatory collapse, tachycardia, bradycardia, arrhythmia, palpitations, chest wall rigidity, hypertension, hypotension, orthostatic hypotension, syncope, circulatory depression, **shock, cardiac arrest**
- **Dermatologic:** Pruritus, urticaria, edema, hemorrhagic urticaria (rare)
- **GI:** *Nausea, vomiting, sweating,* dry mouth, anorexia, constipation, biliary tract spasm; increased colonic motility with chronic ulcerative colitis
- **GU:** Ureteral spasm, spasm of vesical sphincters, urinary retention or hesitancy, oliguria, antidiuretic effect, reduced libido or potency
- **Respiratory:** Suppression of cough reflex, respiratory depression, apnea, **respiratory arrest, laryngospasm, bronchospasm**
- **Other:** Physical tolerance and dependence, psychological dependence

Interactions

✱ **Drug-drug** • Increased likelihood of respiratory depression, hypotension, profound sedation or coma with barbiturate general anesthetics

✱ **Drug-lab test** • Elevated biliary tract pressure may cause increases in plasma amylase, lipase determinations 24 hr after administration

■ Nursing considerations

CLINICAL ALERT!

Name confusion has occurred between *Paregoric* (camphorated tincture of opium) and *Opium Tincture, Deodorized;* use caution.

Assessment

- **History:** Hypersensitivity to opioids, diarrhea caused by poisoning, bronchial asthma, COPD, cor pulmonale, respiratory depression, kyphoscoliosis, acute alcoholism, increased intracranial pressure, acute abdominal conditions, CV disease, supraventricular tachycardias, myxedema, seizure disorders, delirium tremens, cerebral arteriosclerosis, ulcerative colitis, fever, Addison's disease, prostatic hypertrophy, urethral stricture, recent GI or GU surgery, toxic psychosis, renal or hepatic impairment, pregnancy, lactation
- **Physical:** T; skin color, texture, lesions; orientation, reflexes, bilateral grip strength, affect, pupil size; P, auscultation, BP, orthostatic BP, perfusion; R, adventitious sounds; bowel sounds, normal output; frequency and pattern of voiding, normal output; LFTs, renal and thyroid function tests

Interventions

- Give to lactating women 4–6 hr before the next feeding to minimize the amount in milk.
- Reassure patient that addiction is unlikely; most patients who receive opiates for medical reasons do not develop dependence syndromes.

Teaching points

- Take this drug exactly as prescribed.
- Do not take leftover medication for other disorders, and do not let anyone else take the prescription.
- You may experience these side effects: Nausea, loss of appetite (take with food and lie quietly; eat frequent small meals); constipation (use a laxative); dizziness, sedation, drowsiness, impaired visual acuity (avoid driving, performing other tasks that require alertness, visual acuity).
- Report severe nausea, vomiting, constipation, shortness of breath, or difficulty breathing.

▽ oprelvekin

See Appendix W, *Less commonly used drugs.*

▽ orlistat

(ore' lah stat)

Alli, Xenical

PREGNANCY CATEGORY B

Drug classes
Lipase inhibitor
Weight loss drug

Therapeutic actions
Synthetic derivative of lipostatin, a naturally occurring lipase inhibitor or so-called fat blocker. Binds to gastric and pancreatic lipase to prevent the digestion of fats. When taken with fat-containing foods, the fat passes through the intestines unchanged and is not absorbed.

Indications
- Treatment of obesity as part of weight loss program that includes diet and exercise

Contraindications and cautions
- Contraindicated with hypersensitivity to orlistat, pregnancy, lactation, chronic malabsorption syndrome.
- Use cautiously with impaired hepatic function, biliary obstruction, pancreatic disease.

Available forms
Capsules—60 (*Alli*), 120 mg (*Xenical*)

Dosages
Adults
120 mg tid PO with each main meal containing fat. For OTC use, 60 mg PO with each meal containing fat, not exceeding 3 capsules/day.
Pediatric patients
Safety and efficacy not established.

Pharmacokinetics
Not absorbed systemically

Adverse effects
- **Dermatologic:** *Rash, dry skin*
- **GI:** *Dry mouth,* nausea, flatulence, *loose stools,* oily stools, fecal incontinence or urgency
- **Other:** Vitamin deficiency of fat-soluble vitamins (A, D, E, K)

Interactions
✱ **Drug-drug** • Decreased absorption of fat-soluble vitamins • Additive lipid-lowering effects with pravastatin; monitor patient response • Increased risk of bleeding related to decreased vitamin K; when taking with oral anticoagulants, monitor patient closely

■ Nursing considerations
Assessment
- **History:** Hypersensitivity to orlistat, impaired hepatic or pancreatic function, pregnancy, biliary obstruction, lactation
- **Physical:** Weight, T, skin rash, lesions; liver evaluation; LFTs

Interventions
- Ensure that patient is participating in a weight-loss diet and exercise program.
- Administer with meals.
- Arrange for administration of fat-soluble vitamins. Do not administer with orlistat; separate doses.
- Provide sugarless lozenges and frequent mouth care if dry mouth is a problem.
- Ensure ready access to bathroom facilities if diarrhea occurs.

⊗ ***Warning*** Counsel patient about the use of barrier contraceptives while using this drug; pregnancy should be avoided because of the possible risk to the fetus.

Teaching points
- Take this drug with meals that contain fat. Do not take the drug if you do not eat a meal. This drug is not a substitute for a reduced-calorie diet.
- You may need to take a vitamin supplement while you are using this drug. Take the supplement at least 2 hours before or after taking orlistat.
- Do not take this drug during pregnancy. If you think that you are pregnant or you wish to become pregnant, consult your health care provider.
- You may experience these side effects: Dry mouth (suck sugarless lozenges and perform frequent mouth care), nausea, loose stools, flatulence (stay close to the bathroom; this may pass in time).
- Report rash, glossy tongue, vision changes, bruising, changes in stool or urine color.

orphenadrine citrate

(or fen' a dreen)

Banflex, Flexon, Norflex

PREGNANCY CATEGORY C

Drug class

Skeletal muscle relaxant (centrally acting)

Therapeutic actions

Precise mechanisms not known; acts in the CNS; does not directly relax tense skeletal muscles; does not directly affect the motor endplate or motor nerves.

Indications

- Relief of discomfort associated with acute, painful musculoskeletal conditions; as an adjunct to rest, physical therapy, and other measures
- Unlabeled use: 100 mg at bedtime for the treatment of leg cramps

Contraindications and cautions

- Contraindicated with hypersensitivity to orphenadrine, glaucoma, pyloric or duodenal obstruction, stenosing peptic ulcers, achalasia, cardiospasm (megaesophagus), prostatic hypertrophy, bladder neck obstruction, myasthenia gravis, lactation.
- Use cautiously with cardiac decompensation, coronary insufficiency, cardiac arrhythmias, hepatic or renal impairment, pregnancy, allergy to sulfites with some products.

Available forms

SR tablets DNC—100 mg; injection—30 mg/mL; tablets—100 mg

Dosages

Adults

60 mg IV or IM. May repeat every 12 hr. Inject IV over 5 min. Alternatively, give 100 mg PO every morning and evening.

Pediatric patients

Safety and efficacy not established; not recommended.

Geriatric patients

Use caution and regulate dosage carefully; patients older than 60 yr frequently develop increased sensitivity to adverse CNS effects of anticholinergic drugs.

Pharmacokinetics

Route	*Onset*	*Peak*	*Duration*
IM, IV	Rapid	2 hr	4–6 hr
Oral	Rapid	2 hr	4–6 hr

Metabolism: Hepatic; $T_{1/2}$: 14 hr
Distribution: Crosses placenta; enters breast milk
Excretion: Feces, urine

IV FACTS

Preparation: No further preparation is required.
Infusion: Administer slowly IV, each 60 mg over 5 min.

Adverse effects

- **CNS:** *Weakness, headache, dizziness, confusion* (especially in elderly), hallucinations, drowsiness, memory loss, psychosis, agitation, nervousness, delusions, delirium, paranoia, euphoria, depression, paresthesia, blurred vision, pupil dilation, increased intraocular tension
- **CV:** *Tachycardia,* palpitation, transient syncope, hypotension, orthostatic hypotension
- **Dermatologic:** Urticaria, other dermatoses
- **GI:** *Dry mouth, gastric irritation, vomiting, nausea, constipation,* dilation of the colon, paralytic ileus
- **GU:** *Urinary hesitancy and retention,* dysuria, difficulty achieving or maintaining an erection
- **Other:** *Flushing, decreased sweating,* elevated temperature, muscle weakness, cramping

Interactions

✱ **Drug-drug** • Additive anticholinergic effects with other anticholinergic drugs • Additive adverse CNS effects with phenothiazines • Possible masking of the development of persistent extrapyramidal symptoms, tardive dyskinesia in long-term therapy with phenothiazines, haloperidol

■ Nursing considerations

Assessment

- **History:** Hypersensitivity to orphenadrine, glaucoma, pyloric or duodenal obstruction, stenosing peptic ulcers, achalasia, cardiospasm, prostatic hypertrophy, bladder neck obstruction, myasthenia gravis, cardiac dysfunction, hepatic or renal impairment, lactation, pregnancy
- **Physical:** Weight; T; skin color, lesions; orientation, affect, reflexes, bilateral grip strength, vision examination with tonometry; P, BP, orthostatic BP, auscultation; bowel sounds, normal output, liver evaluation; prostate palpation, normal output, voiding pattern; urinalysis, CBC with differential, LFTs, renal function tests, ECG

Interventions

- Ensure that patient is supine during IV injection and for at least 15 min thereafter; assist patient from the supine position after treatment.
- Ensure that patients swallow SR tablets whole, and do not cut, crush, or chew them.

⊗ ***Warning*** Decrease or discontinue drug temporarily if dry mouth is so severe that swallowing or speaking becomes difficult.

⊗ ***Warning*** Give with caution, reduce dosage in hot weather; drug interferes with sweating and body's ability to thermoregulate in hot environments.

- Arrange for analgesics if headache occurs (adjunct for relief of muscle spasm).

Teaching points

- Swallow sustained-release tablets whole; do not cut, crush, or chew them.
- Do not consume alcohol while using this drug.
- You may experience these side effects: Drowsiness, dizziness, blurred vision (avoid driving or engaging in activities that require alertness and visual acuity); dry mouth (suck on sugarless lozenges or ice chips); nausea (eat frequent small meals); difficulty urinating (empty your bladder just before taking the medication); constipation (increase fluid and fiber intake and exercise regularly); headache (request medication).
- Report dry mouth, difficult urination, constipation, headache, or GI upset that persists; rash or itching; rapid heart rate or palpitations; mental confusion; eye pain; fever; sore throat; bruising.

▽ oseltamivir phosphate

*(oz el **tam'** ah ver)*

Tamiflu

PREGNANCY CATEGORY C

Drug classes

Antiviral

Neuraminidase inhibitor

Therapeutic actions

Selectively inhibits influenza virus neuraminidase; by blocking the actions of this enzyme, there is decreased viral release from infected cells, increased formation of viral aggregates, and decreased spread of the virus.

Indications

- Treatment of uncomplicated acute illness due to influenza virus (A or B) in adults and children who have been symptomatic for 2 days or less
- Prevention of naturally occurring influenza A and B in adults and children in close contact with the flu
- Unlabeled use: Treatment of avian flu

Contraindications and cautions

- Contraindicated with allergy to any component of the drug.
- Use cautiously with pregnancy, lactation, asthma, COPD.

Available forms

Capsules—30, 45, 75 mg; powder for oral suspension—12 mg/mL

Dosages

Adults and patients 13 yr and older

- *Treatment:* 75 mg PO bid for 5 days, starting within 2 days of the onset of symptoms.

- *Prevention:* 75 mg/day PO for at least 10 days; begin treatment within 2 days of exposure.

Pediatric patients 1–12 yr

- *Treatment:* 30–75 mg PO bid for 5 days based on weight—use suspension.
- *Prevention:* If patient weighs 15 kg or less, 30 mg/day PO; if 15–23 kg, 45 mg/day PO; if 23–40 kg, 60 mg/day PO; if more than 40 kg, 75 mg/day PO. Continue for 10 days.

Pediatric patients 6–11 mo

- *Treatment:* 25 mg PO bid.
- *Prevention:* 25 mg/day PO for 10 days.

Pediatric patients 3–5 mo

- *Treatment:* 20 mg PO bid.
- *Prevention:* 20 mg/day PO for 10 days.

Pediatric patients younger than 3 mo

- *Treatment:* 12 mg PO bid.
- *Prevention:* Not recommended.

Patients with renal impairment

For creatinine clearance of 30 mL/min or less, use 75 mg/day PO for 5 days, 75 mg PO every other day for prophylaxis.

Pharmacokinetics

Route	*Onset*	*Peak*
Oral	Varies	2.5–6 hr

Metabolism: Hepatic; $T_{1/2}$: 6–10 hr
Distribution: Crosses placenta; may enter breast milk
Excretion: Urine

Adverse effects

- **CNS:** *Headache,* dizziness
- **GI:** *Nausea,* vomiting, *diarrhea, anorexia*
- **Respiratory:** Cough, *rhinitis,* bronchitis
- **Other:** Risk of self-injury and delirium, particularly in children

■ Nursing considerations

Assessment

- **History:** Allergy to any components of the drug, COPD, asthma, pregnancy, lactation
- **Physical:** T; orientation, reflexes; R, adventitious sounds; bowel sounds

Interventions

- Administer within 2 days of the onset of flu symptoms.
- Encourage patient to complete full 5-day course of therapy; advise patient that treatment does not decrease the risk of transmission of the flu to others.
- Start dosage for prevention within 2 days of exposure and continue for at least 10 days.
- Prepare solution by adding 23 mL of water to bottle containing powder; shake well for 15 sec. Shake solution well before each dose. The reconstituted oral suspension should be used within 10 days of preparation.
- Monitor children for self-injury, delirium.

Teaching points

- Take the full course of therapy as prescribed; be advised that this drug does not decrease the risk of transmitting the virus to others.
- Shake solution well before each use; store in refrigerator.
- You may experience these side effects: Nausea, vomiting, loss of appetite, diarrhea; headache, dizziness (use caution if driving an automobile or operating dangerous machinery).
- Report severe diarrhea, severe nausea, worsening of respiratory symptoms.

oxacillin sodium

*(ox a **sill'** in)*

PREGNANCY CATEGORY B

Drug classes

Antibiotic
Penicillinase-resistant penicillin

Therapeutic actions

Bactericidal: Inhibits cell wall synthesis of sensitive organisms, causing cell death.

Indications

- Infections due to penicillinase-producing staphylococci; may be used to initiate treatment when a staphylococci infection is suspected

Contraindications and cautions

- Contraindicated with allergies to penicillins, cephalosporins, or other allergens.
- Use cautiously with renal disorders, pregnancy, lactation (may cause diarrhea or candidiasis in infants).

Available forms

Powder for injection—500 mg; 1, 2 g

Dosages

Maximum recommended dosage is 6 g/day.

Adults and pediatric patients weighing 40 kg or more

250–500 mg every 4–6 hr IM or IV. Up to 1 g every 4–6 hr in severe infections.

Pediatric patients weighing less than 40 kg

Neonates weighing less than 2 kg: 25–50 mg/kg every 12 hr IV or IM.
Neonates weighing 2 kg or more: 25–50 mg/kg every 8 hr IV.
Children weighing less than 40 kg: 50–100 mg/kg/day IV or IM in equally divided doses every 4–6 hr.

Pharmacokinetics

Route	*Onset*	*Peak*	*Duration*
IM	Rapid	30–60 min	4–6 hr
IV	Rapid	15 min	Length of infusion

Metabolism: Hepatic; $T_{1/2}$: 0.5–1 hr
Distribution: Crosses placenta; enters breast milk
Excretion: Bile, urine

IV FACTS

Preparation: Dilute for direct IV administration to a maximum concentration of 1 g/10 mL using sodium chloride injection or sterile water for injection. For IV infusion: Reconstituted solution may be diluted with compatible IV solution: 0.9% sodium chloride injection, 5% dextrose in water or in normal saline, 10% D-fructose in water or in normal saline, lactated Ringer's solution, lactated potassic saline injections, 10% invert sugar in water or in normal saline, 10% invert sugar plus 0.3% potassium chloride in water, Travert's 10% Electrolyte 1, 2, or 3. 0.5–40 mg/mL solutions are stable for up to 12 hr at room temperature. Discard after that time.
Infusion: Give by direct administration slowly to avoid vein irritation, each 1 g over 10 min; infusion—up to 6 hr.
Incompatibilities: Do not mix in the same IV solution as other antibiotics.

Adverse effects

- **CNS:** Lethargy, hallucinations, **seizures**
- **GI:** *Glossitis, stomatitis, gastritis, sore mouth,* "furry" or black "hairy" tongue, *nausea, vomiting, diarrhea,* abdominal pain, bloody diarrhea, enterocolitis, pseudomembranous colitis, nonspecific hepatitis
- **GU:** Nephritis—oliguria, proteinuria, hematuria, casts, azotemia, pyuria
- **Hematologic:** Anemia, thrombocytopenia, leukopenia, neutropenia, prolonged bleeding time (more common than with other penicillinase-resistant penicillins)
- **Hypersensitivity:** *Rash, fever, wheezing,* **anaphylaxis**
- **Local:** *Pain, phlebitis,* thrombosis at injection site
- **Other:** *Superinfections,* sodium overload leading to heart failure

Interactions

✱ **Drug-drug** • Decreased effectiveness with tetracyclines • Inactivation of aminoglycosides in parenteral solutions with oxacillin
✱ **Drug-lab test** • False-positive Coombs' test with IV oxacillin

■ Nursing considerations

Assessment

- **History:** Allergies to penicillins, cephalosporins, or other allergens; renal disorders; pregnancy; lactation
- **Physical:** Culture infection; skin color, lesions; R, adventitious sounds; bowel sounds: CBC, LFTs, renal function tests, serum electrolytes, Hct, urinalysis

Interventions

- Culture infection before treatment; reculture if response is not as expected.
- Continue therapy for at least 2 days after infection has disappeared, usually 7–10 days.
- Reconstitute for IM use to a dilution of 250 mg/1.5 mL using sterile water for injection or sodium chloride injection. Discard after 3 days at room temperature or after 7 days if refrigerated.
- Reconstituted oral solution is stable 3 days at room temperature, 14 days refrigerated.

⊗ ***Warning*** Keep epinephrine, IV fluids, vasopressors, bronchodilators, oxygen, and emergency equipment readily available in case of serious hypersensitivity reaction.

Teaching points

- You may experience these side effects: Upset stomach, nausea, diarrhea (eat frequent small meals), mouth sores (perform frequent mouth care), pain at the injection site.
- Report difficulty breathing, rashes, severe diarrhea, severe pain at injection site, mouth sores.
- Finish entire course of therapy as prescribed.

oxaliplatin

See Appendix W, *Less commonly used drugs.*

oxandrolone

(ox an' droh lone)

Oxandrin

PREGNANCY CATEGORY X

CONTROLLED SUBSTANCE C-III

Drug classes

Anabolic steroid
Hormone

Therapeutic actions

Testosterone analogue with androgenic and anabolic activity; promotes body tissue-building processes; reverses catabolic or tissue-depleting processes; increases Hgb and red cell mass.

Indications

- Relief of bone pain accompanying osteoporosis
- Adjunctive therapy to promote weight gain after weight loss following extensive surgery, chronic infections, trauma
- Offset protein catabolism associated with prolonged use of corticosteroids
- Orphan drug uses: Short stature associated with Turner's syndrome, HIV wasting syndrome, and HIV-associated muscle weakness
- Unlabeled use: Alcoholic hepatitis

Contraindications and cautions

- Contraindicated with known sensitivity to anabolic steroids; prostate, breast cancer; BPH; pituitary insufficiency; MI (contraindicated because of effects on cholesterol); nephrosis; liver disease; hypercalcemia; pregnancy, lactation.
- Use cautiously with HF; cardiac, renal, or liver disease; epilepsy; migraines; diabetes.

Available forms

Tablets—2.5 mg, 10 mg

Dosages

Adults

2.5 mg PO bid–qid; up to 20 mg has been used to achieve the desired effect; 2–4 wk needed to evaluate response.

Pediatric patients

Give a total daily dose of 0.1 mg/kg or less or 0.045 mg/lb or less PO; may be repeated intermittently.

Pharmacokinetics

Route	*Onset*
Oral	Slow

Metabolism: Hepatic; $T_{1/2}$: 9 hr
Distribution: Crosses placenta; enters breast milk
Excretion: Urine

Adverse effects

- **CNS:** *Excitation, insomnia,* chills, toxic confusion
- **Endocrine:** *Virilization: Prepubertal males*—phallic enlargement, hirsutism, increased skin pigmentation; *postpubertal males*—inhibition of testicular function, gynecomastia, testicular atrophy, priapism, baldness, epididymitis, change in libido; *females*—hirsutism, hoarseness, deepening of the voice, clitoral enlargement, menstrual irregularities, baldness; decreased glucose tolerance
- **GI:** Hepatotoxicity, peliosis, **hepatitis** with **liver failure or intra-abdominal hemorrhage; liver cell tumors,** sometimes malignant, *nausea, vomiting, diarrhea, abdominal fullness, loss of appetite, burning of tongue*

O

- **GU:** Possible increased risk of prostatic hypertrophy, carcinoma in geriatric patients
- **Hematologic:** *Blood lipid changes;* iron deficiency anemia, hypercalcemia, altered serum cholesterol levels; *retention of sodium, chloride, water,* potassium, phosphates and calcium
- **Other:** *Acne,* premature closure of the epiphyses, edema

Interactions

✱ Drug-drug • Potentiation of oral anticoagulants with anabolic steroids • Decreased need for insulin, oral hypoglycemia drugs with anabolic steroids

✱ Drug-lab test • Altered glucose tolerance tests • Decrease in thyroid function tests (may persist for 2–3 wk after stopping therapy) • Increased creatinine, creatinine clearance, which may last for 2 wk after therapy

■ Nursing considerations

Assessment

- **History:** Sensitivity to anabolic steroids; prostate or breast cancer; BPH; pituitary insufficiency; MI; nephrosis; liver disease; hypercalcemia; pregnancy; lactation; HF; renal, cardiac, or liver disease, epilepsy, diabetes, migraines
- **Physical:** Skin color, texture; hair distribution pattern; affect, orientation; abdominal examination, liver evaluation; serum electrolytes and cholesterol levels, glucose tolerance tests, thyroid function tests, long-bone X-ray (in children)

Interventions

- Administer with food if GI upset or nausea occurs.

⊗ ***Warning*** Monitor effect on children with long-bone X-rays every 3–6 mo; discontinue drug well before the bone age reaches the norm for the patient's chronologic age because effects may continue for 6 mo after therapy.

- Ensure that women of childbearing age are not pregnant and understand the need to use contraceptives to prevent pregnancy.
- Monitor patient for edema; arrange for diuretic therapy.

⊠ ***Black box warning*** Monitor liver function and serum electrolytes periodically, and consult with physician for corrective measures; risk of peliosis hepatitis, liver cell tumors.

⊠ ***Black box warning*** Measure cholesterol levels periodically in patients who are at high risk for CAD; lipid level may increase.

- Monitor diabetic patients closely because glucose tolerance may change. Adjustments may be needed in insulin, oral hypoglycemic dosage, and diet.

Teaching points

- Take drug with food if nausea or GI upset occurs.
- Diabetic patients need to monitor urine or blood sugar closely because glucose tolerance may change; report any abnormalities to your health care provider for corrective action.
- These drugs do not enhance athletic ability but do have serious effects. They should not be used for increasing muscle strength.
- Periodic blood tests will be needed to monitor drug effects on your body.
- This drug cannot be taken during pregnancy; serious adverse effects can occur. Using barrier contraceptives is advised.
- You may experience these side effects: Nausea, vomiting, diarrhea, burning of the tongue (eat frequent small meals); body hair growth, baldness, deepening of the voice, decrease in libido, impotence (most reversible); excitation, confusion, insomnia (avoid driving, performing tasks that require alertness); swelling of the ankles, fingers (request medication).
- Report ankle swelling, skin color changes, severe nausea, vomiting, hoarseness, body hair growth, deepening of the voice, acne, menstrual irregularities.

▽ oxaprozin

*(oks a **pro'** zin)*

oxaprozin

Apo-Oxaprozin (CAN), Daypro

oxaprozin potassium

Daypro ALTA

PREGNANCY CATEGORY C

Drug classes
Analgesic (nonopioid)
Antipyretic
NSAID

Therapeutic actions
Inhibits prostaglandin synthetase to cause antipyretic and anti-inflammatory effects; the exact mechanism of action is not known.

Indications
- Acute or long-term use in the management of signs and symptoms of osteoarthritis, rheumatoid arthritis, and juvenile rheumatoid arthritis

Contraindications and cautions
- Contraindicated with significant renal impairment, lactation.
- Use cautiously with impaired hearing, allergies, hepatic, CV, and GI conditions, pregnancy.

Available forms
Caplets, tablets—600 mg; tablets—678 mg (*Daypro ALTA* equivalent to 600 mg oxaprozin)

Dosages
Adjust to the lowest effective dose to minimize side effects. Maximum daily dose, 1,800 mg or 26 mg/kg, whichever is lower. Maximum dose for *Daypro ALTA* is 1,200 mg/day.

Adults
- *Osteoarthritis:* 1,200 mg PO once daily; use initial dose of 600 mg with low body weight or milder disease.
- *Rheumatoid arthritis:* 1,200 mg PO once daily.

Pediatric patients 6–16 yr
- *Juvenile rheumatoid arthritis (non-ALTA product only):* 600–1,200 mg/day PO based on body weight.

Pharmacokinetics

Route	Onset	Peak	Duration
Oral	Varies	3–5 hr	24–36 hr
Daypro ALTA	Unknown	2 hr	Unknown

Metabolism: Hepatic; $T_{1/2}$: 42–50 hr

Distribution: Crosses placenta; enters breast milk

Excretion: Feces, urine

Adverse effects
- **CNS:** Dizziness, somnolence, insomnia, fatigue, tiredness, dizziness, tinnitus, ophthalmic effects
- **Dermatologic:** Rash, pruritus, sweating, dry mucous membranes, stomatitis
- **GI:** *Nausea, dyspepsia,* GI pain, *diarrhea,* vomiting, *constipation,* flatulence
- **GU:** Dysuria, renal impairment
- **Hematologic:** Bleeding, platelet inhibition with higher doses
- **Other:** Peripheral edema, **anaphylactoid reactions** to **anaphylactic shock**

■ Nursing considerations
Assessment
- **History:** Renal impairment; impaired hearing; allergies; hepatic, CV, and GI conditions; lactation, pregnancy
- **Physical:** Skin color and lesions; orientation, reflexes, ophthalmologic and audiometric evaluation, peripheral sensation; P, edema; R, adventitious sounds; liver evaluation; CBC, clotting times, LFTs, renal function tests; serum electrolytes, stool guaiac

O

Interventions
⊗ ***Black box warning*** Be aware that patient may be at increased risk for CV events, GI bleeding; monitor accordingly.
- Administer drug with food or after meals if GI upset occurs.
- Arrange for periodic ophthalmologic examination during long-term therapy.

⊗ ***Warning*** If overdose occurs, institute emergency procedures—gastric lavage, induction of emesis, supportive therapy.

Teaching points
- Take drug with food or meals if GI upset occurs.
- Dizziness, drowsiness can occur (avoid driving or using dangerous machinery).
- Report sore throat, fever, rash, itching, weight gain, swelling in ankles or fingers, changes in vision, black tarry stools.

oxazepam

(ox a' ze pam)

Apo-Oxazepam (CAN), Serax

PREGNANCY CATEGORY D

CONTROLLED SUBSTANCE C-IV

Drug classes

Anxiolytic
Benzodiazepine

Therapeutic actions

Exact mechanisms not understood; acts mainly at subcortical levels of the CNS, leaving the cortex relatively unaffected; main sites of action may be the limbic system and reticular formation; benzodiazepines potentiate the effects of GABA, an inhibitory neurotransmitter; anxiolytic effects occur at doses well below those needed to cause sedation, ataxia.

Indications

- Management of anxiety disorders or for short-term relief of symptoms of anxiety; anxiety associated with depression also is responsive
- Management of anxiety, tension, agitation, and irritability in older patients
- Alcoholics with acute tremulousness, inebriation, or anxiety associated with alcohol withdrawal

Contraindications and cautions

- Contraindicated with hypersensitivity to benzodiazepines, tartrazine (in the tablets); psychoses; acute narrow-angle glaucoma; shock; coma; acute alcoholic intoxication with depression of vital signs; pregnancy (risk of congenital malformations, neonatal withdrawal syndrome); labor and delivery ("floppy infant" syndrome); lactation (may cause infants to become lethargic and lose weight).
- Use cautiously with impaired liver or renal function, debilitation.

Available forms

Capsules—10, 15, 30 mg

Dosages

Increase dosage gradually to avoid adverse effects.

Adults

10–15 mg PO or up to 30 mg PO tid–qid, depending on severity of symptoms of anxiety. The higher dosage range is recommended in alcoholics.

Pediatric patients 6–12 yr

Dosage not established.

Geriatric patients or patients with debilitating disease

Initially, 10 mg PO tid. Gradually increase to 15 mg PO tid–qid if needed and tolerated.

Pharmacokinetics

Route	*Onset*	*Peak*
Oral	Slow	2–4 hr

Metabolism: Hepatic; $T_{1/2}$: 5–20 hr
Distribution: Crosses placenta; enters breast milk
Excretion: Urine

Adverse effects

- **CNS:** *Transient, mild drowsiness* (initially), *sedation, depression, lethargy, apathy, fatigue, light-headedness, disorientation,* restlessness, confusion, crying, delirium, headache, slurred speech, dysarthria, stupor, rigidity, tremor, dystonia, vertigo, euphoria, nervousness, difficulty in concentration, vivid dreams, psychomotor retardation, extrapyramidal symptoms, mild paradoxical excitatory reactions during first 2 wk of treatment, visual and auditory disturbances, diplopia, nystagmus, depressed hearing
- **CV:** Bradycardia, tachycardia, **CV collapse,** hypertension and hypotension, palpitations, edema
- **Dermatologic:** Urticaria, pruritus, rash, dermatitis
- **GI:** *Constipation, diarrhea, dry mouth,* salivation, nausea, anorexia, vomiting, difficulty in swallowing, gastric disorders
- **GU:** *Incontinence, urinary retention,* changes in libido, menstrual irregularities
- **Hematologic:** Elevations of blood enzymes, hepatic impairment, blood dyscrasias: Agranulocytosis, leukopenia

- **Other:** *Nasal congestion, hiccups, fever, diaphoresis,* paresthesias, muscular disturbances, gynecomastia, drug dependence with withdrawal syndrome when drug is discontinued (more common with abrupt discontinuation of higher dosage used for longer than 4 mo)

Interactions

✱ **Drug-drug** • Increased CNS depression with alcohol or other CNS depressants • Decreased sedation when given to heavy smokers of cigarettes or if taken concurrently with theophyllines

■ Nursing considerations

Assessment

- **History:** Hypersensitivity to benzodiazepines, tartrazine; psychoses; acute narrow-angle glaucoma; shock; coma; acute alcoholic intoxication; pregnancy; labor and delivery; lactation; impaired liver or renal function, debilitation
- **Physical:** Skin color, lesions; T; orientation, reflexes, affect, ophthalmologic examination; P, BP; R, adventitious sounds; liver evaluation, abdominal examination, bowel sounds, normal output; CBC, LFTs, renal function tests

Interventions

⊗ ***Warning*** Taper dosage gradually after long-term therapy, especially in patients with epilepsy.

Teaching points

- Take this drug exactly as prescribed; do not stop taking drug (during long-term therapy) without consulting health care provider.
- You may experience these side effects: Drowsiness, dizziness (may lessen; avoid driving or engaging in other dangerous activities); GI upset (take with food); depression, dreams, emotional upset, crying.
- Report severe dizziness, weakness, drowsiness that persists, palpitations, swelling of the extremities, visual changes, difficulty voiding, rash or skin lesion.

▽ oxcarbazepine

*(oks car **baz'** e peen)*

Trileptal

PREGNANCY CATEGORY C

Drug class

Antiepileptic

Therapeutic actions

Mechanism of action not understood; antiepileptic activity may be related to its ability to block voltage-sensitive sodium channels, increase potassium conductance, and affect high-voltage activated calcium channels, leading to enhanced membrane stability.

Indications

- As monotherapy or adjunct therapy in the treatment of partial seizures in adults and children 4 yr and older
- Adjunct therapy for children 2 yr and older with epilepsy
- Unlabeled use: Alternative treatment of bipolar disorder, diabetic neuropathy

Contraindications and cautions

- Contraindicated with hypersensitivity to carbamazepine or oxcarbazepine; lactation.
- Use cautiously in the elderly and with hyponatremia, renal or hepatic impairment, pregnancy.

Available forms

Tablets—150, 300, 600 mg; suspension—60 mg/mL

Dosages

Adults

- *Adjunctive therapy:* 300 mg PO bid, may be increased to a total of 1,200 mg PO bid if clinically needed.
- *Conversion to monotherapy:* 300 mg PO bid started while reducing the dose of other antiepileptics; other drugs should be reduced over 3–6 wk while increasing oxcarbazepine over 2–4 wk to maximum of 2,400 mg/day (in divided doses).

- *Starting as monotherapy:* Start with 300 mg PO bid and increase by 300 mg/day every third day until the desired dose of 1,200 mg/day is reached. Some patients may benefit from doses as high as 2,400 mg/day but should be carefully monitored.

Pediatric patients 2–16 yr

- *Adjunctive therapy*

  4–16 yr: 8–10 mg/kg/day PO given in two equally divided doses not to exceed 600 mg/day. Achieve the target dose over 2 wk. Suggested target dosages follow:

Weight (kg)	*Dosage (mg/day)*
20–29	900
29.1–39	1,200
More than 39	1,800

  2–4 yr and more than 20 kg: 8–10 mg/kg/day PO not to exceed 600 mg/day.
  2–4 yr and less than 20 kg: 16–20 mg/kg/day PO not to exceed 600 mg/day.
- *Monotherapy for partial seizures in epileptic children 4–16 yr:* 8–10 mg/kg/day PO in two divided doses. If the patient is taking another antiepileptic, slowly withdraw that drug over 3–6 wk. Then, increase the oxcarbazepine in 10 mg/kg/day increments at weekly intervals to the desired level. If the patient is not taking another antiepileptic, increase the dose by 5 mg/kg/day every third day to the recommended dosage. Recommended dosages by weight:

Weight (kg)	*Dosage (mg/day)*
20	600–900
25–30	900–1,200
35–40	900–1,500
45	1,200–1,500
50–55	1,200–1,800
60–65	1,200–2,100
70 or more	1,500–2,100

Geriatric patients or patients with renal impairment

Use caution, drug may cause confusion, agitation. For creatinine clearance less than 30 mL/min, initiate dosage at one-half the usual starting dose for the indication; increase slowly until desired clinical response is seen; monitor patient carefully.

Pharmacokinetics

Route	*Onset*	*Peak*
Oral	Slow	4–5 hr

Metabolism: Hepatic; $T_{1/2}$: 2 hr, then 9 hr
Distribution: Crosses placenta; enters breast milk
Excretion: Feces, urine

Adverse effects

- **CNS:** *Dizziness, drowsiness, unsteadiness,* disturbance of coordination, confusion, headache, fatigue, visual hallucinations, depression with agitation, behavioral changes in children, suicidal ideation
- **CV:** *Hypotension, hypertension, bradycardia, tachycardia,* atrial fibrillation
- **GI:** *Nausea, vomiting,* gastric distress, abdominal pain, diarrhea, increased liver enzymes
- **GU:** *Impaired fertility,* hematuria, dysuria, priapism, renal calculi
- **Metabolic and nutritional:** Respiratory acidosis, hyperkalemia, *hyponatremia,* thirst
- **Respiratory: Pulmonary edema,** pleural effusion, hypoventilation, *hypoxia,* dyspnea, **bronchospasm**
- **Other:** Fever, hypovolemia, sweating, rigors, acne, alopecia, anaphylactic reactions, angioedema

Interactions

✱ **Drug-drug** • Possible decreased oxcarbazepine effectiveness if combined with phenytoin, carbamazepine, phenobarbital, valproic acid, verapamil; if these combinations are used, monitor patient closely • Decreased effectiveness of felodipine if combined with oxcarbazepine • Decreased effectiveness of hormonal contraceptives if combined with oxcarbazepine; suggest the use of barrier contraceptives if this combination is used • Increased serum levels and risk of toxicity of phenytoin, phenobarbital; if this combination is used, monitor patient closely for signs of toxicity and arrange to decrease drug dosage as needed • Possible increased sedation if combined with alcohol; avoid this combination

■ Nursing considerations
Assessment
- **History:** Hypersensitivity to carbamazepine or oxcarbazepine; hyponatremia; serious dermatologic reactions; renal or hepatic impairment; pregnancy, lactation
- **Physical:** T; skin color, lesions; orientation, affect, reflexes; P, BP, perfusion; ECG; R, adventitious sounds; bowel sounds, normal output; normal urinary output, voiding pattern; LFTs, renal function tests; serum sodium

Interventions
⊗ ***Warning*** Monitor serum sodium prior to and periodically during therapy with oxcarbazepine; serious hyponatremia can occur. Signs and symptoms of hyponatremia include nausea, malaise, headache, lethargy, confusion, and decreased sensation.
- Investigate if patient has a history of hypersensitivity to carbamazepine. Stop drug if signs or symptoms of hypersensitivity occur.
- Give drug with food or milk to prevent GI upset. Arrange for patient to have small, frequent meals if GI upset occurs.

⊗ ***Warning*** Arrange to reduce dosage or discontinue oxcarbazepine, or substitute other antiepileptic, gradually. Abrupt discontinuation of antiepileptic may precipitate status epilepticus.
- Monitor patient carefully when converting to monotherapy from combined therapy or when adding oxcarbazepine to an established regimen.
- Monitor patient for changes in behavior, depression, suicidality.
- Ensure ready access to bathroom facilities if GI effects occur.
- Establish safety precautions if CNS changes occur (use side rails, accompany patient when ambulating).
- Arrange for appropriate counseling for women of childbearing age who wish to become pregnant; using barrier contraceptives is recommended while using this drug.
- Offer support and encouragement for dealing with epilepsy and adverse drug effects; arrange for consultation with support groups for patients with epilepsy as needed.

Teaching points
- Take this drug exactly as prescribed.
- Do not discontinue this drug abruptly or change dosage, except on the advice of your health care provider.
- Avoid the use of alcohol, sleep-inducing, or over-the-counter drugs while you are using this drug; these could cause dangerous effects. If you think that you need one of these preparations, consult your health care provider.
- Use only barrier contraceptives; if you wish to become pregnant while you are taking this drug, you should consult your health care provider. Hormonal contraceptives may be ineffective.
- Blood tests to measure your blood sodium levels will be needed periodically while you are using this drug.
- Wear or carry a medical alert tag at all times so that any emergency medical personnel taking care of you will know that you have epilepsy and are taking antiepileptic medication.
- You may experience these side effects: Drowsiness, dizziness, blurred vision (avoid driving a car or performing other tasks requiring alertness or visual acuity if this occurs); GI upset (take the drug with food or milk and eat frequent small meals).
- Report bruising, unusual bleeding, abdominal pain, yellowing of the skin or eyes, pale-colored feces, darkened urine, impotence, severe central nervous system disturbances, edema, fever, chills, thirst, pregnancy, thoughts of suicide.

O

▽ oxybutynin chloride
(ox i ***byoo'*** *ti nin)*

Apo-Oxybutynin (CAN), Ditropan XL (DNC), Gelnique, Gen-Oxybutynin (CAN), Oxytrol, PMS-Oxybutynin (CAN)

PREGNANCY CATEGORY B

Drug classes
Anticholinergic
Urinary antispasmodic

Therapeutic actions
Acts directly to relax smooth muscle and inhibits the effects of acetylcholine at muscarinic

receptors; reported to be less potent an anticholinergic than atropine but more potent as antispasmodic and devoid of antinicotinic activity at skeletal neuromuscular junctions or autonomic ganglia.

Indications

- Relief of symptoms of bladder instability associated with voiding in patients with uninhibited neurogenic and reflex neurogenic bladder
- ER tablets: Treatment of signs and symptoms of overactive bladder (incontinence, urgency, frequency); treatment of pediatric patients 6 yr and older with symptoms of detrusor overactivity associated with a neurological condition, such as spina bifida (*Ditropan XL*)

Contraindications and cautions

- Contraindicated with allergy to oxybutynin, pyloric or duodenal obstruction, obstructive intestinal lesions or ileus, intestinal atony, megacolon, colitis, obstructive uropathies, glaucoma, myasthenia gravis, CV instability in acute hemorrhage, urinary retention.
- Use cautiously with hepatic, renal impairment; pregnancy; lactation.

Available forms

Tablets—5 mg; syrup—5 mg/5 mL; ER tablets DNC—5, 10, 15 mg; transdermal patch—3.9 mg/day; topical gel—100 mg/mL

Dosages

Adults

5 mg PO bid or tid. Maximum dose is 5 mg qid. ER tablets—5 mg PO daily, up to a maximum of 30 mg/day; transdermal patch—1 patch applied to dry, intact skin on the abdomen, hip, or buttock every 3–4 days (twice weekly); topical gel—apply 1 mL to thigh, abdomen, or upper arm once every 24 hr.

Pediatric patients older than 5 yr

5 mg PO bid. Maximum dose is 5 mg tid.

Pediatric patients older than 6 yr

ER tablets: 5 mg PO daily. Dosage may be adjusted in 5-mg increments up to maximum of 20 mg/day.

Impaired geriatric patients

2.5 mg PO bid or tid.

Pharmacokinetics

Route	*Onset*	*Peak*	*Duration*
Oral	30–60 min	3–6 hr	6–10 hr
Transdermal	24–48 hr	Varies	96 hr

Metabolism: Hepatic; $T_{1/2}$: Unknown
Distribution: Crosses placenta; may enter breast milk
Excretion: Urine

Adverse effects

- **CNS:** *Drowsiness, dizziness, blurred vision,* dilatation of the pupil, cycloplegia, increased ocular tension, weakness, headache
- **CV:** Tachycardia, palpitations, hypertension
- **GI:** *Dry mouth, nausea,* vomiting, constipation, bloated feeling
- **GU:** *Urinary hesitancy,* retention, impotence
- **Hypersensitivity:** Allergic reactions including urticaria, dermal effect
- **Other:** *Decreased sweating,* heat prostration in high environmental temperatures secondary to loss of sweating

Interactions

✱ **Drug-drug** • Decreased effectiveness of phenothiazines with oxybutynin • Decreased effectiveness of haloperidol and development of tardive dyskinesia • Increased toxicity if combined with amantadine, nitrofurantoin

■ Nursing considerations

Assessment

- **History:** Allergy to oxybutynin, intestinal obstructions or lesions, intestinal atony, obstructive uropathies, glaucoma, myasthenia gravis, CV instability in acute hemorrhage, hepatic or renal impairment, pregnancy, lactation
- **Physical:** Skin color, lesions; T; orientation, affect, reflexes; ophthalmologic examination, ocular pressure measurement; P, rhythm, BP; bowel sounds, liver evaluation; LFTs, renal function tests, cystometry

Interventions

- Arrange for cystometry and other diagnostic tests before and during treatment.
- Arrange for ophthalmologic examination before therapy and periodically during therapy.

- Do not cut, crush, or allow patient to chew ER tablets.

Teaching points

- Take this drug as prescribed; do not cut, crush, or chew ER tablets.
- If using the transdermal patch, apply to dry, intact skin on the abdomen, hip, or buttock every 3–4 days (twice weekly). Remove the old system before applying a new one. Select a new site for application of each new system.
- If using the topical gel, apply 1 mL to thigh, abdomen, or upper arm once every 24 hours. Rotate application sites.
- Periodic bladder examinations will be needed during this treatment to evaluate therapeutic response.
- You may experience these side effects: Dry mouth (suck sugarless lozenges and use frequent mouth care); GI upset; blurred vision; drowsiness (avoid driving or performing tasks that require alertness); decreased sweating (avoid high temperatures; serious complications can occur because you will be heat intolerant).
- Report blurred vision, fever, rash, nausea, vomiting.

DANGEROUS DRUG

oxycodone hydrochloride

*(ox i **koe'** done)*

ETH-Oxydose, M-oxy, OxyContin (DNC), OxyFAST, OxyIR, Roxicodone, Roxicodone Intensol, Supeudol (CAN)

PREGNANCY CATEGORY B

CONTROLLED SUBSTANCE C-II

Drug class

Opioid agonist analgesic

Therapeutic actions

Acts as agonist at specific opioid receptors in the CNS to produce analgesia, euphoria, sedation; the receptors mediating these effects are thought to be the same as those mediating the effects of endogenous opioids (enkephalins, endorphins).

Indications

- Relief of moderate to moderately severe pain
- CR tablets: Management of moderate to severe pain when a continuous, around-the-clock analgesic is needed for an extended period of time

Contraindications and cautions

- Contraindicated with hypersensitivity to opioids; diarrhea caused by poisoning (before toxins are eliminated); pregnancy (readily crosses placenta; neonatal withdrawal); labor or delivery (opioids given to the mother can cause respiratory depression in neonate; premature infants are at special risk; may prolong labor); bronchial asthma, COPD, cor pulmonale, respiratory depression, anoxia; kyphoscoliosis; acute alcoholism, increased intracranial pressure, lactation.
- Use cautiously with acute abdominal conditions, CV disease, supraventricular tachycardias, myxedema, seizure disorders, delirium tremens, cerebral arteriosclerosis, ulcerative colitis, fever, Addison's disease, prostatic hypertrophy, urethral stricture, recent GI or GU surgery, toxic psychosis, renal or hepatic impairment.

Available forms

Immediate-release capsules—5 mg; immediate-release tablets—5, 10, 15, 20, 30 mg; CR tablets (DNC)—10, 15, 20, 30, 40, 60, 80, 160 mg; oral solution—5 mg/5 mL; solution concentrate—20 mg/mL

Dosages

Individualize dosage.

Adults

5 mg PO every 6 hr. *OxyIR, OxyFAST,* 5 mg every 3–6 hr. CR (*OxyContin*), 10–20 mg PO every 12 hr.

- *Breakthrough pain:* Immediate-release (*OxyIR*): 5 mg PO every 4 hr.

Pediatric patients

CR is not recommended for pediatric patients. Regular and immediate-release dosage should be individualized based on patient's age and size.

Geriatric patients or impaired adults

Use caution. Respiratory depression may occur in the elderly, the very ill, or those with respiratory problems.

O

Pharmacokinetics

Route	Onset	Peak	Duration
Oral	15–30 min	1 hr	4–6 hr

Metabolism: Hepatic; $T_{1/2}$: 2–3 hr
Distribution: Crosses placenta; enters breast milk
Excretion: Urine

Adverse effects

- **CNS:** *Light-headedness, dizziness, sedation,* euphoria, dysphoria, delirium, insomnia, agitation, anxiety, fear, hallucinations, disorientation, drowsiness, lethargy, impaired mental and physical performance, coma, mood changes, weakness, headache, tremor, seizures, miosis, visual disturbances
- **CV:** Facial flushing, peripheral circulatory collapse, tachycardia, bradycardia, arrhythmia, palpitations, chest wall rigidity, hypertension, hypotension, orthostatic hypotension, syncope, circulatory depression, **shock, cardiac arrest**
- **Dermatologic:** Pruritus, urticaria, edema, hemorrhagic urticaria (rare)
- **GI:** *Nausea, vomiting, sweating* (more common in ambulatory patients and those without severe pain), dry mouth, anorexia, constipation, biliary tract spasm; increased colonic motility in patients with chronic ulcerative colitis
- **GU:** Ureteral spasm, spasm of vesical sphincters, urinary retention or hesitancy, oliguria, antidiuretic effect, reduced libido or potency
- **Respiratory:** Suppression of cough reflex, respiratory depression, apnea, **respiratory arrest, laryngospasm, bronchospasm**
- **Other:** Physical tolerance and dependence, psychological dependence

Interactions

✱ **Drug-drug** • Increased likelihood of respiratory depression, hypotension, profound sedation or coma in patients receiving barbiturate general anesthetics, protease inhibitors

✱ **Drug-lab test** • Elevated biliary tract pressure may cause increases in plasma amylase, lipase; determinations for 24 hr after administration

■ Nursing considerations

Assessment

- **History:** Hypersensitivity to opioids, diarrhea caused by poisoning, pregnancy, labor or delivery, bronchial asthma, COPD, cor pulmonale, respiratory depression, kyphoscoliosis, acute alcoholism, increased intracranial pressure, acute abdominal conditions, CV disease, myxedema, seizure disorders, cerebral arteriosclerosis, ulcerative colitis, fever, Addison's disease, prostatic hypertrophy, urethral stricture, recent GI or GU surgery, toxic psychosis, renal or hepatic impairment, lactation
- **Physical:** T; skin color, texture, lesions; orientation, reflexes, bilateral grip strength, affect, pupil size; P, auscultation, BP, orthostatic BP, perfusion; R, adventitious sounds; bowel sounds, normal output; frequency and pattern of voiding, normal output; ECG; EEG; LFTs, renal and thyroid function tests

Interventions

- Administer to nursing women 4–6 hr before the next feeding to minimize amount in milk.
- Do not crush, break, or allow patient to chew CR preparations.
- Administer immediate-release preparations to cover breakthrough pain.

⊗ ***Black box warning*** *OxyFAST* and *Roxicodone Intensol* are highly concentrated preparations. Use extreme care.

⊗ ***Black box warning*** Be aware that this drug has abuse potential, and monitor patients accordingly.

⊗ ***Warning*** Keep opioid antagonist and facilities for assisted or controlled respiration readily available during parenteral administration.

- Reassure patient that addiction is unlikely; most patients who receive opiates for medical reasons do not develop dependence syndromes.

Teaching points

- Take drug exactly as prescribed. Do not crush, break, or chew controlled-release preparations.

- Do not take any leftover medication for other disorders, and do not let anyone else take the prescription.
- You may experience these side effects: Nausea, loss of appetite (take with food; lie quietly; eat frequent small meals); constipation (use a laxative); dizziness, sedation, drowsiness, impaired visual acuity (avoid driving, performing other tasks that require alertness, visual acuity).
- Report severe nausea, vomiting, constipation, shortness of breath, or difficulty breathing.

oxymetazoline

(ox i met az' oh leen)

Afrin No Drip 12-Hour, Afrin Severe Congestion with Menthol, Afrin 12-Hour Original, Afrin 12-Hour Original Pump Mist, Dristan 12 Hr Nasal, Duramist Plus, Genasal, Nasal Relief, Neo-Synephrine 12 Hour Extra Moisturizing, Nostrilla, 12-hour Nasal, Vicks Sinex 12-Hour Long Acting

PREGNANCY CATEGORY C

Drug class

Nasal decongestant

Therapeutic actions

Acts directly on alpha receptors to produce vasoconstriction of arterioles in nasal passages, which produces a decongestant response; no effect on beta receptors.

Indications

- Topical: Symptomatic relief of nasal and nasopharyngeal mucosal congestion due to colds, hay fever, or other respiratory allergies

Contraindications and cautions

- Contraindicated with allergy to oxymetazoline, angle-closure glaucoma, anesthesia with cyclopropane or halothane, thyrotoxicosis, diabetes, hypertension, CV disorders, women in labor whose BP exceeds 130/80.
- Use cautiously with angina, arrhythmias, prostatic hypertrophy, unstable vasomotor syndrome, lactation.

Available forms

Nasal spray or solution—0.05%

Dosages

Adults and patients older than 6 yr

Two to three sprays of 0.05% solution in each nostril bid morning and evening or every 10–12 hr for up to 3 days.

Pharmacokinetics

Route	*Onset*	*Duration*
Nasal	5–10 min	6–10 hr

Metabolism: Hepatic; $T_{1/2}$: Unknown
Distribution: Crosses placenta; may enter breast milk
Excretion: Urine

Adverse effects

Systemic effects are less likely with topical administration than with systemic administration, but because systemic absorption can take place, the systemic effects should be considered:

- **CNS:** *Fear, anxiety, tenseness, restlessness, headache, light-headedness, dizziness,* drowsiness, tremor, insomnia, hallucinations, psychological disturbances, seizures, CNS depression, weakness, blurred vision, ocular irritation, tearing, photophobia, symptoms of paranoid schizophrenia
- **CV:** Arrhythmias, hypertension resulting in intracranial hemorrhage, **CV collapse** with hypotension, palpitations, tachycardia, precordial pain in patients with ischemic heart disease
- **GI:** *Nausea,* vomiting, anorexia
- **GU:** Constriction of renal blood vessels, *dysuria, vesical sphincter spasm* resulting in difficult and painful urination, urinary retention with prostatism
- **Local:** *Rebound congestion* with topical nasal application
- **Other:** *Pallor,* respiratory difficulty, orofacial dystonia, sweating

Interactions

✱ **Drug-drug** • Severe hypertension with MAOIs, TCAs • Additive effects and increased risk of toxicity if taken with urinary alkalinizers • Decreased vasopressor response with reserpine, methyldopa, urinary acidifiers

■ Nursing considerations

Assessment

- **History:** Allergy to oxymetazoline; angle-closure glaucoma; anesthesia with cyclopropane or halothane; thyrotoxicosis, diabetes, hypertension, CV disorders; prostatic hypertrophy, unstable vasomotor syndrome; lactation, pregnancy
- **Physical:** Skin color, T; orientation, reflexes, peripheral sensation, vision; P, BP, auscultation, peripheral perfusion; R, adventitious sounds; urinary output pattern, bladder percussion, prostate palpation; nasal mucous membrane evaluation

Interventions

⊗ ***Warning*** Monitor CV effects carefully; patients with hypertension may experience changes in BP because of the additional vasoconstriction. If a nasal decongestant is needed, pseudoephedrine is the drug of choice.

Teaching points

- Do not exceed recommended dose. Use proper administration technique for topical nasal application. Avoid prolonged use because underlying medical problems can be disguised. Do not use longer than 3 days.
- Rebound congestion may occur when this drug is stopped; drink plenty of fluids, use a humidifier, and avoid smoke-filled areas to help decrease problems.
- You may experience these side effects: Dizziness, tremor, weakness, restlessness, lightheadedness (avoid driving or operating dangerous equipment); urinary retention (void before taking drug).
- Report nervousness, palpitations, sleeplessness, sweating.

▽ oxymetholone

(ox i ***meth'*** *oh lone)*

Anadrol-50

PREGNANCY CATEGORY X

CONTROLLED SUBSTANCE C-III

Drug classes

Anabolic steroid
Hormone

Therapeutic actions

Testosterone analogue with androgenic and anabolic activity; promotes body tissue-building processes and reverses catabolic or tissue-depleting processes; increases Hgb and red cell mass.

Indications

- Anemias caused by deficient red cell production
- Acquired or congenital aplastic anemia
- Myelofibrosis and hypoplastic anemias due to myelotoxic drugs
- Unlabeled use: HIV-associated wasting

Contraindications and cautions

- Contraindicated with known sensitivity to oxymetholone or anabolic steroids, prostate or breast cancer, BPH, pituitary insufficiency, MI, nephrosis, liver disease, hypercalcemia, pregnancy, lactation.
- Use cautiously with diabetes; seizure disorders; migraines; hepatic, cardiac, or renal disease; HF.

Available forms

Tablets—50 mg

Dosages

Adults and children

1–5 mg/kg/day PO. Usual effective dose is 1–2 mg/kg/day. Give for a minimum trial of 3–6 mo. Following remission, patients may be maintained without the drug or on a lower daily dose. Continuous therapy is usually needed in cases of congenital aplastic anemia.

Pediatric patients

Use with extreme caution due to risk of serious disruption of growth and development; weigh benefits and risks.

Pharmacokinetics

Route	*Onset*
Oral	Rapid

Metabolism: Hepatic; $T_{1/2}$: 9 hr

Distribution: Crosses placenta; enters breast milk
Excretion: Urine

Adverse effects

- **CNS:** *Excitation, insomnia,* chills, toxic confusion
- **Endocrine:** *Virilization: Prepubertal males*—phallic enlargement, hirsutism, increased skin pigmentation; *postpubertal males*—inhibition of testicular function, gynecomastia, testicular atrophy, priapism, baldness, epididymitis, change in libido; *females*—hirsutism, hoarseness, deepening of the voice, clitoral enlargement, menstrual irregularities, baldness; decreased glucose tolerance
- **GI:** Hepatotoxicity, peliosis, **hepatitis with liver failure or intra-abdominal hemorrhage; liver cell tumors,** sometimes malignant and fatal, *nausea, vomiting, diarrhea, abdominal fullness, loss of appetite, burning of tongue*
- **GU:** Possible increased risk of prostatic hypertrophy, carcinoma in geriatric patients
- **Hematologic:** *Blood lipid changes:* Decreased HDL and sometimes increased LDL; iron deficiency anemia; hypercalcemia; altered serum cholesterol levels; *retention of sodium, chloride, water,* potassium, phosphates, and calcium
- **Other:** *Acne,* premature closure of the epiphyses, edema

Interactions

✱ **Drug-drug** • Potentiation of oral anticoagulants with anabolic steroids • Decreased need for insulin, oral hypoglycemia drugs
✱ **Drug-lab test** • Altered glucose tolerance tests • Decrease in thyroid function tests, which may persist for 2–3 wk after therapy • Increased creatinine, decreased creatinine clearance, which may last for 2 wk after therapy

■ Nursing considerations

Assessment

- **History:** Known sensitivity to oxymetholone or anabolic steroids; prostate or breast cancer; BPH; pituitary insufficiency; MI; nephrosis; liver disease; hypercalcemia; pregnancy; lactation, HF; cardiac, renal, or hepatic disease; migraines; seizures; diabetes
- **Physical:** Skin color, texture; hair distribution pattern; affect, orientation; abdominal examination, liver evaluation; serum electrolytes and cholesterol levels, glucose tolerance tests, thyroid function tests, long-bone X-ray (in children)

Interventions

- Administer with food if GI upset or nausea occurs.

⊗ ***Warning*** Monitor effect on children with long-bone X-rays every 3–6 mo; discontinue drug well before the bone age reaches the norm for the patient's chronologic age because effects may continue for 6 mo after therapy.

- Monitor for edema; arrange for diuretic therapy as needed.

⊠ ***Black box warning*** Monitor liver function, serum electrolytes during therapy, and consult with physician for corrective measures; peliosis hepatis, liver cell tumors can occur.

⊠ ***Black box warning*** Measure cholesterol levels in patients who are at high risk for CAD; lipid levels may increase.

- Caution patients that this drug cannot be used during pregnancy; advise patient to use barrier contraceptives.
- Monitor patients with diabetes closely because glucose tolerance may change. Adjust insulin, oral hypoglycemic dosage, and diet.

Teaching points

- Take with food if nausea or GI upset occurs.
- Patients with diabetes need to monitor urine sugar closely because glucose tolerance may change; report any abnormalities to your health care provider, so corrective action can be taken.
- This drug cannot be taken during pregnancy; use barrier contraceptives while using this drug.
- These drugs do not enhance athletic ability but do have serious effects and should not be used for increasing muscle strength.
- You may experience these side effects: Nausea, vomiting, diarrhea, burning of the tongue (eat frequent small meals); body hair

growth, baldness, deepening of the voice, decrease in libido, impotence (most reversible); excitation, confusion, insomnia (avoid driving, performing tasks that require alertness); swelling of the ankles, fingers (request medication).
- Report ankle swelling, skin color changes, severe nausea, vomiting, hoarseness, body hair growth, deepening of the voice, acne, menstrual irregularities in women.

DANGEROUS DRUG

oxymorphone hydrochloride

(ox i mor' fone)

Opana, Opana ER (DNC)

PREGNANCY CATEGORY C

CONTROLLED SUBSTANCE C-II

Drug class

Opioid agonist analgesic

Therapeutic actions

Acts as agonist at specific opioid receptors in the CNS to produce analgesia, euphoria, sedation; the receptors mediating these effects are thought to be the same as those mediating the effects of endogenous opioids (enkephalins, endorphins).

Indications

- Relief of moderate to moderately severe acute pain (immediate-release form)
- Parenterally (injection only) for preoperative medication, support of anesthesia, obstetric analgesia
- Relief of moderate to severe pain in patients who need around-the-clock opioid treatment for extended time (ER form)
- Relief of anxiety in patients with pulmonary edema associated with left ventricular dysfunction (parenteral)
- Relief of moderate to severe pain

Contraindications and cautions

- Contraindicated with hypersensitivity to opioids, diarrhea caused by poisoning (before toxins are eliminated), pregnancy (readily crosses placenta; neonatal withdrawal), labor or delivery (opioids given to the mother can cause respiratory depression of neonate; premature infants are at special risk; may prolong labor), bronchial asthma, COPD, cor pulmonale, respiratory depression, anoxia, kyphoscoliosis, acute alcoholism, increased intracranial pressure, lactation.
- Use cautiously with acute abdominal conditions, CV disease, supraventricular tachycardias, myxedema, seizure disorders, delirium tremens, cerebral arteriosclerosis, ulcerative colitis, fever, Addison's disease, prostatic hypertrophy, urethral stricture, recent GI or GU surgery, toxic psychosis, renal or hepatic impairment.

Available forms

Injection—1 mg/mL; tablets—5, 10 mg; ER tablets (DNC)—5, 7.5, 10, 15, 20, 30, 40 mg

Dosages

Adults

Oral

For immediate-release form, 10–20 mg PO every 4–6 hr. For ER tablets, 5 mg PO every 12 hr; may be increased in 5- to 10-mg increments every 3–7 days to cover pain.

IV

Initially, 0.5 mg.

Subcutaneous or IM

Initially, 1–1.5 mg every 4–6 hr as needed. For analgesia during labor, 0.5–1 mg IM.

Pediatric patients

Safety and efficacy not established for children younger than 12 yr.

Geriatric patients or impaired adults

Use caution; respiratory depression may occur in the elderly, the very ill, and those with respiratory problems.

Pharmacokinetics

Route	*Onset*	*Peak*	*Duration*
Oral (ER)	15–30 min	60 min	8–10 hr
Oral (immediate-release)	5–10 min	1 hr	3–6 hr
IV	5–10 min	15–60 min	3–6 hr
IM, Subcut.	10–15 min	30–60 min	3–6 hr

Metabolism: Hepatic; $T_{1/2}$: 7–9 hr
Distribution: Crosses placenta; enters breast milk
Excretion: Urine

IV FACTS

Preparation: No further preparation needed.
Infusion: Inject slowly over 5 min directly into vein or into tubing of running IV.

Adverse effects

- **CNS:** *Light-headedness, dizziness, sedation,* euphoria, dysphoria, delirium, insomnia, agitation, anxiety, fear, hallucinations, disorientation, drowsiness, lethargy, impaired mental and physical performance, coma, mood changes, weakness, headache, tremor, seizures, miosis, visual disturbances
- **CV:** Facial flushing, peripheral circulatory collapse, tachycardia, bradycardia, arrhythmia, palpitations, chest wall rigidity, hypertension, hypotension, orthostatic hypotension, syncope, circulatory depression, **shock, cardiac arrest**
- **Dermatologic:** Pruritus, urticaria, edema, hemorrhagic urticaria (rare)
- **GI:** *Nausea, vomiting, sweating* (more common in ambulatory patients and those without severe pain), dry mouth, anorexia, constipation, biliary tract spasm; increased colonic motility in patients with chronic ulcerative colitis
- **GU:** Ureteral spasm, spasm of vesical sphincters, urinary retention or hesitancy, oliguria, antidiuretic effect, reduced libido or potency
- **Local:** Pain at injection site, tissue irritation and induration (subcutaneous injection)
- **Respiratory:** Suppression of cough reflex, respiratory depression, apnea, **respiratory arrest, laryngospasm, bronchospasm**
- **Other:** Physical tolerance and dependence, psychological dependence

Interactions

✱ **Drug-drug** • Increased likelihood of respiratory depression, hypotension, profound sedation or coma in patients receiving barbiturate general anesthetics or other CNS depressants • Risk of severe increase in serum drug level and potentially fatal overdose if combined with alcohol; avoid this combination

✱ **Drug-lab test** • Elevated biliary tract pressure may cause increases in plasma amylase, lipase; determinations for 24 hr after administration of opioids

■ Nursing considerations

Assessment

- **History:** Hypersensitivity to opioids, diarrhea caused by poisoning, pregnancy, labor or delivery, bronchial asthma, COPD, cor pulmonale, respiratory depression, kyphoscoliosis, acute alcoholism, increased intracranial pressure, acute abdominal conditions, CV disease, myxedema, seizure disorders, delirium tremens, cerebral arteriosclerosis, ulcerative colitis, fever, Addison's disease, prostatic hypertrophy, urethral stricture, recent GI or GU surgery, toxic psychosis, renal or hepatic impairment
- **Physical:** T; skin color, texture, lesions; orientation, reflexes, bilateral grip strength, affect, pupil size; P, auscultation, BP, orthostatic BP, perfusion; R, adventitious sounds; bowel sounds, normal output; frequency and pattern of voiding, normal output; ECG; EEG; LFTs, renal and thyroid function tests

Interventions

⊗ ***Black box warning*** Make sure that patient swallows ER tablets whole. Cutting, crushing, or chewing them could cause rapid release and fatal overdose.

⊗ ***Black box warning*** Note that ER form has abuse potential; monitor patient accordingly. Drug is indicated only for around-the-clock use over an extended time. Drug is not to be given PRN.

⊗ ***Black box warning*** Patient must not consume alcohol in any form while taking oxycodone to avoid risk of serious increase in serum drug level and potentially fatal overdose.

⊗ ***Warning*** Keep opioid antagonist and facilities for assisted or controlled respiration readily available during parenteral administration.

⊗ ***Warning*** Use caution when injecting subcutaneously into chilled areas of the body or in patients with hypotension or in shock; impaired perfusion may delay absorption; with repeated doses, an excessive amount may be absorbed when circulation is restored.

O

- Reassure patient that addiction is unlikely; most patients who receive opiates for medical reasons do not develop dependence syndromes.
- Give to breast-feeding women 4–6 hr before the next feeding to minimize amount in milk; use is generally not advised in breast-feeding women because of risk of respiratory depression in the baby.

Teaching points

- Take this drug exactly as prescribed. If taking ER tablets, swallow them whole; do not cut, crush, or chew them.
- Do not consume alcohol or take medications that contain alcohol while taking oxycodone; doing so increases the risk of serious or fatal reactions.
- Do not take leftover medication for other disorders, and do not let anyone else take the prescription.
- You may experience these side effects: Nausea, loss of appetite (take drug with food and lie quietly; eat frequent small meals); constipation (use a laxative); dizziness, sedation, drowsiness, impaired visual acuity (avoid driving, performing other tasks that require alertness, visual acuity).
- Report severe nausea, vomiting, constipation, shortness of breath or difficulty breathing.

DANGEROUS DRUG

oxytocin

*(ox i **toe'** sin)*

Pitocin

PREGNANCY CATEGORY X

Drug classes

Hormone
Oxytocic

Therapeutic actions

Synthetic form of an endogenous hormone produced in the hypothalamus and stored in the posterior pituitary; stimulates the uterus, especially the gravid uterus just before parturition, and causes myoepithelium of the lacteal glands to contract, which results in milk ejection in lactating women.

Indications

- Antepartum: To initiate or improve uterine contractions to achieve early vaginal delivery; stimulation or reinforcement of labor in selected cases of uterine inertia; management of inevitable or incomplete abortion; second trimester abortion
- Postpartum: To produce uterine contractions during the third stage of labor and to control postpartum bleeding or hemorrhage
- Lactation deficiency
- Unlabeled uses: To evaluate fetal distress (oxytocin challenge test), treatment of breast engorgement

Contraindications and cautions

- Contraindicated with significant cephalopelvic disproportion, unfavorable fetal positions or presentations, obstetric emergencies that favor surgical intervention, prolonged use in severe toxemia, uterine inertia, hypertonic uterine patterns, induction or augmentation of labor when vaginal delivery is contraindicated, previous cesarean section, pregnancy.
- Use cautiously with renal impairment.

Available forms

Injection—10 units/mL

Dosages

Adjust dosage based on uterine response.

Adults

- *Induction or stimulation of labor:* Initial dose of no more than 0.5–2 milliunits/min (0.0005–0.002 units/min) by IV infusion through an infusion pump. Increase the dose in increments of no more than 1–2 milliunits/min at 30- to 60-min intervals until a contraction pattern similar to normal labor is established. Rates exceeding 9–10 milliunits/min are rarely required. Discontinue in event of uterine hyperactivity, fetal distress.
- *Control of postpartum uterine bleeding:*

IV

Add 10–40 units to 1,000 mL of a nonhydrating diluent, infuse at a rate to control uterine atony.

IM

Administer 10 units after delivery of the placenta.

- *Treatment of incomplete or inevitable abortion:* IV infusion of 10 units of oxytocin with 500 mL physiologic saline solution or 5% dextrose in physiologic saline infused at a rate of 10–20 milliunits (20–40 drops)/min. Do not exceed 30 units in 12 hr because of risk of water intoxication.

Pharmacokinetics

Route	Onset	Duration
IV	Immediate	60 min
IM	3–5 min	2–3 hr

Metabolism: Hepatic; $T_{1/2}$: 1–6 min
Distribution: Crosses placenta; enters breast milk
Excretion: Urine

IV FACTS

Preparation: Add 1 mL (10 units) to 1,000 mL of 0.9% aqueous sodium chloride or other IV fluid; the resulting solution will contain 10 milliunits/mL (0.01 units/mL).
Infusion: Infuse via constant infusion pump to ensure accurate control of rate; rate determined by uterine response; begin with 1–2 mL/min and increase at 15- to 60-min intervals.
Compatibilities: Compatible at a concentration of 5 units/L in dextrose–Ringer's combinations; dextrose–lactated Ringer's combinations; dextrose–saline combinations; dextrose 2%, 5%, and 10% in water; fructose 10% in water; Ringer's injection; lactated Ringer's injection; sodium chloride 0.45% and 0.9% injection; and 1/6M sodium lactate.
Incompatibilities: Do not combine in solution with fibrinolysin or heparin.

Adverse effects

- **CV:** *Cardiac arrhythmias,* PVCs, hypertension, subarachnoid hemorrhage
- **Fetal effects:** *Fetal bradycardia,* neonatal jaundice, low Apgar scores
- **GI:** *Nausea, vomiting*
- **GU:** Postpartum hemorrhage, uterine rupture, pelvic hematoma, *uterine hypertonicity,* spasm, tetanic contraction, rupture of the uterus with excessive dosage or hypersensitivity
- **Hypersensitivity: Anaphylactic reaction**
- **Other:** Maternal and fetal deaths when used to induce labor or in first or second stages of labor; **afibrinogenemia; severe water intoxication** with seizures and coma, **maternal death** (associated with slow oxytocin infusion over 24 hr; oxytocin has antidiuretic effects)

■ Nursing considerations

Assessment

- **History:** Significant cephalopelvic disproportion, unfavorable fetal positions or presentations, severe toxemia, uterine inertia, hypertonic uterine patterns, previous cesarean section
- **Physical:** Fetal heart rate (continuous monitoring is recommended); fetal positions; fetal-pelvic proportions; uterine tone; timing and rate of contractions; breast examination; orientation, reflexes; P, BP, edema; R, adventitious sounds; CBC, bleeding studies, urinary output

Interventions

⊠ ***Black box warning*** Reserve for medical use, not elective induction.

- Ensure fetal position and size and absence of complications that are contraindicated with oxytocin before therapy.

⊗ ***Warning*** Ensure continuous observation of patient receiving IV oxytocin for induction or stimulation of labor; fetal monitoring is preferred. A physician should be immediately available to deal with complications if they arise.

- Regulate rate of oxytocin delivery to establish uterine contractions that are similar to normal labor; monitor rate and strength of contractions; discontinue drug and notify physician at any sign of uterine hyperactivity or spasm.

⊗ ***Warning*** Monitor maternal BP during oxytocin administration; discontinue drug and notify physician with any sign of hypertensive emergency.

- Monitor neonate for jaundice.

Teaching points

- The patient receiving parenteral oxytocin is usually receiving it as part of an immediate

C

medical situation, and the drug teaching should be incorporated into the teaching about delivery. The patient needs to know the name of the drug and what she can expect after it is administered.

DANGEROUS DRUG

paclitaxel

(pak leh tax' ell)

Abraxane, Onxol, Taxol

PREGNANCY CATEGORY D

Drug class

Antineoplastic

Therapeutic actions

Inhibits the normal dynamic reorganization of the microtubule network that is essential for dividing cells; leads to cell death in rapidly dividing cells.

Indications

- *Onxol* and *Taxol:* Treatment of metastatic carcinoma of the ovary after failure of first-line or subsequent therapy
- *Abraxane, Onxol,* and *Taxol:* Treatment of breast cancer after failure of combination therapy
- *Taxol:* First-line treatment of non–small-cell lung cancer
- *Taxol:* Second-line treatment of AIDS-related Kaposi's sarcoma
- Unlabeled uses: Treatment of advanced head and neck cancer, previously untreated extensive-stage small-cell lung cancer, adenocarcinoma of the upper GI tract, hormone-refractory prostate cancer, leukemias

Contraindications and cautions

- Contraindicated with hypersensitivity to paclitaxel or drug formulated with polyoxethylated castor oil, bone marrow depression, severe neurologic toxicity, lactation, pregnancy.
- Use cautiously with cardiac conduction defects, severe hepatic impairment.

Available forms

Injection—6 mg/mL; powder for injection—100 mg

Dosages

Adults

- *Ovarian cancer:* In previously untreated patients, 135 mg/m^2 IV over 24 hr *or* 175 mg/m^2 IV over 3 hr every 3 wk followed by 75 mg/m^2 IV cisplatin (*Taxol* only). In previously treated patients, 135 mg/m^2 *or* 175 mg/m^2 IV over 3 hr every 3 wk. Do not repeat the IV until the neutrophil count is at least 1,500 $cells/mm^3$ and platelet count is at least 100,000 $cells/mm^3$.
- *Breast cancer:* 175 mg/m^2 IV over 3 hr every 3 wk for four courses after failure of chemotherapy (*Taxol* only); 175 mg/m^2 IV over 3 hr every 3 wk after initial chemotherapy failure or relapse within 6 mo; or 260 mg/m^2 IV over 30 min every 3 wk (*Abraxane*).
- *AIDS-related Kaposi's sarcoma:* 135 mg/m^2 IV over 3 hr every 3 wk *or* 100 mg/m^2 IV over 3 hr every 2 wk. Do not administer *Taxol* if neutrophil count is less than 1,000 cells/mm^3.
- *Non–small-cell-lung cancer:* 135 mg/m^2 IV over 24 hr followed by 75 mg/m^2 cisplatin IV every 3 wk. Reduce dose by 20% if neutrophil count is less than 500 $cells/mm^3$ for a week or longer.

Pediatric patients

Safety and efficacy not established.

Pharmacokinetics

Route	*Onset*	*Duration*
IV	Rapid	6–12 hr

Metabolism: Hepatic; $T_{1/2}$: 13–20 hr
Distribution: Crosses placenta; enters breast milk
Excretion: Bile

IV FACTS

Preparation: Use extreme caution when handling drug; dilute before infusion in 0.9% sodium chloride, 5% dextrose injection, 5% dextrose and 0.9% sodium chloride injection, 5% dextrose in Ringer's injection to a concentration of 0.3–1.2 mg/mL; stable at room temperature for 27 hr. Refrigerate unopened vials; avoid use of PVC infusion bags and tubing.
Infusion: Administer over 3 hr or 24 hr through an in-line filter not greater than 0.22 mcg. Do not use a filter with *Abraxane.*

Y-site compatibility: May be given with fluconazole.

Adverse effects

- **CNS:** Peripheral sensory neuropathy, mild to severe
- **CV:** Bradycardia, hypotension, severe CV events
- **GI:** *Nausea, vomiting,* mucositis, anorexia, elevated liver enzymes
- **Hematologic: Bone marrow depression, infection**
- **Other: Hypersensitivity reactions,** *myalgia, arthralgia, alopecia*

Interactions

✱ **Drug-drug** • Increased myelosuppression with cisplatin • Increased paclitaxel effects with ketoconazole, verapamil, diazepam, quinidine, dexamethasone, cyclosporine, teniposide, etoposide, vincristine, testosterone

■ Nursing considerations

CLINICAL ALERT!
Name confusion has occurred between *Taxol* (paclitaxel) and *Taxotere* (docetaxel). Serious adverse effects can occur; use extreme caution.

Assessment

- **History:** Hypersensitivity to paclitaxel, castor oil; bone marrow depression; cardiac conduction defects; severe hepatic impairment; pregnancy; lactation
- **Physical:** Neurologic status, T; P, BP, peripheral perfusion; skin color, texture, hair distribution; abdominal examination, mucous membranes; LFTs, renal function tests, CBC

Interventions

⊗ ***Black box warning*** Do not administer drug unless blood counts are within acceptable parameters.

⊗ ***Warning*** Handle drug with great care; gloves are recommended. If drug comes in contact with skin, wash immediately with soap and water.

⊗ ***Black box warning*** When using *Onxol* or *Taxol,* premedicate with one of the following drugs to prevent severe hypersensitivity reactions: Oral dexamethasone 20 mg, 12 hr and 6 hr before paclitaxel, 10 mg if AIDS-related Kaposi's sarcoma; diphenhydramine 50 mg IV 30–60 min before paclitaxel; and cimetidine 300 mg IV or ranitidine 50 mg IV 30–60 min before paclitaxel.

- Monitor BP and pulse during administration.
- Obtain blood counts before and at least monthly during treatment.
- Monitor patient's neurologic status frequently during treatment.
- Advise patient to avoid pregnancy; serious fetal harm can occur; advise using barrier contraceptives.

Teaching points

- This drug must be given over a 30-minute, 3-hour, or 24-hour period once every 3 weeks. Mark a calendar noting drug days.
- Have regular blood tests and neurologic examinations while receiving this drug.
- Avoid pregnancy while you are taking this drug, serious fetal harm can occur; using barrier contraceptives is advised.
- You may experience these side effects: Nausea and vomiting (if severe, request antiemetics; frequent small meals also may help); weakness, lethargy (frequent rest periods will help); increased susceptibility to infection (avoid crowds and exposure to diseases); numbness and tingling in the fingers or toes (avoid injury to these areas; use care with tasks requiring precision); loss of hair (obtain a wig or other head covering; keep the head covered at extremes of temperature).
- Report severe nausea and vomiting; fever, chills, sore throat; unusual bleeding or bruising; numbness or tingling in your fingers or toes; chest pain.

palifermin

See Appendix W, *Less commonly used drugs.*

paliperidone

*(pal ah **peer'** ah dohn)*

Invega (DNC), Invega Sustenna

PREGNANCY CATEGORY C

P

Drug classes
Atypical antipsychotic
Benzisoxazole

Therapeutic actions
Mechanism of action not completely understood; is the major active metabolite of risperidone. Blocks dopamine and serotonin receptors in the brain and depresses the RAS. Antihistaminic and alpha-adrenergic blocking activity may contribute to some therapeutic and adverse effects.

Indications
- Treatment of schizophrenia; acute and long-term maintenance treatment of schizophrenia; as monotherapy or as adjunct to mood stabilizers or antidepressants

Contraindications and cautions
- Contraindicated with hypersensitivity to any component of the drug or to risperidone, lactation, and in elderly patients with dementia-related psychosis.
- Use cautiously with prolonged QT interval and with other drugs that prolong QT interval; pregnancy; history of arrhythmias, GI disorders, seizures, hypotension; diabetes mellitus; CV disease; renal impairment; risk of aspiration; and in elderly patients.

Available forms
ER tablets (DNC)—3, 6, 9 mg; injection—39/0.25 mL, 78 mg/0.25 mL, 117 mg/0.75 mL, 156 mg/mL, 234 mg/1.5 mL

Dosages
Adults
6 mg/day PO in the morning; may be adjusted to a maximum 12 mg/day PO if warranted and tolerated by the patient. Increases of 3 mg/day at intervals of at least 5 days are suggested. Parenteral—234 mg IM, followed by 156 mg IM in 1 wk, both injections in the deltoid. 117 mg IM 1 wk later in gluteal or deltoid site. Maintenance dose—39–234 mg IM once per month in deltoid or gluteal site.

Pediatric patients
Safety and efficacy not established.

Patients with renal impairment
In mild renal impairment (creatinine clearance 50–80 mL/min), maximum dosage 6 mg/day; or 156 mg IM, followed by 117 mg IM in 1 wk (both in deltoids), then monthly injections of 78 mg IM in deltoid or gluteal site. In severe renal impairment (creatinine clearance 10–50 mL/min), maximum dosage 3 mg/day. IM route not recommended.

Pharmacokinetics

Route	*Onset*	*Peak*
Oral	Gradual	24 hr

Metabolism: Hepatic; $T_{1/2}$: 23 hr
Distribution: Crosses placenta; enters breast milk
Excretion: Urine

Adverse effects
- **CNS:** *Headache, dizziness, akathisia, somnolence,* dystonia, *extrapyramidal disorders,* hypertonia, tremor, *parkinsonism,* anxiety, blurred vision, tardive dyskinesia
- **CV:** *Tachycardia,* arrhythmia, palpitations, hypotension, *orthostatic hypotension,* prolonged QT interval
- **GI:** Dyspepsia, nausea, dry mouth, salivary hypersecretion
- **Respiratory:** Cough
- **Other:** Fever, fatigue, pain, **increased mortality in geriatric patients with dementia-related psychosis, neuroleptic malignant syndrome,** hyperglycemia, hyperprolactinemia

Interactions
✱ **Drug-drug** • Risk of increased CNS depression if combined with alcohol and other central-acting depressants; use caution if this combination cannot be avoided • Potential for decreased effectiveness of levodopa or dopamine agonist; monitor patient closely and adjust dosage as needed • Risk of severe orthostatic hypotension if combined with other drugs that cause orthostatic hypotension; monitor patient closely and adjust dosage as needed

■ Nursing considerations
Assessment
- **History:** Hypersensitivity to any component of paliperidone or risperidone; pregnancy; lactation; dementia-related psychosis

in elderly patients; prolonged QT interval or use of other drugs known to prolong it; history of arrhythmias, GI disorders, hypotension, or seizures; diabetes mellitus; CV disease; renal impairment; risk of aspiration
- **Physical:** Orientation, affect, reflexes; BP, standing BP, P; renal function tests; blood glucose; ECG

Interventions

⊗ ***Black box warning*** Avoid use in elderly patients with dementia-related psychosis; increased risk of CV death. Drug is not approved for this use.
- Limit amount of drug dispensed to patients with suicidal ideation.
- Do not cut, crush, or allow patient to chew tablets; give with adequate liquids to ensure swallowing.
- Advise patient that the tablet matrix is insoluble and that it is normal to see tablets in the stool.
- Monitor patient's body temperature, and rule out infection if fever occurs; risk of neuroleptic malignant hyperthermia.
- Monitor patient regularly for hyperglycemia.
- Advise patient to avoid excessive heat and dehydration, which could aggravate orthostatic hypotension.
- Advise patient to use contraception while on this drug; advise nursing mothers to find another method of feeding the baby while on this drug.

Teaching points

- Take this drug in the morning; swallow tablet whole with a full glass of water. Do not cut, crush, or chew the tablet. If you miss a dose, do not double the following dose; instead, take a dose as soon as you remember and continue with your usual dose the following morning.
- Do not be concerned if you see tablets in your stool. This drug is in a matrix system that allows slow release throughout the day; the matrix will pass in your stool.
- This drug enters breast milk and could have effects on a nursing baby; if you are nursing a baby you should find another method of feeding the baby while you are on this drug.
- It is not known how this drug could affect a fetus. If you are pregnant or decide to become pregnant while on this drug, consult with your health care provider; use of contraception is advised.
- This drug interacts with some other drugs and could cause serious side effects; tell any health care provider who is taking care of you that you are on this drug.
- Avoid drinking alcoholic beverages while on this drug.
- You may experience these side effects: Impaired judgment, thinking, or motor skills, (do not drive a car or operate any dangerous machinery while on this drug, and avoid making any important decisions until you are sure how this drug is affecting you), low blood pressure on standing (stand up slowly, make sure you are steady before moving, avoid excessive heat exposure and dehydration).
- Report fever; suicidal thoughts; severe dizziness; increased thirst, hunger, or urination; anxiety; rapid or irregular heartbeat.

▽ palivizumab

(pa live ah zoo' mab)

Synagis

PREGNANCY CATEGORY C

Drug classes

Antiviral
Monoclonal antibody

Therapeutic actions

A murine and human monoclonal antibody produced by recombinant DNA technology specific to an antigenic site of the RSV; has neutralizing effects on the RSV.

Indications

- Prevention of serious lower respiratory tract disease caused by RSV in pediatric patients at high risk for RSV disease

Contraindications and cautions

- Contraindicated with allergy to palivizumab or any murine product.
- Use cautiously with fever (antipyretics should be used to decrease fever before beginning therapy); previous administration

of palivizumab (antibodies frequently develop, causing a risk of serious reactions on repeat administration); pregnancy, history of bleeding disorders.

Available forms

Injection—50 mg/0.5 mL, 100 mg/mL

Dosages

Administer IM only.

Pediatric patients

15 mg/kg IM as a single injection, once a month during RSV season, with first dose given before start of RSV season. Give injection preferably in anterolateral aspect of thigh; do not use gluteal muscle because of risk of damaging sciatic nerve.

Pharmacokinetics

Route	*Onset*	*Peak*
IM	Slow	2–7 days

Metabolism: Tissue; $T_{1/2}$: 18 days
Excretion: Unknown

Adverse effects

- **CNS:** Malaise
- **GI:** Nausea, vomiting, gastroenteritis
- **Respiratory:** URI, pharyngitis, otitis media
- **Other:** Increased susceptibility to infection; **risk of severe anaphylactoid reaction,** especially with repeated administrations, *fever, chills*

Interactions

✱ Drug-drug ⊗ ***Warning*** Reduce dosage of other immunosuppressive agents; severe immunosuppression can lead to increased susceptibility to infection and increased risk of lymphomas.

■ Nursing considerations

Assessment

- **History:** Allergy to palivizumab or any murine product; previous administration of palivizumab; bleeding disorders
- **Physical:** T, body weights; P, BP; R, adventitious sounds; CBC

Interventions

- Monitor WBC levels and circulating T cells periodically during therapy.
- Monitor for any sign of RSV infection; do not use during acute RSV infection, use only for prophylaxis.
- Protect patient from exposure to infections and maintain sterile technique for invasive procedures.
- Arrange for nutritional consult if nausea and vomiting are persistent.

Teaching points

- Protect your child from exposure to infection while he is using this drug; people may wear masks and rubber gloves when caring for your child; visitors may have to be limited.
- Report fever, fussiness, other infections; difficulty breathing.

▽ palonosetron hydrochloride

(pal on os' e tron)

Aloxi

PREGNANCY CATEGORY B

Drug classes

Antiemetic
Selective serotonin receptor antagonist

Therapeutic actions

Selectively binds to serotonin receptors in the CTZ, blocking the nausea and vomiting caused by the release of serotonin by mucosal cells during chemotherapy, radiotherapy, or surgical invasion, an action that stimulates the CTZ and causes nausea and vomiting.

Indications

- Prevention of acute and delayed nausea and vomiting associated with initial and repeat courses of moderately and highly emetogenic chemotherapy
- Prevention of postoperative nausea and vomiting for up to 24 hr after surgery (IV)

Contraindications and cautions

- Contraindicated with allergy to palonosetron or any of its components.
- Use cautiously with known prolonged QT interval or high risk for prolongation of QT

interval (hypokalemia, hypomagnesemia, diuretic use, antiarrhythmic use) pregnancy, lactation.

Available forms

Injection—0.25 mg/5 mL, 0.075 mg/1.5 mL; capsules—0.5 mg

Dosages

Adults

- *Chemotherapy-induced nausea and vomiting:* 0.25 mg IV as a single dose over 30 sec, given 30 min before the start of chemotherapy, or 5 mg PO 1 hr before start of chemotherapy.
- *Postoperative nausea and vomiting:* 0.075 mg IV as a single dose over 10 sec, given immediately before induction of anesthesia.

Pediatric patients

Safety and efficacy not established.

Pharmacokinetics

Route	*Onset*	*Peak*
IV	Immediate	End of infusion
Oral	Rapid	5 hr

Metabolism: Hepatic; $T_{1/2}$: 40 hr
Distribution: May cross placenta; may enter breast milk
Excretion: Feces, urine

IV FACTS

Preparation: No further preparation is needed; solution should be clear and free of particulate matter before use. Store at room temperature; protect from light.
Infusion: Infuse over 30 sec (chemotherapy-induced nausea and vomiting) or over 10 sec (postoperative nausea and vomiting); flush the infusion line with normal saline before and after administration.
Compatibilities: Do not mix in solution with any other drugs.

Adverse effects

- **CNS:** *Headache,* somnolence, drowsiness, sedation, paresthesia, anxiety, insomnia
- **CV:** Tachycardia, bradycardia, hypotension, other arrhythmias, vein distention
- **GI:** Diarrhea, *constipation,* abdominal pain, dyspepsia, dry mouth, hiccups, flatulence
- **Other:** Fever, pruritus, flulike symptoms, fatigue

■ Nursing considerations

Assessment

- **History:** Allergy to palonosetron, pregnancy, lactation, electrolyte abnormality, risk for prolonged QT interval
- **Physical:** Orientation, reflexes, affect; skin evaluation; cardiac rhythm, P, BP; bowel sounds; T

Interventions

- Provide mouth care and sugarless lozenges to suck to help alleviate nausea and dry mouth.
- Establish safety precautions (side rails, assistance with ambulation, proper lighting) if CNS or visual effects occur.
- Provide appropriate analgesics for headache.

Teaching points

- This drug is given IV or orally just before you receive your chemotherapy or before surgery. It will help decrease nausea and vomiting.
- You may experience these side effects: Lack of sleep, drowsiness (use caution if driving or performing tasks that require alertness); constipation; headache (appropriate medication will be provided).
- Report severe headache, fever, numbness or tingling, severe constipation, dizziness.

P

pamidronate disodium

(pah mih' dro nate)

Aredia

PREGNANCY CATEGORY D

Drug classes

Bisphosphonate
Calcium regulator

Therapeutic actions

Slows normal and abnormal bone resorption without inhibiting bone formation and mineralization.

Indications

- Treatment of hypercalcemia associated with malignancy

- Treatment of moderate to severe Paget's disease
- Treatment of osteolytic lesions in breast cancer patients receiving chemotherapy and hormonal therapy
- Treatment of osteolytic bone lesions of multiple myeloma
- Unlabeled uses: Postmenopausal osteoporosis, hyperparathyroidism, prostatic carcinoma, immobilization-related hypercalcemia to prevent fractures and bone pain, osteoporosis with spinal cord injury

Contraindications and cautions

- Contraindicated with allergy to pamidronate disodium or bisphosphonates.
- Use cautiously with renal failure, enterocolitis, pregnancy, lactation.

Available forms

Powder for injection—30, 90 mg; injection—3, 6, 9 mg/mL

Dosages

Adults

- *Hypercalcemia:* 60–90 mg IV given over 4–24 hr as a single dose. Do not exceed 90 mg in a single dose.
- *Paget's disease:* 30 mg/day IV as a 4-hr infusion on 3 consecutive days for a total dose of 90 mg. Do not exceed 90 mg in a single dose.
- *Osteolytic bone lesions:* 90 mg IV as a 2-hr infusion every 3–4 wk. For bone lesions caused by multiple myeloma, give as 4-hr infusion once monthly. Do not exceed 90 mg in single dose.

Pediatric patients

Safety and efficacy not established.

Patients with renal impairment

Do not exceed single dose of 90 mg.

Pharmacokinetics

Route	*Onset*	*Duration*
IV	Rapid	72 hr

Metabolism: Hepatic; $T_{1/2}$: 1.6 hr, then 27.3 hr
Distribution: Crosses placenta; may enter breast milk
Excretion: Urine

IV FACTS

Preparation: Reconstitute by adding 10 mL sterile water for injection to each vial; allow drug to dissolve. For treatment of malignancy-associated hypercalcemia, may be further diluted in 1,000 mL sterile 0.45% or 0.9% sodium chloride or 5% dextrose injection; stable for 24 hr at room temperature.
Infusion: Infuse over 2–24 hr (90-mg dose); over 4 hr (30–60-mg dose).
Incompatibilities: Do not mix with calcium-containing infusions, such as Ringer's; give in a single IV infusion and keep line separate from all other drugs.

Adverse effects

- **CNS:** Headache, insomnia
- **GI:** *Nausea, diarrhea*
- **Musculoskeletal:** *Increased or recurrent bone pain* at pagetic sites, focal osteomalacia, osteonecrosis of the jaw (cancer patients)
- **Other:** Fever, fatigue

■ Nursing considerations

Assessment

- **History:** Allergy to pamidronate disodium or any bisphosphonates, renal failure, enterocolitis, lactation
- **Physical:** Skin lesions, color, T; muscle tone, bone pain; bowel sounds; urinalysis, serum calcium

Interventions

- Provide saline hydration before administration.
- Monitor serum calcium levels before, during, and after therapy. Consider retreatment if hypercalcemia recurs, but allow at least 7 days between treatments.
- Do not give foods high in calcium, vitamins with mineral supplements, or antacids high in metals within 2 hr of dosing.
- Advise a dental examination and completion of any needed preventive care before beginning therapy in cancer patients. Avoid any dental work during therapy.
- Maintain adequate nutrition, particularly intake of calcium and vitamin D.
- Monitor patients with renal impairment carefully; arrange for reduction of dosage if glomerular filtration rate is reduced.

⊗ **Warning** Keep calcium readily available in case hypocalcemic tetany develops.

Teaching points

- Do not take foods high in calcium, antacids, or vitamins with minerals within 2 hours of receiving this drug.
- You should have a dental examination and complete any needed dental care before beginning therapy if you are being treated for cancer.
- You may experience these side effects: Nausea, diarrhea, recurrent bone pain.
- Report twitching, muscle spasms, dark urine, severe diarrhea.

▽ pancrelipase

*(pan kre **ly'** pase)*

Creon 5, 10, 20, 25 (CAN); Creon Delayed-Release Capsules (DNC); Kutrase; Ku-Zyme; Ku-Zyme HP; Lipram 4500; Lipram-PN10, 16, 20; Lipram-UL12, 18, 20; Palcaps 10 (DNC); PAN-2400 Caps; Pancrease MT 4 (DNC), 10 (DNC), 16 (DNC), 20 (DNC); Pancrecarb MS-4 (DNC), MS-8 (DNC), MS-16 (DNC); Pangestyme CN-10, 20; Pangestyme EC; Pangestyme MT 16; Pangestyme UL 12,18, 20; Panokase Tab, Plaretase 8000 Tab, Ultrase Capsules, Ultrase MT 12, 18, 20; Viokase 8, 16; Viokase Powder, Zenpep (DNC)

PREGNANCY CATEGORY C

Drug class

Digestive enzyme

Therapeutic actions

Replacement of pancreatic enzymes: Helps to digest and absorb fat, proteins, and carbohydrates.

Indications

- Replacement therapy in patients with deficient exocrine pancreatic secretions, cystic fibrosis, chronic pancreatitis, postpancreatectomy, ductal obstructions, pancreatic insufficiency, steatorrhea or malabsorption syndrome, and postgastrectomy
- Presumptive test for pancreatic function

Contraindications and cautions

- Contraindicated with allergy to any component, pork products; acute pancreatitis; acute exacerbations of chronic pancreatitis.
- Use cautiously with pregnancy, lactation.

Available forms

Capsules—4,000, 5,000, 8,000, 12,000, 16,000, 18,000, 20,000 units; DR capsules (DNC)—4,000, 5,000, 8,000, 10,000, 12,000, 16,000, 18,000, 20,000 units; powder—16,800 unit; tablets—8,000, 16,000 units; DR capsules (*Zenpep*) (DNC)—5,000, 10,000, 15,000, 20,000 units

Dosages

Adults

Capsules and tablets

4,000–20,000 units PO with each meal and with snacks, usually 1–3 capsules or tablets before or with meals and snacks. May be increased to 8 capsules or tablets in severe cases. 500 units/kg/meal to maximum of 2,500 units/kg/meal (*Zenpep*). Patients with pancreatectomy or obstruction, 8,000–16,000 units PO lipase at 2-hr intervals, may be increased to 64,000–88,000 units.

Powder

0.7 g PO with meals.

Pediatric patients 7–12 yr

4,000–12,000 units PO lipase with each meal and with snacks.

Pediatric patients 4 yr to younger than 12 yr

500 units/kg/meal to maximum of 2,500 units/kg/meal (*Zenpep*).

Pediatric patients 1–6 yr

4,000–8,000 units PO lipase with each meal and 4,000 units with snacks.

Pediatric patients 1 to younger than 4 yr

1,000 units/kg/meal to maximum of 2,500 units/kg/meal (*Zenpep*).

Pediatric patients 6 mo–1 yr

2,000 units lipase PO per meal; 2,000–4,000 units per feeding (*Zenpep*).

Pharmacokinetics
Generally no systemic absorption.

Adverse effects
- **GI:** *Nausea, abdominal cramps, diarrhea*
- **GU:** Hyperuricosuria, hyperuricemia with extremely high doses
- **Hypersensitivity:** Asthma with inhalation of fine-powder concentrates in sensitized individuals

■ Nursing considerations
Assessment
- **History:** Allergy to any component, pork products; pregnancy; lactation
- **Physical:** R, adventitious sounds; abdominal examination, bowel sounds; pancreatic function tests

Interventions
- Administer before or with meals and snacks.

⊗ ***Warning*** Avoid inhaling or spilling powder on hands because it may irritate skin or mucous membranes.

⊗ ***Warning*** Dosages above recommended range may result in colonic strictures, especially in patients with cystic fibrosis.

- Be aware that *Zenpep* is not interchangeable with other pancrelipase preperations.
- Do not crush or let patient chew the enteric-coated capsules; drug will not survive acid environment of the stomach.

Teaching points
- Take drug before or with meals and snacks.
- Do not crush or chew the enteric-coated capsules; swallow whole. *Zenpep* capsules may be opened and sprinkled on food if swallowing capsule is difficult.
- Do not inhale powder dosage forms; severe reaction can occur.
- You may experience these side effects: Abdominal discomfort, diarrhea.
- Report joint pain, swelling, soreness; difficulty breathing; GI upset.

▽ panitumumab
See Appendix W, *Less commonly used drugs*.

▽ pantoprazole
*(pan **toe'** pray zol)*

Panto IV (CAN), Pantoloc (CAN), Protonix (DNC), Protonix IV

PREGNANCY CATEGORY B

Drug classes
Antisecretory drug
Proton pump inhibitor

Therapeutic actions
Gastric acid-pump inhibitor: Suppresses gastric acid secretion by specific inhibition of the hydrogen-potassium ATPase enzyme system at the secretory surface of the gastric parietal cells; blocks the final step of acid production.

Indications
- Oral: Short-term (8 wk or less) and long-term treatment of GERD
- Maintenance healing of erosive esophagitis
- Long-term treatment of pathological hypersecretory conditions
- IV: Short-term (7–10 days) treatment of GERD in patients unable to continue oral therapy
- IV: Treatment of pathological hypersecretory conditions associated with Zollinger-Ellison syndrome and other neoplastic conditions
- Unlabeled use: Treatment of duodenal ulcer

Contraindications and cautions
- Contraindicated with hypersensitivity to any proton pump inhibitor or any drug components.
- Use cautiously with pregnancy, lactation.

Available forms
DR tablet (DNC)—20, 40 mg; granules for oral suspension—40 mg/packet; powder for injection—40 mg/vial

Dosages
Adults
40 mg PO daily for maintenance healing of erosive esophagitis for 8 wk or less. The 8-wk course may be repeated if healing has not occurred; give continually for hypersecretory disorders; 40 mg/day IV for 7–10 days. Up to

240 mg/day PO or IV has been used for severe hypersecretory syndromes.

Pediatric patients younger than 18 yr
Safety and efficacy not established.

Patients with hepatic impairment
Use caution and monitor patient closely.

Pharmacokinetics

Route	*Onset*	*Peak*
Oral	1 hr	3–5 hr
IV	Rapid	3–5 hr

Metabolism: Hepatic; $T_{1/2}$: 1.5 hr
Distribution: Crosses placenta; may enter breast milk
Excretion: Bile, urine

IV FACTS

Preparation: Reconstitute with 10 mL 0.9% sodium chloride; may then be further diluted with 100 mL 5% dextrose injection, 0.9% sodium chloride injection or lactated Ringer's, final concentration 0.4 mg/mL; reconstituted solution can be stored 2 hr, dilution up to 12 hr at room temperature. Avoid use of spiked IV system adapters with vials.
Infusion: Infuse over at least 15 min using in-line filter.
Incompatibilities: Do not mix with or administer through the same line as other IV solutions.

Adverse effects

- **CNS:** *Headache, dizziness,* asthenia, vertigo, insomnia, apathy, anxiety, paresthesias, dream abnormalities
- **Dermatologic:** Rash, inflammation, urticaria, pruritus, alopecia, dry skin
- **GI:** *Diarrhea, abdominal pain, nausea, vomiting,* constipation, dry mouth, tongue atrophy
- **Respiratory:** *URI symptoms,* cough, epistaxis, pneumonia
- **Other:** Cancer in preclinical studies, back pain, fever, vitamin B_{12} deficiency

Interactions

✱ **Drug-drug** • Fewer drug interactions reported than with other proton pump inhibitors

■ Nursing considerations

Assessment

- **History:** Hypersensitivity to any proton pump inhibitor or any drug components, pregnancy, lactation
- **Physical:** Skin lesions; T; reflexes, affect; urinary output, abdominal examination; respiratory auscultation

Interventions

- Administer once or twice a day. Caution patient to swallow tablets whole; not to cut, chew, or crush.

⊗ ***Warning*** Arrange for further evaluation of patient after 4 wk of therapy for gastroesophageal reflux disorders. Symptomatic improvement does not rule out gastric cancer; gastric cancer did occur in preclinical studies.

- Maintain supportive treatment as appropriate for underlying problem.
- Switch patients on IV therapy to oral dosage as soon as possible.
- Provide additional comfort measures to alleviate discomfort from GI effects and headache.

Teaching points

- Take the drug once or twice a day. Swallow the tablets whole—do not chew, cut, or crush them.
- Arrange to have regular medical follow-up care while you are using this drug.
- Maintain all of the usual activities and restrictions that apply to your condition. If this becomes difficult, consult your health care provider.
- You may experience these side effects: Dizziness (avoid driving a car or performing hazardous tasks); headache (consult your health care provider if these become bothersome; medications may be available to help); nausea, vomiting, diarrhea (proper nutrition is important; consult a dietitian to maintain nutrition; stay near a bathroom); symptoms of upper respiratory tract infection, cough (this is a drug effect; do not self-medicate; consult your health care provider if this becomes uncomfortable).
- Report severe headache, worsening of symptoms, fever, chills, blurred vision, periorbital pain.

paricalcitol

See Appendix W, *Less commonly used drugs*.

paroxetine

(pah rox' a teen)

paroxetine hydrochloride

Apo-Paroxetine (CAN), CO Paroxetine (CAN), Gen-Paroxetine (CAN), Novo-Paroxetine (CAN), Paxil, Paxil CR (DNC), ratio-Paroxetine (CAN)

paroxetine mesylate

Pexeva

PREGNANCY CATEGORY C

Drug class

Antidepressant

Therapeutic actions

Potentiates serotonergic activity in the CNS, resulting in antidepressant effect.

Indications

- Treatment of major depressive disorder
- Treatment of OCD
- Treatment of panic disorders
- Treatment of social anxiety disorder (social phobia)
- Treatment of generalized anxiety disorder
- Treatment of PTSD
- Treatment of PMDD
- Unlabeled uses: Treatment of hot flashes, diabetic neuropathy

Contraindications and cautions

- Contraindicated with use of MAOI or thioridazine.
- Use cautiously in the elderly; with renal or hepatic impairment, pregnancy, lactation, suicidal patients.

Available forms

Tablets—10, 20, 30, 40 mg; CR tablets (DNC)—12.5, 25, 37.5 mg; suspension—10 mg/5 mL

Dosages

Adults

- *Depression:* 20 mg/day PO as a single daily dose. Range, 20–50 mg/day. Or 25–62.5 mg/day CR tablet.
- *OCD:* 20 mg/day PO as a single dose, may increase in 10-mg/day increments; do not exceed 60 mg/day.
- *Panic disorder:* 10 mg/day, increase in increments of 10 mg/wk; usual range, 10–60 mg/day. Or 12.5–75 mg/day CR tablet; do not exceed 75 mg/day.
- *Social anxiety disorder:* 20 mg/day PO as a single dose in the morning. Or, 12.5 mg/day PO CR form. May increase up to 60 mg/day or 37.5 mg/day CR form.
- *Generalized anxiety disorder:* 20 mg/day PO as a single daily dose. Range, 20–50 mg/day.
- *PMDD:* 12.5 mg/day PO as a single dose in the morning. Range, 12.5–25 mg/day. May be given daily or just during the luteal phase of the cycle.
- *PTSD:* 20 mg/day as a single dose. Range, 20–50 mg/day PO.
- *Switching to or from an MAOI:* At least 14 days should elapse between discontinuation of MAOI and initiation of paroxetine therapy; similarly, allow 14 days between discontinuing paroxetine and beginning MAOI.

Pediatric patients

Safety and efficacy not established.

Geriatric patients or patients with renal or hepatic impairment

10 mg/day PO; do not exceed 40 mg/day. Or 12.5 mg/day CR tablet; do not exceed 50 mg/day.

Pharmacokinetics

Route	Onset
Oral	Slow

Metabolism: Hepatic; $T_{1/2}$: 24 hr

Distribution: Crosses placenta; enters breast milk

Excretion: Urine

Adverse effects

- **CNS:** *Somnolence, dizziness, insomnia, tremor, nervousness, headache,* anxiety, paresthesia, blurred vision

- **CV:** Palpitations, vasodilation, orthostatic hypotension, hypertension
- **Dermatologic:** *Sweating,* rash, redness
- **GI:** *Nausea, dry mouth, constipation, diarrhea,* anorexia, flatulence, vomiting
- **GU:** *Ejaculatory disorders, male genital disorders,* urinary frequency
- **Respiratory:** Yawns, pharyngitis, cough
- **Other:** *Asthenia*

Interactions

✱ **Drug-drug** • Increased paroxetine levels and toxicity with cimetidine, MAOIs • Decreased therapeutic effects of phenytoin, digoxin • Decreased effectiveness of paroxetine with phenobarbital, phenytoin • Increased serum levels and possible toxicity of procyclidine, tryptophane, warfarin • Risk of serotonin syndrome (hypertension, hyperthermia, mental status changes) if used with other SSRIs

✱ **Drug-alternative therapy** • Increased sedative-hypnotic effects with St. John's wort

■ Nursing considerations

Assessment

- **History:** Hypersensitivity to paroxetine, renal or hepatic impairment, seizure disorder, pregnancy, lactation
- **Physical:** Orientation, reflexes; P, BP, perfusion; R, adventitious sounds; bowel sounds, normal output; urinary output; liver evaluation; LFTs, renal function tests

Interventions

⊠ ***Black box warning*** Be alert for increased suicidality in children, adolescents, and young adults; monitor accordingly.

- Administer once a day in the morning.
- Shake suspension well before using.
- Ensure that patient swallows CR tablets whole; do not cut, crush, or chew.
- Limit amount of drug given to potentially suicidal patients.
- Abruptly discontinuing the drug may result in discontinuation symptoms (agitation, palpitations); consider tapering.
- Advise patient to avoid using if pregnant or lactating.

Teaching points

- Take this drug exactly as directed and as long as directed. Shake suspension well before using. Swallow controlled-release tablets whole; do not cut, crush, or chew.
- Abruptly stopping the drug without tapering the dose may cause symptoms including agitation and palpitations.
- This drug should not be taken during pregnancy or when nursing a baby; using barrier contraceptives is advised.
- You may experience these side effects: Drowsiness, dizziness, tremor (use caution and avoid driving or performing other tasks that require alertness); GI upset (frequent small meals, frequent mouth care may help); alterations in sexual function.
- Report severe nausea, vomiting; palpitations; blurred vision; excessive sweating; thoughts of suicide.

▽ pazopanib

See Appendix X, *Less commonly used drugs.*

▽ pegaptanib

See Appendix X, *Less commonly used drugs.*

▽ pegaspargase

See Appendix X, *Less commonly used drugs.*

▽ pegfilgrastim (G-CSF conjugate)

*(peg fill **grass'** stim)*

Neulasta

Pregnancy Category C

Drug class

Colony-stimulating factor

Therapeutic actions

Covalent conjugate of the human granulocyte colony-stimulating factor (filgrastim) produced by recombinant DNA technology; has a longer duration of action than filgrastim; increases the production of neutrophils within the bone marrow with little effect on the production of other hematopoietic cells.

P

Indications

- To decrease the incidence of infection in patients with nonmyeloid malignancies receiving myelosuppressive anticancer drugs associated with a significant incidence of severe febrile neutropenia

Contraindications and cautions

- Contraindicated with hypersensitivity to *Escherichia coli* products, filgrastim.
- Use cautiously with sickle cell disease, pregnancy, lactation.

Available forms

Injection—10 mg/mL in prefilled syringes

Dosages

Adults

6 mg subcutaneously as a single dose once per chemotherapy cycle. Do not give in the period 14 days before and 24 hr after administration of cytotoxic chemotherapy.

Pediatric patients

Safety and efficacy not established.

Pharmacokinetics

Route	Peak	Duration
Subcut.	8 hr	Varies

Metabolism: Unknown; $T_{1/2}$: 15–80 hr
Distribution: Crosses placenta; may enter breast milk
Excretion: Unknown

Adverse effects

- **CNS:** *Headache, generalized weakness, fatigue, dizziness, insomnia*
- **Dermatologic:** *Alopecia,* rash, *mucositis*
- **GI:** *Nausea, vomiting, stomatitis, anorexia, diarrhea, constipation, taste perversion, dyspepsia, abdominal pain*
- **Respiratory: Acute respiratory distress syndrome**
- **Other: Splenic rupture,** aggravation of sickle cell disease, *fever, arthralgia, peripheral edema, myalgia, bone pain, granulocytopenic allergic reactions* (anaphylaxis, rash, urticaria), *increased LDH, alkaline phosphatase, uric acid*

Interactions

✷ **Drug-drug** • Risk of increased effects if combined with lithium; if this combination is used, monitor neutrophil counts frequently

■ Nursing considerations

CLINICAL ALERT!
Name confusion has been reported between *Neulasta* (pegfilgrastim) and *Neumega* (oprelvekin); use caution.

Assessment

- **History:** Hypersensitivity to *E. coli* products, filgrastim; sickle cell disease; pregnancy, lactation
- **Physical:** Skin color, lesions, hair; T; orientation, affect; abdominal examination, status of mucous membranes; CBC, platelets

Interventions

- Obtain CBC and platelet count prior to and twice weekly during therapy.

⊗ ***Warning*** Administer no earlier than 24 hr after cytotoxic chemotherapy and not in the period of 14 days before the administration of chemotherapy.

- Give one injection with each course of chemotherapy.
- Store in refrigerator; allow to warm to room temperature before use; if syringe is at room temperature for 48 hr or longer, discard. Use each syringe for one dose.
- Do not shake syringe before use. Protect syringe from light. Make sure the syringe is free of particulate matter and that the solution is not discolored before using.
- Monitor patient for any sign of infection and arrange for appropriate treatment.
- Protect patient from exposure to infection.
- Provide appropriate comfort and supportive measures for headache, bone pain, or GI discomfort.
- Arrange for patient to obtain wig or other head covering if alopecia occurs; cover head at extremes of temperature.
- Arrange for small frequent meals if nausea and vomiting are a problem.
- Offer support and encouragement to deal with pain, discomfort, and hair loss.

Teaching points

- This drug will be given by subcutaneous injection once with each cycle of your chemotherapy.
- Avoid exposure to infection while you are receiving this drug (avoid crowds and people with known infections).
- Keep appointments for frequent blood tests to evaluate effects of drug on your blood count.
- You may experience these side effects: Bone pain (analgesia may be ordered), nausea and vomiting (eat frequent small meals), loss of hair (you may want to arrange for appropriate head covering; it is very important to cover head in extreme temperatures).
- Report fever, chills, severe bone pain, sore throat, weakness, pain or swelling at injection site.

peginterferon alfa-2a

See Appendix W, *Less commonly used drugs*.

peginterferon alfa-2b

See Appendix W, *Less commonly used drugs*.

pegvisomant

See Appendix W, *Less commonly used drugs*.

pemetrexed

See Appendix W, *Less commonly used drugs*.

penbutolol sulfate

*(pen **byoo'** toe lole)*

Levatol

PREGNANCY CATEGORY C

Drug classes

Antihypertensive
Beta-adrenergic blocker

Therapeutic actions

Competitively blocks beta-adrenergic receptors in the heart and juxtaglomerular apparatus, reducing the influence of the sympathetic nervous system on these tissues; decreasing the excitability of the heart, cardiac output, and release of renin; and lowering BP.

Indications

- Treatment of mild to moderate hypertension, alone or as part of combination therapy

Contraindications and cautions

- Contraindicated with sinus bradycardia, bronchial asthma, second- or third-degree heart block, cardiogenic shock, HF, lactation.
- Use cautiously with renal failure, diabetes or thyrotoxicosis, asthma, COPD, impaired hepatic function, pregnancy.

Available forms

Tablets—20 mg

Dosages

Adults

Usual starting dose, maintenance dose, and dose used in combination with other antihypertensives: 20 mg PO daily. Doses of 40–80 mg daily have been used but with no additional antihypertensive effect.

Pediatric patients

Safety and efficacy not established.

Pharmacokinetics

Route	*Onset*	*Peak*	*Duration*
Oral	Varies	2–3 hr	20 hr

Metabolism: Hepatic; $T_{1/2}$: 5 hr
Distribution: Crosses placenta; enters breast milk
Excretion: Urine

Adverse effects

- **Allergic reactions:** Pharyngitis, erythematous rash, fever, sore throat, **laryngospasm,** respiratory distress
- **CNS:** Dizziness, vertigo, tinnitus, fatigue, emotional depression, paresthesias, sleep disturbances, hallucinations, disorientation, memory loss, slurred speech
- **CV:** *Bradycardia, HF, cardiac arrhythmias, sinoatrial or AV nodal block, tachycardia,* peripheral vascular insufficiency, claudication, **CVA, pulmonary edema,** hypotension

P

- **Dermatologic:** Rash, pruritus, sweating, dry skin
- **EENT:** Eye irritation, dry eyes, conjunctivitis, blurred vision
- **GI:** *Gastric pain, flatulence, constipation, diarrhea, nausea, vomiting,* anorexia, ischemic colitis, mesenteric arterial thrombosis, retroperitoneal fibrosis, hepatomegaly, acute hepatitis
- **GU:** *Impotence, decreased libido,* Peyronie's disease, dysuria, nocturia, frequent urination, renal arterial thrombosis
- **Musculoskeletal:** Joint pain, arthralgia, muscle cramp
- **Respiratory: Bronchospasm,** dyspnea, cough, bronchial obstruction, nasal stuffiness, rhinitis, pharyngitis (less likely than with propranolol)
- **Other:** *Decreased exercise tolerance, development of ANA,* hyperglycemia or hypoglycemia, elevated serum transaminase, alkaline phosphatase, and LDH

Interactions

✱ **Drug-drug** • Increased effects and adverse effects with verapamil, other calcium channel blockers • Decreased effects with epinephrine • Increased risk of peripheral ischemia, even gangrene, with ergot alkaloids (dihydroergotamine, methysergide, ergotamine) • Prolonged hypoglycemic effects of insulin • Increased first-dose response to prazosin • Paradoxical hypertension when clonidine is given with beta-blockers; increased rebound hypertension when clonidine is discontinued in patients on beta-blockers • Decreased hypertensive effect if given with NSAIDs (piroxicam, indomethacin, ibuprofen) • Decreased bronchodilator effects of theophylline and decreased bronchial and cardiac effects of sympathomimetics with penbutolol

✱ **Drug-lab test** • Possible false results with glucose or insulin tolerance tests

■ Nursing considerations

Assessment

- **History:** Sinus bradycardia, heart block, cardiogenic shock, HF, renal failure, diabetes or thyrotoxicosis, asthma or COPD, impaired hepatic function, lactation, pregnancy
- **Physical:** Weight, skin condition, neurologic status, P, BP, ECG, respiratory status, renal and thyroid function tests, blood and urine glucose

Interventions

- Give drug once a day. Monitor response and maintain at lowest possible dose.

⊗ *Warning* Do not discontinue drug abruptly after long-term therapy (hypersensitivity to catecholamines may have developed, causing exacerbation of angina, MI, and ventricular arrhythmias; taper drug gradually over 2 wk with monitoring).

- Consult with physician about withdrawing drug if patient is to undergo surgery (withdrawal is controversial).

Teaching points

- Do not stop taking this drug unless instructed to do so by your health care provider.
- Avoid driving or dangerous activities if dizziness or drowsiness occurs.
- Report difficulty breathing, night cough, swelling of extremities, slow pulse, confusion, depression, rash, fever, sore throat.

▽ penicillamine

See Appendix W, *Less commonly used drugs*.

▽ penicillin G benzathine

*(pen i **sill'** in)*

Bicillin L-A, Permapen

PREGNANCY CATEGORY B

Drug classes

Antibiotic
Penicillin antibiotic

Therapeutic actions

Bactericidal: Inhibits synthesis of cell wall of sensitive organisms, causing cell death.

Indications

- Severe infections caused by sensitive organisms (streptococci)
- URI caused by sensitive streptococci

- Treatment of syphilis, bejel, congenital syphilis, pinta, yaws
- Prophylaxis of rheumatic fever and chorea

Contraindications and cautions

- Contraindicated with allergies to penicillins, cephalosporins, or other allergens.
- Use cautiously with renal disorders, pregnancy, lactation (may cause diarrhea or candidiasis in the infant).

Available forms

Injection—600,000, 1.2 million, 2.4 million units/dose

Dosages

Adults

- *Streptococcal infections (including otitis media, URIs of mild to moderate severity):* 1.2 million units IM as a single dose.
- *Early syphilis:* 2.4 million units IM as a single dose.
- *Syphilis lasting longer than 1 yr:* 7.2 million units given as 2.4 million units IM weekly for 3 wk.
- *Yaws, bejel, pinta:* 1.2 million units IM as a single dose.
- *Erysipeloid:* 1.2 million units IM as a single dose.
- *Prophylaxis of rheumatic fever or chorea:* 1.2 million units IM every month; alternatively, 600,000 units every 2 wk.

Pediatric patients

- *Streptococcal infections (including otitis media, URIs of mild to moderate severity): Children weighing less than 60 lb:* 300,000–600,000 units IM as a single injection. *Older children:* 900,000 units IM as a single injection.
- *Congenital syphilis: Children younger than 2 yr:* 50,000 units/kg body weight. *Children 2 to 12 yr:* Adjust dosage based on adult schedule.

Pharmacokinetics

Route	*Onset*	*Peak*	*Duration*
IM	Slow	12–24 hr	Days

Metabolism: Hepatic; $T_{1/2}$: 30–60 min
Distribution: Crosses placenta; enters breast milk
Excretion: Urine

Adverse effects

- **CNS:** Lethargy, hallucinations, seizures
- **GI:** *Glossitis, stomatitis, gastritis, sore mouth,* furry tongue, black "hairy" tongue, *nausea, vomiting, diarrhea,* abdominal pain, bloody diarrhea, enterocolitis, pseudomembranous colitis, nonspecific hepatitis
- **GU:** Nephritis
- **Hematologic:** Anemia, thrombocytopenia, leukopenia, neutropenia, prolonged bleeding time (more common than with other penicillinase-resistant penicillins)
- **Hypersensitivity:** *Rash, fever, wheezing,* **anaphylaxis**
- **Local:** *Pain, phlebitis,* thrombosis at injection site, Jarisch-Herxheimer reaction when used to treat syphilis
- **Other:** *Superinfections,* sodium overload, leading to heart failure

Interactions

✷ **Drug-drug** • Decreased effectiveness of penicillin G benzathine with tetracyclines • Inactivation of parenteral aminoglycosides (amikacin, gentamicin, kanamycin, neomycin, tobramycin); separate administration times

■ Nursing considerations

Assessment

- **History:** Allergies to penicillins, cephalosporins, other allergens; renal disorders; pregnancy, lactation
- **Physical:** Culture infection; skin color, lesions; R, adventitious sounds; bowel sounds: CBC, LFTs, renal function tests, serum electrolytes, Hct, urinalysis

Interventions

⊗ ***Warning*** Drug is not for IV use. Do not inject or admix with other IV solutions. Inadvertent IV administration has caused cardiorespiratory arrest and death.

- Culture infection before beginning treatment; reculture if response is not as expected.
- Give by IM route only.
- Continue therapy for at least 2 days after infection has disappeared, usually 7–10 days.
- Give IM injection in upper outer quadrant of the buttock. In infants and small children, the midlateral aspect of the thigh may be preferred.

Teaching points
- You will need to receive a full course of drug therapy.
- You may experience these side effects: Nausea, vomiting, diarrhea, mouth sores, pain at injection sites.
- Report difficulty breathing, rashes, severe diarrhea, severe pain at injection site, mouth sores, unusual bleeding or bruising.

penicillin G potassium
(pen i sill' in)

penicillin G potassium (aqueous)
Pfizerpen

penicillin G sodium

PREGNANCY CATEGORY B

Drug classes
Antibiotic
Penicillin antibiotic

Therapeutic actions
Bactericidal: Inhibits synthesis of cell wall of sensitive organisms, causing cell death.

Indications
- Treatment of severe infections caused by sensitive organisms—streptococci, pneumococci, staphylococci, *Neisseria gonorrhoeae, Treponema pallidum,* meningococci, *Actinomyces israelii, Clostridium perfringens* and *tetani, Leptotrichia buccalis* (Vincent's disease), *Spirillum minus* or *Streptobacillus moniliformis, Listeria monocytogenes, Fusobacterium fusiformisans, Pasteurella multocida, Erysipelothrix insidiosa, Escherichia coli, Enterobacter aerogenes, Alcaligenes faecalis, Salmonella, Shigella, Proteus mirabilis, Corynebacterium diphtheriae, Bacillus anthracis*
- Treatment of syphilis, gonococcal infections
- Unlabeled use: Treatment of Lyme disease

Contraindications and cautions
- Contraindicated with allergy to penicillins, cephalosporins, imipenem, beta-lactamase inhibitors, other allergens.
- Use cautiously with renal disease, pregnancy, lactation (may cause diarrhea or candidiasis in the infant).

Available forms
Injection—1, 2, 3 million units/50 mL; powder for injection—5, 20 million units/vial

Dosages
Adults
- *Meningococcal meningitis:* 1–2 million units every 2 hr IM or by continuous IV infusion of 20–30 million units/day.
- *Actinomycosis:* 1–6 million units/day IM in divided doses every 4–6 hr for 6 wk or IV for cervicofacial cases; 10–20 million units/day IV for thoracic and abdominal diseases.
- *Clostridial infections:* 20 million units/day in divided doses every 4–6 hr IM or IV with antitoxin therapy.
- *Fusospirochetal infections (Vincent's disease):* 5–10 million units/day IM or IV in divided doses every 4–6 hr.
- *Rat-bite fever:* 12–15 million units/day IM or IV in divided doses every 4–6 hr for 3–4 wk.
- *Listeria infections:* 15–20 million units/day IM or IV in divided doses every 4–6 hr for 2 or 4 wk (meningitis or endocarditis, respectively).
- *Pasteurella infections:* 4–6 million units/day IM or IV in divided doses every 4–6 hr for 2 wk.
- *Erysipeloid endocarditis:* 12–20 million units/day IM or IV in divided doses every 4–6 hr for 4–6 wk.
- *Diphtheria (adjunctive therapy with antitoxin to prevent carrier state):* 2–3 million units/day IM or IV in divided doses every 4–6 hr for 10–12 days.
- *Anthrax:* Minimum of 5 million units/day IM or IV in divided doses.
- *Serious streptococcal infections:* 5–24 million units/day in divided doses every 4–6 hr.

- *Syphilis:* 18–24 million units/day IV every 4–6 hr for 10 days followed by benzathine penicillin G 2.4 million units IM weekly for 3 wk.
- *Gonorrhea:* 10 million units/day IV every 4–6 hr until improvement occurs.

Pediatric patients

- *Meningitis:* 250,000 units/kg/day IM or IV in divided doses every 4 hr for 7–14 days.
- *Streptococcal infections:* 150,000 units/kg/day IV or IM every 4–6 hr.
  Infants older than 7 days: 75,000 units/kg/day IV in divided doses every 8 hr.
- *Meningitis:* 200,000–300,000 units/kg/day IV every 6 hr.
  Infants younger than 7 days: 50,000 units/kg/day IV in divided doses every 12 hr.
- *Group B streptococcus:* 100,000 units/kg/day IV.

Pharmacokinetics

Route	*Onset*	*Peak*
IM, IV	Rapid	15–30 min

Metabolism: Hepatic; $T_{1/2}$: 30–60 min
Distribution: Crosses placenta; enters breast milk
Excretion: Urine

IV FACTS

Preparation: Prepare solution using sterile water for injection, isotonic sodium chloride injection, or 5% dextrose injection. Loosen powder in vial; reconstitute with vial held horizontally. Shake vigorously. Do not use with carbohydrate solutions at alkaline pH; do not refrigerate powder; sterile solution is stable for 1 wk refrigerated. IV solutions are stable at 24 hr at room temperature. Discard solution after 24 hr.
Infusion: Administer doses of 10–20 million units by slow infusion.
Incompatibilities: Do not mix with aminoglycosides, amphotericin B, bleomycin, chlorpromazine, cytarabine, hydroxyzine, methylprednisolone, prochlorperazine, promethazine.

Adverse effects

- **CNS:** Lethargy, hallucinations, seizures
- **GI:** *Glossitis, stomatitis, gastritis, sore mouth,* furry tongue, black "hairy" tongue, *nausea, vomiting, diarrhea,* abdominal pain, bloody diarrhea, enterocolitis, pseudomembranous colitis, nonspecific hepatitis
- **GU:** Nephritis—oliguria, proteinuria, hematuria, casts, azotemia, pyuria
- **Hematologic:** Anemia, thrombocytopenia, leukopenia, neutropenia, prolonged bleeding time
- **Hypersensitivity reactions:** *Rash, fever, wheezing,* anaphylaxis
- **Local:** *Pain, phlebitis,* thrombosis at injection site, Jarisch-Herxheimer reaction when used to treat syphilis
- **Other:** *Superinfections;* sodium overload, leading to HF

Interactions

✷ **Drug-drug** • Decreased effectiveness of penicillin G with tetracyclines • Inactivation of parenteral aminoglycosides (amikacin, gentamicin, kanamycin, neomycin, streptomycin, tobramycin)

✷ **Drug-lab test** • False-positive Coombs' test (IV)

■ Nursing considerations

Assessment

- **History:** Allergy to penicillins, cephalosporins, imipenem, beta-lactamase inhibitors, other allergens, renal disease, lactation, pregnancy
- **Physical:** Culture infection; skin rashes, lesions; R, adventitious sounds; bowel sounds, normal output; CBC, LFTs, renal function tests, serum electrolytes, Hct, urinalysis; skin test with benzylpenicylloyl-polylysine if hypersensitivity reactions to penicillin have occurred

Interventions

- Culture infection before beginning treatment; reculture if response is not as expected.
- Use the smallest volume possible for IM injection to avoid pain and discomfort.
- Continue treatment for 48–72 hr after the patient is asymptomatic.

⊗ ***Warning*** Monitor serum electrolytes and cardiac status if penicillin G is given by IV infusion. Sodium or potassium preparations have been associated with severe electrolyte imbalances.

P

- Explain the reason for parenteral administration; offer support and encouragement to deal with therapy.

⊗ **Warning** Keep epinephrine, IV fluids, vasopressors, bronchodilators, oxygen, and emergency equipment readily available in case of serious hypersensitivity reaction.

- Arrange for corticosteroids or antihistamines for skin reactions.

Teaching points

- This drug must be given by injection for severe infections.
- You may experience these side effects: Upset stomach, nausea, vomiting (eat frequent small meals); sore mouth (frequent mouth care may help); diarrhea; pain or discomfort at the injection site.
- Report unusual bleeding, sore throat, rash, hives, fever, severe diarrhea, difficulty breathing.

▽penicillin G procaine (penicillin G procaine, aqueous, APPG)

*(pen i **sill'** in)*

Wycillin

PREGNANCY CATEGORY B

Drug classes

Antibiotic
Penicillin (long-acting, parenteral)

Therapeutic actions

Bactericidal: Inhibits cell wall synthesis of sensitive organisms, causing cell death.

Indications

- Treatment of moderately severe infections caused by sensitive organisms—streptococci, pneumococci, staphylococci, meningococci, *Actinomyces israelii, Clostridium perfringens* and *tetani, Leptotrichia buccalis* (Vincent's disease), *Spirillum minus, Streptobacillus moniliformis, Listeria monocytogenes, Pasteurella multocida, Erysipelothrix insidiosa, Escherichia coli, Enterobacter aerogenes, Alcaligenes faecalis, Salmonella, Shigella, Proteus mirabilis, Corynebacterium diphtheriae, Bacillus anthracis*
- Treatment of specific STDs

Contraindications and cautions

- Contraindicated with allergies to penicillins, cephalosporins, procaine, or other allergens.
- Use cautiously with renal disorders, pregnancy, lactation (may cause diarrhea or candidiasis in the infant).

Available forms

Injection—600,000, 1,200,000 units/dose

Dosages

Adults

- *Moderately severe infections caused by sensitive strains of streptococci, pneumococci, staphylococci:* Minimum of 600,000–1 million units/day IM.
- *Bacterial endocarditis (group A streptococci):* 600,000–1 million units/day IM.
- *Fusospirochetal infections:* 600,000–1 million units/day IM.
- *Rat-bite fever:* 600,000–1 million units/day IM.
- *Erysipeloid:* 600,000–1 million units/day IM.
- *Diphtheria:* 300,000–600,000 units/day IM with antitoxin.
- *Diphtheria carrier state:* 300,000 units/day IM for 10 days.
- *Anthrax:* 600,000–1 million units/day IM.
- *Syphilis (negative spinal fluid):* 600,000 units/day IM for 8 days.
- *Late syphilis:* 600,000 units/day for 10–15 days.
- *Neurosyphilis:* 2.4 million units/day IM with 500 mg probenecid PO qid for 10–14 days, followed by 2.4 million units IM benzathine penicillin G following completion of treatment regimen.

Pediatric patients

- *Congenital syphilis in patients weighing less than 32 kg:* 50,000 units/kg per day IM for 10 days.
- *Group A streptococcal and staphylococcal pneumonia in patients weighing less than 27 kg:* 300,000 units/day/IM.

Pharmacokinetics

Route	Onset	Peak	Duration
IM	Varies	4 hr	15–20 hr

Metabolism: Hepatic; $T_{1/2}$: 30–60 min
Distribution: Crosses placenta; enters breast milk
Excretion: Urine

Adverse effects

- **CNS:** Lethargy, hallucinations, seizures
- **GI:** *Glossitis, stomatitis, gastritis, sore mouth,* furry tongue, black "hairy" tongue, *nausea, vomiting, diarrhea,* abdominal pain, bloody diarrhea, enterocolitis, pseudomembranous colitis, nonspecific hepatitis
- **GU:** Nephritis—oliguria, proteinuria, hematuria, casts, azotemia, pyuria
- **Hematologic:** Anemia, thrombocytopenia, leukopenia, neutropenia, prolonged bleeding time
- **Hypersensitivity:** *Rash, fever, wheezing,* **anaphylaxis**
- **Local:** *Pain, phlebitis,* thrombosis at injection site, Jarisch-Herxheimer reaction when used to treat syphilis
- **Other:** *Superinfections;* sodium overload, leading to HF

Interactions

✱ **Drug-drug** • Decreased effectiveness of penicillin G procaine with tetracyclines • Inactivation of parenteral aminoglycosides (amikacin, gentamicin, kanamycin, neomycin, streptomycin, tobramycin)

■ Nursing considerations

Assessment

- **History:** Allergies to penicillins, cephalosporins, procaine, other allergens, renal disorders, pregnancy, lactation
- **Physical:** Culture infection; skin color, lesions; R, adventitious sounds; bowel sounds: CBC, LFTs, renal function tests, serum electrolytes, Hct, urinalysis

Interventions

- Culture infection before beginning treatment; reculture if response is not as expected.
- Administer by IM route only.
- Continue therapy for at least 2 days after infection has disappeared, usually 7–10 days.
- Administer IM injection in upper outer quadrant of the buttock. In infants and small children, the midlateral aspect of the thigh may be preferred.

Teaching points

- This drug can be given only by IM injection.
- You may experience these side effects: Nausea, vomiting, diarrhea, mouth sores, pain at injection sites.
- Report difficulty breathing, rashes, severe diarrhea, severe pain at injection site, mouth sores, unusual bleeding or bruising.

▽ penicillin V (penicillin V potassium)

*(pen i **sill'** in)*

Apo-Pen-VK (CAN), Nu-Pen-VK (CAN), Veetids

PREGNANCY CATEGORY B

Drug classes

Antibiotic
Penicillin (acid stable)

Therapeutic actions

Bactericidal: Inhibits cell wall synthesis of sensitive organisms, causing cell death.

Indications

- Mild to moderately severe infections caused by sensitive organisms—streptococci, pneumococci, staphylococci, fusospirochetes
- Unlabeled uses: Prophylactic treatment of children with sickle cell anemia, mild to moderate anaerobic infections, Lyme disease, postexposure anthrax prophylaxis

Contraindications and cautions

- Contraindicated with allergies to penicillins, cephalosporins, or other allergens.
- Use cautiously with renal disorders, pregnancy, lactation (may cause diarrhea or candidiasis in the infant).

Available forms

Tablets—250, 300, 500 mg; powder for oral solution—125, 250, 300 mg/5 mL

P

Dosages

Adults and patients older than 12 yr

- *Fusospirochetal infections:* 250–500 mg every 6–8 hr PO.
- *Streptococcal infections (including otitis media, URIs of mild to moderate severity, scarlet fever, erysipelas):* 125–250 mg every 6–8 hr PO for 10 days.
- *Pneumococcal infections:* 250–500 mg every 6 hr PO until afebrile for 48 hr.
- *Staphylococcal infections of skin and soft tissues:* 250–500 mg every 6–8 hr PO.
- *Prevention of recurrence of rheumatic fever/chorea:* 125–250 mg twice daily.
- *Lyme disease:* 500 mg PO qid for 10–20 days.
- *Mild, uncomplicated cutaneous anthrax:* 200–500 mg PO qid.

Adults and patients older than 9 yr

- *Anthrax prophylaxis:* 7.5 mg/kg PO qid.

Pediatric patients younger than 12 yr

15–62.5 mg/kg/day PO given every 6–8 hr. Calculate doses according to weight.

- *Sickle cell anemia as prophylaxis of* S. pneumoniae *septicemia:* 250 mg PO bid; 3 mo–5 yr: 125 mg PO bid.
- *Mild, uncomplicated cutaneous anthrax in children older than 2 yr:* 25–50 mg/kg daily in two or four divided doses.

Pediatric patients younger than 9 yr

- *Anthrax prophylaxis:* 50 mg/kg/day PO in four divided doses.

Pharmacokinetics

Route	*Onset*	*Peak*
Oral	Varies	60 min

Metabolism: Hepatic; $T_{1/2}$: 30 min
Distribution: Crosses placenta; enters breast milk
Excretion: Urine

Adverse effects

- **CNS:** Lethargy, hallucinations, seizures
- **GI:** *Glossitis, stomatitis, gastritis, sore mouth,* furry tongue, black "hairy" tongue, *nausea, vomiting, diarrhea,* abdominal pain, bloody diarrhea, enterocolitis, pseudomembranous colitis, nonspecific hepatitis
- **GU:** Nephritis—oliguria, proteinuria, hematuria, casts, azotemia, pyuria
- **Hematologic:** Anemia, thrombocytopenia, leukopenia, neutropenia, prolonged bleeding time
- **Hypersensitivity reactions:** *Rash, fever, wheezing,* **anaphylaxis** (sometimes fatal)
- **Other:** *Superinfections;* sodium overload leading to HF; potassium poisoning—hyperreflexia, coma, cardiac arrhythmias, **cardiac arrest** (potassium preparations)

Interactions

✱ **Drug-drug** • Decreased effectiveness with tetracyclines

■ Nursing considerations

Assessment

- **History:** Allergies to penicillins, cephalosporins, or other allergens; renal disorders; pregnancy; lactation
- **Physical:** Culture infection; skin color, lesions; R, adventitious sounds; bowel sounds: CBC, LFTs, renal function tests, serum electrolytes, Hct, urinalysis

Interventions

- Culture infection before beginning treatment; reculture if response is not as expected.
- Continue therapy for at least 2 days after infection has disappeared, usually 7–10 days.
- Do not administer oral drug with milk, fruit juices, or soft drinks; a full glass of water is preferred; this oral penicillin is less affected by food than other penicillins.

Teaching points

- Avoid self-treating other infections with this antibiotic because it is specific for the infection being treated. Complete the full course of drug therapy.
- You may experience these side effects: Nausea, vomiting, diarrhea, mouth sores.
- Report difficulty breathing, rashes, severe diarrhea, mouth sores, unusual bleeding, or bruising.

pentamidine isethionate

*(pen **ta'** ma deen ess **thye'** oh nate)*

Parenteral: Pentacarinat, Pentam 300

Inhalation: NebuPent

PREGNANCY CATEGORY C

Drug class

Antiprotozoal

Therapeutic actions

Antiprotozoal activity in susceptible *Pneumocystis carinii* pneumonia infections; mechanism of action is not fully understood, but the drug interferes with nuclear metabolism and inhibits the synthesis of DNA, RNA, phospholipids, and proteins, which lead to cell death.

Indications

- Treatment of *P. carinii* pneumonia, especially in patients who do not respond to therapy with the less toxic trimethoprim-sulfamethoxazole combination (injection)
- Inhalation: Prevention of *P. carinii* pneumonia in high-risk, HIV-infected patients
- Unlabeled use (injection): Treatment of trypanosomiasis, visceral leishmaniasis

Contraindications and cautions

If the diagnosis of *P. carinii* pneumonia has been confirmed, there are no absolute contraindications to the use of this drug.

- Contraindicated with history of anaphylactic reaction to inhaled or parenteral pentamidine isethionate (inhalation therapy), lactation.
- Use cautiously with hypotension, hypertension, hypoglycemia, hyperglycemia, hypocalcemia, leukopenia, thrombocytopenia, anemia, hepatic or renal impairment, pregnancy.

Available forms

Injection—300 mg/vial; powder for injection—300 mg; aerosol—300 mg

Dosages

Adults and pediatric patients

Parenteral

4 mg/kg once a day for 14–21 days by deep IM injection or IV infusion over 60 min.

Inhalation

300 mg once every 4 wk administered through the *Respirgard II* nebulizer.

Pharmacokinetics

Route	*Onset*
IM	Slow
Inhalation	Rapid

Metabolism: $T_{1/2}$: 6.4–9.4 hr

Distribution: Crosses placenta; enters breast milk

Excretion: Urine

IV FACTS

Preparation: Prepare solution by dissolving contents of 1 vial in 3–5 mL of sterile water for injection or 5% dextrose injection; do not use saline for reconstitution. Dilute the calculated dose further in 50–250 mL of 5% dextrose solution; solutions of 1 and 2.5 mg/mL in 5% dextrose are stable at room temperature for up to 24 hr. Protect from light.

Infusion: Infuse the diluted solution over 60–120 min.

Y-site incompatibility: Do not mix with foscarnet or fluconazole.

Adverse effects

Parenteral

- **CV:** *Hypotension,* tachycardia
- **GI:** *Nausea, anorexia*
- **GU:** *Elevated serum creatinine,* **acute renal failure**
- **Hematologic:** *Leukopenia, hypoglycemia,* thrombocytopenia, hypocalcemia, elevated LFTs
- **Local:** *Pain, abscess at injection site*
- **Other: Stevens-Johnson syndrome,** *fever, rash,* **severe hypotension,** hypoglycemia, and cardiac arrhythmias

Inhalation

- **CNS:** *Fatigue, dizziness,* headache, tremors, confusion, anxiety, memory loss, seizures, insomnia, drowsiness

P

- **CV:** Tachycardia, hypotension, hypertension, palpitations, syncope, vasodilatation
- **GI:** *Metallic taste in mouth, anorexia, nausea, vomiting,* gingivitis, dyspepsia, oral ulcer, gastritis, hypersalivation, dry mouth, melena, colitis, abdominal pain
- **Respiratory:** *Shortness of breath, cough, pharyngitis, congestion,* **bronchospasm,** rhinitis, laryngitis, **laryngospasm,** hyperventilation, pneumothorax
- **Other:** *Rash, night sweats, chills*

■ Nursing considerations

Assessment

- **History:** History of anaphylactic reaction to inhaled or parenteral pentamidine isethionate, hypotension, hypertension, hypoglycemia, hyperglycemia, hypocalcemia, leukopenia, thrombocytopenia, anemia, hepatic or renal impairment, pregnancy, lactation
- **Physical:** Skin lesions, color; T; reflexes, affect (inhalation); BP, P, baseline ECG; BUN, serum creatinine, blood glucose, CBC, platelet count, LFTs, serum calcium

Interventions

⊗ ***Warning*** Monitor patient closely during administration; fatalities have been reported.

- Arrange for these tests to be performed before, during, and after therapy: Daily BUN, daily serum creatinine, daily blood glucose; regular CBC, platelet counts, LFTs, serum calcium; periodic ECG.

⊗ ***Warning*** Position patient in supine position before parenteral administration to protect patient if BP changes.

- Reconstitute for inhalation: Dissolve contents of 1 vial in 6 mL of sterile water for injection. Use only sterile water. Saline cannot be used, precipitates will form. Place entire solution in nebulizer reservoir. Solution is stable for 48 hr in original vial at room temperature if protected from light. Do not mix with other drugs.
- Administer inhalation using the *Respirgard II* nebulizer. Deliver the dose using a flow rate of 5–7 L/min and an air or oxygen source set at 40–50 PSI until the chamber is empty (30–45 min).
- For IM use: Prepare IM solution by dissolving contents of 1-g vial in 3 mL of sterile water for injection; protect from light. Discard any unused portions. Inject deeply into large muscle group. Inspect injection site regularly; rotate injection sites.
- Instruct patient and significant other in the reconstitution of inhalation solutions and administration for outpatient use.

Teaching points

- Parenteral drug can be given only IV or IM and must be given every day. Inhalation drug must be given using the *Respirgard II* nebulizer. Prepare the solution as instructed by your health care provider, using only sterile water for injection. Protect the medication from exposure to light. Use freshly reconstituted solution. The drug must be used once every 4 weeks. Prepare a calendar with drug days marked as a reminder. Do not mix any other drugs in the nebulizer.
- Have frequent blood tests and blood pressure checks because this drug may cause many changes in your body.
- You may feel weak and dizzy with sudden position changes; take care to change position slowly.
- If using the inhalation, metallic taste and GI upset may occur. Frequent small meals and mouth care may help.
- Report pain at injection site, confusion, hallucinations, unusual bleeding or bruising, weakness, fatigue.

DANGEROUS DRUG

▽ pentazocine

(pen taz' oh seen)

pentazocine hydrochloride with naloxone hydrochloride, 0.5 mg

Oral: Talwin NX

pentazocine lactate

Parenteral: Talwin

PREGNANCY CATEGORY C

CONTROLLED SUBSTANCE C-IV

Drug class

Opioid agonist-antagonist analgesic

Therapeutic actions

Pentazocine acts as an agonist at specific (kappa) opioid receptors in the CNS to produce analgesia, sedation; acts as an agonist at sigma opioid receptors to cause dysphoria, hallucinations; acts at mu opioid receptors to antagonize the analgesic and euphoric activities of some other opioid analgesics. Has lower abuse potential than morphine, other pure opioid agonists; the oral preparation contains the opioid antagonist naloxone, which has poor bioavailability when given orally and does not interfere with the analgesic effects of pentazocine but serves as a deterrent to the unintended IV injection of solutions made from the oral tablets.

Indications

- Oral and parenteral: Relief of moderate to severe pain
- Parenteral: Preanesthetic medication and as supplement to surgical anesthesia

Contraindications and cautions

- Contraindicated with hypersensitivity to opioids, sulfites (oral and parenteral), naloxone (oral form); pregnancy (neonatal withdrawal); lactation.
- Use cautiously with physical dependence on an opioid analgesic (can precipitate a withdrawal syndrome); bronchial asthma, COPD, cor pulmonale, respiratory depression, anoxia, increased intracranial pressure; acute MI with hypertension, left ventricular failure or nausea and vomiting; renal or hepatic impairment; labor or delivery (opioids given to the mother can cause neonatal respiratory depression; premature infants are especially at risk; may prolong labor).

Available forms

Injection—30 mg/mL; tablets—25, 50 mg

Dosages

Adults

Oral

Initially, 50 mg every 3–4 hr. Increase to 100 mg if needed. Do not exceed a total dose of 600 mg/24 hr.

Parenteral

30 mg IM, subcutaneously, or IV. May repeat every 3–4 hr. Doses exceeding 30 mg IV or 60 mg IM or subcutaneously are not recommended. Do not exceed 360 mg/24 hr. Give subcutaneously only when necessary; repeat injections should be given IM.

- *Patients in labor:* A single 30-mg IM dose is most common. A 20-mg IV dose given 2–3 times at 2- to 3-hr intervals relieves pain when contractions become regular.

Pediatric patients younger than 12 yr

Not recommended.

Geriatric patients or impaired adults

Use caution; respiratory depression may occur in the elderly, the very ill, and those with respiratory problems. Dosage may need to be reduced.

Pharmacokinetics

Route	*Onset*	*Peak*	*Duration*
Oral, IM, Subcut.	15–30 min	1–3 hr	3 hr
IV	2–3 min	15 min	3 hr

Metabolism: Hepatic; $T_{1/2}$: 2–3 hr
Distribution: Crosses placenta; enters breast milk
Excretion: Feces, urine

IV FACTS

Preparation: No further preparation is required.
Infusion: Inject directly into vein or into tubing of actively running IV; infuse slowly, each 5 mg over 1 min.
Incompatibilities: Do not mix in same syringe as barbiturates; precipitate will form.

Adverse effects

- **CNS:** *Light-headedness, dizziness, sedation, euphoria,* dysphoria, delirium, insomnia, agitation, anxiety, fear, hallucinations, disorientation, drowsiness, lethargy, impaired mental and physical performance, coma, mood changes, weakness, headache, tremor, seizures, miosis, visual disturbances
- **CV:** Facial flushing, peripheral circulatory collapse, tachycardia, bradycardia, arrhythmia, palpitations, chest wall rigidity,

P

hypertension, hypotension, orthostatic hypotension, syncope, circulatory depression, **shock, cardiac arrest**

- **Dermatologic:** Pruritus, urticaria, edema
- **GI:** *Nausea, vomiting, sweating* (more common in ambulatory patients and those without severe pain), dry mouth, anorexia, constipation, biliary tract spasm; increased colonic motility in patients with chronic ulcerative colitis
- **GU:** Ureteral spasm, spasm of vesical sphincters, urinary retention or hesitancy, oliguria, antidiuretic effect, reduced libido or potency
- **Local:** Pain at injection site, tissue irritation and induration (subcutaneous injection)
- **Respiratory:** Suppression of cough reflex, respiratory depression, apnea, respiratory arrest, **laryngospasm, bronchospasm**
- **Other:** Physical tolerance and dependence, psychological dependence (**the oral form has been especially abused in combination with tripelennamine—"Ts and Blues"—with serious and fatal consequences;** addition of naloxone to oral formulation may decrease this abuse)

Interactions

✱ **Drug-drug** • Increased likelihood of respiratory depression, hypotension, profound sedation, or coma with barbiturate general anesthetics • Precipitation of withdrawal syndrome in patients previously given other opioid analgesics, including morphine, methadone (note that this applies to the parenteral preparation without naloxone and to the oral preparation that includes naloxone)

■ Nursing considerations

Assessment

- **History:** Hypersensitivity to opioids, naloxone (oral form), sulfites (oral and parenteral); physical dependence on an opioid analgesic; pregnancy; labor or delivery; lactation; respiratory disease; anoxia; increased intracranial pressure; acute MI; renal or hepatic impairment
- **Physical:** T; skin color, texture, lesions; orientation, reflexes, bilateral grip strength, affect, pupil size; P, auscultation, BP, orthostatic BP, perfusion; R, adventitious sounds; bowel sounds, normal output; frequency and pattern of voiding, normal output; LFTs, renal function tests, CBC with differential

Interventions

⊗ ***Black box warning*** Be aware that *Talwin NX* is for oral use only; it can be lethal if injected.

- Do not mix parenteral pentazocine in same syringe as barbiturates; precipitate will form.

⊗ ***Warning*** Keep opioid antagonist, equipment for assisted or controlled respiration readily available during parenteral administration.

⊗ ***Warning*** Use caution when injecting subcutaneously into chilled areas of the body or in patients with hypotension or in shock; impaired perfusion may delay absorption; with repeated doses, an excessive amount may be absorbed when circulation is restored.

⊗ ***Warning*** Withdraw drug gradually if it has been given for 4 or 5 days, especially to emotionally unstable patients or those with a history of drug abuse; a withdrawal syndrome sometimes occurs in these circumstances.

- Reassure patient that addiction is unlikely; most patients who receive opiates for medical reasons do not develop dependence syndromes.

Teaching points

- Take drug exactly as prescribed.
- Avoid alcohol, antihistamines, sedatives, tranquilizers, and over-the-counter drugs while taking this drug.
- Do not take any leftover medication for other disorders, and do not let anyone else take the prescription.
- You may experience these side effects: Nausea, loss of appetite (take drug with food, lie quietly, eat frequent small meals); constipation (a laxative may help); dizziness, sedation, drowsiness, impaired visual acuity (avoid driving or performing other tasks that require alertness, visual acuity).
- Report severe nausea, vomiting, constipation, shortness of breath or difficulty breathing.

pentetate calcium trisodium (Ca-DTPA), pentetate zinc trisodium (Zn-DTPA)

See Appendix W, *Less commonly used drugs*.

DANGEROUS DRUG

pentobarbital (pentobarbital sodium)

*(pen toe **bar'** bi tal)*

Nembutal

PREGNANCY CATEGORY D

CONTROLLED SUBSTANCE C-II

Drug classes
Antiepileptic
Barbiturate
Hypnotic
Sedative or hypnotic

Therapeutic actions
General CNS depressant; barbiturates inhibit impulse conduction in the ascending RAS, depress the cerebral cortex, alter cerebellar function, depress motor output, and can produce excitation, sedation, hypnosis, anesthesia, and deep coma; at anesthetic doses, has antiseizure activity.

Indications
- Sedative
- Preanesthetic in pediatric patients
- Antiepileptic, in anesthetic doses, for emergency control of certain acute seizure episodes (eg, status epilepticus, eclampsia, meningitis, tetanus, toxic reactions to strychnine or local anesthetics)

Contraindications and cautions
- Contraindicated with hypersensitivity to barbiturates, manifest or latent porphyria, marked liver impairment, nephritis, severe respiratory distress, previous addiction to sedative-hypnotic drugs, pregnancy (fetal damage, neonatal withdrawal syndrome), lactation.
- Use cautiously with acute or chronic pain (paradoxical excitement or masking of important symptoms), seizure disorders (abrupt discontinuation of daily doses can result in status epilepticus), fever, hyperthyroidism, diabetes mellitus, severe anemia, pulmonary or cardiac disease, status asthmaticus, shock, uremia.

Available forms
Injection—50 mg/mL

Dosages
Adults
Use only when prompt action is imperative.
IV: Give by slow IV injection, not to exceed 50 mg/min. Initial dose is 100 mg in a 70-kg adult. Wait at least 1 min for full effect. Base dosage on response. Additional small increments may be given up to a total of 200–500 mg. Minimize dosage in seizure states to avoid compounding the depression that may follow seizures.
IM: Inject deeply into a muscle mass. Usual adult dose is 150–200 mg. Do not exceed a volume of 5 mL at any site due to tissue irritation.
Pediatric patients
Use caution; barbiturates may produce irritability, aggression, inappropriate tearfulness.
IV: Reduce initial adult dosage on basis of age, weight, and patient's condition.
IM: Dosage frequently ranges from 25–80 mg or 2–6 mg/kg. Do not exceed 100 mg.
Geriatric patients or those with debilitating disease
Reduce dosage and monitor closely. May produce excitement, depression, or confusion.

Pharmacokinetics

Route	Onset	Duration
IM, IV	Rapid	2–3 hr

Metabolism: Hepatic; $T_{1/2}$: 15–50 hr
Distribution: Crosses placenta; enters breast milk
Excretion: Urine

IV FACTS
Preparation: No further preparation is required.
Infusion: Infuse slowly, each 50 mg over 1 min; monitor patient response to dosage.
Incompatibilities: Do not combine with chlorpheniramine, codeine, ephedrine, erythromycin, hydrocortisone, insulin, norepinephrine,

P

penicillin G, potassium, phenytoin, promazine, vancomycin.

Adverse effects

- **CNS:** *Somnolence, agitation, confusion, hyperkinesia, ataxia, vertigo, CNS depression, nightmares, lethargy, residual sedation (hangover), paradoxical excitement, nervousness, psychiatric disturbance, hallucinations, insomnia, anxiety, dizziness, thinking abnormality*
- **CV:** *Bradycardia, hypotension, syncope*
- **GI:** *Nausea, vomiting, constipation, diarrhea, epigastric pain*
- **Hypersensitivity:** Rashes, angioneurotic edema, serum sickness, morbiliform rash, urticaria; rarely, exfoliative dermatitis, **Stevens-Johnson syndrome**
- **Local:** *Pain, tissue necrosis at injection site,* gangrene; arterial spasm with inadvertent intra-arterial injection; thrombophlebitis; permanent neurologic deficit if injected near a nerve
- **Respiratory:** *Hypoventilation, apnea, respiratory depression,* **laryngospasm, bronchospasm, circulatory collapse**
- **Other:** Tolerance, psychological and physical dependence; **withdrawal syndrome**

Interactions

✱ **Drug-drug** • Increased CNS depression with alcohol • Decreased effects of these drugs: Oral anticoagulants, corticosteroids, hormonal contraceptives and estrogens, beta-adrenergic blockers (especially propranolol, metoprolol), theophylline, metronidazole, doxycycline, phenylbutazones, quinidine

■ Nursing considerations

Assessment

- **History:** Hypersensitivity to barbiturates, manifest or latent porphyria, marked liver impairment, nephritis, severe respiratory distress, previous addiction to sedative-hypnotic drugs, acute or chronic pain, seizure disorders, pregnancy, lactation, fever, hyperthyroidism, diabetes mellitus, severe anemia, pulmonary or cardiac disease, shock, uremia
- **Physical:** Weight; T; skin color, lesions, injection site; orientation, affect, reflexes; P, BP, orthostatic BP; R, adventitious sounds; bowel sounds, normal output, liver evaluation; LFTs, renal function tests, blood and urine glucose, BUN

Interventions

⊗ ***Warning*** Do not administer intra-arterially; may produce arteriospasm, thrombosis, or gangrene.

- Administer IV doses slowly.
- Administer IM doses deep in a muscle mass.

⊗ ***Warning*** Do not use parenteral form if solution is discolored or contains a precipitate.

⊗ ***Warning*** Monitor injection sites carefully for irritation and extravasation (IV use); solutions are alkaline and very irritating to the tissues.

- Monitor P, BP, and respiration carefully during IV administration.

⊗ ***Warning*** Taper dosage gradually after repeated use, especially in patients with epilepsy.

Teaching points

- This drug will make you drowsy and less anxious.
- Do not try to get up after you have received this drug (request assistance to sit up or move about).

▽pentosan polysulfate sodium

See Appendix W, *Less commonly used drugs*.

▽pentostatin (2′ deoxycoformycin [DCF])

See Appendix W, *Less commonly used drugs*.

▽pentoxifylline

*(pen tox **ih'** fi leen)*

Apo-Pentoxifilline SR (CAN) DNC, Nu-Pentoxifylline SR (CAN) DNC, ratio-Pentoxifylline (CAN), Trental DNC

PREGNANCY CATEGORY C

Drug classes
Hemorrheologic drug
Xanthine

Therapeutic actions
Reduces RBC aggregation and local hyperviscosity, decreases platelet aggregation, decreases fibrinogen concentration in the blood; precise mechanism of action is not known.

Indications
- Intermittent claudication, to improve function and symptoms
- Unlabeled use: Cerebrovascular insufficiency to improve psychopathologic symptoms, diabetic vascular disease, aphthous stomatitis

Contraindications and cautions
- Contraindicated with allergy to pentoxifylline or methylxanthines (eg, caffeine, theophylline; drug is a dimethylxanthine derivative); recent cerebral or retinal hemorrhage.
- Use cautiously with pregnancy, lactation.

Available forms
CR tablets DNC—400 mg; ER tablets DNC—400 mg

Dosages
Adults
400 mg tid PO with meals. Decrease to 400 mg bid if adverse side effects occur. Continue for at least 8 wk.
Pediatric patients
Safety and efficacy not established.

Pharmacokinetics

Route	Onset	Peak
Oral	Varies	60 min

Metabolism: Hepatic; $T_{1/2}$: 0.4–1.6 hr
Distribution: Crosses placenta; enters breast milk
Excretion: Urine

Adverse effects
- **CNS:** *Dizziness, headache,* tremor, anxiety, confusion
- **CV:** Angina, chest pain, arrhythmia, hypotension, dyspnea
- **Dermatologic:** Brittle fingernails, pruritus, rash, urticaria
- **GI:** *Dyspepsia, nausea,* vomiting
- **Hematologic:** Pancytopenia, purpura, thrombocytopenia

Interactions
✱ **Drug-drug** • Increased therapeutic and toxic effects of theophylline when combined; monitor closely and adjust dosage as needed

■ Nursing considerations
Assessment
- **History:** Allergy to pentoxifylline or methylxanthines, pregnancy, lactation
- **Physical:** Skin color, T; orientation, reflexes; P, BP, peripheral perfusion; CBC

Interventions
- Monitor patient for angina and arrhythmias.
- Administer drug with meals.
- Caution patient to swallow tablets whole and not to cut, crush, or chew them.

Teaching points
- Take drug with meals. Swallow tablets whole; do not cut, crush, or chew.
- This drug helps the signs and symptoms of claudication, but additional therapy is sometimes needed.
- Dizziness may occur as a result of therapy; avoid driving and operating dangerous machinery; take precautions to prevent injury.
- Report chest pain, flushing, loss of consciousness, twitching, numbness, and tingling.

P

perindopril erbumine
(pur in' doh pril)

Aceon

PREGNANCY CATEGORY C
(FIRST TRIMESTER)

PREGNANCY CATEGORY D
(SECOND AND THIRD TRIMESTERS)

Drug classes
ACE inhibitor
Antihypertensive

Therapeutic actions
Renin, synthesized by the kidneys, is released into the circulation where it acts on a plasma

precursor to produce angiotensin I, which is converted by ACE to angiotensin II—a potent vasoconstrictor that also causes release of aldosterone from the adrenals. Perindopril blocks the conversion of angiotensin I to angiotensin II, leading to decreased BP, decreased aldosterone secretion, a small increase in serum potassium levels, and sodium and fluid loss.

Indications

- Treatment of hypertension, alone or in combination with other antihypertensive
- Treatment of patients with stable coronary artery disease to reduce the risk of CV mortality and nonfatal MI

Contraindications and cautions

- Contraindicated with allergy to any ACE inhibitor, pregnancy, history of ACE inhibitors–associated angioedema.
- Use cautiously with impaired renal function, HF, salt or volume depletion, lactation.

Available forms

Tablets—2, 4, 8 mg

Dosages

Adults

Hypertension: 4 mg PO daily; may be titrated to a maximum of 16 mg/day.
CV disease: 4 mg/day PO for 2 wk; increase to a maintenance dose of 8 mg/day PO.

Pediatric patients

Safety and efficacy not established.

Geriatric patients

Maximum daily dosage should not exceed 8 mg/day.

Patients with renal impairment

For creatinine clearance greater than 30 mL/min, give initial dose of 2 mg/day PO. Maximum dose, 8 mg/day. For creatinine clearance of 30 mL/min or less, do not administer drug.

Pharmacokinetics

Route	Onset	Peak
Oral	1 hr	3–7 hr

Metabolism: Hepatic; $T_{1/2}$: 30–120 hr
Distribution: Crosses placenta; enters breast milk
Excretion: Urine

Adverse effects

- **CNS:** *Headache, dizziness, insomnia, fatigue,* paresthesias
- **CV:** *Orthostatic hypotension,* tachycardia, angina pectoris, MI, Raynaud's syndrome, HF (severe hypotension in salt- or volume-depleted patients)
- **GI:** *Gastric irritation, nausea, diarrhea,* aphthous ulcers, peptic ulcers, dysgeusia, cholestatic jaundice, hepatocellular injury, anorexia, constipation
- **GU:** *Proteinuria,* renal insufficiency, renal failure, polyuria, oliguria, frequency of urination
- **Hematologic:** Neutropenia, agranulocytosis, thrombocytopenia, hemolytic anemia, **pancytopenia**
- **Other:** *Angioedema* (particularly of the face, extremities, lips, tongue, larynx; death has been reported with **airway obstruction**—greater risk in black patients); *cough,* muscle cramps, impotence

Interactions

✱ **Drug-drug** • Decreased antihypertensive effects if taken with indomethacin • Risk of increased lithium levels if taken with potassium-sparing diuretics

■ Nursing considerations

Assessment

- **History:** Allergy to any ACE inhibitor; impaired renal function; HF; salt or volume depletion; pregnancy, lactation ACE inhibitor–associated angioedema
- **Physical:** Skin color, lesions, turgor; T; P, BP, peripheral perfusion; mucous membranes, bowel sounds, liver evaluation; urinalysis, LFTs, renal function tests, CBC and differential

Interventions

⊗ ***Warning*** Keep epinephrine readily available in case of angioedema of the face or neck region; if patient has difficulty breathing, consult with physician and administer epinephrine as appropriate.

⊗ ***Warning*** Alert surgeon and mark the patient's chart with notice that perindopril is being taken. The angiotensin II formation subsequent to compensatory renin release during surgery will be blocked. Hypotension may be reversed with volume expansion.

- Monitor patients on diuretic therapy for excessive hypotension; the diuretic can be stopped 2–3 days before beginning therapy with perindopril and reintroduced slowly, monitoring patient response.
- Monitor patient closely in any situation that may lead to a fall in BP secondary to reduction in fluid volume—excessive perspiration and dehydration, vomiting, diarrhea—as excessive hypotension may occur.
- Arrange for reduced dosage in patients with impaired renal function.

⊗ ***Black box warning*** Caution patient that this drug can cause serious fetal injury; advise using barrier contraceptives.

Teaching points

- Take this drug once a day; it may be taken with meals. Do not stop taking the medication without consulting your health care provider.
- Use caution with any condition that may lead to a drop in blood pressure—diarrhea, sweating, vomiting, dehydration. If lightheadedness or dizziness should occur, consult your health care provider.
- Avoid the use of over-the-counter medications while you are on this drug—especially avoid cough, cold, or allergy medications that may contain ingredients that will interact with this drug. If you feel that you need one of these preparations, consult your health care provider.
- Avoid pregnancy while using this drug; serious fetal injury could occur. Using barrier contraceptives is advised; if pregnancy should occur, stop drug and notify your health care provider.
- You may experience these side effects: GI upset, loss of appetite, change in taste perception (these may be limited effects that will pass; taking the drug with meals may help); mouth sores (frequent mouth care may help); rash; fast heart rate; dizziness, light-headedness (this usually passes after the first few days of therapy; if it occurs, change position slowly and limit your activities to ones that do not require alertness and precision); headache, fatigue, sleeplessness.
- Report mouth sores, sore throat, fever, chills, swelling of the hands, feet, irregular heartbeat, chest pains, swelling of the face, eyes, lips, tongue, difficulty breathing.

▽phenazopyridine hydrochloride (phenylazodiaminopyridine hydrochloride)

*(fen az oh **peer'** i deen)*

Azo-Standard, Baridium, Geridium, Phenazo (CAN), Prodium, Pyridium, Pyridium Plus, Urogesic, UTI Relief

PREGNANCY CATEGORY B

Drug class

Urinary analgesic

Therapeutic actions

An azo dye that is excreted in the urine and exerts a direct topical analgesic effect on urinary tract mucosa; exact mechanism of action is not understood.

Indications

- Symptomatic relief of pain, urgency, burning, frequency, and discomfort related to irritation of the lower urinary tract mucosa caused by infection, trauma, surgery, endoscopic procedures, passage of sounds or catheters

Contraindications and cautions

- Contraindicated with allergy to phenazopyridine, renal insufficiency.
- Use cautiously with pregnancy, lactation.

Available forms

Tablets—95, 97.2, 100, 200 mg

Dosages

Adults

200 mg PO tid after meals. Do not exceed 2 days if used with antibacterial agent.

Pediatric patients 6–12 yr

12 mg/kg/day divided into three doses PO for no longer than 2 days.

P

Pharmacokinetics

Route	Onset
Oral	Rapid

Metabolism: Hepatic; $T_{1/2}$: Unknown
Distribution: Crosses placenta; may enter breast milk
Excretion: Urine

Adverse effects

- **CNS:** *Headache*
- **Dermatologic:** *Rash,* yellowish tinge to skin or sclera, pruritus
- **GI:** *GI disturbances*
- **Hematologic:** Methemoglobinemia, hemolytic anemia
- **Other:** Renal and hepatic toxicity, *yellow-orange discoloration of urine*

Interactions

✱ **Drug-lab test** • Interference with colorimetric laboratory test procedures

■ Nursing considerations

Assessment

- **History:** Allergy to phenazopyridine, renal insufficiency, pregnancy
- **Physical:** Skin color, lesions; urinary output; normal GI output, bowel sounds, liver palpation; urinalysis, LFTs, renal function tests, CBC

Interventions

- Give after meals to avoid GI upset.
- Warn patient drug may stain contact lenses.
- Do not give longer than 2 days if being given with antibacterial agent for treatment of UTI.
- Alert patient that urine may turn reddish-orange and may stain fabric.

⊗ ***Warning*** Discontinue drug if skin or sclera become yellowish, a sign of drug accumulation.

Teaching points

- Take drug after meals to avoid GI upset.
- Urine may be reddish-orange (normal effect; urine may stain fabric). Contact lenses may be permanently stained.
- Report yellowish staining of skin or eyes, headache, unusual bleeding or bruising, fever, sore throat.

▽ phenelzine sulfate

(fen' el zeen)

Nardil

PREGNANCY CATEGORY C

Drug classes

Antidepressant
MAOI

Therapeutic actions

Irreversibly inhibits MAO, an enzyme that breaks down biogenic amines, such as epinephrine, norepinephrine, and serotonin, thus allowing these biogenic amines to accumulate in neuronal storage sites. According to the biogenic amine hypothesis, this accumulation of amines is responsible for the clinical efficacy of MAOIs as antidepressants.

Indications

- Treatment of patients with depression characterized as atypical, nonendogenous, or neurotic; patients who are unresponsive to other antidepressive therapy; and patients in whom other antidepressive therapy is contraindicated
- Unlabeled uses: Treatment of bulimia, PTSD, chronic migraine not responsive to standard treatment, social anxiety disorders

Contraindications and cautions

- Contraindicated with hypersensitivity to any MAOI, pheochromocytoma, HF, history of liver disease or abnormal LFTs, severe renal impairment, confirmed or suspected cerebrovascular defect, CV disease, hypertension, history of headache, suicidal ideation.
- Use cautiously with seizure disorders; hyperthyroidism; impaired hepatic, renal function; psychiatric patients (agitated or schizophrenic patients may show excessive stimulation; bipolar patients may shift to hypomanic or manic phase); patients scheduled for elective surgery; pregnancy; lactation.

Available forms

Tablets—15 mg

Dosages

Adults

Initially, 15 mg PO tid. Increase dosage to at least 60 mg/day at a rapid pace consistent with patient tolerance. Many patients require therapy at 60 mg/day for at least 4 wk before response. Some patients may require 90 mg/day. After maximum benefit is achieved, reduce dosage slowly over several weeks. Maintenance may be 15 mg/day or every other day.

Pediatric patients younger than 16 yr

Not recommended.

Geriatric patients

Patients older than 60 yr are more prone to develop adverse effects; adjust dosage accordingly.

Pharmacokinetics

Route	Onset	Peak	Duration
Oral	Slow	1 hr	48–96 hr

Metabolism: Hepatic; $T_{1/2}$: 12 hr
Distribution: Crosses placenta; enters breast milk
Excretion: Urine

Adverse effects

- **CNS:** *Dizziness, vertigo, headache, overactivity, hyperreflexia, tremors, muscle twitching, mania, hypomania, jitteriness, confusion, memory impairment, insomnia, weakness, fatigue, drowsiness, restlessness, overstimulation, increased anxiety, agitation, blurred vision, sweating,* akathisia, ataxia, coma, euphoria, neuritis, repetitious babbling, chills, glaucoma, nystagmus, suicidal thoughts
- **CV: Hypertensive crises** (sometimes fatal, sometimes with intracranial bleeding, usually attributable to ingestion of contraindicated food or drink containing tyramine; see drug-food interactions below; symptoms include some or all of the following: Occipital headache, which may radiate frontally; palpitations; neck stiffness or soreness; nausea; vomiting; sweating; dilated pupils; photophobia; tachycardia or bradycardia; chest pain); *orthostatic hypotension, sometimes associated with falling; disturbed cardiac rate and rhythm,* palpitations, tachycardia
- **Dermatologic:** Minor skin reactions, spider telangiectases, photosensitivity
- **GI:** *Constipation, diarrhea, nausea, abdominal pain, edema, dry mouth, anorexia, weight changes*
- **GU:** Dysuria, incontinence, urinary retention, sexual disturbances
- **Other:** Hematologic changes, black tongue, hypernatremia

Interactions

✱ **Drug-drug** ⊗ ***Warning*** Hypertensive crisis, coma, severe seizures with TCAs (eg, imipramine, desipramine). Note: MAOIs and TCAs have been used successfully in some patients resistant to therapy with single agents; however, case reports indicate that the combination can cause serious and potentially fatal side effects.

• Increased sympathomimetic effects (hypertensive crisis) with sympathomimetic drugs (norepinephrine, epinephrine, dopamine, dobutamine, levodopa, ephedrine, carbamazepine), amphetamines, other anorexiants, local anesthetic solutions containing sympathomimetic • Additive hypoglycemic effect with insulin, oral sulfonylureas • Increased hypotensive effects with beta blockers, anesthetics, thiazide diuretics • Increased risk of adverse interaction with meperidine, dextromethorphan • Risk of serotonin syndrome if combined with SSRIs or other serotonergic agents

✱ **Drug-food** ⊗ ***Warning*** Tyramine (and other pressor amines) contained in foods are normally broken down by MAO enzymes in the GI tract; in the presence of MAOIs, these vasopressors may be absorbed in high concentrations; in addition, tyramine releases accumulated norepinephrine from nerve terminals; thus, hypertensive crisis may occur when the following foods that contain tyramine or other vasopressors are ingested by a patient on an MAOI: Dairy products (blue, camembert, cheddar, mozzarella, parmesan, romano, roquefort, Stilton cheeses; sour cream; yogurt); meats, fish (liver, pickled herring, fermented sausages—bologna, pepperoni, salami; caviar; dried fish; other fermented or spoiled meat or fish); undistilled beverages (imported beer, ale; red wine, especially Chianti; sherry; coffee, tea, colas containing caffeine; chocolate drinks); fruits and

P

vegetables (avocado, fava beans, figs, raisins, bananas); yeast extracts; soy sauce; chocolate.

✷ **Drug-alternative therapy** • May cause headaches, manic episodes if combined with ginseng therapy

■ Nursing considerations

Assessment

- **History:** Hypersensitivity to any MAOI; pheochromocytoma; HF; abnormal LFTs; severe renal impairment; cerebrovascular defect; CV disease, hypertension; history of headache; seizure disorders; hyperthyroidism; impaired hepatic, renal function; psychiatric disorder; elective surgery; pregnancy, lactation; suicidal ideation
- **Physical:** Weight; T; skin color, lesions; orientation, affect, reflexes, vision; P, BP, orthostatic BP, auscultation, perfusion; bowel sounds, normal output, liver evaluation; urine flow, normal output; thyroid palpation; LFTs, renal and thyroid function tests, urinalysis, CBC, ECG, EEG

Interventions

⊗ ***Black box warning*** Be aware of an increased risk of suicidality in children, adolescents, and young adults; monitor patients accordingly.

- Limit amount of drug that is available to suicidal patients.
- Monitor BP and orthostatic BP carefully; arrange for more gradual increase in dosage in patients who show tendency for hypotension.

⊗ ***Warning*** Have periodic LFTs during therapy; discontine drug at first sign of hepatic impairment or jaundice.

⊗ ***Warning*** Discontinue drug and monitor BP carefully if patient reports unusual or severe headache.

⊗ ***Warning*** Keep phentolamine or another alpha-adrenergic blocking drug readily available in case hypertensive crisis occurs.

- Provide a diet that is low in tyramine-containing foods.

Teaching points

- Take drug exactly as prescribed. Do not stop taking this drug abruptly or without consulting your health care provider.
- Avoid ingestion of tyramine-containing foods while you are taking this drug and for 2 weeks afterward (patient and significant other should receive a list of such foods).
- Avoid alcohol; other sleep-inducing drugs; all over-the-counter drugs, including nose drops, cold and hay fever remedies; and appetite suppressants. Many of these contain substances that could cause serious or even life-threatening problems.
- You may experience these side effects: Dizziness, weakness or fainting when arising from a horizontal or sitting position (transient; change position slowly); drowsiness, blurred vision (reversible; if severe, avoid driving or performing tasks that require alertness); nausea, vomiting, loss of appetite (frequent small meals, frequent mouth care may help); memory changes, irritability, emotional changes, nervousness (reversible).
- Report headache, rash, darkening of the urine, pale stools, yellowing of the eyes or skin, fever, chills, sore throat, thoughts of suicide, and any other unusual symptoms.

DANGEROUS DRUG

▽ phenobarbital

*(fee noe **bar'** bi tal)*

phenobarbital

Oral preparations: Bellatal, Solfoton

phenobarbital sodium

Parenteral: Luminal Sodium, PMS-Phenobarbital (CAN)

PREGNANCY CATEGORY D

CONTROLLED SUBSTANCE C-IV

Drug classes

Antiepileptic
Barbiturate (long acting)
Hypnotic
Sedative

Therapeutic actions

General CNS depressant; barbiturates inhibit impulse conduction in the ascending RAS, depress the cerebral cortex, alter cerebellar function, depress motor output, and can produce excitation, sedation, hypnosis, anesthesia, and deep coma; at subhypnotic doses, has antiseizure activity, making it suitable for long-term use as an antiepileptic.

Indications

- Oral or parenteral: Sedative
- Oral or parenteral: Hypnotic, treatment of insomnia for up to 2 wk
- Oral: Long-term treatment of generalized tonic-clonic and cortical focal seizures
- Oral: Emergency control of certain acute seizures (eg, those associated with status epilepticus, eclampsia, meningitis, tetanus, and toxic reactions to strychnine or local anesthetics)
- Parenteral: Preanesthetic
- Parenteral: Treatment of generalized tonic-clonic and cortical focal seizures
- Parenteral: Emergency control of acute seizures (tetanus, eclampsia, epilepticus)

Contraindications and cautions

- Contraindicated with hypersensitivity to barbiturates, manifest or latent porphyria, marked liver impairment, nephritis, severe respiratory distress, previous addiction to sedative-hypnotic drugs (may be ineffective and may contribute to further addiction), pregnancy (fetal damage, neonatal withdrawal syndrome).
- Use cautiously with acute or chronic pain (drug may cause paradoxical excitement or mask important symptoms); seizure disorders (abrupt discontinuation of daily doses can result in status epilepticus); lactation (secreted in breast milk; drowsiness in nursing infants); fever, hyperthyroidism, diabetes mellitus, severe anemia, pulmonary or cardiac disease, status asthmaticus, shock, uremia, impaired liver or renal function, debilitation.

Available forms

Tablets—15, 16, 30, 60, 90, 100 mg; capsules—16 mg; elixir—15 mg/5 mL, 20 mg/5 mL; injection—30, 60, 65, 130 mg/mL

Dosages

Adults

Oral

- *Sedation:* 30–120 mg/day in two to three divided doses. No more than 400 mg per 24 hr.
- *Hypnotic:* 100–200 mg at bedtime.
- *Antiepileptic:* 60–200 mg/day.

IM or IV

- *Sedation:* 30–120 mg/day IM or IV in two to three divided doses.
- *Preoperative sedation:* 100–200 mg IM, 60–90 min before surgery.
- *Hypnotic:* 100–320 mg IM or IV.
- *Acute seizures:* 200–320 mg IM or IV repeated in 6 hr if needed.

Pediatric patients

Oral

- *Sedation:* 2 mg/kg/dose PO tid. 8–32 mg/dose.
- *Hypnotic:* Determine dosage using age and weight charts.
- *Antiepileptic:* 3–6 mg/kg/day.

IM or IV

- *Preoperative sedation:* 1–3 mg/kg IM or IV 60–90 min before surgery.
- *Antiepileptic:* 4–6 mg/kg/day for 7–10 days to a blood level of 10–15 mcg/mL or 10–15 mg/kg/day IV or IM.
- *Status epilepticus:* 15–20 mg/kg IV over 10–15 min.

Geriatric patients or patients with debilitating disease or renal or hepatic impairment

Reduce dosage and monitor closely—may produce excitement, depression, or confusion.

Pharmacokinetics

Route	Onset	Duration
Oral	30–60 min	10–16 hr
IM, Subcut.	10–30 min	4–6 hr
IV	5 min	4–6 hr

Metabolism: Hepatic; $T_{1/2}$: 79 hr; 110 hr (children)
Distribution: Crosses placenta; enters breast milk
Excretion: Urine

P

IV FACTS

Preparation: No further preparation is needed.

Infusion: Infuse very slowly, each 60 mg over 1 min, directly IV or into tubing or running IV; inject partial dose and observe for response before continuing. It may require at least 15 min to achieve peak levels in brain tissue. Avoid overdosing by observing effects before continued dosing.

Incompatibilities: Do not combine with chlorpromazine, ephedrine, hydralazine, hydrocortisone, hydroxyzine, insulin, levorphanol, meperidine, morphine, norepinephrine, pentazocine, procaine, promethazine, streptomycin, vancomycin.

Adverse effects

- **CNS:** *Somnolence, agitation, confusion, hyperkinesia, ataxia, vertigo, CNS depression, nightmares, lethargy, residual sedation (hangover), paradoxical excitement, nervousness, psychiatric disturbance, hallucinations, insomnia, anxiety, dizziness, thinking abnormality*
- **CV:** *Bradycardia, hypotension, syncope*
- **GI:** *Nausea, vomiting, constipation, diarrhea, epigastric pain*
- **Hypersensitivity:** Rashes, angioneurotic edema, serum sickness, morbiliform rash, urticaria; rarely, exfoliative dermatitis, **Stevens-Johnson syndrome**
- **Local:** *Pain, tissue necrosis at injection site,* gangrene; arterial spasm with inadvertent intra-arterial injection; thrombophlebitis; permanent neurologic deficit if injected near a nerve
- **Respiratory: Hypoventilation, apnea, respiratory depression, laryngospasm, bronchospasm, circulatory collapse**
- **Other:** Tolerance, psychological and physical dependence, **withdrawal syndrome**

Interactions

✱ **Drug-drug** • Increased serum levels and therapeutic and toxic effects with valproic acid • Increased CNS depression with alcohol • Increased risk of neuromuscular excitation and hypotension with barbiturate anesthetic • Decreased effects of the following drugs: theophyllines, oral anticoagulants, beta blockers, doxycycline, corticosteroids, hormonal contraceptives and estrogens, metronidazole, phenylbutazones, quinidine, felodipine, fenoprofen

■ Nursing considerations

Assessment

- **History:** Hypersensitivity to barbiturates, manifest or latent porphyria, marked liver impairment, nephritis, severe respiratory distress, previous addiction to sedative-hypnotic drugs, pregnancy, acute or chronic pain, seizure disorders, lactation, fever, hyperthyroidism, diabetes mellitus, severe anemia, cardiac disease, shock, uremia, impaired liver or renal function, debilitation
- **Physical:** Weight; T; skin color, lesions; orientation, affect, reflexes; P, BP, orthostatic BP; R, adventitious sounds; bowel sounds, normal output, liver evaluation; LFTs, renal function tests, blood and urine glucose, BUN

Interventions

⊠ ***Black box warning*** Risk of suicidal ideation is increased; monitor patient accordingly.

- Monitor patient responses, blood levels (as appropriate) if any interacting drugs listed above are given with phenobarbital; suggest alternative means of contraception to women using hormonal contraceptives.

⊗ ***Warning*** Do not give intra-arterially; may produce arteriospasm, thrombosis, or gangrene.

- Administer IV doses slowly at no more than 60 mg/min.
- Administer IM doses deep in a large muscle mass (gluteus maximus, vastus lateralis) or other areas where there is little risk of encountering a nerve trunk or major artery.

⊗ ***Warning*** Monitor injection sites carefully for irritation, extravasation (IV use). Solutions are alkaline and very irritating to the tissues. Inject 0.5% procaine at affected site if extravasation occurs; apply heat to area.

- Monitor P, BP, and respiration carefully during IV administration.
- Arrange for periodic lab tests of hematopoietic, renal, and hepatic systems during long-term therapy.

⊗ ***Warning*** Taper dosage gradually after repeated use, especially in patients with epilepsy. When changing from one antiepileptic to another, taper dosage of the drug being discontinued while increasing the dosage of the replacement drug.

Teaching points

- This drug will make you drowsy and less anxious; do not try to get up after you have received this drug (request assistance to sit up or move around).
- Take this drug exactly as prescribed; this drug is habit forming; its effectiveness in facilitating sleep disappears after a short time.
- Do not take this drug longer than 2 weeks (for insomnia), and do not increase the dosage without consulting your health care provider.
- Do not reduce the dosage or discontinue this drug (when used for epilepsy); abrupt discontinuation could result in a serious increase in seizures.
- Wear a medical alert tag so that emergency medical personnel will know you have epilepsy and are taking this medication.
- Avoid pregnancy while taking this drug; use a means of contraception other than hormonal contraceptives.
- You may experience these side effects: Drowsiness, dizziness, hangover, impaired thinking (may lessen after a few days; avoid driving or engaging in dangerous activities); GI upset (take drug with food); dreams, nightmares, difficulty concentrating, fatigue, nervousness (reversible).
- Report severe dizziness, weakness, drowsiness that persists, rash or skin lesions, fever, sore throat, mouth sores, easy bruising or bleeding, nosebleed, petechiae, pregnancy, thoughts of suicide.

DANGEROUS DRUG

▽ phentolamine mesylate

(fen tole' a meen)

Rogitine (CAN)

PREGNANCY CATEGORY C

Drug classes

Alpha-adrenergic blocker
Diagnostic agent

Therapeutic actions

Competitively blocks postsynaptic $alpha_1$-adrenergic receptors, decreasing sympathetic tone on the vasculature, dilating blood vessels, and lowering arterial BP (no longer used to treat essential hypertension because it also blocks presynaptic $alpha_2$-adrenergic receptors that are believed to mediate a feedback inhibition of further norepinephrine release; this accentuates the reflex tachycardia caused by the lowering of BP); use of phentolamine injection as a test for pheochromocytoma depends on the premise that a greater BP reduction will occur with pheochromocytoma than with other etiologies of hypertension.

Indications

- Pheochromocytoma: Prevention or control of hypertensive episodes that may result from stress or manipulation during preoperative preparation and surgical excision
- Pharmacologic test for pheochromocytoma (urinary assays of catecholamines, other biochemical tests have largely supplanted the phentolamine test)
- Prevention and treatment of dermal necrosis and sloughing following IV administration or extravasation of norepinephrine or dopamine
- Unlabeled use: Treatment of hypertensive crises secondary to interactions between MAOIs and sympathomimetic amines, or secondary to rebound hypertension on withdrawal of clonidine, propranolol, or other antihypertensives

Contraindications and cautions

- Contraindicated with hypersensitivity to phentolamine or related drugs, evidence of CAD (MI, angina, coronary insufficiency).
- Use cautiously with pregnancy, lactation.

Available forms

Powder for injection—5 mg

Dosages

Adults

- *Prevention or control of hypertensive episodes in pheochromocytoma:* For use in

P

preoperative reduction of elevated BP, inject 5 mg IV or IM 1–2 hr before surgery. Repeat if necessary. Administer 5 mg IV during surgery as indicated to control paroxysms of hypertension, tachycardia, respiratory depression, seizures, or other effects of epinephrine toxicity.

- *Prevention of tissue necrosis and sloughing following extravasation of IV dopamine:* Infiltrate 10–15 mL of 0.9% sodium chloride injection containing 5–10 mg of phentolamine mesylate.
- *Prevention of tissue necrosis and sloughing following extravasation of IV norepinephrine:* 10 mg phentolamine added to each liter of IV fluids containing norepinephrine.
- *Diagnosis of pheochromocytoma:* See the manufacturer's recommendations. This test should be used only to confirm evidence and after the risks have been carefully considered.

Pediatric patients

- *Prevention or control of hypertensive episodes in pheochromocytoma:* For use in preoperative reduction of elevated BP, inject 1 mg IV or IM 1–2 hr before surgery. Repeat if necessary. Administer 1 mg IV during surgery as indicated to control paroxysms of hypertension, tachycardia, respiratory depression, seizures.
- *Prevention of tissue necrosis and sloughing following extravasation of IV dopamine:* Use 0.1–0.2 mg/kg up to maximum of 10 mg.

Pharmacokinetics

Route	*Onset*	*Peak*	*Duration*
IM	Rapid	20 min	30–45 min
IV	Immediate	2 min	15–30 min

Metabolism: Unknown; $T_{1/2}$: 19 min
Distribution: Unknown
Excretion: Urine

IV FACTS

Preparation: Reconstitute by adding 1 mL of sterile water for injection to the vial, producing a solution of 5 mg/mL.
Infusion: Inject slowly directly into vein or into tubing of actively running IV, each 5 mg over 1 min.

Adverse effects

- **CNS:** *Weakness, dizziness*
- **CV:** *Acute and prolonged hypotensive episodes,* orthostatic hypotension, **MI,** cerebrovascular spasm, cerebrovascular occlusion, *tachycardia, arrhythmias*
- **GI:** *Nausea,* vomiting, diarrhea
- **Other:** Flushing, nasal stuffiness

Interactions

✱ **Drug-drug** • Decreased vasoconstrictor and hypertensive effects of epinephrine, ephedrine

■ Nursing considerations

Assessment

- **History:** Hypersensitivity to phentolamine or related drugs, evidence of CAD, pregnancy
- **Physical:** Orientation, affect, reflexes; ophthalmologic examination; P, BP, orthostatic BP, supine BP, perfusion, edema, auscultation; bowel sounds, normal output

Interventions

- Change positions slowly.
- Monitor BP response and HR carefully.

Teaching points

- Report dizziness, palpitations.

DANGEROUS DRUG

▽ phenylephrine hydrochloride

(fen ill ef' rin)

Parenteral: Neo-Synephrine
Oral: AH-chew D, Sudafed PE
Oral drops: Little Colds Decongestant for Infants & Children, PediaCare Children's Decongestant
Topical OTC nasal decongestants: Little Noses Gentle Formula, Neo-Synephrine, Rhinall, Vicks Sinex Ultra Fine Mist
Strips: Sudafed PE Quick-Dissolve, Thin Strips Decongestant; Triaminic Thin Strips Cold, Triaminic Infant

Ophthalmic preparations (0.12% solutions are OTC):
AK-Dilate, Mydfrin, Neo-Synephrine, Relief

PREGNANCY CATEGORY C

Drug classes
Alpha-adrenergic agonist
Nasal decongestant
Ophthalmic vasoconstrictor or mydriatic
Sympathomimetic amine
Vasopressor

Therapeutic actions
Powerful postsynaptic alpha-adrenergic receptor stimulant that causes vasoconstriction and increased systolic and diastolic BP with little effect on the beta receptors of the heart. Topical application causes vasoconstriction of the mucous membranes, which in turn relieves pressure and promotes drainage of the nasal passages. Topical ophthalmic application causes contraction of the dilator muscles of the pupil (mydriasis), vasoconstriction, and increased outflow of aqueous humor.

Indications
Parenteral
- Treatment of vascular failure in shock, shocklike states, drug-induced hypotension, or hypersensitivity
- To overcome paroxysmal supraventricular tachycardia
- To prolong spinal anesthesia
- Vasoconstrictor in regional anesthesia
- To maintain an adequate level of BP during spinal and inhalation anesthesia

Nasal solution and oral
- Symptomatic relief of nasal and nasopharyngeal mucosal congestion due to the common cold, sinusitis, hay fever, or other respiratory allergies
- Adjunctive therapy of middle ear infections by decreasing congestion around the eustachian ostia

Ophthalmic solution
- 10% solution: Decongestant and vasoconstrictor and for pupil dilation in uveitis, wide-angle glaucoma, and surgery
- 2.5% solution: Decongestant and vasoconstrictor and for pupil dilation in uveitis, open-angle glaucoma in conjunction with miotics, refraction, ophthalmoscopic examination, diagnostic procedures, and before intraocular surgery
- 0.12% solution: Decongestant to provide temporary relief of minor eye irritations caused by hay fever, colds, dust, wind, smog, or hard contact lenses

Contraindications and cautions
- Contraindicated with hypersensitivity to phenylephrine or sulfites; severe hypertension, ventricular tachycardia; narrow-angle glaucoma.
- Use cautiously with thyrotoxicosis, diabetes, hypertension, CV disorders; prostatic hypertrophy, unstable vasomotor syndrome; lactation, pregnancy.

Available forms
Chewable tablets—10 mg; tablets—10 mg; oral drops—2.5 mg/mL, 7.5 mg/5 mL; strips—1.25, 2.5, 10 mg; nasal solution—0.125%, 0.25%, 0.5%, 1%; ophthalmic solution—0.12%, 2.5%, 10%; injection—10 mg/mL

Dosages
Parenteral preparations may be given IM, subcutaneously, by slow IV injection, or as a continuous IV infusion of dilute solutions; for supraventricular tachycardia and emergency use, give by direct IV injection.

Adults

Parenteral
- *Mild to moderate hypotension (adjust dosage on basis of BP response):* 1–10 mg subcutaneously or IM; do not exceed an initial dose of 5 mg. A 5-mg IM dose should raise BP for 1–2 hr. Or for IV use, 0.1–0.5 mg IV. Initial dose should not exceed 0.5 mg. Do not repeat more often than every 10–15 min. 0.5 mg IV should raise the pressure for 15 min.
- *Severe hypotension and shock:* For continuous infusion, add 10 mg to 500 mL of dextrose injection or sodium chloride injection. Start infusion at 100–180 mcg/min (based on a drop factor of 20 drops/mL; this would be 100–180 drops/min). When BP is stabilized, maintain at 40–60 mcg/min. If prompt vasopressor response is not obtained, add 10-mg increments to infusion bottle.

P

- *Spinal anesthesia:* 2–3 mg subcutaneously or IM 3–4 min before injection of spinal anesthetic.
- *Hypotensive emergencies during anesthesia:* Give 0.2 mg IV. Do not exceed 0.5 mg/dose.
- *Prolongation of spinal anesthesia:* Addition of 2–5 mg to the anesthetic solution increases the duration of motor block by as much as 50%.
- *Vasoconstrictor for regional anesthesia:* 1:20,000 concentration (add 1 mg of phenylephrine to every 20 mL of local anesthetic solution).
- *Paroxysmal supraventricular tachycardia:* Rapid IV injection (within 20–30 sec) is recommended. Do not exceed an initial dose of 0.5 mg. Subsequent doses should not exceed the preceding dose by more than 0.1–0.2 mg and should never exceed 1 mg. Use only after other treatments have failed.

Nasal solution

- *Nasal congestion:* 2–3 sprays or drops of the 0.25% or 0.5% solution in each nostril every 3–4 hr. In severe cases, the 0.5% or 1% solution may be needed; 10 mg PO bid–qid.

Ophthalmic solution

- *Vasoconstriction and pupil dilation:* 1 drop of 2.5% or 10% solution on the upper limbus. May be repeated in 1 hr. Precede instillation with a local anesthetic to prevent tearing and dilution of the drug solution.
- *Uveitis to prevent posterior synechiae:* 1 drop of the 2.5% or 10% solution on the surface of the cornea with atropine.
- *Glaucoma:* 1 drop of 10% solution on the upper surface of the cornea repeated as often as necessary and in conjunction with miotics in patients with wide-angle glaucoma.
- *Intraocular surgery:* 2.5% or 10% solution may be instilled in the eye 30–60 min before the operation.
- *Refraction:* 1 drop of a cycloplegic drug followed in 5 min by 1 drop of phenylephrine 2.5% solution and in 10 min by another drop of the cycloplegic.
- *Ophthalmoscopic examination:* 1 drop of 2.5% phenylephrine solution in each eye. Mydriasis is produced in 15–30 min and lasts for 1–3 hr.
- *Minor eye irritation:* 1–2 drops of the 0.12% solution in eye bid–qid as needed.

Oral

- *Nasal congestion:* 1 to 2 tablets every 4 hr. Strips: 1 strip every 4 hr; do not exceed 6 strips in 24 hr. Place 1 strip on tongue and let dissolve. Liquid: 10 mL every 6 hr.

Pediatric patients

Parenteral

- *Hypotension during spinal anesthesia:* 0.5–1 mg/25 lb subcutaneously or IM.

Nasal solution

- *Nasal congestion:*
  2–6 yr: 2–3 drops of 0.125% solution in each nostril every 4 hr, prn.
  Older than 6 yr: 1–2 sprays of the 0.25% solution in each nostril no more than every 4 hr.

Ophthalmic solution

- *Refraction:* 1 drop of atropine sulfate 1% in each eye. Follow in 10–15 min with 1 drop of phenylephrine 2.5% solution and in 5–10 min with a second drop of atropine. Eyes will be ready for refraction in 1–2 hr.

Oral

- *Nasal congestion:*
  Children 2–5 yr: 1 dropperful of 0.25% oral drops every 4 hr; do not exceed 6 doses in 24 hr.
  Children 6–11 yr: 1 tablet every 4 hr.

Geriatric patients

These patients are more likely to experience adverse reactions; use with caution.

Pharmacokinetics

Route	*Onset*	*Duration*
IV	Immediate	15–20 min
IM, Subcut.	10–15 min	30–120 min

Topical form is generally not absorbed systemically.

Metabolism: Hepatic and tissue; $T_{1/2}$: 47–100 hr

Distribution: Crosses placenta; enters breast milk

Excretion: Unknown

IV FACTS

Preparation: Inject directly for emergency use as a 1 mg/mL solution; dilute phenylephrine 1 mg/L is compatible with dextrose-Ringer's combinations; dextrose-lactated

Ringer's combinations; dextrose-saline combinations; dextrose 2.5%, 5%, and 10% in water; Ringer's injection; lactated Ringer's injection; 0.45% and 0.9% sodium chloride injection; 1/6 M sodium lactate injection.
Infusion: Give single dose over 20–30 sec to 1 min. Determine actual rate of continuous infusion using an infusion pump by patient response. For infusion, add 10 mg phenylephrine to 500 mg of diluent.

Adverse effects

Adverse effects are less likely with topical administration.

Systemic administration

- **CNS:** *Fear, anxiety, tenseness, restlessness, headache, light-headedness, dizziness,* drowsiness, tremor, insomnia, hallucinations, psychological disturbances, seizures, CNS depression, weakness, blurred vision, ocular irritation, tearing, photophobia, symptoms of paranoid schizophrenia
- **CV: Cardiac arrhythmias**
- **GI:** *Nausea,* vomiting, anorexia
- **GU:** Constriction of renal blood vessels and *decreased urine formation* (initial parenteral administration), *dysuria, vesical sphincter spasm* resulting in difficult and painful urination, urinary retention in males with prostatism
- **Local:** Necrosis and sloughing if extravasation occurs with IV use
- **Other:** *Pallor,* respiratory difficulty, orofacial dystonia, sweating

Nasal solution

- **EENT:** *Blurred vision,* ocular irritation, tearing, photophobia
- **Local:** *Rebound congestion, local burning and stinging,* sneezing, dryness, contact dermatitis

Ophthalmic solutions

- **CNS:** *Headache, browache, blurred vision,* photophobia, difficulty with night vision, *pigmentary (adrenochrome) deposits in the cornea, conjunctiva,* or lids if applied to damaged cornea
- **Local:** *Transitory stinging on initial instillation*
- **Other:** Rebound miosis, decreased mydriatic response in older patients; significant BP elevation in compromised elderly patients with cardiac problems

Interactions

✱ **Drug-drug** ⊗ ***Warning*** Severe headache, hypertension, hyperpyrexia, possibly resulting in hypertensive crisis with MAOIs (isocarboxazid, phenelzine, tranylcypromine). Do not administer sympathomimetic amines to patients on MAOIs.
• Increased sympathomimetic effects with TCAs (eg, imipramine) • Excessive hypertension with furazolidone • Decreased antihypertensive effect of methyldopa • Potential for serious arrhythmias with halogenated hydrocarbon anesthetics

■ Nursing considerations

Assessment

- **History:** Hypersensitivity to phenylephrine; severe hypertension, ventricular tachycardia; narrow-angle glaucoma; thyrotoxicosis; diabetes; CV disorders; prostatic hypertrophy; unstable vasomotor syndrome; pregnancy; lactation; sulfite sensitivity
- **Physical:** Skin color, T; orientation, reflexes, affect, peripheral sensation, vision, pupils; BP, P, auscultation, peripheral perfusion; R, adventitious sounds; urinary output, bladder percussion, prostate palpation; ECG

Interventions

⊗ ***Warning*** Protect parenteral solution from light; do not administer unless solution is clear; discard unused portion.

⊗ ***Warning*** Keep an alpha-adrenergic blocking agent readily available in case of severe reaction or overdose.

⊗ ***Warning*** Infiltrate area of extravasation with phentolamine (5–10 mg in 10–15 mL of saline), using a fine hypodermic needle; usually effective if area is infiltrated within 12 hr of extravasation.

- Monitor P, BP continuously during parenteral administration.
- Ensure than patient is hydrated during therapy.
- Do not administer ophthalmic solution that has turned brown or contains precipitates; prevent prolonged exposure to air and light.

- Administer ophthalmic solution as follows: Have patient lie down or tilt head backward and look at ceiling. Hold dropper above eye; drop medicine inside lower lid while patient is looking up. Do not touch dropper to eye, fingers, or any surface. Have patient keep eye open and avoid blinking for at least 30 sec. Apply gentle pressure with fingers to inside corner of the eye for about 1 min. Caution patient not to close eyes tightly and not to blink more often than usual.
- Do not administer other eye drops for at least 5 min after phenylephrine.
- Do not administer nasal decongestant for longer than 3–5 days.
- Do not administer ophthalmic solution for longer than 72 hr.
- Monitor BP and cardiac response regularly in patients with any CV disorders.
- Use topical anesthetics if ophthalmic preparations are painful and burning.
- Monitor CV effects carefully; patients with hypertension who take this drug may experience changes in BP because of the additional vasoconstriction. If a nasal decongestant is needed, pseudoephedrine is the drug of choice.

Teaching points

- Do not exceed recommended dose. Demonstrate proper use of topical nasal and ophthalmic preparations to your health care provider.
- Avoid prolonged use, because underlying medical problems can be disguised. Usual limit is 3–5 days for nasal decongestant, 72 hours for ophthalmic preparations.
- You may experience these side effects: Dizziness, drowsiness, fatigue, apprehension (use caution if driving or performing tasks that require alertness); *nasal solution*—burning or stinging when first used (transient); *ophthalmic solution*—slight stinging when first used (usually transient); blurring of vision.
- Report nervousness, palpitations, sleeplessness, sweating; *ophthalmic solution*—severe eye pain, vision changes, floating spots, eye redness or sensitivity to light, headache.

phenytoin (diphenylhydantoin, phenytoin sodium)

(fen' i toe in)

Dilantin-125, Dilantin Infatab, Dilantin Injection, Dilantin Kapseals, Phenytek

PREGNANCY CATEGORY D

Drug classes

Antiarrhythmic, group 1b
Antiepileptic
Hydantoin

Therapeutic actions

Has antiepileptic activity without causing general CNS depression; stabilizes neuronal membranes and prevents hyperexcitability caused by excessive stimulation; limits the spread of seizure activity from an active focus; also effective in treating cardiac arrhythmias, especially those induced by cardiac glycosides; antiarrhythmic properties are very similar to those of lidocaine; both are class IB antiarrhythmics.

Indications

- Control of grand mal (tonic-clonic) and psychomotor seizures
- Prevention and treatment of seizures occurring during or following neurosurgery
- Parenteral administration: Control of status epilepticus of the grand mal type
- Unlabeled uses: Antiarrhythmic, particularly in arrhythmias induced by cardiac glycosides (IV preparations); treatment of trigeminal neuralgia (tic douloureux)

Contraindications and cautions

- Contraindicated with hypersensitivity to hydantoins, sinus bradycardia, sinoatrial block, Stokes-Adams syndrome, pregnancy (data suggest an association between antiepileptic use and an elevated incidence of birth defects; however, do not discontinue antiepileptic therapy in pregnant women who are receiving such therapy to prevent major seizures; stopping drug is likely to precipitate status epilepticus, with attendant hypoxia and risk to both mother and fetus), lactation.

- Use cautiously with acute intermittent porphyria, hypotension, severe myocardial insufficiency, diabetes mellitus, hyperglycemia.

Available forms

Chewable tablets—50 mg; oral suspension—125 mg/5 mL; ER capsules—30, 100, 200, 300 mg; injection—50 mg/mL

Dosages

Adults

Phenytoin sodium, parenteral

- *Status epilepticus:* 10–15 mg/kg by slow IV. For maintenance, 100 mg PO or IV every 6–8 hr. Higher doses may be required. Do not exceed an infusion rate of 50 mg/min. Follow each IV injection with an injection of sterile saline through the same needle or IV catheter to avoid local venous irritation by the alkaline solution. Continuous IV infusion is not recommended.
- *Neurosurgery (prophylaxis):* 100–200 mg IM every 4 hr during surgery and the postoperative period (IM route is not recommended because of erratic absorption, pain, and muscle damage at the injection site).
- *IM therapy in a patient previously stabilized on oral dosage:* Increase dosage by 50% over oral dosage. When returning to oral dosage, decrease dose by 50% of the original oral dose for 1 wk to prevent excessive plasma levels due to continued absorption from IM tissue sites. Avoid IM route of administration if possible due to erratic absorption and pain and muscle damage at injection site.

Phenytoin and phenytoin sodium, oral

Individualize dosage. Determine serum levels for optimal dosage adjustments. The clinically effective serum level is usually between 10 and 20 mcg/mL.

- *Loading dose (hospitalized patients without renal or liver disease):* Initially, 1 g of phenytoin capsules (phenytoin sodium, prompt) is divided into three doses (400 mg, 300 mg, 300 mg) and given every 2 hr. Normal maintenance dosage is then instituted 24 hr after the loading dose with frequent serum determinations.
- *No previous treatment:* Start with 100 mg tid PO. Satisfactory maintenance dosage is usually 300–400 mg/day. An increase to 600 mg/day may be needed.
- *Single daily dosage (phenytoin sodium, extended):* If seizure control is established with divided doses of three 100-mg extended phenytoin sodium capsules per day, once-a-day dosage with 300 mg PO may be considered. Do not use prompt phenytoin capsules, suspension, or chewable tablets for once-daily dosing.

Pediatric patients

Phenytoin sodium, parenteral

- *Status epilepticus:* Administer phenytoin IV. Determine dosage according to weight in proportion to dose for a 70-kg adult (see adult dosage earlier on this page; see Appendix I, *Recommended pediatric immunizations*). Pediatric dosage may be calculated on the basis of 250 mg/m^2. Dosage for infants and children also may be calculated on the basis of 10–15 mg/kg, given in divided doses of 5–10 mg/kg. For neonates, 15–20 mg/kg in divided doses of 5–10 mg/kg is recommended.

Phenytoin and phenytoin sodium, oral

Children not previously treated: Initially, 5 mg/kg/day in two to three equally divided doses. Subsequent dosage should be individualized to a maximum of 300 mg/day. Daily maintenance dosage is 4–8 mg/kg. Children older than 6 yr may require the minimum adult dose of 300 mg/day.

Geriatric patients and patients with hepatic impairment

Use caution and monitor for early signs of toxicity; phenytoin is metabolized in the liver.

Pharmacokinetics

Route	*Onset*	*Peak*	*Duration*
Oral	Slow	2–12 hr	6–12 hr
IV	1–2 hr	Rapid	12–24 hr

Metabolism: Hepatic; $T_{1/2}$: 6–24 hr
Distribution: Crosses placenta; enters breast milk
Excretion: Urine

P

IV FACTS

Preparation: Administration by IV infusion is not recommended because of low solubility of drug and likelihood of precipitation; however, this may be feasible if proper precautions are observed. Use suitable vehicle of 0.9% sodium chloride or lactated Ringer's injection, appropriate concentration (less than 6.7 mg/mL); prepare immediately before administration, and use an in-line filter.

Infusion: Infuse slowly in small increments, each 25–50 mg over 1–5 min; infuse flush immediately after drug to reduce the risk of damage to vein and tissues.

Incompatibilities: Do not combine with other medications in solution.

Y-site incompatibility: Do not give with amphotericin B, ciprofloxacin, clarithromycin, diltiazem, enalaprilat, fentanyl, gatifloxacin, heparin, heparin with hydrocortisone, hydromorphone, linezolid, methadone, morphine, potassium, propofol, sufentanil, theophylline, vitamin B complex with C.

Adverse effects

Some adverse effects are related to plasma concentrations, as follows:

Plasma Concentration	*Adverse Effects*
5–10 mcg/mL	Some therapeutic effects
10–20 mcg/mL	Usual therapeutic range
More than 20 mcg/mL	Far-lateral nystagmus risk
More than 30 mcg/mL	Ataxia is usually seen
More than 40 mcg/mL	Significantly diminished mental capacity

- **CNS:** *Nystagmus, ataxia, dysarthria, slurred speech, mental confusion, dizziness, drowsiness, insomnia, transient nervousness, motor twitchings, fatigue, irritability, depression, numbness, tremor, headache,* photophobia, diplopia, conjunctivitis, suicidal ideation
- **CV: CV collapse,** hypotension (when administered rapidly IV; not to exceed 50 mg/min)
- **Dermatologic:** Dermatologic reactions, scarlatiniform, morbilliform, maculopapular, urticarial and nonspecific rashes; serious and sometimes fatal dermatologic reactions—**bullous, exfoliative, or purpuric dermatitis, lupus erythematosus, and Stevens-Johnson syndrome,** toxic epidermal necrolysis, hirsutism, alopecia, coarsening of the facial features, enlargement of the lips, Peyronie's disease
- **GI:** *Nausea,* vomiting, diarrhea, constipation, *gingival hyperplasia,* toxic hepatitis, **liver damage,** sometimes fatal; hypersensitivity reactions with hepatic involvement, including hepatocellular degeneration and fatal hepatocellular necrosis
- **GU:** Nephrosis
- **Hematologic: Hematopoietic complications,** sometimes fatal: thrombocytopenia, leukopenia, granulocytopenia, agranulocytosis, pancytopenia; macrocytosis and megaloblastic anemia that usually respond to folic acid therapy; eosinophilia, monocytosis, leukocytosis, simple anemia, hemolytic anemia, aplastic anemia, hyperglycemia
- **IV use complications:** Hypotension, transient hyperkinesia, drowsiness, nystagmus, circumoral tingling, vertigo, nausea, CV collapse, CNS depression
- **Respiratory:** Pulmonary fibrosis, acute pneumonitis
- **Other:** Lymph node hyperplasia, sometimes progressing to **frank malignant lymphoma,** monoclonal gammopathy and multiple myeloma (prolonged therapy), polyarthropathy, osteomalacia, weight gain, chest pain, periarteritis nodosa

Interactions

✱ **Drug-drug** • Increased pharmacologic effects with allopurinol, benzodiazepines, chloramphenicol, cimetidine, disulfiram, ethanol (acute ingestion), isoniazid, metronidazole, miconazole, omeprazole, phenacemide, phenylbutazone, sulfonamides, trimethoprim • Complex interactions and effects when phenytoin and valproic acid are given together; phenytoin toxicity with apparently normal serum phenytoin levels; decreased plasma levels of valproic acid; breakthrough seizures when the two drugs are given together • Decreased pharmacologic effects with antineoplastics, diazoxide, ethanol (chronic ingestion), folic acid, loxapine, nitrofurantoin, pyridoxime, sucralfate, rifampin, theophylline (applies only to oral hydantoins, absorption of which is decreased) • Increased pharmacologic effects and toxicity with amiodarone, chloramphenicol, fluconazole, isoniazid • Increased pharmacologic effect of primidone • Increased hepatotoxicity with acetaminophen • Decreased pharmacologic effects of amiodarone, cardiac glycosides, corticosteroids, cyclosporine, disopyramide, doxycycline, estrogens, furosemide, haloperidol, levodopa, methadone, metyra-pone, mexiletine, phenothiazide, sulfonylureas, hormonal contraceptives, quinidine, atracurium, pancuronium, vecuronium, carbamazepine, diazoxide • Severe hypotension and bradycardia when IV phenytoin is given with dopamine

✱ **Drug-lab test** • Interference with the metyrapone and the 1-mg dexamethasone tests for at least 7 days

✱ **Drug-food** • Enteral tube feedings may delay absorption of drug. Provide a 2-hr window between *Dilantin* doses and tube feedings

■ Nursing considerations

Assessment

- **History:** Hypersensitivity to hydantoins, sinus bradycardia, AV heart block, Stokes-Adams syndrome, acute intermittent porphyria, hypotension, severe myocardial insufficiency, diabetes mellitus, hyperglycemia, pregnancy, lactation
- **Physical:** T; skin color, lesions; lymph node palpation; orientation, affect, reflexes, vision examination; P, BP; R, adventitious sounds; bowel sounds, normal output, liver evaluation; periodontal examination; LFTs, urinalysis, CBC and differential, blood proteins, blood and urine glucose, EEG, ECG

Interventions

- Use only clear parenteral solutions; a faint yellow color may develop, but this has no effect on potency. If the solution is refrigerated or frozen, a precipitate might form, but it will dissolve if the solution is allowed to stand at room temperature. Do not use solutions that have haziness or a precipitate.

⊗ **Warning** Administer IV slowly to prevent severe hypotension and venous irritation; the margin of safety between full therapeutic and toxic doses is small. Continually monitor patient's cardiac rhythm and check BP frequently and regularly during IV infusion. Suggest use of fosphenytoin sodium if IV route is needed.

- Monitor injection sites carefully; drug solutions are very alkaline and irritating.

⊗ **Warning** Monitor for therapeutic serum levels of 10–20 mcg/mL.

- Give oral drug with or without food in a consistent manner. Give with food if patient complains of GI upset.
- Recommend that the oral phenytoin prescription be filled with the same brand each time; differences in bioavailability have been documented.
- Suggest that adult patients who are controlled with 300-mg extended phenytoin capsules try once-a-day dosage to increase compliance and convenience.

⊗ **Warning** Reduce dosage, discontinue phenytoin, or substitute other antiepileptic gradually; abrupt discontinuation may precipitate status epilepticus.

- Phenytoin is ineffective in controlling absence (petit mal) seizures. Patients with combined seizures will need other medication for their absence seizures.

⊗ **Warning** Discontinue drug if rash, depression of blood count, enlarged lymph nodes, hypersensitivity reaction, signs of liver damage, or Peyronie's disease (induration of the corpora cavernosa of the penis) occurs. Institute another antiepileptic promptly.

- Monitor hepatic function periodically during long-term therapy; monitor blood counts and urinalysis monthly.
- Monitor blood or urine sugar of patients with diabetes mellitus regularly. Adjustment of dosage of hypoglycemic patients may be needed because antiepileptic may inhibit insulin release and induce hyperglycemia.
- Monitor patient for suicidality, thoughts of suicide; patient may be at increased risk.

⊗ **Warning** Have lymph node enlargement occurring during therapy evaluated carefully. Lymphadenopathy that simulates Hodgkin's lymphoma has occurred. Lymph node hyperplasia may progress to lymphoma.

- Monitor blood proteins to detect early malfunction of the immune system (eg, multiple myeloma).
- Arrange instruction in proper oral hygiene technique for long-term patients to prevent development of gum hyperplasia.

P

Teaching points

- Take this drug exactly as prescribed, with food to reduce GI upset, or without food—but maintain consistency in the manner in which you take it. Be especially careful not to miss a dose if you are on once-a-day therapy.
- Do not discontinue this drug abruptly or change dosage, except on the advice of your health care provider.
- Maintain good oral hygiene (regular brushing and flossing) to prevent gum disease; arrange frequent dental checkups to prevent serious gum disease.
- Arrange for frequent checkups to monitor your response to this drug.
- Monitor your blood or urine sugar regularly, and report any abnormality to your health care provider if you have diabetes.
- This drug is not recommended for use during pregnancy. It is advisable to use some form of contraception other than hormonal contraceptives.
- Wear or carry a medical alert tag so that any emergency medical personnel will know that you have epilepsy and are taking antiepileptic medication.
- You may experience these side effects: Drowsiness, dizziness, confusion, blurred vision (avoid driving or performing other tasks requiring alertness or visual acuity; alcohol may intensify these effects); GI upset (take drug with food, eat frequent small meals).
- Report rash, severe nausea or vomiting, drowsiness, slurred speech, impaired coordination (ataxia), swollen glands, bleeding, swollen or tender gums, yellowish discoloration of the skin or eyes, joint pain, unexplained fever, sore throat, unusual bleeding or bruising, persistent headache, malaise, any indication of an infection or bleeding tendency, abnormal erection, pregnancy, thoughts of suicide.

pilocarpine hydrochloride

See Appendix W, *Less commonly used drugs*.

pimozide

See Appendix W, *Less commonly used drugs*.

pindolol

(pin' doe lole)

Apo-Pindol (CAN), Gen-Pindolol (CAN), Nu-Pindol (CAN), Visken

PREGNANCY CATEGORY B

Drug classes

Antihypertensive
Beta-adrenergic blocker (nonselective)

Therapeutic actions

Competitively blocks beta-adrenergic receptors but also has some intrinsic sympathomimetic activity; however, the mechanism by which it lowers BP is unclear, because it only slightly decreases resting cardiac output and inconsistently affects plasma renin levels.

Indications

- Management of hypertension, alone or with other drugs, especially diuretics
- Unlabeled use: Treatment of fibromyalgia

Contraindications and cautions

- Contraindicated with sinus bradycardia, second- or third-degree heart block, cardiogenic shock, HF, bronchial asthma, severe COPD, pregnancy (embryotoxic in preclinical studies), lactation.
- Use cautiously with diabetes, thyrotoxicosis.

Available forms

Tablets—5, 10 mg

Dosages

Adults

Initially, 5 mg PO bid. Adjust dosage as needed in increments of 10 mg/day at 3- to 4-wk intervals to a maximum of 60 mg/day. Usual maintenance dose is 5 mg tid.

Pediatric patients

Safety and efficacy not established.

Pharmacokinetics

Route	*Onset*
Oral	Varies

Metabolism: Hepatic; $T_{1/2}$: 3–4 hr
Distribution: Crosses placenta; enters breast milk
Excretion: Urine

Adverse effects

- **Allergic reactions:** Pharyngitis, erythematous rash, fever, sore throat, **laryngospasm,** respiratory distress
- **CNS:** *Dizziness,* vertigo, tinnitus, *fatigue,* emotional depression, paresthesias, sleep disturbances, hallucinations, disorientation, memory loss, slurred speech
- **CV:** *Bradycardia, HF, cardiac arrhythmias, sinoatrial or AV nodal block, tachycardia,* peripheral vascular insufficiency, claudication, **CVA,** pulmonary edema, hypotension
- **Dermatologic:** Rash, pruritus, sweating, dry skin
- **EENT:** Eye irritation, dry eyes, conjunctivitis, blurred vision
- **GI:** *Gastric pain, flatulence, constipation, diarrhea, nausea, vomiting,* anorexia, ischemic colitis, renal and mesenteric arterial thrombosis, retroperitoneal fibrosis, hepatomegaly, acute pancreatitis
- **GU:** *Impotence, decreased libido,* Peyronie's disease, dysuria, nocturia, urinary frequency
- **Musculoskeletal:** Joint pain, arthralgia, muscle cramp
- **Respiratory: Bronchospasm,** dyspnea, cough, bronchial obstruction, nasal stuffiness, rhinitis, pharyngitis (less likely than with propranolol)
- **Other:** *Decreased exercise tolerance, development of ANAs,* hyperglycemia or hypoglycemia, elevated serum transaminase, alkaline phosphatase, and LDH

Interactions

✱ **Drug-drug** • Increased effects with verapamil • Decreased effects with indomethacin, ibuprofen, naproxen, piroxicam, sulindac • Prolonged hypoglycemic effects of insulin • Peripheral ischemia possible if pindolol combined with ergot alkaloids • Initial hypertensive episode followed by bradycardia with epinephrine • Increased first-dose response to prazosin • Increased serum levels and toxic effects with lidocaine • Paradoxical hypertension when clonidine is given with beta blockers; increased rebound hypertension when clonidine is discontinued in patients on beta-blockers • Decreased bronchodilator effects of theophyllines

✱ **Drug-lab test** • Possible false results with glucose or insulin tolerance tests

■ Nursing considerations

CLINICAL ALERT!
Name confusion has been reported between pindolol and *Plendil* (felodipine); use caution.

Assessment

- **History:** Sinus bradycardia, second- or third-degree heart block, cardiogenic shock, HF, diabetes, thyrotoxicosis, asthma, pregnancy, lactation
- **Physical:** Weight, skin condition, neurologic status, P, BP, ECG, respiratory status, renal and thyroid function, blood and urine glucose

Interventions

⊗ ***Warning*** Do not discontinue drug abruptly after long-term therapy (hypersensitivity to catecholamines may have developed, causing exacerbation of angina, MI, and ventricular arrhythmias). Taper drug gradually over 2 wk with monitoring.

- Consult with physician about withdrawing drug if patient is to undergo surgery (withdrawal is controversial).

Teaching points

- Do not stop taking this drug unless instructed to do so by your health care provider.
- Avoid driving or dangerous activities if you are drowsy or dizzy.
- Report difficulty breathing, night cough, swelling of extremities, slow pulse, confusion, depression, rash, fever, sore throat.

DANGEROUS DRUG

▽ pioglitazone

(pie oh ***glit'*** *ah zohn)*

Actos, Apo-Pioglitazone (CAN), ratio-Pioglitazone (CAN)

PREGNANCY CATEGORY C

P

Drug classes

Antidiabetic
Thiazolidinedione

Therapeutic actions

Resensitizes tissues to insulin; stimulates insulin receptor sites to lower blood glucose and improve the action of insulin; decreases hepatic gluconeogenesis and increases insulin-dependent muscle glucose uptake.

Indications

- Monotherapy as an adjunct to diet and exercise to improve glucose control in patients with type 2 diabetes
- As part of combination with a sulfonylurea, metformin, or insulin when diet, exercise plus a single agent alone does not result in adequate glycemic control in type 2 diabetes

Contraindications and cautions

- Contraindicated with allergy to any thiazolidinedione, type 1 diabetes, ketoacidosis, New York Heart Association Class III or IV HF, lactation.
- Use cautiously with advanced heart disease, liver failure, pregnancy.

Available forms

Tablets—15, 30, 45 mg

Dosages

Adults

15–30 mg daily as a single oral dose; if adequate response is not seen, dosage may be increased to a maximum 45 mg daily PO.

- *Combination therapy with sulfonylurea or metformin:* 15–30 mg daily PO added to the established dose of the other agent; if hypoglycemia occurs, reduce the dose of the other agent.
- *Combination therapy with insulin:* Initiate pioglitazone at 15 or 30 mg while maintaining insulin dose. Decrease insulin dose by 10%–25% if hypoglycemic or if glucose is less than 100 mg/dL.

Pediatric patients

Safety and efficacy not established.

Patients with hepatic impairment

Use caution and monitor patient closely. Do not administer if ALT exceeds 2.5 times the upper limit of normal.

Pharmacokinetics

Route	*Onset*	*Peak*
Oral	Rapid	2–4 hr

Metabolism: Hepatic; $T_{1/2}$: 3–7 hr
Distribution: Crosses placenta; enters breast milk
Excretion: Feces, urine

Adverse effects

- **CNS:** *Headache, pain, myalgia*
- **CV:** Fluid retention, HF
- **Endocrine: Hypoglycemia, hyperglycemia,** *aggravated diabetes*
- **GI:** Diarrhea, liver injury
- **Respiratory:** Sinusitis, URI, rhinitis
- **Other:** *Infections, fatigue,* tooth disorders

Interactions

✱ **Drug-drug** • Decreased effectiveness of hormonal contraceptives, which may result in ovulation and risk of pregnancy; suggest the use of an alternative method of birth control or consider a higher dose of the contraceptive

✱ **Drug-alternative therapy** • Increased risk of hypoglycemia if taken with juniper berries, ginseng, garlic, fenugreek, coriander, dandelion root, celery

■ Nursing considerations

CLINICAL ALERT!
Name confusion has been reported between *Actos* (pioglitazone) and *Actonel* (risedronate); use caution.

Assessment

- **History:** Allergy to any thiazolidinedione, type 1 diabetes, ketoacidosis, serious hepatic impairment, advanced heart disease, pregnancy, lactation
- **Physical:** T; orientation, reflexes, peripheral sensation; R, adventitious sounds; liver evaluation; LFTs, blood glucose, CBC

Interventions

- Monitor baseline LFTs before beginning therapy and periodically during therapy.
- Monitor urine or blood glucose levels frequently to determine effectiveness of drug and dosage being used.

⊗ ***Black box warning*** Thiazolidinediones cause or worsen HF in some patients, and pioglitazone is not recommended for patients with symptomatic heart failure (contraindicated in New York Heart Association Class III and IV HF). After starting or increasing pioglitazone, watch carefully for signs or symptoms of HF. If they develop, manage HF according to current standards of care. Pioglitazone may be reduced or discontinued.

- Administer without regard to meals.
- Arrange for consultation with dietitian to establish weight loss program and dietary control as appropriate.
- Arrange for thorough diabetic teaching program to include disease, dietary control, exercise, signs and symptoms of hypoglycemia and hyperglycemia, avoidance of infection, hygiene.

Teaching points

- Do not discontinue this medication without consulting your health care provider; continue with your diet and exercise program for diabetes control.
- Take this drug without regard to meals. If a dose is missed, it may be taken at the next scheduled time. If dose is missed for an entire day, do not take a double dose the next day.
- Monitor urine or blood very closely for glucose and ketones as prescribed while adjusting to drug.
- Use barrier contraceptives if currently using hormonal contraceptives; these contraceptives may be ineffective if combined with pioglitazone.
- Report fever, sore throat, unusual bleeding or bruising, rash, dark urine, light-colored stools, hypoglycemic or hyperglycemic reactions, swelling, difficulty breathing.

▽ pirbuterol acetate

*(peer **byoo'** ter ole)*

Maxair Autohaler

PREGNANCY CATEGORY C

Drug classes

Antasthmatic
Beta$_2$-selective adrenergic agonist
Bronchodilator
Sympathomimetic

Therapeutic actions

Relatively selective beta-adrenergic stimulator; acts at beta$_2$-adrenergic receptors to cause bronchodilation (and vasodilation); at higher doses, beta$_2$-selectivity is lost, and the drug also acts at beta$_1$ receptors to cause typical sympathomimetic cardiac effects.

Indications

- Prophylaxis and treatment of reversible bronchospasm, including asthma; alone or in combination with theophylline or corticosteroid therapy

Contraindications and cautions

- Contraindicated with hypersensitivity to pirbuterol, tachyarrhythmias, general anesthesia with halogenated hydrocarbons or cyclopropane, unstable vasomotor system disorders, hypertension.
- Use cautiously with coronary insufficiency, history of CVA, COPD with degenerative heart disease, hyperthyroidism, history of seizure disorders, psychoneurosis, pregnancy, lactation.

Available forms

Aerosol—0.2 mg/actuation

Dosages

Adults and pediatric patients older than 12 yr

Two inhalations (0.4 mg) repeated every 4–6 hr. One inhalation (0.2 mg) may be sufficient. Do not exceed a total daily dose of 12 inhalations.

Pediatric patients younger than 12 yr

Safety and efficacy not established.

Pharmacokinetics

Route	*Onset*	*Duration*
Inhalation	5 min	5 hr

P

Metabolism: Hepatic and tissue; $T_{1/2}$: 2 hr
Distribution: Crosses placenta; may enter breast milk
Excretion: Urine

Adverse effects

- **CNS:** *Restlessness, apprehension,* anxiety, fear, CNS stimulation, hyperkinesia, *insomnia,* tremor, drowsiness, *irritability,* weakness, vertigo, headache
- **CV:** Cardiac arrhythmias, tachycardia, palpitations, PVCs (rare), anginal pain (less likely with this drug than with bronchodilator doses of a nonselective beta-agonist [ie, isoproterenol]), changes in BP, sweating, pallor, flushing
- **GI:** *Nausea,* vomiting, heartburn, unusual or bad taste in mouth
- **Hypersensitivity:** Immediate hypersensitivity (allergic) reactions
- **Respiratory:** Respiratory difficulties, pulmonary edema, coughing, **bronchospasm,** paradoxical airway resistance with repeated, excessive use of inhalation preparations

Interactions

✷ **Drug-drug** • Increased sympathomimetic effects when given with other sympathomimetic drugs

■ Nursing considerations

CLINICAL ALERT!
Name confusion has been reported between *Maxair* (pirbuterol) and *Maxalt* (rizatriptan); use extreme caution.

Assessment

- **History:** Hypersensitivity to pirbuterol, tachyarrhythmias, general anesthesia with halogenated hydrocarbons or cyclopropane, unstable vasomotor system disorders, hypertension, coronary insufficiency, history of CVA, COPD, hyperthyroidism, seizure disorders, psychoneurosis, pregnancy, lactation
- **Physical:** Weight, skin color, T, turgor; orientation, reflexes, affect; P, BP; R, adventitious sounds; blood and urine glucose, serum electrolytes, LFTs, thyroid function tests, ECG, CBC

Interventions

- Use smallest dose for least time; drug tolerance can occur with prolonged use.

⊗ ***Warning*** Keep a beta-adrenergic blocker (a cardioselective beta blocker, such as atenolol, should be used in patients with respiratory distress) readily available in case cardiac arrhythmias occur.

- Do not exceed recommended dosage; administer during second half of inspiration, because the airways are wider and distribution is more extensive.

Teaching points

- Do not exceed recommended dosage; adverse effects or loss of effectiveness may result. Read product instructions and consult your health care provider if you have any questions.
- If inhalations fail to provide relief, consult your health care provider immediately.
- You may experience these side effects: Drowsiness, dizziness, fatigue, apprehension (use caution if driving or performing tasks that require alertness); nausea, heartburn, change in taste (eat frequent small meals); sweating, flushing, rapid heart rate.
- Report chest pain, dizziness, insomnia, weakness, tremor or irregular heart beat, difficulty breathing, productive cough, failure to respond to usual dosage.

▽ piroxicam

(peer ox' i kam)

Apo-Piroxicam (CAN), Feldene, Gen-Piroxicam (CAN)

PREGNANCY CATEGORY C

Drug class

NSAID (oxicam derivative)

Therapeutic actions

Anti-inflammatory, analgesic, and antipyretic activities related to inhibition of prostaglandin synthesis; exact mechanisms of action are not known.

Indications
- Relief of the signs and symptoms of acute and chronic rheumatoid arthritis and osteoarthritis
- Unlabeled uses: Dysmenorrhea, postoperative and postpartum pain

Contraindications and cautions
- Contraindicated with hypersensitivity to piroxicam or any other NSAID, for perioperative pain in CABG surgery, lactation.
- Use cautiously in the elderly and with renal, hepatic, CV, GI conditions; pregnancy; HF.

Available forms
Capsules—10, 20 mg

Dosages
Adults
Single daily dose of 20 mg PO. Dose may be divided. Steady-state blood levels are not achieved for 7–12 days. Therapeutic response occurs early but progresses over several wk; do not evaluate for 2 wk.
Pediatric patients
Safety and efficacy not established.

Pharmacokinetics

Route	Onset	Peak
Oral	1 hr	3–5 hr

Metabolism: Hepatic; $T_{1/2}$: 50 hr
Distribution: Crosses placenta; enters breast milk
Excretion: Urine

Adverse effects
- **CNS:** *Headache, dizziness, somnolence, insomnia,* fatigue, tiredness, dizziness, tinnitus, ophthalmologic effects
- **Dermatologic:** *Rash,* pruritus, sweating, dry mucous membranes, stomatitis
- **GI:** *Nausea, dyspepsia, GI pain,* diarrhea, vomiting, *constipation,* flatulence
- **GU:** Dysuria, renal impairment
- **Hematologic:** Bleeding, platelet inhibition with higher doses, neutropenia, eosinophilia, leukopenia, pancytopenia, aplastic anemia, thrombocytopenia, agranulocytosis, granulocytopenia, decreased Hgb or Hct, bone marrow depression, menorrhagia
- **Respiratory:** Dyspnea, hemoptysis, pharyngitis, **bronchospasm,** rhinitis
- **Other:** Peripheral edema, **anaphylactoid reactions to anaphylactic shock**

Interactions
✱ **Drug-drug** • Increased serum lithium levels and risk of toxicity • Decreased antihypertensive effects of beta blockers • Decreased therapeutic effects with cholestyramine

■ Nursing considerations
Assessment
- **History:** Allergies; renal, hepatic, CV, GI conditions; history of ulcers; pregnancy; lactation
- **Physical:** Skin color and lesions; orientation, reflexes, ophthalmologic and audiometric evaluation, peripheral sensation; P, edema; R, adventitious sounds; liver evaluation; CBC, clotting times, LFTs, renal function tests; serum electrolytes, stool guaiac

Interventions
⊠ ***Black box warning*** Be aware that patient may be at increased risk for CV event, GI bleeding; monitor accordingly.
- Give drug with food or milk if GI upset occurs.
- Arrange for periodic ophthalmologic examination during long-term therapy.

⊗ ***Warning*** If overdose occurs, institute emergency procedures (gastric lavage, induction of emesis, supportive therapy).

Teaching points
- Take drug with food or meals if GI upset occurs.
- You may experience these side effects: Dizziness, drowsiness (avoid driving or using dangerous machinery).
- Report sore throat, fever, rash, itching, weight gain, swelling in ankles or fingers, changes in vision, black, tarry stools.

▽ pitavastatin
*(pih **ta'** vah **sta'** tin)*

Livalo

PREGNANCY CATEGORY X

P

Drug classes
Antihyperlipidemic
HMG-CoA reductase inhibitor

Therapeutic actions
Inhibits HMG-CoA reductase, the enzyme that catalyzes the first step in the cholesterol synthesis pathway, resulting in a decrease in serum cholesterol, serum LDLs (associated with increased risk of CAD), and increased serum HDLs (associated with decreased CAD risk); increases hepatic LDL recapture sites and enhances reuptake and catabolism of LDL; lowers triglyceride levels.

Indications
- As adjunctive therapy to exercise and diet to reduce elevated total cholesterol, LDLs, apolipoprotein B, and triglycerides and increase HDL in patients with primary hyperlipidemia and mixed dyslipidemia

Contraindications and cautions
- Contraindicated with hypersensitivity to components of drug, active liver disease, concurrent use of cyclosporine, pregnancy, lactation.
- Use cautiously with advanced age, renal impairment, hypothyroidism, concurrent use of fibrates.

Available forms
Tablets—1, 2, 4 mg

Dosages
Adults
Starting dosage, 2 mg/day PO; may increase to a maximum of 4 mg/day.
Pediatric patients
Safety and efficacy not established.
Patients with moderate to end-stage renal impairment on hemodialysis
1 mg/day PO; maximum dosage is 2 mg/day.

Pharmacokinetics

Route	*Onset*	*Peak*
Oral	Rapid	1 hr

Metabolism: Hepatic; $T_{1/2}$: 12 hr
Distribution: Crosses placenta; enters breast milk
Excretion: Feces

Adverse effects
- **CNS:** Headache
- **GI:** Liver enzyme abnormalities, diarrhea, constipation
- **Respiratory:** Nasal pharyngitis
- **Other: Rhabdomyolysis,** *back pain,* myalgia, flulike symptoms, rash

Interactions
✱ **Drug-drug** • Increased serum levels and risk of toxicity with cyclosporine, lopinavir/ritonavir; avoid these combinations • Increased serum levels and risk of toxic effects with erythromycin; limit dosage to 1 mg/day if this combination is used • Increased serum levels and risk of toxic effects with rifampin; limit dosage to 2 mg/day if this combination is used • Potential increased risk of myopathy if taken with fibrates, niacin; if this combination is used, monitor patient closely and use caution • Increased risk of liver damage if taken with large amounts of alcohol; monitor patient closely

■ Nursing considerations
Assessment
- **History:** Hypersensitivity to components of drug, active liver disease, renal impairment, hypothyroidism, history of other drugs being used
- **Physical:** Weight; reflexes; R; LFTs, lipid profile

Interventions
- Obtain LFTs before beginning therapy, at 12 wk following start of therapy or with dosage elevations, then semiannually.
- Administer at any time of day, without regard to food.
- Ensure that patient continues a diet and exercise program.
- Suggest the use of contraceptive measures for women of childbearing age.
- Advise patient to select another method of feeding the baby if nursing.
- Advise patient to promptly notify health care provider if unexplained muscle pain, tenderness, or weakness occurs.

Teaching points

- Take this drug once a day without regard to food, exactly as prescribed.
- Continue the diet and exercise program prescribed for lowering your lipid levels.
- If you miss a dose, take the next dose as soon as you remember. Do not take more than the prescribed amount each day.
- This drug could harm a fetus; the use of contraceptive measures is recommended. If you become pregnant or wish to become pregnant, consult your health care provider.
- It is not known how this drug affects a nursing baby. Because of the potential for serious adverse effects in an infant, you should use another method of feeding the baby while you are taking this drug.
- You will need periodic blood tests to monitor your lipid levels and your liver.
- You may experience these side effects: Headache, muscle aches, runny nose.
- Report unexplained muscle pain, tenderness, or weakness; fever; changes in color of urine or stool.

plasma protein fraction

Plasmanate, Plasma-Plex, Plasmatein, Protenate

PREGNANCY CATEGORY C

Drug classes

Blood product
Plasma protein

Therapeutic actions

Maintains plasma colloid osmotic pressure and carries intermediate metabolites in the transport and exchange of tissue products; important in the maintenance of normal blood volume.

Indications

- Supportive treatment of shock due to burns, trauma, surgery, and infections
- Hypoproteinemia–nephrotic syndrome, hepatic cirrhosis, toxemia of pregnancy, postoperative patients, tuberculous patients, acute respiratory distress syndrome (ARDS), renal dialysis
- Acute liver failure
- Sequestration of protein-rich fluids
- Hyperbilirubinemia and erythroblastosis fetalis as an adjunct to exchange transfusions

Contraindications and cautions

- Contraindicated with allergy to albumin, severe anemia, cardiac failure, normal or increased intravascular volume, current use of cardiopulmonary bypass.
- Use cautiously with hepatic or renal failure, pregnancy.

Available forms

Injection—5%

Dosages

Administer by IV infusion only. Contains 130–160 mEq sodium/L. Do not give more than 250 g in 48 hr; if it seems that more is required, patient probably needs whole blood or plasma.

Adults

- *Hypovolemic shock:* 250–500 mL as an initial dose. Do not exceed 10 mL/min. Adjust dosage based on patient response. Do not exceed 5–8 mL/min as plasma volume approaches normal.
- *Hypoproteinemia:* Daily doses of 1,000–1,500 mL are appropriate. Do not exceed 5–8 mL/min. Adjust infusion rate based on patient response.

Pediatric patients

- *Hypovolemic shock:* Infuse a dose of 6.6–33 mL/kg at 5–10 mL/min. Dose may be repeated depending on patient's response.

Pharmacokinetics

Route	*Duration*
IV	Stays in the intravascular space

Metabolism: $T_{1/2}$: Unknown
Excretion: Unknown

IV FACTS

Preparation: No further preparation required; discard within 4 hr of entering a bottle; store at room temperature; do not use if there is sediment in the bottle. Do not freeze.
Infusion: Regulate based on patient response. Do not exceed 10 mL/min.

P

Compatibilities: Administer in combination with or through the same administration set as the usual IV solutions of saline or carbohydrates.
Incompatibilities: Do not use with alcohol or protein hydrolysates; precipitates may form.

Adverse effects

- **CV:** *Hypotension,* HF, **pulmonary edema following rapid infusion**
- **Hypersensitivity:** Fever, chills, changes in BP, flushing, nausea, vomiting, changes in respiration, rashes

■ Nursing considerations

Assessment

- **History:** Allergy to albumin, severe anemia, cardiac failure, normal or increased intravascular volume, current use of cardiopulmonary bypass, renal or hepatic failure, pregnancy
- **Physical:** Skin color, lesions; T; P, BP, peripheral perfusion; R, adventitious sounds; LFTs, renal function tests, Hct, serum electrolytes

Interventions

- Administer by IV infusion only, without regard to blood group or type.
- Consider the need for whole blood based on the patient's clinical condition; this infusion only provides symptomatic relief of the patient's hypoproteinemia.
- Monitor BP during infusion; discontinue if hypotension occurs.

⊗ ***Warning*** Stop infusion if headache, flushing, fever, or changes in BP occur. Arrange to treat reaction with antihistamines. If a plasma protein is still needed, try material from a different lot number.

- Monitor patient's clinical response and adjust infusion rate accordingly.

Teaching points

- Rate will be adjusted based on your response, so constant monitoring is needed.
- Report headache, nausea, vomiting, difficulty breathing, back pain.

plerixafor

See Appendix W, *Less commonly used drugs*.

poly-L-lactic acid

See Appendix W, *Less commonly used drugs*.

DANGEROUS DRUG

polymyxin B sulfate

*(pol i **mix'** in)*

Ophthalmic: Polymyxin B Sulfate Sterile

PREGNANCY CATEGORY C

Drug class

Antibiotic

Therapeutic actions

Bactericidal: Has surfactant (detergent) activity that allows it to penetrate and disrupt the cell membranes of susceptible gram-negative bacteria, causing cell death; not effective against *Proteus* species.

Indications

- Acute infections caused by susceptible strains of *Pseudomonas aeruginosa, Haemophilus influenzae, Escherichia coli, Aerobacter aerogenes, Klebsiella pneumoniae* when less toxic drugs are ineffective or contraindicated
- Ophthalmic preparations: Infections of the eye caused by susceptible strains of *P. aeruginosa*
- Intrathecal: Meningeal infections caused by *P. aeruginosa*

Contraindications and cautions

- Contraindicated with allergy to polymyxins (polymyxin B, colistin, colistimethate).
- Use cautiously with renal disease, pregnancy, lactation.

Available forms

Injection—500,000 units/vial; ophthalmic solution—500,000 units

Dosages

Adults

IV

15,000–25,000 units/kg/day may be given every 12 hr. Do not exceed 25,000 units/kg/day.

IM

25,000–30,000 units/kg/day divided and given at 4- to 6-hr intervals.

Intrathecal

50,000 units once daily for 3–4 days; then 50,000 units every other day for at least 2 wk after cultures of CSF are negative, and glucose content is normal.

Ophthalmic

1–3 drops of 0.1–0.25% concentration (10,000–25,000 units/mL) in infected eye every hour, increasing the intervals as response warrants.

Pediatric patients

IV

Infants: Up to 40,000 units/kg/day.
Older than 2 yr: Use adult dosage.

IM

Infants: Up to 40,000 units/kg/day; doses as high as 45,000 units/kg/day have been used in cases of sepsis caused by *P. aeruginosa.*
Older than 2 yr: Use adult dosage.

Intrathecal

Younger than 2 yr: 20,000 units once daily for 3–4 days or 25,000 units once every other day. Continue with 25,000 units once every other day for at least 2 wk after cultures of CSF are negative and glucose content is normal.
Older than 2 yr: Use adult dosage.

Ophthalmic

Use adult dosage.

Geriatric patients or patients with renal failure

Reduce dosage from the recommended dose, and follow renal function tests during therapy.

Pharmacokinetics

Route	*Onset*	*Peak*
IV	Rapid	Unknown
IM	Gradual	2 hr

Metabolism: $T_{1/2}$: 4.3–6 hr
Distribution: Does not cross placenta
Excretion: Urine

IV FACTS

Preparation: Dissolve 500,000 units in 300–500 mL of D_5W. Dissolve 500,000 units in 2 mL sterile distilled water or sodium chloride injection, or 1% procaine hydrochloride solution; refrigerate and discard any unused portion after 72 hr.
Infusion: Administer by continuous IV drip using an infusion pump.
Incompatibilities: Do not mix with amphotericin B, chloramphenicol, heparin, magnesium sulfate, tetracycline.

Adverse effects

- **CNS:** Neurotoxicity—*facial flushing, dizziness, ataxia, drowsiness,* paresthesias
- **Dermatologic:** Rash, urticaria
- **GU: Nephrotoxicity**
- **Local:** *Pain at IM injection site; thrombophlebitis at IV injection sites; irritation, burning, stinging, itching, blurring of vision* (ophthalmic preparations)
- **Respiratory: Apnea** (high dosage)
- **Other:** Drug fever, superinfections

Interactions

✷ **Drug-drug** • Increased neuromuscular blockade, apnea, and muscular paralysis when given with nondepolarizing neuromuscular blocking drugs • Increased risk of respiratory paralysis and renal impairment when given with aminoglycosides

P

■ Nursing considerations

Assessment

- **History:** Allergy to polymyxins, renal disease, lactation
- **Physical:** Site of infection, skin color, lesions; orientation, reflexes, speech; R; urinary output; urinalysis, serum creatinine, renal function tests

Interventions

⊗ ***Black box warning*** Monitor the patient's renal function carefully. Be aware that neurotoxicity can result in respiratory paralysis; monitor accordingly.

- Store drug solutions in refrigerator, and discard any unused portion after 72 hr.
- For intrathecal use: Dissolve 500,000 units in 10 mL sterile physiologic saline for a concentration of 50,000 units/mL.

- For ophthalmic use: Reconstitute powder with 20–50 mL of diluent.
- Culture infection before beginning therapy.
- Monitor renal function tests during therapy.
- Monitor for superinfection.
- Do not use IM route routinely; severe pain occurs at injection site.

Teaching points

- Administer ophthalmic preparation as follows: Tilt head back; place medication into eyelid and close eyes; gently hold the inner corner of the eye for 1 minute. Do not touch dropper to the eye. Ophthalmic preparation must be refrigerated. Discard any unused solution after 72 hours.
- You may experience these side effects: Vertigo, dizziness, drowsiness, slurring of speech (avoid driving or using hazardous equipment); numbness, tingling of the tongue, extremities (decrease the dosage); superinfections (frequent hygiene measures will help; request medications); burning, stinging, blurring of vision (ophthalmic; transient).
- Report difficulty breathing, rash or skin lesions, pain at injection site or IV site, change in urinary voiding patterns, fever, flulike symptoms, changes in vision, severe stinging or itching (ophthalmic).

▽ poractant alfa (DDPC, natural lung surfactant; porcine origin)

*(poor **ak'** tant)*

Curosurf

PREGNANCY CATEGORY NR

Drug class

Lung surfactant

Therapeutic actions

A natural porcine compound containing lipids and apoproteins that reduce surface tension and allow expansion of the alveoli; replaces the surfactant missing in the lungs of neonates suffering from RDS.

Indications

- Rescue treatment of infants who have developed RDS
- Unlabeled uses: Severe meconium aspiration syndrome; respiratory failure caused by group B streptococcal infection in neonates

Contraindications and cautions

- Because poractant is used as an emergency drug in acute respiratory situations, the benefits usually outweigh any possible risks.
- Use cautiously with any known family history of allergy to porcine products.

Available forms

Suspension for intratracheal instillation: 1.5, 3 mL

Dosages

⊗ ***Warning*** Accurate determination of birth weight is essential for determining appropriate dosage. Poractant is instilled into the trachea using a catheter inserted into the endotracheal tube.

Administer entire contents of vial (2.5 mL/kg birth weight) intratracheally, giving one-half of the dose into each bronchi. Administer the first dose as soon as possible after the diagnosis of RDS is made and when the patient is on the ventilator. Up to 2 subsequent doses of 1.25 mL/kg birth weight at 12-hr intervals may be needed. Maximum total dose is 5 mL/kg (sum of initial and 2 repeat doses).

Pharmacokinetics

Route	*Onset*	*Peak*
Intratracheal	Immediate	3 hr

Metabolism: Normal surfactant metabolic pathways; $T_{1/2}$: 25 hr
Distribution: Lung tissue
Excretion: Unknown

Adverse effects

- **CNS:** Seizures
- **CV: Patent ductus arteriosus, intraventricular hemorrhage,** *hypotension, bradycardia, flushing*
- **Hematologic:** *Hyperbilirubinemia, thrombocytopenia*

- **Respiratory: Pneumothorax,** *pulmonary air leak,* pulmonary hemorrhage (more often seen with infants weighing less than 700 g), *apnea,* pneumomediastinum, emphysema, endotracheal tube blockage, oxygen desaturation
- **Other:** *Sepsis, nonpulmonary infections*

■ Nursing considerations

Assessment

- **History:** Time of birth, exact birth weight
- **Physical:** T, color; R, adventitious sounds, oximeter, endotracheal tube position and patency, chest movement; ECG, P, BP, peripheral perfusion, arterial pressure (desirable); oxygen saturation, blood gases, CBC; muscular activity, facial expression, reflexes

Interventions

- Arrange for appropriate assessment and monitoring of critically ill infant.
- Monitor ECG and transcutaneous oxygen saturation continually during administration.
- Ensure that endotracheal tube is in the correct position, with bilateral chest movement and lung sounds.
- Arrange for staff to preview teaching videotape, available from the manufacturer, before regular use to cover all of the technical aspects of administration.
- Suction the infant immediately before administration, but do not suction for 2 hr after administration unless clinically necessary.
- Warm vial to room temperature before using, up to 24 hr. No other warming methods should be used. Gently turn vial upside down to obtain uniform suspension. Do not shake vial.
- Store drug in refrigerator. Protect from light. Enter drug vial only once. Discard remaining drug after use.
- Insert 5 French catheter into the endotracheal tube; do not instill into the main stream bronchus.
- Instill dose slowly; inject one-fourth of dose over 2–3 sec; remove catheter and reattach infant to ventilator for at least 30 sec or until stable; repeat procedure administering one-fourth of dose at a time.
- Do not suction infant for 1 hr after completion of full dose; do not flush catheter.
- Continually monitor patient color, lung sounds, ECG, oximeter and blood gas readings during administration and for at least 30 min following administration.
- Maintain appropriate interventions for critically ill infant.
- Offer support and encouragement to parents.

Teaching points

- Parents of the critically ill infant will need a comprehensive teaching and support program. Details of drug effects and administration are best incorporated into the comprehensive program.

porfimer sodium

See Appendix W, *Less commonly used drugs.*

posaconazole

*(pahs ah **kon'** ah zall)*

Noxafil

PREGNANCY CATEGORY C

Drug class

Antifungal (triazole)

Therapeutic actions

Inhibits the synthesis of ergosterol, a key component of the fungal cell membrane; this inhibition leads to inability of the fungus to form the fungal cell wall and results in cell death.

Indications

- Prophylaxis of invasive *Aspergillus* and *Candida* infections in patients 13 yr and older who are at risk of developing these infections because they are immunosuppressed because of prolonged neutropenia from antineoplastic chemotherapy, graft-versus-host disease secondary to bone marrow transplants, or hematologic malignancies
- Treatment of oropharyngeal candidiasis including cases refractory to itraconazole or fluconazole

P

Contraindications and cautions

- Contraindicated with hypersensitivity to any component of the drug and with concurrent use of ergot alkaloids or drugs that are CYP3A4 substrates (terfenadine, pimozide, halofantrine, or quinidine).
- Use cautiously with liver impairment, concurrent use of cyclosporine, prolonged QT interval, pregnancy, lactation.

Available forms

Oral suspension—40 mg/mL

Dosages

Adults and children 13 yr and older

Prevention: 200 mg (5 mL) PO tid. Give with a full meal or liquid nutritional supplement.
Treatment: Loading dose of 100 mg (2.5 mL) PO bid on day 1; then 100 mg/day PO for 13 days. For refractory infection, 400 mg (10 mL) PO bid, with duration based on patient response.

Patients with hepatic impairment

Use cautiously and monitor closely.

Pharmacokinetics

Route	*Onset*	*Peak*
Oral	Rapid	3–5 hr

Metabolism: Hepatic; $T_{1/2}$: 20–66 hr
Distribution: May cross placenta; may pass into breast milk
Excretion: Feces

Adverse effects

- **CNS:** *Headache, dizziness, insomnia,* anxiety
- **CV:** *Hypotension, hypertension, tachycardia*
- **GI:** *Diarrhea, nausea, vomiting, abdominal pain, constipation, mucositis, dyspepsia, anorexia, liver enzyme changes*
- **Hematologic:** *Anemia, neutropenia, hypokalemia, hypomagnesemia, hyperglycemia,* hypocalcemia, *thrombocytopenia*
- **Respiratory:** *Cough, dyspnea, epistaxis*
- **Other:** *Rash, fever, fatigue,* weakness, infections

Interactions

✱ **Drug-drug** • Decreased serum levels and loss of effectiveness if combined with rifabutin, phenytoin, cimetidine; avoid these combinations • Potential for increased serum levels and increased risk of toxicity of cyclosporine, sirolimus, tacrolimus, rifabutin, midazolam, phenytoin if combined with posaconazole; monitor patient closely and reduce dosages as appropriate • Increased serum levels of ergots and risk of ergotism; this combination is contraindicated • Increased serum levels of astemizole, terfenadine, pimozide, quinidine, leading to risk of prolonged QT interval and potentially fatal arrhythmias; avoid this combination • Increased serum levels of vincristine, vinblastine, and potential neurotoxicity; reduce dosage of these drugs and monitor patient closely • Potential for increased levels of statins, leading to possible rhabdomyolysis; reduce dosage of statins if used concurrently • Potential for increased levels of calcium channel blockers, sirolimus; reduce dosage and monitor patient closely

■ Nursing considerations

Assessment

- **History:** Hypersensitivity to any component of the drug; concurrent use of ergot alkaloids or drugs that are CYP3A4 substrates (terfenadine, pimozide, halofantrine, or quinidine); liver impairment; concurrent use of cyclosporine; prolonged QT interval; pregnancy, lactation
- **Physical:** T; orientation; reflexes; skin; BP; R, adventitious sounds; abdominal examinations; LFTs, culture of infected area, CBC, serum electrolytes, ECG

Interventions

- Culture infected area prior to starting drug; drug can be started before results are known, but appropriate adjustments in treatment should be made when culture results are evaluated.
- Give with a full meal or nutritional supplement. If patient is not able to eat a full meal or tolerate oral nutritional supplement, consider a different antifungal agent,

or monitor carefully for breakthrough fungal infections.
- Shake bottle well before use. Use the measuring spoon provided for accuracy.
- Periodically monitor LFTs to make sure hepatotoxicity does not occur.
- Obtain a baseline ECG and monitor any patient at risk for proarrhythmias or prolonged QT interval.
- Suggest the use of contraceptive measures while using this drug; the potential effects on a fetus are not known.
- Advise nursing mothers to use another method of feeding the baby while on this drug.
- Provide supportive measures for GI effects as needed.

Teaching points

- This drug must be taken three times a day (prevention) or twice a day (treatment) with a full meal or nutritional supplement (*Ensure* for example). If you are unable to eat, contact your health care provider.
- Store the bottle at room temperature, and shake it well before each use. To measure your dose accurately, use the spoon that comes with the bottle.
- Tell your health care provider about any other drugs you take; this drug can interact with many other drugs, and appropriate precautions will need to be taken.
- It is very important to maintain your fluid and food intake, which will help healing. Notify your health care provider if nausea or vomiting prevents this.
- You may need blood tests to evaluate the effects of the drug on your body.
- It is not known how this drug could affect a fetus. If you are pregnant or decide to become pregnant while on this drug, consult your health care provider; use of contraceptive measures is advised.
- It is not known how this drug could affect a nursing baby. If you are nursing a baby, you should select another method of feeding.
- You may experience these side effects: Headache, nausea, diarrhea (consult your health care provider; medications may be available to help).
- Report severe diarrhea or vomiting, fever that persists, changes in color of stool or urine, palpitations.

DANGEROUS DRUG

potassium salts

(po ***tass'*** *ee um)*

potassium acetate

potassium chloride

Oral: Apo-K (CAN), Cena-K, Effer-K, Gen-K, Kaon-Cl, Kay Ciel, Kaylixir, K-Dur 10, K-Dur 20, K-Lor, K-Tab, Klor-Con DNC, Klor-Con 10 DNC, Klor-Con M 10 DNC, Klor-Con M 15 DNC, Klor-Con M 20 DNC, Klorvess, Klotrix DNC, K+ 10, Micro-K Extencaps DNC, Potasalan, Ten K

Injection: Potassium Chloride

potassium gluconate

Kaon, K-G Elixir, Tri-K

PREGNANCY CATEGORY C

Drug class

Electrolyte

Therapeutic actions

Principal intracellular cation of most body tissues, participates in a number of physiologic processes—maintaining intracellular tonicity; transmission of nerve impulses; contraction of cardiac, skeletal, and smooth muscle; maintenance of normal renal function; also plays a role in carbohydrate metabolism and various enzymatic reactions.

Indications

- Prevention and correction of potassium deficiency; when associated with alkalosis, use potassium chloride; when associated with acidosis, use potassium acetate, bicarbonate, citrate, or gluconate
- IV: Treatment of cardiac arrhythmias due to cardiac glycosides

Contraindications and cautions

- Contraindicated with allergy to tartrazine, aspirin (tartrazine is found in some preparations marketed as *Kaon-Cl, Klor-Con*); therapy with potassium-sparing diuretics or aldosterone-inhibiting agents; severe renal impairment with oliguria, anuria, azotemia;

P

untreated Addison's disease; hyperkalemia; adynamia episodica hereditaria; acute dehydration; heat cramps; GI disorders that delay passage in the GI tract.
- Use cautiously with cardiac disorders, especially if treated with cardiac glycosides, pregnancy, lactation.

Available forms

Liquids—20, 40 mEq/15 mL; powders—15, 20, 25 mEq/packet; effervescent tablets—20, 25, 50 mEq; CR tablets (DNC)—8, 10, 15, 20 mEq; CR capsules (DNC)—8, 10 mEq; tablets—99, 500, 595 mg; injection—2, 10, 20, 30, 40, 60, 90 mEq

Dosages

Individualize dosage based on patient response using serial ECG and electrolyte determinations in severe cases.

Adults

Oral

- *Prevention of hypokalemia:* 16–24 mEq/day PO.
- *Treatment of potassium depletion:* 40–100 mEq/day PO.

IV

⊗ ***Warning*** Do not administer undiluted. Dilute in dextrose solution to 40–80 mEq/L. Use the following as a guide to administration:

Serum Potassium	*Maximum Infusion Rate*	*Maximum Concentration*	*Maximum 24-hr Dose*
More than 2.5 mEq/L	10 mEq/hr	40 mEq/L	200 mEq
Less than 2 mEq/L	40 mEq/hr	80 mEq/L	400 mEq

Pediatric patients

- *Replacement:* 3 mEq/kg/day or 40 mEq/m^2/day PO or IV.

Geriatric patients or patients with renal impairment

Carefully monitor serum potassium concentration and reduce dosage appropriately.

Pharmacokinetics

Route	*Onset*	*Peak*
Oral	Slow	1–2 hr
IV	Rapid	End of infusion

Metabolism: Cellular; $T_{1/2}$: Unknown
Distribution: Crosses placenta; enters breast milk
Excretion: Urine

IV FACTS

Preparation: Do not administer undiluted potassium IV; dilute in dextrose solution to 40–80 mEq/L; in critical states, potassium chloride can be administered in saline.
Infusion: Adjust dosage based on patient response at a maximum of 10 mEq/L; do not exceed 20 mEq/hr.
Incompatibility: Do not mix with amphotericin B.
Y-site incompatibilities: Do not give with amphotericin B, azithromycin, diazepam, ergotamine, phenytoin.

Adverse effects

- **Dermatologic:** Rash
- **GI:** *Nausea, vomiting, diarrhea, abdominal discomfort,* GI obstruction, GI bleeding, GI ulceration or perforation
- **Hematologic:** Hyperkalemia—increased serum potassium, ECG changes (peaking of T waves, loss of P waves, depression of ST segment, prolongation of QTc interval)
- **Local:** Tissue sloughing, local necrosis, local phlebitis, and venospasm with injection

Interactions

✱ **Drug-drug** • Increased risk of hyperkalemia with potassium-sparing diuretics, salt substitutes using potassium

■ Nursing considerations

Assessment

- **History:** Allergy to tartrazine, aspirin; severe renal impairment; untreated Addison's disease; hyperkalemia; adynamia episodica hereditaria; acute dehydration; heat cramps; GI disorders that cause delay in passage in the GI tract; cardiac disorders; lactation
- **Physical:** Skin color, lesions, turgor; injection sites; P, baseline ECG; bowel sounds, abdominal examination; urinary output; serum electrolytes, serum bicarbonate

Interventions

- Arrange for serial serum potassium levels before and during therapy.
- Administer liquid form to any patient with delayed GI emptying.
- Administer oral drug after meals or with food and a full glass of water to decrease GI upset.
- Caution patient not to chew or crush tablets; have patient swallow tablet whole.
- Mix or dissolve oral liquids, soluble powders, and effervescent tablets completely in 3–8 oz of cold water, juice, or other suitable beverage, and have patient drink it slowly.
- Arrange for further dilution or dose reduction if GI effects are severe.
- Agitate prepared IV solution to prevent "layering" of potassium; do not add potassium to an IV bag in the hanging position.
- Monitor IV injection sites regularly for necrosis, tissue sloughing, and phlebitis.
- Monitor cardiac rhythm carefully during IV administration.
- Caution patient that expended wax matrix capsules will be found in the stool.
- Caution patient not to use salt substitutes.

Teaching points

- Take drug after meals or with food and a full glass of water to decrease GI upset. Do not chew or crush tablets, swallow tablets whole. Mix or dissolve oral liquids, soluble powders, and effervescent tablets completely in 3–8 ounces of cold water, juice, or other suitable beverage, and drink it slowly. Take the drug as prescribed; do not take more than prescribed.
- Do not use salt substitutes.
- You may find wax matrix capsules in the stool. The wax matrix is not absorbed in the GI tract.
- Have periodic blood tests and medical evaluation.
- You may experience these side effects: Nausea, vomiting, diarrhea (taking the drugs with meals, diluting them further may help).
- Report tingling of the hands or feet, unusual tiredness or weakness, feeling of heaviness in the legs, severe nausea, vomiting, abdominal pain, black or tarry stools, pain at IV injection site.

▽pralatrexate

See Appendix W, *Less commonly used drugs*.

▽pralidoxime chloride (2-PAM)

*(pra li **dox'** eem)*

Protopam Chloride

PREGNANCY CATEGORY C

Drug class

Antidote

Therapeutic actions

Reactivates cholinesterase (mainly outside the CNS) inactivated by phosphorylation due to organophosphate pesticide or related compound. Relieves respiratory muscle paralysis related to organophosphate toxicity.

Indications

- Antidote in poisoning due to organophosphate pesticides and chemicals with anticholinesterase activity
- IM use as an adjunct to atropine in poisoning by nerve agents having anticholinesterase activity (autoinjector)
- Control of overdose by anticholinesterase drugs used to treat myasthenia gravis

Contraindications and cautions

- Contraindicated with concomitant use of theophylline, morphine, aminophylline, and succinylcholine and allergy to any component of drug.
- Use cautiously with impaired renal function, myasthenia gravis, pregnancy, lactation.

Available forms

Injection—1 g

Dosages

Adults

- *Organophosphate poisoning:* In absence of cyanosis, give atropine 2–4 mg IV. If cyanosis is present, give 2–4 mg atropine IM while improving ventilation; repeat every 5–10 min until signs of atropine toxicity appear. Maintain atropinization for at least 48 hr. *Give*

P

pralidoxime concomitantly: Inject an initial dose of 1–2 g pralidoxime IV, preferably as a 15- to 30-min infusion in 100 mL of saline. After 1 hr, give a second dose of 1–2 g IV if muscle weakness is not relieved. Give additional doses cautiously. If IV administration is not feasible or if pulmonary edema is present, give IM or subcutaneously.

- *Anticholinesterase (eg, neostigmine, pyridostigmine, ambenonium) overdose:* 1–2 g IV followed by increments of 250 mg every 5 min.
- *Exposure to nerve agents:* Administer atropine and pralidoxime as soon as possible after exposure. Use the autoinjectors, giving the atropine first; repeat both atropine and pralidoxime after 15 min. If symptoms exist after an additional 15 min, repeat injections. If symptoms persist after third set of injections, seek medical help.

Pediatric patients

- *Organophosphate poisoning:* 20–40 mg/kg IV per dose given as above.

Pharmacokinetics

Route	*Onset*	*Peak*
IV	Rapid	5–15 min
IM	Rapid	10–20 min

Metabolism: Hepatic; $T_{1/2}$: 0.8–2.7 hr
Distribution: May cross placenta; may enter breast milk
Excretion: Urine

IV FACTS

Preparation: Dilute 1–2 g pralidoxime in 100 mL saline.
Infusion: Administer over 15–30 min.

Adverse effects

- **CNS:** *Dizziness, blurred vision, diplopia, headache,* drowsiness, nausea, impaired accommodation
- **CV:** Tachycardia
- **Hematologic:** *Transient AST, ALT, CPK elevations*
- **Local:** *Mild to moderate pain at the injection site* 40–60 min after IM injection
- **Respiratory:** Hyperventilation
- **Other:** Muscular weakness

■ Nursing considerations

Assessment

- **History:** Allergy to any component of drug, impaired renal function, myasthenia gravis, lactation, pregnancy
- **Physical:** Reflexes, orientation, vision examination, muscle strength; P, auscultation, baseline ECG; liver evaluation; LFTs, renal function tests

Interventions

- Remove secretions, maintain patent airway, and provide artificial ventilation as needed for acute organophosphate poisoning; then begin drug therapy.
- Institute treatment as soon as possible after exposure to the poison.

⊗ ***Warning*** Remove clothing; thoroughly wash hair and skin with sodium bicarbonate or alcohol as soon as possible after dermal exposure to organophosphate poisoning.

- Use IV sodium thiopental or diazepam if seizures interfere with respiration after organophosphate poisoning.

⊗ ***Warning*** Administer by slow IV infusion; tachycardia, laryngospasm, muscle rigidity have occurred with rapid injection. Do not exceed injection rate of 200 mg/min.

Teaching points

- Discomfort may be experienced at IM injection site. If you receive the autoinjector, you need to understand the indications and proper use of the mechanism, review the signs and symptoms of poisoning.
- Report blurred or double vision, dizziness, nausea.

▽ pramipexole dihydrochloride

*(pram ah **pex'** ole)*

Mirapex

PREGNANCY CATEGORY C

Drug classes

Antiparkinsonian
Dopamine receptor agonist

Therapeutic actions

Stimulates dopamine receptors in the striatum, leading to decrease in parkinsonian symptoms thought to be related to low dopamine levels.

Indications

- Treatment of the signs and symptoms of idiopathic Parkinson's disease
- Treatment of moderate to severe primary restless leg syndrome
- Unlabeled use: Treatment of fibromyalgia

Contraindications and cautions

- Contraindicated with hypersensitivity to pramipexole.
- Use cautiously with symptomatic hypotension, impaired renal function, pregnancy, lactation.

Available forms

Tablets—0.125, 0.25, 0.5, 0.75, 1, 1.5 mg

Dosages

Adults

- *Parkinson's disease:* Increase dosage gradually from a starting dose of 0.125 mg PO tid for 1 wk; wk 2—0.25 mg PO tid; wk 3—0.5 mg PO tid; wk 4—0.75 mg PO tid; wk 5—1 mg PO tid; wk 6—1.25 mg PO tid; wk 7—1.5 mg PO tid. If used in combination with levodopa, consider levodopa dose reduction.
- *Restless leg syndrome:* Initially, 0.125 mg/day PO taken 2–3 hr before bedtime; dose may be increased every 4–7 days, if needed, to 0.25 mg/day and maximum of 0.5 mg/day.

Pediatric patients

Safety and efficacy not established.

Patients with renal impairment

CrCl (mL/min)	*Starting Dose*	*Maximum Dose*
More than 60	0.125 mg PO tid	1.5 mg PO tid
35–59	0.125 mg PO bid	1.5 mg PO bid
15–34	0.125 mg PO daily	1.5 mg PO daily
Less than 15	Safety and efficacy not established; data not available	

Pharmacokinetics

Route	*Onset*	*Peak*
Oral	Varies	2 hr

Metabolism: Hepatic; $T_{1/2}$: 8 hr
Distribution: May cross placenta; may enter breast milk
Excretion: Urine

Adverse effects

- **CNS:** *Headache, dizziness, insomnia,* **somnolence,** hallucinations, confusion, amnesia, extrapyramidal syndrome
- **CV:** Orthostatic hypotension, hypertension, arrhythmia, palpitations, hypotension, tachycardia
- **GI:** *Nausea, constipation,* anorexia, dysphagia
- **Other:** Peripheral edema, decreased weight, *asthenia,* fever

Interactions

✱ Drug-drug • Increase in levodopa levels and effects if combined • Increase in levels with cimetidine, ranitidine, diltiazem, triamterene, verapamil, quinidine, quinine, and drugs eliminated via renal secretion • Decreased effectiveness with dopamine antagonists

■ Nursing considerations

Assessment

- **History:** Hypersensitivity to pramipexole, symptomatic hypotension, impaired renal function, pregnancy, lactation
- **Physical:** Reflexes, affect; T, BP, P, peripheral perfusion; abdominal examination, normal output; auscultation, R; urinary output, renal function tests

Interventions

⊗ ***Warning*** Administer with extreme caution to patients with a history of hypotension, hallucinations, confusion, or dyskinesias.

- Administer with food if GI upset becomes a problem.

⊗ ***Warning*** Do not discontinue abruptly; taper gradually over at least 1 wk.

- Monitor patient while adjusting drug to establish therapeutic dosage. Dosage of levodopa and carbidopa may need to be

P

reduced accordingly to balance therapeutic effects.
- Provide safety precautions as needed if hallucinations occur (more common with elderly).

Teaching points
- For Parkinson's disease, take this drug exactly as prescribed, three times per day, with breakfast, lunch, and dinner. Continue to take your levodopa and carbidopa if prescribed. The dosage of levodopa may need to be decreased after a few days of therapy. The dosage of pramipexole will be slowly increased over a 7-week period. Write your dose down and follow this pattern.
- For restless leg syndrome, take the dose daily 2–3 hours before bedtime. Dosage may be increased as needed.
- Do not stop taking this drug without consulting your health care provider; serious side effects could occur. The drug should be tapered over at least 1 week.
- Avoid becoming pregnant while using this drug; using barrier contraceptives is advised. If you think you are pregnant, notify your health care provider.
- You may experience these side effects: Dizziness, light-headedness, insomnia (avoid driving or operating dangerous machinery); nausea (take drug with meals); edema; weight loss; low blood pressure (change positions slowly; use caution in extremes of heat or exertion); hallucinations (safety precautions may be needed); falling asleep while engaged in activities of daily living (use caution to avoid injury).
- Report severe nausea, severe swelling, sweating, hallucinations, dizziness, fainting.

DANGEROUS DRUG

pramlintide acetate
(pram' lin tyde)

Symlin

PREGNANCY CATEGORY C

Drug classes
Amylinomimetic
Antidiabetic

Therapeutic actions
A synthetic analogue of human amylin, a hormone produced by the beta cells in the pancreas that helps to control glucose levels in the postprandial period; modulates gastric emptying, causes a feeling of fullness or satiety, prevents the postprandial rise in serum glucagon levels all leading to lower serum glucose levels.

Indications
- Adjunct treatment in patients with type 1 diabetes who use mealtime insulin and who have failed to achieve desired glucose control despite optimal insulin therapy
- Adjunct treatment in type 2 diabetes patients who use mealtime insulin and who have failed to achieve desired glucose control despite optimal insulin therapy with or without a concurrent sulfonylurea or metformin

Contraindications and cautions
- Contraindicated with known hypersensitivity to pramlintide or any of its components, gastroparesis, hypoglycemia unawareness.
- Use cautiously with pregnancy, lactation.

Available forms
Solution for injection—0.6 mg/mL

Dosages
Adults
- *Type 2 diabetes:* Initially, 60 mcg by subcutaneous injection immediately prior to major meals. Dose may be increased to 120 mcg if needed and tolerated. Dosage of oral drugs and insulins will need to be reduced, usually by 50% based on patient response.
- *Type 1 diabetes:* Initially, 15 mcg by subcutaneous injection immediately before major meals, titrate at 15 mcg increments to a maintenance dose of 30 or 60 mcg as tolerated. Dosage of insulins will need to be reduced by 50% and the patient must be monitored closely to achieve optimal glucose control.

Pharmacokinetics

Route	*Onset*	*Peak*
Subcut.	Rapid	21 min

Metabolism: Renal; $T_{1/2}$: 48 min
Distribution: May cross placenta; may pass into breast milk
Excretion: Urine

Adverse effects

- **CNS:** Dizziness, headache, fatigue
- **GI:** *Nausea,* anorexia, *vomiting,* abdominal pain
- **Respiratory:** Cough, pharyngitis
- **Other: Hypoglycemia,** injection site reaction

Interactions

✱ **Drug-drug** • Risk of delayed absorption of oral medications because of effects on gastric emptying; if rapid effect is needed, take oral medication 1 hr prior to or 2 hr after pramlintide • Risk of combined effects on gastric emptying if combined with anticholinergic drugs or drugs that slow intestinal absorption of nutrients; avoid this combination

■ Nursing considerations

Assessment

- **History:** Hypersensitivity to pramlintide or any of its components, gastroparesis, hypoglycemia unawareness, pregnancy, lactation
- **Physical:** Orientation, reflexes, affect; abdominal examination; injection site; blood glucose levels

Interventions

⊗ ***Black box warning*** Be aware that severe hypoglycemia has been associated with combined use of insulin, pramlintide; monitor accordingly.

- Inject subcutaneously before each major meal of the day; inject it into a site that is more than 2 inches away from the site of insulin injection.
- Do not combine in syringe with insulin.
- Maintain other antidiabetic drugs, diet and exercise regimen for control of diabetes.
- Administer oral medications at least 1 hr before or 2 hr after administering pramlintide.
- Monitor serum glucose levels and HbA_{1c} levels frequently to evaluate effectiveness of drug on controlling glucose levels.
- Arrange for thorough diabetic teaching program to include disease, dietary control, exercise, signs and symptoms of hypoglycemia and hyperglycemia, avoidance of infection and hygiene.

Teaching points

- This drug is given subcutaneously. Use sterile technique. Dispose of syringes appropriately.
- Do not use any solution that appears cloudy; do not combine this drug in syringe with insulin.
- Inject it into a site on your thigh or abdomen. Rotate injection sites periodically; inject into a site that is at least 2 inches away from the site of your insulin injection.
- Store unopened vials in the refrigerator. Opened bottles may be kept at room temperature. Throw away any out-of-date bottles.
- Inject this drug before any major meal that you are eating; do not use if you are not going to be eating; if you forget a dose, do not inject after you have eaten.
- Be aware that alcohol consumption can change your blood glucose levels and may alter your response to this drug.
- Do not take this drug if you are not able to eat or if you plan to skip a meal or if your blood sugar is too low.
- Do not change the dosage of this drug without consulting your health care provider.
- It is not known how this drug affects a pregnancy. If you think you are pregnant or would like to become pregnant, consult your health care provider.
- It is not known how this drug could affect a nursing baby. If you are nursing a baby, consult your health care provider.
- You will need to regularly monitor your blood glucose levels. Your health care provider may change the dose of pramlintide or your other antidiabetic drugs, based on your blood glucose response.
- It is important that you follow the diet, exercise, and drug guidelines related to your disease.
- Review the signs and symptoms of hypoglycemia; be prepared to treat hypoglycemia with fast-acting sugar or glucagon.
- Do not drive a car or operate potentially dangerous machinery until you are aware of how pramlintide will affect your blood sugar. Low

blood sugar can cause dizziness and changes in thinking.

- This drug affects how fast your stomach empties, which may affect other drugs you may be taking. Consult your health care provider about the need to change the timing of drug administration.
- You may experience these side effects: Injection site reactions (proper injection and rotation of injection sites should help; if problems occur, consult your health care provider); hypoglycemia (use fast-acting sugars or glucagons if this occurs; proper use and eating of meals should prevent this effect); nausea (this usually passes after a few days).
- Report hypoglycemic reactions; redness, pain or swelling at injection sites; stomach pain; vomiting.

▽ prasugrel

(pra' soo grel)

Effient

PREGNANCY CATEGORY B

Drug class

Platelet inhibitor

Therapeutic actions

Inhibits platelet activation and aggregation by irreversibly binding to the $P2Y_{12}$ class of ADP receptors on platelets.

Indications

- To reduce the risk of thrombotic cardiovascular events (including stent thrombosis) in patients with acute coronary syndrome who are to be managed with percutaneous coronary intervention, including patients with unstable angina or non-ST-elevation MI and patients with ST-elevation MI who will be managed with primary or delayed percutaneous coronary intervention

Contraindications and cautions

- Contraindicated with hypersensitivity to components of drug, active pathological bleeding, history of TIA or stroke, patients likely to undergo CABG surgery.
- Use cautiously with age 75 yr and older, body weight less than 60 kg, bleeding tendency, use of drugs that increase risk of bleeding, pregnancy, lactation.

Available forms

Tablets—5, 10 mg

Dosages

Adults

Loading dose: 60 mg PO as single dose, then 10 mg/day PO without regard to food; use 5 mg/day in patients weighing less than 60 kg. Patient should also be receiving aspirin (75–325 mg/day).

Pediatric patients

Safety and efficacy not established.

Pharmacokinetics

Route	*Onset*	*Peak*
Oral	Rapid	30 min

Metabolism: Hepatic; $T_{1/2}$: 2–15 hr

Distribution: May cross placenta; may enter breast milk

Excretion: Urine, feces

Adverse effects

- **CNS:** *Headache,* dizziness
- **CV:** *Hypertension,* hypotension, peripheral edema, atrial fibrillation, bradycardia
- **GI:** Nausea, diarrhea
- **Hematologic:** *Hypercholesterolemia, hyperlipidemia,* leukopenia
- **Respiratory:** Dyspnea, cough
- **Other: Bleeding, thrombotic thrombocytopenic purpura,** rash, fever, fatigue, pain, **risk of thrombotic episodes if stopped prematurely**

Interactions

✱ Drug-drug • Increased risk of bleeding if combined with warfarin or prolonged use of NSAIDs; monitor patient closely and adjust dosage as appropriate

■ Nursing considerations

Assessment

- **History:** Hypersensitivity to components of drug, active pathological bleeding, history of TIA or stroke, planned or anticipated CABG surgery, pregnancy, lactation, age, body weight under 60 kg, bleeding tendency, use of drugs that increase the risk of bleeding

- **Physical:** Weight; T; skin—color, lesions; orientation, affect; P, BP, periphery evaluation for edema; R, adventitious sounds

Interventions

⊗ ***Black box warning*** There is a risk of serious to fatal bleeding with drug administration; do not use with active bleeding or history of TIA or stroke. Risk increases in patients older than 75 yr, patients weighing less than 60 kg, patients with bleeding tendency, and patients taking warfarin or NSAIDs. Do not use in patients who are likely candidates for CABG surgery; if patients taking drug require CABG, stop prasugrel at least 7 days before surgery. Suspect bleeding in patient who becomes hypotensive and has undergone invasive procedures. If possible, control bleeding without discontinuing prasugrel; premature discontinuation increases risk of thrombotic episodes.

- Administer loading dose and then give once a day without regard to food.
- Patient should also be taking aspirin once a day. Check with health care provider.
- Advise patient to use contraceptive measures because it is not known if drug affects a fetus.
- Advise patient to select another method of feeding the baby if nursing; it is not known if drug enters breast milk.
- Limit invasive procedures; be aware that patient may experience prolonged bleeding if undergoing invasive procedures.
- Protect patient from injury; risk of bruising and bleeding is increased.
- Do not discontinue drug prematurely because of increased risk of thrombotic events.
- Alert surgeons that patient is taking drug; if possible, drug should be discontinued at least 7 days before surgery.

Teaching points

- Take this drug exactly as prescribed, once a day without regard to food.
- If you forget a dose, take the next dose at the regular time. Do not attempt to make up or double doses unless you have been instructed to do so by your health care provider.
- Do not run out of this drug or stop taking this drug for any reason. If you stop taking the drug, immediately contact your health care provider because serious events could occur.
- Keep a list of all drugs you are taking, including over-the-counter drugs and herbal therapies, so your health care provider can adjust dosages as needed.
- Inform all your health care providers, including your dentist and surgeons, that you are taking this drug. Because this drug makes you bleed longer, appropriate measures will be needed if invasive procedures are planned.
- You should carry or wear a Medical Alert card to alert people who may care for you during an emergency that you are taking this drug.
- It is not known if this drug affects a fetus; the use of contraceptive measures is advised.
- It is not known if this drug enters breast milk. If you are nursing a baby, you should use another method of feeding the baby.
- You may experience these side effects: Increased bleeding and bruising (take extra precautions to avoid injury; be aware that if you are injured, it will take longer to stop bleeding), nausea, diarrhea (small, frequent meals may help; consult your health care provider if this becomes too uncomfortable); rash, fatigue.
- Rarely, a serious disorder called thrombotic thrombocytopenic purpura can occur. Notify your health care provider immediately if you experience fever, weakness, purple skin patches, yellowing of the skin or eyes, extreme paleness, mental changes.
- Report excessive bruising or bruising from no known cause, uncontrollable bleeding, pink or brown urine, red or tarlike stools, coughing up blood or clots, vomiting blood, or vomit that looks like coffee grounds.

▽ pravastatin sodium

*(prah va **sta'** tin)*

Apo-Pravastatin (CAN), CO Pravastatin (CAN), Gen-Pravastatin (CAN), Novo-Pravastatin (CAN), Nu-Pravastatin (CAN), PMS-Pravastatin (CAN), Pravachol, ratio-Pravastatin (CAN)

PREGNANCY CATEGORY X

Drug classes
Antihyperlipidemic
HMG-CoA reductase inhibitor

Therapeutic actions
Inhibits the enzyme HMG-CoA that catalyzes the first step in the cholesterol synthesis pathway, resulting in a decrease in serum cholesterol, serum LDLs (associated with increased risk of CAD), and either an increase or no change in serum HDLs (associated with decreased risk of CAD).

Indications
- Prevention of first MI and reduction of death from CV disease in patients with hypercholesterolemia at risk of first MI
- Adjunct to diet in the treatment of elevated total cholesterol and LDL cholesterol with primary hypercholesterolemia (types IIa and IIb) in patients unresponsive to dietary restriction of saturated fat and cholesterol and other nonpharmacologic measures
- Slow the progression of coronary atherosclerosis in patients with clinically evident CAD to reduce the risk of acute coronary events in hypercholesterolemia patients
- Reduce the risk of CVA or TIA in patients with history of MI and normal cholesterol levels
- Reduce the risk of recurrent MI and death from heart disease in patients with history of MI and normal cholesterol levels
- Treatment of children 8 yr and older with heterozygous familial hypercholesterolemia as an adjunct to diet and exercise

Contraindications and cautions
- Contraindicated with allergy to pravastatin, fungal byproducts, active liver disease, pregnancy, lactation.
- Use cautiously with impaired hepatic function, cataracts, alcoholism.

Available forms
Tablets—10, 20, 40, 80 mg

Dosages
Adults
Initially, 40 mg/day PO given once daily. Adjust dosage every 4 wk based on response. Maximum daily dose is 80 mg. Maintenance doses range from 40–80 mg/day in a single bedtime dose.
- *Concomitant immunosuppressive therapy:* 10 mg PO daily at bedtime to a maximum of 20 mg/day.

Pediatric patients 14–18 yr
40 mg/day PO.

Pediatric patients 8–13 yr
20 mg/day PO.

Geriatric patients and patients with renal or hepatic impairment
10 mg PO once daily at bedtime; may increase up to 20 mg/day.

Pharmacokinetics

Route	*Onset*	*Peak*
Oral	Slow	60–90 min

Metabolism: Hepatic; $T_{1/2}$: 1.8 hr
Distribution: Crosses placenta; enters breast milk
Excretion: Feces, urine

Adverse effects
- **CNS:** *Headache, blurred vision,* dizziness, insomnia, fatigue, muscle cramps, cataracts
- **GI:** *Flatulence, abdominal pain, cramps, constipation, nausea, vomiting,* heartburn
- **Hematologic:** Elevations of CPK, alkaline phosphatase, and transaminases

Interactions
✱ **Drug-drug** • Possible severe myopathy or rhabdomyolysis with cyclosporine, erythromycin, gemfibrozil, niacin • Possible increased digoxin, warfarin levels if combined; monitor patient and decrease dosage as needed • Increased pravastatin levels with itraconazole; avoid this combination • Decreased pravastatin levels if combined with bile acid sequestrants; space at least 4 hr apart

■ Nursing considerations
Assessment
- **History:** Allergy to pravastatin, fungal byproducts; impaired hepatic function; cataracts; pregnancy; lactation
- **Physical:** Orientation, affect, ophthalmologic examination; liver evaluation; lipid studies, LFTs

Interventions
- Ensure that patient is on a cholesterol-lowering diet before and during therapy.
- Caution patient that this drug cannot be used during pregnancy; advise patient to use barrier contraceptives.
- Suggest another method of feeding the infant if patient is nursing.
- Administer drug at bedtime; highest rates of cholesterol synthesis occur between midnight and 5 AM.
- Arrange for periodic ophthalmologic examination to check for cataract development; monitor liver function.

Teaching points
- Take drug at bedtime.
- Continue your cholesterol-lowering diet and exercise program.
- This drug cannot be taken during pregnancy; using barrier contraceptives is advised.
- This drug cannot be taken while nursing; another method of feeding the baby will be needed.
- Have periodic ophthalmic examinations while you are using this drug.
- You may experience these side effects: Nausea (eat frequent small meals); headache, muscle and joint aches and pains (may lessen); sensitivity to sunlight (use sunblock and wear protective clothing).
- Report severe GI upset, changes in vision, unusual bleeding or bruising, dark urine or light-colored stools, muscle pain or weakness.

praziquantel

See Appendix W, *Less commonly used drugs*.

prazosin hydrochloride

(pra' zoe sin)

Apo-Prazo (CAN), Minipress, Novo-Prazin (CAN)

PREGNANCY CATEGORY C

Drug classes
Alpha-adrenergic blocker
Antihypertensive

Therapeutic actions
Selectively blocks postsynaptic $alpha_1$-adrenergic receptors, decreasing sympathetic tone on the vasculature, dilating arterioles and veins, and lowering supine and standing BP; unlike conventional alpha-adrenergic blocking agents (eg, phentolamine), it does not block $alpha_2$ presynaptic receptors, so it does not cause reflex tachycardia.

Indications
- Treatment of hypertension, alone or in combination with other agents
- Unlabeled uses: Refractory HF, management of Raynaud's vasospasm, treatment of bladder outflow obstruction (BPH), pheochromocytoma

Contraindications and cautions
- Contraindicated with hypersensitivity to prazosin, lactation.
- Use cautiously with HF, angina pectoris, renal failure, pregnancy.

Available forms
Capsules—1, 2, 5 mg

Dosages
⊗ ***Warning*** First dose may cause syncope with sudden loss of consciousness. First dose should be limited to 1 mg PO and given at bedtime.

Adults

Initial dosage is 1 mg PO bid–tid. Increase dosage to a total of 20 mg/day given in divided doses. When increasing dosage, give the first dose of each increment at bedtime. Maintenance dosages most commonly range from 6–15 mg/day given in divided doses.
- *Concomitant therapy:* When adding a diuretic or other antihypertensive drug, reduce dosage to 1–2 mg PO tid and then readjust.

Pediatric patients

Safety and efficacy not established.

Pharmacokinetics

Route	Onset	Peak
Oral	Varies	1–3 hr

P

Metabolism: Hepatic; $T_{1/2}$: 2–3 hr
Distribution: Crosses placenta; may enter breast milk
Excretion: Bile, feces, and urine

Adverse effects

- **CNS:** *Dizziness, headache, drowsiness, lack of energy, weakness,* nervousness, vertigo, depression, paresthesia
- **CV:** *Palpitations,* sodium and water retention, increased plasma volume, edema, dyspnea, syncope, tachycardia, orthostatic hypotension
- **Dermatologic:** Rash, pruritus, alopecia, lichen planus
- **EENT:** Blurred vision, reddened sclera, epistaxis, tinnitus, dry mouth, nasal congestion
- **GI:** *Nausea,* vomiting, diarrhea, constipation, abdominal discomfort or pain
- **GU:** Urinary frequency, incontinence, impotence, priapism
- **Other:** Diaphoresis, lupus erythematosus

Interactions

✱ **Drug-drug** • Severity and duration of hypotension following first dose of prazosin may be greater in patients receiving beta-adrenergic blocking drugs (eg, propranolol), verapamil; first dose of prazosin should be only 0.5 mg or less • Increased risk of hypotension with phosphodiesterase-5 inhibitors (sildenafil, tadalafil, vardenafil)

■ Nursing considerations

Assessment

- **History:** Hypersensitivity to prazosin, HF, angina pectoris, renal failure, lactation, pregnancy
- **Physical:** Weight; skin color, lesions; orientation, affect, reflexes; ophthalmologic examination; P, BP, orthostatic BP, supine BP, perfusion, edema, auscultation; R, adventitious sounds; status of nasal mucous membranes; bowel sounds, normal output; voiding pattern, normal output; renal function tests, urinalysis

Interventions

- Administer, or have patient take, first dose just before bedtime to lessen likelihood of first dose effect (syncope), believed due to excessive orthostatic hypotension.
- Have patient lie down and treat patient supportively if syncope occurs; condition is self-limiting.
- Monitor for orthostatic hypotension, which is most marked in the morning and is accentuated by hot weather, alcohol, and exercise.
- Monitor edema and weight in patients with incipient cardiac decompensation, and add a thiazide diuretic to the drug regimen if sodium and fluid retention or signs of impending heart failure occur.

Teaching points

- Take this drug exactly as prescribed. Take the first dose just before bedtime. Do not drive or operate machinery for 4 hours after the first dose.
- You may experience these side effects: Dizziness, weakness (more likely when changing position, in the early morning, after exercise, in hot weather, and with alcohol; some tolerance may occur; avoid driving or engaging in tasks that require alertness; change position slowly, and use caution when climbing stairs; lie down for a while if dizziness persists); GI upset (eat frequent small meals); impotence; dry mouth (sucking on sugarless lozenges, ice chips may help); stuffy nose. Most effects are transient.
- Report frequent dizziness or faintness.

▽ prednisolone

*(pred **niss'** oh lone)*

prednisolone

Oral: Prelone

prednisolone acetate

Ophthalmic solution:
Econopred, Pred Forte, Pred Mild, ratio-Prednisolone (CAN)

prednisolone sodium phosphate

Ophthalmic solution:
Prednisol

Oral:
Hydrocortone, Orapred, Orapred ODT, Pediapred

PREGNANCY CATEGORY C

Drug classes

Anti-inflammatory
Corticosteroid (intermediate acting)
Glucocorticoid
Hormone

Therapeutic actions

Enters target cells and binds to intracellular corticosteroid receptors, thereby initiating many complex reactions that are responsible for its anti-inflammatory and immunosuppressive effects.

Indications

Systemic

- Hypercalcemia associated with cancer
- Short-term management of various inflammatory and allergic disorders, such as rheumatoid arthritis, collagen diseases (eg, SLE), dermatologic diseases (eg, pemphigus), status asthmaticus, and autoimmune disorders
- Hematologic disorders: Thrombocytopenia purpura, erythroblastopenia
- Ulcerative colitis, acute exacerbations of MS and palliation in some leukemias and lymphomas
- Trichinosis with neurologic or myocardial involvement
- Prednisolone has weaker mineralocorticoid activity than hydrocortisone and is not used as physiologic replacement therapy

Ophthalmic

- Inflammation of the lid, conjunctiva, cornea, and globe

Contraindications and cautions

- Contraindicated with infections (especially TB, fungal infections, amebiasis, vaccinia and varicella, and antibiotic-resistant infections), lactation, idiopathic thrombocytopenic purpura.
- Use cautiously with renal or liver disease, hypothyroidism, ulcerative colitis with impending perforation, diverticulitis, active or latent peptic ulcer, inflammatory bowel disease, heart failure, hypertension, thromboembolic disorders, osteoporosis, seizure disorders, diabetes mellitus, pregnancy.

Ophthalmic preparations

- Contraindicated with acute superficial herpes simplex keratitis; fungal infections of ocular structures; vaccinia, varicella, and other viral diseases of the cornea and conjunctiva; ocular TB.

Available forms

Tablets—5 mg; rapidly dissolving tablets—10, 15, 30 mg; oral syrup—15 mg/5 mL, 5 mg/5 mL; ophthalmic suspension—0.12%, 1%; oral suspension—5, 15 mg/5 mL

Dosages

Adults

Individualize dosage, depending on severity of condition and patient's response. Administer daily dose before 9 AM to minimize adrenal suppression. If long-term therapy is needed, consider alternate-day therapy. After long-term therapy, withdraw drug slowly to avoid adrenal insufficiency. For maintenance therapy, reduce initial dose in small increments at intervals until the lowest dose that maintains satisfactory clinical response is reached.

Oral

Prednisolone: 5–60 mg/day.

- *Acute exacerbations of MS:* 200 mg/day for 1 wk, followed by 80 mg every other day for 1 mo.

Adults and pediatric patients

Ophthalmic

Prednisolone acetate: 2 drops qid. For *Pred Mild* or *Pred Forte,* 1–2 drops bid–qid during first 48 hr; then dosing frequency may be increased if necessary.

Prednisolone sodium phosphate: 1–2 drops up to every hr during the day and every 2 hr during the night. After a favorable response, reduce to 1 drop every 4 hr. Later, further reduction to 1 drop 3–4 times daily may suffice.

Pediatric patients

Individualize dosage depending on severity of condition and patient's response rather than by strict adherence to formulae that correct adult doses for age or weight. Carefully observe growth and development in infants and children on prolonged therapy.

P

Oral suspension

0.14–2 mg/kg/day PO in three to four divided doses.

- *Nephrotic syndrome:* 60 mg/m²/day PO in three divided doses for 4 wk. Then single doses for 4 wk. Alternatively, 40 mg/m²/day PO.

Pharmacokinetics

Route	*Onset*	*Peak*	*Duration*
Oral	Varies	1–2 hr	1–1.5 days

Metabolism: Hepatic; $T_{1/2}$: 3.5 hr
Distribution: Crosses placenta; enters breast milk
Excretion: Urine

Adverse effects

Effects depend on dose, route, and duration of therapy. The following are primarily associated with systemic absorption.

- **CNS:** *Vertigo, headache,* paresthesias, insomnia, seizures, psychosis, cataracts, increased IOP, glaucoma (long-term therapy), *euphoria, depression*
- **CV:** Hypotension, **shock,** hypertension and HF secondary to fluid retention, thromboembolism, thrombophlebitis, fat embolism, cardiac arrhythmias
- **Electrolyte imbalance:** *Na+ and fluid retention,* hypokalemia, hypocalcemia
- **Endocrine:** Amenorrhea, irregular menses, growth retardation, decreased carbohydrate tolerance, diabetes mellitus, cushingoid state (long-term effect), increased blood sugar, increased serum cholesterol, decreased T_3 and T_4 levels, HPA suppression with systemic therapy longer than 5 days
- **GI:** Peptic or esophageal ulcer, pancreatitis, abdominal distention, nausea, vomiting, *increased appetite, weight gain* (long-term therapy)
- **Hypersensitivity:** Hypersensitivity or anaphylactoid reactions
- **Musculoskeletal:** Muscle weakness, steroid myopathy, loss of muscle mass, osteoporosis, spontaneous fractures (long-term therapy)
- **Other:** *Immunosuppression, aggravation, or masking of infections; impaired wound healing;* thin, fragile skin; petechiae, ecchymoses, purpura, striae; subcutaneous fat atrophy

Ophthalmic solutions

- **Local:** Infections, especially fungal; glaucoma, cataracts with long-term therapy
- **Other:** Systemic absorption and adverse effects (see above) with prolonged use

Interactions

✱ **Drug-drug** • Increased therapeutic and toxic effects of prednisolone with ketoconazole • Increased therapeutic and toxic effects of estrogens, including hormonal contraceptives • Risk of severe deterioration of muscle strength in myasthenia gravis patients who also are receiving ambenonium, edrophonium, neostigmine, pyridostigmine • Decreased steroid blood levels with barbiturates, phenytoin, rifampin • Decreased effectiveness of salicylates

✱ **Drug-lab test** • False-negative nitroblue tetrazolium test for bacterial infection • Suppression of skin test reactions

■ Nursing considerations

Assessment

- **History:** Infections; renal or liver disease; hypothyroidism; ulcerative colitis with impending perforation; diverticulitis; active or latent peptic ulcer; inflammatory bowel disease; HF; hypertension; thromboembolic disorders; osteoporosis; seizure disorders; diabetes mellitus; pregnancy; lactation. Ophthalmic: Acute superficial herpes simplex keratitis; fungal infections of ocular structures; vaccinia, varicella, and other viral diseases of the cornea and conjunctiva; ocular TB
- **Physical:** Weight, T, reflexes and grip strength, affect and orientation, P, BP, peripheral perfusion, prominence of superficial veins, R, adventitious sounds, serum electrolytes, blood glucose

Interventions

- Administer once-a-day doses before 9 AM to mimic normal peak corticosteroid blood levels.
- Increase dosage when patient is subject to stress.
- Have patient place orally disintegrating tablet in mouth, let dissolve, and then swallow.

⊗ ***Warning*** Taper doses when discontinuing high-dose or long-term therapy to avoid adrenal insufficiency.

⊗ ***Warning*** Do not give live virus vaccines with immunosuppressive doses of corticosteroids.

Teaching points

Systemic

- Take once-daily doses before 9 AM; if using orally dissolving tablet, place in mouth, let dissolve, and then swallow.
- Do not stop taking the drug without consulting your health care provider.
- Avoid exposure to infections.
- Report unusual weight gain, swelling of the extremities, muscle weakness, black or tarry stools, fever, prolonged sore throat, colds or other infections, worsening of the disorder for which the drug is being taken.

Ophthalmic preparations

- Learn the proper administration technique: Shake suspension well before each use. Lie down or tilt head backward, and look at ceiling. Pull lower eyelid down to form a pocket. Drop suspension inside lower eyelid while looking up. After instilling eye drops, release lower lid, but do not blink for at least 30 seconds; apply gentle pressure to the inside corner of the eye for 1 minute. Do not close eyes tightly, and try not to blink more often than usual. Do not touch dropper to eye, fingers, or any surface. Wait at least 5 minutes before using any other eye preparations.
- Eyes may be sensitive to bright light; sunglasses may help.
- Report worsening of the condition, pain, itching, swelling of the eye, failure of the condition to improve after 1 week.

▽ prednisone

(pred' ni sone)

Apo-Prednisone (CAN), Novo-Prednisone (CAN), Prednisone Intensol Concentrate, Sterapred DS, Sterapred, Winpred (CAN)

PREGNANCY CATEGORY C

Drug classes

Corticosteroid (intermediate acting)
Glucocorticoid
Hormone

Therapeutic actions

Enters target cells and binds to intracellular corticosteroid receptors, initiating many complex reactions that are responsible for its anti-inflammatory and immunosuppressive effects.

Indications

- Replacement therapy in adrenal cortical insufficiency
- Hypercalcemia associated with cancer
- Short-term management of various inflammatory and allergic disorders, such as rheumatoid arthritis, collagen diseases (eg, SLE), dermatologic diseases (eg, pemphigus), status asthmaticus, and autoimmune disorders
- Hematologic disorders: Thrombocytopenia purpura, erythroblastopenia
- Ulcerative colitis, acute exacerbations of MS and palliation in some leukemias and lymphomas
- Trichinosis with neurologic or myocardial involvement

Contraindications and cautions

- Contraindicated with infections, especially tuberculosis, fungal infections, amebiasis, vaccinia and varicella, and antibiotic-resistant infections; lactation.
- Use cautiously with renal or liver disease, hypothyroidism, ulcerative colitis with impending perforation, diverticulitis, active or latent peptic ulcer, inflammatory bowel disease, heart failure, hypertension, thromboembolic disorders, osteoporosis, seizure disorders, diabetes mellitus, hepatic disease, pregnancy (monitor infants for adrenal insufficiency).

Available forms

Tablets—1, 2.5, 5, 10, 20, 50 mg; oral solution—5 mg/5 mL, 5 mg/mL

Dosages

Adults

Individualize dosage depending on severity of condition and patient's response. Administer daily dose before 9 AM to minimize adrenal suppression. If long-term therapy is needed, consider alternate-day therapy. After long-term therapy, withdraw drug slowly to avoid adrenal insufficiency. Initial dose, 5–60 mg/day PO. For maintenance therapy, reduce initial dose in small increments at intervals until lowest dose that maintains satisfactory clinical response is reached. For acute exacerbations of MS, 200 mg/day PO for 1 wk, then 80 mg PO every other day for 1 month.

Pediatric patients

- *Physiologic replacement:* 0.05–2 mg/kg/day PO or 4–5 mg/m^2/day PO in equal divided doses every 12 hr.
- *Other indications:* Individualize dosage depending on severity of condition and the patient's response rather than by strict adherence to formulae that correct adult doses for age or body weight. Carefully observe growth and development in infants and children on prolonged therapy.

Pharmacokinetics

Route	Onset	Peak	Duration
Oral	Varies	1–2 hr	1–1.5 days

Metabolism: Hepatic; $T_{1/2}$: 3.5 hr
Distribution: Crosses placenta; enters breast milk
Excretion: Urine

Adverse effects

- **CNS:** *Vertigo, headache,* paresthesias, insomnia, seizures, psychosis, cataracts, increased IOP, glaucoma (long-term therapy), *euphoria, depression*
- **CV:** Hypotension, **shock,** hypertension and HF secondary to fluid retention, thromboembolism, thrombophlebitis, fat embolism, cardiac arrhythmias
- **Electrolyte imbalance:** *Sodium and fluid retention,* hypokalemia, hypocalcemia
- **Endocrine:** Amenorrhea, irregular menses, growth retardation, decreased carbohydrate tolerance, diabetes mellitus, cushingoid state (long-term effect), increased blood sugar, increased serum cholesterol, decreased T_3 and T_4 levels, HPA suppression with systemic therapy longer than 5 days
- **GI:** Peptic or esophageal ulcer, pancreatitis, abdominal distention, nausea, vomiting, *increased appetite, weight gain* (long-term therapy)
- **Hypersensitivity:** Hypersensitivity or anaphylactoid reactions
- **Musculoskeletal:** Muscle weakness, steroid myopathy, loss of muscle mass, osteoporosis, spontaneous fractures (long-term therapy)
- **Other:** *Immunosuppression, aggravation or masking of infections; impaired wound healing;* thin, fragile skin; petechiae, ecchymoses, purpura, striae; subcutaneous fat atrophy

Interactions

✱ **Drug-drug** • Increased therapeutic and toxic effects with troleandomycin, ketoconazole • Increased therapeutic and toxic effects of estrogens, including hormonal contraceptives • Risk of severe deterioration of muscle strength in myasthenia gravis patients who also are receiving ambenonium, edrophonium, neostigmine, pyridostigmine • Decreased steroid blood levels with barbiturates, phenytoin, rifampin • Decreased effectiveness of salicylates

✱ **Drug-lab test** • False-negative nitroblue tetrazolium test for bacterial infection • Suppression of skin test reactions

■ Nursing considerations

Assessment

- **History:** Infections, renal or liver disease, hypothyroidism, ulcerative colitis with impending perforation, diverticulitis, active or latent peptic ulcer, inflammatory bowel disease, HF, hypertension, thromboembolic disorders, osteoporosis, seizure disorders, diabetes mellitus, hepatic disease, lactation
- **Physical:** Weight, T, reflexes and grip strength, affect and orientation, P, BP, peripheral perfusion, prominence of superficial veins, R, adventitious sounds, serum electrolytes, blood glucose

Interventions

- Administer once-a-day doses before 9 AM to mimic normal peak corticosteroid blood levels.
- Increase dosage when patient is subject to stress.

⊗ ***Warning*** Taper doses when discontinuing high-dose or long-term therapy to avoid adrenal insufficiency.

⊗ ***Warning*** Do not give live virus vaccines with immunosuppressive doses of corticosteroids.

Teaching points

- Do not stop taking the drug without consulting your health care provider; take once-daily doses at about 9 AM.
- Avoid exposure to infections.
- Report unusual weight gain, swelling of the extremities, muscle weakness, black or tarry stools, fever, prolonged sore throat, colds or other infections, worsening of the disorder for which the drug is being taken.

▽ pregabalin

(pray gab' ah lin)

Lyrica

PREGNANCY CATEGORY C

CONTROLLED SUBSTANCE V

Drug classes

Analgesic
Antiepileptic
Calcium channel modulator

Therapeutic actions

Binds to alpha$_2$-delta sites on the nerves in the CNS, which reduces the calcium influx into the cell and decreases the release of neurotransmitters into the synaptic cleft, resulting in less stimulation of the nerve; in lab studies, it also increases the transport and density of GABA, which is known to suppress nerve activity.

Indications

- Management of acute pain associated with diabetic peripheral neuropathy
- Management of postherpetic neuralgia
- Adjunct therapy of adult patients with partial onset seizures
- Management of fibromyalgia
- Unlabeled uses: Treatment of generalized anxiety disorders

Contraindications and cautions

- Contraindicated with known hypersensitivity to pregabalin or any component of the drug, lactation.
- Use cautiously with diabetes, HF, pregnancy.

Available forms

Capsules—25, 50, 75, 100, 150, 200, 225, 300 mg

Dosages

Adults

- *Neuropathic pain:* 100 mg PO tid.
- *Postherpetic neuralgia:* 75–150 mg PO bid or 50–100 mg PO tid as needed to control pain; may be adjusted up to a maximum dose of 600 mg/day.
- *Epilepsy:* 150–600 mg/day PO, divided into two to three doses.
- *Fibromyalgia:* 75 mg PO bid. May be increased within 1 wk to 150 mg PO bid. Maximum dose, 450 mg/day.

Pediatric patients

Safety and efficacy not established.

Patients with renal impairment

If creatinine clearance is 60 mL/min or greater, 150–600 mg/day in two to three divided doses; if creatinine clearance is 30–60 mL/min, 75–300 mg/day in two to three divided doses; if creatinine clearance is 15–30 mL/min, 25–150 mg/day in one dose or divided into two doses; if creatinine clearance is less than 15 mL/min, 25–75 mg/day as one dose.

Pharmacokinetics

Route	*Onset*	*Peak*
Oral	Rapid	1.5 hr

Metabolism: None; $T_{1/2}$: 6.3 hr
Distribution: May cross placenta; may pass into breast milk
Excretion: Urine

Adverse effects

- **CNS:** *Dizziness, somnolence, neuropathy,* ataxia, vertigo, confusion, euphoria, incoordination, vision abnormalities, tremors, thinking abnormalities, suicidal ideation
- **GI:** *Dry mouth, constipation,* flatulence

P

- **Other:** *Peripheral edema, weight gain,* hypoglycemia, back pain, chest pain, *infection, creatine kinase elevations,* loss of fertility (male), **angioedema**

Interactions

✷ **Drug-drug** • Increased risk of sedation and dizziness if combined with CNS depressants, alcohol • Increased incidence of weight gain if combined with pioglitazone, rosiglitazone; monitor patient weight and blood glucose if this combination is used

■ Nursing considerations

Assessment

- **History:** Lactation, pregnancy, diabetes, heart failure, allergy to pregabalin
- **Physical:** Weight; orientation, reflexes, affect, vision; renal function tests, blood glucose level

Interventions

⊗ ***Black box warning*** Risk of suicidal ideation is increased; monitor patient accordingly.

- Do not administer this drug after a fatty or large meal, absorption can be affected.
- Do not stop taking this drug suddenly; dosage should be adjusted to avoid adverse effects.
- Provide safety measures if dizziness, somnolence, changes in thinking occur.
- Monitor weight gain and fluid retention; adjust treatment for diabetes, HF accordingly.
- Encourage women of childbearing age to use barrier contraceptives while on this drug because the effects of the drug on a fetus are not known.
- Advise women who are nursing to find another method of feeding the baby, it is not known if this drug can affect a nursing baby.
- Advise men who plan to father a child that in animal studies, this drug affected fertility and was related to birth defects in the offspring of male animals taking the drug. The decision to take the drug may be affected by this information.

Teaching points

- Take this drug exactly as prescribed. Do not increase the dose without consulting your health care provider.
- Do not stop taking this drug suddenly; serious adverse effects could occur.
- Do not share this drug with anyone else. Carefully dispose of any unused or outdated drug.
- Do not take this drug with or immediately after a high fat or heavy meal. This could interfere with the absorption and effectiveness of the drug.
- It is not known how this drug would affect a pregnancy. If you think you are pregnant or would like to become pregnant, consult your health care provider. You should use contraceptive measures while taking this drug.
- This drug should not be taken while nursing a baby. If you are nursing a baby, another method of feeding the baby should be used while using this drug.
- Do not drink alcohol while you are using this drug.
- If you are a man who wants to father a child, discuss this with your health care provider; this drug caused animals to be less fertile and caused some birth defects in the offspring of males taking this drug.
- You may experience these side effects: Dizziness, sleepiness, changes in thinking and alertness (do not drive a car, operate potentially dangerous equipment, or make important legal decisions if this occurs); dry mouth (sucking on sugarless lozenges, frequent mouth care may help).
- Report rash; changes in vision; weight gain; swelling in feet, legs, face, or tongue; increased bleeding; fever; sudden pain; weakness; or thoughts of suicide.

▽ primidone

(pri' mi done)

Apo-Primidone (CAN), Mysoline

PREGNANCY CATEGORY D

Drug classes

Anticonvulsant
Antiepileptic

Therapeutic actions

Mechanism of action not understood; primidone and its two metabolites, phenobarbital and phenylethylmalonamide, all have antiepileptic activity.

Indications

- Control of grand mal, psychomotor, or focal epileptic seizures, either alone or with other antiepileptics; may control grand mal seizures refractory to other antiepileptics
- Unlabeled use: Treatment of benign familial tremor (essential tremor)—750 mg/day

Contraindications and cautions

- Contraindicated with hypersensitivity to phenobarbital and primidone, porphyria, lactation (somnolence and drowsiness may occur in nursing newborns).
- Use cautiously with pregnancy (association between use of antiepileptics and an elevated incidence of birth defects; however, do not discontinue antiepileptic therapy in pregnant women who are receiving such therapy to prevent major seizures; discontinuing medication is likely to precipitate status epilepticus, with attendant hypoxia and risk to both mother and fetus; to prevent neonatal hemorrhage, primidone should be given with prophylactic vitamin K_1 therapy for 1 mo before and during delivery).

Available forms

Tablets—50, 250 mg

Dosages

Adults

- *Regimen for patients who have received no previous therapy:* Days 1–3, 100–125 mg PO at bedtime; days 4–6, 100–125 mg bid; days 7–9, 100–125 mg tid; day 10–maintenance, 250 mg tid. The usual maintenance dosage is 250 mg tid–qid. If required, increase dosage to 250 mg five to six times daily, but do not exceed dosage of 500 mg qid (2 g/day).
- *Regimen for patients already receiving other antiepileptics:* Start primidone at 100–125 mg PO at bedtime. Gradually increase to maintenance level as the other drug is gradually decreased. Continue this regimen until satisfactory dosage level is achieved for the combination, or the other medication is completely withdrawn. When use of primidone alone is desired, the transition should not be completed in less than 2 wk.

Pediatric patients

- *Regimen for patients who have received no previous therapy:*
  Younger than 8 yr: Days 1–3, 50 mg PO at bedtime; days 4–6, 50 mg bid; days 7–9, 100–125 mg bid; day 10–maintenance, 250 mg tid. The usual maintenance dosage is 125–250 mg tid or 10–25 mg/kg/day in divided doses.
  Older than 8 yr: Use adult dosage.

Pharmacokinetics

Route	*Onset*	*Peak*
Oral	Varies	3–7 hr

Metabolism: Hepatic; $T_{1/2}$: 3–24 hr
Distribution: Crosses placenta; enters breast milk
Excretion: Urine

Adverse effects

- **CNS:** *Ataxia, vertigo, fatigue, hyperirritability,* emotional disturbances, nystagmus, diplopia, drowsiness, personality deterioration with mood changes and paranoia, suicidal ideation, tolerance
- **GI:** *Nausea, anorexia,* vomiting
- **GU:** Sexual impotence
- **Hematologic:** Megaloblastic anemia that responds to folic acid therapy, thrombocytopenia
- **Other:** Morbilliform skin eruptions

Interactions

✱ **Drug-drug** • Toxicity with phenytoins • Increased CNS effects, impaired hand-eye coordination, and death may occur with acute alcohol ingestion • Decreased serum concentrations of primidone and increased serum concentrations of carbamazepine if taken concurrently • Decreased serum concentrations with acetazolamide • Increased levels with isoniazid, nicotinamide, succinimides

■ Nursing considerations

Assessment

- **History:** Hypersensitivity to phenobarbital, porphyria, pregnancy, lactation, suicidal ideation

P

- **Physical:** Skin color, lesions; orientation, affect, reflexes, vision examination; bowel sounds, normal output; CBC and SMA-12, EEG

Interventions

⊠ ***Black box warning*** Risk of suicidal ideation is increased. Monitor patient accordingly.

⊗ ***Warning*** Reduce dosage, discontinue primidone, or substitute other antiepileptic gradually; abrupt discontinuation may precipitate status epilepticus.

- Arrange for patient to have CBC and SMA-12 test every 6 mo during therapy.
- Arrange for folic acid therapy if megaloblastic anemia occurs; primidone does not need to be discontinued.
- Obtain counseling for women of childbearing age who wish to become pregnant.

⊗ ***Warning*** Evaluate for therapeutic serum levels—5–12 mcg/mL for primidone.

Teaching points

- Take this drug exactly as prescribed; do not discontinue this drug abruptly or change dosage, except on the advice of your health care provider.
- Arrange for frequent checkups, including blood tests, to monitor your response to this drug. Keep all appointments for checkups.
- Use contraception at all times. If you wish to become pregnant while you are taking this drug, you should consult your health care provider.
- Wear a medical alert tag at all times so that emergency medical personnel will know that you have epilepsy and are taking antiepileptic medication.
- You may experience these side effects: Drowsiness, dizziness, muscular incoordination (transient; avoid driving or performing other tasks requiring alertness); vision changes (avoid performing tasks that require visual acuity); GI upset (take drug with food or milk, eat frequent small meals).
- Report rash, joint pain, unexplained fever, pregnancy, thoughts of suicide.

▽ probenecid

*(proe **ben'** e sid)*

Benuryl (CAN)

PREGNANCY CATEGORY B

Drug classes

Antigout drug
Uricosuric drug

Therapeutic actions

Inhibits the renal tubular reabsorption of urate, increasing the urinary excretion of uric acid, decreasing serum uric acid levels, retarding urate deposition, and promoting resorption of urate deposits; also inhibits the renal tubular reabsorption of most penicillins and cephalosporins.

Indications

- Treatment of hyperuricemia associated with gout and gouty arthritis (adults)
- Adjuvant to therapy with penicillins or cephalosporins, for elevation and prolongation of plasma levels of the antibiotic

Contraindications and cautions

- Contraindicated with allergy to probenecid, blood dyscrasias, uric acid kidney stones, acute gouty attack.
- Use cautiously with peptic ulcer, acute intermittent porphyria, G6PD deficiency, chronic renal insufficiency, in patients with sulfa allergy, lactation, pregnancy.

Available forms

Tablets—0.5 g

Dosages

Adults

- *Gout:* 0.25 g PO bid for 1 wk; then 0.5 g PO bid. For maintenance, continue dosage that maintains the normal serum uric acid levels. When no attacks occur for 6 mo or longer, decrease the daily dosage by 0.5 g every 6 mo.
- *Penicillin or cephalosporin therapy:* 2 g/day PO in divided doses.

- *Gonorrhea treatment:* Single 1-g dose PO 30 min before penicillin administration.

Pediatric patients

- *Penicillin or cephalosporin therapy: Younger than 2 yr:* Do not use.
  2–14 yr: 25 mg/kg PO initial dose, then 40 mg/kg/day divided in four doses.
  Children 50 kg or greater: Use adult dosage.
- *Gonorrhea treatment in children less than 45 kg:* 23 mg/kg PO in one single dose 30 min before penicillin administration.

Geriatric patients or patients with renal impairment

1 g/day PO may be adequate. Daily dosage may be increased by 0.5 g every 4 wk. Probenecid may not be effective in chronic renal insufficiency when GFR less than 30 mL/min.

Pharmacokinetics

Route	*Onset*	*Peak*
Oral	Varies	2–4 hr

Metabolism: Hepatic; $T_{1/2}$: 5–78 hr
Distribution: Crosses placenta; may enter breast milk
Excretion: Urine

Adverse effects

- **CNS:** *Headache*
- **GI:** *Nausea, vomiting, anorexia,* sore gums
- **GU:** *Urinary frequency,* exacerbation of gout and uric acid stones
- **Hematologic:** Anemia, hemolytic anemia
- **Hypersensitivity:** Reactions including **anaphylaxis,** dermatitis, pruritus, fever
- **Other:** Blushing, dizziness

Interactions

✱ **Drug-drug** • Decreased effectiveness with salicylates • Decreased renal excretion and increased serum levels of methotrexate, dyphylline • Increased pharmacologic effects of thiopental, acyclovir, allopurinol, benzodiazepines, clofibrate, dapsone, NSAIDs, sulfonamides, zidovudine, rifampin

✱ **Drug-lab test** • False-positive test for urine glucose if using Benedict's test, *Clinitest* (use *Clinistix*) • Falsely high determination of theophylline levels • Inhibited excretion of urinary 17-ketosteroids, phenolsulfonphthalein, sulfobromophthalein

■ Nursing considerations

CLINICAL ALERT!
Name confusion has been reported between probenecid and *Procanbid* (procainamide); use extreme caution.

Assessment

- **History:** Allergy to probenecid, blood dyscrasias, uric acid kidney stones, acute gouty attack, peptic ulcer, acute intermittent porphyria, G6PD deficiency, chronic renal insufficiency, pregnancy, lactation
- **Physical:** Skin lesions, color; reflexes, gait; liver evaluation, normal output, gums; urinary output; CBC, LFTs, renal function tests, urinalysis

Interventions

- Administer drug with meals or antacids if GI upset occurs.
- Encourage patient to drink 2.5 to 3 L/day of fluids to decrease the risk of renal stone development.
- Check urine alkalinity; urates crystallize in acid urine; sodium bicarbonate or potassium citrate may be ordered to alkalinize urine.
- Arrange for regular medical follow-up and blood tests.
- Double-check any analgesics ordered for pain; salicylates should be avoided.

Teaching points

- Take the drug with meals or antacids if GI upset occurs.
- You may experience these side effects: Headache (monitor lighting, temperature, noise; consult your health care provider if severe); dizziness (change position slowly; avoid driving or operating dangerous machinery); exacerbation of gouty attack or renal stones (drink plenty of fluids—2.5–3 liters per day); nausea, vomiting, loss of appetite (take drug with meals or request antacids).
- Report flank pain, dark urine or blood in urine, acute gout attack, unusual fatigue or lethargy, unusual bleeding or bruising.

DANGEROUS DRUG

procainamide hydrochloride

*(proe **kane'** a myde)*

Procanbid DNC, Pronestyl

PREGNANCY CATEGORY C

Drug class

Antiarrhythmic

Therapeutic actions

Type IA antiarrhythmic: Decreases rate of diastolic depolarization (decreases automaticity) in ventricles, decreases the rate of rise and height of the action potential, increases fibrillation threshold.

Indications

- Treatment of documented ventricular arrhythmias judged to be life-threatening
- Unlabeled use: Conversion of atrial fibrillation or flutter to sinus rhythm

Contraindications and cautions

- Contraindicated with allergy to procaine, procainamide, or similar drugs; second- or third-degree heart block (unless electrical pacemaker operative); SLE; torsades de pointes; lactation.
- Use cautiously with myasthenia gravis, hepatic or renal disease, pregnancy, blood dyscrasias, HF.

Available forms

Capsules—250, 375, 500 mg; ER tablets DNC—250, 500, 750, 1,000 mg; injection—100, 500 mg/mL

Dosages

Adults

Oral

50 mg/kg/day PO in divided doses every 3 hr. Maintenance dose of 50 mg/kg/day (ER) in divided doses every 6 hr, starting 2–3 hr after last dose of standard oral preparation. If using *Procanbid,* give 50 mg/kg/day in divided doses every 12 hr.

Body Weight	*Standard Preparation*	*ER Preparation*
40–50 kg	250 mg every 3 hr	500 mg every 6 hr
60–70 kg	375 mg every 3 hr	750 mg every 6 hr
80–90 kg	500 mg every 3 hr	1,000 mg every 6 hr
More than 100 kg	625 mg every 3 hr	1,250 mg every 6 hr

IM

0.5–1 g every 4–8 hr until oral therapy can be started.

IV

- Direct IV injection: Dilute in 5% dextrose injection. Give 100 mg every 5 min at a rate not to exceed 25–50 mg/min (maximum dose 1 g).
- IV infusion: 500–600 mg as a loading dose over 25–30 min, then 2–6 mg/min. Monitor very closely.

Pediatric patients

Oral

15–50 mg/kg/day divided in three to six divided doses; maximum, 4 g/day.

IM

20–30 mg/kg/day divided every 4–6 hr; maximum 4 g/day.

IV

Loading dose, 3–6 mg/kg per dose over 5 min; maintenance, 20–80 mcg/kg/min per continuous infusion; maximum, 100 mg/day dose or 2 g/day. 2–5 mg/kg (maximum 100 mg) repeated as necessary every 5–10 min; or, 15 mg/kg given over 30–60 min, followed by maintenance infusion.

Pharmacokinetics

Route	*Onset*	*Peak*	*Duration*
Oral	30 min	90–120 min	3–4 hr
IV	Immediate	20–60 min	3–4 hr
IM	10–30 min	15–60 min	3–4 hr

Metabolism: Hepatic; $T_{1/2}$: 2.5–4.7 hr

Distribution: Crosses placenta; enters breast milk

Excretion: Urine

IV FACTS

Preparation: Dilute the 100- or 500-mg/mL dose in D_5W. For loading dose, dilute 1 g in 50 mL D_5W. For maintenance infusion, dilute 1 g in 250 or 500 mL D_5W.

Infusion: Slowly inject directly into vein or into tubing of actively running IV, 100 mg every 5 min, not faster than 25–50 mg/min; maintenance doses should be given by continual IV infusion with a pump to maintain rate—first 500–600 mg over 25–30 min, then 2–6 mg/min.

Adverse effects

- **CNS:** Mental depression, giddiness, seizures, confusion, psychosis
- **CV:** *Hypotension,* cardiac conduction disturbances
- **Dermatologic:** *Rash,* pruritus, urticaria
- **GI:** *Anorexia, nausea,* vomiting, bitter taste, diarrhea
- **Hematologic:** Granulocytopenia
- **Other:** Lupus syndrome, fever, chills

Interactions

✱ **Drug-drug** • Increased levels with cimetidine, ranitidine, quinolones, thioridazine, ziprasidone, trimethoprim, amiodarone, and other antiarrhythmics; monitor for toxicity

■ Nursing considerations

CLINICAL ALERT!

Name confusion has been reported between *Procanbid* and probenecid; use extreme caution.

Assessment

- **History:** Allergy to procaine, procainamide, or similar drugs; second- or third-degree heart block (unless electrical pacemaker operative); myasthenia gravis; hepatic or renal disease; SLE; torsades de pointes; pregnancy; lactation
- **Physical:** Weight, skin color, lesions; bilateral grip strength; P, BP, auscultation, ECG, edema; bowel sounds, liver evaluation; urinalysis, LFTs, renal function tests, CBC

Interventions

⊗ ***Black box warning*** Administer only to patients with life-threatening arrhythmias; serious proarrhythmias may occur.

- Monitor patient response carefully, especially when beginning therapy.
- Reduce dosage in patients weighing less than 120 lb.
- Reduce dosage in patients with hepatic or renal failure.
- Dosage adjustment may be needed when procainamide is given with other antiarrhythmics, antihypertensives, cimetidine, or alcohol.
- Check to see that patients with supraventricular tachyarrhythmias have been digitalized before giving procainamide.
- Differentiate the ER form from the regular preparation.
- Monitor cardiac rhythm and BP frequently if IV route is used.

⊗ ***Black box warning*** Arrange for periodic ECG monitoring and determination of ANA titers when on long-term therapy; blood dyscrasias may occur.

- Arrange for frequent monitoring of blood counts.
- Give dosages at evenly spaced intervals, around-the- clock; determine a schedule that will minimize sleep interruption.

⊗ ***Warning*** Evaluate for safe and effective serum drug levels: 4–10 mcg/mL.

Teaching points

- Take this drug at evenly spaced intervals, around-the-clock. Do not take double doses; do not skip doses; take exactly as prescribed. You may need an alarm clock to wake you up to take the drug. The best schedule for you will be determined to decrease sleep interruption as much as possible. Do not chew the extended-release tablets.
- You will require frequent monitoring of cardiac rhythm.
- Do not stop taking this drug for any reason without consulting your health care provider.
- Return for regular follow-up visits to check your heart rhythm and blood counts.
- You may experience these side effects: Nausea, loss of appetite, vomiting (eat frequent small meals); small wax cores may be passed in the stool (from extended-release tablet); rash (use careful skin care).
- Report joint pain, stiffness; sore mouth, throat, gums; fever, chills; cold or flulike symptoms; extensive rash, sensitivity to the sun.

procarbazine hydrochloride

See Appendix W, *Less commonly used drugs*.

prochlorperazine

*(proe klor **per'** a zeen)*

prochlorperazine

Rectal suppositories: Compazine, Compro

prochlorperazine edisylate

Oral syrup, injection: Compazine

prochlorperazine maleate

Oral tablets and sustained-release capsules: Compazine DNC

PREGNANCY CATEGORY C

Drug classes

Antiemetic
Antipsychotic
Anxiolytic
Dopaminergic blocker
Phenothiazine (piperazine)

Therapeutic actions

Mechanism of action not fully understood: Antipsychotics block postsynaptic dopamine receptors in the brain, but this may not be necessary and sufficient for antipsychotic activity; depresses the RAS, including the parts of the brain involved with wakefulness and emesis; anticholinergic, antihistaminic (H_1), and alpha-adrenergic blocking activity also may contribute to some of its therapeutic (and adverse) actions.

Indications

- Management of manifestations of psychotic disorders
- Control of severe nausea and vomiting
- Short-term treatment of nonpsychotic anxiety (not drug of choice)

Contraindications and cautions

- Contraindicated with hypersensitivity to phenothiazines, coma or severe CNS depression, bone marrow depression, blood dyscrasia, circulatory collapse, subcortical brain damage, Parkinson's disease, liver damage, cerebral arteriosclerosis, coronary disease, congenital long-QT syndrome, severe hypotension or hypertension, history of cardiac arrhythmias.
- Use cautiously with elderly patients, respiratory disorders, glaucoma, prostatic hypertrophy, epilepsy, breast cancer (elevations in prolactin may stimulate a prolactin-dependent tumor), thyrotoxicosis, peptic ulcer, decreased renal function, myelography within previous 24 hr or scheduled within 48 hr, exposure to heat or phosphorous insecticides, pregnancy, lactation, children younger than 12 yr, especially those with chickenpox, CNS infections (children are especially susceptible to dystonias that may confound the diagnosis of Reye's syndrome).

Available forms

Tablets—5, 10, 25 mg; spansules (SR capsules) DNC—10, 15 mg; syrup—5 mg/5 mL; injection—5 mg/mL; suppositories—2.5, 5, 25 mg

Dosages

Adults

- *Psychotic disturbances:* Initially, 5–10 mg PO tid or qid. Gradually increase dosage every 2–3 days as needed up to 50–75 mg/day for mild or moderate disturbances, 100–150 mg/day for more severe disturbances. For immediate control of severely disturbed adults, 10–20 mg IM repeated every 2–4 hr (every hour for resistant cases); switch to oral therapy as soon as possible.
- *Antiemetic:* For control of severe nausea and vomiting, 5–10 mg PO tid–qid; 15 mg (SR) on arising; 10 mg (SR) every 12 hr; 25 mg rectally bid; or 5–10 mg IM initially, repeated every 3–4 hr up to 40 mg/day.
- *Nausea, vomiting related to surgery:* 5–10 mg IM 1–2 hr before anesthesia or during and after surgery (may repeat once in 30 min); 5–10 mg IV 15 min before anesthesia or during and after surgery (may repeat once); or as IV infusion, 20 mg/L of

isotonic solution added to infusion 15–30 min before anesthesia.

- *Nonpsychotic anxiety:* 5 mg PO tid or qid. For spansules, one 15-mg spansule on arising or one 10-mg spansule every 12 hr. Do not give more than 20 mg/day or for longer than 12 wk.

Pediatric patients

Do not use in pediatric surgery.

Less than 9 kg or younger than 2 yr: Generally not recommended.

Psychotic disturbances: 2–12 yr: 2.5 mg PO or rectally bid–tid. Do not give more than 10 mg on first day. Increase dosage according to patient response; total daily dose usually does not exceed 20 mg (2–5 yr) or 25 mg (6–12 yr).

Younger than 12 yr: 0.132 mg/kg by deep IM injection. Switch to oral dosage as soon as possible (usually after one dose).

- *Antiemetic for control of severe nausea and vomiting:*

Oral or rectal

More than 20 lb or older than 2 yr:

9.1–13.2 kg: 2.5 mg daily–bid, not to exceed 7.5 mg/day.

13.6–17.7 kg: 2.5 mg bid–tid, not to exceed 10 mg/day.

18.2–38.6 kg: 2.5 mg tid or 5 mg bid, not to exceed 15 mg/day.

IM

18.2–38.6 kg: 0.132 mg/kg IM (usually only one dose).

Pharmacokinetics

Route	*Onset*	*Duration*
Oral	30–40 min	3–4 hr
SR	30–40 min	10–12 hr
Rectal	60–90 min	3–4 hr
IM	10–20 min	3–4 hr
IV	Immediate	3–4 hr

Metabolism: Hepatic; $T_{1/2}$: Unknown

Distribution: Crosses placenta; enters breast milk

Excretion: Urine

IV FACTS

Preparation: Dilute 20 mg in not less than 1 L of isotonic solution.

Infusion: Inject 5–10 mg directly IV 15–30 min before induction (may be repeated once), or infuse dilute solution 15–30 min before induction; do not exceed 5 mg/mL/min.

Adverse effects

- **Autonomic:** Dry mouth, salivation, nasal congestion, nausea, vomiting, anorexia, fever, pallor, flushed facies, sweating, constipation, paralytic ileus, urinary retention, incontinence, polyuria, enuresis, priapism, ejaculation inhibition, male impotence
- **CNS:** *Drowsiness, dizziness,* insomnia, vertigo, headache, weakness, tremor, ataxia, slurring, cerebral edema, seizures, exacerbation of psychotic symptoms, extrapyramidal syndromes—*pseudoparkinsonism; dystonias; akathisia,* tardive dyskinesia, potentially irreversible; **NMS**
- **CV:** Hypotension, orthostatic hypotension, hypertension, tachycardia, bradycardia, cardiac arrest, heart failure, cardiomegaly, **refractory arrhythmias,** pulmonary edema
- **EENT:** Glaucoma, *photophobia, blurred vision,* miosis, mydriasis, deposits in the cornea and lens (opacities), pigmentary retinopathy
- **Endocrine:** Lactation, breast engorgement, galactorrhea; SIADH; amenorrhea, menstrual irregularities; gynecomastia; changes in libido; hyperglycemia or hypoglycemia; glycosuria; hyponatremia; pituitary tumor with hyperprolactinemia; inhibition of ovulation, infertility, pseudopregnancy; reduced urinary levels of gonadotropins, estrogens, progestins
- **Hematologic:** Eosinophilia, leukopenia, leukocytosis, anemia; **aplastic anemia; hemolytic anemia;** thrombocytopenic or nonthrombocytopenic purpura; pancytopenia
- **Hypersensitivity:** Jaundice, urticaria, angioneurotic edema, laryngeal edema, photosensitivity, eczema, asthma, anaphylactoid reactions, exfoliative dermatitis
- **Respiratory: Bronchospasm, laryngospasm,** dyspnea; suppression of cough reflex and potential for aspiration
- **Other:** *Urine discolored pink to red-brown*

Interactions

✱ **Drug-drug** • Additive CNS depression with alcohol • Additive anticholinergic effects and

P

possibly decreased antipsychotic efficacy with anticholinergic drugs • Increased likelihood of seizures with metrizamide • Increased chance of severe neuromuscular excitation and hypotension with barbiturate anesthetics (methohexital, thiamylal, phenobarbital, thiopental) • Decreased antihypertensive effect of guanethidine

✱ **Drug-lab test** • False-positive pregnancy tests (less likely if serum test is used) • Increase in PBI, not attributable to an increase in thyroxine • False-positive PKU test results

■ Nursing considerations

Assessment

- **History:** Coma or severe CNS depression; bone marrow depression; circulatory collapse; subcortical brain damage; Parkinson's disease; liver damage; cerebral arteriosclerosis; coronary disease; severe hypotension or hypertension; respiratory disorders; allergy to phenothiazines; glaucoma, prostatic hypertrophy; epilepsy; breast cancer; thyrotoxicosis; peptic ulcer, decreased renal function; myelography within previous 24 hr or scheduled within 48 hr; exposure to heat or phosphorous insecticides; pregnancy; lactation; age younger than 12 yr
- **Physical:** Weight, T; reflexes, orientation, IOP; P, BP, orthostatic BP; R, adventitious sounds; bowel sounds and normal output; liver evaluation; urinary output, prostate size; CBC; urinalysis; LFTs, renal and thyroid function tests

Interventions

- Do not change brand names of oral preparations; bioavailability differences have been documented.
- Do not allow patient to crush or chew SR capsules.
- Do not administer subcutaneously because of local irritation.
- Give IM injections deeply into the upper outer quadrant of the buttock.
- Avoid skin contact with oral solution; contact dermatitis may occur.

⊗ ***Warning*** Discontinue drug if serum creatinine or BUN become abnormal or if WBC count is depressed.

- Elderly patients may be more sensitive to antidopaminergic and anticholinergic effects; monitor accordingly.
- Monitor elderly patients for dehydration, and institute remedial measures promptly; sedation and decreased sensation of thirst related to CNS effects of drug can lead to severe dehydration.
- Consult physician regarding appropriate warning of patient or patient's guardian about tardive dyskinesias.
- Consult physician about dosage reduction, use of anticholinergic antiparkinsonians (controversial) if extrapyramidal effects occur.

Teaching points

- Take drug exactly as prescribed.
- Do not crush or chew sustained-release capsules.
- Avoid contacting skin with drug solutions.
- Maintain fluid intake, and use precautions against heatstroke in hot weather.
- Avoid exposure to ultraviolet or sunlight to prevent photosensitivity. Use sunscreen and protective clothing.
- Avoid driving or engaging in other dangerous activities if dizziness, drowsiness, or vision changes occur.
- Report sore throat, fever, unusual bleeding or bruising, rash, weakness, tremors, impaired vision, dark urine (expect pink or reddish-brown urine), pale stools, yellowing of the skin or eyes.

▽ progesterone

(proe ***jess'*** *ter own)*

Progesterone in oil (parenteral):
Progesterone aqueous

Progesterone
Crinone, Prochieve (vaginal gel), Prometrium

Vaginal insert: Endometrin

PREGNANCY CATEGORY B

PREGNANCY CATEGORY D (INJECTION)

Drug classes

Hormone
Progestin

Therapeutic actions

Endogenous female progestational substance; transforms proliferative endometrium into secretory endometrium; inhibits the secretion of pituitary gonadotropins, which prevents follicular maturation and ovulation; inhibits spontaneous uterine contractions; may have some estrogenic, anabolic, or androgenic activity.

Indications

- Treatment of primary and secondary amenorrhea
- Treatment of abnormal uterine bleeding
- Prevention of endometrial hyperplasia
- Treatment of endometrial hyperplasia in non-hysterectomized women who are receiving conjugated estrogens
- Vaginal: To support embryo implantation and early pregnancy by supplementation of corpus luteal function as part of an assisted reproductive technology treatment program for infertile women younger than 35 yr
- Gel: Infertility, as part of assisted reproductive technology for infertile women
- Unlabeled uses: Treatment of PMS, prevention of premature labor and habitual abortion in the first trimester, treatment of menorrhagia (intrauterine system)

Contraindications and cautions

- Contraindicated with allergy to progestins, thrombophlebitis, thromboembolic disorders, cerebral hemorrhage or history of these conditions, hepatic disease, carcinoma of the breast or genital organs, undiagnosed vaginal bleeding, missed abortion, diagnostic test for pregnancy, pregnancy (fetal abnormalities, including masculinization of the female fetus have occurred), lactation, PID, venereal disease, postpartum endometritis, pelvic surgery, uterine or cervical carcinoma (intrauterine system).
- Use cautiously with epilepsy, migraine, asthma, cardiac dysfunction, renal impairment, lactation.

Available forms

Injection—50 mg/mL; vaginal gel—45 mg (4%), 90 mg (8%); capsules—100, 200 mg; vaginal insert—100 mg

Dosages

Administer parenteral preparation by IM route only.

Adults

- *Amenorrhea:* 5–10 mg/day IM for 6–8 consecutive days. Expect withdrawal bleeding 48–72 hr after the last injection. Or use 400 mg PO in the evening for 10 days. Spontaneous normal cycles may follow.
- *Secondary amenorrhea:* Using 4% gel, 45 mg every other day to maximum of 6 doses. For women who do not respond, trial of 8% gel to maximum of 6 doses.
- *Uterine bleeding:* 5–10 mg/day IM for six doses. Bleeding should cease within 6 days. If estrogen is being given, begin progesterone after 2 wk of estrogen therapy. Discontinue injections when menstrual flow begins.
- *Endometrial hyperplasia:* 200 mg/day PO for 12 days per 28-day cycle in combination with a daily conjugated estrogen.
- *Infertility:* 90 mg vaginally daily in women requiring progesterone supplementation; 90 mg vaginally bid for replacement—continue for 10–12 wk into pregnancy if it occurs.
- *Support for implantation:* 100 mg inserted vaginally two to three times daily starting at oocyte retrieval and continuing for up to 10 wk.

Pharmacokinetics

Route	*Onset*	*Peak*	*Duration*
Oral	Varies	1–2 hr	Unknown
IM	Varies	Unknown	Unknown
Vaginal gel	Slow	Unknown	25–50 hr

Metabolism: Hepatic; $T_{1/2}$: 8–9 hr on steady-state

Distribution: Crosses placenta; enters breast milk

Excretion: Urine, bile

Adverse effects

Parenteral and oral

- **CNS:** Sudden, partial, or complete loss of vision, proptosis, diplopia, migraine,

P

precipitation of acute intermittent porphyria, mental depression, pyrexia, insomnia, somnolence, *dizziness*

- **CV:** Thrombophlebitis, cerebrovascular disorders, retinal thrombosis, **pulmonary embolism**
- **Dermatologic:** Rash with or without pruritus, acne, melasma or chloasma, alopecia, hirsutism, *photosensitivity*
- **GI:** Cholestatic jaundice, nausea, *abdominal cramping, constipation*
- **GU:** *Breakthrough bleeding, spotting, change in menstrual flow, amenorrhea, changes in cervical erosion and cervical secretions, breast tenderness* and secretion, transient increase in sodium and chloride excretion
- **Other:** Fluid retention, edema, *change in weight,* effects similar to those seen with hormonal contraceptives, breast pain

Oral contraceptives

- **CV:** Increased BP, **thromboembolic and thrombotic disease**
- **Endocrine:** Decreased glucose tolerance
- **GI:** Hepatic adenoma

Vaginal gel

- **CNS:** *Somnolence, headache,* nervousness, depression
- **GI:** *Constipation,* nausea, diarrhea
- **Other:** *Breast enlargement,* nocturia, perineal pain

Interactions

✱ **Drug-lab test** • Inaccurate tests of hepatic and endocrine function

✱ **Drug-food** • Decreased metabolism and risk of toxic effects if combined with grapefruit juice; avoid this combination

■ Nursing considerations

Assessment

- **History:** Allergy to progestins, thrombophlebitis, thromboembolic disorders, cerebral hemorrhage, hepatic disease, carcinoma of the breast or genital organs, undiagnosed vaginal bleeding, missed abortion, epilepsy, migraine, asthma, cardiac dysfunction, renal impairment, PID, venereal disease, postpartum endometritis, pelvic surgery, uterine or cervical carcinoma, pregnancy, lactation
- **Physical:** Skin color, lesions, turgor; hair; breasts; pelvic examination; orientation, affect; ophthalmologic examination; P, auscultation, peripheral perfusion, edema; R, adventitious sounds; liver evaluation; LFTs, renal function tests, glucose tolerance; Papanicolaou (Pap) test

Interventions

- Arrange for pretreatment and periodic (at least annual) history and physical examination, including BP, breasts, abdomen, pelvic organs, and a Pap test.
- Arrange for insertion of intrauterine system during or immediately after menstrual period to ensure that the patient is not pregnant; arrange to have patient reexamined after first month menses to ensure that system has not been expelled.

⊗ ***Black box warning*** Do not use progestins for the prevention of CV disease. Drug is not effective for this use; risk of CV disease may actually be increased.

⊗ ***Black box warning*** Caution patient before therapy of the need to prevent pregnancy during treatment and to obtain frequent medical follow-up.

- Administer parenteral preparations by IM injection only.

⊗ ***Warning*** Discontinue medication and consult physician if sudden partial or complete loss of vision occurs; discontinue if papilledema or retinal vascular lesions are present on examination.

⊗ ***Warning*** Discontinue drug and consult physician at the first sign of thromboembolic disease—leg pain, swelling, peripheral perfusion changes, shortness of breath.

Teaching points

- This drug can be given IM; it will be given daily for the specified number of days, or inserted vaginally and can remain for 1 year (as appropriate), or inserted vaginally using the applicator system one to two times per day; or given orally for 10 days.
- If used for fertility program, continue vaginal gel or insert 10–12 weeks into pregnancy until placental autonomy is achieved.
- Do not drink grapefruit juice while using this drug.

- This drug should not be taken during pregnancy (except vaginal gel); serious fetal abnormalities have been reported. If you may be pregnant, consult your health care provider immediately.
- Perform a monthly breast self-examination while using this drug.
- You may experience these side effects: Sensitivity to light (avoid exposure to the sun; use sunscreen and protective clothing); dizziness, sleeplessness, depression (use caution if driving or performing tasks that require alertness); rash, skin color changes, loss of hair; fever; nausea.
- Report pain or swelling and warmth in the calves, acute chest pain or shortness of breath, sudden severe headache or vomiting, dizziness or fainting, visual disturbances, numbness or tingling in the arm or leg.

Vaginal gel or insert

- Report severe headache, abnormal vaginal bleeding or discharge, acute calf or chest pain, fever.

DANGEROUS DRUG

promethazine hydrochloride

(proe meth' a zeen)

Phenadoz, Phenergan, Promethegan

PREGNANCY CATEGORY C

Drug classes

Antiemetic
Antihistamine
Anti–motion-sickness drug
Dopaminergic blocker
Phenothiazine
Sedative-hypnotic

Therapeutic actions

Selectively blocks histamine-1 receptors, diminishing the effects of histamine on cells of the upper respiratory tract and eyes and decreasing the sneezing, mucus production, itching, and tearing that accompany allergic reactions in sensitized people exposed to antigens; blocks cholinergic receptors in the vomiting center that are believed to mediate the nausea and vomiting caused by gastric irritation, by input from the vestibular apparatus (motion sickness, nausea associated with vestibular neuritis), and by input from the chemoreceptor trigger zone (drug- and radiation-induced emesis); depresses the RAS, including the parts of the brain involved with wakefulness.

Indications

- Symptomatic relief of perennial and seasonal allergic rhinitis, vasomotor rhinitis, allergic conjunctivitis; mild, uncomplicated urticaria and angioedema; amelioration of allergic reactions to blood or plasma; dermatographism, adjunctive therapy (with epinephrine and other measures) in anaphylactic reactions
- Treatment and prevention of motion sickness; prevention and control of nausea and vomiting associated with anesthesia and surgery
- Preoperative, postoperative, or obstetric sedation
- Adjunct to analgesics to control postoperative pain
- Adjunctive IV therapy with reduced amounts of meperidine or other opioid analgesics in special surgical situations, such as repeated bronchoscopy, ophthalmic surgery, or in poor-risk patients

Contraindications and cautions

- Contraindicated with hypersensitivity to antihistamines or phenothiazines, coma or severe CNS depression, bone marrow depression, vomiting of unknown cause, concomitant therapy with MAOIs, lactation (lactation may be inhibited).
- Use cautiously with lower respiratory tract disorders (may cause thickening of secretions and impair expectoration), glaucoma, prostatic hypertrophy, CV disease or hypertension, breast cancer, thyrotoxicosis, pregnancy (jaundice and extrapyramidal effects in infants; drug may inhibit platelet aggregation in neonate if taken by mother within 2 wk of delivery), children (antihistamine overdose may cause hallucinations, seizures, and death), a child with a history of sleep apnea, a family history of SIDS, or Reye's syndrome (may mask the symptoms of Reye's syndrome and contribute to its development),

P

the elderly (more likely to cause dizziness, sedation, syncope, toxic confusional states, hypotension, and extrapyramidal effects).

Available forms

Tablets—12.5, 25, 50 mg; syrup—6.25, 25 mg/5 mL; suppositories—12.5, 25, 50 mg; injection—25, 50 mg/mL

Dosages

Adults

- *Allergy:* Average dose is 25 mg PO or by rectal suppository, preferably at bedtime. If needed, 12.5 mg PO before meals and at bedtime; 25 mg IM or IV for serious reactions. May repeat within 2 hr if needed.
- *Motion sickness:* 25 mg PO bid. Initial dose should be scheduled 30–60 min before travel; repeat in 8–12 hr if needed. Thereafter, give 25 mg on arising and before evening meal.
- *Nausea and vomiting:* 25 mg PO; repeat doses of 12.5–25 mg as needed, every 4–6 hr. Give rectally or parenterally if oral dosage is not tolerated. 12.5–25 mg IM or IV, not to be repeated more frequently than every 4–6 hr.
- *Sedation:* 25–50 mg PO, IM, or IV.
- *Preoperative use:* 50 mg PO the night before, or 50 mg with an appropriately reduced dose of meperidine and the required amount of belladonna alkaloid.
- *Postoperative sedation and adjunctive use with analgesics:* 25–50 mg PO, IM, or IV.
- *Labor:* 50 mg IM or IV in early stages. When labor is established, 25–75 mg with a reduced dose of opioid. May repeat once or twice at 4-hr intervals. Maximum dose within 24 hr is 100 mg.

Pediatric patients older than 2 yr

- *Allergy:* 25 mg PO at bedtime or 6.25–12.5 mg tid.
- *Motion sickness:* 12.5–25 mg PO or rectally bid.
- *Nausea and vomiting:* 0.5 mg/lb of body weight IM every 4–6 hr as needed.
- *Sedation:* 12.5–25 mg PO or 12.5–25 mg PO or rectally at bedtime.
- *Preoperative use:* 0.5 mg/lb of body weight PO in combination with an appropriately reduced dose of meperidine and the required amount of an atropine-like drug.
- *Postoperative sedation and adjunctive use with analgesics:* 12.5–25 mg PO, IM, IV or rectally.

Pharmacokinetics

Route	*Onset*	*Duration*
Oral	20 min	12 hr
IM	20 min	12 hr
IV	3–5 min	12 hr

Metabolism: Hepatic; $T_{1/2}$: 9–16 hr
Distribution: Crosses placenta; enters breast milk
Excretion: Urine

IV FACTS

Preparation: Dilute to a concentration no greater than 25 mg/mL.
Infusion: Infuse no faster than 25 mg/min.
Incompatibilities: Do not combine with aminophylline, chloramphenicol, heparin, hydrocortisone, pentobarbital, thiopental.
Y-site incompatibilities: Do not give with foscarnet, heparin, hydrocortisone, potassium chloride.

Adverse effects

- **CNS:** *Dizziness, drowsiness, poor coordination, confusion, restlessness, excitation,* seizures, tremors, headache, blurred vision, diplopia, vertigo, tinnitus
- **CV:** Hypotension, palpitations, bradycardia, tachycardia, extrasystoles
- **Dermatologic:** Urticaria, rash, photosensitivity, chills
- **GI:** *Epigastric distress,* nausea, vomiting, diarrhea, constipation
- **GU:** *Urinary frequency, dysuria,* urinary retention, decreased libido, impotence
- **Hematologic:** Hemolytic anemia, hypoplastic anemia, thrombocytopenia, leukopenia, agranulocytosis, pancytopenia
- **Respiratory:** *Thickening of bronchial secretions;* chest tightness; dry mouth, nose, and throat; respiratory depression; suppression of cough reflex, potential for aspiration
- **Other:** Tingling, heaviness and wetness of the hands

Interactions

✱ **Drug-drug** • Additive anticholinergic effects with anticholinergic drugs • Increased frequency and severity of neuromuscular excitation and hypotension with methohexital, thiamylal, phenobarbital anesthetic, thiopental • Enhanced CNS depression with alcohol

■ Nursing considerations

Assessment

- **History:** Hypersensitivity to antihistamines or phenothiazines, severe CNS depression, bone marrow depression, vomiting of unknown cause, concomitant therapy with MAOIs, lactation, lower respiratory tract disorders, glaucoma, prostatic hypertrophy, CV disease or hypertension, breast cancer, thyrotoxicosis, pregnancy, history of sleep apnea or a family history of SIDS, child with Reye's syndrome
- **Physical:** Weight, T; reflexes, orientation, IOP; P, BP, orthostatic BP; R, adventitious sounds; bowel sounds and normal output, liver evaluation; urinary output, prostate size; CBC; urinalysis; LFTs, renal and thyroid function tests

Interventions

⊗ ***Black box warning*** Do not give to children younger than 2 yr because of risk of fatal respiratory depression; use lowest effective dose and caution in children 2 yr and older.

- Give IM injections deep into muscle.
- Do not administer subcutaneously; tissue necrosis may occur.

⊗ ***Black box warning*** Do not administer intra-arterially; arteriospasm and gangrene of the limb may result. Do not administer subcutaneously into an artery or under the skin; drug may leach into tissue and cause serious injury. If IV route is used, limit drug concentration and rate of administration and ensure open IV line.

⊗ ***Warning*** Reduce dosage of barbiturates given concurrently with promethazine by at least one-half; arrange for dosage reduction of opioid analgesics given concomitantly by one-fourth to one-half.

Teaching points

- Take drug exactly as prescribed.
- Avoid using alcohol.
- Avoid driving or engaging in other dangerous activities if dizziness, drowsiness, or vision changes occur.
- Avoid prolonged exposure to sun, or use a sunscreen or covering garments.
- Maintain fluid intake, and use precautions against heatstroke in hot weather.
- Report sore throat, fever, unusual bleeding or bruising, rash, weakness, tremors, impaired vision, dark urine, pale stools, yellowing of the skin or eyes.

DANGEROUS DRUG

▽ propafenone hydrochloride

(proe ***paf'*** *a non)*

Apo-Propafenone (CAN), Gen-Propafenone (CAN), Rythmol, Rhythmol SR

PREGNANCY CATEGORY C

Drug class

Antiarrhythmic

Therapeutic actions

Class IC antiarrhythmic: Local anesthetic effects with a direct membrane stabilizing action on the myocardial membranes; refractory period is prolonged with a reduction of spontaneous automaticity and depressed trigger activity.

Indications

- Treatment of documented life-threatening ventricular arrhythmias; reserve use for those patients in whom the benefits outweigh the risks
- To prolong the time to recurrence of symptomatic atrial fibrillation in patients with structural heart disease (ER)
- Unlabeled uses: Treatment of supraventricular tachycardias, including atrial fibrillation associated with Wolff-Parkinson-White syndrome

Contraindications and cautions

- Contraindicated with hypersensitivity to propafenone, uncontrolled HF, cardiogenic shock, cardiac conduction disturbances in

P

the absence of an artificial pacemaker, bradycardia, marked hypotension, bronchospastic disorders, manifest electrolyte imbalance, pregnancy (teratogenic in preclinical studies), lactation.
- Use cautiously with hepatic, renal impairment; elevated ANA.

Available forms

Tablets—150, 225, 300 mg; ER capsules—225, 325, 425 mg

Dosages

Adults

Adjust on the basis of response and tolerance. Initiate with 150 mg PO every 8 hr (450 mg/day). Dosage may be increased at a minimum of 3- to 4-day intervals to 225 mg PO every 8 hr (675 mg/day) and if necessary, to 300 mg PO every 8 hr (900 mg/day). Do not exceed 900 mg/day. Decrease dosage with significant widening of the QRS complex or with AV block; ER capsules—initially, 225 mg PO every 12 hr titrate at 5-day intervals to maximum 425 mg every 12 hr.

Pediatric patients

Safety and efficacy not established.

Geriatric patients

Use with caution; increase dose more gradually during the initial phase of treatment.

Pharmacokinetics

Route	*Onset*	*Peak*
Oral	Varies	3.5 hr
ER	Unknown	3–8 hr

Metabolism: Hepatic; $T_{1/2}$: 2–10 hr
Distribution: Crosses placenta; enters breast milk
Excretion: Urine

Adverse effects

- **CNS:** *Dizziness, headache, weakness, fatigue, blurred vision,* abnormal dreams, speech or vision disturbances, coma, confusion, depression, memory loss, numbness, paresthesias, psychosis/mania, seizures, tinnitus, vertigo
- **CV:** *First-degree AV block, intraventricular conduction disturbances,* HF, atrial flutter, AV dissociation, **cardiac arrest,** sick sinus syndrome, sinus pause, sinus arrest, supraventricular tachycardia, *bradycardia, angina*
- **Dermatologic:** Alopecia, pruritus
- **GI:** *Unusual taste, nausea, vomiting, constipation,* dyspepsia, cholestasis, gastroenteritis, hepatitis
- **Hematologic:** *Agranulocytosis,* anemia, granulocytopenia, leukopenia, purpura, thrombocytopenia, positive ANA
- **Musculoskeletal:** Muscle weakness, leg cramps, muscle pain

Interactions

✱ **Drug-drug** • Increased serum levels of propafenone and risk of increased toxicity with quinidine, cimetidine, ritonavir, SSRIs • Increased serum levels of digoxin, warfarin, cyclosporine, beta blockers

■ Nursing considerations

Assessment

- **History:** Hypersensitivity to propafenone, uncontrolled HF, cardiogenic shock, cardiac conduction disturbances in the absence of an artificial pacemaker, bradycardia, marked hypotension, bronchospastic disorders, manifest electrolyte imbalance, hepatic or renal impairment, pregnancy, lactation
- **Physical:** Reflexes, affect; BP, P, ECG, peripheral perfusion, auscultation; abdomen, normal function; LFTs, renal function tests; CBC, Hct, electrolytes; ANA

Interventions

⊗ ***Warning*** Monitor patient response carefully, especially when beginning therapy. Increase dosage at minimum of 3- to 4-day intervals only.
- Reduce dosage with renal or hepatic impairment and with marked previous myocardial damage.
- Increase dosage slowly in patients with myocardial dysfunction; renal or hepatic impairment.

⊠ ***Black box warning*** Arrange for periodic ECG monitoring to monitor effects on cardiac conduction; risk of serious proarrhythmias.

Teaching points
- Take the drug every 8 hours around-the-clock; determine a schedule that will interrupt sleep the least.
- Frequent monitoring of ECG will be needed to adjust dosage or determine effects of drug on cardiac conduction.
- Do not stop taking this drug for any reason without consulting your health care provider.
- Avoid pregnancy while using this drug; use of barrier contraceptives is advised.
- You may experience these side effects: Dizziness, headache (avoid driving or performing hazardous tasks); headache, weakness (request medications; rest periods may help); nausea, vomiting, unusual taste (maintain proper nutrition; take drug with meals); constipation.
- Report swelling of the extremities, difficulty breathing, fainting, palpitations, vision changes, chest pain.

propantheline bromide

See Appendix W, *Less commonly used drugs*.

DANGEROUS DRUG

propoxyphene
*(proe **pox'** i feen)*

propoxyphene hydrochloride (dextropropoxyphene)
Darvon

propoxyphene napsylate
Darvon-N

PREGNANCY CATEGORY C

CONTROLLED SUBSTANCE C-IV

Drug class
Opioid agonist analgesic

Therapeutic actions
Acts as agonist at specific opioid receptors in the CNS to produce analgesia, euphoria, sedation; the receptors mediating these effects are thought to be the same as those mediating the effects of endogenous opioids (enkephalins, endorphins).

Indications
- Relief of mild to moderate pain

Contraindications and cautions
- Contraindicated with hypersensitivity to opioids, pregnancy (neonatal withdrawal has occurred; neonatal safety not established), labor or delivery (especially when delivery of a premature infant is expected; opioids given to mother can cause respiratory depression of neonate; may prolong labor), lactation, suicidal or addiction-prone patients.
- Use cautiously with renal or hepatic impairment; emotional depression; excessive alcohol use; use of antianxiety, antidepressant drugs.

Available forms
Capsules—65 mg; tablets—100 mg

Dosages
Adults
Propoxyphene hydrochloride
65 mg PO every 4 hr as needed. Do not exceed 390 mg/day.
Propoxyphene napsylate
100 mg PO every 4 hr as needed. Do not exceed 600 mg/day.
Pediatric patients
Not recommended.
Geriatric patients or adults with hepatic or renal impairment
Use caution; reduced dosage may be needed.

Pharmacokinetics

Route	Onset	Peak
Oral	30–60 min	2–2.5 hr

Metabolism: Hepatic; $T_{1/2}$: 6–12 hr
Distribution: Crosses placenta; enters breast milk
Excretion: Urine

Adverse effects
- **CNS:** Headache, weakness, *dizziness, sedation,* light-headedness, euphoria, dysphoria, minor visual disturbances

P

- **Dermatologic:** Rashes
- **GI:** *Nausea, vomiting,* constipation, abdominal pain, hepatic impairment
- **Other:** Tolerance and dependence, psychological dependence

Interactions

✱ **Drug-drug** • Increased likelihood of respiratory depression, hypotension, profound sedation, or coma with barbiturate general anesthetics • Increased serum levels and toxicity of carbamazepine • Decreased absorption and serum levels with charcoal

■ Nursing considerations

Assessment

- **History:** Hypersensitivity to opioids, pregnancy, lactation, renal or hepatic impairment, emotional depression
- **Physical:** Skin color, texture, lesions; orientation, reflexes, affect; bowel sounds, normal output; LFTs, renal function tests

Interventions

⊗ ***Black box warning*** Do not use in suicidal or addiction-prone patients; advise patient to limit consumption of alcohol; fatalities have been reported.

- Administer to lactating women 4–6 hr before the next feeding to minimize the amount in milk.

⊗ ***Black box warning*** Limit amount of drug dispensed to depressed, emotionally labile, or potentially suicidal patients; propoxyphene intake alone or with other CNS depressants has been associated with deaths.

⊗ ***Warning*** Keep opioid antagonist and facilities for assisted or controlled respiration readily available in case respiratory depression occurs.

- Give drug with milk or food if GI upset occurs.
- Reassure patient about addiction liability; most patients who receive opiates for medical reasons do not develop dependence syndromes.

Teaching points

- Take drug exactly as prescribed.
- Do not take leftover medication for other disorders, and do not let anyone else take the prescription.
- Avoid alcohol intake while using this drug.
- You may experience these side effects: Nausea, loss of appetite (take drug with food, eat frequent small meals); constipation (request laxative); dizziness, sedation, drowsiness, impaired visual acuity (avoid driving or performing other tasks that require alertness, visual acuity).
- Report severe nausea, vomiting, constipation, shortness of breath or difficulty breathing, thoughts of suicide.

DANGEROUS DRUG

▽ propranolol hydrochloride

(proe ***pran'*** *oh lol)*

Apo-Propranolol (CAN), Inderal, Inderal LA, InnoPran XL, Propranolol Intensol

PREGNANCY CATEGORY C

Drug classes

Antianginal
Antiarrhythmic
Antihypertensive
Beta-adrenergic blocker (nonselective)

Therapeutic actions

Competitively blocks beta-adrenergic receptors in the heart and juxtaglomerular apparatus, decreasing the influence of the sympathetic nervous system on these tissues, the excitability of the heart, cardiac workload and oxygen consumption, and the release of renin and lowering BP; has membrane-stabilizing (local anesthetic) effects that contribute to its antiarrhythmic action; acts in the CNS to reduce sympathetic outflow and vasoconstrictor tone. The mechanism by which it prevents migraine headaches is unknown.

Indications

- Hypertension alone or with other drugs, especially diuretics
- Angina pectoris caused by coronary atherosclerosis
- Idiopathic hypertrophic subaortic stenosis to manage associated stress-induced angina, palpitations, and syncope

- Cardiac arrhythmias, especially supraventricular tachycardia, and ventricular tachycardias induced by cardiac glycosides or catecholamines
- Prevention of reinfarction in clinically stable patients 5–21 days after MI
- Pheochromocytoma, an adjunctive therapy after treatment with an alpha-adrenergic blocker to manage tachycardia before or during surgery or if the pheochromocytoma is inoperable
- Prophylaxis for migraine headache
- Treatment of essential tremor, familial or hereditary
- Unlabeled uses: Recurrent GI bleeding in cirrhotic patients, schizophrenia, tardive dyskinesia, acute panic symptoms, anxiety, HF

Contraindications and cautions

- Contraindicated with allergy to beta-blocking agents, sinus bradycardia, second- or third-degree heart block, cardiogenic shock, HF, bronchial asthma, bronchospasm, COPD, pregnancy (neonatal bradycardia, hypoglycemia, and apnea, and low birth weight with long-term use during pregnancy), lactation.
- Use cautiously with hypoglycemia and diabetes, thyrotoxicosis, hepatic impairment, Raynaud's disease.

Available forms

ER capsules—60, 80, 120, 160 mg; tablets—10, 20, 40, 60, 80, 90 mg; SR capsules—60, 80, 120, 160 mg; injection—1 mg/mL; oral solution—4, 8 mg/mL; concentrated oral solution—80 mg/mL

Dosages

Adults

Oral

- *Hypertension:* 40 mg regular propranolol bid or 80 mg SR or ER daily initially; usual maintenance dose, 120–240 mg/day given bid or tid or 120–160 mg SR or ER daily (maximum dose, 640 mg/day).
- *Angina:* 80–320 mg/day divided bid, tid, or qid or 80 mg SR or ER daily initially; gradually increase dosage at 3- to 7-day intervals; usual maintenance dose, 160 mg/day (maximum dose, 320 mg/day).
- *IHSS:* 20–40 mg tid or qid or 80–160 mg SR or ER daily.
- *Arrhythmias:* 10–30 mg tid or qid.
- *MI:* 180–240 mg/day given tid or qid (maximum dose, 240 mg/day).
- *Pheochromocytoma:* Preoperatively, 60 mg/day for 3 days in divided doses; inoperable tumor, 30 mg/day in divided doses.
- *Migraine:* 80 mg/day daily (SR or ER) or in divided doses; usual maintenance dose, 160–240 mg/day.
- *Essential tremor:* 40 mg bid; usual maintenance dose, 120 mg/day (maximum dose, 320 mg/day).

Parenteral

⊗ **Warning** IV dose is markedly less than oral because of first-pass effect with oral propranolol.

- *Life-threatening arrhythmias:* 1–3 mg IV with careful monitoring, not to exceed 1 mg/min; may give second dose in 2 min, but then do not repeat for 4 hr.

Pediatric patients

Safety and efficacy not established.

Pharmacokinetics

Route	*Onset*	*Peak*	*Duration*
Oral	20–30 min	60–90 min	6–12 hr
IV	Immediate	1 min	4–6 hr

Metabolism: Hepatic; $T_{1/2}$: 3–5 hr; 8–11 hr (SR form)

Distribution: Crosses placenta; enters breast milk

Excretion: Urine

IV FACTS

Preparation: No further preparation is needed.

Infusion: Inject directly IV or into tubing of running IV; do not exceed 1 mg/min.

Adverse effects

- **Allergic reactions:** Pharyngitis, erythematous rash, fever, sore throat, **laryngospasm,** respiratory distress
- **CNS:** Dizziness, vertigo, tinnitus, *fatigue,* emotional depression, paresthesias, sleep disturbances, hallucinations, disorientation, memory loss, slurred speech

P

- **CV:** *Bradycardia, HF, cardiac arrhythmias, sinoatrial or AV nodal block,* peripheral vascular insufficiency, claudication, **CVA, pulmonary edema,** hypotension
- **Dermatologic:** Rash, pruritus, sweating, dry skin
- **EENT:** Eye irritation, dry eyes, conjunctivitis, blurred vision
- **GI:** *Gastric pain, flatulence, constipation, diarrhea, nausea, vomiting,* anorexia, ischemic colitis, renal and mesenteric arterial thrombosis, retroperitoneal fibrosis, hepatomegaly, acute pancreatitis
- **GU:** *Impotence, decreased libido,* Peyronie's disease, dysuria, nocturia, frequency
- **Musculoskeletal:** Joint pain, arthralgia, muscle cramp
- **Respiratory: Bronchospasm,** dyspnea, cough, bronchial obstruction, nasal stuffiness, rhinitis, pharyngitis
- **Other:** *Decreased exercise tolerance, development of ANAs,* hyperglycemia or hypoglycemia, elevated serum transaminase, alkaline phosphatase, and LDH

Interactions

✱ **Drug-drug** • Increased effects with verapamil • Decreased effects with indomethacin, ibuprofen, piroxicam, sulindac, barbiturates • Prolonged hypoglycemic effects of insulin • Initial hypertensive episode followed by bradycardia with epinephrine • Increased first-dose response to prazosin • Increased serum levels and toxic effects with lidocaine, cimetidine • Increased serum levels of propranolol and phenothiazines, hydralazine if the two drugs are taken concurrently • Paradoxical hypertension when clonidine is given with beta blockers; increased rebound hypertension when clonidine is discontinued in patients on beta blockers • Decreased serum levels and therapeutic effects with methimazole, propylthiouracil • Decreased bronchodilator effects of theophyllines • Decreased antihypertensive effects with NSAIDs (ie, ibuprofen, indomethacin, piroxicam, sulindac), rifampin

✱ **Drug-lab test** • Interference with glucose or insulin tolerance tests, glaucoma screening tests

■ Nursing considerations

Assessment

- **History:** Allergy to beta-blocking agents, sinus bradycardia, second- or third-degree heart block, cardiogenic shock, HF, bronchial asthma, bronchospasm, COPD, hypoglycemia and diabetes, thyrotoxicosis, hepatic impairment, pregnancy, lactation, peripheral vascular disease
- **Physical:** Weight, skin color, lesions, edema, T; reflexes, affect, vision, hearing, orientation; BP, P, ECG, peripheral perfusion; R, auscultation; bowel sounds, normal output, liver evaluation; bladder palpation; LFTs, thyroid function tests; blood and urine glucose

Interventions

⊗ ***Black box warning*** Do not discontinue drug abruptly after long-term therapy (hypersensitivity to catecholamines may have developed, causing exacerbation of angina, MI, and ventricular arrhythmias). Taper drug gradually over 2 wk with monitoring.

⊗ ***Warning*** Ensure that alpha-adrenergic blocker has been given before giving propranolol when treating patients with pheochromocytoma; endogenous catecholamines secreted by the tumor can cause severe hypertension if vascular beta receptors are blocked without concomitant alpha blockade.

- Consult with physician about withdrawing drug if patient is to undergo surgery (withdrawal is controversial).
- Provide continuous cardiac and regular BP monitoring with IV form. Change to oral form as soon as possible.
- Give oral drug with food to facilitate absorption.

Teaching points

- Take this drug with meals. Do not discontinue the medication abruptly; abrupt discontinuation can cause worsening of your disorder.
- If you have diabetes, the normal signs of hypoglycemia (tachycardia) may be blocked by this drug; monitor your blood or urine glucose carefully; eat regular meals, and take your diabetic medication regularly.
- You may experience these side effects: Dizziness, drowsiness, light-headedness, blurred

vision (avoid driving or performing hazardous tasks); nausea, loss of appetite (eat frequent small meals); nightmares, depression (request change of your medication); sexual impotence.
- Report difficulty breathing, night cough, swelling of extremities, slow pulse, confusion, depression, rash, fever, sore throat.

propylthiouracil (PTU)

*(proe pill thye oh **yoor'** a sill)*

Propyl-Thyracil (CAN)

PREGNANCY CATEGORY D

Drug class
Antithyroid drug

Therapeutic actions
Inhibits the synthesis of thyroid hormones; partially inhibits the peripheral conversion of T_4 to T_3, the more potent form of thyroid hormone.

Indications
- Hyperthyroidism
- Unlabeled use: Reduces mortality associated with alcoholic liver disease

Contraindications and cautions
- Contraindicated with allergy to antithyroid drugs, pregnancy (can induce hypothyroidism or cretinism in the fetus; use only if absolutely necessary and when mother has been informed about potential harm to the fetus; if antithyroid drug is needed, this is the drug of choice).
- Use cautiously with lactation (if antithyroid drug is needed, this is the drug of choice).

Available forms
Tablets—50 mg

Dosages
Administered usually in three equal doses every 8 hr.

Adults
- Initially, 300 mg/day PO, up to 400–900 mg/day in severe cases. For maintenance, 100–150 mg/day.

Pediatric patients

Neonates: 5–10 mg/kg/day; divided doses every 8 hr.

6–10 yr: Initially, 50–150 mg/day PO or 5–7 mg/kg/day.

10 yr and older: Initially, 150–300 mg/day PO or 5–7 mg/kg/day. Maintenance is determined by the needs of the patient.

Pharmacokinetics

Route	*Onset*
Oral	Varies

Metabolism: Hepatic; $T_{1/2}$: 1–2 hr
Distribution: Crosses placenta; enters breast milk
Excretion: Urine

Adverse effects
- **CNS:** *Paresthesias, neuritis, vertigo, drowsiness,* neuropathies, depression, headache
- **CV:** Vasculitis, periarteritis
- **Dermatologic:** *Skin rash, urticaria,* pruritus, skin pigmentation, exfoliative dermatitis, lupus-like syndrome, loss of hair
- **GI:** *Nausea, vomiting, epigastric distress,* loss of taste, jaundice, hepatitis, **severe liver injury**
- **GU:** Nephritis
- **Hematologic:** Agranulocytosis, granulocytopenia, thrombocytopenia, hypoprothrombinemia, bleeding, aplastic anemia
- **Other:** Arthralgia, myalgia, edema, lymphadenopathy, drug fever

Interactions
✱ **Drug-drug** • Increased risk of bleeding with oral anticoagulants • Alterations in theophylline, metoprolol, propranolol, cardiac glycoside clearance, serum levels and effects as patient moves from hyperthyroid state to euthyroid state

■ Nursing considerations

CLINICAL ALERT!

Name confusion has occurred between propylthiouracil and *Purinethol* (mercaptopurine). Serious adverse effects can occur; use extreme caution.

P

Assessment

- **History:** Allergy to antithyroid drugs, pregnancy, lactation
- **Physical:** Skin color, lesions, pigmentation; orientation, reflexes, affect; liver evaluation; CBC, differential, PT; LFTs, renal function tests, thyroid function tests

Interventions

⊗ ***Warning*** Drug has been associated with severe liver injury; limit use, especially in children.

- Administer drug in three equally divided doses at 8-hr intervals; schedule to maintain the patient's sleep pattern.
- Arrange for regular, periodic blood tests to monitor bone marrow depression and bleeding tendencies.

⊗ ***Warning*** Advise medical personnel doing surgical procedures that this patient is using this drug and is at greater risk for bleeding problems.

Teaching points

- Take this drug around-the-clock at 8-hour intervals.
- This drug must be taken for a prolonged period to achieve the desired effects.
- You may experience these side effects: Dizziness, weakness, vertigo, drowsiness (use caution if operating a car or dangerous machinery); nausea, vomiting, loss of appetite (eat frequent small meals); rash, itching.
- Report fever, sore throat, unusual bleeding or bruising, headache, general malaise.

protamine sulfate

(proe' ta meen)

PREGNANCY CATEGORY C

Drug class

Heparin antagonist

Therapeutic actions

Strongly basic proteins found in salmon sperm; protamines form stable salts with heparin, which results in the immediate loss of anticoagulant activity; administered when heparin has not been given; protamine has weak anticoagulant activity.

Indications

- Treatment of heparin overdose

Contraindications and cautions

- Contraindicated with allergy to protamine sulfate or fish products.
- Use cautiously with pregnancy, lactation.

Available forms

Injection—10 mg/mL

Dosages

Dosage is determined by the amount of heparin in the body and the time that has elapsed since the heparin was given; the longer the interval, the smaller the dose required.

Adults and pediatric patients

1 mg IV neutralizes 90 USP units of heparin derived from lung tissue or 115 USP units of heparin derived from intestinal mucosa.

Pharmacokinetics

Route	*Onset*	*Duration*
IV	5 min	2 hr

Metabolism: Degraded in body; $T_{1/2}$: Unknown

Distribution: Crosses placenta; may enter breast milk

Excretion: Unknown

IV FACTS

Preparation: Administer injection undiluted; if dilution is needed, use 5% dextrose in water or saline; refrigerate any diluted solution. Do not store diluted solution; no preservatives are added. Reconstitute powder for injection with 5 mL bacteriostatic water for injection with benzyl alcohol added to the 50-mg vial (25 mL to the 250-mg vial); stable at room temperature for 72 hr.

Infusion: Administer very slowly IV over at least 10 min; do not exceed 50 mg in any 10-min period; do not give more than 100 mg over a 2-hr period. Guide dosing with coagulation studies.

Incompatibilities: Do not mix in lines with incompatible antibiotics, including many penicillins and cephalosporins.

Adverse effects
- **CV:** *Hypotension*
- **GI:** *Nausea, vomiting*
- **Hypersensitivity:** Anaphylactoid reactions—dyspnea, flushing, hypotension, bradycardia, **anaphylaxis**

■ Nursing considerations
Assessment
- **History:** Allergy to protamine sulfate or fish products, pregnancy, lactation
- **Physical:** Skin color, T; orientation, reflexes; P, BP, auscultation, peripheral perfusion; R, adventitious sounds; plasma thrombin time

Interventions
⊗ ***Warning*** Keep emergency equipment for resuscitation and treatment of shock readily available in case of anaphylactoid reaction.

⊗ ***Warning*** Monitor coagulation studies to adjust dosage, and screen for heparin rebound and response to drug.

Teaching points
- Report shortness of breath, difficulty breathing, flushing, feeling of warmth, dizziness, lack of orientation, numbness, tingling.

▽ protein C concentrate

See Appendix W, *Less commonly used drugs*.

▽ protriptyline hydrochloride
*(proe **trip'** ti leen)*

Vivactil

PREGNANCY CATEGORY C

Drug class
TCA (secondary amine)

Therapeutic actions
Mechanism of action unknown; the TCAs are structurally related to the phenothiazine antipsychotic drugs (eg, chlorpromazine), but in contrast to the phenothiazines, TCAs inhibit the presynaptic reuptake of the neurotransmitters norepinephrine and serotonin; anticholinergic at CNS and peripheral receptors; the relation of these effects to clinical efficacy is unknown.

Indications
- Relief of symptoms of depression (endogenous depression most responsive; unlike other TCAs, protriptyline is "activating" and may be useful in withdrawn and anergic patients)
- Unlabeled use: Treatment of obstructive sleep apnea

Contraindications and cautions
- Contraindicated with hypersensitivity to any tricyclic drug, concomitant therapy with an MAOI, recent MI, myelography within previous 24 hr or scheduled within 48 hr, pregnancy (limb reduction abnormalities), lactation.
- Use cautiously with EST; preexisting CV disorders (eg, severe coronary heart disease, progressive HF, angina pectoris, paroxysmal tachycardia); angle-closure glaucoma, increased IOP, urinary retention, ureteral or urethral spasm; seizure disorders (TCAs lower the seizure threshold); hyperthyroidism (predisposes to CVS toxicity, including cardiac arrhythmias); impaired hepatic, renal function; psychiatric patients (schizophrenic or paranoid patients may exhibit a worsening of psychosis); patients with bipolar disorder (may shift to hypomanic or manic phase); elective surgery (TCAs should be discontinued as long as possible before surgery).

Available forms
Tablets—5, 10 mg

Dosages
Adults

15–40 mg/day PO in three to four divided doses initially. May gradually increase to 60 mg/day if necessary. Do not exceed 60 mg/day. Make increases in dosage in the morning dose.

Pediatric patients

Not recommended; may increase risk of suicidal ideation.

P

Geriatric patients and adolescents

Initially, 5 mg tid PO. Increase gradually if needed. Monitor CV system closely if dose exceeds 20 mg/day.

Pharmacokinetics

Route	Onset	Peak
Oral	Slow	8–12 hr

Metabolism: Hepatic; $T_{1/2}$: 67–89 hr
Distribution: Crosses placenta; enters breast milk
Excretion: Urine

Adverse effects

- **CNS:** *Sedation and anticholinergic (atropine-like) effects*—dry mouth, blurred vision, disturbance of accommodation for near vision, mydriasis, increased IOP, *confusion* (especially in elderly), *disturbed concentration,* hallucinations, disorientation, decreased memory, feelings of unreality, delusions, anxiety, nervousness, restlessness, agitation, panic, insomnia, nightmares, hypomania, mania, exacerbation of psychosis, drowsiness, weakness, fatigue, headache, numbness, tingling, paresthesias of extremities, uncoordination, motor hyperactivity, akathisia, ataxia, tremors, peripheral neuropathy, extrapyramidal symptoms, *seizures,* speech blockage, dysarthria, tinnitus, altered EEG
- **CV:** *Orthostatic hypotension,* hypertension, syncope, tachycardia, palpitations, **MI,** arrhythmias, heart block, precipitation of HF, **CVA**
- **Endocrine:** Elevated or depressed blood sugar; elevated prolactin levels; inappropriate ADH secretion
- **GI:** *Dry mouth, constipation,* paralytic ileus, *nausea,* vomiting, anorexia, epigastric distress, diarrhea, flatulence, dysphagia, peculiar taste, increased salivation, stomatitis, glossitis, parotid swelling, abdominal cramps, black tongue
- **GU:** Urinary retention, delayed micturition, dilation of the urinary tract, gynecomastia, testicular swelling; breast enlargement, menstrual irregularity and galactorrhea; increased or decreased libido; impotence
- **Hematologic:** Bone marrow depression, including agranulocytosis; eosinophilia; purpura; thrombocytopenia; leukopenia
- **Hypersensitivity:** Skin rash, pruritus, vasculitis, petechiae, photosensitization, edema (generalized or of face and tongue), drug fever
- **Withdrawal:** Symptoms with abrupt discontinuation of prolonged therapy: Nausea, headache, vertigo, nightmares, malaise
- **Other:** Nasal congestion, excessive appetite, weight change, sweating, alopecia, lacrimation, hyperthermia, flushing, chills

Interactions

✷ **Drug-drug** • Increased TCA levels and pharmacologic effects with cimetidine, fluoxetine, ranitidine • Altered response, including arrhythmias and hypertension with sympathomimetics • Risk of severe hypertension with clonidine • Hyperpyretic crises, severe seizures, hypertensive episodes, and deaths with MAOIs • Increased CNS effects with alcohol; avoid this combination

■ Nursing considerations

Assessment

- **History:** Hypersensitivity to any tricyclic drug; concomitant therapy with an MAOI; recent MI; myelography within previous 24 hr or scheduled within 48 hr; pregnancy; lactation; EST; preexisting CV disorders; angle-closure glaucoma, increased IOP, urinary retention, ureteral or urethral spasm; seizure disorders; hyperthyroidism; impaired hepatic, renal function; psychiatric disorder; bipolar disorders; elective surgery
- **Physical:** Weight; T; skin color, lesions; orientation, affect, reflexes, vision and hearing; P, BP, orthostatic BP, perfusion; bowel sounds, normal output, liver evaluation; urine flow, normal output; usual sexual function, frequency of menses, breast and scrotal examination; LFTs, urinalysis, CBC, ECG

Interventions

⊗ ***Black box warning*** Limit drug access for depressed and potentially suicidal patients; increased risk of suicidality in children, adolescents, and young adults; monitor accordingly.

⊗ ***Warning*** Reduce dosage if minor side effects develop; discontinue if serious side effects occur.

- Arrange for CBC if patient develops fever, sore throat, or other sign of infection.

Teaching points

- Take drug exactly as prescribed; do not stop taking this drug abruptly or without consulting your health care provider.
- Avoid alcohol and other sleep-inducing or over-the-counter drugs.
- Avoid prolonged exposure to sunlight or sunlamps; use a sunscreen or protective garments.
- You may experience these side effects: Headache, dizziness, drowsiness, weakness, blurred vision (reversible; take safety measures if severe; avoid driving or performing tasks that require alertness); nausea, vomiting, loss of appetite, dry mouth (frequent small meals, frequent mouth care, and sucking sugarless candies may help); nightmares, inability to concentrate, confusion; changes in sexual function; fetal abnormalities (avoid pregnancy, use contraceptive measures).
- Report dry mouth, difficulty in urination, excessive sedation, thoughts of suicide.

▽ pseudoephedrine

(soo dow e ***fed'*** *rin)*

pseudoephedrine hydrochloride (d-isoephedrine hydrochloride)

Cenafed, Congestaid, Decofed, Efidac/24 DNC, Eltor (CAN), Genaphed, Sudafed, Triaminic Allergy Congestion and others, Unifed

pseudoephedrine sulfate

Drixoral Non-Drowsy Formula, ElixSure Children's Congestion

PREGNANCY CATEGORY C

Drug classes

Nasal decongestant
Sympathomimetic amine

Therapeutic actions

Effects are mediated by alpha-adrenergic receptors; causes vasoconstriction in mucous membranes of nasal passages, resulting in their shrinkage, which promotes drainage and improves ventilation.

Indications

- Temporary relief of nasal congestion caused by the common cold, hay fever, other respiratory allergies
- Nasal congestion associated with sinusitis
- Promotes nasal or sinus drainage
- Relief of eustachian tube congestion

Contraindications and cautions

- Contraindicated with MAOI therapy, allergy or idiosyncrasy to sympathomimetic amines, severe hypertension, and CAD.
- Use cautiously with hyperthyroidism, diabetes mellitus, arteriosclerosis, ischemic heart disease, increased IOP, prostatic hypertrophy, lactation, pregnancy.

Available forms

Tablets—30, 60 mg; CR tablets DNC—240 mg; ER tablets DNC—120 mg; chewable tablets—15 mg; capsules—30, 60 mg; liquid—15, 30 mg/5 mL; drops—7.5 mg/0.8 mL; syrup—15 mg/5 mL; suspension—50 mg/5 mL

Dosages

Adults and children older than 12 yr

60 mg every 4–6 hr PO (ER, 120 mg PO every 12 hr; 240 mg/day CR); do not exceed 240 mg in 24 hr.

Pediatric patients 6–12 yr

30 mg every 4–6 hr PO; do not exceed 120 mg in 24 hr.

Pediatric patients 2–5 yr

15 mg as syrup every 4–6 hr PO; do not exceed 60 mg in 24 hr.

Pediatric patients 2 yr and younger

Consult physician.

Geriatric patients

These patients are more likely to experience adverse reactions; use with caution.

Pharmacokinetics

Route	*Onset*	*Duration*
Oral	30 min	4–6 hr

Metabolism: Hepatic; $T_{1/2}$: 7 hr
Distribution: Crosses placenta; enters breast milk
Excretion: Urine

Adverse effects

- **CNS:** *Fear, anxiety, tenseness, restlessness, headache, light-headedness, dizziness, drowsiness, tremors,* insomnia, hallucinations, psychological disturbances, prolonged psychosis, **seizures,** CNS depression, weakness, blurred vision, ocular irritation, tearing, photophobia, orofacial dystonia
- **CV:** *Hypertension, arrhythmias,* CV collapse with hypotension, palpitations, tachycardia, precordial pain
- **Dermatologic:** *Pallor,* sweating
- **GI:** *Nausea, vomiting,* anorexia
- **GU:** Dysuria, urinary retention in BPH
- **Respiratory:** Respiratory difficulty

Interactions

✱ **Drug-drug** • Increased hypertension with MAOIs, guanethidine, furazoladine • Increased duration of action with urinary alkalinizers (potassium citrate, sodium citrate, sodium lactate, tromethamine, sodium acetate, sodium bicarbonate) • Decreased therapeutic effects and increased elimination of pseudoephedrine with urinary acidifiers (ammonium chloride, sodium acid phosphate, potassium phosphate) • Decreased antihypertensive effects of methyldopa

■ Nursing considerations

Assessment

- **History:** Allergy or idiosyncrasy to sympathomimetic amines, severe hypertension and CAD, hyperthyroidism, diabetes mellitus, arteriosclerosis, increased IOP, prostatic hypertrophy, pregnancy, lactation
- **Physical:** Skin color, T; reflexes, affect, orientation, peripheral sensation, vision; BP, P, auscultation; R, adventitious sounds; urinary output, bladder percussion, prostate palpation

Interventions

⊗ ***Warning*** Administer cautiously to patients with CV disease, diabetes mellitus, hyperthyroidism, increased IOP, hypertension, and to patients older than 60 yr who may have increased sensitivity to sympathomimetic amines.

- Avoid prolonged use; underlying medical problems may be causing the congestion.
- Do not cut, crush, or allow patient to chew ER tablets.
- Monitor CV effect carefully; hypertensive patients who take this drug may experience changes in BP because of the additional vasoconstriction. However, if a nasal decongestant is needed, pseudoephedrine is the drug of choice.

Teaching points

- Do not exceed the recommended daily dose; serious overdose can occur. Use caution when using more than one over-the-counter preparation because many of these drugs contain pseudoephedrine, and unintentional overdose may occur.
- Do not cut, crush, or chew ER tablets.
- Avoid prolonged use because underlying medical problems can be disguised.
- You may experience these side effects: Dizziness, restlessness, light-headedness, tremors, weakness (avoid driving or performing hazardous tasks).
- Report palpitations, nervousness, sleeplessness, sweating.

▽ pyrantel pamoate

*(pi **ran'** tel)*

Combantrin (CAN), Pin-Rid, Pin-X, Reese's Pinworm

PREGNANCY CATEGORY C

Drug class

Anthelmintic

Therapeutic actions

A depolarizing neuromuscular blocking agent that causes spastic paralysis of *Enterobius vermicularis* and *Ascaris lumbricoides.* Also effective against *Ancyclostoma duodenale* (hookworm).

Indications
- Treatment of enterobiasis (pinworm infection)
- Treatment of ascariasis (roundworm infection)
- Unlabeled use: Hairworm

Contraindications and cautions
- Contraindicated with allergy to pyrantel pamoate.
- Use cautiously with pregnancy, lactation, hepatic disease.

Available forms
Capsules—180 mg; tablets—62.5 mg; oral suspension—50 mg/mL; liquid—50 mg/mL

Dosages
Adults and pediatric patients older than 2 yr
11 mg/kg (5 mg/lb) PO as a single oral dose. Maximum total dose of 1 g.
Pediatric patients younger than 2 yr
Safety and efficacy not established.

Pharmacokinetics

Route	*Onset*	*Peak*
Oral	Slow	1–3 hr

Metabolism: Hepatic; $T_{1/2}$: 47–100 hr
Distribution: Crosses placenta; may enter breast milk
Excretion: Feces, urine

Adverse effects
- **CNS:** Headache, dizziness, drowsiness, insomnia
- **Dermatologic:** Rash
- **GI:** *Anorexia, nausea, vomiting, abdominal cramps, diarrhea,* gastralgia, tenesmus, transient elevation of AST

Interactions
✱ **Drug-drug** • Pyrantel and piperazine are antagonistic in *Ascaris;* avoid concomitant use • Increases theophylline concentrations; monitor patient closely

■ Nursing considerations
Assessment
- **History:** Allergy to pyrantel pamoate, pregnancy, lactation, hepatic impairment
- **Physical:** Skin color, lesions; orientation, affect; bowel sounds; AST levels

Interventions
- Culture for ova and parasites.
- Administer drug with fruit juice or milk; ensure that entire dose is taken at once.
- Treat all family members (pinworm infestations).
- Disinfect toilet facilities after patient use (pinworms).
- Launder bed linens, towels, nightclothes, and undergarments (pinworms) daily.

Teaching points
- Take the entire dose at once. Drug may be taken with fruit juice or milk.
- Pinworms are easily transmitted; all family members should be treated for complete eradication.
- Strict handwashing and hygiene measures are important. Launder undergarments, bed linens, nightclothes daily; disinfect toilet facilities daily and bathroom floors periodically (pinworm).
- You may experience these side effects: Nausea, abdominal pain, diarrhea (eat frequent small meals); drowsiness, dizziness, insomnia (avoid driving and using dangerous machinery).
- Report rash, joint pain, severe GI upset, severe headache, dizziness.

P

▽ pyrazinamide
*(peer a **zin'** a myde)*

Tebrazid (CAN)

PREGNANCY CATEGORY C

Drug class
Antituberculotic

Therapeutic actions
Bacteriostatic or bacteriocidal against *Mycobacterium tuberculosis;* mechanism of action is unknown.

Indications
- Initial treatment of active TB in adults and children when combined with other antituberculotics

- Treatment of active TB after treatment failure with primary drugs
- Treatment of drug-resistant TB as part of an individualized regimen

Contraindications and cautions

- Contraindicated with allergy to pyrazinamide, acute hepatic disease, lactation, acute gout.
- Use cautiously with diabetes mellitus, acute intermittent porphyria, pregnancy.

Available forms

Tablets—500 mg

Dosages

Adults and pediatric patients

15–30 mg/kg/day PO, given once a day; do not exceed 2 g/day. Always use with up to four other antituberculotics; administer for the first 2 mo of a 6-mo treatment program. 50–70 mg/kg PO twice weekly may increase compliance and is being studied as an alternative dosing schedule. Patients with HIV infection may require a longer course of therapy.

Pharmacokinetics

Route	*Onset*	*Peak*
Oral	Rapid	2 hr

Metabolism: Hepatic; $T_{1/2}$: 9–10 hr
Distribution: Crosses placenta; enters breast milk
Excretion: Urine

Adverse effects

- **Dermatologic:** Rashes, photosensitivity
- **GI:** *Hepatotoxicity, nausea, vomiting,* diarrhea, anorexia
- **Hematologic:** Sideroblastic anemia, thrombocytopenia, adverse effects on clotting mechanism or vascular integrity
- **Other:** Active gout

Interactions

✱ **Drug-lab test** • False readings on *Acetest, Ketostix* urine tests

■ Nursing considerations

Assessment

- **History:** Allergy to pyrazinamide, acute hepatic disease, gout, diabetes mellitus, acute intermittent porphyria, pregnancy, lactation
- **Physical:** Skin color, lesions; joint status; T; liver evaluation; LFTs, serum and urine uric acid levels, blood and urine glucose, CBC

Interventions

- Administer only in conjunction with other antituberculotics.
- Administer once a day.
- Arrange for follow-up of LFTs (AST, ALT) prior to and every 2–4 wk during therapy.

⊗ ***Warning*** Discontinue drug if liver damage or hyperuricemia in conjunction with acute gouty arthritis occurs.

Teaching points

- Take this drug once a day; it will need to be taken with your other tuberculosis drugs.
- Take this drug regularly; avoid missing doses. Do not discontinue this drug without first consulting your health care provider.
- Have regular, periodic medical checkups, including blood tests to evaluate the drug effects.
- You may experience these side effects: Loss of appetite, nausea, vomiting (take drug with food); rash, sensitivity to sunlight (avoid exposure to the sun).
- Report fever, malaise, loss of appetite, nausea, vomiting, darkened urine, yellowing of skin and eyes, severe pain in great toe, instep, ankle, heel, knee, or wrist.

▽ pyridostigmine bromide

*(peer id oh **stig'** meen)*

Mestinon, Mestinon Timespan DNC

PREGNANCY CATEGORY C

Drug classes

Antidote
Antimyasthenic
Cholinesterase inhibitor

Therapeutic actions

Increases the concentration of acetylcholine at the sites of cholinergic transmission and prolongs and exaggerates the effects of acetylcholine by reversibly inhibiting the enzyme acetylcholinesterase, thus facilitating transmission at the skeletal neuromuscular junction.

Indications

- Treatment of myasthenia gravis
- Parenteral: Antidote for nondepolarizing neuromuscular junction blockers (eg, tubocurarine) after surgery
- To increase survival after exposure to sarin "nerve gas" poisoning in conjunction with protective measures

Contraindications and cautions

- Contraindicated with hypersensitivity to anticholinesterases; adverse reactions to bromides; intestinal or urogenital tract obstruction, peritonitis, lactation.
- Use cautiously with asthma, peptic ulcer, bradycardia, cardiac arrhythmias, recent coronary occlusion, vagotonia, hyperthyroidism, epilepsy, pregnancy (given IV near term, drug may stimulate uterus and induce premature labor).

Available forms

Tablets—60 mg ER tablets DNC—180 mg; syrup—60 mg/5 mL; injection—5 mg/mL

Dosages

Adults

Oral

- *Symptomatic control of myasthenia gravis:* Average dose is 600 mg given over 24 hr; range, 60–1,500 mg, spaced to provide maximum relief. ER tablets, average dose is 180–540 mg daily or bid. Individualize dosage, allowing at least 6 hr between doses. Optimum control may require supplementation with the more rapidly acting syrup or regular tablets.
- *Military personnel who face the threat of sarin nerve gas:* 30 mg PO every 8 hr starting several hr before exposure; stop drug if exposure occurs.

Parenteral

- *To supplement oral dosage preoperatively and postoperatively, during labor, during myasthenic crisis, etc:* Give 1/30 the oral dose IM or very slowly IV. May be given 1 hr before second stage of labor is complete (enables patient to have adequate strength and protects neonate in immediate postnatal period).
- *Antidote for nondepolarizing neuromuscular blockers:* Give atropine sulfate 0.6–1.2 mg IV immediately before slow IV injection of pyridostigmine 0.1–0.25 mg/kg. 10–20 mg pyridostigmine usually suffices. Full recovery usually occurs within 15 min but may take 30 min.

Pediatric patients

Oral

- *Symptomatic control of myasthenia gravis:* 7 mg/kg/day divided into five or six doses.

Parenteral

- *Neonates who have myasthenic mothers and who have difficulty swallowing, sucking, breathing:* 0.05–0.15 mg/kg IM. Change to syrup as soon as possible.

Pharmacokinetics

Route	Onset	Duration
Oral	20–30 min	3–6 hr
IM	15 min	2–4 hr
IV	5 min	2–4 hr

Metabolism: Hepatic and tissue; $T_{1/2}$: 1.9–3.7 hr

Distribution: Crosses placenta; enters breast milk

Excretion: Urine

IV FACTS

Preparation: No further preparation is required.

Infusion: Infuse very slowly, each 0.5 mg over 1 min for myasthenia gravis, each 5 mg over 1 min as a muscle relaxant agonist, directly into vein or into tubing of actively running IV of $D_{25}W$, 0.9% sodium chloride, lactated Ringer's solution, or $D_{25}W$ and lactated Ringer's solution.

Adverse effects

- **CNS:** Seizures, dizziness, dysarthria, dysphonia, drowsiness, headache, loss of consciousness
- **CV:** *Bradycardia, cardiac arrhythmias,* AV block and nodal rhythm, **cardiac arrest,** decreased cardiac output leading to hypotension, syncope

P

- **Dermatologic:** Diaphoresis, flushing, skin rash, urticaria
- **EENT:** *Lacrimation, miosis,* spasm of accommodation, diplopia, conjunctival hyperemia
- **GI:** *Salivation, dysphagia, nausea, vomiting, increased peristalsis, abdominal cramps,* flatulence, diarrhea
- **GU:** *Urinary frequency and incontinence,* urinary urgency
- **Local:** Thrombophlebitis after IV use
- **Peripheral:** Skeletal muscle weakness, fasciculations, muscle cramps, arthralgia
- **Respiratory:** *Increased pharyngeal and tracheobronchial secretions,* **laryngospasm, bronchospasm,** bronchiolar constriction, dyspnea, respiratory muscle paralysis, central respiratory paralysis, **anaphylaxis**

Interactions

✱ **Drug-drug** • Decreased effectiveness with profound muscular depression with corticosteroids • Increased and prolonged neuromuscular blockade with succinylcholine

■ Nursing considerations

Assessment

- **History:** Hypersensitivity to anticholinesterases, adverse reactions to bromides, intestinal or urogenital tract obstruction, peritonitis, lactation, asthma, peptic ulcer, cardiac arrhythmias, recent coronary occlusion, vagotonia, hyperthyroidism, epilepsy, pregnancy
- **Physical:** Bowel sounds, normal output; urinary frequency, voiding pattern, normal output; R, adventitious sounds; P, auscultation, BP; reflexes, bilateral grip strength, ECG; thyroid function tests; skin color, texture, lesions

Interventions

- Administer IV slowly.
- Overdose with anticholinesterase drugs can cause muscle weakness (cholinergic crisis) that is difficult to differentiate from myasthenic weakness; administration of atropine may mask the parasympathetic effects of anticholinesterase overdose and further confound the diagnosis.

⊗ ***Warning*** Keep atropine sulfate readily available as an antidote and antagonist to pyridostigmine in case of cholinergic crisis or unusual sensitivity to pyridostigmine.

⊗ ***Warning*** Discontinue drug and consult physician if excessive salivation, emesis, frequent urination, or diarrhea occurs.

- Have patient swallow ER tablets whole; do not cut, crush, or allow patient to chew ER tablets.
- Decrease dosage of drug if excessive sweating or nausea occurs.

Teaching points

- Take drug exactly as prescribed. Your health care provider should teach you and your significant other about drug effects, signs and symptoms of myasthenia gravis, the fact that muscle weakness may be related both to drug overdose and to exacerbation of the disease, and the importance of reporting muscle weakness promptly to the nurse or physician for proper evaluation.
- Do not cut, crush, or chew ER tablets.
- You may experience these side effects: Blurred vision, difficulty with far vision, difficulty with dark adaptation (use caution while driving, especially at night, or performing hazardous tasks in reduced light); increased urinary frequency, abdominal cramps; sweating (avoid hot or excessively humid environments).
- Report muscle weakness, nausea, vomiting, diarrhea, severe abdominal pain, excessive sweating, excessive salivation, frequent urination, urinary urgency, irregular heartbeat, difficulty breathing.

quazepam

(kwa' ze pam)

Doral

PREGNANCY CATEGORY X

CONTROLLED SUBSTANCE C-IV

Drug classes

Benzodiazepine
Sedative-hypnotic

Therapeutic actions

Exact mechanisms of action not understood; acts mainly at subcortical levels of the CNS, leaving the cortex relatively unaffected; main sites of action may be the limbic system and mesencephalic reticular formation; benzodiazepines potentiate the effects of GABA, an inhibitory neurotransmitter.

Indications

- Insomnia characterized by difficulty in falling asleep, frequent nocturnal awakenings, or early morning awakening
- Recurring insomnia or poor sleeping habits
- Acute or chronic medical situations requiring restful sleep

Contraindications and cautions

- Contraindicated with hypersensitivity to benzodiazepines, established or suspected sleep apnea, psychoses, acute narrow-angle glaucoma, shock, coma, acute alcoholic intoxication with depression of vital signs, pregnancy (congenital malformations, neonatal withdrawal syndrome), labor and delivery ("floppy infant" syndrome), lactation (infants become lethargic and lose weight).
- Use cautiously with elderly patients, impaired liver or renal function, debilitation, depression, suicidal tendencies.

Available forms

Tablets—7.5, 15 mg

Dosages

Adults

Initially, 15 mg PO at bedtime. May reduce to 7.5 mg at bedtime in some patients.

Pediatric patients

Not for use in patients younger than 18 yr.

Geriatric patients or patients with debilitating disease

Attempt to reduce nightly dosage after the first one or two nights of therapy.

Pharmacokinetics

Route	*Onset*	*Peak*
Oral	Varies	2 hr

Metabolism: Hepatic; $T_{1/2}$: 41 hr
Distribution: Crosses placenta; enters breast milk
Excretion: Urine

Adverse effects

- **CNS:** Transient, mild drowsiness initially; sedation; depression; lethargy; apathy; fatigue; light-headedness; disorientation; restlessness; confusion; crying; delirium; headache; slurred speech; dysarthria; stupor; rigidity; tremor; dystonia; vertigo; euphoria; nervousness; difficulty in concentration; vivid dreams; psychomotor retardation; extrapyramidal symptoms; mild paradoxical excitatory reactions during first 2 wk of treatment (especially in psychiatric patients, aggressive children, and with high dosage); visual and auditory disturbances; diplopia; nystagmus; depressed hearing; nasal congestion; complex sleep-related behaviors
- **CV:** *Bradycardia, tachycardia,* CV collapse, hypertension and hypotension, palpitations, edema
- **Dependence:** *Drug dependence with withdrawal syndrome* when drug is discontinued (more common with abrupt discontinuation of higher dosage used for longer than 4 mo)
- **Dermatologic:** Pruritus, skin rash, dermatitis
- **GI:** *Constipation, diarrhea,* dry mouth, salivation, nausea, anorexia, vomiting, difficulty in swallowing, gastric disorders, elevations of blood enzymes, hepatic impairment, jaundice
- **GU:** Incontinence, changes in libido, urinary retention, menstrual irregularities
- **Hematologic:** Decreased Hct (primarily with long-term therapy), blood dyscrasias (agranulocytosis, leukopenia, neutropenia)
- **Other: Anaphylaxis, angioedema,** hiccups, fever, diaphoresis, paresthesias, muscular disturbances, gynecomastia

Interactions

✱ **Drug-drug** • Increased CNS depression with alcohol • Increased pharmacologic effects with cimetidine, disulfiram, hormonal contraceptives • Decreased sedative effects with theophylline, aminophylline • Decreased sedative effects with smoking

■ Nursing considerations

Assessment

- **History:** Hypersensitivity to benzodiazepines, psychoses, acute narrow-angle glaucoma,

shock, coma, acute alcoholic intoxication, pregnancy, labor and delivery, lactation, impaired liver or renal function, debilitation, depression, suicidal tendencies
- **Physical:** Skin color, lesions; T; orientation, reflexes, affect, ophthalmologic examination; P, BP; R, adventitious sounds; liver evaluation, abdominal examination, bowel sounds, normal output; CBC, LFTs, renal function tests

Interventions

⊗ ***Warning*** Ensure that patient is not pregnant before use; recommend the use of barrier contraceptives.
- Monitor liver and renal function and CBC during long-term therapy.

⊗ ***Warning*** Taper dosage gradually after long-term therapy, especially in patients with epilepsy, to prevent refractory seizures.

Teaching points

- Take drug exactly as prescribed.
- Do not stop taking this drug (in long-term therapy) without consulting your health care provider.
- This drug should not be used during pregnancy; using barrier contraceptives is advised.
- You may experience these side effects: Drowsiness, dizziness (may lessen; avoid driving or engaging in other dangerous activities); allergic reaction; GI upset (take with water); depression, dreams, complex sleep disorders, emotional upset, crying; nocturnal sleep may be disturbed for several nights after discontinuing the drug.
- Report severe dizziness, weakness, drowsiness that persists, complex sleep-related behaviors, rash or skin lesions, palpitations, swelling of the extremities, visual changes, difficulty voiding, allergic reaction.

▽ quetiapine fumarate

*(kwe **tie'** ah peen)*

Seroquel, Seroquel XR

Pregnancy Category C

Drug classes

Antipsychotic
Dibenzothiazepine

Therapeutic actions

Mechanism of action not fully understood: Blocks dopamine and serotonin receptors in the brain; also acts as a receptor antagonist at histamine and adrenergic receptor sites (which may contribute to the adverse effects of orthostatic hypotension and somnolence).

Indications

- Treatment of schizophrenia in patients older than 18 yr
- Short-term treatment of acute manic or depressive episodes associated with bipolar I disorder, as monotherapy or in combination with lithium or divalproex
- Maintenance treatment of bipolar disorder
- Management of alcohol dependence

Contraindications and cautions

- Contraindicated with coma or severe CNS depression, allergy to quetiapine, lactation.
- Use cautiously with CV disease, hypotension, hepatic impairment, seizures, exposure to extreme heat, autonomic instability, tardive dyskinesia, dehydration, thyroid disease, pregnancy.

Available forms

Tablets—25, 50, 100, 200, 300, 400 mg; ER tablets—200, 300, 400 mg

Dosages

Adults

- *Schizophrenia:* 25 mg PO bid. Increase in increments of 25–50 mg bid–tid on days 2 and 3; dosage range by day 4: 300–400 mg/day in two to three divided doses. Further increases can be made at no less than 2-day intervals. Maximum dose, 800 mg/day. For ER tablets, 300 mg PO once daily in the evening; range, 400–800 mg/day.
- *Manic episodes:* 100 mg/day PO divided bid on day 1; increase to 400 mg/day PO in bid divided doses by day 4 using 100-mg/day increments. Range, 400–800 mg/day given in divided doses.

- *Depressive episodes:* 100 mg PO once daily at bedtime; increase to desired dose of 300 mg/day by day 4.

Pediatric patients

Not recommended for patients younger than 18 yr.

Geriatric or debilitated patients or patients with hepatic impairment

Use lower doses starting with 25 mg/day and increase dosage more gradually than in other patients. For schizophrenia, when stabilized on 200 mg/day, patient may be switched to ER tablets.

Pharmacokinetics

Route	*Onset*	*Peak*	*Duration*
Oral	Slow	1.5 hr	Unknown

Metabolism: Hepatic; $T_{1/2}$: 6 hr
Distribution: Crosses placenta; enters breast milk
Excretion: Feces, urine

Adverse effects

- **Autonomic:** Dry mouth, salivation, nasal congestion, nausea, vomiting, anorexia, fever, pallor, flushed facies, sweating, constipation
- **CNS:** *Drowsiness,* insomnia, vertigo, *headache,* weakness, tremor, tardive dyskinesias, **NMS**
- **CV:** Hypotension, *orthostatic hypotension,* syncope
- **Hematologic:** Increased ALT, total cholesterol and triglycerides
- **Other:** Risk of development of diabetes mellitus

Interactions

✱ **Drug-drug** • CNS effects potentiated by alcohol, CNS depressants • Effects decreased with phenytoin, thioridazine, carbamazepine, phenobarbital, rifampin, glucocorticoids; monitor patient closely and adjust dosages appropriately when these drugs are added to or discontinued from regimen • Increased effects of antihypertensives, lorazepam • Decreased effects of levodopa, dopamine antagonists • Potential for heatstroke and intolerance with drugs that affect temperature regulation (anticholinergics); use extreme caution and monitor patient closely

■ Nursing considerations

Assessment

- **History:** Coma or severe CNS depression, allergy to quetiapine, lactation, pregnancy, CV disease, hypotension, hepatic impairment, seizures, exposure to extreme heat, autonomic instability, tardive dyskinesia, dehydration, thyroid disease, suicidal tendencies
- **Physical:** Body weight, T; reflexes, orientation, IOP; P, BP, orthostatic BP; R, adventitious sounds; CBC, urinalysis, LFTs, renal and thyroid function tests

Interventions

⊗ ***Black box warning*** Do not use this drug to treat elderly patients with dementia-related psychosis; it causes increased risk of CV mortality, including stroke, MI.

⊗ ***Black box warning*** Increased risk of suicidality in children, adolescents, and young adults; not approved for use in children. Monitor patients accordingly.

⊗ ***Warning*** Administer small quantity to any patient with suicidal ideation.

- Make sure patient does not cut, crush, or chew ER tablets; they must be swallowed whole.
- Administer ER tablet once daily in the evening.
- Monitor elderly patients for dehydration and institute remedial measures promptly; sedation and decreased sensation of thirst related to CNS effects of drug can lead to severe dehydration.
- Monitor patient closely in any setting that would promote overheating.
- Regularly monitor patient for signs and symptoms of diabetes mellitus.
- Consult physician about dosage reduction and use of anticholinergic antiparkinsonians (controversial) if extrapyramidal effects occur.

Teaching points

- Take this drug exactly as prescribed.
- Take extended-release tablet once daily in the evening. Do not cut, crush, or chew tablets; they must be swallowed whole.
- This drug should not be used during pregnancy; using barrier contraceptives is advised.
- Maintain fluid intake and use precautions against heatstroke in hot weather.

Q

- You may experience these side effects: Dizziness, drowsiness, fainting (avoid driving or engaging in other dangerous activities); dry mouth, nausea, loss of appetite (frequent mouth care, frequent small meals, and increased fluid intake may help).
- Report sore throat, fever, unusual bleeding or bruising, rash, weakness, tremors, dark-colored urine, pale stools, yellowing of the skin or eyes, suicidal thoughts.

▽quinapril hydrochloride

(kwin' ah pril)

Accupril

PREGNANCY CATEGORY C (FIRST TRIMESTER)

PREGNANCY CATEGORY D (SECOND AND THIRD TRIMESTERS)

Drug classes

ACE inhibitor
Antihypertensive

Therapeutic actions

Quinapril blocks ACE from converting angiotensin I to angiotensin II, a powerful vasoconstrictor, leading to decreased BP, decreased aldosterone secretion, a small increase in serum potassium levels, and sodium and fluid loss; increased prostaglandin synthesis also may be involved in the antihypertensive action.

Indications

- Treatment of hypertension alone or in combination with thiazide-type diuretics
- Adjunctive therapy in the management of HF with cardiac glycosides, diuretics, and beta-adrenergic blockers

Contraindications and cautions

- Contraindicated with allergy to quinapril or other ACE inhibitors, pregnancy, angioedema.
- Use cautiously with impaired renal function, unilateral or bilateral renal artery stenosis, salt or volume depletion, lactation.

Available forms

Tablets—5, 10, 20, 40 mg

Dosages

Adults

- *Hypertension:* Initial dose, 10 or 20 mg PO daily. Maintenance dose, 20–80 mg/day PO as a single dose or two divided doses. Patients on diuretics should discontinue the diuretic 2–3 days before beginning benazepril therapy. If BP is not controlled, add diuretic slowly. If diuretic cannot be discontinued, begin quinapril therapy with 5 mg and monitor carefully for hypotension.
- *HF:* Initial dose, 5 mg PO bid. Dose may be increased as needed to relieve symptoms; usual range, 10–20 mg PO bid; increase doses at weekly intervals until effective dose is reached.

Pediatric patients

Safety and efficacy not established.

Geriatric patients or patients with renal impairment

Initial dose: 10 mg if creatinine clearance greater than 60 mL/min, 5 mg if creatinine clearance 30–60 mL/min, 2.5 mg if creatinine clearance 10–30 mL/min.

Pharmacokinetics

Route	*Onset*	*Peak*	*Duration*
Oral	1 hr	1 hr	24 hr

Metabolism: Hepatic; $T_{1/2}$: 2 hr
Distribution: Crosses placenta; enters breast milk
Excretion: Urine

Adverse effects

- **CV:** Angina pectoris, orthostatic hypotension in salt- or volume-depleted patients, palpitations
- **Dermatologic:** Rash, pruritus, diaphoresis, flushing, photosensitivity
- **GI:** Elevated LFTs, pancreatitis
- **Respiratory:** *Cough*
- **Other:** Angioedema, arthralgia

Interactions

✱ **Drug-drug** • Increased lithium levels • Decreased tetracycline absorption. Separate drugs by 1–2 hr • Risk of hyperkalemia if combined with potassium-sparing diuretics

■ Nursing considerations

Assessment

- **History:** Allergy to quinapril, other ACE inhibitors; impaired renal function; HF; salt or volume depletion; lactation, pregnancy
- **Physical:** Skin color, lesions, turgor; T; P, BP, peripheral perfusion; mucous membranes, bowel sounds, liver evaluation; urinalysis, LFTs, renal function tests, CBC and differential

Interventions

⊗ ***Warning*** Alert surgeon and mark the patient's chart with notice that quinapril is being taken; the angiotensin II formation subsequent to compensatory renin release during surgery will be blocked; hypotension may be reversed with volume expansion.

⊠ ***Black box warning*** Caution patient that this drug should not be used during pregnancy; advise patient to use barrier contraceptives.

- Monitor patient closely in any situation that may lead to a fall in BP secondary to reduction in fluid volume (excessive perspiration and dehydration, vomiting, diarrhea) because excessive hypotension may occur.

Teaching points

- Do not stop taking the medication without consulting your health care provider.
- Be careful in any situation that may lead to a drop in blood pressure (diarrhea, sweating, vomiting, dehydration); if light-headedness or dizziness occurs, consult your health care provider.
- This drug should not be used during pregnancy; using barrier contraceptives is advised.
- You may experience these side effects: GI upset, loss of appetite (transient); light-headedness (usually transient; change position slowly and limit activities to those that do not require alertness and precision); dry cough (not harmful).
- Report mouth sores; sore throat, fever, chills; swelling of the hands, feet; irregular heartbeat, chest pains; swelling of the face, eyes, lips, tongue; difficulty breathing; persistent cough.

DANGEROUS DRUG

quinidine

(qwin' i deen)

quinidine gluconate DNC

quinidine sulfate DNC

PREGNANCY CATEGORY C

Drug class

Antiarrhythmic

Therapeutic actions

Type IA antiarrhythmic: Decreases automaticity in ventricles, decreases height and rate of rise of action potential, decreases conduction velocity, increases fibrillation threshold.

Indications

- Treatment of atrial arrhythmias, paroxysmal or chronic ventricular tachycardia without heart block
- Maintenance therapy after electrocardioversion of atrial fibrillation or atrial flutter
- Treatment of life-threatening *Plasmodium falciparum* infections when IV therapy (quinidine gluconate) is indicated

Contraindications and cautions

- Contraindicated with allergy or idiosyncrasy to quinidine, second- or third-degree heart block, myasthenia gravis, pregnancy (neonatal thrombocytopenia), lactation, thrombocytopenic purpura, in patients with diseases that might be adversely affected by an anticholinergic agent.
- Use cautiously with renal disease, especially renal tubular acidosis, HF, hepatic insufficiency.

Available forms

Tablets—200, 300 mg; SR tablets DNC—300, 324 mg; injection—80 mg/mL

Dosages

Quinidine gluconate contains 62% anhydrous quinidine alkaloid. Quinidine sulfate contains 83% anhydrous quinidine alkaloid.

Q

Adults

Administer a test dose of 200 mg PO or 200 mg IM to test for idiosyncratic reaction. Maintenance therapy, 200–300 mg tid or qid PO or 300–600 mg every 8 hr or every 12 hr if SR form is used.

PO

- *Paroxysmal supraventricular arrhythmias:* 400–600 mg PO every 2–3 hr until paroxysm is terminated.

IM

- *Acute tachycardia:* 600 mg IM quinidine gluconate, followed by 400 mg every 2 hr until rhythm is stable.

IV

330 mg quinidine gluconate injected slowly IV at rate of 1 mL/min of diluted solution (10 mL of quinidine gluconate injection diluted to 50 mL with 5% glucose).

Pediatric patients

300 mg/kg/24 hr PO in five equally divided doses; 2–10 mg/kg/dose IV every 3–6 hr has been used, but this route is not recommended.

Patients with hepatic or renal impairment

Reduce dosage and monitor patient closely.

Pharmacokinetics

Route	*Onset*	*Duration*
Oral	1–3 hr	6–8 hr
IM	30–90 min	6–8 hr
IV	Rapid	6–8 hr

Metabolism: Hepatic; $T_{1/2}$: 6–7 hr
Distribution: Crosses placenta; enters breast milk
Excretion: Feces, urine

IV FACTS

Preparation: Dilute 800 mg quinidine gluconate in 50 mL 5% dextrose injection.
Infusion: Inject slowly at rate of 1 mL/min.
Y-site incompatibility: Do not inject with furosemide.

Adverse effects

- **CNS:** Vision changes (photophobia, blurring, loss of night vision, diplopia)
- **CV: Cardiac arrhythmias,** cardiac conduction disturbances, including heart block, hypotension
- **GI:** Nausea, vomiting, diarrhea, liver toxicity
- **Hematologic:** Hemolytic anemia, hypoprothrombinemia, thrombocytopenic purpura, agranulocytosis, lupus erythematosus-like syndrome (resolves after withdrawal)
- **Hypersensitivity:** Rash, flushing, urticaria, angioedema, respiratory arrest
- **Other:** *Cinchonism* (tinnitus, headache, nausea, dizziness, fever, tremor, visual disturbances)

Interactions

✱ **Drug-drug** • Increased effects and increased risk of toxicity with cimetidine, amiodarone, verapamil • Increased cardiac depressant effects with sodium bicarbonate • Decreased levels with phenobarbital, hydantoins, rifampin, sucralfate • Increased neuromuscular blocking effects of depolarizing and nondepolarizing neuromuscular blocking agents, succinylcholine • Increased digoxin levels and toxicity • Increased effect of oral anticoagulants and bleeding • Decreased levels with phenobarbital, hydantoins, rifampin, sucralfate • Increased neuromuscular blocking effects of depolarizing and nondepolarizing neuromuscular blocking agents, succinylcholine • Increased digoxin levels and toxicity • Increased effect of oral anticoagulants and bleeding • Increased effects of TCAs

✱ **Drug-food** • Decreased metabolism and increased risk of toxic effects if combined with grapefruit juice; avoid this combination

✱ **Drug-lab test** • Quinidine serum levels are inaccurate if the patient is also taking triamterene

■ Nursing considerations

Assessment

- **History:** Allergy or idiosyncrasy to quinidine, second- or third-degree heart block, myasthenia gravis, renal disease, HF, hepatic insufficiency, pregnancy, lactation
- **Physical:** Skin color, lesions; orientation, cranial nerves, bilateral grip strength, reflexes; P, BP, auscultation, ECG, edema; bowel sounds, liver evaluation; urinalysis, LFTs, renal function tests; CBC

Interventions

- Monitor response carefully, especially when beginning therapy.
- Reduce dosage in patients with hepatic or renal failure.
- Reduce dosage with digoxin; monitor digoxin levels closely.
- Adjust dosage if phenobarbital, hydantoin, or rifampin is added or discontinued.
- Check to see that patients with atrial flutter or fibrillation have been digitalized before starting quinidine.
- Differentiate the SR form from the regular form. Make sure SR form is not cut, crushed, or chewed.
- Monitor cardiac rhythm carefully, and frequently monitor BP if given IV or IM.
- Arrange for periodic ECG monitoring when on long-term therapy.
- Monitor blood counts, liver function tests frequently during long-term therapy.

⊗ ***Warning*** Evaluate for safe and effective serum drug levels: 2–6 mcg/mL.

Teaching points

- Take this drug exactly as prescribed. Do not chew the sustained-release tablets. If GI upset occurs, take drug with food. Do not drink grapefruit juice while using this drug.
- You will need frequent cardiac rhythm monitoring and blood tests.
- Wear a medical alert tag stating that you are using this drug.
- Return for regular follow-up visits to check your heart rhythm and blood counts.
- You may experience these side effects: Nausea, loss of appetite, vomiting (eat frequent small meals); dizziness, light-headedness, vision changes (do not drive or operate dangerous machinery); rash (use skin care).
- Report sore mouth, throat, or gums, fever, chills, cold or flulike symptoms, ringing in the ears, severe vision disturbances, headache, unusual bleeding or bruising.

▽quinine sulfate

See Appendix W, *Less commonly used drugs*.

▽rabeprazole sodium

*(rab **beh'** pray zol)*

Aciphex (DNC)

PREGNANCY CATEGORY B

Drug classes

Antisecretory drug
Proton pump inhibitor

Therapeutic actions

Gastric acid-pump inhibitor: Suppresses gastric acid secretion by specific inhibition of the hydrogen and potassium ATPase enzyme system at the secretory surface of the gastric parietal cells; blocks the final step of acid production.

Indications

- Healing and maintenance of erosive or ulcerative GERD; 4–8 wk therapy; may use additional 8 wk as needed
- Short-term treatment of GERD in children 12 yr and older
- Treatment of daytime and nighttime heartburn and other symptoms of GERD
- Healing of duodenal ulcers as short-term treatment of less than 4 wk
- Treatment of pathological hypersecretory conditions (eg, Zollinger-Ellison syndrome, multiple adenomas, systemic mastocytosis)
- Unlabeled use: Treatment of gastric ulcers

Contraindications and cautions

- Contraindicated with hypersensitivity to any proton pump inhibitor or any drug components.
- Use cautiously with pregnancy, lactation.

Available forms

DR tablet (DNC)—20 mg

Dosages

Adults

- *Healing of GERD:* 20 mg PO daily for 4–8 wk.
- *Maintenance of GERD:* 20 mg daily PO.
- *Healing of duodenal ulcer:* 20 mg PO daily for up to 4 wk.
- *Pathological hypersecretory conditions:* 60 mg PO daily to bid for as long as clinically indicated.

R

Pediatric patients 12 yr and older: 20 mg/day PO for up to 8 wk.

Patients with hepatic impairment Use extreme caution with severe hepatic impairment.

Pharmacokinetics

Route	*Onset*	*Peak*
Oral	1 hr	3–5 hr

Metabolism: Hepatic; $T_{1/2}$: 1.5 hr
Distribution: Crosses placenta; may enter breast milk
Excretion: Feces, urine

Adverse effects

- **CNS:** *Headache, dizziness,* asthenia, vertigo, insomnia, apathy, anxiety, paresthesias, dream abnormalities
- **Dermatologic:** Rash, inflammation, urticaria, pruritus, alopecia, dry skin
- **GI:** *Diarrhea, abdominal pain, nausea, vomiting,* constipation, dry mouth, tongue atrophy
- **Respiratory:** *URI symptoms,* cough, epistaxis
- **Other:** Cancer in preclinical studies, back pain, fever

Interactions

✱ **Drug-drug** ⊗ ***Warning*** Risk of severe hypoglycemia if combined with both gemfibrozil and itraconazole; avoid this combination • Increased serum levels and potential increase in toxicity of benzodiazepines when taken concurrently • Risk of hypoglycemia if combined with gemfibrozil; use caution if this combination is used and monitor patient closely

■ Nursing considerations

Assessment

- **History:** Hypersensitivity to any proton pump inhibitor or any drug components, pregnancy, lactation
- **Physical:** Skin lesions; body T; reflexes, affect; urinary output, abdominal examination; respiratory auscultation

Interventions

- Administer once a day. Caution patient to swallow tablets whole, not to cut, crush, or chew.
- Symptomatic improvement does not rule out gastric cancer.
- If administering antacids, they may be administered concomitantly with rabeprazole.
- Maintain supportive treatment as appropriate for underlying problem.
- Provide additional comfort measures to alleviate discomfort such as from GI effects or headache.

Teaching points

- Take the drug once a day. Swallow the tablets whole—do not chew, cut, or crush. This drug will need to be taken for up to 4 weeks (in short-term therapy) or for a prolonged period depending on the condition being treated.
- Arrange to have regular medical follow-up while you are using this drug.
- Maintain all of the usual activities and restrictions that apply to your condition. If this becomes difficult, consult your health care provider.
- You may experience these side effects: Dizziness (avoid driving a car or performing hazardous tasks); headache (consult your health care provider if these become bothersome; medications may be available to help); nausea, vomiting, diarrhea (proper nutrition is important, consult a dietitian to maintain nutrition; ensure ready access to bathroom facilities); symptoms of upper respiratory tract infection, cough (it may help to know that this is a drug effect, do not self-medicate, consult your health care provider if this becomes uncomfortable).
- Report severe headache, worsening of symptoms, fever, chills.

▽ raloxifene hydrochloride

*(rah **lox'** i feen)*

Evista

PREGNANCY CATEGORY X

Drug class

Selective estrogen receptor modulator

Therapeutic actions
Increases bone mineral density without stimulating endometrium in women; modulates effects of endogenous estrogen at specific receptor sites.

Indications
- Prevention and treatment of osteoporosis in postmenopausal women
- Reduction of risk of invasive breast cancer in postmenopausal women with osteoporosis and a high risk of invasive breast cancer
- Unlabeled uses: uterine leiomyoma, pubertal gynecomastia, prevention of bone loss in men with prostate cancer

Contraindications and cautions
- Contraindicated with allergy to raloxifene, pregnancy, lactation, active or history of DVT, pulmonary embolism, or retinal vein thrombosis.
- Use cautiously with history of smoking, venous thrombosis.

Available forms
Tablets—60 mg

Dosages
Adults
60 mg PO daily.

Pharmacokinetics

Route	*Onset*	*Peak*
Oral	Varies	4–7 hr

Metabolism: Hepatic; $T_{1/2}$: 27.7 hr
Distribution: Crosses placenta; enters breast milk
Excretion: Feces

Adverse effects
- **CNS:** Depression, insomnia, vertigo, neuralgia, hypoesthesia
- **CV: Venous thromboembolism**
- **Dermatologic:** *Hot flashes, skin rash*
- **GI:** *Nausea, vomiting,* food distaste
- **GU:** Vaginal bleeding, vaginal discharge
- **Other:** Peripheral edema

Interactions
✱ **Drug-drug** • Increased risk of bleeding with oral anticoagulants; monitor PT or INR closely • Decreased raloxifene absorption if taken with cholestyramine; avoid this combination

■ Nursing considerations
Assessment
- **History:** Allergy to raloxifene, pregnancy, lactation, smoking, history of venous thrombosis
- **Physical:** Skin lesions, color, turgor; pelvic examination; orientation, affect, reflexes; peripheral pulses, edema; LFTs, CBC and differential, bone density

Interventions
- Administer daily without regard to food.
- Arrange for periodic blood counts during therapy.

⊗ ***Warning*** Monitor patient for possible long-term effects, including cancers and thromboses associated with other drugs in this class.

⊗ ***Warning*** Counsel patient about the need to use contraceptive measures to avoid pregnancy while taking this drug; inform patient that serious fetal harm could occur.

- Provide comfort measures to help patient deal with drug effects: Hot flashes (control environmental temperature); headache, depression (monitor light and noise); vaginal bleeding (use good hygiene).

Teaching points
- Take this drug as prescribed.
- This drug can cause serious fetal harm and must not be taken during pregnancy. Contraceptive measures should be used while you are taking this drug. If you become pregnant or would like to become pregnant, consult your health care provider immediately.
- You may experience these side effects: Bone pain; hot flashes (staying in cool places may help); nausea, vomiting (eat frequent small meals); weight gain; dizziness, headache, light-headedness (use caution if driving or performing tasks that require alertness).
- Report marked weakness, sleepiness, mental confusion, pain or swelling of the legs, shortness of breath, blurred vision.

raltegravir

(rahl teh' gra veer)

Isentress

PREGNANCY CATEGORY C

Drug classes

Antiviral drug
Integrase inhibitor

Therapeutic action

Inhibits the virus-specific enzyme integrase, an encoded enzyme needed for viral replication. Blocking this enzyme prevents formation of HIV-1 provirus and leads to decreased viral load and increased active CD4 cells.

Indications

- In combination with other antivirals for the treatment of HIV-1 infection in treatment-experienced adults with evidence of viral replication and HIV-1 strains resistant to multiple antiretroviral drugs
- **NEW INDICATION:** In combination with other antivirals for treatment of HIV-1 infection in treatment-naive adults

Contraindications and cautions

- Contraindicated with hypersensitivity to any component of drug, treatment-naïve adults, children, lactation.
- Use cautiously with patients taking strong inducers of uridine disphosphate glucuronsyltransferase 1A1, patients at risk for rhabdomyolysis or myopathy, pregnant patients.

Available forms

Tablets—400 mg

Dosages

Adults

400 mg PO bid taken with other antivirals and without regard to food. If given with rifampin, 800 mg PO bid without regard to food.

Pharmacokinetics

Route	*Onset*	*Peak*
Oral	Rapid	3 hr

Metabolism: Hepatic; $T_{1/2}$: 9 hr
Distribution: May cross placenta; may enter breast milk
Excretion: Feces, urine

Adverse effects

- **CNS:** *Headache,* dizziness
- **GI:** *Nausea, diarrhea,* abdominal pain, vomiting
- **Other:** *Fever,* rhabdomyolysis, immune reconstitution syndrome

Interactions

✱ **Drug-drug** • Decreased serum levels of raltegravir if combined with rifampin; monitor patient and adjust dosage if this combination must be used

✱ **Drug-drug** • Potential for loss of effectiveness if combined with St. John's wort; avoid this combination

■ Nursing considerations

Assessment

- **History:** Hypersensitivity to raltegravir or any of its components; risk for myopathy or rhabdomyolysis, pregnancy, lactation
- **Physical:** T; orientation; abdominal examination, LFTs, HIV testing

Interventions

- Make sure patient is taking other antiviral drugs when taking this drug.
- Administer without regard to food.
- Encourage women of childbearing age to use barrier contraceptives while on this drug because drug effects on fetus are not known.
- Advise women who are nursing to find another method of feeding the baby; potential effects on the baby are not known.
- Explain that drug does not cure disease and that there is still a risk of transmitting HIV to others.
- Maintain all other therapies related to the HIV infection.

Teaching points

- This drug does not cure HIV. It works with other antiviral drugs to decrease the amount of virus in your body.
- To prevent the spread of HIV, take precautions to avoid exposing others to your blood

and body fluids, and use condoms during sex.
- If you miss a dose, take it as soon as you remember and resume your regular schedule. If you don't remember until it's almost time to take the next dose, skip the missed dose and continue your usual schedule. Do not take two tablets at the same time to make up for a skipped dose. Do not take more than two doses each day.
- Do not let your prescription run out. If you stop taking this drug temporarily, the virus could become resistant to antiviral drugs, decreasing the effectiveness of antiviral treatment and increasing your viral load.
- You will need regular health care, including blood tests, to monitor the effects of this drug on your body.
- It is not known how this drug could affect a fetus. If you are pregnant or decide to become pregnant while on this drug, consult with your health care provider.
- It is not known how this drug could affect a nursing baby. If you are nursing a baby, you should select another feeding method.
- You may experience these side effects: Headache (consult your health care provider, medication may be available to help); nausea (small, frequent meals may help); diarrhea (it may lessen with time, but alert your health care provider if it becomes severe).
- Report signs of infection; unexplained muscle pain, tenderness, or weakness; severe diarrhea; headache that will not go away.

▽ramelteon

*(rah **mell'** tee on)*

Rozerem

PREGNANCY CATEGORY C

Drug classes
Melatonin receptor agonist
Sedative-hypnotic

Therapeutic actions
Agonist at melatonin receptor sites believed to contribute to sleep promotion and thought to be involved in the maintenance of circadian rhythm underlying the normal sleep-wake cycle.

Indications
Treatment of insomnia characterized by difficulty with sleep onset

Contraindications and cautions
- Contraindicated with known hypersensitivity to any component of the drug, severe hepatic impairment, concurrent use of fluvoxamine, lactation, severe sleep apnea, severe COPD.
- Use cautiously with moderate hepatic impairment, pregnancy.

Available forms
Tablets—8 mg

Dosages
Adults
8 mg PO taken within 30 min of going to bed.
Pediatric patients
Safety and efficacy not established.
Patients with hepatic impairment
- *Severe hepatic impairment:* Not recommended.
- *Moderate hepatic impairment:* Use with caution.
- *Concurrent use of CYP1A2 inhibitors:* Use with caution.

Pharmacokinetics

Route	*Onset*	*Peak*
Oral	Rapid	0.5–1.5 hr

Metabolism: Hepatic; $T_{1/2}$: 2-5 hr
Distribution: May cross placenta; may pass into breast milk
Excretion: Feces, urine

R

Adverse effects
- **CNS:** Dizziness, somnolence, depression, insomnia, *headache,* complex sleep disorders
- **GI:** Nausea, diarrhea
- **GU:** Decreased testosterone levels (decreased libido, fertility issues), increased prolactin levels (galactorrhea, amenorrhea, problems with fertility)
- **Respiratory:** URIs
- **Other:** Influenza, arthralgia, myalgia, decreased cortisol levels, **anaphylaxis, angioedema**

Interactions

✱ Drug-drug • Risk of severe increase in serum levels and toxicity of ramelteon if combined with fluvoxamine; avoid this combination • Increased serum levels and risk of adverse effects if combined with potent CYP inhibitors (ketoconazole, fluconazole, itraconazole, clarithromycin, nefazodone, troleandomycin, ritonavir, nelfinavir); monitor patient and adjust dosages as needed

■ Nursing considerations

Assessment

- **History:** Hypersensitivity to any component of the drug, hepatic impairment, concurrent use of fluvoxamine, lactation, severe sleep apnea, severe COPD, pregnancy
- **Physical:** Orientation, reflexes, affect; R, adventitious sounds; abdominal examination; chest examination

Interventions

- Administer drug 30 min before patient is going to bed; encourage no other activities after the patient takes the drug.
- Monitor patients using drug for suicidal ideation.
- Do not administer this drug after a fatty or large meal, absorption can be affected.
- Encourage women of childbearing age to use barrier contraceptives while on this drug; effects of the drug on a fetus are not known.
- Advise women who are nursing to find another method of feeding the baby, it is not known if this drug can affect a nursing baby.

Teaching points

- Take this drug exactly as prescribed, 30 minutes before going to bed. Do not use it longer than advised by your health care provider.
- Do not take this drug unless you are about to get into bed and are able to get 8 or more hours of sleep before you need to be alert again; after taking the drug, limit activities to those involved with getting ready for bed.
- Do not take this drug with or immediately after a high-fat or heavy meal. This could interfere with the absorption and effectiveness of the drug.
- Do not combine this drug with other sleep drugs, including over-the-counter products.
- It is not known how this drug would affect a pregnancy. If you think you are pregnant or would like to become pregnant, consult your health care provider.
- This drug should not be taken while nursing a baby. If you are nursing a baby, another method of feeding the baby should be used while you are using this drug.
- Consult your health care provider if you experience worsening of your insomnia or if you develop any new behavioral signs or symptoms, such as complex sleep-related behaviors.
- You may experience these side effects: Allergic reaction, swelling, changes in thinking, alertness (do not drive a car, operate potentially dangerous equipment, or make important legal decisions the day after you take this drug); headache (consult your health care provider for potential pain medications if this occurs); unpleasant taste, nausea (frequent mouth care, frequent small meals may help); cessation of your period (women), enlargement of breasts, fertility problems.
- Report depression, thoughts of suicide or disturbing thoughts, cessation of menses or breast enlargement or engorgement in women, decreased libido, problems with fertility.

▽ramipril

(ra ***mi'*** *pril)*

Altace

PREGNANCY CATEGORY C
(FIRST TRIMESTER)

PREGNANCY CATEGORY D
(SECOND AND THIRD TRIMESTERS)

Drug classes

ACE inhibitor
Antihypertensive

Therapeutic actions

Ramipril blocks ACE from converting angiotensin I to angiotensin II, a powerful vasoconstrictor, leading to decreased BP, decreased aldosterone secretion, a small increase in serum potassium levels, and sodium and fluid loss;

increased prostaglandin synthesis also may be involved in the antihypertensive action.

Indications

- Treatment of hypertension alone or in combination with thiazide-type diuretics
- Treatment of HF in stable patients in the first few days after MI
- To decrease the risk of MI, CVA, death from CV disease in patients 55 yr and older who are at risk for developing CAD

Contraindications and cautions

- Contraindicated with allergy to ramipril, pregnancy (embryocidal in preclinical studies).
- Use cautiously with impaired renal function, HF, salt or volume depletion, lactation.

Available forms

Capsules—1.25, 2.5, 5, 10 mg

Dosages

Adults

- *Hypertension:* Initial dose, 2.5 mg PO daily. Adjust dosage according to BP response, usually 2.5–20 mg/day as a single dose or in two equally divided doses. Discontinue diuretic 2–3 days before beginning therapy; if not possible, administer initial dose of 1.25 mg.
- *HF:* Initial dose, 2.5 mg PO bid; if patient becomes hypotensive, 1.25 mg PO bid may be used while adjusting up to target dose of 5 mg PO bid; increase dose every 3 wk until target dose is reached.
- *Decrease risk of CV events:* Initial dose, 2.5 mg PO once daily for 1 wk, then 5 mg PO once daily for next 3 wk; for maintenance, 10 mg PO daily.

Pediatric patients

Safety and efficacy not established.

Geriatric patients

Greater sensitivity to drug effects is possible.

Patients with renal impairment

Excretion is reduced in renal failure. Use smaller initial dose: 25% of normally used dose is suggested; for hypertension, 1.25 mg PO daily in patients with creatinine clearance less than 40 mL/min; dosage may be titrated upward until pressure is controlled or a maximum of 5 mg/day.

Pharmacokinetics

Route	Onset	Peak	Duration
Oral	1–2 hr	1–4 hr	24 hr

Metabolism: Hepatic; $T_{1/2}$: 13–17 hr
Distribution: Crosses placenta; enters breast milk
Excretion: Feces, urine

Adverse effects

- **CV:** *Tachycardia,* angina pectoris, HF, MI, Raynaud's syndrome, hypotension in salt- or volume-depleted patients, syncope
- **Dermatologic:** *Rash,* pemphigoid-like reaction, *pruritus,* photosensitivity, erythema multiforme, **Stevens-Johnson syndrome**
- **GI:** *Gastric irritation, aphthous ulcers, dysgeusia,* cholestatic jaundice, hepatocellular injury, anorexia, constipation, pancreatitis
- **GU:** *Proteinuria,* renal insufficiency, renal failure, polyuria, oliguria, urinary frequency
- **Hematologic:** Neutropenia, agranulocytosis, thrombocytopenia, hemolytic anemia, **pancytopenia,** hyperkalemia
- **Other:** *Cough,* malaise, dry mouth, **angioedema**

Interactions

✱ **Drug-drug** • Exacerbation of cough if taken with capsaicin • Increased serum levels and increased toxicity with lithium; monitor patient closely

✱ **Drug-food** • Rate of absorption is reduced with food

✱ **Drug-lab test** • False-positive test for urine acetone

■ Nursing considerations

Assessment

- **History:** Allergy to ramipril, impaired renal function, HF, salt or volume depletion, pregnancy, lactation
- **Physical:** Skin color, lesions, turgor; T; P, BP, peripheral perfusion; mucous membranes, bowel sounds, liver evaluation; urinalysis, LFTs, renal function tests, CBC and differential

Interventions

⊗ ***Black box warning*** Do not use during pregnancy; risk of fetal harm. Advise use of a contraceptive.

- Discontinue diuretic for 2–3 days before beginning therapy, if possible, to avoid severe hypotensive effect.
- Open capsules and sprinkle contents over a small amount of applesauce or mix in applesauce or water if patient has difficulty swallowing capsules. Mixture is stable for 24 hr at room temperature and 48 hr if refrigerated.

⊗ ***Warning*** Alert surgeon and mark chart that ramipril is being used; the angiotensin II formation subsequent to compensatory renin release during surgery will be blocked; hypotension may be reversed with volume expansion.

- Monitor patient closely for falling BP secondary to reduction in fluid volume (excessive perspiration and dehydration, vomiting, diarrhea) because excessive hypotension may occur.
- Reduce dosage in patients with impaired renal function.

Teaching points

- Do not stop taking without consulting your health care provider.
- Be careful in any situation that may lead to a drop in blood pressure (diarrhea, sweating, vomiting, dehydration); if dizziness or light-headedness occurs, consult your health care provider.
- Avoid becoming pregnant while taking this drug; use of a contraceptive is advised.
- You may experience these side effects: GI upset, loss of appetite, change in taste perception (transient); mouth sores (frequent mouth care may help); rash; fast heart rate; dizziness, light-headedness (transient; change position slowly, and limit your activities to those that do not require alertness and precision).
- Report mouth sores; sore throat, fever, chills; swelling of the hands, feet; irregular heartbeat, chest pains; swelling of the face, eyes, lips, tongue; difficulty breathing.

▽ranibizumab

See Appendix W, *Less commonly used drugs*.

▽ranitidine hydrochloride

*(ra **nye'** te deen)*

Apo-Ranitidine (CAN), CO Ranitidine (CAN), Gen-Ranitidine (CAN), Novo-Ranidine, (CAN), Nu-Ranit (CAN), PMS-Ranitidine (CAN), ratio-Ranitidine (CAN), Zantac, Zantac EFFERdose, Zantac GELdose, Zantac 75, Zantac 150

PREGNANCY CATEGORY B

Drug class

Histamine-2 (H_2) antagonist

Therapeutic actions

Competitively inhibits the action of histamine at the H_2 receptors of the parietal cells of the stomach, inhibiting basal gastric acid secretion and gastric acid secretion that is stimulated by food, insulin, histamine, cholinergic agonists, gastrin, and pentagastrin.

Indications

- Short-term treatment of active duodenal ulcer
- Maintenance therapy for duodenal ulcer at reduced dosage
- Short-term treatment and maintenance therapy of active, benign gastric ulcer
- Short-term treatment of GERD
- Pathologic hypersecretory conditions (eg, Zollinger-Ellison syndrome) (adults only)
- Treatment of erosive esophagitis
- Treatment of heartburn, acid indigestion, sour stomach

Contraindications and cautions

- Contraindicated with allergy to ranitidine, lactation.
- Use cautiously with impaired renal or hepatic function, pregnancy.

Available forms

Tablets—75, 150, 300 mg; capsules—150, 300 mg; effervescent tablets and granules—25, 150 mg; syrup—15 mg/mL; injection—1, 25 mg/mL

Dosages

Adults

- *Active duodenal ulcer:* 150 mg bid PO for 4–8 wk. Alternatively, 300 mg PO once daily at bedtime or 50 mg IM or IV every 6–8 hr *or* by intermittent IV infusion, diluted to 100 mL and infused over 15–20 min. Do not exceed 400 mg/day.
- *Maintenance therapy, duodenal ulcer:* 150 mg PO at bedtime.
- *Maintenance therapy, gastric ulcer:* 150 mg PO at bedtime.
- *Active gastric ulcer:* 150 mg bid PO *or* 50 mg IM or IV every 6–8 hr.
- *Pathologic hypersecretory syndrome:* 150 mg bid PO. Individualize the dose with patient's response. Do not exceed 6 g/day.
- *GERD, esophagitis, benign gastric ulcer:* 150 mg bid PO.
- *Treatment of heartburn, acid indigestion:* 75 mg PO as needed.

Pediatric patients 1 mo–16 yr

Injection: 2–4 mg/kg/day IV or IM every 6–8 hr to a maximum of 50 mg every 6–8 hr.

Geriatric patients or patients with impaired renal function

For creatinine clearance less than 50 mL/min, accumulation may occur; use lowest dose possible, 150 mg every 24 hr PO or 50 mg IM or IV every 18–24 hr. Dosing may be increased to every 12 hr if patient tolerates it and blood levels are monitored.

Pharmacokinetics

Route	*Onset*	*Peak*	*Duration*
Oral	Varies	1–3 hr	8–12 hr
IM	Rapid	15 min	8–12 hr
IV	Immediate	5–10 min	8–12 hr

Metabolism: Hepatic; $T_{1/2}$: 2–3 hr
Distribution: Crosses placenta; enters breast milk
Excretion: Urine

▼ IV FACTS

Preparation: For IV injection, dilute 50 mg in 0.9% sodium chloride injection, 5% or 10% dextrose injection, lactated Ringer's solution, 5% sodium bicarbonate injection to a volume of 20 mL; solution is stable for 48 hr at room temperature. For intermittent IV, use as follows: Dilute 50 mg in 100 mL of 5% dextrose injection or other compatible solution.
Infusion: Inject over 5 min or more; for intermittent infusion, infuse over 15–20 min; continuous infusion, 6.25 mg/hr.
Incompatibility: Do not mix with amphotericin B.

Adverse effects

- **CNS:** *Headache,* malaise, dizziness, somnolence, insomnia, vertigo
- **CV:** Tachycardia, bradycardia, PVCs (rapid IV administration)
- **Dermatologic:** *Rash,* alopecia
- **GI:** *Constipation, diarrhea, nausea, vomiting, abdominal pain,* hepatitis, increased ALT levels
- **GU:** Gynecomastia, impotence or decreased libido
- **Hematologic:** Leukopenia, granulocytopenia, thrombocytopenia, pancytopenia
- **Local:** *Pain at IM site, local burning or itching at IV site*
- **Other:** Arthralgias

Interactions

✱ **Drug-drug** • Increased effects of warfarin, TCAs; monitor patient closely and adjust dosage as needed

■ Nursing considerations

CLINICAL ALERT!
Name confusion has been reported between *Zantac* (ranitidine) and *Zyrtec* (cetirizine); use caution.

Assessment

- **History:** Allergy to ranitidine, impaired renal or hepatic function, lactation, pregnancy
- **Physical:** Skin lesions; orientation, affect; pulse, baseline ECG; liver evaluation, abdominal examination, normal output; CBC, LFTs, renal function tests

Interventions

- Administer oral drug with meals and at bedtime.
- Decrease doses in renal and liver failure.
- Provide concurrent antacid therapy to relieve pain.

R

- Administer IM dose undiluted, deep into large muscle group.
- Arrange for regular follow-up, including blood tests, to evaluate effects.

Teaching points

- Take drug with meals and at bedtime. Therapy may continue for 4–6 weeks or longer.
- If you also are using an antacid, take it exactly as prescribed, being careful of the times of administration.
- Have regular medical follow-up care to evaluate your response.
- You may experience these side effects: Constipation or diarrhea (request aid from your health care provider); nausea, vomiting (take drug with meals); enlargement of breasts, impotence or decreased libido (reversible); headache (adjust lights and temperature and avoid noise).
- Report sore throat, fever, unusual bruising or bleeding, tarry stools, confusion, hallucinations, dizziness, severe headache, muscle or joint pain.

▽ranolazine

(ran oh' lah zeen)

Ranexa DNC

PREGNANCY CATEGORY C

Drug classes

Antianginal
Piperazineacetamide

Therapeutic actions

Antianginal, anti-ischemic. Mechanism of action is not known. Prolongs the QT interval; does not decrease HR or BP; decreases myocardial workload.

Indications

- Treatment of chronic angina as first-line therapy or in patients who have not responded adequately to other antianginal drugs; used with amlodipine, beta blockers, nitrates

Contraindications and cautions

- Contraindicated with hypersensitivity to any component of the drug; preexisting QT prolongation, concurrent use of QT-interval prolonging drugs; hepatic impairment; concurrent use of potent or moderately potent CYP3A inhibitors, including diltiazem; lactation.
- Use cautiously with severe renal impairment, history of ventricular tachycardia, pregnancy.

Available forms

ER tablets DNC—500, 1,000 mg

Dosages

Adults

500 mg PO bid; may be increased to maximum of 1,000 mg bid.

Pediatric patients

Safety and efficacy not established.

Patients with hepatic impairment

Not recommended with mild, moderate, or severe hepatic impairment.

Pharmacokinetics

Route	*Onset*	*Peak*
Oral	Rapid	2–5 hr

Metabolism: Hepatic; $T_{1/2}$: 7 hr
Distribution: May cross placenta; may pass into breast milk
Excretion: Urine, feces

Adverse effects

- **CNS:** *Dizziness, headache,* tinnitus, vertigo
- **CV:** Palpitations, peripheral edema, **prolonged QT interval**
- **GI:** *Nausea, constipation,* dry mouth, vomiting, abdominal pain
- **Respiratory:** Dyspnea

Interactions

✱ **Drug-drug** • Risk of increased serum level and toxicity of ranolazine if combined with ketoconazole, diltiazem, verapamil, macrolide antibiotics, HIV protease inhibitors; avoid these combinations • Risk of increased serum digoxin level if taken concurrently; digoxin dosage may need to be decreased • Monitor patients receiving TCAs; antipsychotics or other drugs known to prolong QT interval concurrently; may need lower doses of these drugs

✱ **Drug-food** • Risk of toxic effects if combined with grapefruit juice; avoid drinking grapefruit juice while on ranolazine

■ Nursing considerations

Assessment

- **History:** Allergy to any component of the tablet, preexisting QT-interval prolongation, concurrent use of QT-interval prolonging drugs, hepatic impairment, concurrent use of potent or moderately potent CYP3A inhibitors, renal failure, pregnancy, lactation.
- **Physical:** Orientation, reflexes; BP; respiratory evaluation; baseline ECG, LFTs, and renal function tests

Interventions

- Obtain baseline ECG, LFTs, and renal function tests before starting therapy.
- Ensure that patient swallows tablets whole; do not cut, crush, or let patient chew the tablets.
- Ensure that patient continues to use other prescribed antianginal medications.
- Advise patient to avoid grapefruit juice and grapefruit products while using this drug.
- Suggest use of contraceptive measures while taking this drug; potential effects on a fetus are not known.
- Advise nursing mothers that another method of feeding the baby will be needed while taking this drug.
- Provide safety measures if dizziness and light-headedness occur.

Teaching points

- Take this drug twice a day. Swallow the tablet whole; do not cut, crush, or chew it.
- If you miss a dose of the daily medication, take it as soon as you remember and then return to your usual routine. Do not take more than two doses in one day.
- Do not take this drug for an acute anginal attack; this drug helps chronic chest pain. Continue to use your other angina drugs as prescribed.
- You may be asked to have periodic ECGs and blood tests to monitor the effects of this drug on your body.
- Do not consume grapefruit juice or grapefruit products while taking this drug.
- It is not known how this drug could affect a nursing baby. If you are nursing a baby, you should select another method of feeding the baby.
- It is not known how this drug could affect a fetus. If you are pregnant or decide to become pregnant while on this drug, consult your health care provider.
- You may experience these side effects: Dizziness, light-headedness (if this occurs, avoid driving a car or operating dangerous machinery); headache, constipation (consult your health care provider because medications may be available to help).
- Report palpitations, fainting spells, severe constipation.

▽ rasagiline

(raz ah' gah leen)

Azilect

PREGNANCY CATEGORY C

Drug classes

Antiparkinsonian
MAO type B inhibitor

Therapeutic actions

Inhibits MAO type B (found mostly in the CNS), leading to increased levels of dopamine at the synapse particularly in areas of the brain responsible for controlling movement and coordination; much less effect in the periphery leads to fewer peripheral adverse effects.

Indications

- Treatment of signs and symptoms of idiopathic Parkinson's disease as initial monotherapy and as adjunct therapy with levodopa

Contraindications and cautions

- Contraindicated with known hypersensitivity to any component of the drug; concurrent use of meperdine, tramadol, methadone, propoxyphere, detromethorphan, sympathomimetic amines, MAOIs, SSRIs, TCAs; elective surgery; pheochromocytomas; diets rich in tyramine; severe hepatic insufficiency.

R

- Use cautiously with mild hepatic insufficiency, pregnancy, lactation, use of other CYP1A2 inhibitors.

Available forms
Tablets—0.5, 1 mg

Dosages
Adults
Initial monotherapy: 1 mg/day PO.
Adjunct therapy with levodopa: 0.5 mg/day PO; if response is insufficient, may increase to 1 mg/day PO. In some patients, levodopa dose may need to be decreased. Monitor patient response closely.
Patients with hepatic impairment
In mild hepatic impairment, 0.5 mg/day PO; not recommended in moderate to severe hepatic impairment.
Patients taking CYP1A2 inhibitors (such as ciprofloxacin)
0.5 mg/day PO.
Pediatric patients
Safety and efficacy not established.

Pharmacokinetics

Route	*Onset*	*Peak*
Oral	Rapid	1 hr

Metabolism: Hepatic; $T_{1/2}$: 3 hr
Distribution: May cross placenta; may pass into breast milk
Excretion: Urine

Adverse effects
- **CNS:** *Headache,* conjunctivitis, depression, paresthesia, vertigo
- **CV:** *Hypotension*
- **GI:** *Dyspepsia, dry mouth,* gastroenteritis
- **Respiratory:** Rhinitis
- **Other:** *Arthralgia,* flulike symptoms, fever, arthritis, malaise, neck pain, weight loss, bruising, **melanoma**

Interactions
✱ Drug-drug ⊗ ***Warning*** Risk of severe reaction if combined with meperidine or other analgesics including tramadol, propoxyphene, methadone; avoid these combinations. • Risk of psychosis or bizarre behavior when combined with dextromethorphan, mirtazapine, cyclobenzaprine; avoid these combinations • Risk of hypertensive crisis if combined with sympathomimetic amines, MAOIs; avoid these combinations • Risk of hyperpyrexia when combined with some antidepressants (SSRIs, TCAs); monitor patient closely if these combinations are used • Risk of increased rasagiline levels in patients taking other CYP1A2 inhibitors, such as ciprofloxacin; reduce dose of rasagiline if this combination is used
✱ Drug-alternative therapy ⊗ ***Warning*** Risk of serious reaction if combined with St. John's wort; avoid this combination.
✱ Drug-food ⊗ ***Warning*** Risk of hypertensive crisis with ingestion of tyramine-rich foods or beverages or dietary supplements containing amines.

■ Nursing considerations
Assessment
- **History:** Allergy to any component of the drug; concurrent use of meperidine, tramadol, methadone, propoxyphene, dextromethorphan, sympathomimetic amines, MAOIs, SSRIs, TCAs, other CYP1A2 inhibitors; elective surgery; pheochromocytomas; diets rich in tyramine; hepatic insufficiency; pregnancy, lactation
- **Physical:** T; skin evaluation, lesions; orientation, reflexes, grip strength, gait; BP; LFTs

Interventions
- Obtain LFTs and skin evaluation, preferably by a dermatologist, before and periodically during therapy.

⊗ ***Warning*** Ensure that patient has a list of tyramine-containing foods and understands the importance of avoiding them; hypertensive crisis could occur.

- Ensure that patient continues to use other medications for Parkinson's disease as prescribed.
- Instruct patient and a significant other in the warning signs of a hypertensive crisis.
- Advise patient to avoid use of any other medications, including OTC products and herbal therapies, without consulting a health care provider.
- Provide safety measures if dizziness and lightheadedness occur.

Teaching points

- Take this drug once a day as prescribed.
- If you miss a dose of the daily medication, take it as soon as you remember and then return to your usual routine. Do not take more than one dose in one day.
- Inspect your skin regularly for lesions, moles, and other changes. Melanoma occurs more often in patients with Parkinson's disease. Consult a dermatologist for a baseline report and periodically during therapy.
- If you also take levodopa, you may experience a worsening of your tremor and a drop in blood pressure when you stand. Notify your health care provider if this occurs; a dosage adjustment may be possible.
- You will need to avoid large amounts of food rich in tyramine while taking this drug and for 2 weeks after finishing it. Tyramine-containing foods and beverages include aged or smoked meats or fish, aged cheeses, concentrated yeast extract, and beers and wines that have not been pasteurized.
- It is not known how this drug could affect a fetus. If you are pregnant or decide to become pregnant while on this drug, consult your health care provider.
- It is not known how this drug could affect a nursing baby. If you are nursing a baby, consult your health care provider.
- This drug interacts with many other drugs and could cause serious side effects; do not take any other drug, including over-the-counter drugs and herbal therapies, until you have checked with your health care provider.
- You may experience these side effects: Vertigo, light-headedness (avoid driving a car or operating dangerous machinery); headache (consult your health care provider; medications may be available to help); dry mouth, upset stomach (frequent mouth care, sugar-free lozenges may help).
- Report severe headache, dizziness, blurred vision, difficulty thinking, changes in your skin, chest pain, worsening of your condition.

rasburicase

See Appendix X, *Less commonly used drugs*.

DANGEROUS DRUG

repaglinide

*(re **pag'** lah nyde)*

Prandin

PREGNANCY CATEGORY C

Drug classes

Antidiabetic
Meglitinide

Therapeutic actions

Closes potassium channels in the beta cells of the pancreas, which causes the opening of calcium channels and a resultant increase in insulin release; highly selective for beta cells in the pancreas. Glucose-lowering abilities depend on the existence of functioning beta cells in the pancreas.

Indications

- Adjunct to diet and exercise to lower blood glucose in patients with type 2 diabetes mellitus whose hyperglycemia cannot be managed by diet and exercise alone
- Combination therapy with metformin or thiazolidinediones to lower blood glucose in patients whose hyperglycemia cannot be controlled by diet and exercise plus monotherapy with any of the following agents alone: Metformin, sulfonylureas, or thiazolidinediones

Contraindications and cautions

- Contraindicated with hypersensitivity to the drug, diabetic ketoacidosis, type 1 diabetes.
- Use cautiously with renal or hepatic impairment, pregnancy, lactation.

Available forms

Tablets—0.5, 1, 2 mg

Dosages

Adults

0.5–4 mg PO taken tid or qid 15–30 min (usually within 15 min) before meals; determine dosage based on patient response; maximum dose is 16 mg/day. Monitor patient regularly and adjust dosage as needed, waiting 1 wk between dose adjustments to assess patient response.

Pediatric patients
Safety and efficacy not established.

Patients with renal or hepatic impairment
For severe renal impairment, use starting dose of 0.5 mg PO and titrate carefully. Use cautiously with hepatic impairment; monitor closely.

Pharmacokinetics

Route	Onset	Peak
Oral	Rapid	1 hr

Metabolism: Hepatic; $T_{1/2}$: 1 hr
Distribution: May cross placenta; may enter breast milk
Excretion: Feces, urine

Adverse effects
- **CNS:** *Headache,* paresthesias
- **Endocrine:** *Hypoglycemia*
- **GI:** Nausea, diarrhea, constipation, vomiting, dyspepsia
- **Respiratory:** *URI,* sinusitis, rhinitis, bronchitis

Interactions
✱ **Drug-drug** ⊗ ***Warning*** Risk of severe hypoglycemia if combined with both gemfibrozil and itraconazole; avoid this combination. • Risk of hypoglycemia if combined with gemfibrozil; use caution; monitor patient closely

✱ **Drug-alternative therapy** • Increased risk of hypoglycemia if taken with juniper berries, ginseng, garlic, fenugreek, coriander, dandelion root, celery

■ Nursing considerations
Assessment
- **History:** Hypersensitivity to the drug, diabetic ketoacidosis, type 1 diabetes, renal or hepatic impairment, pregnancy, lactation
- **Physical:** Skin color, lesions; T; orientation, reflexes, peripheral sensation; R, adventitious sounds; liver evaluation, bowel sounds; blood glucose, LFTs, renal function tests

Interventions
- Administer drug before meals; if a patient skips or adds a meal, the dosage should be skipped or added appropriately.
- Monitor urine or serum glucose levels frequently to determine effectiveness of drug and dosage being used.
- Arrange for consult with dietitian to establish weight loss program and dietary control as appropriate.
- Arrange for thorough diabetic teaching program to include disease, dietary control, exercise, signs and symptoms of hypoglycemia and hyperglycemia, avoidance of infection, hygiene.

Teaching points
- Do not discontinue this medication without consulting your health care provider.
- Take this drug before meals (three to four times a day); if you skip a meal, skip the dose; if you add a meal, take a dose before that meal also.
- Monitor urine or blood for glucose and ketones as prescribed.
- Return for regular follow-up and monitoring of your response to the drug and possible need for dosage adjustment.
- Continue diet and exercise program established for control of diabetes.
- Know the signs and symptoms of hypoglycemia and hyperglycemia and appropriate treatment as indicated; report the occurrence of either to your health care provider.
- You may experience these side effects: Headache, increased upper respiratory infections, nausea.
- Report fever, sore throat, unusual bleeding or bruising, severe abdominal pain.

▽ribavirin
*(rye ba **vye'** rin)*

Copegus, Rebetol, RibaPak, Ribasphere, Ribatab, Virazole

PREGNANCY CATEGORY X

Drug class
Antiviral

Therapeutic actions
Antiviral activity against RSV, influenza virus, hepatitis C virus, and HSV; mechanism of action is not known.

Indications

- Aerosol: Treatment of carefully selected hospitalized infants and children with severe RSV infection of lower respiratory tract
- Oral: Treatment of chronic hepatitis C in combination with peginterferon alfa 2a (*Pegasys*) or interferon alfa-2b (*Intron A*) in patients 3 yr or older with compensated liver disease untreated with or refractory to alfa interferon therapy
- With *Pegasys*, treatment of adults with hepatitis C who have compensated liver disease and no previous alfa interferon therapy
- Orphan drug use: Treatment of hemorrhagic fever with renal syndrome
- Unlabeled use for aerosol: Treatment of some influenza A and B infections
- Unlabeled uses of oral preparation: Treatment of some viral diseases, including herpes genitalis, measles, Lassa fever

Contraindications and cautions

- Contraindicated with allergy to drug product, COPD, pregnancy or male whose female partner is pregnant (causes fetal damage), lactation.
- Use cautiously with renal impairment, respiratory dysfunction.

Available forms

Capsules—200 mg; oral solution—40 mg/mL; powder for aerosol reconstitution—6 g/100 mL vial; tablets—200, 400, 600 mg

Dosages

Adults

Weighing 75 kg or less: Two 200-mg capsules PO in the AM, three 200-mg capsules PO in the PM with *Intron A,* 3 million international units subcutaneously three times per wk; or with 180 mcg *Pegasys* subcutaneously per wk for 48 wk.
Weighing more than 75 kg: Three 200-mg capsules PO in AM, three 200-mg capsules PO in PM with 3 million international units *Intron A,* subcutaneously three times per wk; or with 180 mcg *Pegasys* subcutaneously per wk for 48 wk.

Pediatric patients

Aerosol

For use only with small-particle aerosol generator. Check operating instructions carefully. Dilute aerosol powder to 20 mg/mL and deliver for 12–18 hr/day for at least 3 but not more than 7 days.

Oral

15 mg/kg/day PO in divided doses AM and PM. Children 25 kg or more who cannot swallow tablets may use oral solution. Give with interferon alfa-2b (*Intron A*), 3 million international units/m^2, subcutaneously three times per wk.

Patients with anemia as manifested by decrease in Hgb

No cardiac disease, Hgb less than 10 g/dL: Decrease to 600 mg daily (one 200-mg capsule in AM; two 200-mg capsules in PM); 7.5 mg/kg/day PO for children.
No cardiac disease, Hgb less than 8.5 g/dL: Discontinue ribavirin.
Cardiac disease, Hgb decreased by 2 g/dL or more during any 4-wk period of treatment: Decrease to 600 mg daily (one 200-mg capsule in AM; two 200-mg capsules in PM); 7.5 mg/kg/day PO for children.
Cardiac history, Hgb less than 12 g/dL after 4 wk of decreased dose: Discontinue ribavirin.
Patients with hepatitis C and HIV coinfection: 800 mg/day PO ribavirin with 180 mcg *Pegasys* by subcutaneous injection once each wk for 48 wk.
Patients with renal impairment: Do not use if creatinine clearance is less than 50 mL/min.

Pharmacokinetics

Route	Onset	Peak
Aerosol	Slow	60–90 min

Metabolism: Cellular; $T_{1/2}$: 9.5 hr (aerosol)
Distribution: Crosses placenta; enters breast milk
Excretion: Feces, urine

Adverse effects

- **CNS:** Depression, suicidal behavior, nervousness
- **CV: Cardiac arrest,** hypotension
- **Dermatologic:** Rash
- **Hematologic:** Anemia
- **Respiratory:** *Deteriorating respiratory function,* pneumothorax, apnea, bacterial pneumonia
- **Other:** Conjunctivitis, testicular lesions

R

Interactions

✱ **Drug-drug** • Decreased levels of ribavirin when given with antacids; avoid with nucleoside reverse transcriptase inhibitors

■ Nursing considerations

Assessment

- **History:** Allergy to drug product, COPD, pregnancy, lactation
- **Physical:** Skin rashes, lesions; P, BP, auscultation; R, adventitious sounds; Hct

Interventions

- Ensure proper use of small-particle aerosol generator; check operating instructions carefully.
- Ensure that water used as diluent contains no other substance.
- Replace solution in the unit every 24 hr.
- Store reconstituted solution at room temperature.
- For patients on mechanical ventilators, clean and check tubing to prevent accumulation of drug and malfunction of the machine.

⊗ ***Black box warning*** Inhaled form of drug is not for use in adults; testicular lesions, birth defects can occur.

⊗ ***Black box warning*** Ribavirin monotherapy is not effective for the treatment of chronic hepatitis C and should not be used alone for this indication.

⊗ ***Black box warning*** Use of this drug makes patients at high risk for hemolytic anemia, which could lead to MI; do not use in patients with significant or unstable CV disease.

⊗ ***Black box warning*** Monitor respiratory status frequently; pulmonary deterioration and death have occurred during and shortly after treatment with inhalation product.

⊗ ***Black box warning*** Risk of significant fetal defects exists. Caution women to avoid pregnancy while using this drug; use of barrier contraceptives is advised; male partners of pregnant women should not take this drug.

⊗ ***Warning*** Use extreme caution in adults with history of depression or psychiatric disorders.

- Monitor BP and P frequently.

Teaching points

- Explain the use of small-particle aerosol generator to patient or family.
- Take capsules or tablets in morning and evening; mark calendar with days to inject *Intron A* or *Pegasys* as appropriate.
- Avoid pregnancy while taking this drug; using barrier contraceptives is advised; male partners of pregnant women should avoid intercourse.
- Report depression, suicidal ideation, difficulty breathing, muscle pain, dizziness, confusion, shortness of breath (pediatric patients).

▽ rifabutin

See Appendix W, *Less commonly used drugs*.

▽ rifampin

(rif' am pin)

Rifadin, Rimactane, Rofact (CAN)

PREGNANCY CATEGORY C

Drug classes

Antibiotic
Antituberculotic (first-line)

Therapeutic actions

Inhibits DNA-dependent RNA polymerase activity in susceptible bacterial cells.

Indications

- Treatment of pulmonary TB in conjunction with at least one other effective antituberculotic
- *Neisseria meningitidis* carriers, for asymptomatic carriers to eliminate meningococci from nasopharynx; not for treatment of meningitis
- Unlabeled uses: Infections caused by *Staphylococcus aureus* and *Staphylococcus epidermis*, usually in combination therapy; gram-negative bacteremia in infancy; Legionella (*Legionella pneumophila*) not responsive to erythromycin; leprosy (in combination with dapsone); prophylaxis of meningitis caused by *Haemophilus influenzae*

Contraindications and cautions

- Contraindicated with allergy to any rifamycin, acute hepatic disease, lactation.
- Use cautiously with pregnancy (teratogenic effects have been reported in preclinical studies; safest antituberculous regimen for use in pregnancy is considered to be rifampin, isoniazid, and ethambutol).

Available forms

Capsules—150, 300 mg; powder for injection—600 mg

Dosages

Adults

- *Pulmonary TB:* 10 mg/kg/day; not to exceed 600 mg in a single daily dose PO or IV (used in conjunction with other antituberculotics). Continue therapy until bacterial conversion and maximal improvement occur.
- *Meningococcal carriers:* 600 mg PO or IV once daily for 4 consecutive days or 600 mg every 12 hr for 2 days.

Pediatric patients

- *Pulmonary TB:*
  Older than 5 yr: 10–20 mg/kg/day PO or IV not to exceed 600 mg/day.
- *Meningococcal carriers:*
  Younger than 1 mo: 5 mg/kg PO or IV every 12 hr for 2 days.
  Older than 1 mo: 10 mg/kg PO or IV every 12 hr for 2 days, do not exceed 600 mg/dose.

Pharmacokinetics

Route	*Onset*	*Peak*
Oral	Varies	1–4 hr
IV	Rapid	End of infusion

Metabolism: Hepatic; $T_{1/2}$: 3–5.1 hr
Distribution: Crosses placenta; enters breast milk
Excretion: Bile, urine

IV FACTS

Preparation: Reconstitute by transferring 10 mL sterile water for injection to vial containing 600 mg rifampin; swirl gently. Resultant fluid contains 60 mg/mL; stable at room temperature. Further mix with 500–1,000 mL of dextrose 5% or sterile saline.
Infusion: Infuse over 30–180 min, depending on volume.

Adverse effects

- **CNS:** *Headache, drowsiness, fatigue, dizziness,* inability to concentrate, mental confusion, generalized numbness, ataxia, muscle weakness, visual disturbances, exudative conjunctivitis
- **Dermatologic:** *Rash,* pruritus, urticaria, pemphigoid reaction, flushing, reddish-orange discoloration of body fluids—tears, saliva, urine, sweat, sputum
- **GI:** *Heartburn, epigastric distress,* anorexia, nausea, vomiting, gas, cramps, diarrhea, pseudomembranous colitis, pancreatitis, *elevations of liver enzymes,* hepatitis
- **GU:** Hemoglobinuria, hematuria, renal insufficiency, **acute renal failure,** menstrual disturbances
- **Hematologic:** *Eosinophilia, thrombocytopenia, transient leukopenia,* hemolytic anemia, decreased Hgb, hemolysis
- **Other:** Pain in extremities, osteomalacia, myopathy, fever, *flulike symptoms*

Interactions

✱ Drug-drug • Increased incidence of rifampin-related hepatitis with isoniazid • Decreased concentrations of itraconazole • Decreased effectiveness of metoprolol, propranolol, antiarrhythmics, benzodiazepine, buspirone, cyclosporine, digoxin, doxycycline, fluoroquinolones, nifedipine, zolpidem, quinidine, corticosteroids, hormonal contraceptives, methadone, oral anticoagulants, oral sulfonylureas, theophyllines, phenytoin, cyclosporine, ketoconazole, verapamil
✱ Drug-lab test • Rifampin inhibits standard assays for serum folate and vitamin B_{12}

■ Nursing considerations

Assessment

- **History:** Allergy to any rifamycin, acute hepatic disease, pregnancy, lactation
- **Physical:** Skin color, lesions; T; gait, muscle strength; orientation, reflexes, ophthalmologic examination; liver evaluation; CBC, LFTs, renal function tests, urinalysis

Interventions

- Administer on an empty stomach, 1 hr before or 2 hr after meals.
- Administer in a single daily dose.
- Consult pharmacist for rifampin suspension for patients unable to swallow capsules.
- Prepare patient for the reddish-orange coloring of body fluids (urine, sweat, sputum, tears, feces, saliva); soft contact lenses may be permanently stained; advise patients not to wear them during therapy.

⊗ ***Warning*** Arrange for follow-up visits for liver and renal function tests, CBC, and ophthalmologic examinations.

Teaching points

- Take drug in a single daily dose. Take on an empty stomach, 1 hour before or 2 hours after meals.
- Take this drug regularly; avoid missing any doses; do not discontinue this drug without consulting your health care provider.
- Have periodic medical checkups, including eye examinations and blood tests, to evaluate the drug effects.
- You may experience these side effects: Reddish orange coloring of body fluids (tears, sweat, saliva, urine, feces, sputum; stain will wash out of clothing, but soft contact lenses may be permanently stained; do not wear them); nausea, vomiting, epigastric distress; skin rashes or lesions; numbness, tingling, drowsiness, fatigue (use caution if driving or operating dangerous machinery; use precautions to avoid injury).
- Report fever, chills, muscle and bone pain, excessive tiredness or weakness, loss of appetite, nausea, vomiting, yellowing of skin or eyes, unusual bleeding or bruising, skin rash or itching.

▽ rifapentine

*(rif ah **pin'** ten)*

Priftin

PREGNANCY CATEGORY C

Drug classes

Antibiotic
Antituberculotic

Therapeutic actions

Inhibits DNA-dependent RNA polymerase activity in susceptible strains of *Mycobacterium tuberculosis,* causing cell death.

Indications

- Treatment of pulmonary TB in conjunction with at least one other effective antituberculotic
- Orphan drug use: Prophylaxis and treatment of *Mycobacterium avium* complex in patients with AIDS

Contraindications and cautions

- Contraindicated with allergy to any rifamycin, acute hepatic disease.
- Use cautiously with pregnancy (teratogenic effects have been reported in preclinical studies), lactation, hepatic impairment.

Available forms

Tablets—150 mg

Dosages

Adults

- *TB, intensive phase:* 600 mg PO twice weekly with an interval of at least 72 hr between doses; continue for 2 mo. Always give rifapentine in combination with other antituberculotics.
- *Continuation phase:* 600 mg PO once a wk for 4 mo in combination with other agents to which the organism is susceptible.

Pediatric patients

Safety and efficacy not established in patients younger than 12 yr.

Pharmacokinetics

Route	*Onset*	*Peak*
Oral	Slow	5–6 hr

Metabolism: Hepatic; $T_{1/2}$: 13.19 hr
Distribution: May cross placenta; may enter breast milk
Excretion: Feces, urine

Adverse effects

- **CNS:** *Headache, dizziness*
- **Dermatologic:** Pruritus, acne
- **GI:** Nausea, vomiting, diarrhea, cramps
- **GU:** *Pyuria, proteinuria, hematuria*

- **Hematologic:** *Hyperuricemia,* liver enzyme elevations
- **Other:** Pain, arthralgia, *reddish discoloration of body fluids*

Interactions

✱ **Drug-drug** • Decreased effectiveness of protease inhibitors; use extreme caution if this combination is needed; try to avoid this combination • Decreased effectiveness of rifampin if taken with p-aminosalicylic acid, ketoconazole—give the drugs at least 8–12 hr apart • Decreased effectiveness of metoprolol, propranolol, quinidine, corticosteroids, hormonal contraceptives, methadone, oral anticoagulants, oral sulfonylureas, theophyllines, phenytoin, cyclosporine, ketoconazole, verapamil if taken concurrently with rifapentine; monitor patient carefully and adjust dosage as needed

✱ **Drug-lab test** • Rifapentine inhibits standard assays for serum folate and vitamin B_{12}

■ Nursing considerations

Assessment

- **History:** Allergy to any rifamycin, acute hepatic disease, pregnancy, lactation
- **Physical:** Skin color, lesions; T; gait, muscle strength; orientation, reflexes, CBC, LFTs, renal function tests, urinalysis

Interventions

- Administer on an empty stomach, 1 hr before 2 hr after meals; if GI upset is severe, drug may be taken with food.
- Always use in combination with other antituberculotics.
- Prepare patient for the reddish orange coloring of body fluids (urine, sweat, sputum, tears, feces, saliva); soft contact lenses may be permanently stained, patients should be advised not to wear them during drug therapy.
- Recommend the use of barrier contraceptives while using this drug; hormonal contraceptives may be ineffective.
- Provide small, frequent meals if GI upset occurs.
- Provide skin care if dermatologic effects occur.

Teaching points

- Take drug along with any other prescribed antituberculotics. Take on an empty stomach—1 hour before or 2 hours after meals. If your stomach is very upset by the drug, it may be taken with food.
- Take this drug regularly; avoid missing any doses; do not discontinue this drug without consulting your health care provider. Make sure doses are at least 72 hours apart.
- Avoid pregnancy while taking this drug, using barrier contraceptives is advised.
- Arrange to have periodic medical checkups, which will include blood tests to evaluate the drug effects.
- You may experience these side effects: Reddish orange coloring of body fluids (tears, sweat, saliva, urine, feces, sputum; this is an expected occurrence and is not dangerous, do not be alarmed—stain will wash out of clothing but soft contact lenses may be permanently stained, do not wear them when on this drug); nausea, vomiting, epigastric distress (consult your health care provider if any of these become too uncomfortable); skin rashes or lesions (consult your health care provider for appropriate skin care).
- Report fever, chills, muscle and bone pain, excessive tiredness or weakness, loss of appetite, yellowing of skin or eyes, unusual bleeding or bruising, skin rash or itching.

▽ rifaximin

*(reh **facks'** ah men)*

Xifaxan (DNC)

PREGNANCY CATEGORY C

Drug classes

Antibiotic
Antidiarrheal

Therapeutic actions

A structural analogue of rifampin; binds to bacterial DNA-dependent RNA polymerase and inhibits bacterial RNA synthesis. Ninety-seven percent passes through the GI tract unchanged; affects *Escherichia coli* in the GI tract; cause of most traveler's diarrhea.

Indications
- Treatment of patients 12 yr or older with traveler's diarrhea caused by noninvasive strains of *E. coli*
- Unlabeled uses: Hepatic encephalopathy, IBS

Contraindications and cautions
- Contraindicated with allergy to rifaximin, rifampin, or any component of the drug; diarrhea complicated by fever or blood in the stool or caused by pathogens other than *E. coli;* lactation.
- Use cautiously with pregnancy.

Available forms
Tablets (DNC)—200 mg

Dosages
Adults and patients 12 yr and older
200 mg PO tid for 3 days.
Pediatric patients younger than 12 yr
Safety and efficacy not established.

Pharmacokinetics

Route	
Oral	Not absorbed systemically

Metabolism: None; $T_{1/2}$: 5.4–6.2 hr
Distribution: May cross placenta; may enter breast milk
Excretion: Feces

Adverse effects
- **CNS:** Headache, dizziness
- **GI:** Diarrhea, flatulence, abdominal pain, rectal tenesmus, defecation urgency, constipation, vomiting, **pseudomembranous colitis**
- **Respiratory:** Rhinitis, cough, dyspnea, pharyngitis, bronchitis
- **Skin:** Allergic dermatitis, rash, urticaria, pruritus
- **Other:** *Fever,* angioneurotic edema

■ Nursing considerations
Assessment
- **History:** Allergy to rifaximin, rifampin or any component of the drug, diarrhea complicated by fever or blood in the stool or caused by pathogens other than *E. coli,* lactation, pregnancy
- **Physical:** Skin lesions; orientation, reflexes; abdominal examination

Interventions
- Administer three times a day with or without food; ensure that the tablet is swallowed whole.

⊗ ***Warning*** Do not administer if the patient has diarrhea complicated by fever or blood in the stool.

- Administer only to patients with traveler's diarrhea caused by *E. coli;* this drug is not effective for systemic bacterial infections because it is not absorbed.
- Encourage the use of barrier contraceptives during treatment with this drug; it is not known if this drug crosses the placenta.
- Find another method of feeding the baby if patient is nursing; it is not known if this enters breast milk.
- Discontinue drug if diarrhea persists for longer than 24–48 hr or worsens.
- Maintain other measures appropriate for traveler's diarrhea—avoidance of local water, pushing fluids to maintain hydration.

Teaching points
- Take this drug three times a day, with or without food, for the treatment of traveler's diarrhea.
- Swallow the tablet whole; do not cut, crush, or chew the tablets.
- If you forget a dose, take it as soon as you remember and return to your usual regimen. Do not make up doses and do not take more than three doses in 24 hours.
- Do not use this drug to treat any infection other than traveler's diarrhea; it is not absorbed into the bloodstream and is not effective in treating other infections.
- Stop taking the drug and notify your health care provider if a fever develops or blood in the diarrhea occurs, or if the diarrhea persists or worsens after 24–48 hours.
- Avoid pregnancy while taking this drug; if you suspect that you are pregnant, consult your health care provider.
- You should find another method of feeding the baby if you are nursing; it is not known if this drug enters breast milk.

- You may experience these side effects: Dizziness (if this occurs, do not drive a car or operate heavy machine until you know how you will be affected), flatulence, abdominal pain, nausea (try to maintain your hydration drinking bottled water or beverages).
- Report bloody diarrhea, fever, worsening diarrhea.

rilonacept

See Appendix W, *Less commonly used drugs*.

riluzole

See Appendix W, *Less commonly used drugs*.

rimantadine hydrochloride

*(ri **man'** ta deen)*

Flumadine

PREGNANCY CATEGORY C

Drug class
Antiviral

Therapeutic actions
Synthetic antiviral agent that inhibits viral replication, possibly by preventing the uncoating of the virus.

Indications
- Prophylaxis and treatment of illness caused by influenza A virus in adults
- Prophylaxis against influenza A virus in children

Contraindications and cautions
- Contraindicated with allergy to amantadine, rimantadine; lactation.
- Use cautiously with seizures, liver or renal disease, pregnancy.

Available forms
Tablets—100 mg; syrup—50 mg/5 mL

Dosages
Adults and patients older than 10 yr
- *Prophylaxis:* 100 mg/day PO bid.
- *Treatment:* Same dose as above; start treatment as soon after exposure as possible, continuing for 7 days from initial onset of symptoms.

Geriatric patients in nursing homes and patients with severe renal or hepatic impairment
Dose of 100 mg PO daily is recommended.

Pharmacokinetics

Route	*Onset*	*Peak*
Oral	Slow	6 hr

Metabolism: $T_{1/2}$: 25.4 hr
Distribution: May cross placenta; may enter breast milk
Excretion: Urine

Adverse effects
- **CNS:** *Light-headedness, dizziness, insomnia,* confusion, irritability, ataxia, psychosis, depression, hallucinations, seizures
- **CV:** HF, orthostatic hypotension, dyspnea
- **GI:** *Nausea,* anorexia, constipation, dry mouth

Interactions
✱ Drug-drug • Decreased effectiveness with acetaminophen, aspirin • Increased serum levels and effects with cimetidine • Intranasal influenza virus vaccine may interfere with rimantadine; do not vaccinate for 48 hr after rimantadine therapy is complete; do not administer rimantadine for 2 wk after intranasal influenza vaccine administration.

■ Nursing considerations
Assessment
- **History:** Allergy to amantadine, rimantadine; seizures; liver or renal disease; lactation
- **Physical:** Orientation, vision, speech, reflexes; BP, orthostatic BP, P, auscultation, perfusion, edema; R, adventitious sounds; urinary output; BUN, creatinine clearance

Interventions
- Administer full course of drug to achieve the beneficial antiviral effects. Initiate therapy

R

for treatment within 48 hr of onset of symptoms and continue for 7 days.

Teaching points

- You may experience these side effects: Drowsiness, blurred vision (use caution in driving or using dangerous equipment); dizziness, light-headedness (avoid sudden position changes); irritability or mood changes (common; if severe, request a drug change).
- Report swelling of the fingers or ankles, shortness of breath, difficulty urinating, tremors, slurred speech, difficulty walking.

risedronate sodium

*(rah **sed'** dro nate)*

Actonel

PREGNANCY CATEGORY C

Drug class

Bisphosphonate

Therapeutic actions

Affects osteoclast activity by reducing the enzymatic and transport processes that lead to resorption of the bone and by inhibiting the osteoclast proton pump, leading to a rate of bone turnover near normal in patients with Paget's disease.

Indications

- Treatment of Paget's disease of bone in patients with alkaline phosphatase at least two times the upper limit of normal, those who are symptomatic, those at risk for future complications
- Treatment and prevention of osteoporosis in postmenopausal women
- Treatment and prevention of glucocorticoid-induced osteoporosis
- To increase bone mass in men with osteoporosis

Contraindications and cautions

- Contraindicated with allergy to bisphosphonates; severe renal disease, hypocalcemia, inability to stand or sit upright for at least 30 min.
- Use cautiously with renal impairment, lactation, pregnancy.

Available forms

Tablets—5, 30, 35, 75, 150 mg

Dosages

Adults

- *Treatment and prevention of postmenopausal osteoporosis:* 5 mg PO once daily taken in an upright position with 6–8 oz of water at least 30 min before or after any other beverage or food. For postmenopausal osteoporosis, may switch to 35-mg tablet taken PO once per wk or 75 mg PO taken on 2 consecutive days each mo (total of 2 tablets per mo) or one 150-mg tablet PO per mo.
- *Treatment or prevention of glucocorticoid osteoporosis:* 5 mg/day PO.
- *Paget's disease:* 30 mg PO once daily for 2 mo taken in an upright position with 6–8 oz of plain water at least 30 min before or after any other beverage or food; may retreat after at least a 2-mo posttreatment period if indicated.
- *To increase bone mass in men with osteoporosis:* 35 mg PO once/wk.

Pediatric patients

Safety and efficacy not established.

Patients with renal impairment

Not recommended with creatinine clearance less than 30 mL/min; no dosage adjustment is needed if creatinine clearance greater than 30 mL/min.

Pharmacokinetics

Route	*Onset*	*Peak*
Oral	Rapid	1 hr

Metabolism: Not metabolized; $T_{1/2}$: Initial half-life: 1.5 hr; terminal half-life: 48 hr
Distribution: May cross placenta; may enter breast milk
Excretion: Urine

Adverse effects

- **CNS:** *Headache,* paresthesia, *dizziness*
- **CV:** Chest pain, edema, hypertension
- **EENT:** Glaucoma, conjunctivitis, cataract

- **GI:** *Nausea, diarrhea, dyspepsia,* abdominal pain, *anorexia*
- **Skeletal:** *Increased or recurrent bone pain,* osteonecrosis
- **Other:** *Arthralgia,* bone pain, leg cramps, *rash*

Interactions
✱ **Drug-drug** • Absorption of risedronate decreased by calcium, aspirin, aluminum, magnesium; avoid these drugs for 2 hr before to 2 hr after taking risedronate

■ Nursing considerations
Assessment
- **History:** Allergy to bisphosphonates, renal failure, hypocalcemia, pregnancy, lactation
- **Physical:** Muscle tone, bone pain; bowel sounds; eye examination; urinalysis, serum calcium; orientation, affect

Interventions
⊗ ***Warning*** Administer with a full glass of plain (not mineral) water, at least 30 min before or after any other beverage, food, or medication; have patient remain in an upright position for at least 30 min to decrease the incidence of GI effects. Patients taking weekly dose should mark calendar as a reminder.

- Monitor serum calcium levels before, during, and after therapy.

⊗ ***Warning*** Ensure at least a 2-mo rest period after 2-mo course of treatment if retreatment is required for Paget's disease.

- Ensure adequate vitamin D and calcium intake.
- Provide comfort measures if bone pain returns.

Teaching points
- Take this drug with a full glass of water (plain water, not mineral water), at least 30 minutes before or after any other beverage, foods, or medication; remain in an upright position for at least 30 minutes to decrease the GI side effects of the drug. If taking a once-weekly dose, mark a calendar as a reminder.
- Maintain adequate vitamin D and calcium intake while you are using this drug.
- You may experience these side effects: Nausea, diarrhea; bone pain, headache (analgesics may be available to help); rash (appropriate skin care will be suggested).
- Report twitching, muscle spasms, dark-colored urine, edema, bone pain, rash, difficulty swallowing.

▽ risperidone
*(ris **peer'** i dohn)*

Risperdal, Risperdal Consta, Risperdal M-TAB

PREGNANCY CATEGORY C

Drug classes
Antipsychotic
Benzisoxazole

Therapeutic actions
Mechanism of action not fully understood: Blocks dopamine and serotonin receptors in the brain, depresses the RAS; anticholinergic, antihistaminic, and alpha-adrenergic blocking activity may contribute to some of its therapeutic and adverse actions.

Indications
- Treatment of schizophrenia
- Delaying relapse in long-term treatment of schizophrenia
- Short-term treatment of acute manic or mixed episodes associated with bipolar 1 disorder; alone or in combination with lithium or valproate (oral only)
- **NEW INDICATION:** Long-acting injection used as monotherapy or as adjunct to lithium or valproate for maintenance treatment of bipolar 1 disorder (*Risperdal Consta*)
- Treatment of irritability (aggression, self-injury, temper tantrums, quickly changing moods) associated with autistic disorders in children and adolescents
- Unlabeled uses: Treatment of OCD refractory to SSRIs; treatment of tics in Tourette syndrome

Contraindications and cautions
- Contraindicated with hypersensitivity to risperidone, lactation.

R

- Use cautiously with CV disease, pregnancy, renal or hepatic impairment, hypotension.

Available forms

Tablets—0.25, 0.5, 1, 2, 3, 4 mg; oral solution—1 mg/mL; orally disintegrating tablets—0.5, 1, 2, 3, 4 mg; powder for injection—12.5, 25, 37.5, 50 mg

Dosages

Adults

Schizophrenia

- *Initial treatment:* 1 mg PO bid; then gradually increase with daily dosage increments of 1 mg bid on the second and third days to a target dose of 3 mg PO bid by the third day. Range, 4–8 mg/day or 25 mg IM every 2 wk; do not exceed 50 mg IM every 2 wk.
- *Reinitiation of treatment:* Follow initial dosage guidelines, using extreme care due to increased risk of severe adverse effects with reexposure.
- *Switching from other antipsychotics:* Minimize the overlap period and discontinue other antipsychotic before beginning risperidone therapy.
- *Delaying relapse time in long-term treatment:* 3 mg PO bid.

Bipolar 1 disorder

- *Long-term maintenance:* 25–30 mg IM every 2 wk.

Bipolar mania

- 2–3 mg/day PO as a once daily dose; range 1–6 mg/day.

Pediatric patients wtih irritability associated with autistic disorder

Initially, 0.25 mg/day PO for patients weighing less than 20 kg or 0.5 mg/day for patients 20 kg or more. After at least 4 days, may increase to 0.5 mg/day for patients less than 20 kg or 1 mg/day for patients 20 kg or more. Maintain dosage for at least 14 days; may then increase in increments of 0.25 mg/day (less than 20 kg) or 0.5 mg/day (20 kg or more) at 2-wk intervals. Dose may be divided; give at bedtime if somolence occurs.

Geriatric patients or patients with renal or hepatic impairment

Initial dose of 0.5 mg PO bid or 25 mg IM every 2 wk; monitor patient for adverse effects and response.

Pharmacokinetics

Route	Onset	Peak	Duration
Oral	Varies	3–17 hr	Weeks

Metabolism: Hepatic; $T_{1/2}$: 20 hr
Distribution: Crosses placenta; enters breast milk
Excretion: Feces, urine

Adverse effects

- **CNS:** *Insomnia, anxiety, agitation, headache,* somnolence, aggression, dizziness, tardive dyskinesias
- **CV:** Orthostatic hypotension, **arrhythmias**
- **Dermatologic:** Rash, dry skin, seborrhea, photosensitivity
- **GI:** *Nausea, vomiting, constipation,* abdominal discomfort, dry mouth, increased saliva
- **Respiratory:** Rhinitis, coughing, sinusitis, pharyngitis, dyspnea
- **Other:** Chest pain, arthralgia, back pain, fever, **NMS,** diabetes mellitus, hyperglycemia

Interactions

✷ **Drug-drug** • Increased therapeutic and toxic effects with clozapine • Decreased therapeutic effect with carbamazepine • Decreased effectiveness of levodopa

■ Nursing considerations

Assessment

- **History:** Allergy to risperidone, lactation, CV disease, pregnancy, renal or hepatic impairment, hypotension
- **Physical:** T, weight; reflexes, orientation; P, BP, orthostatic BP; R, adventitious sounds; bowel sounds, normal output, liver evaluation; CBC, urinalysis, LFTs, renal function tests

Interventions

⊠ ***Black box warning*** Do not use drug to treat geriatric patients with dementia; it increases risk of CV mortality; drug is not approved for this use.

⊗ ***Warning*** Maintain seizure precautions, especially when initiating therapy and increasing dosage.

⊗ ***Warning*** Administer oral solution directly from calibrated pipette or mix oral solution with 3–4 oz of water, coffee, orange juice, or low-fat milk. Do not mix with cola or tea.

- Open blister units of orally disintegrating tablets individually; do not push tablet through the foil. Use dry hands to remove tablet—immediately place on tongue. Do not allow patient to chew tablet.

⊗ ***Warning*** Monitor patient regularly for signs and symptoms of diabetes mellitus.

- Monitor T. If fever occurs, rule out underlying infection, and consult physician for appropriate comfort measures.
- Advise patient to use contraception during drug therapy.

⊗ ***Warning*** Follow guidelines for discontinuation or reinstitution of the drug carefully.

Teaching points

- Dosage will be increased gradually to achieve most effective dose. Do not take more than your prescribed dosage. Do not make up missed doses; contact your health care provider if this occurs. Do not stop taking this drug suddenly; gradual reduction of dosage is needed to prevent side effects.
- Mix oral solution in 3–4 ounces of water, coffee, orange juice, or low-fat milk. Do not mix with cola or tea.
- Remove orally disintegrating tablet with dry hands. Do not push tablet through foil. Immediately place tablet on tongue; do not split or chew tablet. The tablet will disintegrate within seconds and you can then swallow.
- If receiving IM doses, mark your calendar for every-2-week injections.
- This drug cannot be taken during pregnancy. If you think you are pregnant or wish to become pregnant, consult your health care provider.
- You may experience these side effects: Drowsiness, dizziness, sedation, seizures (avoid driving, operating machinery, or performing tasks that require concentration); dizziness, faintness on arising (change positions slowly; use caution); increased salivation (reversible); constipation; sensitivity to the sun (use a sunscreen or protective clothing).
- Report lethargy, weakness, fever, sore throat, malaise, mouth ulcers, palpitations, increased thirst, increased urination, increased hunger.

▽ritonavir

*(ri **ton'** ah veer)*

Norvir

PREGNANCY CATEGORY B

Drug class

Antiretroviral

Therapeutic actions

Antiviral activity; inhibits HIV protease activity, leading to decrease in production of HIV particles.

Indications

- Treatment of HIV infection in combination with other antiretrovirals

Contraindications and cautions

- Contraindicated with allergy to ritonavir, use of certain drugs (see Interactions).
- Use cautiously with pregnancy, hepatic impairment, lactation.

Available forms

Capsules—100 mg; oral solution—80 mg/mL

Dosages

Adults

600 mg PO bid with food.

Pediatric patients

Start at 250 mg/m^2 PO bid and increase by 50 mg/m^2 twice daily at 2–3 day intervals, to maximum of 400 mg/m^2 PO bid; do not exceed 600 mg bid. Use in combination with other antiretrovirals.

Pharmacokinetics

Route	*Onset*	*Peak*
Oral	Rapid	2–4 hr

Metabolism: Hepatic; $T_{1/2}$: 3–5 hr
Distribution: May cross placenta; may enter breast milk
Excretion: Feces, urine

R

Adverse effects

- **CNS:** *Asthenia, peripheral and circumoral paresthesias,* anxiety, dreams, headache, dizziness, hallucinations, personality changes
- **CV:** Hemorrhage, hypotension, syncope, tachycardia
- **Dermatologic:** Acne, dry skin, contact dermatitis, rash
- **GI:** *Nausea, vomiting, diarrhea, anorexia, abdominal pain, taste perversion,* dry mouth, hepatitis, hepatic impairment, dehydration
- **GU:** Dysuria, hematuria, nocturia, pyelonephritis
- **Respiratory:** Apnea, dyspnea, cough, rhinitis
- **Other:** Hypothermia, chills, back pain, chest pain, edema, cachexia

Interactions

✱ **Drug-drug** ⊗ ***Black box warning*** Potentially large increase in serum concentration of alfuzosin, amiodarone, astemizole, bepridil, bupropion, clozapine, ergotamine, flecainide, meperidine, pimozide, piroxicam, propafenone, propoxyphene, quinidine, rifabutin, terfenadine, voriconazole; potential for serious arrhythmias, seizures, and fatal reactions; do not administer ritonavir with any of these drugs.

⊗ ***Black box warning*** Potentially large increases in serum concentration of these sedatives and hypnotics: Alprazolam, clonazepam, diazepam, estazolam, flurazepam, midazolam, triazolam, zolpidem; extreme sedation and respiratory depression could occur; do not administer ritonavir with any of these drugs.

✱ **Drug-food** • Absorption increased by presence of food; taking drug with food is strongly recommended • Decreased metabolism and risk of toxic effects if combined with grapefruit juice; avoid this combination

✱ **Drug-alternative therapy** • Decreased effectiveness if taken with St. John's wort

■ Nursing considerations

CLINICAL ALERT!

Name confusion has been reported between *Retrovir* (zidovudine) and ritonavir; use caution.

Assessment

- **History:** Allergy to ritonavir, hepatic impairment, pregnancy, lactation
- **Physical:** T; orientation, reflexes; BP, P, peripheral perfusion; R, adventitious sounds; bowel sounds; skin color, perfusion; LFTs

Interventions

- Capsules and oral solution should be stored in refrigerator; solution should be left at room temperature if used within 30 days; protect from light and extreme heat.
- Administer with meals or food to increase absorption.

⊗ ***Black box warning*** Carefully screen drug history to avoid potentially dangerous or life-threatening drug interactions.

Teaching points

- Take this drug with meals or food; store capsules in refrigerator. Taste of solution may be improved if mixed with chocolate milk, *Ensure,* or *Advera* 1 hour before taking. Do not drink grapefruit juice while using this drug.
- Take the full course of therapy as prescribed; do not take double doses if one is missed; do not change dosage without consulting your health care provider. Always take in combination with your other HIV drugs.
- This drug does not cure HIV infection; long-term effects are not yet known; continue to take precautions as the risk of transmission is not reduced by this drug.
- Do not take any other drugs, prescription or over-the-counter, without consulting your health care provider; this drug interacts with many other drugs and serious problems can occur.
- You may experience these side effects: Nausea, vomiting, loss of appetite, diarrhea, abdominal pain, headache, dizziness, numbness, tingling.
- Report severe diarrhea, severe nausea, personality changes, changes in color of urine or stool, fever, chills.

▽ rituximab

See Appendix W, *Less commonly used drugs*.

rivastigmine tartrate
*(riv ah **stig**' meen)*

Exelon, Exelon Oral Solution, Exelon Patch

PREGNANCY CATEGORY B

Drug classes
Alzheimer's disease drug
Cholinesterase inhibitor

Therapeutic actions
Centrally acting, selective, long-acting reversible cholinesterase inhibitor; causes elevated acetylcholine levels in the cortex, which slows the neuronal degradation that occurs in Alzheimer's disease.

Indications
- Treatment of mild to moderate dementia of the Alzheimer's type
- Treatment of mild to moderate dementia associated with Parkinson's disease
- Unlabeled use: Treatment of behavioral effects of Lewy-body dementia

Contraindications and cautions
- Contraindicated with hypersensitivity to rivastigmine.
- Use cautiously with sick sinus syndrome, GI bleeding, seizures, asthma, COPD, pregnancy, lactation.

Available forms
Capsules—1.5, 3, 4.5, 6 mg; oral solution with dosing syringe—2 mg/mL; transdermal patch—4.6 mg/24 hr, 9.5 mg/24 hr

Dosages
Adults
- *Alzheimer's disease:* Initial dosage, 1.5 mg PO bid with food. If tolerated, may adjust to higher doses at 1.5-mg intervals every 2 wks. Usual range, 6–12 mg/day; should not exceed 12 mg/day. If dose is not tolerated, stop drug for several doses and then restart at the same or a lower level. For transdermal patch, initially one 4.6-mg/24 hr patch once/day; after 4 or more wk, may be increased to one 9.5-mg/24 hr patch.
- *Parkinson's dementia:* 3–12 mg/day PO in divided doses bid. Initial dose, 1.5 mg PO bid; increase every 4 wk based on patient tolerance. For transdermal patch, initially one 4.6-mg/24 hr patch once/day; after 4 or more wk, may be increased to one 9.5-mg/24 hr patch.

Pediatric patients
Safety and efficacy not established.

Pharmacokinetics

Route	*Onset*	*Peak*	*Duration*
Oral	Varies	1.4–2.6 hr	12 hr

Metabolism: Hepatic; $T_{1/2}$: 1 hr
Distribution: Crosses placenta; may enter breast milk
Excretion: Urine

Adverse effects
- **CNS:** *Insomnia, fatigue,* dizziness, confusion, ataxia, insomnia, somnolence, tremor, agitation, depression, anxiety, abnormal thinking, syncope
- **CV:** Bradycardia
- **GI:** *Nausea, vomiting, diarrhea, dyspepsia, anorexia, abdominal pain,* flatulence, constipation

Interactions
✱ **Drug-drug** • Increased effects and risk of toxicity if theophylline, cholinesterase inhibitors taken concurrently • Decreased effects of anticholinergics taken concurrently • Increased risk of GI bleeding if taken with NSAIDs

R

■ Nursing considerations
Assessment
- **History:** Allergy to rivastigmine; pregnancy, lactation; sick sinus syndrome; GI bleeding; seizures; asthma; COPD
- **Physical:** Orientation, affect, reflexes; BP, P; abdominal examination; LFTs, renal function tests

Interventions
- Establish baseline functional profile to follow evaluation of drug effectiveness.
- Administer with food in the morning and evening to decrease GI discomfort.

- Mix solution with water, fruit juice, or soda to improve compliance. Dosage of capsules and solution is interchangeable.
- Apply patch to clean, dry skin once daily. Rotate application sites, and remove old patch before applying new one.
- Monitor patient for weight loss, diarrhea, arrhythmias before use and periodically with prolonged use.
- Provide small, frequent meals if GI upset is severe.
- Provide patient safety measures if CNS effects occur.

⊗ ***Warning*** Notify surgeons that patient is on rivastigmine, exaggerated muscle relaxation may occur if succinylcholine-type drugs are used.

Teaching points

- Take drug exactly as prescribed, take with food to decrease GI upset. Solution may be swallowed directly from the syringe or mixed in a small glass of water, cold fruit juice, or soda. In cold fruit juice or soda, mixture is stable up to 4 hours at room temperature.
- Patch should be applied to clean, dry skin. Rotate sites, and remove old patch before applying a new one.
- This drug does not cure the disease but may slow down the degeneration associated with the disease.
- Dosage changes may be needed to achieve the best drug levels.
- You may experience these side effects: Nausea, vomiting (eat frequent small meals) insomnia, fatigue, confusion (use caution if driving or performing tasks that require alertness).
- Report severe nausea, vomiting, changes in stool or urine color, diarrhea, changes in neurologic functioning, palpitations.

▽rizatriptan

*(rih zah **trip'** tan)*

Maxalt, Maxalt-MLT

PREGNANCY CATEGORY C

Drug classes

Antimigraine drug
Serotonin selective agonist

Therapeutic actions

Binds to serotonin receptors to cause vascular constrictive effects on cranial blood vessels, causing the relief of migraine in selected patients whose migraines are caused by vasodilation.

Indications

- Treatment of acute migraine attacks with or without aura

Contraindications and cautions

- Contraindicated with allergy to rizatriptan, active CAD, Prinzmetal's angina, uncontrolled hypertension; recent (within 24 hr) treatment with another 5-HT agonist or an ergotamine-containing or ergot type medication; hemiplegic or basilar migraine.
- Use cautiously with hepatic impairment, dialysis, pregnancy, lactation.

Available forms

Tablets—5, 10 mg; orally disintegrating tablets—5, 10 mg

Dosages

Adults

5 or 10 mg at onset of headache; may repeat in 2 hr if needed. Wait 2 hr between doses. Maximum dose, 30 mg/day.

Pediatric patients younger than 18 yr

Safety and efficacy not established.

Patients with hepatic or renal impairment

Use lowest possible dose, monitor patient closely.

Pharmacokinetics

Route	*Onset*	*Peak*
Oral	Rapid	1 hr

Metabolism: Hepatic; $T_{1/2}$: 2 hr
Distribution: May cross placenta; may enter breast milk
Excretion: Feces, urine

Adverse effects
- **CNS:** *Dizziness, vertigo, weakness, somnolence, paresthesias*
- **CV:** BP increase, palpitations, chest pain
- **GI:** Dry mouth, nausea
- **Other:** *Chest, jaw, or throat pressure*

Interactions
✱ **Drug-drug** ⊗ ***Warning*** Prolonged vasoactive reactions when taken concurrently with ergot-containing drugs; do not use within 24 hr of each other or other serotonin agonist. • Risk of severe effects if taken with or within 2 wk of discontinuation of an MAOI • Risk of increased serum levels and toxic effects with propanolol; recommend 5-mg dose no more than three doses per 24 hr period

✱ **Drug-food** • Food will delay peak onset by 1 hr

■ Nursing considerations

CLINICAL ALERT!
Name confusion has occurred between *Maxalt* (rizatriptan) and *Maxair* (pirbuterol). Use caution.

Assessment
- **History:** Allergy to rizatriptan, active CAD, Prinzmetal's angina, uncontrolled hypertension, hepatic impairment, dialysis, pregnancy, lactation
- **Physical:** Skin color and lesions; orientation, reflexes, peripheral sensation; P, BP; LFTs, renal function tests

Interventions
- Administer to relieve acute migraine, not as a prophylactic measure.
- Have patient place orally disintegrating tablet on tongue and swallow with or without water.
- Establish safety measures if CNS or visual disturbances occur.
- Control environment as appropriate to help relieve migraine (lighting, temperature, noise).

⊗ ***Warning*** Monitor BP of patients with possible CAD; discontinue at any sign of angina, prolonged high BP, or other adverse signs.

Teaching points
- Take drug exactly as prescribed, at the onset of headache or aura; dosage may be repeated in 2 hours if needed. Place orally disintegrating tablet on tongue and allow to dissolve before eating or drinking.
- This drug should not be taken during pregnancy; if you suspect that you are pregnant, consult your health care provider and stop using drug.
- Continue to do anything that normally helps you during a migraine, such as controlling lighting or noise.
- Contact your health care provider immediately if you experience chest pain or pressure that is severe or does not go away.
- You may experience these side effects: Dizziness, drowsiness (avoid driving or the use of dangerous machinery while using this drug); numbness, tingling, feelings of tightness or pressure.
- Report feelings of heat, flushing, tiredness, feelings of sickness, chest pain.

▽ romidepsin

See Appendix W, *Less commonly used drugs*.

▽ romiplostim

See Appendix W, *Less commonly used drugs*.

▽ ropinirole hydrochloride

*(row **pin'** ah roll)*

Requip, Requip XL DNC

PREGNANCY CATEGORY C

Drug classes
Antiparkinsonian
Dopamine receptor agonist

Therapeutic actions
Acts as a non-ergot dopamine agonist acting directly on postsynaptic dopamine receptors of neurons in the brain, mimicking the effects of the neurotransmitter dopamine, which is thought to be deficient in parkinsonism.

R

Indications

- Treatment of idiopathic Parkinson's disease in the early stages as well as in the late stages (immediate-release or ER)
- Treatment of moderate to severe primary restless leg syndrome

Contraindications and cautions

- Contraindicated with hypersensitivity to ropinirole, severe ischemic heart disease or peripheral vascular disease, lactation.
- Use cautiously with dyskinesia, orthostatic hypotension, hepatic or renal impairment, pregnancy, history of sleep disorders or somnolence.

Available forms

Tablets—0.25, 0.5, 1, 2, 3, 4, 5 mg; ER tablets (DNC)—2, 4, 6, 8, 12 mg

Dosages

Adults

- *Parkinson's disease:* Initially, 0.25 mg PO tid for 1st wk; 0.5 mg PO tid for 2nd wk; 0.75 mg PO tid for 3rd wk; 1 mg PO tid for 4th wk. May increase by 1.5 mg/day at 1-wk intervals to 9 mg/day, then by up to 3 mg/day at 1-wk intervals to a maximum dose of 24 mg/day. ER tablets: Initially, 2 mg/day PO; after 1–2 wk, may increase by 2 mg/day; titrate with weekly increases of 2 mg/day to a maximum of 24 mg/day.
- *Restless leg syndrome:* 0.25 mg/day PO, 1–3 hr before bed; after 2 days, increase to 0.5 mg/day PO; after 1 week to 1 mg/day PO. Week 3, increase to 1.5 mg/day; week 4—2 mg/day, week 5—2.5 mg/day; week 6—3 mg/day; week 7—4 mg/day PO if needed to control symptoms.

Pediatric patients

Safety and efficacy not established.

Geriatric patients

Elderly are at higher risk for development of hallucinations; monitor closely and adjust dosage more slowly.

Pharmacokinetics

Route	*Onset*	*Peak*	*Duration*
Oral	Varies	1–2 hr	8 hr
ER	Varies	6–10 hr	16 hr

Metabolism: Hepatic; $T_{1/2}$: 6 hr
Distribution: Crosses placenta; enters breast milk
Excretion: Urine

Adverse effects

- **CNS:** *Dizziness, somnolence, insomnia, hypokinesia or hyperkinesia,* syncope, asthenia, confusion, hallucinations (more common in the elderly), abnormal vision, tremor, anxiety, paresthesias, aggravated parkinsonism
- **CV:** *Orthostatic hypotension,* edema
- **GI:** *Nausea, constipation*
- **Other:** Fatigue, infections, sweating, pharyngitis, pain, arthralgia

Interactions

✱ **Drug-drug** • Increased effects of levodopa; consider decreasing levodopa dose • Increased CNS depression with alcohol, CNS depressants • Monitor and adjust ropinirole dose if estrogen is added to or discontinued from regimen • Increased effects with ciprofloxacin

■ Nursing considerations

Assessment

- **History:** Hypersensitivity to ropinirole, severe ischemic heart disease or peripheral vascular disease, pregnancy, lactation, dyskinesia, orthostatic hypotension, hepatic or renal impairment
- **Physical:** Skin T, color, lesions; orientation, affect, reflexes, bilateral grip strength; vision examination including visual fields; P, BP, orthostatic BP, auscultation; liver evaluation; LFTs, renal function tests

Interventions

- Administer drug with food if GI upset becomes a problem. Ensure that patient does not cut, crush, or chew ER tablets.
- Monitor patient for orthostatic hypotension and establish safety precautions if needed (use side rails, accompany patient).

⊗ ***Warning*** Withdraw gradually over 1 wk to avoid serious side effects.

- Monitor patient carefully and adjust dosage more slowly if patient has hypotension or dyskinesias.

- Monitor elderly patients for the development of hallucinations; provide appropriate safety measures as needed.

⊗ ***Warning*** Start adjustment of drug over again if drug has been discontinued and is being restarted.

- Monitor hepatic and renal function periodically during therapy.

Teaching points

- Take this drug exactly as prescribed; take with food if GI upset occurs. Dosage will change gradually over several weeks. Do not cut, crush, or chew ER tablets.
- Do not discontinue this drug without consulting your health care provider; drug must be stopped gradually to prevent serious adverse effects.
- You may experience these side effects: Drowsiness, dizziness, confusion (avoid driving or engaging in activities that require alertness); nausea (take drug with meals; eat frequent small meals); dizziness or faintness when you get up (change position slowly, exercise caution when climbing stairs); headache, nasal stuffiness (consult your health care provider; there may be medication for these).
- Report fainting, light-headedness, dizziness; black, tarry stools; hallucinations; falling asleep during activities of daily living.

DANGEROUS DRUG

▽ rosiglitazone maleate

*(roh zee **glit'** ah zohn **mal'** ee ate)*

Avandia

PREGNANCY CATEGORY C

Drug classes

Antidiabetic
Thiazolidinedione

Therapeutic actions

Resensitizes tissues to insulin; decreases hepatic gluconeogenesis and increases insulin-dependent muscle glucose uptake.

Indications

- Monotherapy as an adjunct to diet and exercise to improve glucose control in patients with type 2 diabetes
- As part of combination with metformin or a sulfonylurea when diet, exercise, and either agent alone does not result in adequate glycemic control in type 2 diabetes
- Unlabeled uses: Increased ovulation frequency in women with polycystic ovary syndrome; reduction of in-stent restenosis in patients with diabetes

Contraindications and cautions

- Contraindicated with allergy to any thiazolidinedione, type 1 diabetes, ketoacidosis, New York Heart Association Class III or IV HF, lactation.
- Use cautiously with advanced heart disease, liver failure, HF (not recommended in symptomatic HF), pregnancy.

Available forms

Tablets—2, 4, 8 mg

Dosages

Adults

4 mg as a single oral dose or divided into two doses; if adequate response is not seen in 8–12 wk, may be increased to 8 mg daily PO.

- *Combination therapy with metformin:* 4 mg daily PO added to the established dose of metformin; may be increased after 12 wk to 8 mg daily PO.

Pediatric patients

Safety and efficacy not established.

Patients with hepatic impairment

Use caution and monitor patient closely. Do not administer with active liver disease or if ALT exceeds 2.5 times the upper limit of normal.

R

Pharmacokinetics

Route	*Onset*	*Peak*
Oral	Rapid	1.3–3.5 hr

Metabolism: Hepatic; $T_{1/2}$: 3–4 hr
Distribution: Crosses placenta; enters breast milk
Excretion: Feces, urine

Adverse effects

- **CNS:** *Headache, pain*
- **CV: HF**
- **Endocrine: Hypoglycemia, hyperglycemia**

- **GI:** Diarrhea, **liver injury**
- **Respiratory:** Sinusitis, URI, rhinitis, dyspnea
- **Other:** *Infections, fatigue, accidental injury,* edema

Interactions

✱ **Drug-drug** • Risk of increased serum levels if combined with gemfibrozil; monitor patient and adjust dosage as needed

■ Nursing considerations

Assessment

- **History:** Allergy to any thiazolidinedione, type 1 diabetes, ketoacidosis, serious hepatic impairment, advanced heart disease, pregnancy, lactation
- **Physical:** T; orientation, reflexes, peripheral sensation; R, adventitious sounds; liver evaluation; LFTs, blood glucose, CBC

Interventions

⊗ ***Black box warning*** Drug may cause or worsen HF, angina, or MI in some patients; observe patient closely, and stop drug if necessary; do not use in patients with symptomatic HF.

- Monitor serum glucose levels frequently to determine effectiveness of drug and dosage being used.
- Monitor baseline LFTs before beginning therapy and periodically during therapy.
- Administer without regard to meals.
- Arrange for consult with dietitian to establish weight loss program and dietary control as appropriate.
- Arrange for thorough diabetic teaching program to include disease, dietary control, exercise, signs and symptoms of hypoglycemia and hyperglycemia, avoidance of infection, hygiene.

Teaching points

- Do not discontinue drug without consulting your health care provider; continue diet and exercise program for diabetes control.
- Take this drug with meals if desired. If dose is missed, it may be taken at the next meal. If dose is missed for an entire day, do not double dose the next day.
- Monitor urine or blood for glucose and ketones as prescribed; watch very closely while adjusting to drug.
- Report fever, sore throat, bleeding or bruising, rash, dark urine, light-colored stools, hypoglycemic or hyperglycemic reactions, swelling, difficulty breathing.

▽ rosuvastatin calcium

(row sue' va sta tin)

Crestor

PREGNANCY CATEGORY X

Drug classes

Antihyperlipidemic drug
HMG-CoA reductase inhibitor (statin)

Therapeutic actions

A fungal metabolite that inhibits the enzyme (HMG-CoA) that catalyzes the first step in the cholesterol synthesis pathway, resulting in a decrease in serum cholesterol, serum LDLs (associated with increased risk of coronary artery disease) and either an increase or no change in serum HDLs (associated with decreased risk of coronary artery disease).

Indications

- As an adjunct to diet in the treatment of elevated total cholesterol and LDL cholesterol and triglyceride levels in patients with primary hypercholesterolemia (familial and nonfamilial), and in patients with mixed dyslipidemia
- Adjunct to diet to slow atherosclerosis progression in patients with elevated cholesterol
- As an adjunct to diet for the treatment of patients with elevated serum triglyceride levels
- To reduce LDL-C, total cholesterol, and ApoB in patients with homozygous familiar hypercholesterolemia as an adjunct to other lipid-lowering treatments or if such treatments are not available
- Treatment of patients with primary dysbetalipoproteinemia

NEW INDICATION: Treatment of children 10–17 yr (girls must be postmenarchal) with heterozygous familial hypercholesterolemia when diet therapy fails

Contraindications and cautions

- Contraindicated with allergy to any component of the product, active liver disease or persistent elevated serum transaminases, pregnancy, lactation.
- Use cautiously with impaired hepatic function, alcoholism, renal impairment, advanced age, hypothyroidism.

Available forms

Tablets—5, 10, 20, 40 mg

Dosages

Adults

- *Hypercholesteremia and mixed dyslipidemia:* 5–40 mg daily PO. Usual starting dose is 10 mg daily with titration based on serum lipid levels, monitored every 2–4 wk until desired level is achieved.
- *Homozygous familial hypercholesterolemia:* 20 mg daily PO with a maximum 40 mg per day.
- *In combination with cyclosporine:* 5 mg daily PO.
- *In combination with other lipid-lowering drugs:* 10 mg daily PO.

Asian patients

5 mg PO once daiy. Risk of serious side effects if dose increase is needed to control lipid levels.

Pediatric patients 10–17 yr

5–20 mg/day PO.

Patients with renal impairment

5 mg daily PO; do not exceed 10 mg per day.

Pharmacokinetics

Route	Onset	Peak
Oral	Slow	3–5 hr

Metabolism: Hepatic metabolism; $T_{1/2}$: 19 hr
Distribution: Crosses placenta; enters breast milk
Excretion: Feces

Adverse effects

- **CNS:** *Headache,* dizziness, insomnia, hypertonia, paresthesia, depression, anxiety, vertigo, neuralgia
- **CV:** Hypertension, angina pectoris, vasodilatation, palpitation, peripheral edema
- **GI:** *Nausea,* dyspepsia, *diarrhea,* constipation, gastroenteritis, vomiting, flatulence, periodontal abscess, gastritis, **liver failure**
- **Respiratory:** *Pharyngitis, rhinitis, sinusitis,* cough, dyspnea, pneumonia
- **Other:** Arthritis, arthralgia, **rhabdomyolysis, myopathy,** *flulike symptoms*

Interactions

✱ **Drug-drug** ⊗ ***Warning*** Possible increased serum levels and risk of toxicity if taken with cyclosporine, gemfibrozil, lopinavir/ritonavir; adjust dosage accordingly and monitor patient; 10 mg/day is suggested maximum dosage.
- Increased risk of bleeding with coumarin anticoagulants; lower dose and monitor bleeding levels frequently to establish correct dosage
- Decreased absorption if taken with aluminum or magnesium hydroxide antacids; if this combination is used, take the antacid at least 2 hr after the rosuvastatin

■ Nursing considerations

Assessment

- **History:** Allergy to any component of the product, liver disease or persistent elevated serum transaminases, pregnancy, lactation, alcoholism, renal impairment, advanced age, hypothyroidism
- **Physical:** Orientation, affect, P, BP, R, adventitious sounds; liver evaluation; lipid studies, LFTs, renal function tests

Interventions

- Establish baseline serum lipid levels and liver function test results before beginning therapy.
- Arrange for proper consultation about need for diet and exercise changes.
- Administer drug at bedtime (highest rates of cholesterol synthesis occur between midnight and 5 AM).
- Arrange for regular follow-up during long-term therapy.
- Monitor patient closely for signs of muscle injury, especially at higher doses, in Asian patients, and when used in combination with gemfibrozil or cyclosporine.
- Provide comfort measures to deal with headache, muscle cramps, or nausea.
- Advise women of childbearing age that this drug is contraindicated during pregnancy; advise the use of barrier contraceptives.

R

- Suggest an alternate means of feeding the baby to any nursing mother who is prescribed this drug.
- Offer support and encouragement to deal with disease, diet, drug therapy, and follow-up care.

Teaching points

- Take drug at bedtime.
- Institute appropriate diet and exercise changes that need to be made.
- If you miss a dose, take the next dose as soon as you remember and begin again the next day. Do not take two doses in 1 day.
- Avoid pregnancy while taking this drug; using a barrier contraceptive is advised.
- If you are also taking antacids, take the antacid at least 2 hours after your rosuvastatin.
- Stop the drug and contact your health care provider immediately if you experience unexplained muscle pain, tenderness, or weakness with fever or malaise.
- You may experience these side effects: Nausea (eat frequent small meals); headache, flulike symptoms (analgesics may help).
- Report severe GI upset, unusual bleeding or bruising, dark urine or light-colored stools, unexplained muscle pain, tenderness, or weakness.

▽ rufinamide

See Appendix W, *Less commonly used drugs*.

▽ sacrosidase

See Appendix W, *Less commonly used drugs*.

▽ saliva substitute

*(sa **lye'** vah)*

Entertainer's Secret, Moi-Stir, Moi-Stir Swabsticks, MouthKote, Numoisyn, Salivart

PREGNANCY CATEGORY UNKNOWN

Drug class

Saliva substitute

Therapeutic actions

Contains electrolytes and carboxymethylcellulose as a thickening agent to serve as a substitute for saliva in dry mouth syndromes.

Indications

- Management of dry mouth and throat in xerostomia and hyposalivation caused by CVA, medications (including those that cause dysfunction of the salivary glands), radiation therapy, chemotherapy, Sjögren syndrome, Bell palsy, HIV/AIDS, lupus, aging, emotional factors, hoarse voice, scratchy throat, salivary gland disorders, other illnesses

Contraindications and cautions

- Contraindicated with hypersensitivity to carboxymethylcellulose, parabens, components of the preparation.
- Use cautiously with renal failure, HF, hypertension, pregnancy.

Available forms

Solution; lozenges; swab sticks

Dosages

Adults

Spray for one-half second or apply to oral mucosa.

Pediatric patients

Safety and efficacy not established.

Pharmacokinetics

No general systemic absorption. Electrolytes may be absorbed and dealt with in normal electrolyte pathways.

Adverse effects

Other: Excessive absorption of electrolytes (elevated magnesium, sodium, potassium)

■ Nursing considerations

Assessment

- **History:** Allergy to carboxymethylcellulose, parabens, HF, hypertension, renal failure
- **Physical:** BP, P, auscultation, edema; renal function tests; mucosa evaluation

Interventions

- Give for dry mouth and throat.

- Have patient try to swish saliva substitute around mouth following application.
- Monitor patient while eating; swallowing may be impaired and additional therapy required.

Teaching points

- Apply the drug as instructed; swish it around in your mouth after application.
- Use as needed for dry mouth and throat.
- Take care when eating because swallowing may be difficult; additional therapy may be needed.
- Report swelling, headache, irregular heartbeat, leg cramps, failure to relieve discomfort of dry mouth and throat.

salmeterol xinafoate

*(sal **mee'** ter ol ze inn ah **foh'** ate)*

Serevent Diskus

PREGNANCY CATEGORY C

Drug classes

Antasthmatic

$Beta_2$-selective adrenergic agonist

Therapeutic actions

Long-acting agonist that binds to $beta_2$ receptors in the lungs, causing bronchodilation; also inhibits the release of inflammatory mediators in the lung, blocking swelling and inflammation.

Indications

- Maintenance therapy for asthma and prevention of bronchospasm in patients 4 yr and older with reversible obstructive airway disease including nocturnal asthma
- Long-term maintenance treatment of bronchospasm related to COPD
- Prevention of exercise-induced bronchospasm in patients 4 yr and older

Contraindications and cautions

- Contraindicated with hypersensitivity to salmeterol, acute asthma attack, worsening or deteriorating asthma (life-threatening), acute airway obstruction.
- Use cautiously with pregnancy, lactation.

Available forms

Inhalation powder—50 mcg (*Diskus*)

Dosages

Adults and patients 12 yr and older

- *Asthma or bronchospasm:* 1 inhalation (50 mcg) bid.
- *Exercise-induced asthma:* 1 inhalation 30 min or more before exertion.
- *COPD:* 1 inhalation (50 mcg) bid.

Pediatric patients 4–12 yr

- *Asthma or bronchospasm:* 1 inhalation (50 mcg) bid, 12 hr apart.
- *Prevention of exercise-induced asthma:* 1 inhalation 30 min or more before exercising.

Pharmacokinetics

Route	*Onset*	*Peak*	*Duration*
Inhalation	13–20 min	3–4 hr	7.5–17 hr

Metabolism: Hepatic; $T_{1/2}$: Unknown
Distribution: May cross placenta; may enter breast milk
Excretion: Feces, urine

Adverse effects

- **CNS:** *Headache, tremor,* dizziness
- **CV:** *Tachycardia, palpitations,* hypertension
- **Respiratory:** Worsening of asthma, difficulty breathing, **bronchospasm; asthma related deaths (risk higher in black than white patients)**
- **Other:** Pain

Interactions

✱ **Drug-drug** • Risk of severe bronchospasm if combined with beta blockers; use a cardioselective beta blocker and monitor patient closely if this combination is used • Potential for worsened hypokalemia and ECG abnormalities if combined with diuretics; monitor patient very closely • Administer with extreme caution to patients being treated with MAOIs or TCAs, or within 2 wk of discontinuation of such agents because the action of salmeterol may be potentiated by these agents

■ Nursing considerations

Assessment

- **History:** Allergy to salmeterol, pregnancy, acute asthma attack, worsening asthma, lactation
- **Physical:** R, adventitious sounds; P, BP, ECG; orientation, reflexes; LFTs

Interventions

⊗ ***Black box warning*** Ensure that drug is not used to treat acute asthma or with worsening or deteriorating asthma (risk of death).

- Instruct in the proper use of *Diskus.*
- Have patients who experience exercise-induced asthma use it 30–60 min before activity.
- Arrange for periodic evaluation of respiratory condition.

Teaching points

- Use the pressurized metered-dose inhaler as instructed. Shake well before using. Use only twice a day. If drug is to be used periodically for exercise-induced asthma, use 30–60 minutes before activity.
- To gain full therapeutic benefit in the treatment of reversible airway obstruction, administer twice a day (morning and evening).
- Obtain periodic evaluations of your respiratory problem.
- You may experience these side effects: Headache (request analgesics); tremors (use care in performing dangerous tasks); fast heartbeat, palpitations (monitor activity; rest frequently).
- Report severe headache, irregular heartbeat, worsening of asthma, difficulty breathing.

▽ salsalate (salicylsalicylic acid)

(sal' sa layt)

Amigesic, Argesic-SA, Artha-G, Disalcid, Marthritic, Salflex, Salsitab

Pregnancy Category C

Drug classes

Analgesic (nonopioid)
Anti-inflammatory
Antirheumatic
NSAID
Salicylate

Therapeutic actions

Analgesic and antirheumatic effects are attributable to the ability to inhibit the synthesis of prostaglandins, important mediators of inflammation; antipyretic effects are not fully understood, but salicylates probably act in the thermoregulatory center of the hypothalamus to block the effects of endogenous pyrogen by inhibiting the synthesis of the prostaglandin intermediary; after absorption, this drug is hydrolyzed into two molecules of salicylic acid; insoluble in gastric secretions, it is not absorbed in the stomach, but in the small intestine; reported to cause fewer GI adverse effects than aspirin.

Indications

- Relief of mild to moderate pain
- Relief of symptoms of various inflammatory conditions—rheumatic fever, rheumatoid arthritis, osteoarthritis

Contraindications and cautions

- Contraindicated with allergy to salicylates or NSAIDs, bleeding disorders, impaired hepatic or renal function, GI ulceration (less of a problem with salsalate than with other anti-inflammatories), lactation and perioperatively in patients undergoing coronary artery bypass graft surgery.
- Use cautiously in pregnancy; and in children and teenagers with influenza or chickenpox—use of salicylates in these patients may be associated with the development of Reye's syndrome. This acute, life-threatening condition, characterized by vomiting, lethargy, and belligerence, may progress to delirium and coma and has a mortality rate of 20%–30%.

Available forms

Capsules—500, 750 mg; tablets—500, 750 mg

Dosages

Adults

3,000 mg/day PO given in divided doses.

Pediatric patients
Safety and efficacy not established.

Pharmacokinetics

Route	*Onset*	*Peak*	*Duration*
Oral	10–30 min	1–3 hr	3–6 hr

Metabolism: Hepatic; $T_{1/2}$: 2–3 hr (15–30 hr with large doses over extended periods)
Distribution: Crosses placenta; enters breast milk
Excretion: Urine

Adverse effects

- **Acute salicylate toxicity:** Respiratory alkalosis, hyperpnea, tachypnea, hemorrhage, excitement, confusion, asterixis, pulmonary edema, seizures, tetany, metabolic acidosis, fever, coma, **CV collapse, renal and respiratory failure**
- **CNS:** *Headache, dizziness, somnolence, insomnia,* fatigue, tiredness, dizziness, tinnitus, ophthalmologic effects
- **Dermatologic:** *Rash,* pruritus, sweating, dry mucous membranes, stomatitis
- **GI:** *Nausea, dyspepsia, GI pain,* diarrhea, vomiting, *constipation,* flatulence
- **GU:** Dysuria, renal impairment
- **Hematologic:** Bleeding, platelet inhibition with higher doses, neutropenia, eosinophilia, leukopenia, pancytopenia, thrombocytopenia, agranulocytosis, granulocytopenia, aplastic anemia, decreased Hgb or Hct, bone marrow depression, menorrhagia
- **Respiratory:** Dyspnea, hemoptysis, pharyngitis, **bronchospasm,** rhinitis
- **Salicylism:** Dizziness, tinnitus, difficulty hearing, nausea, vomiting, diarrhea, mental confusion, lassitude (dose-related)
- **Other:** Peripheral edema, **anaphylactoid reactions** to **anaphylactic shock**

Interactions

✱ **Drug-drug** • Increased risk of GI ulceration with corticosteroids and alcohol • Increased risk of salicylate toxicity with carbonic anhydrase inhibitors • Increased toxicity of carbonic anhydrase inhibitors, valproic acid • Decreased serum salicylate levels with corticosteroids, antacids, urine alkalinizers (sodium acetate, sodium bicarbonate, sodium citrate, sodium lactate, tromethamine) • Increased methotrexate levels and toxicity • Greater glucose-lowering effect of sulfonylureas, insulin with large doses of salicylates • Decreased uricosuric effect of probenecid, sulfinpyrazone • Decreased diuretic effect of spironolactone

✱ **Drug-lab test** • Salicylate competes with thyroid hormone for binding to plasma proteins, which may be reflected in a depressed plasma T_4 value • False-negative readings for urine glucose by glucose oxidase method and copper reduction method • Interference with urine 5-HIAA determinations by fluorescent methods but not by nitrosonaphthol colorimetric method • Interference with urinary ketone determination by ferric chloride method • Falsely elevated urine VMA levels with most tests; false decrease in VMA using the Pisano method • Serum uric acid levels are elevated by salicylate levels less than 10 mg/dL and decreased by levels greater than 10 mg/dL

■ Nursing considerations

Assessment

- **History:** Allergy to salicylates or NSAIDs, bleeding disorders, impaired hepatic or renal function, GI ulceration, lactation, pregnancy
- **Physical:** Skin color and lesions; eighth cranial nerve function, orientation, reflexes, affect; P, BP, perfusion; R, adventitious sounds; liver evaluation and bowel sounds; CBC, urinalysis, stool guaiac, LFTs, renal function tests

Interventions

⊠ ***Black box warning*** Patient may be at increased risk for GI bleeding and CV events; monitor accordingly.

- Administer drug with food or after meals if GI upset occurs.
- Administer drug with a full glass of water to reduce risk of tablet or capsule lodging in the esophagus.

⊗ ***Warning*** Institute emergency procedures if overdose occurs: Gastric lavage, induction of emesis, activated charcoal, supportive therapy.

- Provide further comfort measures to reduce pain, fever, and inflammation.

Teaching points

- Take the drug with food or after meals if GI upset occurs.

- Report ringing in the ears, dizziness, confusion, abdominal pain, rapid or difficult breathing, nausea, vomiting.

sapropterin dihydrochloride

See Appendix W, *Less commonly used drugs*.

saquinavir mesylate

*(sa **kwen'** a veer)*

Invirase

PREGNANCY CATEGORY B

Drug classes

Antiviral
Protease inhibitor

Therapeutic actions

Protease inhibitor, which in combination with nucleoside analogues is effective in HIV infections with changes in surrogate markers.

Indications

- Treatment of HIV infection in combination with other antiretrovirals
- **NEW INDICATION:** Unlabeled use: Postexposure prophylaxis following occuptional exposure to HIV

Contraindications and cautions

- Contraindicated with life-threatening allergy to any component, severe hepatic impairment.
- Use cautiously with hepatic impairment, pregnancy, lactation, hemophilia, diabetes.

Available forms

Capsules—200 mg; tablets—500 mg

Dosages

Adults and patients older than 16 yr

1,000 mg bid with ritonavir 100 mg bid given together within 2 hr after a meal or with lopinavir 400 mg/ritonavir 100 mg PO bid (tablets); 1,000 mg bid PO with lopinavir 400 mg ritonavir 100 mg PO bid (capsules).

Pediatric patients younger than 16 yr

Safety and efficacy not established.

Patients with hepatic impairment

Reduce dose and monitor hepatic function tests. Drug is contraindicated with severe hepatic impairment.

Pharmacokinetics

Route	Onset	Peak
Oral	Slow	Unknown

Metabolism: Hepatic; $T_{1/2}$: 3–6 hr
Distribution: May cross placenta; may enter breast milk
Excretion: Feces

Adverse effects

- **CNS:** *Headache,* insomnia, myalgia, malaise, dizziness, paresthesia, fatigue
- **GI:** *Nausea, GI pain, diarrhea,* anorexia, vomiting, dyspepsia
- **Metabolic:** Fat redistribution may occur (central obesity, buffalo hump, cushingoid appearance)
- **Other:** *Asthenia,* elevated CPK, elevated triglycerides, cholesterol

Interactions

✱ **Drug-drug** • Decreased effectiveness with rifampin, rifabutin, phenobarbital, phenytoin, dexamethasone, carbamazepine, nevirapine • Increased saquinavir plasma concentrations with clarithromycin, indinavir, ritonavir, nelfinavir, delavirdine, ketoconazole • Increased sildenafil concentrations when coadministered with saquinavir • Potential for serious to life-threatening reactions with ergot derivatives, midazolam, triazolam, antiarrhythmics, rifampin • Risk of serious hepatic toxicity if combined with HMG-CoA inhibitors (statins); avoid this combination and, if use is required, monitor LFTs regularly

✱ **Drug-food** • Decreased metabolism and risk of toxic effects if combined with grapefruit juice, garlic capsules; avoid these combinations

✱ **Drug-alternative therapy** • Decreased effectiveness if combined with St. John's wort

■ Nursing considerations

CLINICAL ALERT!
Name confusion has occurred between *Invirase* (saquinavir) and *Inversine* (mecamylamine); and between saquinavir and *Sinequan;* use caution.

Assessment

- **History:** Life-threatening allergy to any component; impaired hepatic function, pregnancy, lactation, diabetes, hemophilia
- **Physical:** T; affect, reflexes, peripheral sensation; bowel sounds, liver evaluation; LFTs, CPK levels, abdominal examination

Interventions

⊗ ***Black box warning*** Capsules and tablets are not interchangeable; use tablets only when combined with ritonavir. If saquinavir is the only protease inhibitor in a treatment regimen, use capsules.

- Administer within 2 hr after a full meal.
- Monitor patient for signs of opportunistic infections that will need to be treated appropriately.
- Administer the drug concurrently with a nucleoside analogue.
- Offer support and encouragement to the patient to deal with the diagnosis as well as the effects of drug therapy and the high expense of treatment.

Teaching points

- Take drug as prescribed; take within 2 hours of a full meal; take concurrently with other prescribed medication. Do not drink grapefruit juice while using this drug.
- Store drug at room temperature; use by expiration date.
- These drugs are not a cure for AIDS or AIDS-related complex; opportunistic infections may occur and regular medical care should be sought to deal with the disease.
- The long-term effects of this drug are not yet known.
- This drug combination does not reduce the risk of transmission of HIV to others by sexual contact or blood contamination—use appropriate precautions.
- You may experience these side effects: Nausea, loss of appetite, change in taste (eat frequent small meals); dizziness, loss of feeling (take appropriate precautions).
- Report extreme fatigue, lethargy, severe headache, severe nausea, vomiting, difficulty breathing, rash, changes in color of urine or stool.

▽ sargramostim (granulocyte macrophage colony–stimulating factor, GM-CSF)

*(sar **gram'** oh stim)*

Leukine

PREGNANCY CATEGORY C

Drug class

Colony-stimulating factor

Therapeutic actions

Human GM-CSF produced by recombinant DNA technology; increases the proliferation and differentiation of hematopoietic progenitor cells; can activate mature granulocytes and macrophages.

Indications

- Myeloid reconstitution after autologous bone marrow transplantation and allogenic bone marrow transplantation
- Treatment of neutropenia associated with bone marrow transplantation failure or engraftment delay
- Induction chemotherapy in AML to shorten neutrophil recovery time
- Acceleration of myeloid recovery in patients with non-Hodgkin's lymphoma, acute lymphoblastic leukemia, and Hodgkin's lymphoma undergoing autologous bone marrow transplantation
- Mobilization of hematopoietic progenitor cells for collection by leukapheresis and to accelerate myeloid reconstitution following peripheral blood progenitor cell (PBPC) transplantation
- Unlabeled uses: Treatment of myelodysplastic syndrome, decreases nadir of leukopenia related to myelosuppression of chemotherapy, corrects neutropenia in aplastic anemia patients, decreases transplant-associated organ system damage, promotes early grafting

S

Contraindications and cautions

- Contraindicated with hypersensitivity to yeast products, excessive leukemic myeloid blasts in bone marrow or peripheral blood; in neonates (benzyl alcohol is a constituent of *Leukine* liquid and bacteriostatic water for injection diluent and should not be administered to neonates because of association with fatal "gasping syndrome").
- Use cautiously with renal or hepatic failure, lactation, concomitant use with chemotherapy and radiation therapy or within 24 hours preceding or following chemotherapy or radiation therapy, pregnancy.

Available forms

Powder for injection—250 mcg

Dosages

Adults

- *Myeloid reconstitution after autologous or allogenic bone marrow transplantation:* 250 mcg/m²/day for 21 days as a 2-hr IV infusion beginning 2–4 hr after the autologous bone marrow infusion and not less than 24 hr after the last dose of chemotherapy and radiation therapy. Patient should not receive sargramostim until post-marrow infusion ANC is less than 500 cells/mm³. Continue until ANC is greater than 1,500 cells/mm³ for 3 consecutive days. If severe adverse reactions occur, decrease dose by 50% or stop drug. If patient has blast cells or disease progression, stop drug immediately.
- *Bone marrow transplantation failure or engraftment delay:* 250 mcg/m²/day for 14 days as a 2-hr IV infusion; the dose can be repeated after 7 days off therapy if engraftment has not occurred. If engraftment still does not occur, third dose of 500 mcg/m²/day may be administered for 14 days after another 7 days off therapy.
- *Neutrophil recovery following chemotherapy in AML:* 250 mcg/m²/day IV over 4 hr starting on about day 11 or 4 days after chemotherapy induction.
- *Mobilization of PBPC:* 250 mcg/m²/day IV over 24 hr or subcutaneously once daily; continue throughout harvesting.
- *Post-PBPC transplant:* 250 mcg/m²/day IV over 24 hr or subcutaneously once daily beginning immediately after infusion of progenitor cells; continue until ANC is greater than 1,500 cells/mm³ for 3 consecutive days.

Pediatric patients

Safety and efficacy not established.

Pharmacokinetics

Route	Peak	Duration
IV	2 hr or more	6 hr
Subcut.	1–3 hr	12 hr

Metabolism: Unknown; $T_{1/2}$ (IV): 60 min; subcutaneous: 162 min
Distribution: May cross placenta; may enter breast milk
Excretion: Unknown

IV FACTS

Preparation: Reconstitute powder with 1 mL sterile water for injection; gently swirl contents to avoid foaming; do not shake, and avoid excessive agitation. Resulting solution should be clear, colorless, and isotonic. Do not reenter vial; discard any unused portion. Dilute in 0.9% sodium chloride injection; administer within 6 hr; refrigerate until ready to use.
Infusion: ⊗ ***Warning*** Infuse over 2 hr; do not use an in-line membrane filter; do not mix with any other medication or in any other diluent (except if albumin is needed for final concentration; see package label).
Incompatibilities: Do not mix with any solution other than 0.9% sodium chloride. Do not add to any other medications.

Adverse effects

- **CNS:** Headache, *fever,* generalized weakness, fatigue, *malaise, asthenia*
- **CV:** Edema
- **Dermatologic:** *Alopecia,* rash, mucositis
- **GI:** *Nausea, vomiting,* stomatitis, anorexia, *diarrhea,* constipation
- **Other:** *Bone pain,* generalized pain, sore throat, cough, arthralgia

Interactions

✱ **Drug-drug** • Drugs that may potentiate the myeloproliferative effects of sargramostim, such as lithium and corticosteroids, should be used with caution

■ Nursing considerations

Assessment

- **History:** Hypersensitivity to yeast products; pregnancy, lactation, excessive leukemic myeloid blasts in bone marrow or peripheral blood, renal or hepatic failure
- **Physical:** Skin color, lesions, hair; T; abdominal examination, status of mucous membranes; blood counts, platelets, body weight and hydration status

Interventions

- Obtain CBC and platelet count prior to and twice weekly during therapy.

⊗ ***Warning*** Administer no less than 24 hr after cytotoxic chemotherapy and within 2–4 hr of bone marrow infusion.

- Administer daily as a 2-hr infusion.

⊗ ***Warning*** Store in refrigerator; do not freeze or shake. Use powder within 6 hr of mixing. If using powder, use each vial for one dose; do not reenter vial. Discard any unused drug.

- Do not shake vial before use.

Teaching points

- This drug must be taken as long as needed.
- Avoid exposure to infection (avoid crowds, visitors with infections).
- This drug should not be taken during pregnancy; using barrier contraceptives is advised.
- Frequent blood tests will be needed to evaluate drug effects.
- You may experience these side effects: Nausea and vomiting (eat frequent small meals); loss of hair (obtain appropriate head covering; cover head in temperature extremes); fever (request medication).
- Report fever, chills, sore throat, weakness, pain or swelling at injection site, difficulty breathing, chills.

DANGEROUS DRUG

saxagliptin

(sacks ah **glip'** *ten)*

Onglyza

PREGNANCY CATEGORY B

Drug classes

Antidiabetic drug
DPP—4 (dipeptidyl peptidase–4) enzyme inhibitor

Therapeutic actions

Slows the inactivation of the incretin hormones, increasing these hormone levels and prolonging their activity. The incretin hormones stimulate insulin release in response to a meal and help regulate glucose homeostasis throughout the day. This increases and prolongs insulin release and reduces hepatic glucose production to help achieve glycemic control.

Indications

- As an adjunct to diet and exercise to improve glycemic control in adults with type 2 diabetes

Contraindications and cautions

- Contraindicated with history of serious hypersensitivity reactions to saxagliptin.
- Use cautiously with moderate or severe renal impairment, concurrent use of strong CYP3A inhibitors, pregnancy, lactation.

Available forms

Tablets—2.5, 5 mg

Dosages

Adults

2.5–5 mg/day PO without regard to meals.

Pediatric patients

Safety and efficacy not established.

Patients with renal impairment

2.5 mg/day PO for moderate to severe renal impairment (CrCl 50 mL/min or less).

Pharmacokinetics

Route	Onset	Peak
Oral	Moderate	2 hr

Metabolism: Hepatic; $T_{1/2}$: 2.5–3 hr
Distribution: May cross placenta; enters breast milk
Excretion: Feces, urine

Adverse effects

- **CNS:** *Headache,* dizziness
- **GI:** Abdominal pain, gastroenteritis, vomiting
- **GU:** *UTI*
- **Respiratory:** *URI,* nasopharyngitis
- **Other:** Hypoglycemia

S

Interactions

✱ **Drug-drug** • Risk of increased plasma levels and toxicity if combined with strong CYP3A4/5 inhibitors (atazanavir, clarithromycin, ketoconazole, indinavir, itraconazole, nefazodone, nelfinavir, ritonavir, saquinavir, telithromycin); if this combination is used, limit saxagliptin dosage to 2.5 mg/day

✱ **Drug-alternative therapies** • Increased risk of hypoglycemia if taken with celery, coriander, dandelion root, fenugreek, garlic, ginseng, juniper berries

■ Nursing considerations

Assessment

- **History:** Hypersensitivity to component of drug, renal impairment, pregnancy, lactation
- **Physical:** R, adventitious sounds; renal function tests; blood glucose, HbA1c levels

Interventions

- Monitor blood glucose and HbA1c levels before and periodically during therapy.
- Monitor renal function tests before and periodically during therapy.
- Ensure that patient continues diet and exercise program for management of type 2 diabetes.
- If appropriate, ensure that patient continues use of other prescribed drugs to manage type 2 diabetes.
- Arrange for thorough diabetic teaching program, including diet, exercise, signs and symptoms of hypoglycemia and hyperglycemia, and safety measures to avoid infections and injuries.

Teaching points

- Take this drug once a day, with or without food.
- If you forget a dose, take it as soon as you remember; then begin your usual dosage the next day. Do not make up skipped doses and do not take more than one dose each day.
- Maintain your blood glucose level as directed by your health care provider.
- Continue the diet and exercise program designed for the treatment of your type 2 diabetes. Continue other drugs you may be using to treat your diabetes if instructed to do so by your health care provider.
- Arrange for periodic monitoring of your fasting blood glucose and glycosylated hemoglobin levels.
- Know that your health care provider will request periodic blood tests to monitor your kidney function.
- It is not known how this drug affects a fetus. If you are pregnant or thinking about becoming pregnant, discuss this with your health care provider.
- This drug does enter breast milk, but it is not known how this could affect a nursing baby. If you are nursing a baby, discuss this with your health care provider.
- During times of stress (surgery, infection, injury), the needs of your body change. Consult your health care provider immediately if you experience stress. The dosage of your antidiabetic drugs and the actual drugs that are needed may change.
- Report the use of herbal or over-the-counter therapies or other prescription drugs to your health care provider; many of these may change your glucose level and dosage adjustments will be needed,
- Report signs and symptoms of infection, uncontrolled glucose level, severe headache, increased stress, trauma.

▽ scopolamine hydrobromide (hyoscine HBr)

*(skoe **pol'** a meen)*

Oral, Parenteral: Scopace, Scopolamine HBr

Transdermal system: Transderm-Scop

Ophthalmic solution: Isopto Hyoscine Ophthalmic

PREGNANCY CATEGORY C

Drug classes

Anticholinergic
Antiemetic
Anti–motion-sickness drug
Antimuscarinic
Antiparkinsonian

Antispasmodic
Belladonna alkaloid
Parasympatholytic

Therapeutic actions

Mechanism of action as anti–motion-sickness drug not understood; antiemetic action may be mediated by interference with cholinergic impulses to the vomiting center (CTZ); has sedative and amnesia-inducing properties; blocks effects of acetylcholine at muscarinic cholinergic receptors that mediate effects of parasympathetic postganglionic impulses, thus depressing salivary and bronchial secretions, inhibiting vagal influences on the heart, relaxing the GI and GU tracts, inhibiting gastric acid secretion, relaxing the pupil of the eye (mydriatic effect), and preventing accommodation for near vision (cycloplegic effect).

Indications

- Transdermal system: Prevention and control of nausea and vomiting associated with motion sickness and recovery from surgery
- Adjunctive therapy with antacids and histamine-2 antihistamines in peptic ulcer supportive treatment of functional GI disorders (diarrhea, pylorospasm, hypermotility, IBS, spastic colon, acute enterocolitis, pancreatitis, infant colic)
- Preanesthetic medication to control bronchial, nasal, pharyngeal, and salivary secretions; prevent bronchospasm and laryngospasm; block cardiac vagal inhibitory reflexes during induction of anesthesia and intubation; produce sedation
- Induction of obstetric amnesia with analgesics calming delirium
- Treatment of postencephalitic parkinsonism and paralysis agitans; relief of symptoms in spastic states
- Ophthalmic solution: Diagnostically to produce mydriasis and cycloplegia
- Ophthalmic solution: Preoperative and postoperative states in the treatment of iridocyclitis

Contraindications and cautions

- Contraindicated with hypersensitivity to anticholinergic drugs; glaucoma; adhesions between iris and lens; stenosing peptic ulcer, pyloroduodenal obstruction, paralytic ileus, intestinal atony, severe ulcerative colitis, toxic megacolon, symptomatic prostatic hypertrophy, bladder neck obstruction; bronchial asthma, COPD, cardiac arrhythmias, tachycardia, myocardial ischemia; impaired metabolic, liver, or renal function (increased likelihood of adverse CNS effects); myasthenia gravis; pregnancy (causes respiratory depression in neonates, contributes to neonatal hemorrhage); lactation.
- Use cautiously with Down syndrome, brain damage, spasticity, hypertension, hyperthyroidism; glaucoma or tendency to glaucoma (ophthalmic solution).

Available forms

Tablets—0.4 mg; injection—0.3, 0.4, 0.86, 1 mg/mL; transdermal system—1.5 mg; ophthalmic solution—0.25%

Dosages

Adults

Oral

0.4–0.8 mg PO daily; may be increased with caution.

Transdermal system

- *Motion sickness:* Apply one transdermal system to the postauricular skin at least 4 hr before antiemetic effect is required. Scopolamine 1 mg will be delivered over 3 days. If continued effect is needed, replace system every 3 days.

Parenteral

0.32–0.65 mg subcutaneously or IM. May give IV after dilution in sterile water for injection. May repeat if needed up to qid.

Ophthalmic solution

- *Refraction:* Instill 1–2 drops into the eye or eyes 1 hr before refracting.
- *Uveitis:* Instill 1–2 drops into the eye or eyes up to qid.

Pediatric patients

Oral

Do not use oral scopolamine in children younger than 6 yr unless directed by physician.

Transdermal system

Do not use transdermal system in children.

Parenteral

0.006 mg/kg subcutaneously, IM or IV; maximum dose is 0.3 mg. 6 mo–3 yr: 0.1–0.15 mg IM or IV. 3 yr–6 yr: 0.2–0.3 mg IM or IV.

S

Antiemetic
0.006 mg/kg subcutaneously.

Geriatric patients
More likely to cause serious adverse reactions, especially CNS reactions; use lowest possible dose and monitor patient closely.

Pharmacokinetics

Route	*Onset*	*Peak*	*Duration*
Oral	Unknown	1 hr	8–10 hr
IM, Subcut.	30 min	1 hr	4–6 hr
IV	10 min	1 hr	2–4 hr
Transdermal	4–5 hr	24 hr	72 hr
Ophthalmic	10–20 min	30–45 min	Days

Metabolism: Hepatic; $T_{1/2}$: 8 hr
Distribution: Crosses placenta; enters breast milk
Excretion: Urine

IV FACTS

Preparation: Dilute in sterile water for injection.
Infusion: Inject directly into vein or into tubing of actively running IV; inject slowly over 5–10 min.

Adverse effects

- **CNS:** *Pupil dilation, photophobia, blurred vision, headache, drowsiness,* dizziness, mental confusion, excitement, restlessness, hallucinations, delirium in the presence of pain
- **CV:** Palpitations, tachycardia
- **GI:** *Dry mouth, constipation,* paralytic ileus, altered taste perception, nausea, vomiting, dysphagia, heartburn
- **GU:** *Urinary hesitancy and retention,* impotence
- **Hypersensitivity: Anaphylaxis,** urticaria, other dermatologic effects
- **Other:** Suppression of lactation, flushing, fever, *nasal congestion, decreased sweating*

Interactions

✱ **Drug-drug** • Decreased antipsychotic effectiveness of haloperidol • Decreased effectiveness of phenothiazines, but increased incidence of paralytic ileus • Increased CNS depression with alcohol

■ Nursing considerations

Assessment

- **History:** Hypersensitivity to anticholinergic drugs; glaucoma; adhesions between iris and lens; stenosing peptic ulcer, pyloroduodenal obstruction, intestinal atony, severe ulcerative colitis, symptomatic prostatic hypertrophy, bladder neck obstruction; bronchial asthma, COPD; cardiac arrhythmias, myocardial ischemia; impaired metabolic, liver, or renal function; myasthenia gravis; Down syndrome; brain damage, spasticity; hypertension; hyperthyroidism; pregnancy; lactation
- **Physical:** Skin color, lesions, texture; T; orientation, reflexes, bilateral grip strength; affect; ophthalmic examination; P, BP; R, adventitious sounds; bowel sounds, normal output; urinary output, prostate palpation; LFTs, renal function tests, ECG

Interventions

- Ensure adequate hydration; provide environmental control (temperature) to prevent hyperpyrexia.

Teaching points

- Take as prescribed, 30–60 minutes before meals. Avoid excessive dosage.
- Avoid hot environments. You will be heat intolerant, and dangerous reactions may occur.
- Avoid alcohol; serious sedation could occur.
- When using transdermal system, take care to wash hands thoroughly after handling patch and dispose of patch properly to avoid contact with children and pets. Remove the old patch before applying a new one.
- You may experience these side effects: Dizziness, sedation, drowsiness (use caution driving or performing tasks that require alertness); constipation (ensure adequate fluid intake, proper diet); dry mouth (sugarless lozenges, frequent mouth care may help; may lessen); blurred vision, sensitivity to light (reversible, avoid tasks that require acute vision; wear sunglasses); impotence (reversible); difficulty urinating (empty bladder before taking drug).
- Report rash, flushing, eye pain, difficulty breathing, tremors, loss of coordination, irregular heartbeat, abdominal distention,

hallucinations, severe or persistent dry mouth, difficulty urinating, constipation, sensitivity to light.

DANGEROUS DRUG

secobarbital sodium
*(see koe **bar'** bi tal)*

Seconal Sodium

PREGNANCY CATEGORY D

CONTROLLED SUBSTANCE C-II

Drug classes
Antiepileptic
Barbiturate (short-acting)
Sedative-hypnotic

Therapeutic actions
General CNS depressant; barbiturates inhibit impulse conduction in the ascending RAS, depress the cerebral cortex, alter cerebellar function, depress motor output, and can produce excitation (especially with subanesthetic doses with pain), sedation, hypnosis, anesthesia, and deep coma; at anesthetic doses, has antiepileptic activity.

Indications
- Intermittent use as a sedative, hypnotic, or preanesthetic medication

Contraindications and cautions
- Contraindicated with hypersensitivity to barbiturates; manifest or latent porphyria; marked liver impairment; nephritis; severe respiratory distress, respiratory disease with dyspnea, obstruction, or cor pulmonale; previous addiction to sedative-hypnotic drugs (drug may be ineffective, and use may contribute to further addiction); pregnancy (readily crosses placenta and has caused fetal damage, neonatal withdrawal syndrome).
- Use cautiously with acute or chronic pain (drug may cause paradoxical excitement or mask important symptoms); seizure disorders (abrupt discontinuation of daily doses can result in status epilepticus); lactation (has caused drowsiness in nursing infants); fever, hyperthyroidism, diabetes mellitus, severe anemia, pulmonary or cardiac disease, status asthmaticus, shock, uremia; impaired liver or renal function, debilitation.

Available forms
Capsules—100 mg

Dosages
Adults

Adjust dosage on basis of age, weight, condition.
- *Preoperative sedation:* 200–300 mg PO 1–2 hr before surgery.
- *Bedtime hypnotic:* 100 mg PO at bedtime; do not use longer than 2 wk.

Pediatric patients

⊗ ***Warning*** Barbiturates may produce irritability, excitability, inappropriate tearfulness, and aggression.
- *Preoperative sedation:* 2–6 mg/kg PO 1–2 hr before surgery; maximum dose, 100 mg.

Geriatric patients or patients with debilitating disease

Reduce dosage and monitor closely. May produce excitement, depression, or confusion.

Patients with hepatic or renal impairment

Reduce dosage.

Pharmacokinetics

Route	*Onset*	*Duration*
Oral	10–15 min	3–4 hr

Metabolism: Hepatic; $T_{1/2}$: 15–40 hr
Distribution: Crosses placenta; enters breast milk
Excretion: Urine

Adverse effects
- **CNS:** *Somnolence, agitation, confusion, hyperkinesia, ataxia, vertigo, CNS depression, nightmares, lethargy, residual sedation (hangover), paradoxical excitement, nervousness, psychiatric disturbance, hallucinations, insomnia, anxiety, dizziness, thinking abnormality,* complex sleep disorders
- **CV:** *Bradycardia, hypotension, syncope*
- **GI:** *Nausea, vomiting, constipation, diarrhea, epigastric pain*
- **Hypersensitivity:** Rashes, angioneurotic edema, serum sickness, morbilliform rash,

S

urticaria; rarely, exfoliative dermatitis, **Stevens-Johnson syndrome**
- **Respiratory:** *Hypoventilation, apnea, respiratory depression,* **laryngospasm, bronchospasm,** circulatory collapse
- **Other:** Tolerance, psychological and physical dependence; **anaphylaxis, angioedema, withdrawal syndrome**

Interactions

✱ **Drug-drug** • Increased CNS depression with alcohol • Increased renal toxicity with methoxyflurane • Decreased effects of oral anticoagulants, corticosteroids, hormonal contraceptives and estrogens, metronidazole, metoprolol, propranolol, doxycycline, oxyphenbutazone, phenylbutazone, quinidine with barbiturates • Decreased theophylline serum levels and effectiveness secondary to increased clearance • Decreased bioavailability of verapamil

■ Nursing considerations

Assessment

- **History:** Hypersensitivity to barbiturates; manifest or latent porphyria; nephritis; severe respiratory distress; previous addiction to sedative-hypnotic drugs; pregnancy; acute or chronic pain; seizure disorders; lactation; fever, hyperthyroidism, diabetes mellitus, severe anemia, pulmonary or cardiac disease, shock, uremia; impaired liver or renal function, debilitation
- **Physical:** Weight; T; skin color, lesions; orientation, affect, reflexes; P, BP, orthostatic BP; R, adventitious sounds; bowel sounds, normal output, liver evaluation; LFTs, renal function tests, blood and urine glucose, BUN

Interventions

⊗ ***Warning*** Monitor patient for anaphylaxis, angioedema, blood levels with the above interacting drugs; suggest alternatives to hormonal contraceptives.

- Do not use as a bedtime hypnotic for longer than 2 wk.
- Stay with children who have received preoperative sedation.

⊗ ***Warning*** Taper dosage gradually after repeated use, especially in patients who have epilepsy, to avoid refractory seizures.

Teaching points

- Do not use this drug with alcohol.
- Do not use this drug during pregnancy; use of barrier contraceptives is recommended.
- If you are nursing a baby, you should use another method of feeding the baby.
- Do not stand or sit up after you have received this drug (request assistance if you must sit up or move about).
- This drug will make you drowsy (or induce sleep) and make you less anxious. This drug may cause allergic reaction, swelling, complex sleep-related behaviors.

▽ secretin

See Appendix W, *Less commonly used drugs*.

▽ selegiline hydrochloride

*(se **leh'** ge leen)*

Apo-Selegiline (CAN), Carbex, Eldepryl, Emsam, Gen-Selegiline (CAN), Zelapar

Pregnancy Category C

Drug classes

Antidepressant
Antiparkinsonian
MAO type B inhibitor

Therapeutic actions

Mechanism of action not completely understood; inhibits MAO type B activity; may have other mechanisms of increasing dopaminergic activity.

Indications

- Adjunct in management of patients with Parkinson's disease whose response to levodopa and carbidopa has decreased
- Treatment of major depressive disorder (*Emsam*)

Contraindications and cautions

- Contraindicated with hypersensitivity to any component of the drug, pregnancy, lacta-

tion, concurrent use of carbamazepine or oxcarbazine.
- Use cautiously with geriatric patients.

Available forms

Capsules—5 mg; tablets—5 mg; orally disintegrating tablets—1.25 mg; transdermal system—6 mg/24 hr, 9 mg/24 hr, 12 mg/24 hr

Dosages

Adults

- *Parkinson's disease:* 10 mg/day PO in divided doses of 5 mg each taken at breakfast and lunch. After 2–3 days, attempt to decrease dose of levodopa and carbidopa; reductions of 10%–30% are typical. If using orally disintegrating tablet, 1.25 mg/day PO in the morning before breakfast. Place tablet on top of tongue; avoid food or beverage for 5 min. May be increased after 6 wk to 2.5 mg/day. Patient should be under close supervision because of risk of altered mental state.
- *Depression:* Apply one patch (*Emsam*) daily to dry, intact skin on upper torso, upper thigh, or outer surface of upper arm. Start with 6-mg/24-hr system and increase to maximum of 12 mg/24 hr if needed and tolerated.

Pediatric patients

Not recommended for children younger than 16 yr.

Geriatric patients

Maximum dose of transdermal system, 6 mg/24 hr. Use with caution and carefully monitor for orthostatic BP changes.

Pharmacokinetics

Route	Onset	Peak
Oral	Rapid	30–120 min

Metabolism: Hepatic; $T_{1/2}$: 20.5 hr
Distribution: Crosses placenta; enters breast milk
Excretion: Urine

Adverse effects

- **CNS:** *Headache, dizziness, light-headedness, confusion, hallucinations, dyskinesias, vivid dreams,* increased tremor, loss of balance, restlessness, depression, drowsiness, disorientation, apathy, blurred vision, diplopia
- **CV:** Orthostatic hypotension, hypertension, arrhythmia, palpitations, hypotension, tachycardia
- **Dermatologic:** Increased sweating, diaphoresis, facial hair development, hair loss, hematoma, rash, photosensitivity
- **GI:** *Nausea, vomiting, abdominal pain, dry mouth,* constipation, rectal bleeding, heartburn, diarrhea, anorexia
- **GU:** Slow urination, transient nocturia, prostatic hypertrophy, urinary hesitancy, urine retention
- **Other: Asthma**

Interactions

✱ **Drug-drug** • Severe adverse effects to fatalities if combined with meperidine, fluoxetine: Avoid these combinations • Use extreme caution with opioid analgesics • Concurrent use of carbamazepine, oxcarbazepine is contraindicated

✱ **Drug-food** • Avoid tyramine-rich foods and beverages starting on first day of therapy with 9- or 12-mg patch; continue to avoid for 2 wk after reduction to 6-mg patch or discontinuation of 9- or 12-mg patch

■ Nursing considerations

Assessment

- **History:** Hypersensitivity to any component of drug; pregnancy, lactation
- **Physical:** Skin color, lesions; orientation, affect, reflexes; BP, standing BP, P; abdominal examination; prostate examination (males)

Interventions

⊗ ***Black box warning*** Risk of suicidality in children, adolescents, and young adults is increased; monitor accordingly.

- Administer oral drug only as adjunct to levodopa and carbidopa in patients whose symptoms are deteriorating; administer twice daily with breakfast and lunch.
- Limit oral drug to 10 mg/day; larger doses may lead to loss of MAO type B specificity and increase risk of severe hypertensive reactions.
- Dispense least amount of drug possible, especially with depressed patients.

- Administer orally disintegrating tablet by placing on patient's tongue; do not allow food or beverages for 5 min.
- Apply dermal patch to dry, intact skin on upper torso, upper thigh, or outer upper arm. Replace every 24 hr; remove the old patch before applying a new one.
- Monitor the patient for improvement in Parkinson's disease symptoms; if symptoms improve after 2–3 days, begin reducing dosage of levodopa and carbidopa.
- Provide safety measures if dizziness and lightheadedness occur.
- Provide small, frequent meals if GI upset is a problem.
- Provide ice, sugarless lozenges to suck and frequent mouth care if dry mouth is an issue.
- Maintain usual program for treatment of patients with Parkinson's disease.

Teaching points

- Take the oral drug twice a day, with breakfast and lunch. Continue to take your levodopa and carbidopa; the dosage may be decreased in a few days. Do not exceed 10 milligrams per day, serious effects could occur; maintain all of your usual activities and restrictions related to your Parkinson's disease.
- If using orally disintegrating tablets, place on your tongue and allow to dissolve; do not eat or drink anything for 5 minutes; do this in the morning before breakfast.
- If using the patch, apply to your upper torso, upper thigh, or outer upper arm on dry, intact skin; replace the patch every 24 hours; always remove the old patch before applying a new one.
- It is not known how this drug could affect a fetus, if you are pregnant or decide to become pregnant while on this drug, consult your health care provider.
- It is not known how this drug could affect a nursing baby. If you are nursing a baby, consult your health care provider.
- This drug interacts with some other drugs, and this interaction could cause serious side effects; tell any health care provider who is taking care of you that you are on this drug.
- You may experience these side effects: Dizziness, drowsiness, anxiety, disorientation (do not drive a car or operate any dangerous machinery while on this drug; avoid making any important decisions); dry mouth (frequent mouth care, sugarless lozenges may help); nausea, vomiting (it is important to try to maintain your fluid intake and nutrition, let your health care provider know if this becomes difficult).
- Report severe headache, mood changes, confusion, sleep disturbances, dizziness on rising, fainting.

▽sertraline hydrochloride

(sir' trah leen)

Apo-Sertraline (CAN), Novo-Sertraline (CAN), ratio-Sertraline (CAN), Zoloft

PREGNANCY CATEGORY C

Drug classes

Antidepressant
SSRI

Therapeutic actions

Acts as an antidepressant by inhibiting CNS neuronal uptake of serotonin; blocks uptake of serotonin with little effect on norepinephrine, muscarinic, histaminergic, and alpha$_1$-adrenergic or dopaminergic receptors.

Indications

- Treatment of major depressive disorder
- Treatment of OCD
- Treatment of panic disorder with or without agoraphobia
- Treatment of PTSD; long-term use to prevent relapse and sustain symptom improvement
- Treatment of PMDD
- Treatment of social anxiety disorder (social phobia)
- Unlabeled uses: Nocturnal enuresis, hot flashes, cholestatic pruritus

Contraindications and cautions

- Contraindicated with hypersensitivity to sertraline.

- Use cautiously with impaired hepatic or renal function, lactation, pregnancy.

Available forms

Tablets—25, 50, 100, 150, 200 mg; oral concentrate—20 mg/mL

Dosages

Adults

- *Major depressive disorder and OCD:* Administer once a day, morning or evening. 50 mg PO daily; may be increased to up to 200 mg/day; dosage increases should not occur at intervals less than 1 wk.
- *Panic disorder and PTSD:* 25 mg PO daily. After 1 wk increase to 50 mg once daily.
- *PMDD:* 50 mg/day PO daily or just during luteal phase of menstrual cycle.
- *Social anxiety disorder:* 25 mg/day PO; increase to 50 mg/day after 1 wk. Range, 50–200 mg/day.

Pediatric patients

- OCD:
  6–12 yr: 25 mg PO once daily. May be increased slowly as needed.
  13–17 yr: 50 mg PO once daily. May be increased slowly as needed to maximum of 200 mg/day.

Geriatric patients or patients with hepatic impairment

Give a lower or less frequent dose. Use response as dosage guide.

Pharmacokinetics

Route	Onset	Peak
Oral	Slow	4.5–8.4 hr

Metabolism: Hepatic; $T_{1/2}$: 26 hr (104–active metabolite)
Distribution: Crosses placenta; may enter breast milk
Excretion: Feces, urine

Adverse effects

- **CNS:** *Headache, nervousness, drowsiness, anxiety, tremor, dizziness, insomnia,* lightheadedness, agitation, sedation, abnormal gait, psychosis, seizures, *vision changes, fatigue*
- **CV:** Hot flashes, palpitations, chest pain
- **Dermatologic:** *Sweating,* rash, pruritus, acne, contact dermatitis
- **GI:** *Nausea,* vomiting, *diarrhea, dry mouth,* anorexia, dyspepsia, constipation, taste changes, flatulence, gastroenteritis, dysphagia, gingivitis
- **GU:** *Painful menstruation,* sexual dysfunction, frequency, cystitis, impotence, urgency, vaginitis
- **Respiratory:** URIs, pharyngitis, cough, dyspnea, bronchitis, *rhinitis*
- **Other:** Fever, back pain, thirst

Interactions

✱ **Drug-drug** ⊗ ***Warning*** Serious, sometimes fatal, reactions with MAOI; allow at least 14 days to elapse between MAOI and sertraline use.

⊗ ***Warning*** Possible risk of increased QTc interval if combined with pimozide; do not use together.

- Increased serum levels of sertraline with cimetidine

✱ **Drug-food** • Increased rate of absorption with food

✱ **Drug-alternative therapy** • Increased risk of severe reaction if combined with St. John's wort

■ Nursing considerations

Assessment

- **History:** Hypersensitivity to sertraline, impaired hepatic or renal function, lactation, pregnancy
- **Physical:** Weight; T; skin rash, lesions; reflexes, affect; bowel sounds, liver evaluation; P, peripheral perfusion; urinary output, LFTs, renal function tests

Interventions

⊗ ***Black box warning*** Risk of suicidality is increased in children, adolescents and young adults; monitor accordingly.

- Use lower dose in elderly patients and with hepatic or renal impairment.
- Dilute oral concentrate in 4 oz water, ginger ale, lemon-lime soda, lemonade, or orange juice only; administer immediately after diluting.

⊗ ***Warning*** Establish suicide precautions for severely depressed patients. Limit number of tablets given at any time.

- Give drug once a day, morning or evening.

- Increase dosage at intervals of not less than 1 wk.
- Counsel patient to use nonhormonal contraceptives; pregnancy should be avoided due to risk to fetus.

Teaching points

- Take this drug once a day, at the same time, morning or evening; do not exceed the prescribed dose. It may take 4–6 weeks to see any improvement.
- Dilute concentrate immediately before use in 4 ounces of water, ginger ale, lemon-lime soda, lemonade, or orange juice only.
- Consult your health care provider if you think that you are pregnant or wish to become pregnant.
- You may experience these side effects: Dizziness, drowsiness, nervousness, insomnia (avoid driving or performing hazardous tasks); nausea, vomiting (eat frequent small meals); dry mouth (suck sugarless lozenges; perform frequent mouth care); excessive sweating (monitor temperature; avoid overheating).
- Report rash, mania, seizures, edema, difficulty breathing, increased depression, thoughts of suicide.

sevelamer hydrochloride

See Appendix W, *Less commonly used drugs*.

sibutramine hydrochloride

*(sib **buh'** trah meen)*

Meridia

PREGNANCY CATEGORY C

CONTROLLED SUBSTANCE C-IV

Drug classes

Anorexiant
Weight-loss drug

Therapeutic actions

Inhibits the reuptake of norepinephrine, 5-HT, and dopamine; these effects act to suppress the appetite and decrease depression; is nonsedating, non-anticholinergic and has no central depressant effects.

Indications

- Management of obesity, including weight loss and maintenance of weight loss, in conjunction with a reduced-calorie diet

Contraindications and cautions

- Contraindicated with hypersensitivity to sibutramine; pregnancy; anorexia nervosa, bulemia nervosa; and in patients receiving MAOIs or centrally acting appetite-suppressant drugs.
- Use cautiously with impaired renal or hepatic function, hypertension, arrhythmias.

Available forms

Capsules—5, 10, 15 mg

Dosages

Adults

Initial dose, 10 mg PO daily; may increase after 4 wk to up to 15 mg PO daily as tolerated; 5-mg dose may be used if patient cannot tolerate 10-mg dose.

Pediatric patients

Safety and efficacy not established in patients younger than 16 yr.

Pharmacokinetics

Route	*Onset*	*Peak*
Oral	Slow	3–4 hr

Metabolism: Hepatic; $T_{1/2}$: 1.1 hr for parent drug; 14–16 hr for metabolites
Distribution: Crosses placenta; may enter breast milk
Excretion: Feces, urine

Adverse effects

- **CNS:** *Headache, nervousness, sleep difficulties*
- **CV:** Hypertension, tachycardia, arrhythmias
- **Dermatologic:** *Rash, dry skin*
- **GI:** *Dry mouth,* nausea, anorexia, *constipation*
- **Other: Neuroleptic malignant syndrome**

Interactions

✱ **Drug-drug** ⊗ ***Warning*** Serious and potentially fatal reactions if taken with MAOIs; avoid this combination.

• Risk of increased CNS effects if taken with alcohol, CNS stimulants • Risk of serotonin syndrome if combined with other serotogenic agents • Increased risk of toxicity with agents that may raise BP or increase HR

■ Nursing considerations

Assessment

- **History:** Hypersensitivity to sibutramine; impaired hepatic or renal function; lactation; pregnancy; hypertension; arrhythmias
- **Physical:** Weight, T; skin rash, lesions; reflexes, affect; liver evaluation; P, BP, ECG, peripheral perfusion; LFTs, renal function tests

Interventions

- Ensure that patient is participating in a weight loss and exercise program.

⊗ ***Warning*** Establish suicide precautions for severely depressed patients. Dispense only a small number of capsules at a time to these patients.

- Patient may be at increased risk for neuroleptic malignant syndrome; monitor accordingly.
- Administer drug once a day, in the morning or in the evening.
- Increase dosage after 4 wk if adequate response is not achieved.
- Provide sugarless lozenges and frequent mouth care if dry mouth is a problem.
- Counsel patient about the use of nonhormonal contraceptives while using this drug; pregnancy should be avoided because of the possible risk to the fetus.

Teaching points

- Take this drug once a day, at the same time each day, in the morning or in the evening; do not exceed the prescribed dose.
- Use together with diet and exercise to lose weight.
- Do not take this drug during pregnancy. If you think that you are pregnant or wish to become pregnant, consult your health care provider.
- Limit your alcohol consumption while using this drug.
- You may experience these side effects: Dizziness, drowsiness, nervousness, insomnia (avoid driving or performing hazardous tasks); dry mouth (sucking sugarless lozenges and frequent mouth care may help); dry skin, rash (provide skin care as recommended).
- Report rash, mania, seizures, edema, difficulty breathing, palpitations.

▽sildenafil citrate

*(sill **den'** ah fill)*

Revatio, Viagra

PREGNANCY CATEGORY B

Drug classes

Impotence drug
Phosphodiesterase inhibitor

Therapeutic actions

Selectively inhibits cGMP-specific phosphodiesterase type 5. The mechanism of penile erection involves the release of nitric oxide into the corpus cavernosum of the penis during sexual stimulation. Nitrous oxide activates cGMP, which causes smooth muscle relaxation, allowing the flow of blood into the corpus cavernosum. Sildenafil prevents the breakdown of cGMP by phosphodiesterase, leading to increased cGMP levels and prolonged smooth muscle relaxation, promoting the flow of blood into the corpus cavernosum and decreasing pressure in the pulmonary bed.

Indications

- Treatment of ED in the presence of sexual stimulation
- Treatment of pulmonary arterial hypertension to improve exercise ability

Contraindications and cautions

- Contraindicated with allergy to any component of the tablet, concomitant use of nitrates; contraindicated for women or children if used for sexual dysfunction.
- Use cautiously with hepatic or renal impairment; with anatomic deformation of the penis; with known cardiac disease (effects of sexual activity need to be evaluated).

Available forms

Tablets—20 mg (*Revatio*); 25, 50, 100 mg (*Viagra*); single use vial for injection—10 mg/12.5 mL (*Revatio*)

Dosages

Adults

ED: 50 mg PO taken 1 hr before anticipated sexual activity; range, 25–100 mg PO. May be taken 30 min–4 hr before sexual activity. Limit use to once per day (*Viagra*).
Pulmonary arterial hypertension: 20 mg PO tid, at least 4–6 hr apart and without regard to food (*Revatio*); or 10 mg by IV bolus tid (*Revatio*).

Pediatric patients

Not intended for use in children.

Geriatric patients

For patients older than 65 yr, start with 25 mg PO when used for erectile dysfunction.

Patients with renal or hepatic impairment

Patients with hepatic impairment or creatinine clearance less than 30 mL/min may have increased serum levels; start dose at 25 mg PO (*Viagra*); no dosage adjustment needed for *Revatio*.

Pharmacokinetics

Route	Onset	Peak
Oral	Rapid	30–120 min

Metabolism: Hepatic; $T_{1/2}$: 4 hr
Distribution: Not intended for use in women, no clear studies on crossing the placenta or entering breast milk (*Viagra*)
Excretion: Feces, urine

IV FACTS

Preparation: Use as provided; solution should be clear and colorless. Store at room temperature. Single use only.
Infusion: Administer as IV bolus into actively running line or by direct IV injection.

Adverse effects

- **CNS:** *Headache,* abnormal vision, dizziness, nasal congestion, ischemic optic neuropathy, sudden loss of hearing
- **CV:** *Flushing*
- **GI:** *Dyspepsia,* diarrhea
- **Other:** UTI, rash

Interactions

✱ **Drug-drug** ⊗ ***Warning*** Possible severe hypotension and serious cardiac events if combined with nitrates or alpha adrenergic blockers; this combination must be avoided. • Possible increased sildenafil levels and effects if taken with cimetidine, amlodipine, erythromycin, protease inhibitors; monitor patient and reduce dosage as needed

✱ **Drug-food** • Decreased rate of absorption and onset of action if taken with a high-fat meal • Decreased metabolism and risk of toxic effects if combined with grapefruit juice; avoid this combination • Use with alcohol may result in decrease in BP, orthostatic hypotension

■ Nursing considerations

Assessment

- **History:** Allergy to any component of the tablet; hepatic or renal impairment; with anatomical deformation of the penis, known cardiac disease; concomitant use of nitrates
- **Physical:** Orientation, affect; skin color, lesions; P, BP, ECG, LFTs, renal function tests

Interventions

- Ensure diagnosis of pulmonary arterial hypertension (*Revatio*). Reserve IV use for patients unable to take oral form.
- Ensure diagnosis of ED and determine underlying causes and other appropriate treatment (*Viagra*).
- Advise patient that drug does not work in the absence of sexual stimulation. Limit use to once per day (*Viagra*).
- Remind patient that drug does not protect against STDs and appropriate measures should be taken.

⊗ ***Warning*** Advise patient to never take this drug with nitrates; serious and even fatal complications can occur.

⊗ ***Warning*** Advise patients receiving HIV medications that there is an increased risk of sildenafil-associated adverse drug reactions, including hypotension, visual changes, and priapism. Do not exceed 25 mg of sildenafil in 48 hr.

⊗ ***Warning*** Advise patients not to take this drug within 4 hr of an alpha blocker.

Teaching points

- For erectile dysfunction, take this drug 30 minutes to 4 hours before anticipated sexual activity. The usual timing is 1 hour. The drug will have no effect in the absence of sexual stimulation.
- If taking this drug for pulmonary arterial hypertension take three times a day; make sure the doses are 4–6 hours apart.
- Onset of drug effects will be slowed if taken with a high-fat meal; plan accordingly. Avoid drinking grapefruit juice if using this drug.
- This drug will not protect you from sexually transmitted diseases; use appropriate precautions.
- Stop the drug and call your health care provider immediately if you experience sudden loss of vision.
- Do not take this drug if you are taking any nitrates; serious side effects and even death can occur.
- You may experience these side effects: Headache, dizziness, rash, flushing.
- Report difficult or painful urination, rash, dizziness, palpitations, loss of vision or hearing.

silodosin

*(sill oh **do'** zin)*

Rapaflo

PREGNANCY CATEGORY B

Drug classes

Alpha$_1$-adrenergic blocker
BPH drug

Therapeutic actions

Blocks the smooth muscle alpha$_1$-adrenergic receptors in the prostate, prostatic capsule, prostatic urethra, and bladder neck, leading to bladder and prostate relaxation and improved urine flow in cases of BPH.

Indications

- Treatment of signs and symptoms of BPH

Contraindications and cautions

- Contraindicated with known hypersensitivity to any component of the drug, lactation, pregnancy, severe renal impairment, severe hepatic impairment, concurrent use of strong cytochrome P450 inhibitors.
- Use cautiously in patients with hypotension, prostate cancer, cataract surgery, moderate renal impairment.

Available forms

Capsules: 4, 8 mg

Dosages

Adults

8 mg/day PO once daily with a meal.

Pediatric

Safety and efficacy not established.

Patients with renal impairment

With severe renal impairment (creatinine clearance of 30 mL/min or less), drug is contraindicated; with moderate renal impairment (creatinine clearance of 30–50 mL/min), 4 mg/day PO once daily with a meal.

Patients with hepatic impairment

With severe hepatic impairment (Child-Pugh score of 10 or more), drug is contraindicated. With mild to moderate hepatic impairment, no dosage adjustment is needed.

Pharmacokinetics

Route	*Onset*	*Peak*
Oral	Rapid	2–3.5 hr

Metabolism: Hepatic; $T_{1/2}$: 5–20 hr
Distribution: May cross placenta; may enter breast milk (not indicated for use in women)
Excretion: Feces, urine

Adverse effects

- **CNS:** *Dizziness, headache,* insomnia
- **CV:** Orthostatic hypotension
- **GI:** Diarrhea, impaired hepatic function
- **GU:** *Retrograde ejaculation, abnormal ejaculate*
- **Respiratory:** Nasopharyngitis, nasal congestion, sinusitis
- **Other:** Pruritus, purpura, intraoperative floppy iris syndrome with cataract surgery

S

Interactions

✱ **Drug-drug** • Increased risk of elevated silodosin serum levels and toxicity if combined with strong cytochrome 450 inhibitors (ketoconazole, clarithromycin, itraconazole, ritonavir); this combination is contraindicated • Increased risk of hypotension if combined with other alpha blockers; if this combination is used, monitor patient closely and adjust dosages as needed • Risk of increased serum levels if combined with cyclosporine; avoid this combination

■ Nursing considerations

Assessment

- **History:** Known hypersensitivity to any component of the drug, lactation, pregnancy, renal impairment, hepatic impairment, concurrent use of strong cytochrome P450 inhibitors, hypotension, prostate cancer, cataract surgery
- **Physical:** Orientation, affect, reflexes; skin color, lesions; BP, orthostatic BP, status of nasal mucosa; prostate examination, voiding pattern, normal output; LFTs, renal function tests, PSA level

Interventions

- Ensure that patient does not have prostate cancer before beginning therapy.
- Administer drug once a day with a meal.
- If patient is to undergo cataract surgery, there is a risk of floppy iris syndrome occurring. Surgeon should be alerted to the use of the drug, even if the drug has been discontinued; the patient may require additional surgical intervention.
- Provide safety measures if CNS effects occur.
- Monitor patient carefully for orthostatic hypotension; dizziness and syncope may occur. Establish safety precautions as needed. (Use side rails and provide assistance with ambulation.)

Teaching points

- Take this drug exactly as prescribed, once a day with a meal.
- Tell your surgeon that you are taking or have taken this drug if you are considering cataract surgery.
- You may experience these side effects: Headache (medications may be available to help); dizziness, weakness, which may become less over time (this is more likely when you are changing positions, after exercise, in hot weather, and after consuming alcohol; do not drive or operate hazardous machinery if this occurs; change position slowly, use caution when climbing stairs, lie down if the dizziness becomes severe); abnormal ejaculation, ejaculate with little to no semen (this is reversible when the drug is discontinued).
- Report fainting, changes in the color of stool or urine, severe dizziness, worsening of symptoms, rash.

▽ simethicone

(sigh meth' ih kohn)

Flatulex, Gas-X, Genasyme Drops, Mylanta Gas Relief, Mylicon, Ovol (CAN), Phazyme, Phazyme 95, Phazyme 125, Phazyme Quick Dissolve

PREGNANCY CATEGORY UNKNOWN

Drug class

Antiflatulent

Therapeutic actions

Defoaming action disperses and prevents the formation of mucus-surrounded gas pockets in the GI tract; changes the surface tension of gas bubbles in the stomach and small intestine, enabling the bubbles to coalesce, allowing gas to be more easily freed by belching or flatus.

Indications

- Relief of symptoms of pressure, bloating, and fullness from excess gas in the digestive tract; postoperative gaseous distention and pain, use in endoscopic examination; air swallowing; functional dyspepsia; spastic or irritable colon; diverticulosis
- Unlabeled use: Treatment of colic in infants

Contraindications and cautions

- Contraindicated with allergy to components of the product.

Available forms

Chewable tablets—40, 80, 125, 130, 150 mg; tablets—60, 95 mg; capsules—125, 180 mg; drops—40 mg/0.6 mL

Dosages

Adults

Oral

- *Capsules:* 125 mg PO qid, after each meal and at bedtime.
- *Tablets:* 40–125 mg PO qid, after each meal and at bedtime.
- *Drops:* 40–80 mg PO qid up to 500 mg/day, after each meal and at bedtime.

Pediatric patients 2–12 yr

40 mg PO qid after each meal and at bedtime.

Pediatric patients younger than 2 yr

20 mg PO qid after each meal and at bedtime; up to 240 mg/day.

Pharmacokinetics

Not absorbed systemically; excreted unchanged in feces

Adverse effects

- **GI:** Nausea, vomiting, *diarrhea,* constipation, belching, passing of flatus

■ Nursing considerations

Assessment

- **History:** Hypersensitivity to simethicone
- **Physical:** Bowel sounds, normal output

Interventions

- Give after each meal and at bedtime.
- Shake drops thoroughly before each use.
- Add drops to 30 mL cool water, infant formula, or other liquid to ease administration to infants.
- Ensure chewable tablets are chewed thoroughly before swallowing.

Teaching points

- Take drug after each meal and at bedtime; chew chewable tablets thoroughly before swallowing; shake drops bottle before administration. Parents may want to add drops to 30 milliliters of cool water, infant formula, or other liquid to ease administration.
- You may experience increased belching and passing of flatus as gas disperses.
- Report extreme abdominal pain, worsening of condition being treated, vomiting.

▽simvastatin

(sim va ***stah'*** *tin)*

Apo-Simvastatin (CAN), CO Simvastatin (CAN), Gen-Simvastatin (CAN), Novo-Simvastatin (CAN), PMS-Simvastatin (CAN), ratio-Simvastatin (CAN), Zocor

PREGNANCY CATEGORY X

Drug classes

Antihyperlipidemic
HMG-CoA reductase inhibitor

Therapeutic actions

Inhibits HMG-CoA reductase, the enzyme that catalyzes the first step in the cholesterol synthesis pathway, resulting in a decrease in serum cholesterol, serum LDLs, and either an increase or no change in serum HDLs.

Indications

- Adjunct to diet in the treatment of elevated total cholesterol and LDL cholesterol with primary hypercholesterolemia (types IIa and IIb) in those unresponsive to dietary restriction of saturated fat and cholesterol and other nonpharmacologic measures
- To reduce the risk of coronary disease, mortality, and CV events, including CVA, TIA, MI, and reduction in need for bypass surgery and angioplasty in patients with coronary heart disease and hypercholesterolemia
- Treatment of patients with isolated hypertriglyceridemia
- Treatment of type III hyperlipoproteinemia
- Treatment of adolescents 10–17 yr with heterozygous familial hypercholesterolemia

Contraindications and cautions

- Contraindicated with allergy to simvastatin, fungal byproducts; active liver disease or unexplained, persistent elevations of serum transaminases; pregnancy, lactation.
- Use cautiously with impaired hepatic and renal function, cataracts.

Available forms

Tablets—5, 10, 20, 40, 80 mg; orally disintegrating tablets—10, 20, 40, 80 mg

Dosages

Adults

- *Hyperlipidemia:* Initially, 20 mg PO; up to 80 mg PO daily in the evening. Usual range, 5–80 mg/day. Maximum dose, 80 mg/day. Adjust at 4-wk intervals.
- *Prevention of coronary events:* 20–40 mg PO once daily in the evening.
- *Familial hypercholesterolemia:* 40 mg/day PO in the evening, or 80 mg/day divided into doses of 20 mg, 20 mg, and 40 mg in the evening.
- *Combination therapy:* Do not combine with other statins; if used with fibrates or niacin, do not exceed 10 mg/day; regular dose if combined with bile acid sequestrants. Combined with cyclosporine, start with 5 mg/day; do not exceed 10 mg/day. Combination with amiodarone or verapamil, dose should not exceed 20 mg/day.

Pediatric patients 10–17 yr

10 mg/day PO in the evening. Range, 10–40 mg/day based on response.

Patients with renal impairment

Starting dose, 5 mg/day PO; increase dose slowly, monitoring response.

Pharmacokinetics

Route	Onset	Peak
Oral	Slow	1.3–2.4 hr

Metabolism: Hepatic; $T_{1/2}$: 3 hr
Distribution: Crosses placenta; enters breast milk
Excretion: Feces, urine

Adverse effects

- **CNS:** *Headache,* asthenia, sleep disturbances
- **GI:** *Flatulence, diarrhea, abdominal pain, cramps, constipation, nausea,* dyspepsia, heartburn, **liver failure**
- **Respiratory:** Sinusitis, pharyngitis
- **Other: Rhabdomyolysis, acute renal failure**, arthralgia, myalgia

Interactions

✱ **Drug-drug** ⊗ ***Warning*** Increased risk of myopathy and rhabdomyolysis with clarithromycin, erythromycin, HIV protease inhibitors, itraconazole, ketoconazole, nefazodone; avoid concomitant use or suspend therapy during treatment with clarithromycin, erythromycin, itraconazole, and ketoconazole. • Increased risk of myopathy and rhabdomyolysis with amiodarone, verapamil; do not exceed 20 mg simvastatin daily • Increased risk of myopathy and rhabdomyolysis with cyclosporine, fibrates, niacin; monitor patient closely if use together cannot be avoided. Do not exceed 10 mg simvastatin daily • Digoxin levels may increase slightly; closely monitor plasma digoxin levels at the start of simvastatin therapy • Increased risk for hepatotoxicity with hepatotoxic drugs; avoid concurrent use • Simvastatin may slightly enhance anticoagulant effect of warfarin; monitor PT and INR at the start of therapy and during dose adjustment

✱ **Drug-food** • Decreased metabolism and risk of toxic effects if combined with grapefruit juice; avoid this combination

■ Nursing considerations

Assessment

- **History:** Allergy to simvastatin, fungal byproducts; impaired hepatic function; pregnancy; lactation
- **Physical:** Orientation, affect; liver evaluation, abdominal examination; lipid studies, LFTs

Interventions

- Ensure that patient has tried a cholesterol-lowering diet regimen for 3–6 mo before beginning therapy.
- Give in the evening; highest rates of cholesterol synthesis are between midnight and 5 AM.
- Advise patient that this drug cannot be taken during pregnancy; advise patient to use barrier contraceptives.
- Arrange for regular follow-up during long-term therapy. Consider reducing dose if cholesterol falls below target.

Teaching points

- Take drug in the evening. Do not drink grapefruit juice while using this drug.
- Have periodic blood tests.
- This drug cannot be taken during pregnancy; using barrier contraceptives is recommended.
- You may experience these side effects: Nausea (eat frequent small meals); headache, muscle and joint aches and pains (may lessen); sensitivity to light (use a sunscreen and wear protective clothing).
- Report severe GI upset, changes in vision, unusual bleeding or bruising, dark urine or light-colored stools, fever, muscle pain, or soreness.

sirolimus

See Appendix W, *Less commonly used drugs*.

DANGEROUS DRUG

sitagliptin phosphate

(sit ah **glip'** *ten)*

Januvia

PREGNANCY CATEGORY B

Drug classes

Antidiabetic drug

DPP-4 (dipeptidyl peptidase-4) enzyme inhibitor

Therapeutic actions

Slows the inactivation of the incretin hormones, increasing these hormone levels and prolonging their activity. The incretin hormones stimulate insulin release in response to a meal and help to regulate glucose homeostasis throughout the day. This increases and prolongs insulin release and reduces hepatic glucose production to help achieve glycemic control.

Indications

- Adjunct to diet and exercise to improve glycemic control in patients with type 2 diabetes mellitus, as monotherapy or with other oral antidiabetics

Contraindications and cautions

- Contraindicated with history of serious hypersensitivity reactions to sitagliptin.
- Use cautiously with renal insufficiency, concurrent use of other drugs known to cause hypoglycemia, pregnancy, lactation.

Available forms

Tablets—25, 50, 100 mg

Dosages

Adults

100 mg/day PO as monotherapy or combined with metformin, pioglitazone, rosiglitazone, or other oral drugs.

Pediatric patients

Safety and efficacy not established.

Patients with renal impairment

With creatinine clearance of 30–50 mL/min, 50 mg/day PO; with creatinine clearance less than 30 mL/min, 25 mg/day PO.

Pharmacokinetics

Route	Onset	Peak
Oral	Rapid	1–4 hr

Metabolism: Unchanged; $T_{1/2}$: 12.4 hr

Distribution: May cross placenta; may enter breast milk

Excretion: Urine

Adverse effects

- **CNS:** *Headache*
- **Respiratory:** *Nasopharyngitis, URIs*
- **Other:** Hypoglycemia

Interactions

✱ **Drug-drug** • Risk of hypoglycemia when combined with other drugs or herbal remedies known to cause hypoglycemia; monitor patient closely and adjust dosages as needed

■ Nursing considerations

Assessment

- **History:** Renal impairment, pregnancy, lactation
- **Physical:** R, adventitious sounds; blood sugar, HbA_{1C}, renal function tests

Interventions

- Monitor blood glucose levels and HbA_{1C} before and periodically during therapy.

S

- Ensure that patient continues exercise and diet program for management of type 2 diabetes.
- Monitor baseline renal function tests before and periodically during therapy.
- Ensure that patient continues with appropriate use of other drugs to manage type 2 diabetes if indicated.
- Arrange for thorough diabetic teaching program to include diet, exercise, signs and symptoms of hypoglycemia and hyperglycemia, safety measures to avoid infections, injuries.

Teaching points

- This drug should be taken once a day, with or without food.
- If you forget a dose of the drug, take it as soon as you remember, then begin your usual dosage the next day. Do not make up skipped doses or take more than one dose each day.
- Monitor your blood glucose levels as directed by your health care provider.
- Continue the diet and exercise program designed for the treatment of your type 2 diabetes; continue any other drugs used to treat your diabetes if instructed to do so by your health care provider.
- Arrange for periodic monitoring of your fasting blood sugar and glycosylated hemoglobin levels.
- It is not known if this drug could affect a fetus. If you are pregnant or are thinking about becoming pregnant, consult your health care provider.
- It is not known how this drug could affect a nursing baby; discuss the use of this drug during breast-feeding with your health care provider.
- During times of stress (surgery, infection, injury), your body's needs change. Consult your health care provider immediately if you experience times of stress; your dosage or drug choices may need to change.
- Report any other drug, herbal remedies, or over-the-counter medications you may be using to your health care provider; many of these are known to alter your glucose levels, and dosage adjustments may be needed.
- Report fever or signs of infection, uncontrolled glucose levels, severe headache, stress, or trauma.

▽ sodium bicarbonate

(soe' dee um)

Parenteral: Neut

Prescription and OTC preparations: Bell/ans

PREGNANCY CATEGORY C

Drug classes

Antacid
Electrolyte
Systemic alkalinizer
Urinary alkalinizer

Therapeutic actions

Increases plasma bicarbonate; buffers excess hydrogen ion concentration; raises blood pH; reverses the clinical manifestations of acidosis; increases the excretion of free base in the urine, effectively raising the urinary pH; neutralizes or reduces gastric acidity, resulting in an increase in the gastric pH, which inhibits the proteolytic activity of pepsin.

Indications

- Treatment of metabolic acidosis, with measures to control the cause of the acidosis
- Adjunctive treatment in severe diarrhea with accompanying loss of bicarbonate
- Treatment of certain drug intoxications, hemolytic reactions that require alkalinization of the urine; prevention of methotrexate nephrotoxicity by alkalinization of the urine
- Minimization of uric acid crystalluria in gout, with uricosuric agents
- Minimization of sulfonamide crystalluria
- Oral: Symptomatic relief of upset stomach from hyperacidity associated with peptic ulcer, gastritis, peptic esophagitis, gastric hyperacidity, hiatal hernia
- Oral: Prophylaxis of GI bleeding, stress ulcers, aspiration pneumonia
- To reduce the incidence of chemical phlebitis and patient discomfort due to vein irritation at or near the infusion site by raising the pH of IV acid solutions

Contraindications and cautions

- Contraindicated with allergy to components of preparations; low serum chloride (secondary to vomiting, continuous GI suction, diuretics associated with hypochloremic alkalosis); metabolic and respiratory alkalosis; hypocalcemia (alkalosis may precipitate tetany).
- Use cautiously with impaired renal function, HF, edematous or sodium-retaining states, oliguria or anuria, potassium depletion (may predispose to metabolic alkalosis), pregnancy, lactation.

Available forms

Injection—0.5, 0.6, 0.9, 1.0 mEq/mL; neutralizing additive solution—0.48, 0.5 mEq/mL; tablets—325, 520, 650 mg

Dosages

Adults

- *Urinary alkalinization:* Initially, 3,900 mg; then 1,300–2,600 mg every 4 hr.
- *Antacid:* 300 mg–2 g daily to qid PO, usually 1–3 hr after meals and at bedtime.
  - *60 yr and older:* 1 or 2 tablets every 4 hr; maximum, 12 tablets/24 hr.
  - *Younger than 60 yr:* 1–4 tablets every 4 hr; maximum, 24 tablets/24 hr.
- *Adjunct to advanced CV life support during CPR:* Although no longer routinely recommended, inject either 300–500 mL of a 5% solution or 200–300 mEq of a 7.5% or 8.4% solution as rapidly as possible. Base further doses on subsequent blood gas values. Alternatively for adults, 1 mEq/kg dose, then repeat 0.5 mEq/kg every 10 min.
- *Severe metabolic acidosis:* Dose depends on blood carbon dioxide content, pH, and patient's clinical condition. Generally, administer 90–180 mEq/L IV during first hr, then adjust PRN.

Adults and adolescents

- *Less urgent metabolic acidosis:* 2–5 mEq/kg as a 4–8 hr IV infusion. May be added to IV fluids, with rate and dosage determined by arterial blood gases and estimation of base deficit.

Pediatric patients

1 to 2 mEq/kg (1 mL/kg of an 8.4% solution) by slow IV or intraosseous injection.

Younger than 2 yr: Use 4.2% solution. Don't exceed 8 mEq/kg daily.

- *Metabolic acidosis:*
  Younger children—Use caution, and base dosage on blood gases and calculation of base deficit.
  Older children—Follow adult recommendation.
- *Urinary alkalinization:* 84–840 mg/kg PO daily.

Geriatric patients or patients with renal impairment

Reduce dosage and carefully monitor base deficit, serum electrolytes, and clinical response.

Pharmacokinetics

Route	*Onset*	*Peak*	*Duration*
Oral	Rapid	30 min	1–3 hr
IV	Immediate	Rapid	Unknown

Metabolism: $T_{1/2}$: Unknown
Distribution: Crosses placenta; enters breast milk
Excretion: Urine

IV FACTS

Preparation: Direct IV push requires no further preparation; continuous infusion may be diluted in saline, dextrose, and dextrose and saline solutions.
Infusion: Administer by IV direct injection slowly; continuous infusion should be regulated with close monitoring of electrolytes and response, 2–5 mEq/kg over 4–8 hr.
Incompatibilities: Avoid solutions containing calcium; precipitation may occur.
Y-site incompatibilities: Do not give with inamrinone, verapamil, calcium. Norepinephrine and dobutamine are also incompatible.

Adverse effects

- **GI:** Gastric rupture following ingestion
- **Hematologic:** *Systemic alkalosis* (headache, nausea, irritability, weakness, tetany, confusion), hypokalemia secondary to intracellular shifting of potassium, hypernatremia
- **Local:** Chemical cellulitis, tissue necrosis, ulceration and sloughing at the site of infiltration (parenteral)

Interactions

✱ **Drug-drug** • Increased pharmacologic effects of anorexiants, flecainide, mecamylamine, quinidine, sympathomimetics with oral sodium bicarbonate • Increased half-lives and duration of effects of amphetamines, ephedrine, pseudoephedrine due to alkalinization of urine • Decreased pharmacologic effects of lithium, salicylates, sulfonylureas, methotrexate, doxycycline, and other tetracyclines

■ Nursing considerations

Assessment

- **History:** Allergy to components of preparations, low serum chloride, metabolic and respiratory alkalosis, hypocalcemia, impaired renal function, HF, edematous or sodium-retaining states, oliguria or anuria, potassium depletion, pregnancy
- **Physical:** Skin color, turgor; injection sites; P, rhythm, peripheral edema; bowel sounds, abdominal examination; urinary output; serum electrolytes, serum bicarbonate, arterial blood gases, urinalysis, renal function tests

Interventions

⊗ ***Warning*** Monitor arterial blood gases, and calculate base deficit when administering parenteral sodium bicarbonate. Adjust dosage based on response. Administer slowly, and do not attempt complete correction within the first 24 hr; risk of systemic alkalosis is increased.

- Give parenteral preparations by IV route.

⊗ ***Warning*** Check serum potassium levels before IV administration; risk of metabolic acidosis is increased in states of hypokalemia, requiring reduction of sodium bicarbonate. Monitor IV injection sites carefully; if infiltration occurs, promptly elevate the site, apply warm soaks, and if needed, arrange for the local injection of lidocaine or hyaluronidase to prevent sloughing.

- Have patient chew oral tablets thoroughly before swallowing, and follow them with a full glass of water.
- Do not give oral sodium bicarbonate within 1–2 hr of other oral drugs to reduce risk of drug interactions.
- Monitor cardiac rhythm carefully during IV administration.

Teaching points

- Chew oral tablets thoroughly, and follow with a full glass of water. Do not take within 1–2 hours of any other drugs to decrease risk of drug interactions.
- Have periodic blood tests and medical evaluations.
- Report irritability, headache, tremors, confusion, swelling of extremities, difficulty breathing, black or tarry stools, pain at IV injection site (parenteral form).

▽sodium ferric gluconate complex

See Appendix W, *Less commonly used drugs*.

▽sodium fluoride

(soe' dee um)

ACT, Fluor-A-Day (CAN), Fluorinse, Fluoritab, Flura, Flura-Drops, Flura-Loz, Gel Kam, Gel-Tin, Karidium, Karigel, Karigel-N, Luride, MouthKote F/R, Pediaflor, Pharmaflur, Pharmaflur df, Pharmaflur 1.1, Phos-Flur, PreviDent 5000 Plus, Stop, Thera-Flur-N Gel-Drops

PREGNANCY CATEGORY C

Drug classes

Mineral
Trace element

Therapeutic actions

Acts systemically before tooth eruption and topically after tooth eruption to increase tooth resistance to acid dissolution and promote remineralization of teeth and inhibit caries formation by microbes.

Indications

- Prevention of dental caries
- Unlabeled use: Prevention of osteoporosis

Contraindications and cautions

- Contraindicated in areas where fluoride content of drinking water exceeds 0.7 parts per million (ppm), with low-sodium or sodium-free diets, hypersensitivity to fluoride. Do not use in children younger than 3 yr when the fluoride content of drinking water is 0.3 ppm or more. Do not use 1 mg/5 mL (as a supplement) in children younger than 6 yr.
- Use cautiously with pregnancy, lactation.

Available forms

Chewable tablets—0.25, 0.5, 1 mg; tablets—1 mg; drops—0.125, 0.25, 0.5 mg/mL; lozenges—1 mg; solution—0.2 mg/mL; rinse—0.02%, 0.04%, 0.09%, 0.2%; gel—0.1%, 0.5%, 1.2%, 1.23%

Dosages

Adults

Rinse or topical rinse

10 mL once daily or weekly; swish around teeth and spit out.

Gel or cream

Apply thin ribbon to toothbrush or mouth tray for 1 min; brush, rinse, and spit out.

Pediatric patients

Oral

- Fluoride content of drinking water less than 0.3 ppm:
  6 mo–3 yr: 0.25 mg PO daily.
  3–6 yr: 0.5 mg PO daily.
  6–16 yr: 1 mg PO daily.
- Fluoride content of drinking water 0.3–0.6 ppm:
  6 mo–3 yr: None.
  3–6 yr: 0.25 mg PO daily.
  6–16 yr: 0.5 mg PO daily.
- Fluoride content of drinking water more than 0.6 ppm: None.

Rinse or topical rinse

6–12 yr: 5–10 mL/day.
Older than 12 yr: 10 mL/day; have patient swish around teeth for 1 min and spit out.

Gel

Apply 4–6 drops on applicator. Put applicator over teeth and bite down for 6 min. Have patient spit out excess gel.

Pharmacokinetics

Route	*Onset*
Oral	Unknown

Metabolism: $T_{1/2}$: Unknown
Distribution: Crosses placenta; enters breast milk
Excretion: Feces, sweat, urine

Adverse effects

- **Dermatologic:** Eczema, atopic dermatitis, urticaria, rash
- **Other:** Gastric distress, headache, weakness, staining of teeth (with stannous fluoride rinse)

Interactions

✱ **Drug-food** • Milk, dairy products may decrease absorption; avoid simultaneous use

■ Nursing considerations

Assessment

- **History:** Fluoride content of drinking water; low-sodium or sodium-free diets; hypersensitivity to fluoride; pregnancy, lactation
- **Physical:** Skin color, turgor; state of teeth and gums

Interventions

- Do not give within 1 hr of milk or dairy products.
- Tablets may be chewed, swallowed whole, or added to drinking water or juice.
- Give drops undiluted, or with fluids or food.
- Ensure that patient has brushed and flossed teeth before using rinse and that patient expectorates fluid; it should not be swallowed.
- Ensure that patients using cream or gel rinse thoroughly and spit out fluid.
- Monitor teeth, and arrange for dental consultation if mottling of teeth occurs.

⊗ ***Warning*** Monitor patient for signs of overdose (salivation, nausea, abdominal pain, vomiting, diarrhea, irritability, seizures, respiratory arrest); forced diuresis, gastric lavage, or supportive measures may be required.

Teaching points

- Take this drug as prescribed; chew tablets, swallow whole, or add to drinking water or fruit juice.

- Dilute drops in fluids or food, or take undiluted.
- Brush and floss before using rinse; swish around mouth and spit out liquid; do not eat, drink, or rinse out mouth for 30 minutes after use. If using cream or gel, apply thin ribbon to toothbrush, brush, rinse thoroughly and spit.
- Avoid using milk or dairy products and this drug within 1 hour of each other.
- Arrange to have regular dental examinations.
- Report increased salivation, nausea, abdominal pain, diarrhea, irritability, mottling of teeth.

sodium hyaluronate

See Appendix W, *Less commonly used drugs*.

sodium oxybate

(soe' dee um)

Xyrem

PREGNANCY CATEGORY B

CONTROLLED SUBSTANCE C-III

Drug classes
Anticataplectic
CNS depressant

Therapeutic actions
CNS depressant, its mechanism of action in affecting cataplexy is not understood.

Indications
- Treatment of excessive daytime sleepiness and cataplexy in patients with narcolepsy
- Unlabeled uses: Fibromyalgia pain, fatigue

Contraindications and cautions
- Contraindicated with hypersensitivity to any component of the drug, succinic semialdehyde dehydrogenase deficiency, concomitant treatment with sedative-hypnotics.
- Use cautiously with respiratory dysfunction, depression, pregnancy, lactation.

Available forms
Solution—500 mg/mL

Dosages
Adults

4.5 g/day PO divided into two equal doses of 2.25 g. Administer drug at bedtime and again 2.5–4 hr later. Doses may be increased no more than every 1–2 wk to a maximum of 9 g/day in increments of 1.5 g/day (0.75 g/dose).

Pediatric patients younger than 16 yr

Safety and efficacy not established.

Patients with hepatic impairment

Reduce initial dose by half, and adjust dosage to effect while watching closely for adverse reactions.

Pharmacokinetics

Route	*Onset*	*Peak*
Oral	Varies	0.5–1.25 hr

Metabolism: Hepatic; $T_{1/2}$: 0.5–1 hr
Distribution: Crosses placenta; may enter breast milk
Excretion: Lungs, urine

Adverse effects
- **CNS:** *Headache, dizziness, somnolence,* sleepwalking, nervousness, confusion, depression, abnormal dreams, asthenia, muscle weakness, loss of consciousness, insomnia
- **GI:** *Diarrhea, nausea,* vomiting, abdominal pain, dyspepsia
- **GU:** Urinary incontinence
- **Respiratory:** *URI symptoms, pharyngitis,* sinusitis, rhinitis, **respiratory depression**
- **Other:** *Flulike symptoms,* accidental injury, back pain, infections

Interactions
✱ **Drug-drug** • Risk for serious CNS depression if combined with any sedative-hypnotic drug, including alcohol; avoid this combination

■ Nursing considerations
Assessment
- **History:** Hypersensitivity to any component of the drug, succinic semialdehyde dehy-

drogenase deficiency, concomitant treatment with sedative-hypnotic agents, respiratory dysfunction, depression, pregnancy, lactation
- **Physical:** T; reflexes, affect, orientation; R, respiratory auscultation; LFTs

Interventions

⊗ ***Black box warning*** Counsel patient that this drug is also known as GHB, a drug known for abuse. The patient will be asked to view an educational program, agree to the safety measures to ensure that only the patient has access to the drug, and agree to return for follow-up at least every 3 mo.

- Dilute each dose with 60 mL water in the child-resistant dosing cups. Prepare both the bedtime dose and the repeat dose at the same time.
- Encourage patient to refrain from eating for at least 2 hr before going to bed and taking the drug.

⊗ ***Warning*** Administer first dose of the day when the patient is in bed. Patient should stay in bed after taking the dose. The second dose should be given 2½–4 hr later, with the patient sitting up in bed. After taking the second dose, the patient should lie in bed.

- Encourage patient to avoid driving or performing tasks that require alertness for at least 6 hr after taking the drug.
- Do not administer any sedative or hypnotic drugs to a patient who is taking sodium oxybate.
- Provide safety precautions for storage and dispensing of the drug.

Teaching points

- Prepare two doses of the drug in the evening before going to bed. Add 60 milliliters (4 measuring tablespoons) water to the dose· of the drug. Place the doses in the child-resistant dosing cups provided with the drug. Take the first dose when you first go to bed. Place the second dose in easy reach from your bed, but out of the reach of children or pets. Set your alarm to take the second dose 2½–4 hours later. Sit up in bed and take the dose. Lie back down and go back to sleep.
- Avoid eating for at least 2 hours before going to bed. Food will interfere with the actions of this drug.
- Take special precautions to ensure the safety of this drug. It is a controlled substance and cannot be shared with or given to any other person. The drug should be locked up and secured from other people and from children. Keep the drug in the original bottle. When the bottle is empty, remove the label, wash out the bottle and throw the bottle away.
- You may experience these side effects: Dizziness (avoid driving a car or performing hazardous tasks for at least 6 hours after taking the drug); headache (medications may be available to help); nausea, vomiting, diarrhea (proper nutrition is important, consult a dietitian to maintain nutrition); symptoms of upper respiratory tract infection, cough (do not self-medicate; consult your health care provider if this becomes uncomfortable); urinary incontinence or bedwetting (consult your health care provider if this occurs).
- Report fever, difficulty breathing, bed-wetting, confusion, depression, pregnancy.

▽sodium phenylacetate/sodium benzoate

See Appendix W, *Less commonly used drugs*.

▽sodium polystyrene sulfonate

(soe' dee um)

Kayexalate, Kionex, SPS

PREGNANCY CATEGORY C

Drug class

Potassium-removing resin

Therapeutic actions

An ion exchange resin that releases sodium ions in exchange for potassium ions as it passes along the intestine after oral administration or is retained in the colon after enema, thus reducing elevated serum potassium levels; action is limited and unpredictable.

Indications

- Treatment of hyperkalemia

Contraindications and cautions

- Contraindicated with allergy to any component of the drug, obstructive bowel, severe hypertension, severe HF, marked edema (risk of sodium overload).
- Use cautiously with severe hyperkalemia; may need other definitive measures.

Available forms

Suspension—15 g/60 mL; powder 4.1 mEq/g

Dosages

Adults

Oral

15–60 g/day, best given as 15 g daily to qid. May be given as suspension with water or syrup (20–100 mL). Often given with sorbitol to combat constipation. May be introduced into stomach via nasogastric tube.

Enema

30–50 g every 6 hr given in appropriate vehicle and retained for 30–60 min or as long as possible.

Pediatric patients

Give lower doses, using the exchange ratio of 1 mEq potassium/g resin as the basis for calculation; a dose of approximately 1 g/kg every 6 hr has been recommended.

Pharmacokinetics

Route	*Onset*
Oral	2–12 hr
Rectal	Very long

Excretion: Feces

Adverse effects

- **GI:** *Constipation,* fecal impaction, *gastric irritation, anorexia, nausea, vomiting*
- **Hematologic:** *Hypokalemia,* electrolyte abnormalities (particularly decrease in calcium and magnesium)

Interactions

✱ **Drug-drug** • Risk of metabolic alkalosis with nonabsorbable cation-donating antacids (eg, magnesium hydroxide, aluminum carbonate)

■ Nursing considerations

Assessment

- **History:** Severe hypertension, severe HF; marked edema
- **Physical:** Orientation, reflexes; P, auscultation, BP, baseline ECG, peripheral edema; bowel sounds, abdominal examination; serum electrolytes

Interventions

- Administer resin through plastic stomach tube, or mixed with a diet appropriate for renal failure.
- Give powder form of resin in an oral suspension with a syrup base to increase palatability.
- Administer as an enema after first giving a cleansing enema; insert a soft, large (French 28) rubber tube into the rectum for a distance of about 20 cm; with the tip well into the sigmoid colon, tape into place. Suspend the resin in 100 mL sorbitol or 20% dextrose in water at body temperature, introduce by gravity, keeping the particles in suspension by stirring. Flush with 50–100 mL fluid and clamp the tube, leaving it in place. If back leakage occurs, elevate hips or have patient assume the knee-chest position. Retain suspension for at least 30 min (several hours is preferable), then irrigate the colon with a non–sodium-containing solution at body temperature; 2 quarts of solution may be necessary to remove the resin. Drain the return constantly through a Y-tube connection.

⊗ ***Warning*** Prepare fresh suspensions for each dose. Do not store beyond 24 hr. Do not heat suspensions; this may alter the exchange properties.

- Monitor patient and consider use of other measures (IV calcium, sodium bicarbonate, or glucose and insulin) in cases of severe hyperkalemia, with rapid tissue breakdown: burns, renal failure.
- Monitor serum electrolytes (potassium, sodium, calcium, magnesium) regularly, and arrange to counteract disturbances.
- Arrange for treatment of constipation with 10–20 mL of 70% sorbitol every 2 hr or as needed to produce two watery stools per day. Establish a bowel training program.

Teaching points

- This drug is often used in emergencies. Drug instruction should be incorporated within general emergency instructions.
- Frequent blood tests will be needed to monitor drug effect.
- You may experience these side effects: GI upset, constipation.
- Report confusion, irregular heartbeats, constipation, severe GI upset.

solifenacin succinate

*(sole ah **fen'** ah sin **suck'** sin ate)*

VESIcare (ONC)

PREGNANCY CATEGORY C

Drug classes

Muscarinic receptor antagonist
Urinary antispasmodic

Therapeutic actions

Counteracts smooth muscle spasm of the urinary tract by relaxing the detrusor and other smooth muscles through action at the muscarinic parasympathetic receptors.

Indications

- Treatment of overactive bladder with symptoms of urge urinary incontinence, urgency, and urinary frequency

Contraindications and cautions

- Contraindicated with allergy to drug or any component of the drug, severe hepatic impairment, urine retention, gastric retention, uncontrolled narrow-angle glaucoma, lactation.
- Use cautiously with presence of bladder outflow obstruction, GI obstructive disorders, decreased GI motility, controlled narrow-angle glaucoma, reduced renal or hepatic function, congenital or acquired QT prolongation, pregnancy.

Available forms

Tablets (ONC)—5, 10 mg

Dosages

Adults

5 mg/day PO, swallowed whole with water. May be increased to 10 mg/day if desired effect is not seen.

Pediatric patients

Safety and efficacy not established.

Patients with severe renal or moderate hepatic impairment

Do not exceed 5 mg/day PO.

Pharmacokinetics

Route	Onset	Peak
Oral	Slow	3–8 hr

Metabolism: Hepatic: $T_{1/2}$: 45–68 hr
Distribution: May cross placenta, may enter breast milk
Excretion: Feces, urine

Adverse effects

- **CNS:** Dizziness, blurred vision, dry eyes
- **GI:** *Dry mouth, constipation,* nausea, dyspepsia, upper abdominal pain, vomiting
- **GU:** Urinary retention
- **Respiratory:** Cough
- **Other:** Fatigue, lower limb edema

Interactions

✱ Drug-drug ⊗ ***Warning*** There is a risk of prolonged QT interval and potential serious cardiac arrhythmias if combined with other drugs that prolong QT interval; monitor patient closely.

- Risk of increased serum levels and toxic effects if combined with ketoconazole; if this combination is used, monitor patient and consider lowering dose of solifenacin; maximum dose of 5 mg daily with ketoconazole or other potent CYP3A4 inhibitors

■ Nursing considerations

Assessment

- **History:** Allergy to drug or any component of the drug, urinary retention, gastric retention, uncontrolled narrow-angle glaucoma, lactation, bladder outflow obstruction, GI obstructive disorders, decreased GI motility, reduced renal or hepatic function, congenital or acquired QT prolongation, pregnancy

S

- **Physical:** Orientation, affect, reflexes, ophthalmic examination, ocular pressure measurement; P; bowel sounds, oral mucous membranes; baseline ECG, LFTs, renal function tests, bladder residual volume

Interventions

- Arrange for definitive treatment of underlying medical conditions that may be causing overactive bladder.
- Ensure that patient does not cut, crush, or chew tablets.
- Provide sugarless lozenges for patient to suck and frequent mouth care if dry mouth is a serious problem.
- Provide frequent small meals if GI upset occurs.
- Establish bowel program if constipation is a problem.
- Arrange for ophthalmic examination before beginning therapy and periodically during therapy.
- Establish safety precautions if CNS effects occur.
- Measure post-void residual urine volume if patient has difficulty voiding.

Teaching points

- Take drug once a day with water. Swallow whole, do not cut, crush or chew tablet. Take with or without food.
- Be aware that this drug is meant to relieve the symptoms you are experiencing; other medications may be used to treat the cause of the symptoms.
- You may not be able to sweat normally while on this drug; use caution in any situation that could lead to overheating.
- Consult your health care provider if you become pregnant or want to become pregnant; it is not known if this drug affects the fetus.
- If you are nursing a baby, another method of feeding the baby should be used while you are on this drug.
- You may experience these side effects: Dry mouth, GI upset (sucking on sugarless lozenges and frequent mouth care may help); drowsiness, blurred vision (avoid driving or performing tasks that require alertness while on this drug); constipation (medication may be available to help).
- Report inability to void, fever, blurring of vision, severe constipation.

▽ somatropin

*(soe ma **troe'** pin)*

Accretropin, Genotropin, Genotropin Miniquick, Humatrope, HumatroPen, Norditropin, Nutropin, Nutropin AQ, Omnitrope, Saizen, Serostim, Serostim LQ, Tev-Tropin, Zorbtive

PREGNANCY CATEGORY C

PREGNANCY CATEGORY B (GENOTROPIN, SAIZEN, SEROSTIM)

Drug class

Hormone

Therapeutic actions

Hormone of recombinant DNA origin; contains the identical amino acid sequence of pituitary-derived human growth hormone; therapeutically equivalent to endogenous growth hormone; stimulates skeletal (linear) growth, growth of internal organs, protein synthesis, many other metabolic processes required for normal growth.

Indications

- All but *Serostim:* Long-term treatment of children with growth failure due to lack of adequate endogenous growth hormone secretion
- *Nutropin* and *Nutropin AQ:* Treatment of children with growth failure related to chronic renal failure, chronic renal insufficiency, up to the time of renal transplantation
- *Accretropin, Genotropin, Norditropin, Nutropin, Nutropin AQ,* and *Humatrope:* Treatment of girls suffering from Turner's syndrome
- *Serostim, Serostim LQ:* Treatment of AIDS wasting and cachexia to increase lean body mass and improve physical endurance
- *Genotropin:* Long-term treatment of children with growth failure due to Prader-Willi syndrome (PWS)

- *Genotropin:* Long-term treatment of growth failure in children of small gestational age (SGA) who do not catch up by 2 yr
- *Genotropin, Norditropin, Nutropin, Nutropin AQ, Humatrope, Omnitrope, Saizen:* Growth hormone deficiency (GHD) in adults
- *Humatrope:* Treatment of short stature or growth failure in children with short stature-homeobox (SHOX)-containing gene deficiency whose epiphyses have not closed.

NEW INDICATION: *Humatrope:* Treatment of short stature in children of SGA who do not manifest catch-up growth by 2–4 yr

- *Humatrope, Nutropin, Nutropin AQ:* Long-term treatment of idiopathic short stature in pediatric patients whose epiphyses are not closed and for whom diagnostic evaluation excludes other causes treatable by other means
- *Norditropin:* Treatment of short stature in children with Noonan syndrome or Turner's syndrome
- Treatment of short stature in children who are SGA who do not catch up by 2–4 yr
- *Norditropin:* Treatment of adults with severe GHD
- *Saizen:* Replacement of endogenous growth hormone in adults with GHD who have GHD alone or in combination with multiple hormone deficiencies as a result of pituitary disease, hypothalamic disease, surgery, radiation therapy, or trauma or who had GHD as a child and who have had continued GHD established as an adult

Contraindications and cautions

- Contraindicated with known sensitivity to somatropin, benzyl alcohol, glycerin (*Humatrope*), closed epiphyses, underlying cranial lesions, neoplasms, diabetic retinopathy, acute illness secondary to complications of open-heart surgery, abdominal surgeries, accidental trauma.
- Use cautiously with pregnancy, lactation.

Available forms

Powder for injection—varies for each brand

Dosages

Individualize dosage based on response.

Adults

Genotropin

0.04–0.08 mg/kg/wk subcutaneously divided into 6–7 injections.

Serostim

Weighing less than 35 kg: 0.1 mg/kg subcutaneously daily at bedtime.

Weighing 35–45 kg: 4 mg subcutaneously daily.

Weighing 45–55 kg: 5 mg subcutaneously daily.

Weighing more than 55 kg: 6 mg subcutaneously daily.

Serostim LQ

0.1 mg/kg/day subcutaneously to a maximum 6 mg; patients at increased risk for adverse effects can try 0.1 mg/kg every other day.

Humatrope

Up to 0.006 mg/kg/day subcutaneously; may increase to 0.0125 mg/kg/day.

Nutropin

Up to 0.006 mg/kg/day subcutaneously up to 0.025 mg/kg/day in patients younger than 35 yr and 0.0125 mg/kg/day in patients older than 35 yr.

Nutropin AQ

0.006 mg/kg/day subcutaneously to a maximum dose of 0.025 mg/kg/day for patients younger than 35 yr or 0.0125 mg/kg/day for patients older than 35 yr. Increase dose in 0.1-mg increments.

Norditropin

Up to 0.004 mg/kg/day subcutaneously; may be increased to 0.016 mg/kg/day over 6 wk if needed.

Saizen

0.005 mg/kg/day by subcutaneous injection; may be increased up to 0.01 mg/kg/day after 4 wk depending on response and tolerance. Titration should be based on age and gender adjusted serum growth factor levels.

Omnitrope

0.04 mg/kg/wk subcutaneously as a daily divided dose given in the evening; increase at 4- to 8-wk intervals to a maximum of 0.08 mg/kg/wk.

Pediatric patients

Accretropin

- *GHD:* 0.18–0.3 mg/kg/wk subcutaneously divided into daily doses.
- *Turner's syndrome:* 0.36 mg/kg/wk subcutaneously divided into daily doses.

S

Humatrope

0.18–0.3 mg/kg/wk subcutaneously or IM divided into doses given three times/wk or six times/wk for GHD.

- *Turner's syndrome:* Up to 0.375 mg/kg/wk subcutaneously divided into equal doses given either daily or on 3 alternate days.
- *Short stature with SHOX:* 0.35 mg/kg by subcutaneous injection each week, divided into equal daily doses.

Nutropin or Nutropin AQ

- *GHD:* 0.3 mg/kg/wk subcutaneously up to 0.7 mg/kg/wk in divided daily injections.
- *Chronic renal insufficiency:* 0.35 mg/kg/wk subcutaneously divided into daily doses.
- *Turner's syndrome:* up to 0.375 mg/kg/wk subcutaneously divided into equal doses given either daily or on 3 alternate days.

Omnitrope

0.16–0.24 mg/kg/wk subcutaneously divided into daily doses.

Saizen

0.06 mg/kg subcutaneously or IM three times/wk.

Norditropin

0.024–0.034 mg/kg subcutaneously, six to seven times/wk.

- *Noonan syndrome:* Up to 0.066 mg/kg/day subcutaneously.
- *Turner's syndrome:* Up to 0.067 mg/kg/day subcutaneously.

Tev-Tropin

Up to 0.1 mg/kg subcutaneously three times per wk.

Genotropin

0.24 mg/kg/wk subcutaneously for PWS divided into six to seven doses; 0.16–0.24 mg/kg/wk subcutaneously for GHD divided into six to seven doses; 0.48 mg/kg/wk for SGA.

Pharmacokinetics

Route	*Onset*	*Peak*
IM, Subcut.	Varies	3–7.5 hr

Metabolism: Hepatic; $T_{1/2}$: 1.7–4.2 hr
Distribution: Crosses placenta; enters breast milk
Excretion: Feces, urine

Adverse effects

- **Endocrine:** Hypothyroidism, insulin resistance
- **Hematologic:** *Development of antibodies to growth hormone*
- **Other:** Swelling, joint pain, muscle pain, carpal tunnel syndrome, increased growth of preexisting nevi, headache, injection site pain

Interactions

✱ **Drug-drug** • Use caution in combination with drugs metabolized by CYP450 liver enzymes

■ Nursing considerations

Assessment

- **History:** Known sensitivity to somatropin, closed epiphyses, underlying cranial lesions
- **Physical:** Height; weight; thyroid function tests, glucose tolerance tests, growth hormone levels

Interventions

- Administer drug IM or subcutaneously as appropriate.
- Divide total dose into smaller increments given six to seven times/wk for smaller patients unable to tolerate injections.
- Reconstitute drug following manufacturer's instructions; do not shake; do not inject if solution is cloudy or contains particles.
- Refrigerate vials; reconstituted vials should be used within 7 days; do not freeze drug.
- Arrange for tests of glucose tolerance, thyroid function, and growth hormone antibodies. Arrange for treatment as indicated.

Teaching points

- This drug must be given IM or subcutaneously (depending on drug). It can be given in six to seven smaller doses if needed. Dispose of syringes properly.
- You may experience these side effects: Sudden growth, increased appetite; decreased thyroid function (fatigue, malaise, hair loss, dry skin—request hormone).
- Report lack of growth, increased hunger, thirst, increased and frequent voiding, fatigue, dry skin, intolerance to cold.

somatropin, rDNA origin

See Appendix W, *Less commonly used drugs*.

sorafenib tosylate

See Appendix W, *Less commonly used drugs*.

sotalol hydrochloride

(soh' tal lole)

Apo-Sotalol (CAN), Betapace, Betapace AF, Gen-Sotalol (CAN), PMS-Sotalol (CAN), ratio-Sotalol (CAN)

PREGNANCY CATEGORY B

Drug classes

Antiarrhythmic, classes II and III
Beta-adrenergic blocker

Therapeutic actions

Blocks beta-adrenergic receptors of the sympathetic nervous system in the heart and juxtaglomerular apparatus (kidney), thus decreasing the excitability of the heart, decreasing cardiac output and oxygen consumption.

Indications

- Treatment of life-threatening ventricular arrhythmias; because of proarrhythmic effects, use for less than life-threatening arrhythmias, even symptomatic ones, is not recommended
- *Betapace AF:* Maintenance of normal sinus rhythm—to delay the time to recurrence of atrial fibrillation or flutter in patients with symptomatic atrial fibrillation or flutter who are currently in sinus rhythm

Contraindications and cautions

- Contraindicated with bronchial asthma (*Betapace*), sinus bradycardia (HR less than 45 beats/min), second, or third-degree heart block (PR interval greater than 0.24 sec), cardiogenic shock, uncontrolled HF, lactation, congenital or acquired long QT syndromes, hypokalemia and hypomagnesemia.
- Use cautiously with diabetes or thyrotoxicosis, hepatic or renal impairment, sick sinus syndrome, recent MI, pregnancy.

Available forms

Tablets—80, 120, 160, 240 mg

Dosages

Adults

Initial dose, 80 mg PO bid. Adjust gradually, every 3 days, until appropriate response occurs; may require 240–320 mg/day (*Betapace*); up to 120 mg bid (*Betapace AF*).

Pediatric patients older than 2 yr with normal renal function

30 mg/m^2 tid. Can titrate to a maximum of 60 mg/m^2. Allow 36 hr between increments.

Pediatric patients younger than 2 yr

See manufacturer's instructions.

Geriatric patients or patients with renal impairment

Betapace

For creatinine clearance less than 10 mL/min, individualize dose based on response. See table below for dosing intervals.

CrCl (mL/min)	*Dosing Intervals*
More than 60	12 hr
30–59	24 hr
10–29	36–48 hr

Betapace AF

Betapace AF is contraindicated for creatinine clearance less than 40 mL/min. See table below for dosing intervals.

CrCl (mL/min)	*Dosing Intervals*
More than 60	12 hr
40–59	24 hr

S

Pharmacokinetics

Route	*Onset*	*Peak*
Oral	Varies	3–4 hr

Metabolism: $T_{1/2}$: 12 hr
Distribution: Crosses placenta; enters breast milk
Excretion: Urine

Adverse effects

- **Allergic reactions:** Pharyngitis, erythematous rash, fever, sore throat, **laryngospasm, respiratory distress**

- **CNS:** Dizziness, vertigo, tinnitus, fatigue, emotional depression, paresthesias, sleep disturbances, hallucinations, disorientation, memory loss, slurred speech
- **CV:** *HF, cardiac arrhythmias, SA or AV nodal block,* peripheral vascular insufficiency, claudication, **CVA, pulmonary edema,** hypotension
- **Dermatologic:** Rash, pruritus, sweating, dry skin
- **EENT:** Eye irritation, dry eyes, conjunctivitis, blurred vision
- **GI:** *Gastric pain, flatulence, constipation, diarrhea, nausea, vomiting,* anorexia
- **GU:** *Impotence, decreased libido,* Peyronie's disease, dysuria, nocturia, frequent urination
- **Musculoskeletal:** Joint pain, arthralgia, muscle cramp
- **Respiratory: Bronchospasm,** dyspnea, cough, bronchial obstruction, nasal stuffiness, rhinitis
- **Other:** *Decreased exercise tolerance, development of antinuclear antibodies,* hyperglycemia or hypoglycemia, elevated serum transaminase

Interactions

✱ **Drug-drug** • Possible increased effects with verapamil • Increased risk of orthostatic hypotension with prazosin • Possible increased BP lowering effects with aspirin, bismuth subsalicylate, magnesium salicylate, sulfinpyrazone, hormonal contraceptives • Decreased antihypertensive effects with NSAIDs, clonidine • Possible increased hypoglycemic effect of insulin • Risk of potentially fatal arrhythmias if combined with drugs that increase QTc interval (class I and III antiarrhythmics, phenothiazines, TCAs, bepridil, certain oral macrolides, certain quinolone antibiotics) • Possible reduction of efficacy when given with antacids containing aluminum oxide and magnesium hydroxide

✱ **Drug-lab test** • Possible false results with glucose or insulin tolerance tests (oral)

■ Nursing considerations

Assessment

- **History:** Sinus bradycardia; second- or third-degree heart block; cardiogenic shock, HF; asthma, COPD; pregnancy, lactation; diabetes or thyrotoxicosis; prolonged QTc interval, bronchial asthma
- **Physical:** Weight; skin condition; neurologic status; P, BP, ECG; respiratory status, renal and thyroid function tests, blood and urine glucose

Interventions

- Take this drug on an empty stomach.

⊗ ***Black box warning*** Do not give drug for ventricular arrhythmias unless the patient is unresponsive to other antiarrhythmics and has a life-threatening ventricular arrhythmia. Monitor patient response carefully; proarrhythmic effect can be pronounced.

- Maintain patient on continuous cardiac monitoring for at least 3 days when initiating therapy.

⊗ ***Warning*** Do not discontinue drug abruptly after long-term therapy. Taper drug gradually over 2 wk with monitoring (abrupt withdrawal may cause serious beta-adrenergic rebound effects).

- Discontinue other antiarrhythmics gradually, allowing for two to three plasma half-lives of the drug before starting sotalol. After discontinuing amiodarone, do not start sotalol until QTc interval is normalized.
- Consult with physician about withdrawing drug if patient is to undergo surgery (withdrawal is controversial).

Teaching points

- Take drug on an empty stomach.
- Do not stop taking unless told to do so by your health care provider.
- Avoid driving or dangerous activities if dizziness or weakness occurs.
- You may experience these side effects: Dizziness, light-headedness, loss of appetite, nightmares, depression, sexual impotence.
- Report difficulty breathing, night cough, swelling of extremities, slow pulse, confusion, depression, rash, fever, sore throat.

spironolactone
(speer on oh ***lak'*** *tone)*

Aldactone, Novospiroton (CAN)

PREGNANCY CATEGORY C

Drug classes
Aldosterone antagonist
Potassium-sparing diuretic

Therapeutic actions
Competitively blocks the effects of aldosterone in the renal tubule, causing loss of sodium and water and retention of potassium.

Indications
- Diagnosis and maintenance of primary hyperaldosteronism
- Adjunctive therapy in edema associated with HF, nephrotic syndrome, hepatic cirrhosis when other therapies are inadequate or inappropriate
- Treatment of hypokalemia or prevention of hypokalemia in patients who would be at high risk if hypokalemia occurred (eg, patients receiving cardiac glycosides), patients with cardiac arrhythmias
- Essential hypertension, usually in combination with other drugs
- Unlabeled uses: Treatment of hirsutism because of its antiandrogenic properties, palliation of symptoms of PMS, treatment of familial male precocious puberty, short-term treatment of acne vulgaris

Contraindications and cautions
- Contraindicated with allergy to spironolactone, hyperkalemia, renal disease, anuria, amiloride or triamterene use.
- Use cautiously with pregnancy, lactation.

Available forms
Tablets—25, 50, 100 mg

Dosages
Adults
- *Edema:* Initially, 100 mg/day (range 25–200 mg/day) when given as the sole agent; continue at least 5 days; then adjust dosage or add another diuretic or both.
- *Diagnosis of hyperaldosteronism:* 400 mg/day PO for 3–4 wk (long test). Correction of hypokalemia and hypertension are presumptive evidence of primary hyperaldosteronism. 400 mg/day PO for 4 days (short test). If serum potassium increases but decreases when drug is stopped, presumptive diagnosis can be made.
- *Maintenance therapy for hyperaldosteronism:* 100–400 mg/day PO.
- *Essential hypertension:* 50–100 mg/day PO. May be combined with other diuretics.
- *Hypokalemia:* 25–100 mg/day PO.

Pediatric patients
- Safety and efficacy not established.

Pharmacokinetics

Route	*Onset*	*Peak*	*Duration*
Oral	24–48 hr	48–72 hr	48–72 hr

Metabolism: Hepatic; $T_{1/2}$: 20 hr
Distribution: Crosses placenta; enters breast milk
Excretion: Feces, urine

Adverse effects
- **CNS:** *Dizziness, headache, drowsiness,* fatigue, ataxia, confusion
- **Dermatologic:** *Rash,* urticaria
- **GI:** *Cramping, diarrhea,* dry mouth, thirst, vomiting
- **GU:** Impotence, irregular menses, amenorrhea, postmenopausal bleeding
- **Hematologic:** Hyperkalemia, hyponatremia, agranulocytosis
- **Other:** Carcinogenic in animals, *deepening of the voice, hirsutism, gynecomastia*

Interactions
✱ **Drug-drug** • Increased hyperkalemia with potassium supplements, ACE inhibitors, diets rich in potassium • Decreased diuretic effect with salicylates • Decreased hypoprothrombinemic effect of anticoagulants • Increased hypotensive effect with diuretics and other hypotensive drugs, especially ganglionic blockers

✱ **Drug-food** • Increased absorption when taken with food

✱ **Drug-lab test** • Interference with radioimmunoassay for digoxin; false increase in serum digoxin levels • Interference with fluorometric determinations of plasma and urinary cortisol

✱ **Drug-alternative therapy** • Decreased effectiveness if combined with licorice therapy

■ Nursing considerations

Assessment

- **History:** Allergy to spironolactone, hyperkalemia, renal disease, pregnancy, lactation
- **Physical:** Skin color, lesions, edema; orientation, reflexes, muscle strength; P, baseline ECG, BP; R, pattern, adventitious sounds; liver evaluation, bowel sounds; urinary output patterns, menstrual cycle; CBC, serum electrolytes, renal function tests, urinalysis

Interventions

⊗ ***Black box warning*** Drug has been shown to be a tumorigen with chronic toxicity in rats; avoid unnecessary use of this drug.

- Mark calendars of edema outpatients as reminders of alternate-day or 3- to 5-day/wk therapy.
- Give daily doses early so that increased urination does not interfere with sleep.
- Measure and record regular weight to monitor mobilization of edema fluid.
- Avoid giving food rich in potassium.
- Arrange for regular evaluation of serum electrolytes and BUN.

Teaching points

- Record alternate-day therapy on a calendar, or prepare dated envelopes. Take the drug early because of increased urination.
- Weigh yourself on a regular basis, at the same time and in the same clothing, and record the weight on your calendar.
- Avoid foods that are rich in potassium (fruits, *Sanka*); avoid licorice.
- You may experience these side effects: Increased volume and frequency of urination; dizziness, confusion, feeling faint on arising, drowsiness (avoid rapid position changes, hazardous activities such as driving, using alcohol); increased thirst (suck on sugarless lozenges; use frequent mouth care); changes in menstrual cycle, deepening of the voice, impotence, enlargement of the breasts can occur (reversible).
- Report weight change of more than 3 pounds in 1 day, swelling in your ankles or fingers, dizziness, trembling, numbness, fatigue, enlargement of breasts, deepening of voice, impotence, muscle weakness, or cramps.

▽ stavudine (d4T)

(stay vyoo' deen)

Zerit XR

Pregnancy Category C

Drug classes

Antiviral
Nucleoside reverse transcriptase inhibitor

Therapeutic actions

Inhibits replication of some retroviruses, including HIV, HTLV III, LAV, and ARV.

Indications

- Treatment of HIV-1 infection in combination with other antiretroviral therapy

Contraindications and cautions

- Contraindicated with life-threatening allergy to any component, lactation.
- Use cautiously with compromised bone marrow, impaired renal or hepatic function, or risk factors for liver disease, pregnancy.

Available forms

ER capsules—37.5, 50, 75, 100 mg

Dosages

Adults

ER

Weighing less than 60 kg: 75 mg/day PO once daily.

Weighing 60 kg or more: 100 mg/day PO once daily.

Pediatric patients

ER form not recommended.

Patients with renal impairment

CrCl (mL/min)	Weighing 60 kg or more	Weighing less than 60 kg
More than 50	40 mg every 12 hr	30 mg every 12 hr
26–50	20 mg every 12 hr	15 mg every 12 hr
10–25	20 mg/day	15 mg/day

Patients with persistent peripheral neuropathy

Dose may be resumed at 50% of normal after temporary withdrawal.

Pharmacokinetics

Route	Onset	Peak
Oral	Varies	60–90 min

Metabolism: Unknown; $T_{1/2}$: 30–60 min
Distribution: Crosses placenta; may enter breast milk
Excretion: Urine

Adverse effects

- **CNS:** *Headache,* insomnia, myalgia, *asthenia,* malaise, dizziness, paresthesia, somnolence, motor weakness, peripheral neuropathy
- **GI:** *Nausea, GI pain, diarrhea,* anorexia, vomiting, dyspepsia, **hepatomegaly with steatosis, pancreatitis**
- **Hematologic:** *Agranulocytopenia,* severe anemia requiring transfusions
- **Other:** *Fever,* diaphoresis, dyspnea, *rash,* taste perversion, **lactic acidosis,** body fat redistribution

Interactions

✱ **Drug-drug** • Increased risk of fatal or nonfatal pancreatitis if combined with didanosine; monitor closely • Increased risk of lactic acidosis, severe hepatomegaly when taken with other nucleoside analogues, such as zidovudine, doxorubicin, ribavirin

■ Nursing considerations

Assessment

- **History:** Life-threatening allergy to any component; compromised bone marrow; impaired renal or hepatic function; pregnancy, lactation
- **Physical:** Skin rashes, lesions, texture; T; affect, reflexes, peripheral sensation; bowel sounds, liver evaluation; LFTs, renal function tests, CBC and differential

Interventions

⊠ ***Black box warning*** Monitor patient closely for pancreatitis throughout therapy; fatal and nonfatal pancreatitis have occurred.

- Monitor hematologic indices every 2 wk during therapy.

⊗ ***Warning*** Monitor neurologic function. If neuropathy occurs, discontinue. Restart at 50% dose when neuropathy resolves.

- Give every 12 hr, around-the-clock; schedule dose so it will not interrupt sleep.

⊠ ***Black box warning*** Monitor LFTs; lactic acidosis and severe hepatomegaly may occur.

Teaching points

- Take drug once each day. Do not share this drug; take exactly as prescribed.
- Stavudine is not a cure for AIDS; opportunistic infections may occur; regular medical care should be sought to deal with the disease.
- Always take this drug in combination with other HIV drugs.
- Frequent blood tests are needed; results may indicate a need to decrease or discontinue drug temporarily.
- Stavudine does not reduce the risk of HIV transmission by sexual contact or blood contamination; use appropriate precautions.
- This drug should be used during pregnancy only if the potential benefit justifies the potential risk; using barrier contraceptives is advised.
- You may experience these side effects: Nausea, loss of appetite, change in taste (eat frequent small meals); dizziness, loss of feeling (take precautions); headache, fever, muscle aches.
- Report extreme fatigue, lethargy, severe headache, severe nausea, vomiting, difficulty breathing, rash, numbness or tingling in feet or hands.

S

▽ streptomycin sulfate

See Appendix W, *Less commonly used drugs.*

streptozocin

See Appendix W, *Less commonly used drugs.*

succimer (DMSA)

(sux' i mer)

Chemet

PREGNANCY CATEGORY C

Drug classes

Antidote
Chelate

Therapeutic actions

Forms water-soluble chelates with lead, leading to increased urinary excretion of lead.

Indications

- Treatment of lead poisoning in children with blood levels greater than 45 mcg/dL (not for prophylactic use)
- Orphan drug use: Prevention of cystine kidney stones in patients with homozygous cystinuria
- Unlabeled use: Treatment of other heavy metal poisonings (mercury, arsenic)

Contraindications and cautions

- Contraindicated with allergy to succimer, pregnancy (teratogenic and embryotoxic), lactation.
- Use cautiously with impaired renal or hepatic function.

Available forms

Capsules—100 mg

Dosages

Pediatric patients

Starting dose of 10 mg/kg or 350 mg/m^2 every 8 hr PO for 5 days; reduce dosage to 10 mg/kg or 350 mg/m^2 every 12 hr PO for 2 wk (therapy runs for 19 days).

Pharmacokinetics

Route	*Onset*	*Peak*
Oral	Varies	1–2 hr

Metabolism: Hepatic; $T_{1/2}$: 2 days
Distribution: Crosses placenta; may enter breast milk
Excretion: Feces, urine

Adverse effects

- **CNS:** Drowsiness, dizziness, sleepiness, otitis media, watery eyes
- **Dermatologic:** Papular rash, herpetic rash, mucocutaneous eruptions, pruritus
- **GI:** *Nausea, vomiting,* diarrhea, severe transaminases, metallic taste in mouth, loss of appetite
- **GU:** Decreased urination, voiding difficulty
- **Hematologic:** Neutropenia, increased platelets, intermittent eosinophilia
- **Other:** *Back, stomach, flank, head, rib pain;* chills; fever; flulike symptoms

Interactions

✱ **Drug-drug** • High risk of toxicity with other chelating agents (EDTA)
✱ **Drug-lab test** • False-positive tests of urine ketones using *Ketostix* • False decrease in serum uric acid, CPK

■ Nursing considerations

Assessment

- **History:** Allergy to succimer; lactation, pregnancy; renal or hepatic impairment
- **Physical:** Weight; orientation, affect; liver evaluation; urinalysis; LFTs, renal function tests; serum lead levels

Interventions

- Test serum blood levels before therapy and monitor weekly.
- Monitor serum transaminase level prior to and weekly during treatment.
- Identify the source of lead and facilitate its removal; succimer is not prophylactic to prevent lead poisoning.
- Ensure that patient continues therapy for full 19 days.
- For children unable to swallow capsules: Separate capsules and give medicated beads on a small amount of soft food or by spoon followed by fruit drink.
- All patients undergoing treatment should be adequately hydrated.

Teaching points

- For children unable to swallow capsules: Separate capsules and give medicated beads on a small amount of soft food or by spoon followed by fruit drink.
- Ensure child maintains good fluid intake.
- You may experience these side effects: Nausea, vomiting, loss of appetite (eat frequent small meals); abdominal, back, rib, flank pain (request medication).
- Report rash, difficulty breathing, difficulty walking, tremors.

sucralfate

*(soo **kral'** fayt)*

Apo-Sucralfate (CAN), Carafate, Sulcrate (CAN)

PREGNANCY CATEGORY B

Drug class

Antiulcer drug

Therapeutic actions

Forms an ulcer-adherent complex at duodenal ulcer sites, protecting the ulcer against acid, pepsin, and bile salts, thereby promoting ulcer healing; also inhibits pepsin activity in gastric juices.

Indications

- Short-term treatment of duodenal ulcers, up to 8 wk
- Maintenance therapy for duodenal ulcer at reduced dosage after healing
- Orphan drug use: Treatment of oral and esophageal ulcers due to radiation, chemotherapy, and sclerotherapy
- Unlabeled uses: Accelerates healing of gastric ulcers, long-term treatment of gastric ulcers, treatment of reflux and peptic esophagitis, treatment of NSAID or aspirin-induced GI symptoms and GI damage, prevention of stress ulcers in critically ill patients

Contraindications and cautions

- Contraindicated with allergy to sucralfate, chronic renal failure or dialysis (buildup of aluminum may occur with aluminum-containing products).
- Use cautiously with pregnancy, lactation.

Available forms

Tablets—1 g; suspension—1 g/10 mL

Dosages

Adults

- *Active duodenal ulcer:* 1 g PO qid on an empty stomach (1 hr before meals and at bedtime). Continue treatment for 4–8 wk.
- *Maintenance:* 1 g PO bid.

Pediatric patients

Safety and efficacy not established.

Pharmacokinetics

Route	Onset	Duration
Oral	30 min	5 hr

Minimal systemic absorption

Adverse effects

- **CNS:** Dizziness, sleeplessness, vertigo
- **Dermatologic:** Rash, pruritus
- **GI:** *Constipation,* diarrhea, nausea, indigestion, gastric discomfort, dry mouth
- **Other:** Back pain

Interactions

✱ **Drug-drug** • Decreased serum levels and effectiveness of phenytoin, ciprofloxacin, norfloxacin, digoxin, ketoconazole, tetracycline, theophylline, penicillamine, warfarin, levothyroxine, quinidine; separate administration by 2 hr • Risk of aluminum toxicity with aluminum-containing antacids

■ Nursing considerations

Assessment

- **History:** Allergy to sucralfate; chronic renal failure or dialysis; pregnancy, lactation
- **Physical:** Skin color, lesions; reflexes, orientation; mucous membranes, normal output

Interventions

- Give drug on an empty stomach, 1 hr before or 2 hr after meals and at bedtime.
- Monitor pain; use antacids to relieve pain.
- Administer antacids between doses of sucralfate, not within 30 min before or after sucralfate doses.

S

Teaching points

- Take the drug on an empty stomach, 1 hour before or 2 hours after meals and at bedtime.
- If you are also taking antacids for pain relief, do not take antacids 30 minutes before or after taking sucralfate.
- You may experience these side effects: Dizziness, vertigo (avoid driving or operating dangerous machinery); indigestion, nausea (eat frequent small meals); dry mouth (use frequent mouth care, suck on sugarless lozenges); constipation (request aid).
- Report severe gastric pain.

DANGEROUS DRUG

sufentanil citrate

*(soo **fen'** ta nil)*

Sufenta

PREGNANCY CATEGORY C

CONTROLLED SUBSTANCE C-II

Drug class

Opioid agonist analgesic

Therapeutic actions

Acts at specific opioid receptors, causing analgesia, respiratory depression, physical depression, euphoria.

Indications

- Analgesic adjunct to maintain balanced general anesthesia
- Primary anesthetic with 100% oxygen to induce and maintain anesthesia in major surgical procedures
- Epidural analgesia with bupivacaine during labor and delivery

Contraindications and cautions

- Contraindicated with known sensitivity to sufentanil, pregnancy.
- Use cautiously with obesity, hepatic disease, head injury, diabetes, arrhythmias, lactation, severe debilitation, renal or pulmonary disease.

Available forms

Injection—50 mcg/mL

Dosages

Individualize dosage; monitor vital signs routinely.

Adults

- *Adjunct to general anesthesia:* 1–2 mcg/kg IV initially; 10–25 mcg for maintenance; not to exceed 1 mcg/kg/hr of expected surgical time.
- *With oxygen and skeletal muscle relaxant for anesthesia:* 8–30 mcg/kg IV initially; supplement with doses of 0.5–10 mcg/kg IV; not to exceed 30 mcg/kg for the procedure.
- *Epidural analgesia:* 10–15 mcg via epidural administration with 10 mL bupivacaine 0.125%; may repeat twice at 1-hr or longer intervals (total of three doses).

Pediatric patients 2–12 yr

- *With oxygen and skeletal muscle relaxant for anesthesia:* 10–25 mcg/kg IV initially; supplement with doses of 25–50 mcg IV.

Pharmacokinetics

Route	*Onset*	*Duration*
IV	Immediate	5 min
Epidural	10 min	1.7 hr

Metabolism: Hepatic; $T_{1/2}$: 2.7 hr
Distribution: Crosses placenta; enters breast milk
Excretion: Urine

IV FACTS

Preparation: Protect vials from light.
Infusion: Give slowly over 1–2 min by direct injection or into running IV tubing.

Adverse effects

- **CNS:** *Sedation, clamminess, sweating, headache, vertigo, floating feeling, dizziness, lethargy, confusion, light-headedness,* nervousness, unusual dreams, agitation, euphoria, hallucinations, delirium, insomnia, anxiety, fear, disorientation, impaired mental and physical performance, coma, mood changes, weakness, headache, tremor, seizures
- **CV:** Palpitations, change in BP, circulatory depression, **cardiac arrest, shock,** tachycardia, bradycardia, arrhythmia

- **Dermatologic:** Rash, hives, pruritus, flushing, warmth, sensitivity to cold
- **EENT:** Diplopia, blurred vision
- **GI:** *Nausea, vomiting,* dry mouth, anorexia, constipation, biliary tract spasm
- **GU:** Ureteral spasm, spasm of vesical sphincters, urinary retention or hesitancy, oliguria, antidiuretic effect, reduced libido or potency
- **Local:** Phlebitis following IV injection, pain at injection site
- **Respiratory:** Slow, shallow respiration, apnea, suppression of cough reflex, **laryngospasm, bronchospasm**
- **Other:** Physical tolerance and dependence; psychological dependence; skeletal muscle rigidity, possibly requiring neuromuscular blocker

Interactions

✱ **Drug-drug** • Potentiation of effects with general anesthetics, opiate agonists, tranquilizers, sedatives, hypnotics (barbiturates) • Increased risk of hypotension and bradycardia if given with beta blockers, calcium channel blockers

✱ **Drug-food** • Decreased metabolism and risk of toxic effects if combined with grapefruit juice; avoid this combination

✱ **Drug-lab test** • Elevated biliary tract pressure may cause increases in plasma amylase, lipase; determinations of these levels may be unreliable for 24 hr after administration of opioids

■ Nursing considerations

CLINICAL ALERT!

Name confusion has occurred between sufentanil and fentanyl; use extreme caution.

Assessment

- **History:** Hypersensitivity to sufentanil or opioids; physical dependence on an opioid analgesic; pregnancy, lactation; COPD; increased intracranial pressure; acute MI, biliary tract surgery; renal or hepatic impairment
- **Physical:** Orientation, reflexes, bilateral grip strength, affect; pupil size, vision; pulse, auscultation, BP; R, adventitious sounds; bowel sounds, normal output; LFTs, renal function tests

Interventions

- Give to lactating women 4–6 hr before the next feeding to minimize the amount in milk.
- Ensure that patient avoids grapefruit juice while using this drug.

⊗ ***Warning*** Provide opioid antagonist, keep equipment for assisted or controlled respiration readily available during parenteral administration.

Teaching points

- Incorporate teaching about drug into preoperative or postoperative teaching program.
- You may experience these side effects: Dizziness, sedation, drowsiness, impaired visual acuity (ask for assistance to move); nausea, loss of appetite (lie quietly, eat frequent small meals); constipation (use a laxative).
- Report severe nausea, vomiting, palpitations, shortness of breath or difficulty breathing.

sulfadiazine

*(sul fa **dye'** a zeen)*

PREGNANCY CATEGORY C

PREGNANCY CATEGORY D (LABOR AND DELIVERY)

Drug classes

Antibiotic

Sulfonamide

Therapeutic actions

Bacteriostatic: Competitively antagonizes PABA, an essential component of folic acid synthesis in gram-negative and gram-positive bacteria; prevents cell replication.

Indications

- Treatment of acute infections caused by susceptible organisms: UTIs, chancroid, inclusion conjunctivitis, trachoma, nocardiosis, toxoplasmosis (with pyrimethamine), malaria (as adjunctive therapy for chloroquine-resistant strains of *Plasmodium falciparum*), acute otitis media (due to *Haemophilus influenzae* when used with penicillin or erythromycin), *H. influenzae* meningitis (as adjunctive therapy with par-

S

enteral streptomycin), meningococcal meningitis, rheumatic fever
- Orphan drug use: With pyrimethamine for treatment of *Toxoplasma gondii* encephalitis in patients with AIDS

Contraindications and cautions
- Contraindicated with allergy to sulfonamides, sulfonylureas, thiazides; pregnancy (teratogenic; may cause kernicterus); lactation (risk of kernicterus, diarrhea, rash).
- Use cautiously with impaired renal or hepatic function, G6PD deficiency, porphyria.

Available forms
Tablets—500 mg

Dosages
Adults
Loading dose, 2–4 g PO. Maintenance, 2–4 g/day PO in three to six divided doses.
- Prevention of recurrent attacks of rheumatic fever (not for initial therapy of streptococcal infections):
  Weight less than 30 kg: 0.5 g/day PO.
  Weight more than 30 kg: 1 g/day PO.
- *Toxoplasmosis:* 1–1.5 g qid in combination with pyrimethamine for 3–4 wk.
- *For suppressive or maintenance therapy in HIV patients:* 0.5–1 g every 6 hr PO with oral pyrimethamine and leucovorin.

Pediatric patients
Younger than 2 mo: Not recommended except to treat congenital toxoplasmosis.
Older than 2 mo: Initial dose, 75 mg/kg PO. Maintenance, 150 mg/kg/day PO in four to six divided doses with a maximum dose of 6 g/day.
- *Toxoplasmosis:* 100–200 mg/kg daily in combination with pyrimethamine for 3–4 wk.
- For suppressive or maintenance therapy in HIV patients:
  Infants and children: 85–120 mg/kg daily in two to four divided doses with oral pyrimethamine and leucovorin.
  Adolescents: 0.5–1 g every 6 hr PO with oral pyrimethamine and leucovorin.

Pharmacokinetics

Route	*Onset*	*Peak*
Oral	Varies	3–6 hr

Metabolism: Hepatic; $T_{1/2}$: Unknown
Distribution: Crosses placenta; enters breast milk
Excretion: Urine

Adverse effects
- **CNS:** *Headache,* peripheral neuropathy, mental depression, seizures, ataxia, hallucinations, tinnitus, vertigo, insomnia, hearing loss, drowsiness, transient lesions of posterior spinal column, transverse myelitis
- **Dermatologic:** *Photosensitivity,* cyanosis, petechiae, alopecia
- **GI:** *Nausea, emesis, abdominal pains,* diarrhea, bloody diarrhea, anorexia, pancreatitis, stomatitis, impaired folic acid absorption, hepatitis, **hepatocellular necrosis**
- **GU:** *Crystalluria, hematuria,* proteinuria, nephrotic syndrome, toxic nephrosis with oliguria and anuria, oligospermia, infertility
- **Hematologic:** *Agranulocytosis,* aplastic anemia, thrombocytopenia, leukopenia, hemolytic anemia, hypoprothrombinemia, methemoglobinemia, megaloblastic anemia
- **Hypersensitivity: Stevens-Johnson syndrome,** generalized skin eruptions, epidermal necrolysis, urticaria, serum sickness, pruritus, exfoliative dermatitis, anaphylactoid reactions, periorbital edema, conjunctival and scleral redness, photosensitization, arthralgia, allergic myocarditis, transient pulmonary changes with eosinophilia, decreased pulmonary function
- **Other:** Drug fever, chills, periarteritis nodosum

Interactions
✱ **Drug-drug** • Increased risk of hypoglycemia when tolbutamide, tolazamide, glyburide, glipizide, acetohexamide, chlorpropamide are taken concurrently • Increased risk of phenytoin toxicity with sulfonamides • Risk of hemorrhage when combined with oral anticoagulants • Increased risk of nephrotoxicity with cyclosporine and decreased cyclosporine effect

✱ **Drug-lab test** • False-positive urinary glucose tests using Benedict's method

■ Nursing considerations
Assessment
- **History:** Allergy to sulfonamides, sulfonylureas, thiazides; pregnancy, lactation; impaired renal or hepatic function; G6PD deficiency
- **Physical:** T; skin color, lesions; culture of infected site; orientation, reflexes, affect, peripheral sensation; R, adventitious sounds; mucous membranes, bowel sounds, liver evaluation; LFTs, renal function tests, CBC and differential, urinalysis

Interventions
- Arrange for culture and sensitivity tests of infection before therapy; repeat cultures if response is not as expected.
- Administer drug on an empty stomach, 1 hr before or 2 hr after meals, with a full glass of water.

⊗ ***Warning*** Ensure adequate fluid intake; sulfadiazine is very insoluble and may cause crystalluria if high concentrations occur in the urine; alkalinization of the urine may be necessary.

⊗ ***Warning*** Discontinue drug immediately if hypersensitivity reaction occurs.

Teaching points
- Complete full course of therapy.
- Take the drug on an empty stomach, 1 hour before or 2 hours after meals, with a full glass of water.
- Drink 8 glasses of water per day.
- This drug is specific to this disease; do not self-treat any other infection.
- You may experience these side effects: Sensitivity to sunlight (use sunscreens; wear protective clothing); dizziness, drowsiness, difficulty walking, loss of sensation (avoid driving or performing tasks that require alertness); nausea, vomiting, diarrhea; loss of fertility.
- Report blood in the urine, rash, ringing in the ears, difficulty breathing, fever, sore throat, chills.

▽ sulfasalazine
*(sul fa **sal'** a zeen)*

Azulfidine, Azulfidine EN-Tabs DNC, PMS-Sulfasalazine (CAN), PMS-Sulfasalazine EC (CAN), Salazopyrin EN-Tabs (CAN)

PREGNANCY CATEGORY B

Drug classes
Anti-inflammatory
Antirheumatic
Sulfonamide

Therapeutic actions
Bacteriostatic: Competitively antagonizes PABA, an essential component of folic acid synthesis in susceptible gram-negative and gram-positive bacteria; one-third of the oral dose is absorbed from the small intestine; remaining two-thirds passes into the colon where it is split into 5-aminosalicylic acid and sulfapyridine; most of the sulfapyridine is absorbed; the 5-aminosalicylic acid acts locally as an anti-inflammatory agent.

Indications
- Treatment of ulcerative colitis
- DR: Treatment of rheumatoid arthritis (RA) in patients intolerant or unresponsive to other anti-inflammatories
- *Azulfidine EN-Tabs:* Treatment of children 6–16 yr with juvenile rheumatoid arthritis, (JRA) involving five joints, who have not responded adequately to salicylates or other NSAIDs
- Unlabeled uses: Crohn's disease, ankylosing spondylitis, psoriatic arthritis

Contraindications and cautions
- Contraindicated with allergy to sulfonamides, sulfonylureas, thiazides, salicylates; pregnancy (teratogenic may cause kernicterus); lactation (risk of kernicterus, diarrhea, rash); intestinal or urinary obstruction; porphyria; and in pediatric patients younger than 2 yr.
- Use cautiously with impaired renal or hepatic function, G6PD deficiency, blood dyscrasias.

Available forms

Tablets—500 mg; DR tablets DNC—500 mg

Dosages

Administer around-the-clock; dosage intervals should not exceed 8 hr. Give after meals.

Adults

- *Ulcerative colitis:* Initial therapy, 3–4 g/day PO in evenly divided doses. Initial doses of 1–2 g/day PO may lessen adverse GI effects. Doses of more than 4 g/day increase risk of toxicity. Maintenance, 2 g/day PO in evenly spaced doses (500 mg qid).
- *Adult RA:* 2 g daily in two evenly divided doses.

Pediatric patients

- *Ulcerative colitis:* For children 6 yr or older, initial therapy, 40–60 mg/kg/24 hr PO in three to six divided doses. Maintenance therapy, 30 mg/kg/24 hr PO in four equally divided doses. Maximum dosage, 2 g/day.
- *JRA—polyarticular course:* For children 6 yr or older, 30–50 mg/kg daily in two evenly divided doses. Maximum, 2 g/day.

Pharmacokinetics

Route	*Onset*	*Peak*
Oral	Varies	1.5–6 hr, 6–24 hr metabolite

Metabolism: Hepatic; $T_{1/2}$: 5–10 hr
Distribution: Crosses placenta; enters breast milk
Excretion: Urine

Adverse effects

- **CNS:** *Headache,* peripheral neuropathy, mental depression, seizures, ataxia, hallucinations, tinnitus, vertigo, insomnia, hearing loss, drowsiness, transient lesions of posterior spinal column, transverse myelitis
- **Dermatologic:** Photosensitivity, cyanosis, petechiae, alopecia
- **GI:** *Nausea, emesis, abdominal pains,* diarrhea, bloody diarrhea, *anorexia,* pancreatitis, stomatitis, impaired folic acid absorption, hepatitis, **hepatocellular necrosis**
- **GU:** *Crystalluria, hematuria,* proteinuria, nephrotic syndrome, toxic nephrosis with oliguria and anuria, *oligospermia,* infertility
- **Hematologic:** *Agranulocytosis,* aplastic anemia, thrombocytopenia, leukopenia, hemolytic anemia, hypoprothrombinemia, methemoglobinemia, megaloblastic anemia
- **Hypersensitivity: Stevens-Johnson syndrome,** generalized skin eruptions, epidermal necrolysis, urticaria, serum sickness, pruritus, exfoliative dermatitis, anaphylactoid reactions, periorbital edema, conjunctival and scleral redness, photosensitization, arthralgia, allergic myocarditis, transient pulmonary changes with eosinophilia, decreased pulmonary function
- **Other:** Drug fever, chills, periarteritis nodosum

Interactions

✷ **Drug-drug** • Decreased absorption of digoxin with lessened therapeutic effect; monitor patient, space doses at least 2 hr apart • Increased risk of folate deficiency, monitor for signs of folate deficiency

■ Nursing considerations

Assessment

- **History:** Allergy to sulfonamides, sulfonylureas, thiazides, salicylates; pregnancy; lactation; impaired renal or hepatic function; G6PD deficiency; porphyria
- **Physical:** T; skin color, lesions; culture of infected site; orientation, reflexes, affect, peripheral sensation; R, adventitious sounds; mucous membranes, bowel sounds, liver evaluation; LFTs, renal function tests, CBC and differential, urinalysis

Interventions

- Administer drug after meals or with food to prevent GI upset. Administer it around-the-clock.
- Ensure that patient swallows tablets whole; do not cut, crush, or chew.

⊗ ***Warning*** Ensure adequate fluid intake; sulfasalazine is very insoluble and may cause crystalluria if high concentrations occur in the urine; alkalinization of the urine may be needed.

⊗ ***Warning*** Discontinue drug immediately if hypersensitivity reaction occurs.

Teaching points

- Complete full course of therapy. Swallow tablets whole; do not cut, crush, or chew.
- Take the drug with food or meals to decrease GI upset.
- Drink eight glasses of water per day.
- You may experience these side effects: Sensitivity to sunlight (use sunscreen, wear protective clothing); dizziness, drowsiness, difficulty walking, loss of sensation (avoid driving or performing tasks that require alertness); nausea, vomiting, diarrhea; loss of fertility; yellow-orange urine.
- Report blood in the urine, rash, ringing in the ears, difficulty breathing, fever, sore throat, chills.

sulindac

*(sul **in'** dak)*

Apo-Sulin (CAN), Clinoril

PREGNANCY CATEGORY B (FIRST AND SECOND TRIMESTERS)

PREGNANCY CATEGORY D (THIRD TRIMESTER)

Drug classes

Analgesic
Antipyretic
NSAID

Therapeutic actions

Anti-inflammatory, analgesic, and antipyretic activities largely related to inhibition of prostaglandin synthesis; exact mechanisms of action are not known.

Indications

- Acute or long-term use to relieve signs and symptoms of osteoarthritis, rheumatoid arthritis, acute gouty arthritis
- Acute or long-term use in relief of signs and symptoms of ankylosing spondylitis, acute painful shoulder

Contraindications and cautions

- Contraindicated for perioperative pain in coronary artery bypass graft (CABG) surgery and in pregnancy, lactation.
- Use cautiously with patients for whom acute asthmatic attacks, urticaria, or rhinitis are precipitated by aspirin or other NSAIDs, renal, hepatic, CV, and GI conditions.

Available forms

Tablets—150, 200 mg

Dosages

Do not exceed 400 mg/day.

Adults

- *Rheumatoid arthritis or osteoarthritis, ankylosing spondylitis:* Initial dose of 150 mg bid PO. Individualize dosage.
- *Acute painful shoulder, acute gouty arthritis:* 200 mg bid PO. After adequate response, reduce dosage. Acute painful shoulder usually requires 7–14 days of therapy; acute gouty arthritis, 7 days.

Pediatric patients

Safety and efficacy not established.

Patients with hepatic or renal impairment

Reduce dosage.

Pharmacokinetics

Route	Onset	Peak	Duration
Oral	Varies	2–4 hr	10–12 hr

Metabolism: Hepatic; $T_{1/2}$: 7.8 hr (parent drug), 16.4 hr (active metabolite)
Distribution: Crosses placenta; enters breast milk
Excretion: Feces, urine

Adverse effects

- **CNS:** *Headache, dizziness, somnolence, insomnia,* fatigue, tiredness, dizziness, tinnitus, ophthalmologic effects
- **CV:** Heart failure
- **Dermatologic:** *Rash,* pruritus, sweating, dry mucous membranes, stomatitis
- **GI:** *Nausea, dyspepsia, GI pain,* diarrhea, vomiting, *constipation,* flatulence, anorexia
- **GU:** Dysuria, renal impairment, pancreatitis
- **Hematologic:** Bleeding, platelet inhibition with higher doses, neutropenia, eosinophilia, leukopenia, pancytopenia, thrombocytopenia, agranulocytosis, granulocytopenia, aplastic anemia, decreased Hgb or Hct, bone marrow depression, menorrhagia

S

- **Respiratory:** Dyspnea, hemoptysis, pharyngitis, **bronchospasm,** rhinitis
- **Other:** Peripheral edema, **anaphylactoid reactions** to **fatal anaphylactic shock**

Interactions

✱ **Drug-drug** • Increased serum lithium levels and risk of toxicity • Decreased antihypertensive effects of beta blockers • Decreased therapeutic effects of bumetanide, furosemide, ethacrynic acid

✱ **Drug-food** • Decreased rate and extent of absorption when taken with food

■ Nursing considerations

Assessment

- **History:** Allergies; renal, hepatic, CV, and GI conditions; pregnancy; lactation
- **Physical:** Skin color and lesions; orientation, reflexes, ophthalmologic and audiometric evaluation, peripheral sensation; P, edema; R, adventitious sounds; liver evaluation; CBC, clotting times, LFTs, renal function tests; serum electrolytes, stool guaiac

Interventions

⊠ ***Black box warning*** Be aware that patient may be at increased risk for CV events, GI bleeding; monitor accordingly. Drug is contraindicated for treating perioperative pain in CABG surgery.

- Give with food or milk if GI upset occurs.
- Arrange for periodic ophthalmologic examination during long-term therapy.

⊗ ***Warning*** If overdose occurs, institute emergency procedures—gastric lavage, induction of emesis, supportive therapy.

Teaching points

- Take with food or meals if GI upset occurs.
- Take only the prescribed dosage.
- You may experience these side effects: Dizziness, drowsiness (avoid driving or using dangerous machinery).
- Report sore throat, fever, rash, itching, weight gain, swelling in ankles or fingers, changes in vision, black, tarry stools.

▽ sumatriptan succinate

*(sue mah **trip'** tan)*

Apo-Sumatriptan (CAN), Gen-Sumatriptan (CAN), Imitrex, Novo-Sumatriptan (CAN), Novo-Sumatriptan DF (CAN), PMS-Sumatriptan (CAN), ratio-Sumatriptan (CAN), Sumavel DosePro

PREGNANCY CATEGORY C

Drug classes

Antimigraine drug (triptan)
Serotonin-selective agonist

Therapeutic actions

Binds to serotonin receptors to cause vascular constrictive effects on cranial blood vessels, causing the relief of migraine in selective patients.

Indications

- Treatment of acute migraine attacks with or without aura (oral, nasal, subcutaneously)

Contraindications and cautions

- Contraindicated with allergy to sumatriptan, cerebrovascular or peripheral vascular syndromes, severe hepatic impairment, MAOIs, uncontrolled hypertension, hemiplegic migraine, pregnancy, CAD
- Use cautiously with the elderly, lactation, renal function impairment.

Available forms

Tablets—25, 50, 100 mg; injection—4 mg/0.5 mL, 6 mg/0.5 mL; nasal spray—5 mg/0.1 mL, 20 mg/0.1 mL; needle-free injection system—4, 6 mg

Dosages

Adults

Oral

25, 50, or 100 mg; additional doses may be repeated in 2 hr or more; up to a maximum of 200 mg/day.

Subcutaneous

6 mg, may be repeated in 1 hr. Maximum, 12 mg/24 hr. Autoinjector is available.

Intranasal

5, 10, or 20 mg into one nostril or 10 mg divided into two doses of 5 mg, one in each nostril, may be repeated after 2 hr. Maximum, 40 mg/24 hr.

Pediatric patients

Safety and efficacy not established.

Patients with hepatic impairment

Maximum single dose, 50 mg.

Pharmacokinetics

Route	*Onset*	*Peak*
Subcut.	Varies	5–20 min
Oral	60–90 min	2–4 hr
Injection	Rapid	90 min

Metabolism: Hepatic; $T_{1/2}$: 115 min
Distribution: Crosses placenta; enters breast milk
Excretion: Urine, feces (tablets)

Adverse effects

- **CNS:** *Dizziness, vertigo,* headache, anxiety, malaise or fatigue, *weakness, myalgia*
- **CV:** *BP alterations, tightness or pressure in chest,* **shock**
- **GI:** Abdominal discomfort, dysphagia
- **Local:** *Injection site discomfort,* nose and throat discomfort (nasal spray)
- **Other:** *Tingling, warm/hot sensations, burning sensation, feeling of heaviness, pressure sensation, numbness, feeling of tightness,* feeling strange, cold sensation

Nasal spray

- **GI:** Bad taste in mouth, nausea

Interactions

✱ **Drug-drug** • Prolonged vasoactive reactions with ergot-containing drugs (should not be used within 24 hr of each other) • Increased serum levels and toxicity of sumatriptan with MAOIs; avoid this combination and for 2 wk after MAOI discontinuation

✱ **Drug-alternative therapy** • Increased risk of severe reaction if combined with St. John's wort therapy

■ Nursing considerations

Assessment

- **History:** Allergy to sumatriptan; active CAD; uncontrolled hypertension; hemiplegic migraine; pregnancy, lactation
- **Physical:** Skin color and lesions; orientation, reflexes, peripheral sensation; P, BP; LFTs, renal function tests

Interventions

- Administer to relieve acute migraine, not as a prophylactic measure.
- Administer as subcutaneous injection just below the skin as soon as possible after symptoms begin.
- Repeat injection only after 1 hr if relief is not obtained; only 2 injections may be given each 24 hr.
- Administer PO with fluids; may repeat in 2 hr if no relief.
- Repeat nasal spray after 2 hr if headache returns or does not respond.
- Monitor BP of patients with possible CAD; discontinue at any sign of angina, prolonged high BP.

Teaching points

- Learn to use the autoinjector; injection may be repeated only after 1 hour if relief is not obtained; do not administer more than two injections in 24 hours.
- Inject just below the skin as soon as possible after onset of migraine; this drug is for an acute attack only, not for use to prevent attacks. Dispose of needles and syringes appropriately.
- Administer nasal spray as a single dose; repeat if needed only after 2 hours.
- Take oral drug with fluids, may be repeated in 2 hours if no relief or return of headache.
- This drug should not be taken during pregnancy; if you suspect that you are pregnant, consult your health care provider and stop using drug.
- Contact your health care provider immediately if you experience severe or continuous chest pain or pressure.
- You may experience these side effects: Dizziness, drowsiness (avoid driving or the use of dangerous machinery); numbness, tingling, feelings of tightness or pressure.

- Report feelings of heat, flushing, tiredness, feelings of sickness, swelling of lips or eyelids.

sunitinib

See Appendix W, *Less commonly used drugs.*

tacrine hydrochloride (tetrahydroamino-acridine, THA)

(tay' krin)

Cognex

PREGNANCY CATEGORY C

Drug classes

Alzheimer's disease drug
Cholinesterase inhibitor

Therapeutic actions

Centrally acting reversible cholinesterase inhibitor, leading to elevated acetylcholine levels in the cortex, which slows the neuronal degradation that occurs in Alzheimer's disease.

Indications

- Treatment of mild to moderate dementia of the Alzheimer's type

Contraindications and cautions

- Contraindicated with allergy to tacrine or acridine derivatives, previous tacrine-associated jaundice, pregnancy, increased serum bilirubin greater than 3 mg/dL.
- Use cautiously with renal or hepatic disease, bladder obstruction, seizure conditions, sick sinus syndrome, GI bleeding, anesthesia, lactation, asthma.

Available forms

Capsules—10, 20, 30, 40 mg

Dosages

Adults

10 mg PO qid; maintain this dose for 4 wk with regular monitoring of transaminase levels; after 4 wk, increase dose to 20 mg PO qid; if patient is tolerant to drug and transaminase levels are within normal limits, increase at 4-wk intervals at 10-mg increases to a total of 120–160 mg/day.

Pediatric patients

Safety and efficacy not established.

Patients with hepatic impairment

For ALT levels greater than 3 but less than 5 times the upper level of normal, reduce dose by 40 mg/day; adjust up if levels improve. For ALT levels greater than 5 times the upper level of normal, stop treatment. Rechallenge if levels become normal.

Pharmacokinetics

Route	*Onset*	*Peak*
Oral	Varies	1–2 hr

Metabolism: Hepatic; $T_{1/2}$: 2–4 hr
Distribution: Crosses placenta; may enter breast milk
Excretion: Urine

Adverse effects

- **CNS:** *Headache, fatigue, dizziness, confusion,* ataxia, insomnia, somnolence, tremor, agitation, depression, anxiety, abnormal thinking
- **CV:** Chest pain
- **Dermatologic:** *Rash,* flushing, purpura
- **GI:** *Nausea, vomiting, diarrhea, dyspepsia, anorexia, abdominal pain,* flatulence, constipation, **hepatotoxicity**
- **GU:** Urinary frequency, UTIs
- **Respiratory:** *Rhinitis,* URIs, coughing

Interactions

✱ Drug-drug • Increased effects and risk of toxicity of theophylline, cholinesterase inhibitors • Decreased effects of anticholinergics • Increased effects with cimetidine
✱ Drug-food • Decreased absorption and serum levels of tacrine if taken with food

■ Nursing considerations

Assessment

- **History:** Allergy to tacrine or acridine derivatives; previous tacrine-associated jaundice, pregnancy, renal or hepatic disease, bladder obstruction, seizure conditions, sick sinus syndrome, GI bleed, anesthesia, lactation, asthma

- **Physical:** Orientation, affect, reflexes; BP, P; R, adventitious sounds; urinary output; abdominal examination; LFTs, renal function tests; serum transaminase levels

Interventions

- Arrange for regular transaminase level determination before and during therapy.

⊗ ***Warning*** Use with great care in patients with any history of hepatic impairment.

- Administer around-the-clock at regular intervals for best results.
- Give on an empty stomach, 1 hr before or 2 hr after meals.
- Administer with meals only if severe GI upset occurs.
- Decrease dose and slowly discontinue drug if side effects become severe.

⊗ ***Warning*** Notify surgeons that patient is on tacrine; exaggerated muscle relaxation may occur if succinylcholine-type drugs are used.

⊗ ***Warning*** Do not suddenly discontinue high doses of drug.

- Monitor for any signs of neurologic change or deterioration; drug does not stop the disease but slows the degeneration.

Teaching points

- Take drug exactly as prescribed, around-the-clock. Work with your health care provider to establish a schedule that is least disruptive. Do not take more than the prescribed dose.
- Take drug on an empty stomach, 1 hour before or 2 hours after meals. If severe GI upset occurs, drug may be taken with meals.
- This drug does not cure the disease but is thought to slow down the degeneration associated with the disease.
- Arrange for regular blood tests and follow-up visits while adjusting to this drug.
- You may experience these side effects: Nausea, vomiting (eat frequent small meals); dizziness, confusion, light-headedness (use caution if driving or performing tasks that require alertness).
- Report nausea, vomiting, changes in stool or urine color, diarrhea, rash, changes in neurologic functioning, yellowing of eyes or skin.

▽tacrolimus (FK 506)

(tack row' lim us)

Prograf, Protopic

PREGNANCY CATEGORY C

Drug classes

Immunomodulator
Immunosuppressant

Therapeutic actions

Immunosuppressant; inhibits T-lymphocyte activation; exact mechanism of action not known but binds to intracellular protein, which may prevent the generation of nuclear factor of activated T cells and suppress the immune activation and response of T cells.

Indications

- Prophylaxis for organ rejection in liver or kidney transplants and allogenic heart transplants in conjunction with adrenal corticosteroids
- Topical: Short-term and intermittent long-term treatment of moderate to severe atopic dermatitis when other therapies are not effective or contraindicated
- Unlabeled uses: Prevention and treatment of graft-versus-host disease after hematopoietic stem cell transplantation; Crohn's disease; rheumatoid arthritis

Contraindications and cautions

- Contraindicated with allergy to tacrolimus, hypersensitivity to HCO-60 polyoxyl 60 hydrogenated castor oil (IV form), pregnancy, lactation.
- Use cautiously with impaired renal function, hyperkalemia, malabsorption, impaired hepatic function.

Available forms

Capsules—0.5, 1, 5 mg; injection—5 mg/mL; ointment—0.03%, 0.1%

Dosages

Adults

Oral

- *Kidney transplant:* 0.2 mg/kg/day divided every 12 hr.

- *Liver transplant:* 0.10–0.15 mg/kg/day divided every 12 hr; administer initial dose no sooner than 6 hr after transplant. If transferring from IV, give first dose 8–12 hr after discontinuing IV infusion. Adjust dosage based on clinical assessment of rejection tolerance of drug.
- *Heart transplant:* 0.075 mg/kg/day PO or IV in two divided doses given every 12 hr. Give first dose no sooner than 6 hr after transplant. If therapy starts with IV route, switch to oral route as soon as possible, 8–12 hr after discontinuing IV infusion.

Parenteral

For patients unable to take capsules, 0.03–0.05 mg/kg/day (liver or kidney transplant) or 0.01 mg/kg/day (heart transplant) as continuous IV infusion begun no sooner than 6 hr after transplant. Switch to oral drug as soon as possible.

Topical

Apply thin layer of 0.03% or 0.1% ointment to affected area bid. Rub in gently and completely. Stop drug when signs and symptoms resolve.

Pediatric patients

Children require the larger dose; begin treatment at higher end of recommended adult dose.

Oral

- *Liver transplant:* 0.15–0.20 mg/kg/day.

Parenteral

- *Liver transplant:* 0.03–0.05 mg/kg/day.

Topical

2–15 yr: Apply thin layer of 0.03% ointment bid. Rub in gently and completely. Stop drug when signs and symptoms resolve.
Younger than 2 yr: Not recommended.

Patients with hepatic or renal impairment

Start with lowest possible dose; delay therapy up to 48 hr in patients with postoperative oliguria.

Pharmacokinetics

Route	*Onset*	*Peak*
Oral	Varies	1.5–3.5 hr
IV	Rapid	1–2 hr

Metabolism: Hepatic; $T_{1/2}$: 11.7–18.8 hr (IV)
Distribution: Crosses placenta; enters breast milk
Excretion: Urine, feces

IV FACTS

Preparation: Dilute IV solution immediately before use; use 0.9% sodium chloride injection or 5% dextrose injection to a concentration between 0.004 and 0.02 mg/mL. Do not store in a PVC container; discard after 24 hr.
Infusion: Give by continuous IV infusion using an infusion pump.

Adverse effects

- **CNS:** *Tremor, headache, insomnia,* paresthesias
- **CV:** Hypertension
- **GI: Hepatotoxicity,** *constipation, diarrhea, nausea, vomiting,* anorexia
- **GU:** *Renal impairment,* nephrotoxicity, UTI, oliguria
- **Hematologic:** Leukopenia, anemia, hyperkalemia, hypokalemia, hyperglycemia, hypomagnesemia
- **Other:** Abdominal pain, fever, asthenia, back pain, ascites, neoplasias, increased susceptibility to infection, lymphoma development, diabetes mellitus, hypercholesterolemia, **anaphylaxis**

Interactions

✱ **Drug-drug** • Increased risk of nephrotoxicity with other nephrotoxic agents (cyclosporine) • Risk of severe myopathy or rhabdomyolysis with any HMG-CoA inhibitor • Increased risk of toxicity with metoclopramide, nicardipine, cimetidine, clarithromycin, erythromycin, calcium channel blockers • Decreased therapeutic effect with carbamazepine, phenobarbital, phenytoin, rifamycins
✱ **Drug-food** • Decreased metabolism and risk of toxic effects if combined with grapefruit juice; avoid this combination
✱ **Drug-alternative therapy** • Decreased therapeutic effect with St. John's wort

■ Nursing considerations

Assessment

- **History:** Allergy to tacrolimus or polyoxyethylated castor oil; impaired renal function; malabsorption; lactation, pregnancy
- **Physical:** T; skin color, lesions; BP, peripheral perfusion; liver evaluation, bowel sounds, gum evaluation; LFTs, renal function tests, CBC, potassium, glucose

Interventions

⊗ ***Black box warning*** Protect patient from infection. Risk of infection, lymphoma is high; monitor closely.

- Use parenteral administration only if patient is unable to take the oral drug; transfer to oral drug as soon as possible.
- Apply thin layer of ointment to affected area; do not use occlusive dressings; do not apply to wet skin; encourage patient to avoid exposure to sunlight.

⊗ ***Warning*** Monitor renal and LFTs before and periodically during therapy; marked decreases in function may require dosage changes or discontinuation.

- Monitor tacrolimus blood concentrations.
- Monitor liver function and hematologic tests to determine dosage.

Teaching points

- Avoid infections; avoid crowds and people with infections. Also avoid having vaccinations while taking this drug. Notify your health care provider at once if you injure yourself.
- Do not drink grapefruit juice while using this drug.
- This drug should not be taken during pregnancy. If you think that you are pregnant or you want to become pregnant, consult your health care provider.
- Arrange to have periodic blood tests to monitor drug response and effects.
- Do not discontinue without consulting your health care provider. Continue use of topical ointment for 1 week after resolution of the infection.
- If you are using the topical form, avoid sunlight, use sunscreen and protective clothing.
- You may experience these side effects: Nausea, vomiting (take drug with food); diarrhea; headache (request analgesics).
- Report unusual bleeding or bruising, fever, sore throat, mouth sores, tiredness.

▽tadalafil

*(tah **dal'** ah fill)*

Adcirca, Cialis

PREGNANCY CATEGORY B

Drug classes

Impotence drug
Phosphodiesterase-5 inhibitor

Therapeutic actions

Selectively inhibits cyclic guanosine monophosphate (cGMP) specific phosphodiesterase type 5. The mechanism of penile erection involves the release of nitric oxide into the corpus cavernosum of the penis during sexual stimulation. Nitrous oxide activates cGMP, which causes smooth muscle relaxation allowing the flow of blood into the corpus cavernosum. Tadalafil prevents the breakdown of cGMP by phosphodiesterase, leading to increased cGMP levels and prolonged smooth muscle relaxation, thus promoting the flow of blood into the corpus cavernosum, relaxation of pulmonary muscle cells, and vasodilation of the pulmonary vascular bed.

Indications

- Treatment of ED in the presence of sexual stimulation (*Cialis*)
- Once daily for treatment of ED in men who anticipate having sex more than twice weekly (*Cialis*)
- **NEW INDICATION:** Treatment of pulmonary arterial hyertension, to improve exercise tolerance (*Adcirca*)

Contraindications and cautions

- Contraindicated with allergy to any component of the tablet, concurrent use of nitrates or alpha blockers; contraindicated for use in women or children.
- Use cautiously with hepatic or renal impairment; with anatomical deformation of the penis, with known cardiac disease (effects of sexual activity need to be evaluated), congenital prolonged QT interval, unstable angina; hypotension (systolic pressure less than 90 mm Hg); uncontrolled hypertension (BP higher than 170/110 mm Hg); severe hepatic impairment; end-stage renal disease with dialysis; hereditary degenerative retinal disorders.

Available forms

Tablets—2.5, 5, 10, 20 mg (*Cialis*); 20 mg (*Adcirca*)

T

Dosages

Adults

Erectile dysfunction: 10 mg PO taken before anticipated sexual activity; range 5–20 mg PO. Limit use to once per day.

For once-daily use: 2.5 mg/day PO without regard to food. May be increased to 5 mg/day PO based on patient response.

Pulmonary arterial hypertension: 40 mg/day PO without regard to food, given as a once-daily dose. Do not divide.

Pediatric patients

Not intended for use in children.

Patients receiving itraconazole, ketoconazole, ritonavir

Do not exceed one 10-mg dose in 72-hr period.

Patients with renal impairment

For creatinine clearance 31–50 mL/min, initial dose not to exceed 5 mg PO daily or 10 mg PO every 48 hr.; no further adjustment needed for once-daily use. For creatinine clearance less than 30 mL/min, 5 mg PO every 72 hr; once-daily use not recommended (*Cialis*).

Patients with hepatic impairment

For Child-Pugh class A or B, maximum dosage should not exceed 10 mg PO daily. Use caution with once-daily use; Child-Pugh class C not recommended (*Cialis*).

Pharmacokinetics

Route	Onset	Peak
Oral	Rapid	0.5–6 hr

Metabolism: Hepatic, $T_{1/2}$: 17.5 hr
Distribution: Not intended for use in women
Excretion: Feces, urine

Adverse effects

- **CNS:** *Headache,* abnormal vision, changes in color vision, fatigue, ischemic optic neuropathy, sudden loss of hearing
- **CV:** *Flushing,* angina, chest pain, hypertension, hypotension, **MI,** palpitation, postural hypotension, tachycardia
- **GI:** *Dyspepsia,* diarrhea, abdominal pain, dry mouth, esophagitis, gastritis, GERD, nausea, abnormal liver function test results
- **GU:** Abnormal erection, spontaneous erection, priapism
- **Respiratory:** Rhinitis, sinusitis, dyspnea, epistaxis, pharyngitis, nasal congestion
- **Other:** Flulike symptoms, edema, pain, rash, sweating, **Stevens-Johnson syndrome,** myalgia

Interactions

✱ **Drug-drug** ⊗ ***Warning*** Possible severe hypotension and serious cardiac events if combined with nitrates, alpha blockers; this combination is contraindicated.
• Possible increased tadalafil levels and effects if taken with ketoconazole, itraconazole, erythromycin; monitor patient and reduce dosage as needed • Increased tadalafil serum levels if combined with indinavir, ritonavir; if these drugs are being used, limit tadalafil dose to 10 mg in a 72-hr period • Reduced tadalafil levels and effectiveness if combined with rifampin • Risk for increased cardiac effects, decreased BP, or flushing if combined with alcohol; warn patient of this possibility if patient uses alcohol

✱ **Drug-food** • Possible increased tadalafil levels if taken with grapefruit juice

■ Nursing considerations

Assessment

- **History:** Allergy to any component of the tablet; concurrent use of nitrates or alpha blockers; unstable angina, hypotension, uncontrolled hypertension; severe hepatic impairment; end-stage renal disease with dialysis; hereditary degenerative retinal disorders; anatomical deformation of the penis; cardiac disease; congenital prolonged QT interval
- **Physical:** Orientation, affect; skin color, lesions; R, adventitious sounds; P, BP, ECG, LFTs, renal function tests

Interventions

- Ensure diagnosis of ED and determine underlying causes and other appropriate treatment.
- Advise patient with ED that drug does not work without sexual stimulation. Limit use to once per day.
- Remind patient with ED that drug does not protect against STDs and appropriate measures should be taken.
- Ensure that patient with pulmonary arterial hypertension takes dose all at once, once a day.

⊗ ***Warning*** Tell patient to never take this drug with nitrates or alpha-adrenergic blockers; serious, even fatal complications can occur.

- Warn patient of the risk of lowered BP or dizziness if drug is taken with alcohol.

Teaching points

- If you are taking this drug for erectile dysfunction, take the drug before anticipated sexual activity. The drug will stay in your body for up to 3 days. The drug will have no effect unless there is sexual stimulation. If you anticipate sexual activity more than twice per week, daily dosing should be considered.
- If you are taking this drug for erectile dysfunction, this drug will not protect you from sexually transmitted diseases; use appropriate precautions.
- If you are taking this drug for pulmonary arterial hypertension, this drug will help to increase your ability to exercise. Take the drug once a day; do not split the dose.
- Do not take this drug if you are taking any nitrates, alpha blockers, or other drugs for treating erectile dysfunction; serious side effects and even death can occur.
- Many drugs may interact with tadalafil; always consult your health care provider before taking any drug, including over-the-counter drugs and herbal therapies. Dosage adjustments may be needed.
- Stop taking the drug and contact your health care provider if you experience sudden loss of vision.
- Combining this drug with alcohol could cause dizziness, loss of blood pressure, or increased flushing.
- You may experience these side effects: Headache, dizziness, upset stomach, runny nose, muscle pains. These side effects should go away within a couple of hours. If side effects persist, consult your health care provider.
- Report difficult or painful urination, vision changes, fainting, erection that persists for longer than 4 hours (if this occurs, seek medical assistance as soon as possible), sudden loss of vision or hearing.

▽talc, USP

See Appendix W, *Less commonly used drugs.*

DANGEROUS DRUG

▽tamoxifen citrate

*(ta **mox'** i fen)*

Apo-Tamox (CAN), Gen-Tamoxifen (CAN), Soltamox, Tamofen (CAN)

PREGNANCY CATEGORY D

Drug classes

Antiestrogen
Antineoplastic

Therapeutic actions

Potent antiestrogenic effects: Competes with estrogen for binding sites in target tissues, such as the breast.

Indications

- Treatment of metastatic breast cancer in women and men; in premenopausal women with metastatic breast cancer, tamoxifen is an alternative to oophorectomy or ovarian irradiation
- Treatment of node-positive breast cancer in postmenopausal women following total mastectomy or segmental mastectomy, axillary dissection, and breast irradiation
- Treatment of axillary node-negative breast cancer in women following total mastectomy or segmental mastectomy, axillary dissection, and breast irradiation
- Reduction in risk of invasive breast cancer in women with ductal carcinoma in situ (DCIS) following breast surgery and radiation
- Reduction in occurrence of contralateral breast cancer in patients receiving adjuvant tamoxifen therapy for breast cancer
- Reduction in incidence of breast cancer in women at high risk for breast cancer
- Unlabeled uses: Treatment of mastalgia; useful for decreasing size and pain of gynecomastia; treatment of McCune-Albright syndrome and precocious puberty in girls 2–10 yr; malignant carcinoid tumor, carcinoid syndrome

Contraindications and cautions

- Contraindicated with allergy to tamoxifen, pregnancy, lactation, women who require concomitant coumarin-type anticoagulation therapy or in women with a history of DVT or PE.

- Use cautiously in women with a history of thromboembolic events.

Available forms

Tablets—10, 20 mg; oral solution—10 mg/5 mL

Dosages

Adults

- *Breast cancer:* 20–40 mg/day PO for 5 yr. Dosages of more than 20 mg/day should be given in divided doses, morning and evening.
- *Reduction in breast cancer incidence:* 20 mg/day PO for 5 yr.
- *DCIS:* 20 mg/day PO for 5 yr.

Pharmacokinetics

Route	*Onset*	*Peak*
Oral	Varies	4–7 hr

Metabolism: Hepatic; $T_{1/2}$: 7–14 days
Distribution: Crosses placenta; may enter breast milk
Excretion: Feces

Adverse effects

- **CNS:** Depression, light-headedness, dizziness, headache, corneal opacity, decreased visual acuity, retinopathy, **CVA**
- **Dermatologic: Stevens-Johnson syndrome,** *hot flashes, rash*
- **GI:** *Nausea, vomiting,* food distaste, alterations in liver enzymes
- **GU:** *Vaginal bleeding, vaginal discharge, menstrual irregularities,* pruritus vulvae, endometrial cancer, uterine sarcoma
- **Hematologic:** Hypercalcemia, especially with bone metastases, thrombocytopenia, leukopenia, anemia, **DVT**
- **Other:** Peripheral edema; increased bone and tumor pain and local disease (initially seen with a good tumor response, usually subsides); cancer in animal studies, changes in LFTs, **PE**

Interactions

✱ **Drug-drug** • Increased risk of bleeding with oral anticoagulants • Increased serum levels with bromocriptine • Increased risk of thromboembolic events if given with cytotoxic agents

✱ **Drug-food** • Decreased metabolism and risk of toxic effects if combined with grapefruit juice; avoid this combination

✱ **Drug-lab test** • Possible increase in calcium levels, T4 levels without hyperthyroidism

■ Nursing considerations

Assessment

- **History:** Allergy to tamoxifen, pregnancy, lactation, previous DVT or PE
- **Physical:** Skin lesions, color, turgor; pelvic examination; orientation, affect, reflexes; ophthalmologic examination; peripheral pulses, edema; LFTs, CBC and differential, estrogen receptor evaluation of tumor cells

Interventions

⊗ ***Black box warning*** Alert women with DCIS and those at high risk for breast cancer of risks for serious to potentially fatal drug effects; discuss benefits versus risks.

- Administer bid, in the morning and the evening.
- Arrange for periodic blood counts.
- Arrange for initial ophthalmologic examination and periodic examinations if visual changes occur.
- Counsel patient to use contraception while taking this drug; inform patient that serious fetal harm could occur.
- Decrease dosage if adverse effects become severe.

Teaching points

- For doses greater than 20 milligrams, take the drug twice a day, in the morning and evening. Do not drink grapefruit juice while using this drug.
- This drug can cause serious fetal harm and must not be taken during pregnancy. Contraceptive measures should be used. If you become pregnant or you want to become pregnant, consult your health care provider immediately. Avoid nursing a baby during therapy.
- Have regular gynecologic examinations during therapy.
- You may experience these side effects: Bone pain; hot flashes (staying in cool places may help); nausea, vomiting (eat frequent small

meals); weight gain; menstrual irregularities; dizziness, headache, light-headedness (use caution if driving or performing tasks that require alertness).

- Report marked weakness, sleepiness, mental confusion, pain or swelling of the legs, shortness of breath, blurred vision.

tamsulosin hydrochloride

*(tam soo **low'** sin)*

Flomax DNC

PREGNANCY CATEGORY B

Drug class
Alpha-adrenergic blocker (peripherally acting)

Therapeutic actions
Blocks the smooth muscle $alpha_1$-adrenergic receptors in the prostate, prostatic capsule, prostatic urethra, and bladder neck, leading to relaxation of the bladder and prostate and improving the flow of urine in cases of BPH.

Indications
- Treatment of the signs and symptoms of BPH
- Unlabeled use: Adjunct in managing ureteral stones

Contraindications and cautions
- Contraindicated with hypersensitivity to tamsulosin, prostate cancer, pregnancy, lactation.
- Use cautiously with hypotension, sulfa hypersensitivity.

Available forms
Capsules DNC—0.4 mg

Dosages
Adults
0.4 mg PO daily 30 min after the same meal each day; if response is not satisfactory in 2–4 wk, dosage may be increased to 0.8 mg PO daily 30 min after the same meal each day. If therapy is interrupted for any reason for several days, resume dosing at 0.4 mg PO daily.

Pediatric patients
Safety and efficacy not established.

Pharmacokinetics

Route	*Onset*	*Peak*
Oral	Varies	4–6 hr

Metabolism: Hepatic; $T_{1/2}$: 9–15 hr
Distribution: May cross placenta; enters breast milk
Excretion: Feces, urine

Adverse effects
- **CNS:** *Somnolence, insomnia,* headache, dizziness
- **CV:** *Orthostatic hypotension,* syncope
- **GI:** *Nausea,* dyspepsia
- **GU:** *Abnormal ejaculation, decreased libido,* increased urinary frequency
- **Other:** Cough, sinusitis, rhinitis, *increased risk of intraoperative floppy iris syndrome with cataract surgery*

Interactions
✱ **Drug-drug** • Increased hypotensive effects with other alpha-adrenergic antagonists, sildenafil, tadalafil, vardenafil • Risk of increased toxic effects of cimetidine

■ Nursing considerations

CLINICAL ALERT!
Name confusion has occurred between *Flomax* (tamsulosin) and *Fosamax* (alendronate); use caution.

Assessment
- **History:** Allergy to tamsulosin or sulfa drugs; pregnancy, lactation; prostatic cancer; hypotension
- **Physical:** Body weight; skin color, lesions; orientation, affect, reflexes; ophthalmologic examination; P, BP, orthostatic BP; R, adventitious sounds, status of nasal mucous membranes; voiding pattern, normal output, urinalysis

Interventions
- Ensure that patient does not have prostatic cancer before beginning treatment.
- Administer once a day, 30 min after the same meal each day.
- Resume therapy at 0.4 mg daily if therapy is interrupted for several days for any reason.

T

- Ensure that patient does not crush, chew, or open capsule. Capsule should be swallowed whole.
- Monitor patient carefully for orthostatic hypotension; chance of orthostatic hypotension, dizziness, and syncope is high with the first dose. Establish safety precautions as appropriate.
- Alert surgeon that patient is on this drug if patient is going to have cataract surgery; increased risk of intraoperative floppy iris syndrome may require additional surgical intervention

Teaching points

- Take this drug exactly as prescribed, once a day. Do not chew, crush, or open capsules; capsules must be swallowed whole. Use care when beginning therapy; the chance of dizziness or syncope is greatest at that time. Change position slowly to avoid increased dizziness. Take the drug 30 minutes after the same meal each day.
- This drug should not be combined with drugs used to treat erectile dysfunction.
- Tell your surgeon that you are taking this drug if you are considering cataract surgery.
- You may experience these side effects: Dizziness, weakness (more likely when you change position, in the early morning, after exercise, in hot weather, and when you have consumed alcohol; some tolerance may occur after you have taken the drug for a while; avoid driving or engaging in tasks that require alertness; change position slowly, use caution in climbing stairs, lie down if dizziness persists); GI upset (eat frequent small meals); impotence (discuss this with your health care provider); stuffy nose. Most of these effects will disappear gradually with continued therapy.
- Report frequent dizziness or fainting, worsening of symptoms.

▽tapentadol

*(tah **pen**' tah dohl)*

Nucynta

PREGNANCY CATEGORY C

Drug classes

Opioid receptor analgesic (mu specific)
Norepinephrine reuptake inhibitor

Therapeutic actions

Binds to and activates μ-opioid receptors in the CNS, inhibiting transmission of pain at the spinal cord, and affects activity in parts of the brain that control how pain is perceived; analgesic properties are enhanced by the blocking of norepinephrine reuptake at the nerve synapse, increasing concentration of norepinephrine in the synaptic cleft.

Indications

- Relief of moderate to severe pain in patients 18 yr and older

Contraindications and cautions

- Contraindicated with known hypersensitivity to any component of the drug, increased intracranial pressure, impaired consciousness or coma, significant respiratory depression, acute or severe bronchial asthma, hypercapnia, paralytic ileus, within 14 days of MAOI use, pregnancy.
- Use cautiously with elderly or debilitated patients, asthma, COPD, severe obesity, sleep apnea syndrome, myxedema, CNS depression, lactation, pancreatic or biliary tract disease, hepatic or renal impairment, seizure disorders.

Available forms

Tablets–50, 75, 100 mg

Dosages

Adults

50–100 mg PO every 4–6 hr.

Pediatric patients

Safety and efficacy not established.

Geriatric or debilitated patients

Use caution. Start with the smallest dose and evaluate response.

Pharmacokinetics

Route	*Onset*	*Peak*
Oral	Rapid	1 hr

Metabolism: Hepatic; $T_{1/2}$: Unknown

Distribution: May cross placenta; may enter breast milk
Excretion: Urine

Adverse effects

- **CNS:** *Drowsiness, dizziness,* changes in thinking, *headache*
- **GI:** *Nausea, vomiting,* constipation
- **Respiratory:** Respiratory depression
- **Other:** Drug abuse

Interactions

✱ **Drug-drug** • Risk of increased CNS depression (which could lead to respiratory depression) if combined with general anesthetics, opioids, phenothiazines, sedatives, hypnotics, alcohol; if these combinations are used, monitor patient closely and adjust dosages as needed • Risk of potentially life-threatening serotonin syndrome if combined with SSRIs, TCAs, triptans, other norepinephrine reuptake inhibitors or with MAOIs; use within 14 days of MAOIs is contraindicated; if other combinations are used, patient should be strictly monitored and dosage adjustments made as needed
Drug-alternative therapy • Risk of serotonin syndrome if combined with St. John's wort; advise patient to avoid this combination

■ Nursing considerations

Assessment

- **History:** Hypersensitivity to any component of the drug; acute or severe bronchial asthma, COPD, hypercapnia; MAOI use within 14 days; severe obesity, sleep apnea syndrome; myxedema, CNS depression, seizure disorders; increased intracranial pressure; pancreatic or biliary tract disease, paralytic ileus; hepatic or renal impairment; pregnancy, lactation
- **Physical:** Orientation, affect, pain evaluation; R, adventitious sounds; bowel sounds; LFTs, renal function tests

Interventions

- Assess for pain before beginning therapy and periodically during therapy.
- Dispense the least amount of drug feasible; risk of abuse exists.
- Institute safety measures (use side rails, assist with ambulation); drug increases risk of dizziness and drowsiness.
- Provide frequent small meals if GI upset is a problem.

Teaching points

- Take this drug exactly as prescribed; do not increase dosage without consulting with the health care provider.
- You may experience these side effects: Headache (medication may be available to help); nausea and vomiting (frequent small meals may help); dizziness and drowsiness (avoid driving a car or operating hazardous machinery until you know how this drug will affect you).
- This drug may enter breast milk and could affect your baby if you are breast-feeding. Allow 3-4 hours to pass before nursing your baby if you are taking this drug. Consider an alternate method of feeding your baby or an alternate pain medication.
- Be aware that alcohol may increase the sedation effects of this drug; avoid this combination.
- This drug may interact with many other medications. Tell your health care provider about every medication you are taking.
- Do not use St. John's wort while you are taking this drug; serious side effects can occur.
- Report severe nausea and vomiting, shortness of breath, rash.

▽tegaserod maleate

See Appendix W, *Less commonly used drugs.*

▽telbivudine

See Appendix W, *Less commonly used drugs.*

▽telithromycin

*(tell ith roe **mye**´ sin)*

Ketek DNC

PREGNANCY CATEGORY C

Drug classes

Antibiotic
Ketolide

T

Therapeutic actions

Bacteriostatic or bactericidal in susceptible bacteria; binds to sites on bacterial ribosomes, causing change in protein function, leading to cell death.

Indications

- Only for treatment of mild to moderately severe community-acquired pneumonia caused by *Streptococcus pneumoniae* (including multi-drug resistant strains), *Haemophilus influenzae, Moraxella catarrhalis, Chlamydophilia pneumoniae, Mycoplasma pneumoniae* in patients 18 yr and older

Contraindications and cautions

- Contraindicated with allergy to telithromycin, to any component of the drug or to any macrolide antibiotic; congenital QT prolongation, proarrhythmic conditions (hypokalemia), significant bradycardia; concurrent use of pimozide, class Ia or III antiarrhythmics, simvastatin, lovastatin, atorvastatain; myasthenia gravis; history of hepatitis or jaundice.
- Use cautiously with renal or hepatic impairment, pregnancy, lactation.

Available forms

Tablets (DNC)—300, 400 mg

Dosages

Adults

Give 800 mg once daily PO for 7–10 days.

Pediatric patients

Safety and efficacy not established.

Patients with renal impairment

In patients with creatinine clearance less than 30 mL/min, including those on dialysis, give 600 mg PO once daily for 7–10 days after dialysis session is complete. In patients with creatinine clearance less than 30 mL/min and hepatic impairment, give 400 mg PO once daily for 7–10 days.

Pharmacokinetics

Route	Onset	Peak
Oral	Rapid	0.5–4 hr

Metabolism: Hepatic metabolism; $T_{1/2}$: 10 hr
Distribution: May cross placenta; passes into breast milk
Excretion: Feces, urine

Adverse effects

- **CNS:** Headache, dizziness, vertigo
- **CV: Prolonged QT interval, torsades de pointes**
- **GI:** *Diarrhea,* nausea, vomiting, taste alterations, loose stools, **pseudomembranous colitis,** hepatic impairment
- **Other:** *Superinfections,* hypersensitivity reactions ranging from rash to **anaphylaxis,** visual disturbances

Interactions

✱ **Drug-drug** ⊗ ***Warning*** Risk of increased serum levels and potentially serious adverse effects if combined with pimozide, simvastatin, lovastatin, atorvastatin, midazolam; avoid these combinations.
• Risk of increased exposure to metoprolol if given in combination, caution should be used • Risk of increased levels of digoxin; if this combination is used, monitor serum digoxin levels regularly and adjust dosage accordingly • Risk of decreased telithromycin levels and loss of therapeutic effect if combined with rifampin, phenytoin, carbamazepine, phenobarbital; suggest use of a different antibiotic if these drugs are used • Risk of increased GI effects of theophylline if taken together, separate doses by at least 1 hr if these two drugs are used

■ Nursing considerations

Assessment

- **History:** Known allergy to telithromycin, to any component of the drug, or to any macrolide antibiotic; congenital QT prolongation, proarrhythmic conditions, significant bradycardia; concurrent use of pimozide, class Ia or III antiarrhythmics, simvastatin, lovastatin, atorvastatin; myasthenia gravis; renal or hepatic impairment; pregnancy; lactation
- **Physical:** Site of infection, skin color, lesions; orientation, affect; baseline ECG, GI output, bowel sounds, liver evaluation;

culture and sensitivity tests of infection, LFTs, renal function tests

Interventions

⊗ ***Black box warning*** Contraindicated for use in patients with myasthenia gravis; life-threatening respiratory failure may occur.

- Culture site of infection before beginning therapy; make sure drug is used only as indicated.
- Administer at about the same time each day, without regard to food.
- Make sure that the tablet is swallowed whole, do not cut, crush, or allow the patient to chew the tablet.
- Monitor liver function in patients on prolonged therapy.
- Institute appropriate hygiene measures and arrange treatment if superinfections occur.
- If GI upset occurs provide frequent, small meals; encourage patient to maintain fluid intake and nutrition.
- Establish safety measures (eg, accompany patient, side rails) if CNS changes occur.

Teaching points

- Take this drug at about the same time each day, without regard to food. Do not cut, crush or chew the tablets; they must be swallowed whole.
- If you miss a dose, take the next dose as soon as you remember and then again about that time the next day; do not take more than one dose per day.
- Avoid quickly looking between objects in the distance and objects nearby if you are having visual difficulties.
- Take the full, prescribed dose of *Ketek*. Do not use the drug after the expiration date and do not save tablets for future use.
- You may experience these side effects: Nausea, diarrhea, discomfort (eat frequent small meals), headache (analgesics may be available to help, consult with your health care provider), dizziness (do not drive a car or operate hazardous machinery if this occurs).
- Report persistent or bloody diarrhea, visual disturbances that interfere with your daily activities, fainting, yellow color to the eyes or skin.

▽telmisartan

(tell mah sar' tan)

Micardis

PREGNANCY CATEGORY C (FIRST TRIMESTER)

PREGNANCY CATEGORY D (SECOND AND THIRD TRIMESTERS)

Drug classes

Angiotensin II receptor antagonist
Antihypertensive

Therapeutic actions

Selectively blocks the binding of angiotensin II to specific tissue receptors found in the vascular smooth muscle and adrenal gland; this action blocks the vasoconstriction effect of the renin-angiotensin system, as well as the release of aldosterone, leading to decreased BP.

Indications

- Treatment of hypertension, alone or in combination with other antihypertensives

Contraindications and cautions

- Contraindicated with hypersensitivity to telmisartan, pregnancy (use during the second or third trimester can cause injury or death to the fetus), lactation.
- Use cautiously with hepatic or biliary impairment, hypovolemia.

Available forms

Tablets—20, 40, 80 mg

Dosages

Adults

Usual starting dose, 40 mg PO daily. Adjust dosage based on patient response. Maximum dose, 80 mg/day. If response is still not as expected, a diuretic should be added.

Pediatric patients

Safety and efficacy not established.

Pharmacokinetics

Route	*Onset*	*Peak*	*Duration*
Oral	Rapid	0.5–1 hr	24 hr

T

Metabolism: Hepatic; $T_{1/2}$: 24 hr
Distribution: May cross placenta; may enter breast milk
Excretion: Feces

Adverse effects

- **CNS:** *Light-headedness, headache, dizziness,* muscle weakness
- **CV:** Hypotension, palpitations
- **Dermatologic:** Rash, dermatitis, eczema, urticaria, pruritus
- **GI:** Constipation, flatulence, gastritis, vomiting, dry mouth, dental pain
- **GU:** Decreased renal function
- **Respiratory:** Asthma, dyspnea, epistaxis, cough
- **Other:** Back pain, gout

Interactions

✱ **Drug-drug** • Increased serum levels and risk of toxicity of digoxin if combined

■ Nursing considerations

Assessment

- **History:** Hypersensitivity to telmisartan; pregnancy, lactation; hepatic or biliary impairment; hypovolemia
- **Physical:** Skin lesions, turgor; T; orientation, reflexes, affect; BP; R, respiratory auscultation; LFTs

Interventions

- Administer without regard to meals.

⊗ ***Black box warning*** Ensure that patient is not pregnant before beginning therapy. Suggest the use of barrier birth control while using telmisartan; fetal injury and deaths have been reported.

- Find an alternate method of feeding the baby if given to a nursing mother. Depression of the renin-angiotensin system in infants is potentially very dangerous.

⊗ ***Warning*** Alert the surgeon and mark the patient's chart with notice that telmisartan is being taken. The blockage of the renin-angiotensin system following surgery can produce problems. Hypotension may be reversed with volume expansion.

- If BP control does not reach desired levels, diuretics or other antihypertensives may be added to telmisartan. Monitor patient's BP carefully.
- Monitor patient closely in any situation that may lead to a decrease in BP secondary to reduction in fluid volume—excessive perspiration, dehydration, vomiting, diarrhea—excessive hypotension can occur.

Teaching points

- Take drug without regard to meals. Do not stop taking this drug without consulting your health care provider.
- Use a barrier method of birth control while taking this drug; if you become pregnant or want to become pregnant, consult your health care provider.
- You may experience these side effects: Dizziness (avoid driving a car or performing hazardous tasks); headache (medications may be available to help); nausea, vomiting, diarrhea (proper nutrition is important, consult with your dietitian to maintain nutrition); symptoms of upper respiratory tract infection; cough (do not self-medicate, consult your health care provider if this becomes uncomfortable).
- Report fever, chills, dizziness, pregnancy.

▽ temazepam

(te maz' e pam)

Apo-Temazepam (CAN), CO Temazepam (CAN), Gen-Temazepam (CAN), Novo-Temazepam (CAN), PMS-Temazepam (CAN), ratio-Temazepam (CAN), Restoril

PREGNANCY CATEGORY X

CONTROLLED SUBSTANCE C-IV

Drug classes

Benzodiazepine
Sedative-hypnotic

Therapeutic actions

Exact mechanisms of action not understood; acts mainly at subcortical levels of the CNS, leaving the cortex relatively unaffected; main sites of action may be the limbic system and mesencephalic reticular formation; benzodiazepines potentiate the effects of GABA, an inhibitory neurotransmitter.

Indications

- Insomnia characterized by difficulty falling asleep, frequent nocturnal awakenings, or early morning awakening
- Recurring insomnia or poor sleeping habits
- Acute or chronic medical situations requiring restful sleep

Contraindications and cautions

- Contraindicated with hypersensitivity to benzodiazepines, psychoses, acute narrow-angle glaucoma, shock, coma, acute alcoholic intoxication with depression of vital signs, pregnancy (risk of congenital malformations, neonatal withdrawal syndrome), labor and delivery ("floppy infant" syndrome), lactation (infants may become lethargic and lose weight).
- Use cautiously with impaired liver or renal function, debilitation, depression, suicidal tendencies.

Available forms

Capsules—7.5, 15, 22.5, 30 mg

Dosages

Adults

15–30 mg PO before bedtime.

Pediatric patients

Not for use in patients younger than 18 yr.

Geriatric or debilitated patients

Initially, 7.5 mg PO; adjust dosage, increasing if needed.

Pharmacokinetics

Route	Onset	Peak
Oral	Varies	1.2–1.6 hr

Metabolism: Hepatic; $T_{1/2}$: 10–20 hr
Distribution: Crosses placenta; enters breast milk
Excretion: Urine

Adverse effects

- **CNS:** *Transient, mild drowsiness initially; sedation, depression, lethargy, apathy, fatigue, light-headedness, disorientation, restlessness, confusion,* crying, delirium, headache, slurred speech, dysarthria, stupor, rigidity, tremor, dystonia, vertigo, euphoria, nervousness, difficulty concentrating, vivid dreams, psychomotor retardation, extrapyramidal symptoms, *mild paradoxical excitatory reactions during first 2 wk of treatment* (especially in psychiatric patients, aggressive children, and with high dosage), visual and auditory disturbances, diplopia, nystagmus, depressed hearing, nasal congestion, complex sleep-related behaviors
- **CV:** *Bradycardia, tachycardia,* **CV collapse,** hypertension and hypotension, palpitations, edema
- **Dependence:** *Drug dependence with withdrawal syndrome* when drug is discontinued
- **Dermatologic:** Urticaria, pruritus, rash, dermatitis
- **GI:** *Constipation, diarrhea,* dry mouth, salivation, nausea, anorexia, vomiting, difficulty in swallowing, gastric disorders, elevations of blood enzymes; hepatic impairment, jaundice
- **GU:** *Incontinence, urinary retention, changes in libido,* menstrual irregularities
- **Hematologic:** Decreased Hct (primarily with long-term therapy), blood dyscrasias
- **Other:** Hiccups, fever, diaphoresis, paresthesias, muscular disturbances, gynecomastia, **anaphylaxis, angioedema**

Interactions

✱ **Drug-drug** • Increased CNS depression with alcohol and other CNS depressants (eg, barbiturates, opioids) • Decreased sedative effects with theophylline, aminophylline, dyphylline

■ Nursing considerations

Assessment

- **History:** Hypersensitivity to benzodiazepines; psychoses; acute narrow-angle glaucoma; shock, coma; acute alcoholic intoxication; pregnancy, lactation; impaired liver or renal function, debilitation; depression, suicidal tendencies
- **Physical:** Skin color, lesions; T; orientation, reflexes, affect, ophthalmologic examination; P, BP; R, adventitious sounds; liver evaluation, abdominal examination, bowel sounds, normal output; CBC, LFTs, renal function tests

Interventions

⊗ ***Warning*** Taper dosage gradually after long-term therapy, especially in patients with epilepsy, to prevent refractory seizures.

- Caution patient to avoid pregnancy while taking this drug; advise patient to use barrier contraceptives.

Teaching points

- Take drug exactly as prescribed.
- During long-term therapy, do not stop taking this drug without consulting your health care provider.
- Do not drink alcohol or use other CNS depressants while on this drug.
- Avoid pregnancy while taking this drug; serious fetal harm could occur. Using contraceptive measures is advised.
- Nocturnal sleep may be disturbed for several nights after discontinuing the drug.
- You may experience these side effects: Drowsiness, dizziness (may lessen; avoid driving or engaging in other dangerous activities); swelling, allergic reaction; GI upset (take drug with water); depression, dreams, emotional upset, crying, complex sleep-related behaviors, allergic reaction, or swelling.
- Report severe dizziness, allergies, weakness, drowsiness that persists, rash or skin lesions, palpitations, swelling of extremities, visual changes, difficulty voiding, sleep disorders.

temozolomide

See Appendix W, *Less commonly used drugs.*

temsirolimus

See Appendix W, *Less commonly used drugs.*

DANGEROUS DRUG

tenecteplase

*(teh **nek'** ti plaze)*

TNKase

PREGNANCY CATEGORY C

Drug class

Thrombolytic enzyme

Therapeutic actions

Enzyme that converts plasminogen to the enzyme plasmin (fibrinolysin), which degrades fibrin clots; lyses thrombi and emboli; is most active at the site of the clot and causes little systemic fibrinolysis.

Indications

- Reduction of mortality associated with acute MI

Contraindications and cautions

- Contraindicated with allergy to tenecteplase; active internal bleeding; history of CVA; intracranial or intraspinal surgery or trauma (within 2 mo); intracranial neoplasm, arteriovenous malformation, or aneurysm; known bleeding diathesis; severe uncontrolled hypertension.
- Use cautiously with recent major surgery, previous puncture of noncompressible vessels, cerebrovascular disease, recent GI or GU bleeding, recent trauma, hypertension, high likelihood of left heart thrombus, acute pericarditis, subacute bacterial endocarditis, hemostatic defects (including those secondary to severe hepatic or renal disease), severe hepatic impairment, pregnancy, diabetic hemorrhagic retinopathy or other hemorrhagic ophthalmic conditions, septic thrombophlebitis or occluded AV cannula at seriously infected site, advanced age, patients currently receiving oral anticoagulants, recent use of GP IIb/IIIa inhibitors, any other condition in which bleeding constitutes a significant hazard or would be particularly difficult to manage because of its location.

Available forms

Powder for injection—50 mg

Dosages

Adults

⊗ ***Warning*** Do not exceed 50 mg/dose. Initiate treatment as soon as possible after onset of acute MI. Administer as IV bolus over 5 sec. Dose is based on weight:

Less than 60 kg: 30 mg.

60–69 kg: 35 mg.

70–79 kg: 40 mg.

80–89 kg: 45 mg.
90 kg or more: 50 mg.

Pediatric patients

Safety and efficacy not established.

Geriatric patients

Dosage adjustment is not recommended, but elderly patients have an increased risk of adverse effects. Monitor closely for early signs of bleeding.

Pharmacokinetics

Route	*Onset*	*Peak*
IV	Immediate	5–10 min

Metabolism: Hepatic; $T_{1/2}$: 90–130 min
Distribution: Crosses placenta; may enter breast milk
Excretion: Bile

IV FACTS

Preparation: Reconstitute using the supplied 10-cc syringe with twinpack dual cannula device and 10 mL sterile water for injection. Do not shake. Slight foaming is normal and should dissipate if left standing for 10 min. Reconstituted solution is 5 mg/mL. Use immediately or may be refrigerated for up to 8 hr.
Infusion: Infuse as a bolus injection over 5 sec. Flush any dextrose-containing lines with saline before injecting and after administration. Discard any leftover solution.
Incompatibilities: Do not add other medications to infusion solution.

Adverse effects

- **CV:** Cardiac arrhythmias with coronary reperfusion, hypotension, AV block, **MI,** cardiogenic shock, cholesterol embolization (eg, livedo reticularis, "purple toe" syndrome, acute renal failure, pancreatitis, hypertension)
- **Hematologic: Bleeding,** particularly at venous or arterial access sites; GI bleeding; intracranial hemorrhage
- **Other:** Urticaria, nausea, vomiting, fever, allergic reactions

Interactions

✱ **Drug-drug** • Increased risk of hemorrhage if used with heparin or oral anticoagulants, aspirin, dipyridamole, ticlopidine, clopidogrel; monitor patient very closely if these combinations are used • Decreased effectiveness if combined with aminocaproic acid

✱ **Drug-lab test** • During tenecteplase therapy, results of coagulation tests or measures of fibrinolytic activity may be unreliable unless specific precautions are taken to prevent *in vitro* artifacts

■ Nursing considerations

Assessment

- **History:** Allergy to tenecteplase; active internal bleeding; recent (within 2 mo) CVA; intracranial or intraspinal surgery or neoplasm; recent major surgery, obstetrical delivery, organ biopsy, or rupture of a noncompressible blood vessel; recent serious GI bleed; recent serious trauma, including CPR; SBE; hemostatic defects; cerebrovascular disease; early-onset, type 1 diabetes; severe uncontrolled hypertension; liver disease; pregnancy, lactation
- **Physical:** Skin color, T, lesions; orientation, reflexes; P, BP, peripheral perfusion, baseline ECG; R, adventitious sounds; liver evaluation, Hct, platelet count, thrombin time (TT), aPTT, PT/INR

Interventions

⊗ ***Warning*** Arrange to discontinue concurrent heparin and tenecteplase if serious bleeding occurs.

- Arrange for regular monitoring of coagulation studies.

⊗ ***Warning*** Apply pressure or pressure dressings or both to control superficial bleeding (at invaded or disturbed areas); avoid IM injections, invasive procedures, and excessive handling of the patient.

- Avoid any arterial invasive procedures during therapy.
- Arrange for typing and cross-matching of blood in case serious blood loss occurs and whole blood transfusions are required.
- Monitor patient for signs of bleeding; provide safety procedures to avoid injury.

Teaching points

- This drug can only be given IV and you will need to be closely monitored during drug treatment.

T

- You may experience these side effects: Tendency to bleed easily (use caution to avoid injury, use electric razor, a soft toothbrush, use caution with sharp objects), strict bed rest will help to decrease the risk of bleeding. If bleeding does occur, apply pressure to the site until bleeding stops.
- Report bruising or bleeding; blood in urine, stool, or with coughing; bleeding gums; changes in vision; difficulty breathing, chest pain.

▽tenofovir disoproxil fumarate

*(te **noe'** fo veer)*

Viread

PREGNANCY CATEGORY B

Drug classes

Antiviral
Nucleotide reverse transcriptase inhibitor

Therapeutic actions

Antiviral activity; inhibits HIV reverse transcriptase activity, leading to a blocking of HIV reproduction.

Indications

- Treatment of HIV-1 infection in combination with other antiretrovirals
- Treatment of chronic hepatitis B in adults

Contraindications and cautions

- Contraindicated with allergy to tenofovir or any other components of the product, chronic hepatitis B.
- Use cautiously in pregnancy, hepatic or renal impairment, lactation.

Available forms

Tablets—300 mg

Dosages

Adults

300 mg/day PO without regard to food.

Pediatric patients

Safety and efficacy not established.

Patients with renal impairment

Adjust dosage as follows:

CrCl (mL/min)	*Dose*
50 or more	300 mg every 24 hr
30–49	300 mg every 48 hr
10–29	300 mg twice a wk
Hemodialysis	300 mg every wk or after a total of about 12 hr of dialysis

Pharmacokinetics

Route	*Onset*	*Peak*
Oral	Rapid	45–75 min

Metabolism: Unknown; $T_{1/2}$: 17 hr
Distribution: May cross placenta; may enter breast milk
Excretion: Urine

Adverse effects

- **CNS:** *Headache, asthenia*
- **GI:** *Nausea, vomiting, diarrhea,* anorexia, abdominal pain, *flatulence,* **severe hepatomegaly with steatosis**
- **Metabolic: Lactic adicosis, sometimes severe**

Interactions

✱ **Drug-drug** • Increased concentration and toxicity of didanosine if used concurrently; decrease didanosine dose to 250 mg in patients weighing more than 60 kg • Increased tenofovir concentrations with atazanavir and lopinavir; monitor patient closely • Risk of decreased atazanavir levels if combined with tenofovir; administer 300 mg atazanavir with 100 mg ritonavir only; do not administer atazanavir alone • Avoid use with other combination drugs that include tenofovir.

✱ **Drug-food** • Increased bioavailability if combined with food; tenofovir can be taken without regard to meals

■ Nursing considerations

Assessment

- **History:** Allergy to tenofovir, renal or hepatic impairment, pregnancy, lactation
- **Physical:** T, orientation, reflexes, abdominal examination, LFTs, renal function tests

Interventions

- Administer with other antiretrovirals; do not use as monotherapy.

⊠ ***Black box warning*** Monitor hepatic function closely; risk of lactic acidosis and severe hepatic toxicity.

⊠ ***Black box warning*** Severe exacerbation of hepatitis B has occurred when anti–hepatitis B therapy is discontinued. Monitor patient for several months if drug is discontinued.

- Monitor patients with hepatic or renal problems for possible adverse effects.

⊗ ***Warning*** Withdraw drug and monitor patient if signs or symptoms of lactic acidosis or hepatotoxicity develop, including hepatomegaly and steatosis. These are more common in women, obesity, and prolonged tenofovir use.

- Encourage women of childbearing age to use barrier contraceptives while taking this drug because the effects of the drug on the fetus are not known.
- Advise women who are nursing to find another method of feeding the baby.

Teaching points

- Take this drug once a day without regard to meals or food.
- Take the full course of therapy as prescribed; always take in combination with other antivirals; if you miss a dose, take it as soon as you remember and then take the next dose at the usual time. If it is almost time for the next dose when you remember, just take the next dose. Do not take any double doses.
- This drug does not cure HIV infection; long-term effects are not yet known; continue to take precautions because the risk of transmission is not reduced by this drug.
- Avoid pregnancy while taking this drug; using barrier contraceptives is advised.
- Do not take any other drug, prescription or over-the-counter, without consulting your health care provider; this drug interacts with other drugs and serious problems can occur.
- You may experience these side effects: Nausea, vomiting, loss of appetite, diarrhea, abdominal pain, headache (try to maintain nutrition and fluid intake as much as possible; eat frequent small meals); redistribution of fat on the body (arms and legs may become thin, a "buffalo hump" may develop on the back of the neck, and fat may be distributed in the breasts and along the trunk).
- Report severe diarrhea, jaundice, changes in color of stool or urine, rapid respirations.

▽terazosin hydrochloride

(ter ay' zoe sin)

Apo-Terazocin (CAN), Hytrin, Novo-Terazocin (CAN), PMS-Terazocin (CAN), ratio-Terazocin (CAN)

Pregnancy Category C

Drug classes

Alpha$_1$-adrenergic blocker
Antihypertensive

Therapeutic actions

Drug selectively blocks postsynaptic alpha$_1$-adrenergic receptors, decreasing sympathetic tone on the vasculature, dilating arterioles and veins, and lowering supine and standing BP; unlike conventional alpha-adrenergic blocking agents (eg, phentolamine), it does not also block alpha$_2$ presynaptic receptors, does not cause reflex tachycardia. Relaxes the smooth muscle by blocking alpha$_1$-adrenergic receptors in the bladder neck and prostate thereby improving the symptoms of BPH.

Indications

- Treatment of symptomatic BPH
- Treatment of hypertension alone or in combination with other drugs
- Unlabeled uses: Symptomatic treatment of chronic abacterial prostatitis, ureteral stones

Contraindications and cautions

- Contraindicated with hypersensitivity to terazosin and during lactation.
- Use cautiously in patients taking other antihypertensives, HF, renal failure, pregnancy.

Available forms

Tablets, capsules—1, 2, 5, 10 mg

Dosages

Adults

Adjust dose and dosing interval (12 or 24 hr) individually.

- *Hypertension:* Initial dose, 1 mg PO at bedtime. Do not exceed 1 mg; strictly adhere to this regimen to avoid severe hypotensive reactions. Slowly increase dose to achieve desired BP response. Usual range, 1–5 mg PO daily. Up to 20 mg/day has been beneficial. Monitor BP 2–3 hr after dosing to determine maximum effect. If response is diminished after 24 hr, consider increasing dosage or use a twice daily regimen. If drug is not taken for several days, restart with initial 1-mg dose.
- *BPH:* Initial dose, 1 mg PO at bedtime. Increase to 2, 5, or 10 mg PO daily. 10 mg/day for 4–6 wk may be required to assess benefit. If drug is not taken for several days, restart with the initial dose.

Pediatric patients

Safety and efficacy not established.

Pharmacokinetics

Route	*Onset*	*Peak*
Oral	Varies	1 hr

Metabolism: Unknown; $T_{1/2}$: 12 hr
Distribution: Crosses placenta; may enter breast milk
Excretion: Feces, urine

Adverse effects

- **CNS:** *Dizziness, headache, drowsiness, lack of energy, weakness, somnolence,* nervousness, vertigo, depression, paresthesia
- **CV:** *Palpitations,* sodium and water retention, increased plasma volume, *edema,* syncope, tachycardia, *orthostatic hypotension,* angina
- **Dermatologic:** Rash, pruritus, alopecia
- **EENT:** Blurred vision, reddened sclera, floppy iris syndrome during cataract surgery, epistaxis, tinnitus, dry mouth, nasal congestion
- **GI:** *Nausea,* vomiting, diarrhea, constipation, abdominal discomfort or pain
- **GU:** Urinary frequency, incontinence, impotence, priapism
- **Respiratory:** *Dyspnea, nasal congestion, sinusitis*
- **Other:** Diaphoresis, **allergic anaphylaxis**

Interactions

✱ **Drug-drug** • Risk of marked hypotension with drugs used to treat ED; use caution

■ Nursing considerations

Assessment

- **History:** Hypersensitivity to terazosin; HF; renal failure; pregnancy, lactation
- **Physical:** Weight; skin color, lesions; orientation, affect, reflexes; ophthalmologic examination; P, BP, orthostatic BP, supine BP, perfusion, edema, auscultation; R, adventitious sounds, status of nasal mucous membranes; bowel sounds, normal output; voiding pattern, urinary output; renal function tests, urinalysis

Interventions

⊗ ***Warning*** Administer or have patient take first dose just before bedtime to lessen likelihood of first dose effect, syncope due to excessive orthostatic hypotension.

⊗ ***Warning*** Have patient lie down, and treat supportively if syncope occurs; condition is self-limiting.

- Monitor patient for orthostatic hypotension, which is most marked in the morning, and is accentuated by hot weather, alcohol, exercise.
- Monitor edema and weight in patients with incipient cardiac decompensation, and add a thiazide diuretic to the drug regimen if sodium and fluid retention, signs of impending HF, occur.

Teaching points

- Take this drug exactly as prescribed. Take the first dose just before bedtime. Do not drive or operate machinery for 12 hours after the first dose.
- Use caution if you are using drugs to treat erectile dysfunction; dizziness, low blood pressure can occur.
- You may experience these side effects: Dizziness, weakness (more likely when changing position, in early morning, after exercise, in hot weather, and with alcohol use; some tolerance may occur after taking the drug for a while, but avoid driving or engaging in tasks that require alertness; change position slowly; use caution when climbing stairs; lie down

for a while if dizziness persists); GI upset (eat frequent small meals); impotence; dry mouth (suck on sugarless lozenges or ice chips); stuffy nose. Most effects will gradually disappear.
- Report frequent dizziness or faintness.

▽terbinafine hydrochloride

(ter bin' ah feen)

Apo-Terbinafine (CAN), CO Terbinafine (CAN), Gen Terbinafine (CAN), Lamisil, Lamisil Oral Granules, PMS-Terbinafine (CAN)

PREGNANCY CATEGORY B

Drug classes
Allylamine
Antifungal

Therapeutic actions
A synthetic allylamine that is thought to block squalene oxidase, thus preventing the biosynthesis of ergosterol, an essential component of fungal cell walls.

Indications
- Treatment of tinea capitis in patients 4 yr and older (oral granules)
- Treatment of onychomycosis of the toenail or fingernail caused by dermatophytes

Contraindications and cautions
- Contraindicated with allergy to any component of the product, hepatic failure, pregnancy, lactation.
- Use cautiously with hepatic impairment, renal impairment, immunodeficiency.

Available forms
Tablets—250 mg; oral granules—125, 187.5 mg

Dosages
Adults
- *Fingernail onychomycosis:* 250 mg/day PO for 6 wk.
- *Toenail onychomycosis:* 250 mg/day PO for 12 wk.
- *Tinea capitis:* 250 mg/day PO for 6 wk.

Pediatric patients

Tinea capitis

Weight less than 25 kg: 125 mg/day PO for 6 wk.
25–35 kg: 187.5 mg/day PO for 6 wk.
Weight more than 35 kg: 250 mg/day PO for 6 wk.

Pharmacokinetics

Route	Onset	Peak
Oral	Moderate	2 hr

Metabolism: Hepatic metabolism, $T_{1/2}$: 36 hr
Distribution: May cross placenta; enters breast milk
Excretion: Urine

Adverse effects
- **CNS:** Headache, taste disturbance, visual disturbance
- **Dermatological: Rash,** *pruritus,* urticaria
- **GI:** Diarrhea, abdominal pain, dyspepsia, nausea, flatulence, **hepatic failure,** liver enzyme abnormalities, taste disturbances

Interactions
✱ **Drug-drug** • Decreased effectiveness of terbinafine if combined with rifampin, cyclosporine • Increased serum levels and risk of toxicity if combined with cimetidine • Increased serum levels of dextromethorphan and risk of toxicity if combined with terbinafine; monitor patient closely if this combination must be used

■ Nursing considerations

CLINICAL ALERT!
Name confusion has been reported between *Lamisil* (terbinafine) and *Lamictal* (lamotrigine); use extreme caution.

Assessment
- **History:** Allergy to any component of the product, hepatic or renal impairment, immunodeficiency, pregnancy, lactation
- **Physical:** Skin evaluation; liver examination, bowel sounds; T; nail specimen culture, LFTs

Interventions
- Obtain nail culture or biopsy to confirm the diagnosis of onychomycosis before beginning therapy.

- Suggest waiting until after delivery instead of using this drug during pregnancy or lactation; effects on the fetus are not known.
- Suggest an alternative method of feeding the infant if this drug is prescribed for a nursing mother.
- For oral granules, sprinkle entire packet of granules on a spoonful of nonacidic food, such as mashed potatoes. Have patient swallow entire spoonful without chewing.

⊗ ***Black box warning*** Monitor the patient regularly for any sign of hepatic impairment; liver failure can occur.

- Discontinue drug if a skin rash appears, or with hepatic failure.
- Provide appropriate analgesics for headache.

Teaching points

- Take this drug for the full recommended course of treatment.
- If using oral granules, sprinkle entire packet on a spoonful of nonacidic food, such as mashed potatoes. Then swallow entire spoonful without chewing.
- You may experience these side effects: Headache (medication will be arranged), diarrhea, abdominal pain, nausea (eat frequent small meals).
- Report persistent nausea, lack of appetite, yellowing of the eyes or skin, dark urine or pale stools.
- Report skin rash to your health care provider immediately.

▽terbutaline sulfate

*(ter **byoo'** ta leen)*

Brethine

PREGNANCY CATEGORY B

Drug classes

Antasthmatic
$Beta_2$-selective adrenergic agonist
Bronchodilator
Sympathomimetic
Tocolytic drug

Therapeutic actions

In low doses, acts relatively selectively at $beta_2$-adrenergic receptors to cause bronchodilation and relax the pregnant uterus; at higher doses, $beta_2$ selectivity is lost and the drug acts at $beta_1$ receptors to cause typical sympathomimetic cardiac effects.

Indications

- Prophylaxis and treatment of bronchial asthma and reversible bronchospasm that may occur with bronchitis and emphysema in patients 12 yr and older
- Unlabeled use: Tocolytic to prevent preterm labor

Contraindications and cautions

- Contraindicated with hypersensitivity to terbutaline; tachyarrhythmias, tachycardia caused by digoxin toxicity; general anesthesia with halogenated hydrocarbons or cyclopropane, which sensitize the myocardium to catecholamines; unstable vasomotor system disorders; labor and delivery (may inhibit labor; parenteral use of beta-adrenergic agonists can accelerate fetal heart beat, cause hypoglycemia, hypokalemia, and pulmonary edema in the mother and hypoglycemia in the neonate); lactation.
- Use cautiously with diabetes, coronary insufficiency, CAD, history of CVA, COPD patients who have developed degenerative heart disease, hyperthyroidism, history of seizure disorders, psychoneurotic individuals, hypertension.

Available forms

Tablets—2.5, 5 mg; injection—1 mg/mL

Dosages

Adults and patients older than 15 yr

Oral

5 mg at 6-hr intervals tid during waking hours. If side effects are pronounced, reduce to 2.5 mg tid. Do not exceed 15 mg/day.

Parenteral

0.25 mg subcutaneously into lateral deltoid area. If no significant improvement in 15–30 min, give another 0.25-mg dose. Do not exceed 0.5 mg/4 hr. If patient fails to respond to second 0.25-mg dose within 15–30 min, other therapeutic measures should be considered.

Pediatric patients

Oral

12–15 yr: 2.5 mg tid. Do not exceed 7.5 mg/24 hr.

Younger than 12 yr: Not recommended.

Geriatric patients

Patients older than 60 yr are more likely to experience side effects. Use with extreme caution.

Pharmacokinetics

Route	*Onset*	*Peak*	*Duration*
Subcut.	5–15 min	30–60 min	1.5–4 hr
Oral	30 min	2–3 hr	4–8 hr

Metabolism: Tissue; $T_{1/2}$: 2–4 hr
Distribution: May cross placenta; enters breast milk
Excretion: Urine

Adverse effects

- **CNS:** *Restlessness, apprehension, anxiety, fear,* CNS stimulation, hyperkinesia, insomnia, tremor, drowsiness, irritability, weakness, vertigo, headache, seizures
- **CV:** *Cardiac arrhythmias, palpitations,* anginal pain (less likely with bronchodilator doses of this drug than with bronchodilator doses of a nonselective beta agonist [isoproterenol]), changes in BP and ECG
- **GI:** *Nausea,* vomiting, heartburn, unusual or bad taste in mouth
- **Respiratory:** *Respiratory difficulties,* **pulmonary edema,** *coughing,* **bronchospasm**
- **Other:** Sweating, pallor, flushing, muscle cramps, elevated LFTs

Interactions

✱ **Drug-drug** • Increased likelihood of cardiac arrhythmias with halogenated hydrocarbon anesthetics (halothane), cyclopropane • Risk of hypokalemia if combined with diuretics • Increased risk of hypokalemia and ECG changes with MAOIs and TCAs • Do not administer with other sympathomimetics, theophylline

■ Nursing considerations

CLINICAL ALERT!

Due to similar packaging, terbutaline injection has been confused with methergine injection (methylergonovine maleate); use extreme caution.

Assessment

- **History:** Hypersensitivity to terbutaline; tachyarrhythmias; general anesthesia with halogenated hydrocarbons or cyclopropane; unstable vasomotor system disorders; hypertension; CAD; history of CVA; COPD patients who have developed degenerative heart disease; hyperthyroidism; history of seizure disorders; psychoneurotic individuals; pregnancy; labor and delivery; lactation
- **Physical:** Weight; skin color, T, turgor; orientation, reflexes; P, BP; R, adventitious sounds; blood and urine glucose; serum electrolytes; LFTs, thyroid function tests; ECG

Interventions

- Use minimal doses for minimal periods of time; drug tolerance can occur with prolonged use.

⊗ ***Warning*** Keep a beta blocker (a cardioselective beta blocker, such as atenolol, should be used in patients with respiratory distress) readily available in case cardiac arrhythmias occur.

- Do not exceed recommended dosage.

Teaching points

- Do not exceed recommended dosage; adverse effects or loss of effectiveness may result. Read product instructions; consult your health care provider if you have any questions.
- You may experience these side effects: Weakness, dizziness, inability to sleep (use caution when driving or performing activities that require alertness); nausea, vomiting (eat frequent small meals); fast heart rate, anxiety.
- Report chest pain, dizziness, insomnia, weakness, tremor or irregular heartbeat, failure to respond to usual dosage.

▽ teriparatide

See Appendix X, *Less commonly used drugs.*

testosterone
(tess ***toss'*** *ter ohn)*

testosterone
Transdermal patch: Androderm
Transdermal gel: AndroGel 1%, Testim
Testosterone pellets: Testopel Pellets
Testosterone buccal: Striant

testosterone cypionate (long-acting)
Depo-Testosterone

testosterone enanthate (long-acting)
Delatestryl

PREGNANCY CATEGORY X

CONTROLLED SUBSTANCE C-III

Drug classes
Androgen
Hormone

Therapeutic actions
Primary natural androgen; responsible for growth and development of male sex organs and the maintenance of secondary sex characteristics; administration of exogenous testosterone increases the retention of nitrogen, sodium, potassium, phosphorus; decreases urinary excretion of calcium; increases protein anabolism and decreases protein catabolism; stimulates the production of RBCs.

Indications
- Replacement therapy in hypo-gonadism—primary hypogonadism, hypogonadotropic hypogonadism, delayed puberty (men)
- Testosterone enanthate only: Inoperable breast cancer, metastatic mammary cancer

Contraindications and cautions
- Contraindicated with known sensitivity to androgens; prostate or breast cancer in men; pregnancy; lactation; serious cardiac, hepatic, or renal disease. *Androderm* contraindicated for use in women.
- Use cautiously with MI.

Available forms
Transdermal system—2.5, 5 mg/24 hr; transdermal gel, 1%; pellets—75 mg; testosterone enanthate injection—200 mg/mL; buccal system—30 mg; testosterone cypionate injection—100, 200 mg/mL

Dosages
Adults
- *Carcinoma of the breast and metastatic mammary cancer:* 200–400 mg IM (testosterone enanthate) every 2–4 wk.
- *Male hypogonadism (replacement therapy):* 50–400 mg testosterone cypionate or testosterone enanthate every 2–4 wk given IM, or 150–450 mg testosterone enanthate pellets implanted subcutaneously every 3–6 mo.
- *Inoperable carcinoma of the breast:* 200–400 mg testosterone enanthate given IM every 2–4 wk.
- *Males with delayed puberty:* 50–200 mg IM (testosterone enanthate) every 2–4 wk for a limited duration (4–6 mo) or 150 mg pellets subcutaneously every 3–6 mo (testosterone pellets).
- *Primary hypogonadism, hypogonadotropic hypogonadism in males:* Testosterone patch, initially 6 mg/day system applied to scrotal skin; then 4-mg/day system (*Androderm*); testosterone gel—5 mg/day (preferably in the morning) applied to clean, dry, intact skin of the shoulders, upper arms, or abdomen (*AndroGel* or *Testim*); apply one buccal system (30 mg) to gum region bid (morning and evening); rotate sites; usual position is above incisor on either side of mouth (*Striant*).

Pharmacokinetics

Route	*Onset*	*Duration*
IM	Slow	1–3 days
IM cypionate	Slow	2–4 wk
IM enanthate	Slow	2–4 wk
Dermal	Rapid	24 hr
Buccal	Rapid	12 hr

Metabolism: Hepatic; $T_{1/2}$: 10–100 min; up to 8 days (cypionate)
Distribution: Crosses placenta; may enter breast milk
Excretion: Feces, urine

Adverse effects

- **CNS:** *Dizziness, headache, sleep disorders, fatigue,* tremor, sleeplessness, generalized paresthesia, sleep apnea syndrome
- **Dermatologic:** *Rash,* dermatitis, anaphylactoid reactions, acne
- **Endocrine:** *Androgenic effects* (acne, edema, mild hirsutism, decrease in breast size, deepening of the voice, oily skin or hair, weight gain, clitoral hypertrophy or testicular atrophy), *hypoestrogenic effects* (flushing, sweating, vaginitis, nervousness, emotional lability), gynecomastia in males
- **GI:** *Nausea,* hepatic impairment; **hepatocellular carcinoma**
- **GU:** Fluid retention, decreased urinary output, changes in libido
- **Hematologic:** *Polycythemia; leukopenia;* hypercalcemia; altered serum cholesterol levels; retention of sodium, chloride, water, potassium, phosphates, and calcium
- **Other:** Chills, premature closure of the epiphyses, hypercalcemia

Interactions

✱ **Drug-food** • Decreased metabolism and risk of toxic effects if combined with grapefruit juice; avoid this combination

✱ **Drug-lab test** • Altered glucose tolerance tests • With no evidence of clinical thyroid dysfunction, decrease in thyroid function tests, which may persist for 2–3 wk after therapy • Increased creatinine, creatinine clearance, which may last for 2 wk after therapy

■ Nursing considerations

Assessment

- **History:** Known sensitivity to androgens, prostate or breast cancer in males, cardiac disease, renal disease, liver disease, pregnancy, lactation
- **Physical:** Skin color, lesions, texture; hair distribution pattern; injection site; affect, orientation, peripheral sensation; abdominal examination, liver evaluation; serum electrolytes, serum cholesterol levels, LFTs, glucose tolerance tests, thyroid function tests, long-bone X-ray (in children)

Interventions

- Apply dermal patch to clean, dry skin as directed. Do not use chemical depilatories. *Androderm* is to be applied to nonscrotal skin on back, abdomen, upper arms. Remove the old patch before applying a new one.

⊗ ***Black box warning*** There is a risk of toxic effects (enlarged genitalia, greater-than-normal bone age) in children exposed to patients using transdermal form (*AndroGel, Testim*). Patient should wash hands after applying drug and cover treated area with clothing to reduce exposure.

- Apply buccal system to gum region above incisor on either side of mouth; rotate sites (*Striant*). Place rounded side of buccal system against gum and hold firmly in place for 30 sec to ensure adhesion. If system falls off during 12-hr period, remove old system and replace with new system.
- Inject testosterone deeply into gluteal muscle.
- Shake vials well before use; crystals will redissolve.
- Do not administer frequently; these drugs are absorbed slowly; testosterone enanthate and cypionate are long acting and provide therapeutic effects for about 4 wk.
- Monitor effect on children with long-bone X-rays every 3–6 mo during therapy; discontinue drug well before the bone age reaches the norm for the patient's chronologic age.
- Monitor patient for edema; arrange for diuretic therapy as needed.
- Monitor liver function and serum electrolytes periodically during therapy, and consult with physician for corrective measures as needed.
- Periodically measure cholesterol levels in patients who are at high risk for CAD.
- Monitor patients with diabetes closely because glucose tolerance may change; adjustments may be needed in insulin, oral hypoglycemic dosage, and diet.
- Periodically monitor urine and serum calcium during treatment of disseminated breast carcinoma and metastatic mammary cancer, and arrange for appropriate treatment or discontinuation of the drug.
- Monitor elderly men for prostatic hypertrophy and carcinoma.

- Advise female patients, especially pregnant patients, that they should avoid contact with application site of testosterone gel as well as transdermal patches.

⊗ ***Warning*** Discontinue drug and arrange for consultation if abnormal vaginal bleeding occurs.

Teaching points

- The injection forms of this drug can only be given by IM injection. Mark a calendar indicating days for injection. If using the dermal patch, apply the patch to dry, clean skin as directed. *Androderm* is to be applied to nonscrotal skin on your back, abdomen, or upper arm. Remove the old patch before applying a new one. *AndroGel* is to be applied to skin of the shoulders and upper arms. Do not shower or swim for at least 1 hour after application of gel. Wash hands after applying gel. Cover area with clothing if you are in contact with children because children can experience adverse effects if exposed to the gel.
- Apply buccal system to gum region above incisor on either side of mouth; rotate sites. Check to make sure system remains in place after brushing teeth, using mouthwash, eating, and drinking.
- Avoid grapefruit juice while using this drug.
- This drug cannot be taken during pregnancy; serious fetal effects could occur. Women should use contraceptive measures.
- Patients with diabetes should monitor serum glucose closely because glucose tolerance may change; report any abnormalities to prescriber, so corrective action can be taken.
- You may experience these side effects: Body hair growth, baldness, deepening of the voice, loss of libido, impotence (reversible); excitation, confusion, insomnia (avoid driving or performing tasks that require alertness); swelling of the ankles, fingers (request medication).
- Report ankle swelling; nausea; vomiting; yellowing of skin or eyes; unusual bleeding or bruising; penile swelling or pain; hoarseness, body hair growth, deepening of the voice, acne, menstrual irregularities, pregnancy.

▽tetrabenazine

*(tet ra **ben'** ah zeen)*

Xenazine

PREGNANCY CATEGORY C

Drug classes

Monoamine depletor
Anti-chorea drug

Therapeutic actions

Inhibits monoamine transport systems, resulting in a decreased uptake of the monoamines dopamine, serotonin, norepinephrine, and histamine into synaptic vesicles and a depletion of monoamine stores; exact mechanism of action of effects on chorea are not understood.

Indications

- Treatment of chorea associated with Huntington's disease

Contraindications and cautions

- Contraindicated with active suicidality, untreated or inadequately treated depression, impaired hepatic function, concurrent use of MAOIs or reserpine.
- Use cautiously with prolonged QT interval, pregnancy, lactation.

Available forms

Tablets—12.5, 25 mg

Dosages

Adults

12.5 mg/day PO in the morning; after 1 week, increase to 12.5 mg PO bid; may be slowly titrated as needed to a maximum dose of 100 mg/day in divided doses.

Pediatric patients

Safety and efficacy not established.

Pharmacokinetics

Route	*Onset*	*Peak*
Oral	Slow	2 hr

Metabolism: Hepatic; $T_{1/2}$: 4–8 hr, then 2–4 hr (active metabolite)

Distribution: May cross placenta; may enter breast milk
Excretion: Urine

Adverse effects

- **CNS:** *Sedation, insomnia, depression, anxiety,* irritability, obsessive reaction, *akathisia*, parkinsonism, dizziness, headache, unsteady gait
- **GI:** *Nausea*, vomiting, decreased appetite
- **Respiratory:** *URI*, shortness of breath, bronchitis
- **Other:** *Fatigue*

Interactions

✱ **Drug-drug** • Risk of increased serum levels and toxicity if given with any potent CYP2D6 inhibitor (fluoxetine, paroxetine, quinidine); dosage of tetrabenazine should be halved if combined with any of these drugs • Increased risk of prolonged QT interval if combined with any other drugs that prolong QT interval (antipsychotics, antiarrhythmics); avoid this combination • Increased sedation if combined with alcohol or other sedating drugs • Increased adverse reactions if combined with dopamine agonists; monitor patient carefully • Increased risk of serious adverse effects if taken with MAOIs, reserpine; avoid this combination; at least 20 days should elapse and chorea symptoms should return before switching a patient from these drugs to tetrabenazine

■ Nursing considerations

Assessment

- **History:** Active suicidality, untreated or inadequately treated depression; impaired hepatic function; concurrent use of MAOIs, reserpine; prolonged QT interval; pregnancy, lactation
- **Physical:** T; orientation, affect; R, adventitious sounds; CBC with platelet counts, peripheral blood smear, ECG, LFTs

Interventions

⊗ ***Black box warning*** There is an increased risk of depression and suicidality with drug administration; monitor patient accordingly.

- Tell patient and his family that there is a risk of increased suicidal ideation and increased depression while on this drug. Discuss signs to watch for and tell them whom to notify if these effects occur.
- Establish a baseline of patient's chorea symptoms to evaluate drug's effectiveness and to create guidelines for dosing.
- Inform patient that motor function changes, including Parkinson-like symptoms, and sedation and confusion may occur. Advise patient to avoid driving, operating dangerous machinery, or making important decisions until the effects of the drug on the patient are known.
- Advise the use of contraceptive measures while on this drug.
- Encourage nursing mothers to find a different method of feeding the baby while on this drug.

Teaching points

- Take this drug once a day in the morning initially. Your dosage will be adjusted over time to determine the dosage that is most effective for you; when your maintenance dosage is determined, you may need to take the drug two to three times a day.
- Be aware that this drug may increase signs and symptoms of depression and may lead to thoughts of suicide. You and a significant other should be aware of these signs (withdrawal, irritability, inability to sleep, aggression, anxiety) and should report them to your health care provider immediately if they occur.
- Always tell your health care provider about other drugs or alternative therapies that you might be using or that you might stop using. This drug can be affected by many other drugs, and your dosage may need to be adjusted.
- It is not known whether this drug affects an unborn baby. If you wish to become pregnant, discuss this wish with your health care provider. If you should become pregnant while taking this drug, consult with your health care provider.
- It is not known how this drug affects a nursing baby. Because of the potential for adverse effects to the infant, another method of feeding the baby should be used while you are on this drug.
- Be aware that alcohol or use of any other CNS depressants, such as sleeping aids, may

increase the sedative effects of this drug; avoid these combinations.

- You may experience these side effects: Sedation, drowsiness, changes in level of alertness (do not drive a car or operate dangerous machinery and do not make important decisions until you know how this drug will affect you); changes in motor function with tremors, Parkinson-like symptoms. (This is an effect of the drug; if it becomes too uncomfortable, discuss this problem with your health care provider; your dosage may need to be adjusted.)
- Report tremors, restlessness, thoughts of suicide, increased depression, inability to stay alert, sudden behavioral changes.

tetracycline hydrochloride

(tet ra sye' kleen)

Apo-Tetra (CAN), Nu-Tetra (CAN), Sumycin

PREGNANCY CATEGORY D

Drug classes

Antibiotic
Tetracycline

Therapeutic actions

Bacteriostatic: Inhibits protein synthesis of susceptible bacteria, preventing cell replication.

Indications

Systemic administration

- Infections caused by rickettsiae; *Mycoplasma pneumoniae;* agents of psittacosis, ornithosis, lymphogranuloma venereum and granuloma inguinale; *Borrelia recurrentis, Haemophilus ducreyi, Yersinia pestis, Yersinia tularensis, Bartonella bacilliformis, Bacteroides, Vibrio cholerae, Campylobacter fetus, Brucella, Escherichia coli, Enterobacter aerogenes, Shigella, Acinetobacter calcoaceticus, Haemophilus influenzae, Klebsiella,* trachoma
- When penicillin is contraindicated, infections caused by *Neisseria gonorrhoeae, Treponema pallidum, Treponema pertenue, Listeria monocytogenes, Clostridium, Bacillus anthracis, Fusobacterium fusiforme, Actinomyces*
- Adjunct to amebicides in acute intestinal amebiasis
- Uncomplicated urethral, endocervical, or rectal infections in adults caused by *Chlamydia trachomatis*
- Adjunctive therapy for severe acne

Contraindications and cautions

Systemic administration and dermatologic solution

- Contraindicated with allergy to any of the tetracyclines, pregnancy (toxic to the fetus), lactation (causes damage to the teeth of infant).
- Use cautiously with hepatic or renal impairment.

Available forms

Capsules—250, 500 mg; oral suspension—125 mg/5 mL

Dosages

Adults

Systemic administration

1–2 g/day PO in two to four equal doses. Up to 500 mg PO qid.

- *Brucellosis:* 500 mg PO qid for 3 wk with 1 g streptomycin bid IM the first wk and daily the second wk.
- *Syphilis:* 30–40 g PO in divided doses over 10–15 days (*Sumycin*); 500 mg PO qid for 15–30 days (all others).
- *Uncomplicated gonorrhea:* 500 mg every 6 hr PO for 7 days.
- *Gonococcal urethritis:* 500 mg every 4–6 hr for 4–6 days.
- *Uncomplicated urethral, endocervical, or rectal infections with chlamydia trachomatis:* 500 mg qid PO for at least 7 days.
- *Severe acne:* 1 g/day PO in divided doses; then 125–500 mg/day.

Pediatric patients older than 8 yr

Oral

25–50 mg/kg/day PO in four equal doses.

Pharmacokinetics

Route	Onset	Peak
Oral	Varies	2–4 hr

Topical: No general systemic absorption.

Metabolism: $T_{1/2}$: 6–12 hr
Distribution: Crosses placenta; enters breast milk
Excretion: Feces, urine

Adverse effects

Systemic administration

- **Dermatologic:** *Phototoxic reactions, rash,* exfoliative dermatitis
- **GI:** *Discoloring and inadequate calcification of primary teeth of fetus if used by pregnant women, discoloring and inadequate calcification of permanent teeth if used during period of dental development,* fatty liver, liver failure, *anorexia, nausea, vomiting, diarrhea, glossitis, dysphagia,* enterocolitis, esophageal ulcers, esophagitis
- **Hematologic:** Hemolytic anemia, thrombocytopenia, neutropenia, eosinophilia, leukocytosis, leukopenia
- **Hypersensitivity:** Reactions from urticaria to **anaphylaxis,** including intracranial hypertension
- **Other:** *Superinfections,* local irritation at parenteral injection sites

Interactions

✱ **Drug-drug** • Decreased absorption with calcium salts, magnesium salts, zinc salts, aluminum salts, bismuth salts, iron, urinary alkalinizers, food, dairy products, charcoal • Increased digoxin toxicity • Increased nephrotoxicity with methoxyflurane • Decreased effectiveness of hormonal contraceptives, although rare, has been reported with a risk of breakthrough bleeding or pregnancy • Decreased activity of penicillins

■ Nursing considerations

Assessment

- **History:** Systemic administration and dermatologic solution: Allergy to any of the tetracyclines; hepatic or renal impairment; pregnancy, lactation
- **Physical:** Systemic administration, topical dermatologic solution: Site of infection, skin color, lesions; R, adventitious sounds; bowel sounds, output, liver evaluation; urinalysis, BUN, LFTs, renal function tests. Dermatologic ointment: Site of infection

Interventions

- Administer oral medication on an empty stomach, 1 hr before or 2–3 hr after meals. Do not give with antacids. If antacids must be used, give them 3 hr after the dose of tetracycline.
- Culture infection before beginning drug therapy; many resistant strains have been identified.
- Do not administer during pregnancy; drug is toxic to the fetus.

⊗ ***Warning*** Do not use outdated drugs; degraded drug is highly nephrotoxic and should not be used.

- Arrange for regular renal function tests with long-term therapy.

Teaching points

- Take the drug throughout the day for best results. The drug should be taken on an empty stomach, 1 hour before or 2–3 hours after meals, with a full glass of water. Do not take the drug with food, dairy products, iron preparations, or antacids.
- Finish your complete prescription; if any is left, discard it immediately. Never take an outdated tetracycline product.
- There have been reports of pregnancy occurring when taking tetracycline with hormonal contraceptives. To be certain of avoiding pregnancy, use an additional type of contraceptive.
- This drug should not be used during pregnancy; using barrier contraceptives is advised.
- You may experience these side effects: Stomach upset, nausea (reversible); superinfections in the mouth, vagina (frequent washing may help this problem; if severe, request medication); sensitivity of the skin to sunlight (use protective clothing and sunscreen).
- Report severe cramps, watery diarrhea, rash or itching, difficulty breathing, dark urine or light-colored stools, yellowing of the skin or eyes.

▽ tetrahydrozoline hydrochloride

*(tet rah hi **draz'** oh leen)*

Tyzine, Tyzine Pediatric

OTC ophthalmic preparation: Geneye, Geneye Extra, Murine Plus, Optigene 3

PREGNANCY CATEGORY C

Drug classes
Alpha agonist
Nasal decongestant
Ophthalmic decongestant
Ophthalmic vasoconstrictor and mydriatic

Therapeutic actions
Acts directly on alpha receptors to produce vasoconstriction of arterioles in nasal passages, which produces a decongestant response; no effect on beta receptors; dilates pupils; increases flow of aqueous humor, vasoconstricts in eyes.

Indications
- Topical: Symptomatic relief of nasal and nasopharyngeal mucosal congestion due to the common cold, hay fever, or other respiratory allergies
- Ophthalmic: Temporary relief of redness, burning, and irritation due to dryness of the eye or discomfort due to minor irritations or to exposure to wind or sun

Contraindications and cautions
- Contraindicated with allergy to tetrahydrozoline, angle-closure glaucoma, anesthesia with cyclopropane or halothane, thyrotoxicosis, diabetes, hypertension, CV disorders, women in labor whose BP exceeds 130/80 mm Hg, concurrent MAOI use.
- Use cautiously with angina, arrhythmias, prostatic hypertrophy, unstable vasomotor syndrome, lactation.

Available forms
Nasal solution—0.05%, 0.1%; nasal spray—0.1%; ophthalmic solution—0.05%, 0.1%

Dosages
Adults
Nasal
2–4 drops of 0.1% solution in each nostril three to four times/day; *or* 3–4 sprays in each nostril every 4 hr as needed.
Ophthalmic
Instill 1–2 drops into eye or eyes up to four times/day.
Pediatric patients
Nasal
2–6 yr: 2–3 drops of 0.05% solution in each nostril every 4–6 hr as needed, but not more frequently than every 3 hr.
6 yr and older: Use adult dosage.
Ophthalmic
Safety and efficacy not established.

Pharmacokinetics

Route	*Onset*	*Duration*
Nasal	5–10 min	6–10 hr
Ophthalmic: No general systemic absorption.		

Metabolism: Hepatic; $T_{1/2}$: Unknown
Distribution: Crosses placenta; may enter breast milk
Excretion: Urine

Adverse effects
- **CNS:** *Fear, anxiety, tenseness, restlessness, headache, light-headedness, dizziness,* drowsiness, tremor, insomnia, hallucinations, psychological disturbances, seizures, CNS depression, weakness, blurred vision, ocular irritation, tearing, photophobia
- **CV:** Arrhythmias, hypertension resulting in intracranial hemorrhage, **CV collapse with hypotension,** palpitations, tachycardia, precordial pain in patients with ischemic heart disease
- **GI:** *Nausea,* vomiting, anorexia
- **GU:** Constriction of renal blood vessels, *dysuria, vesical sphincter spasm,* resulting in difficult and painful urination, urinary retention in males with prostatism
- **Local:** *Rebound congestion* with topical nasal application, burning, stinging, sneezing, dryness
- **Other:** *Pallor,* respiratory difficulty, orofacial dystonia, sweating

Interactions

✱ **Drug-drug** • Severe hypertension when taken with MAOIs, TCAs, furazolidone • Additive effects increase risk of toxicity with urinary alkalinizers • Decreased vasopressor response with reserpine, methyldopa, urinary acidifiers • Decreased hypotensive action of guanethidine

■ Nursing considerations

Assessment

- **History:** Allergy to tetrahydrozoline; narrow-angle glaucoma; anesthesia with cyclopropane or halothane; thyrotoxicosis, diabetes, hypertension, CV disorders; prostatic hypertrophy, unstable vasomotor syndrome; lactation; pregnancy
- **Physical:** Skin color, T; orientation, reflexes, peripheral sensation, vision; P, BP, auscultation, peripheral perfusion; R, adventitious sounds; urinary output pattern, bladder percussion, prostate palpation; nasal mucous membrane evaluation

Interventions

- Do not administer ophthalmic solution if it is cloudy or changes color.

⊗ ***Warning*** Monitor CV effects carefully; patients with hypertension who take this drug may experience changes in BP because of the additional vasoconstriction. If an oral nasal decongestant is needed, pseudoephedrine is the drug of choice.

Teaching points

- Do not exceed recommended dose. Demonstrate proper administration technique for topical nasal application and administration of eye drops. Remove contact lenses before using eyedrops. Avoid prolonged use because underlying medical problems can be disguised.
- Rebound congestion may occur when this drug is stopped; drink plenty of fluids, use a humidifier, avoid smoke-filled areas, limit use to 72 hours.
- You may experience these side effects: Dizziness, weakness, restlessness, light-headedness, tremor (avoid driving or operating dangerous equipment); urinary retention (empty bladder before taking drug).
- Report nervousness, palpitations, sleeplessness, sweating, blurred vision.

▽thalidomide

See Appendix W, *Less commonly used drugs.*

▽theophylline

(thee off' i lin)

Immediate-release capsules, tablets: Elixophyllin, Slo-Phyllin

Timed-release capsules: Theo-24 DNC

Timed-release tablets: Theochron DNC, Uniphyl DNC

PREGNANCY CATEGORY C

Drug classes

Bronchodilator
Xanthine

Therapeutic actions

Relaxes bronchial smooth muscle, causing bronchodilation and increasing vital capacity that has been impaired by bronchospasm and air trapping; actions may be mediated by inhibition of phosphodiesterase, which increases the concentration of cyclic adenosine monophosphate; in concentrations that may be higher than those reached clinically, it also inhibits the release of slow-reacting substance of anaphylaxis and histamine.

Indications

- Symptomatic relief or prevention of bronchial asthma and reversible bronchospasm associated with chronic bronchitis and emphysema
- Unlabeled use of 2 mg/kg/day to maintain serum concentrations between 3 and 5 mcg/mL: Treatment of apnea and bradycardia of prematurity

Contraindications and cautions

- Contraindicated with hypersensitivity to any xanthines, peptic ulcer, active gastritis, pregnancy (neonatal tachycardia, jitteriness, and withdrawal apnea), underlying seizure disorders (unless receiving appropriate antiepileptic).

T

- Use cautiously with cardiac arrhythmias, acute myocardial injury, HF, cor pulmonale, severe hypertension, severe hypoxemia, renal or hepatic disease, hyperthyroidism, alcoholism, labor (may inhibit uterine contractions), lactation, status asthmaticus.

Available forms

CR tablets DNC—400, 450, 600 mg; ER capsules DNC—100, 125, 200, 300, 400, 450 mg; elixir—80 mg/15 mL; injection—0.8, 1.6, 2, 3.2, 4 mg/mL

Dosages

Maintain serum levels in the therapeutic range of 10–15 mcg/mL; base dosage on lean body mass.

Anhydrous Theophylline Content in Theophylline Derivatives (these products are more water soluble than anhydrous theophylline)

Drug	*Anhydrous Theophylline Content*
aminophylline anhydrous	85.7%
aminophylline hydrous	78.9%
theophylline monohydrate	90.7%

Adults and children weighing more than 45 kg without risk of impaired excretion

- *Elixophyllin:* Initially, 300 mg/day PO in divided doses every 6–8 hr. After 3 days, may be increased to 400 mg/day PO in divided doses every 6–8 hr. After 3 more days may be increased to 600 mg/day PO in divided doses every 6–8 hr if tolerated and needed.
- *ER capsule:* Initially, 300 mg/day PO in divided doses every 8–12 hr. After 3 days, may be increased to 400 mg/day PO in divided doses every 8–12 hr. After 3 more days, may be increased to 600 mg/day PO in divided doses every 8–12 hr if tolerated and needed.
- *Theo-24, Uniphyl:* Initially, 300–400 mg/day PO once every 24 hr. After 3 days, may be increased to 400–600 mg/day PO once every 24 hr. After 3 more days, may be increased based on theophylline level to stay within safe range.

Adults and children with risk factors for impaired clearance, geriatric patients, patients for whom monitoring serum theophylline levels is not feasible

- *Elixophyllin: Children 1–15 yr:* Final dose should not exceed 16 mg/kg/day up to a maximum 400 mg/day. *Patients 16 yr and older and geriatric patients:* Final dose should not exceed 400 mg/day.
- *Theo-24, Uniphyl: Children 12–15 yr:* Final dose should not exceed 16 mg/kg/day up to a maximum 400 mg/day. *Patients older than 16 yr and geriatric patients:* Final dose should not exceed 400 mg/day.

Adults

Parenteral

Check serum levels after 24 hr when changing IV doses.

- *Nonsmokers ages 16–60 yr:* 0.4 mg/kg/hr.
- *Patients with HF, liver function impairment, sepsis, organ failure:* 0.2 mg/kg/hr IV.
- *Geriatric patients:* 0.3 mg/kg/hr IV.
- *Dosage adjustment based on serum theophylline levels during long-term therapy:* Serum theophylline levels less than 10 mcg/mL are too low, levels of 10–15 mcg/mL are within normal limits, and levels greater than 20 mcg/mL are too high.
  Serum theophylline level 5–10 mcg/mL: Increase dose by about 25% at 3-day intervals until desired response or serum level occurs.
  Serum theophylline level 10–20 mcg/mL: Maintain dosage; recheck at 6- to 12-mo intervals.
  Serum theophylline level 20–25 mcg/mL: Decrease dose by about 25%; recheck level in 3 days.
  Serum theophylline level 25–30 mcg/mL: Skip next dose, and decrease subsequent doses by 25%; recheck level after 3 days.
  Serum theophylline level greater than 30 mcg/mL: Skip next two doses and decrease later doses by 50%. Recheck level after 3 days.
- *Measurement of serum theophylline levels during chronic therapy:* Measure serum theophylline in blood sample drawn 1–2 hr after administration of immediate-release

preparations, 5–9 hr after administration of most timed-release products.

Pediatric patients

Oral

Premature infants younger than 24 days: 1 mg/kg PO every 12 hr.

Premature infants 24 days and older: 1.5 mg/kg PO every 12 hr.

Full-term infants and infants up to 26 wk: Total dose in mg = [(0.2 × age in weeks) + 5] × body weight in kilograms, divided into three equal doses every 8 hr.

Infants 26 wk and older: Total dose in mg = [(0.2 × age in weeks) + 5] × body weight in kilograms, divided into four equal doses every 6 hr.

Parenteral

Neonates 24 days and younger: 1 mg/kg every 12 hr.

Neonates older than 24 days: 1.5 mg/kg every 12 hr.

Infants: mg/hr = 0.008 × age in weeks + 0.21.

Children 1–9 yr: 0.8 mg/kg/hr.

Children 9–12 yr: 0.7 mg/kg/hr.

Children 12–16 yr who smoke cigarettes or marijuana: 0.7 mg/kg/hr.

Children 12–16 yr who are nonsmokers: 0.5 mg/kg/hr.

Pediatric patients weighing less than 45 kg without risk of impaired clearance

Elixophyllin: Initially, 12–14 mg/kg/day PO up to a maximum 300 mg/day PO in divided doses every 4–6 hr. After 3 days, may be increased to 16 mg/kg/day PO up to a maximum 400 mg/day PO in divided doses every 4–6 hr. After 3 more days, may be increased to 20 mg/kg/day PO up to a maximum 600 mg/day PO in divided doses every 4–6 hr if tolerated and needed.

ER capsule: Initially, 12–14 mg/kg/day PO up to a maximum 300 mg/day PO in divided doses every 8–12 hr. After 3 days, may be increased to 16 mg/kg/day PO up to a maximum 400 mg/day PO in divided doses every 8–12 hr. After 3 more days, may be increased to 20 mg/kg/day PO up to a maximum 600 mg/day PO in divided doses every 8–12 hr if tolerated and needed.

Theo-24, Uniphyl: Initially, 12–14 mg/kg/day PO up to a maximum 300 mg/day PO once every 24 hr. After 3 days, may be increased to 16 mg/kg/day PO up to a maximum 400 mg/day PO once every 24 hr. After 3 more days, may be increased to 20 mg/kg/day PO up to a maximum 600 mg/day PO once every 24 hr if tolerated and needed.

Pharmacokinetics

Route	Onset	Peak
Oral	Varies	2 hr
IV	Immediate	End of infusion

Metabolism: Hepatic; $T_{1/2}$: 3–15 hr (nonsmokers) or 4–5 hr (smokers)

Distribution: Crosses placenta; enters breast milk

Excretion: Urine

IV FACTS

Preparation: Prepare using sterile technique. Drug provided in 5% dextrose solution. Store at room temperature.

Infusion: Titrate based on patient response. Do not exceed 17 mg/hr. Monitor serum concentration.

Incompatibilities: Do not add any other drugs to solution.

Adverse effects

- **CNS:** *Irritability (especially children), restlessness,* dizziness, headache, seizures, muscle twitching, severe depression, stammering speech, abnormal behavior characterized by withdrawal, mutism, and unresponsiveness alternating with hyperactive periods
- **CV:** Palpitations, sinus tachycardia, ventricular tachycardia, **life-threatening ventricular arrhythmias,** circulatory failure
- **GI:** *Loss of appetite,* hematemesis, epigastric pain, gastroesophageal reflux during sleep
- **GU:** Proteinuria, increased excretion of renal tubular cells and RBCs; diuresis (dehydration), urinary retention in men with prostate enlargement
- **Respiratory:** Tachypnea, **respiratory arrest**
- **Serum theophylline levels less than 20 mcg/mL:** 20 mcg/mL: Adverse effects uncommon

T

- **Serum theophylline levels greater than 20–25 mcg/mL:** *Nausea, vomiting, diarrhea, headache, insomnia, irritability* (75% of patients)
- **Serum theophylline levels greater than 35 mcg/mL:** Hyperglycemia, hypotension, cardiac arrhythmias, tachycardia (greater than 10 mcg/mL in premature newborns); seizures, brain damage, **death**
- **Other:** Fever, flushing, hyperglycemia, SIADH, rash, increased AST

Interactions

✱ **Drug-drug** • Increased effects and toxicity with cimetidine, erythromycin, troleandomycin, ciprofloxacin, norfloxacin, ofloxacin, hormonal contraceptives, ticlopidine, ranitidine • Possibly decreased effects with rifampin • Increased serum levels and risk of toxicity in hypothyroid patients, decreased levels in patients who are hyperthyroid; monitor patients on thioamides, thyroid hormones for changes in serum levels as patients become euthyroid • Increased cardiac toxicity with halothane • Decreased effects in patients who are cigarette smokers (1–2 packs/day); theophylline dosage may need to be increased 50%–100% • Decreased effects with barbiturates, charcoal • Decreased effects of phenytoins, benzodiazepines, and theophylline preparations • Decreased effects of nondepolarizing neuromuscular blockers • Mutually antagonistic effects of beta blockers and theophylline preparations

✱ **Drug-food** • Theophylline elimination is increased by a low-carbohydrate, high-protein diet and by charcoal-broiled beef • Theophylline elimination is decreased by a high-carbohydrate, low-protein diet • Food may alter bioavailability, absorption of timed-release theophylline preparations; these may rapidly release their contents with food and cause toxicity. Timed-release forms should be taken on an empty stomach

✱ **Drug-lab test** • Interference with spectrophotometric determinations of serum theophylline levels by furosemide, probenecid, theobromine; coffee, tea, cola beverages, chocolate, acetaminophen cause falsely high values • Alteration in assays of uric acid, urinary catecholamines, plasma free fatty acids

✱ **Drug-alternative therapy** • Decreased effectiveness if taken with St. John's wort

■ Nursing considerations

Assessment

- **History:** Hypersensitivity to any xanthines; peptic ulcer, active gastritis; status asthmaticus; cardiac arrhythmias, acute myocardial injury, HF, cor pulmonale; severe hypertension; severe hypoxemia; renal or hepatic disease; hyperthyroidism; pregnancy, lactation
- **Physical:** Skin color, texture, lesions; reflexes, bilateral grip strength, affect; P, auscultation, BP, perfusion; R, adventitious sounds; bowel sounds, normal output; frequency, voiding pattern, normal urinary output; ECG; EEG; LFTs, renal and thyroid function tests

Interventions

- Caution patient not to chew or crush enteric-coated timed-release preparations.
- Give liquid dosage forms in divided doses. Give with food if GI effects occur.
- Do not give timed-release preparations with food; these should be given on an empty stomach, 1 hr before or 2 hr after meals.
- Advise patients that this drug should not be used during pregnancy; using barrier contraceptives is recommended.

⊗ ***Warning*** Monitor results of serum theophylline level determinations carefully, and reduce dosage if serum levels exceed therapeutic range of 10–15 mcg/mL.

- Monitor carefully for clinical signs of adverse effects, particularly if serum theophylline levels are not available.

⊗ ***Warning*** Keep diazepam readily available to treat seizures.

Teaching points

- Take this drug exactly as prescribed. If a timed-release product is prescribed, take it on an empty stomach, 1 hour before or 2 hours after meals. Do not chew or crush timed-release preparations; it may be necessary for you to take this drug around-the-clock for adequate control of asthma attacks.
- Avoid excessive intake of coffee, tea, cocoa, cola beverages, and chocolate. These con-

tain theophylline-related substances that may increase your side effects.
- Smoking cigarettes or other tobacco products may markedly influence the effects of theophylline. It is preferable not to smoke while you are taking this drug. Notify your health care provider if you change your smoking habits while you are taking this drug; it may be necessary to change your drug dosage.
- Have frequent blood tests to monitor drug effects and ensure safe and effective dosage.
- Do not use this drug during pregnancy; using barrier contraceptives is advised.
- You may experience these side effects: Nausea, loss of appetite (take drug with food if taking immediate-release or liquid dosage forms); difficulty sleeping, depression, emotional lability.
- Report nausea, vomiting, severe GI pain, restlessness, seizures, irregular heartbeat.

DANGEROUS DRUG

▽thioguanine (TG, 6-Thioguanine)

*(thye oh **gwah'** neen)*

Lanvis (CAN), Tabloid

PREGNANCY CATEGORY D

Drug classes
Antimetabolite
Antineoplastic

Therapeutic actions
Tumor-inhibiting properties, probably due to interference with a number of steps in the synthesis and use of purine nucleotides, which are normally incorporated into DNA and RNA.

Indications
- Remission induction, consolidation, and maintenance therapy of acute nonlymphocytic leukemias—usually used in combination therapy

Contraindications and cautions
- Contraindicated with allergy to thioguanine, prior resistance to thioguanine or mercaptopurine, hematopoietic depression, pregnancy (potential mutagen and teratogen), lactation.
- Use cautiously with impaired hepatic or renal function.

Available forms
Tablets—40 mg

Dosages
Adults and pediatric patients
Total dose may be given at one time. Initial dosage, 2 mg/kg/day PO daily for 4 wk. If no clinical improvement is seen and there are no toxic effects, increase dose to 3 mg/kg/day. If complete hematologic remission is obtained, institute maintenance therapy. No adjustment of dosage is needed if used as part of combination therapy.

Pharmacokinetics

Route	Onset	Peak
Oral	Slow	8 hr

Metabolism: Hepatic; $T_{1/2}$: 11 hr
Distribution: Crosses placenta; may enter breast milk
Excretion: Urine

Adverse effects
- **GI: Hepatotoxicity,** *nausea, vomiting, anorexia,* diarrhea, stomatitis
- **Hematologic:** *Bone marrow suppression, immunosuppression, hyperuricemia* due to rapid lysis of malignant cells
- **Other:** Fever, weakness, cancer, chromosomal aberrations

■ Nursing considerations
Assessment
- **History:** Allergy to thioguanine, prior resistance to thioguanine; hematopoietic depression; impaired hepatic function; pregnancy, lactation
- **Physical:** Skin color; mucous membranes, liver evaluation, abdominal examination; CBC, differential, Hgb, platelet counts; LFTs; serum uric acid

Interventions
- Evaluate hematopoietic status before and frequently during therapy.

⊗ ***Warning*** Discontinue drug therapy if platelet count is less than 50,000 or polymorphonuclear granulocyte count is less than 1,000; consult physician for dosage adjustment.

⊗ ***Warning*** Arrange for discontinuation of this drug at any sign of hematologic or hepatic toxicity; consult physician.

- Ensure that patient is not pregnant before administration.

⊗ ***Warning*** Ensure that patient is well hydrated before and during therapy to minimize adverse effects of hyperuricemia; allopurinol and drugs to alkalinize the urine are sometimes prescribed.

- Administer as a single daily dose.

Teaching points

- Drink adequate fluids while you are using this drug; drink at least 8–10 glasses of fluid each day.
- This drug may cause miscarriages and birth defects. Both men and women who receive this drug should be using a reliable form of contraception. Discuss with your health care provider how long you should wait to conceive a child after therapy ends.
- Have frequent, regular medical follow-up visits, including frequent blood tests to assess drug effects.
- You may experience these side effects: Mouth sores (use frequent mouth care); nausea, vomiting, loss of appetite (eat frequent small meals); increased susceptibility to infection (avoid crowds and infections).
- Report fever, chills, sore throat, unusual bleeding or bruising, yellow discoloration of the skin or eyes, abdominal pain, flank pain, joint pain, swelling of the feet or legs.

DANGEROUS DRUG

▽thiotepa (triethylenethiophosphoramide, TESPA, TSPA)

*(thye oh **tep'** ah)*

Thioplex

PREGNANCY CATEGORY D

Drug classes

Alkylating drug
Antineoplastic

Therapeutic actions

Cytotoxic: Disrupts the bonds of DNA, causing cell death; cell cycle nonspecific.

Indications

- Treatment of adenocarcinoma of the breast, ovary
- Superficial papillary carcinoma of the urinary bladder
- Controlling intracavity effusions secondary to diffuse or localized neoplastic disease of various serosal cavities
- Treatment of lymphoma, including Hodgkin's lymphoma (no longer a drug of choice)

Contraindications and cautions

- Contraindicated with allergy to thiotepa, hematopoietic depression, pregnancy, lactation.
- Use cautiously with impaired hepatic or renal function, concomitant therapy with other alkylating agents or irradiation.

Available forms

Powder for injection—15, 30 mg

Dosages

Adults

IV

0.3–0.4 mg/kg at 1- to 4-wk intervals.

Intratumor

Drug is diluted in sterile water to a concentration of 10 mg/mL, then 0.6–0.8 mg/kg is injected directly into the tumor after a local anesthetic is injected through the same needle. Maintenance doses of 0.07–0.8 mg/kg every 1–4 wk depending on patient's condition.

Intracavity

0.6–0.8 mg/kg through the same tube that is used to remove fluid from the cavity.

Intravesical

Dehydrate patient with papillary carcinoma of the bladder for 8–12 hr prior to treatment. Then instill 60 mg in 30–60 mL of sodium chloride injection into the bladder by catheter. Retain for 2 hr. If patient is unable to retain

60 mL, give the dose in 30 mL. Repeat once a week for 4 wk.

Pharmacokinetics

Route	*Onset*
IV	Gradual

Metabolism: Hepatic; $T_{1/2}$: 109 min
Distribution: Crosses placenta; may enter breast milk
Excretion: Urine

IV FACTS

Preparation: Reconstitute powder with sterile water for injection. 1.5 mL of diluent gives a drug concentration of 5 mg/0.5 mL of solution. May be further diluted with sodium chloride injection, dextrose injection, dextrose and sodium chloride injection, Ringer's injection, lactated Ringer's injection. Store powder in the refrigerator, reconstituted solution is stable for 8 hr if refrigerated. Sterile water for injection produces an isotonic solution, other diluents may produce a hypertonic solution that may cause mild to moderate discomfort on injection. ⊗ ***Warning*** Check solution before use; solution should be clear to slightly opaque; grossly opaque solutions or solutions with precipitates should not be used.
Infusion: Administer IV dose directly and rapidly, 60 mg over 1 min. There is no need for slow IV drip or the use of large volumes of fluid.

Adverse effects

- **CNS:** *Dizziness,* headache, blurred vision
- **Dermatologic:** Hives, rash, weeping from subcutaneous lesions, contact dermatitis at injection site, alopecia
- **GI:** *Nausea, vomiting,* anorexia
- **GU:** *Amenorrhea, interference with spermatogenesis,* dysuria, urinary retention
- **Hematologic:** *Hematopoietic toxicity*
- **Other:** Febrile reactions, cancer, fatigue

■ Nursing considerations

Assessment

- **History:** Allergy to thiotepa; hematopoietic depression; impaired renal or hepatic function; concomitant therapy with other alkylating agents or irradiation; pregnancy, lactation
- **Physical:** Weight; skin color, lesions; T; orientation, reflexes; CBC, differential; urinalysis; LFTs, renal function tests

Interventions

- Ensure that patient is not pregnant before administration; advise the use of barrier contraceptives.
- Arrange for blood tests to evaluate bone marrow function before therapy, weekly during therapy, and for at least 3 wk after therapy.
- Mix solution with 2% procaine hydrochloride, 1:1,000 epinephrine hydrochloride, or both for local use into single or multiple sites.
- Reduce dosage with renal or hepatic impairment and for bone marrow depression.

Teaching points

- This drug can be given only parenterally. Prepare a calendar of treatment days.
- This drug should not be taken during pregnancy; use birth control while you are being treated with this drug. If you become pregnant, consult your health care provider.
- Have regular medical follow-up visits, including blood tests, to assess drug effects.
- You may experience these side effects: Nausea, vomiting, loss of appetite (request an antiemetic; eat frequent small meals); dizziness, headache (use special safety precautions to prevent falls or injury); amenorrhea in women, change in sperm production.
- Report unusual bleeding or bruising, fever, chills, sore throat, stomach or flank pain, severe nausea and vomiting, skin rash or hives.

T

▽thiothixene (thiothixene hydrochloride)

*(thye oh **thix'** een)*

Navane

PREGNANCY CATEGORY C

Drug classes

Antipsychotic
Dopaminergic blocker
Thioxanthene

Therapeutic actions

Mechanism of action not fully understood: Blocks postsynaptic dopamine receptors in the brain, but this may not be necessary and sufficient for antipsychotic activity.

Indications

- Management of schizophrenia

Contraindications and cautions

- Contraindicated with coma or severe CNS depression, blood dyscrasia, circulatory collapse, subcortical brain damage, Parkinson's disease, liver damage, cerebral arteriosclerosis, coronary disease, severe hypotension or hypertension, pregnancy, lactation.
- Use cautiously with respiratory disorders ("silent pneumonia"); glaucoma, prostatic hypertrophy; epilepsy or history of epilepsy (drug lowers seizure threshold); breast cancer; thyrotoxicosis (severe neurotoxicity); peptic ulcer, decreased renal function; myelography within previous 24 hr or scheduled within 48 hr; exposure to heat or phosphorous insecticides; children younger than 12 yr, especially those with chickenpox, CNS infections (children are especially susceptible to dystonias that may confound the diagnosis of Reye's syndrome).

Available forms

Capsules—1, 2, 5, 10, 20 mg

Dosages

Full clinical effects may require 6 wk–6 mo of therapy.

Adults

Initially, 2 mg PO tid (mild conditions) or 5 mg bid (more severe conditions). Increase dose as needed; the usual optimum dose is 20–30 mg/day. May increase to 60 mg/day, but further increases rarely increase beneficial response.

Pediatric patients

Not recommended for children younger than 12 yr.

Geriatric or debilitated patients

Use lower doses and increase more gradually.

Pharmacokinetics

Route	*Onset*	*Duration*
Oral	Slow	12 hr

Metabolism: Hepatic; $T_{1/2}$: 34 hr
Distribution: Crosses placenta; enters breast milk
Excretion: Bile, feces

Adverse effects

- **Autonomic:** *Dry mouth, salivation, nasal congestion, nausea,* vomiting, anorexia, fever, pallor, flushed facies, sweating, constipation, paralytic ileus, urinary retention, incontinence, polyuria, enuresis, priapism, ejaculation inhibition, male impotence
- **CNS:** *Drowsiness,* insomnia, vertigo, headache, weakness, tremor, ataxia, slurring, cerebral edema, seizures, exacerbation of psychotic symptoms, extrapyramidal syndromes—*pseudoparkinsonism; dystonias; akathisia,* tardive dyskinesias, potentially irreversible NMS; extrapyramidal symptoms, hyperthermia, **autonomic disturbances** (rare, but 20% fatal)
- **CV:** Hypotension, orthostatic hypotension, hypertension, tachycardia, bradycardia, cardiac arrest, HF, cardiomegaly, **refractory arrhythmias** (some fatal), pulmonary edema
- **EENT:** Glaucoma, *photophobia, blurred vision,* miosis, mydriasis, deposits in the cornea and lens (opacities), pigmentary retinopathy
- **Endocrine:** Lactation, breast engorgement, galactorrhea; SIADH; amenorrhea, menstrual irregularities; gynecomastia; changes in libido; hyperglycemia or hypoglycemia; glycosuria; hyponatremia; pituitary tumor with hyperprolactinemia; inhibition of ovulation, infertility, pseudopregnancy; reduced urinary levels of gonadotropins, estrogens, progestins
- **Hematologic:** Eosinophilia, leukopenia, leukocytosis, anemia, **aplastic anemia,** hemolytic anemia, thrombocytopenic or nonthrombocytopenic purpura, pancytopenia
- **Hypersensitivity:** Jaundice, urticaria, angioneurotic edema, laryngeal edema, pho-

tosensitivity, eczema, asthma, anaphylactoid reactions, exfoliative dermatitis

- **Respiratory: Bronchospasm, laryngospasm,** dyspnea, suppression of cough reflex and potential for aspiration
- **Other:** *Urine discolored pink to red-brown*

Interactions

✱ **Drug-drug** • Decreased effects with carbamazepine • Possible increased CNS effects with CNS agents such as alcohol • Risk of decreased blood pressure with antihypertensives

✱ **Drug-lab test** • False-positive pregnancy tests (less likely if serum test is used) • Increase in PBI not attributable to an increase in thyroxine

■ Nursing considerations

CLINICAL ALERT!

Name confusion has been reported between *Navane* (thiothixene) and *Norvasc* (amlodipine). Use caution.

Assessment

- **History:** Severe CNS depression; blood dyscrasia; circulatory collapse; subcortical brain damage; Parkinson's disease; liver damage; cerebral arteriosclerosis; coronary disease, severe hypotension or hypertension; respiratory disorders; glaucoma; prostatic hypertrophy; epilepsy; breast cancer; thyrotoxicosis; peptic ulcer; decreased renal function; myelography within previous 24 hr or scheduled within 48 hr; exposure to heat, phosphorous insecticides; pregnancy, lactation; chickenpox; CNS infections
- **Physical:** Weight, T; reflexes, orientation, IOP; P, BP, orthostatic BP; R, adventitious sounds; bowel sounds and normal output, liver evaluation; urinary output, prostate size; CBC, urinalysis, LFTs, renal and thyroid function tests

Interventions

⊗ ***Black box warning*** Risk of death increases if antipsychotics are used to treat elderly patients with dementia-related psychosis; drug is not approved for this use.

⊗ ***Warning*** Discontinue drug if serum creatinine or BUN becomes abnormal or if WBC count is depressed.

- Monitor elderly patients for dehydration, and institute remedial measures promptly; sedation and decreased sensation of thirst related to CNS effects can lead to severe dehydration.
- Consult physician regarding appropriate warning of patient or patient's guardian about tardive dyskinesias.
- Consult physician about dosage reduction, use of anticholinergic antiparkinsonians (controversial) if extrapyramidal effects occur.

Teaching points

- Take drug exactly as prescribed.
- Avoid driving or engaging in other dangerous activities if drowsiness, tremor, weakness, or vision changes occur.
- Avoid prolonged exposure to sun or use a sunscreen or covering garments.
- Maintain fluid intake, and use precautions against heatstroke in hot weather.
- Report sore throat, fever, unusual bleeding or bruising, rash, weakness, tremors, impaired vision, dark urine (pink or reddish brown urine is to be expected), pale stools, yellowing of the skin or eyes.

▽ thyroid, desiccated

(thye' roid)

Armour Thyroid, Bio-Throid, Nature-Throid, Thyroid USP, Westhroid

PREGNANCY CATEGORY A

Drug class

Thyroid hormone preparation (contains T_3 and T_4 in their natural state and ratio)

Therapeutic actions

Increases the metabolic rate of body tissues, increasing oxygen consumption, respiratory and heart rate; rate of fat, protein, and carbohydrate metabolism; and growth and maturation; exact mechanism of action is not known.

Indications

- Replacement therapy in hypothyroidism
- Treatment of thyroid cancer
- Treatment or prevention of various types of euthyroid goiters
- Treatment of thyrotoxicosis with antithyroid drugs to prevent goitrogenesis and hypothyroidism and thyrotoxicosis during pregnancy
- Diagnostic use in suppression tests

Contraindications and cautions

- Contraindicated with allergy to active or extraneous constituents of drug; thyrotoxicosis and acute MI uncomplicated by hypothyroidism.
- Use cautiously with Addison's disease (treatment of hypoadrenalism with corticosteroids should precede thyroid therapy), pregnancy, lactation, myxedema, allergy to pork products, CV disease.

Available forms

Capsules—7.5, 15, 30, 60, 90, 120, 150, 180, 240 mg; tablets—15, 16.25, 30, 32.4, 32.5, 60, 64.8, 65, 90, 120, 129.6, 130, 180, 194.4, 195, 240, 300 mg

Dosages

Adults

- *Hypothyroidism:* Initially, 30 mg/day PO, increased by 15 mg/day every 2–3 wk. Usual maintenance dose is 60–120 mg PO daily.

Geriatric patients or patients with heart disease or longstanding hypothyroidism

Initially, 15 mg/day.

Pediatric patients

15 mg PO daily. May increase dosage at 2-wk intervals.

0–6 mo: 7.5–30 mg/day PO.
6–12 mo: 30–45 mg/day PO.
1–5 yr: 45–60 mg/day PO.
6–12 yr: 60–90 mg/day PO.
Older than 12 yr: 90 mg/day PO.

Pharmacokinetics

Route	Onset	Peak
Oral	Varies	4 hr

Metabolism: Liver, kidney, and tissue; $T_{1/2}$: 1–2 days (T_{13}), 6–7 days (T_4)

Distribution: Does not readily cross placenta; minimally enters breast milk

Excretion: Feces, urine

Adverse effects

All adverse effects are rare at therapeutic doses.

- **Dermatologic:** Partial loss of hair in first few months of therapy in children
- **Endocrine:** Hyperthyroidism (palpitations, elevated pulse pressure, tachycardia, arrhythmias, angina pectoris, cardiac arrest; tremors, headache, nervousness, insomnia; nausea, diarrhea, changes in appetite; weight loss, menstrual irregularities, sweating, heat intolerance, fever)
- **Hypersensitivity:** Allergic skin reactions

Interactions

✱ **Drug-drug** • Decreased absorption with cholestyramine and antacids; give 4 hr apart from thyroid • Increased risk of bleeding with warfarin • Decreased effectiveness of cardiac glycosides with thyroid replacement • Alterations in theophylline clearance occur in hypothyroid patients; if thyroid state changes during therapy, monitor patient carefully • Possible decreased effects with estrogen products

■ Nursing considerations

Assessment

- **History:** Allergy to active or extraneous constituents of drug or bovine or porcine products; thyrotoxicosis; acute MI uncomplicated by hypothyroidism; Addison's disease; lactation
- **Physical:** Skin lesions, color, T, texture; T; muscle tone, orientation, reflexes; P, auscultation, baseline ECG, BP; R, adventitious sounds; thyroid function tests

Interventions

- Monitor response carefully when beginning therapy, and adjust dosage accordingly.
- Administer as a single daily dose before breakfast with a full glass of water.
- Arrange for regular, periodic blood tests of thyroid function.
- Monitor cardiac response throughout therapy. Reduce dose if angina occurs.

Teaching points

- Take as a single dose before breakfast with a full glass of water.
- This drug replaces a very important hormone and will need to be taken for life. Do not discontinue this drug without consulting your health care provider; serious problems can occur.
- Wear or carry a medical alert tag to alert emergency medical personnel that you are using this drug.
- Nausea and diarrhea may occur (dividing the dose may help).
- Have periodic blood tests and medical evaluations while you are using this drug. Keep your scheduled appointments.
- Report headache, chest pain, palpitations, fever, weight loss, sleeplessness, nervousness, irritability, unusual sweating, intolerance to heat, diarrhea.

▽tiagabine hydrochloride

(tye ag' ah bine)

Gabitril Filmtabs

PREGNANCY CATEGORY C

Drug class

Antiepileptic

Therapeutic actions

Increases GABA levels in the brain, which may result in antiseizure effects. GABA is the major inhibitory neurotransmitter in the CNS; tiagabine binds to GABA reuptake sites, preventing its reuptake, and increases levels in the presynaptic neurons and the glia.

Indications

- Adjunctive therapy in patients older than 12 yr with partial seizures

Contraindications and cautions

- Contraindicated with hypersensitivity to tiagabine, hepatic disease or significant hepatic impairment.
- Use cautiously with pregnancy, lactation, and the elderly.

Available forms

Tablets—2, 4, 12, 16 mg

Dosages

Adults

4 mg PO daily for 1 wk; may be increased by 4–8 mg/wk until desired response is seen; maximum dose, 56 mg/day in two to four divided doses. Usual maintenance dose is 32–56 mg daily.

Pediatric patients 12–18 yr

4 mg PO daily for 1 wk; may be increased to 8 mg/day in two divided doses for 1 wk; then increased by 4–8 mg/wk up to a maximum of 32 mg/day in two to four divided doses.

Pediatric patients younger than 12 yr

Not recommended.

Pharmacokinetics

Route	*Onset*	*Peak*
Oral	Rapid	30–60 min

Metabolism: Hepatic; $T_{1/2}$: 7–9 hr
Distribution: Crosses placenta; may enter breast milk
Excretion: Feces, urine

Adverse effects

- **CNS:** *Dizziness, asthenia, somnolence,* nervousness, tremor, concentration difficulties
- **Dermatologic: Serious rash**
- **EENT:** Possible long-term ophthalmic effects
- **GI:** *GI upset, pain, nausea*
- **GU:** Irregular menses, secondary amenorrhea, dysuria, incontinence

Interactions

✱ **Drug-drug** • Decreased serum levels with carbamazepine, phenytoin, primidone; phenobarbital, adjustment in tiagabine dosage may be needed • Possible interaction with valproate; monitor patient closely • Increased CNS depression if combined with other CNS depressants (alcohol, hypnotics)

■ Nursing considerations

Assessment

- **History:** Hypersensitivity to tiagabine; hepatic disease or significant hepatic impairment; pregnancy, lactation

T

- **Physical:** Weight; skin color, lesions; orientation, eye examination, affect, reflexes; LFTs

Interventions

⊗ ***Black box warning*** Risk of suicidal ideation is increased; monitor patient accordingly.

- Give drug with food.
- Reduce dosage and adjust more slowly if patient is not on concomitant phenytoin, phenobarbital, or carbamazepine.
- Provide frequent skin care if dermatologic effects occur.

⊗ ***Warning*** Avoid abrupt discontinuation; serious side effects could occur.

- Establish safety precautions (use side rails, accompany patient) if CNS changes occur.
- Arrange for appropriate counseling for women of childbearing age who wish to become pregnant.

Teaching points

- Take this drug exactly as prescribed. If you miss a dose, take it as soon as you remember; do not double doses.
- Do not discontinue this drug abruptly or change dosage, except on the advice of your health care provider.
- Avoid the use of alcohol and sleep-inducing or over-the-counter drugs while you are using this drug; these preparations could cause dangerous effects. If you feel that you need one of these preparations, consult your health care provider.
- Use contraceptives at all times. If you want to become pregnant while you are taking this drug, consult your health care provider.
- Wear a medical alert bracelet at all times so that any emergency medical personnel will know that you have epilepsy and are taking antiepileptic medication.
- You may experience these side effects: Drowsiness (avoid driving or performing other tasks requiring alertness); GI upset (take the drug with food or milk; eat frequent small meals).
- Report bruising, yellowing of the skin or eyes, pale-colored feces, rash, pregnancy, vision changes, thoughts of suicide.

▽ticlopidine hydrochloride

*(tye **kloh'** pih deen)*

Apo-ticlopidine (CAN), Gen-Ticlopidine (CAN), Nu-Ticlopidine (CAN), Ticlid

PREGNANCY CATEGORY B

Drug class

Antiplatelet

Therapeutic actions

Interferes with platelet membrane function by inhibiting fibrinogen binding and platelet-platelet interactions; inhibits platelet aggregation and prolongs bleeding time; effect is irreversible for life of the platelet.

Indications

- Reduces risk of thrombotic CVA in patients who have experienced CVA precursors and in patients who have had a completed thrombotic CVA; reserve use for patients who are intolerant to aspirin therapy because side effects may be life-threatening
- Prevention of acute stent thrombosis in coronary arteries; used with antiplatelet doses of aspirin
- Unlabeled uses: Intermittent claudication, chronic arterial occlusion, subarachnoid hemorrhage, uremic patients with AV shunts or fistulas, open-heart surgery, coronary artery bypass grafts, primary glomerulonephritis, sickle cell disease

Contraindications and cautions

- Contraindicated with allergy to ticlopidine, neutropenia, thrombocytopenia, history of thrombotic thrombocytopenic purpura (TTP), hemostatic disorders, bleeding ulcer, intracranial bleeding, severe liver disease, lactation.
- Use cautiously with renal disorders, pregnancy, elevated cholesterol, recent trauma.

Available forms

Tablets—250 mg

Dosages
Adults
250 mg PO bid with food.
Pediatric patients
Safety and efficacy not established for patients younger than 18 yr.

Pharmacokinetics

Route	*Onset*	*Peak*
Oral	Rapid	2 hr

Metabolism: Hepatic; $T_{1/2}$: 12.6 hr, then 4–5 days
Distribution: Crosses placenta; enters breast milk
Excretion: Feces, urine

Adverse effects
- **CNS:** Dizziness
- **GI:** *Diarrhea, nausea, vomiting, abdominal pain,* flatulence, dyspepsia, anorexia
- **Hematologic: Neutropenia, TTP,** bleeding
- **Local:** *Pain, phlebitis,* thrombosis at injection site
- **Other:** Rash, purpura

Interactions
✱ **Drug-drug** • Decreased effectiveness of digoxin • Increased serum levels and effects of theophylline, aspirin, NSAIDs • Increased effects with cimetidine • Decreased absorption with antacids
✱ **Drug-food** • Increased availability with food

■ Nursing considerations
Assessment
- **History:** Allergy to ticlopidine; neutropenia, thrombocytopenia; hemostatic disorders; bleeding ulcer, intracranial bleeding; severe liver disease; renal disorders; pregnancy, lactation, elevated cholesterol; recent trauma
- **Physical:** Skin color, lesions; orientation; bowel sounds, normal output; CBC, LFTs, renal function tests, serum cholesterol

Interventions
⊠ ***Black box warning*** Monitor WBC count before use and frequently while initiating therapy; if neutropenia is present or occurs, discontinue drug immediately.

- Administer with food or just after eating to minimize GI irritation and increase absorption.
- Monitor patient for any sign of excessive bleeding (eg, bruises, dark stools), and monitor bleeding times.
- Provide increased precautions against bleeding during invasive procedures; bleeding will be prolonged.

⊗ ***Warning*** Mark chart of patient receiving drug to alert medical personnel of increased risk of bleeding in cases of surgery or dental surgery.

Teaching points
- Take drug with meals or just after eating.
- You will need regular blood tests to monitor your response to this drug.
- It may take longer than normal to stop bleeding; avoid contact sports, use electrical razors; apply pressure for extended periods to bleeding sites.
- Notify dentist or surgeon that you are using this drug before invasive procedures.
- You may experience these side effects: Upset stomach, nausea, diarrhea, loss of appetite (eat frequent small meals).
- Report fever, chills, sore throat, rash, bruising, bleeding, dark stools or urine.

▽ tigecycline
*(tye gah **sigh'** klin)*

Tygacil

PREGNANCY CATEGORY D

Drug classes
Antibiotic
Glycylcycline

Therapeutic actions
Inhibits protein translation on ribosomes in specific bacteria, leading to inhibition of bacterial cell growth and cell death; mechanism is not used by many resistant strains.

Indications
- Treatment of complicated skin and skin structure infections caused by susceptible strains of *Escherichia coli, Enterococcus*

faecalis (vancomycin-susceptible strains only), *Staphylococcus aureus* (methicillin-susceptible and resistant strains), *Streptococcus agalactiae, Streptococcus anginosus, Streptococcus pyogenes, Bacteroides fragilis, Klebsiella pneumoniae, Enterobacter cloacae*
- Treatment of adults with community-acquired pneumonia
- Treatment of intra-abdominal infections caused by *Citrobacter freundii, Enterobacter cloacae, E. coli, Klebsiella oxytoca, Klebiella pneumoniae, Enteroccus faecalis* (vancomycin susceptible strains only), *S. anginosus, B. fragilis, Bacteroides thetaiotaomicron, Bacteroides uniformis, Bacteroides vulgatus, Clostridium perfringens, Peptostreptococcus micros*

Contraindications and cautions
- Contraindicated with hypersensitivity to tigecycline or any of its components, pregnancy.
- Use cautiously with allergy to tetracycline antibiotics, lactation.

Available forms
Powder for reconstitution for injection—50 mg/5 mL vial

Dosages
Adults
100 mg IV, followed by 50 mg IV every 12 hr. *Tygacil* should be infused over 30–60 min. Therapy should continue for 5–14 days, based on patient response and bacterial progress.
- *Severe hepatic impairment (Child-Pugh C):* 100 mg IV, followed by 25 mg IV every 12 hr. Patient should be monitored closely.

Pharmacokinetics

Route	Onset	Peak
IV	Rapid	End of infusion

Metabolism: Minimal metabolism: $T_{1/2}$: 27–42 hr
Distribution: May cross placenta; may pass into breast milk
Excretion: Feces, urine

IV FACTS
Preparation: Reconstitute with 5.3 mL 0.9% sodium chloride or 5% dextrose to yield 10 mg/mL. Gently swirl vial until drug dissolves, withdraw 5 mL of solution and immediately add to 100 mL IV bag for infusion. Reconstituted solution should be orange to yellow in color. Solution should be clear with no particulate matter. If particulate matter or discoloration (green to black) is seen, discard solution. Reconstituted solution is stable for up to 6 hr at room temperature, 24 hr if refrigerated, or up to 48 hr if refrigerated in IV bag.
Infusion: Infuse over 30–60 min; flush the tubing of any running IV with 0.9% sodium chloride injection or 5% dextrose injection before and after infusing *Tygacil.*
Y-site incompatibilities: Amphotericin B, chlorpromazine, methyprednisolone, voriconazole, diazepam.
Y-site compatibilities: Dobutamine, dopamine, lactated Ringer's solution, lidocaine, potassium chloride, ranitidine, theophylline, morphine.

Adverse effects
- **CNS:** Dizziness, insomnia, *headache*
- **CV:** Hypotension, hypertension, phlebitis, peripheral edema
- **GI:** *Diarrhea,* **pseudomembranous colitis,** dyspepsia, *nausea, vomiting,* constipation, liver enzyme elevations
- **Respiratory:** Cough, dyspnea
- **Other:** Pruritus, rash, sweating, fever, pain, suppressed bone marrow, superinfections, photosensitivity

Interactions
✱ **Drug-drug** • Possible decreased effectiveness of oral contraceptives; suggest use of barrier contraceptives during treatment • Possible alteration in effects of warfarin if taken in combination; monitor patient closely and follow coagulation tests closely

■ Nursing considerations
Assessment
- **History:** Hypersensitivity to tigecycline or any of its components, pregnancy, allergy to tetracycline antibiotics, lactation

- **Physical:** T; orientation, reflexes; BP, peripheral pulses; abdominal examination; skin color, lesions; R, chest sounds; LFTs; culture and sensitivity of infected site

Interventions

- Perform culture and sensitivity tests to assure that this is the most appropriate antibiotic for the infection being treated.
- Advise the use of barrier contraceptives during therapy.
- Suggest another method of feeding the baby if patient is nursing a baby during therapy.
- Provide comfort measures and possible analgesics for headache and pain.
- Encourage frequent, small meals if GI effects are uncomfortable.

Teaching points

- You will receive *Tygacil* as an IV infusion over 30–60 minutes every 12 hours for 5–14 days.
- Tests will be run to make sure that this is the most appropriate antibiotic for your particular infection.
- It is not known how this drug could affect a nursing baby. If you are nursing a baby, another method of feeding the baby should be selected.
- It is not known how this drug could affect a fetus, if you are pregnant or decide to become pregnant while on this drug, consult your health care provider. Use of barrier contraceptives is advised; this drug may block the effects of hormone contraceptives.
- You may experience these side effects: Nausea, vomiting, and diarrhea (these symptoms may lessen over time; if they become bothersome, talk to your health care provider about possible treatments); sensitivity to light (use a sunscreen and wear protective clothing and sunglasses if you have to be exposed to sunlight).
- Report bloody diarrhea, unrelenting diarrhea, rash, swelling of the extremities, discomfort at the injection site.

tiludronate disodium

See Appendix W, *Less commonly used drugs.*

timolol maleate

(tim' oh lol)

Apo-Timol (CAN), Apo-Timop (CAN), Betimol, Blocadren, Gen-Timolol (CAN), Istalol, PMS-Timolol (CAN), Timoptic, Timoptic-XE

PREGNANCY CATEGORY C

Drug classes

Antiglaucoma drug
Antihypertensive
Beta-adrenergic blocker

Therapeutic actions

Competitively blocks beta-adrenergic receptors in the heart and juxtaglomerular apparatus, decreasing the influence of the sympathetic nervous system on these tissues and decreasing the excitability of the heart, decreasing cardiac output and oxygen consumption, decreasing the release of renin, and lowering BP; reduces IOP by decreasing the production of aqueous humor and possibly by increasing aqueous humor outflow.

Indications

- Hypertension, used alone or in combination with other antihypertensives, especially thiazide-type diuretics
- Prevention of reinfarction in MI patients who are hemodynamically stable
- Prophylaxis of migraine
- Ophthalmic solution: Reduction of IOP in chronic open-angle glaucoma, some patients with secondary glaucoma, aphakic patients with glaucoma ocular hypertension

Contraindications and cautions

- Contraindicated with sinus bradycardia (HR less than 45 beats/min), second- or third-degree heart block (PR interval greater than 0.24 sec), cardiogenic shock, HF, asthma, COPD, pregnancy, lactation.
- Use cautiously with diabetes or thyrotoxicosis (timolol can mask the usual cardiac signs of hypoglycemia and thyrotoxicosis).

Available forms

Tablets—5, 10, 20 mg; ophthalmic solution, gel—0.25%, 0.5%

Dosages

Adults

Oral

- *Hypertension:* Initially, 10 mg bid. Increase dosage at 1-wk intervals to a maximum of 60 mg/day divided into two doses, as needed. Usual maintenance dose is 20–40 mg/day given in two divided doses.
- *Prevention of reinfarction in MI (long-term prophylaxis in patients who survived the acute phase):* 10 mg bid PO within 1–4 wk of infarction.
- *Migraine:* 10 mg PO bid; during maintenance, the 20 mg/day may be given as a single dose. May be increased to a maximum of 30 mg/day in divided doses or decreased to 10 mg/day. Discontinue if satisfactory response is not obtained after 6–8 wk.

Ophthalmic

Initially, 1 drop of 0.25% solution bid into the affected eye or eyes. Adjust dosage on basis of response to 1 drop of 0.5% solution bid or 1 drop of 0.25% solution daily. When replacing other agents, make change gradually and individualize dosage. One drop in the affected eye each morning (*Istalol*).

Pediatric patients

Safety and efficacy not established.

Pharmacokinetics

Route	*Onset*	*Peak*
Oral	Varies	1–2 hr
Ophthal	Rapid	1–5 hr

Metabolism: Hepatic; $T_{1/2}$: 3–4 hr
Distribution: Crosses placenta; enters breast milk
Excretion: Urine

Adverse effects

Oral

- **Allergic reactions:** Pharyngitis, erythematous rash, fever, sore throat, **laryngospasm,** respiratory distress
- **CNS:** Dizziness, vertigo, tinnitus, fatigue, emotional depression, paresthesias, sleep disturbances, hallucinations, disorientation, memory loss
- **CV:** *HF, cardiac arrhythmias, sinoatrial or AV nodal block,* peripheral vascular insufficiency, claudication, **CVA, pulmonary edema,** hypotension, chest pain
- **Dermatologic:** Rash, pruritus, sweating, dry skin
- **EENT:** Eye irritation, dry eyes, conjunctivitis, blurred vision
- **GI:** *Gastric pain, flatulence, constipation, diarrhea, nausea, vomiting,* anorexia, ischemic colitis, renal and mesenteric arterial thrombosis, retroperitoneal fibrosis, hepatomegaly, acute pancreatitis
- **GU:** *Impotence, decreased libido,* Peyronie's disease, dysuria, nocturia, frequent urination
- **Musculoskeletal:** Joint pain, arthralgia, muscle cramp
- **Respiratory: Bronchospasm,** dyspnea, cough, bronchial obstruction, nasal stuffiness, rhinitis, pharyngitis (less likely than with propranolol)
- **Other:** *Decreased exercise tolerance, development of ANA,* hyperglycemia or hypoglycemia, elevated serum transaminase

Ophthalmic

- **Local:** Ocular irritation, decreased corneal sensitivity, visual refractive changes, diplopia, ptosis, tearing

Interactions

✱ **Drug-drug** • Increased effects with verapamil • Increased risk of orthostatic hypotension with prazosin • Decreased antihypertensive effects with NSAIDs • Risk of rebound hypertension following clonidine withdrawal • Decreased elimination of theophyllines with resultant decrease in expected actions of both drugs when taken concurrently • Peripheral ischemia and possible gangrene with ergotamine, methysergide, dihydroergotamine • Increased risk of hypoglycemia and masked signs of hypoglycemia with insulin • Hypertension followed by severe bradycardia with epinephrine • All of the above may occur with ophthalmic timolol; in addition, additive effects are possible with oral beta blockers

✱ **Drug-lab test** • Possible false results with glucose or insulin tolerance tests (oral)

■ Nursing considerations

Assessment

- **History:** Sinus bradycardia, second- or third-degree heart block, cardiogenic shock, HF, asthma, COPD, pregnancy, lactation, diabetes or thyrotoxicosis
- **Physical:** Weight, skin condition, neurologic status, P, BP, ECG, respiratory status, renal and thyroid function, blood and urine glucose

Interventions

⊗ ***Warning*** Do not discontinue the drug abruptly after long-term therapy (hypersensitivity to catecholamines may have developed, causing exacerbation of angina, MI, and ventricular arrhythmias). Taper drug gradually over 2 wk with monitoring.

- Consult with surgeon about withdrawal if patient is to undergo surgery (withdrawal is controversial).

Teaching points

- Do not stop taking this drug unless instructed to do so by your health care provider.
- Avoid driving or dangerous activities if dizziness or shaking occurs.
- If using ophthalmic form, administer eye drops properly to minimize systemic absorption.
- Report difficulty breathing, night cough, swelling of extremities, slow pulse, confusion, depression, rash, fever, sore throat.

▽tinidazole

*(teh **nid'** ah zol)*

Tindamax

PREGNANCY CATEGORY C

Drug classes

Antiprotozoal
Nitroimidazole

Therapeutic actions

Antiprotozoal; mechanism of action against *Giardia, Entamoeba* species is not known.

Indications

- Treatment of trichomoniasis caused by *Trichomonas vaginitis*
- Treatment of giardiasis caused by *Giardia duodenalisi* or *G. lamblia* in patients 3 yr and older
- Treatment of amebiasis and amebic liver abscess caused by *Entamoeba histolytica* patients 3 yr and older
- Treatment of bacterial vaginosis in non-pregnant adult women

Contraindications and cautions

- Contraindicated with allergy to tinidazole, any component of the drug, or other nitroimidazoles; the first trimester of pregnancy; lactation.
- Use cautiously with second or third trimester of pregnancy, history of blood dyscrasias, CNS disorders, hepatic impairment.

Available forms

Tablets—250, 500 mg

Dosages

Adults

- *Trichomoniasis, giardiasis:* Single dose of 2 g PO taken with food.
- *Amebiasis:* 2 g/day PO for 3 days, taken with food.
- *Amebic liver abscess:* 2 g/day PO for 3–5 days, taken with food.
- *Bacterial vaginosis:* 2 g/day PO for 2 days or 1 g/day PO for 5 days.

Pediatric patients older than 3 yr

- *Giardiasis:* Single dose of 50 mg/kg PO (up to 2 g) taken with food.
- *Amebiasis:* 50 mg/kg/day PO (up to 2 g/day) for 3 days, taken with food.
- *Amebic liver abscess:* 50 mg/kg/day PO (up to 2 g/day) for 3–5 days, taken with food.

Pharmacokinetics

Route	*Onset*	*Peak*
Oral	Rapid	1.6 hr

Metabolism: Hepatic metabolism; $T_{1/2}$: 12–14 hr
Distribution: Crosses placenta; passes into breast milk
Excretion: Feces, urine

Adverse effects

- **CNS:** Weakness, fatigue, malaise, dizziness, headache, drowsiness, **seizures,** peripheral neuropathy

T

- **GI:** Metallic taste, nausea, anorexia, dyspepsia, cramps, vomiting, constipation, diarrhea, stomatitis
- **GU:** Darkened urine
- **Other:** *Transient neutropenia, transient leukopenia,* superinfections (*Candida*)

Interactions

✱ Drug-drug ⊗ *Warning* Risk of severe adverse effects if combined with alcohol; advise patient to avoid intake of alcohol while on tinidazole and for 3 days after treatment.
• Possibility of increased effects of oral anticoagulants; monitor the patient and adjust dosage of oral anticoagulant appropriately for up to 8 days after stopping tinidazole therapy
• Risk of psychotic reactions if combined with disulfiram; avoid this combination and avoid use within 2 wk of tinidazole therapy • Potential for increased serum levels of lithium if taken concurrently; monitor patient for any sign of lithium intoxication • Potential risk for increased serum levels of cyclosporine, tacrolimus, IV phenytoin, 5-FU if taken with tinidazole; monitor patients for potential toxicity and decrease dosage appropriately • Potential for decreased effectiveness of tinidazole if combined with cholestyramine or oxytetracycline
• Potential for increased serum levels and risk of toxicity if combined with cimetidine, ketoconazole, other CYP3A4 inhibitors; monitor patient closely

■ Nursing considerations

Assessment

- **History:** Allergy to tinidazole or any component of the drug or to other nitroimidazoles, pregnancy, lactation, history of blood dyscrasias, CNS disorders, hepatic impairment
- **Physical:** Orientation, affect, reflexes; GI mucosa, output, bowel sounds, liver evaluation; CBC, LFTs, renal function tests

Interventions

⊠ ***Black box warning*** Avoid use unless clearly needed; tinidiazole is carcinogenic in laboratory animals.

- Administer with food to decrease GI side effects.
- Institute appropriate hygiene measures and arrange treatment if superinfections occur.
- If GI upset occurs provide frequent small meals; encourage patient to maintain fluid intake and nutrition.
- Establish safety measures (eg, accompany patient, side rails) if CNS changes occur.
- Suggest another method of feeding the baby if patient is nursing.
- Recommend the use of contraceptive measures while using this drug.

Teaching points

- Take this drug exactly as prescribed, complete the full course of the therapy and do not use this drug to treat any other infections.
- If you miss a dose, take the next dose as soon as you remember; do not take more than the prescribed dose each day.
- Take the drug with food to help decrease GI side effects.
- Be aware that your urine may become dark; this is a drug effect.
- Do not drink alcohol while taking this drug and for three days following completion of the treatment; serious adverse effects could occur.
- This drug should not be used during pregnancy or while nursing; use of contraceptives is recommended while on this drug. If you are nursing, you should select another method of feeding the baby.
- You may experience these side effects: Nausea, diarrhea, metallic taste (frequent small meals, frequent mouth care may help); headache (analgesics may be available to help, consult your health care provider); dizziness (do not drive a car or operate hazardous machinery if this occurs).
- Report vaginal itching, white patches in the mouth, numbness or tingling of the extremities.

DANGEROUS DRUG

▽ tinzaparin sodium

(ten zah' pear in)

Innohep

PREGNANCY CATEGORY B

Drug classes

Anticoagulant
Low–molecular-weight heparin

Therapeutic actions
Low–molecular-weight heparin that inhibits thrombus and clot formation by blocking factor Xa and factor IIa, preventing the formation of clots.

Indications
- Treatment of acute, symptomatic deep vein thrombosis with or without pulmonary emboli when given with warfarin sodium
- Unlabeled use: Prevention of DVT in patients undergoing surgery at risk for thromboembolic complications

Contraindications and cautions
- Contraindicated with hypersensitivity to any tinzaparin, sulfites, benzyl alcohol, heparin, pork products; history of heparin-induced thrombocytopenia; uncontrolled bleeding.
- Use cautiously with pregnancy or lactation, history of GI bleed, elderly patients with renal insufficiency.

Available forms
Injection—20,000 international units/mL

Dosages
Adults
175 international units/kg/day subcutaneously given once daily for 6 days or more and until the patient has been successfully anticoagulated with warfarin (INR 2 or higher for 2 consecutive days).
Pediatric patients
Safety and efficacy not established.

Pharmacokinetics

Route	*Onset*	*Peak*	*Duration*
Subcut.	2–3 hr	4–5 hr	12 hr

Metabolism: Cellular; $T_{1/2}$: 3–4 hr
Distribution: May cross placenta, may enter breast milk
Excretion: Urine

Adverse effects
- **Hematologic: Hemorrhage;** *bruising;* thrombocytopenia; elevated AST, ALT levels; hyperkalemia
- **Hypersensitivity:** Chills, fever, urticaria, asthma
- **Other:** Fever; pain; local irritation; hematoma; erythema at site of injection; **increased risk of death in elderly patients with renal insufficiency**

Interactions
✱ **Drug-drug** • Increased bleeding tendencies with oral anticoagulants, salicylates, penicillins, cephalosporins, antiplatelets
✱ **Drug-lab test** • Increased AST, ALT levels
✱ **Drug-alternative therapy** • Increased risk of bleeding if combined with chamomile, garlic, ginger, ginkgo, and ginseng therapy

■ Nursing considerations
Assessment
- **History:** Recent surgery or injury; sensitivity to heparin, low–molecular-weight heparins, pork products; pregnancy, lactation; recent GI bleed
- **Physical:** Peripheral perfusion, R, stool guaiac test, PTT, INR or other tests of blood coagulation, platelet count, renal function tests

Interventions
- Arrange to begin warfarin therapy within 1–3 days of starting tinzaparin.

⊗ ***Warning*** Increased risk of death in elderly patients with renal insufficiency. A different anticoagulant should be considered in these situations.

⊗ ***Warning*** Give deep subcutaneous injections; do not give by IM or IV injection.

⊠ ***Black box warning*** Use extreme caution with spinal or epidural anesthesia; risk of spinal hematoma and neurologic damage exists.

- Administer by deep subcutaneous injection; patient should be lying down; alternate administration between the left and right anterolateral and left and right posterolateral abdominal wall. Introduce the whole length of the needle into a skin fold held between the thumb and forefinger; hold the skin fold throughout the injection.
- Apply pressure to all injection sites after needle is withdrawn; inspect injection sites for signs of hematoma.
- Do not massage injection sites.

- Do not mix with other injections or infusions.
- Store at room temperature; fluid should be clear, colorless to pale yellow.
- Provide for safety measures (electric razor, soft toothbrush) to prevent injury to patient who is at risk for bleeding.
- Check patient for signs of bleeding and monitor blood tests.

⊗ ***Warning*** Keep protamine sulfate (tinzaparin antidote) readily available in case of overdose. Each milligram of protamine sulfate (1% solution) neutralizes 100 international units of tinzaparin. Give very slowly IV over 10 min.

Teaching points

- This drug must be given subcutaneously (cannot be taken orally).
- Arrange for periodic blood tests that will be needed to monitor your response to this drug.
- Be careful to avoid injury while you are using this drug: Use an electric razor, avoid activities that might lead to injury.
- Report nose bleed, bleeding of the gums, unusual bruising, black or tarry stools, cloudy or dark urine, abdominal or lower back pain, severe headache.

▽tiopronin

See Appendix W, *Less commonly used drugs.*

▽tiotropium bromide

*(tye oh **troh'** pee um)*

Spiriva

PREGNANCY CATEGORY C

Drug classes

Anticholinergic
Antimuscarinic
Bronchodilator

Therapeutic actions

Competitively antagonistic at muscarinic receptor sites; causes smooth muscle relaxation, leading to bronchodilation.

Indications

- Long-term once-daily maintenance treatment of bronchospasm associated with COPD, including chronic bronchitis and emphysema

Contraindications and cautions

- Contraindicated with allergy to atropine or its derivatives, ipratropium or any component of the product.
- Use cautiously with narrow-angle glaucoma, prostatic hyperplasia, bladder neck obstruction, moderate to severe renal impairment (creatinine clearance of 50 mL/min or less), pregnancy, lactation.

Available forms

Powder for inhalation—18 mcg supplied with *Handihaler* inhalation device

Dosages

Adults

Inhalation of the contents of one capsule per day using the *Handihaler* inhalation device.

Pediatric patients

Safety and efficacy not established.

Pharmacokinetics

Route	*Onset*	*Peak*
Inhalation	Rapid	5 min

Metabolism: $T_{1/2}$: 5–6 days
Distribution: May cross placenta; may enter breast milk
Excretion: Urine, feces

Adverse effects

- **CNS:** *Blurred vision*
- **CV:** Edema
- **GI:** *Dry mouth,* constipation, abdominal pain, dyspepsia, vomiting
- **Respiratory:** Epistaxis, pharyngitis, rhinitis, *sinusitis, URI,* cough
- **Other:** Myalgia, rash, infections, *accidents,* candidiasis, UTI, flulike symptoms, arthritis

Interactions

✱ **Drug-drug** • Risk of increased adverse effects if combined with other anticholinergics; avoid this combination

■ Nursing considerations
Assessment
- **History:** Allergy to atropine or its derivatives, ipratropium, or any component of the product; narrow-angle glaucoma; prostatic hyperplasia, bladder neck obstruction, severe renal impairment; pregnancy, lactation
- **Physical:** Orientation, vision, IOP; skin evaluation; cardiac rhythm, bowel sounds; R, adventitious sounds

Interventions
- Do not use this drug for acute respiratory problems.
- Instruct patient in the proper use of the *Handihaler* inhalation device.
- Do not use any other drugs in the *Handihaler* inhalation device.

⊗ ***Warning*** Evaluate patient for glaucoma; discontinue drug at first sign of developing glaucoma—eye pain, blurred vision, visual halos with red eye and corneal edema.

- Have patient void before using medication if urinary retention is a problem.

Teaching points
- Administer this drug once daily using the provided *Handihaler* inhalation device. Do not use this device for any other drugs. Do not swallow capsules.
- Keep the capsule in the foil blister pack until ready to use; discard any capsules inadvertently opened and left exposed to the air.
- Follow the directions that come with the *Handihaler* for proper administration of the drug and cleaning of the device.
- Avoid getting the inhalation powder in your eyes; if this occurs, gently wash the eye.
- Use this drug for maintenance of your COPD. Do not use it if you have acute trouble breathing.
- Empty your bladder before using this drug if you have a problem with urinary retention.
- You may experience these side effects: Dry mouth (drink plenty of fluids; suck sugarless lozenges); constipation (consult your health care provider); blurred vision (avoid driving a car or operating hazardous machinery).
- Report eye pain, eye discomfort, blurred vision, visual halos or colored images along with red eye (consult your health care provider immediately), urinary retention, difficulty urinating.

▽tipranavir
(tip ran' ah veer)

Aptivus DNC

PREGNANCY CATEGORY C

Drug classes
Antiviral drug
Protease inhibitor

Therapeutic actions
Inhibits virus specific processing of polyproteins, leading to the inability to produce mature virions and decreasing virus levels.

Indications
- Along with ritonavir, as combination treatment of patients infected with HIV, with evidence of viral replication who are treatment-experienced or have HIV-1 strains resistant to multiple protease inhibitors

Contraindications and cautions
- Contraindicated with known hypersensitivity tipranavir or any of its components, moderate to severe hepatic insufficiency (Child-Pugh class B or C).
- Use cautiously with diabetes mellitus, hypergylcemia, known allergy to sulfonamides, hemophilia, hepatits B or C infection, pregnancy, lactation.

Available forms
Capsules DNC—250 mg; solution—100 mg/mL

Dosages
Adults

500 mg/day PO in combination with 200 mg ritonavir, taken with food.

Pediatric patients ages 2–18 yr

14 mg/kg with 6 mg/kg of ritonavir PO bid (375 mg/m^2 with 150 mg/m^2 ritonavir PO bid). Maximum dose, 500 mg/day with 200 mg ritonavir.

T

Pharmacokinetics

Route	Onset	Peak
Oral	Slow	2.9 hr

Metabolism: Hepatic: $T_{1/2}$: 4.8–6 hr
Distribution: May cross placenta; may pass into breast milk
Excretion: Feces, urine

Adverse effects

- **CNS:** Depression, insomnia, headache
- **GI:** *Nausea,* vomiting, abdominal pain, *diarrhea,* potentially fatal liver impairment
- **Respiratory:** Cough, bronchitis
- **Other:** Skin rash, flulike symptoms, fever, malaise, increased cholesterol, triglycerides

Interactions

✱ **Drug-drug** • Potential for serious to life-threatening reactions if combined with amiodarone, bepridil, flecainide, propafenone, quinidine, astemizole, terfenadine, rifampin, dihydroergotamine, ergonovine, ergotamine, methylergonovine, lovastatin, simvastatin, pimozide, midazolam, triazolam; avoid these combinations • Potential for decreased serum levels of didanosine if combined; space doses of didanosine and tipranavir and ritonavir by at least 2 hr • Potential for decreased serum levels of amprenavir, lopinavir, saquinavir if combined with tipranavir and ritonavir; avoid this combination • Potential for increased serum levels of itraconazole, ketoconazole, voriconazole if used in combination with tipranavir and ritonavir; avoid high doses, monitor patient closely • Potential for adverse effects if combined with calcium channel blockers; use caution and monitor patient closely • Potential for increased levels of desipramine if used in combination; dosage reduction of desipramine and careful patient monitoring is recommended • Potential for disulfiram-like reaction if combined with disulfiram, metronidazole; monitor patient • Risk of increased levels of oral antidiabetic drugs, leading to potential for hypoglycemia; monitor glucose levels closely and adjust dosages as needed • Risk of increased tipranavir levels and atorvastatin levels if these two drugs are combined; start with lowest possible dose of atorvastatin and monitor patient closely • Risk of increased serum levels and toxic effects of cyclosporine, sirolimus, tacrolimus if used in combination; monitor serum levels closely and adjust dosages as needed • Possible decreased levels of meperidine, methadone if combined with tipranavir and ritonavir; monitor patient and adjust dosages as needed • Risk of decreased serum levels of hormonal contraceptives, leading to lack of effectiveness, and ethinyl estradiol; alternate forms of birth control should be used; monitor women on replacement therapy for low levels of estrogen • Risk of increased serum levels and adverse effects of sildenafil, tadalafil, vardenafil; use extreme caution, start at lowest possible doses and limit use to every 48 hr (sildenafil) or 72 hr (tadalafil, vardenafil) • Risk of increased serum levels of SSRIs; monitor patient and adjust dosage as needed • Potential for unpredictable effects of warfarin when used in combination; monitor bleeding times carefully and adjust dosages as needed
✱ **Drug-alternative therapy** • Potential for loss of effectiveness if combined with St. John's wort; avoid this combination

■ Nursing considerations

Assessment:

- **History:** Hypersensitivity to tipranavir or any of its components, moderate to severe hepatic insufficiency, diabetes mellitus, hyperglycemia, known allergy to sulfonamides, hemophilia, hepatits B or C infection, pregnancy, lactation
- **Physical** T; orientation; skin color, lesions; abdominal examination, LFTs, HIV testing, blood counts

Interventions

⊗ ***Black box warning*** Assess liver function before and periodically during therapy; increased risk of hepatotoxicity in patients with hepatitis. Administration of tipranavir with ritonavir has caused fatal and nonfatal intracranial hemorrhage; monitor patient carefully.

- Make sure that the patient also takes ritonavir when taking this drug.
- Make sure that the patient swallows capsules whole; do not cut, crush, or allow the patient to chew the capsules.
- Administer ritonavir and tipranavir with food.

- Before beginning therapy, assess the patient's drug regimen for numerous, potential drug interactions.
- Withdraw drug and monitor patient if patient develops signs of lactic acidosis or hepatotoxicity, including hepatomegaly and steatosis.
- Encourage women of childbearing age to use barrier contraceptives while on this drug because the effects of the drug on a fetus are not known.
- Advise women who are nursing to find another method of feeding the baby; potential effects on the baby are not known.
- Advise patient that this drug does not cure the disease and there is still a risk of transmitting the disease to others.
- Maintain all other therapies related to the HIV infection.

Teaching points

- This drug is not a cure for HIV. It works with ritonavir to decrease the number of viruses in your body.
- You should still take precautions to prevent the spread of HIV; do not share any personal items that may have blood or body fluids on them; use barrier contraceptives if having intercourse.
- Always take tipranavir with ritonavir; take these drugs with food.
- Do not cut, crush, or chew the capsules; swallow capsules whole.
- Store opened bottles of these capsules in the refrigerator; do not use this drug after the expiration date on the bottle. Do not refrigerate or freeze oral solution.
- If you forget a dose of the drug, take that dose along with your ritonavir as soon as you remember, then take your next dose at the usual time. Do not take more than one dose each day.
- This drug interacts with many other drugs; make sure to tell all health care providers that you are taking this drug.
- You will need to have regular health care, including blood tests, to monitor the effects of this drug on your body.
- It is not known how this drug could affect a nursing baby. If you are nursing a baby, another method of feeding the baby should be selected while you are taking this drug.
- It is not known how this drug could affect a fetus, if you are pregnant or want to become pregnant while on this drug, consult your health care provider.
- You may experience these side effects: Headache (consult your health care provider, medication may be available to help); nausea (eating frequent small meals may help); diarrhea (this may lessen with time; alert your health care provider if this becomes severe); liver injury (this could be serious; stop taking the drug and alert your health care provider if you experience yellowing of your skin or eyes, tea-colored urine, general tiredness, pale stools, pain or sensitivity on your right side).
- Report yellowing of the skin or eyes, general malaise and flulike symptoms, changes in the color of your urine or stool, right-sided pain or tenderness.

▽tirofiban hydrochloride

*(tye row **fye'** ban)*

Aggrastat

PREGNANCY CATEGORY B

Drug classes

Antiplatelet
Glycoprotein IIb/IIIa inhibitor

Therapeutic actions

Inhibits platelet aggregation by binding to the platelet receptor glycoprotein, which prevents the binding of fibrinogen and other adhesive ligands to the platelet.

Indications

- Treatment of acute coronary syndrome in combination with heparin
- Prevention of cardiac ischemic complications in patients undergoing elective, emergency, or urgent percutaneous coronary intervention

Contraindications and cautions

- Contraindicated with allergy to any component of this product, bleeding diathesis, hemorrhagic CVA, active or abnormal bleeding or CVA within 30 days, uncontrolled or

T

severe hypertension, major surgery within 4 wk, low platelet count, aortic aneurysm, aortic dissection, acute pericarditis.
- Use cautiously with pregnancy, lactation, renal insufficiency, the elderly, platelet count less than 150,000/mm^3, dialysis.

Available forms

Injection concentrate—250 mcg/mL; injection—50 mcg/mL

Dosages

Adults

0.4 mcg/kg/min IV infusion over 30 min, then continue at rate of 0.1 mcg/kg/min.

Pediatric patients

Not recommended.

Patients with renal impairment

Use one-half the recommended adult dosage and monitor patient closely.

Pharmacokinetics

Route	*Onset*	*Peak*	*Duration*
IV	15 min	30 min	4–8 hr

Metabolism: Tissue; $T_{1/2}$: 2 hr
Distribution: Crosses placenta; may enter breast milk
Excretion: Feces, urine

IV FACTS

Preparation: Withdraw and discard 100 mL from a 500-mL bag of sterile 0.9% sodium chloride or D_5W; replace this volume with 100 mL tirofiban injection (two-50 mL vials) or remove 50 mL from 250-mL bag of sterile 0.9% sodium chloride or D_5W; replace this volume with 50 mL tirofiban injection; doing so will provide a concentration of 50 mcg/mL; mix well prior to administration. Protect from light; discard any remaining solution 24 hr after beginning of infusion. Premixed tirofiban is available in *IntraVia* containers at a concentration of 50 mcg/mL. To open, tear off dust cover; squeeze bag to ensure that no leaks occur—if fluid leaks out, discard solution as sterility has been compromised.
Infusion: Infuse loading dose of 0.4 mcg/kg/min over 30 min; continue infusion at rate of 0.1 mcg/kg/min.

Incompatibilities: Do not mix in solution with diazepam. May be given in same IV line as heparin, dopamine, lidocaine, potassium chloride, and famotidine.

Adverse effects

- **CNS:** *Dizziness,* weakness, syncope, flushing
- **CV:** Bradycardia
- **GI:** Nausea, GI distress, constipation, diarrhea
- **Other:** *Bleeding, hypotension,* edema, pain

Interactions

✱ **Drug-drug** • Increased risk of bleeding when combined with aspirin, warfarin, NSAIDs, antiplatelets, heparin; monitor patient closely

✱ **Drug-alternative therapy** • Increased risk of bleeding if combined with chamomile, garlic, ginger, ginkgo and ginseng, turmeric, horse chestnut seed, green tea leaf, grape seed extract, feverfew, don quai; monitor patient closely

■ Nursing considerations

CLINICAL ALERT!
Name confusion has been reported with *Aggrastat* (tirofiban) and argatroban. Use extreme caution.

Assessment

- **History:** Allergy to any component of this product; bleeding diathesis; hemorrhagic CVA; active, abnormal bleeding or CVA within 30 days; uncontrolled or severe hypertension; major surgery within 6 wk; dialysis; low platelet count; aortic aneurysm; aortic dissection; pregnancy; lactation; renal impairment
- **Physical:** Skin color, T, lesions; orientation, reflexes, affect; P, BP, orthostatic BP, baseline ECG, peripheral perfusion; respiratory rate, adventitious sounds, aPTT, PT, active clotting time, CBC

Interventions

- Use tirofiban in conjunction with heparin.
- To minimize patient's blood loss, use as few arterial and venous punctures, IM injections, catheterizations, and intubations as possible.

⊗ ***Warning*** Avoid the use of noncompressible IV access sites to prevent excessive, uncontrollable bleeding.

- Arrange for baseline and periodic CBC, PT, aPTT, and active clotting time. Maintain aPTT between 50–70 sec; and active bleeding time between 300 and 350 sec.
- Properly care for femoral access site to minimize bleeding. Document aPTT of less than 45 sec, and stop heparin for 3–4 hr before pulling sheath.

Teaching points

- This drug is given to minimize blood clotting and cardiac damage. It must be given IV.
- You will be monitored closely and your blood will be tested periodically to monitor the effects of this drug on your body.
- You may experience these side effects: Dizziness, light-headedness, bleeding.
- Report light-headedness, palpitations, pain at IV site, bleeding.

▽ tizanidine

*(tis **an'** i deen)*

Apo-Tizanidine (CAN), Zanaflex

PREGNANCY CATEGORY C

Drug classes

Antispasmodic
Sympatholytic (centrally acting)

Therapeutic actions

Centrally acting alpha$_2$-agonist; antispasmodic effect thought to be a result of indirect depression of polysynaptic reflexes by blocking the excitatory actions of spinal interneurons.

Indications

- Acute and intermittent management of increased muscle tone associated with spasticity

Contraindications and cautions

- Contraindicated with hypersensitivity to tizanidine, concomitant use of fluroxamine, ciprofloxacin.
- Use cautiously with hepatic or renal impairment, hypotension, pregnancy, lactation.

Available forms

Tablets—2, 4 mg; capsules—2, 4, 6 mg

Dosages

Adults

4 mg/day PO, increased in 2- to 4-mg increments as needed over 2–4 wk. Usual maintenance dose is 8 mg PO every 6–8 hr; maximum dose, 36 mg/day in divided doses.

Pediatric patients

Safety and efficacy not established.

Patients with renal impairment

Use lower doses, monitor response.

Pharmacokinetics

Route	*Onset*	*Peak*	*Duration*
Oral	30–60 min	1–2 hr	3–6 hr

Metabolism: Hepatic; $T_{1/2}$: 2.7–4.2 hr
Distribution: Crosses placenta; may enter breast milk
Excretion: Urine

Adverse effects

- **CNS:** *Drowsiness, sedation, dizziness, asthenia,* headache, hallucinations, somnolence
- **CV:** *Hypotension, orthostatic hypotension,* bradycardia
- **GI:** *Dry mouth, constipation,* anorexia, malaise, nausea, vomiting, parotid pain, parotitis, mild transient abnormalities in LFTs

Interactions

✱ **Drug-drug** • Potential risk of increased depression with alcohol, baclofen, other CNS depressants • Possible increased effects with hormonal contraceptives; monitor patient and decrease tizanidine dose • Do not use in combination with other alpha$_2$-adrenergic agonists

■ Nursing considerations

Assessment

- **History:** Hypersensitivity to tizanidine, clonidine; hepatic or renal impairment; hypotension; pregnancy, lactation
- **Physical:** Mucous membranes—color, lesions; orientation, affect; P, BP, orthostatic BP; perfusion; liver evaluation; LFTs, renal function tests

Interventions

- Administer drug every 6–8 hr around-the-clock for best effects.
- Adjust drug dosage slowly, which helps to decrease side effects.
- Continue all supportive measures used for spinal cord–injured or neurologically damaged patients.
- Provide sugarless lozenges or ice chips, as appropriate, if dry mouth or altered taste occurs.
- Establish safety precautions if CNS or hypotensive changes occur (use side rails, accompany patient when ambulating).
- Attempt to lower dose if side effects become severe or intolerable.

Teaching points

- Take this drug exactly as prescribed. It is important that you not miss doses. Consult your health care provider to determine a schedule that will not interfere with rest.
- Continue all other supportive measures for your condition.
- You may experience these side effects: Drowsiness, dizziness, light-headedness, headache, weakness (use caution while driving or performing tasks that require alertness or physical dexterity); dry mouth (suck on sugarless lozenges or ice chips); GI upset (eat frequent small meals); dizziness, light-headedness when changing position (rise slowly, use caution when transferring).
- Report changes in urine or stool, severe dizziness or passing out, changes in vision, difficulty swallowing.

tobramycin sulfate

*(toe bra **mye'** sin)*

Parenteral: generic
Nebulizer solution: TOBI
Ophthalmic: Defy, Tobrex Ophthalmic

PREGNANCY CATEGORY D (INJECTION, INHALATION)

PREGNANCY CATEGORY B (OPHTHALMIC)

Drug class

Aminoglycoside antibiotic

Therapeutic actions

Bactericidal: Inhibits protein synthesis in susceptible strains of gram-negative bacteria; mechanism of lethal action is not fully understood, but functional integrity of bacterial cell membrane appears to be disrupted.

Indications

- Parenteral: Serious infections caused by susceptible strains of *Pseudomonas aeruginosa, Proteus species, Providencia species, Escherichia coli, Klebsiella-Enterobacter-Serratia* group, *Citrobacter* species, and staphylococci (including *Staphylococcus aureus*)
- Staphylococcal infections when penicillin is contraindicated or when the bacteria are not susceptible
- Serious, life-threatening, gram-negative infections when susceptibility studies have not been completed (sometimes concurrent penicillin or cephalosporin therapy)
- Nebulizer solution: Management of cystic fibrosis patients with *P. aeruginosa*
- Ophthalmic: Treatment of superficial ocular infections due to susceptible strains of organisms

Contraindications and cautions

- Contraindicated with allergy to aminoglycosides, pregnancy, lactation.
- Use cautiously with patients who are elderly or who have diminished hearing, decreased renal function, dehydration, neuromuscular disorders (myasthenia gravis, parkinsonism, infant botulism), herpes, vaccinia, varicella, mycobacterial infections, fungal infections.

Available forms

Injection—10, 40 mg/mL, 80 mg/100 mL normal saline; powder for injection—1.2 g; nebulizer solution—300 mg/5 mL; ophthalmic solution—0.3%; ophthalmic ointment—3 mg/g

Dosages

IM or IV

Doses based on ideal body weight.

Adults

3 mg/kg/day in three equal doses every 8 hr. Up to 5 mg/kg/day in three to four equal doses can be used in life-threatening infections, but reduce to 3 mg/kg/day as soon as possible. Do not exceed 5 mg/kg/day unless serum levels are monitored.

Pediatric patients older than 1 wk

6–7.5 mg/kg/day in three to four equally divided doses.

Premature infants or neonates 1 wk and younger

Up to 4 mg/kg/day in two equal doses every 12 hr.

Geriatric patients or patients with renal failure

Reduce dosage, and carefully monitor serum drug levels and renal function tests throughout treatment. Reduced dosage nomogram is available; check manufacturer's information.

Adults and children 6 yr and older

Nebulizer solution

300 mg bid. Administer in 28-day cycles: 28 days on, 28 days of rest. Inhale over 10–15 min.

Ophthalmic solution

- *Mild to moderate infection:* One or two drops into conjunctival sac of affected eye or eyes every 4 hr.
- *Severe infection:* Two drops into conjunctival sac of affected eye or eyes hourly until improvement occurs.

Ophthalmic ointment

One-half-inch ribbon bid–tid.

- *Severe infection:* One-half inch every 3–4 hr.

Pharmacokinetics

Route	*Onset*	*Peak*
IM, IV	Rapid	30–90 min
Ophthalmologic	Rapid	Unknown
Inhalation	Rapid	20 min

Metabolism: Minimal hepatic; $T_{1/2}$: 2–3 hr
Distribution: Crosses placenta; enters breast milk
Excretion: Urine

IV FACTS

Preparation: Dilute vials of solution for injection. Usual volume of diluent is 50–100 mL of 9% sodium chloride injection or 5% dextrose injection (less for children). Reconstitute powder for injection with sterile water for injection according to manufacturer's instructions.
Infusion: Infuse over 20–60 min.
Incompatibilities: Do not premix with other drugs; administer other drugs separately.

Adverse effects

- **CNS:** Ototoxicity, vestibular paralysis, confusion, disorientation, depression, lethargy, nystagmus, visual disturbances, headache, *numbness, tingling,* tremor, paresthesias, muscle twitching, seizures, muscular weakness, neuromuscular blockade
- **CV:** Palpitations, hypotension, hypertension
- **EENT:** Localized ocular toxicity and hypersensitivity reactions; *lid itching, swelling;* conjunctival erythema; punctate keratitis
- **GI:** Hepatic toxicity, *nausea, vomiting, anorexia,* weight loss, stomatitis, increased salivation
- **GU:** *Nephrotoxicity*
- **Hematologic:** Agranulocytosis, *leukemoid reaction,* granulocytosis, leukopenia, leukocytosis, thrombocytopenia, eosinophilia, pancytopenia, anemia, hemolytic anemia, increased or decreased reticulocyte count, electrolyte disturbances
- **Hypersensitivity:** *Purpura, rash,* urticaria, exfoliative dermatitis, itching
- **Local:** *Pain, irritation, arachnoiditis at IM injection sites*
- **Other:** Fever, apnea, splenomegaly, joint pain, *superinfections*

Interactions

✱ **Drug-drug** • Increased ototoxic, nephrotoxic, neurotoxic effects with other aminoglycosides, potent diuretics • Increased neuromuscular blockade and muscular paralysis with anesthetics, nondepolarizing neuromuscular blocking drugs, succinylcholine • Potential inactivation of both drugs if mixed with beta-lactam-type antibiotics • Increased bactericidal effect with penicillins, cephalosporins, carbenicillin, ticarcillin

■ Nursing considerations

Assessment

- **History:** Allergy to aminoglycosides, diminished hearing, decreased renal function, dehydration, neuromuscular disorders, lactation, pregnancy, infections (ophthalmic solutions)
- **Physical:** Weight; renal function, eighth cranial nerve function; state of hydration; hepatic function, CBC; skin color and lesions; orientation and affect; reflexes; bilateral grip strength; bowel sounds

Interventions

⊗ ***Black box warning*** Injection may cause serious ototoxicity, nephrotoxicity, and neurotoxicity. Monitor patient closely for changes in renal and CNS function.

- Arrange culture and sensitivity tests of infection before beginning therapy.

⊗ ***Warning*** Limit duration of treatment to short term to reduce the risk of toxicity; usual duration of treatment is 7–14 days.

- Use ophthalmologic tobramycin only when indicated by sensitivity tests; use of ophthalmologic tobramycin may cause sensitization that will contraindicate the systemic use of tobramycin or other aminoglycosides in serious infections.
- Monitor total serum concentration of tobramycin if ophthalmologic solution or inhaled tobramycin is used concurrently with parenteral aminoglycosides.
- Administer IM dose by deep IM injection.
- Administer nebulizer solution for 28 days; followed by 28 days of rest; have patient in upright position, inhale over 10–15 min.
- Ensure that patient is well hydrated before and during therapy.

Teaching points

Parenteral

- Report hearing changes, dizziness, pain at injection site.

Ophthalmic solution

- Tilt head back; place medication into conjunctival sac, and close eye; apply light finger pressure on lacrimal sac for 1 minute.
- Solution may cause blurring of vision or stinging on administration.
- Report severe stinging, itching, or burning.

Nebulizer solution

- Inhale over 10–15 minutes while in an upright position.
- Mark calendar with 28 days of using drug followed by 28 days without using drug.
- Store drug in refrigerator; do not expose to intense light.

▽tolazamide

See Appendix W, *Less commonly used drugs.*

▽tolbutamide

See Appendix W, *Less commonly used drugs.*

▽tolcapone

*(toll **kap'** own)*

Tasmar

PREGNANCY CATEGORY C

Drug classes

Antiparkinsonian
COMT inhibitor

Therapeutic actions

Selectively and reversibly inhibits COMT, an enzyme that eliminates biologically active catecholamines including dopa, dopamine, norepinephrine, epinephrine; when given with levodopa, tolcapone's inhibition of COMT is believed to increase the plasma concentrations and duration of action of levodopa.

Indications

- Adjunct with levodopa and carbidopa in the treatment of the signs and symptoms of idiopathic Parkinson's disease

Contraindications and cautions

- Contraindicated with hypersensitivity to drug or its components, lactation, liver disease, patients with a history of nontraumatic rhabdomyolysis or hyperpyrexia and confusion.
- Use cautiously with hypertension, hypotension, or renal impairment, pregnancy.

Available forms

Tablets—100, 200 mg

Dosages

Adults

Initial maintenance dosage, 100 mg PO tid. Maximum daily dose, 600 mg. 200 mg tid is more associated with liver enzyme elevation and is only recommended when benefit outweighs risk. However, 200 mg tid can be used if benefit is justified. If patient does not show a clinical benefit within 3 wk of treatment with 200 mg tid, tolcapone should be discontinued.

Pediatric patients

Safety and efficacy not established.

Patients with renal or hepatic impairment

Discontinue drug if liver enzyme values are greater than 2x upper limit of normal. Patients with moderate to severe hepatic impairment should not exceed 100 mg PO tid; patients with liver enzyme values greater than the upper limit of normal at initiation should not receive this drug. Use caution in patients with renal impairment.

Pharmacokinetics

Route	Onset	Peak
Oral	Varies	2 hr

Metabolism: Hepatic; $T_{1/2}$: 2–3 hr

Distribution: Crosses placenta; enters breast milk

Excretion: Feces, urine

Adverse effects

- **CNS:** *Disorientation, confusion,* memory loss, *hallucinations,* psychoses, agitation, nervousness, delusions, delirium, paranoia, euphoria, excitement, *light-headedness, dizziness,* depression, drowsiness, weakness, giddiness, paresthesia, heaviness of the limbs, numbness of fingers
- **CV:** Hypotension, orthostatic hypotension
- **Dermatologic:** Rash, urticaria, other dermatoses
- **GI:** Acute suppurative parotitis, *nausea, vomiting,* diarrhea, epigastric distress, flatulence, **fulminant and possibly fatal liver failure**
- **Respiratory:** URIs, dyspnea, sinus congestion
- **Other:** Muscular weakness, muscular cramping

Interactions

✱ **Drug-drug** • Risk of serious reaction if combined with MAOIs; avoid this combination

■ Nursing considerations

Assessment

- **History:** Hypersensitivity to drug or its components; hypertension, hypotension; hepatic or renal impairment; pregnancy, lactation
- **Physical:** Weight; T; skin color, lesions; orientation, affect, reflexes, bilateral grip strength, visual examination; P, BP, orthostatic BP, auscultation; bowel sounds, normal output, liver evaluation; urinary output, voiding pattern, LFTs, renal function tests

Interventions

- Administer in conjunction with levodopa and carbidopa. Monitor patient response; customary levodopa dosage may need to be decreased.

⊗ ***Black box warning*** Risk of potentially fatal acute fulminant liver failure exists. Monitor LFTs before and every 2 wk during therapy; discontinue drug at any sign of liver damage; use drug for patients no longer responding to other therapies.

- Provide sugarless lozenges or ice chips to suck if dry mouth is a problem.
- Give with meals if GI upset occurs; give before meals to patients bothered by dry mouth; give after meals if drooling is a problem or if drug causes nausea.

⊗ ***Warning*** Avoid abrupt withdrawal of drug, which can lead to more serious complications. Taper drug slowly over 2 wk if possible.

- Advise patient to use barrier contraceptives; serious birth defects can occur while using this drug. Advise nursing mothers to use another means of feeding the baby because drug can enter breast milk and adversely affect the infant.
- Establish safety precautions if CNS, vision changes, hallucinations, or hypotension occurs (eg, use side rails, accompany patient when ambulating).
- Provide additional comfort measures appropriate to patient with parkinsonism.

Teaching points

- Take this drug exactly as prescribed. Take in conjunction with your levodopa and carbidopa. Do not stop this drug suddenly; it must be tapered over 2 weeks.
- Use barrier contraceptives while using this drug, serious birth defects can occur. Do not nurse your baby while using this drug; the drug enters breast milk and can adversely affect the baby.
- You may experience these side effects: Drowsiness, dizziness, confusion, blurred vision (avoid driving a car or engaging in activities that require alertness and visual acuity if these occur; rise slowly when changing positions to help decrease dizziness); nausea (eat frequent small meals); dry mouth (suck sugarless lozenges or ice chips); hallucinations (it may help to know that this is a side effect of the drug; use care and have someone stay with you if this occurs); constipation (if maintaining adequate fluid intake and exercising regularly do not help, consult your health care provider).
- Report constipation, rapid or pounding heartbeat, confusion, eye pain, hallucinations, rash, changes in color of urine or stools, fever, chills, fatigue, yellowing of skin or eyes.

tolmetin sodium

(tole' met in)

PREGNANCY CATEGORY C

PREGNANCY CATEGORY D (3RD TRIMESTER)

Drug class

NSAID

Therapeutic actions

Anti-inflammatory, analgesic, and antipyretic activities largely related to inhibition or prostaglandin synthesis; exact mechanisms of action are not known.

Indications

- Treatment of acute flares and long-term management of rheumatoid arthritis and osteoarthritis
- Treatment of juvenile rheumatoid arthritis in patients older than 2 yr

Contraindications and cautions

- Contraindicated in patients with hypersensitivity to the drug or any of its components, in patients who have had reactions to aspirin or other NSAIDs, and with lactation.
- Use cautiously with allergies, renal, hepatic, CV and GI conditions, coagulation defects, patients taking anticoagulants, pregnancy.

Available forms

Tablets—200, 600 mg; capsules—400 mg

Dosages

Adults

Do not exceed 1,800 mg/day. Doses exceeding 1.8 g daily have not been studied. Subsequent dosing adjustment based on response and tolerance after 1–2 wk.

- *Rheumatoid arthritis or osteoarthritis:* Initial dose, 400 mg PO tid (1,200 mg/day) preferably including dose on arising and at bedtime. Maintenance dose, 600–1,800 mg/day in three to four divided doses for rheumatoid arthritis; 600–1,600 mg/day in three to four divided doses for osteoarthritis.

Pediatric patients 2 yr and older

Initially, 20 mg/kg/day PO in three to four divided doses; when control has been achieved, the usual dose is 15–30 mg/kg/day. Do not exceed 30 mg/kg/day.

Pharmacokinetics

Route	*Onset*	*Peak*
Oral	Varies	30–60 min

Metabolism: Hepatic; $T_{1/2}$: 2–7 hr
Distribution: Crosses placenta; enters breast milk
Excretion: Urine

Adverse effects

- **CNS:** *Headache, dizziness, somnolence, insomnia,* fatigue, tiredness, dizziness, tinnitus, *ophthalmologic effects,* weakness
- **Dermatologic:** *Rash,* pruritus, sweating, dry mucous membranes, stomatitis

- **GI:** *Nausea, dyspepsia, GI pain, diarrhea,* vomiting, constipation, flatulence
- **GU:** Dysuria, renal impairment, including renal failure, interstitial nephritis, hematuria
- **Hematologic:** Bleeding, platelet inhibition with higher doses, neutropenia, eosinophilia, *leukopenia,* pancytopenia, thrombocytopenia, agranulocytosis, granulocytopenia, aplastic anemia, decreased Hgb or Hct, bone marrow depression, *menorrhagia*
- **Respiratory:** Dyspnea, hemoptysis, pharyngitis, **bronchospasm,** rhinitis
- **Other:** Peripheral edema, **anaphylactoid reactions** to **fatal anaphylactic shock**

Interactions

✱ Drug-lab test • False-positive tests for proteinuria using acid precipitation tests; no interference has been reported with dye-impregnated reagent strips

■ Nursing considerations

Assessment

- **History:** Allergies; renal, hepatic, CV, and GI conditions; pregnancy, lactation
- **Physical:** Skin color, lesions; orientation, reflexes, ophthalmologic and audiometric evaluation, peripheral sensation; P, edema; R, adventitious sounds; liver evaluation; CBC, clotting times, LFTs, renal function tests; serum electrolytes, stool guaiac

Interventions

- Administer with milk if GI upset occurs; do not give with food—bioavailability is decreased by up to 16%.
- Use antacids other than sodium bicarbonate if GI upset occurs.
- Arrange for periodic ophthalmologic examination during long-term therapy.

⊗ ***Warning*** If overdose occurs, institute emergency procedures—gastric lavage, induction of emesis, supportive therapy.

⊗ ***Black box warning*** Be aware that patient may be at increased risk for CV event, GI bleeding; monitor accordingly.

Teaching points

- Take drug on an empty stomach; may be taken with milk or antacids other than sodium bicarbonate if GI upset occurs.
- Take only the prescribed dosage.
- You may experience these side effects: Dizziness, drowsiness (avoid driving or using dangerous machinery).
- Report sore throat, fever, rash, itching, weight gain, swelling in ankles or fingers; changes in vision; black, tarry stools.

▽ tolterodine tartrate

(toll tear' oh deen)

Detrol, Detrol LA DNC

PREGNANCY CATEGORY C

Drug class

Antimuscarinic

Therapeutic actions

Competitively blocks muscarinic receptor sites; bladder contraction is mediated by muscarinic receptors—blocking these receptors decreases bladder contraction.

Indications

- Treatment of overactive bladder in patients with symptoms of urinary frequency, urgency or incontinence

Contraindications and cautions

- Contraindicated with urinary retention, uncontrolled narrow-angle glaucoma, gastric retention, allergy to the drug or any of its components.
- Use cautiously with renal or hepatic impairment, pregnancy, lactation.

Available forms

Tablets—1, 2 mg; ER capsules DNC—2, 4 mg

Dosages

Adults

2 mg PO bid, may be lowered to 1 mg PO bid based on individual response; ER capsules—4 mg PO taken once daily; may be lowered to 2 mg once daily based on response.

Pediatric patients

Safety and efficacy not established.

Patients with hepatic and renal impairment

Reduce dosage to 1 mg PO bid (2 mg daily ER capsules) and monitor patient.

T

Pharmacokinetics

Route	Onset	Duration
Oral	1–2 hr	6–8 hr

Metabolism: Hepatic; $T_{1/2}$: 1.9–3.7 hr
Distribution: Crosses placenta; enters breast milk
Excretion: Urine

Adverse effects

- **CNS:** *Blurred vision,* headache, dizziness, somnolence
- **Dermatologic:** Pruritus, rash, erythema, dry skin
- **GI:** *Nausea, vomiting, constipation, dyspepsia,* flatulence, *dry mouth,* abdominal pain
- **GU:** *Dysuria,* urinary retention; impotence, UTIs
- **Other:** Weight gain, pain, fatigue, acute myopia and secondary angle closure glaucoma (pain, visual changes, redness, increased IOP)

Interactions

✱ Drug-drug • Risk of increased serum levels and toxicity if given with drugs that inhibit CYP2D6 (such as fluoxetine); reduce dose to 1 mg PO bid (2 mg daily ER capsules)

■ Nursing considerations

Assessment

- **History:** Urinary retention, uncontrolled narrow-angle glaucoma, allergy to the drug or any of its components, renal or hepatic impairment, pregnancy, lactation
- **Physical:** Bowel sounds, normal output; normal urinary output, prostate palpation; IOP, vision; LFTs, renal function tests; skin color, lesions, texture; weight

Interventions

- Ensure that patient does not cut, crush, or chew ER forms.
- Provide frequent small meals if GI upset is severe.
- Provide frequent mouth hygiene or skin care if dry mouth or skin occurs.
- Arrange for safety precautions if blurred vision occurs.
- Monitor bowel function and arrange for bowel program if constipation occurs.

Teaching points

- Take drug exactly as prescribed. Do not cut, crush, or chew ER forms.
- You may experience these side effects: Constipation (ensure adequate fluid intake, proper diet; consult your health care provider if this becomes a problem); dry mouth (suck sugarless lozenges, practice frequent mouth care; this effect sometimes lessens over time); blurred vision (it may help to know that these are drug effects that will go away when you discontinue the drug; avoid tasks that require acute vision); difficulty in urination (it may help to empty the bladder immediately before taking each dose of drug).
- Report rash, flushing, eye pain, difficulty breathing, tremors, loss of coordination, irregular heartbeat, palpitations, headache, abdominal distention.

▽ tolvaptan

See Appendix W, *Less commonly used drugs.*

▽ topiramate

*(toe **pie'** rah mate)*

Gen-Topiramate (CAN), PMS-Topiramate (CAN), ratio-Topiramate (CAN), Topamax DNC

PREGNANCY CATEGORY C

Drug classes

Antiepileptic
Antimigraine

Therapeutic actions

Mechanism of action not understood; antiepileptic effects may be due to the actions of blocking sodium channels in neurons with sustained depolarization; increasing GABA activity at receptors, thus potentiating the effects of this inhibitory neurotransmitter; and blocking excitatory neurotransmitters at neuron receptor sites.

Indications

- Monotherapy for the treatment of patients 10 yr and older with partial onset or primary generalized tonic-clonic seizures
- Adjunctive therapy for partial-onset seizure treatment in adults and children 2–16 yr
- Adjunctive therapy for seizures associated with Lennox-Gastaut syndrome in adults and children older than 2 yr
- Adjunctive therapy for primary generalized tonic-clonic seizures in adults and children 2–16 yr
- Prophylaxis of migraine headaches in adults
- Unlabeled uses: Cluster headaches, infantile spasms, alcohol dependence, bulimia nervosa, weight loss

Contraindications and cautions

- Contraindicated with hypersensitivity to any component of the drug.
- Use cautiously with pregnancy (use only if benefits outweigh potential risks to fetus), lactation, renal or hepatic impairment, renal stones, glaucoma.

Available forms

Tablets DNC—25, 50, 100, 200 mg; sprinkle capsules—15, 25 mg

Dosages

Adults 17 yr and older

- *Migraine prophylaxis:* Initially, 25 mg PO in the evening for 1 wk; week 2—25 mg PO bid, morning and evening; week 3—25 mg PO in the morning and 50 mg PO in the evening; week 4—50 mg PO morning and evening.
- *Seizure disorder:* 200–400 mg PO daily in two divided doses. Therapy should be initiated at a dose of 25–50 mg/day titrated up in increments of 25–50 mg/wk.

Patients 10 yr and older

- *Monotherapy:* 25 mg PO bid, titrating to maintenance dose of 200 mg PO bid over 6 wk. Week 1—25 mg bid; week 2—50 mg bid; week 3—75 mg bid; week 4—100 mg bid; week 5—150 mg bid; week 6—200 mg bid.

Pediatric patients 2–16 yr

5–9 mg/kg/day PO in two divided doses. Therapy should be initiated at a nightly dose of 25 mg (or less, based on 1–3 mg/kg/day) for the first week. The dose may be titrated up by increments of 1–3 mg/kg/day (administered in two divided doses) at 1–2 wk intervals.

Patients with hepatic or renal impairment

For creatinine clearance less than 70 mL/min, use one-half the usual dose; allow increased time to reach desired level. For patients with hepatic impairment, adjust slowly; monitor patient carefully.

Pharmacokinetics

Route	*Onset*	*Peak*
Oral	Rapid	2 hr

Metabolism: Hepatic; $T_{1/2}$: 21 hr
Distribution: Crosses placenta; enters breast milk
Excretion: Urine
Removed by hemodialysis: Supplemental dose may be needed

Adverse effects

- **CNS:** *Ataxia, somnolence, dizziness, nystagmus,* nervousness, anxiety, tremor, speech impairment, paresthesias, confusion, depression
- **GI:** *Nausea, dyspepsia,* anorexia, vomiting
- **GU:** Dysmenorrhea, renal stones
- **Hematologic:** Leukopenia
- **Respiratory:** *URI,* pharyngitis, sinusitis
- **Other:** *Fatigue,* rash, acute myopia and secondary angle-closure glaucoma (pain, visual disturbances, pupil dilation, redness, increased IOP), weight loss

Interactions

✱ **Drug-drug** • Increased CNS depression if taken with alcohol or CNS depressants; use extreme caution • Increased risk of renal stone development with carbonic anhydrase inhibitors • Decreased effects of hormonal contraceptives with topiramate; suggest use of barrier contraceptives instead • Decreased serum levels if combined with phenytoin, carbamazepine, valproic acid

■ Nursing considerations

CLINICAL ALERT!
Name confusion has occurred between *Topamax* and *Toprol-XL* (metoprolol); use caution.

Assessment

- **History:** Hypersensitivity to any component of the drug; pregnancy, lactation; renal or hepatic impairment, renal stones
- **Physical:** Skin color, lesions; orientation, affect, reflexes, vision examination; R, adventitious sounds; LFTs, renal function tests

Interventions

⊗ *Warning* Reduce dosage; discontinue or substitute other antiepileptic gradually; abrupt discontinuation may precipitate status epilepticus.

⊗ *Warning* There is an increased risk of suicidality with drug administration; monitor patient accordingly.

⊗ *Warning* Stop the drug immediately and arrange for appropriate consultations at first sign of blurred vision, periorbital edema, or redness.

- Administer with food if GI upset occurs.
- Caution patient not to chew or break tablets because of bitter taste.
- Have patient swallow sprinkle capsules whole or by carefully opening capsule and sprinkling onto a soft food. Swallow this immediately; do not allow it to be chewed.
- Encourage patients with a history of renal stone development to maintain adequate fluid intake while using this drug.
- Suggest using barrier contraceptives to patients taking this drug.
- Arrange for consultation with appropriate epilepsy support groups as needed.

Teaching points

- Take this drug exactly as prescribed. Do not break or chew tablets; they have a very bitter taste. Sprinkle capsule may also be swallowed whole. If using sprinkle capsules, open carefully and sprinkle onto soft food and swallow immediately; do not chew.
- Do not discontinue this drug abruptly or change dosage except on the advice of your health care provider.
- Arrange for frequent check-ups to monitor your response to this drug. It is very important that you keep all appointments for check-ups.
- Wear or carry medical identification at all times so that any emergency medical personnel will know that you have epilepsy and are taking antiepileptic medication.
- Avoid using alcohol while you are taking this drug; serious sedation could occur.
- You may experience these side effects: Drowsiness, dizziness, sleepiness (avoid driving or performing other tasks that require alertness; symptoms may occur initially but usually disappear with continued therapy); vision changes (avoid performing tasks that require visual acuity); GI upset (take drug with food; eat frequent small meals).
- Report fatigue, vision changes, speech problems, personality changes, thoughts of suicide.

▽topotecan hydrochloride

See Appendix W, *Less commonly used drugs.*

DANGEROUS DRUG

▽toremifene citrate

(tore em' ah feen)

Fareston

PREGNANCY CATEGORY D

Drug classes

Antineoplastic
Estrogen receptor modulator

Therapeutic actions

Binds to estrogen receptors, has anti-estrogen effects, and inhibits growth of estrogen receptorpositive and estrogen receptor-negative breast cancer cell lines.

Indications

- Treatment of advanced breast cancer in postmenopausal women with estrogen receptor–positive disease or estrogen-receptor unknown tumors

Contraindications and cautions

- Contraindicated with allergy to toremifene, history of thromboembolic disorder, pregnancy, lactation.

- Use cautiously with history of hypercalcemia, hepatic impairment, pre-existing endometrial hyperplasia.

Available forms

Tablets—60 mg

Dosages

Adults

60 mg PO daily; continue until disease progression occurs.

Pharmacokinetics

Route	*Onset*	*Peak*
Oral	Rapid	1–6 hr

Metabolism: Hepatic; $T_{1/2}$: 5–6 days
Distribution: Crosses placenta; enters breast milk
Excretion: Feces, urine

Adverse effects

- **CNS:** Depression, light-headedness, *dizziness,* headache, hallucinations, vertigo
- **Dermatologic:** *Hot flashes, skin rash*
- **GI:** *Nausea, vomiting,* food distaste
- **GU:** Vaginal bleeding, vaginal discharge
- **Other:** Peripheral edema, hypercalcemia, cataracts, sweating, thrombophlebitis, pulmonary embolism

Interactions

✸ **Drug-drug** • Increased risk of bleeding if taken with oral anticoagulants; monitor the patient's INR

■ Nursing considerations

Assessment

- **History:** Allergy to toremifene, pregnancy, lactation, hypercalcemia, hepatic impairment, thromboembolism history and pre-existing endometrial hyperplasia
- **Physical:** Skin lesions, color, turgor; pelvic examination; orientation, affect, reflexes; BP, peripheral pulses, edema; LFTs, serum electrolytes

Interventions

- Administer daily without regard to food.
- Counsel patient about the need to use contraceptive measures while taking this drug; inform patient that serious fetal harm could occur.
- Provide comfort measures to help patient deal with drug effects: Hot flashes (control temperature of environment); headache, depression (monitor light and noise); vaginal bleeding (use hygiene measures).

Teaching points

- Take this drug as prescribed.
- This drug can cause serious fetal harm and must not be taken during pregnancy. Barrier contraceptives should be used while you are taking this drug. If you become pregnant or decide that you want to become pregnant, consult your health care provider immediately.
- You may experience these side effects: Hot flashes (stay in cool places); nausea, vomiting (eat frequent small meals); weight gain; dizziness, headache, light-headedness (use caution if driving or performing tasks that require alertness).
- Report marked weakness, sleepiness, mental confusion, changes in color of urine or stool, rash, vision changes.

▽torsemide

(tor' seh myde)

Demadex

PREGNANCY CATEGORY B

Drug classes

Loop (high-ceiling) diuretic
Sulfonamide

Therapeutic actions

Inhibits the reabsorption of sodium and chloride from the proximal and distal renal tubules and the loop of Henle, leading to a natriuretic diuresis.

Indications

- Treatment of hypertension and edema associated with HF, hepatic cirrhosis, renal failure

Contraindications and cautions

- Contraindicated with allergy to torsemide; known hypersensitivity to sulfonylureas; anuria, severe renal failure; hepatic coma.

- Use cautiously with SLE, electrolyte depletion, gout, diabetes mellitus, lactation, pregnancy.

Available forms

Tablets—5, 10, 20, 100 mg; injection—10 mg/mL

Dosages

Adults

⊗ ***Warning*** Do not exceed 200 mg/day.

- *HF:* 10–20 mg PO or IV daily. Dose may be titrated upward by doubling the dose until desired results are seen. Do not exceed 200 mg/day.
- *Chronic renal failure:* 20 mg PO or IV daily. Dose may be titrated upward by doubling the dose until desired results are seen. Do not exceed 200 mg/day.
- *Hepatic failure:* 5–10 mg PO or IV daily. Do not exceed 40 mg/day.
- *Hypertension:* 5 mg PO daily. May be increased to 10 mg if response is not sufficient.

Pediatric patients

Safety and efficacy not established.

Pharmacokinetics

Route	*Onset*	*Peak*	*Duration*
Oral	60 min	60–120 min	6–8 hr
IV	10 min	60 min	6–8 hr

Metabolism: Hepatic; $T_{1/2}$: 210 min
Distribution: Crosses placenta; may enter breast milk
Excretion: Urine

IV FACTS

Preparation: May be given direct IV over 2 min or diluted in solution with D_5W, 0.9% sodium chloride, 0.45% sodium chloride. Discard unused solution after 24 hr.
Infusion: Give by direct injection slowly, over 1–2 min. Further diluted in solution, give slowly, each 200 mg over 2 min.

Adverse effects

- **CNS:** *Asterixis, dizziness,* vertigo, paresthesias, confusion, fatigue, nystagmus, *weakness, headache, drowsiness,* fatigue, blurred vision, tinnitus, irreversible hearing loss
- **CV:** *Orthostatic hypotension,* volume depletion, cardiac arrhythmias, thrombophlebitis
- **GI:** *Nausea, anorexia, vomiting, diarrhea,* gastric irritation and pain, dry mouth, acute pancreatitis, jaundice, polydipsia
- **GU:** *Polyuria, nocturia,* glycosuria, renal failure
- **Hematologic:** *Hypokalemia,* leukopenia, anemia, thrombocytopenia, hyperuricemia, hypoglycemia
- **Local:** *Pain, phlebitis at injection site*
- **Other:** Muscle cramps and muscle spasms, weakness, arthritic pain, fatigue, hives, photosensitivity, rash, pruritus, sweating, nipple tenderness, impotence

Interactions

✱ Drug-drug • Decreased diuresis and natriuresis with NSAIDs • Increased risk of cardiac glycoside toxicity (secondary to hypokalemia) • Increased risk of ototoxicity with aminoglycoside antibiotics, cisplatin, ethacrynic acid

■ Nursing considerations

Assessment

- **History:** Allergy to torsemide, sulfonylurea; electrolyte depletion; anuria; severe renal failure; hepatic coma; SLE; gout; diabetes mellitus; lactation, pregnancy
- **Physical:** Skin color, lesions; edema; orientation, reflexes, hearing; pulses, baseline ECG, BP, orthostatic BP, perfusion; R, pattern, adventitious sounds; liver evaluation, bowel sounds; urinary output patterns; CBC, serum electrolytes, blood sugar, LFTs, renal function tests, uric acid, urinalysis

Interventions

- Administer with food or milk to prevent GI upset.
- Mark calendars or other reminders of drug days if intermittent therapy is optimal for treating edema.
- Administer single daily doses early in the day so increased urination will not disturb sleep.
- Avoid IV use if oral use is at all possible.
- Measure and record regular weights to monitor fluid changes.

- Monitor serum electrolytes, hydration, and liver function during long-term therapy.
- Provide diet rich in potassium or give supplemental potassium.

Teaching points

- Record alternate-day or intermittent therapy on a calendar or dated envelopes.
- Take the drug early in the day so increased urination will not disturb sleep.
- Take the drug with food or meals to prevent GI upset.
- Weigh yourself on a regular basis, at the same time and in the same clothing, and record the weight on your calendar.
- You may experience these side effects: Increased volume and frequency of urination; dizziness, feeling faint on arising, drowsiness (avoid rapid position changes, driving a car and other hazardous activities, and alcohol consumption); sensitivity to sunlight (use sunglasses and sunscreen; wear protective clothing when outdoors); increased thirst (suck sugarless lozenges; practice frequent mouth care); loss of body potassium (a potassium-rich diet, or even a potassium supplement, will be needed).
- Report weight change of more than 3 pounds in 1 day; swelling in ankles or fingers; unusual bleeding or bruising; nausea, dizziness, trembling, numbness, fatigue; muscle weakness or cramps.

▽tositumomab and iodine I-131 tositumomab

See Appendix W, *Less commonly used drugs.*

DANGEROUS DRUG

▽tramadol hydrochloride

(tram' ah doll)

Ryzolt DNC, Ultram, Ultram ER DNC

Pregnancy Category C

Drug classes

Analgesic (centrally acting)
Opioid analgesic

Therapeutic actions

Binds to mu-opioid receptors and inhibits the reuptake of norepinephrine and serotonin; causes many effects similar to the opioids—dizziness, somnolence, nausea, constipation—but does not have the respiratory depressant effects.

Indications

- Relief of moderate to moderately severe pain
- Relief of moderate to severe chronic pain in adults who need around-the-clock treatment for extended periods (ER tablets)
- Unlabeled uses: Premature ejaculation; restless leg syndrome

Contraindications and cautions

- Contraindicated with allergy to tramadol or opioids or acute intoxication with alcohol, opioids, or psychoactive drugs.
- Use cautiously with pregnancy, lactation; seizures; concomitant use of CNS depressants, MAOIs, SSRIs, TCAs; renal impairment; hepatic impairment.

Available forms

Tablets—50 mg; ER tablets DNC—100, 200, 300 mg

Dosages

Adults

Patients who require rapid analgesic effect: 50–100 mg PO every 4–6 hr; do not exceed 400 mg/day.

Patients with moderate to moderately severe chronic pain: Initiate at 25 mg/day in the morning, and titrate in 25-mg increments every 3 days to reach 100 mg/day. Then, increase in 50-mg increments every 3 days to reach 200 mg/day. After titration, 50–100 mg every 4–6 hr; do not exceed 400 mg/day. Alternatively, 100-mg ER tablet once daily, titrated by 100-mg increments every 5 days; do not exceed 300 mg/day.

Pediatric patients

Safety and efficacy not established.

Geriatric patients or patients with hepatic or renal impairment

Older than 75 yr: Do not exceed 300 mg/day. *Patients with cirrhosis:* 50 mg every 12 hr. ER tablets should not be used in severe hepatic impairment (Child-Pugh class C).

T

Patients with creatinine clearance less than 30 mL/min: 50–100 mg PO every 12 hr. Maximum 200 mg/day. ER tablets should not be used in patients with creatinine clearance less than 30 ml/min.

Pharmacokinetics

Route	*Onset*	*Peak*
Oral	1 hr	2 hr

Metabolism: Hepatic; $T_{1/2}$: 6–7 hr
Distribution: Crosses placenta; enters breast milk
Excretion: Urine

Adverse effects

- **CNS:** *Sedation, dizziness or vertigo, headache,* confusion, dreaming, sweating, anxiety, **seizures**
- **CV:** *Hypotension,* tachycardia, bradycardia
- **Dermatologic:** *Sweating,* pruritus, rash, pallor, urticaria
- **GI:** *Nausea, vomiting,* dry mouth, constipation, flatulence
- **Other:** Potential for abuse, **anaphylactoid reactions**

Interactions

✱ **Drug-drug** • Decreased effectiveness with carbamazepine • Increased risk of tramadol toxicity with MAOIs or SSRIs

■ Nursing considerations

Assessment

- **History:** Hypersensitivity to tramadol; pregnancy; acute intoxication with alcohol, opioids, psychotropic drugs or other centrally acting analgesics; lactation; seizures; concomitant use of CNS depressants or MAOIs; renal or hepatic impairment; past or present history of opioid addiction
- **Physical:** Skin color, texture, lesions; orientation, reflexes, bilateral grip strength, affect; P, auscultation, BP; bowel sounds, normal output; LFTs, renal function tests

Interventions

- Control environment (temperature, lighting) if sweating or CNS effects occur.
- Ensure that patient does not cut, crush, or chew ER tablets.

⊗ ***Warning*** Limit use in patients with past or present history of addiction to or dependence on opioids.

Teaching points

- Do not cut, crush, or chew ER tablets; swallow them whole.
- You may experience these side effects: Dizziness, sedation, drowsiness, impaired visual acuity (avoid driving or performing tasks that require alertness); nausea, loss of appetite (lie quietly, eat frequent small meals).
- Report severe nausea, dizziness, severe constipation.

▽ trandolapril

*(tran **dole'** ah pril)*

Mavik

PREGNANCY CATEGORY C (FIRST TRIMESTER)

PREGNANCY CATEGORY D (SECOND AND THIRD TRIMESTERS)

Drug classes

ACE inhibitor
Antihypertensive

Therapeutic actions

Blocks ACE from converting angiotensin I to angiotensin II, a powerful vasoconstrictor, leading to decreased BP, decreased aldosterone secretion, a small increase in serum potassium levels, and sodium and fluid loss; increased prostaglandin synthesis may also be involved in the antihypertensive action.

Indications

- Treatment of hypertension, alone or in combination with other antihypertensives
- Treatment of post-MI patients with evidence of left-ventricular dysfunction and symptoms of HF
- Unlabeled use: Diabetic nephropathy

Contraindications and cautions

- Contraindicated with allergy to ACE inhibitors, history of ACE-associated angioedema.
- Use cautiously with impaired renal function, HF, CAD, salt or volume depletion, surgery, pregnancy, lactation, renal artery stenosis.

Available forms

Tablets—1, 2, 4 mg

Dosages

Adults

- *Hypertension:* African-American patients: 2 mg PO daily. All other patients: 1 mg PO daily. For maintenance, 2–4 mg/day. Maximum, 8 mg.
- *Patients on diuretics:* To prevent hypotension, stop diuretic 2–3 days before beginning trandolapril. Resume diuretic only if BP is not controlled. If diuretic cannot be discontinued, start at 0.5 mg PO daily and adjust upward as needed.
- *HF post-MI:* May start therapy 3 to 5 days after the MI. 1 mg/day PO; adjust to a target of 4 mg/day.

Pediatric patients

Safety and efficacy not established.

Patients with renal or hepatic impairment

0.5 mg PO daily, adjust at 1-wk intervals to control BP; usual range is 2–4 mg PO daily.

Pharmacokinetics

Route	*Peak*	*Duration*
Oral	3–4 hr	24 hr

Metabolism: $T_{1/2}$: 14–16 hr
Distribution: Crosses placenta; enters breast milk
Excretion: Feces, urine

Adverse effects

- **CNS:** Headache, fatigue
- **CV:** *Tachycardia,* angina pectoris, **MI,** HF, Raynaud's syndrome, hypotension in salt- or volume-depleted patients
- **Dermatologic:** *Rash*
- **GI:** *Diarrhea,* GI upset
- **GU:** Renal insufficiency, renal failure, polyuria, oliguria, urinary frequency, UTI
- **Other:** *Cough, dizziness,* malaise, dry mouth

Interactions

✱ **Drug-drug** • Excessive hypotension may occur with diuretics; monitor closely • Hyperkalemia may occur with potassium supplements, potassium-sparing diuretics, salt substitutes; monitor serum potassium levels • Potential increase in lithium levels if taken concurrently; decreased lithium dose may be needed

■ Nursing considerations

Assessment

- **History:** Allergy to ACE inhibitors, impaired renal or hepatic function, CAD, HF, salt or volume depletion, surgery, pregnancy, lactation
- **Physical:** Skin color, lesions, turgor; T; P, BP, peripheral perfusion; mucous membranes, bowel sounds, liver evaluation; urinalysis, LFTs, renal function tests, CBC and differential

Interventions

⊗ ***Black box warning*** Ensure that patient is not pregnant before administering; advise patient to use barrier contraceptives.

- Administer once a day at same time each day.

⊗ ***Warning*** Alert surgeon and mark the patient's chart with notice that trandolapril is being taken; angiotensin II formation subsequent to compensatory renin release during surgery will need to be blocked; hypotension may be reversed with volume expansion.

- Monitor patient closely in any situation that may lead to fall in BP secondary to reduction in fluid volume—excessive perspiration and dehydration, vomiting, diarrhea—as excessive hypotension may occur.
- Reduce dosage in patients with impaired renal or hepatic function.

⊗ ***Warning*** Discontinue immediately if laryngeal edema, angioedema, or jaundice occurs.

Teaching points

- Take drug once a day at generally the same time each day. Do not stop taking this medication without consulting your health care provider.
- This drug cannot be used during pregnancy; using barrier contraceptives is recommended.

- Be careful in situations that may lead to drop in blood pressure (diarrhea, sweating, vomiting, dehydration); if light-headedness or dizziness occurs, consult your health care provider.
- While taking this drug, avoid using over-the-counter medications, especially cough, cold, or allergy medications; they may contain ingredients that will interact with this drug. If you feel that you need one of these preparations, consult your health care provider.
- You may experience these side effects: GI upset, diarrhea (limited effects that will pass); dizziness, light-headedness (usually passes after first few days; change position slowly and limit your activities to those that do not require alertness and precision); cough (can be very irritating and does not respond to cough suppressants; notify health care provider if very uncomfortable).
- Report sore throat, fever, chills; swelling of the hands or feet; irregular heartbeat, chest pains; swelling of the face, eyes, lips, tongue; difficulty breathing; yellowing of skin.

tranexamic acid

See Appendix W, *Less commonly used drugs.*

tranylcypromine sulfate

*(tran ill **sip'** roe meen)*

Parnate

Pregnancy Category C

Drug classes
Antidepressant
MAOI

Therapeutic actions
Irreversibly inhibits MAO, an enzyme that breaks down biogenic amines, such as epinephrine, norepinephrine, and serotonin, allowing these biogenic amines to accumulate in neuronal storage sites; according to the biogenic amine hypothesis, this accumulation of amines is responsible for the clinical efficacy of MAOIs as antidepressants.

Indications
- Treatment of adult outpatients with a major depressive episode without melancholia; efficacy in endogenous depression has not been established
- Unlabeled uses: Migraine headache, panic disorder, social anxiety disorder, bipolar depression, Alzheimer's disease, Parkinson's disease

Contraindications and cautions
- Contraindicated with hypersensitivity to any MAOI; pheochromocytoma, HF; history of liver disease or abnormal LFTs; severe renal impairment; confirmed or suspected cerebrovascular defect; CV disease, hypertension; history of headache (headache is an indicator of hypertensive reaction to drug); myelography within previous 24 hr or scheduled within 48 hr; lactation; patients scheduled for elective surgery (MAOIs should be discontinued 10 days before surgery).
- Use cautiously with seizure disorders; hyperthyroidism; impaired hepatic, renal function; psychiatric patients (agitated or schizophrenic patients may show excessive stimulation; bipolar patients may shift to hypomanic or manic phase); pregnancy or in women of childbearing age.

Available forms
Tablets—10 mg

Dosages
Adults
Usual effective dose is 30 mg/day PO in divided doses. If no improvement is seen within 2–3 wk, increase dosage in 10 mg/day increments every 1–3 wk. May be increased to a maximum of 60 mg/day.
Pediatric patients
Not recommended for patients younger than 16 yr.
Geriatric patients
Patients older than 60 yr are more prone to develop side effects; use with caution.

Pharmacokinetics

Route	*Onset*	*Duration*
Oral	Rapid	3–5 days

Metabolism: Hepatic; $T_{1/2}$: Unknown
Distribution: Crosses placenta; enters breast milk
Excretion: Urine

Adverse effects

- **CNS:** *Dizziness, vertigo, headache, overactivity, hyperreflexia, tremors, muscle twitching, mania, hypomania, jitteriness, confusion, memory impairment, insomnia, weakness, fatigue, drowsiness, restlessness, overstimulation, increased anxiety, agitation, blurred vision, sweating,* akathisia, ataxia, coma, euphoria, neuritis, repetitious babbling, chills, glaucoma, nystagmus
- **CV: Hypertensive crises, sometimes fatal,** sometimes with intracranial bleeding, usually attributable to tyramine ingestion (see Drug–food interactions); symptoms include occipital headache, which may radiate frontally; palpitations; neck stiffness or soreness; nausea; vomiting; sweating (sometimes with fever, cold and clammy skin); dilated pupils; photophobia; tachycardia or bradycardia; chest pain; *orthostatic hypotension, sometimes associated with falling; disturbed cardiac rate and rhythm,* palpitations, tachycardia
- **Dermatologic:** Minor skin reactions, spider telangiectases, photosensitivity
- **GI:** *Constipation, diarrhea, nausea, abdominal pain, edema, dry mouth, anorexia, weight changes*
- **GU:** Dysuria, incontinence, urinary retention, sexual disturbances
- **Other:** Hematologic changes, black tongue, hypernatremia

Interactions

✱ Drug-drug ⊗ *Warning* Potentially dangerous hypotension with general anesthetics; avoid this combination.
• Increased sympathomimetic effects (hypertensive crisis) with sympathomimetic drugs (norepinephrine, epinephrine, dopamine, dobutamine, levodopa, ephedrine), amphetamines, other anorexiants, local anesthetic solutions containing sympathomimetics • Hypertensive crisis, coma, severe seizures with TCAs (eg, imipramine, desipramine) • Additive hypoglycemic effect with insulin, oral sulfonylureas (eg, tolbutamide) • Increased risk of adverse interactive actions with meperidine • Reduce dose of barbiturates if given with MAOIs • Toxic levels of buspirone and bupropion if combined with MAOIs; separate use by 10 or 14 days, respectively • Increased hypertension effects with carbamazepine, levodopa • Risk of hypotension with thiazide diuretics • Serious, sometimes fatal, reactions with SSRIs; separate use by 5 wk with fluoxetine, 2 wk with sertraline and paroxetine

✱ Drug-food ⊗ *Warning* Tyramine (and other pressor amines) contained in foods are normally broken down by MAO enzymes in the GI tract; in the presence of MAOIs, these vasopressors may be absorbed in high concentrations; in addition, tyramine releases accumulated norepinephrine from nerve terminals; thus, hypertensive crisis may occur when the following foods that contain tyramine or other vasopressors are ingested by a patient on an MAOI: Dairy products (blue, camembert, cheddar, mozzarella, parmesan, Romano, Roquefort, Stilton cheeses; sour cream; yogurt); meats, fish (liver, pickled herring, fermented sausages [bologna, pepperoni, salami], caviar, dried fish, other fermented or spoiled meat or fish); undistilled beverages (imported beer, ale; red wine, especially Chianti; sherry; coffee, tea, colas containing caffeine; chocolate drinks); fruits, vegetables (avocado, fava beans, figs, raisins, bananas, yeast extracts, soy sauce, chocolate).

■ Nursing considerations

Assessment

- **History:** Hypersensitivity to any MAOI; pheochromocytoma; HF; abnormal LFTs; severe renal impairment; confirmed or suspected cerebrovascular defect; CV disease, hypertension; history of headache; myelography within previous 24 hr or scheduled within 48 hr; lactation; seizure disorders; hyperthyroidism; impaired hepatic, renal function; psychiatric disorder; scheduled elective surgery; pregnancy
- **Physical:** Weight; T; skin color, lesions; orientation, affect, reflexes, vision; P, BP, orthostatic BP, perfusion; bowel sounds, normal output, liver evaluation; urine flow,

normal output; LFTs, renal function tests, urinalysis, CBC, ECG, EEG

Interventions

⊠ ***Black box warning*** Limit amount of drug available to suicidal patients; possible increased risk of suicidality in children, adolescents, and young adults; monitor accordingly.

- Monitor BP and orthostatic BP carefully; arrange for more gradual increase in dosage initially in patients who show tendency for hypotension.

⊗ ***Warning*** Arrange for periodic LFTs during therapy; discontinue drug at first sign of hepatic impairment or jaundice.

- Monitor BP carefully (and if appropriate, discontinue drug) if patient reports unusual or severe headache.

⊗ ***Warning*** Keep phentolamine or another alpha-adrenergic blocking drug readily available in case of hypertensive crisis.

Teaching points

- Take drug exactly as prescribed.
- Do not stop taking drug abruptly or without consulting your health care provider.
- Avoid ingesting tyramine-containing foods or beverages while using this drug and for 10 days afterward (patient and significant other should receive a list of such foods and beverages; see Appendix D, *Important dietary guidelines for patient teaching*).
- You may experience these side effects: Dizziness, weakness or fainting when arising from a horizontal or sitting position (transient; change position slowly); drowsiness, blurred vision (reversible; safety measures may need to be taken if severe; avoid driving or performing tasks that require alertness); nausea, vomiting, loss of appetite (frequent small meals, frequent mouth care may help); nightmares, confusion, inability to concentrate, emotional changes; changes in sexual function.
- Report headache, rash, darkening of the urine, pale stools, yellowing of the eyes or skin, fever, chills, sore throat, or any other unusual symptoms, thoughts of suicide.

DANGEROUS DRUG

▽trastuzumab

*(trass too **zoo'** mab)*

Herceptin

PREGNANCY CATEGORY D

Drug classes

Antineoplastic
Monoclonal antibody

Therapeutic actions

Humanoid anticlonal antibody to the human epidermal growth factor receptor 2 (HER2) protein. This protein is often overexpressed in patients with aggressive, metastatic breast cancer.

Indications

- Treatment of metastatic breast cancer with tumors that overexpress HER2 protein (a genetic defect) as a first-line therapy in combination with paclitaxel and as a single agent in second- and third-line therapy
- Adjunct treatment of patients with HER2-overexpressing breast cancer in combination with doxorubicin, cyclophosphamide, and paclitaxel

Contraindications and cautions

- Contraindicated with allergy to trastuzumab or any component of the drug, breast cancers without HER2 overexpression.
- Use cautiously with known cardiac disease, bone marrow depression, lactation, pregnancy.

Available forms

Powder for injection—440 mg

Dosages

Adults

Initially, 4 mg/kg IV once by IV infusion over 90 min. For maintenance, 2 mg/kg IV once weekly over at least 30 min as tolerated. Do not exceed 500 mg/dose.

Combination therapy: After completion of doxorubicin and cyclophosphamide therapy, give trastuzumab weekly for 52 wk. During the first 12 wk, give trastuzumab with paclitaxel.

Pharmacokinetics

Route	Onset	Duration
IV	Slow	Days

Metabolism: Tissue; $T_{1/2}$: 2–9 days
Distribution: Crosses placenta, may enter breast milk

IV FACTS

Preparation: Reconstitute powder with diluent provided; dilute in 250 mL 0.9% sodium chloride injection. Solution should be colorless to pale yellow. Solution is stable for 28 days after reconstitution with diluent provided. Must write expiration date on vial (28 days after reconstitution).
Infusion: Infuse initial dose over 90 min; maintenance doses may be infused over 30 min.
Incompatibilities: Do not mix with any other drug solution or add any other drugs to the IV line.

Adverse effects

- **CNS:** Malaise, headache, tremor, insomnia, paresthesia
- **CV: Serious cardiac toxicity**
- **GI:** Vomiting, nausea, *diarrhea, abdominal pain*
- **Other:** *Anemia,* pain, edema, *increased susceptibility to infection, leukopenia, local reaction at infusion site, infusion reaction* (flushing, sweating, chills, fever), *fever, chills,* hypersensitivity reactions, myalgia, rash, pulmonary toxicity

■ Nursing considerations

Assessment

- **History:** Allergy to trastuzumab or any component of the product; known cardiac disease, bone marrow depression; pregnancy, lactation
- **Physical:** T; P, BP; R, adventitious sounds; baseline ECG; orientation, affect, CBC with differential, tumor testing for HER2 status

Interventions

⊗ ***Black box warning*** Monitor patient at time of infusion and provide comfort measures and analgesics as appropriate if infusion reaction occurs.

⊗ ***Black box warning*** Monitor cardiac status, especially if patient is receiving chemotherapy. Keep emergency equipment readily available if cardiac toxicity occurs; cardiomyopathy may occur.

⊗ ***Black box warning*** Monitor patient for possibly severe pulmonary toxicity, especially within 24 hours of infusion. Discontinue at signs or symptoms of respiratory involvement.

- Protect patient from exposure to infections and maintain sterile technique for invasive procedures.

Teaching points

- This drug is given IV to help fight your breast cancer. It will be given once a week. Mark a calendar with return dates for repeat infusion.
- Avoid infection while you are using this drug; stay away from crowded areas and people with known infections.
- You may experience these side effects: Discomfort, sweating, fever during infusion (comfort measures and analgesics may help); diarrhea, nausea, abdominal pain.
- Report chest pain, difficulty breathing, chills, fever.

▽trazodone hydrochloride

See Appendix W, *Less commonly used drugs.*

▽treprostinil sodium

*(tra **pros'** tin ill)*

Remodulin, Tyvaso

PREGNANCY CATEGORY B

Drug classes

Endothelin receptor antagonist
Prostacyclin analogue (vasodilating drug)

Therapeutic actions

Specifically blocks receptor sites for endothelin (ET_A and ET_B) in the endothelium and vascular smooth muscles; these endothelins are elevated in plasma and lung tissue of patients with pulmonary arterial hypertension; also inhibits platelet aggregation.

T

Indications

- Treatment of pulmonary arterial hypertension in patients with class II–class IV symptoms, to improve exercise ability and to decrease the rate of clinical worsening
- To diminish the rate of deterioration in patients undergoing transition from epoprostenol (*Flolan*)

Contraindications and cautions

- Contraindicated with allergy to treprostinil or any component of the drug.
- Use cautiously in elderly patients and with hepatic or renal impairment, lactation, pregnancy.

Available forms

Multi-use vials—1, 2.5, 5, 10 mg/mL; solution for inhalation—0.6 mg/mL

Dosages

Adults

Administered by continuous subcutaneous infusion. Initially the rate is 1.25 nanograms/kg/min. If this initial dose cannot be tolerated, the infusion rate should be reduced to 0.625 nanograms/kg/min. Rate is increased in increments of no more than 1.25 nanograms/kg/min/wk for the first 4 wk, then by 2.5 nanograms/kg/min/wk. Do not exceed 40 nanograms/kg/min. Dosage is based on clinical response and patient tolerance. Abrupt withdrawal or significant decrease in dosage may result in worsening symptoms. See the manufacturer's instructions for infusion weight charts.

- *Transition from Flolan:* Base rate of change on individual patient response. Start *Remodulin* infusion at 10% of starting *Flolan* dose. Decrease *Flolan* to 80% starting dose and increase *Remodulin* dose to 30% starting *Flolan* dose. Decrease *Flolan* dose to 60% starting and increase *Remodulin* dose to 50% starting *Flolan* dose. Decrease *Flolan* dose to 40% starting dose and increase *Remodulin* dose to 70% starting *Flolan* dose. Decrease *Flolan* dose to 20% starting dose and increase *Remodulin* dose to 90% starting *Flolan* dose. Decrease *Flolan* dose to 5% starting dose and increase *Remodulin* dose to 110% starting *Flolan* dose. Discontinue *Flolan* and continue *Remodulin* dose at 110% of *Flolan* starting dose plus an additional 5–10% as needed.
- *Inhalation:* Initially, 3 breaths (18 mcg), using *Tyvaso* Inhalation System, per treatment session; 4 sessions per day, approximately 4 hr apart during waking hours. Increase by additional 3 breaths per session at 1- to 2-wk intervals if needed and tolerated. Maintenance dose, 9 breaths (54 mcg) per session.

Pediatric patients

Safety and efficacy not established.

Patients with hepatic impairment

Decrease initial dose to 0.625 nanograms/kg/min and increase slowly.

Pharmacokinetics

Route	Onset	Peak
Subcut.	Gradual	10 hr

Metabolism: Hepatic; $T_{1/2}$: 2–4 hr
Distribution: Crosses placenta; may enter breast milk
Excretion: Feces, urine

Adverse effects

- **CNS:** *Headache,* dizziness
- **CV:** Vasodilation, edema, hypotension, dyspnea, chest pain
- **GI:** *Nausea, diarrhea,* vomiting
- **Skin:** Pruritus, *rash*
- **Other:** *Pain at injection site, local reaction at infusion site,* increased bleeding, *jaw pain*

Interactions

✱ **Drug-drug** • Potential for increased hypotensive effects if combined with other drugs that decrease BP; monitor patient carefully • Potential for increased bleeding tendencies if combined with drugs that alter blood clotting or inhibit platelets

■ Nursing considerations

Assessment

- **History:** Allergy to treprostinil or any component of the drug, hepatic or renal impairment, pregnancy, lactation, advanced age

- **Physical:** Skin color, lesions; injection site; orientation, BP; LFTs, renal function tests, CBC

Interventions

- Evaluate the patient for the ability to accept, place, and care for a subcutaneous catheter and to use a continuous infusion pump.
- Ensure that patient is reevaluated weekly for possible adjustments in dosage.
- Inspect solution to make sure no particulate matter is present before use. Use vial within 14 days of initial introduction into the vial.
- Monitor injection site for any sign of reaction of infection.
- When giving drug through inhalation route, administer only through the *Tyvaso* Inhalation System. Administer undiluted as supplied.

⊗ ***Warning*** Monitor patients who are discontinuing treprostinil; tapering of dose may be needed to avoid sudden worsening of disease.

- Provide analgesics as appropriate for patients who develop headache or injection site pain.
- Monitor patient's functional level to note improvement in exercise tolerance.
- Maintain other measures used to treat pulmonary arterial hypertension.

Teaching points

- This drug must be given by a continuous subcutaneous infusion pump. It may be needed for prolonged periods, possibly years. The pump is lightweight and attached to a catheter that goes into your skin. You will need to care for the insertion site and set and monitor the pump. It is recommended to have a significant other who is also able to care for and maintain the site and the pump as a backup for you.
- If receiving this drug by inhalation, use undituted only through the *Tyvaso* Inhalation System.
- This drug should not be taken during pregnancy; using a barrier contraceptive is advised.
- Keep a chart of your exercise tolerance to help monitor improvement in your condition.
- This drug should not be discontinued abruptly. It must be tapered. Notify your health care provider if anything happens to prevent you from getting your continuous infusion of the drug.
- Continue your usual procedures for treating your pulmonary arterial hypertension.
- You will need to be followed closely to determine the correct dose of the drug that is best for your situation.
- You may experience these side effects: Headache (analgesics may help); stomach upset (taking with food); pain at the injection site (analgesics may also help, monitor the site for any sign of redness, heat, or swelling).
- Report swelling of the extremities, dizziness, chest pain, fever, changes in the appearance of the catheter insertion site.

DANGEROUS DRUG

▽tretinoin (retinoic acid)

(tret' i noyn)

Altinac, Atralin, Avita, Renova, Retin-A, Retin-A Micro, Stieva-A (CAN), Vesanoid DNC

PREGNANCY CATEGORY D

Drug classes

Antineoplastic
Retinoid (topical form)

Therapeutic actions

Induces cell differentiation and decreases proliferation of acute promyelocytic leukemia cells, leading to an initial maturation of the primitive promyelocytes, followed by a repopulation of the bone marrow and peripheral blood by normal hematopoietic cells in patients achieving complete remission; exact mechanism of action is not understood. Acne: decreased cohesiveness and increased turnover of follicular epithelial cells, decreasing comedones.

Indications

- Induction of remission in acute promyelocytic leukemia (APL)
- Topical treatment of acne vulgaris
- Adjunctive agent for use in mitigation of fine wrinkles, mottled hyperpigmentation in select patients (topical)

- Unlabeled uses: Hyperpigmentation of photoaged skin, postinflammatory hyperpigmentation, facial actinic keratoses (topical)

Contraindications and cautions

- Contraindicated with allergy to retinoids or parabens, suicidal tendencies, pregnancy, lactation.
- Use cautiously with liver disease, hypercholesterolemia, hypertriglyceridemia.

Available forms

Capsule (DNC)—10 mg; cream—0.02%, 0.025%, 0.05%, 0.1%; gel—0.025%, 0.01%, 0.04%, 0.05%, 0.1%

Dosages

Adults

Oral

45 mg/m²/day PO administered in two evenly divided doses until complete remission is documented; discontinue therapy 30 days after complete remission is obtained or after 90 days, whichever comes first.

Topical

Apply once a day before bedtime. Cover entire affected area lightly, avoiding mucous membranes.

Pediatric patients

Not recommended for use.

Pharmacokinetics

Route	*Onset*	*Peak*
Oral	Slow	1–2 hr

Metabolism: Hepatic; $T_{1/2}$: 0.5–2 hr
Distribution: Crosses placenta; may enter breast milk
Excretion: Feces, urine

Adverse effects

- **CNS:** *Fever, headache,* **pseudotumor cerebri** (papilledema, headache, nausea, vomiting, visual disturbances), *earache, visual disturbances, malaise, sweating,* suicidal ideation
- **CV:** Arrhythmias, flushing, hypotension, heart failure, **MI, cardiac arrest**
- **Dermatologic:** *Skin fragility, dry skin, pruritus, rash,* thinning hair, peeling of palms and soles, skin infections, photosensitivity, nail brittleness, petechiae
- **GI:** *Hemorrhage, nausea, vomiting, abdominal pain,* anorexia, inflammatory bowel disease
- **GU:** Renal insufficiency, dysuria, frequency, enlarged prostate
- **Hematologic: Rapid and evolving leukocytosis,** *decreased liver function, elevated lipids, elevated liver enzymes*
- **Musculoskeletal:** Skeletal hyperostosis, arthralgia, *bone and joint pain* and stiffness
- **Respiratory: Retinoic acid-APL syndrome** (fever, dyspnea, weight gain, pulmonary infiltrates, pleural or pericardial effusion, hypotension may progress to death)

Interactions

✱ **Drug-drug** • Increased risk of high serum levels and toxicity with ketoconazole • Combination therapy with hydroxyurea may lead to massive cell lysis and bone marrow necrosis • Increased risk of skin irritability if topically used with keratolytic agents (sulfur, resorcinol, benzoyl peroxide, salicylic acid); avoid this combination

■ Nursing considerations

Assessment

- **History:** Allergy to retinoids or parabens; pregnancy, lactation; liver disease; hypercholesterolemia, hypertriglyceridemia; suicidal tendencies
- **Physical:** Skin color, lesions, turgor, texture; joints—range of motion; orientation, reflexes, affect, ophthalmologic examination; mucous membranes, bowel sounds; R, adventitious sounds, auscultation; serum triglycerides, HDL, sedimentation rate, CBC and differential, urinalysis, pregnancy test, chest X-ray

Interventions

⊗ ***Black box warning*** Ensure that patient is not pregnant before administering; arrange for a pregnancy test within 2 wk of beginning therapy. Advise patient to use two forms of contraception during treatment and for 1 mo after treatment is discontinued.

⊠ **Black box warning** There is a risk of rapid leukocytosis (40% of patients); notify physician immediately if this occurs.

⊠ **Black box warning** This drug should only be used under the supervision of an experienced practitioner or in an institution experienced with its use.

⊗ **Warning** Monitor patient for any suicidal ideation or tendencies. The risk of suicide should be explained, the Medguide brochure should be given, and the patient must sign the release affirming that he or she understands the potential risk.

- Oral tretinoin is for induction of remission only; arrange for consolidation or maintenance chemotherapy for acute promyelocytic leukemia after induction therapy.
- Arrange for baseline recording of serum lipids and triglyceride levels, LFTs, chest X-ray, CBC with differential and coagulation profile; monitor for changes frequently.

⊠ **Black box warning** Discontinue drug and notify physician if LFTs are greater than five times upper range of normal, pulmonary infiltrates appear, or patient has difficulty breathing; serious side effects can occur.

⊗ **Warning** Discontinue drug if signs of papilledema occur; consult a neurologist for further care.

⊠ **Black box warning** Monitor patient for retinoic acid-APL syndrome (fever, dyspnea, acute respiratory distress, weight gain, pulmonary infiltrates, pleural and pericardial effusion, multiorgan failure). Endotracheal intubation and mechanical ventilation may be required.

⊗ **Warning** Discontinue drug if visual disturbances occur, and arrange for an ophthalmologic examination.

⊗ **Warning** Discontinue drug if abdominal pain, rectal bleeding, or severe diarrhea occurs, and consult with physician.

- Monitor triglycerides during therapy; if elevations occur, institute other measures to lower serum triglycerides—reduce weight, dietary fat; exercise; increase intake of insoluble fiber; decrease alcohol consumption.

⊗ **Warning** Keep high-dose steroids readily available in case of severe leukocytosis or liver damage.

- Administer drug with meals; do not crush capsules.
- Do not administer vitamin supplements that contain vitamin A.
- Maintain supportive care appropriate for patients with APL (eg, monitor for and treat infections, prophylaxis for bleeding).
- Topical form should be applied lightly to entire area before bed. Clean area thoroughly before use.

Teaching points

- Take the oral drug with meals; do not crush capsules.
- Frequent blood tests will be needed to evaluate the drug's effects on your body.
- This drug has been associated with severe birth defects and miscarriages; it should not be used by pregnant women. Use contraceptives during treatment and for 1 month after treatment is discontinued. If you think you are pregnant, consult your health care provider immediately.
- You will not be permitted to donate blood while using this drug because of its possible effects on the fetus of a blood recipient.
- Avoid the use of vitamin supplements containing vitamin A; serious toxic effects may occur. Limit alcohol consumption. You may also need to limit your intake of fats and increase exercise to limit the drug's effects on blood triglyceride levels.
- At bedtime, clean affected area well and apply topical form lightly to entire area.
- You may experience these side effects: Dizziness, lethargy, headache, visual changes (avoid driving or performing tasks that require alertness); sensitivity to the sun (avoid sunlamps, exposure to the sun; use sunscreens and protective clothing); diarrhea, abdominal pain, loss of appetite (take drug with meals); dry mouth (suck sugarless lozenges); eye irritation and redness, inability to wear contact lenses; dry skin, itching, redness.
- Report headache with nausea and vomiting, difficulty breathing, severe diarrhea or rectal bleeding, visual difficulties, suicidal ideas or feelings.

triamcinolone
*(trye am **sin'** oh lone)*

triamcinolone acetonide
IM, intra-articular, or soft-tissue injection; respiratory inhalant; dermatologic ointment, cream, lotion, aerosol: AllerNaze, Azmacort, Flutex, Kenalog, Nasacort AQ, Oracort (CAN), Triacet, Triderm

triamcinolone hexacetonide
Intra-articular, intralesional injection: Aristospan Intra-articular, Aristospan Intralesional

PREGNANCY CATEGORY C

Drug classes
Corticosteroid (intermediate acting)
Glucocorticoid
Hormone

Therapeutic actions
Enters target cells and binds to cytoplasmic receptors, thereby initiating many complex reactions that are responsible for its anti-inflammatory and immunosuppressive effects.

Indications
- Systemic: Hypercalcemia associated with cancer
- Short-term management of inflammatory and allergic disorders such as rheumatoid arthritis, collagen diseases (eg, SLE), dermatologic diseases (eg, pemphigus), status asthmaticus, and autoimmune disorders
- Hematologic disorders: Thrombocytopenia purpura, erythroblastopenia
- Ulcerative colitis, acute exacerbations of MS, and palliation in some leukemias and lymphomas
- Trichinosis with neurologic or myocardial involvement
- Pulmonary emphysema with bronchial spasm or edema; diffuse interstitial pulmonary fibrosis; with diuretics in HF with refractory edema and in cirrhosis with refractory ascites
- Postoperative dental inflammatory reactions
- Intra-articular, soft-tissue administration for conditions such as arthritis, psoriatic plaques
- Respiratory inhalant: Control of bronchial asthma requiring corticosteroids in conjunction with other therapy
- Prophylactic therapy in the maintenance treatment of asthma (bid use)
- Dermatologic preparations: To relieve inflammatory and pruritic manifestations of dermatoses that are steroid responsive
- Nasal spray: Treatment of seasonal and perennial allergic-rhinitis symptoms in patients 6 yr and older

Contraindications and cautions
- Contraindicated with infections, especially TB, fungal infections, amebiasis, vaccinia and varicella, and antibiotic-resistant infections; lactation.
- Use cautiously with pregnancy (teratogenic in preclinical studies), renal or liver disease, hypothyroidism, ulcerative colitis with impending perforation, diverticulitis, active or latent peptic ulcer, inflammatory bowel disease, heart failure, hypertension, thromboembolic disorders, osteoporosis, seizure disorders, diabetes mellitus.

Available forms
Injection—5, 20, 25, 40 mg/mL; aerosol—100 mcg/actuation; topical ointment—0.025, 0.05, 0.1, 0.5%; cream—0.25, 0.1, 0.5%; lotion—0.025, 0.1%; nasal spray—50, 55 mcg/actuation

Dosages
Adults
Systemic
Individualize dosage, depending on the severity of the condition and the patient's response. Administer daily dose before 9 AM to minimize adrenal suppression. If long-term therapy is needed, consider alternate-day therapy. After long-term therapy, withdraw drug slowly to avoid adrenal insufficiency. For maintenance therapy, reduce initial dose in small increments at intervals until the lowest effective dose is reached.

IM (triamcinolone acetonide)
2.5–100 mg/day.

Respiratory inhalant (triamcinolone acetonide)
200 mcg released with each actuation delivers about 100 mcg to the patient. Two inhalations tid–qid, not to exceed 16 inhalations/day.

Nasal spray
Two sprays (220 mcg total dose) in each nostril daily—maximum of four sprays/day.

Adults and pediatric patients

Intra-articular, intralesional
Dose will vary with joint or soft-tissue site to be injected.

- *Triamcinolone acetonide:* 2.5–15 mg.
- *Triamcinolone diacetate:* 5–40 mg intra-articular; 5–48 mg intralesional; do not use more than 12.5 mg per injection site or 25 mg per lesion.
- *Triamcinolone hexacetonide:* 2–20 mg intra-articular; up to 0.5 mg/square inch of affected area intralesional.

Topical dermatologic preparations
Apply sparingly to affected area bid–qid.

Pediatric patients

Systemic
Individualize dosage, depending on the severity of the condition and the patient's response rather than by formulae that correct adult doses for age or body weight. Carefully observe growth and development in infants and children on prolonged therapy.

Respiratory inhalant (triamcinolone acetonide)
200 mcg released with each actuation delivers about 100 mcg to the patient.
6–12 yr: One or two inhalations tid–qid, not to exceed 12 inhalations/day.

Nasal spray
6–12 yr: One spray in each nostril once per day (100–110 mcg dose), maximum dose two sprays/nostril/day.

Topical dermatologic preparations
Apply low-potency form sparingly to affected area bid–qid.

Pharmacokinetics

Route	*Onset*	*Peak*	*Duration*
IM	24–48 hr	8–10 hr	1–6 wk

Metabolism: Hepatic; $T_{1/2}$: 2–5 hr
Distribution: Crosses placenta; enters breast milk
Excretion: Urine

Adverse effects

Effects depend on dose, route, and duration of therapy.

- **CNS:** *Vertigo, headache,* paresthesias, insomnia, seizures, psychosis, cataracts, increased IOP, glaucoma (long-term therapy)
- **CV:** Hypotension, shock, hypertension and heart failure secondary to fluid retention, thromboembolism, thrombophlebitis, fat embolism, cardiac arrhythmias
- **Electrolyte imbalance:** *Sodium and fluid retention,* hypokalemia, hypocalcemia
- **Endocrine:** Amenorrhea, irregular menses, growth retardation, decreased carbohydrate tolerance, diabetes mellitus, cushingoid state (long-term effect), increased blood sugar, increased serum cholesterol, decreased T_3 and T_4 levels, HPA suppression with systemic therapy longer than 5 days
- **GI:** Peptic or esophageal ulcer, pancreatitis, abdominal distention, nausea, vomiting, *increased appetite, weight gain* (long-term therapy)
- **Hypersensitivity:** Hypersensitivity or anaphylactoid reactions
- **Musculoskeletal:** Muscle weakness, steroid myopathy, loss of muscle mass, osteoporosis, spontaneous fractures (long-term therapy)
- **Other:** *Immunosuppression, aggravation, or masking of infections; impaired wound healing;* thin, fragile skin; petechiae, ecchymoses, purpura, striae; subcutaneous fat atrophy

Intra-articular

- **Local:** Osteonecrosis, tendon rupture, infection

Intralesional (face and head)

- **Local:** Blindness (rare)

Respiratory inhalants

- **Local:** Oral, laryngeal, and pharyngeal irritation; fungal infections

Topical dermatologic ointments, creams, sprays

- **Local:** Local burning, irritation, acneiform lesions, striae, skin atrophy

T

Interactions

✱ Drug-drug • Risk of severe deterioration of muscle strength when given to myasthenia gravis patients who are also receiving ambenonium, edrophonium, neostigmine, pyridostigmine • Decreased steroid blood levels with barbiturates, phenytoin, rifampin • Decreased effectiveness of salicylates, oral antidiabetics

✱ Drug-lab test • False-negative nitroblue-tetrazolium test for bacterial infection • Suppression of skin test reactions

■ Nursing considerations

Assessment

- **History:** Infections; renal or liver disease; hypothyroidism; ulcerative colitis with impending perforation; diverticulitis; active or latent peptic ulcer; inflammatory bowel disease; HF; hypertension; thromboembolic disorders; osteoporosis; seizure disorders; diabetes mellitus; pregnancy; lactation
- **Physical:** Weight, T; reflexes and grip strength, affect and orientation, P, BP, peripheral perfusion, prominence of superficial veins; R, adventitious sounds; serum electrolytes, blood glucose

Interventions

- Administer once-a-day doses before 9 AM to mimic normal peak corticosteroid blood levels.
- Increase dosage when patient is subject to stress.

⊗ ***Warning*** Taper doses when discontinuing high-dose or long-term therapy to allow adrenal recovery.

- Do not give live virus vaccines with immunosuppressive doses of corticosteroids.

⊗ ***Warning*** Taper systemic steroids carefully during transfer to inhalational steroids; deaths caused by adrenal insufficiency have occurred.

- Use caution when occlusive dressings or tight diapers cover affected area; these can increase systemic absorption when using topical preparations.
- Avoid prolonged use of topical preparations near the eyes, in genital and rectal areas, and in skin creases.

Teaching points

- Do not stop taking the drug without consulting your health care provider.
- Avoid exposure to infections.
- Report unusual weight gain, swelling of the extremities, muscle weakness, black or tarry stools, fever, prolonged sore throat, colds or other infections, worsening of your disorder.

Intra-articular administration

- Do not overuse joint after therapy, even if pain is gone.

Respiratory inhalant

- Do not use during an acute asthmatic attack or to manage status asthmaticus.
- Do not use with systemic fungal infections.
- Do not use more often than prescribed.
- Do not stop using this drug without consulting your health care provider.
- Administer inhalational bronchodilator drug first, if also receiving bronchodilator therapy; rinse mouth after use.

Nasal spray

- Do not spray in eyes.
- Prime pump before first use and again if not used for more than 2 weeks.

Topical dermatologic preparations

- Apply drug sparingly, avoid contact with eyes.
- Report irritation or infection at the site of application.

▽ triamterene

*(trye **am'** ter een)*

Dyrenium

PREGNANCY CATEGORY C

Drug class

Potassium-sparing diuretic

Therapeutic actions

Inhibits sodium reabsorption in the renal distal tubule, causing loss of sodium and water and retention of potassium.

Indications

- Edema associated with HF, nephrotic syndrome, hepatic cirrhosis; steroid-induced edema, edema from secondary hyperaldosteronism (alone or with other diuretics for added diuretic or antikaliuretic effects), hypertension

Contraindications and cautions

- Contraindicated with allergy to triamterene, hyperkalemia, renal disease (except nephrosis), liver disease, lactation.
- Use cautiously with diabetes mellitus, hyperuricemia, pregnancy.

Available forms

Capsules—50, 100 mg

Dosages

Adults

Edema: 100 mg bid PO if used alone after meals. Reduce dosage if added to other diuretic or antihypertensive therapy. Maintenance dosage should be individualized, may be as low as 100 mg every other day. Do not exceed 300 mg/day.

Hypertension: Start with 25 mg PO once daily; usual dose 50–100 mg/day.

Pediatric patients

Safety and efficacy not established.

Pharmacokinetics

Route	Onset	Peak	Duration
Oral	2–4 hr	3 hr	7–9 hr

Metabolism: Hepatic; $T_{1/2}$: 3 hr

Distribution: Crosses placenta; enters breast milk

Excretion: Urine

Adverse effects

- **CNS:** *Headache,* drowsiness, fatigue, *weakness*
- **Dermatologic:** Rash, photosensitivity
- **GI:** *Nausea, anorexia, vomiting, dry mouth,* diarrhea
- **GU:** Renal stones, interstitial nephritis
- **Hematologic: Hyperkalemia**, blood dyscrasias

Interactions

✱ **Drug-drug** • Increased hyperkalemia with potassium supplements, diets rich in potassium, ACE inhibitors, other potassium-sparing diuretics • Increased serum levels and possible toxicity with cimetidine, indomethacin, lithium • Increased risk of amantadine toxicity

✱ **Drug-lab test** • Interference with fluorescent measurement of serum quinidine levels

■ Nursing considerations

Assessment

- **History:** Allergy to triamterene, hyperkalemia, renal or liver disease, diabetes mellitus, pregnancy, lactation
- **Physical:** Skin color, lesions, edema; orientation, reflexes, muscle strength; pulses, baseline ECG, BP; R, pattern, adventitious sounds; liver evaluation, bowel sounds; urinary output patterns; CBC, serum electrolytes, blood sugar, LFTs, renal function tests, urinalysis

Interventions

- Administer with food or milk if GI upset occurs.
- Mark calendars or provide other reminders of drug days for outpatients if alternate-day or 3- to 5-day/wk therapy is optimal for treating edema.
- Administer early in the day so that increased urination does not disturb sleep.
- Measure and record regular weights to monitor mobilization of edema fluid.
- Arrange for regular evaluation of serum electrolytes and BUN.

Teaching points

- Record alternate-day therapy on a calendar, or make dated envelopes. Take the drug early in the day as increased urination will occur. The drug may be taken with food or meals if GI upset occurs.
- Weigh yourself on a regular basis, at the same time and in the same clothing, and record the weight on your calendar.
- You may experience these side effects: Increased volume and frequency of urination; drowsiness (avoid rapid position changes; do not engage in hazardous activities such as driving a car; this problem is often made worse by the use of alcohol); avoid foods that are rich in potassium (eg, fruits, *Sanka*); sensitivity to sunlight and bright lights (wear sunglasses; use sunscreens and protective clothing).

- Report weight change of more than 3 pounds in 1 day, swelling in ankles or fingers, fever, sore throat, mouth sores, unusual bleeding or bruising, dizziness, trembling, numbness, fatigue.

triazolam

*(trye **ay**' zoe lam)*

Apo-Triazo (CAN), Gen-Triazolam (CAN), Halcion

PREGNANCY CATEGORY X

CONTROLLED SUBSTANCE C-IV

Drug classes

Benzodiazepine
Sedative-hypnotic

Therapeutic actions

Exact mechanisms of action not understood; acts mainly at subcortical levels of the CNS, leaving the cortex relatively unaffected; main sites of action may be the limbic system and mesencephalic reticular formation; benzodiazepines potentiate the effects of GABA, an inhibitory neurotransmitter.

Indications

- Insomnia characterized by difficulty falling asleep, frequent nocturnal awakenings, or early morning awakening (short-term use: 7–10 days)
- Acute or chronic medical situations requiring restful sleep

Contraindications and cautions

- Contraindicated with hypersensitivity to benzodiazepines; pregnancy (risk of congenital malformations, neonatal withdrawal syndrome); labor and delivery ("floppy infant" syndrome); lactation (infants may become lethargic and lose weight).
- Use cautiously with impaired liver or renal function, debilitation, depression, suicidal tendencies.

Available forms

Tablets—0.125, 0.25 mg

Dosages

Adults

0.125–0.5 mg PO before retiring.

Pediatric patients

Not for use in patients younger than 18 yr.

Geriatric or debilitated patients

Initially, 0.125–0.25 mg PO. Adjust as needed and tolerated.

Pharmacokinetics

Route	*Onset*	*Peak*
Oral	Varies	30 min–2 hr

Metabolism: Hepatic; $T_{1/2}$: 1.5–5.5 hr
Distribution: Crosses placenta; enters breast milk
Excretion: Urine

Adverse effects

- **CNS:** *Transient, mild drowsiness initially; sedation, depression, lethargy,* apathy, fatigue, *light-headedness, disorientation, restlessness, confusion,* crying, delirium, headache, slurred speech, dysarthria, stupor, rigidity, tremor, dystonia, vertigo, euphoria, nervousness, difficulty in concentration, vivid dreams, psychomotor retardation, extrapyramidal symptoms; *mild paradoxical excitatory reactions during first 2 wk of treatment* (especially in psychiatric patients, aggressive children, and with high dosage), visual and auditory disturbances, diplopia, nystagmus, depressed hearing, nasal congestion, retrograde amnesia, "traveler's amnesia," complex sleep-related behaviors
- **CV:** *Bradycardia, tachycardia,* CV collapse, hypertension and hypotension, palpitations, edema
- **Dependence:** *Drug dependence with withdrawal syndrome* when drug is discontinued (more common with abrupt discontinuation of higher dosage used for longer than 4 mo)
- **Dermatologic:** Urticaria, pruritus, rash, dermatitis
- **GI:** *Constipation, diarrhea,* dry mouth, salivation, nausea, anorexia, vomiting, difficulty in swallowing, gastric disorders, elevations of blood enzymes—hepatic impairment, jaundice

- **GU:** *Incontinence, changes in libido, urine retention,* menstrual irregularities
- **Hematologic:** Decreased Hct, blood dyscrasias
- **Other:** Hiccups, fever, diaphoresis, paresthesias, muscular disturbances, gynecomastia, **anaphylaxis, angioedema**

Interactions

✱ **Drug-drug** ⊗ ***Warning*** Potentially serious to fatal reactions with ketoconazole, itraconazole; avoid this combination.
• Increased CNS depression and sedation with alcohol, cimetidine, omeprazole, disulfiram, hormonal contraceptives • Decreased sedative effects with theophylline, aminophylline, dyphylline, oxtriphylline
✱ **Drug-food** • Decreased metabolism and risk of toxic effects if combined with grapefruit juice; avoid this combination

■ Nursing considerations

Assessment

- **History:** Hypersensitivity to benzodiazepines; pregnancy, lactation; impaired liver or renal function; debilitation; depression, suicidal tendencies
- **Physical:** Skin color, lesions; T; orientation, reflexes, affect, ophthalmologic examination; P, BP; R, adventitious sounds; liver evaluation, abdominal examination, bowel sounds, normal output; CBC, LFTs, renal function tests

Interventions

- Arrange for periodic blood counts, urinalyses, and blood chemistry analyses with protracted treatment.
- Caution women of childbearing age to avoid pregnancy; using barrier contraceptives is advised.

⊗ ***Warning*** Taper dosage gradually after long-term therapy, especially in patients with epilepsy.

Teaching points

- Take drug exactly as prescribed. Do not drink grapefruit juice while using this drug.
- Do not stop taking drug (in long-term therapy) without consulting your health care provider.
- Avoid alcohol and sleep-inducing and over-the-counter drugs.
- Avoid pregnancy while taking this drug; using contraceptives is advised; serious fetal harm could occur.
- You may experience these side effects: Drowsiness, dizziness (may lessen; avoid driving or engaging in hazardous activities); allergic reaction, swelling; GI upset (take drug with food); depression, dreams, emotional upset, crying; sleep disturbance for several nights after discontinuing the drug, complex sleep-related behaviors.
- Report severe dizziness, allergies, weakness, drowsiness that persists, rash or skin lesions, palpitations, swelling of extremities, visual changes, difficulty voiding, sleep disorders.

▽ trientine hydrochloride

See Appendix W, *Less commonly used drugs.*

▽ trihexyphenidyl hydrochloride

*(trye hex ee **fen'** i dill)*

Apo-Trihex (CAN)

PREGNANCY CATEGORY C

Drug class

Antiparkinsonian (anticholinergic type)

Therapeutic actions

Has anticholinergic activity in the CNS that is believed to help normalize the hypothesized imbalance of cholinergic and dopaminergic neurotransmission created by the loss of dopaminergic neurons in the basal ganglia of the brain of parkinsonism patients; reduces severity of rigidity and reduces to a lesser extent the akinesia and tremor that characterize parkinsonism; less effective overall than levodopa; peripheral anticholinergic effects suppress secondary symptoms of parkinsonism, such as drooling.

T

Indications

- Adjunct in the treatment of parkinsonism (postencephalitic, arteriosclerotic, and idiopathic)
- Adjuvant therapy with levodopa for the treatment of Parkinson's disease
- Control of drug-induced extrapyramidal disorders

Contraindications and cautions

- Contraindicated with hypersensitivity to trihexyphenidyl; glaucoma, especially angle-closure glaucoma; pyloric or duodenal obstruction, stenosing peptic ulcers, achalasia (megaesophagus); myasthenia gravis; lactation.
- Use cautiously with cardiac arrhythmias, hypertension, hypotension, hepatic or renal impairment, alcoholism, chronic illness, people who work in hot environment, pregnancy, prostatic hypertrophy or bladder neck obstructions.

Available forms

Tablets—2, 5 mg; elixir—2 mg/5 mL

Dosages

Adults

Tablets

- *Parkinsonism:* 1 mg PO the first day. Increase by 2-mg increments at 3- to 5-day intervals until a total of 6–10 mg is given daily. Postencephalitic patients may require 12–15 mg/day. Tolerated best if daily dose is divided into three (or four) doses administered at mealtimes (and bedtime).
- *Concomitant use with levodopa:* Usual dose of each may need to be reduced; however, trihexyphenidyl has been shown to decrease bioavailability of levodopa. Adjust dosage on basis of response. 3–6 mg/day PO of trihexyphenidyl is usually adequate.
- *Concomitant use with other anticholinergics:* Gradually substitute trihexyphenidyl for all or part of the other anticholinergic and reduce dosage of the other anticholinergic gradually.
- *Drug-induced extrapyramidal symptoms:* Initially, 1 mg PO. Dose of tranquilizer may need to be reduced temporarily to expedite control of extrapyramidal symptoms. Adjust dosage of both drugs subsequently to maintain ataractic effect without extrapyramidal reactions. Usual dose 5–15 mg daily. If reactions are not controlled in a few hours, progressively increase subsequent doses until control is achieved.

Pediatric patients

Safety and efficacy not established.

Geriatric patients

Patients older than 60 yr often develop increased sensitivity to the CNS effects of anticholinergic drugs.

Pharmacokinetics

Route	Onset	Peak	Duration
Oral	1 hr	2–3 hr	6–12 hr

Metabolism: Hepatic; $T_{1/2}$: 5.6–10.2 hr
Distribution: Crosses placenta; enters breast milk
Excretion: Urine

Adverse effects

- **CNS** (some CNS effects are characteristic of centrally acting anticholinergics): *Disorientation, confusion,* memory loss, hallucinations, psychoses, agitation, nervousness, delusions, delirium, paranoia, euphoria, excitement, *light-headedness, dizziness,* depression, drowsiness, weakness, giddiness, paresthesia, heaviness of the limbs, numbness of fingers, *blurred vision, mydriasis,* diplopia, increased intraocular tension, angle-closure glaucoma
- **CV:** Tachycardia, palpitations, hypotension, orthostatic hypotension
- **Dermatologic:** Rash, urticaria, other dermatoses
- **GI:** *Dry mouth, constipation,* dilation of the colon, paralytic ileus, acute suppurative parotitis, nausea, vomiting, epigastric distress
- **GU:** *Urinary retention,* urinary hesitancy, dysuria, difficulty achieving or maintaining an erection
- **Other:** Muscular weakness, muscular cramping, *flushing, decreased sweating,* elevated T

Interactions

✱ **Drug-drug** • Additive adverse CNS effects; toxic psychosis with phenothiazines • Possible

masking of the development of persistent extrapyramidal symptoms, tardive dyskinesia, in patients on long-term therapy with antipsychotics, such as phenothiazines, haloperidol
- Decreased therapeutic efficacy of antipsychotics (phenothiazines, haloperidol)

■ Nursing considerations

Assessment

- **History:** Hypersensitivity to trihexyphenidyl; glaucoma; pyloric or duodenal obstruction, stenosing peptic ulcers; achalasia; prostatic hypertrophy or bladder neck obstructions; myasthenia gravis, tachycardia, cardiac arrhythmias; hypertension, hypotension; hepatic or renal impairment; alcoholism; chronic illness; work environment; pregnancy, lactation
- **Physical:** Weight, T; skin color, lesions; orientation, affect, reflexes, bilateral grip strength, visual examination, including tonometry; P, BP, orthostatic BP, auscultation; bowel sounds, normal output, liver evaluation; urinary output, voiding pattern, prostate palpation; LFTs, renal function tests

Interventions

⊗ ***Warning*** Decrease dosage or discontinue drug temporarily if dry mouth is so severe that swallowing or speaking becomes difficult.

- Give with caution and arrange dosage reduction in hot weather; drug interferes with sweating and ability of body to maintain body heat equilibrium; anhidrosis and fatal hyperthermia have occurred.
- Ensure that patient voids before receiving each dose if urinary retention is a problem.

Teaching points

- Take this drug exactly as prescribed.
- Use caution in hot weather (this drug makes you more susceptible to heat prostration).
- You may experience these side effects: Drowsiness, dizziness, confusion, blurred vision (avoid driving or engaging in activities that require alertness and visual acuity); nausea (eat frequent small meals); dry mouth (suck sugarless lozenges or ice chips); painful or difficult urination (emptying the bladder immediately before each dose may help); constipation (if maintaining adequate fluid intake and exercising regularly do not help, consult your health care provider).
- Report difficult or painful urination, constipation, rapid or pounding heartbeat, confusion, eye pain, or rash.

▽trimethobenzamide hydrochloride

*(trye meth oh **ben'** za myde)*

Oral preparations: Tigan

Parenteral preparations: Tigan

PREGNANCY CATEGORY C

Drug class

Antiemetic (anticholinergic)

Therapeutic actions

Mechanism of action not understood; antiemetic action may be mediated through the CTZ; impulses to the vomiting center do not appear to be affected.

Indications

- Control of nausea and vomiting

Contraindications and cautions

- Contraindicated with allergy to trimethobenzamide, benzocaine, or similar local anesthetics; uncomplicated vomiting in children (drug may contribute to development of Reye's syndrome or unfavorably influence its outcome; extrapyramidal effects of drugs may obscure diagnosis of Reye's syndrome); pregnancy.
- Use cautiously with lactation; acute febrile illness, appendicitis, encephalitis, gastroenteritis, dehydration, electrolyte imbalance, especially when these occur in children, the elderly, or debilitated; narrow-angle glaucoma; stenosing peptic ulcer; symptomatic prostatic hypertrophy; bronchial asthma; bladder neck obstruction; pyloroduodenal obstruction; cardiac arrhythmias; recent use of CNS-acting drugs (phenothiazine, barbiturates, belladonna alkaloids).

Available forms

Capsules—300 mg; injection—100 mg/mL

Dosages
Adults
Oral
- *Nausea and vomiting:* 300 mg tid–qid.
- *Postoperative nausea/vomiting or for treatment of gastroenteritis:* 300 mg tid–qid.

Parenteral
200 mg IM tid–qid.

Pediatric patients
Not recommended.

Geriatric patients
More likely to cause serious adverse reactions in elderly patients; use with caution.

Pharmacokinetics

Route	Onset	Duration
Oral	10–40 min	3–4 hr
IM	15 min	2–3 hr

Metabolism: Hepatic; $T_{1/2}$: Unknown
Distribution: Crosses placenta; enters breast milk
Excretion: Urine

Adverse effects
- **CNS:** Parkinsonlike symptoms, coma, seizures, opisthotonus, depression, disorientation, *dizziness, drowsiness, headache, blurred vision*
- **CV:** Hypotension
- **GI:** Diarrhea
- **Hematologic:** Blood dyscrasias, jaundice
- **Hypersensitivity:** Allergic-type skin reactions
- **Local:** *Pain following IM injections*

■ Nursing considerations
Assessment
- **History:** Allergy to trimethobenzamide, benzocaine, or similar local anesthetics; uncomplicated vomiting in children; pregnancy, lactation; acute febrile illness, encephalitis, gastroenteritis, dehydration, electrolyte imbalance; narrow-angle glaucoma; stenosing peptic ulcer; symptomatic prostatic hypertrophy; bronchial asthma; bladder neck obstruction; pyloroduodenal obstruction; cardiac arrhythmias
- **Physical:** Skin color, lesions, texture; T; orientation, reflexes, affect; vision examination; P, BP; R, adventitious sounds; bowel sounds; prostate palpation; CBC, serum electrolytes

Interventions
- Administer IM injections deep into upper outer quadrant of the gluteal region.
- Ensure adequate hydration.

Teaching points
- Take as prescribed. Avoid excessive dosage.
- Avoid alcohol while taking this drug; serious sedation could occur.
- You may experience these side effects: Dizziness, sedation, drowsiness (use caution if driving or performing tasks that require alertness); diarrhea; blurred vision (reversible).
- Report difficulty breathing, tremors, loss of coordination, sore muscles or muscle spasms, unusual bleeding or bruising, sore throat, visual disturbances, irregular heartbeat, yellowing of the skin or eyes.

▽ trimethoprim (TMP)
*(trye **meth'** oh prim)*

Primsol, Proloprim, Trimpex

PREGNANCY CATEGORY C

Drug class
Antibacterial

Therapeutic actions
Inhibits folic acid reduction to tetrahydrofolate in susceptible bacteria; the bacterial enzyme involved in this reaction is more readily inhibited than the mammalian enzyme.

Indications
- Uncomplicated UTIs caused by susceptible strains of *Eschirichia coli, Proteus mirabilis, Klebsiella pneumoniae, Enterobacter* species, and coagulase-negative *Staphylococcus* species, including *S. saprophyticus*
- Treatment of acute otitis media due to susceptible strains of *Streptococcus pneumoniae* and *Haemophilus influenzae* in children

- Unlabeled uses: With dapsone for treatment of initial episodes of *Pneumocystis jiroveci (carinii)* pneumonia in patients who cannot tolerate co-trimoxazole; treatment and prevention of traveler's diarrhea

Contraindications and cautions

- Contraindicated with allergy to trimethoprim, pregnancy (teratogenic in preclinical studies), megaloblastic anemia due to folate deficiency.
- Use cautiously with hepatic or renal impairment, lactation.

Available forms

Tablets—100, 200 mg; solution—50 mg/5 mL

Dosages

Adults

100 mg PO every 12 hr or 200 mg every 24 hr for 10–14 days for acute uncomplicated UTIs.

Pediatric patients

- *Otitis media:* 10 mg/kg/day in divided doses every 12 hr for 10 days.

Geriatric patients or patients with renal impairment

For creatinine clearance of 15–30 mL/min, 50 mg PO every 12 hr; for creatinine clearance less than 15 mL/min, not recommended.

Pharmacokinetics

Route	*Onset*	*Peak*
Oral	Varies	1–4 hr

Metabolism: Hepatic; $T_{1/2}$: 8–10 hr
Distribution: Crosses placenta; enters breast milk
Excretion: Urine

Adverse effects

- **Dermatologic:** *Rash,* pruritus, exfoliative dermatitis
- **GI:** *Epigastric distress,* nausea, vomiting, glossitis
- **Hematologic:** Thrombocytopenia, leukopenia, neutropenia, megaloblastic anemia, methemoglobinemia, elevated serum transaminase and bilirubin, increased BUN and serum creatinine levels
- **Other:** Fever

■ Nursing considerations

Assessment

- **History:** Allergy to trimethoprim, megaloblastic anemia due to folate deficiency, renal or hepatic impairment, pregnancy, lactation
- **Physical:** Skin color, lesions; T; status of mucous membranes; CBC; LFTs, renal function tests

Interventions

- Perform culture and sensitivity tests before beginning drug therapy.
- Protect the 200-mg tablets from exposure to light.
- Arrange for regular, periodic blood counts during therapy.

⊗ ***Warning*** Discontinue drug and consult with physician if any significant reduction in any formed blood element occurs.

Teaching points

- Take the full course of the drug; take all the tablets prescribed.
- Have periodic medical checkups, including blood tests.
- You may experience these side effects: Epigastric distress, nausea, vomiting (eat frequent small meals); rash (consult your health care provider for appropriate skin care).
- Report fever, sore throat, unusual bleeding or bruising, dizziness, headaches, rash.

▽ trimipramine maleate

(trye mi' pra meen)

Apo-Trimip (CAN), Surmontil

PREGNANCY CATEGORY C

T

Drug class

TCA (tertiary amine)

Therapeutic actions

Mechanism of action unknown; the TCAs are structurally related to the phenothiazine antipsychotics (eg, chlorpromazine); TCAs inhibit the presynaptic reuptake of the neurotransmitters norepinephrine and serotonin; anticholinergic at CNS and peripheral receptors;

the relation of these effects to clinical efficacy is unknown.

Indications

- Relief of symptoms of depression (endogenous depression most responsive); sedative effects of tertiary amine TCAs may be helpful in patients whose depression is associated with anxiety and sleep disturbance
- Unlabeled use: Duodenal ulcers

Contraindications and cautions

- Contraindicated with hypersensitivity to any tricyclic drug, concomitant therapy with an MAOI, recent MI, myelography within previous 24 hr or scheduled within 48 hr, pregnancy (limb reduction abnormalities may occur), lactation.
- Use cautiously with EST; preexisting CV disorders (eg, severe CAD, progressive HF, angina pectoris, paroxysmal tachycardia); angle-closure glaucoma, increased IOP; urinary retention, ureteral or urethral spasm (anticholinergic effects of TCAs may exacerbate these conditions); seizure disorders (TCAs lower the seizure threshold); hyperthyroidism (predisposes to CVS toxicity, including cardiac arrhythmias); impaired hepatic, renal function; psychiatric patients (schizophrenic or paranoid patients may exhibit a worsening of psychosis); patients with bipolar disorder (may shift to hypomanic or manic phase); elective surgery (TCAs should be discontinued as long as possible before surgery).

Available forms

Capsules—25, 50, 100 mg

Dosages

Adults

- *Hospitalized patients:* Initially, 100 mg/day PO in divided doses. Gradually increase to 200 mg/day as required. If no improvement in 2–3 wk, increase to a maximum dose of 250–300 mg/day.
- *Outpatients:* Initially, 75 mg/day PO in divided doses. May increase to 150 mg/day. Do not exceed 200 mg/day. Total daily dosage may be administered at bedtime. Maintenance dose is 50–150 mg/day given as a single dose at bedtime. After satisfactory response, reduce to lowest effective dosage. Continue therapy for 3 mo or longer to lessen possibility of relapse.

Pediatric patients 12 yr and older

50 mg/day PO with gradual increases up to 100 mg/day.

Pediatric patients younger than 12 yr

Not recommended.

Geriatric patients

50 mg/day PO with gradual increases up to 100 mg/day PO.

Pharmacokinetics

Route	*Onset*	*Peak*
Oral	Varies	2 hr

Metabolism: Hepatic; $T_{1/2}$: 7–30 hr
Distribution: Crosses placenta; enters breast milk
Excretion: Feces, urine

Adverse effects

- **CNS:** *Sedation and anticholinergic (atropine-like) effects; confusion* (especially in elderly), *disturbed concentration,* hallucinations, disorientation, decreased memory, feelings of unreality, delusions, anxiety, nervousness, restlessness, agitation, panic, insomnia, nightmares, hypomania, mania, exacerbation of psychosis, drowsiness, weakness, fatigue, headache, numbness, tingling, paresthesias of extremities, incoordination, motor hyperactivity, akathisia, ataxia, tremors, peripheral neuropathy, extrapyramidal symptoms, *seizures,* speech blockage, dysarthria, tinnitus, altered EEG, suicidal ideation
- **CV:** *Orthostatic hypotension,* hypertension, syncope, tachycardia, palpitations, **MI,** arrhythmias, heart block, **precipitation of HF, CVA**
- **Endocrine:** Elevated or depressed blood sugar, elevated prolactin levels, SIADH secretion
- **GI:** *Dry mouth, constipation,* paralytic ileus, *nausea,* vomiting, anorexia, epigastric distress, diarrhea, flatulence, dysphagia, peculiar taste in mouth, increased salivation, stomatitis, glossitis, parotid swelling, abdominal cramps, black tongue, hepatitis,

jaundice (rare), elevated transaminase, altered alkaline phosphatase
- **GU:** Urinary retention, delayed micturition, dilation of the urinary tract, gynecomastia, testicular swelling; breast enlargement, menstrual irregularity and galactorrhea; increased or decreased libido; impotence
- **Hematologic:** Bone marrow depression including agranulocytosis; eosinophilia, purpura, thrombocytopenia, leukopenia
- **Hypersensitivity:** Rash, pruritus, vasculitis, petechiae, photosensitization, edema (generalized, facial, tongue), drug fever
- **Withdrawal:** Symptoms with abrupt discontinuation of prolonged therapy: Nausea, headache, vertigo, nightmares, malaise
- **Other:** Nasal congestion, excessive appetite, weight gain or loss, sweating, alopecia, lacrimation, hyperthermia, flushing, chills

Interactions

✱ **Drug-drug** • Increased TCA levels and pharmacologic (especially anticholinergic) effects with cimetidine, fluoxetine, ranitidine • Risk of arrhythmias and hypertension with sympathomimetics • Risk of severe hypertension with clonidine • Risk of life-threatening cardiac arrhythmias if combined with clarithromycin, fluoroquinolone antibiotics; avoid this combination • Hyperpyretic crises, severe seizures, hypertensive episodes and deaths with MAOIs. *Note:* MAOIs and TCAs have been used successfully in some patients resistant to therapy with single agents; however, case reports indicate that the combination can cause serious and potentially fatal adverse effects

■ Nursing considerations

Assessment

- **History:** Hypersensitivity to any tricyclic drug; concomitant therapy with an MAOI; recent MI; myelography within previous 24 hr or scheduled within 48 hr; pregnancy; lactation; EST; preexisting CV disorders; angle-closure glaucoma, increased IOP; urinary retention, ureteral or urethral spasm; seizure disorders; hyperthyroidism; impaired hepatic, renal function; psychiatric disorders; bipolar disorder; elective surgery
- **Physical:** Weight; T; skin color, lesions; orientation, affect, reflexes, vision and hearing; P, BP, orthostatic BP, perfusion; bowel sounds, normal output, liver evaluation; urine flow, normal output; usual sexual function, frequency of menses, breast and scrotal examination; LFTs, urinalysis; CBC, ECG

Interventions

⊠ ***Black box warning*** Ensure that depressed and potentially suicidal patients have access to limited quantities of the drug. Monitor patients for suicidal ideation, especially when beginning therapy or changing doses; high risk of suicidality in children, adolescents, and young adults.

- Administer major portion of dose at bedtime if drowsiness or severe anticholinergic effects occur.

⊗ ***Warning*** Reduce dosage if minor side effects develop; discontinue if serious side effects occur.

- Arrange for CBC if patient develops fever, sore throat, or other sign of infection.

Teaching points

- Take drug exactly as prescribed.
- Do not stop taking this drug abruptly or without consulting your health care provider.
- Avoid alcohol, other sleep-inducing drugs, and over-the-counter drugs.
- Avoid prolonged exposure to sunlight or sunlamps; use a sunscreen or protective garments.
- You may experience these side effects: Headache, dizziness, drowsiness, weakness, blurred vision (reversible; safety measures may need to be taken if severe; avoid driving or performing tasks that require alertness); nausea, vomiting, loss of appetite, dry mouth (eat frequent small meals; practice frequent mouth care; suck sugarless candies); nightmares, inability to concentrate, confusion; changes in sexual function.
- Report dry mouth, difficulty in urination, excessive sedation.

DANGEROUS DRUG

▽ triptorelin pamoate

(trip toe rell' in)

Trelstar Depot, Trelstar LA

PREGNANCY CATEGORY X

T

Drug classes
Antineoplastic
Hormone
LHRH analogue

Therapeutic actions
An analogue of LHRH; causes a decrease in FSH and LH levels, leading to a suppression of ovarian and testicular hormone production, which causes decreased levels of estrogens (in women) and testosterone (in men); after continuous use, a sustained decrease in FSH and LH levels occurs.

Indications
- Palliative treatment of advanced prostatic cancer when orchiectomy or estrogen administration are not indicated or are unacceptable to the patient
- Treatment of advanced-stage prostatic cancer

Contraindications and cautions
- Contraindicated with pregnancy, lactation, hypersensitivity to LHRH or any component.
- Use cautiously with urinary tract obstructions, metastatic vertebral lesions.

Available forms
Powder for depot injection—3.75 mg, 11.25 mg

Dosages
Adults
- *Palliative treatment:* 3.75 mg depot injection IM once monthly into buttock.
- *Treatment:* 11.25 mg injection IM every 3 mo into buttock.

Pediatric patients
Safety and efficacy not established.

Pharmacokinetics

Route	Onset	Peak
IM	Slow	1–3 hr

Metabolism: Hepatic; $T_{1/2}$: 2.8–4 hr
Distribution: Crosses placenta; may enter breast milk
Excretion: Bile, urine

Adverse effects
- **CNS:** Insomnia, dizziness, lethargy, anxiety, depression, headache
- **CV:** HF, edema, hypertension, arrhythmia, chest pain
- **GI:** Nausea, anorexia
- **GU:** *Hot flashes, sexual dysfunction, decreased erections, lower urinary tract symptoms*
- **Other:** *Bone pain,* rash, sweating, cancer, **anaphylaxis, angioedema**

Interactions
✷ **Drug-drug** • Do not administer with drugs that increase prolactin production—antipsychotics, metoclopramide; risk of severe hyperprolactinemia

■ Nursing considerations
Assessment
- **History:** Pregnancy, lactation, hypersensitivity to LHRH or other LHRH drugs
- **Physical:** Skin T, lesions; reflexes, affect; BP, P; urinary output; serum testosterone levels, PSA levels

Interventions
- Reconstitute with 2 mL sterile water for injection. Shake well. Withdraw the entire contents of the vial into the syringe and inject immediately.
- Monitor testosterone and PSA levels prior to and periodically during therapy.
- Ensure repeat injection each month or every 3 mo—it is important to keep as close to this schedule as possible.
- Offer appropriate comfort measures (eg, temperature control, analgesics) to help patient cope with hot flashes, urinary retention, and bone pain. Most likely to occur at initiation of therapy.

Teaching points
- This drug must be injected each month or every 3 months.
- Do not take this drug if pregnant; if you are pregnant or want to become pregnant, consult your health care provider.
- You may experience these side effects: Hot flashes (staying in a cool place may help you to cope with this effect); sexual dysfunction, such as regression of sex organs, impaired fertility, decreased erections (it may help to know that these are drug effects; if

these become worrisome, consult your health care provider); bone pain, urinary retention, blood in the urine (these effects usually resolve within the first week of treatment; analgesics may be ordered to help you cope with the pain).
- Report chest pain, rapid heartbeat, numbness or tingling, breast pain, difficulty breathing, unresolved nausea and vomiting, signs of infection at the injection site.

▽trospium chloride

(troz' pee um)

Sanctura, Sanctura XR DNC

PREGNANCY CATEGORY C

Drug classes
Antimuscarinic
Antispasmodic

Therapeutic actions
Competitively blocks muscarinic receptor sites; bladder contraction is mediated by muscarinic receptors—blocking these receptors decreases bladder contraction, relieving bladder spasm.

Indications
- Urinary incontinence, urgency, and frequency caused by overactive bladder

Contraindications and cautions
- Contraindicated with allergy to trospium or any component of the drug; presence of or risk for urinary retention, gastric retention, uncontrolled narrow-angle glaucoma.
- Use cautiously with renal or hepatic impairment, ulcerative colitis, intestinal atony, myasthenia gravis, bladder or gastric outlet obstruction, pregnancy, lactation.

Available forms
Tablets—20 mg; ER capsules DNC—60 mg

Dosages
Adults younger than 75 yr
20 mg PO bid taken on an empty stomach, at least 1 hr before meals. Alternatively, 60 mg ER tablet PO once/day.

Adults 75 yr and older
Monitor patient response and adjust dosage down to 20 mg/day.

Pediatric patients
Safety and efficacy not established.

Patients with renal impairment
For creatinine clearance less than 30 mL/min, 20 mg/day PO given at bedtime.

Pharmacokinetics

Route	*Onset*	*Peak*
Oral	Slow	5–6 hr

Metabolism: Hepatic metabolism; $T_{1/2}$: 20 hr
Distribution: May cross placenta; passes into breast milk
Excretion: Feces, urine

Adverse effects
- **CNS:** *Headache,* dry eyes, dizziness, blurred vision
- **GI:** *Dry mouth, constipation,* abdominal pain, dyspepsia, flatulence, vomiting
- **GU:** Urinary retention
- **Other:** *Fatigue,* decreased sweating

Interactions
✱ **Drug-drug** • Increased risk of adverse effects if combined with any other anticholinergic drugs; if this combination is used, monitor patient carefully and adjust dosages accordingly • Potential for altered excretion of other drugs eliminated by tubular secretion (digoxin, morphine, metformin, tenfovir, procainamide, pancuronium, vancomycin); if any of these drugs are given concurrently, monitor patient carefully for increased adverse effects or decreased therapeutic effects of both drugs and adjust dosages accordingly

T

■ Nursing considerations
Assessment
- **History:** Allergy to trospium or any component of the drug; presence of or risk for urinary retention, gastric retention, uncontrolled narrow-angle glaucoma, renal or hepatic impairment, ulcerative colitis, intestinal atony, myasthenia gravis, bladder or gastric outlet obstruction; pregnancy, lactation

- **Physical:** Orientation, affect, vision, IOP; GI output, bowel sounds, liver evaluation; normal urinary output, prostate palpation; LFTs, renal function tests

Interventions

- Administer drug on an empty stomach, at least 1 hr before meal. Ensure that patient does not cut, crush, or chew ER form.
- Provide frequent small meals if GI upset is severe.
- Establish safety measures (eg, accompany patient, use side rails) if vision changes occur.
- Provide frequent mouth hygiene and sugarless lozenges if dry mouth is a problem.
- Monitor bowel function and arrange for appropriate bowel program if constipation occurs.

Teaching points

- Take this drug twice a day on an empty stomach, at least 1 hour before your next meal. Do not cut, crush, or chew ER form.
- If you miss a dose, take the next dose as soon as you remember and then again about that time the next day; do not take more than two doses per day.
- Know that you may be at higher risk for developing heat-related problems—sweating may be decreased so your body will not be able to cool off. Avoid excessive heat if at all possible; if you are in a hot environment drink plenty of fluids.
- You may experience these side effects: Dry mouth (sucking on sugarless lozenges and frequent mouth care may help); GI upset, nausea (frequent small meals may help); headache (analgesics may be available to help, consult with your health care provider); dizziness (do not drive a car or operate hazardous machinery if this occurs); urinary retention (emptying your bladder before taking the medicine may help); constipation (if this becomes a problem, consult your health care provider for appropriate remedies).
- Report inability to urinate, abdominal pain, severe constipation, fever.

▽urea

(yoor ee' a)

Ureaphil

PREGNANCY CATEGORY C

Drug class

Osmotic diuretic

Therapeutic actions

Elevates the osmolarity of the glomerular filtrate, hindering the reabsorption of water and leading to a loss of water, sodium, and chloride; creates an osmotic gradient in the eye between plasma and ocular fluids, reducing IOP.

Indications

- Reduction of intracranial pressure and treatment of cerebral edema
- Reduction of elevated IOP
- Unlabeled use: Induction of abortion when used by intra-amniotic injection

Contraindications and cautions

- Contraindicated with active intracranial bleeding (except during craniotomy), severe renal or hepatic disease, marked dehydration.
- Contraindicated for infusion into veins of the lower extremities of elderly patients.
- Use cautiously with pregnancy, lactation.

Available forms

Injection—40 g/150 mL

Dosages

Adults

Slow (over 1–2.5 hr) IV infusion of 30% solution only, 1–1.5 g/kg. Do not exceed 120 g/day or 1.5 g/kg.

Pediatric patients

0.5–1.5 g/kg IV. As little as 0.1 g/kg may be adequate in children younger than 2 yr.

Pharmacokinetics

Route	*Onset*	*Peak*	*Duration*
IV	30–45 min	60 min	5–6 hr

Metabolism: $T_{1/2}$: Unknown
Distribution: Crosses placenta; enters breast milk
Excretion: Urine

IV FACTS

Preparation: For 135 mL of a 30% solution of sterile urea, mix one 40-g vial with 105 mL of 5% or 10% dextrose injection or 10% invert sugar in water; each mL of a 30% solution provides 300 mg of urea; use only fresh solution; discard any solution within 24 hr after reconstitution.
Infusion: Administer 30% solution by slow IV infusion; do not exceed 4 mL/min.
Incompatibilities: Do not administer urea through the same IV set as blood or blood products.

Adverse effects

- **CNS:** *Dizziness, headache,* syncope, disorientation
- **GI:** *Nausea, vomiting*
- **Hematologic:** Hyponatremia, hypokalemia
- **Local:** Tissue necrosis if extravasation occurs at IV site
- **Other:** Thrombophlebitis, febrile response, hypervolemia if improperly administered

■ Nursing considerations

Assessment

- **History:** Active intracranial bleeding, marked dehydration, hepatic or renal disease, pregnancy, lactation
- **Physical:** Skin color, edema; orientation, reflexes, muscle strength, pupillary reflexes; pulses, BP, perfusion; R, pattern, adventitious sounds; urinary output patterns; serum electrolytes, urinalysis, LFTs, renal function tests

Interventions

- Do not infuse into veins of lower extremities of elderly patients.
- Monitor urinary output carefully.
- Monitor BP regularly and carefully.
- Monitor serum electrolytes periodically.
- Monitor intracranial pressure when appropriate.
- Use an indwelling catheter in comatose patients.

Teaching points

- This drug can only be given IV.
- You may experience these side effects: Increased urination, GI upset (eat frequent small meals); dry mouth (suck sugarless lozenges); headache, blurred vision (use caution when moving around; ask for assistance).
- Report pain at the IV site, severe headache, chest pain.

urofollitropin, purified

See Appendix W, *Less commonly used drugs*.

ursodiol (ursodeoxycholic acid)

(ur soe ***dye'*** *ole)*

Actigall, URSO, URSO 250, URSO DS (CAN), URSO Forte

PREGNANCY CATEGORY B

Drug class

Gallstone-solubilizing drug

Therapeutic actions

A naturally occurring bile acid that suppresses hepatic synthesis of cholesterol and inhibits intestinal absorption of cholesterol, leading to a decreased cholesterol concentration in the bile and a bile that is cholesterol solubilizing and not cholesterol precipitating.

Indications

- Treatment of selected patients with radiolucent, noncalcified gallstones in gallbladders for whom elective surgery is contraindicated
- Prevention of gallstone formation in obese patients experiencing rapid weight loss
- Treatment of primary biliary cirrhosis (tablets only)
- Unlabeled uses: Cholestasis-associated pruritus, primary sclerosing cholangitis

U

Contraindications and cautions

- Contraindicated with allergy to bile salts, hepatic impairment, calcified stones, radiopaque stones or radiolucent bile pigment stones, unremitting acute cholecystitis, cholangitis, biliary obstruction, gallstone pancreatitis, biliary GI fistula (cholecystectomy required), pregnancy.

- Use cautiously with lactation.

Available forms

Capsules—300 mg; tablets—250, 500 mg (*URSO*)

Dosages

Adults

- *Solubilization of gallstones:* 8–10 mg/kg/day PO given in two to three divided doses. Resolution of the gallstones requires months of therapy; condition needs to be monitored with ultrasound at 6-mo and 1-yr intervals.
- *Treatment of biliary cirrhosis:* 13–15 mg/kg/day PO administered in two to four divided doses with food; readjust dosage based on patient response (*URSO*).
- *Prevention of gallstones:* 300 mg PO bid or 8–10 mg/kg/day PO in two to three divided doses.

Pediatric patients

Safety and efficacy not established.

Pharmacokinetics

Route	Onset	Peak
Oral	Varies	Days

Metabolism: Hepatic; $T_{1/2}$: Unknown
Distribution: Crosses placenta; may enter breast milk
Excretion: Feces

Adverse effects

- **CNS:** Headache, fatigue, anxiety, depression, sleep disorder
- **Dermatologic:** Pruritus, rash, urticaria, dry skin, sweating, hair thinning
- **GI:** *Diarrhea,* cramps, heartburn, constipation, nausea, vomiting, anorexia, epigastric distress, dyspepsia, flatulence, abdominal pain
- **Respiratory:** Rhinitis, cough
- **Other:** Back pain, arthralgia, myalgia

Interactions

✱ **Drug-drug** • Absorption decreased if taken with bile acid sequestering agents (cholestyramine, colestipol), aluminum-based antacids

■ Nursing considerations

Assessment

- **History:** Allergy to bile salts, hepatic impairment, calcified stones, radiopaque stones or radiolucent bile pigment stones, unremitting acute cholecystitis, cholangitis, biliary obstruction, gallstone pancreatitis, biliary-GI fistula, pregnancy, lactation
- **Physical:** Liver evaluation, abdominal examination; affect, orientation; skin color, lesions; LFTs, hepatic and biliary radiological studies, biliary ultrasound

Interventions

- Assess patient carefully for suitability of ursodiol therapy. Alternative therapy should be reviewed before using ursodiol.
- Give drug in two to three divided doses.
- Do not administer drug with aluminum-based antacids. If such drugs are needed, administer 2–3 hr after ursodiol.
- Schedule patients for periodic oral cholecystograms or ultrasonograms to evaluate drug effectiveness at 6-mo intervals until resolution, then every 3 mo to monitor stone formation. Stones recur within 5 yr in more than 50% of patients. If gallstones appear to have dissolved, continue treatment for 3 mo and perform follow-up ultrasound.
- Monitor LFTs periodically. Carefully assess patient if any change in liver function occurs.

Teaching points

- Take drug two to four times a day. Take the drug as long as prescribed. It may be needed for a long time.
- This drug may dissolve your gallstones; it does not "cure" the problem that caused the stones, and in many cases, the stones can recur. Medical follow-up care is important.
- Arrange to receive periodic X-rays or ultrasound tests of your gallbladder; you also will need periodic blood tests to evaluate your response to this drug. Keep follow-up appointments.
- Do not take with any aluminum-based antacids.
- You may experience these side effects: Diarrhea; rash (skin care may help); headache, fatigue (request analgesics).

- Report gallstone attacks (abdominal pain, nausea, vomiting), yellowing of the skin or eyes.

ustekinumab

See Appendix W, *Less commonly used drugs.*

valacyclovir hydrochloride

(val ah ***sye'*** *kloe ver)*

Valtrex

PREGNANCY CATEGORY B

Drug class

Antiviral

Therapeutic actions

Antiviral activity; inhibits viral DNA replication and deactivates viral DNA polymerase.

Indications

- Treatment of herpes zoster (shingles)
- Episodic treatment of first-episode or recurrent genital herpes in immunocompetent patients
- Suppression of recurrent episodes of genital herpes in HIV patients
- Reduction of risk of heterosexual transmission of genital herpes to healthy partners when combined with safe sex practices
- Treatment of cold sores (herpes labialis) in healthy adults and adolescents
- Unlabeled use: Prevention of cytomegalovirus in patients with renal transplantation

Contraindications and cautions

- Contraindicated with allergy to valacyclovir or acyclovir.
- Use cautiously with pregnancy, renal impairment, thrombotic thrombocytopenic purpura, lactation.

Available forms

Tablets—500 mg, 1 g

Dosages

Adults

- *Herpes zoster:* 1 g tid PO for 7 days; most effective if started within 48 hr of onset of symptoms (rash).
- *Genital herpes:* 1 g PO bid for 7–10 days for initial episode.
- *Episodic treatment of recurrent genital herpes:* 500 mg PO bid for 3 days or 1 g/day for 5 days.
- *Suppression of recurrent episodes of genital herpes:* 1 g PO daily; patients with history of less than nine episodes in 1 yr may respond to 500 mg PO daily.
- *Suppression of recurrent episodes in HIV-infected patients:* 500 mg PO bid for 5–10 days.
- *Reduction of risk of transmission:* 500 mg/day PO for the source partner. For HIV-positive patients, 500 mg PO bid.
- *Cold sores:* 2 g PO bid for 1 day.

Pediatric patients

Safety and efficacy not established. Dosages that have been used:

- *Chickenpox:* Children 2–18 yr: 20 mg/kg PO tid for 5 days. Maximum dose, 1 g tid.
- *Cold sores:* Children 12 yr and older: 2 g PO every 12 hr for one day.

Patients with renal impairment

Dosage adjustment variations by indication and CrCl

Indication	*CrCl 30–49*	*CrCl 10–29*	*CrCl less than 10*
Herpes zoster	1 g every 12 hr	1 g every 24 hr	500 mg every 24 hr
Genital herpes			
–initial treatment	1 g every 12 hr	1 g every 24 hr	500 mg every 24 hr
–recurrent episodes	500 mg every 12 hr	500 mg every 24 hr	500 mg every 24 hr
–suppressive therapy	1g every 24 hr	500 mg every 24 hr	500 mg every 24 hr
–suppressive therapy for 9 or fewer episodes	500 mg every 24 hr	500 mg every 48 hr	500 mg every 48 hr

Pharmacokinetics

Route	*Onset*	*Peak*
Oral	Rapid	3 hr

V

Metabolism: Not metabolized; $T_{1/2}$: 2.5–3.3 hr
Distribution: Crosses placenta; enters breast milk
Excretion: Feces, urine

Adverse effects

- **CNS:** Headache, dizziness
- **GI:** *Nausea, vomiting,* diarrhea, anorexia
- **GU:** Acute renal failure

Interactions

✱ **Drug-drug** • Decreased rate of effectiveness with probenecid, cimetidine

■ Nursing considerations

CLINICAL ALERT!
Name confusion has been reported with *Valtrex* (valacyclovir) and *Valcyte* (valganciclovir); use caution.

Assessment

- **History:** Allergy to valacyclovir, acyclovir; renal disease; lactation; thrombotic thrombocytopenic purpura; pregnancy
- **Physical:** Orientation; urinary output; abdominal examination, normal output; BUN, creatinine clearance

Interventions

- Begin treatment within 48–72 hr of onset of symptoms of shingles.
- Administer without regard to meals; administer with meals to decrease GI upset, if needed.
- Provide appropriate analgesics for headache and discomfort of shingles.
- Advise continued use of safe sex practices.

Teaching points

- Take this drug without regard to meals; if GI upset is a problem, take with meals.
- Take the full course of therapy as prescribed.
- Avoid contact with lesions and avoid intercourse when lesions or symptoms are present to avoid infecting others.
- Start therapy at first sign of an episode when treating recurrent herpes.
- You may experience these side effects: Nausea, vomiting, loss of appetite, diarrhea, headache, dizziness.
- Report severe diarrhea, nausea, headache, worsening of the shingles.

▽ valganciclovir hydrochloride

*(val gan **sigh'** kloe veer)*

Valcyte DNC

PREGNANCY CATEGORY C

Drug class

Antiviral

Therapeutic actions

Antiviral activity; inhibits viral DNA replication in cytomegalovirus (CMV).

Indications

- Treatment of CMV retinitis in patients with AIDS
- Prevention of CMV infection in high-risk kidney-pancreas, kidney, and heart transplant patients
- **NEW INDICATION:** Prevention of CMV infection in pediatric patients with kidney or heart transplant at high risk for CMV infection

Contraindications and cautions

- Contraindicated with hypersensitivity to valganciclovir, ganciclovir, or acyclovir; lactation.
- Use cautiously in the elderly; with cytopenia, history of cytopenic reactions, impaired renal function, bone marrow suppression, hemodialysis, pregnancy.

Available forms

Tablets DNC—450 mg; oral solution—50 mg/5 mL

Dosages

Adults

900 mg PO bid for 21 days; maintenance, 900 mg PO daily.

- *Prevention of CMV:* 900 mg daily initiated within 10 days of transplantation and continued for 100 days after transplantation

Pediatric patients 4 mo–16 yr

Dose in mg = 7 × BSA × CrCl. Maximum dose, 900 mg/day. May use oral solution or tablets.

Patients with renal impairment

Do not administer to patients on hemodialysis. For patients with renal impairment, see the following table:

CrCl (mL/min)	*Initial Dose*	*Maintenance Dose*
60 or more	900 mg PO bid	900 mg/day PO
40–59	450 mg PO bid	450 mg/day PO
25–39	450 mg PO daily	450 mg PO every other day
10–24	450 mg PO every 2 days	450 mg PO twice weekly

Pharmacokinetics

Route	*Onset*	*Peak*
Oral	Slow	1–3 hr

Metabolism: Hepatic transformation to ganciclovir; $T_{1/2}$: 4 hr
Distribution: Crosses placenta; may enter breast milk
Excretion: Urine

Adverse effects

- **CNS:** *Headache, insomnia,* neuropathy, paresthesias, confusion, hallucinations
- **GI:** *Nausea, vomiting,* anorexia, *diarrhea,* abdominal pain
- **Hematologic:** *Neutropenia, anemia,* thrombocytopenia
- **Other:** *Fever,* retinal detachment

Interactions

✱ **Drug-drug** ⊗ ***Warning*** Use with extreme caution with cytotoxic drugs because the accumulation effect could cause severe bone marrow depression and other GI and dermatologic problems.
⊗ ***Warning*** Extreme drowsiness and risk of bone marrow depression if taken with zidovudine; avoid this combination.
• Increased valganciclovir effects if taken with probenecid • Increased risk of seizures if taken concurrently with imipenem-cilastatin

■ Nursing considerations

CLINICAL ALERT!
Name confusion has been reported with *Valcyte* (valganciclovir) and *Valtrex* (valacyclovir); use caution.

Assessment

- **History:** Hypersensitivity to valganciclovir, ganciclovir, or acyclovir; cytopenia; history of cytopenic reactions; impaired renal function; pregnancy; lactation
- **Physical:** T, orientation, reflexes, urinary output, CBC, BUN, creatinine clearance

Interventions

- Administer drug with food to maximize absorption and to decrease GI upset.

⊗ ***Warning*** Do not exceed the recommended dosage or frequency; note that valganciclovir cannot be substituted for ganciclovir capsules on a one-to-one basis.

- Arrange for decreased dosage in patients with impaired renal function.

⊠ ***Black box warning*** Arrange for CBC before beginning therapy and at least weekly thereafter. Consult with physician and arrange for reduced dosage if WBC count or platelets fall. Toxicity includes granulocytopenia, anemia, and thrombocytopenia.

⊗ ***Warning*** Consult with pharmacy for proper disposal of unused tablets. Precautions are required for disposal of nucleoside analogues. Do not cut, crush, or chew tablets. Avoid handling broken tablets.

- Arrange for periodic ophthalmic examinations during therapy. Drug is not a cure of the disease and deterioration may occur.
- Provide comfort measures for patients who develop fever, rash, or headache.
- Advise patients that valganciclovir can decrease sperm production in men and cause birth defects in the fetus. Advise the patient to use some form of contraception during valganciclovir therapy. Men receiving valganciclovir therapy should use some form of barrier contraception during and for at least 90 days after therapy.

Black box warning Advise patient that valganciclovir has caused cancer and fetal damage in animals and that risk is possible in humans.

- Maintain support therapy and program for AIDS patients who are receiving this drug as part of their overall treatment plan.

Teaching points

- Take this drug with food to help the absorption of the drug and possibly decrease GI upset. Swallow tablets whole. Do not cut, crush, or chew them.
- Drink 2 to 3 liters of water each day while taking this drug, unless otherwise instructed by your health care provider.
- Make appointments for frequent blood tests that will need to be done to determine the effects of the drug on your blood count and to determine the appropriate dosage needed. It is important that you keep appointments for these tests.
- Arrange for periodic eye examinations (every 4–6 weeks) during therapy to evaluate progress of the disease. This drug is not a cure for your retinitis.
- If you are also receiving zidovudine, the two drugs cannot be given concomitantly; severe adverse effects may occur.
- If you think you are pregnant or want to become pregnant, consult your health care provider. Use contraception during drug therapy. Male patients should use barrier contraceptives during drug therapy and for at least 90 days after therapy.
- You may experience these side effects: Decreased blood count leading to susceptibility to infection (frequent blood tests will be needed; avoid crowds and exposure to disease as much as possible); birth defects and decreased sperm production (drug cannot be taken during pregnancy); sedation, dizziness, confusion (avoid driving or operating dangerous machinery if these effects occur).
- Report bruising, bleeding, infection, extreme fatigue, edema.

valproic acid

(val proe' ik)

valproic acid

Apo-Valproic Acid (CAN), Gen-Valproic (CAN), PMS-Valproic Acid (CAN), ratio-Valproic (CAN), Stavzor

Capsules: Depakene DNC

sodium valproate

Syrup: Depakene

valproate acid

Injection: Depacon

divalproex sodium

Tablets, enteric coated: Depakote DNC, Depakote ER DNC, Depakote Sprinkle, Divalproex, Epival (CAN)

PREGNANCY CATEGORY D

Drug class

Antiepileptic

Therapeutic actions

Mechanism of action not understood: Antiepileptic activity may be related to the metabolism of the inhibitory neurotransmitter, GABA; divalproex sodium is a compound containing equal proportions of valproic acid and sodium valproate.

Indications

- *Valproic acid:* Sole and adjunctive therapy in simple (petit mal) and complex absence seizures; acute treatment of manic episodes associated with bipolar disorder; prophylaxis of migraine headaches; adjunctive therapy for multiple seizure disorders
- *Depakote ER:* Treatment of epilepsy in children 10 yr and older; treatment of acute manic or mixed episodes associated with bipolar disorder, with or without psychotic features
- *Depakote ER:* Treatment of bipolar mania
- *Depakote, Depakote ER:* Prophylaxis of migraine headaches

- *Divalproex, sodium valproate injection:* Treatment of complex partial seizures as monotherapy or with other antiepileptics
- Unlabeled uses: Adjunct in symptom management of schizophrenia, treatment of aggressive outbursts in children with ADHD, organic brain syndrome

Contraindications and cautions

- Contraindicated with hypersensitivity to valproic acid, hepatic disease, or significant hepatic impairment.
- Use cautiously with children younger than 18 mo; children younger than 2 yr, especially with multiple antiepileptics, congenital metabolic disorders, severe seizures accompanied by severe mental retardation, organic brain disorders (higher risk of developing fatal hepatotoxicity); pregnancy (fetal neural tube defects; do not discontinue to prevent major seizures; discontinuing such medication is likely to precipitate status epilepticus, hypoxia and risk to both mother and fetus); lactation.

Available forms

Capsules—250 mg; DR capsules DNC—125, 250, 500 mg; syrup—250 mg/5 mL; DR tablets DNC—125, 250, 500 mg; sprinkle capsules—125 mg; injection—100 mg/mL; ER tablets DNC—250, 500 mg

Dosages

Adults

Dosage is expressed as valproic acid equivalents. Initial dose is 10–15 mg/kg/day PO, increasing at 1-wk intervals by 5–10 mg/kg/day until seizures are controlled or side effects preclude further increases. Maximum recommended dosage is 60 mg/kg/day PO. If total dose exceeds 250 mg/day, give in divided doses.

- *Acute mania or bipolar disorder:* Initially, 25 mg/kg/day PO once daily. Dose should be increased rapidly to achieve the lowest therapeutic dose. Maximum dose 60 mg/kg/day PO (*Depakote ER* only).
- *Bipolar mania:* 750 mg PO daily in divided doses; do not exceed 60 mg/kg/day (*Divalproex DR* tablets only).
- *Migraine:* 250 mg PO bid; up to 1,000 mg/day has been used (*Divalproex DR* tablets); 500 mg ER tablet once a day.

Pediatric patients 10 yr and older

10–15 mg/kg/day PO.

Pediatric patients 10 yr and younger

Use extreme caution. Fatal hepatotoxicity has occurred. Children younger than 2 yr are especially susceptible. Monitor all children carefully.

Pharmacokinetics

Route	*Onset*	*Peak*
Oral	Varies	1–4 hr
IV	Rapid	1 hr

Metabolism: Hepatic; $T_{1/2}$: 6–16 hr
Distribution: Crosses placenta; enters breast milk
Excretion: Urine

IV FACTS

Preparation: Dilute vial in 5% dextrose injection, 0.9% sodium chloride injection or lactated Ringer's injection. Stable for 24 hr at room temperature. Discard unused portions.
Infusion: Administer over 60 min, not more than 20 mg/min. Do not use more than 14 days; switch to oral products as soon as possible.

Adverse effects

- **CNS:** *Sedation,* tremor (may be dose-related), emotional upset, depression, psychosis, aggression, hyperactivity, behavioral deterioration, weakness, suicidality
- **Dermatologic:** Transient increases in hair loss, rash, petechiae
- **GI:** *Nausea, vomiting, indigestion,* diarrhea, abdominal cramps, constipation, anorexia with weight loss, increased appetite with weight gain, **life-threatening pancreatitis, hepatic failure**; elevated liver enzyme, serum bilirubin
- **GU:** Irregular menses, secondary amenorrhea
- **Hematologic:** Altered bleeding time; thrombocytopenia; bruising; hematoma formation; frank hemorrhage; relative lymphocytosis; hypofibrinogenemia; leukopenia, eosinophilia, anemia, bone marrow suppression

Interactions

✱ **Drug-drug** • Increased serum phenobarbital, primidone, ethosuximide, diazepam, zidovudine levels • Complex interactions with phenytoin; breakthrough seizures have occurred with the combination of valproic acid and phenytoin • Increased serum levels and toxicity with salicylates, cimetidine, chlorpromazine, erythromycin, felbamate • Decreased effects with carbamazepine, rifampin, lamotrigine • Decreased serum levels with charcoal • Increased sedation with alcohol, other CNS depressants

✱ **Drug-lab test** • False interpretation of urine ketone test

■ Nursing considerations

CLINICAL ALERT!

Confusion has occurred between DR *Depakote* and *Depakote ER*. Dosage is very different and serious adverse effects can occur; use extreme caution.

Assessment

- **History:** Hypersensitivity to valproic acid; hepatic impairment; pregnancy, lactation
- **Physical:** Weight; skin color, lesions; orientation, affect, reflexes; bowel sounds, normal output; CBC and differential, bleeding time tests, LFTs, serum ammonia level, exocrine pancreatic function tests, EEG

Interventions

- Give drug with food if GI upset occurs; substitution of the enteric-coated formulation also may be of benefit; have patient swallow ER tablet whole; do not cut, crush, or chew.
- Be aware that patient may be at increased risk for suicidal ideation and suicidality; monitor accordingly.

⊗ ***Warning*** Reduce dosage, discontinue, or substitute other antiepileptics gradually; abrupt discontinuation of all antiepileptics may precipitate absence seizures.

⊠ ***Black box warning*** Arrange for frequent LFTs; discontinue drug immediately with suspected or apparent significant hepatic impairment; continue LFTs to determine if hepatic impairment progresses in spite of drug discontinuation.

⊗ ***Warning*** Arrange for patient to have platelet counts, bleeding time determination before therapy, periodically during therapy, and prior to surgery. Monitor patient carefully for clotting defects (bruising, blood-tinged toothbrush). Discontinue if there is evidence of hemorrhage, bruising, or disorder of hemostasis.

- Monitor ammonia levels, and discontinue if there is clinically significant elevation in level.
- Monitor serum levels of valproic acid and other antiepileptics given concomitantly, especially during the first few weeks of therapy. Adjust dosage on the basis of these data and clinical response.

⊠ ***Black box warning*** Arrange for counseling for women of childbearing age who wish to become pregnant; drug may be teratogenic.

⊠ ***Black box warning*** Discontinue the drug at any sign of pancreatitis; life-threatening pancreatitis has occurred.

⊗ ***Warning*** Evaluate for therapeutic serum levels—usually 50–100 mcg/mL.

Teaching points

- Take this drug exactly as prescribed. Do not chew tablets or capsules before swallowing them. Swallow them whole to prevent local irritation of mouth and throat. *Depakote Sprinkle* tablets may be opened and sprinkled on applesauce or pudding.
- Do not discontinue this drug abruptly or change dosage, except on the advice of your health care provider.
- Avoid alcohol and sleep-inducing and over-the-counter drugs. These could cause dangerous effects.
- Have frequent checkups, including blood tests, to monitor your drug response. Keep all appointments for checkups.
- Use contraceptive techniques at all times. If you want to become pregnant, consult your health care provider.
- Wear a medical ID tag to alert emergency medical personnel that you have epilepsy and are taking antiepileptic medication.
- If you have diabetes, this drug may interfere with urine tests for ketones.

- You may experience these side effects: Drowsiness (avoid driving or performing other tasks requiring alertness; take at bedtime); GI upset (take with food or milk, eat frequent small meals; if problem persists, substitute enteric-coated drug); transient increase in hair loss.
- Report bruising, pink stain on the toothbrush, yellowing of the skin or eyes, pale feces, rash, pregnancy, abdominal pain with nausea, vomiting, anorexia, thoughts of suicide.

valsartan

(val sar' tan)

Diovan

PREGNANCY CATEGORY C (FIRST TRIMESTER)

PREGNANCY CATEGORY D (SECOND AND THIRD TRIMESTERS)

Drug classes

Angiotensin II receptor blocker
Antihypertensive

Therapeutic actions

Selectively blocks the binding of angiotensin II to specific tissue receptors found in the vascular smooth muscle and adrenal gland; this action blocks the vasoconstricting effect of the renin–angiotensin system as well as the release of aldosterone, leading to decreased BP; may prevent the vessel remodeling associated with the development of atherosclerosis.

Indications

- Treatment of hypertension, alone or in combination with other antihypertensives
- Treatment of HF in patients who are intolerant of ACE inhibitors
- Reduction in CV mortality in stable patients with left ventricular failure or left ventricular dysfunction following MI

Contraindications and cautions

- Contraindicated with hypersensitivity to valsartan, pregnancy (use during second or third trimester can cause injury or even death to fetus), lactation.
- Use cautiously with hepatic or renal impairment, hypovolemia.

Available forms

Tablets—40, 80, 160, 320 mg

Dosages

Adults

- *Hypertension:* 80 mg PO daily; range 80–320 mg/day.
- *HF:* Starting dose is 40 mg bid, titration to 80 mg and 160 mg bid should be done to the highest dose, as tolerated by the patient. Maximum daily dose is 320 mg daily given in divided doses. May be given in combination with other antihypertensives. Consider dosage reduction if used with diuretics.
- *Post-MI left ventricular dysfunction:* Start as early as 12 hr post-MI; 20 mg PO bid, may increase after 7 days to 40 mg PO bid; titrate to 160 mg PO bid if tolerated.

Pediatric patients 6–16 yr

- *Hypertension:* Starting dosage, 1.3 mg/kg PO once daily (up to 40 mg). Target dosage, 1.3–2.7 mg/kg PO once daily (40–160 mg/day.

Patients with severe hepatic or renal impairment

Exercise caution and monitor patient frequently.

Pharmacokinetics

Route	*Onset*	*Peak*
Oral	Varies	2–4 hr

Metabolism: Hepatic; $T_{1/2}$: 6 hr
Distribution: Crosses placenta; enters breast milk
Excretion: Feces, urine

Adverse effects

- **CNS:** *Headache, dizziness,* syncope, muscle weakness
- **CV:** Hypotension
- **Dermatologic:** Rash, inflammation, urticaria, pruritus, alopecia, dry skin
- **GI:** *Diarrhea, abdominal pain, nausea,* constipation, dry mouth, dental pain
- **Respiratory:** *URI symptoms, cough,* sinus disorders
- **Other:** Back pain, fever, gout, hyperkalemia

■ Nursing considerations

Assessment

- **History:** Hypersensitivity to valsartan; pregnancy, lactation; hepatic or renal impairment; hypovolemia
- **Physical:** Skin lesions, turgor; T; reflexes, affect; BP; R, respiratory auscultation; LFTs, renal function tests

Interventions

- Administer without regard to meals.

⊠ ***Black box warning*** Ensure that patient is not pregnant before beginning therapy; suggest use of barrier birth control while using drug; fetal injury and deaths have been reported.

- Find alternative method of feeding infant if drug is being given to nursing mother. Depression of renin-angiotensin system in infants is potentially very dangerous.

⊗ ***Warning*** Alert surgeon and mark the patient's chart that valsartan is being given. Blockage of renin-angiotensin system following surgery can produce problems. Hypotension may be reversed with volume expansion.

- Monitor patient closely in any situation that may lead to decrease in BP secondary to reduction in fluid volume—excessive perspiration, dehydration, vomiting, diarrhea—because excessive hypotension can occur.

Teaching points

- Take this drug without regard to meals. Do not stop taking drug without consulting your health care provider.
- Use a barrier method of birth control while using this drug; if you become pregnant or want to become pregnant, consult your health care provider.
- You may experience these side effects: Dizziness (avoid driving or performing hazardous tasks); headache (medications may be available to help); nausea, vomiting, diarrhea (proper nutrition is important; consult a dietitian); symptoms of upper respiratory tract infection, cough (do not self-medicate; consult your health care provider if this becomes uncomfortable).
- Report fever, chills, dizziness, pregnancy.

▽ vancomycin hydrochloride

*(van koe **mye'** sin)*

Vancocin, Vancoled

PREGNANCY CATEGORY C

PREGNANCY CATEGORY B (PULVULES)

Drug class

Antibiotic

Therapeutic actions

Bactericidal: Inhibits cell wall synthesis of susceptible organisms, causing cell death.

Indications

- Parenteral: Potentially life-threatening infections not treatable with other less toxic antibiotics
- Severe staphylococci infections in patients who cannot receive or have failed to respond to penicillins and cephalosporins
- Prevention of bacterial endocarditis in penicillin-allergic patients undergoing dental, upper respiratory, GI, or GU surgery or invasive procedures
- Oral: Staphylococcal enterocolitis and antibiotic-associated pseudomembranous colitis caused by *Clostridium difficile*

Contraindications and cautions

- Contraindicated with allergy to vancomycin.
- Use cautiously with hearing loss, renal impairment, pregnancy, lactation.

Available forms

Pulvules—125, 250 mg; powder for oral solution—1, 10 g; powder for injection—500 mg; 1, 5, 10 g

Dosages

Adults

500 mg–2 g/day PO in three or four divided doses for 7–10 days; 500 mg IV every 6 hr or 1 g IV every 12 hr.

- *Pseudomembranous colitis caused by* C. difficile: 500 mg to 2 g/day PO in three to four divided doses for 7–10 days or 125 mg PO tid–qid.

Pediatric patients

40 mg/kg/day PO in three to four divided doses for 7–10 days. 10 mg/kg/dose IV every 6 hr. Do not exceed 2 g/day.

- *Premature and full-term neonates:* Use with caution because of incompletely developed renal function. Initial dose of 15 mg/kg, followed by 10 mg/kg every 12 hr in first week of life and every 8 hr thereafter up to age of 1 mo.
- *Pseudomembranous colitis caused by* C. difficile: 40 mg/kg/day in four divided doses PO for 7–10 days. Do not exceed 2 g/day.

Geriatric patients or patients with renal failure

Monitor dosage and serum levels very carefully. Dosage nomogram is available for determining the dose according to creatinine clearance (see manufacturer's insert).

Pharmacokinetics

Route	*Onset*	*Peak*
Oral	Varies	Varies
IV	Rapid	End of infusion

Metabolism: $T_{1/2}$: 4–6 hr
Distribution: Crosses placenta; may enter breast milk
Excretion: Urine

IV FACTS

Preparation: Not for IM administration. Reconstitute with 10 mL sterile water for injection; 500 mg/mL concentration results. Dilute reconstituted solution with 100–200 mL of 0.9% sodium chloride injection or D_5W for intermittent infusion. For continuous infusion (use only if intermittent therapy is not possible), add 2–4 (1–2 g) vials reconstituted solution to sufficiently large volume of 0.9% sodium chloride injection or D_5W to permit slow IV drip of the total daily dose over 24 hr. Refrigerate reconstituted solution; stable over 14 days. Further diluted solution is stable for 24 hr.

Infusion: For intermittent infusion, infuse every 6 hr over at least 60 min, no faster than 1,000 mg/hr, to avoid irritation, hypotension, throbbing back and neck pain. Give continuously slowly over 24 hr.

Incompatibilities: Do not mix with amobarbital, chloramphenicol, dexamethasone, heparin, barbiturates, warfarin.

Y-site incompatibility: Do not give with foscarnet.

Adverse effects

- **CNS:** *Ototoxicity*
- **CV:** Hypotension (IV administration)
- **Dermatologic:** *Urticaria,* macular rashes
- **GI:** *Nausea*
- **GU:** *Nephrotoxicity*
- **Hematologic:** Eosinophilia, neutropenia
- **Other:** Superinfections; **"red neck** or **red man syndrome"** (sudden and profound fall in BP, fever, chills, paresthesias, erythema of the neck and back)

Interactions

✱ **Drug-drug** • Increased neuromuscular blockade with atracurium, pancuronium, tubocurarine, vecuronium • Increased risk of ototoxicity or nephrotoxicity when administered with other ototoxic or nephrotoxic drugs (aminoglycosides, amphotericin B, bacitracin, cisplatin)

■ Nursing considerations

Assessment

- **History:** Allergy to vancomycin, hearing loss, renal impairment, pregnancy, lactation
- **Physical:** Site of infection, skin color, lesions; orientation, reflexes, auditory function; BP, perfusion; R, adventitious sounds; CBC, LFTs, renal function tests, auditory tests

Interventions

- Oral solution: Add 115 mL distilled water to contents of 10-g container. Each 6 mL of solution will contain 500 mg vancomycin. Alternatively, dilute the contents of 500-mg vial for injection in 30 mL of water for oral or nasogastric tube administration.

⊗ ***Warning*** Observe the patient very closely when giving parenteral solution, particularly the first doses; "red man" syndrome can occur (see adverse effects); slow administration decreases the risk of adverse effects.

- Culture site of infection before beginning therapy.

- Monitor renal function tests with prolonged therapy.

⊗ ***Warning*** Evaluate for safe serum levels; concentrations of 60–80 mcg/mL are toxic.

Teaching points

- This drug is available only in the IV and oral forms.
- Do not stop taking this drug without notifying your health care provider.
- Take the full prescribed course of this drug.
- You may experience these side effects: Nausea (eat frequent small meals); changes in hearing; superinfections in the mouth, vagina (frequent hygiene measures will help).
- Report ringing in the ears, loss of hearing, difficulty voiding, rash, flushing.

▽ vardenafil hydrochloride

*(var **den'** ah fill)*

Levitra

PREGNANCY CATEGORY B

Drug classes

Impotence drug
Phosphodiesterase type 5 inhibitor

Therapeutic actions

Selectively inhibits cyclic guanosine monophosphate (cGMP) specific phosphodiesterase type 5. The mechanism of penile erection involves the release of nitric oxide into the corpus cavernosum of the penis during sexual stimulation. Nitrous oxide activates cGMP, which causes smooth muscle relaxation allowing the flow of blood into the corpus cavernosum. Vardenafil prevents the breakdown of cGMP by phosphodiesterase, leading to increased cGMP levels and prolonged smooth muscle relaxation promoting the flow of blood into the corpus cavernosum.

Indications

- Treatment of ED occurring in the presence of sexual stimulation
- Unlabeled use: Raynaud phenomenon

Contraindications and cautions

- Contraindicated with allergy to any component of the tablet, concurrent use of nitrates or alpha blockers.
- Contraindicated for women or children.
- Use cautiously with hepatic or renal impairment; with anatomic deformation of the penis, with known cardiac disease (effects of sexual activity need to be evaluated), congenital prolonged QT interval, unstable angina; hypotension (systolic pressure less than 90 mm Hg); uncontrolled hypertension (greater than 170/110 mm Hg), severe hepatic impairment; end-stage renal disease with dialysis; hereditary degenerative retinal disorders.

Available forms

Tablets—2.5, 5, 10, 20 mg

Dosages

Adults

5–10 mg PO taken 1 hr before anticipated sexual activity; range 5–20 mg PO. Limit use to once per day.

Pediatric patients

Not intended for use in children.

Geriatric patients and those with moderate hepatic impairment

Starting dose of 5 mg PO is suggested.

Pharmacokinetics

Route	*Onset*	*Peak*
Oral	Rapid	30–120 min

Metabolism: Hepatic, $T_{1/2}$: 4–5 hr
Distribution: Not intended for use in women, no clear studies on crossing the placenta or entering breast milk
Excretion: Feces

Adverse effects

- **CNS:** *Headache,* abnormal vision, dizziness, hypertonia, insomnia, somnolence, vertigo, ischemic optic neuropathy, sudden hearing loss
- **CV:** *Flushing,* angina, chest pain, hypertension, hypotension, **MI,** palpitation, postural hypotension, tachycardia
- **GI:** *Dyspepsia,* diarrhea, abdominal pain, dry mouth, esophagitis, gastritic, GERD

- **GU:** Abnormal ejaculation, priapism
- **Respiratory:** Rhinitis, sinusitis, dyspnea, epistaxis, pharyngitis
- **Other:** Flulike symptoms, edema, pain, rash, sweating

Interactions

✱ Drug-drug ⊗ ***Warning*** Possible severe hypotension and serious cardiac events if combined with nitrates, alpha blockers; this combination must be avoided.

- Possible increased vardenafil levels and effects if taken with ketoconazole, itraconazole, erythromycin; monitor patient and reduce dosage as needed, usually to 2.5 mg/day PO
- Increased vardenafil serum level if combined with indinavir, ritonavir; if these drugs are being used, limit vardenafil dose to 2.5 mg in a 24-hr period

■ Nursing considerations

Assessment

- **History:** Allergy to any component of the tablet, concurrent use of nitrates or alpha blockers; unstable angina, hypotension, uncontrolled hypertension; severe hepatic impairment; end-stage renal disease with dialysis; hereditary degenerative retinal disorders; anatomical deformation of the penis; cardiac disease, congenital prolonged QT interval
- **Physical:** Orientation, affect; skin color, lesions; R, adventitious sounds; P, BP, ECG, LFTs, renal function tests; hearing, vision examinations

Interventions

- Ensure diagnosis of ED and determine underlying causes and other appropriate treatment.
- Advise patient that drug does not work without sexual stimulation. Limit use to once per day.
- Teach patient to contact health care provider about any loss of vision or hearing.
- Remind patient that drug does not protect against STDs and appropriate measures should be taken.

⊗ ***Warning*** Advise patient to never take this drug with nitrates or alpha blockers; serious and even fatal complications can occur.

Teaching points

- Take this drug 60 minutes before anticipated sexual activity. The drug will have no effect unless there is sexual stimulation.
- This drug will not protect you from sexually transmitted diseases; use appropriate precautions.
- Do not take this drug if you are taking any nitrates or alpha blockers; serious side effects or death can occur.
- Many drugs may interact with vardenafil; always consult your health care provider before taking any drug, including over-the-counter drugs and herbal therapies; dosage adjustments may be needed.
- You may experience these side effects: Headache, dizziness, upset stomach, runny nose; these side effects should go away within a couple of hours. If side effects persist, consult your health care provider.
- Stop drug and consult your health care provider immediately if you experience sudden loss of vision or hearing.
- Report difficult or painful urination, vision changes, fainting, erection that persists for longer than 4 hours, sudden loss of vision.

▽ varenicline tartrate

*(var **en'** ah klin)*

Chantix

PREGNANCY CATEGORY C

Drug classes

Nicotine receptor antagonist
Smoking deterrent

Therapeutic actions

Selectively binds with specific neuronal nicotinic acetylcholine receptors; acts as an agonist at these sites while preventing nicotine binding to these receptors. This mechanism is thought to aid in smoking cessation.

Indications

- Aid to smoking cessation treatment

Contraindications and cautions

- Contraindicated with hypersensitivity to any component of the drug, lactation.
- Use cautiously with pregnancy.

Available forms

Capsules—0.5, 1 mg

Dosages

Adults

The patient should pick a date to stop smoking and begin drug therapy 1 wk before that date.

Days 1–3, 0.5 mg/day PO; days 4–7, 0.5 mg PO bid; day 8 until the end of treatment, 1 mg PO bid. Drug should be taken after eating with a full glass of water. Treatment should last 12 wk; patients who successfully quit smoking in that time may benefit from another 12 wk to increase the likelihood of long-term abstinence. Patients who fail to quit smoking during the 12 wk or who relapse after treatment can be treated again when factors leading to failed attempt have been identified and addressed.

Pediatric patients

Not recommended for children younger than 18 yr.

Patients with severe renal impairment

Initially, 0.5 mg/day PO; titrate to 0.5 mg PO bid. If on dialysis, 0.5 mg/day.

Pharmacokinetics

Route	*Onset*	*Peak*
Oral	Rapid	3–4 hr

Metabolism: Minimal; $T_{1/2}$: 24 hr
Distribution: May cross placenta; may enter breast milk
Excretion: Unchanged in urine

Adverse effects

- **CNS:** *Headache, insomnia, abnormal dreams,* somnolence, lethargy, dysgeusia, behavioral changes, suicidal ideation, agitation, depression
- **Dermatologic:** Rash
- **GI:** *Nausea,* abdominal pain, *flatulence,* dyspepsia, *vomiting, constipation,* dry mouth, GERD, increased appetite, anorexia
- **Respiratory:** Rhinorrhea, dyspnea, URIs
- **Other:** Fatigue, malaise, asthenia

■ Nursing considerations

Assessment

- **History:** Hypersensitivity to any component of drug; lactation, pregnancy; smoking history
- **Physical:** Orientation, affect, reflexes; R, breath sounds; abdominal examination

Interventions

⊗ ***Black box warning*** There is a risk of serious mental health events, including changes in behavior, depressed mood, hostility, and suicidal thoughts, with drug administration; monitor patient accordingly.

- Instruct patient to pick a day to quit smoking; drug therapy should begin 1 wk before that date.
- Administer drug after patient has eaten, with a full glass of water.
- Provide patient with educational materials and support for smoking cessation.
- Encourage patient to continue efforts at smoking cessation even if a lapse occurs.
- Provide safety measures if insomnia, lethargy occur.
- Suggest use of contraceptive measures; help patient select another method of feeding the baby if she is nursing during drug therapy.
- Consider a second 12-wk course of therapy if patient is successful at smoking cessation to improve the chances of continued abstinence.
- Monitor patient for behavioral changes and suicidal ideation; stop drug and get medical attention if these effects occur.

Teaching points

- This drug reacts with nicotine receptors in your brain to decrease your desire for nicotine and will alter your reaction to nicotine when you do smoke, making it less desirable. You should have support for your efforts to stop smoking.
- You will take *Chantix* after eating with a full glass of water. The dose will need to be adjusted.
- Select a day to stop smoking. Begin taking *Chantix* 1 week before that day. Days 1–3 of

that week, you will take 0.5 mg (white tablet) once each day. Days 4–7, you will take 0.5 mg twice a day, once in the morning and once in the evening. From day 8 until you are finished with treatment, you will take 1 mg (blue tablet) twice a day, once in the morning and once in the evening. The course of treatment is usually 12 weeks. If you have good success, you may have another 12-week course to help increase the chances of long-term success.

- If you forget a dose of the drug, take it as soon as you remember; if you remember close to the time for your next dose, just take that dose. Do not double the dose.
- If you have a relapse, keep taking the drug and continue to try to stop smoking.
- It is not known if this drug could affect a fetus. If you are pregnant or are thinking about becoming pregnant, consult your health care provider before using this drug; you should not smoke when you are pregnant.
- It is not known how this drug could affect a nursing baby. If you are nursing a baby, use another method of feeding the baby during drug treatment.
- Stop drug and seek medical help if agitation, depression, or thoughts of suicide occur.
- You may experience these side effects: nausea, insomnia (when starting therapy; they should pass as your body adjusts to the drug; if they should become severe, contact your health care provider).
- Report severe constipation, severe vomiting, failure to quit smoking, behavioral changes, thoughts of suicide.

▽venlafaxine hydrochloride

(vin lah ***facks'*** *in)*

Effexor, Effexor XR DNC

PREGNANCY CATEGORY C

Drug classes

Antidepressant
Anxiolytic

Therapeutic actions

Potentiates the neurotransmitter activity in the CNS; inhibits serotonin, norepinephrine, and dopamine reuptake leading to prolonged stimulation at neuroreceptors.

Indications

- Treatment of major depressive disorder
- Treatment of generalized anxiety disorder (ER only)
- Treatment of social anxiety disorder (ER only)
- Treatment of panic disorder, with or without agoraphobia (ER only)
- Unlabeled uses: PMDD, hot flushes, autism, pain

Contraindications and cautions

- Contraindicated with allergy to venlafaxine, use of MAOIs within last 14 days.
- Use cautiously with pregnancy, lactation, patients whose underlying medical condition might be compromised by increased heart rate (hyperthyroidism, HF, recent MI).

Available forms

Tablets—25, 37.5, 50, 75, 100, 150, 225 mg; ER capsules DNC—37.5, 75, 150 mg

Dosages

Adults

- *Depression:* Starting dose, 75 mg/day PO in two to three divided doses (or once a day, ER capsule) taken with food. May be increased at intervals of no less than 4 days up to 225 mg/day to achieve desired effect; maximum dose 375 mg/day in three divided doses.
- *Transfer to or from MAOI:* At least 14 days should elapse from the discontinuation of the MAOI and the starting of venlafaxine; allow at least 7 days to elapse from the stopping of venlafaxine to the starting of an MAOI.
- *Generalized anxiety disorder/social anxiety:* 75–225 mg/day PO should be taken on a daily basis, not as needed (ER only).
- *Panic disorder:* 37.5 mg/day PO for 7 days, then increase based on patient response to 75 mg/day for 7 days, and then 75 mg/day weekly increases to a maximum of 225 mg/day (ER only).

Pediatric patients

Safety and efficacy not established.

V

Patients with renal or hepatic impairment

For patients with creatinine clearance of 10–70 mL/min, reduce dosage by 25%–50%. For patients on dialysis, reduce dosage by 50% (give after dialysis completion on dialysis days). For patients with hepatic impairment, reduce total daily dose by 50%, and increase very slowly to achieve desired effect.

Pharmacokinetics

Route	*Onset*	*Duration*
Oral	Slow	48 hr

Metabolism: Hepatic; $T_{1/2}$: 1.3–2 hr
Distribution: Crosses placenta; may enter breast milk
Excretion: Urine

Adverse effects

- **CNS:** *Somnolence, dizziness, insomnia, nervousness,* anxiety, tremor, dreams
- **CV:** Vasodilation, hypertension, tachycardia
- **Dermatologic:** *Sweating,* rash, pruritus
- **GI:** *Nausea, constipation, anorexia,* diarrhea, vomiting, dyspepsia, *dry mouth,* flatulence
- **GU:** *Abnormal ejaculation,* impotence, urinary frequency
- **Other:** *Headache, asthenia,* infection, chills, chest pain

Interactions

✱ **Drug-drug** • Increased serum levels and risk of toxicity with MAOIs (within last 14 days), cimetidine • Serotonin syndrome may occur if combined with trazodone • Increased sedation with alcohol

✱ **Drug-alternative therapy** • Increased sedation and hypnotic effects with St. John's wort

■ Nursing considerations

Assessment

- **History:** Allergy to venlafaxine; use of MAOIs within last 14 days; pregnancy, lactation
- **Physical:** Skin color, T, lesions; reflexes, gait, sensation, cranial nerve evaluation; mucous membranes, abdominal examination, normal output; P, BP, peripheral perfusion

Interventions

- Limit amount of drug available; increased risk of successful suicide attempts with this antidepressant.
- Give with food to decrease GI effects. Ensure that patient swallows ER capsules whole; do not allow patient to cut, crush, or chew them.
- Advise patient to use contraceptives.

⊗ ***Black box warning*** Monitor patients for suicidal ideation, especially when beginning therapy or changing dosage; high risk in children, adolescents, and young adults.

Teaching points

- Take with food to decrease GI upset. Do not cut, crush, or chew capsules; swallow capsules whole.
- Avoid alcohol while using this drug.
- This drug cannot be taken during pregnancy; use birth control. If you become pregnant, consult your health care provider.
- You may experience these side effects: Loss of appetite, nausea, vomiting, dry mouth (use frequent mouth care; eat frequent small meals; suck sugarless lozenges); constipation (request bowel program); dizziness, drowsiness, tremor (avoid driving or operating dangerous machinery).
- Report rash, hives, increased depression, thoughts of suicide, pregnancy.

DANGEROUS DRUG

▽ verapamil hydrochloride

(ver ap' a mill)

Apo-Verap (CAN), Apo-Verap SR (DNC) (CAN), Calan, Calan SR (DNC), Covera-HS, Gen-Verapamil (CAN), Gen-Verapamil SR (DNC) (CAN), Isoptin SR (DNC), Nu-Verap (CAN), Verelan (DNC), Verelan PM (DNC)

PREGNANCY CATEGORY C

Drug classes

Antianginal
Antiarrhythmic
Antihypertensive
Calcium channel blocker

Therapeutic actions

Inhibits the movement of calcium ions across the membranes of cardiac and arterial muscle cells; calcium is involved in the generation of the action potential in specialized automatic and conducting cells in the heart, in arterial smooth muscle, and in excitation-contraction coupling in cardiac muscle cells; inhibition of transmembrane calcium flow results in the depression of impulse formation in specialized cardiac pacemaker cells, slowing of the velocity of conduction of the cardiac impulse, the depression of myocardial contractility, and the dilation of coronary arteries and arterioles and peripheral arterioles; these effects lead to decreased cardiac work, decreased cardiac energy consumption, and in patients with vasospastic (Printzmetal's) angina, increased delivery of oxygen to myocardial cells.

Indications

- Angina pectoris due to coronary artery spasm (Printzmetal's variant angina)
- Effort-associated angina
- Chronic stable angina
- Unstable, crescendo, preinfarction angina
- Essential hypertension
- Parenteral: Treatment of supraventricular tachyarrhythmias
- Parenteral: Temporary control of rapid ventricular rate in atrial flutter or atrial fibrillation

Contraindications and cautions

- Contraindicated with allergy to verapamil; sick sinus syndrome, except with ventricular pacemaker; heart block (second- or third-degree); hypotension; pregnancy, lactation.
- Use cautiously with idiopathic hypertrophic subaortic stenosis, cardiogenic shock, severe HF, impaired renal or hepatic function, and in patients with atrial flutter or atrial fibrillation and an accessory to bypass tract.

Available forms

Tablets—40, 80, 120 mg; SR tablets DNC—120, 180, 240 mg; ER tablets DNC—120, 180, 240 mg; injection—2.5 mg/mL; ER capsules DNC—100, 120, 180, 200, 240, 300, 360 mg

Dosages

Adults

Oral

Immediate-release

- *Angina:* 80–120 mg PO tid. Doses of 40 mg PO tid may be used. Maintenance 240–480 mg daily.
- *Arrhythmias:* 240–480 mg/day in divided doses.
- *In digitalized adults:* 240–320 mg/day.
- *Hypertension:* 40 mg to 80 mg PO tid.

ER

- *Capsules:* 120–240 mg/day PO in the morning. Titrate dose to a maximum 480 mg/day.
- *Tablets:* 120–180 mg/day PO in the morning. Titrate to maximum 240 mg every 12 hr.

SR

- 120–180 mg/day PO. Titrate up to a maximum 480 mg PO in the morning.

Parenteral

IV use only. Initial dose, 5–10 mg over 2 min; may repeat dose of 10 mg 30 min after first dose if initial response is inadequate.

Pediatric patients

IV

1 yr and younger: Initial dose, 0.1–0.2 mg/kg over 2 min.

1–15 yr: Initial dose, 0.1–0.3 mg/kg over 2 min. Do not exceed 5 mg. Repeat above dose 30 min after initial dose if response is not adequate. Repeat dose should not exceed 10 mg.

Geriatric patients or patients with renal impairment

Reduce dosage, and monitor patient response carefully. Give IV doses over 3 min to reduce risk of serious side effects. Administer IV doses very slowly, over 2 min.

Pharmacokinetics

Route	Onset	Peak	Duration
Oral	30 min	1–2.2 hr	3–7 hr
IV	1–5 min	3–5 min	2 hr

Metabolism: Hepatic; $T_{1/2}$: 3–7 hr
Distribution: Crosses placenta; enters breast milk
Excretion: Urine

IV FACTS

Preparation: No further preparation required.

V

Infusion: Infuse very slowly over 2–3 min.
Y-site incompatibilities: Do not give with albumin, ampicillin, nafcillin, oxacillin, sodium bicarbonate, amphotericin B, hydralazine, aminophylline.

Adverse effects

- **CNS:** *Dizziness,* vertigo, emotional depression, sleepiness, *headache*
- **CV:** *Peripheral edema, hypotension,* arrhythmias, bradycardia; AV heart block
- **GI:** *Nausea,* constipation
- **Other:** Muscle fatigue, diaphoresis, rash

Interactions

✱ **Drug-drug** ⊗ ***Warning*** Risk of serious cardiac effects with IV beta blockers; do not give these drugs within 48 hr before or 24 hr after IV verapamil.
• Increased cardiac depression with beta blockers • Additive effects of verapamil and digoxin to slow AV conduction • Increased serum levels of digoxin, carbamazepine, prazosin, quinidine • Increased respiratory depression with atracurium, pancuronium, tubocurarine, vecuronium • Decreased effects with calcium, rifampin
✱ **Drug-food** • Decreased metabolism and risk of toxic effects if combined with grapefruit juice; avoid this combination

■ Nursing considerations

Assessment

- **History:** Allergy to verapamil; sick sinus syndrome; heart block; IHSS; cardiogenic shock, severe HF; hypotension; impaired hepatic or renal function; pregnancy, lactation
- **Physical:** Skin color, edema; orientation, reflexes; P, BP, baseline ECG, peripheral perfusion, auscultation; R, adventitious sounds; liver evaluation, normal output; LFTs, renal function tests, urinalysis

Interventions

⊗ ***Warning*** Monitor patient carefully (BP, cardiac rhythm, and output) while drug is being titrated to therapeutic dose. Dosage may be increased more rapidly in hospitalized patients under close supervision.

- Ensure that patient swallows SR or ER tablets whole; patient should not cut, crush, or chew them.
- Monitor BP very carefully with concurrent doses of antihypertensives.
- Monitor cardiac rhythm regularly during stabilization of dosage and periodically during long-term therapy.
- Administer SR or ER form in the morning with food to decrease GI upset.
- Protect IV solution from light.
- Monitor patients with renal or hepatic impairment carefully for possible drug accumulation and adverse reactions.

Teaching points

- Take extended- or sustained-release form in the morning with food; swallow it whole; do not cut, crush, or chew it. Do not drink grapefruit juice while using this drug.
- You may experience these side effects: Nausea, vomiting (eat frequent small meals); headache (adjust lighting, noise, and temperature; request medication); dizziness, sleepiness (avoid driving or operating dangerous equipment); emotional depression (reversible); constipation (request aid).
- Report irregular heart beat, shortness of breath, swelling of the hands or feet, pronounced dizziness, nausea, constipation.

▽ verteporfin

See Appendix W, *Less commonly used drugs*.

▽ vigabatrin

See Appendix W, *Less commonly used drugs*.

DANGEROUS DRUG

▽ vinblastine sulfate (VLB)

*(vin **blas'** teen)*

Velban

PREGNANCY CATEGORY D

Drug classes

Antineoplastic
Mitotic inhibitor

Therapeutic actions
Affects cell energy production required for mitosis, has antimitotic effect and causes abnormal mitotic figures.

Indications
- Palliative treatment for lymphocytic lymphoma, histiocytic lymphoma, generalized Hodgkin's lymphoma (stages III and IV), mycosis fungoides, advanced testicular carcinoma, Kaposi's sarcoma, Letterer-Siwe disease
- Treatment of choriocarcinoma, breast cancer unresponsive to other therapies
- Hodgkin's lymphoma (advanced) alone or in combination therapies
- Advanced testicular germinal-cell cancers alone or in combination therapy

Contraindications and cautions
- Contraindicated with allergy to vinblastine, leukopenia, acute infection, pregnancy, lactation.
- Use cautiously with liver disease.

Available forms
Powder for injection—10 mg; injection—1 mg/mL

Dosages
⊗ ***Warning*** Do not administer more than once a wk because of leukopenic response.

Adults

Initial dose, 3.7 mg/m^2 as a single IV dose, followed at weekly intervals by increasing doses at 1.8 mg/m^2 increments; a conservative regimen follows:

Week	*Dose (mg/m^2)*
First wk	3.7
Second wk	5.5
Third wk	7.4
Fourth wk	9.25
Fifth wk	11.1

Use these increments until a maximum dose of 18.5 mg/m^2 is reached; do not increase dose after WBC count is reduced to 3,000/mm^3.

- *Maintenance therapy:* When dose produces WBC count of 3,000/ mm^3, use a dose one increment smaller for weekly maintenance. Do not give another dose until WBC count is 4,000/ mm^3 even if 7 days have passed. Duration of therapy depends on disease and response; up to 2 yr may be needed.

Pediatric patients

Initial dose, 2.5 mg/m^2 as a single IV dose, followed at weekly intervals by increasing doses at 1.25 mg/m^2 increments; a conservative regimen follows:

Week	*Pediatric Dose (mg/m^2)*
First wk	2.5
Second wk	3.75
Third wk	5
Fourth wk	6.25
Fifth wk	7.5

Use these increments until a maximum dose of 12.5 mg/m^2 is reached; do not increase dose after WBC count is reduced to 3,000/mm^3.

Patients with hepatic impairment

For serum bilirubin exceeding 3 mg/dL, decrease dose by 50%.

Pharmacokinetics

Route	*Onset*
IV	Slow

Metabolism: Hepatic; $T_{1/2}$: 3.7 min, then 1.6 hr, then 24.8 hr

Distribution: Crosses placenta; enters breast milk

Excretion: Bile

IV FACTS
Preparation: Add 10 mL of sodium chloride injection preserved with phenol or benzyl alcohol to the vial for a concentration of 1 mg/mL. Refrigerate drug; opened vials are stable for 28 days when refrigerated.

Infusion: Inject into tubing of a running IV or directly into the vein over 1 min or as a prolonged infusion over up to 96 hr. Rinse syringe and needle with venous blood prior to withdrawing needle from vein (to minimize extravasation). Do not inject into an extremity with poor circulation or repeatedly into the same vein.

Y-site incompatibility: Do not give with furosemide.

Adverse effects
- **CNS:** Numbness, paresthesias, peripheral neuritis, mental depression, loss of deep

tendon reflexes, *headache*, seizures, malaise, *weakness*, dizziness

- **Dermatologic:** Topical epilation (loss of hair), vesiculation of the skin
- **GI:** *Nausea, vomiting,* pharyngitis, vesiculation of the mouth, ileus, *diarrhea,* constipation, *anorexia,* abdominal pain, rectal bleeding, hemorrhagic enterocolitis
- **GU:** Aspermia
- **Hematologic:** Leukopenia
- **Local:** *Local cellulitis,* phlebitis, sloughing if extravasation occurs
- **Other:** Pain in tumor site

Interactions

✱ Drug-drug • Decreased serum concentrations of phenytoins • Risk of toxicity if combined with erythromycin

✱ Drug-food • Decreased metabolism and risk of toxic effects if combined with grapefruit juice; avoid this combination

■ Nursing considerations

CLINICAL ALERT!

Confusion has occurred between vinblastine and vincristine; use extreme caution if giving either drug.

Assessment

- **History:** Allergy to vinblastine, leukopenia, acute infection, liver disease, pregnancy, lactation
- **Physical:** Weight; hair; T; reflexes, gait, sensation, orientation, affect; mucous membranes, abdominal examination, rectal examination; CBC, LFTs, serum albumin

Interventions

- Ensure that patient is not pregnant before administering; advise patients to use contraceptive measures.

⊗ ***Black box warning*** Do not administer IM or subcutaneously due to severe local reaction and tissue necrosis. Fatal if given intrathecally. Use extreme caution.

⊗ ***Black box warning*** Watch for irritation and infiltration; extravasation causes tissue damage and necrosis. If it occurs, discontinue injection immediately, and give remainder of dose in another vein. Consult physician to arrange for hyaluronidase injection into local area, after which apply moderate heat to disperse drug and minimize pain.

⊗ ***Warning*** Avoid contact with the eyes; if contact occurs, immediately wash thoroughly with water.

- Consult with physician if antiemetic is needed for severe nausea and vomiting.
- Check CBC before each dose.

Teaching points

- Prepare a calendar for dates to return for treatment and drug therapy. Avoid grapefruit juice while you are using this drug.
- This drug should not be used during pregnancy. Use birth control. If you become pregnant, consult your health care provider.
- Have regular blood tests to monitor the drug's effects.
- You may experience these side effects: Loss of appetite, nausea, vomiting, mouth sores (use frequent mouth care; eat frequent small meals; maintain nutrition; request an antiemetic); constipation (a bowel program may be ordered); malaise, weakness, dizziness, numbness and tingling (avoid injury); loss of hair, rash (obtain a wig; keep the head covered in extremes of temperature).
- Report severe nausea, vomiting, pain or burning at injection site, abdominal pain, rectal bleeding, fever, chills, acute infection.

DANGEROUS DRUG

▽vincristine sulfate (LCR, VCR)

*(vin **kris'** teen)*

Oncovin, Vincasar PFS

PREGNANCY CATEGORY D

Drug classes

Antineoplastic
Mitotic inhibitor

Therapeutic actions

Mitotic inhibitor: Arrests mitotic division at the stage of metaphase; exact mechanism of action unknown.

Indications

- Acute leukemia
- Hodgkin's lymphoma, non-Hodgkin's lymphoma, rhabdomyosarcoma, neuroblastoma, Wilms' tumor as part of combination therapy

Contraindications and cautions

- Contraindicated with allergy to vincristine, leukopenia, acute infection, pregnancy, lactation, demyelinating form of Charcot-Marie-Tooth syndrome.
- Use cautiously with neuromuscular disease, diabetes insipidus, hepatic impairment.

Available forms

Injection—1 mg/mL

Dosages

Adults

1.4 mg/m^2 IV at weekly intervals.

Pediatric patients

1.5–2 mg/m^2 IV weekly.

- *Weight less than 10 kg or body surface area less than 1 m^2:* 0.05 mg/kg once per wk.

Geriatric patients or patients with hepatic impairment

For serum bilirubin exceeding 3 mg/dL, reduce dosage by 50%.

Pharmacokinetics

Route	*Onset*	*Peak*
IV	Varies	15–30 min

Metabolism: Hepatic; $T_{1/2}$: 5 min, then 2.3 hr, then 85 hr

Distribution: Crosses placenta; enters breast milk

Excretion: Feces, urine

▼IV FACTS

Preparation: No further preparation required; drug should be refrigerated.

Infusion: Inject solution directly into vein or into the tubing of a running IV infusion.

Y-site incompatibility: Do not give with furosemide.

Adverse effects

- **CNS:** *Ataxia, cranial nerve manifestations;* foot drop, headache, seizures, bladder neuropathy, paresthesias, sensory impairment, *neuritic pain, muscle wasting,* SIADH, optic atrophy, transient cortical blindness, ptosis, diplopia, photophobia
- **GI:** *Constipation,* oral ulcerations, abdominal cramps, vomiting, diarrhea, intestinal necrosis
- **GU:** Acute uric acid nephropathy, polyuria, dysuria
- **Hematologic:** *Leukopenia*
- **Local:** Local irritation, cellulitis if extravasation occurs
- **Other:** *Weight loss, loss of hair,* fever, **death** with serious overdose

Interactions

✱ **Drug-drug** • Decreased serum levels and therapeutic effects of digoxin • If L-asparaginase is administered first, the hepatic clearance of vincristine may be reduced. Give vincristine 12–24 hr before L-asparaginase to minimize toxicity

✱ **Drug-food** • Decreased metabolism and risk of toxic effects if combined with grapefruit juice; avoid this combination

■ Nursing considerations

CLINICAL ALERT!

Confusion has occurred between vincristine and vinblastine; use extreme caution if giving either drug.

Assessment

- **History:** Allergy to vincristine, leukopenia, acute infection, neuromuscular disease, diabetes insipidus, hepatic impairment, pregnancy, lactation
- **Physical:** Weight; hair; T; reflexes, gait, sensation, cranial nerve evaluation, ophthalmic examination; mucous membranes, abdominal examination; CBC, serum sodium, LFTs, urinalysis

Interventions

- Ensure that patient is not pregnant before administering; using barrier contraceptives is advised.
- Tell patient to avoid grapefruit juice while being treated with this drug.

⊠ ***Black box warning*** Do not administer IM or subcutaneously due to severe local reaction and tissue necrosis. Do not give intrathecally; drug is fatal if given intrathecally. Use extreme caution.

⊗ ***Black box warning*** Watch for irritation and infiltration; extravasation causes tissue damage and necrosis. If extravasation occurs, discontinue injection immediately and give remainder of dose in another vein. Consult with physician to arrange for hyaluronidase injection into local area, and apply heat to disperse the drug and to minimize pain.

- Arrange for wig or suitable head covering if hair loss occurs; ensure that patient's head is covered in extremes of temperature.
- Monitor urine output and serum sodium; if SIADH occurs, consult with physician, and arrange for fluid restriction and perhaps a potent diuretic. Dispose of excretions properly.

Teaching points

- Prepare a calendar of dates to return for treatment and additional therapy.
- Avoid grapefruit juice while you are using this drug.
- This drug cannot be taken during pregnancy; use birth control. If you become pregnant, consult your health care provider.
- Have regular blood tests to monitor the drug's effects.
- You may experience these side effects: Loss of appetite, nausea, vomiting, mouth sores (frequent mouth care, frequent small meals may help; maintain nutrition; request an antiemetic); constipation (bowel program may be ordered); sensitivity to light (wear sunglasses; avoid bright lights); numbness, tingling, change in style of walking (reversible; may persist for up to 6 weeks); hair loss (transient; obtain a wig or other suitable head covering; keep the head covered at extremes of temperature).
- Report change in frequency of voiding; swelling of ankles, fingers, and so forth; changes in vision; severe constipation, abdominal pain.

DANGEROUS DRUG

vinorelbine tartrate

(vin oh ***rel'*** *been)*

Navelbine

PREGNANCY CATEGORY D

Drug classes

Antineoplastic
Mitotic inhibitor

Therapeutic actions

Affects cell energy production required for mitosis; has antimitotic effect, prevents the formation of microtubules and leads to cell death; cell cycle specific.

Indications

- First-line treatment of ambulatory patients with unresectable advanced non–small-cell lung cancer
- Treatment of stage IV non–small-cell lung cancer alone or with cisplatin
- Treatment of stage III non–small-cell lung cancer with cisplatin
- Unlabeled uses: Breast cancer, ovarian cancer, Hodgkin's lymphoma, desmoid tumors and fibromatosis, advanced Kaposi's sarcoma

Contraindications and cautions

- Contraindicated with allergy to vinca alkaloids, pretreatment granulocyte counts of 1,000 cells/mm^3 or less, pregnancy, lactation.
- Use cautiously with liver disease.

Available forms

Injection—10 mg/mL

Dosages

Adults

⊗ ***Warning*** Do not administer more than once a wk because of leukopenic response.

- *Monotherapy:* Initial dose, 30 mg/m^2 as single IV dose; repeat once a wk until progression of disease or toxicity limits use.
- *With cisplatin:* 25 mg/m^2 in combination with cisplatin 100 mg/m^2 given every 4 wk, or 30 mg/m^2 with cisplatin 120 mg/m^2 given on days 1 and 29, then every 6 wk.

Patients with hepatic impairment
If total serum bilirubin concentration is 2.1–3 mg/dL, reduce dose to 50% of starting dose; if greater than 3 mg/dL, reduce to 25% of starting dose.

Pharmacokinetics

Route	*Onset*
IV	Slow

Metabolism: Hepatic; $T_{1/2}$: 22–66 hr
Distribution: Crosses placenta; enters breast milk
Excretion: Bile, feces

IV FACTS

Preparation: Dilute for 50- or 10-mg solution. Supplied as single-use vials only. Discard after withdrawing solution.
Infusion: Inject into tubing of a running IV or directly into the vein over 6–10 min. Rinse syringe and needle with venous blood prior to withdrawing needle from vein (to minimize extravasation). Do not inject into an extremity with poor circulation or repeatedly into the same vein. Follow with 150–250 ml saline or dextrose to decrease phlebitis. If administered via IV piggyback, should be done via central access.

Adverse effects

- **CNS:** Numbness, paresthesias (less common than with other vinca alkaloids); headache, weakness, dizziness
- **Dermatologic:** Topical epilation (loss of hair), vesiculation of the skin
- **GI:** Nausea, vomiting, pharyngitis, vesiculation of the mouth, ileus, diarrhea, constipation, anorexia, abdominal pain, *increased liver enzymes*
- **Hematologic: Granulocytopenia, leukopenia**
- **Local:** Local cellulitis, phlebitis, sloughing with extravasation
- **Other:** Myalgia, arthralgia

Interactions

✱ **Drug-drug** • Acute pulmonary reactions with mitomycin • Increased risk of granulocytopenia with cisplatin • Risk of neuropathies if combined or given sequentially with paclitaxel; monitor patient closely

■ Nursing considerations

Assessment

- **History:** Allergy to vinca alkaloids, leukopenia, acute infection, liver disease, pregnancy, lactation
- **Physical:** Weight; hair; T; reflexes, gait, sensation, orientation, affect; mucous membranes, abdominal examination; CBC, LFTs, serum albumin

Interventions

- Ensure that patient is not pregnant before use; advise patient to use barrier contraceptives.

⊠ ***Black box warning*** Do not administer IM or subcutaneously—severe local reaction and tissue necrosis occur. Fatal if given intrathecally. Use extreme caution.

⊠ ***Black box warning*** Watch for irritation and infiltration; extravasation can cause tissue damage and necrosis. If extravasation should occur, discontinue injection immediately and consult physician to arrange for hyaluronidase injection into local area, after which apply moderate heat to disperse drug and minimize pain.

⊗ ***Warning*** Avoid contact with the eyes; if contact occurs, immediately wash thoroughly with water.

- Consult with physician if antiemetic is needed for severe nausea and vomiting.

⊠ ***Black box warning*** Check CBC before each dose; severe granulocytosis is possible. Adjust or delay dose as appropriate.

Teaching points

- Prepare a calendar for dates to return for treatment and additional therapy.
- This drug should not be used during pregnancy. Use birth control. If you become pregnant, consult your health care provider.
- Have regular blood tests to monitor the drug's effects.
- You may experience these side effects: Loss of appetite, nausea, vomiting, mouth sores (frequent mouth care, frequent small meals may help; maintain nutrition; request an antiemetic); constipation (bowel program may be ordered); malaise, weakness, dizziness, numbness and tingling (avoid injury); loss of hair, rash (obtain a wig; keep the head covered in extremes of temperature).

- Report severe nausea, vomiting, pain or burning at injection site, abdominal pain, rectal bleeding, fever, chills, acute infection.

voriconazole

*(vor ah **kon'** ah zole)*

Vfend

PREGNANCY CATEGORY D

Drug class

Triazole antifungal

Therapeutic actions

Inhibits fungal ergosterol biosynthesis leading to cell membrane rupture and cell death in susceptible fungi.

Indications

- Treatment of invasive aspergillosis
- Treatment of serious fungal infections caused by *Scedosporium apiospermum, Pseudallescheria boydii,* and *Fusarium* species in patients intolerant of or refractory to other therapy
- Treatment of esophageal candidiasis
- **NEW INDICATION:** Treatment of candidemia in nonneutropenic patients with disseminated skin infections and abdominal, kidney, bladder wall, and wound infections

Contraindications and cautions

- Contraindicated with hypersensitivity to voriconazole, treatment with other drugs that could prolong the QTc interval, severe hepatic impairment, galactose intolerance, and in patients taking the following drugs: Ergot alkaloids, sirolimus, rifabutin, rifampin, carbamazepine, and long-acting barbiturates.
- Use cautiously with known allergies to other azoles, pregnancy, lactation.

Available forms

Tablets—50, 200 mg; powder for injection—200 mg to be reconstituted to 10 mg/mL; powder for oral suspension—40 mg/mL

Dosages

Adults

Loading dose of 6 mg/kg IV every 12 hr for two doses, then 3–4 mg/kg IV every 12 hr or 200 mg PO every 12 hr. Switch to oral dose as soon as patient is able:

Weight less than 40 kg: 100 mg PO every 12 hr; may increase to 150 mg PO every 12 hr if needed.

Weight of 40 kg or more: 200 mg PO every 12 hr; may increase to 300 mg PO every 12 hr if needed.

- *Esophageal candidiasis:* 200–300 mg PO every 12 hr (reduce to 100–150 mg PO every 12 hr if weight is less than 40 kg) for 14 days or for at least 7 days following symptom resolution.

Pediatric patients younger than 12 yr

Safety and efficacy not established.

Pharmacokinetics

Route	*Peak*	*Duration*
Oral	1–2 hr	96 hr
IV	Onset of infusion	96 hr

Metabolism: Hepatic; $T_{1/2}$: 24 hr

Distribution: Crosses placenta; may enter breast milk

Excretion: Urine

IV FACTS

Preparation: Reconstitute powder with 19 mL of water for injection, resulting solution contains 10 mg/mL. Shake the vial until powder is dissolved. Further dilute *Vfend* to obtain a concentration of 5 mg/mL using 0.9% sodium chloride, lactated Ringer's solution, 5% dextrose and lactated Ringer's solution, 5% dextrose and 0.45% sodium chloride, 5% dextrose, 5% dextrose and 20 mEq potassium chloride, 0.45% sodium chloride, 5% dextrose and 0.9% sodium chloride. Do not use if solution is not clear or if it contains particulate matter. Use immediately after reconstitution. Discard any unused solution.

Infusion: Infuse over 1–2 hr at no more than 3 mg/kg/hr.

Incompatibilities: Do not infuse with parenteral nutrition, blood products, electrolyte supplements, any alkaline solution, other drug infusions.

Adverse effects

- **CNS:** Headache, *visual disturbance,* hallucinations, dizziness
- **CV:** Tachycardia, BP changes, vasodilation, chest pain, peripheral edema, prolonged QTc interval
- **GI:** Nausea, vomiting, diarrhea, dry mouth, abnormal LFTs, abdominal pain
- **Hematologic:** Anemia, thrombocytopenia, leukopenia
- **Other:** *Fever,* chills, rash, pruritus, **anaphylactic reaction, Stevens-Johnson syndrome**

Interactions

✱Drug-drug ⊗ ***Warning*** Decreased serum levels and effectiveness of voriconazole if combined with rifampin, rifabutin, carbamazepine, phenobarbital, mephobarbital; avoid these combinations.

⊗ ***Warning*** Increased serum levels of sirolimus, terfenadine, pimozide, quinidine, ergot alkaloids if taken with voriconazole; avoid these combinations.

⊗ ***Warning*** Increased plasma concentration of ergot alkaloids, which may lead to ergotism; avoid this combination.

• Possible alterations in serum levels and effectiveness of warfarin, tacrolimus, statins, oral anticoagulants, benzodiazepine, calcium channel blockers, sulfonylureas, vincristine, vinblastine, when taken with voriconazole; patients should be monitored closely and appropriate dosage adjustments made • Altered serum levels and risk of adverse effects from both drugs when voriconazole is taken concomitantly with phenytoin, omeprazole, protease inhibitors; patients should be monitored frequently and appropriate dosage adjustments made • Increased plasma levels of cyclosporine; reduce cyclosporine dose to one-half of the starting dose and monitor cyclosporine blood levels frequently; after voriconazole therapy ends, increase cyclosporine dose as needed

✱Drug alternative therapy • Risk of increased serum levels and toxicity if combined with St. John's wort; this combination is contraindicated

■ Nursing considerations

Assessment

- **History:** Hypersensitivity to *Escherichia coli* products, filgrastim, sickle cell disease, pregnancy, lactation
- **Physical:** Skin color, lesions, hair; T; orientation, affect; abdominal examination, status of mucous membranes; LFTs, renal function tests, CBC, platelets

Interventions

- Obtain baseline liver function before beginning therapy and repeat during the course of therapy. Stop drug at first sign of significant liver toxicity.

⊗ ***Warning*** Check patient's medications carefully before beginning drug therapy; voriconazole is associated with many drug interactions.

- Administer oral drug on an empty stomach, at least 1 hr before or 2 hr after meals.
- Monitor vision changes. Advise patient not to drive at night or perform potentially hazardous tasks because of possible visual disturbances.
- Protect patient from exposure to strong sunlight while using this drug.
- Women of childbearing age should be advised to use barrier contraceptives while using this drug because of the risk of fetal death or abnormalities.
- Provide appropriate comfort and supportive measures for headache or GI discomfort.
- Arrange for frequent small meals if nausea and vomiting are a problem.

Teaching points

- This drug will be started by IV infusion and then you will switch to an oral form.
- Take the drug on an empty stomach 1 hour before or 2 hours after a meal.
- Avoid exposure to strong sunlight while you are using this drug.
- Do not use St. John's wort while taking this drug.
- Women of childbearing age should use barrier contraceptives while using this drug; it has been associated with fetal abnormalities.
- Tell any other health care provider that you see that you are taking this drug; it has been associated with many drug interactions when

taken with other drugs. Adjustments may be needed.

- You may experience these side effects: Nausea and vomiting (eat frequent small meals); headache, fever (analgesics may be available that will help); visual changes (do not drive at night, avoid performing potentially hazardous tasks while on this drug).
- Report fever, chills, changes in color of stool or urine, visual disturbances.

vorinostat

See Appendix W, *Less commonly used drugs.*

DANGEROUS DRUG

warfarin sodium

(war' far in)

Apo-Warfarin (CAN), Coumadin, Gen-Warfarin (CAN)

PREGNANCY CATEGORY X

Drug classes

Coumarin derivative
Oral anticoagulant

Therapeutic actions

Interferes with the hepatic synthesis of vitamin K–dependent clotting factors (factors II-prothrombin, VII, IX, and X), resulting in their eventual depletion and prolongation of clotting times.

Indications

- Venous thrombosis and its extension, treatment, and prophylaxis
- Treatment of thromboembolic complications of atrial fibrillation with embolization, and cardiac valve replacement
- Pulmonary embolism, treatment, and prophylaxis
- Prophylaxis of systemic embolization after acute MI

Contraindications and cautions

- Contraindicated with allergy to warfarin; SBE; hemorrhagic disorders; TB; hepatic diseases; GI ulcers; renal disease; indwelling catheters, spinal puncture; aneurysm; diabetes; visceral carcinoma; uncontrolled hypertension; severe trauma (including recent or contemplated CNS, eye surgery; recent placement of IUD); threatened abortion, menometrorrhagia; pregnancy (fetal damage and death); lactation (suggest using heparin if anticoagulation is required).
- Use cautiously with HF; diarrhea; fever; thyrotoxicosis; senile, psychotic, or depressed patients.

Available forms

Tablets—1, 2, 2.5, 3, 4, 5, 6, 7.5, 10 mg; powder for injection—5 mg, reconstitutes to 2 mg/mL

Dosages

Adjust dosage according to the one-stage PT to achieve and maintain 1.5–2.5 times the control value or prothrombin activity 20%–30% of normal; PT ratio of 1.3–1.5 or INR of 2–3. IV use is reserved for situations in which oral warfarin is not feasible. Dosages are the same for oral and IV forms.

Adults

Initially, 2–5 mg/day PO. Adjust dosage according to PT response. For maintenance, 2–10 mg/day PO based on PT ratio or INR.

Geriatric patients

Lower doses are usually needed; begin with smaller doses than those recommended for adults, and closely monitor PT ratio or INR.

Pharmacokinetics

Route	*Peak*	*Duration*
Oral	1.5–3 days	2–5 days

Metabolism: Hepatic; $T_{1/2}$: 1–2.5 days
Distribution: Crosses placenta; enters breast milk
Excretion: Feces, urine

IV FACTS

Preparation: Reconstitute vial with 2.7 mL of sterile water. Protect from light. Use within 4 hr of reconstitution.
Infusion: Inject slowly over 1–2 min; switch to oral preparation as soon as possible.

Adverse effects

- **Dermatologic:** *Alopecia, urticaria, dermatitis*
- **GI:** *Nausea,* vomiting, anorexia, abdominal cramping, diarrhea, retroperitoneal hematoma, hepatitis, jaundice, mouth ulcers
- **GU:** Priapism, nephropathy, red-orange urine
- **Hematologic:** Granulocytosis, leukopenia, eosinophilia; **hemorrhage**—GI or urinary tract bleeding (hematuria, dark stools; paralytic ileus, intestinal obstruction from hemorrhage into GI tract); petechiae and purpura, bleeding from mucous membranes; hemorrhagic infarction, vasculitis, skin necrosis; adrenal hemorrhage and resultant adrenal insufficiency; compressive neuropathy secondary to hemorrhage near a nerve
- **Other:** Fever, "purple toes" syndrome

Interactions

✱ **Drug-drug** • Increased bleeding tendencies with salicylates, chloral hydrate, clofibrate, disulfiram, chloramphenicol, metronidazole, cimetidine, ranitidine, co-trimoxazole, sulfinpyrazone, quinidine, quinine, thyroid drugs, glucagon, danazol, erythromycin, androgens, amiodarone, cefamandole, cefotetan, cefazolin, cefoxitin, ceftriaxone, meclofenamate, mefenamic acid, famotidine, nizatidine, nalidixic acid • Decreased anticoagulation effect may occur with barbiturates, griseofulvin, rifampin, phenytoin, carbamazepine, vitamin K, vitamin E, cholestyramine, aminoglutethimide, ethchlorvynol • Altered effects with methimazole, propylthiouracil • Increased activity and toxicity of phenytoin when taken with oral anticoagulants

✱ **Drug-lab test** • Red-orange discoloration of alkaline urine may interfere with some lab tests

✱ **Drug-alternative therapy** • Increased risk of bleeding if combined with angelica, cat's claw, chamomile, chondroitin, feverfew, garlic, ginkgo, goldenseal, grape seed extract, green leaf tea, horse chestnut seed, psyllium, and tumeric

■ Nursing considerations

Assessment

- **History:** Allergy to warfarin; SBE; hemorrhagic disorders; TB; hepatic diseases; GI ulcers; renal disease; indwelling catheters, spinal puncture; aneurysm; diabetes; visceral carcinoma; uncontrolled hypertension; severe trauma; threatened abortion, menometrorrhagia; pregnancy; lactation; HF; diarrhea; fever; thyrotoxicosis; senility, psychosis, or depression
- **Physical:** Skin lesions, color, T; orientation, reflexes, affect; P, BP, peripheral perfusion, baseline ECG; R, adventitious sounds; liver evaluation, bowel sounds, normal output; CBC, urinalysis, guaiac stools, PT, LFTs, renal function tests

Interventions

- Genetic testing can help to determine reasonable dosage. Decreased clearance occurs with CYP2C9*2 and CYP2C9*3 variant alleles.
- Do not use drug if patient is pregnant (heparin is anticoagulant of choice); advise patient to use contraceptives.
- Monitor PT ratio or INR regularly to adjust dosage.
- Administer IV form to patients stabilized on *Coumadin* who are not able to take oral drug. Dosages are the same. Return to oral form as soon as feasible.
- Do not change brand names once stabilized; bioavailability may be a problem.

⊠ ***Black box warning*** Evaluate patient regularly for signs of blood loss (petechiae, bleeding gums, bruises, dark stools, dark urine). Maintain PT ratio of 1.3–1.5, 1.5–2 with mechanical prosthetic valves or recurrent systemic embolism; INR ratio of 2–3, 3–4.5 with mechanical prosthetic valves or recurrent systemic emboli; risk of serious to fatal bleeding exists.

- Do not give patient any IM injections.

⊗ ***Warning*** Double check all drugs ordered for potential drug interactions; dosage of both drugs may need to be adjusted.

- Use caution when discontinuing other drugs; warfarin dosage may need to be adjusted; carefully monitor PT values.
- Keep vitamin K readily available in case of overdose.
- Arrange for frequent follow-up, including blood tests to evaluate drug effects.

⊗ ***Warning*** Evaluate for therapeutic effects: INR within therapeutic range.

Teaching points

- Many factors may change your body's response to this drug—fever, change of diet, change of environment, other medications. Your dosage may have to be changed repeatedly. Write down changes that are prescribed.
- Do not start or stop taking any medication without consulting your health care provider. Other drugs can affect your anticoagulant; starting or stopping another drug can cause excessive bleeding or interfere with the desired drug effects.
- Carry or wear a medical ID tag to alert emergency medical personnel that you are taking this drug.
- Avoid situations in which you could be easily injured (contact sports, shaving with a straight razor).
- Have periodic blood tests to check on the drug action. These tests are important.
- Use contraception; do not become pregnant while taking this drug.
- You may experience these side effects: Stomach bloating, cramps (transient); loss of hair, rash; orange-red discoloration to the urine (if upsetting, add vinegar to your urine and the color should disappear).
- Report unusual bleeding (from brushing your teeth, excessive bleeding from injuries, excessive bruising), black or bloody stools, cloudy or dark urine, sore throat, fever, chills, severe headaches, dizziness, suspected pregnancy.

▽xylometazoline hydrochloride

*(zye low met **az'** oh leen)*

Otrivin Nasal Drops or Spray, Otrivin Pediatric Nasal Drops

PREGNANCY CATEGORY C

Drug class

Nasal decongestant

Therapeutic actions

Acts directly on alpha receptors to produce vasoconstriction of arterioles in nasal passages, which produces a decongestant response; no effect on beta receptors.

Indications

- Topical: Symptomatic relief of nasal and nasopharyngeal mucosal congestion caused by the common cold, hay fever, or other respiratory allergies

Contraindications and cautions

- Contraindicated with allergy to xylometazoline, angle-closure glaucoma, anesthesia with cyclopropane or halothane, thyrotoxicosis, diabetes, hypertension, CV disorders, women in labor whose BP exceeds 130/80 mm Hg.
- Use cautiously with angina, arrhythmias, prostatic hypertrophy, unstable vasomotor syndrome, lactation, pregnancy.

Available forms

Nasal solution—0.05%, 0.1%

Dosages

Adults and patients 12 yr and older

One or three sprays or 2–3 drops in each nostril every 8–10 hr (0.1% solution).

Pediatric patients 2–12 yr

Two or three drops of 0.05% solution or one spray in each nostril every 8–10 hr (0.05% solution). Do not exceed three doses in 24 hr.

Pharmacokinetics

Route	*Onset*	*Duration*
Nasal	5–10 min	5–6 hr

Metabolism: Hepatic; $T_{1/2}$: Unknown
Distribution: Crosses placenta; may enter breast milk
Excretion: Urine

Adverse effects

Systemic effects are less likely with topical administration than with systemic administration, but because systemic absorption can take place, the systemic effects should be considered.

- **CNS:** *Fear, anxiety, tenseness, restlessness, headache, light-headedness, dizziness,* drowsiness, tremor, insomnia, hallucina-

tions, psychological disturbances, seizures, CNS depression, weakness, blurred vision, ocular irritation, tearing, photophobia, symptoms of paranoid schizophrenia
- **CV:** Arrhythmias, hypertension resulting in intracranial hemorrhage, CV collapse with hypotension, palpitations, tachycardia, precordial pain in patients with ischemic heart disease
- **GI:** *Nausea,* vomiting, anorexia
- **GU:** Constriction of renal blood vessels, *dysuria, vesical sphincter spasm,* resulting in difficult and painful urination; urinary retention in males with prostatism
- **Local:** *Rebound congestion* with topical nasal application
- **Other:** *Pallor,* respiratory difficulty, orofacial dystonia, sweating

Interactions

✱ **Drug-drug** • Severe hypertension with MAOIs, TCAs, furazolidone • Additive effects and increased risk of toxicity with urinary alkalinizers • Decreased vasopressor response with reserpine, methyldopa, urinary acidifiers

■ Nursing considerations

Assessment

- **History:** Allergy to xylometazoline; angle-closure glaucoma; anesthesia with cyclopropane or halothane; thyrotoxicosis, diabetes, hypertension, CV disorders; prostatic hypertrophy, unstable vasomotor syndrome; lactation
- **Physical:** Skin color, T; orientation, reflexes, peripheral sensation, vision; P, BP, auscultation, peripheral perfusion; R, adventitious sounds; urinary output pattern, bladder percussion, prostate palpation; nasal mucous membrane evaluation

Interventions

⊗ ***Warning*** Monitor CV effects carefully in hypertensive patients; change in BP may be from additional vasoconstriction. If a nasal decongestant is needed, pseudoephedrine is the drug of choice.

Teaching points

- Do not exceed recommended dose. Demonstrate proper administration technique for topical nasal application. Avoid prolonged use because underlying medical problems can be disguised.
- Rebound congestion may occur when this drug is stopped; drink plenty of fluids, use a humidifier, avoid smoke-filled areas.
- You may experience these side effects: Dizziness, weakness, light-headedness, restlessness, tremor (avoid driving or operating dangerous equipment); urinary retention (empty bladder before taking drug).
- Report nervousness, palpitations, sleeplessness, sweating.

▽ zafirlukast

*(zah **fur'** luh kast)*

Accolate

PREGNANCY CATEGORY B

Drug classes

Antiasthmatic
Leukotriene receptor antagonist

Therapeutic actions

Selectively and competitively blocks receptor for leukotriene D_4 and E_4, components of SRS-A, thus blocking airway edema, smooth muscle constriction, and cellular activity associated with inflammatory process that contribute to signs and symptoms of asthma.

Indications

- Prophylaxis and long-term treatment of bronchial asthma in adults and children 5 yr and older
- Unlabeled use: Chronic urticaria

Contraindications and cautions

- Contraindicated with hypersensitivity to zafirlukast or any of its components, acute asthma attacks, status asthmaticus.
- Use cautiously in patients who previously required corticosteroid therapy to control asthma; with hepatic or renal impairment; as oral steroid use is decreased; pregnancy; lactation.

Available forms

Tablets—10, 20 mg

Dosages

Adults and patients 12 yr and older

20 mg PO bid on an empty stomach 1 hr before or 2 hr after eating.

Pediatric patients 5–11 yr

10 mg PO bid on an empty stomach.

Pharmacokinetics

Route	*Onset*	*Peak*
Oral	Rapid	3 hr

Metabolism: Hepatic; $T_{1/2}$: 10 hr
Distribution: Crosses placenta; enters breast milk
Excretion: Feces, urine

Adverse effects

- **CNS:** *Headache,* dizziness, myalgia, behavior and mood changes
- **GI:** Nausea, diarrhea, abdominal pain, vomiting, liver enzyme elevation
- **Other:** Generalized pain, fever, accidental injury, infection; **Churg-Strauss syndrome** (eosinophilia, vasculitic rash, pulmonary and cardiac complications) when oral steroid dose is reduced

Interactions

✱ **Drug-drug** • Increased risk of bleeding with warfarin; these patients should have INR done regularly and warfarin dose decreased accordingly • Potential for increased effects and toxicity of calcium channel blockers, cyclosporine • Decreased effectiveness with erythromycin, theophylline • Possible severe reaction when oral steroid dose is reduced while on zafirlukast; monitor patients very closely

✱ **Drug-food** • Bioavailability decreased markedly by presence of food; administer at least 1 hr before or 2 hr after meals

■ Nursing considerations

Assessment

- **History:** Hypersensitivity to zafirlukast; impaired renal or hepatic function; pregnancy, lactation; acute asthma or bronchospasm
- **Physical:** T; orientation, reflexes; R, adventitious sounds; GI evaluation; LFTs, renal function tests

Interventions

- Administer on an empty stomach 1 hr before or 2 hr after meals.
- Ensure that drug is taken continually for optimal effect.

⊗ ***Warning*** Do not administer for acute asthma attack or acute bronchospasm.

⊗ ***Warning*** There is a risk of neuropsychiatric events, mood and behavior changes with drug administration. Monitor patient accordingly; discontinue drug if these occur.

Teaching points

- Take this drug on an empty stomach, 1 hour before or 2 hours after meals.
- Take this drug regularly as prescribed; do not stop taking it during symptom-free periods; do not stop taking it without consulting your health care provider.
- Do not take this drug for acute asthma attack or acute bronchospasm; this drug is not a bronchodilator; routine emergency procedures should be followed during acute attacks.
- Avoid use of over-the-counter medications while using this drug; many of them contain products that can interfere with drug or cause serious side effects. If you think that you need one of these products, consult your health care provider.
- You may experience these side effects: Dizziness (use caution when driving or performing activities that require alertness); nausea, vomiting (eat frequent small meals); headache (analgesics may be helpful).
- Report fever, acute asthma attacks, severe headache.

▽ zaleplon

(zal' ah plon)

Sonata

PREGNANCY CATEGORY C

CONTROLLED SUBSTANCE C-IV

Drug class

Sedative-hypnotic (nonbarbiturate)

Therapeutic actions

Interacts with GABA-B2 receptor complex to cause suppression of neurons leading to sedation and hypnosis.

Indications

- Short-term treatment of insomnia

Contraindications and cautions

- Contraindicated with hypersensitivity to zaleplon, lactation.
- Use cautiously with impaired hepatic or respiratory function, depressed patients, pregnancy, labor and delivery.

Available forms

Capsules—5, 10 mg

Dosages

Adults

10 mg PO at bedtime. Patient must remain in bed for 4 hr after taking the drug. Do not exceed 20 mg/day.

Pediatric patients

Safety and efficacy not established.

Geriatric patients or debilitated patients

5 mg PO at bedtime. Do not exceed 10 mg/day.

Patients with hepatic impairment

Mild to moderate impairment: 5 mg/day

Severe impairment: Not recommended.

Pharmacokinetics

Route	*Onset*	*Peak*
Oral	Rapid	1 hr

Metabolism: Hepatic; $T_{1/2}$: 1 hr

Distribution: Crosses placenta; may enter breast milk

Excretion: Urine

Adverse effects

- **CNS:** Headache, depression, drowsiness, somnolence, abnormal vision, lack of coordination, *short-term memory impairment,* complex sleep-related behaviors
- **GI:** Diarrhea
- **Hypersensitivity:** Generalized allergic reactions; pruritus, rash; **anaphylaxis; angioedema**

Interactions

✱ **Drug-drug** • Increased sedation with alcohol or other CNS depressants; avoid this combination • Risk of increased serum levels and toxicity with cimetidine, rifampin

■ Nursing considerations

Assessment

- **History:** Hypersensitivity to zaleplon, impaired hepatic or respiratory function, pregnancy, labor or delivery, lactation, depression
- **Physical:** T, orientation, affect, reflexes, vision examination; P, BP; bowel sounds, normal output, liver evaluation; LFTs

Interventions

- Do not prescribe or dispense more than 1 month's supply at a time.

⊗ ***Warning*** Limit amount of drug dispensed to depressed patients.

- Administer to patient at bedtime; onset of action is rapid and sleep usually occurs within 20 min; encourage patient to remain in bed for 4 hr after taking drug to ensure patient safety.
- Help patients with prolonged insomnia to seek the cause of their problem and not to rely on drugs for sleep (eg, ingestion of stimulants such as caffeine shortly before bedtime, fear).
- Institute appropriate additional measures for rest and sleep (eg, back rub, quiet environment, warm milk, reading).

Teaching points

- Take this drug exactly as prescribed. Do not exceed prescribed dosage. Long-term use is not recommended. Time your drug dose to allow you to go to bed immediately after taking the drug. Drug effects will be felt for 4 hours; after that time you may safely become active again.
- You may experience these side effects: Drowsiness, allergic reactions, swelling, dizziness, blurred vision (avoid driving a car or performing tasks requiring alertness or visual acuity if these occur); diarrhea (ensure ready access to bathroom facilities), sleep disorders.
- Report rash, sore throat, fever, bruising, allergic reaction, swelling, complex sleep-related behaviors.

zanamivir

(zan am' ah ver)

Relenza

PREGNANCY CATEGORY C

Drug classes

Antiviral
Neuroaminidase inhibitor

Therapeutic actions

Selectively inhibits influenza virus neuroaminidase; by blocking the actions of this enzyme, there is decreased viral release from infected cells, increased formation of viral aggregates, and decreased spread of the virus.

Indications

- Prevention and treatment of uncomplicated acute illness due to influenza virus in adults and children 7 yr and older who have been symptomatic for 2 days
- Prevention of influenza in patients 5 yr and older
- **NEW INDICATION:** Unlabeled use: Treatment of H1N1 infection

Contraindications and cautions

- Contraindicated with allergy to any component of the drug.
- Use cautiously with pregnancy, lactation, asthma, COPD, or severe medical conditions.

Available forms

Powder blister for inhalation—5 mg

Dosages

Adults and children 7 yr and older

Treatment: Two inhalations (one 5-mg blister per inhalation administered with a *Diskhaler* device, for a total of 10 mg) bid at 12 hr intervals for 5 days. Should be started within 2 days of onset of flu symptoms; give two doses on the first treatment day, at least 2 hr apart; subsequent doses should be separated by 12 hr.

Adults and children 5 yr and older

Prevention in community outbreak: Two inhalations (10 mg) per day for 28 days. Dose should be given at about the same time each day.

Prevention in household exposure: Two inhalations (10 mg) per day for 10 days. Dose should be given at about the same time each day.

Pharmacokinetics

Route	*Onset*	*Peak*
Inhalation	Rapid	1–2 hr

Metabolism: Hepatic; $T_{1/2}$: 2.5–5 hr
Distribution: Crosses placenta; may enter breast milk
Excretion: Feces, urine

Adverse effects

- **CNS:** *Headache,* dizziness
- **GI:** *Nausea,* vomiting, *diarrhea, anorexia*
- **Respiratory:** Cough; *rhinitis;* bronchitis; ear, nose, and throat infections; **bronchospasm; serious respiratory effects**
- **Other:** Flulike symptoms, bacterial infections

■ Nursing considerations

Assessment

- **History:** Allergy to any components of the drug; COPD, asthma; pregnancy, lactation
- **Physical:** T; orientation, reflexes; R, adventitious sounds; bowel sounds

Interventions

- Administer using a *Diskhaler* delivery system. Demonstrate use of system to patient.
- Encourage patient to complete full course of therapy; advise patient that risk of transmission of flu to others is not decreased.
- Administer bronchodilators before using zanamivir if they are due at the same time as zanamivir dose.

⊗ ***Warning*** Caution patients with asthma or COPD of the risk of bronchospasm; a fast-acting inhaled bronchodilator should be on hand in case bronchospasm occurs; zanamivir should be discontinued and physician consulted promptly if respiratory symptoms worsen.

Teaching points

- Take this drug every 12 hours, at the same time each day, for as many days as prescribed. Use the *Diskhaler* delivery system provided.
- Take the full course of therapy as prescribed; this drug does not decrease the risk of transmitting the virus to others.
- If a bronchodilator is being used to treat a respiratory problem, the bronchodilator should be used before this drug.
- You may experience these side effects: Nausea, vomiting, loss of appetite, diarrhea; headache, dizziness (use caution if driving or operating dangerous machinery).
- Report severe diarrhea, severe nausea, worsening of respiratory symptoms.

ziconotide

See Appendix W, *Less commonly used drugs*.

zidovudine (azidothymidine, AZT, Compound S)

(zid o ***vew'*** *den)*

Retrovir

PREGNANCY CATEGORY C

Drug class

Antiviral

Therapeutic actions

Thymidine analogue isolated from the sperm of herring; drug is activated to a triphosphate form that inhibits replication of some retroviruses, including HIV, HTLV III, alpha retrovirus, lymphadenopathy-associated virus.

Indications

- Management of certain adult patients with symptomatic HIV infection in combination with other antiretrovirals
- Prevention of maternal–fetal HIV transmission

Contraindications and cautions

- Contraindicated with life-threatening allergy to any component, pregnancy, lactation.
- Use cautiously with compromised bone marrow, impaired renal or hepatic function.

Available forms

Capsules—100 mg; tablets—300 mg; syrup—50 mg/5 mL; injection—10 mg/mL

Dosages

Adults

Oral

- *Symptomatic HIV infection:* 600 mg daily in divided doses as either 200 mg tid or 300 mg bid. Monitor hematologic indices every 2 wk. If significant anemia (Hgb less than 7.5 g/dL, reduction of more than 25%) or reduction of granulocytes more than 50% below baseline occurs, dose interruption is necessary until evidence of bone marrow recovery is seen. If less severe bone marrow depression occurs, a dosage reduction may be adequate.
- *Prevention of maternal–fetal transmission:* 100 mg PO five times/day until the start of labor.

IV

1 mg/kg 5–6 times/day infused over 1 hr.

Pediatric patients 6 wk–12 yr

4 to less than 9 kg: 24 mg/kg/day PO in two to three divided doses.

9 to less than 30 kg: 18 mg/kg/day PO in two to three divided doses.

30 kg and over: 600 mg/day PO in two to three divided doses.

Infants born to HIV-infected mothers

2 mg/kg every 6 hr starting within 12 hr of birth to 6 wk of age or 1.5 mg/kg IV over 30 min every 6 hr.

Pharmacokinetics

Route	*Onset*	*Peak*
Oral	Varies	30–90 min
IV	Rapid	End of infusion

Metabolism: Hepatic; $T_{1/2}$: 30–60 min
Distribution: Crosses placenta; may enter breast milk
Excretion: Urine

IV FACTS

Preparation: Remove desired dose from vial, and dilute in D_5W to a concentration no greater

Z

than 4 mg/mL. Discard after 24 hr. Protect from light.
Infusion: Administer over 60 min; avoid rapid infusion. For a pregnant patient, when labor starts, given to the mother as a single 2 mg/kg dose infused over 1 hr followed by 1 mg/kg/hr given by continuous IV infusion until the umbilical cord is clamped.
Incompatibilities: Do not mix with blood or blood products.

Adverse effects

- **CNS:** *Headache,* insomnia, myalgia, *asthenia,* malaise, dizziness, paresthesias, somnolence
- **GI:** *Nausea, GI pain, diarrhea,* anorexia, vomiting, dyspepsia, lactic acidosis with severe hepatomegaly
- **Hematologic:** *Agranulocytopenia,* severe anemia requiring transfusions
- **Other:** *Fever,* diaphoresis, dyspnea, *rash,* taste perversion

Interactions

✱ **Drug-drug** • Increased risk of hematologic toxicity if combined with nephrotoxic, cytotoxic, or bone marrow suppressing drugs, ganciclovir, interferon alfa • Increased risk of neurotoxicity when used with acyclovir • Severe drowsiness and lethargy with cyclosporine
✱ **Drug-alternative therapy** • Decreased effectiveness if taken with St. John's wort

■ Nursing considerations

CLINICAL ALERT!
Name confusion has been reported between *Retrovir* (zidovudine) and ritonavir; use caution.

Assessment

- **History:** Life-threatening allergy to any component, compromised bone marrow, impaired renal or hepatic function, pregnancy, lactation
- **Physical:** Skin rashes, lesions, texture; T; affect, reflexes, peripheral sensation; bowel sounds, liver evaluation; LFTs, renal function tests, CBC and differential

Interventions

⊗ ***Black box warning*** Monitor hematologic indices every 2 wk; hematologic toxicity has occurred.

- Give the drug around-the-clock; rest periods may be needed during the day due to interrupted sleep.

⊗ ***Black box warning*** Monitor LFTs; lactic acidosis with severe hepatomegaly is possible.

⊗ ***Black box warning*** Patient is at increased risk for symptomatic myopathy; monitor accordingly.

Teaching points

- Take drug every 4 hours, around-the-clock. Use an alarm clock to wake you up at night; rest periods during the day may be needed. Do not share this drug; take exactly as prescribed.
- Zidovudine is not a cure for AIDS or AIDS-related complex; opportunistic infections may occur; obtain continuous medical care.
- Arrange for frequent blood tests; results of blood counts may indicate dosage needs to be decreased or drug discontinued temporarily.
- Zidovudine does not reduce the risk of transmission of HIV to others by sexual contact or blood contamination; use precautions.
- You may experience these side effects: Nausea, loss of appetite, change in taste (eat frequent small meals); dizziness, loss of feeling (use precautions); headache, fever, muscle aches.
- Report extreme fatigue, lethargy, severe headache, severe nausea, vomiting, difficulty breathing, rash.

▽ zileuton

*(zye **loot'** on)*

Zyflo CR (DNC)

PREGNANCY CATEGORY C

Drug classes

Antiasthmatic
Leukotriene formation inhibitor

Therapeutic actions
Selectively and competitively blocks the receptor that inhibits leukotriene formation, thus blocking many of the signs and symptoms of asthma (neutrophil and eosinophil migration, neutrophil and monocyte aggregation, leukocyte adhesion, increased capillary permeability, and smooth muscle contraction). These actions contribute to inflammation, edema, mucus secretion and bronchoconstriction caused by cold air challenge in patients with asthma.

Indications
- Prophylaxis and long-term treatment of asthma in adults and children 12 yr and older

Contraindications and cautions
- Contraindicated with hypersensitivity to zileuton or any of its components, acute asthma attacks, status asthmaticus, pregnancy and lactation, severe hepatic impairment.
- Use cautiously with hepatic impairment.

Available forms
CR tablets DNC—600 mg

Dosages
Adults and patients 12 yr and older
CR tablets, 1,200 mg (2 tablets) PO bid within 1 hr after morning and evening meals for a total daily dose of 2,400 mg.
Patients with hepatic impairment
Use caution; contraindicated if liver enzymes (AST, ALT) three or more times normal.

Pharmacokinetics

Route	*Onset*	*Peak*
Oral	Rapid	1.7 hr

Metabolism: Hepatic; $T_{1/2}$: 2.5 hr
Distribution: Crosses placenta; enters breast milk
Excretion: Unknown

Adverse effects
- **CNS:** *Headache,* dizziness, myalgia, behavior and mood changes
- **GI:** Nausea, diarrhea, abdominal pain, vomiting, **elevation of liver enzymes**
- **Other:** Generalized pain, fever, myalgia

Interactions
✱ **Drug-drug** • Increased effects of propranolol, theophylline, warfarin; monitor patient and decrease dose as appropriate
✱ **Drug-food** • Bioavailability decreased markedly by the presence of food; administer at least 1 hr before or 2 hr after meals

■ Nursing considerations
Assessment
- **History:** Hypersensitivity to zileuton, impaired hepatic function, lactation, pregnancy, acute asthma or bronchospasm
- **Physical:** T; orientation, reflexes; R, adventitious sounds; GI evaluation; LFTs

Interventions
⊗ ***Warning*** Obtain baseline LFTs before beginning therapy; monitor liver enzymes on a regular basis during therapy; discontinue drug and consult prescriber if enzymes rise more than three times normal.
⊗ ***Warning*** There is a risk of neuropsychiatric events, including mood and behavior changes with drug administration. Monitor accordingly; discontinue drug if these occur.
- Administer CR tablets within 1 hour after morning and evening meals. Do not cut, crush, or let patient chew CR tablets.
- Ensure that drug is taken continually for optimal effect.

⊗ ***Warning*** Do not administer for acute asthma attack or acute bronchospasm.

Teaching points
- Take this drug regularly as prescribed; do not stop taking this drug during symptom-free periods; do not stop taking this drug without consulting your health care provider. Continue taking any other antiasthmatics that have been prescribed for you.
- Do not cut, crush, or chew CR tablets; swallow them whole. Take CR tablets within 1 hour after morning and evening meals.
- Do not take this drug for an acute asthma attack or acute bronchospasm; this drug is not a bronchodilator; routine emergency procedures should be followed during acute attacks.

- Avoid the use of over-the-counter drugs while you are using this medication; many of them contain products that can interfere with or cause serious side effects when used with this drug. If you feel that you need one of these products, consult your health care provider.
- You may experience these side effects: Dizziness (use caution when driving or performing activities that require alertness); nausea, vomiting (eat frequent small meals; take drug with food); headache (analgesics may be helpful).
- Report fever, acute asthma attacks, flulike symptoms, lethargy, pruritus, changes in color of urine or stool.

▽ziprasidone

*(zih **praz'** i done)*

Geodon

PREGNANCY CATEGORY C

Drug classes

Atypical antipsychotic
Benzisoxazole

Therapeutic actions

Mechanism of action not fully understood; blocks dopamine and serotonin receptors in the brain, depresses the reticular activating system; effective in suppressing many of the negative aspects of schizophrenia (blunted affect, social withdrawal, lack of motivation, anger).

Indications

- Treatment of schizophrenia and to delay the time and rate of relapse
- Oral: Treatment of acute bipolar mania including manic or mixed episodes associated with bipolar disorder with or without psychotic features; maintenance treatment, used with lithium and valproate
- IM: Rapid control of agitated behavior and psychotic symptoms in patients with acute schizophrenia exacerbations

Contraindications and cautions

- Contraindicated with allergy to ziprasidone, prolonged QTc interval, history of severe cardiac disease.
- Use cautiously with renal or hepatic impairment, CV disease, pregnancy, lactation.

Available forms

Capsules—20, 40, 60, 80 mg; powder for injection—20 mg

Dosages

Adults

- *Schizophrenia:* Initially, 20 mg PO bid with food. Adjust as needed. Effective range, 20–80 mg PO bid.
- *Rapid control of agitated behavior:* 10–20 mg IM; doses of 10 mg may be repeated every 2 hr; doses of 20 mg may be repeated in 4 hr. Maximum dose, 40 mg/day.
- *Bipolar mania:* 40 mg PO bid with food. May be increased to 60 or 80 mg PO bid with food.

Pediatric patients

Safety and efficacy not established.

Pharmacokinetics

Route	*Onset*	*Peak*	*Duration*
Oral	Varies	1 hr	6–8 hr

Metabolism: Hepatic; $T_{1/2}$: 3 hr
Distribution: Crosses placenta; enters breast milk
Excretion: Urine

Adverse effects

- **CNS:** *Somnolence, drowsiness, sedation, headache,* extrapyramidal reactions
- **CV: Arrhythmias,** hypotension, ECG changes, hypertension, prolonged QTc interval
- **GI:** *Nausea, dyspepsia, constipation,* abdominal discomfort, dry mouth
- **GU:** Polyuria
- **Other:** *Fever,* weight gain (not as likely as with other antipsychotics), rash, risk of development of diabetes mellitus

Interactions

✱ **Drug-drug** ⊗ ***Warning*** Increased risk of severe cardiac arrhythmias if taken with other drugs that prolong the QTc interval.
• Additive hypotension when given with other antihypertensives

✱ **Drug-alternative therapy** • Possibility of increased toxicity if taken with St. John's wort

■ Nursing considerations

Assessment

- **History:** Allergy to ziprasidone, pregnancy, lactation, cardiac disease, hepatic or renal impairment, prolonged QTc interval
- **Physical:** T, weight; reflexes, orientation; P, ECG; bowel sounds, normal output, liver evaluation; normal urine output; urinalysis, LFTs, renal function tests

Interventions

⊗ ***Warning*** Ensure that patient is not pregnant before beginning therapy; advise patient to use contraceptive measures while using this drug.

⊗ ***Black box warning*** Increased risk of death if used in elderly patients with dementia-related psychosis; do not use drug in these patients; drug not approved for this use.

- Obtain baseline ECG to rule out prolonged QTc interval; monitor periodically throughout therapy.
- Monitor weight before beginning therapy and periodically during therapy. Weight gain is not usually a concern with this drug.
- Monitor patient regularly for signs and symptoms of diabetes mellitus.
- Follow patients with renal or hepatic impairment carefully throughout therapy.
- Continue other measures used to deal with schizophrenia.

Teaching points

- This drug cannot be taken during pregnancy. If you think you are pregnant, or want to become pregnant, consult your health care provider.
- You may experience these side effects: Somnolence, drowsiness, dizziness, sedation (avoid driving a car, operating machinery, or performing tasks that require concentration); nausea, dyspepsia (eat frequent small meals); headache (analgesics may be available to help, consult your health care provider).
- Report lethargy, weakness, fever, sore throat, palpitations, return of symptoms.

▽ zoledronic acid

(zoh leh ***droh'*** *nik)*

Reclast, Zometa

PREGNANCY CATEGORY D

Drug classes

Bisphosphonate
Calcium regulator

Therapeutic actions

A bisphonic acid that inhibits bone resorption, possibly by inhibiting osteoclast activity and promoting osteoclast cell apoptosis; this action leads to a decrease in the release of calcium from bone and a decrease in serum calcium.

Indications

- IV treatment of the hypercalcemia of malignancy (*Zometa*)
- Treatment of Paget's disease of bone in men and women (*Reclast*)
- Treatment of postmenopausal osteoporosis (*Reclast*)
- Prevention of new clinical fractures in patients with low-trauma hip fractures (*Reclast*)
- Treatment of patients with multiple myelomas and patients with documented bone metastases from solid tumors in conjunction with standard antineoplastic therapy (*Zometa*)
- Unlabeled use: Prevention of osteopenia in patients with prostate, breast, or ovarian cancer

Contraindications and cautions

- Contraindicated with allergy to any components of the drug or to bisphosphonates; severe renal impairment.
- Use cautiously with renal impairment (do not exceed single doses of 4 mg, and duration of infusion must not be less than 15 min), hepatic impairment, aspirin-sensitive asthmatic patients, pregnancy, or lactation.

Available forms

Injection—4 mg/5 mL; 5 mg/100 mL (*Reclast*)

Dosages

Adults

Zometa: 4 mg IV as a single-dose infusion of not less than 15 min for hypercalcemia of malignancy with albumin-corrected serum calcium levels of 12 mg/dL or greater. Retreatment may be done with 4 mg IV if

Z

needed; a minimum of 7 days should elapse between doses with careful monitoring of serum creatinine levels. Patients with solid tumors should receive 4 mg IV every 3–4 wk to treat bone metastasis.
Reclast: 5 mg IV infused via vented infusion line over at least 15 min. Retreatment may be considered as needed once every 2 yr for osteoporosis.

Pediatric patients

Safety and efficacy not established.

Patients with renal impairment

Zometa: Mild to moderate renal impairment for patients with multiple myeloma and bone metastases from solid tumors (see chart for dosages).

CrCl (mL/min)	*Dose*
More than 60	4 mg
50–60	3.5 mg
40–49	3.3 mg
30–39	3 mg
Less than 30	Contraindicated

Reclast: If creatinine clearance 35 mL/min or greater, 5 mg over at least 15 min. Not recommended for patients with severe renal failure.

Pharmacokinetics

Route	*Onset*	*Peak*
IV	Slow	8 hr

Metabolism: Hepatic; $T_{1/2}$: 0.23 hr then 1.75 hr
Distribution: May cross placenta; may enter breast milk
Excretion: Urine

IV FACTS

Preparation: Withdraw solution, equivalent to 4 mg *Zometa,* further dilute in 100 mL 0.9% sodium chloride, 5% dextrose injection. May be refrigerated and stored for up to 24 hr before the time of the end of the infusion. For *Reclast,* no additional preparation needed; use a vented infusion line.
Infusion: Infuse over no less than 15 min.
Incompatibilities: Do not mix with any other drug solution; always administer via a separate line. Physically incompatible with calcium-containing infusions.

Adverse effects

- **CNS:** Agitation, confusion, *insomnia,* anxiety
- **CV:** *Hypotension*
- **GI:** *Nausea, constipation,* vomiting, diarrhea, abdominal pain, anorexia
- **Hematologic:** Hypophosphatemia, hypokalemia, hypomagnesemia, hypocalcemia
- **Respiratory:** *Dyspnea,* coughing, pleural effusion
- **Other:** *Infections* (UTI, candidiasis), *fever,* progression of cancer, osteonecrosis of the jaw, renal impairment

Interactions

✱ **Drug-drug** • Possible increased risk of hypocalcemia if taken with aminoglycosides, loop diuretics; if this combination is used, monitor serum calcium levels closely

■ Nursing considerations

Assessment

- **History:** Allergy to components of the drug or any bisphosphonate, hepatic or renal impairment, aspirin-sensitive asthma, pregnancy, lactation
- **Physical:** T, BP, R, orientation and affect, adventitious sounds, CBC and electrolytes, renal function tests

Interventions

- Arrange for the patient to have a dental examination and any needed preventive treatments before beginning therapy. Avoid any invasive dental work or surgery while on this drug to decrease risk of osteonecrosis of the jaw.
- Patients with multiple myeloma or bone metastases associated with solid tumors who receive zoledronic acid should also receive 500 mg of elemental calcium daily and a multivitamin containing 400 units of vitamin D daily.
- Make sure that patient is well hydrated before use; vigorous saline hydration to establish a urine output of about 2 L/day is suggested.
- Monitor urinary output and assess patient for hydration status continually.

⊗ ***Warning*** Monitor serum creatinine levels prior to each dose of zoledronic acid;

follow dosage guidelines for any indication of renal toxicity.

⊗ ***Warning*** There is an increased risk of renal impairment and renal failure with drug administration. Check renal function regularly; use caution with other nephrotoxic drugs.

- Ensure that reconstituted solution is infused within 24 hr of reconstitution.
- For *Reclast,* make sure to use a vented infusion line.
- Ensure that drug infuses over not less than 15 min.
- Provide frequent small meals if GI upset occurs.
- Arrange for nutritional consult if nausea and vomiting are persistent.
- Monitor patient for any sign of infection and arrange for appropriate interventions.

Teaching points

- Arrange to have a dental examination and complete any needed treatment before starting this drug.
- This drug must be given by IV infusion; you will be closely monitored prior to and following the infusion.
- If you are returning for infusions every 3–4 weeks or once per year, mark a calendar with your return dates.
- It is important to maintain your fluid levels before using this drug; drink fluids as much as possible to ensure that you are hydrated.
- It is important to take vitamin D and calcium supplements to help prevent osteoporosis and reduce the risk of new fractures.
- Avoid invasive dental procedures and dental surgery.
- You may experience these side effects: Nausea, vomiting (eat frequent small meals); agitation, confusion, anxiety (consult your health care provider if this becomes a problem).
- Report difficulty breathing, muscle pain, tremors, pain at injection site.

▽ zolmitriptan

*(zohl mah **trip'** tan)*

Zomig (ONC), Zomig-ZMT

PREGNANCY CATEGORY C

Drug classes

Antimigraine drug
Serotonin selective agonist

Therapeutic actions

Binds to serotonin receptors to cause vascular constrictive effects on cranial blood vessels, causing the relief of migraine in selected patients.

Indications

- Treatment of acute migraine attacks with or without aura

Contraindications and cautions

- Contraindicated with allergy to zolmitriptan, active CAD, Prinzmetal's angina, pregnancy.
- Use cautiously with the elderly and with lactation.

Available forms

Tablets (ONC)—2.5, 5 mg; nasal spray—5 mg; orally disintegrating tablet—2.5 mg

Dosages

Adults

Oral

For tablets or orally disintegrating tablets, 2.5 mg PO at onset of headache or with beginning of aura; may repeat dose if headache persists after 2 hr; do not exceed 10 mg in 24 hr.

Nasal spray

1 spray in nostril at onset of headache or beginning of aura; may repeat in 2 hr if needed. Maximum dose, 10 mg/24 hr.

Pediatric patients

Safety and efficacy not established.

Patients with hepatic impairment

Use caution; keep doses at 2.5 mg or less. Significant increases in BP can occur.

Pharmacokinetics

Route	*Onset*	*Peak*
Oral	Varies	2–4 hr
Nasal	15 min	2 hr

Metabolism: Hepatic; $T_{1/2}$: 2.5–3.7 hr
Distribution: Crosses placenta; may enter breast milk
Excretion: Feces, urine

Adverse effects

- **CNS:** *Dizziness, vertigo,* headache, anxiety, malaise or fatigue, *weakness, myalgia*
- **CV:** *BP alterations, tightness or pressure in chest*
- **GI:** Abdominal discomfort, dysphagia
- **Other:** *Tingling, warm/hot sensations, burning sensation, feeling of heaviness, pressure sensation, numbness, feeling of tightness,* feeling strange, cold sensation

Interactions

✱ **Drug-drug** ⊗ ***Warning*** Risk of severe effects with an MAOI or within 2 wk of discontinuing an MAOI.
• Prolonged vasoactive reactions with ergot-containing drugs • Increased risk of toxic effects with cimetidine, hormonal contraceptives
• A serotonin syndrome may occur when sibutramine is coadministered

■ Nursing considerations

Assessment

- **History:** Allergy to zolmitriptan, active CAD, Prinzmetal's angina, pregnancy, lactation
- **Physical:** Skin color and lesions; orientation, reflexes, peripheral sensation; P, BP; LFTs, renal function tests

Interventions

- Administer to relieve acute migraine, not as prophylactic measure. Ensure that patient does not cut, crush, or chew tablets.
- Establish safety measures if CNS or visual disturbances occur.
- Control environment as appropriate to help relieve migraine (eg, lighting, temperature).

⊗ ***Warning*** Monitor BP of patients with possible CAD; discontinue at any sign of angina or prolonged high BP.

Teaching points

- Take this drug exactly as prescribed, at the onset of headache or aura.
- Use drug right after removing from blister package. Do not break, crush, or chew tablet. Place orally disintegrating tablet on your tongue and let it dissolve.
- This drug should not be taken during pregnancy; if you suspect that you are pregnant, contact your health care provider and stop using the drug.
- Continue measures that usually help you during a migraine (adjust lighting, noise).
- Contact your health care provider immediately if you experience chest pain or pressure that is severe or does not go away.
- You may experience these side effects: Dizziness, drowsiness (avoid driving or using dangerous machinery); numbness, tingling, feelings of tightness or pressure.
- Report feelings of heat, flushing, tiredness, nausea, swelling of lips or eyelids.

zolpidem tartrate

(zol' pih dem)

Ambien, Ambien CR (DNC), Zolpimist

PREGNANCY CATEGORY B (IMMEDIATE-RELEASE)

PREGNANCY CATEGORY C (ER)

CONTROLLED SUBSTANCE C-IV

Drug class

Sedative-hypnotic (nonbarbiturate)

Therapeutic actions

Modulates GABA receptors to cause suppression of neurons, leading to sedation, anticonvulsant, anxiolytic, and relaxant properties.

Indications

- Short-term treatment of insomnia
- Treatment of insomnia in adults who experience difficulties with sleep onset and sleep maintenance (ER tablets)

Contraindications and cautions

- Contraindicated with hypersensitivity to zolpidem.
- Use cautiously with acute intermittent porphyria, impaired hepatic or renal function, addiction-prone patients, pregnancy, lactation.

Available forms

Tablets—5, 10 mg; ER tablets ONC—6.25, 12.5 mg; orally disintegrating tablets—5, 10 mg; oral spray—5, 10 mg

Dosages

Adults

10 mg PO at bedtime. Do not exceed 10 mg/day. ER tablets—12.5 mg/day PO. Oral spray—Two to three sprays in mouth, over tongue at bedtime.

Pediatric patients

Safety and efficacy not established.

Geriatric patients

Increased chance of confusion, acute brain syndrome; initiate treatment with 5 mg PO or 6.25 mg/day PO ER tablets.

Pharmacokinetics

Route	Onset	Peak
Oral	45 min	1.6 hr

Metabolism: Hepatic; $T_{1/2}$: 2.6 hr
Distribution: Crosses placenta; may enter breast milk
Excretion: Urine

Adverse effects

- **CNS:** Seizures, hallucinations, ataxia, EEG changes, pyrexia, *morning drowsiness, hangover, headache, dizziness,* vertigo, acute brain syndrome and confusion; paradoxical excitation, anxiety, depression, nightmares, dreaming, diplopia, blurred vision, *suppression of REM sleep,* REM rebound when drug is discontinued, complex sleep disorders
- **GI:** Esophagitis, vomiting, *nausea,* diarrhea, constipation
- **Hypersensitivity:** Generalized allergic reactions; pruritus, rash
- **Other:** Flulike symptoms, dry mouth, infection, **anaphylaxis, angioedema**

■ Nursing considerations

Assessment

- **History:** Hypersensitivity to zolpidem, acute intermittent porphyria, impaired hepatic or renal function, addiction-prone, lactation, pregnancy
- **Physical:** T; skin color, lesions; orientation, affect, reflexes, vision examination; P, BP; bowel sounds, normal output, liver evaluation; CBC with differential; LFTs, renal function tests

Interventions

⊗ ***Warning*** Limit amount of drug dispensed to patients who are depressed or suicidal.

⊗ ***Warning*** Withdraw drug gradually if patient has used drug long-term or if patient has developed tolerance. Supportive therapy similar to that for withdrawal from barbiturates may be necessary to prevent dangerous withdrawal symptoms.

- Place orally disintegrating tablet in patient's mouth; have patient swallow tablet with saliva. Do not allow patient to chew, break, or split tablet.
- Prime oral spray before first use by compressing the container five times. Teach the patient proper administration.

Teaching points

- Take this drug exactly as prescribed. Do not exceed prescribed dosage. Long-term use is not recommended.
- If using oral spray, prime container before initial use by compressing the container five times. Hold container upright and aim it directly into your open mouth. Compress the container completely, spraying over your tongue and directly into your mouth. If drug is not used for 14 or more days, prime the container once before using.
- You may experience these side effects: Drowsiness, allergic reaction, swelling, dizziness, blurred vision (avoid driving or performing tasks requiring alertness or visual acuity); GI upset (eat frequent small meals), sleep disorders.
- Report rash, sore throat, fever, bruising, allergic reaction, swelling, complex sleep-related behaviors, thoughts of suicide.

zonisamide

*(zoh **niss'** ah myde)*

Zonegran

PREGNANCY CATEGORY C

Drug class

Antiepileptic

Therapeutic actions

Mechanism of action not fully understood; inhibits voltage-sensitive sodium and calcium channels, stabilizing the neuronal membrane and modulating calcium-dependent presynaptic release of excitatory amino acids; may also have dopaminergic effects.

Indications

- Adjuvant therapy in the treatment of partial seizures in adults with epilepsy

Contraindications and cautions

- Contraindicated with lactation, history of sulfonamide hypersensitivity.
- Use cautiously with impaired hepatic, renal, or cardiac function; pregnancy.

Available forms

Capsules—25, 50, 100 mg

Dosages

Adults

Initial dose, 100 mg PO daily as a single dose—not divided—subsequent doses can be divided; may increase by 100 mg/day every 2 wk to achieve control. Maximum dose, 600 mg/day.

Pediatric patients

Not recommended in patients younger than 16 yr.

Pharmacokinetics

Route	*Onset*	*Peak*
Oral	Rapid	2–6 hr

Metabolism: Hepatic; $T_{1/2}$: 49.7–130 hr
Distribution: Crosses placenta; may enter breast milk
Excretion: Urine

Adverse effects

- **CNS:** *Dizziness,* insomnia, headache, somnolence, *ataxia,* diplopia, blurred vision, nystagmus, *decrease in mental functioning*
- **Dermatologic:** *Rash*
- **GI:** *Nausea,* vomiting, *dry mouth, unusual taste in mouth*
- **Other:** Bone marrow depression, *renal calculi,* oligohidrosis and hyperthermia (pediatric), metabolic acidosis

Interactions

✱ **Drug-drug** • Rapid elimination of zonisamide if taken with enzyme-inducing antiepileptics—carbamazepine, phenytoin, phenobarbital, primidone • Increased levels and potential for toxicity with carbamazepine if taken with zonisamide; adjust dosage and monitor patient carefully

■ Nursing considerations

Assessment

- **History:** Lactation; impaired hepatic, renal, or cardiac function; pregnancy
- **Physical:** Weight; T; skin color, lesions; orientation, affect, reflexes; P, BP, perfusion; bowel sounds, normal output; LFTs, renal function test, CBC

Interventions

⊗ ***Warning*** Monitor drug doses carefully when starting therapy and with each increase in dose; special care will need to be taken when changing the dose or frequency of any other antiepileptic.

⊗ ***Warning*** There is a risk of metabolic acidosis with drug administration. Measure serum bicarbonate level before and periodically during therapy. Alkali therapy is recommended if drug is needed and acidosis occurs.

⊗ ***Warning*** Patient may be at increased risk for suicidal ideation and suicidality; monitor accordingly.

⊗ ***Warning*** Taper drug slowly over a 2-wk period when discontinuing.

- Ensure that patient is well hydrated to prevent formation of renal calculi.
- Provide safety measures if CNS effects occur.

Teaching points

- Take this drug exactly as prescribed. Dosage may be increased slowly.
- Do not discontinue this drug abruptly or change dosage, except on the advice of your health care provider.
- You should wear a medical alert tag at all times so that any emergency medical personnel taking care of you will know that you have epilepsy and are taking antiepileptic medication.
- You may experience these side effects: Dizziness, drowsiness, decreased mental functioning (avoid driving a car or performing other tasks requiring alertness or visual acuity if this occurs); GI upset (taking the drug with food or milk and eating frequent small meals may help); headache (medication can be ordered); rash (skin care and lotions may be helpful).
- Report yellowing of skin, abdominal pain, changes in color of urine or stools, flank pain, painful urination, thoughts of suicide.

Appendices

Appendix A

Alternative and complementary therapies

Many dietary supplements and "natural" remedies are used by the public for self-treatment. These substances, many derived from the folklore of various cultures, commonly contain ingredients that have been identified and that have known therapeutic activities. Some of these substances have unknown mechanisms of action but over the years have been reliably used to relieve specific symptoms. There is an element of the placebo effect in using some of these substances. The power of believing that something will work and that there is some control over the problem is often beneficial in achieving relief from pain or suffering. Some of these substances may contain yet unidentified ingredients, which eventually may prove useful in the modern field of pharmacology. Because these products are not regulated or monitored, there is always a possibility of toxic effects. Some of these products may contain ingredients that interact with prescription drugs. A history of the use of these alternative therapies may explain unexpected reactions to some drugs. Drugs that the substance interacts with are in **bold.**

Substance	Reported uses and possible risks
acidophilus (probiotics)	Oral: prevention or treatment of uncomplicated diarrhea Decreased effectiveness of **warfarin.**
alfalfa	Topical: healing ointment, relief of arthritis pain Oral: treatment of arthritis, hot flashes; strength giving; reduction of cholesterol level Increased risk of bleeding with **warfarin;** increased photosensitivity with **chlorpromazine;** increased risk of hypoglycemia with **antidiabetic drugs;** loss of effectiveness with **hormonal contraceptives** or **hormone replacement**
allspice	Topical: anesthetic for teeth and gums; soothes sore joints and muscles Oral: treatment of indigestion, flatulence, diarrhea, fatigue Risk of seizures with excessive use; decreased **iron** absorption.
aloe leaves	Topical: treatment of burns, healing of wounds Oral: treatment of chronic constipation Caution: Oral use may cause serious hypokalemia; risk of spontaneous abortion if used in third trimester
androstenedione	Oral, spray: anabolic steroid to increase muscle mass and strength Caution: May increase risk of CV disease and certain cancers.
angelica	Oral: "cure all" for gynecologic problems, headaches, backaches, loss of appetite, and GI spasms; increases circulation in the periphery Risk of bleeding if combined with **anticoagulants.**
anise	Oral: relief of dry cough, treatment of flatulence May increase **iron** absorption and cause toxicity.
apple	Oral: control of blood glucose, constipation May interfere with **antidiabetic drugs.**

Substance	Reported uses and possible risks
arnica	Topical: relief of pain from muscle or soft tissue injury Oral: immune system stimulant May decrease effects of **antihypertensives** and increase effects of **anticoagulants** and **platelet drugs;** very toxic to children.
ashwagandha	Oral: to improve mental and physical functioning; general tonic; to protect cells during cancer chemotherapy and radiation therapy May increase bleeding with **anticoagulants;** may interfere with **thyroid replacement** therapy. Discourage use during pregnancy and lactation.
astragalus	Oral: to increase stamina, energy; to improve immune function, resistance to disease; to treat upper respiratory tract infection, common cold May increase effects of **antihypertensives.** Caution against use during fever or acute infection.
barberry	Oral: antidiarrheal, antipyretic, cough suppressant Risk of spontaneous abortion if taken during pregnancy. May increase effects of **antihypertensives, antiarrhythmics.**
basil	Oral: analgesic, anti-inflammatory, hypoglycemic Risk of increased hypoglycemic effects of **antidiabetic drugs.**
bayberry	Topical: to promote wound healing Oral: stimulant, emetic, antidiarrheal May block effects of **antihypertensives.**
bee pollen	Oral: to treat allergies, asthma, impotence, prostatitis; suggested use to decrease cholesterol levels Risk of hyperglycemia; discourage use by diabetic patients or with **antidiabetic drugs.** May cause allergic reaction in patients allergic to bees.
betel palm	Oral: mild stimulant, digestive aid Increased risk of hypertensive crisis with **MAOIs;** blocks heart-rate reduction of **beta blockers, digoxin;** alters effects of **antiglaucoma drugs.**
bilberry	Oral: treatment of diabetes; cardiovascular problems; lowers cholesterol and triglycerides; treatment of diabetic retinopathy; treatment of cataracts, night blindness Increased risk of bleeding with **anticoagulants;** disulfiram-like reaction with **alcohol.**
birch bark	Topical: treatment of infected wounds, cuts Oral: as tea for relief of stomachache Topical form very toxic to children.
blackberry	Oral: as tea for generalized healing; treatment of diabetes Risk of interaction with **antidiabetic drugs.**

(continued)

Substance	Reported uses and possible risks
black cohosh root	Oral: treatment of PMS, menopausal disorders, rheumatoid arthritis Contains estrogen-like components. Caution against use with **hormone replacement therapy** or **hormonal contraceptives;** discourage use during pregnancy and lactation; may lower blood pressure with **sedatives, antihypertensives, anesthetics;** increased risk of fungal infection with **immunosuppressants.**
bromelain	Oral: treatment of inflammation, sports injuries, upper respiratory tract infection, PMS, and adjunctive therapy in cancer treatment May cause nausea, vomiting, diarrhea, menstrual disorders.
burdock	Oral: treatment of diabetes; atropine-like adverse effects, uterine stimulant May increase hypoglycemic effects of **antidiabetic drugs.**
capsicum	Topical: external analgesic Oral: treatment of bowel disorders, chronic laryngitis, peripheral vascular disease May increase bleeding with **warfarin, aspirin;** increases cough with **ACE inhibitors;** increases toxicity with **MAOIs;** increases sedation with **sedatives.**
catnip leaves	Oral: treatment of bronchitis, diarrhea
cat's claw	Oral: treatment of allergies, arthritis; adjunct in the treatment of cancers and AIDS Discourage use during pregnancy and lactation and use by transplant recipients; increased risk of bleeding episodes if taken with oral **anticoagulants;** increased hypotension with **antihypertensives.**
cayenne pepper	Topical: treatment of burns, wounds, relief of toothache
celery	Oral: lowers blood glucose, acts as a diuretic; may cause potassium depletion Advise caution when taken with **antidiabetic drugs.**
chamomile	Topical: treatment of wounds, ulcer, conjunctivitis Oral: treatment of migraines, gastric cramps, relief of anxiety Contains coumarin–closely monitor patients taking **anticoagulants.** May cause depression; monitor patients on **antidepressants.** Cross-reaction with ragweed allergies may occur. Discourage use during pregnancy and lactation.
chaste-tree berry	Oral: progesterone-like effects; used to treat PMS and menopausal problems, and to stimulate lactation Advise caution when taken with **hormone replacement therapy** and **hormonal contraceptives.**
chicken soup	Oral: breaks up respiratory secretions, bronchodilator, relieves anxiety
chicory	Oral: treatment of digestive tract problems, gout; stimulates bile secretions

Substance	Reported uses and possible risks
Chinese angelica (dong quai)	Oral: general tonic; treatment of anemias, PMS, menopause, antihypertensive, laxative Use caution with the flu, hemorrhagic diseases. Monitor patients on **antihypertensives, vasodilators,** or **anticoagulants** for toxic effects. Advise caution when taken with **hormone replacement therapy.**
chondroitin	Oral: treatment of osteoarthritis and related disorders (usually combined with glucosamine) Risk of increased bleeding if combined with **anticoagulants.**
chong cao fungi	Oral: antioxidant; promotes stamina, sexual function Discourage use by children.
coleus forskohlii	Oral: treatment of asthma, hypertension, eczema Urge caution when taken with **antihypertensives** or **antihistamines;** severe additive effects can occur. Discourage use if patient has hypotension or peptic ulcer.
comfrey	Topical: treatment of wounds, cuts, ulcers Oral: gargle for tonsillitis Warn against using with **eucalyptus;** monitor liver function.
coriander	Oral: weight loss, lowers blood glucose Advise caution when taken with **antidiabetic drugs.**
creatine monohydrate	Oral: enhancement of athletic performance Warn against using with **insulin;** do not use with caffeine.
dandelion root	Oral: treatment of liver and kidney problems; decreases lactation (after delivery or with weaning); lowers blood glucose Advise caution when taken with **antidiabetic drugs, antihypertensives,** and **quinolone antibiotics.**
DHEA	Oral: slows aging, improves vigor ("Fountain of Youth"); androgenic side effects Risk of interactions with **alprazolam, calcium channel blockers,** and **antidiabetic drugs.** Screen patients older than 40 yr for hormonally sensitive cancers before use.
di huang	Oral: treatment of diabetes mellitus Risk of hypoglycemia with **antidiabetic drugs.**
dried root bark of lycium Chinese mill	Oral: lowers cholesterol, lowers blood glucose Advise caution with **antidiabetic drugs.**
echinacea (cone flower)	Oral: treatment of colds, flu; stimulates the immune system, attacks viruses; causes immunosuppression if used long-term May be liver toxic. Discourage use longer than 12 wk. Caution against taking with **liver-toxic drugs** or **immunosuppressants.** Discourage use with **antifungals;** serious liver injury could occur. Advise against use by patients with SLE, TB, AIDS.
elder bark and flowers	Topical: gargle for tonsillitis, pharyngitis Oral: treatment of fever, chills

(continued)

Substance	Reported uses and possible risks
ephedra	Oral: increases energy, relieves fatigue May cause serious complications, including death; increased risk of hypertension, stroke, MI; interacts with many drugs; **banned by the FDA.**
ergot	Oral: treatment of migraine headaches, treatment of menstrual problems, hemorrhage Monitor patient who takes ergot with **antihypertensives.**
eucalyptus	Topical: treatment of wounds Oral: decreases respiratory secretions suppresses cough Warn against using with **comfrey;** very toxic in children.
evening primrose	Oral: treatment of PMS, menopause, rheumatoid arthritis, diabetic neuropathy Discourage use with **phenothiazines, antidepressants**–increases risk of seizures; discourage use by those with epilepsy, schizophrenia.
false unicorn root	Oral: treatment of menstrual and uterine problems Advise against use during pregnancy and lactation.
fennel	Oral: treatment of colic, gout, flatulence; enhances lactation Significantly decreases levels of **ciprofloxacin.**
fenugreek	Oral: lowers cholesterol level; reduces blood glucose; aids in healing Advise caution when taken with **antidiabetic drugs, anticoagulants.**
feverfew	Oral: treatment of arthritis, fever, migraine Advise caution when taken with **anticoagulants;** may increase bleeding. Discourage use before or immediately after surgery because of bleeding risk.
fish oil	Oral: treatment of coronary diseases, arthritis, colitis, depression, aggression, attention deficit disorder
gamboge	Oral: appetite suppressant, lowers cholesterol, promotes weight loss Oral use may be unsafe; discourage use.
garlic	Oral: treatment of colds; diuretic; prevention of CAD; intestinal antiseptic; lowers blood glucose; anticoagulant effects; decreases BP Advise caution if patient has diabetes or takes an **oral anticoagulant.** Known to affect blood clotting. Anemia reported with long-term use.
ginger	Oral: treatment of nausea, motion sickness, postoperative nausea (may increase risk of miscarriage) Affects blood clotting. Warn against use with **anticoagulants.**
ginkgo	Oral: vascular dilation; increases blood flow to the brain, improving cognitive function; used in treating Alzheimer's disease; antioxidant Can inhibit blood clotting. Seizures reported with high doses. Warn against use with **anticoagulants, aspirin,** or **NSAIDs.** Can interact with **phenytoin, carbamazepine, phenobarbital, TCAs, MAOIs,** and **antidiabetic drugs;** advise caution.

Substance	Reported uses and possible risks
ginseng	Oral: aphrodisiac, mood elevator, tonic; antihypertensive; decreases cholesterol levels; lowers blood glucose; adjunct in cancer chemotherapy and radiation therapy May cause irritability if combined with **caffeine.** Inhibits clotting. Warn against use with **anticoagulants, aspirin, NSAIDs.** Warn against use for longer than 3 mo. May cause headaches, manic episodes if used with **phenelzine, MAOIs.** Additive effects of **estrogens** and **corticosteroids.** May also interfere with cardiac effects of **digoxin.** Monitor patient closely if he takes these drugs or an **anti-diabetic drug.**
glucosamine	Oral: treatment of osteoarthritis and joint diseases, usually combined with chondroitin Monitor glucose levels in diabetic patients.
goldenrod leaves	Oral: treatment of renal disease, rheumatism, sore throat, eczema May decrease effects of **diuretics** by increasing sodium retention. Advise caution if patient has a history of allergies.
goldenseal	Oral: lowers blood glucose, aids healing; treatment of bronchitis, colds, flulike symptoms, cystitis May cause false-negative test results in those who use such drugs as marijuana and cocaine. Large amounts may cause paralysis. Affects blood clotting; warn against use with **anticoagulants.** May interfere with **antihypertensives, acid blockers, barbiturates.** May increase effects of **sedatives.** Death can result from overdose.
gotu kola	Topical: chronic venous insufficiency Warn against using with **antidiabetic drugs, cholesterol-lowering drugs, sedatives.**
grape seed extract	Oral: treatment of allergies, asthma; improves circulation; decreases platelet aggregation Advise caution with **oral anticoagulants;** may increase bleeding.
green tea leaf	Oral: antioxidant, to prevent cancer and cardiovascular disease, to increase cognitive function (caffeine effects) Advise caution with **oral anticoagulants;** may increase bleeding. May increase BP. Caution against using with milk.
guarana	Oral: decreases appetite, promotes weight loss Advise caution; increases blood pressure, risk of CV events.
guayusa	Oral: lowers blood glucose; promotes weight loss Advise caution with **antihypertensives.** Decreases absorption of **iron.** May decrease clearance of **lithium.**
hawthorn	Oral: treatment of angina, arrhythmias, BP problems; decreases cholesterol Advise caution with **digoxin, ACE inhibitors, CNS depressants;** may potentiate effects.
hop	Oral: sedative; aids healing; alters blood glucose Discourage use with **CNS depressants, antipsychotics.**

(continued)

Substance	Reported uses and possible risks
horehound	Oral: expectorant; treatment of respiratory problems, GI disorders Use caution with **antidiabetic drugs, antihypertensives.**
horse chestnut seed	Oral: treatment of varicose veins, hemorrhoids Advise caution with oral **anticoagulants;** may increase bleeding.
hyssop	Topical: treatment of cold sores, genital herpes, burns, wounds Oral: treatment of coughs, colds, indigestion, and flatulence Warn against use by pregnant patients and those with seizures; toxic in children and pets.
jambul	Oral: treatment of diarrhea, dysentery; lowers blood glucose Use caution with **CNS depressants.**
Java plum	Oral: treatment of diabetes mellitus Advise caution with **antidiabetic drugs.**
jojoba	Topical: promotion of hair growth, relief of skin problems Toxic if ingested.
juniper berries	Oral: increases appetite, aids digestion; diuretic; urinary tract disinfectant; lowers blood glucose level Advise caution when taken with **antidiabetic drugs.** Not for use in pregnancy.
kava	Oral: treatment of nervous anxiety, stress, restlessness; tranquilizer Warn against use with **alprazolam;** may cause coma. Advise against use with Parkinson's disease or history of stroke. Discourage use with **St. John's wort, anxiolytics, alcohol.** Risk of serious liver toxicity.
kudzu	Oral: reduces cravings for **alcohol;** being researched for use with alcoholics Interacts with **anticoagulants, aspirin, antidiabetic drugs, CV drugs.**
lavender	Topical: astringent for minor cuts, burns Oral: treatment of insomnia, restlessness Advise caution with **CNS depressants.** Oil is potentially poisonous.
ledum tincture	Topical: treatment of insect bites, puncture wounds; dissolves some blood clots and bruises
licorice	Oral: prevents thirst, soothes coughs; treats "incurable" chronic fatigue syndrome; treatment of duodenal ulcer. Acts like aldosterone. Blocks **spironolactone** effects. Can lead to **digoxin** toxicity because of effects of lowering aldosterone. Advise extreme caution. Contraindicated with renal or liver disease, hypertension, CAD, pregnancy, lactation. Warn against taking with **thyroid drugs, antihypertensives, hormonal contraceptives.**
ma huang	Oral: treatment of colds, nasal congestion, asthma Contains ephedrine. Warn against use with **antihypertensives, antidiabetic drugs, MAOIs, digoxin.** Serious adverse effects could occur.

Substance	Reported uses and possible risks
mandrake root	Oral: treatment of fertility problems
marigold leaves and flowers	Oral: relief of muscle tension, increases wound healing Advise against use during pregnancy and breast-feeding.
melatonin	Oral: relief of jet lag, treatment of insomnia, jet lag Advise caution with **antihypertensives, benzodiazepines, beta blockers, methamphetamine.**
milk thistle	Oral: treatment of hepatitis, cirrhosis, fatty liver caused by alcohol or drug use May affect metabolism and increase toxicity of **drugs using CP450, CYP3A4,** and **CYP2C9** systems.
milk vetch	Oral: improves resistance to disease; adjunct therapy in cancer chemotherapy and radiation therapy
mistletoe leaves	Oral: promotes weight loss; relief of signs and symptoms of diabetes Advise caution with **antihypertensives, CNS depressants, immunosuppressants.**
momordica charantia (Karela)	Oral: blocks intestinal absorption of glucose; lowers blood glucose; weight loss Advise caution when taken with **antidiabetic drugs.**
nettle	Topical: stimulation of hair growth, treatment of bleeding Oral: treatment of rheumatism, allergic rhinitis; antispasmodic; expectorant Advise against use during pregnancy and breast-feeding. Increases effects of **diuretics.**
nightshade leaves and roots	Oral: stimulates circulatory system; treatment of eye disorders
octacosanol	Oral: treatment of parkinsonism, enhancement of athletic performance Advise against use during pregnancy and lactation; avoid use with **carbidopa-levodopa.**
parsley seeds and leaves	Oral: treatment of jaundice, asthma, menstrual difficulties, urinary infections, conjunctivitis Risk of serotonin syndrome with **SSRIs, lithium, opioids;** increased hypotension with **antihypertensives.**
passionflower vine	Oral: sedative and hypnotic May increase sedation with other **CNS depressants, MAOIs.** Advise against drinking **alcohol** while taking this herb. Tell patient not to use with **anticoagulants.**
peppermint leaves	Oral: treatment of nervousness, insomnia, dizziness, cramps, coughs Topical: rubbed on forehead to relieve tension headaches
psyllium	Oral: treatment of constipation; lowers cholesterol Can cause severe gas and stomach pain; may interfere with nutrient absorption. Avoid use with **warfarin, digoxin, lithium**—absorption of drug may be blocked. Do not combine with **laxatives.**

(continued)

Substance	Reported uses and possible risks
raspberry	Oral: healing of minor wounds; control and treatment of diabetes, GI disorders, upper respiratory disorders Advise caution with **antidiabetic drugs;** disulfiram-like reaction with **alcohol.**
red clover	Oral: estrogen replacement in menopause, suppresses whooping cough, asthma Risk of bleeding wtih **anticoagulants, antiplatelet;** discourage use in pregnancy.
red yeast rice	Oral: cholesterol-lowering agent Increased risk of rhabdomyolysis with **cyclosporine, fibric acid, niacin, lovastatin, grapefruit juice.**
rose hips	Oral: laxative, to boost the immune system and prevent illness Advise caution with **estrogens, iron, warfarin.**
rosemary	Topical: relief of rheumatism, sprains, wounds, bruises, eczema Oral: gastric stimulation, relief of flatulence, stimulation of bile release, relief of colic Disulfiram-like reaction with **alcohol.**
rue extract	Topical: relief of pain associated with sprains, groin pulls, whiplash Advise caution with **antihypertensive drugs, digoxin, warfarin.**
saffron	Oral: treatment of menstrual problems, abortifacient
sage	Oral: lowers BP; lowers blood glucose Advise caution with **antidiabetic drugs, anticonvulsants, alcohol.**
SAM-e (adomet)	Oral: promotion of general well-being and health May cause frequent GI complaints and headache. Risk of serotonin syndrome with **antidepressants.**
sarsaparilla	Oral: treatment of skin disorders, rheumatism Advise caution with **anticonvulsants.**
sassafras	Topical: treatment of local pain, skin eruptions Oral: enhancement of athletic performance, “cure” for syphilis Oil may be toxic to fetus, children, and adults when ingested. Interacts with many drugs.
saw palmetto	Oral: treatment of BPH Warn against use with estrogen-replacement or hormonal contraceptives—may greatly increase adverse effects. May decrease iron absorption. Advise against use with **finasteride;** toxicity could occur.
schisandra	Oral: health tonic, liver protectant; adjunct in cancer chemotherapy and radiation therapy Warn against use during pregnancy; causes uterine stimulation. Advise caution with all **drugs metabolized in the liver.**

Substance	Reported uses and possible risks
squaw vine	Oral: diuretic, tonic, aid in labor and childbirth, treatment of menstrual problems May cause liver toxicity; increased toxicity of **digoxin.** Disulfiram-like reaction with **alcohol.**
St. John's wort	Oral: treatment of depression, PMS symptoms; antiviral Topical: to treat puncture wounds, insect bites, crushed fingers or toes Discourage tyramine-containing foods; hypertensive crisis is possible. Thrombocytopenia has been reported. Can increase sensitivity to light; advise against taking with drugs that cause photosensitivity. Severe photosensitivity can occur in light-skinned people. Serious interactions have been reported with **SSRIs, MAOIs, kava, digoxin, theophylline, AIDS antiviral drugs, sympathomimetics, antineoplastics, hormonal contraceptives.** Advise against these combinations.
sweet violet flowers	Oral: treatment of respiratory disorders; emetic Increases effects of **laxatives.**
tarragon	Oral: weight loss; prevents cancer; lowers blood glucose Advise caution with **antidiabetic drugs.**
tea tree oil	Topical: antifungal, antibacterial; used to treat burns, insect bites, irritated skin, acne; used as a mouthwash
thyme	Topical: as liniment, gargle; to treat wounds Oral: antidiarrheal, relief of bronchitis, laryngitis May increase sensitivity to light; warn against combining with **photosensitivity-causing drugs.** Also warn against combining with **MAOIs** or **SSRIs;** may cause serious adverse effects.
turmeric	Oral: antioxidant, anti-inflammatory; used to treat arthritis May cause GI distress. Warn against use with known biliary obstruction. May cause increased bleeding with oral **anticoagulants, NSAIDs.** Advise caution with **immunosuppressants.**
valerian	Oral: sedative and hypnotic; reduces anxiety, relaxes muscles Can cause severe liver damage. Warn against use with **barbiturates, alcohol, CNS depressants,** or **antihistamines;** can cause serious sedation.
went rice	Oral: cholesterol- and triglyceride-lowering effects Warn against use in pregnancy, liver disease, alcoholism, or acute infection.
white willow bark	Oral: treatment of fevers Advise caution with **anticoagulants, NSAIDs, diuretics.**
xuan shen	Oral: lowers blood glucose; slows heart rate; treatment of HF Advise caution when taken with **antidiabetic drugs.**
yohimbe	Oral: treatment of ED Can affect BP; CNS stimulant; has cardiac effects. Manic episodes have been reported in psychiatric patients. Warn against use with **SSRIs,** tyramine-containing foods. Advise caution with **TCAs.**

APPENDIX B

Preventing miscommunication

Although abbreviations can save time, they also raise the risk of misinterpretation, which can lead to potentially disastrous consequences, especially when dealing with drug administration. To help reduce the risk of being misunderstood, always take the time to write legibly and to spell out anything that could be misread. This caution extends to how you write numbers as well as drug names and other drug-related instructions.

Dosages

When writing a drug dosage, never add a zero **after** a decimal point and always add a zero **before** a decimal point. If you write 1.0 mg instead of the correct 1 mg, the dosage easily could be misread as 10 mg. Likewise, if you write .5 mg instead of the correct 0.5 mg, the dosage could be misread as 5 mg.

Drug names

Be careful with drug names. For instance, if you write $MgSO_4$ as shorthand for magnesium sulfate, you could be misread as meaning morphine sulfate. The opposite is also true; if you write MS or $MS0_4$, meaning morphine sulfate, you could be misread as meaning magnesium sulfate. Instead, make sure to clearly write out all drug names, particularly those that could be dangerous if confused or that could be easily confused.

Common dangerous abbreviations

Try to avoid these common—and dangerous—abbreviations, especially those that appear in color.

Abbreviation	Intended use	Potential misreading	Preferred use
BT	bedtime	May be read as "bid" or twice daily	Spell out "bedtime."
cc	cubic centimeters	May be read as "u" or units	Use "milliliters," abbreviated as "mL" or "ml."
D/C	discharge or discontinue	May lead to premature discontinuation of drug therapy or premature discharge	Spell out "discharge" or "discontinue."
hs	at bedtime	May read as "half-strength"	Spell out "at bedtime."
HS	half-strength	May be read as "at bedtime"	Spell out "half-strength."
IJ	injection	May be read as "IV"	Spell out "injection."
IN	intranasal	May be read as "IM" or "IV"	Spell out "intranasal" or use "NAS."
IU	international unit	May be read as "IV" or "10"	Spell out "international unit."

Abbreviation	Intended use	Potential misreading	Preferred use
µg	microgram	May be read as "mg"	Use "mcg."
o.d. or O.D.	once daily	May be read as "right eye"	Spell out "once daily."
per os	by mouth	May be read as "left eye"	Use "PO" or spell out "orally."
q.d. or QD	daily	May be read as "qid"	Spell out "daily."
q1d	once daily	May be read as "qid"	Spell out "once daily."
qhs	every bedtime	May be read as "qhr" (every hour)	Spell out "nightly."
qn	every night	May be read as "qh" (every hour)	Spell out "nightly" or "at bedtime."
q.o.d. or QOD	every other day	May be read as "q.d." (daily) or "q.i.d." (four times daily)	Spell out "every other day."
SC, SQ	subcutaneous	May be read as "SL" (sublingual) or "5 every"	Spell out "subcutaneous" or use "subcut."
U or u	unit	May be read as "0" (100 instead of 10U)	Spell out "unit."
x7d	for 7 days	May be read as "for seven doses"	Spell out "for 7 days."
o	hour	May be read as a zero	Spell out "hour" or use "hr."

APPENDIX C

Patient teaching to prevent medication errors

Medication errors present a constant risk, particularly for patients who take multiple drugs prescribed by multiple health care providers. Health care settings have many safety checks in place to help avoid medication errors. These checks involve the prescriber of the drug, the pharmacist who dispenses the drug, and the nurse who administers it. The most important safety check of all, however, remains with the patient—who is the only person in the system who has all the pertinent information to prevent medication errors, both inside and outside the health care facility.

When being prescribed medications, patients should learn these key points to reduce the risk of medication errors.

Keep a list

Keep a written list of all the drugs you take, including over-the-counter drugs, herbal products, and other supplements. Make sure the list includes brand names, generic names, the amount you take, and how often you take each product. Then make sure to carry this list with you and show it to all your health care providers, including dentists and emergency personnel.

Know your drugs

Make sure you know the reason why you take each of your drugs. This knowledge will help you understand and describe any issues that might arise about your health status or your treatments.

Follow the directions

Carefully read the label of each of your drugs, and follow the directions for taking it safely. Do not stop taking a drug without first consulting the prescriber.

Store carefully

Always store drugs in a dry place, safely out of the reach of children and pets. Storing drugs in the bathroom, where it is often hot and steamy, can cause them to break down. Also, make sure to keep all drugs in their original, labeled containers.

Speak up

You, the patient, are the most important member of your health care team. Tell your health care providers about your health history, allergies (especially drug allergies), medications, and current health problems. Never be afraid to ask questions about your health or your treatments.

Keep children safe

If you are a parent or a child's caregiver, take these steps to prevent medication errors.

- Keep a list of the child's medications, and take it with you to all health care appointments.
- Never give an adult's medication to a child. Children's bodies process drugs differently than adults' and could place them at increased risk for ill effects.
- Read the label carefully before giving any medication, including an over-the-counter product, to a child. Be especially careful if the child is receiving more than one medication.
- For liquid drugs, measure each dose using a special dose-measuring spoon. Do not use a kitchen spoon to measure medication doses.
- Call your health care provider right away if the child seems to be getting worse or is having trouble with the medication.
- If you have doubts or concerns about how the child is doing, call your health care provider.

APPENDIX D

Important dietary guidelines for patient teaching

Tyramine-rich foods (important to avoid with MAOIs, some antihypertensives)

- Aged cheese
- Avocados
- Bananas
- Beer
- Bologna
- Caffeinated beverages
- Chocolate
- Liver
- Pepperoni
- Pickled fish
- Red wine (Chianti)
- Ripe fruit
- Salami
- Smoked fish
- Yeast
- Yogurt

Potassium-rich foods (important to eat with potassium-wasting diuretics)

- Avocados
- Bananas
- Broccoli
- Cantaloupe
- Dried fruit
- Grapefruit
- Lima beans
- Navy beans
- Nuts
- Oranges
- Peaches
- Potatoes
- Prunes
- Rhubarb
- *Sanka* coffee
- Spinach
- Sunflower seeds
- Tomatoes

Calcium-rich foods (important after menopause, in children, in hypocalcemic states)

- Bok choy
- Broccoli
- Canned salmon
- Canned sardines
- Clams
- Cream soup (made with milk)
- Dairy products
- Milk
- Molasses
- Oysters
- Spinach
- Tofu

Urine acidifiers (important in maintaining excretion of some drugs)

- Cheese
- Cranberries
- Eggs
- Fish
- Grains
- Plums
- Poultry
- Prunes
- Red meat

Urine alkalinizers (important in maintaining excretion of some drugs)

- Apples
- Berries
- Citrus fruit
- Milk
- Vegetables

Iron-rich foods (important in maintaining RBCs)

- Beets
- Cereals
- Dried beans and peas
- Dried fruit
- Enriched grains
- Leafy green vegetables
- Organ meats (liver, heart, kidney)

Low-sodium foods (important in HF, hypertension, fluid overload)

- Egg yolks
- Fresh fruit
- Fresh vegetables
- Grits
- Honey
- Jam and jelly
- Lean meat
- Lima beans
- Macaroons
- Potatoes
- Poultry
- Puffed rice
- Puffed wheat
- Pumpkin
- Red kidney beans
- Sherbet
- Unsalted nuts

High-sodium foods (important to avoid in HF, hypertension, fluid overload)

- Barbecue
- Beer
- Butter
- Buttermilk
- Cake, bread, and other mixes
- Canned seafood
- Canned soup
- Canned spaghetti
- Cookies
- Cured meat
- Fast food
- Microwave dinners
- Pickles
- Prepackaged dinners
- Pretzels
- Sauces
- Sauerkraut
- Snack foods
- Tomato ketchup
- TV dinners

APPENDIX E

Drugs that interact with grapefruit juice

Grapefruit juice inhibits the CYP450 3A4 system in the liver, which can cause a decrease in the metabolism of many drugs. Decreasing the metabolism of the drug can lead to increased serum drug levels and toxicity. If any of these drugs are being given, the patient should avoid the use of grapefruit juice. If a patient has been stabilized on one of these drugs and suddenly begins to develop signs of drug toxicity, ask the patient specifically if he has been drinking grapefruit juice. If a patient is receiving one of these drugs, a key point of patient education should be to avoid the use of grapefruit juice. It takes approximately 48 hr for grapefruit juice to be cleared from the body.

albendazole
alfentanil
amiodarone
amlodipine
atorvastatin
17 beta-estradiol
budesonide
buspirone
caffeine
calcium channel blockers
carbamazepine
carvedilol
cilostazol
clarithromycin
clomipramine
cortisol
cyclophosphamide
cyclosporine A
dextromethorphan
diltiazem
erythromycin
estrogens
etoposide
felodipine
fentanyl
fexofenadine
fluoxetine
fluvastatin
fluvoxamine
indinavir
itraconazole
losartan
lovastatin
methadone
methylprednisolone
nelfinavir
nicardipine
nifedipine
nimodipine
nisoldipine
progesterone
quinidine
ritonavir
saquinavir
scopolamine
sertraline
sildenafil
simvastatin
sirolimus
sufentanil
tacrolimus
tadalafil
tamoxifen
temsirolimus
testosterone
theophylline
triazolam
troleandomycin
verapamil
vinblastine
vincristine
warfarin

Intramuscular and subcutaneous routes of administration

Choosing an IM injection site

When reviewing sites for IM injection, avoid any site that looks inflamed, edematous, or irritated. Also, avoid using a site that contains moles, birthmarks, scar tissue, or other lesions. Then select an appropriate site, such as one of those shown at right, and consider these guidelines:

- The dorsogluteal and ventrogluteal muscles are used most commonly for IM injections.
- The deltoid muscle may be used for injections of 2 mL or less.
- The vastus lateralis muscle is used most commonly in children.
- The rectus femoris may be used in infants.

Dorsogluteal muscle

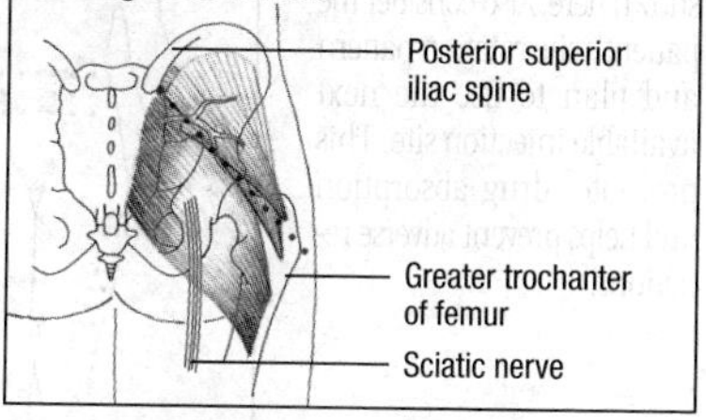

Ventrogluteal muscle

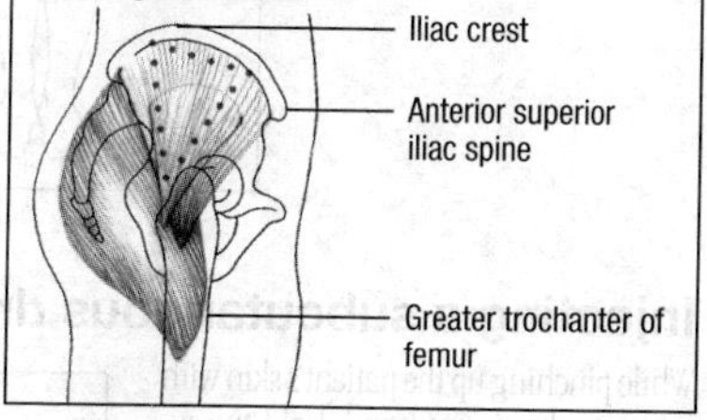

Deltoid muscle

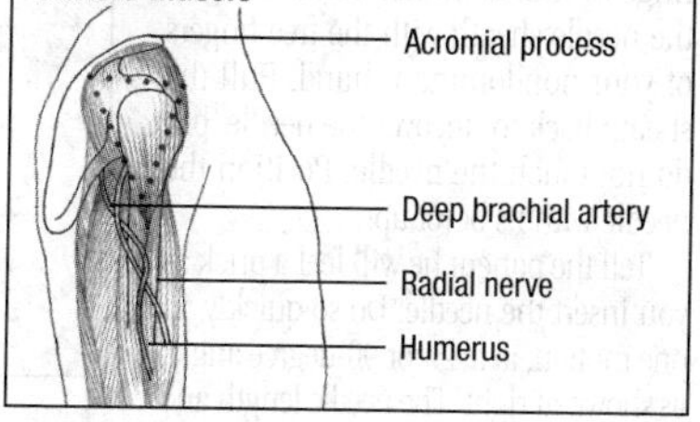

Vastus lateralis and rectus femoris muscles

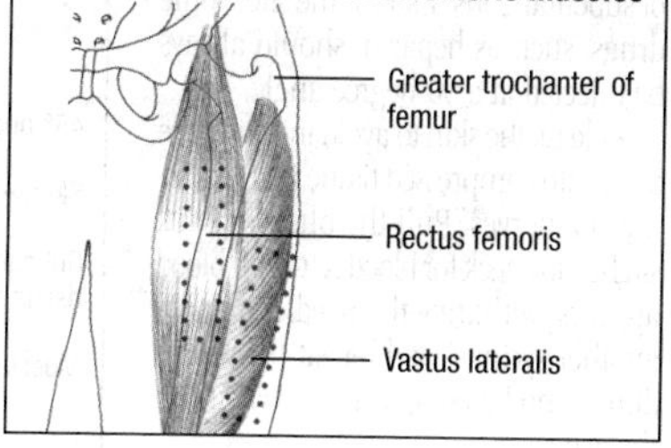

Selecting a subcutaneous injection site

To select an appropriate injection site, consider the available areas for subcutaneous injection. These areas offer sites on the abdomen, upper arms, thighs, shoulders, and lower back, as shown here. Also consider the patient's site rotation pattern and plan to use the next available injection site. This promotes drug absorption and helps prevent adverse reactions.

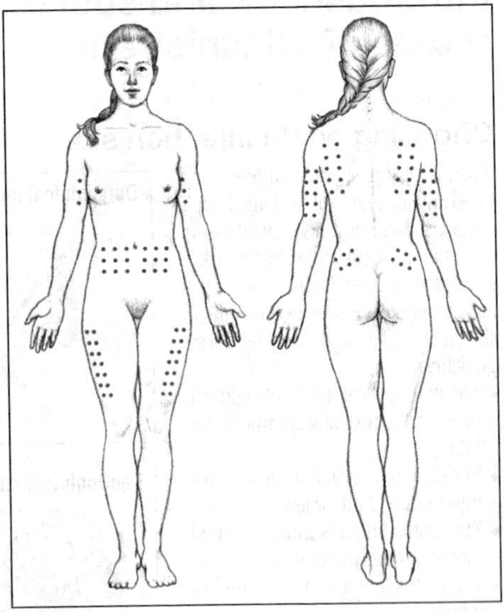

Injecting a subcutaneous drug

While pinching up the patient's skin with your nondominant hand, hold the syringe in your dominant hand and grip the needle sheath with the free fingers of your nondominant hand. Pull the sheath back to uncover the needle, but do not touch the needle. Position the needle with its bevel up.

Tell the patient he will feel a prick as you insert the needle. Do so quickly, in one motion, at a 45- or 90-degree angle, as shown at right. The needle length and the angle you use depend on the amount of subcutaneous tissue at the site. Some drugs, such as heparin, should always be injected at a 90-degree angle.

Release the skin to avoid injecting the drug into compressed tissue and irritating the nerves. Pull the plunger back slightly to check for blood return. If blood appears, withdraw the needle, prepare another syringe, and repeat the procedure. If no blood appears, slowly inject the drug.

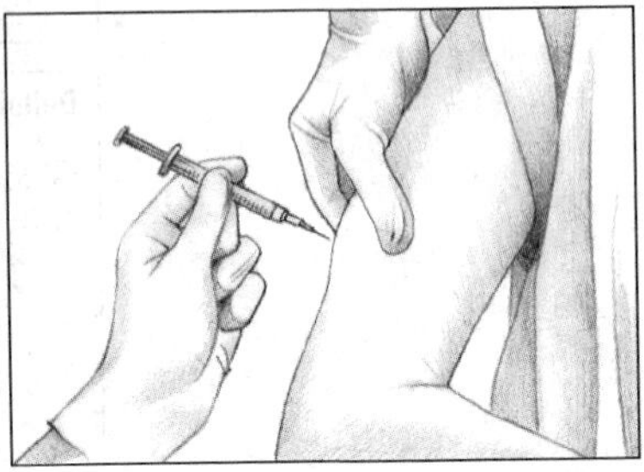

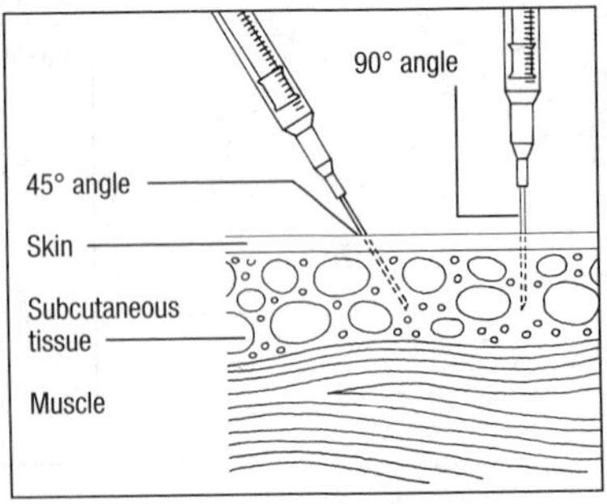

Appendix G

Medication disposal guidelines

The White House Office of National Drug Control Policy, the Department of Health and Human Services, and the Environmental Protection Agency have established guidelines for the proper disposal of unused, unneeded, or expired medications to promote consumer safety and protect the environment. It is important that you know how to properly dispose of medications to block access to them by potential abusers and to protect the water supply and environment from possible contamination. When disposing of medications, follow these guidelines.

Disposing in trash

- Take unused, unneeded, or expired medications out of their original containers.
- Mix the medication with an undesirable substance, such as coffee grounds or used kitty litter, and place it in an impermeable, nondescript container, such as an empty can or a sealable storage bag. These steps help keep the medication from being diverted for illicit use or being accidentally ingested by children or animals.
- Place the closed container in your household trash.

Disposing in toilet

- Flush prescription drugs down the toilet **only** if the accompanying patient information specifically instructs you to do so.

Disposing at a hospital or government-sponsored site

- You may be able to return unused, unneeded, or expired prescription drugs to a pharmaceutical take-back location that offers safe disposal. Many hospitals have such facilities; check with your local hospital, health department or local government.

APPENDIX H

Calculating pediatric dosages

Children typically require different doses of drugs than adults because children's bodies often handle drugs very differently from adults' bodies. The standard drug dosages listed in package inserts and references such as the *Physician's Desk Reference* refer to the adult dosage. In some cases, a pediatric dosage is suggested, but in many cases it will need to be calculated based on the child's age, weight, or body surface area. The following are some standard formulae for calculating the pediatric dose.

Fried's rule

$$\text{Infant's dose (age younger than 1 yr)} = \frac{\text{infant's age (in mo)}}{\text{150 mo}} \times \text{average adult dose}$$

Young's rule

$$\text{Child's dose (ages 1–12 yr)} = \frac{\text{child's age (in yr)}}{\text{child's age (in yr)} + 12} \times \text{average adult dose}$$

Clark's rule

$$\text{Child's dose} = \frac{\text{weight of child (lb)}}{\text{150 lb}} \times \text{average adult dose}$$

Surface area rule

$$\text{Child's dose} = \frac{\text{surface area of child (in square meters)}}{1.73} \times \text{average adult dose}$$

The surface area of a child is determined using a nomogram that determines surface area based on height and weight measurements.

Pediatric dosage calculations should be checked by two persons. Many institutions have procedures for double checking the dosage calculation of those drugs used most frequently in the pediatric area (eg, digoxin).

Recommended pediatric immunizations

Vaccine	Birth	1 mo	2 mo	4 mo	6 mo	12 mo	15 mo	18 mo	19–23 mo	2–3 yr	4–6 yr
Hepatitis B	HepB	HepB			HepB						
Rotavirus			Rota	Rota	Rota						
Diphtheria, tetanus, pertussis			DTaP	DTaP	DTaP		DTaP				DTaP
H. influenzae type b			Hib	Hib	Hib	Hib					
Pneumococcal			PCV	PCV	PCV	PCV				PPSV	
Inactivated poliovirus			IPV	IPV	IPV						IPV
Influenza					Influenza (yearly)						
Measles, mumps, rubella						MMR					MMR
Varicella						Varicella					Varicella
Hepatitis A						HepA (2 doses)				HepA series	
Meningococcal										MCV4	

Vaccine	7–10 yr	11–12 yr	13–18 yr
Tetanus, diphtheria, pertussis		Tdap	Tdap
Human papillomavirus		HPV (3 doses)	HPV series
Meningococcal	MCV	MCV	MCV
Pneumococcal	PPSV		
Influenza	Influenza (yearly)		
Hepatitis A	HepA series		
Hepatitis B	HepB series		
Inactivated Poliovirus	IPV series		
Measles, mumps, rubella	MMR series		
Varicella	Varicella series		

- Range of recommended ages
- Catch up immunization
- Certain high-risk groups

For details on the pediatric immunization schedule see:
http://www.cdc.gov/vaccines/recs/schedules/child-schedule.htm

Recommended adult immunizations

Vaccine	Age				
	19–26 yr	27–49 yr	50–59 yr	60–64 yr	65 yr and older
Tetanus, diphtheria, pertussis (Td/Tdap)	Substitute one-time dose of Tdap for Td booster; then boost with Td every 10 yr				Td booster every 10 yr
Human papillomavirus (HPV)	3 doses (females)				
Varicella	2 doses				
Zoster				1 dose	
Measles, mumps, rubella (MMR)	1 or 2 doses		1 dose		
Influenza			1 dose annually		
Pneumococcal (polysaccharide)	1 or 2 doses				1 dose
Hepatitis A	2 doses				
Hepatitis B	3 doses				
Meningococcal	1 or more doses				

Vaccine	Indication								
	1	2	3a	3b	4	5	6	7	8
Tetanus, diphtheria, pertussis (Td/Tdap)	Td	Substitute one-time dose of Tdap for Td booster; then boost with Td every 10 yr							
Human papilloma virus		3 doses for women through age 26 yr							
Measles, mumps, rubella (MMR)				1 or 2 doses					
Varicella				2 doses					
Influenza	1 dose TIV annually								1 dose TIV or LAIV annually
Pneumococcal (polysaccharide)		1 or 2 doses							
Hepatitis A	2 doses								
Hepatitis B	3 doses								
Meningococcal	1 or more doses								
Zoster					1 dose				

- For all persons in this category who meet the age requirements and who lack evidence of immunity.
- Recommended if some other risk factor is present.
- No recommendations.

Indication key:

1. Pregnancy
2. Immunocompromising conditions (excluding HIV)
3. HIV infection, CD4+ T lymphocyte count a. less than 200 cells/μL b. 200 cells/μL or greater
4. Diabetes, heart disease, chronic pulmonary disease, chronic alcoholism
5. Asplenia (including elective splenectomy and terminal complement component deficiencies)
6. Chronic liver disease
7. Kidney failure, end-stage renal disease, recipients of hemodialysis
8. Health care workers

For more details, see http://www.cdc.gov/vaccines/recs/schedules/adult-schedule.htm

APPENDIX K

Federal drug classifications

FDA pregnancy categories

The FDA has established five categories to indicate the potential for a systemically absorbed drug to cause birth defects. The key differentiation among the categories rests upon the degree (reliability) of documentation and the risk-benefit ratio.

Category A: Adequate studies in pregnant women have not demonstrated a risk to the fetus in the first trimester of pregnancy, and there is no evidence of risk in later trimesters.

Category B: Animal studies have not demonstrated a risk to the fetus but there are no adequate studies in pregnant women. *Or,* animal studies have shown an adverse effect, but adequate studies in pregnant women have not demonstrated a risk to the fetus during the first trimester of pregnancy, and there is no evidence of risk in later trimesters.

Category C: Animal studies have shown an adverse effect on the fetus but there are no adequate studies in humans; the benefits from the use of the drug in pregnant women may be acceptable despite its potential risks. *Or,* there are no animal reproduction studies and no adequate studies in humans.

Category D: There is evidence of human fetal risk, but the potential benefits from the use of the drug in pregnant women may be acceptable despite its potential risks.

Category X: Studies in animals or humans demonstrate fetal abnormalities or adverse reaction; reports indicate evidence of fetal risk. The risk of use in a pregnant woman clearly outweighs any possible benefit.

Regardless of the designated Pregnancy Category or presumed safety, *no* drug should be administered during pregnancy unless it is clearly needed.

DEA schedules of controlled substances

The Controlled Substances Act of 1970 regulates the manufacturing, distribution, and dispensing of drugs that are known to have abuse potential. The DEA is responsible for the enforcement of these regulations. The controlled drugs are divided into five DEA schedules based on their potential for abuse and physical and psychological dependence.

Schedule I *(C-I)*: High abuse potential and no accepted medical use (heroin, marijuana, LSD)

Schedule II *(C-II)*: High abuse potential with severe dependence liability (narcotics, amphetamines, and barbiturates)

Schedule III *(C-III)*: Less abuse potential than Schedule II drugs and moderate dependence liability (nonbarbiturate sedatives, nonamphetamine stimulants, limited amounts of certain narcotics)

Schedule IV *(C-IV)*: Less abuse potential than Schedule III and limited dependence liability (some sedatives, antianxiety agents, and nonnarcotic analgesics)

Schedule V *(C-V)*: Limited abuse potential. Primarily small amounts of narcotics (codeine) used as antitussives or antidiarrheals. Under federal law, limited quantities of certain Schedule V drugs may be purchased without a prescription directly from a pharmacist. The purchaser must be at least 18 years of age and must furnish suitable identification. All such transactions must be recorded by the dispensing pharmacist.

Prescribing physicians and dispensing pharmacists must be registered with the DEA, which also provides forms for the transfer of Schedule I and II substances and establishes criteria for the inventory and prescribing of controlled substances. State and local laws are often more stringent than federal law. In any given situation, the more stringent law applies.

APPENDIX L

Cardiovascular guidelines

Classification of blood lipid levels

Serum level	Low*	Optimal*	Normal or desirable*	Borderline high*	High*	Very high*
Total cholesterol			Less than 200	200–239	240 or more	
LDL cholesterol		Less than 100	100–129	130–159	160–189	190 or more
HDL cholesterol	Less than 40				60 or more	
Triglycerides			Less than 150	150–199	200–499	500 or more

* In mg/dL.
LDL target goal is determined by the presence of other major cardiovascular risk factors (cigarette smoking, hypertension, low HDL, family history of premature CAD, men 45 years or older, women 55 years or older).
For 0–1 risk factor, goal for total cholesterol is 160 mg/dL; for 2 or more risk factors, goal is less than 130 mg/dL; for persons with congestive heart disease or diabetes, goal is less than 100 mg/dL.

From the Third Report of the National Cholesterol Education Program (NCEP) Expert Panel on Detection, Evaluation, and Treatment of High Blood Cholesterol in Adults (Adult Treatment Panel III). U.S. Department of Health and Human Services, National Institutes of Health, National Heart, Lung, and Blood Institute, 2002. Available at http://www.nhlbi.nih.gov/guidelines/cholesterol/atp3full.pdf.

Classification of blood pressure

Category	Systolic blood pressure (mm Hg)		Diastolic blood pressure (mm Hg)
Normal	Less than 120	and	Less than 80
Prehypertension	120–139	or	80–89
Hypertension, Stage 1	140–159	or	90–99
Hypertension, Stage 2	160 or more	or	100 or more

From the Seventh Report of the Joint National Committee on Prevention, Detection, Evaluation, and Treatment of High Blood Pressure (JNC 7). U.S. Department of Health and Human Services, National Institutes of Health, National Heart, Lung, and Blood Institute, 2003.
Available at http://www.nhlbi.nih.gov/guidelines/hypertension/jnc7full.pdf.

APPENDIX M

Normal laboratory values

Test	Conventional units	Systems international units
albumin	3.5–5.0 g/dL	35–50 g/L
aminotransferases		
ALT	7–53 international units/L	0.12–0.88 μkat/L
AST	11–47 international units/L	0.8–0.78 μkat/L
ammonia	15–56 mcg/dL	9–33 μmol/L
amylase	25–115 international units/L	0.42–1.92 μkat/L
bilirubin		
total	0.3–1.1 mg/dL	5.13–18.80 μmol/L
direct	0–0.3 mg/dL	0–5.1 μmol/L
blood gases		
pH	7.35–7.45	7.35–7.45
PO_2	80–105 mm Hg	10.6–14 kPa
PCO_2	35–45 mm Hg	4.7–6 kPa
BUN	8–25 mg/dL	2.9–8.9 mmol/L
calcium		
total	8.6–10.3 mg/dL	2.15–2.58 mmol/L
ionized	4.5–5.1 mg/dL	1.13–1.28 mmol/L
chloride	97–110 mEq/L	97–110 mmol/L
coagulation studies		
bleeding time	2.5–9.5 min	150–570 sec
fibrinogen	150–360 mg/dL	1.5–3. 6 g/L
PTT	21–32 sec	21–32 sec
prothrombin time	8.2–10.3 sec	8.2–10.3 sec
INR	0.9–1.13	0.9–1.13
thrombin time	11.3–18.5 sec	11.3–18.5 sec
creatinine	0.5–1.7 mg/dL	44–150 μmol/L
erythrocyte count		
male	$4.5–5.7 \times 10^6/mm^3$	$4.5–5.7 \times 10^{12}/L$
female	$3.9–5 \times 10^6/mm^3$	$3.9–5 \times 10^{12}/L$
glucose (fasting)	65–109 mg/dL	3.58–6.1 mmol/L
hematocrit		
male	41–50%	138–172 g/L
female	35–46%	120–156 g/L

Always check test results against the values considered normal by the laboratory doing the test. Variations between laboratories are possible.

Test	Conventional units	Systems international units
hemoglobin		
male	13.8–17.2 g/dL	138–172 g/L
female	12–15.6 g/dL	120–156 g/L
hemoglobin A_{1c}	Less than 6% of total Hb	Less than 0.06 of total Hb
iron		
male	45–160 mcg/dL	8.1–31.3 μmol/L
female	30–160 mcg/dL	5.4–31.3 μmol/L
LDH	100–250 international units/L	1.67–4.17 μkat/L
leukocyte count		
total	3.8–9.8 × 10^3/μL	3.8–9.8 × 10^9/L
lymphocytes	1.2–3.3 × 10^3/μL	1.2–3.3 × 10^9/L
mononuclear cells	0.2–0.7 × 10^3/μL	0.2–0.7 × 10^9/L
granulocytes	1.8–6.6 × 10^3/μL	1.8–6.6 × 10^9/L
lipase	10–150 units/L	10–150 units/L
magnesium	1.3–2.2 mEq/L	0.65–1.10 mmol/L
phosphate	2.5–4.5 mg/dL	0.75–1.35 mmol/L
platelet count	140–440 × 10^3/μL	140–440 × 10^9/L
reticulocyte count		
adults	0.5–1.5%	0.005–0.015%
children	2.5–6.5%	
potassium	3.3–4.9 mEq/L	3.3–4.9 mmol/L
sodium	135–145 mEq/L	135–145 mmol/L
uric acid	3–8 mg/dL	179–476 μmol/L

Always check test results against the values considered normal by the laboratory doing the test. Variations between laboratories are possible.

APPENDIX N

Canadian drug information

Narcotics, controlled drugs, benzodiazepines, and other targeted substances

This table summarizes the requirements for prescribing, dispensing, and record-keeping for narcotics, controlled drugs, benzodiazepines, and other targeted substances. This information is not a comprehensive review; the reader is encouraged to seek additional and confirmatory information (eg, Controlled Drugs and Substances Act, Narcotic Control Regulations, parts G and J of the Food and Drug Regulations, Benzodiazepines, and Other Targeted Substances Regulations). *Reviewed 2009 by the Office of Controlled Substances, Health Canada.*

Classification and description	Legal requirements
Narcotic drugs*	
• 1 narcotic (eg, cocaine, codeine, hydromorphone, ketamine, morphine) • 1 narcotic + 1 active non-narcotic ingredient (eg, *Novahistex DH, Tylenol No. 4*) • All narcotics for parenteral use (eg, fentanyl, pethidine) • All products containing hydrocodone, oxycodone, methadone, or pentazocine • Dextropropoxyphene (eg, *Darvon-N, 642*) • Nabilone (ie, Cesamet)	• Written prescription required. • Verbal prescriptions not permitted. • Refills not permitted. • Written prescription may be prescribed to be dispensed in divided portions (part-fills). • For part-fills, copies of prescriptions should be made in reference to the original prescription. Indicate on the original prescription: the new prescription number, the date of the part-fill, the quantity dispensed, and the pharmacist's initials. • Transfers not permitted. • Record and retain all documents pertaining to all transactions for at least 2 years in a manner that permits an audit. • Sales reports required except for dextropropoxyphene, propoxyphene. • Report any loss or theft of narcotic drugs within 10 days to the Office of Controlled Substances at the address indicated on the forms.
Narcotic preparations*	
• Verbal prescription narcotics: 1 narcotic + 2 or more active non-narcotic ingredients in a recognized therapeutic dose (eg, *Fiorinal-C¼, Fiorinal-C½, Robitussin AC, 282, 292, Tylenol No. 2* and *No. 3*) • Exempted codeine compounds: contain codeine up to 8 mg/solid dosage form or 20 mg/30 mL liquid + 2 or more active non-narcotic ingredients (eg, *Atasol-8*).	• Written or verbal prescriptions permitted. • Refills not permitted. • Written or verbal prescriptions may be prescribed to be dispensed in divided portions (part-fills). • For part-fills, copies of prescriptions should be made in reference to the original prescription. Indicate on the original prescription: the new prescription number, the date of the part-fill, the quantity dispensed, and the pharmacist's initials. • Transfers not permitted. • Exempted codeine compounds when dispensed pursuant to a prescription follow the same regulations as for verbal prescription narcotics.

*The products noted are examples only.

Classification and description	Legal requirements
Narcotic preparations* (continued)	
	• Record and retain all documents pertaining to all transactions for at least 2 years, in a manner that permits an audit. • Sales reports not required. • Report any loss or theft of narcotic drugs within 10 days to the Office of Controlled Substances at the address indicated on the forms.
Controlled drugs*	
• Part I Amphetamines (eg, *Dexedrine, Adderall XR*) Methylphenidate (eg, *Biphentin, Concerta, Ritalin*) Pentobarbital (*Nembutal*) Preparations: 1 controlled drug + 1 or more active noncontrolled ingredient(s) in a recognized therapeutic dose (eg, *Bellergal Spacetabs*)	• Written or verbal prescriptions permitted. • Refills not permitted for verbal prescriptions. • Refills permitted for written prescriptions if the prescriber has indicated in writing the number of refills and dates for, or intervals between, refills. • Written or verbal prescriptions may be prescribed to be dispensed in divided portions (part-fills). • For refills and part-fills, copies of prescriptions should be made in reference to the original prescription. Indicate on the original prescription: the new prescription number, the date of the repeat or part-fill, the quantity dispensed, and the pharmacist's initials. • Transfers not permitted. • Record and retain all documents pertaining to all transactions for a period of at least 2 years, in a manner that permits an audit. • Sales reports required except for controlled drug preparations. • Report any loss or theft of controlled drugs within 10 days to the Office of Controlled Substances at the address indicated on the forms.
• Part II Barbiturates (eg, phenobarbital) Butorphanol Diethylpropion (*Tenuate*) Nalbuphine (*Nubain* injection) Preparations: 1 controlled drug + 1 or more active noncontrolled ingredient(s) in a recognized therapeutic dose (eg, *Fiorinal*) • Part III Anabolic steroids including: Nandrolone decanoate (eg, *Deca-Durabolin*) Testosterone (eg, *Androderm*) Testosterone cypionate (eg, *Depo-Testosterone*) Testosterone undercanoate (eg, *Andriol*)	• Written or verbal prescriptions permitted. • Refills permitted for written or verbal prescriptions if the prescriber has authorized in writing or verbally (at the time of issuance) the number of refills and dates for, or intervals between, refills. • Written or verbal prescriptions may be prescribed to be dispensed in divided portions (part-fills). • For refills and part-fills, copies of prescriptions should be made in reference to the original prescription. Indicate on the original prescription: the new prescription number, the date of the repeat or part-fill, the quantity dispensed, and the pharmacist's initials. • Transfers not permitted. • Record and retain all documents pertaining to all transactions for a period of at least 2 years, in a manner that permits an audit. • Sales reports not required. • Report the loss or theft of controlled drugs within 10 days to the Office of Controlled Substances at the address indicated on the forms.

*The products noted are examples only.

Classification and description	Legal requirements
Benzodiazepines and other targeted substances*	
Alprazolam Bromazepam Chlordiazepoxide Clobazam Diazepam Ethchlorvynol Lorazepam Oxazepam Temazepam Triazolam	• Written and verbal prescriptions permitted. • Refills for written or verbal prescriptions permitted if indicated by prescriber and less than 1 yr has elapsed since the day the prescription was issued by the prescriber. • Part-fills permitted as per prescriber's instructions. • For refills or part-fills of prescriptions, record the following information: date of the repeat or part-fill, prescription number, quantity dispensed, and the pharmacist's initials. • Transfer of prescriptions permitted except a prescription that has been already transferred. • Record and retain all documents pertaining to all transactions for a period of at least 2 years, in a manner that permits an audit. • Sales reports not required. • Report any loss or theft of benzodiazepines and other targeted substances within 10 days to the Office of Controlled Substances at the address indicated on the forms.

Adapted with permission from the *Compendium of Pharmaceuticals and Specialties*. Ottawa, Canada: Canadian Pharmacists Association, 2010: pp. A1–A2.

*The products noted are only examples.

Adverse reaction reporting: Pharmaceuticals, biologics, natural health products, radiopharmaceuticals

The following is a description of the Canada Vigilance Program. This information is not intended to present a comprehensive review.

Reviewed 2009 by the Marketed Health Products Directorate, Health Canada (Candace Fisher).

Why report? All marketed health products have benefits and risks. Although health products are tested for safety and efficacy before they are licensed, some adverse reactions* may not become evident until the general population uses a health product under "real life" circumstances. By submitting a suspected adverse reaction report, you are contributing to the ongoing collection of safety and effectiveness information that occurs once health products are marketed. Reported adverse reaction information may contribute to:

- the identification of previously unrecognized rare or serious adverse reactions;
- changes in product safety information or other regulatory actions such as withdrawal of a product from the Canadian market;
- international data regarding benefits, risks, or effectiveness of health products;
- health product safety knowledge that benefits all Canadians.

What to report? Health Canada, through the Canada Vigilance Program, is responsible for collecting and assessing adverse reaction reports for the following health products marketed in Canada: Pharmaceuticals (prescription and nonprescription), biologics (including fractionated blood products as well as therapeutic and diagnostic vaccines), natural health products, and radiopharmaceuticals.

You do not have to be certain that a health product caused the reaction in order to report it. Adverse reaction reports are, for the most part, only suspected associations.

The Canada Vigilance Program wants to know about all suspected adverse reactions, but especially if they are:

- **Unexpected adverse reactions,** regardless of their severity (not consistent with product information or labelling).
- **Serious adverse reactions**†, whether expected or not.
- **Adverse reactions related to recently marketed health products** (on the market for less than 5 years).

How to report to Canada Vigilance? Report any adverse reactions associated with the use of health products to the Canada Vigilance Program by one of the following three ways:

- Call toll-free at 1-866-234-2345
- Report online at www.healthcanada.gc.ca/medeffect
- Complete a Canada Vigilance Reporting Form and:
  - Fax toll-free to 1-866-678-6789 or
  - Mail to Canada Vigilance Program, Health Canada, Postal Locator 0701C, Ottawa, ON K1A 0K9

Postage paid labels, Canada Vigilance Reporting Form, and the adverse reaction reporting guidelines are available on the MedEffect™ Canada Web site at www.healthcanada.gc.ca/medeffect.

About MedEffect™ Canada: MedEffect™ Canada makes it simple and efficient for health professionals and consumers to complete and file adverse reaction reports to the Canada Vigilance Program via Web, phone, fax, or mail and provides centralized access to relevant and reliable health products safety information as it becomes available, in a easy to find, easy to remember location. This includes access to Health Canada's advisories, warnings, and recalls, the Canadian Adverse Reaction Newsletter (CARN), and the Canada Vigilance Online Database.

By subscribing to the MedEffect™ e-Notice you will automatically receive health product advisories warnings and recalls notices as well as the latest issue of the Canadian Adverse Reaction Newsletter by e-mail.

*An adverse reaction is a harmful and unintended response to a health product.
†A serious adverse reaction is one which requires inpatient hospitalization or prolongation of existing hospitalization, causes congenital malformation, results in persistent or significant disability or incapacity, is life-threatening, or results in death. Adverse reactions that require significant medical intervention to prevent one of these outcomes are also considered to be serious.

Adapted with permission from the *Compendium of Pharmaceuticals and Specialties*. Ottawa, Canada: Canadian Pharmacists Association, 2010, p. A9.

Canada Vigilance Regional Offices

British Columbia and Yukon
Canada Vigilance Regional Office–BC and Yukon
400-4595 Canada Way
Burnaby BC V5G 1J9
Email: CanadaVigilance_BC@hc-sc.gc.ca

Alberta and Northwest Territories
Canada Vigilance Regional Office-Alberta and Northwest Territories
Suite 730
9700 Jasper Ave.
Edmonton AB T5J 4C3
Email: CanadaVigilance_AB@hc-sc.gc.ca

Saskatchewan
Canada Vigilance Regional Office-Saskatchewan
4th floor, Room 412
101-22nd Street East
Saskatoon SK S7K 0E1
Email: CanadaVigilance_SK@hc-sc.gc.ca

Manitoba
Canada Vigilance Regional Office-Manitoba
510 Lagimodière Blvd.
Winnipeg MB R2J 3Y1
Email: CanadaVigilance_MB@hc-sc.gc.ca

Ontario and Nunavut
Canada Vigilance Regional Office-Ontario and Nunavut
2301 Midland Ave.
Toronto ON M1P 4R7
Email: CanadaVigilance_ON@hc-sc.gc.ca

Québec
Canada Vigilance Regional Office-Québec
1001 Saint-Laurent St. West
Longueuil QC J4K 1C7
Email: CanadaVigilance_QC@hc-sc.gc.ca

Atlantic
Canada Vigilance Regional Office–Atlantic for New Brunswick, Nova Scotia, Prince Edward Island, Newfoundland, and Labrador
1505 Barrington St., Maritime Centre
Suite 1625, 16th Floor
Halifax NS B3J 3Y6
Email: CanadaVigilance_ATL@hc-sc.gc.ca

Adapted with permission from the *Compendium of Pharmaceuticals and Specialties*. Ottawa, Canada: Canadian Pharmacists Association, 2010, p. A9.

APPENDIX O

Commonly used Canadian drugs

cyproterone acetate

ANDROCUR, CYPRONE, CYPROSTAT, PROCUR, AND OTHERS

Drug class and indications

Androgen receptor antagonist, antineoplastic, contraceptive

Treatment of prostate cancer, BPH, priapism, hypersexuality, hirsutism; hormone therapy for male-to-female transgender patients, hot flashes; part of combination oral contraceptives

Dosages and special alerts

25 mg PO bid. Up to 100 mg/day can be used for BPH, priapism, hypersexuality, hirsutism, hormone therapy for male-to-female transgender persons, hot flashes; 300 mg/day PO or IM for prostate cancer; 2 mg with 35 or 50 mcg/day PO ethinyl estradiol for contraception. Not for use in pregnancy. Monitor for liver toxicity; risk increases with higher doses. Risk of adrenal suppression, depression and mood changes, gynecomastia, and sexual dysfunction in males exists. Dosage should be tapered when discontinuing to allow adrenal function to return and to balance testosterone production.

doxylamine succinate and pyridoxine hydrochloride

DICLECTIN

Drug class and indications

Antinausea drug, antihistamine, vitamin

Prevention of nausea and vomiting in pregnancy

Dosages and special alerts

Two DR tablets (10 mg doxylamine, 10 mg pyridoxine/tablet) PO at bedtime. One tablet in the morning and one tablet midday may be added if needed to control nausea and vomiting. Tablet must be swallowed whole; do not cut, crush, or chew tablet. Drug may cause drowsiness, vertigo, nervousness, disorientation. Warn patient to avoid driving or operating dangerous machinery until the effects of the drug are known. Do not combine with alcohol or other CNS depressants. Not for use in patients with epilepsy.

flunarizine hydrochloride

SIBELIUM

Drug class and indications

Antimigraine drug

Prevention of migraine with or without aura

Dosages and special alerts

10 mg/day PO in the evening. 5 mg/day may be tried in patients who experience adverse effects. Not for treatment of acute migraine. Contraindicated for use in patients with history or depression and in patients with pre-existing extrapyramidal disorders. Not recommended for use in pregnancy. Motor disturbances are very common, but these disturbances do not respond to antiparkinsonian drugs. Effects usually reverse with discontinuation of the drug. Sedation and drowsiness may occur. Warn patient to avoid driving or operating dangerous machinery until the effects of the drug are known.

▽ flupentixol

FLUANXOL

Drug class and indications

Antipsychotic, thioxanthene derivative

Maintenance therapy for chronic schizophrenia in patients whose main manifestations do not include excitement, agitation, or hyperactivity

Dosages and special alerts

IM: 20 mg by deep IM injection; a second dose of 20–40 mg IM may be given in 4 to 10 days. If patient is controlled and tolerates the drug well, maintenance dose is 20–40 mg IM every 2–3 wk.

PO: 1 mg PO tid. May be increased to control symptoms to maintenance dose of 3–6 mg/day. Once stabilized, patients may be switched to IM coverage every 2–3 weeks. Contraindicated with CNS depression, blood dyscrasias, pheochromocytoma, liver damage, renal dysfunction. Do not use to treat severe agitation in psychiatric or psychoneurotic patients or to treat elderly patients with agitation. Use cautiously with pregnancy and lactation. Monitor for sedation and extrapyramidal responses. Warn patient to avoid driving or operating dangerous machinery until the effects of the drug are known.

▽ L-tryptophan

TRYPTAN AND OTHERS

Drug class and indications

Amino acid, sleep aid

To improve sleep and enhance mood

Dosages and special alerts

One or two 500-mg tablets PO at bedtime with food; may be increased to a maximum of eight capsules (4 g) per day. The amino acid is converted to serotonin in the brain to promote natural sleep and improve mood. No known contraindications exist. Few adverse effects reported.

▽ nitrazepam

MOGADON

Drug class and indications

Hypnotic, anticonvulsant, benzodiazepine

Symptomatic relief of transient and short-term insomnia characterized by difficulty falling asleep, frequent nocturnal awakenings, or early morning awakenings for a maximum of 7–10 days. May also be useful for the treatment of myoclonic seizures.

Dosages and special alerts

5–10 mg PO before bedtime for a maximum of 7–10 days. Elderly or debilitated patients should start at 2.5 mg/day and should not exceed 5 mg/day PO. *Children treated for myoclonic seizures (up to 30 kg):* 0.3–1 mg/kg/day PO divided into three doses. Contraindicated with myasthenia gravis, sleep apnea syndrome, known paradoxical reactions to alcohol or sedative medications, hypersensitivity to any benzodiazepine; use extreme caution with history of substance of alcohol abuse. Not recommended during pregnancy. Sedative effects, confusion, and drowsiness are common. Caution patient to avoid driving or operating hazardous machinery. Use of flumazenil (benzodiazepine antagonist) not recommended in patients with epilepsy who are treated with nitrazepam; this combination may precipitate seizures.

▽ petrolatum

Drug class and indications

Emollient, lubricant

To provide a protective barrier to prevent loss of fluid; lubricant to prevent friction and tissue breakdown

Dosages and special alerts

Apply topically to affected areas; used to lubricate and provide a moisture barrier. Apply to intact skin only. Not for ingestion or injection.

▽ zopiclone

IMOVANE, RHOVANE

Drug class and indications

Sedative-hypnotic; cyclopyrrolone derivative

Treatment of insomnia

Dosages and special alerts

7.5 mg PO taken at bedtime. Use cautiously with elderly or debilitated patients, history of depression, pregnancy, lactation and history of substance abuse (may be habit-forming). Monitor for dizziness, sedation, anxiety, nervousness; warn patient to avoid driving or operating hazardous machinery until the effects of the drug are known. Dry mouth, metallic taste may occur; frequent mouth care and sucking sugarless lozenges may help. Be alert for sudden mood changes when drug is stopped.

Appendix P

Topical drugs

Topical drugs are agents that are intended for surface use, not ingestion or injection. They may be very toxic if absorbed into the system, but they serve several purposes when used topically.

Pregnancy Category C

Contraindicated with allergy to these drugs, open wounds, or abrasions.

Adverse effects

Local irritation (common), stinging, burning, dermatitis, toxic effects if absorbed systemically.

Teaching points

Apply sparingly to affected area as directed. Do not use with open wounds or broken skin. Avoid contact with eyes. Report any local irritation, allergic reaction, worsening of condition being treated.

Drug	Selected trade names	Instructions and preparations
Acne, rosacea, and melasma products		
adapalene	*Differin*	Do not use on cuts or any open area. Avoid use on sunburned skin, in combination with other products, or exposure to sun. Apply a thin film to affected area after washing every night at bedtime. Drug is less drying than other products.
alitretinoin	*Panretin*	Used for treatment of lesions of Kaposi's sarcoma. 1% gel; apply as needed to cover lesions twice daily. Inflammation, peeling, redness may occur.
azelaic acid	*Azelex* *Finacea*	Wash and dry skin. Massage a thin layer into affected area twice daily. Wash hands thoroughly after application. Improvement usually occurs within 4 wk. Initial irritation usually occurs but passes with time.
clindamycin	*Clindesse* *Evoclin*	2% vaginal cream for the treatment of bacterial vaginitis; one applicatorful (100 mg) given vaginally at any time of the day. 1% foam used for the treatment of acne vulgaris; apply once daily to affected areas that have been washed and are fully dry.
clindamycin and benzoyl peroxide	*Acanya* *BenzaClin*	Apply gel to affected areas bid. Wash area and pat dry before application.
clindamycin and tretinoin	*Ziana*	Rub pea-size amount over entire face once daily at bedtime. Not for use by patients with colitis.
dapsone	*Aczone Gel*	Apply thin layer of gel to affected areas bid. Closely follow Hgb, reticulocyte count in patients with G6PD deficiencies.

(continued)

Drug	Selected trade names	Instructions and preparations
Acne, rosacea, and melasma products (continued)		
fluocinolone acetonide, hydroquinone, and tretinoin	*Tri-Luma*	Do not use during pregnancy. Apply to depigmented area of melasma once each evening, at least 30 min before bedtime after cleansing and patting dry; avoid occlusive dressings. Use a sunscreen and protective clothing if outside; skin dryness and peeling may occur.
metronidazole	*MetroGel* *MetroLotion* *Noritate*	For treatment of rosacea. Apply cream to affected area bid.
sodium sulfacetamide	*Klaron*	Apply a thin film bid to affected areas. Wash affected area with mild soap and water; pat dry. Avoid use in denuded or abraded areas.
tazarotene	*Tazorac*	Avoid use in pregnancy. Apply thin film once daily in the evening. Do not use with irritants or products with high alcohol content. Drying causes photosensitivity.
tretinoin, 0.025% cream	*Avita*	Apply thin layer once daily. Discomfort, peeling, redness may occur for the first 2–4 wk. Worsened acne may occur in first few wk.
tretinoin, 0.05% cream	*Renova*	Used for removal of fine wrinkles. Apply thin coat in the evening.
tretinoin, gel	*Retin-A* Micro*	Apply to cover once daily after cleansing. Exacerbation of inflammation may occur at first. Therapeutic effects usually seen in first 2 wk.
Analgesics		
capsaicin	*Capsin* *No Pain-HP* *Pain Doctor* *Pain-X* *Qutenza* *R-Gel* *Zostrix* *Zostrix-HP*	Apply not more than tid to qid. Applied locally, provides temporary relief from the pain of osteoarthritis, rheumatoid arthritis, neuralgias. Do not bandage tightly. Stop use and seek health care if condition worsens or persists after 14–28 days. *Qutenza*: Apply patch to relieve pain of postherpetic neuralgia.
Antibiotics		
ciprofloxacin and dexamethasone	*Ciprodex*	Apply drops to ears of child with acute otitis media who has tympanostomy tubes; apply to outer ear canal of patients with acute otitis externa.
mupirocin	*Bactroban*	Used to treat impetigo caused by *Staphylococcus aureus, Streptococcus,* and *Staphylococcus pyogenes.* Apply small amount to affected area tid; may be covered with a gauze dressing. Monitor for signs of superinfection; reevaluate if no clinical response in 3–5 days.

Drug	Selected trade names	Instructions and preparations
Antibiotics (continued)		
mupirocin calcium	*Bactroban Nasal*	Used to eradicate the nasal colonization of methicillin-resistant *S. aureus.* Apply one-half of the ointment from single-use tube between nostrils and apply bid for 5 days.
retapamulin	*Altabax*	Used to treat impetigo. Apply thin layer of ointment to affected area bid for 5 days. May be used on patients 9 mo and older.
Anti–diaper-rash drug		
miconazole, zinc oxide, petrolatum	*Vusion*	Apply gently to diaper area for 7 days. Verify *Candida* infection before beginning treatment. Combine with frequent diaper changes and gentle washing.
Antifungals		
butenafine hydrochloride	*Mentax*	Used to treat intradigital pedia (athlete's foot), tinea corporis, ringworm, tinea cruris. Apply to affected area once a day for 4 wk.
butoconazole nitrate	*Gynazole-1*	Apply intravaginally as one dose. Culture fungus; if no response, reculture. Ensure use of full course of therapy. May cause irritation, burning.
ciclopirox	*Loprox* *Penlac Nail Lacquer*	Used to treat onychomycosis of fingernails and toenails in immunocompromised patients. Apply directly to affected fingernails or toenails.
clotrimazole	*Cruex* *Desenex* *Lotrimin* *Mycelex*	Clean area before applying. Gently massage into affected area up to twice daily. Use for up to 4 wk. Discontinue if irritation, worsening of condition occurs.
econazole nitrate	*Spectazole*	Apply locally once or twice daily. Clean area before applying. Treat for 2–4 wk. Discontinue if irritation, burning, or worsening of condition occurs. For athlete's foot, change socks and shoes at least once a day.
gentian violet		Do not apply to active lesions. Apply locally up to twice daily. May stain skin and clothing.
ketoconazole	*Nizoral*	Apply as shampoo daily. Itching or stinging of the scalp may occur.
naftifine hydrochloride	*Naftin*	Gently massage into affected area twice daily. Avoid occlusive dressings. Wash hands thoroughly after application. Do not use longer than 4 wk.
oxiconazole	*Oxistat*	Apply every day up to twice daily. May be needed for up to 1 mo.

(continued)

Drug	Selected trade names	Instructions and preparations
Antifungals (continued)		
sertaconazole nitrate	*Ertaczo*	Apply to areas between toes affected by tinea pedis and to the surrounding healthy tissue bid for 4 wk.
terbinafine	*Lamisil*	Apply to area bid until clinical signs are improved, 1–4 wk. Do not use occlusive dressings. Report local irritation. Discontinue if local irritation occurs.
tolnaftate	*Absorbine* *Aftate* *Genaspor* *Quinsana Plus* *Tinactin*	Apply small amount bid for 2–3 wk; 4–6 wk may be needed if skin is very thick. Clean skin with soap and water before applying drug, dry thoroughly, wear loose, well-fitting shoes, change socks at least four times a day.
Antihistamine		
azelastine hydrochloride	*Astelin* *Astepro*	Use two sprays per nostril bid. Avoid use of alcohol and OTC antihistamines; dizziness and sedation can occur.
Antipsoriatics		
anthralin	*Dritho-Scalp* *Psoriatec*	Apply every day only to psoriatic lesions. Use protective dressing. Avoid contact with eyes. May stain fabrics, skin, hair, fingernails.
calcipotriene	*Dovonex*	Used as a synthetic vitamin D_2. Use only for disorder prescribed. Apply thin layer once or twice a day. Monitor serum calcium levels with extended use. May cause local irritation.
calcipotriene and betamethasone	*Taclonex* *Taclonex Scalp*	Apply to affected area once daily for up to 4 wk. Maximum, 100 g/wk. Limit treatment area to 30% of body surface. Do not use occlusive dressings on the area.
Antiseborrheics		
chloroxine	*Capitrol*	Do not use on active lesions. Massage into wet scalp; leave lather on for 3 min. May discolor blond, gray, bleached hair.
selenium sulfide	*Selsun Blue*	Massage 5–10 mL into scalp; rest 2–3 min, rinse, repeat. May damage jewelry; remove jewelry before use. Discontinue use if local irritation occurs.
Antiseptics		
benzalkonium chloride	*Benza* *Mycocide NS* *Zephiran*	Mix in solution as needed. Spray for preoperative use; store instruments in solution. Thoroughly rinse detergents and soaps from skin before use. Add antirust tablets for instruments stored in solution; dilute solution as indicated for use.

Drug	Selected trade names	Instructions and preparations
Antiseptics (continued)		
chlorhexidine gluconate	*BactoShield* *Dyna-Hex* *Exidine* *Hibiclens* *Hibistat*	Use for surgical scrub, preoperative skin prep, wound cleansing, preoperative bathing and showering. Scrub or rinse. Leave on for 15 sec; for surgical scrub, leave on for 3 min.
hexachlorophene	*pHisoHex*	Use for surgical wash, scrub. Apply as wash; do not use with burns or on mucous membranes. Rinse thoroughly. Do not use routinely for bathing infants.
iodine		Wash affected area with solution. Solution is highly toxic; avoid occlusive dressings; stains skin and clothing.
povidone iodine	*ACU-dyne* *Betadine* *Betagen* *Etodine* *Iodex* *Minidyne* *Operand* *Polydine*	HIV may be inactivated in this solution. Apply as needed; treated areas may be bandaged. Causes less irritation than iodine and is less toxic.
sodium hypochlorite	*Dakin's solution*	Apply as antiseptic. *Caution:* Chemical burns can occur.
thimerosal	*Aeroaid* *Mersol*	Used preoperatively and as first aid for abrasions, wounds. Apply every day up to three times per day. Contains mercury compound.
Antivirals		
acyclovir	*Zovirax*	Apply 0.5-inch ribbon to affected area and rub in gently six times daily for 7 days.
docosanol	*Abreva*	Used to treat oral and facial herpes simplex cold sores, fever blisters. Apply five times per day for 10 days. Caution patient not to overuse.
imiquimod	*Aldara*	Used to treat external genital warts and perianal warts. Apply a thin layer to warts and rub in three times per wk at bedtime for 16 wk; remove with soap and water after 6–10 hr. For typical nonhyperkeratotic actinic keratoses on face or scalp in immune-compromised patients, apply cream to affected area before bed twice weekly for 16 wk. For topical treatment of superficial basal cell carcinoma in immune-compromised patients, 10–40 mg applied to lesion five times weekly at bedtime for 6 wk.
kunecatechins	*Veregen*	Used to treat external and perianal warts in immunocompetent patients older than 18 yr. Apply to each wart tid for up to 16 wk; do not cover treated area.

(continued)

Drug	Selected trade names	Instructions and preparations
***Antivirals* (continued)**		
penciclovir	*Denavir*	Used to treat cold sores in healthy patients. Reserve use for herpes labialis on lips and face; avoid mucous membranes. Use at first sign of cold sore. Apply thin layer to affected area every 2 hr while awake for 4 days.
Burn treatments		
mafenide	*Sulfamylon*	Apply to a clean, debrided wound, one or two times per day with a gloved hand. Cover burn at all times with drug, reapply as needed. Bathe patient in a whirlpool daily to aid debridement. Continue mafenide until healing occurs; monitor for infection and toxicity—acidosis. May cause marked discomfort on application.
nitrofurazone	*Furacin*	Apply directly to burn or place on gauze; reapply daily. Flushing the dressing with sterile saline facilitates removal. Monitor for signs of superinfections; treat supportively. Rash frequently occurs.
silver sulfadiazine	*Silvadene* *SSD cream* *Thermazene*	Apply once or twice a day to a clean, debrided wound. Use a 1/16-inch thickness. Bathe patient in a whirlpool to aid debridement. Dressings are not necessary but may be used; reapply as needed. Monitor for fungal superinfections.
Corticosteroids		
alclometasone dipropionate	*Aclovate*	Available as ointment and cream in 0.05% concentration.
betamethasone dipropionate	*Diprosone* *Maxivate* *Taro-Sone (CAN)*	Available as ointment, cream, gel, lotion, aerosol in 0.05% concentration.
betamethasone dipropionate augmented	*Diprolene* *Diprolene AF* *Diprosone*	Available as ointment, cream, lotion in 0.05% concentration.
betamethasone valerate	*Betaderm (CAN)* *Beta-Val* *Luxiq, Prevex B (CAN)*	Available as ointment, cream, and lotion in 0.1% concentration.
	Valisone	Available as foam in 0.12% concentration.
ciclesonide	*Alvesco*	Available as 80 mcg and 160 mcg/actuation.
clobetasol propionate	*Clobex*	Available as 0.05% spray.
	Cormax *Dermovate (CAN)* *Olux* *Temovate*	Available as ointment, cream, foam, and gel in 0.05% concentration.

Drug	Selected trade names	Instructions and preparations
Corticosteroids (continued)		
clocortolone pivalate	*Cloderm*	Available as cream in 0.1% concentration.
desonide	*DesOwen*	Available as ointment, lotion, and cream in 0.05% concentration.
	Verdeso	Available as foam in 0.05% concentration.
desoximetasone	*Topicort*	Available as ointment and cream in 0.25% concentration. Available as cream and gel in 0.05% concentration.
dexamethasone	*Aeroseb-Dex* *DecaSpray*	Available as aerosol in 0.01% and 0.04% concentrations.
dexamethasone sodium phosphate		Available as cream in 0.1% concentration.
diflorasone diacetate	*Florone* *Florone E* *Maxiflor* *Psorcon E*	Available as ointment and cream in 0.05% concentration.
fluocinolone acetonide	*Fluonid*	Available as solution in 0.01% concentration.
	Synalar	Available as ointment in 0.025% concentration, as cream in 0.01% and 0.025% concentrations, and as solution in 0.01% concentration.
fluocinonide	*Fluonex* *Lyderm Cream (CAN)*	Available as cream in 0.05% concentration.
	Lidex	Available as ointment, cream, solution, and gel in 0.05% concentration.
	Vanos	Available as cream in 0.1% concentration.
flurandrenolide		Available as ointment, cream, and lotion in 0.05% concentration and as tape containing 4 mcg/cm^2.
fluticasone fumarate	*Veramyst*	Available as nasal spray containing 55 mcg/spray.
fluticasone propionate	*Cutivate*	Available as cream in 0.05% concentration and ointment in 0.005% concentration.
halcinonide	*Halog*	Available as ointment, cream, and solution in 0.1% concentration.
halobetasol propionate	*Ultravate*	Available as ointment and cream in 0.05% concentration.

(continued)

Drug	Selected trade names	Instructions and preparations
Corticosteroids (continued)		
hydrocortisone	*Bactine Hydrocortisone* *Cort-Dome* *Cortizone-5* *Dermolate* *Dermtex HC*	Available as lotion in 0.25%, 0.5%, 1%, 2%, 2.5% concentrations.
	Cortizone-10 *Hycort* *Tegrin-HC*	Available as cream, lotion, ointment, and aerosol in 0.5% concentration.
	Hytone	Available as cream, ointment, and solution at 1% concentration.
hydrocortisone acetate	*Anusol-HC1*	Available as cream in 1% concentration.
	Cortaid *Lanacort-5*	Available as ointment in 0.5% concentration.
	Cortaid with Aloe	Available as cream in 0.5% concentration.
	Corticaine (R_x) *Gynecort* *Lanacort-5*	Available as cream in 0.5% concentration.
hydrocortisone buteprate		Available as cream in 0.1% concentration.
hydrocortisone butyrate	*Locoid*	Available as ointment and cream in 0.1% concentration.
hydrocortisone valerate	*Westcort*	Available as ointment and cream in 0.2% concentration.
mometasone furoate	*Asmanex Twisthaler*	Available as powder for oral inhalation at 220 mcg/actuation; for patients 4 yr and older.
	Elocon	Available as ointment, cream, and lotion in 0.1% concentration.
	Nasonex	Available as nasal spray in 0.2% concentration.
prednicarbate	*Dermatop*	Available as preservative-free cream in 0.1% concentration.
triamcinolone acetonide	*Aristocort*	Available as ointment in 0.1% and 0.5% concentrations and as cream in 0.025% and 0.5% concentrations.
	Flutex, Kenalog	Available as ointment in 0.025% concentration.
	Triacet, Triderm	Available as cream in 0.1% concentration and as lotion in 0.025% and 0.1% concentrations.

Drug	Selected trade names	Instructions and preparations
Emollients		
boric acid ointment	*Borofax*	Relieves burns, itching, irritation. Apply as needed.
dexpanthenol	*Panthoderm*	Relieves itching and aids in healing for mild skin irritations. Apply once or twice daily.
urea	*Aquacare* *Carmol 10* *Carmol 20* *Carmol 40* *Gordon's Urea 40%* *Nutraplus* *Ureacin-10* *Ureacin-20*	Apply bid to qid to area affected; rub in completely. Also used to restore nails (*Gordon's Urea 40%*)—cover with plastic wrap; keep dry and remove in 3–7 days.
vitamins A and D		Relieves minor burns, chafing, skin irritations. Apply locally with gentle massage bid to qid. Consult physician if not improved within 7 days.
zinc oxide	*Borofax Skin Protectant*	Relieves burns, abrasions, diaper rash. Apply as needed.
Estrogen		
estradiol hemihydrate	*Vagifem*	For treatment of atrophic vaginitis. Use one tablet inserted vaginally every day for 2 wk; then one tablet inserted vaginally two times per week. Try to taper every 3–6 months.
Growth factor		
becaplermin	*Regranex*	Increases incidence of healing of diabetic foot ulcers as adjunctive therapy. Apply to diabetic foot ulcers daily; patient must have an adequate blood supply. Risk of cancer increases with prolonged use.
Hair removal product		
eflornithine	*Vaniqa*	Approved for use in women only. Apply to unwanted facial hair bid for up to 24 wk. Do not wash treated areas until at least 4 hr after treatment.
Hemostatics		
absorbable gelatin (also comes in powder form)	*Gelfoam*	To prepare paste, add 3–4 mL sterile saline to contents of jar. Apply sponge dry or saturated with saline. Smear or press paste to cut surface; when bleeding stops, remove excess. Apply sponge and leave in place; it will be absorbed. Assess continually for infection; agent may act as site of infection or abscess formation. Do not use with infection.

(continued)

Drug	Selected trade names	Instructions and preparations
Hemostatics (continued)		
human fibrin sealant	*Artiss* *Evicel*	Spray or drip onto tissue in short bursts (0.1–0.2 mL) to produce a thin, even layer. If hemostasis is not complete, a second layer may be applied. Adjunct to decrease bleeding in vascular and liver surgery or used to adhere to autologous skin grafts for burns (*Artiss*). Monitor patient for anaphylactic reaction.
microfibrillar collagen	*Avitene Hemostat* *Hemopad* *Hemotene*	Use dry. Apply directly to the source of bleeding; apply pressure. Time will vary from 3–5 min depending on the site. Discard any unused product; monitor for infection; do not use with infection. Remove any excess material once bleeding has been controlled.
thrombin	*Thrombinar* *Thrombostat*	Prepare in sterile distilled water or isotonic saline; 100–1,000 units/mL. Mix freely with blood on the surface of injury; contraindicated with any bovine allergies. Watch for any sign of severe allergic reaction in sensitive individuals.
thrombin, recombinant	*Recothrom*	Apply solution directly to bleeding site with absorbable gelatin sponge; amount needed varies with area to be treated. Reserve use for minor bleeding or oozing. Contraindicated with allergy to hamster or snake proteins.
Immune modulator		
pimecrolimus	*Elidel*	Treatment of mild to moderate atopic dermatitis in non-immunocompromised patients older than 2 yr in whom conventional therapy is inappropriate or ineffective. Apply thin layer to affected area bid; discontinue if resolution of disease occurs.
Keratolytics		
podofilox	*Condylox*	Apply every 12 hr for 3 consecutive days. Allow to dry before using area. Dispose of used applicator. May cause burning and discomfort.
podophyllum resin	*Podocon-25* *Podofin*	Applied only by physician. Do not use if wart is inflamed or irritated. Very toxic; use minimum amount possible to avoid absorption.
Local anesthetic/analgesic		
lidocaine/ tetracaine	*Synera*	Dermal analgesia for superficial venous access and dermatological procedures. Apply one patch to intact skin 20–30 min before dermal procedure.
Lotions and solutions		
Burow's solution aluminum acetate	*Domeboro Powder* *Pedi-Boro Soak Paks*	Astringent wet dressing for relief of inflammatory conditions, insect bites, athlete's foot, bruises. Dissolve packet or tablet in pint of water, apply every 15–30 min for 4–8 hr; do not use occlusive dressing or in plastic containers.

Drug	Selected trade names	Instructions and preparations
Lotions and solutions (continued)		
calamine lotion		Relieves itching; pain of poison ivy, poison sumac, poison oak, insect bites, and minor skin irritations. Apply to affected area tid to qid.
hamamelis water	*A-E-R* *Witch Hazel*	Relieves itching and irritation of vaginal infection, hemorrhoids, postepisiotomy discomfort, posthemorrhoidectomy care. Apply locally up to six times per day.
Nasal corticosteroid		
fluticasone propionate	*Flonase*	Used as preventive treatment of asthma, not as primary treatment. May take several weeks to work. Clean nasal spray adapter weekly. *Adult:* Two sprays in each nostril daily. Approved for children 4–11 yr.
	Flovent Diskus *Flovent HFA*	Used as prophylactic treatment of asthma for patients age 4 and older who require a corticosteroid: 88–220 mcg bid using provided inhalation device or nasal inhalation.
Oral preparation		
amlexanox	*Aphthasol*	Apply solution or mucoadhesive disc to each aphthous ulcer qid—after meals, at bedtime, following oral hygiene—for 10 days; consult with dentist if ulcers are not healed within 10 days. May cause local pain.
Pediculicides and scabicides		
benzyl alcohol		5% lotion for treatment of head lice in patients 6 mo and older; not for use in infants. Apply to scalp or hair near scalp.
crotamiton	*Eurax*	For external use. Shake well, and massage into skin of entire body; repeat in 24 hr. Bathe or shower 48 hr after last use. Change bed linens and clothing the next day. Dry-clean contaminated clothing or wash in hot water.
lindane		For external use; not for use in premature neonates. Apply thin layer to entire body; leave on 8–12 hr, then wash thoroughly. Shampoo 1–2 oz into dry hair and leave for 4 min. Reapply after 7 days if signs of live lice recur. Teach hygiene and prevention; treat all contacts. Inform parents that this is a readily communicable disease.
malathion	*Ovide Lotion*	Avoid use with open lesions. Apply to dry hair; leave on 8–12 hr. Repeat in 7–9 days. Change bed linens and clothing. Treat all contacts. Contains flammable alcohol.
permethrin	*Acticin* *Elimite* *Nix*	For external use, including prophylaxis during head lice epidemics. Thoroughly massage into skin (30 g/adult); wash off after 8–14 hr. Shampoo into freshly washed, rinsed, towel-dried hair. Leave on 10 min; rinse. Notify health care provider if rash, itching worsen.

Appendix Q

Ophthalmic drugs

Ophthalmic drugs are intended for direct administration into the conjunctiva of the eye. These drugs are used to treat glaucoma (miotics constrict the pupil and decrease the resistance to aqueous flow), to aid in diagnosis of eye problems (mydriatics dilate the pupil for examination of the retina; cycloplegics paralyze the muscles that control the lens to aid refraction), to treat local ophthalmic infections or inflammation, and to provide relief from the signs and symptoms of allergic reactions.

Pregnancy Category C

Contraindicated in cases of allergy to these drugs. These drugs are seldom absorbed systemically, but caution should be taken with any patient who would have problems with the systemic effects of the drug if it were absorbed systemically.

Adverse effects

Local irritation, stinging, burning, blurring of vision (prolonged when using ointment), tearing; headache.

Dosage

1–2 drops to each eye bid to qid or 0.25–0.5 inch of ointment to each eye is the usual dosage.

Solution or drops

Wash hands thoroughly before administering; do not touch dropper to eye or to any other surface; have patient tilt head backward or lie down and stare upward; gently grasp lower eyelid and pull the eyelid away from the eyeball; instill drop(s) into pouch formed by eyelid; release lid slowly; have patient close eye and look downward; apply gentle pressure to the inside corner of the eye for 3–5 min to retard drainage; do not rub eyes; do not rinse eyedropper. Do not use eyedrops that have changed color; if more than one type of eyedrop is used, separate administration by 5 min.

Ointment

Wash hands thoroughly before administering; hold tube between hands for several minutes to warm the ointment; discard the first cm of ointment when opening the tube for the first time; tilt head backward or lie down and stare upward; gently pull out lower lid to form pouch; place 0.25–0.5 inch of ointment inside the lower lid; have patient close eyes for 1–2 min and roll eyeball in all directions; remove any excess ointment from around eye. If using more than one kind of ointment, wait 10 min before administration.

Teaching points

Teach patient the proper administration technique for the ophthalmic drug ordered; caution patients that transient stinging or burning may occur and that blurring vision may also occur—appropriate safety measures should be taken; sensitivity to sun will occur with mydriatic agents, which cause pupils to dilate; sunglasses may be needed. Report severe eye discomfort, palpitations, nausea, headache.

Drug	Trade names	Usage	Special considerations
apraclonidine	*Iopidine*	To control or prevent postsurgical elevations of IOP in patients after argon-laser eye surgery; short-term adjunct in patients on maximum tolerated therapy who need additional IOP reduction	Monitor for the possibility of vasovagal attack; do not give to patients with allergy to clonidine.
azelastine hydrochloride	*Optivar*	Treatment of ocular itching associated with allergic conjunctivitis	Antihistamine, mast cell stabilizer. *3 yr and older:* 1 drop bid. Rapid onset, 8 hr duration.
bepotastine besilate	*Bepreve*	Treatment of ocular itching associated with allergic rhinitis	Apply twice daily. Not for children younger than 2 yr.
besifloxacin	*Besivance*	Treatment of bacterial conjunctivitis (pinkeye)	1 drop in affected eye tid (6–8 hr apart); use for 7 days.
bimatoprost	*Lumigan*	Treatment of open-angle glaucoma and ocular hypertension	First- or second-line treatment; darkening of iris may occur; 1 drop daily in the evening.
brimonidine tartrate	*Alphagan P*	Treatment of open-angle glaucoma and ocular hypertension	Selective alpha$_2$-antagonist; minimal effects on CV and pulmonary systems; may stain soft contact lenses. Do not use with MAOIs. 1 drop tid.
brimonidine and timolol	*Combigan*	Treatment of IOP	1 drop every 12 hr. Do not use with contact lenses.
brinzolamide	*Azopt*	Decrease IOP in open-angle glaucoma	May be given with other agents; 1 drop tid. Give 10 min apart from other agents.
bromfenac 0.09%	*Xibrom*	Treatment of postsurgical inflammation and reduction of ocular pain in patients who have undergone cataract extraction	1 drop in affected eye bid, beginning 24 hr after surgery and continuing for 2 wk
carbachol	*Carbastat* *Carboptic* *Miostat*	Direct-acting miotic; for treatment of glaucoma; for miosis during surgery	Surgical dose a one-use only portion; 1 or 2 drops up to tid as needed for glaucoma.
cyclopentolate	*AK-Pentolate* *Cyclogyl* *Pentolair*	Mydriasis or cycloplegia in diagnostic procedures	Individuals with dark pigmented irides may require higher doses; compress lacrimal sac for 2–3 min after administration to decrease any systemic absorption.

(continued)

Drug	Trade names	Usage	Special considerations
cyclosporine emulsion 0.05%	*Restasis*	Increases tear production in patients whose tear production is presumed to be suppressed because of ocular inflammation associated with keratoconjunctivitis sicca	1 drop in each eye twice a day, approximately 12 hr apart; remove contact lenses before using.
dexamethasone intravitreal	*Ozurdex*	Extended-release intravitreal injection for treatment of macular edema following branch retinal artery occlusion or central retinal vein occlusion	Monitor for infection, retinal detachment, and increased intraocular pressure after injection. Use cautiously with history of ocular herpes simplex.
diclofenac sodium	*Voltaren*	Photophobia; for use in patients undergoing incisional refractive surgery	Apply 1 drop qid beginning 24 hr after cataract surgery; continue through the first 2 wk postoperatively.
difluprednate	*Durezol*	Anti-inflammatory and analgesic for treatment of postoperative ocular pain and inflammation	Apply 1 drop to affected eye qid beginning 24 hr after surgery and continuing for 2 wk.
dipivefrin	*AKPro* *Propine*	Control of IOP in chronic open-angle glaucoma	1 drop every 12 hr. Monitor closely with tonometry.
dorzolamide	*Trusopt*	Treatment of elevated IOP in patients with ocular hypertension or open-angle glaucoma	A sulfonamide; monitor patients on parenteral sulfonamides for possible additive effects. Children: 1 drop in each eye tid.
dorzolamide 2% and timolol 0.5%	*Cosopt*	Decrease IOP in open-angle glaucoma or ocular hypertension in patients who do not respond to beta blockers alone	Administer 1 drop in affected eye bid. Monitor for cardiac failure; if absorbed, may mask symptoms of hypoglycemia or thyrotoxicosis.
echothiophate		Treatment of open-angle glaucoma, accommodative estropia; irreversible cholinesterase inhibitor; long-acting.	Given only once or twice a day because of long action; tolerance may develop with prolonged use. Usually responds to a rest period.
emedastine	*Emadine*	Temporary relief of signs and symptoms of allergic conjunctivitis	1 drop in affected eye or eyes up to qid. Do not wear contact lenses if eyes are red; may cause headache, blurred vision.
epinastine hydrochloride	*Elestat*	Prevention of itching caused by allergic conjunctivitis	Remove contact lenses before applying. Instill 1 drop in each eye bid for entire time of exposure, even if itching subsides.

Drug	Trade names	Usage	Special considerations
fluocinolone acetonide intravitreal implant	*Retisert*	Treatment of chronic noninfectious uveitis affecting the posterior segment of the eye	1 surgically implanted insert (releases 0.6 mcg per day for approximately 30 mo). May be replaced after 30 mo if needed.
fluorometholone	*Flarex* *Fluor-Op* *FML*	Topical corticosteroid used for treatment of inflammatory conditions of the eye	Improvement should occur within several days, discontinue if no improvement is seen. Monitor IOP if used longer than 10 days. Discontinue if swelling of the eye occurs.
ganciclovir	*Zirgan*	Treatment of acute herpetic keratitis	Apply gel to lower conjunctival sac daily.
gatifloxacin	*Zymar*	Treatment of bacterial conjunctivitis caused by susceptible strains of *Corynebacterium propinquum, Staphylococcus aureus, Staphylococcus epidermidis, Streptococcus mitis, Streptococcus pneumoniae, Haemophilus influenzae*	Contacts should not be worn during these infections; ensure that patient is not allergic to any quinolone antibiotic. Can cause blurred vision.
homatropine	*Homatropine HBr* *Isopto-Homatropine*	Long-acting mydriatic and cycloplegic used for refraction and treatment of inflammatory conditions of the uveal tract or preoperative and postoperative states when mydriasis is required	Individuals with dark pigmented irides may require larger doses; 5–10 min is usually required for refraction.
ketorolac	*Acuvail* (0.45%)	Treatment of pain and inflammation following cataract surgery	Apply to affected eye bid.
ketotifen	*Zaditor*	An antihistamine and mast cell stabilizer; provides temporary relief of itching due to allergic conjunctivitis	Remove contact lenses before use—may be replaced within 10 min.
latanoprost	*Xalatan*	Treatment of open-angle glaucoma or ocular hypertension in patients intolerant or nonresponsive to other agents	Remove contact lenses before and for 15 min after use; allow at least 5 min between this and the use of any other agents; expect burning, blurred vision.
levobunolol	*AKBeta* *Betagan Liquifilm*	Lowering of IOP with chronic, open-angle glaucoma, ocular hypertension	1 or 2 drops bid. Do not combine with other beta blockers.

(continued)

Drug	Trade names	Usage	Special considerations
levofloxacin	*Quixin*	Treatment of bacterial conjunctivitis caused by susceptible bacteria	1 or 2 drops in affected eye every 2 hr while awake, days 1 and 2; then every 4 hr while awake, up to four times per day for days 3 to 7.
lodoxamide tromethamine	*Alomide*	Treatment of vernal conjunctivitis and keratitis for patients older than 2 yr	Patients should not wear contact lenses while using this drug; discontinue if stinging and burning persist after instillation.
loteprednol etabonate	*Alrex (0.2%)*	Treatment of postoperative inflammation after ocular surgery	1 or 2 drops qid beginning 24 hr after surgery and continuing for 2 wk. Shake vigorously before use. Discard after 14 days; prolonged use may cause nerve or eye damage.
	Lotemax (0.5%)	Treatment of steroid-resistant ocular disease	1 or 2 drops qid.
loteprednol etabonate/ tobramycin	*Zylet*	Treatment of steroid-responsive inflammatory ocular conditions where there is a risk of superficial bacterial ocular infection	1 or 2 drops into conjunctival sac every 4 –6 hr; during first 24–48 hr, dose may increase to every 1–2 hr.
metipranolol	*OptiPranolol*	Beta blocker; used in treating chronic open-angle glaucoma and ocular hypertension	Concomitant therapy may be needed; caution patient about possible vision changes.
moxifloxacin	*Vigamox*	Treatment of bacterial conjunctivitis caused by susceptible strains of *Corynebacterium* species, *Micrococcus luteus, Staphylococcus, Staphylococcus aureus, Staphylococcus haemolyticus, Staphylococcus hominis, Staphylococcus warneri, Streptococcus pneumoniae, Streptococcus viridans* group, *Acinetobacter lwoffii, Haemophilus influenzae, Haemophilus parainfluenzae, Chlamydia trachomatis*	Contact lenses should not be worn during these infections; ensure that patient is not allergic to any quinolone antibiotic. Can cause blurred vision.
natamycin	*Natacyn*	Antibiotic used to treat fungal blepharitis, conjunctivitis, and keratitis; drug of choice for *Fusarium sotani* keratitis	Shake well before each use; store at room temperature; failure to improve in 7–10 days suggests a nonsusceptible organism; reevaluate.

Drug	Trade names	Usage	Special considerations
nedocromil sodium	*Alocril*	Treatment of itching of allergic conjunctivitis	Use at regular intervals through the entire allergic season: 1 or 2 drops in each eye bid.
olopatadine hydrochloride	*Patanol*	Mast cell stabilizer and antihistamine; provides fast onset of relief of itching due to conjunctivitis with prolonged action	Not for use with contact lenses; headache is a common adverse effect.
pemirolast potassium	*Alamast*	Prevention of itchy eyes due to allergic conjunctivitis	1 or 2 drops qid.
pilocarpine	*Adsorbocarpine* *Akarpine* *Isopto Carpine* *Pilocar* *Piloptic* *Pilostat*	Chronic and acute glaucoma; treatment of mydriasis caused by drugs; direct-acting miotic drug	Can be stored at room temperature for up to 8 wk, then discard. 1 or 2 drops up to six times per day may be needed, based on patient response.
polydimethyl-siloxane	*AdatoSil 5000*	Treatment of retinal detachments where other therapy is not effective or is inappropriate; primary choice for retinal detachment due to AIDS-related CMV retinitis or viral infection	Monitor for cataracts; must be injected into aqueous humor.
rimexolone	*Vexol*	Corticosteroid; postoperative ocular surgery and for treatment of anterior uveitis	Monitor for signs of steroid absorption.
timolol maleate	*Timoptic XE*	Treatment of elevated IOP in ocular hypertension or open-angle glaucoma	1 drop in affected eye once a day in the morning.
travoprost	*Travatan* *Travatan Z*	Treatment of open-angle glaucoma and ocular hypertension	1 drop in affected eye or eyes each evening; eye discomfort, pain, darkening of iris, growth of eyelashes common.
trifluridine	*Viroptic*	Antiviral; used to treat primary keratoconjunctivitis and recurrent epithelial keratitis due to herpes simplex virus types 1 and 2	Transient burning and stinging may occur; reconsider drug if improvement is not seen within 7 days. Do not administer for longer than 21 days at a time.
tropicamide	*Mydriacyl* *Opticyl* *Tropicacyl*	Mydriatic and cycloplegic; used for refraction	1 or 2 drops of 1% solution; repeat in 5 min. May repeat in 30 min for prolonged effects.

APPENDIX R

Laxatives

Laxative use has been replaced by the use of proper diet and exercise in many clinical situations. Most laxatives are available as OTC preparations and are often abused by people who become dependent on them for GI movement.

Indications

Short-term relief of constipation; to prevent straining; to evacuate the bowel for diagnostic procedures; to remove ingested poisons from the lower GI tract; as adjunct in anthelmintic therapy

Drug	Selected trade names	Type
bisacodyl	*Bisa-Lax* *Dulcolax*	Stimulant
cascara		Stimulant
castor oil	*Emulsoil*	Stimulant
docusate	*Colace* *ex-lax Stool Softener* *Genasoft* *Phillips' Liqui-Gels*	Detergent, softener
glycerin	*Fleet Babylax* *Sani-Supp*	Hyperosmolar agent
lactulose	*Cephulac* *Chronulac* *Constilac* *Constulose*	Hyperosmolar agent
lubiprostone	*Amitiza*	Chloride channel activator
magnesium citrate	*Citrate of Magnesia*	Saline
magnesium hydroxide	*Milk of Magnesia* *MOM* *Philip's MOM*	Saline
magnesium sulfate	*Epsom Salts*	Saline

Pregnancy Category C

Contraindicated in cases of allergy to these drugs, third trimester of pregnancy, acute abdominal pain.

Adverse effects

Excessive bowel activity, perianal irritation, abdominal cramps, *weakness, dizziness,* cathartic dependence

Teaching points

Use as a temporary measure. Swallow tablets whole. Do not take this drug within 1 hr of any other drugs. Report sweating, flushing, muscle cramps, excessive thirst.

Dosage	Onset	Special considerations
10–15 mg PO 2.5 g in water via enema	6–10 hr Rapid	Allergy to tartrazine in *Dulcolax* tablets; may discolor urine.
325–650 mg PO	6–10 hr	
15–30 mL PO	2–6 hr	May be very vigorous; may cause abdominal cramping.
50–250 mg PO	24–72 hr	Gentle; beneficial with anorectal conditions that are painful and with dry or hard feces.
Rectal suppository; 4 mL liquid by rectum	15–30 min	Insert suppository high into rectum, retain 15 min; insert liquid dispenser and apply gentle, steady pressure until all liquid is gone, then remove.
15–30 mL PO	24–48 hr	Also used for treatment of portal system encephalopathy. May be more palatable mixed with fruit juice, water, or milk.
24 mcg PO bid with food	1–2 hr	May cause nausea, diarrhea; also approved for the treatment of IBS with constipation in women 18 yr and older.
1 glassful PO	0.5–3 hr	Reduce pediatric dosage by one-half.
15–30 mL PO	0.5–3 hr	Take with liquids; flavored varieties vary.
5–10 mL PO	0.5–3 hr	Take mixed with glass of water; reduce pediatric dose to 2.5–5 mL in one-half glass of water.

(continued)

Drug	Selected trade names	Type
mineral oil	*Kondremul Plain*	Emollient
polycarbophil	*Equalactin* *FiberCon* *Konsyl Fiber*	Bulk
polyethylene glycol	*MiraLax*	Bulk
polyethylene glycol-electrolyte solution	*CoLyte* *GoLYTELY* *NuLYTELY*	Bulk
polyethylene glycol, sodium sulfate, sodium chloride, potassium chloride, sodium ascorbate, ascorbic acid	*MoviPrep*	Osmotic
psyllium	*Fiberall* *Hydrocil Instant* *Metamucil*	Bulk
senna	*Agoral* *Black-Draught* *Fletcher's Castoria* *Senna-Gen* *Senokot*	Stimulant
sodium chloride, sodium bicarbonate, potassium chloride with bisacodyl tablets	*HalfLytely and Bisacodyl Bowel Prep Kit*	Stimulant Bulk

Dosage	Onset	Special considerations
5–45 mL PO	6–8 hr	Reduce pediatric dose to 5–20 mL. May decrease absorption of fat-soluble vitamins. Use caution to avoid lipid pneumonia with aspiration.
1 g PO 1–4 times per day as needed; do not exceed 6 g per day in adults or 3 g per day in children	12–24 hr	Good with IBS, diverticulitis. Abdominal fullness may occur. Smaller doses more frequently may alleviate discomfort.
Dissolve 17 g in 8 oz water and drink every day for up to 2 wk	48–72 hr	Do not use with bowel obstruction; diarrhea common.
4 L oral solution before GI examination	1 hr	Used as bowel evacuant before GI examinations. Do not use with GI obstruction, megacolon. GI discomfort common.
1 L PO followed by 16 oz of fluid the evening before colonoscopy and repeated the morning of colonoscopy; or 2 L followed by 32 oz of fluid the evening before colonoscopy	1 hr	Maintain hydration. Use caution in patients with history of seizures.
1 tsp or packet in cool water or juice, 1–3 times per day PO in children	12–24 hr	Safest and most physiologic. Ensure that patient has sufficient water to completely swallow dose.
1–8 tablets per day PO at bedtime; suppository by rectum; syrup—10–25 mL PO	6–10 hr	May be very aggressive; abdominal cramps and discomfort may occur.
Swallow 4 bisacodyl tablets; after first bowel movement, or in 6 hr, drink solution at a rate of one 8-oz glass every 10 min to a total of 8 glasses	1–6 hr	Bowel cleansing before colonoscopy.

Appendix S

Combination products by therapeutic class

AMPHETAMINES

dextroamphetamine and amphetamine

Controlled Substance C-II

Adderall (DNC), Adderall XR

Tablets:
1.25 mg (5-mg tablet), 2.5 mg (10-mg tablet), 5 mg (20-mg tablet), or 7.5 mg (30-mg tablet) each of dextroamphetamine sulfate and saccharate, amphetamine aspartate, and sulfate

ER capsules (DNC):
1.25 mg (5-mg capsule), 2.5 mg (10-mg capsule), 3.75 mg (15-mg capsule), 5 mg (20-mg capsule), 6.25 mg (25-mg capsule), or 7.5 mg (30-mg capsule) of each component

Usual adult and pediatric dosage: 5–60 mg PO per day to control symptoms of narcolepsy or ADHD; ER capsules: 10–30 mg per day.

See also **dextroamphetamine.**

ANALGESICS

acetaminophen and codeine

Controlled Substance C-III

Tylenol with Codeine

Elixir:
12 mg codeine, 120 mg acetaminophen/5 mL

Tablets:
No. 2: 15 mg codeine, 300 mg acetaminophen
No. 3: 30 mg codeine, 300 mg acetaminophen
No. 4: 60 mg codeine, 300 mg acetaminophen

Usual adult dosage: One or two tablets PO every 4–6 hr as needed or 15 mL every 4–6 hr.

See also **acetaminophen, codeine.**

aspirin and codeine

Controlled Substance C-III

Empirin with Codeine

Tablets:
No. 3: 30 mg codeine, 325 mg aspirin
No. 4: 60 mg codeine, 325 mg aspirin

Usual adult dosage: One or two tablets PO every 4–6 hr as needed.

See also **aspirin, codeine.**

(DNC) Do not crush.

codeine, aspirin, caffeine, and butalbital

CONTROLLED SUBSTANCE C-III

Fiorinal with Codeine

Capsules:
30 mg codeine, 325 mg aspirin, 40 mg caffeine, 50 mg butabarbital

Usual adult dosage: One or two capsules PO every 4 hr as needed for pain, up to 6 per day.

See also **codeine, aspirin, caffeine, butalbital.**

diclofenac sodium and misoprostol

PREGNANCY CATEGORY X

Arthrotec

Tablets:
'50': 50 mg diclofenac, 200 mcg misoprostol
'75': 75 mg diclofenac, 200 mcg misoprostol

Usual adult dosage:

- *Osteoarthritis: Arthrotec* '50' PO tid; *Arthrotec* '50' or '75' PO bid.
- *Rheumatoid arthritis: Arthrotec* '50' PO tid or qid; *Arthrotec* '50' or '75' PO bid.

See also **diclofenac, misoprostol.**

hydrocodone and aspirin

CONTROLLED SUBSTANCE C-III

Azdone, Damason-P, Lortab ASA

Tablets:
5 mg hydrocodone, 500 mg aspirin

Usual adult dosage: One tablet PO every 4–6 hr as needed.

See also **aspirin.**

hydrocodone bitartrate and acetaminophen

CONTROLLED SUBSTANCE C-III

Anexsia, Ceta-Plus, Co-Gesic, Duocet, Hydrogesic, Lorcet Plus Tablets, Lortab Tablets, Margesic H, Norco, Stagesic, Vicodin, Vicodin ES, Vicodin HP, Zydone

Elixir:
2.5 mg hydrocodone, 167 mg acetaminophen/5 mL

Capsules or tablets:
2.5 mg hydrocodone, 500 mg acetaminophen
5 mg hydrocodone, 500 mg acetaminophen
5, 7.5, 10 mg hydrocodone, 400 mg acetaminophen
7.5 mg hydrocodone, 500 mg acetaminophen
7.5 mg hydrocodone, 650 mg acetaminophen

10 mg hydrocodone, 650 mg acetaminophen

Norco tablets:

5 mg hydrocodone, 325 mg acetaminophen
7.5 mg hydrocodone, 325 mg acetaminophen
10 mg hydrocodone, 325 mg acetaminophen

Usual adult dosage: Check brand-name products to determine specific dosage combinations available. One or two tablets or capsules PO every 4–6 hr, up to 8 per day.

See also **acetaminophen.**

hydrocodone and ibuprofen

CONTROLLED SUBSTANCE C-III

Vicoprofen

Tablets:

2.5 mg hydrocodone, 200 mg ibuprofen
7.5 mg hydrocodone, 200 mg ibuprofen
10 mg hydrocodone, 200 mg ibuprofen

Usual adult dosage: One tablet PO every 4–6 hr as needed.

See also **ibuprofen.**

morphine and naltrexone

CONTROLLED SUBSTANCE C-II

Embeda

ER capsules DNC:

20 mg morphine, 0.8 mg naltrexone
30 mg morphine, 1.2 mg naltrexone
50 mg morphine, 2 mg naltrexone
60 mg morphine, 2.4 mg naltrexone
80 mg morphine, 3.2 mg naltrexone
100 mg morphine, 4 mg naltrexone

Usual adult dosage: One or two tablets PO daily when a continuous, around-the-clock analgesic is needed for a prolonged period; capsules may be opened and sprinkled over applesauce.

See also **morphine, naltrexone.**

naproxen and lansoprazole

Prevacid NapraPAC

Tablet/capsule kits:

375 mg naproxen tablet, 15-mg delayed-release lansoprazole capsule
500 mg naproxen tablet, 15-mg delayed-release lansoprazole capsule

Usual adult dosage: One naproxen tablet and one lansoprazole capsule PO in the morning before eating with a full glass of water, and one naproxen tablet in the evening with a full glass of water. Combination pack is designed to decrease the incidence of GI bleeding in patients on long-term therapy for treatment of arthritis or ankylating spondylosis.

See also **naproxen, lansoprazole.**

DNC Do not crush.

oxycodone and acetaminophen

CONTROLLED SUBSTANCE C-II

Percocet, Roxicet, Roxilox, Tylox

Tylox capsules:
5 mg oxycodone, 500 mg acetaminophen
Tablets:
2.25, 4.5, 5 mg oxycodone, 325 mg acetaminophen
Usual adult dosage: One or two tablets PO every 4–6 hr as needed.
See also **oxycodone, acetaminophen.**

oxycodone and aspirin

CONTROLLED SUBSTANCE C-II

Percodan, Roxiprin

Tablets:
4.5 mg oxycodone, 325 mg aspirin
Usual adult dosage: One or two tablets PO every 6 hr as needed.
See also **oxycodone, aspirin.**

oxycodone and ibuprofen

CONTROLLED SUBSTANCE C-II

Combunox

Tablets:
5 mg oxycodone, 400 mg ibuprofen
Usual adult dosage: One tablet PO every 6 hr as needed for moderate to severe pain. Do not exceed four tablets in 24 hr or use for more than 7 days.
See also **ibuprofen, oxycodone.**

propoxyphene and acetaminophen

Darvocet A500

Tablets:
100 mg propoxyphene, 500 mg acetaminophen
Usual adult dosage: One or two tablets PO every 4–6 hr as needed.
See also **propoxyphene, acetaminophen.**

tramadol hydrochloride and acetaminophen

Ultracet

Tablets:
37.5 mg tramadol, 325 mg acetaminophen

Usual adult dosage: Two tablets PO every 4–6 hr as needed. Do not exceed eight tablets per day. Reduce dosage with geriatric or renally impaired patients.
See also **tramadol, acetaminophen.**

ANTIACNE DRUGS

ethinyl estradiol and norethindrone

Estrostep Fe

Tablets:
1 mg norethindrone, 20 mcg ethinyl estradiol
1 mg norethindrone, 30 mcg ethinyl estradiol
1 mg norethindrone, 35 mcg ethinyl estradiol
Usual adult dosage: One tablet PO each day (21 tablets contain active ingredients and seven are inert).
See also **norethindrone, estradiol.**

norgestimate and ethinyl estradiol

Ortho Tri-Cyclen

Tablets:
0.18 mg norgestimate, 35 mcg ethinyl estradiol (7 tablets)
0.215 mg norgestimate, 35 mcg ethinyl estradiol (7 tablets)
0.25 mg norgestimate, 35 mcg ethinyl estradiol (7 tablets)
Usual adult dosage: For women older than 15 yr: One tablet PO per day.
Birth control agent used cyclically (21 tablets contain active ingredients, 7 are inert).
See also **estradiol.**

ANTIBACTERIALS

amoxicillin and clavulanic acid

Augmentin, Augmentin ES-600, Augmentin XR

Tablets:
'250': 250 mg amoxicillin, 125 mg clavulanic acid
'500': 500 mg amoxicillin, 125 mg clavulanic acid
'875': 875 mg amoxicillin, 125 mg clavulanic acid
Powder for oral suspension:
'125' powder: 125 mg amoxicillin, mg clavulanic acid
'250' powder: 250 mg amoxicillin, 62.5 mg clavulanic acid
'400' powder: 400 mg amoxicillin, 57 mg clavulanic acid
Solution (*Augmentin ES-600*):
600 mg amoxicillin, 42.9 mg clavulanic acid/5 mL
Chewable tablets:
'125': 125 mg amoxicillin, 31.25 mg clavulanic acid
'200': 200 mg amoxicillin, 28.5 mg clavulanic acid
'250': 250 mg amoxicillin, 62.5 mg clavulanic acid
'400': 400 mg amoxicillin, 57 mg clavulanic acid

XR tablets:
1,000 mg amoxicillin, 62.5 mg clavulanic acid

Usual adult dosage: One 250-mg tablet or one 500-mg tablet PO every 8 hr. For severe infections: 875-mg tablet PO every 12 hr. For those with difficulty swallowing, substitute the 125 mg/5 mL or 250 mg/5 mL for the 500-mg tablet or the 200 mg/5 mL or 400 mg/5 mL for the 875-mg tablet.

Usual pediatric dosage: In children weighing less than 40 kg: 20–40 mg amoxicillin/kg PO per day in divided doses every 8 hr (pediatric dosage is based on amoxicillin content) or every 12 hr; 90 mg/kg per day PO oral solution divided every 12 hr (*Augmentin ES-600*).

See also **amoxicillin.** Clavulanic acid protects amoxicillin from breakdown by bacterial beta-lactamase enzymes and is given only in combination with certain antibodies that are broken down by beta-lactamase.

co-trimoxazole (TMP-SMZ)

Bactrim, Bactrim DS, Bactrim Pediatric, Cotrim, Cotrim DS, Cotrim Pediatric, Septra, Septra DS, Sulfatrim

Tablets:
80 mg trimethoprim (TMP), 400 mg sulfamethoxazole (SMZ)
160 mg TMP, 800 mg SMZ

Oral suspension:
40 mg TMP, 200 mg SMZ per 5 mL

IV infusion:
16 mg/mL TMP, 80 mg/mL SMZ per 5 mL
80 mg TMP, 400 mg SMZ per 5 mL

Usual adult dosage:

- *UTIs, shigellosis, acute otitis media:* 160 mg TMP and 800 mg SMZ PO every 12 hr; 8–10 mg/kg per day (based on TMP component) in two to four divided doses every 6, 8, or 12 hr IV. Treat for up to 14 days (UTI) or for 5 days (shigellosis).
- *Acute exacerbations of chronic bronchitis:* 160 mg TMP and 800 mg SMZ PO every 12 hr for 14 days.
- Pneumocystis carinii *pneumonitis*: 20 mg/kg TMP and 100 mg/kg SMZ every 24 hr PO in divided doses every 6 hr; 15–20 mg/kg per day (based on TMP component) in three or four divided doses every 6–8 hr IV. Treat for 14 days.
- *Traveler's diarrhea:* 160 mg TMP and 800 mg SMZ PO every 12 hr for 5 days

Usual pediatric dosage:

- *UTIs, shigellosis, acute otitis media:* 8 mg/kg/day TMP and 40 mg/kg/day SMZ PO in two divided doses every 12 hr; 8–10 mg/kg/day (based on TMP component) in two to four divided doses every 6, 8, or 12 hr IV. Treat for 10–14 days (UTIs and acute otitis media) or for 5 days (shigellosis).
- Pneumocystis carinii *pneumonitis:* 20 mg/kg TMP and 100 mg/kg SMZ every 24 hr PO in divided doses every 6 hr; 15–20 mg/kg per day (based on TMP component) in three to four divided doses every 6–8 hr IV. Treat for 14 days.

Impaired renal function:

CrCl (mL/min)	*Dosage*
More than 30	Use standard dosage.
15–30	Use one-half of standard dosage.
Less than 15	Not recommended.

- Administer IV over 60–90 min. Thoroughly flush IV line after each use; do not refrigerate. IV solution must be diluted before use. See manufacturer's instructions. Do not give IM.

See also **sulfamethoxazole, trimethoprim.**

erythromycin and sulfisoxazole

Granules for oral suspension:

Erythromycin ethylsuccinate (equivalent of 200 mg erythromycin activity) and 600 mg sulfisoxazole per 5 mL when reconstituted according to manufacturer's directions

- Usual dosage for acute otitis media: 50 mg/kg per day erythromycin and 150 mg/kg per day sulfisoxazole PO in divided doses qid for 10 days.
- Administer without regard to meals; refrigerate after reconstitution; use within 14 days.

See also **erythromycin, sulfisoxazole.**

imipenem and cilastatin

Primaxin

Powder for injection (IV):

250 mg imipenem, 250 mg cilastatin
500 mg imipenem, 500 mg cilastatin

Powder for injection (IM):

500 mg imipenem, 500 mg cilastatin

- Follow manufacturer's instructions for reconstituting and diluting the drug.
- Administer each 250- to 500-mg dose by IV infusion over 20–30 min; infuse each 1-g dose over 40–60 min. Give 500–750 mg IM every 12 hr. Do not exceed 1,500 mg/day.
- Dosage recommendations based on imipenem. Initially based on type and severity of infection and later on severity of patient's illness, degree of susceptibility of the pathogens, and patient's age, weight, and creatinine clearance. Dosage for adults with normal renal function is 250 mg to 1 g IV every 6–8 hr, not to exceed 50 mg/kg/day or 4 g/day, whichever is less.
- Dosage for patients with renal impairment is based on creatinine clearance and weight. Consult manufacturer's guidelines.
- Imipenem inhibits cell wall synthesis in susceptible bacteria; cilastatin inhibits the renal enzyme that metabolizes imipenem; these drugs are available **only** in the combined form.

piperacillin sodium and tazobactam sodium

Zosyn

Tazobactam is a beta-lactamase inhibitor used in combination with the broad-spectrum penicillin.

Powder for injection:

2 g piperacillin, 0.25 g tazobactam
3 g piperacillin, 0.375 g tazobactam
4 g piperacillin, 0.5 g tazobactam

Usual adult dosage: 12 g/1.5 g IV given as 3.375 g every 6 hr.

- Recommended for appendicitis, peritonitis, postpartum endometritis and PID, community-acquired pneumonia, nosocomial pneumonia if agent is responsive in sensitivity testing.

- Reduced dosage required for renal impairment or dialysis.
- Administer by IV infusion over 30 min. Reconstitute with 5 mL of suitable diluent per 1 g piperacillin. Discard after 24 hr.

See also **piperacillin.**

quinupristin and dalfopristin

Synercid

New class of drugs available **only** as this combination product.
Streptogramin antibiotics:
500-mg/10-mL vial contains 150 mg quinupristin, 350 mg dalfopristin

- Treatment of life-threatening, susceptible infections associated with vancomycin-resistant *E. faecium* bacteremia (VREF), complicated skin infections due to *S. aureus, S. pyogenes.*
- Skin infections in patients older than 16 yr: 7.5 mg/kg IV every 12 hr for 7 days.
- VREF in patients older than 16 yr: 7.5 mg/kg IV every 8 hr.

⊗ ***Warning*** Dangerous when used with drugs that prolong the QTc interval.

- May cause pseudomembranous colitis.

sulbactam and ampicillin

Unasyn

Powder for injection:
1.5-g vial: 1 g ampicillin, 0.5 g sulbactam
3-g vial: 2 g ampicillin, 1 g sulbactam

Usual adult dosage: 0.5–1 g sulbactam with 1–2 g ampicillin IM or IV every 6–8 hr.
Pediatric dosage:
Less than 40 kg: 300 mg/kg per day IV in divided doses every 6 hr.
40 kg or more: adult dosage, do not exceed 4 g per day.

See also **ampicillin.** Sulbactam inhibits many bacterial penicillinase enzymes, thus broadening the spectrum of ampicillin; sulbactam is also weakly antibacterial alone.

ticarcillin and clavulanic acid

Timentin

Powder for injection, solution for injection:
3.1-g vial (3 g ticarcillin, 0.1 g clavulanic acid)
Administer by IV infusion over 30 min.

- Dosage for 60-kg adults: 3.1 g (3 g ticarcillin, 0.1 g clavulanic acid) IV every 4–6 hr. Dosage for adults less than 60 kg: 200–300 mg ticarcillin/kg per day IV in divided doses every 4–6 hr.
- Urinary tract infections: 3.1 g (3 g ticarcillin, 0.1 g clavulanic acid) IV every 8 hr.
- Pediatric dosage in children 3 mo and older: 3.1 g (3 g ticarcillin, 0.1 g clavulanic acid) IV every 4–6 hr or 200–300 mg/kg per day IV in divided doses every 4–6 hr.
- Geriatric or renal-failure patients: For patients on hemodialysis, give 2 g IV every 12 hr, supplemented with 3.1 g after each dialysis. For patients with renal impairment, give initial loading dose of 3.1 g, then as follows:

CrCl (mL/min)	Dosage
More than 60	3.1 g IV every 4 hr
30–60	2 g IV every 4 hr
10–30	2 g IV every 8 hr
Less than 10	2 g IV every 12 hr
Less than 10 with hepatic disease	2 g IV every 24 hr

- Continue treatment for 2 days after signs and symptoms of infection have disappeared. Usual duration of therapy is 10–14 days.

See also **ticarcillin.** Clavulanic acid protects ticarcillin from breakdown by bacterial beta-lactamase enzymes and is given only in combination with certain antibiotics that are broken down by beta-lactamase.

ANTI-CORONARY ARTERY DISEASE DRUGS

amlodipine besylate and atorvastatin calcium

Caduet

Tablets:
- 2.5 mg amlodipine with 10, 20, or 40 mg atorvastatin
- 5 mg amlodipine with 10, 20, 40, or 80 mg atorvastatin
- 10 mg amlodipine with 10, 20, 40, or 80 mg atorvastatin

Usual adult dosage: One tablet PO every day, taken in the evening. Dosage should be adjusted using the individual products; then switch to appropriate combination product.
See also **amlodipine, atorvastatin.**

ANTIDEPRESSANTS

chlordiazepoxide and amitriptyline

Limbitrol DS 10–25

Tablets:
- 5 mg chlordiazepoxide, 12.5 mg amitriptyline
- 10 mg chlordiazepoxide, 25 mg amitriptyline

Usual adult dosage: 10 mg chlordiazepoxide with 25 mg amitriptyline PO three or four times per day up to six times daily. For patients who do not tolerate higher doses, 5 mg chlordiazepoxide with 12.5 mg amitriptyline PO three or four times per day. Reduce dosage after initial response.
See also **amitriptyline, chlordiazepoxide.**

olanzapine and fluoxetine

Symbyax

Capsules:
- 6 mg olanzapine, 25 mg fluoxetine
- 6 mg olanzapine, 50 mg fluoxetine
- 12 mg olanzapine, 25 mg fluoxetine
- 12 mg olanzapine, 50 mg fluoxetine

Usual adult dosage: One capsule PO daily in the evening.
See also **fluoxetine, olanzapine.**

perphenazine and amitriptyline

Etrafon, Etrafon-A, Etrafon-Forte

Tablets:
- 2 mg perphenazine, 10 mg amitriptyline
- 2 mg perphenazine, 25 mg amitriptyline
- 4 mg perphenazine; 10 mg amitriptyline
- 4 mg perphenazine, 25 mg amitriptyline
- 4 mg perphenazine, 50 mg amitriptyline

Usual adult dosage: 2–4 mg perphenazine with 10–50 mg amitriptyline PO three or four times per day. Reduce dosage after initial response.
See also **amitriptyline, perphenazine.**

ANTIDIABETICS

glipizide and metformin

Metaglip

Tablets:
- 2.5 mg glipizide, 250 mg metformin
- 2.5 mg glipizide, 500 mg metformin
- 5 mg glipizide, 500 mg metformin

Usual adult dosage: One tablet PO per day with a meal; adjust dose based on patient response. Do not exceed maximum dose of 20 mg glipizide with 2,000 mg metformin per day.
See also **glipizide, metformin.**

glyburide and metformin

Glucovance

Tablets:
- 1.25 mg glyburide, 250 mg metformin
- 2.5 mg glyburide, 500 mg metformin
- 5 mg glyburide, 500 mg metformin

Usual adult dosage: One tablet daily PO with a meal, usually in the morning.
Not for initial therapy; drug should be adjusted using the individual products, switching to appropriate dosage of this combination product.
See also **glyburide, metformin.**

pioglitazone and glimepiride

Duetact

Tablets:
- 30 mg pioglitazone with 2 or 4 mg glimepiride

Usual adult dosage: One tablet/day PO with first meal of the day.
See also **pioglitazone, glimepiride.**

▽ pioglitazone and metformin

ACTO*plus* Met DNC

Tablets:
15 mg pioglitazone, 500 mg metformin
15 mg pioglitazone, 850 mg metformin
ER tablets DNC:
5 mg pioglitazone, 1,000 mg metformin
30 mg pioglitazone, 1,000 mg metformin

Usual adult dosage: One tablet PO once or twice a day with meals based on patient response and glycemic control; ER tablets, once a day.
See also **metformin, pioglitazone.**

▽ repaglinide and metformin

PrandiMet

Tablets:
1 mg repaglinide, 500 mg metformin
2 mg repaglinide, 500 mg metformin

Usual adult dosage: 1 tablet PO once a day or in divided doses; titrate as needed for glycemic control.
See also **repaglinide, metformin.**

▽ rosiglitazone and glimepiride

Avandaryl

Tablets:
4 mg rosiglitazone, 1 mg glimepiride
4 mg rosiglitazone, 2 mg glimepiride
4 mg rosiglitazone, 4 mg glimepiride
8 mg rosiglitazone, 2 mg glimepiride
8 mg rosiglitazone, 4 mg glimepiride

Usual adult dosage: 4 mg rosiglitazone with 1 or 2 mg glimepiride PO once daily with first meal of the day. Titrate as needed for glycemic control.
See also **rosiglitazone, glimepiride.**

▽ rosiglitazone and metformin

Avandamet

Tablets:
1 mg rosiglitazone, 500 mg metformin
2 mg rosiglitazone, 500 mg metformin
2 mg rosiglitazone, 1 g metformin

4 mg rosiglitazone, 500 mg metformin
4 mg rosiglitazone, 1 g metformin
Usual adult dosage: 4 mg rosiglitazone with 500 mg metformin, PO once a day or in divided doses. Not for initial therapy; dosage should be adjusted using individual drugs alone and then switching to the appropriate dosage of the combination product. See package insert for details on adjusting dosage based on use of other agents and previous dosage levels.
See also **metformin, rosiglitazone.**

sitagliptin and metformin

Janumet

Tablets:
50 mg sitagliptin, 500 or 1,000 mg metformin
Usual adult dosage: One tablet PO bid with meals; maximum daily dosage 100 mg sitagliptin, 2,000 mg metformin
See also **sitagliptin, metformin.**

ANTIDIARRHEALS

diphenoxylate hydrochloride and atropine sulfate

CONTROLLED SUBSTANCE C-V

Logen, Lomanate, Lomotil, Lonox

Tablets:
2.5 mg diphenoxylate hydrochloride, 0.025 mg atropine sulfate
Liquid:
2.5 mg diphenoxylate hydrochloride, 0.025 mg atropine sulfate/5 mL
- Individualized dosage.

Usual adult dosage: 5 mg PO qid.
- Pediatric initial dosage (use only liquid in children 2–12 yr): 0.3–0.4 mg/kg PO daily in four divided doses.

Age (yr)	*Weight (kg)*	*Dose (mL)*	*Frequency*
2	11–14	1.5–3	4 times daily
3	12–16	2–3	4 times daily
4	14–20	2–4	4 times daily
5	16–23	2.5–4.5	4 times daily
6–8	17–32	2.5–5	4 times daily
9–12	23–55	3.5–5	4 times daily

- Reduce dosage as soon as initial control of symptoms is achieved. Maintenance dosage may be as low as one-fourth of the initial dosage.

See also **atropine sulfate.**

ANTIHYPERTENSIVES

▽aliskiren and hydrochlorothiazide

Tekturna HCT

Tablets:
- 150 mg aliskiren, 12.5 mg hydrochlorothiazide
- 150 mg aliskiren, 25 mg hydrochlorothiazide
- 300 mg aliskiren, 12.5 mg hydrochlorothiazide
- 300 mg aliskiren, 25 mg hydrochlorothiazide

Usual adult dosage: One tablet PO daily.

May be given with other antihypertensives. Should be taken at about the same time each day.
See also **aliskiren, hydrochlorothiazide.**

▽aliskiren and valsartan

Valturna

Tablets:
- 150 mg aliskiren, 160 mg valsartan
- 300 mg aliskiren, 320 mg valsartan

Usual adult dosage: One tablet PO daily.

Indicated when hypertension is not controlled by one drug alone.
See also **aliskiren, valsartan.**

▽amlodipine and benazepril

Lotrel

Capsules:
- 2.5 mg amlodipine, 10 mg benazepril
- 5 mg amlodipine, 10 mg benazepril
- 5 mg amlodipine, 20 mg benazepril
- 5 mg amlodipine, 40 mg benazepril
- 10 mg amlodipine, 20 mg benazepril
- 10 mg amlodipine, 40 mg benazepril

Usual adult dosage: One tablet PO daily in the morning.

Monitor patient for hypotension and adverse effects closely over first 2 wk and regularly thereafter.
See also **amlodipine, benazepril.**

▽amlodipine and olmesartan

Azor

Tablets:
- 5 mg amlodipine, 20 mg olmesartan
- 10 mg amlodipine, 20 mg olmesartan
- 5 mg amlodipine, 40 mg olmesartan
- 10 mg amlodipine, 40 mg olmesartan

Usual adult dosage: One tablet PO daily; titrate based on patient response.
See also **amlodipine, olmesartan.**

amlodipine and valsartan

Exforge

Tablets:
- 5 mg amlodipine, 160 mg valsartan
- 5 mg amlodipine, 320 mg valsartan
- 10 mg amlodipine, 160 mg valsartan
- 10 mg amlodipine, 320 mg valsartan

Usual adult dosage: One tablet PO daily at about the same time each day.
Dosage based on patient response.
See also **amlodipine, valsartan.**

amlodipine, valsartan, and hydrochlorothiazide

Exforge HCT

Tablets:
- 5 mg amlodipine, 160 mg valsartan, 12.5 mg hydrochlorothiazide
- 10 mg amlodipine, 160 mg valsartan, 12.5 mg hydrochlorothiazide
- 5 mg amlodipine, 160 mg valsartan, 25 mg hydrochlorothiazide
- 10 mg amlodipine, 320 mg valsartan, 25 mg hydrochlorothiazide

Usual adult dosage: One tablet PO daily; titrate based on patient response.
See also **amlodipine, hydrochlorothiazide, valsartan.**

atenolol and chlorthalidone

Tenoretic

Tablets:
- 50 mg atenolol, 25 mg chlorthalidone
- 100 mg atenolol, 25 mg chlorthalidone

Usual adult dosage: One tablet PO daily in the morning.
Drug should be adjusted using the individual products, then switched to appropriate dosage.
See also **atenolol, chlorthalidone.**

bisoprolol and hydrochlorothiazide

Ziac

Tablets:
- 2.5 mg bisoprolol, 6.25 mg hydrochlorothiazide
- 5 mg bisoprolol, 6.25 mg hydrochlorothiazide
- 10 mg bisoprolol, 6.25 mg hydrochlorothiazide

Usual adult dosage: One tablet daily PO in morning. Initial dose is 2.5/6.25 mg tablet PO daily.
Dosage should be adjusted within 1 wk; optimal antihypertensive effect may require 2–3 wk.
See also **bisoprolol, hydrochlorothiazide.**

candesartan and hydrochlorothiazide

Atacand HCT

Tablets:
16 mg candesartan, 12.5 mg hydrochlorothiazide
32 mg candesartan, 12.5 mg hydrochlorothiazide
Usual adult dosage: One tablet PO daily in the morning.
Drug should be adjusted using the individual products, then switched to appropriate dosage.
See also **candesartan, hydrochlorothiazide.**

chlorthalidone and clonidine

Clorpres

Tablets:
15 mg chlorthalidone, 0.1 mg clonidine hydrochloride
15 mg chlorthalidone, 0.2 mg clonidine hydrochloride
15 mg chlorthalidone, 0.3 mg clonidine hydrochloride
Usual adult dosage: One or two tablets per day PO in the morning; may be given once or twice daily.
Dosage should be adjusted with the individual products, switching to this combination product when patient's condition is stabilized on the dosage of each drug available in this combination.
See also **clonidine.**

enalapril and hydrochlorothiazide

Vaseretic

Tablets:
5 mg enalapril maleate, 12.5 mg hydrochlorothiazide
10 mg enalapril maleate, 25 mg hydrochlorothiazide
Usual adult dosage: One or two tablets per day PO in the morning.
Dosage should be adjusted with individual products, switching to combination product after patient's condition is stabilized on the dosage of each drug that is available in this combination.
See also **enalapril maleate, hydrochlorothiazide.**

eprosartan and hydrochlorothiazide

Teveten HCT

Tablets:
600 mg eprosartan, 12.5 mg hydrochlorothiazide
600 mg eprosartan, 25 mg hydrochlorothiazide
Usual adult dosage: One tablet PO each day. Dosage should be established with each component alone before using the combination product; if BP is still not controlled, 300 mg eprosartan may be added each evening.
See also **eprosartan mesylate, hydrochlorothiazide.**

fosinopril and hydrochlorothiazide

Monopril-HCT

Tablets:
- 10 mg fosinopril, 12.5 mg hydrochlorothiazide
- 20 mg fosinopril, 12.5 mg hydrochlorothiazide

Usual adult dosage: One tablet PO per day in the morning.
Drug should be adjusted using the individual products, switching to appropriate dosage of this combination product.
See also **fosinopril, hydrochlorothiazide.**

hydrochlorothiazide and benazepril

Lotensin HCT

Tablets:
- 6.25 mg hydrochlorothiazide, 5 mg benazepril
- 12.5 mg hydrochlorothiazide, 10 mg benazepril
- 12.5 mg hydrochlorothiazide, 20 mg benazepril
- 25 mg hydrochlorothiazide, 20 mg benazepril

Usual adult dosage: One tablet per day PO in the morning.
Dosage should be adjusted with the individual products, switching to this combination product once the patient's condition is stabilized.
See also **benazepril, hydrochlorothiazide.**

hydrochlorothiazide and captopril

Capozide

Tablets:
- 15 mg hydrochlorothiazide, 25 mg captopril
- 15 mg hydrochlorothiazide, 50 mg captopril
- 25 mg hydrochlorothiazide, 25 mg captopril
- 25 mg hydrochlorothiazide, 50 mg captopril

Usual adult dosage: One or two tablets PO daily, 1 hr before or 2 hr after meals.
Dosage should be adjusted with individual products, switching to this combination product when patient's condition is stabilized on the dosage of each drug available in this combination.
See also **captopril, hydrochlorothiazide.**

hydrochlorothiazide and propranolol

Inderide

Tablets:
- 25 mg hydrochlorothiazide, 80 mg propranolol hydrochloride

Usual adult dosage: One or two tablets PO bid.
Dosage should be adjusted with individual products, switching to combination product when patient's condition is stabilized on the dosage of each drug available in this combination.
See also **hydrochlorothiazide, propranolol.**

irbesartan and hydrochlorothiazide

Avalide

Tablets:
150 mg irbesartan, 12.5 mg hydrochlorothiazide
300 mg irbesartan, 12.5 mg hydrochlorothiazide
300 mg irbesartan, 25 mg hydrochlorothiazide

Usual adult dosage: One or two tablets per day PO.
Dosage should be adjusted with individual products, switching to combination product when patient's condition is stabilized.
See also **hydrochlorothiazide, irbesartan.**

lisinopril and hydrochlorothiazide

Prinzide, Zestoretic

Tablets:
10 mg lisinopril, 12.5 mg hydrochlorothiazide
20 mg lisinopril, 12.5 mg hydrochlorothiazide
20 mg lisinopril, 25 mg hydrochlorothiazide

Usual adult dosage: One tablet per day PO taken in the morning.
Dosage should be adjusted with individual products, switching to combination product when patient's condition is stabilized.
See also **hydrochlorothiazide, lisinopril.**

losartan and hydrochlorothiazide

Hyzaar

Tablets:
50 mg losartan, 12.5 mg hydrochlorothiazide
100 mg losartan, 12.5 mg hydrochlorothiazide
100 mg losartan, 25 mg hydrochlorothiazide

Usual adult dosage: One tablet per day PO in the morning.
- Not for initial therapy; start using each component and if desired effects are obtained, *Hyzaar* may be used.
- Used to reduce the incidence of CVA in hypertensive patients with left ventricular hypertrophy (not effective for this use in black patients).

See also **hydrochlorothiazide, losartan.**

metoprolol and hydrochlorothiazide

Lopressor HCT

Tablets:
50 mg metoprolol, 25 mg hydrochlorothiazide
100 mg metoprolol, 25 mg hydrochlorothiazide
100 mg metoprolol, 50 mg hydrochlorothiazide

Usual adult dosage: One tablet PO per day.

Drug should be adjusted using the individual products, switching to appropriate dosage of this combination product.
See also **hydrochlorothiazide, metoprolol.**

moexipril and hydrochlorothiazide

Uniretic

Tablets:
- 7.5 mg moexipril, 12.5 mg hydrochlorothiazide
- 15 mg moexipril, 25 mg hydrochlorothiazide

Usual adult dosage: One or two tablets per day 1 hr before or 2 hr after a meal. Not for initial therapy. Adjust dose to maintain appropriate BP.
See also **hydrochlorothiazide, moexipril.**

nadolol and bendroflumethiazide

Corzide

Tablets:
- 40 mg nadolol, 5 mg bendroflumethiazide
- 80 mg nadolol, 5 mg bendroflumethiazide

Usual adult dosage: One tablet PO per day in the morning.
Drug should be adjusted using the individual products, switching to appropriate dosage of this combination product.
See also **bendroflumethiazide, nadolol.**

olmesartan medoxomil and hydrochlorothiazide

Benicar HCT

Tablets:
- 20 mg olmesartan, 12.5 mg hydrochlorothiazide
- 40 mg olmesartan, 12.5 mg hydrochlorothiazide
- 40 mg olmesartan, 25 mg hydrochlorothiazide

Usual adult dosage: One tablet PO per day in the morning.
Establish dosage with each drug individually, then switch to appropriate dosage of the combined product.
See also **hydrochlorothiazide, olmesartan.**

quinapril and hydrochlorothiazide

Accuretic

Tablets:
- 10 mg quinapril, 12.5 mg hydrochlorothiazide
- 20 mg quinapril, 12.5 mg hydrochlorothiazide

Usual adult dosage: One tablet PO per day in the morning.
Drug should be adjusted using the individual products, switching to appropriate dosage of this combination product.
See also **hydrochlorothiazide, quinapril.**

telmisartan and amlodipine

Twynsta

Tablets:
- 40 mg telmisartan, 5 mg amlodipine
- 40 mg telmisartan, 10 mg amlodipine
- 80 mg telmisartan, 5 mg amlodipine
- 80 mg telmisartan, 10 mg amlodipine

Usual adult dosage: One tablet PO daily.
May be used in combination with other drugs.
See also **amlodipine, telmisartan.**

telmisartan and hydrochlorothiazide

Micardis HCT

Tablets:
- 40 mg telmisartan, 12.5 mg hydrochlorothiazide
- 80 mg telmisartan, 12.5 mg hydrochlorothiazide
- 80 mg telmisartan, 25 mg hydrochlorothiazide

Usual adult dosage: One tablet PO per day; may be adjusted up to 160 mg telmisartan and 25 mg hydrochlorothiazide, based on patient's response.
See also **hydrochlorothiazide, telmisartan.**

trandolapril and verapamil

Tarka

Tablets:
- 1 mg trandolapril, 240 mg verapamil
- 2 mg trandolapril, 180 mg verapamil
- 2 mg trandolapril, 240 mg verapamil
- 4 mg trandolapril, 240 mg verapamil

Usual adult dosage: One tablet PO per day, taken with food.
Dosage should be adjusted with the individual products, switching to this combination product when the patient's condition is stabilized on the dosage of each drug available in combination.
Ensure that patient swallows tablet whole. Do not cut, crush, or chew.
See also **trandolapril, verapamil.**

valsartan and hydrochlorothiazide

Diovan HCT

Tablets:
- 80 mg valsartan, 12.5 mg hydrochlorothiazide
- 160 mg valsartan, 12.5 mg hydrochlorothiazide
- 160 mg valsartan, 25 mg hydrochlorothiazide
- 320 mg valsartan, 12.5 mg hydrochlorothiazide
- 320 mg valsartan, 25 mg hydrochlorothiazide

Usual adult dosage: One tablet per day PO.
Not for initial therapy; start using each component first.
See also **hydrochlorothiazide, valsartan.**

ANTIMIGRAINE DRUGS

acetaminophen and caffeine

Migraten

Capsules:
325 mg acetaminophen, 100 mg caffeine
Usual adult dosage: Two capsules at onset of migraine; then one every hour until resolved. Maximum, 5 capsules in 12 hr. For tension headache, one to two capsules every 4 hr, up to 8 capsules per day.
See also **acetaminophen.**

ergotamine and caffeine

Cafergot, Migergot

Tablets:
1 mg ergotamine tartrate, 100 mg caffeine
Suppositories:
2 mg ergotamine tartrate, 100 mg caffeine
Usual adult oral dosage: Two tablets at first sign of attack. Follow with one tablet every 30 min, if needed. Maximum dose is six tablets per attack. Do not exceed 10 tablets per wk.
Usual adult rectal dosage: One suppository at first sign of attack; follow with second dose after 1 hr, if needed. Maximum dose is two per attack. Do not exceed five per wk.
Do not combine this drug with ritonavir, nelfinavir, indinavir, erythromycin, clarithromycin, or troleandomycin—serious vasospasm events could occur.
See also **ergotamine.**

sumatriptan and naproxen sodium

Treximet

Tablets:
85 mg sumatriptan, 500 mg naproxen
Usual adult dosage: One tablet PO at the onset of acute migraine.
See also **naproxen, sumatriptan.**

ANTIPARKINSONIANS

levodopa and carbidopa

Parcopa, Sinemet (DNC), Sinemet CR

Tablets:
100 mg levodopa, 10 mg carbidopa
100 mg levodopa, 25 mg carbidopa
250 mg levodopa, 25 mg carbidopa

Orally disintegrating tablets:
100 mg levodopa, 10 mg carbidopa
100 mg levodopa, 25 mg carbidopa
250 mg levodopa, 25 mg carbidopa
Controlled release tablets DNC:
100 mg levodopa, 25 mg carbidopa
200 mg levodopa, 50 mg carbidopa

Usual adult dosage: Starting dose for patients not presently receiving levodopa: One tablet of 100 mg levodopa/10 mg carbidopa or 100 mg levodopa/25 mg carbidopa PO tid. For patients receiving levodopa: Start combination therapy with the morning dose at least 8 hr after the last dose of levodopa and choose a daily dosage of levodopa and carbidopa that will provide 25% of the previous levodopa daily dose. Dosage must be adjusted based on the patient's clinical response. See manufacturer's directions for adjusting the combination and single-agent drugs. *Orally disintegrating tablets:* Initially, one 100/25-mg tablet PO tid. Place tablet on top of the tongue where it will dissolve within seconds, then have the patient swallow the saliva; no additional liquid is required. Dosage may be increased by one tablet every day or every other day as needed to total daily dose of eight tablets (two tablets qid) as needed to control symptoms.

Carbidopa is available alone only by a specific request to the manufacturer from physicians who have a patient who needs a different dosage of carbidopa than is provided by the fixed combination drug; carbidopa is a peripheral inhibitor of dopa decarboxylase, an enzyme that converts dopa to dopamine, which cannot penetrate the CNS. The addition of carbidopa to the levodopa regimen reduces the dose of levodopa needed and decreases the incidence of certain adverse reactions to levodopa.

See also **carbidopa, levodopa.**

levodopa, carbidopa, and entacapone

Stalevo 50, Stalevo 75, Stalevo 100, Stalevo 125, Stalevo 150, Stalevo 200

Tablets:
50 mg levodopa, 12.5 mg carbidopa, 200 mg entacapone
75 mg levodopa, 18.75 mg carbidopa, 200 mg entacapone
100 mg levodopa, 25 mg carbidopa, 200 mg entacapone
125 mg levodopa, 31.25 mg carbidopa, 200 mg entacapone
150 mg levodopa, 37.5 mg carbidopa, 200 mg entacapone
200 mg levodopa, 50 mg carbidopa, 200 mg entacapone

Usual adult dosage: One tablet every 3–8 hr, based on the patient's clinical response.

See also **carbidopa, entacapone, levodopa.**

ANTIPLATELETS

aspirin and dipyridamole

Aggrenox

Capsules:
25 mg aspirin, 200 mg dipyridamole

Usual adult dosage: One capsule PO bid to decrease risk of CVA in patients with known cerebrovascular disease.

See also **aspirin, dipyridamole.**

DNC Do not crush.

ANTIULCER DRUGS

bismuth subsalicylate, metronidazole, and tetracycline

Helidac

Tablets:
262.4 mg bismuth subsalicylate, 250 mg metronidazole, 500 mg tetracycline hydrochloride
Usual adult dosage: One tablet PO qid for 14 days along with a prescribed histamine-2 antagonist. Indicated for the treatment of active duodenal ulcers associated with *Helicobacter pylori* infection.
See also **bismuth subsalicylate, metronidazole, tetracycline.**

lansoprazole, amoxicillin, and clarithromycin

Prevpac

Daily administration pack:
Two 30-mg lansoprazole capsules, four 500-mg amoxicillin capsules, and two 500-mg clarithromycin tablets.
Usual adult dosage: Divide pack equally to take twice daily, morning and evening for 10–14 days.

ANTIVIRALS

abacavir and lamivudine

Epzicom

Tablets:
600 mg abacavir with 300 mg lamivudine
Usual adult dosage: One tablet PO daily, taken without regard to food and in combination with other antiretroviral drugs.
See also **abacavir, lamivudine.**

abacavir, zidovudine, and lamivudine

Trizivir

Tablets:
300 mg abacavir, 300 mg zidovudine, 150 mg lamivudine
Usual adult dosage: One tablet PO bid.
Carefully monitor patient for hypersensitivity reactions.
See also **abacavir, lamivudine, zidovudine.**

efavirenz, emtricitabine, tenofovir

Atripla

Tablets:
600 mg efavirenz, 200 mg emtricitabine, 300 mg tenofovir
Usual adult dosage: One tablet PO at bedtime on an empty stomach.
Pediatric patients: Not recommended for children younger than 18 yr.
Renal impairment: Not recommended for patients with moderate or severe renal impairment.
See also **efavirenz, emtricitabine, tenofovir.**

emtricitabine and tenofovir disproxil fumarate

Truvada

Tablets:
200 mg emtricitabine with 300 mg tenofovir
Usual adult dosage: One tablet PO daily, taken without regard to food and in combination with other antiretroviral drugs.
See also **emtricitabine, tenofovir.**

lamivudine and zidovudine

Combivir

Tablets:
150 mg lamivudine, 300 mg zidovudine
Usual adult dose: One tablet PO bid.
Not recommended for children or adults weighing less than 50 kg. May be taken with food.
Does not decrease risk of spreading infections; use caution.
See also **lamivudine, zidovudine.**

DIURETICS

amiloride and hydrochlorothiazide

Moduretic

Tablets:
5 mg amiloride, 50 mg hydrochlorothiazide
Usual adult dosage: One or two tablets per day PO with meals.
See also **amiloride, hydrochlorothiazide.**

hydrochlorothiazide and triamterene

Dyazide

Capsules:
25 mg hydrochlorothiazide, 37.5 mg triamterene
Usual adult dosage: One or two capsules PO per day or bid after meals.
See also **hydrochlorothiazide, triamterene.**

Maxzide, Maxzide-25

Tablets:
25 mg hydrochlorothiazide, 37.5 mg triamterene
50 mg hydrochlorothiazide, 75 mg triamterene
Usual adult dosage: One or two tablets PO per day.
See also **hydrochlorothiazide, triamterene**

spironolactone and hydrochlorothiazide

Aldactazide

Tablets:
25 mg spironolactone, 25 mg hydrochlorothiazide
Usual adult dosage: One to eight tablets PO daily.
Tablets:
50 mg spironolactone, 50 mg hydrochlorothiazide
Usual adult dosage: One to four tablets PO daily.
See also **hydrochlorothiazide, spironolactone.**

HEART FAILURE DRUGS

isosorbide dinitrate and hydralazine hydrochloride

BiDil

Tablets:
20 mg isosorbide dinitrate, 37.5 mg hydralazine
Usual adult dosage: One tablet PO tid; may be increased to two tablets tid. For adjunct therapy in self-identified black patients to improve functional survival.
See also **isosorbide dinitrate, hydralazine.**

LIPID-LOWERING DRUGS

ezetimibe and simvastatin

Vytorin

Tablets:
10 mg ezetimibe; 10 mg simvastatin
10 mg ezetimibe; 20 mg simvastatin
10 mg ezetimibe; 40 mg simvastatin
10 mg ezetimibe; 80 mg simvastatin
Usual adult dosage: One tablet PO daily, taken in evening in combination with cholesterol-lowering diet and exercise. Dosage of simvastatin in the combination may be adjusted based on patient response. If given with a bile sequestrant, must be given at least 2 hr before or 4 hr after the bile sequestrant.
See also **ezetimibe, simvastatin.**

▽ niacin and lovastatin

Advicor

Tablets:
500 mg niacin, 20 mg lovastatin
750 mg niacin, 20 mg lovastatin
1,000 mg niacin, 20 mg lovastatin
Usual adult dosage: One tablet daily PO at night.
See also **lovastatin, niacin.**

▽ simvastatin and niacin

Simcor

Tablets:
20 mg simvastatin, 500 mg niacin
20 mg simvastatin, 750 mg niacin
20 mg simvastatin, 1,000 mg niacin
Usual adult dosage: One tablet PO per day; titrate based on lipid levels. Maximum dose 2,000 mg niacin with 40 mg simvastatin per day.
See also **niacin, simvastatin.**

MENOPAUSE DRUGS

▽ drospirenone and estradiol

Angeliq

Tablets:
0.5 mg drospirenone, 1 mg estradiol
Usual adult dosage: One tablet each day PO. Monitor potassium level closely.
See also **estradiol.**

▽ drospirenone and ethinyl estradiol

YAZ

Tablets:
3 mg drospirenone, 0.02 mg ethinyl estradiol
Usual adult dosage: One tablet each day PO. Monitor potassium level closely.
Also approved to treat premenstrual dysphoric disorder, acne.

▽ estradiol and norethindrone (transdermal)

CombiPatch

Patch:
0.05 mg per day estradiol, 0.14 mg per day norethindrone
0.05 mg per day estradiol, 0.25 mg per day norethindrone

Usual adult dosage: Change patch twice a week.
For relief of symptoms of menopause.
See also **estrogens.**

estradiol and norethindrone (oral)

Activella

Tablets:
0.5 mg estradiol, 0.1 mg norethindrone
1 mg estradiol, 0.5 mg norethindrone
Usual adult dosage: One tablet each day.
For treatment of moderate to severe vasomotor symptoms, vulvar and vaginal atrophy, prevention of postmenopausal osteoporosis in women with intact uterus.
See also **estrogens.**

estradiol and norgestimate

Ortho-Prefest

Tablets:
1 mg estradiol, 0.09 mg norgestimate
Usual adult dosage: One tablet per day PO (3 days of pink tablets: estradiol alone; followed by 3 days of white tablets: estradiol and norgestimate combination; continue cycle uninterrupted).
Treatment of moderate to severe symptoms of menopause and prevention of osteoporosis in women with intact uterus.
See also **estradiol.**

estrogen, medroxyprogesterone, and conjugated estrogens

Prempro

Tablets:
0.3 mg conjugated estrogen, 1.5 mg medroxygesterone
0.45 mg conjugated estrogen, 1.5 mg medroxygesterone
0.625 mg conjugated estrogen, 2.5 mg medroxyprogesterone
0.625 mg conjugated estrogen, 5 mg medroxyprogesterone
Usual adult dosage: One tablet per day PO.
For relief of symptoms of menopause and prevention of osteoporosis in women with intact uterus.
See also **estrogen.**

estrogens and medroxyprogesterone

Premphase

Tablets:
0.625 mg conjugated estrogens, 5 mg medroxyprogesterone
Usual adult dosage: One tablet per day PO.
Treatment of moderate to severe symptoms of menopause and prevention of osteoporosis in women with intact uterus.
See also **estrogen, medroxyprogesterone.**

ethinyl estradiol and norethindrone acetate

femHRT

Tablets:
2.5 mcg ethinyl estradiol, 0.5 mg norethindrone acetate
5 mcg ethinyl estradiol, 1 mg norethindrone acetate
Usual adult dosage: One tablet per day PO.
Treatment of signs and symptoms of menopause and prevention of osteoporosis in women with intact uterus.
See also **estradiol, norethindrone.**

OPIOID AGONISTS

buprenorphine and naloxone

CONTROLLED SUBSTANCE C-III

Suboxone

Sublingual tablets:
2 mg buprenorphine, 0.5 mg naloxone
8 mg buprenorphine, 2 mg naloxone
Usual adult dosage: 12–16 mg sublingually once each day following induction with sublingual buprenorphine for treatment of opioid dependence.
See also **buprenorphine, naloxone.**

RESPIRATORY DRUGS

budesonide and formoterol fumarate

Symbicort 80/4.5, Symbicort 160/4.5

Inhalation:
80 mcg budesonide, 4.5 mcg formoterol fumarate
160 mcg budesonide, 4.5 mcg formoterol fumarate
Usual dosage in patients 12 yr and older: Two inhalations bid, morning and evening.
Use for long-term maintenance of asthma, not for acute attacks.
See also **budesonide, formoterol.**

fluticasone and salmeterol

Advair Diskus, Advair HFA

Inhalation:
100 mcg fluticasone, 50 mcg salmeterol
250 mcg fluticasone, 50 mcg salmeterol
500 mcg fluticasone, 50 mcg salmeterol
Usual dosage in patients 12 yr and older: One inhalation bid to manage asthma.

Usual dosage in patients 4–11 yr: One inhalation (100 mcg fluticasone, 50 mcg salmeterol) bid in the morning and evening about 12 hr apart.
See also **fluticasone, salmeterol.**

ipratropium and albuterol

Combivent

Metered-dose inhaler:
18 mcg ipratropium bromide, 90 mcg albuterol
Usual adult dosage: Two inhalations four times per day
Not for use during acute attack.
Use caution with known sensitivity to atropine, soy beans, soya lecithin, peanuts.
Treatment of bronchospasm with COPD in patients who require more than a single bronchodilator.
See also **albuterol, ipratropium.**

loratadine and pseudoephedrine

Claritin-D (OTC)

ER tablets:
5 mg loratadine, 120 mg pseudoephedrine
Usual adult dosage: One tablet PO every 12 hr.
See also **loratadine, pseudoephedrine.**

Claritin-D 24 Hour

ER tablets:
10 mg loratadine, 240 mg pseudoephedrine
Usual adult dosage: One tablet PO every day.
See also **loratadine, pseudoephedrine.**

TENSION HEADACHE DRUGS

butalbital, acetaminophen, and caffeine

Esgic-Plus

Capsules:
50 mg butalbital, 500 mg acetaminophen, 40 mg caffeine
Usual adult dosage: One capsule PO every 4 hr as needed, up to six per day. May be habit-forming; avoid driving and dangerous tasks.
See also **acetaminophen, caffeine.**

APPENDIX T

Frequently used combination products by trade name

Many products are available on the market in combination form. Many of these are OTC preparations. It is helpful to have a guide to the ingredients of these products when instructing patients or assessing for drug interactions. The following is a list of brand names, active ingredients, and common usages for various combination products. Nursing process information can be checked by looking up the active ingredients.

Trade name	Active ingredients	Common usage
Acanya	clindamycin, benzoyl peroxide	Anti-acne drug
Accuretic	quinapril, hydrochlorothiazide	Antihypertensive
Actifed Cold & Allergy	pseudoephedrine, triprolidine	Decongestant, antihistamine
ACTOplus Met	pioglitazone, metformin	Antidiabetic
Adderall	dextroamphetamine sulfate and saccharate, amphetamine aspartate and sulfate	Amphetamine
Adderall XL	dextroamphetamine sulfate and saccharate, amphetamine aspartate and sulfate	Treatment of ADHD
Advair Diskus	fluticasone, salmeterol	Antiasthmatic
Advair HFA	fluticasone, salmeterol	Antiasthmatic
Advicor	niacin, lovastatin	Antihyperlipidemic
Advil Cold and Sinus	ibuprofen, pseudoephedrine	Decongestant, analgesic
Aggrenox	aspirin, dipyridamole	Stroke prevention
Aldactazide	spironolactone, hydrochlorothiazide	Diuretic
Alka-Seltzer Plus Cold & Cough	chlorpheniramine, dextromethorphan, phenylephrine	Decongestant, antihistamine, antitussive
Alka-Seltzer Plus Flu Medicine	dextromethorphan, chlorpheniramine, aspirin	Antitussive, analgesic, decongestant
Allegra-D	pseudoephedrine, fexofenadine	Decongestant, antihistamine
Allegra-D 24 hour	pseudoephedrine, fexofenadine	Decongestant, antihistamine
Allerest Maximum Strength	pseudoephedrine, chlorpheniramine	Decongestant, antihistamine

Trade name	Active ingredients	Common usage
Anacin	aspirin, caffeine	Analgesic
Anacin Aspirin-Free	diphenhydramine, acetaminophen	Analgesic
Anexsia	hydrocodone, acetaminophen	Analgesic
Angeliq	drospirenone, estradiol	Menopause
Antrocol	atropine, phenobarbital	Sedative, GI anticholinergic
Apri	ethinyl estradiol, desogestrel	Hormonal contraceptive
Atacand HCT	candesartan, hydrochlorothiazide	Antihypertensive
Atripla	efavirenz, emtricitabine, tenofovir	Antiviral
Augmentin	amoxicillin, clavulanic acid	Antibiotic
Augmentin ES-600	amoxicillin, clavulanic acid	Antibiotic
Augmentin XR	amoxicillin, clavulanic acid	Antibiotic
Avalide	irbesartan, hydrochlorothiazide	Antihypertensive
Avandamet	rosiglitazone, metformin	Antidiabetic
Avandaryl	rosiglitazone, glimepiride	Antidiabetic
Aviane	estradiol, levonorgestrel	Hormonal contraceptive
Azdone	hydrocodone, aspirin	Analgesic
Azor	amlodipine, olmesartan	Antihypertensive
Bactrim	trimethoprim, sulfamethoxazole	Antibiotic
Bayer Plus Extra Strength	aspirin, calcium carbonate	Analgesic
Bayer Select Maximum Strength Backache	magnesium tetrahydrate, aspirin	Analgesic
Bayer Select Maximum Strength Night Time Pain Relief	acetaminophen, diphenhydramine	Analgesic
Benadryl Allergy & Sinus	diphenhydramine, pseudoephedrine, acetaminophen	Decongestant
Benicar HCT	olmesartan, hydrochlorothiazide	Antihypertensive
BenzaClin	clindamycin, benzoyl peroxide	Anti-acne drug
BiDil	isosorbide dinitrate, hydralazine	Heart failure

(continued)

Trade name	Active ingredients	Common usage
Bromo Seltzer	acetaminophen, sodium bicarbonate, citric acid	Analgesic, antacid
Bronkaid Dual Action	theophylline, ephedrine, guaifenesin	Antiasthmatic
Bufferin	aspirin, magnesium carbonate, calcium carbonate, magnesium oxide	Analgesic, antacid
Caduet	amlodipine, atorvastatin	CAD prevention
Cafergot	ergotamine, caffeine	Antimigraine
Capozide	captopril, hydrochlorothiazide	Antihypertensive
Ceta-Plus	hydrocodone, acetaminophen	Analgesic
Cheracol Plus	codeine, guaifenesin, alcohol	Antitussive, expectorant
Chlor-Trimeton Allergy-D 4-Hr	pseudoephedrine, chlorpheniramine	Antihistamine, decongestant
Chlor-Trimeton Allergy-D 12-H	pseudoephedrine, chlorpheniramine	Antihistamine, decongestant
Ciprodex	ciprofloxacin, dexamethasone	Antibiotic, corticosteroid
Claritin-D 12 Hour	loratadine, pseudoephedrine	Decongestant, antihistamine
Claritin-D 24 Hour	loratadine, pseudoephedrine	Decongestant, antihistamine
Clorpres	chlorthalidone, clonidine	Antihypertensive
Codimal DH	phenylephrine, pyrilamine, hydrocodone	Antitussive, decongestant, antihistamine
Codimal PH	codeine, pyrilamine, phenylephrine	Antitussive, antihistamine, decongestant
Co-Gesic	hydrocodone, acetaminophen	Analgesic
CombiPatch	estrogen, norethindrone	Menopause drug
Combivent	ipratropium, albuterol	Antiasthmatic, COPD drug
Combivir	lamivudine, zidovudine	Antiviral
Combunox	oxycodone, ibuprofen	Analgesic
Comtrex Acute Head Cold & Sinus Pressure Relief	pseudoephedrine, brompheniramine, acetaminophen	Antihistamine, decongestant, analgesic

Trade name	Active ingredients	Common usage
Comtrex Cough & Cold Relief	pseudoephedrine, dextromethorphan, chlorpheniramine, acetaminophen	Decongestant, antitussive, analgesic, antihistamine
Contac Day & Night	pseudoephedrine, diphenhydramine, acetaminophen	Decongestant, antihistamine, analgesic
Coricidin "D" Cold, Flu & Sinus	chlorpheniramine, acetaminophen, pseudoephedrine	Antihistamine, decongestant, analgesic
Coricidin HBP Cold & Flu Tablets	chlorpheniramine, acetaminophen	Antihistamine, analgesic
Corzide	nadolol, bendroflumethiazide	Antihypertensive
Cotrim	trimethoprim, sulfamethoxazole	Antibiotic
Cryselle	ethinyl estradiol, norgestrel	Hormonal contraceptive
Cyclessa	desogestrel, ethinyl estradiol	Hormonal contraceptive
Cyclomydril	cyclopentolate, phenylephrine	Ophthalmic
Cylex	methenamine, sodium salicylate, benzoic acid	Urinary anti-infective
Damason-P	hydrocodone, aspirin	Analgesic
Darvocet A500	propoxyphene, acetaminophen	Analgesic
Deconamine	pseudoephedrine, chlorpheniramine	Antihistamine, decongestant
Dermoplast	benzocaine, menthol, methylparaben	Local anesthetic
Di Gel	magnesium hydroxide, aluminum hydroxide, magnesium carbonate, simethicone	Antacid, anti-gas
Dilaudid Cough Syrup	hydromorphone, guaifenesin	Antitussive
Dimetapp	brompheniramine, pseudoephedrine	Antihistamine, decongestant
Dimetapp Cold & Allergy	pseudoephedrine, brompheniramine	Antihistamine, decongestant
Diovan HCT	valsartan, hydrochlorothiazide	Antihypertensive
Doxidan	docusate, phenolphthalein	Laxative

(continued)

Trade name	Active ingredients	Common usage
Dristan Cold Multi-Symptom	phenylephrine, chlorpheniramine, acetaminophen	Antihistamine, decongestant
Drixoral Allergy Sinus	pseudoephedrine, dexbrompheniramine, acetaminophen	Antihistamine, decongestant
Duetact	pioglitazone, glimepiride	Antidiabetic
Duocet	hydrocodone, acetaminophen	Analgesic
Dyazide	triamterene, hydrochlorothiazide	Diuretic
Embeda	morphine, naltrexone	Analgesic
Empirin with Codeine	aspirin, codeine	Analgesic
Epzicom	abacavir, lamivudine	Antiviral
Esgic Plus	butalbital, acetaminophen, caffeine	Anti–tension headache
Estrostep FE	ethinyl estradiol, norethindrone	Hormonal contraceptive
Etrafon	perphenazine, amitriptyline	Antidepressant
Excedrin Extra Strength	aspirin, acetaminophen, caffeine	Analgesic
Excedrin P.M.	acetaminophen, dimenhydramine	Analgesic
Exforge	amlodipine, valsartan	Antihypertensive
Exforge HCT	amlodipine, valsartan, hydrochlorothiazide	Antihypertensive
Fansidar	sulfadoxine, pyrimethamine	Antimalarial
Femcon Fe	ethinyl estradiol, norethindrone	Hormonal contraceptive
femHRT	ethinyl estradiol, norethindrone	Menopause drug
Fioricet	acetaminophen, butalbital, caffeine	Analgesic
Fiorinal	aspirin, butalbital, caffeine	Analgesic
Fiorinal with Codeine	aspirin, butalbital, caffeine, codeine	Analgesic
Fosamax Plus D	alendronate, cholecalciferol	Osteoporosis
Gaviscon	aluminum hydroxide, magnesium carbonate	Antacid
Gelusil	aluminum hydroxide, magnesium hydroxide, simethicone	Antacid
Glucovance	glyburide, metformin	Antidiabetic

Trade name	Active ingredients	Common usage
Granulex	trypsin, Balsam Peru, castor oil	Topical enzyme
Haley's MO	mineral oil, magnesium hydroxide	Laxative
Helidac	bismuth subsalicylate, metronidazole, tetracycline	Antiulcer
Hydrogesic	hydrocodone, acetaminophen	Analgesic
Hyzaar	losartan, hydrochlorothiazide	Antihypertensive
Inderide	hydrochlorothiazide, propranolol	Antihypertensive
Janumet	sitagliptin, metformin	Antidiabetic
Junel 21 Day 1/20	ethinyl estradiol, norethindrone	Hormonal contraceptive
Junel 21 Day 1.5/30	ethinyl estradiol, norethindrone	Hormonal contraceptive
Junel Fe 1/20	ethinyl estradiol, norethindrone	Hormonal contraceptive
Junel Fe 1.5/30	ethinyl estradiol, norethindrone	Hormonal contraceptive
Kariva	ethinyl estradiol, desogestrel	Hormonal contraceptive
Kondremul Plain	mineral oil, Irish moss, glycerin, acacia	Laxative
Librax	chlordiazepoxide, clidinium	Anticholinergic, antispasmodic
Limbitrol DS 10-25	chlordiazepoxide, amitriptyline	Antidepressant
Logen	diphenoxylate, atropine	Antidiarrheal
Lomanate	diphenoxylate, atropine	Antidiarrheal
Lomotil	diphenoxylate, atropine	Antidiarrheal
Lonox	diphenoxylate, atropine	Antidiarrheal
Lopressor HCT	metoprolol, hydrochlorothiazide	Antihypertensive
Lorcet Plus Tablets	hydrocodone, acetaminophen	Analgesic
Lortab Tablets	hydrocodone, acetaminophen	Analgesic
Lo Seasonique	levonorgestrel, estradiol	Hormonal contraceptive
Lotensin HCT	hydrochlorothiazide, benazepril	Antihypertensive
Lotrel	amlodipine, benazepril	Antihypertensive
Low-Ogestrel	ethinyl estradiol, norgestrel	Hormonal contraceptive

(continued)

Trade name	Active ingredients	Common usage
Lufyllin GG	dyphylline, guaifenesin	Bronchodilator, expectorant
Lybrel	norgestrel, estradiol	Hormonal contraceptive
Malarone	atovaquone, proguanil	Antimalarial
Margesic H	hydrocodone, acetaminophen	Analgesic
Maxitrol	dexamethasone, neomycin, polymyxin B	Ophthalmic
Maxzide	triamterene, hydrochlorothiazide	Diuretic
Maxzide-25	hydrochlorothiazide, triamterene	Diuretic
Metaglip	glipizide, metformin	Antidiabetic
Micardis HCT	telmisartan, hydrochlorothiazide	Antihypertensive
Micrainin	meprobamate, aspirin	Analgesic
Microgestin Fe 1/20	ethinyl estradiol, norethindrone	Hormonal contraceptive
Microgestin Fe 1.5/30	ethinyl estradiol, norethindrone	Hormonal contraceptive
Midol Maximum Strength	acetaminophen, caffeine	Analgesic
Midol Teen	acetaminophen, pamabrom	Analgesic
Migergot	ergotamine, caffeine	Antimigraine
Migraten	acetaminophen, caffeine	Antimigraine
Moduretic	amiloride, hydrochlorothiazide	Diuretic
MonoNessa	ethinyl estradiol, norgestimate	Hormonal contraceptive
Monopril-HCT	fosinopril, hydrochlorothiazide	Antihypertensive
Mucinex DM	guaifenesin, dextromethorphan	Expectorant, cough suppressant
Mycolog-II	triamcinolone, nystatin	Antifungal
Mylagen Gelcaps	magnesium carbonate	Antacid
Mylagen II Liquid	aluminum hydroxide, magnesium hydroxide, simethicone	Antacid
Mylanta	aluminum hydroxide, magnesium hydroxide, simethicone, sorbitol	Antacid
Mylanta Gelcaps	calcium carbonate, magnesium hydroxide	Antacid

Trade name	Active ingredients	Common usage
Necon 1/35E	norethindrone, ethinyl estradiol	Hormonal contraceptive
Necon 1/50	mestranol, norethindrone	Hormonal contraceptive
Necon 7/7/7	ethinyl estradiol, norethindrone	Hormonal contraceptive
Necon 10/11	ethinyl estradiol, norethindrone	Hormonal contraceptive
Neosporin	polymyxin B, neomycin, bacitracin	Antibiotic
Norgesic	orphenadrine, aspirin, caffeine	Skeletal muscle relaxant
NuvaRing	etonogestrel, ethinyl estradiol	Contraceptive ring
NyQuil Cold/Cough Relief	pseudoephedrine, chlorpheniramine, dextromethorphan	Antihistamine, decongestant, antitussive
Ogestrel	ethinyl estradiol, norgestrel	Hormonal contraceptive
Ortho-Cyclen	ethinyl estradiol, norgestimate	Hormonal contraceptive
Ortho-Evra	norgestimate, ethinyl estradiol	Contraceptive patch
Ortho-Novum 1/35	ethinyl estradiol, norethindrone	Hormonal contraceptive
Ortho-Novum 1/50	ethinyl estradiol, norethindrone	Hormonal contraceptive
Ortho-Novum 10/11	ethinyl estradiol, norethindrone	Hormonal contraceptive
Ortho-Prefest	estradiol, norgestimate	Menopause drug
Ortho Tri-Cyclen	norgestimate, ethinyl estradiol	Antiacne drug, hormonal contraceptive
Ortho Tri-Cyclen Lo	ethinyl estradiol, norgestimate	Hormonal contraceptive
Otocort	hydrocortisone, neomycin, polymyxin B	Antibiotic, steroid
Ovcon-50	ethinyl estradiol, ethynodiol diacetate	Hormonal contraceptive
Pamprin	acetaminophen, pamabrom, pyrilamine	Analgesic
Parcopa	levodopa, carbidopa	Antiparkinsonian
Pepcid Complete	famotidine, calcium carbonate, magnesium hydroxide	Antacid
Percocet	oxycodone, acetaminophen	Analgesic
Percodan	oxycodone, aspirin	Analgesic

(continued)

Trade name	Active ingredients	Common usage
Phrenilin	acetaminophen, butalbital	Analgesic, sedative
Polysporin	polymyxin B, bacitracin	Antibiotic
Portia	levonorgestrel, ethinyl estradiol	Hormonal contraceptive
PrandiMet	repaglinide, metformin	Antidiabetic
Premphase	estrogen, medroxyprogesterone	Menopause drug
Prempro	estrogen, medroxyprogesterone	Menopause drug
Premsyn PMS	acetaminophen, pamabrom, pyrilamine	Analgesic
Prevpac	lansoprazole, amoxicillin, clarithro-mycin	Ulcer treatment
Primatene	theophylline, ephedrine	Antiasthmatic
Primaxin	imipenem, cilastin	Antibiotic
Prinzide	lisinopril, hydrochlorothiazide	Antihypertensive
Quasense	levonorgestrel, ethinyl estradiol	Hormonal contraceptive
Repan	acetaminophen, caffeine, butalbital	Analgesic
RID	pyrethrins, piperonyl butoxide	Pediculicide
Rifamate	isoniazid, rifampin	Antituberculotic
Riopan Plus	magaldrate, simethicone	Antacid
Robitussin Allergy & Cough	dextromethorphan, bromphenir-amine, pseudoephedrine	Antitussive, antihistamine, decongestant
Robitussin CF	pseudoephedrine, guaifenesin, alcohol, dextromethorphan	Antitussive, expectorant, decongestant
Robitussin Cold, Sinus & Congestion	acetaminophen, guaifenesin, alcohol, pseudoephedrine	Antitussive, expectorant, decongestant, analgesic
Robitussin DM	guaifenesin, dextromethorphan, alcohol	Antitussive, expectorant
Robitussin PE	pseudoephedrine, guaifenesin, alcohol	Decongestant, expectorant
Rondec	pseudophedrine, carbinoxamine	Antihistamine, decongestant
Roxilox	oxycodone, acetaminophen	Analgesic
Roxiprin	oxycodone, aspirin	Analgesic

Trade name	Active ingredients	Common usage
RuLox Plus	aluminum hydroxide, magnesium hydroxide	Antacid
Ryna	pseudoephedrine, chlorpheniramine	Antihistamine, decongestant
Seasonale	levonorgestrel, ethinyl estradiol	Hormonal contraceptive
Seasonique	levonorgestrel, ethinyl estradiol	Hormonal contraceptive
Sedapap	acetaminophen, butalbital	Analgesic
Senokot-S	senna, docusate	Laxative
Septra DS	trimethoprim, sulfamethoxazole	Antibiotic
Simcor	simvastatin, niacin	Antihyperlipidemic
Sinemet	levodopa, carbidopa	Antiparkinsonian
Sinemet-CR	levodopa, carbidopa	Antiparkinsonian
Sine-Off No Drowsiness	pseudoephedrine, acetaminophen	Decongestant, analgesic
Sinutab	pseudoephedrine, chlorpheniramine, acetaminophen	Decongestant, analgesic, antihistamine
Sprintec	norgestimate, ethinyl estradiol	Oral contraceptive
Stagesic	hydrocodone, acetaminophen	Analgesic
Stalevo	levodopa, carbidopa, entacapone	Antiparkinsonian
Suboxone	buprenorphine, naloxone	Opioid agonist/antagonist
Sudafed Sinus Headache	pseudoephedrine, acetaminophen	Antihistamine, analgesic
Sulfatrim	trimethoprim, sulfamethoxazole	Antibiotic
Symbicort	budesonide, formoterol	Antiasthmatic
Synalgos DC	aspirin, caffeine, dihydrocodeine	Analgesic
Synercid	quinupristin, dalfopristin	Antibiotic
Talacen	pentazocine, acetaminophen	Analgesic
Talwin Compound	aspirin, pentazocine	Analgesic
Tarka	trandolapril, verapamil	Antihypertensive
Tavist Allergy	pseudoephedrine, acetaminophen	Antihistamine, analgesic

(continued)

Trade name	Active ingredients	Common usage
Tekturna HCT	aliskiren, hydrochlorothiazide	Antihypertensive
Tenoretic	atenolol, chlorthalidone	Antihypertensive
Teveten HCT	eprosartan, hydrochlorothiazide	Antihypertensive
TheraFlu Flu & Cold	pseudoephedrine, chlorpheniramine, acetaminophen	Antihistamine, decongestant
TheraFlu Flu, Cold & Cough	pseudoephedrine, chlorpheniramine, dextromethorphan, acetaminophen	Antihistamine, decongestant, antitussive
Timolide	hydrochlorothiazide, timolol	Antihypertensive
TMP-SMZ	trimethoprim, sulfamethoxazole	Antibiotic
Treximet	sumatriptan, naproxen	Antimigraine drug
Triad	acetaminophen, caffeine, butalbital	Analgesic
Triaminic Chest & Nasal Congestion	dextromethorphan, pseudoephedrine	Antitussive, decongestant
Triaminic Cold & Allergy	chlorpheniramine, pseudoephedrine	Antihistamine, decongestant
Triaminic Cold & Cough	chlorpheniramine, pseudoephedrine, dextromethorphan	Antihistamine, decongestant, antitussive
Tri-Legest FE	estradiol, norethindrone	Hormonal contraceptive
Trivora-28	ethinyl estradiol, levonorgestrel	Hormonal contraceptive
Trizivir	abacavir, zidovudine, lamivudine	Antiviral, AIDS drug
Truvada	emtricitabine, tenofovir	Antiviral
Twynsta	amlodipine, telmisartan	Antihypertensive
Tylenol Flu	acetaminophen, pseudoephedrine, dextromethorphan	Antitussive, decongestant, analgesic
Tylenol Multi-Symptom	acetaminophen, pseudoephedrine, dextromethorphan, guaifenesin	Antitussive, decongestant, expectorant, analgesic
Tylenol with Codeine	acetaminophen, codeine	Analgesic
Tylox	oxycodone, acetaminophen	Analgesic
Ultracet	tramadol, acetaminophen	Analgesic
Unasyn	ampicillin, sulbactam	Antibiotic
Uniretic	moexipril, hydrochlorothiazide	Antihypertensive

Trade name	Active ingredients	Common usage
Valturna	aliskiren, valsartan	Antihypertensive
Vaseretic	enalapril, hydrochlorothiazide	Antihypertensive
Vicks Cough Relief	dextromethorphan, benzocaine	Antitussive, local anesthetic
Vicks DayQuil	dextromethorphan, pseudoephedrine, acetaminophen	Antitussive, decongestant
Vicks 44 Cough Relief	dextromethorphan, benzocaine	Antitussive
Vicks NyQuil Multi-Symptom	dextromethorphan, doxylamine, pseudoephedrine, acetaminophen	Antihistamine, antitussive, decongestant, analgesic
Vicodin	hydrocodone, acetaminophen	Analgesic
Vicoprofen	hydrocodone, ibuprofen	Analgesic
Vytorin	ezetimibe, simvastatin	Lipid-lowering drug
Yasmin	drospirenone, ethinyl estradiol	Hormonal contraceptive
YAZ	drospirenone, ethinyl estradiol	Menopause, PMDD
Zestoretic	lisinopril, hydrochlorothiazide	Antihypertensive
Ziac	bisoprolol, hydrochlorothiazide	Antihypertensive
Zosyn	piperacillin, tazobactam	Antibiotic
Zovia 1/35E	ethinyl estradiol, ethynodiol diacetate	Hormonal contraceptive
Zovia 1/50E	ethinyl estradiol, ethynodiol diacetate	Hormonal contraceptive
Zydone	hydrocodone, acetaminophen	Analgesic
Zyrtec-D	cetirizine, pseudoephedrine	Antihistamine, decongestant

APPENDIX U

Hormonal contraceptives

Usual dosage for oral contraceptives: Take one tablet PO daily for 21 days, beginning within 5 days of the first day of menstrual bleeding (day 1 of the cycle is the first day of menstrual bleeding). Inert tablets or no tablets are taken for the next 7 days. Then start a new course of 21 days.

Suggested measures for missed doses of oral contraceptives:

One tablet missed: Take tablet as soon as possible, or take two tablets the next day.

Two consecutive tablets missed: Take two tablets daily for the next 2 days, then resume the regular schedule.

Three consecutive tablets missed: Begin a new cycle of tablets 7 days after the last tablet was taken; use an additional method of birth control until the start of the next menstrual period.

Postcoital contraception ("morning after" pills): Safe and effective for emergency contraception. Dosing regimen starts within 72 hr of unprotected intercourse with a follow-up dose of the same number of pills 12 hr after the first dose.

Ovral: two white tablets
Nordette: four light orange tablets
Lo/Ovral: four white tablets
Triphasil: four yellow tablets

Plan B: 0.75 mg levonorgestrel; take one tablet within 72 hr of sexual intercourse, take the second tablet 12 hr later.

Plan B One-Step: 1.5 mg levonorgestrel; take one tablet within 72 hr of unprotected sexual intercourse. Available OTC for patients 17 yr and older.

Oral contraceptives

Trade name	Combination
Monophasic	
Alesse, Aviane, Lessina	20 mcg estradiol and 0.10 mg levonorgestrel
Apri, Desogen, Ortho-Cept, Reclipsen	30 mcg ethinyl estradiol and 0.15 mg desogestrel
Balziva, Femcon Fe chewable tablets, Ovcon-35, Zenchent	35 mcg ethinyl estradiol and 0.4 mg norethindrone
Brevicon, Modicon, Necon 0.5/35	35 mcg ethinyl estradiol (estrogen) and 0.5 mg norethindrone (progestin)
Cryselle, Lo/Ovral, Low-Ogestrel	30 mcg ethinyl estradiol (estrogen) and 0.3 mg norgestrel
Kelnor 1/35, Zovia 1/35E	35 mcg ethinyl estradiol (estrogen) and 1 mg ethynodiol diacetate (progestin)
Zovia 1/50E	50 mcg ethinyl estradiol (estrogen) and 1 mg ethynodiol diacetate (progestin)

Trade name	Combination
Monophasic (continued)	
Jolessa, Levora 0.15/30, Nordette, Portia	30 mcg ethinyl estradiol (estrogen) and 0.15 mg levonorgestrel (progestin)
Junel Fe 1/20, Junel 21 Day 1/20, Loestrin 21 1/20, Loestrin Fe 21 1/20, Microgestin Fe 1/20	20 mcg ethinyl estradiol (estrogen) and 1 mg norethindrone (progestin)
Junel Fe 1.5/30, Junel 21 Day 1.5/30, Loestrin 21 1.5/30, Loestrin Fe 1.5/30, Microgestin Fe 1.5/30	30 mcg ethinyl estradiol (estrogen) and 1.5 mg norethindrone acetate (progestin)
Kariva, Mircette	20 mcg ethinyl estradiol (estrogen) and 0.15 mg desogestrel (proestin)
Lessina, Lutera, Sronyx	0.10 mg levonorgestrel and 0.02 mg ethinyl estradiol
Lo Seasonique	0.1 mg levonorgestrel and 0.02 mg ethinyl estradiol (84 tablets); 0.01 mg ethinyl estradiol (7 tablets)
Lybrel	0.09 mg levonorgestrel and 0.02 mg ethinyl estradiol in continual use to eliminate menstrual periods
MonoNessa, Ortho-Cyclen, Sprintec	35 mcg ethinyl estradiol (estrogen) and 0.25 mg norgestimate (progestin)
Necon 1/35, Norinyl 1+35, Ortho-Novum 1/35	35 mcg ethinyl estradiol (estrogen) and 1 mg norethindrone (progestin)
Necon 1/50, Norinyl 1+50	50 mcg mestranol (estrogen) and 1 mg norethindrone (progestin)
Ogestrel, Ovral-28	50 mcg ethinyl estradiol (estrogen) and 0.5 mg norgestrel (progestin)
Ortho-Novum 1/50, Ovcon-50	50 mcg ethinyl estradiol (estrogen) and 1 mg norethindrone acetate (progestin)
Quasense, Seasonale, Seasonique	0.15 levonorgestrel and 0.03 mg ethinyl estradiol taken as 84 days active tablets, 7 days inactive
Solia	30 mcg ethinyl estradiol and 0.15 mg desogestrel
Yasmin	3 mg drospirenone (progestin) and 30 mcg ethinyl estradiol (estrogen); must monitor potassium levels
Biphasic	
Necon 10/11, Ortho-Novum 10/11	phase 1—10 tablets: 0.5 mg norethindrone and 35 mcg ethinyl estradiol;
	phase 2—11 tablets: 1 mg norethindrone and 35 mcg ethinyl estradiol

(continued)

Trade name	Combination
Triphasic	
Aranelle, Leena, Tri-Norinyl	phase 1—7 tablets, 0.5 mg norethindrone (progestin) and 35 mcg ethinyl estradiol (estrogen); phase 2—9 tablets, 1 mg norethindrone (progestin) and 35 mcg ethinyl estradiol (estrogen); phase 3—5 tablets, 0.5 mg norethindrone (progestin) and 35 mcg ethinyl estradiol (estrogen)
Cesia, Cyclessa, Velivet	phase 1—7 tablets, 0.1 mg desogestrel and 25 mcg ethinyl estradiol; phase 2—7 tablets, 0.125 mg desogestrel and 25 mcg ethinyl estradiol; phase 3—7 tablets, 0.15 mg desogestrel and 25 mcg ethinyl estradiol
Enpresse, Triphasil	phase 1—6 tablets, 0.05 mg levonorgestrel (progestin) and 30 mcg ethinyl estradiol (estrogen); phase 2—5 tablets, 0.075 mg levonorgestrel (progestin) and 40 mcg ethinyl estradiol (estrogen); phase 3—10 tablets, 0.125 mg levonorgestrel (progestin) and 30 mcg ethinyl estradiol (estrogen)
Estrostep Fe	phase 1—5 tablets, 1 mg norethindrone and 20 mcg ethinyl estradiol; phase 2—7 tablets, 1 mg norethindrone and 30 mcg ethinyl estradiol; phase 3—9 tablets, 1 mg norethindrone and 35 mcg ethinyl estradiol
Ortho-Novum 7/7/7, Necon 7/7/7	phase 1—7 tablets, 0.5 mg norethindrone (progestin) and 35 mcg ethinyl estradiol (estrogen); phase 2—7 tablets, 0.75 mg norethindrone (progestin) and 35 mcg ethinyl estradiol (estrogen); phase 3—7 tablets, 1 mg norethindrone (progestin) and 35 mcg ethinyl estradiol (estrogen)
Ortho Tri-Cyclen, TriNessa, Tri-Previfem, Tri-Sprintec	phase 1—7 tablets, 0.18 mg norgestimate and 35 mcg ethinyl estradiol; phase 2—7 tablets, 0.215 mg norgestimate and 35 mcg ethinyl estradiol; phase 3—7 tablets, 0.25 mg norgestimate and 35 mcg ethinyl estradiol
Ortho Tri-Cyclen Lo	phase 1—7 tablets, 0.18 mg norgestimate and 25 mcg ethinyl estradiol; phase 2—7 tablets, 0.215 mg norgestimate and 25 mcg ethinyl estradiol; phase 3—7 tablets, 0.25 mg norgestimate and 25 mcg ethinyl estradiol

Trade name	Combination
Triphasic (continued)	
Trivora-28	phase 1—6 tablets, 0.5 mg levonorgestrel (progestin) and 30 mcg ethinyl estradiol (estrogen); phase 2—5 tablets, 0.075 mg levonorgestrel (progestin) and 40 mcg ethinyl estradiol (estrogen); phase 3—10 tablets, 0.125 mg levonorgestrel (progestin) and 30 mcg ethinyl estradiol (estrogen)

Implantable system

Trade name	Combination
Implanon	68 mg etonogestrel implanted subdermally in inner aspect of non-dominant upper arm. Left in place for no longer than 3 yr and then must be removed. New implants may then be inserted.

Injectable contraceptives

Trade name	Combination
Depo-Provera	150 mg medroxyprogesterone Give 1-mL injection deep IM, repeated every 3 mo.

Intrauterine systems

Trade name	Combination
Mirena	52 mg levonorgestrel inserted into the uterus for up to 5 yr. (Also approved to treat heavy menstrual bleeding in women using an intrauterine system for contraception.)

Transdermal system

Trade name	Combination
Ortho Evra	6 mg norelgestromin, 0.75 ethinyl estradiol in a patch form, which releases 150 mcg norelgestromin and 20 mcg ethinyl estradiol each 24 hr for 1 wk. Patch is applied on the same day of the wk for 3 consecutive wk, followed by a patch-free week.

Vaginal ring

Trade name	Combination
NuvaRing	0.12 mg etonogestrel (progestin), 0.015 mg ethinyl estradiol (estrogen) per day; insert ring into vagina on or before the 5th day of menstrual period; remove after 3 wk. Insert new ring after 1-wk rest.

Commonly used biologicals

diphtheria and tetanus toxoids, combined, adsorbed (DT, Td) (available in adult and pediatric preparations)

Therapeutic actions

Contains reduced dose of inactivated diphtheria toxin and full dose of inactivated tetanus toxin to provide adequate immunization in adults without the severe sensitivity reactions caused when full pediatric doses of diphtheria toxoid are given to adults.

Indications

- Active immunization of adults and children 7 yr and older against diphtheria and tetanus. *Trivalent DTP* is preferred for use in most children; DT can be used for children 6 wk and older when pertussis vaccine is contraindicated.

Adverse effects

Fretfulness; drowsiness; anorexia; vomiting; transient fever; malaise; generalized aches and pains; edema of injection area with redness, swelling, induration, pain (may persist for a few days); hypersensitivity reactions.

Dosage

Two primary IM doses of 0.5 mL each given at 4- to 8-wk intervals, followed by a third 0.5-mL IM dose given in 6–12 mo. Routine booster of 0.5 mL IM every 10 yr for maintenance of immunity.

Nursing considerations

- Use caution in pregnant women. **Pregnancy Category C**—safety not established.
- Defer administration of routine immunizing or booster doses in case of acute infection.
- Arrange to interrupt immunosuppressive therapy if emergency booster doses of *Td* are required after injury.
- Not for treatment of acute tetanus or diphtheria infections.
- Administer by IM injection only; avoid subcutaneous or IV injection. Deltoid muscle is the preferred site. Do not administer into the same site more than once.

⊗ ***Warning*** Arrange for epinephrine 1:1,000 to be immediately available at time of injection in case of hypersensitivity reactions.

- Provide comfort measures to help patient cope with discomforts of injection: analgesics, warm soaks for injection site, small meals, environmental control—temperature, stimuli.
- Provide patient with written record of immunization and reminder of when booster injection is needed.

diphtheria and tetanus toxoids and acellular pertussis vaccine, adsorbed (DTaP)

Adacel, Boostrix, Daptacel, Infanrix, Tripedia

Therapeutic actions

Provides detoxified diphtheria and tetanus toxins and acellular pertussis vaccine to stimulate an immunologic response in children leading to an active immunity against these diseases.

Indications

- Primary immunization of children 6 wk and older–7 yr. Induction of immunity against diphtheria, tetanus, and pertussis. Immunization of adults against pertussis.

Adverse effects

Hypersensitivity reactions; erythema, induration, redness, pain, swelling of the injection area; nodule at the injection site, which may persist for several weeks; temperature elevations, malaise, chills, irritability, fretfulness, drowsiness, anorexia, vomiting, persistent crying; rarely—fatal reactions.

Dosage

- As primary immunization: 3 IM doses of 0.5 mL at 4- to 8-wk intervals. Start doses by 6–8 wk of age; finish by 7th birthday. Use the same vaccine for all three doses.
- Fourth dose: 0.5 mL IM at 15–20 mo, at least 6 mo after previous dose.
- Fifth dose: 0.5 mL IM at 4–6 yr or preferably before entry into school (*Infanrix, Tripedia, Daptacel*). If fourth dose was given after the 4-yr birthday, the preschool dose may be omitted.
- Booster injections: 10–18 yr (*Boostrix*) 0.5 mL IM; 11–64 yr (*Adacel*) 0.5 mL IM. Allow at least 5 yr between last of the series and booster dose.

Nursing considerations

- Do not use for treatment of acute tetanus, diphtheria, or whooping cough infections.
- Do not administer primary series to any person 7 yr or older.
- Do not attempt routine immunization with DTaP if the child has a personal history of CNS disease or convulsions.
- Do not administer DTaP after recent blood transfusions or receipt of immune globulin, in immunodeficiency disorders or with immunosuppressive therapy, or to patients with malignancy.
- Question the parent concerning occurrence of any signs or symptoms of adverse reactions after the previous dose before administering a repeat dose of the vaccine. If temperature higher than 39°C (103°F), convulsions with or without fever, alterations of consciousness, focal neurologic signs, screaming episodes, shock, collapse, somnolence, or encephalopathy has occurred, DTP is contraindicated and diphtheria and tetanus toxoids without pertussis should be used for immunization.
- Administer by IM injection only. Avoid subcutaneous or IV injection. Midlateral muscle of the thigh is the preferred site for infants; deltoid muscle is the preferred site for older children. Do not administer at same site more than once.

⊗ ***Warning*** Arrange for epinephrine 1:1,000 to be immediately available at time of injection in case of hypersensitivity reactions.

- DTaP products are not generically equivalent and are not interchangeable. Use vaccines from the same manufacturer for at least the first three doses.
- Provide comfort measures and teach parents to provide comfort measures to help the patient cope with the discomforts of the injection: analgesics, warm soaks for injection site, small meals, environmental control—temperature, stimuli.

- Provide parent with written record of immunization and reminder of when booster injection is needed.

diphtheria and tetanus toxoids, acellular pertussis, and *Haemophilus influenzae* type b conjugate vaccines (DTaP-HIB)

TriHIBit

Therapeutic actions

Contains diphtheria and tetanus toxoids and acellular pertussis vaccine along with *H. influenzae* type b conjugates to stimulate active immune response against these diseases in children who have received the vaccine.

Indications

- Active immunization of children ages 15–18 mo who have been immunized against diphtheria, tetanus, and pertussis with three doses consisting of diphtheria and tetanus toxoids and whole cell pertussis (DTP) or DTaP vaccine and three doses or fewer of *ActHIB* within the first year of birth for prevention of invasive diseases caused by *H. influenzae* or by diphtheria, tetanus, and pertussis.

Adverse effects

Hypersensitivity reactions: erythema, induration, redness, pain, swelling of the injection area; nodule at the injection site, which may persist for several wk; temperature elevations, malaise, chills, irritability, fretfulness, drowsiness, anorexia, vomiting, persistent crying; rarely—fatal reactions.

Dosage

- **First, second, and third doses at 2, 4, and 6 mo:** *ActHIB* reconstituted with normal saline solution or DTP, 0.5 mL given IM.
- **Fourth dose at 15–18 mo:** *ActHIB* reconstituted with DTP or *Tripedia* (*TriHIBit*) or with normal saline solution, 0.5 mL given IM.
- **Fifth dose at age 4–6 yr:** *Tripedia* or DTP, 0.5 mL given IM.

Nursing considerations

- Do not administer to children younger than age 15 mo.
- Do not administer if patient is febrile.
- To reconstitute, agitate *Tripedia* vial, withdraw 0.6 mL, inject into *ActHIB* vial, and agitate vial. Solution should appear whitish in color. Administer within 30 min of reconstitution.
- Give by IM injection, preferably into the gluteal area.
- Provide comfort measures and teach parents to provide comfort measures to help the patient cope with the discomforts of the injection: analgesics, rest, decongestants.
- Provide parents with written record of immunization and reminder that the flu vaccine is needed every yr just before the flu season.

diphtheria and tetanus toxoids and acellular pertussis adsorbed, hepatitis B (recombinant), and inactivated poliovirus vaccine combined

Pediarix

Therapeutic actions

Contains diphtheria and tetanus toxoids, acellular pertussis vaccine, recombinant antigenic hepatitis B vaccine and inactivated poliovirus vaccine in one injection to stimulate active immunity against these diseases in children who have received all doses of the vaccine.

Indications

- Active immunization against diphtheria, tetanus, pertussis, hepatitis B virus, and poliomyelitis caused by poliovirus Types 1, 2, and 3 as a three-dose primary series in infants born to HBsAg-negative mothers.

Adverse effects

Hypersensitivity reactions: erythema, induration, redness, pain, swelling of the injection area; nodule at the injection site, which may persist for several weeks; temperature elevations, malaise, chills, irritability, fretfulness, drowsiness, anorexia, vomiting, persistent crying; rarely—fatal reactions.

Dosage

- Infants with hepatitis B surface antigen (HBsAG)–negative mothers, three 0.5-mL doses IM given at 6- to 8- (preferably 8-) wk intervals beginning at 2 mo.
- Children previously vaccinated with one dose of hepatitis B vaccine should receive the three-dose series.
- Children previously vaccinated with one or more doses of *Infanrix* or *IPV: Pediarix* may be used to complete the series.

Nursing considerations

- Administer only to children of HbsAg-negative mothers.
- Do not administer to children with immunodeficiency, immunosuppression, or malignancy.
- Do not administer to any person younger than 6 wk or older than 7 yr.
- Do not administer if patient is febrile.
- Administer by IM injection only; avoid subcutaneous or IV injection. Midlateral muscle of the thigh is the preferred site for infants; deltoid muscle is the preferred site for older children.
- Shake the vial vigorously to suspend the drug; do not use if particles are apparent; do not re-enter the vial; discard any unused portion.
- Do not administer into the same site more than once.

⊗ ***Warning*** Arrange for epinephrine 1:1,000 to be immediately available at time of injection because of risk of hypersensitivity reactions.

- Provide comfort measures and teach parents to provide comfort measures to help the patient cope with the discomforts of the injection: analgesics, warm soaks for the injection site, small meals, environmental control—temperature, stimuli.
- Provide parents with written record of immunization and reminder of when booster injections are needed.
- Do not use this drug as a booster injection after the completion of the three-shot series; use appropriate single vaccines for boosters.

diphtheria and tetanus toxoids and acellular pertussis adsorbed and inactivated poliovirus vaccine

Kinrix

Therapeutic actions

Contains diphtheria and tetanus toxoids, acellular pertussis, and inactivated poliovirus in one injection to stimulate active immunity against these diseases in children.

Indications

- Active immunization against diphtheria, tetanus, pertussis, and poliomyelitis as the fifth dose in the diphtheria, tetanus, acellular pertussis series and the fourth dose in the inactivated poliovirus series in children 4–6 yr whose previous immunizations have been with *Infanrix* or *Pediarix* for the first three doses and *Infanrix* for the fourth dose.

Adverse effects

Hypersensitivity reactions; local reactions at injection site, including warmth, redness, swelling, pain; headache; nausea; myalgia; fever; URI symptoms.

Dosage

One IM injection of 0.5 mL.

Nursing considerations

- Drug is contraindicated with severe allergic reaction to any other vaccine, encephalopathy, and progressive neurologic diseases.
- Ensure that patient has received other immunizations in the series before administration.
- Use cautiously in patients with latex allergy.
- Children at high risk for seizures should receive an antipyretic at time of administration.
- Do not administer if patient is febrile or shows signs of active infection.
- Do not mix in syringe with other vaccines; administer at different sites than other vaccines.
- Provide comfort measures and teach parents to provide comfort measures (analgesics, antipyretics, warm packs to injection site, small meals, environmental control of temperature and stimuli) to help patient cope with effects of the injection.
- Provide parents with a written record of the immunization.

diphtheria and tetanus toxoids and acellular pertussis adsorbed, inactivated poliovirus vaccine, and *Haemophilus* b conjugate (tetanus toxoid conjugate) vaccine

Pentacel

Therapeutic actions

Contains diphtheria and tetanus toxoids, acellular pertussis, inactivated poliovirus and *Haemophilus* b conjugate vaccine in one injection to stimulate active immunity against these diseases in children.

Indications

- Primary active immunization of children between 6 wk and 4 yr against diphtheria, tetanus, pertussis, poliomyelitis, and *H. influenza* b.

Adverse effects
Hypersensitivity reactions; local reactions at injection site, including warmth, redness, swelling, pain; headache; nausea; myalgia; fever; URI symptoms.

Dosage
Four-dose series of IM injections of 0.5 mL beginning as early as 6 wk and then every 4–8 wk. A booster dose of *Daptacel* should be given at 4–6 yr.

Nursing considerations
- Contraindicated with severe allergic reaction to any other vaccine, encephalopathy, progressive neurologic diseases.
- Children at high risk for seizures should receive an antipyretic at time of administration.
- Do not administer if patient is febrile or shows signs of active infection.
- Do not mix in syringe with other vaccines; administer at different sites than other vaccines.
- Provide comfort measures and teach parents to provide comfort measures (analgesics, antipyretics, warm packs to injection site, small meals, environmental control of temperature and stimuli) to help patient cope with effects of the injection.
- Provide parents with a written record of the immunization and a date to return for the second dose in the series.

▽ *Haemophilus* b conjugate vaccine
ActHIB, Hiberix, HibTITER, Liquid PedvaxHIB

Therapeutic actions
Provides antigenic combination of *Haemophilus* b conjugate vaccine to stimulate an immunologic response in children, leading to an active immunity against these diseases.

Indications
- Active immunization of infants and children against *H. influenzae* b for primary immunization and routine recall; 2–71 mo (*HibTITER*, *PedvaxHIB*), 2–18 mo (*ActHIB* with DPT), or 15–18 mo (*ActHIB* with *Tripedia*).

Adverse effects
Hypersensitivity reactions; erythema, induration, redness, pain, swelling of the injection area; nodule at the injection site, which may persist for several weeks; temperature elevations, malaise, chills, irritability, fretfulness, drowsiness, anorexia, vomiting, persistent crying; rarely—fatal reactions.

Dosage
ActHIB: Reconstitute with DTP, *Tripedia*, or saline.
- *2–6 mo:* 3 IM injections of 0.5 mL at 2, 4, and 6 mo; 0.5 mL at 15–18 mo and DPT alone at 4–6 yr.
- *7–11 mo:* 2 IM injections of 0.5 mL at 8-wk intervals; booster dose at 15–18 mo.
- *12–14 mo:* 0.5 mL IM with a booster 2 mo later.
- *15–18 mo:* 0.5 mL IM, booster of *Tripedia* at 4–6 yr.

Hiberix
- *15 mo–4 yr:* Booster dose: 0.5 mL IM as a single dose.

HibTITER
- *2–6 mo:* 3 separate IM injections of 0.5 mL at 2-mo intervals.
- *7–11 mo:* 2 IM injections of 0.5 mL; give 2 mo apart.
- *12–14 mo:* 0.5 mL IM.

Booster dose at 15 mo or older but not less than 2 mo from last dose. Unvaccinated children 15–71 mo: 0.5 mL IM.

PedvaxHIB

- *2–14 mo:* 2 IM injections of 0.5 mL at 2 mo of age and 2 mo later; 0.5-mL booster at 12 mo (if 2 doses complete before 12 mo, not less than 2 mo after last dose).
- *15 mo or older:* 0.5 mL IM, single injection.

Nursing considerations

- Do not administer to children with immunodeficiency, immunosuppression, or malignancy.
- Do not administer to adults.
- Do not administer in the presence of febrile illness.
- Administer by IM injection only. Avoid subcutaneous or IV injection. Midlateral muscle of the thigh is the preferred site for infants; deltoid muscle is the preferred site for older children. Do not administer at same site more than once.

⊗ ***Warning*** Arrange for epinephrine 1:1,000 to be immediately available at time of injection in case of hypersensitivity reaction.

- Provide comfort measures and teach parents to provide comfort measures to help patient cope with the discomforts of the injection: analgesics, warm soaks for injection site, small meals, environmental control—temperature, stimuli.
- Provide parents with written record of immunization and reminder of when booster injection is needed.
- Conjugate vaccines can be given simultaneously with other routine vaccines using separate sites and syringes.

▽ *Haemophilus* b conjugate vaccine with hepatitis B surface antigen (recombinant)

Comvax

Therapeutic actions

Provides antigenic hepatitis B vaccine to stimulate an immunologic response in children, leading to an active immunity against the disease.

Indications

- Active immunization of infants, 6 wk–15 mo and children against hepatitis B, for primary immunization and routine recall for ages 2–15 mo.

Adverse effects

Hypersensitivity reactions: erythema, induration, redness, pain, swelling of the injection area; nodule at the injection site, which may persist for several weeks; temperature elevations, malaise, chills, irritability, fretfulness, drowsiness, anorexia, vomiting, persistent crying; rarely—fatal reactions.

Dosage

- Infants with hepatitis B surface antigen (HBsAg)–negative mothers: Three 0.5-mL IM doses at 2, 4, and 12–15 mo.
- Children previously vaccinated with one or more doses of hepatitis B vaccine or *Haemophilus* b vaccine: 0.5-mL IM doses at 2, 4, and 12–15 mo.

Nursing considerations

- Administer only to children of HBsAg-negative mothers.
- Do not administer to children with immunodeficiency, immunosuppression, or malignancy.

- Do not administer to adults.
- Do not administer if patient has febrile illness.
- Administer by IM injection only. Avoid subcutaneous or IV injection. Midlateral muscle of the thigh is the preferred site for infants; deltoid muscle is the preferred site for older children.
- Do not administer into same site more than once.

⊗ ***Warning*** Arrange for epinephrine 1:1,000 to be immediately available at time of injection because of risk of hypersensitivity reactions.

- Provide comfort measures and teach parents to provide comfort measures to help patient cope with the discomforts of the injection: analgesics, warm soaks for injection site, small meals, environmental control—temperature, stimuli.
- Provide parents with written record of immunization and reminder of when booster injection is needed.
- Conjugate vaccines can be given simultaneously with other routine vaccines, using separate sites and syringes.

▷ hepatitis A vaccine, inactivated

Havrix, Vaqta

Therapeutic actions

Contains hepatitis A antigen that stimulates production of specific antibodies against hepatitis A virus (HAV), which protects against HAV infection. The immunity does not protect against hepatitis caused by other agents.

Indications

- Active immunization of adults and children 12 mo and older against disease caused by HAV in situations that warrant immunization (eg, travel, institutionalization); used with immune globulin for immediate and long-term protection against hepatitis A.

Adverse effects

Transient fever; edema of injection area with redness, swelling, induration, pain (may persist for a few days); upper respiratory illness, headache, rash.

Dosage

- Adults: *Havrix*—1440 ELISA units (1 mL) IM; same dose booster in 6–12 mo. *Vaqta*—50 units (1 mL) IM; same dose booster in 6–18 mo.
- Pediatric patients 12 mo–18 yr: 25 units/0.5 mL IM with a repeat dose in 6–18 mo. (*Vaqta*); 720 ELISA units (0.5 mL) IM; repeat dose in 6–12 mo (*Havrix*).

Nursing considerations

- Use caution in pregnancy. **Pregnancy Category C**—safety not established.
- Defer administration in case of acute infection.
- Administer by IM injection only. Deltoid muscle is the preferred site; do not give in the gluteal site.

⊗ ***Warning*** Arrange for epinephrine 1:1,000 to be immediately available at time of injection in case of hypersensitivity reaction.

- Provide comfort measures to help patient cope with the discomforts of the injection (analgesics, warm soaks for injection site, small meals, environmental control of temperature and stimuli).
- Provide patient with written record of immunization and timing for booster immunization.

hepatitis A inactivated and hepatitis B recombinant vaccine

Twinrix

Therapeutic actions

Provides inactivated hepatitis A antigens that stimulate production of specific antibodies against hepatitis A virus (HAV), which protect against hepatitis A, and inactivated human hepatitis B surface antigen particles, which stimulate active immunity and production of antibodies against hepatitis B surface antigens.

Indications

- Active immunization against disease caused by HAV and hepatitis B virus in persons 18 yr and older who want protection against or are at high risk of exposure to the viruses.

Adverse effects

Soreness, swelling, erythema, warmth, induration at injection site; malaise, fatigue, headache, nausea, vomiting, dizziness; myalgia, arthralgia, rash, low-grade fever; pharyngitis, rhinitis, cough; lymphadenopathy; hypotension; dysuria.

Dosage

- Three doses (1 mL by IM injection) given on a 0-, 1-, and 6-month schedule.
- Accelerated dosage: Four doses (1 mL by IM injection) on days 0, 7, 21, and 30, followed by booster dose at 12 mo.
- Safety for use in patients younger than 18 yr not established.

Nursing considerations

- Do not administer to any patient with a known hypersensitivity to hepatitis A vaccine or hepatitis B vaccine or any components used in the solution.
- Use cautiously with bleeding disorders, immunosuppression, pregnancy, and lactation. **Pregnancy Category C**—safety not established.
- Postpone injection in the presence of moderate to severe illness.
- Administer IM, preferably in the deltoid region. Do not administer in the gluteal region.
- Shake vial or syringe well before withdrawal; observe for any particulate matter or discoloration. Should appear as a white, homogenous, turbid suspension; discard if it appears otherwise.
- Administer drug as provided; do not dilute.
- Provide comfort measures—analgesics, antipyretics, care of injection site—to help patient cope with the effects of the injection.
- Provide patient with a written record of the immunization and the dates that repeat vaccinations and antibody tests are needed.

hepatitis B immune globulin (HBIG)

HepaGam B, HyperHEP B S/D, Nabi-HB

Therapeutic actions

Globulin contains a high titer of antibody to hepatitis B surface antigen (HBsAg), providing a passive immunity to HBsAg.

Indications

- Postexposure prophylaxis following parenteral exposure (accidental "needle-stick"), direct mucous membrane contact (accidental splash), or oral ingestion (pipetting accident) involving

HBsAg-positive materials such as blood, plasma, serum, or sexual exposure to an HbsAg-positive person.
- Prophylaxis in infants born to HBsAg-positive mothers.
- Adjunct to hepatitis B vaccine when rapid achievement of protective levels of antibodies is desirable.
- Prevention of hepatitis B recurrence after liver transplant in HBsAg-positive transplant recipients (HepaGam B).

Adverse effects
Hypersensitivity reactions; tenderness, muscle stiffness at the injection site; urticaria, angioedema; fever, chills, nausea, vomiting, chest tightness.

Dosage
- Perinatal exposure: 0.5 mL IM within 12 hr of birth; repeat dose at 1 mo and 6 mo after initial dose.
- Percutaneous exposure: 0.06 mL/kg IM immediately (within 7 days) and repeat 28–30 days after exposure. Usual adult dose is 3–5 mL.
- Individuals at high risk of infection: 0.06 mL/kg IM at same time (but at a different site) as hepatitis B vaccine is given.
- *HepaGam B* after liver transplant: 20,000 international units IV at 2 mL/min. Give first dose with liver transplant and then daily on days 1–7, every 2 wk from day 14 through 12 wk, and monthly from month 4 onward.
- Sexual exposure: A single dose of 0.06 mL/kg IM within 14 days of last sexual contact.

Nursing considerations
- Do not administer to patients with history of allergic response to gamma globulin or with anti–immunoglobulin A antibodies.
- Use caution in pregnant women. **Pregnancy Category C**—safety not established. Use only if benefits outweigh potential unknown risks to the fetus.
- HBIG may be administered at the same time or up to 1 mo preceding hepatitis B vaccination without impairing the active immune response from the vaccination.
- Administer IM in the deltoid region or anterolateral aspect of upper thigh. Do not administer IV.
- Administer the appropriate dose as soon after exposure as possible (within 7 days is preferable); repeat 28–30 days after exposure.

⊗ ***Warning*** Have epinephrine 1:1,000 immediately available at time of injection in case of anaphylactic reaction.
- Provide comfort measures to help patient deal with discomfort of drug therapy—analgesics, antipyretics, environmental control.

▽ hepatitis B vaccine
Engerix-B, Recombivax HB

Therapeutic actions
Provides inactivated human hepatitis B surface antigen particles to stimulate active immunity and production of antibodies against hepatitis B surface antigens using surface antigen produced by yeast.

Indications
- Immunization against infection caused by all known subtypes of hepatitis B virus, especially those at high risk for infection—health care personnel, military personnel identified to be at risk, prisoners, users of illicit drugs, populations with high incidence (Eskimos,

Indochinese refugees, Haitian refugees), morticians and embalmers, persons at increased risk because of their sexual practices (repeated STDs, homosexually active males, prostitutes), patients in hemodialysis units, patients requiring frequent blood transfusions, residents of mental institutions, household contacts of people with persistent hepatitis B antigenemia.
- All infants, adolescents 11–12 yr, and older unvaccinated adolescents at high risk.

Adverse effects

Soreness, swelling, erythema, warmth, induration at injection site; malaise, fatigue, headache, nausea, vomiting, dizziness; myalgia, arthralgia, rash; low-grade fever, pharyngitis, rhinitis, cough; lymphadenopathy; hypotension; dysuria.

Dosage

- *Birth–10 yr:* Initial dose—0.5 mL IM, followed by 0.5 mL IM at 1 mo and 6 mo after initial dose.
- *11–19 yr:* 0.5 mL IM, followed by 0.5 mL IM at 1 mo and 6 mo after initial dose.
- *Adults:* Initial dose—1 mL IM, followed by 1 mL IM at 1 mo and 6 mo after initial dose, all types.
- *Dialysis or predialysis patients:* Initial dose—40 mcg IM; repeat dose at 1 mo, 2 mo, and 6 mo after initial dose (*Engerix-B*). Or, 40 mcg IM; repeat dose at 1 mo and 6 mo (*Recombivax HB*).
- Revaccination (a booster dose should be considered with anti-HBs levels less than 10 milli-international units/mL 1–2 mo after third dose). *Children younger than 10 yr:* 10 mcg. *Adults and patients older than 10 yr:* 20 mcg. *Hemodialysis patients (when antibody testing indicates need):* two 20-mcg doses.

Nursing considerations

- Do not administer to any patient with known hypersensitivity to any component of the vaccine or allergy to yeast.
- Use caution in pregnant or nursing women. **Pregnancy Category C**—safety not established. Use only if clearly needed and benefits outweigh potential unknown effects.
- Use caution in any patient with active infection. Delay use of vaccine if possible. Use with caution in any patient with compromised cardiopulmonary status or patients in whom a febrile or systemic reaction could present a significant risk.
- Administer IM, preferably in the deltoid muscle in adults or the anterolateral thigh muscle in infants and small children. Do not administer IV or intradermally; subcutaneous route may be used in patients who are at high risk for hemorrhage following IM injection, but increased incidence of local effects has been noted.
- Shake vaccine container well before withdrawing solution; no dilution is needed. Use vaccine as supplied. Vaccine appears as a slightly opaque, white suspension. Refrigerate vials; do not freeze.

⊗ ***Warning*** Have epinephrine 1:1,000 immediately available at time of injection in case of severe anaphylactic reaction.

- Provide comfort measures—analgesics, antipyretics, care of injection site—to help patient cope with effects of the drug.
- Provide patient or parent with a written record of the immunization and dates that repeat injections and antibody tests are needed.

▽human papillomavirus recombinant vaccine, bivalent types 16 and 18

Cervarix

Therapeutic actions

Human papillomavirus capsid proteins that generate the formation of immunoglobulin G–neutralizing antibodies directed against those strains of human papillomavirus.

Indications

- Prevention of diseases caused by oncogenic human papillomavirus types 16 and 18 in young girls and women ages 10–25 yr, including cervical cancer, cervical intraepithelial neoplasia grade 2 or worse, adenocarcinoma in situ, and cervical intraepithelial neoplasia grade 1.

Adverse effects

Injection site reactions (pain, redness, swelling), fatigue, headache, myalgia, GI symptoms, arthralgia, syncope.

Dosage

Three doses of 0.5 mL IM given at 0, 1, and 6 months.

Nursing considerations

- Do not administer to anyone with immunodeficiency/suppression or malignancy.
- Do not administer with antiviral medications or other immunizations or immune suppressants.
- Do not administer if patient has febrile illness or active infection.
- Do not administer to patient with known allergy to components of drug or to latex.
- Do not administer to women who are pregnant unless the benefit clearly outweighs the risk.

⊗ ***Warning*** Have epinephrine 1:1000 immediately available at time of injection in case of anaphylactic reaction.

- Observe patient for 15 minutes following vaccine administration; syncope is common and may occur with any dose of the series.
- Provide comfort measures (analgesics, rest, decongestants) to help patient cope with discomforts of immunization.
- Ensure that patient understands the importance of regular cervical cancer screening throughout life.
- Provide patient with written record of immunization; give patient a reminder for return dates to complete the series.

▽human papillomavirus recombinant vaccine, quadrivalent

Gardasil

Therapeutic actions

Noninfectious, recombinant virus particles that stimulate antibody production to human papillomavirus types 6, 11, 16, and 18; providing humoral immunity to virus that cause such diseases as cervical cancer, genital warts, cervical adenocarcinoma in situ, cervical intraepithelial neoplasia, vulvar intraepithelial neoplasia, vaginal intraepithelial neoplasia, cervical intraepithelial neoplasia.

Indications

- Prevention of diseases caused by human papillomavirus types 6, 11, 16, and 18 in young girls and women ages 9–26 yr, including cervical cancer, precancerous genital lesions, genital warts, and vaginal and vulvar cancer.
- Prevention of genital warts caused by human papillomavirus types 6 and 11 in men and boys 9–26 yr.

Adverse effects

Injection site reactions (redness, warmth, swelling, bruising, pain), dizziness, diarrhea, nasal congestion, myalgia, arthralgia, fever, fainting.

Dosage

- Three separate IM injections of 0.5 mL each, second dose 2 mo after the initial dose and last dose 6 mo after the first dose; for girls and women 9–26 yr.

Nursing considerations

- Do not administer to anyone with immunodeficiency/suppression or malignancy.
- Do not administer with any antiviral drugs or with other immunizations or immune suppressants.
- Do not administer if patient has febrile illness or active infection.
- Do not administer to patient allergic to any component of the drug; do not repeat injections in patients who experience hypersensitivity reactions.
- Do not administer to women who are pregnant. **Pregnancy Category B.**
- Administer by IM injection in the deltoid or upper thigh. Shake well before using; do not use if drug is discolored or contains particulate matter.

⊗ ***Warning*** Have epinephrine 1:1,000 immediately available at time of injection in case of anaphylactic reaction.

- Have patient remain seated or lying down for 15 min after vaccination for safety; fainting, twitching, and seizurelike activity have occurred.
- Provide comfort measures (analgesics, rest, decongestants) to help the patient cope with discomforts of immunization.
- Ensure that patients understand the importance of regular cervical cancer screening throughout life.
- Provide patient with written record of immunization and reminders for second and third injections.

▽ immune globulin intramuscular (IG; gamma globulin; IGIM)

GamaSTAN S/D

immune globulin intravenous (IGIV)

Carimune NF, Flebogamma 5%, Gammagard Liquid, Gamunex, Iveegam EN, Octagam, Privigen

immune globulin subcutaneous (IGSC, SCIG)

Vivaglobin

Therapeutic actions

Contains human globulin (16.5% IM, 5% IV), which provides passive immunity through the presence of injected antibodies. IM gamma globulin involves a 2- to 5-day delay before adequate serum levels are obtained. IV gamma globulin provides immediate antibody levels. Mechanism of action in idiopathic thrombocytopenic purpura not determined.

Indications

- Prophylaxis after exposure to hepatitis A, measles (rubeola), varicella, rubella; IM route is preferred.
- Prophylaxis for patients with immunoglobulin deficiency—subcutaneously, IM; IV if immediate increase in antibodies is necessary.
- Idiopathic thrombocytopenic purpura. IV route has produced temporary increase in platelets in emergency situations (*Carimune NF, Gamunex*).
- Kawasaki syndrome (*Iveegam EN*).
- Primary immune deficient diseases (*Octagam, Vivaglobin*).
- Primary humoral immunodeficiencies (*Flebogamma, Iveegam EN*).
- Maintenance treatment of patients with primary immunodeficiencies (*Carimune NF*).
- Treatment of chronic inflammatory demyelinating polyneuropathy (*Gamunex*).

Adverse effects

Tenderness, muscle stiffness at injection site; urticaria, angioedema, nausea, vomiting, chills, fever, chest tightness; anaphylactic reactions, precipitous fall in blood pressure—more likely with IV administration. Risk of acute renal failure with IV products.

Dosage

- Hepatitis A: 0.02 mL/kg IM for household and institutional contacts. Persons traveling to areas where hepatitis A is common: 0.02 mL/kg IM if staying less than 2 mo; 0.06 mL/kg IM repeated every 5 mo for prolonged stay.
- Measles (rubeola): 0.25 mL/kg IM if exposed less than 6 days previously; immunocompromised child exposed to measles: 0.5 mL/kg to a maximum of 15 mL IM given immediately.
- Varicella: 0.6–1.2 mL/kg IM given promptly if zoster immune globulin is unavailable.
- Rubella: 0.55 mL/kg IM given to those pregnant women who have been exposed to rubella and will not consider a therapeutic abortion may decrease likelihood of infection and fetal damage.
- Immunoglobulin deficiency: Initial dosage of 1.3 mL/kg IM, followed in 3–4 wk by 0.66 mL/kg IM every 3–4 wk; some patients may require more frequent injections.
- *Carimune NF:* 0.2 g/kg IV once a mo.
- *Octagam/Flebogamma:* 300–600 mg/kg IV every 3–4 wk.
- Patients with primary immune deficiency: 100–200 mg/kg subcutaneously every week. Adjust dosage based on patient's response.

Nursing considerations

⊠ ***Black box warning*** Risk of renal dysfunction, renal failure, or death exists. Monitor patient accordingly.

- Do not administer to patients with history of allergy to gamma globulin or antiimmunoglobulin A antibodies.
- Use IM gamma globulin with caution in patients with thrombocytopenia or any coagulation disorder that would contraindicate IM injections. Use only if benefits outweigh risks.
- Use with caution in pregnant women. **Pregnancy Category C**—safety not established.
- Administer 2 wk before or 3 mo after immune globulin administration because antibodies in the globulin preparation may interfere with the immune response to the vaccination.

⊗ ***Warning*** Have epinephrine 1:1,000 immediately available at time of injection in case of anaphylactic reaction, which is more likely with IV immune globulin, large IM doses, and repeated injections.

- Refrigerate drug; do not freeze. Discard partially used vials.
- Administer IM preparation by IM injection only; do not administer subcutaneously or intradermally.
- Check manufacturer's guidelines before using any immune globulin.
- Administer IV preparation with extreme caution.
- Do not mix immune globulin with any other medications.
- Monitor patient's vital signs continuously and observe for any symptoms during IV administration. Adverse effects appear to be related to the rate of infusion.
- Provide comfort measures or teach patient to provide comfort measures—analgesics, antipyretics, warm soaks to injection site—to help patient to cope with the discomforts of drug therapy.
- Provide patient with written record of injection and dates for follow-up injections as needed.

▽ influenza A (H1N1) 2009 monovalent vaccine

Therapeutic actions
Inactivated type A influenza (H1N1 variant) virus antigens that stimulate production of antibodies specific to the antigens used.

Indications
- Active immunization against influenza caused by pandemic (H1N1) 2009 virus.

Adverse effects
Injection site reactions (redness, warmth, swelling, bruising, pain), headache, diarrhea, rhinitis, fever, flulike syndrome.

Dosage
0.5 mL IM as a single injection.

Nursing considerations
- Do not administer to anyone with immunodeficiency/suppression or malignancy.
- Do not administer with antiviral medications or other immunizations or immune suppressants.
- Caution patient who has just received the vaccine to avoid people who are immune suppressed; the disease could be transmitted to them and they could become ill.
- Do not administer to patient with febrile illness or active, untreated tuberculosis.
- Do not administer to patients with known allergy to components of drug, eggs or chicken protein, neomycin, or polymyxin or to those who have had a life-threatening reaction to influenza vaccine.
- Do not administer to women who are pregnant unless the benefit clearly outweighs the risk.
- Administer by IM injection; inspect solution for particulate matter or discoloration.

⊗ ***Warning*** Have epinephrine 1:1000 immediately available at time of injection in case of anaphylactic reaction.

- Provide comfort measures (analgesics, rest, decongestants) to help patient cope with discomforts of the immunization.
- Provide patient with written record of immunization.

▽influenza A (H1N1) 2009 monovalent vaccine live, intranasal

Therapeutic actions

Live, attenuated type A influenza (H1N1 variant) virus antigens that stimulate production of antibodies specific to the antigens used.

Indications

- Active immunization of patients ages 2–49 yr against influenza caused by pandemic (H1N1) 2009 virus.

Adverse effects

Runny nose, nasal complications, fever, sore throat, decreased appetite, irritability, muscle aches, headache, lethargy.

Dosage

Children and adults 10–49 yr: 0.2 mL (0.1 mL in each nostril).
Children 2–9 yr: Two doses of 0.2 mL each (0.1 mL in each nostril) approximately 1 month apart.

Nursing considerations

- Do not administer to anyone with immunodeficiency/suppression or malignancy.
- Do not administer with antiviral medications or other immunizations or immune suppressants.
- Caution patient who has just received vaccine to avoid people who are immune suppressed; the disease could be transmitted to them and they could become ill.
- Do not administer to patient with febrile illness or active, untreated tuberculosis,
- Do not administer to patients with known allergy to components of drug, eggs or chicken protein, gentamicin, gelatin, or arginine or to those who have had a life-threatening reaction to influenza vaccine.
- Do not administer to patients with asthma or to children younger than 5 yr with recurrent wheezing, which could be exacerbated by the vaccination.
- Do not administer to women who are pregnant unless the benefit clearly outweighs the risk.

⊗ **Warning** Have epinephrine 1:1000 immediately available at time of injection in case of anaphylactic reaction.

- Provide comfort measures (analgesics, rest, decongestants) to help patient cope with discomforts of the immunization.
- Provide patient with written record of immunization. If patient is 2–9 yr, give parents a reminder to return for second dose.

▽influenza virus vaccine

Agriflu, Alfuria, Fluarix, FluLaval, Fluvirin, Fluzone, Fluzone High Dose

Therapeutic actions

Inactivated influenza virus antigens stimulate an active immunity through the production of antibodies specific to the antigens used; the antigens used vary from yr to yr depending on which influenza virus strains are anticipated to be prevalent.

Indications

- Prophylaxis for people at high risk of developing complications from infection with influenza virus, including adults and children with chronic cardiovascular or pulmonary disorders, chronic metabolic disorders, renal impairment, anemia, immunosuppression, asthma; residents of long-term care facilities; medical personnel with extensive contact with high-risk patients, to prevent their transmitting the virus to these patients; children on long-term aspirin therapy who are at high risk of developing Reye's syndrome; people who provide essential community services (to decrease the risk of disruption of services).

- Active immunization against influenza caused by influenza virus types A and B in children 6 mo and older (*Fluzone*), children 4 yr and older (*Fluvirin*), children 3–17 yr and adults (*Fluarix*), adults 18 yr and older (*FluLaval*), adults 65 yr and older at high risk for complications (*Fluzone High Dose*).
- Priority active immunization in patients at high risk for influenza complications when dosages are limited.

Adverse effects

Tenderness, redness, and induration at the injection site; fever, malaise, myalgia; allergic responses—flare, wheal, respiratory symptoms; Guillain-Barré syndrome.

Dosage

- *6–35 mo:* Split virus or purified surface antigen only—0.25 mL IM repeated in 4 wk.
- *3–8 yr:* Split virus or purified surface antigen only—0.5 mL IM repeated in 4 wk.
- *9 yr and older:* Split virus or purified surface antigen—0.5 mL IM.
- *18 yr and older (Fluarix):* 0.5 mL IM using the prefilled syringe. Shake the syringe before use.

Nursing considerations

- Do not administer to patients with sensitivities to eggs, chicken, chicken feathers, or chicken dander. If an allergic condition is suspected, administer a scratch test or an intradermal injection (0.05–0.1 mL) of vaccine diluted 1:100 in sterile saline. A wheal greater than 5 mm justifies withholding immunization.
- Do not administer to patient with a hypersensitivity to any component of the vaccine or history of Guillain-Barré syndrome.
- Do not administer to infants and children at the same time as diphtheria, tetanus toxoid, and pertussis vaccine (DTP) or within 14 days after measles virus vaccine.
- Delay administration in the presence of acute respiratory disease or other active infection or acute febrile illness.
- Use caution in pregnant women. **Pregnancy Category C**—safety not established. Delay use until the second or third trimester to minimize concern over possible teratogenicity.
- Monitor patient for enhanced drug effects and possible toxicity of theophylline, warfarin sodium for as long as 3 wk after vaccine injection.
- Administer IM only. The deltoid muscle is preferred for adults and older children, the anterolateral aspect of the thigh for infants and younger children.
- Consider the possible need for amantadine for therapeutic use for patients in high-risk groups who develop illness compatible with influenza during a period of known influenza A activity in the community.

⊗ ***Warning*** Have epinephrine 1:1,000 immediately available at time of injection in case of anaphylactic reaction.

- Provide comfort measures or teach patient to provide comfort measures—analgesics, antipyretics, warm soaks to injection site—to help patient cope with effects of the drug.
- Provide patient with written record of vaccination and dates of second injection as appropriate.
- Do not use vaccine supplies remaining from previous years for current year vaccination.

influenza virus vaccine, H5N1

H5N1

Therapeutic actions

Contains inactivated type A influenza virus H5N1, which induces antibodies against this viral strain and blocks attachment of the virus to respiratory cells.

Indications

- Active immunization of persons 18–64 yr at increased risk of exposure to H5N1 influenza (avian flu) virus.

Adverse effects

Hypersensitivity reactions; injection site reactions, including warmth, redness, swelling, pain; headache; nausea; fever; symptoms of URI.

Dosage

- *Adults 18–64 yr:* 1 mL IM into deltoid muscle of upper arm, followed by 1 mL IM 21–35 days later.

Nursing considerations

- Virus is grown in chicken eggs; use caution in patients allergic to chickens.
- Use caution in pregnant women; vaccine is **Pregnancy Category C.** Use only if potential benefit outweighs risk to fetus.
- Do not mix in syringe with other vaccines or inject at same site as other vaccines.
- Provide comfort measures as needed, such as analgesics, antipyretics, and warm packs to injection site.
- Give patient a written record of the vaccination and a date to return for the second dose.

influenza virus vaccine, live, intranasal

FluMist

Therapeutic actions

Contains attenuated virus reassortants of the three most commonly encountered viruses each year, as determined by the US Public Health Service; administered intranasally, these antigens produce a protective immunity against these strains.

Indications

- Active immunization for prevention of disease caused by influenza A and B viruses in healthy children, adolescents, and adults 2–49 yr.

Adverse effects

Irritability, *headache;* vomiting; sore throat, *runny nose, cough;* fever, chills, muscle aches, decreased activity, tiredness.

Dosage

- *2–8 yr, not previously vaccinated:* Two doses (0.2 mL each) intranasally, given as one spray (0.1 mL) per nostril, at least 1 month apart.
- *2–8 yr, previously vaccinated:* One dose (0.2 mL) intranasally, given as one spray (0.1 mL) per each nostril.
- *9–49 yr:* One dose (0.5 mL) intranasally each flu season.

- *5–8 yr not previously vaccinated with* FluMist: Two doses (0.5 mL each), given 60 days apart ± 14 days.
- *5–8 yr previously vaccinated with* FluMist: One dose (0.5 mL) per flu season.

Nursing considerations

- Do not administer to anyone with immunodeficiency, immunosuppression, or malignancy.
- Do not administer with any antiviral drugs or with other immunizations.
- Do not administer to a patient with febrile illness.
- Do not administer with aspirin or aspirin-related products in children; these products could mask Reye's syndrome.
- Do not administer to women who are pregnant or nursing a baby. **Pregnancy Category C.**
- Administer this vaccine as one spray in the nostril.
- Provide comfort measures and teach patients to provide comfort measures to help the patient cope with the discomforts of the immunization (analgesics, rest, decongestants).
- Caution patients that they may be able to transmit influenza after they have received the vaccine; they should avoid close contact with any people who may be immunocompromised.
- Provide parents with written record of immunization and reminder that the vaccine is needed every year just before flu season.

measles (rubeola) virus vaccine, live, attenuated

Attenuvax

Therapeutic actions

Attenuated measles virus produces a modified measles infection and stimulates an active immune reaction with antibodies to the measles virus.

Indications

- Immunization against measles (rubeola) immediately after exposure to natural measles; more effective if given before exposure—children 15 mo and older (immunization with trivalent MMR vaccine is the preferred product for routine vaccinations).
- Revaccination for children immunized before age 12 mo or vaccinated with inactivated vaccine alone.
- Prophylaxis for high school or college age persons in epidemic situations or for adults in isolated communities where measles is not endemic.

Adverse effects

Moderate fever, rash; high temperature (less common); febrile convulsions, Guillain-Barré syndrome, ocular palsies (less common); burning or stinging wheal or flare at injection site.

Dosage

Inject the total volume of the reconstituted vaccine or 0.5 mL of multi-dose vial subcutaneously into the outer aspect of the upper arm; dose is the same for all patients.

Nursing considerations

- Do not administer to patients with a history of anaphylactic hypersensitivity to neomycin (contained in injection), to patients with immune deficiency conditions (immunosuppressive therapy with corticosteroids, antineoplastics; neoplasms; immunodeficiency states), to patients receiving immune serum globulin.
- Do not administer to pregnant women. **Pregnancy Category C**—advise patients to avoid pregnancy for 3 mo following vaccination. If measles exposure occurs during pregnancy, provide passive immunity with immune serum globulin.

- Use caution if administering to children with history of febrile convulsions, cerebral injury, or other conditions in which stress due to fever should be avoided.
- Use caution if administering to patient with a history of sensitivity to eggs, chicken, chicken feathers.
- Do not administer within 1 mo of immunization with other live virus vaccines; may be administered concurrently with monovalent or trivalent polio vaccine, rubella vaccine, mumps vaccine.
- Do not administer for at least 3 mo following blood or plasma transfusions or administration of serum immune globulin.
- Monitor for possible depression of tuberculin skin sensitivity; administer test before or simultaneously with vaccine.
- Administer with a sterile syringe free of preservatives, antiseptics, and detergents for each injection (these may inactivate the live virus vaccine). Use a 23-gauge, ⅝-inch needle.
- Refrigerate unreconstituted vial; protect from exposure to light. Use only the diluent supplied with the vaccine and reconstitute just before using. Discard reconstituted vaccine if not used within 8 hr.

⊗ ***Warning*** Have epinephrine 1:1,000 immediately available at time of injection in case of anaphylactic reaction.

- Provide comfort measures or teach patient or parent to provide comfort measures to help patient to cope with the discomforts of drug therapy: analgesics, antipyretics, warm soaks to injection site.
- Provide patient or parent with a written record of immunization.

▽ measles, mumps, rubella vaccine, live (MMR)

M-M-R II

Therapeutic actions

Attenuated measles, mumps, and rubella viruses produce a modified infection and stimulate an active immune reaction with antibodies to these viruses.

Indications

- Immunization against measles, mumps, rubella in children older than 15 mo and adults.

Adverse effects

Moderate fever, rash, burning or stinging wheal or flare at injection site, high temperature; less common: febrile convulsions, Guillain-Barré syndrome, ocular palsies.

Dosage

0.5 mL reconstituted vaccine subcutaneously into the outer aspect of the upper arm. Dose is the same for all patients. Booster dose is recommended on entry into school and again at entry into junior high school.

Nursing considerations

- Do not administer to patients with a history of anaphylactic hypersensitivity to neomycin (contained in injection), to patients with immune deficiency conditions (immunosuppressive therapy with corticosteroids, antineoplastics; neoplasms; immunodeficiency states), to patients receiving immune serum globulin.
- Do not administer to pregnant women. **Pregnancy Category C**—advise patients to avoid pregnancy for 3 mo following vaccination. If measles exposure occurs during pregnancy, provide passive immunity with immune serum globulin.

- Use caution if administering to children with history of febrile convulsions, cerebral injury, or other conditions in which stress due to fever should be avoided.
- Use caution if administering to patient with a history of sensitivity to eggs, chicken, chicken feathers.
- Do not administer within 1 mo of immunization with other live virus vaccines; may be administered concurrently with monovalent or trivalent polio vaccine, rubella vaccine, mumps vaccine.
- Do not administer for at least 3 mo following blood or plasma transfusions or administration of serum immune globulin.
- Monitor for possible depression of tuberculin skin sensitivity. Administer the test before or simultaneously with the vaccine.
- Administer with a sterile syringe free of preservatives, antiseptics, and detergents for each injection (these may inactivate the live virus vaccine). Use a 25-gauge, ⅝-inch needle.
- Refrigerate unreconstituted vial. Protect from exposure to light. Use only the diluent supplied with the vaccine and reconstitute just before using. Discard reconstituted vaccine if not used within 8 hr.

⊗ ***Warning*** Have epinephrine 1:1,000 immediately available at time of injection in case of anaphylactic reaction.

- Provide comfort measures or teach patient or parent to provide comfort measures to help patient cope with the discomforts of drug therapy (analgesics, antipyretics, warm soaks to injection site).
- Provide patient or parent with a written record of immunization.
- Trivalent measles, mumps, and rubella vaccine is the vaccination of choice for routine vaccinations. Another combination—rubella and mumps vaccine (*Biavax II*)—is used for specific situations.

▽ measles, mumps, rubella, and varicella virus vaccine, live

ProQuad

Therapeutic actions

Attenuated measles, mumps, rubella, and varicella viruses produce a modified infection and stimulate an active immune reaction with antibodies to these viruses.

Indications

- Active immunization of children ages 12 mo–12 yr, for the prevention of measles, mumps, rubella, and varicella virus infections.

Adverse effects

Irritability; diarrhea, fever, chills, muscle aches, injection site reactions; less common—fever, convulsions, ocular palsies.

Dosage

0.5 mL by subcutaneous injection; allow 1 mo to elapse between the administration of any vaccine containing measles antigens and the administration of *ProQuad*; if a second varicella vaccine is needed, allow 3 mo between administration of the two doses.

Nursing considerations

- Do not administer to anyone with immunodeficiency/suppression or malignancy.
- Do not administer with any antiviral medications or with other immunizations or immune suppressants.

- Do not administer in the presence of febrile illness or with active, untreated TB.
- Do not administer to a patient with known allergy to any component of the drug, gelatin, or neomycin.
- Do not administer with aspirin or aspirin-related products in children. These products could mask the presence of Reye's syndrome; advise parents not to use aspirin for 6 wk following the vaccination.
- Do not administer to women who are pregnant or nursing. **Pregnancy Category C**—safety not established.
- Administer by subcutaneous injection only; inspect solution for particulate matter.
- Administer immediately after reconstituting with provided sterile water.

⊗ ***Warning*** Have epinephrine 1:1,000 immediately available at time of injection in case of anaphylactic reaction.

- Provide comfort measures or teach parents to provide comfort measures to help the patient cope with the discomforts of the immunization (analgesics, rest, decongestants).
- Provide parents with written record of immunization.

▽ mumps virus vaccine, live

Mumpsvax

Therapeutic actions

Viral antigen stimulates active immunity through production of antibodies to the mumps virus.

Indications

- Immunization against mumps in children older than 12 mo and adults. (Trivalent measles, mumps, and rubella vaccine is the drug of choice for routine vaccinations.)

Adverse effects

Fever, parotitis, orchitis; purpura and allergic reactions such as wheal and flare at injection site; febrile seizures, unilateral nerve deafness, encephalitis—rare; anaphylactic reactions.

Dosage

Inject total volume (0.5 mL) of reconstituted vaccine subcutaneously into the outer aspect of the upper arm; each dose contains not less than 20,000 $TCID_{50}$ (Tissue Culture Infectious Doses) of mumps virus vaccine. (Vaccine is available only in single-dose vials of diluent.)

Nursing considerations

⊠ ***Black box warning*** Be aware that the trivalent measles, mumps, and rubella vaccine is preferred.

- Do not administer to patients with history of hypersensitivity to neomycin (each single-dose vial of vaccine contains 25 mcg neomycin); immune deficiency conditions. **Pregnancy Category C**—advise patient to avoid pregnancy for 3 mo after vaccination.
- Use caution if administering to a patient with history of allergy to eggs, chicken, or chicken feathers.
- Delay administration in the presence of active infection.
- Do not administer within 1 mo of immunization with other live virus vaccines, but it may be administered concurrently with live monovalent or trivalent polio vaccine, live rubella vaccine, live measles vaccine.
- Do not administer for at least 3 mo following blood or plasma transfusions or administration of serum immune globulin.
- Monitor for possible depression of tuberculin skin sensitivity; administer test before or simultaneously with the vaccine.

- Administer with a sterile syringe free of preservatives, antiseptics, and detergents for each injection (these may inactivate the live virus vaccine). Use a 25-gauge, ⅝-inch needle.
- Refrigerate unreconstituted vial. Protect from exposure to light.
- Use only the diluent supplied with the vaccine and reconstitute just before using. Discard reconstituted vaccine if not used within 8 hr.

⊗ **Warning** Have epinephrine 1:1,000 immediately available at time of injection in case of anaphylactic reaction.

- Provide comfort measures or teach patient or parent to provide comfort measures to help patient cope with the discomforts of drug therapy (analgesics, antipyretics, warm soaks to injection site).
- Provide patient or parent with a written record of vaccination.

pneumococcal vaccine, polyvalent

Pneumovax 23

Therapeutic actions

Polysaccharide capsules of the 23 most prevalent or invasive pneumococcal types stimulate active immunity through antipneumococcal antibody production against the capsule types contained in the vaccine.

Indications

- Immunization against pneumococcal pneumonia and bacteremia caused by the types of pneumococci included in the vaccine, specifically in children older than 2 yr and adults with chronic illnesses or who are immunocompromised and at increased risk for pneumococcal infections.
- Prophylaxis in children 2 yr and older with asymptomatic or symptomatic HIV infections.
- Prophylaxis in community groups at high risk for pneumococcal infections—institutionalized persons, groups in an area of outbreak, patients at high risk of influenza complications, including pneumococcal infection.

Adverse effects

Erythema, induration, soreness at injection site; fever, myalgia; acute febrile reactions, rash, arthralgia (less common); paresthesias, acute radiculoneuropathy (rare); anaphylactic reaction.

Dosage

One 0.5-mL dose subcutaneously or IM. Not recommended for children younger than 2 yr.

Nursing considerations

- Do not administer to patients with hypersensitivity to any component of the vaccine or with previous immunization with any polyvalent pneumococcal vaccine.
- Do not administer less than 10 days before or during treatment for Hodgkin's lymphoma.
- Use caution if administering to patients who are nursing or pregnant. **Pregnancy Category C**—safety not established.
- Use caution if administering to patients with cardiac, pulmonary disorders; systemic reaction could pose a significant risk.
- May be administered concomitantly with influenza virus vaccine by separate injection in the other arm.
- Administer subcutaneously or IM only, preferably in the deltoid muscle or lateral mid-thigh; do not give IV.
- Refrigerate vials. Use directly as supplied; do not dilute (reconstitution is not necessary).

⊗ **Warning** Have epinephrine 1:1,000 immediately available at time of injection in case of anaphylactic reaction.

- Provide or teach patient to provide appropriate comfort measures—analgesics, antipyretics, warm soaks to injection site—to help patient to cope with effects of the drug therapy.
- Provide patient with written record of immunization and caution patient not to have another polyvalent pneumococcal vaccine injection.

▽ pneumococcal 7-valent conjugate vaccine (diphtheria CRM_{197} protein)

Prevnar

Therapeutic actions

Stimulates active immunity against disease caused by *Streptococcus pneumoniae* by introduction of seven capsular serotypes.

Indications

- Prevention of invasive *S. pneumoniae* disease in infants and toddlers; for use in all children younger than 23 mo. For high-risk populations age 24–59 mo, including children with sickle cell anemia, HIV, functional or anatomic asplenia, other immunocompromised conditions, and Native Americans and Alaskan natives.
- Active immunization of infants and toddlers against otitis media caused by vaccine serotypes.
- Prevention of otitis media caused by resistant strains.

Adverse effects

Fretfulness; drowsiness; anorexia; vomiting; transient fever; malaise; generalized aches and pains; edema of injection area with redness, swelling, induration, pain (may persist for a few days); hypersensitivity reactions.

Dosage

0.5 mg IM, preferably injected in the anterolateral aspect of the thigh in infants and the deltoid muscle of the upper arm in older children.

- *7–11 mo:* Three doses with two doses at least 4 wk apart and last dose at older than 1 yr of age.
- *12–23 mo:* Two doses spaced at least 2 mo apart.
- *24 mo–9 yr:* One dose.

Nursing considerations

- Defer administration of routine immunizing or booster doses in case of acute infection or febrile illness.
- Not for treatment of acute pneumococcal infections.
- Shake vigorously before use. Do not use if a uniform suspension is not attained.
- Administer by IM injection only; avoid subcutaneous or IV injection. Do not inject vaccine in gluteal area.

⊗ **Warning** Arrange for epinephrine 1:1,000 to be immediately available at time of injection because of risk of hypersensitivity reactions.

- Provide comfort measures to help patient cope with the discomforts of the injection (analgesics, warm soaks for injection site, small meals, environmental control of temperature and stimuli).
- Provide parent with written record of immunization and reminder of when additional injections are needed.

poliovirus vaccine, inactivated (IPV, Salk)

IPOL

Therapeutic actions

Inactivated, attenuated sterile suspension of three types of poliovirus used to produce antibody response against poliomyelitis infection.

Indications

- Prevention of poliomyelitis caused by poliovirus types 1, 2, and 3 as routine immunization of infants and children.

Adverse effects

Local reaction at site of injection within 48 hr.

Dosage

- *Children:* 0.5 mL subcutaneously at 2 mo, 4 mo, and 6–18 mo. A booster dose is needed at time of entry into elementary school.
- *Adults:* Not usually needed in adults in the United States; if unimmunized adult is exposed, is traveling to a high-risk area, or is a household contact of children receiving IPV (inactivated poliovirus vaccine; Salk vaccine) immunization is recommended. 0.5 mL subcutaneously: two doses given at 1- to 2-mo intervals and a third dose given 6–12 mo later. Previously vaccinated adults at risk for exposure should receive a 0.5-mL dose of this drug.

Nursing considerations

- Do not administer to patients with known hypersensitivity to streptomycin or neomycin (each dose contains less than 25 mcg of each).
- Defer administration in the presence of persistent vomiting or diarrhea and in patients with acute illness or any advanced debilitating condition.
- Do not administer to any patient with immune deficiency conditions; do not administer shortly after immune serum globulin (ISG) unless necessary because of travel or exposure; if given with or shortly after ISG dose should be repeated after 3 mo.
- Use caution if administering to pregnant patients. **Pregnancy Category C**—safety not established; use only if clearly needed and benefits outweigh potential unknown effects on the fetus.
- Refrigerate vaccine. Do not freeze.
- Provide patient or parent with a written record of the vaccination and information on when additional doses are needed.

RH_o (D) immune globulin

HyperRHO S/D Full Dose, RhoGAM

RH_o (D) immune globulin micro-dose

HyperRHO S/D Minidose, MICRhoGAM

RH_o (D) immune globulin IV (human) (RH_o D IGIV)

Rhophylac, WinRho SDF

Therapeutic actions

Suppresses the immune response of nonsensitized Rh_0-negative individuals who receive Rh_0-positive blood as the result of a fetomaternal hemorrhage or a transfusion accident; each vial of Rh_0-immune globulin completely suppresses immunity to 15 mL of Rh-positive packed RBCs (about 30 mL whole blood); each vial of Rh_0 immune globulin micro-dose suppresses immunity to 2.5 mL Rh-positive packed RBCs.

Indications

- Prevention of sensitization to the Rh_0 factor.
- To prevent hemolytic disease of the newborn (erythroblastosis fetalis) in a subsequent pregnancy—mother must be Rh_0 negative; mother must not be previously sensitized to Rh_0 factor; infant must be Rh_0 positive and direct antiglobulin negative—used at full-term delivery, for incomplete pregnancy, for antepartum prophylaxis in case of abortion or ectopic pregnancy.
- To prevent Rh_0 sensitization in Rh_0-negative patients accidentally transfused with Rh_0-positive blood.
- To raise platelet count in Rh_0-positive adults with intact spleen and immune thrombocytopenic purpura (ITP).

Adverse effects

Pain and soreness at injection site.

Dosage

- *Postpartum prophylaxis:* One vial IM or IV (*WinRho SDF*) within 72 hr of delivery.
- *Antepartum prophylaxis:* One vial IM or IV (*WinRho SDF*) at 28 wk gestation and one vial within 72 hr after an Rh-incompatible delivery to prevent Rh isoimmunization during pregnancy.
- *Following amniocentesis, miscarriage, abortion, ectopic pregnancy at or beyond 13 wk gestation:* One vial IM or IV.
- *Transfusion accidents:* Multiply the volume in mL of Rh-positive whole blood administered by the Hct of the donor unit and divide this volume (in mL) by 15 to obtain the number of vials to be administered. If results of calculation are a fraction, administer the next whole number of vials.
- *ITP:* 250 international units/kg IV at 2 mL/15–60 sec.
- *Spontaneous abortion, induced abortion, or termination of ectopic pregnancy up to and including 12 wk gestation (unless the father is Rh negative):* One vial micro-dose IM given as soon as possible after termination of pregnancy.

Nursing considerations

- Rh_0 globulin is not needed in Rh_0-negative mothers if the father can be determined to be Rh_0 negative.
- Do not administer to the Rh_0-positive postpartum infant, to an Rh_0-positive individual, to an Rh_0-negative individual previously sensitized to the Rh_0 antigen (if it is not known whether a woman is Rh_0 sensitized, administer the Rh_0 globulin).
- Before administration, determine the infant's blood type and arrange for a direct antiglobulin test using umbilical cord, venous, or capillary blood; confirm that the mother is Rh_0 negative.

⊗ **Warning** Do not administer *HyperRHO S/D, RhoGam* IV; administer IM within 72 hr after Rh_0-incompatible delivery, miscarriage, abortion, or transfusion.

- For IM use, prepare one vial dose by withdrawing entire contents of vial; inject entire contents.
- For IM use, prepare two or more vial doses using 5- to 10-mL syringes. Withdraw contents from the vials to be administered at one time and inject. Contents of the total number of vials may be injected as a divided dose at different injection sites at the same time, or the total dosage may be divided and injected at intervals, as long as the total dose is administered within 72 hr postpartum or after a transfusion accident.

- Refrigerate vials; do not freeze.
- Provide appropriate comfort measures if injection sites are painful.
- Reassure patient and explain what has been given and why; the patient needs to know what was given in the event of future pregnancies.

rotavirus vaccine, live, oral pentavalent

Rotarix, RotaTeq

Therapeutic actions

Live, reassortant rotaviruses that replicate in the small intestine and stimulate an active immunity to prevent rotavirus gastroenteritis.

Indications

- Prevention of rotavirus gastroenteritis in infants and children.

Adverse effects

Irritability; diarrhea, vomiting, fever, pneumonia, gastroenteritis, UTI.

Dosage

- Three ready-to-use liquid pouch doses (2 mL each) PO starting at age 6–12 wk, with subsequent doses at 4–10 wk intervals (third dose should not be given after age 32 wk) (*RotaTeq*).
- Two doses of 1 mL each PO beginning at age 6 wk. Allow 4 wk before the second dose. Series must be completed by age 24 wk (*Rotarix*).

Nursing considerations

- Do not administer to anyone with immunodeficiency, immunosuppression, or malignancy.
- Do not administer in the presence of febrile illness.
- Do not administer to a patient with a known allergy to any component of the drug.
- Do not administer to women who are pregnant or nursing. **Pregnancy Category C.**
- Do not have close contact with people with malignancies or who are immune compromised; live virus may shed.
- Provide comfort measures or teach parents to provide comfort measures to help patient cope with discomforts of immunization. Provide analgesics, fluids, and limited diet.
- Provide parents with written record of immunization.

rubella virus vaccine, live

Meruvax II

Therapeutic actions

Live virus stimulates active immunity through development of antibodies against the rubella virus.

Indications

- Immunization against rubella—children 12 mo of age to puberty, adolescent and adult males, nonpregnant adolescent and adult females, rubella-susceptible women in the postpartum period, leukemia patients in remission whose chemotherapy has been terminated for at least 3 mo, susceptible persons traveling abroad.
- Revaccination of children vaccinated at younger than 12 mo.

Adverse effects

Burning, stinging at injection site; regional lymphadenopathy, urticaria, rash, malaise, sore throat, fever, headache, polyneuritis—symptoms similar to natural rubella; arthritis, arthralgia—often 2–4 wk after receiving the vaccine.

Dosage

Inject total volume of reconstituted vaccine subcutaneously into the outer aspect of the upper arm; each dose contains not less than 1,000 $TCID_{50}$ (Tissue Culture Infectious Doses) of rubella.

Nursing considerations

⊗ ***Black box warning*** Be aware that the measles, mumps, and rubella vaccine is preferred for immunization.

- Do not administer to patients with a history of anaphylactic hypersensitivity to neomycin (each dose contains 25 mcg neomycin), to patients with immune deficiency conditions, to patients receiving immune serum globulin or blood transfusions.
- Do not administer to pregnant women. **Pregnancy Category C**—advise patients to avoid pregnancy for 3 mo following vaccination.
- Defer administration in the presence of acute respiratory or other active infections; susceptible children with mild illnesses may be vaccinated.
- Do not administer within 1 mo of immunization with other live virus vaccines, except that rubella vaccine may be administered concurrently with live monovalent or trivalent polio vaccine, live measles virus vaccine, live mumps vaccine.
- Do not administer for at least 3 mo following blood or plasma transfusions or administration of serum immune globulin.
- Monitor for possible depression of tuberculin skin sensitivity; administer the test before or simultaneously with the vaccine.
- Refrigerate vials and protect from light. Reconstitute using only the diluent supplied with the vial; use as soon as possible after reconstitution; discard reconstituted vaccine if not used within 8 hr.
- Provide or instruct patient to provide appropriate comfort measures to help patient cope with the adverse effects of the drug—analgesics, antipyretics, fluids, rest.
- Provide patient or parent with a written record of immunization; advise that revaccination is not necessary.

▽ rubella and mumps virus vaccine, live

Biavax II

Therapeutic actions

Viral antigens stimulate active immunity against rubella and mumps through production of antibodies to both the rubella and mumps viruses.

Indications

- Simultaneous immunization against rubella and mumps in children older than 12 mo, preferably at 15 mo.

Adverse effects

Fretfulness; drowsiness; anorexia; vomiting; transient fever; malaise; generalized aches and pains; edema of injection area with redness, swelling, induration, pain (may persist for a few days); hypersensitivity reactions

Dosage
0.5 mg subcutaneously preferably injected in the outer aspect of the upper arm. Booster doses at the age of entry into kindergarten and again in junior high school are preferably done using a trivalent measles, mumps, and rubella vaccine.

Nursing considerations
- Defer administration of routine immunizing or booster doses in case of acute infection.
- Use only the diluent supplied to reconstitute. Protect from light. Discard after 8 hr.
- Not for treatment of acute infections.
- Administer by subcutaneous injection only; not for IM or IV injection.

⊗ ***Warning*** Arrange for epinephrine 1:1,000 to be immediately available at time of injection in case of hypersensitivity reaction.

- Provide comfort measures to help patient cope with the discomforts of the injection (analgesics, warm soaks for injection site, small meals, environmental control of temperature and stimuli).
- Provide parent with written record of immunization and reminder of when additional injections are needed.

smallpox vaccine
Dryvax

Therapeutic actions
A live-virus preparation of vaccinia virus prepared from calf lymph, which stimulates immunity and cellular hypersensitivity to the smallpox virus.

Indications
- Active immunization against smallpox disease.

Adverse effects
Fever, regional lymphadenopathy, malaise; generalized rashes (erythematous, urticarial nonspecific) spread of inoculation to sites other than site administered; rarely: Stevens-Johnson syndrome or other severe reactions including encephalitis, encephalopathy, progressive vaccinia, eczema vaccinatum with severe disability or death.

Dosage
- Primary vaccination: Using the vaccinating needle, two or three punctures into a prepared, dried area on the upper deltoid muscle or the posterior aspect of the arm over the triceps muscle onto which a drop of the live vaccine has been placed. Inspect the site for reaction after 6–8 days; if a major reaction has occurred, the site will scab over and heal, leaving a scar. If a mild or equivocal reaction has occurred, review the vaccination technique and repeat the process using 15 punctures into the area where a drop of vaccine has been placed.

Nursing considerations
- Follow the procedure for reconstitution of the vaccine precisely. Date vial and store only up to 15 days.
- Using strict sterile technique and wearing protective gloves, follow guidelines for use of the vaccine: clean and dry area, place one drop of vaccine on the area, and use the supplied bifurcated needle to puncture the skin enough to see blood appear.
- Dispose of the needles and vaccine appropriately.
- Do not administer if the patient has a febrile illness.
- Do not administer by IM, subcutaneous, or IV routes.

- Do not administer to anyone with allergies to any component of the vaccine, including polymyxin B sulfate, dihydrostreptomycin, chlortetracycline, or neomycin.
- Do not administer to anyone with eczema or with a past history of eczema or those with household contact with people who have eczema or exfoliative skin conditions.
- Do not administer to anyone taking systemic corticosteroids or immunosuppressive drugs or who is immunocompromised.
- Do not administer to anyone who is pregnant or to household contacts of anyone who is pregnant. **Pregnancy Category C.**
- Provide comfort measures and teach parents to provide comfort measures to help the patient cope with the discomforts of the injection: analgesics, small meals, environmental control (of temperature and stimuli).
- Leave the vaccination area uncovered, or cover the area with a loose bandage until the scab has fallen off and the area is healing. Do not use salves or lotions on the site. Caution the patient not to touch or scratch the area. Strict handwashing technique is advised after changing the dressing or touching the area. Bandages should be disposed of properly to avoid contact with other areas or other people.
- Arrange for the patient to have the site inspected 6–8 days after the inoculation. If a major reaction does not occur, the patient should be revaccinated.
- Provide parents with written record of immunization and reminder of when booster injection is needed.

typhoid vaccine

Typhim Vi, Typhoid Vaccine HP, Vivotif Berna

Therapeutic actions

Contains live attenuated strains of typhoid bacteria; produces a humoral antibody response against the causative agent of typhoid fever. Precise mechanism of action is not understood.

Indications

- Active immunization against typhoid fever (*Typhim Vi, Vivotif Berna*).
- Immunization of adults and children against disease caused by *Salmonella typhi* (routine immunization is not recommended in the United States but is recommended for travelers, workers in microbiology fields, or those who may come into household contact with typhoid fever).

Adverse effects

Transient fever; edema of injection area with redness, swelling, induration, pain (may persist for a few days); headache, malaise.

Dosage

- Parenteral (*HP*). *Older than 10 yr:* 2 doses of 0.5 mL subcutaneously at intervals of 4 wk or longer. *10 yr or younger:* Two doses of 0.25 mL subcutaneously at 4-wk or longer intervals.
- Booster dose (given every 3 yr in cases of continued exposure). *Older than 10 yr:* 0.5 mL subcutaneously or 0.1 mL intradermally. *6 mo–10 yr:* 0.25 mL subcutaneously or 0.1 mL intradermally.
- Parenteral (*Typhim Vi*). *Children 2 yr and older:* 0.5 mL IM; booster dose every 2 yr: 0.5 mL IM.
- Oral (*Vivotif Berna*). *Patients older than 6 yr:* One capsule on days 1, 3, 5, and 7 taken 1 hr before a meal with a cold or lukewarm drink. There are no data on the need for a booster dose at this time; 4 capsules on alternating days—once every 5 yr is suggested.
- Complete vaccine regimen 1–2 wk before potential exposure.

Nursing considerations

- Use caution with pregnancy. **Pregnancy Category C**—safety not established.
- Defer administration in case of acute infection, GI illness, nausea, vomiting.
- Have patient swallow capsules whole; do not chew. All four doses must be taken to ensure antibody response.
- Administer *Typhim Vi* parenteral doses by IM injection; deltoid muscle is the preferred site. *Typhoid Vaccine HP* is administered subcutaneously. Booster doses may be given intradermally.

⊗ ***Warning*** Arrange for epinephrine 1:1,000 to be immediately available at time of injection because of risk of hypersensitivity reactions.

- Provide comfort measures to help patient cope with the discomforts of the injection (analgesics, warm soaks for injection site, small meals, environmental control of temperature and stimuli).
- Provide patient with written record of immunization and information on booster immunization if appropriate.
- Vaccines must be kept refrigerated. Do not freeze injectable products.

varicella virus vaccine, live

Varivax

Therapeutic actions

Contains live attenuated varicella virus obtained from human or guinea pig cell cultures. Varicella virus causes chickenpox in children and adults. Vaccine produces an active immunity to the virus; longevity of immunity is not known.

Indications

- Active immunization of adults and children 12 mo or older against chickenpox (varicella).

Adverse effects

Transient fever; edema of injection area with redness, swelling, induration, pain (may persist for a few days); upper respiratory illness, cough, rash.

Dosage

- *Adult and patients 13 yr and older:* 0.5 mL subcutaneously in the deltoid area followed by 0.5 mL 4–8 wk later.
- *Children 1–12 yr:* Single 0.5-mL dose subcutaneously.

Nursing considerations

- Use caution with allergy to neomycin or gelatin; use caution in pregnancy. **Pregnancy Category C**—safety not established.
- Defer administration in case of acute infection and for at least 5 mo after plasma transfusion or receipt of immune globulin, other immunizations.
- Do not administer salicylates for up to 6 wk after immunization; cases of Reye's syndrome have been reported.
- Use reconstituted vaccine within 30 min. Only use diluent supplied.
- Administer by subcutaneous injection. Outer aspect of upper arm is preferred site.

⊗ ***Warning*** Arrange for epinephrine 1:1,000 to be immediately available at time of injection because of risk of hypersensitivity reactions.

- Provide comfort measures to help patient cope with the discomforts of the injection (analgesics, warm soaks for injection site, small meals, environmental control of temperature and stimuli).

- Provide patient with written record of immunization. It is not known whether booster immunization will be needed.

zoster vaccine, live

Zostavax

Therapeutic actions

Attenuated, live varicella-zoster virus causes a boost in the varicella-zoster virus immunity in older individuals; stimulating production of their own varicella-zoster virus antibodies. Herpes zoster, which causes shingles, is a reactivation of the varicella-zoster virus that causes chickenpox.

Indications

Prevention of herpes zoster (shingles) in patients older than 60 yr.

Adverse effects

Injection site reactions (redness, warmth, swelling, bruising, pain), headache, diarrhea, rhinitis, fever, flulike symptoms.

Dosage

One injection of the single-dose vaccine by subcutaneous injection in the upper arm. Vaccine should be frozen and reconstituted, using the supplied diluent, immediately after removal from the freezer; administer immediately after reconstituting.

Nursing considerations

- Do not administer to anyone with immunodeficiency/suppression or malignancy.
- Do not administer with any antiviral medications or with other immunizations or immune suppressants.
- Caution patient to avoid people who are immune suppressed after they receive the vaccine; the disease could be transmitted to them and they could become ill.
- Do not administer in the presence of febrile illness or with active, untreated tuberculosis.
- Do not administer to a patient with known allergy to any component of the drug, gelatin, or neomycin.
- Do not administer to women who are pregnant; recommend use of contraceptive measures at time of vaccination and for 3 mo after the injection. **Pregnancy Category C**—safety not established.
- Administer by subcutaneous injection only; inspect solution for particulate matter.
- Administer immediately after reconstituting with provided diluent.

⊗ ***Warning*** Have epinephrine 1:1,000 immediately available at time of injection in case of anaphylactic reaction.

- Provide comfort measures to help the patient cope with the discomforts of the immunization—analgesics, rest, decongestants.
- Provide patient with written record of immunization.

Other biologicals

Name	Indications	Instructions
Immune globulins		
anti-thymocyte globulin (*Thymoglobulin*)	Treatment of renal transplant acute rejection in conjunction with immunosuppression.	1.5 mg/kg/day for 7–14 days as 6-hr IV infusion for first dose and at least 4 hr each subsequent dose. Store in refrigerator and use within 4 hr of reconstitution.
botulism immune globulin (*BabyBIG*)	Treatment of patients younger than 1 yr with infant botulism caused by toxin A or B.	1 mL/kg as a single IV infusion as soon as diagnosis has been made.
cytomegalovirus immune globulin IV (CMV-IGIV) (*CytoGam*)	Attenuation of primary CMV disease following renal, lung, liver, pancreas, and heart transplant.	15 mg/kg IV over 30 min, increase to 30 mg/kg IV for 30 min, then 60 mg/kg IV to a maximum of 150 mg/kg. Infuse at 72 hr, 2 wk, and then 4, 6, 8, 12, and 16 wk. Monitor for allergic reactions. Use within 6 hr of entering vial. Administer through an IV line with an in-line filter (15 micron).
lymphocyte, immune globulin (*Atgam*)	Management of allograft rejection in renal transplants; treatment of aplastic anemia.	10–30 mg/kg/day IV adult transplant; 5–25 mg/kg/day IV pediatric transplant, 10–20 mg/kg/day IV for 8–14 days for aplastic anemia. Stable for up to 12 hr after reconstitution. Administer a skin test prior to administration of first dose.
rabies immune globulin (*HyperRab S/D, Imogam Rabies-HT*)	Passive protection against rabies in nonimmunized patients with exposure to rabies.	20 international units/kg IM as single dose at same time as rabies vaccine. Infuse wound area if possible. Never give in same site as vaccine. Refrigerate vial.
tetanus immune globulin (*BayTet*)	Passive immunization against tetanus, useful at time of injury.	250 units IM. Do not give IV. Arrange proper medical care of wound.
vaccina immune globulin IV (*VIGIV*)	Treatment or modification of vaccina infections.	2 mL/kg (100 mg/kg) IV.
varicella-zoster immune globulin (*Varicella-Zoster Immune Globulin*)	Passive immunity for immunosuppressed patients with significant exposure to varicella.	125 units/10 kg IM to a maximum of 625 units. Administer within 96 hr of exposure to chickenpox. Not for use in nonimmunosuppressed individuals. Give no more than 2.5 mL at a single site.

Name	Indications	Instructions
Antitoxins and antivenins		
antivenin (crotalidae) polyvalent	Neutralize the venom of pit vipers, including rattlesnakes, copperheads.	20–40 mL IV; up to 100–150 mL IV in severe cases. Removal of venom should be done at once; antivenin to rare breeds of snake may be available from the CDC.
antivenin (micrurus fulvius)	Neutralize the venom of coral snakes in the United States.	30–50 mL by slow IV injection. Give first 1 to 2 mL over 3–5 min and observe for allergic reaction. Flush with IV fluids after antivenin has been infused. May require up to 100 mL.
Black Widow spider species antivenin (*Antivenin Latrodectus mactans*)	Treatment of symptoms of Black Widow spider bites.	2.5 mL IM; may be given IV in 10–50 mL saline over 15 min. Ensure supportive therapy and use of muscle relaxants.
crotalidae polyvalent immune fab (ovine) (*CroFab*)	Treatment of rattlesnake bites.	4–6 vials IV; may be repeated based on patient response. Dilute each vial with 10 mL sterile water, then with 250 mL 0.9% sodium chloride. Give each 250 mL over 60 min. Contains specific antibody fragments that bind to four different rattlesnake toxins. Removal of venom should be done at once. Monitor patient carefully for hypersensitivity reaction. Most effective if given within first 6 hr after snake bite.
Bacterial vaccines		
BCG (*TICE BCG*)	Exposure to TB of skin test—negative infants and children; treatment of groups with high rates or TB; travel to areas with high rates of endemic TB.	0.2–0.3 mL percutaneous using a sterile multipuncture disc. Refrigerate, protect from light; keep the vaccination site clean until reaction disappears.
meningococcal polysaccharide diphtheria toxoid conjugate vaccine (*Menactra*)	Active immunization of patients 2–55 yr to prevent invasive meningococcal disease caused by *N. meningitidis* subgroups A, C, Y, and W-135.	0.5 mL IM; need for booster is not known. Monitor for injection site reaction.
meningococcal polysaccharide vaccine (*Menomune-A/C/Y/W-135*)	Prevention of meningitis in patients at risk in epidemic or highly endemic areas; prophylaxis for college freshmen living in dormitories.	0.5 mL subcutaneously. May revaccinate with 0.5 mL in high-risk patients. Consider revaccination within 3–5 yr. Reconstitute with diluent provided.

Name	Indications	Instructions
Viral vaccines		
Japanese encephalitis vaccine (*JE-VAX*)	Active immunization in persons older than 1 yr who will reside or travel in areas where it is endemic or epidemic.	3 subcutaneous doses of 1 mL given at days 0, 7, and 30; children 1–3 yr: three subcutaneous doses of 0.5 mL. Refrigerate vial. Do not remove rubber stopper. Do not travel within 10 days of vaccination.
Japanese encephalitis vaccine, inactivated, adsorbed (*Ixiaro*)	Active immunization for prevention of disease caused by Japanese encephalitis virus (JEV) in patients 17 yr and older	2 doses of 0.5 mL each IM, given 28 days apart. Series should be completed at least 1 week before exposure to JEV. Contains protamine sulfate; not for use in pregnant or nursing women.
rabies vaccine (*Imovax Rabies, RabAvert*)	Preexposure rabies immunization for patients in high-risk area; postexposure antirabies regimen in conjunction with rabies immunoglobulin.	Preexposure: 1 mL IM on days 0, 7, and 21 or 28. Postexposure: 1 mL IM on days 0, 3, 7, 14, and 28. Refrigerate. If titers are low, booster may be needed.
yellow fever vaccine (*YF-Vax*)	Immunization of travelers to endemic areas.	0.5 mL subcutaneously. Booster dose suggested every 10 yr. Use cautiously with allergy to chicken or egg products.

Appendix W

Less commonly used drugs

abatacept

Orencia

Drug class and indications

Immune modulator, antiarthritic

Reduction of the signs and symptoms, including major clinical response, slowing the progression of structural damage, and improving physical function in adult patients with moderately to severely active rheumatoid arthritis who have had an inadequate response to one or more disease-modifying antirheumatic drugs, as monotherapy or in combination with other drugs other than tumor necrosis factor (TNF) antagonists.

Reduction of signs and symptoms of moderately active polyarticular juvenile idiopathic arthritis in children 6 yr and older as monotherapy or in combination with methotrexate.

Dosages and special alerts

Adults: Less than 60 kg: 500 mg IV over 30 min, repeated at 2 and 4 wk, then every 4 wk. 60–100 kg: 750 mg IV over 30 min, repeated at 2 and 4 wk, then every 4 wk. More than 100 kg: 1 g IV over 30 min, repeated at 2 and 4 wk, then every 4 wk. Pediatric patients: Less than 75 kg: 10 mg/kg IV over 30 min repeated at 2 and 4 wk, then every 4 wk. Maximum dose: 1,000 mg. 75–100 kg: 750 mg IV over 30 min, repeated at 2 and 4 wk, then every 4 wk. More than 100 kg: 1,000 mg IV over 30 min, repeated at 2 and 4 wk, then every 4 wk. Risk of serious infection with TNF antagonists; do not give with live vaccines.

acitretin

Soriatane

Drug class and indications

Antipsoriatic agent; retinoic acid

Treatment of severe psoriasis.

Dosages and special alerts

25–50 mg/day PO with the main meal. Numerous adverse effects. Stop drug when lesions resolve. Do not crush capsules. Do not allow patient to donate blood. Monitor vision periodically; protect patient from sun exposure. ⊗ ***Black box warning*** Pregnancy category X; do not give to pregnant women.

adalimumab

Humira

Drug class and indications

Antiarthritic, monoclonal antibody

Reduction of the signs and symptoms of and inhibition of the progression of structural damage in adults with moderately to severely active rheumatoid arthritis and in children 4 yr and older with moderately to severely active polyarticular rheumatoid arthritis.

Reduction of the signs and symptoms of active arthritis in patients with psoriatic arthritis.

Reduction of the signs and symptoms of active ankylosing spondylitis.

Dosages and special alerts

Adults: 40 mg subcutaneously every other wk, may be increased to 40 mg subcutaneously every wk in patients not on methotrexate. Pediatric patients ages 4–17 yr: Weighing 15 to less than 30 kg: 20 mg subcutaneously every other wk. Weighing 30 kg or more: 40 mg subcutaneously every other wk. Use cautiously with immunosuppressants; severe infection can occur. Avoid use in pregnancy. Monitor for CNS effects, demyelinating disease has been reported. ⊗ ***Black box warning*** High risk of infection.

adenosine

Adenocard, Adenoscan

Drug class and indications

Antiarrhythmic, diagnostic agent

Conversion to sinus rhythm of paroxysmal supraventricular tachycardias (*Adenocard*); with thallium, assessment of patients with suspected CAD (*Adenoscan*).

Dosages and special alerts
Conversion of arrhythmias in patients weighing more than 50 kg: 6 mg by rapid IV bolus; for repeat dose, use 12 mg by IV bolus within 1–2 min. May be repeated a second time. *Patients weighing less than 50 kg:* 0.05–0.1 mg/kg as rapid IV bolus, may give another bolus in 1–2 min, increased by 0.05–0.1 mg/kg. Maximum single dose, 0.3 mg/kg. *Cardiac assessment:* 140 mcg/kg/min IV, infused over 6 min. Inject thallium at 3 min. Maintain emergency equipment on standby, and monitor continually. Have methylxanthines available as antidote.

agalsidase beta
Fabrazyme

Drug class and indications
Enzyme
Treatment of Fabry's disease.

Dosages and special alerts
1 mg/kg body weight IV every 2 wk; infused at a rate of no more than 0.25 mg/min. Infusion reactions are common; antipyretics and corticosteroids are given before the infusion; fever and chills may occur later. Continue regular regimen for treatment of Fabry's disease.

DANGEROUS DRUG
aldesleukin
Proleukin

Drug class and indications
Antineoplastic
Metastatic renal cell carcinoma in adults. Treatment of adult metastatic melanoma.

Dosages and special alerts
600,000 international units/kg IV every 8 hr, given over 15 min as two 50-day cycles; total of 14 doses, followed by 9 days of rest, then 14 more doses; can be retreated after 7 wk if tumor shrinkage occurs. Monitor for capillary leak syndrome with third spacing of fluids and hypotension; GI bleeding has been reported.

alefacept
Amevive

Drug class and indications
Immunosuppressant
Treatment of adults with moderate to severe chronic plaque psoriasis who are candidates for systemic therapy or phototherapy.

Dosages and special alerts
7.5 mg as an IV bolus once a wk or 15 mg IM given once a wk; recommended course is 12 weekly injections. An additional 12-wk course may be initiated if CD4+ T lymphocytes are within normal range and 12 wk have passed since first course. Patient has increased risk of infection; monitor closely.

DANGEROUS DRUG
alemtuzumab
Campath

Drug class and indications
Monoclonal antibody, antineoplastic
Treatment of B cell chronic lymphocytic leukemia in patients treated with alkylating agents who have failed fludarabine therapy.

Dosages and special alerts
3 mg/day as a 2-hr IV infusion, increase up to 30 mg/day as a 2-hr infusion three times weekly, every other day for 12 wk. Premedicate with diphenhydramine and acetaminophen. Ensure that the patient is well hydrated. ⊗ ***Black box warning*** Monitor patient for bone marrow suppression, infusion reactions. Prophylactic antibiotic and antiviral therapy may be used to prevent serious infections.

alglucosidase alfa
Myozyme

Drug class and indications
Enzyme, Pompe's disease drug

To improve ventilator-free survival in patients with infantile-onset Pompe's disease.

Dosages and special alerts

20 mg/kg by IV infusion administered over 4 hr, every 2 wk. Because of a high risk of infusion reaction, infusion should be started as 1mg/kg/hr and then increased by 2 mg/kg/hr every 30 min, based on patient tolerance, to a maximum of 7 mg/kg/hr. Do not infuse in solution with any other drug. Monitor carefully for hypersensitivity reaction, cardiorespiratory failure.

alpha$_1$-proteinase inhibitor

Aralast, Prolastin, Prolastin C, Zemaira

Drug class and indications

Blood product

Aralast/Prolastin

Treatment of congenital alpha$_1$-antitrypsin deficiency, chronic treatment of adults with early evidence of panacinar emphysema.

Zemaira

Chronic augmentation and maintenance therapy in patients with alpha$_1$-proteinase inhibitor deficiency and clinical evidence of emphysema.

Dosages and special alerts

Aralast/Prolastin

60 mg/kg IV once a wk to achieve functional levels of alpha$_1$-proteinase inhibitor in lower respiratory tract. Monitor for possible hepatitis related to the use of human blood products.

Prolastin C

0.08 mL/Kg/min IV once a wk.

Zemaira

60 mg/kg IV weekly, infused over 15 min. Monitor for any sign of hypersensitivity reactions; drug should be discontinued if these occur. Warn the patient that product is made from human plasma and possible viral infection could occur—rash, drowsiness, chills, and joint pain should be reported immediately.

DANGEROUS DRUG

altretamine

Hexalen

Drug class and indications

Antineoplastic

Used as a single agent for the palliative treatment of patients with persistent or recurrent ovarian cancer following first-line treatment with cisplatin or alkylating agents.

Dosages and special alerts

260 mg/m^2/day PO given for 14 or 21 consecutive days of a 28-day cycle given as divided doses with meals and at bedtime. Consider an antiemetic or decreased dose if severe nausea or vomiting occur. ⊗ ***Black box warning*** Monitor blood counts and neurological status frequently; risk of cytopenias, infections.

alvimopan

Entereg

Drug class and indications

Peripheral mu-opioid receptor antagonist

To accelerate upper and lower GI recovery following partial large- or small-bowel resection surgery with primary anastomosis.

Dosages and special alerts

12 mg PO given 30 min to 5 hr before surgery followed by 12 mg PO bid for up to 7 days to a maximum of 15 doses. For use in hospitalized patients only. Contraindicated in patients with more than 7 consecutive days of opioid therapy before treatment. Patients recently exposed to opioids will be more sensitive to drug effects and may experience nausea, vomiting, and diarrhea. Not recommended for patients with severe hepatic or renal disease. Risk of MI exists.

ambrisentan

Letairis

Drug class and indications

Endothelin receptor antagonist, antihypertensive

Treatment of pulmonary artery hypertension in patients with class II or III symptoms to improve exercise capacity and delay clinical worsening.

Dosages and special alerts
Initially, 5 mg/day PO; may be increased to 10 mg/day if needed and tolerated. Not recommended with moderate to severe hepatic impairment; risk of severe liver injury. Pregnancy category X; use of two forms of contraception advised. Available only through Letairis Access Program. ⊗ ***Black box warning*** Potential for severe liver injury; not for use in pregnancy.

amifostine

Ethyol

Drug class and indications
Cytoprotective drug

Reduction of renal toxicity associated with repeated administration of cisplatin in patients with advanced ovarian cancer; reduction of incidence of xerostomia in patients receiving radiation for head and neck cancer.

Unlabeled use: Protection of lung fibroblasts from effects of paclitaxel.

Dosages and special alerts
910 mg/m² IV daily as a 15-min infusion. Start within 30 min of starting chemotherapy. Monitor BP carefully; severe hypotension has been reported.

aminolevulinic acid hydrochloride

Levulan Kerastick

Drug class and indications
Photosensitizer

Treatment of nonkeratotic actinic keratoses of the face and scalp.

Dosages and special alerts
Must be applied in timing with blue light photodynamic illuminator; clean and dry area to be treated, break ampule, and apply solution with applicator provided. Light treatment must be done within the next 14–18 hr. One application of solution and one dose illumination per treatment site per 8-wk treatment session.

antihemophilic factor, recombinant

Advate, Xyntha

Drug class and indications
Antihemophilia drug

Prevention and control of bleeding episodes in hemophilia A; perioperative management of patients with hemophilia A.

Dosages and special alerts
Dosage is based on serum factor VIII level needed and body weight. See manufacturer's details. Antihemophilic factor required (international units) = body wt (kg) × desired factor VIII increase (% of normal) × 0.5.

antithrombin, recombinant

ATryn

Drug class and indications
Coagulation inhibitor

Prevention of perioperative and peripartum thromboembolic events in patients with hereditary antithrombin (AT) deficiency.

Dosages and special alerts
Loading dose given as a 15-min IV infusion based on AT level and body weight; maintenance dose given by continuous IV infusion to maintain AT activity levels between 80% and 120% of normal; perioperative: 100 − baseline AT ÷ 2.3 (for loading dose) or 10.2 (for maintenance) × body weight in kg; pregnant women: 100 − baseline AT ÷ 1.3 (loading dose) or 5.4 (maintenance) × body weight in kg. Contraindicated with allergy to goats or goat products; risk of hemorrhage and injection site reactions. Coagulation parameters must be followed closely.

DANGEROUS DRUG

antithrombin III

Thrombate III

Drug class and indications

Coagulation inhibitor

Treatment of patients with hereditary antithrombin III deficiency in connection with surgical or obstetric procedures or when they have thromboembolism.

Replacement therapy in congenital antithrombin III deficiency.

Dosages and special alerts

Dosage units = desired antithrombin level (%)—baseline ATIII level (%) × body weight (kg) divided by 1.4 every 2–8 days. Dosage varies greatly; frequent blood tests are needed.

apomorphine

Apokyn

Drug class and indications

Dopamine agonist, antiparkinsonism drug

Intermittent treatment of hypomobility, "off" episodes (drug wearing off) caused by advanced Parkinson's disease.

Dosages and special alerts

2 mg by subcutaneous injection, increased slowly while monitoring BP to achieve control; maximum dose 6 mg. Give 300 mg trimethobenzamide PO tid from 3 days before starting apomorphine to completion of at least 2 mo of therapy. Monitor patient for prolonged QT interval. GI effects common.

DANGEROUS DRUG

argatroban

Argatroban

Drug class and indications

Anticoagulant

Prophylaxis or treatment of thrombosis in heparin-induced thrombocytopenia; as an anticoagulant in patients at risk of heparin-induced thrombocytopenia undergoing percutaneous coronary intervention (PCI).

Dosages and special alerts

Dilute to concentration of 1 mg/mL; administer 2 mcg/kg/min as a continuous infusion. Monitor aPTT, usually achieves desired level within 1–3 hr; adjust dose of infusion to maintain a steady state aPPT that is 1.5–3 times the initial baseline value; do not exceed 10 mcg/kg/hr. Reduce initial dose to 0.5 mcg/kg/min with hepatic impairment. With PCI—25 mcg/kg/min with a bolus of 350 mcg/kg over 3–5 min. Excessive bleeding and hemorrhage may occur; monitor patient carefully for any sign of excess bleeding, decrease infusion rate or stop drug if excessive bleeding occurs.

DANGEROUS DRUG

arsenic trioxide

Trisenox

Drug class and indications

Antineoplastic

Induction and remission of acute promyelocytic leukemia in patients refractory to retinoid or anthracycline chemotherapy and whose leukemia is characterized by t(15;17) translocation or PML/RAR-alpha gene expression.

Dosages and special alerts

Induction: 0.15 mg/kg/day IV until bone marrow remission (maximum, 60 doses). Consolidation: 0.15 mg/kg/day IV starting 3–6 wk after completion of induction (maximum, 25 doses over 5 wk). Cardiac and CNS toxicity common; baseline and weekly ECG; biweekly electrolytes, CBC with differential and clotting profiles advised.

Avoid seafood and many alternative therapies (arsenic in many of these). Advise patient to avoid pregnancy, driving, or dangerous activities. ⊠ ***Black box warning*** Drug can be highly toxic and carcinogenic.

auranofin

Ridaura

Drug class and indications

Gold compound, antirheumatic

Management of adults with active classic or definite rheumatoid arthritis who have insufficient response to or intolerance to NSAIDs.

Dosages and special alerts
3 mg PO bid or 6 mg/day PO as a single dose; after 6 mo may be increased to 3 mg PO tid; do not exceed 9 mg/day. Monitor lung function, renal status, and blood counts. Protect patient from sunlight and UV exposure; systemic corticosteroids can be used for mild reactions. ⊗ ***Black box warning*** Discontinue drug at first sign of toxicity; severe bone marrow suppression, renal toxicity, and diarrhea are possible.

DANGEROUS DRUG

azacitidine

Vidaza

Drug class and indications
Antineoplastic
Treatment of myelodysplastic syndrome including refractory anemias and chronic myelomonocytic leukemia.

Dosages and special alerts
75 mg/m^2/day by subcutaneous injection for 7 days every 4 wk; patients should receive at least four cycles. May be increased to 100 mg/m^2/day if no benefit after two cycles. Premedicate for nausea and vomiting. Monitor blood counts and adjust dosage as needed. Pregnancy should be avoided, and men taking this drug should not father children.

basiliximab

Simulect

Drug class and indications
Immunosuppressant, monoclonal antibody
Prophylaxis of acute rejection in renal transplant patients in combination with cyclosporine and corticosteroids.

Dosages and special alerts
Two doses of 20 mg IV with the first dose 2 hr before transplant, then 4 days after transplant. Drug must be given in combination with other immunosuppressant drugs. GI effects common.

DANGEROUS DRUG

BCG intravesical

TheraCys, Tice BCG

Drug class and indications
Antineoplastic
Treatment and prophylaxis for carcinoma in situ of the urinary bladder; prophylaxis of primary or recurrent Ta and T1 papillary tumors following transurethral resection; administered intravesically only.

Dosages and special alerts
Do not drink fluids for 4 hr before treatment; empty bladder before treatment. Instill 1 ampule, diluted as indicated in saline solution by catheter, allow to flow slowly. Have patient lie down for first hr, turning side to side, and then stay upright for 1 hr. Try to retain solution for 2 hr, and void retained solution trying not to splash liquid. Increase fluid intake for next few days. Monitor patient for local discomfort and reactions and for bone marrow depression and infection. ⊗ ***Black box warning*** Take precautions when handling drug; infection can occur.

DANGEROUS DRUG

bevacizumab

Avastin

Drug class and indications
Monoclonal antibody, antineoplastic
Used with 5-fluorouracil for first-line or second-line treatment of patients with metastatic carcinoma of the colon or rectum.
Used with paclitaxel and carboplatin for first-line treatment of unresectable, locally advanced recurrent or metastatic nonsquamous, non–small-cell lung cancer.
With paclitaxel for the treatment of metastatic HER2-negative breast cancer in patients who have not had chemotherapy.
NEW INDICATION: Treatment of glioblastoma multiforme with progression following standard therapy.
NEW INDICATION: Treatment of metastatic renal cell carcinoma with interferon-alfa.

Dosages and special alerts
For colon cancer, 5–10 mg/kg as an IV infusion every 14 days until disease progression is detected. First infusion over 90 min; second over 60 min; then infuse over 30 min. For lung cancer, 15 mg/kg as an IV infusion every 3 wk. For breast cancer: 10 mg/kg as an IV infusion every 14 days. Monitor blood counts and nutritional state. Patient may need treatment for constipation.

DANGEROUS DRUG

bexarotene
Targretin

Drug class and indications
Antineoplastic
Treatment of the cutaneous manifestations of cutaneous T-cell lymphoma in patients refractory to at least one other systemic therapy.

Dosages and special alerts
300 mg/m^2 PO daily; may be increased to 400 mg/m^2 PO daily. Risk of serious pancreatitis, photosensitivity. ⊗ ***Black box warning*** Pregnancy category X.

bicalutamide
Casodex

Drug class and indications
Antiandrogen
Treatment of advanced prostatic carcinoma in combination with LHRH analogue.

Dosages and special alerts
50 mg/day PO at the same time each day. Monitor liver function regularly. Administer only with LHRH analogue.

DANGEROUS DRUG

bivalirudin
Angiomax

Drug class and indications
Anticoagulant; thrombin inhibitor
Anticoagulation of patients undergoing percutaneous transluminal angioplasty who have unstable angina and who are receiving aspirin.
Treatment of patients with, or at risk for heparin-induced thrombocytopenia and thrombosis syndromes who are undergoing percutaneous cardiac intervention.

Dosages and special alerts
0.75 mg/kg IV bolus, then 1.75 mg/kg/hr IV for duration of procedure; infusion can be continued for 4 hr after procedure. After 4 hr, IV infusion of 0.2 mg/kg/hr may be used for up to 20 hr, if needed. Reduce dosage with renal impairment. Give with aspirin. Monitor for excessive bleeding, which would indicate need to discontinue drug.

DANGEROUS DRUG

bortezomib
Velcade

Drug class and indications
Antineoplastic
Treatment of multiple myeloma or mantle cell lymphoma in patients who have received at least one prior therapy, or in those previously untreated.

Dosages and special alerts
1.3 mg/m^2/dose IV twice weekly for 2 wk (days 1, 4, 8, and 11) followed by a 10-day rest (days 12–21); then repeat the cycle. Monitor for peripheral neuropathies and thrombocytopenia; provide appropriate safety measures.

botulinum toxin type B
Myobloc

Drug class and indications
Skeletal muscle relaxant, direct acting
Reduction of the severity of abnormal head position and neck pain associated with cervical dystonia.

Dosages and special alerts
2,500–5,000 units IM, injected locally into affected muscles. Blocks cholinergic transmission between the nerve and muscle. Monitor for lack of muscle function, infection at injection site. ⊗ ***Black box warning*** Not for use in treatment of muscle spasms or

cerebral palsy. Risk of botulinum toxicity if drug spreads from area of injection.

C1 inhibitor (human)

Cinryze

Drug class and indications

Proteinase inhibitor, blood product

Routine prophylaxis against angioedema attacks in adults and adolescents with hereditary angioedema.

Dosages and special alerts

1,000 units IV every 3–4 days at rate of 1 mL/min. Monitor for immediate, potentially life-threatening hypersensitivity reactions (have epinephrine readily available). Associated risks include thrombotic events in patients with risk factors for thrombosis and potential for infectious agents in product because it is made from human plasma.

canakinumab

Ilaris

Drug class and indications

Interleukin blocker

Treatment of cryopyrin-associated periodic syndrome in patients 4 yr and older, including familial cold autoinflammatory syndrome.

Treatment of Muckle-Wells syndrome.

Dosages and special alerts

40 kg and more: 150 mg by subcutaneous injection; 15–40 kg: 2 mg/kg by subcutaneous injection; children 15–40 kg with inadequate response: dose may be increased to 3 mg/kg. Injections are given every 8 wk. Patient may be at increased risk for infections. Do not give live vaccines to patient using this drug. URI symptoms are most common adverse effect.

caspofungin acetate

Cancidas

Drug class and indications

Echinocandin, antifungal

Treatment of invasive aspergillosis in patients who are unresponsive to or who cannot tolerate standard therapy.

Treatment of esophageal candidiasis.

Treatment of candidemia and other *Candida* infections.

Empirical treatment when fungal infection is suspected in febrile and neutropenic patients.

Dosages and special alerts

Single loading dose of 70 mg IV, followed by daily IV infusion of 50 mg/day for at least 14 days. No loading dose is given for esophageal candidiasis. Monitor for IV complications. Use with cyclosporin is not recommended.

cellulose sodium phosphate (CSP)

Calcibind

Drug class and indications

Antilithic, resin exchange drug

Absorptive hypercalciuria type 1 (recurrent calcium oxalate or calcium phosphate stones).

Dosages and special alerts

15 g/day PO (5 g with each meal) in patients with urinary calcium exceeding 300 mg/day; reduce to 10 g/day PO (5 g with supper and 2.5 g with other meals) when urinary calcium falls to less than 150 mg/day. Caution patient to continue diet to moderate calcium oxalate intake; give supplemental magnesium gluconate while giving this drug; suspend powder in water, soft drink, or fruit juice and give 1 hr before the meal; urge patient to increase fluid intake.

certolizumab pegol

Cimzia

Drug class and indications

Tumor necrosis factor blocker, immune modulator

Reduction of the signs and symptoms of Crohn's disease; maintenance of clinical response in adult patients with moderately to severely active disease who responded inadequately to conventional therapy.

NEW INDICATION: Treatment of moderately to severely active rheumatoid arthritis in adults.

Dosages and special alerts

400 mg subcutaneously, repeated at wk 2 and 4; if clinical response occurs, maintenance dose of 400 mg subcutaneously every 4 wk. Associated risks include serious infections, malignancies, and CNS demyelinating disorder. Prescreen for TB and hepatitis B and monitor patient closely.

cetrorelix acetate

Cetrotide

Drug class and indications

Fertility drug

Inhibition of premature LH surges in women undergoing controlled ovarian stimulation.

Dosages and special alerts

3 mg subcutaneously given with gonadotropins when serum estradiol levels show appropriate stimulation; if HCG is not given within 4 days, continue giving 0.25 mg/day subcutaneously until HCG is given or 0.25 mg subcutaneously morning or evening of stimulation day 5, or morning of stimulation day 6, continue daily until HCG is given. Patient or significant other should learn to give subcutaneous injections using the proper technique. Given only as part of overall fertility program.

DANGEROUS DRUG

cetuximab

Erbitux

Drug class and indications

Monoclonal antibody, antineoplastic

Monotherapy or in combination with irinotecan for the treatment of advanced epidermal growth factor receptor-expressing colorectal carcinoma.

With radiation for the treatment of locally or regionally advanced squamous cell carcinoma of the head and neck.

Monotherapy for recurrent or metastatic squamous cell cancer of the head and neck after failure of platinum therapy.

Dosages and special alerts

400 mg/m^2 IV as a loading dose, infused over 120 min; weekly maintenance of 250 mg/m^2 IV infused over 60 min. Premedication with an antihistamine is recommended. Monitor for acute infusion reaction; interstitial pulmonary disease and dermatologic toxicity.

cevimeline hydrochloride

Evoxac

Drug class and indications

Parasympathomimetic

Treatment of symptoms of dry mouth in patients with Sjögren's syndrome.

Dosages and special alerts

30 mg PO tid; administer with food if GI upset is severe; monitor swallowing; monitor patient for dehydration and provide supportive therapy.

chenodiol

Chenix

Drug class and indications

Gallstone solubilizer

Treatment of selected patients with radiolucent gallstones in well-opacifying gallbladders when elective surgery is contraindicated.

Dosages and special alerts

13–16 mg/kg/day in two doses, AM and PM. Start with 250 mg PO bid for 2 wk, then increase by 250 mg/day each wk. Monitor liver function carefully. Discontinue if hepatitis occurs; caution patient to use barrier contraceptives and avoid pregnancy.

chlorpropamide

Drug class and indications
Antidiabetic, sulfonylurea (first generation)

Adjunct to diet to lower blood glucose level in patients with type 2 diabetes mellitus.

Dosages and special alerts
250 mg/day PO. For maintenance therapy, 100–250 mg/day; do not exceed 750 mg/day. Not for pediatric use. May increase risk of CV events. Watch for possible hypoglycemia.

choline magnesium trisalicylate
Tricosal

Drug class and indications
NSAID, salicylate, antipyretic, analgesic

Treatment of osteoarthritis, rheumatoid arthritis; relief of moderate pain, fever.

Dosages and special alerts
Adults: For arthritis, 1.5–2.5 g/day PO in divided doses; do not exceed 4.5 g/day. For pain or fever, 2–3 g/day PO in divided doses. Pediatric patients: Base dosage on patient's age; see manufacturer's guidelines. Usually 217.5–652.5 mg PO every 4 hr as needed. GI effects common; give with meals to decrease them. Dizziness can also occur.

chorionic gonadotropin alfa (recombinant)
Ovidrel

Drug class and indications
Fertility drug

Induction of ovulation in infertile females who have been pretreated with FSH.

Induction of final follicular maturation and early luteinization in infertile women who have undergone pituitary desensitization and who have been appropriately pretreated with FSH.

Dosages and special alerts
250 mcg subcutaneously given 1 day following the last dose of a follicle-stimulating agent. Administer only when adequate follicular development has occurred. Do not administer if there is an excessive ovarian response. Inject into stomach area. Alert patient to risk of multiple births; patient should report shortness of breath, sudden abdominal pain, nausea, vomiting.

cidofovir
Vistide

Drug class and indications
Antiviral

Treatment of CMV retinitis in AIDS patients.

Dosages and special alerts
5 mg/kg IV infused over 1 hr once per wk for 2 wk; then 5 mg/kg IV every 2 wk. Probenecid must be given orally, 2 g PO before dose and 1 g at 2 and 8 hr after each dose. Maintain hydration. ⊗ ***Black box warning*** Monitor renal function closely; renal toxicity is common. Monitor neutrophils.

DANGEROUS DRUG

clofarabine
Clolar

Drug class and indications
Antimetabolite, antineoplastic

Treatment of patients ages 1–21 yr with ALL after at least two relapses from other regimens.

Dosages and special alerts
52 mg/m² by IV infusion over 2 hr daily for 5 consecutive days; repeat every 2–6 wk, based on recovery of baseline function. GI toxicity, bone marrow suppression, risk of infection are common.

coagulation factor VIIa (recombinant)
NovoSeven

Drug class and indications
Antihemophilic

Treatment of bleeding episodes in hemophilia A or B patients with inhibitors to factor VIII or factor IX.

Dosages and special alerts
90 mcg/kg as an IV bolus every 2 hr until hemostasis is achieved; continue dosing at 3- to 6-hr intervals after hemostasis in severe bleeds. Monitor for early signs of hypersensitivity reactions (hives, wheezing, hypotension, anaphylaxis).

cosyntropin
Cortrosyn

Drug class and indications
Diagnostic agent
Diagnostic tests of adrenal function.

Dosages and special alerts
0.25–0.75 mg IV or IM or as an IV infusion of 0.04 mg/hr. Monitor for seizures, anaphylactoid reactions, excessive adrenal effects. Monitor plasma and urinary corticosteroid levels to determine adrenal function.

cromolyn sodium
Crolom, Nalcrom (CAN), NasalCrom

Drug class and indications
Antiallergy drug
Prevention and treatment of allergic rhinitis, allergy eye disorders (ophthalmic).

Dosages and special alerts
1 spray in each nostril three to six times a day, as needed, or 1 to 2 drops in each eye four to six times a day as needed. Do not wear soft contact lenses if using ophthalmic preparation. Encourage continued use for optimal effects.

daclizumab
Zenapax

Drug class and indications
Immunosuppressive monoclonal antibody
Prophylaxis of acute rejection in renal transplant patients in combination with cyclosporine and corticosteroids.

Dosages and special alerts
1 mg/kg IV—5 doses, with the first dose within 24 hr of transplant, remaining doses within 14 days. Protect patient from infections and invasive procedures; GI effects common.

dapsone

Drug class and indications
Leprostatic
Treatment of Hansen's disease.
Treatment of dermatitis herpetiformis.

Dosages and special alerts
50–100 mg/day PO (leprosy). 50 mg/day PO (dermatitis herpetiformis); 50–300 mg/day has been used. Children should not receive more than 100 mg/day. Monitor patients for bone marrow suppression and for the development of resistance if relapse occurs. Give with food to decrease GI upset. Drug will need to be used for prolonged time.

darunavir
Prezista

Drug class and indications
Antiviral, protesase inhibitor
Treatment of adults with advanced HIV disease with progression of disease following antiretroviral treatment; used with 100 mg ritonavir and combinations of other HIV drugs.

Dosages and special alerts
600 mg PO bid with ritonavir 100 mg PO bid with food. Interacts with many other drugs; check drug regimen carefully before starting therapy. Monitor patient for rash, bone marrow suppression. Watch for increased bleeding in patients with hemophilia and glucose alterations in diabetics.

DANGEROUS DRUG

dasatinib
Sprycel

Drug class and indications
Kinase inhibitor, antineoplastic
Treatment of adults in all phases of CML (chronic, accelerated, or myeloid or lymphoid

blast phase) with resistance or intolerance to prior treatment, given with imatinib.

Treatment of adults with Philadelphia chromosome–positive acute lymphoblastic leukemia with resistance or tolerance to prior therapy.

Dosages and special alerts
140 mg/day PO in two equally divided doses, one morning and one evening, without food. Tablets should be swallowed whole, not cut, crushed, or chewed. Monitor patient for edema, excessive bleeding, bone marrow suppression. Advise use of barrier contraceptives for both men and women using the drug.

DANGEROUS DRUG

daunorubicin citrate
DaunoXome

Drug class and indications
Antineoplastic

First-line treatment of advanced HIV-associated Kaposi's sarcoma.

Dosages and special alerts
40 mg/m^2 IV, infused over 1 hr; repeat every 2 wk. Decrease dose with renal or hepatic impairment. Monitor for extravasation; severe damage can occur. Do not use during pregnancy. ⊗ ***Black box warning*** Cardiac toxicity possible; monitor ECG and enzymes, and decrease dosage as needed.

DANGEROUS DRUG

decitabine
Dacogen

Drug class and indications
Antineoplastic antibiotic

Treatment of patients with myelodysplastic syndromes.

Dosages and special alerts
15 mg/m^2 IV, infused over 3 hr every 8 hr for 3 days. Repeat cycle every 6 wk for at least four cycles; may be continued as long as it benefits the patient. Premedicate patient with antiemetics. Monitor patient carefully for GI disturbances, bone marrow suppression.

deferasirox
Exjade

Drug class and indications
Chelate

Treatment of chronic iron overload due to blood transfusion (transfusional hemosiderosis) in patients 2 yr and older.

Dosages and special alerts
20 mg/kg/day PO. Therapy should be started when a patient has evidence of chronic iron overload as with transfusions of 100 mL/kg packed red cells. Maintenance: monthly serum ferritin levels should be drawn and dosage adjusted in steps of 5–10 mg/kg. If serum ferritin levels fall below 500 mcg/L, consider stopping therapy. Do not exceed 30 mg/kg/day. Monitor for changes in vision and hearing, liver toxicity.

deferoxamine mesylate
Desferal

Drug class and indications
Chelate

Treatment of acute iron toxicity and chronic iron overload.

Dosages and special alerts
Acute toxicity: 1 g IM or IV, followed by 0.5 g every 4 hr for 2 doses, then every 4–12 hr based on patient response.

Chronic overload: 0.5–1 g IM qid; 2 g IV with each unit of blood or 20–40 mg/kg/day as a continuous subcutaneous infusion over 8–24 hr. IM preferred for acute intoxication; slow IV infusion for chronic overload. Monitor serum iron levels. Note that injection can be very painful.

degarelix
Degarelix for Injection

Drug class and indications
GnRH receptor antagonist, antineoplastic

Treatment of advanced prostate cancer.

Dosages and special alerts
Initially, 240 mg by subcutaneous injection, given as two separate 120-mg injections, followed by maintenance dose of 80 mg subcutaneously every 28 days. Pregnancy category X. Risk of prolonged QT interval. Injection site reactions, hot flashes, weight gain are common.

denileukin diftitox

Ontak

Drug class and indications
Biological protein

Treatment of cutaneous T-cell lymphoma in patients whose cells express the CD25 component of the IL-2-receptor.

Dosages and special alerts
Adults: 9 or 18 mcg/kg/day IV over at least 15 min for 5 consecutive days every 21 days. Monitor for capillary leak syndrome.
⊗ ***Black box warning*** Severe hypersensitivity reactions may occur; have life-support equipment available.

DANGEROUS DRUG

desirudin

Iprivask

Drug class and indications
Anticoagulant; thrombin inhibitor

Prevention of DVT in patients undergoing elective hip replacement.

Dosages and special alerts
15 mg every 12 hr by subcutaneous injection, initial dose given 5–15 min before surgery but after induction of anesthesia; give for 9–12 days. Administer by deep subcutaneous injection; alternate sites. Monitor blood clotting daily and protect from injury.

DANGEROUS DRUG

dexmedetomidine hydrochloride

Precedex

Drug class and indications
Sedative, hypnotic

Sedation of initially intubated and mechanically ventilated patients during treatment in an ICU setting.

Dosages and special alerts
1 mcg/kg infused over 10 min, then 0.2–0.7 mcg/kg/hr using a controlled infusion device for up to 24 hr; drug is not indicated for use longer than 24 hr.

dexrazoxane

Totect

Drug class and indications
Lyopilizate

Treatment of extravasation resulting from IV anthracycline chemotherapy.

Dosages and special alerts
Given IV once daily for 3 days. *Day 1:* 1,000 mg/m^2; maximum dose, 2,000 mg. *Day 2:* 1,000 mg/m^2; maximum dose, 2,000 mg. *Day 3:* 500 mg/m^2; maximum dose, 1,000 mg. Infuse over 1–2 hr. Reduce dose by 50% in patients with creatinine clearance less than 40 mL/min. Monitor patient for bone marrow supression, fever, and pain and burning at injection site. Do not give to pregnant women or nursing mothers.

dihydroergotamine mesylate

D.H.E. 45, Migranal

Drug class and indications
Ergot derivative, antimigraine drug

Acute treatment of migraine headaches with or without aura; acute treatment of cluster headache (parenteral).

Dosages and special alerts
1 mg IM, IV, or subcutaneously at first sign of headache; may repeat at 1-hr intervals for a total of 3 mg. Or one spray (0.5 mg) in each nostril followed by another spray in each nostril 15 min later for a total of 3 mg. Be aware of possible coronary artery vasoconstriction. Numbness, tingling are common. If patient has nausea or vomiting, give drug with an antiemetic.

dimercaprol

BAL in Oil

Drug class and indications
Antidote, chelate

Treatment of arsenic, gold, mercury poisoning.

Treatment of acute lead poisoning when used with calcium edetate disodium.

Treatment of acute mercury poisoning if used within the first 1–2 hr.

Dosages and special alerts
2.5–5 mg/kg IM qid for 2 days, taper to bid for 10 days. Can cause severe renal damage; alkalinize urine to increase chelated complex excretion. Use extreme caution with children.

dipyridamole

Dipridacot (CAN), Persantine

Drug class and indications
Antianginal, antiplatelet, diagnostic agent

With warfarin to prevent thromboembolism in patients with prosthetic heart valves; diagnostic aid to assess CAD in patients unable to exercise.

Dosages and special alerts
75–100 mg PO qid to prevent thromboembolism. For CAD, 0.142 mg/kg/min IV, infused over 4 min. Continually monitor patient receiving IV form. Give oral drug at least 1 hr before meals. Warn patient about possible light-headedness.

dornase alfa

Pulmozyme

Drug class and indications
Cystic fibrosis drug

Management of respiratory symptoms of cystic fibrosis in conjunction with other drugs; treatment of advanced cystic fibrosis.

Dosages and special alerts
2.5 mg daily through a nebulizer; may increase to 2.5 mg bid in patients 5 yr or older. Store drug in the refrigerator. Make sure the patient knows how to use the nebulizer properly. Continue other treatments for cystic fibrosis.

doxercalciferol

Hectorol

Drug class and indications
Vitamin D analogue

Reduction of elevated intact parathyroid hormone (iPTH) levels in the management of secondary hyperparathyroidism in patients undergoing chronic renal dialysis; secondary hyperparathyroidism in patients with stage 3 or 4 chronic kidney disease who do not need dialysis.

Dosages and special alerts
With dialysis: 10 mcg three times per wk at dialysis. Maximum, 20 mcg three times per wk. Regulate dose by iPTH levels. Monitor carefully for hypercalcemia (arrhythmias, seizures, calcifications). Without dialysis: 1 mcg PO daily; adjust dosage based on PTH levels. Maximum dose, 3.5 mcg/day.

droperidol

Inapsine

Drug class and indications
General anesthetic

Dosages and special alerts
2.5 mg IM or IV. Use caution with renal or hepatic failure. Monitor patient for hypotension. Onset 3–10 min, recovery 2–4 hr; patient may have drowsiness, chills, or hallucinations during recovery. ⊗ ***Black box warning*** May prolong QT interval; monitor appropriately.

eculizumab

Soliris

Drug class and indications
Monoclonal antibody, complement inhibitor

Treatment of patients with paroxysmal nocturnal hemoglobinuria to reduce hemolysis.

Dosages and special alerts
600 mg IV over 35 min every 7 days for first 4 wk, followed by 900 mg IV as fifth dose 7 days later, and then 900 mg IV every 14 days. Patient must have had recent meningococcal vaccine before starting therapy; drug increases risk of infection. Monitor patient for early signs of meningococcal infection. Stopping drug can cause serious hemolysis; must monitor patient for 8 wk after stopping drug.

eltrombopag

Promacta

Drug class and indications
Thrombopoietin receptor agonist

Treatment of chronic immune idiopathic thrombocytopenic purpura in patients who have insufficient response to conventional therapies, including splenectomy.

Dosages and special alerts
50 mg PO once daily; may be increased to a maximum 75 mg/day. Patients of eastern Asian ancestry or with mild to moderate hepatic dysfunction should be started on 25 mg/day PO. May increase the risk of bone marrow–related malignancies; monitor CBC carefully. ⊗ ***Black box warning*** Risk of severe to fatal hepatotoxicity exists; monitor patient very closely and adjust dosage or discontinue drug if liver enzymes start to rise. Drug available only through limited distribution programs.

DANGEROUS DRUG

epirubicin hydrochloride

Ellence

Drug class and indications
Antineoplastic, antibiotic

Adjunctive therapy in patients with evidence of axillary node tumor involvement after resection of primary breast cancer.

Dosages and special alerts
100–120 mg/m^2 IV given in repeated 3- to 4-wk cycles, all on day 1; given with cyclophosphamide and 5-fluorouracil. Premedicate with antiemetics and antibiotics; encourage patient to drink plenty of fluids. Alert patient that hair loss may occur. ⊗ ***Black box warning*** Cardiac toxicity can occur; obtain baseline ECG. Monitor for bone marrow suppression. Severe local cellulitis can occur with extravasation; discontinue immediately if burning or stinging occurs.

epoprostenol sodium (prostacyclin, PGX, PGI_2)

Flolan

Drug class and indications
Prostaglandin

Treatment of primary pulmonary hypertension in patients unresponsive to standard therapy.

Dosages and special alerts
2 ng/kg/min with increases in increments of 2 ng/kg as tolerated using a portable infusion pump through a central venous catheter; 20–40 ng/kg/min common dosage after 6 mo of continuous therapy. Teach patient and significant other the proper maintenance and use of infusion pump, ensure that therapy is continuous. Headache, muscle aches, and pains are common.

ergotamine tartrate

Ergomar

Drug class and indications
Ergot derivative, antimigraine drug

Prevention or abortion of vascular headaches, such as migraine and cluster headaches.

Dosages and special alerts
One tablet (2 mg) under the tongue soon after the first symptoms, with subsequent doses at 30-min intervals. Do not exceed 3 tablets/day or 10 mg/week. Nausea and numbness and tingling are common. CV effects, including chest pain, may occur. Drug is pregnancy category X.

DANGEROUS DRUG

erlotinib

Tarceva

Drug class and indications

Monoclonal antibody, antineoplastic

Treatment of patients with locally advanced or metastatic non–small-cell lung cancer after failure of at least one course of chemotherapy.

In combination with gemcitabine for first-line treatment of locally advanced, unresectable, or metastatic pancreatic cancer.

Dosages and special alerts

Non–small-cell lung cancer: 150 mg/day PO on an empty stomach. Monitor for potentially serious interstitial lung disease. GI effects are common.

Pancreatic cancer: 100 mg/day PO on an empty stomach with IV gemcitabine.

Risk of GI perforation, Stevens-Johnson syndrome, ocular disorders.

ethacrynic acid

Edecrin

Drug class and indications

Loop, high ceiling diuretic

Treatment of edema associated with HF, cirrhosis, renal disease; acute pulmonary edema; ascites associated with malignancy, idiopathic edema, lymphedema; short-term management of congenital heart disease in children.

Dosages and special alerts

50–200 mg/day PO, based on patient response. IV use in adults: 50 mg IV run slowly over several min to a maximum of 100 mg. Oral use in children, 25 mg/day, adjust in 25 mg increments as needed. Give oral dose with food or milk. Monitor weight and output regularly. Monitor potassium levels and provide replacement as needed.

everolimus

Afinitor

Drug class and indications

Kinase inhibitor, antineoplastic

Treatment of advanced renal cell carcinoma after failure with sunitinib or sorafenib.

Dosages and special alerts

10 mg PO once daily with food. May be decreased to 5 mg/day to manage adverse effects or with moderate hepatic impairment. Pregnancy category D; fetal harm can occur. Risk of pneumonitis, serious to fatal infections, oral ulcerations, and elevations in blood glucose, lipid, and serum creatinine levels. Patients must be monitored very closely. Avoid use with strong CYP3A4 inhibitors; increase dose to a maximum 20 mg/day if drug must be given with strong CYP3A4 inducers. Do not give live vaccines to patient taking this drug.

DANGEROUS DRUG

exemestane

Aromasin

Drug class and indications

Antineoplastic

Treatment of advanced breast cancer in postmenopausal women whose disease has progressed following tamoxifen therapy.

Dosages and special alerts

25 mg PO every day with meals. May be antagonized by estrogens. Avoid use during premenopause or with renal or hepatic impairment. Hot flashes, GI upset, anxiety, depression, headache are common.

ferumoxytol

Feraheme

Drug class and indications

Iron replacement product

Treatment of iron deficiency anemia in adults with chronic renal failure.

Dosages and special alerts
500 mg IV, followed by 500 mg IV 3-8 days later depending on patient response. Infuse as undiluted injection at 30 mg/sec (1 mL/sec). May be readministered if indicated by persistent or recurrent anemia. Risk of iron overload; blood pressure changes are common. Monitor patient carefully for possible hypersensitivity reactions for 30 min after infusion. Drug is a superparamagnetic iron oxide that can alter MRI results and interpretation for up to 3 mo following administration; does not interfere with CAT scans or regular X-rays.

fibrinogen concentrate, human

RiaSTAP

Drug class and indications
Coagulation factor

Treatment of acute bleeding episodes in patients with congenital fibrinogen deficiency, including afibrinogenemia and hypofibrinogenemia.

Dosages and special alerts
70 mg/kg by slow IV injection, not to exceed 5 mL/min; dosage adjusted to a target fibrinogen level of 100 mg/dL. Risk of thrombotic events, severe hypersensitivity reactions. Drug is prepared from pooled human plasma; patient should be aware of potential infection risk.

DANGEROUS DRUG

floxuridine

FUDR

Drug class and indications
Antimetabolite, antineoplastic

Palliative management of GI adenocarcinoma metastatic to the liver that is incurable by surgery or other means.

Dosages and special alerts
0.1–0.6 mg/kg/day per intra-arterial infusion; continue until adverse effects occur, and resume when adverse effects resolve. Monitor bone marrow status; warn patient of possible severe GI effects.

fludrocortisone acetate

Florinef Acetate

Drug class and indications
Corticosteroid, hormone, mineralocorticoid

Partial replacement therapy in primary and secondary adrenocortical insufficiency.

Treatment of salt-losing adrenogenital syndrome with glucocorticoid therapy.

Dosages and special alerts
Adrenocortical insufficiency: 0.1 mg/day PO; may decrease to 0.05 mg/day PO if hypertension occurs. Salt-losing adrenogenital syndrome: 0.1–0.2 mg/day PO. Always use in conjunction with glucocorticoid therapy. Risk of increased fluid volume, headaches, tendon contractures. Discontinue at any sign of overdose (hypertension, edema, excessive weight gain, increased heart size). If infants or children are maintained on long-term therapy, monitor growth and development closely.

follitropin alfa

Gonal-F

Drug class and indications
Fertility drug

Induction of ovulation, stimulation, and development of multiple follicles for in vitro fertilization.

Also used to increase spermatogenesis in men with hypogonadism.

Dosages and special alerts
Ovulation induction: 75 international units/day subcutaneously, increase by 37.5 international units/day after 14 days; may increase again after 7 days; do not exceed 35 days of treatment.
Follicle development: 150 international units/day subcutaneously on days 2 or 3 and continue for 10 days. In patients whose endogenous gonadotropin levels are suppressed, initiate at 225 international units/day subcutaneously. Adjust dose after 5 days based on patient response; dosage should be adjusted no more than every 3–5 days and by no more than 75–150 international units at each

adjustment. Maximum, 450 international units/day; then give 5,000–10,000 units HCG.
Spermatogenesis: 150 international units subcutaneously three times per wk in conjunction with HCG. May increase to 300 international units three times per wk, as needed. May administer up to 18 mo for adequate effect. Pregnancy category X. Explain risk of multiple births; risk of arterial thromboembolism.

follitropin beta

Follistim, Puregon (CAN)

Drug class and indications

Fertility drug

Induction of ovulation, stimulation and development of multiple follicles for in vitro fertilization.

Dosages and special alerts

Ovulation induction: 75 international units/day subcutaneously, increase by 37.5 international units/day after 14 days; do not exceed 35 days of treatment.
Follicle development: 150–225 international units/day subcutaneously or IM for at least 4 days of treatment. Adjust dose based on ovarian response; then give 5,000–10,000 international units. HCG: maintenance dosage of 375–600 international units/day subcutaneously or IM may be necessary. Drug is pregnancy category X. Give subcutaneously in navel or abdomen. Warn patients of risk of multiple births.

fomepizole

Antizol

Drug class and indications

Antidote

Antidote for antifreeze (ethylene glycol) poisoning or for use in suspected poisoning.

Antidote for methanol poisoning.

Dosages and special alerts

15 mg/kg loading dose followed by doses of 10 mg/kg every 12 hr for 12 doses given as a slow IV infusion over 30 min. Start immediately after diagnosis is made. Headache, nausea, and dizziness are common. Consider hemodialysis as added therapy.

galsulfase

Naglazyme

Drug class and indications

Enzyme

Treatment of patients with mucopolysaccharidosis VI to improve walking and stair climbing capacity.

Dosages and special alerts

1 mg/kg once weekly by IV infusion, diluted and infused over 4 hr. Patient should receive antihistamine with or without an antipyretic 30–60 min before the infusion begins.

ganirelix acetate

Antagon

Drug class and indications

Fertility drug

Inhibition of premature LH surges in women undergoing controlled ovarian overstimulation as part of a fertility program.

Dosages and special alerts

250 mcg subcutaneously once daily starting on day 2 or 3 of the cycle. Drug is pregnancy category X. Teach patient to administer subcutaneous injections. Abdominal pain is a common adverse effect.

DANGEROUS DRUG

gefitinib

Iressa

Drug class and indications

Antineoplastic

Monotherapy for treatment of patients with locally advanced or metastatic non–small-cell lung cancer who have been receiving the drug and have been doing well. No longer available for initiating therapy.

Dosages and special alerts

250 mg/day PO with or without food. Monitor pulmonary function; potentially fatal

interstitial lung disease possible. Eye pain and corneal erosion also reported.

DANGEROUS DRUG

gemtuzumab ozogamicin

Mylotarg

Drug class and indications
Monoclonal antibody, antineoplastic

Treatment of CD33-positive AML in the first relapse in patients 60 yr and older who are not candidates for cytotoxic chemotherapy.

Dosages and special alerts
9 mg/m^2 IV over 2 hr for a total of 2 doses given 14 days apart. Administer diphenhydramine, acetaminophen before each dose. Ensure patient is hydrated; GI problems, fever common. Monitor vital signs for 4 hr following infusion. ⊗ ***Black box warning*** Protect patient from infection; bone marrow suppression is common.

glatiramer acetate

Copaxone

Drug class and indications
MS drug

Reduction of frequency of relapses in patients with relapsing or remitting MS.
NEW INDICATION: Treatment of patients who have experienced a first clinical episode of MS and who have MRI features consistent with MS.

Dosages and special alerts
20 mg/day by subcutaneous injection; rotate injection sites. Photosensitivity may occur.

gold sodium thiomalate

Aurolate

Drug class and indications
Gold compound, antirheumatic

Treatment of selected, early cases of adult and juvenile rheumatoid arthritis.

Dosages and special alerts
Weekly IM injections: 10 mg IM wk 1, 25 mg IM wk 2 and 3; then 25–50 mg/wk IM to a total dose of 1 g. Maintenance injections of 25–50 mg IM every other wk for 2–30 wk, may change to every third or fourth wk if response is adequate. Pediatric dosing: 10 mg IM test dose, then 1 mg/kg/wk IM; do not exceed 50 mg/dose. Injection reactions are common. Protect patient from sunlight and UV exposure; systemic corticosteroids can be used to manage mild reactions. ⊗ ***Black box warning*** Monitor lung, renal function and blood counts; discontinue at first sign of toxicity.

gonadorelin hydrochloride

Factrel

Drug class and indications
Diagnostic agent

Evaluation of functional capacity and response of the gonadotropes of the anterior pituitary.

Testing for suspected gonadotropin deficiency.

Evaluating residual activity following pituitary removal or irradiation.

Dosages and special alerts
100 mg subcutaneously or IV; in females, perform test days 1–7 of the menstrual cycle; have patient report any difficulty breathing.

DANGEROUS DRUG

histrelin implant

Vantas

Drug class and indications
Gonadotrophic-releasing hormone used as antineoplastic.

Palliative treatment of advanced prostate cancer.

Dosages and special alerts
One implant inserted subcutaneously and left in for 12 mo. May be removed and a new implant inserted after 12 mo. Monitor for insertion site reactions.

hyaluronic acid derivatives

Euflexxa, Hyalgan, Orthovisc, Supartz, Synvisc

Drug class and indications

Glycosamine polysaccharide

Treatment of pain in osteoarthritis of the knee in patients who have failed to respond to other therapies.

Dosages and special alerts

2 mL by intra-articular injection in knee once weekly for a total of 3–5 injections. Use caution with latex allergies. Joint swelling may occur; avoid strenuous activities or prolonged weight bearing for 48 hr. Headache may occur.

hyaluronidase

Amphadase, Hylenex, Vitrase

Drug class and indications

Enzyme

Used to increase absorption and dispersion of injected drugs.

For hypodermoclysis.

Used as an adjunct in subcutaneous urography for improving the resorption of radiopaque agents.

Dosages and special alerts

Absorption of injected drugs: Adults: Add 150 units of hyaluronidase to the injection solution. Pediatric patients: Add 150 units of hyaluronidase to the injection solution, may be added to small amounts up to 200 mL. Do not administer with dopamine or alpha adrenergic drugs. Monitor the patient for local reactions.
Hypodermoclysis: Adults: 150 units injected under the skin, close to the clysis. Pediatric patients younger than 3 yr: limit single clysis to 200 mL; premature infants or during the neonatal period: do not exceed 25 mL/kg at a rate no greater than 2 mL/min. Use care to avoid overhydration by controlling rate and volume. Do not administer with dopamine or alpha adrenergic drugs. Monitor the patient for local reactions.
Adjunct to subcutaneous urography: 75 units injected subcutaneously over each scapula, followed by injection of the contrast media at the same sites.

hydroflumethiazide

Drug class and indications

Thiazide diuretic (available in combination products only)

Treatment of hypertension; adjunct therapy for edema associated with HF, cirrhosis, renal impairment, corticosteroid or estrogen therapy.

Dosages and special alerts

Hypertension: 50–100 mg/day PO.
Edema: Initially, 50 mg PO bid; maintenance, 25–50 mg/day PO.
Give early in the day so increased urination will not affect sleep; give with food or meals to decrease GI upset.

hydroxocobalamin

Cyanokit

Drug class and indications

Antidote

Treatment of known or suspected cyanide poisoning.

Dosages and special alerts

5 g (2 vials) by IV infusion over 15 min; a second dose may be given if needed by IV infusion over 15–120 min, based on patient condition. Warn patient that urine will be red for up to 5 wk after treatment. Skin and mucous membranes may be red up to 2 wk after treatment; protect from sun exposure during this period.

hydroxyethyl starch in sodium chloride

Voluven

Drug class and indications

Colloid, plasma expander

Treatment and prophylaxis of hypovolemia.

Dosages and special alerts
Begin infusion slowly to monitor patient for anaphylactic reaction; base daily dosage and rate of infusion on patient's blood loss, hemodynamics, and hemodilution effects. Up to 50 mL/kg/day (3,500 mL for a 70-kg patient). For children, 7–25 mL/kg/day has been used. Monitor patient very closely, and adjust rate based on response. Watch for hypervolemia and anaphylactoid reactions.

hylan b gel

Hylaform

Drug class and indications
Polysaccharide, cosmetic drug

Correction of moderate to severe facial wrinkles or folds.

Dosages and special alerts
Injected into the dermal layer to correct wrinkles or folds; may need to be repeated over time. Monitor for infection. Avoid sun exposure immediately after injection.

DANGEROUS DRUG

ibritumomab

Zevalin

Drug class and indications
Monoclonal antibody, antineoplastic

Treatment of patients with relapsed or refractory low-grade follicular transformed B-cell non-Hodgkin's lymphoma.

NEW INDICATION: Treatment of patients with previously untreated follicular non-Hodgkin lymphoma who experience relapse to first-line therapy.

Dosages and special alerts
Single infusion of 250 mg/m^2 rituximab preceding a fixed dose of 5 mCi/kg ibritumomab as a 10-min IV push. Administer a second cycle 7–9 days later. Premedicate with acetaminophen and diphenhydramine before each rituximab infusion. Monitor for severe cytopenia, severe infusion reactions, severe cutaneous reactions.

idursulfase

Elaprase

Drug class and indications
Enzyme, Hunter's syndrome drug

Treatment of patients with Hunter's syndrome (mucopolysaccharidosis II).

Dosages and special alerts
0.5 mg/kg IV every week, infused over 1–3 hr. First infusion should be at 8 mL/hour (must be diluted in 100 mL of 0.9% sodium chloride injection) for the first 15 min; then increase by 8 mL/hr at 15-min intervals if patient tolerates infusion; do not exceed 100 mL/hr. Risk of serious anaphylactoid reactions; start therapy slowly, and monitor patient closely. Drug improves walking capacity.

iloprost

Ventavis

Drug class and indications
Vasodilator

Treatment of pulmonary arterial hypertension in patients with New York Heart Association class III to IV symptoms to improve composite endpoints.

Dosages and special alerts
2.5 mcg inhaled using the *ProDose* or *I-neb AAD system*. May be increased to 5 mcg; repeat inhalation 6–9 times/day while awake. Maximum dose 45 mcg/day. Monitor exercise and activity tolerances.

infliximab

Remicade

Drug class and indications
Monoclonal antibody

Used to reduce the signs and symptoms of moderate to severe Crohn's disease in adults and children who do not respond adequately to conventional therapy.

Treatment of rheumatoid arthritis (RA) together with methotrexate as a first-line therapy.

Treatment of patients with fistulizing Crohn's disease.

Used to reduce signs and symptoms, inhibit structural damage, and improve physical functioning of active arthritis in patients with psoriatic arthritis.

Used to reduce the signs and symptoms, and decrease the corticosteroid use in patients with moderately to severely active ulcerative colitis.

Dosages and special alerts

5 mg/kg IV over 2 hr given once (Crohn's disease). May repeat dose with fistulating or psoriatic arthritis disease at 2 wk and 6 wk after first dose, then every 8 wk with psoriatic arthritis or Crohn's disease. 3 mg/kg IV followed by 3 mg/kg at 2 and 6 wk, then every 8 wk (RA). 5 mg/kg IV at 0, 2, and 6 wk for induction, followed by 5 mg/kg IV every 8 wk for maintenance (ulcerative colitis). Do not use in patients with allergy to mouse protein. Discontinue if lupus-like reaction occurs. ⊗ ***Black box warning*** There is an increased risk of malignancies and infections; monitor patient closely.

insoluble Prussian blue

Radiogardase

Drug class and indications

Ferric hexacyanoferrate

Treatment of patients with known or suspected contamination with radioactive cesium or radioactive or nonradioactive thallium to increase their rates of elimination.

Dosages and special alerts

Adults and children 12 yr and older: 3 g PO tid. Children 2–12 yr: 1 g PO tid. Prevent constipation; stool will be blue. If capsules cannot be swallowed, contents may be added to food and eaten. Alert patient that teeth and mouth may become blue. Protect others from contamination by flushing toilet several times with each use, washing hands carefully, and cleaning up any spilled urine, blood, or feces.

interferon alfacon-1

Infergen

Drug class and indications

Interferon, immune modulator

Treatment of chronic hepatitis C in patients 18 yr and older with compensated liver disease and HCV antibodies.

Dosages and special alerts

9 mcg by subcutaneous injection three times per wk for 24 wk; at least 48 hr should separate doses. Monitor for possible severe adverse reactions. Monitor for suicidal ideation and take appropriate precautions. Tell female patients to use contraceptives. Treat nausea and vomiting as needed.

interferon alfa-n3

Alferon LDO, Alferon N

Drug class and indications

Alferon LDO

Immunomodulator

Treatment of condylomata acuminata (venereal and genital warts).

Alferon N

Interferon, antiviral

Treatment of phase I/II ARC, AIDS, asymptomatic AIDS.

Dosages and special alerts

Alferon LDO

0.05 mL per wart two times per wk for 8 wk. Maximum 0.5 mL per treatment session.

Alferon N

Investigational drug with this indication; orphan drug status.

iron sucrose

Venofer

Drug class and indications

Iron salt

Treatment of iron deficiency anemia in patients undergoing chronic hemodialysis or peritoneal dialysis who are receiving supplemental erythropoietin therapy and nondialysis dependent chronic renal failure patients with or without erythropoietin.

Dosages and special alerts
100 mg (5 mL) IV, one to three times per wk, during dialysis. Administer slowly, 1 mL over 2–5 min. Non-dialysis patients receive 1,000 mg IV over 14 days given as 200 mg IV on 5 different days. Serious to fatal hypersensitivity reactions have occurred. Administer test dose and monitor patient carefully during administration.

isocarboxazid
Marplan

Drug class and indications
MAOI
Treatment of depression (not a first choice for initial treatment).

Dosages and special alerts
Up to 40 mg PO daily. Dosage can usually be reduced after 3–4 wk because drug effects are cumulative. Not a first-line treatment for depression because of potential for serious adverse effects and food interactions. Might be useful in patients unable to tolerate newer and safer antidepressants. Patient must be given list of tyramine-containing foods.

ivermectin
Stromectol

Drug class and indications
Anthelmintic
Treatment of intestinal strongyloidiasis.
Treatment of onchocerciasis.

Dosages and special alerts
Strongyloidiasis: 200 mcg/kg PO as a single dose.
Onchocerciasis: 150 mcg/kg PO as a single dose; may be repeated in 3–12 mo if needed. Give with a full glass of water. Nausea and vomiting very common. Instruct patient to use barrier contraceptives while on this drug.

ixabepilone
Ixempra

Drug class and indications
Antineoplastic, microtubule inhibitor
As monotherapy or with capecitabine for the treatment of metastatic or locally advanced breast cancer after failure of anthracycline and a taxane.

Dosages and special alerts
40 mg/m^2 IV infused over 3 hr every 3 wk. Premedicate with corticosteroids. ⊗ ***Black box warning*** Severe liver failure possible; monitor for bone marrow suppression, neuropathies, cardiac effects.

lanreotide acetate
Somatuline Depot

Drug class and indications
Hormone, growth hormone (GH) inhibitor
Long-term treatment of acromegaly in patients who have had inadequate response to or cannot be treated with surgery or raditaion therapy.

Dosages and special alerts
Initially, 90 mg (range, 60–120 mg) subcutaneously every 4 wk for 3 mo; adjust dosage based on GH or insulin growth factor-1 level. Reduce dose with renal or hepatic impairment. Risk of gallstones, thyroid suppression, hypoglycemia, hyperglycemia, bradycardia. Monitor GH and insulin growth factor-1 serum levels to establish dosage.

lanthanum carbonate
Fosrenol

Drug class and indications
Phosphate binder
Reduction of serum phosphate levels in patients with end stage renal disease.

Dosages and special alerts
750–1,500 mg/day PO in divided doses taken with meals. Titrate to achieve desired serum

phosphate levels. Chew tablets thoroughly. GI upset may occur.

DANGEROUS DRUG

lapatinib

Tykerb

Drug class and indications

Kinase inhibitor, antineoplastic

With capecitabine, for treatment of patients with advanced or metastatic breast cancer whose tumors overexpress HER2 and who have received treatment including an anthracycline, a taxane, and trastuzumab.

Dosages and special alerts

1,250 mg (5 tablets) PO once daily on days 1–21. On days 1–14, given with capecitabine 2,000 mg/m^2/day PO in two doses about 12 hr apart. Give in repeating 21-day cycle. Reduce lapatinib dosage to 750 mg/day PO with severe hepatic impairment. Stop drug if left ventricular ejection fraction (LVEF) is grade 2 or higher or it falls below lower limit of normal; may be restarted at 1,000 mg/day after at least 2 wk if LVEF returns to normal. Monitor heart function. Rash and GI upset common. Numerous drug interactions possible; avoid grapefruit juice.

laronidase

Aldurazyme

Drug class and indications

Enzyme

Treatment of patients with Hurler and Hurler-Scheie forms of mucopolysaccharidosis 1 and for patients with Scheie form who have moderate to severe symptoms.

Dosages and special alerts

0.58 mg/kg IV, infused over 3–4 hr, once each wk. Infusion reaction common, antipyretic and antihistamine given 60 min before infusion helps; regular follow-up essential; drug improves respiratory function and walking capacity.

lenalidomide

Revlimid

Drug class and indications

Immune modulator, antianemic

Treatment of patients with transfusion-dependent anemia due to low or intermediate-1-risk myelodysplastic syndromes associated with a deletion of 5q cytogenetic abnormality with or without additional cytogenetic abnormalities.

Treatment of multiple myeloma, with dexamethasone, in patients who have received at least one other therapy.

Dosages and special alerts

Patients with anemia: 10 mg/day PO with water. Dosage may need to be lowered based on patient response and blood counts. Female patients must be tested to ensure that they are not pregnant and must agree to use two forms of contraception while using this drug. Male patients must agree to use contraceptive measures while using this drug.
Patients with multiple myeloma: 25 mg/day PO on days 1–21 of a 28-day cycle with dexamethasone 40 mg/day PO on days 1–4, 9–12, and 17–20 for first four cycles; for remaining cycles, given only on days 1–4.
Patients with renal impairment: Patient should be monitored closely and dosage adjusted downward as needed. Associated with serious birth defects; only dispensed through the Revassist Program and requires frequent pregnancy tests and signed agreement of understanding of risks; risk of PE, DVTs. Patient cannot donate blood or sperm.

DANGEROUS DRUG

lepirudin

Refludan

Drug class and indications

Anticoagulant

Treatment of heparin-induced thrombocytopenia associated with thromboembolic disease; a rare allergic reaction to heparin; directly inhibits thrombin.

Dosages and special alerts
0.4 mg/kg initial IV bolus followed by a continuous infusion of 0.15 mg/kg for 2–10 days. Monitor for bleeding from any sites; watch for hepatic injury. Reduce dosage with renal failure. Increased risk of bleeding if combined with chamomile, garlic, ginger, ginkgo, or ginseng therapy.

levoleucovorin

Drug class and indications
Folate analogue, rescue drug

To diminish the toxicity and counteract the effects of impaired methotrexate elimination and of inadvertent overdosage of folic acid antagonists after high-dose methotrexate therapy in osteosarcoma.

Dosages and special alerts
Serum methotrexate level of 10 micromolars at 24 hr, one micromolar at 48 hr, and less than 0.2 micromolar at 72 hr after methotrexate administration: 7.5 mg IV every 6 hr for 60 hr. (Ten doses starting at 24 hr after start of methotrexate.)
Serum methotrexate level remaining about 0.2 micromolar at 72 hr and more than 0.05 micromolar at 96 hr after methotrexate administration: Continue 7.5 mg IV every 6 hr until the methotrexate level is less than 0.05 micromolar.
Serum methotrexate level of 50 micromolars or more at 24 hr or 5 micromolars or more at 48 hr after administration, or a 100% or greater increase in serum creatinine level at 24 hr after methotrexate administration: 75 mg IV every 3 hr until methotrexate is less that 1 micromolar. Then 7.5 mg IV every 3 hr until methotrexate is less than 0.5 micromolar.
Inadvertent methotrexate overdose: 7.5 mg IV every 6 hr beginning within 24 hr of overdosage. Continue until methotrexate levels are within nontoxic range. Administer slowly because of high calcium levels in solution.

lincomycin hydrochloride
Lincocin

Drug class and indications
Lincosamide antibiotic

Treatment of serious infections that are responsive to lincomycin, when less toxic antibiotics are not effective.

Dosages and special alerts
Adult: 500 mg PO every 6–8 hr, or 600 mg IM every 12–24 hr, or 600 mg–1 g IV every 8–12 hr. Pediatric: 30–60 mg/kg/day PO, or 10 mg/kg IM every 12–24 hr, or 10–20 mg/kg/day IV in divided doses. Serious colitis can occur; have metronidazole or vancomycin and corticosteroids available; monitor for stomatitis.

lutropin
Luveris

Drug class and indications
Luteinizing hormone, fertility drug

Used in combination with *Gonal-f* to stimulate follicle development in hypogonadotropic hypogonadal women as part of a fertility regimen.

Dosages and special alerts
75 international units subcutaneously daily with 75–150 international units *Gonal-f* for up to 14 days per cycle. Monitor for ovarian overstimulation; there is a risk for multiple births.

mecasermin
Increlex

Drug class and indications
Insulin growth factor-1

Long-term treatment of growth failure in children with severe primary insulin growth factor-1 deficiency or with growth hormone gene deletion who have developed neutralizing antibodies to growth hormone.

Dosages and special alerts

Dosage is based on individual response and glucose levels. Initially, 0.04–0.08 mg/kg (40–80 mcg/kg) bid by subcutaneous injection; may be increased by 0.04 mg/kg per dose to a maximum dose of 0.12 mg/kg bid. Hypoglycemia is common, monitor patient and ensure that patient eats after administration; tonsillar hypertrophy is common.

mesna

Mesnex

Drug class and indications

Cytoprotective drug

Prophylaxis to reduce the incidence of ifosfamide-induced hemorrhagic cystitis.

Unlabeled use: Reduction of the incidence of cyclophosphamide-induced hemorrhagic cystitis.

Dosages and special alerts

20% ifosfamide dose IV at the time of ifosfamide injection and at 4 and 8 hr after that. Timing needs to be exact. Monitor for any signs of bladder hemorrhage.

methazolamide

GlaucTabs

Drug classes and indications

Glaucoma drug, carbonic anhydrase inhibitor

Adjunct treatment of chronic open angle glaucoma, secondary glaucoma.

Preoperative use in acute angle-closure glaucoma where delay in surgery is desired to lower IOP.

Dosages and special alerts

50–100 mg PO bid or tid as needed to achieve best results. Administer with food if GI upset is a problem. Arrange for regular evaluation of IOP.

methoxsalen

Oxsoralen-Ultra, Uvadex

Drug class and indications

Psoralen

Symptomatic treatment of severe disabling psoriasis refractory to other forms of therapy; repigmentation of vitiliginous skin.

Treatment of cutaneous cell lymphoma.

Unlabeled use: With ultraviolet A radiation (UVAR), treatment of mycosis fungoides.

Orphan drug use: With UVAR photophoresis to treat diffuse systemic sclerosis; prevention of acute rejection of cardiac allografts.

Dosages and special alerts

Oral: Dosage varies with weight; dosing must be timed to coincide with UV light exposure. Do not expose patient to additional UV light. GI effects are very common.

methsuximide

Celontin

Drug class and indications

Antiepileptic, succinimide

Control of absence seizures when refractory to other drugs.

Dosages and special alerts

300 mg/day PO for the first wk; may increase to a maximum of 1.2 g/day as needed. Reduce dosage slowly, do not stop suddenly. Discontinue drug if rash, altered blood count, unusual depression or aggression occurs. May be used with other antiepileptic drugs. Increased risk of suicidality.

methylnaltrexone bromide

Relistor

Drug class and indications

Opioid receptor antagonist, laxative

Treatment of opioid-induced constipation in patients with advanced illness receiving palliative care when response to laxative therapy has not been sufficient.

Dosages and special alerts

Dosage depends on weight. 38–less than 62 kg: 8 mg by subcutaneous injection every other day. 62–114 kg: 12 mg by subcutaneous injection every other day. If weight falls outside the above limits: 0.15 mg/kg per dose by subcutaneous injection every other day. Reduce dose by one-half with severe renal impairment. Monitor for severe diarrhea.

metyrosine

Demser

Drug class and indications

Enzyme inhibitor

Preoperative preparation for surgery for pheochromocytoma.

Management of pheochromocytoma when surgery is contraindicated.

Chronic treatment of malignant pheochromocytoma.

Dosages and special alerts

250–500 mg PO qid. Preoperative: 2–3 g/day PO for 5–7 days. Maximum, 4 g/day. Ensure a liberal intake of fluids. Severe diarrhea may occur; use antidiarrheals if needed.

miglustat

Zavesca

Drug class and indications

Enzyme inhibitor

Treatment of adult patients with mild to moderate type I Gaucher's disease for whom enzyme replacement is not a therapeutic option.

Dosages and special alerts

100 mg PO tid at regular intervals. Monitor for diarrhea, weight loss, and tremor; dosage may need to be reduced. Drug is pregnancy category X and it may also alter men's fertility. Caution patient about tremor development.

milnacipran

Savella

Drug class and indications

Selective serotonin and norepinephrine reuptake inhibitor

Management of fibromyalgia in adults.

Dosages and special alerts

Initially, 12.5 mg/day PO; increase over 1 wk to recommended dose of 50 mg PO bid. Doses up to 200 mg/day have been used. ⊗ ***Black box warning*** Increased risk of suicidality; monitor patient accordingly. Avoid use with MAO inhibitors and in patients with uncontrolled narrow-angle glaucoma. Serotonin syndrome has been reported. Headache, nausea, constipation, dizziness, insomnia, dry mouth, and palpitations are common.

DANGEROUS DRUG

mitotane

Lysodren

Drug class and indications

Antineoplastic

Treatment of inoperable hormone-secreting or hormone-non-secreting adrenal cortical carcinomas.

Dosages and special alerts

2–6 g/day PO in divided doses tid to qid, slowly increased to 9–10 g/day; if no benefits are seen by 3 mo, consider another form of treatment. Birth defects have been reported with use; suggest use of contraceptives. ⊗ ***Black box warning*** Discontinue temporarily in times of severe stress; adrenal hormone replacement may be needed in times of stress.

nefazodone

Drug class and indications

Antidepressant

Treatment of depression.

Dosages and special alerts

200 mg/day PO in divided doses, may be increased at 1-wk intervals to 300–600 mg/day. Limit available doses for severely depressed patients, and take suicide precautions. Use caution to assure at least 14 days between MAOI and nefazodone use and at least 7 days between stopping nefazodone and starting MAOIs. ⊗ ***Black box warning*** Watch for signs of hepatic impairment, and stop drug

immediately if they occur. Increased risk of suicidality, suicidal ideation.

DANGEROUS DRUG

nelarabine

Arranon

Drug class and indications

Antimitotic drug, antineoplastic

Treatment of patients with T-cell acute lymphoblastic leukemia and T-cell lymphoblastic lymphoma whose disease has not responded to or has relapsed following treatment with at least two chemotherapy regimens.

Dosages and special alerts

Adults: 1,500 mg/m^2 IV over 2 hr on days 1, 3, and 5; repeat every 21 days. Pediatric patients: 650 mg/m^2 IV over 1 hr daily for 5 consecutive days; repeat every 21 days. Bone marrow suppression common. ⊗ ***Black box warning*** Watch for neurologic toxicity, including neuropathies and demyelination disorders.

nesiritide

Natrecor

Drug class and indications

Human B-type natriuretic peptide, vasodilator

Treatment of patients with acutely decompensated HF with dyspnea at rest or with minimal activity.

Dosages and special alerts

2 mcg/kg IV bolus followed by a continuous infusion of 0.01 mcg/kg/min for no longer than 48 hr. Monitor patient continuously. Discontinue if serious hypotension occurs, which could worsen condition. Maintain hydration. Replace any reconstituted solution every 24 hr.

nilotinib

Tasigna

Drug class and indications

Kinase inhibitor, antineoplastic

Treatment of chronic phase and accelerated phase Philadelphia chromosome–positive CML in adults resistant to or intolerant of prior therapy that included imatinib.

Dosages and special alerts

400 mg PO bid, about 12 hr apart, without food. Dosage may need adjustment based on myelosuppression during therapy. Watch for prolonged QT interval, bone marrow suppression, and possible liver toxicity.

nimodipine

Drug class and indications

Calcium channel blocker

Improvement of neurologic deficits due to spasm following a subarachnoid hemorrhage (SAH) from ruptured congenital intracranial aneurysm.

Dosages and special alerts

60 mg PO every 4 hr, beginning within 96 hr of SAH for 21 consecutive days. Monitor for cardiac effects (arrhythmias, hypotension). If patient is unable to take oral medications, remove contents of capsule using a needle and empty contents into nasogastric tube; flush with 30 mL normal saline.

nitazoxanide

Alinia

Drug class and indications

Antiprotozoal

Treatment of diarrhea caused by *Cryptosporidium parvum* in patients 1 yr and older.

Treatment of *Giardia lamblia* in pediatric patients 1–11 yr.

Dosages and special alerts

Patients 12–47 mo: 5 mL (100 mg nitazoxanide) PO every 12 hr for 3 days. Patients 4–11 yr: 10 mL (200 mg nitazoxanide) PO every 12 hr for 3 days. Patients 12 yr and older: 500 mg (tablet or suspension) PO every 12 hr for 3 days taken with food. Obtain stool for ova and parasite testing before beginning therapy. To reconstitute, tap bottle until all powder flows freely; add about 24 mL of water to bottle and shake vigorously to suspend powder; add remaining 24 mL of water and shake vigorously again. Use cautiously with diabetic patients; suspension contains sucrose. Give drug with food. Advise parents to use good hand-washing technique and to dispose of diapers properly, when appropriate.

ofatumumab

Arzerra

Drug class and indications

Cytotoxic monoclonal antibody, antineoplastic

Treatment of chronic lymphocytic leukemia refractory to standard therapy.

Dosages and special alerts

12 doses given by IV infusion using the following schedule: 300 mg, followed in 1 wk by 2,000 mg/wk for seven doses, followed 4 wk later by 2,000 mg every 4 wk for four doses. Premedicate patient with acetaminophen, antihistamines, and IV corticosteroids. Infusion reaction is common; bone marrow suppression and infections, including progressive multifocal leukoencephalopathy and activation of hepatitis B, can occur; rash and GI effects are most common.

olsalazine sodium

Dipentum

Drug class and indications

Anti-inflammatory

Maintenance of remission of ulcerative colitis in patients intolerant to sulfasalazine.

Dosages and special alerts

1 g/day PO, divided into two doses. Give with meals. Monitor patient for renal impairment. Abdominal pain common.

omalizumab

Xolair

Drug class and indications

Monoclonal antibody, antiasthmatic

To decrease asthma exacerbation in patients 12 yr and older with moderate to severe persistent asthma who have a positive skin test to a perennial airborne allergen, who are not controlled by inhaled corticosteroids.

Dosages and special alerts

150–375 mg by subcutaneous injection every 2–4 wk, based on body weight and pretreatment immunoglobulin E levels. Discontinue and arrange for appropriate therapy at first sign of severe allergic reaction. Solution is thick; complete injection may take 5–10 sec. Do not use during pregnancy or lactation.

oprelvekin

Neumega

Drug class and indications

Interleukin

Prevention of severe thrombocytopenia and reduction of platelet transfusions following myelosuppressive chemotherapy in patients with nonmyeloid malignancies at high risk to develop severe thrombocytopenia.

Dosages and special alerts

50 mcg/kg/day subcutaneously starting 1 day after chemotherapy and continuing for 14–21 days or until platelet count is at least 50,000 cells/mm^3. Protect patient from exposure to infection; urge the use of contraceptives. ⊗ ***Black box warning*** Drug may cause severe allergic reaction, including anaphylaxis.

DANGEROUS DRUG

oxaliplatin

Eloxatin

Drug class and indications

Antineoplastic

Treatment of patients with metastatic carcinoma of the colon or rectum whose disease has progressed during or within 6 mo of completion of first-line therapy with 5-fluorouracil (5-FU)/leucovorin (LV) and irinotecan; first-line therapy for advanced colorectal cancer with 5-FU and LV.

Dosages and special alerts
85 mg/m^2 IV infusion in 250–500 mL D_5W with leucovorin 200 mg/m^2 in D_5W both given over 2 hr followed by 5-FU 400 mg/m^2 IV bolus over 2–4 min, followed by 5-FU 600 mg/m^2 IV infusion in 500 mL D_5W as a 22-hr continuous infusion on day 1, then leucovorin 200 mg/m^2 IV infusion over 2 hr followed by 5-FU 400 mg/m^2 bolus given over 2–4 min, followed by 5-FU 600 mg/m^2 IV infusion in 500 mL D_5W as a 22-hr continuous infusion on day 2; repeat cycle every 2 wk. Premedicate with antiemetics and dexamethasone. Monitor for potentially dangerous anaphylactic reactions.

palifermin

Kepivance

Drug class and indications
Keratinocyte growth factor

To decrease the incidence and duration of severe oral mucositis in patients with hematologic malignancies receiving myelotoxic chemotherapy requiring hematopoietic stem cell support.

Dosages and special alerts
60 mcg/kg/day by IV bolus infusion for 3 consecutive days before and 3 consecutive days after chemotherapy regimen. Monitor for rash and mouth changes such as taste alteration.

DANGEROUS DRUG

panitumumab

Vectibix

Drug class and indications
Monoclonal antibody, antineoplastic

Treatment of epidermal growth factor receptor–expressing metastatic colorectal carcinoma with disease progressing with or after chemotherapy regimens containing fluoropyrimidine, cisplatin, and irinotecan.

Dosages and special alerts
6 mg/kg IV over 60 min every 14 days; doses larger than 1,000 mg should be given over 90 min. Dosage should be adjusted in patients experiencing infusion reactions or severe adverse reactions. ⊠ ***Black box warning*** Monitor patient for possibly severe infusion reactions, dermatological toxicity, pulmonary fibrosis.

paricalcitol

Zemplar

Drug class and indications
Vitamin

Prevention and treatment of secondary hyperparathyroidism associated with chronic renal failure.

Dosages and special alerts
0.04–0.1 mcg/kg injected during dialysis, not more often than every other day. Patients not on dialysis: 1–2 mcg/day PO or 2–4 mcg PO three times a wk, based on parathyroid levels. Monitor for hypercalcemia, treat appropriately. Ensure adherence to dietary regimen and use of calcium supplements.

pazopanib

Votrient

Drug class and indications
Kinase inhibitor, antineoplastic

Treatment of advanced renal cell carcinoma.

Dosages and special alerts
800 mg/day PO without food (at least 1 hr before or 2 hr after meals). Not for use with severe hepatic impairment; limit to 200 mg/day with moderate hepatic impairment. Prolongs QT interval. Fatal hemorrhagic events have been reported. Arterial thrombotic events, some fatal; GI perforations and fistulas; hypertension; hypothyroidism; and proteinuria have occurred. Pregnancy Category D; advise use of contraceptives. Diarrhea, depigmentation of hair, and GI effects are common. Patient must be monitored very carefully.

pegaptanib

Macugen

Drug class and indications
Monoclonal antibody

Treatment of neovascular (wet) age-related macular degeneration.

Dosages and special alerts
0.3 mg once every 6 wk by intravitreous injection into the affected eye. Monitor for vision changes, eye infection, retinal detachment, and traumatic cataract.

DANGEROUS DRUG

pegaspargase

Oncaspar

Drug class and indications
Antineoplastic

Treatment of ALL in patients hypersensitive to native forms of L-asparaginase or as a component of a multi-drug regimen.

Dosages and special alerts
2,500 international units/m^2 IM or IV every 14 days. Associated with pancreatitis, bone marrow depression, and renal toxicity. Monitor patient closely. Save IV use for extreme situations. IM use is preferred.

peginterferon alfa-2a

Pegasys

Drug class and indications
Interferon

Treatment of adults with hepatitis C who have compensated liver disease and who have not been treated with interferon alfa.

Dosages and special alerts
180 mcg subcutaneously once each wk for 48 wk. Adjust dosage with low neutrophil counts, low platelet counts, and for patients on dialysis or who have impaired liver function. Interstitial pneumonitis has been reported; monitor lung function closely. Cardiac dysfunction and hepatic impairment can occur. Protect patient from exposure to infection.

peginterferon alfa-2b

Peg-Intron

Drug class and indications
Interferon

Treatment of patients older than 18 yr with chronic hepatitis C, who have not received alpha interferon and who have compensated liver function.

■ **NEW INDICATION:** Treatment of hepatitis C in patients who have not received interferons; given with ribavirin.

Unlabeled use: Renal carcinoma.

Dosages and special alerts
1 mcg/kg subcutaneously once per wk for 1 yr; flulike symptoms common. Monitor bone marrow and liver function.

pegvisomant

Somavert

Drug class and indications
Human growth hormone analogue

Treatment of acromegaly in patients who have had no adequate response to surgery or radiation and other standard therapies or patients for whom these therapies are not appropriate.

Dosages and special alerts
40 mg by subcutaneous injection as a loading dose; then 10 mg/day by subcutaneous injection. Local reactions to the injection are common; rotate sites regularly and monitor for infection. Monitor liver function and blood glucose levels regularly.

DANGEROUS DRUG

pemetrexed

Alimta

Drug class and indications
Antifolate antineoplastic given with cisplatin

Treatment of patients with malignant mesothelioma whose disease is unresectable or who are not candidates for surgery.

Treatment of locally advanced or metastatic non–small-cell lung cancer as a single agent after prior chemotherapy or with cisplatin for first-line treatment.

Dosages and special alerts
500 mg/m² IV infused over 10 min on day 1, followed by 75 mg/m² cisplatin (treatment of mesothelioma only) IV over 2 hr; repeat cycle every 21 days. Pretreat with corticosteroid, folic acid, and vitamin B_{12}. Monitor for bone marrow suppression and GI effects.

penicillamine

Cuprimine, Depen

Drug classes and indications
Chelate, antirheumatic

Treatment of severe, active rheumatoid arthritis when other therapies fail, Wilson's disease, cystinuria when other measures fail.

Dosages and special alerts
125–250 mg/day PO; may be increased to 1 g/day if needed. Serious bone marrow suppression, myasthenic syndrome, polymyositis can occur; discontinue if drug fever occurs; Monitor patient closely; push fluids with cystinuria.

pentetate calcium trisodium (Ca-DTPA)

penetate zinc trisodium (Zn-DTPA)

Drug class and indications
Chelate

Treatment of patients with known or suspected internal contamination with plutonium, americium, or curium, to increase rates of elimination.

Dosages and special alerts
1 g Ca-DTPA IV followed in 24 hr by 1 g Zn-DTPA IV using a slow IV push over 3–4 min. Pediatric patients: 14 mg/kg/day IV (not to exceed 1 g/dose), first using Ca-DTPA, then switching to Zn-DTPA 24 hr after initial dose. Use precautions for handling wastes to avoid contamination of others. Nursing mothers should express breast milk and dispose of it properly. Encourage hydration to improve elimination of the radioactive materials.

pentosan polysulfate sodium

Elmiron

Drug class and indications
Bladder protectant

Relief of bladder pain associated with interstitial cystitis.

Dosages and special alerts
100 mg PO tid on an empty stomach. May cause loss of hair (suggest wearing a wig); increased bleeding (is a low–molecular-weight heparin).

DANGEROUS DRUG

pentostatin (2' deoxycoformycin [DCF])

Nipent

Drug class and indications
Antineoplastic; antibiotic

Treatment of adults with alpha interferon refractory hairy cell leukemia, chronic lymphocytic leukemia, cutaneous T-cell lymphoma, peripheral T-cell lymphoma.

Dosages and special alerts
4 mg/m² IV every other wk, decrease to 2 mg/m² with renal impairment. Hydrate patient before each dose and monitor closely. ⊗ ***Black box warning*** Associated with fatal pulmonary toxicity and bone marrow depression.

pilocarpine hydrochloride

Salagen

Drug class and indications
Parasympathomimetic; mouth and throat product

Treatment of symptoms of xerostomia from salivary gland dysfunction caused by radiation therapy for cancer of the head and neck.

Dosages and special alerts

5–10 mg PO tid. Can cause blurred vision, parasympathomimetic effects. Monitor susceptible patients carefully.

pimozide

Orap

Drug class and indications

Antipsychotic; diphenylbutylpiperidine

Suppression of severely compromising motor or phonic tics in patients with Tourette syndrome who have not responded to other therapy.

Dosages and special alerts

1–2 mg/day PO; up to a maximum of 10 mg/day. Monitor for prolonged QTc interval. Has been associated with severe cardiac complications; may cause dizziness, sedation, Parkinson-like symptoms.

plerixafor

Mozobil

Drug class and indications

Hematopoietic stem cell mobilizer

Mobilization of hematopoietic stem cells to the peripheral blood for collection and subsequent autologous transplantation in patients with non-Hodgkin lymphoma and multiple myeloma in combination with a granulocyte-colony stimulating factor (G-CSF).

Dosages and special alerts

Start therapy after patient has received G-CSF once daily for 4 days; 0.24 mg/kg by subcutaneous injection, repeated for up to 4 consecutive days. Administer approximately 11 hours before apheresis. In severe renal impairment, reduce dose to 0.16 mg/kg. May mobilize leukemic cells; do not use in leukemia. Monitor blood counts and watch for potential splenic rupture. Headache, dizziness, nausea, vomiting, and injection site reactions are common.

poly-L-lactic acid

Sculptra

Drug classes and indications

Polymer, cosmetic device

Restoration and correction of the signs of lipoatrophy in patients with HIV syndrome.

Dosages and special alerts

0.1–0.2 mL injected intradermally at each injection site. Up to 20 injections per cheek may be needed; re-treat periodically. Do not use if any sign of skin infection is present. Apply ice packs to area immediately after injection and for first 24 hr; massage injection sites daily.

DANGEROUS DRUG

porfimer sodium

Photofrin

Drug class and indications

Antineoplastic

Photodynamic therapy for palliation of patients with completely or partially obstructing esophageal cancer or transitional cancer who cannot be treated with laser alone, transitional cell carcinoma in situ of urinary bladder, endobronchial non–small-cell lung cancer.

Dosages and special alerts

2 mg/kg IV given as a slow injection over 3–5 min; must be followed in 40–50 hr and again in 96–120 hr by laser therapy. Monitor for pleural effusion and respiratory complications. Avoid any contact with the drug. Protect patient from exposure to light for 30 days after treatment.

pralatrexate

Folotyn

Drug class and indications

Folate analogue metabolic inhibitor, antineoplastic

Treatment of relapsed or refractory peripheral T-cell lymphoma.

Dosages and special alerts
30 mg/m² as an IV push over 3–5 min once weekly for 6 wk in a 7-wk cycle. Patient should also receive vitamin B_{12}, 1 mg IM every 8–10 wk, and folic acid, 1–1.25 mg/day PO. Pregnancy Category X. Bone marrow suppression is common. Mucositis can be severe; dosage may need to be modified.

praziquantel
Biltricide

Drug class and indications
Anthelmintic

Treatment of Schistosoma infections, liver flukes.

Orphan drug use: treatment of neurocysticercosis.

Dosages and special alerts
3 doses of 20–25 mg/kg PO as a one-day treatment; allow 4–6 hr between doses. Administer with food. Do not cut, crush, or chew tablets; swallow whole. GI upset is common.

DANGEROUS DRUG

procarbazine hydrochloride
Matulane

Drug class and indications
Antineoplastic

Used in combination with other antineoplastics for treatment of stage III and IV Hodgkin's lymphoma (part of MOPP chemotherapy regimen).

Dosages and special alerts
2–4 mg/kg/day PO for the first wk, and then 4–6 mg/kg/day PO. Maintenance dosage: 1–2 mg/kg/day. Monitor bone marrow and adjust dosage accordingly. Stress need for barrier contraceptives. Advise patient to avoid alcohol and foods high in tyramine.

propantheline bromide
Pro-Banthine

Drug class and indications
Anticholinergic, antimuscarinic, parasympatholytic, antispasmodic

Adjunct therapy in the treatment of peptic ulcer.

Unlabeled uses: antisecretory and antispasmodic.

Dosages and special alerts
7.5–15 mg PO 30 min before meals and at bedtime. Pediatric patients: 1.5 mg/kg/day PO in divided doses tid to qid as an antisecretory or 2–3 mg/kg/day PO in divided doses every 4–6 hr and at bedtime as an antispasmodic. Not approved for peptic ulcer. Monitor patient's hydration. Control environment to prevent hyperpyrexia. Encourage patient to void before each dose because urine retention can occur.

DANGEROUS DRUG

protein C concentrate (human)
Ceprotin

Drug class and indications
Blood product, anticoagulant

Replacement therapy for patients with severe congenital protein C deficiency to prevent and treat venous thrombosis and purpura fulminans.

Dosages and special alerts
Initially, 100–120 international units/kg by IV injection. Then 60–80 international units/kg IV every 6 hr for three more doses. Maintenance dose, 45–60 international units/kg IV every 6–12 hr based on patient response. Monitor patient closely for possibly severe allergic reaction. Risk of disease transmission in blood products.

quinine sulfate
Qualaquin

Drug class and indications
Cinchonan, antimalarial

Treatment of uncomplicated *Plasmodium falciparum* malaria.

Dosages and special alerts
648 mg (two capsules) PO every 8 hr for 7 days. Not for use in children. Reduce dosage with severe renal impairment. Cinchonism causes vision changes, dizziness, sweating, tinnitus, headache, progressing to GI problems. Use caution with prolonged QT interval. Not for treating nocturnal leg cramps.

ranibizumab
Lucentis

Drug class and indications
Monoclonal antibody, ophthalmic agent
Treatment of patients with neovascular (wet) age-related macular degeneration.

Dosages and special alerts
0.5 mg (0.05 mL) by intravitreal injection once every mo; may be changed to once every 3 mo after the first four injections if monthly injections are not feasible. Monitor patient carefully for detached retina, increased IOP. Patient should be anesthesized before injection and should receive antibiotic treatment.

rasburicase
Elitek

Drug class and indications
Enzyme
Initial management of plasma uric acid levels in patients with leukemia, lymphoma, and solid tumor malignancies who are receiving anti-cancer therapy expected to result in tumor lysis and subsequent elevation of plasma uric acid.

Dosages and special alerts
0.15 or 0.2 mg/kg IV as a single daily infusion over 30 min for 5 days. Chemotherapy should be started 4–24 hr after the first dose. Blood drawn to monitor uric acid levels must be collected in pre-chilled, heparinized vials and kept in an ice-water bath. Analysis must be done within 4 hr.

rifabutin
Mycobutin

Drug class and indications
Antibiotic
Prevention and treatment of disseminated *Mycobacterium avium* complex disease in patients with advanced HIV infection.

Dosages and special alerts
Adults: 300 mg PO daily. Children: 5 mg/kg/day. GI effects, bone marrow depression common. Body fluids turn a reddish-orange; contact lenses may be stained. Do not use with active TB.

rilonacept
Arcalyst

Drug class and indications
Interleukin blocker, anti-inflammatory drug
Treatment of cryopyrin-associated periodic syndromes, including familial cold autoinflammatory syndrome and Muckle-Wells syndrome in adults and children 12 yr and older.

Dosages and special alerts
Adults: Loading dose of 320 mg given as two 160-mg (2-mL) subcutaneous injections given at different sites; then once-weekly subcutaneous injections of 160 mg (2 mL). Pediatric patients 12–17 yr: Loading dose of 4.4 mg/kg up to a maximum of 320 mg subcutaneously. May be given in divided doses if necessary; then once-weekly injections of 2.2 mg/kg up to a maximum 160 mg. Monitor lipid levels. Risk of severe infection exists.

riluzole
Rilutek

Drug class and indications
Amyotrophic lateral sclerosis (ALS) drug
Treatment of ALS; extends survival time or time to tracheostomy.
Orphan drug use: Treatment of Huntington's disease.

Dosages and special alerts
50 mg PO every 12 hr. Slows disease but does not cure it. Take on an empty stomach at the same time each day. Protect drug from light. Commonly causes nausea and vomiting.

DANGEROUS DRUG

rituximab

Rituxan

Drug class and indications
Antineoplastic, monoclonal antibody

First-line treatment or treatment of relapsed or refractory, low-grade or follicular CD20-positive non-Hodgkin's B-cell lymphoma.

With methotrexate, to reduce signs and symptoms of moderately to severely active rheumatoid arthritis in patients with inadequate response to tumor necrosis factor antagonists.

Dosages and special alerts
Lymphoma in adults: 375 mg/m^2 IV, once weekly for four or eight doses.
Arthritis: Two 1,000-mg infusions separated by 2 wk, given with methotrexate.
Premedicate patient with acetaminophen and diphenhydramine to decrease fever, chills associated with infusion. Protect patient from exposure to infection. Monitor for reactivation of hepatitis B; discontinue use if viral hepatitis occurs. ⊗ ***Black box warning*** Fatal infusion reactions, severe cutaneous reactions, and tumor lysis syndrome are possible.

romidepsin

Istodax

Drug class and indications
Histone deacetylase inhibitor, antineoplastic

Treatment of patients with cutaneous T-cell lymphoma who have received at least one prior systemic therapy.

Dosages and special alerts
14 mg/m^2 IV over a 4-hr period on days 1, 8, and 15 of a 28-day cycle. Repeat every 28 days if patient tolerates drug and benefits from it effects. Pregnancy category D. Associated with ECG changes, including prolonged QT interval. Binds to estrogen receptors and may cause fetal harm. May negate effects of hormonal contraceptives; use of barrier contraceptives is advised. May cause GI upset and bone marrow depression.

romiplostim

Nplate

Drug class and indications
Thrombopoietin receptor agonist

Treatment of thrombocytopenia in patients with chronic immune thrombocytopenic purpura who have insufficient response to corticosteroids, immunoglobulins, or splenectomy.

Dosages and special alerts
1 mcg/kg by subcutaneous injection once a wk; adjust dosage in increments of 1 mcg/kg to achieve platelet count of 50×10^9. Maximum weekly dose is 10 mcg/kg. Risk of thrombosis, reticulin deposition in the bone marrow, and hematologic malignancies. Patient must be enrolled in the *Nplate NEXUS* program; drug must be administered by a health care provider enrolled in the program. Not for use in pregnant or nursing women.

rufinamide

Banzel

Drug class and indications
Antiepileptic, sodium channel blocker

Adjunctive treatment of seizures associated with Lennox-Gastaut syndrome in adults and children 4 yr and older.

Dosages and special alerts
Adults: Initially, 400–800 mg/day PO in two equally divided doses. Increase to a target 3,200 mg/day PO in two equally divided doses. Pediatric patients age 4 and older: Initially, 10 mg/kg/day PO in two equally divided doses to a target of 45 mg/kg/day or 3,200 mg/day, whichever is less. Monitor for suicidal ideation and mood changes. Hormonal contraceptives may not be effective if combined with this drug.

sacrosidase

Sucraid

Drug class and indications

Enzyme

Oral replacement of genetically determined sucrase deficiency.

Dosages and special alerts

15 kg or less: 1 mL or 22 drops per meal or snack. More than 15 kg: 2 mL or 44 drops per meal or snack. Do not use in patients with known allergy to yeast. Refrigerate bottle; discard 4 wk after opening.

sapropterin dihydrochloride

Kuvan

Drug class and indications

Coenzyme factor, phenylalanine reducer

With diet, to reduce blood phenylalanine level in patients with hyperphenylalinemia caused by tetrahydrobiopterin-responsive phenylketonuria.

Dosages and special alerts

4 yr and older: Starting dose 10 mg/kg/day PO once daily. May be adjusted to 5–20 mg/kg/day based on blood phenylalanine level. Dissolve tablets in water or apple juice and have patient drink within 15 min. Monitor phenylalanine level and adjust dosage as needed. Must be used with dietary restrictions.

secretin

ChiRhoStim

Drug class and indications

Diagnostic agent

Stimulation of pancreatic secretions to aid in the diagnosis of pancreatic exocrine dysfunction.

Stimulation of gastrin secretion to aid in the diagnosis of gastrinoma.

Dosages and special alerts

0.2–0.4 mcg/kg IV over 1 min.

sevelamer hydrochloride

Renagel

Drug class and indications

Calcium-phosphate binder

Reduction of serum phosphorus levels in hemodialysis patients in end-stage renal disease.

Dosages and special alerts

One to four tablets with each meal based on serum phosphorus levels; may be increased by one tablet per meal to achieve desired serum phosphorus level. Does not cause increase in calcium levels.

sirolimus

Rapamune

Drug class and indications

Immunosuppressant

Prophylaxis for organ rejection in renal transplants in conjunction with adrenal corticosteroids and cyclosporine.

Dosages and special alerts

Dosage based on weight. Less than 40 kg: Loading dose of 3 mg/m^2 then 1 mg/m^2/day PO. 40 kg or more: Loading dose of 6 mg PO as soon after transplant as possible, and then daily dose of 2 mg PO in combination with cyclosporine and corticosteroids. Monitor liver and renal function closely; changes could indicate need to change dose or discontinue drug. ⊗ ***Black box warning*** Drug is associated with these risks: Increased susceptibility to infections, graft loss and hepatic artery thrombosis with liver transplant, bronchial anastomotic dehiscence in lung transplants.

sodium ferric gluconate complex

Ferrlecit

Drug class and indications

Iron product

Treatment of iron deficiency in patients undergoing chronic hemodialysis who are also receiving erythropoietin therapy.

Dosages and special alerts
Test dose: 2 mL diluted in 50 mL 0.9% sodium chloride for injection, given IV over 60 min. Adults: 10 mL diluted in 100 mL 0.9% sodium chloride for injection given IV over 60 min. Most patients will initially require 8 doses given at sequential dialysis sessions, then periodic use based on hematocrit. Flushing and hypertension are common effects.

sodium hyaluronate

Hyalgan

Drug class and indications
Hyaluronic acid derivative

Treatment of pain in osteoarthritis of the knee in patients who have failed to respond to conservative therapy and analgesics.

Dosages and special alerts
2 mL by intra-articular injection once a wk for 5 wk. Do not use in any other joint; remove effusions. Before injection, use strict aseptic technique. Avoid any weight bearing after injection.

sodium phenylacetate/ sodium benzoate

Ammonul

Drug class and indications
Urea substitute, ammonia reducer

Adjunctive therapy in the treatment of hyperammonemia and associated encephalopathy in patients with deficiencies in enzymes associated with the urea cycle.

Dosages and special alerts
0–20 kg: 2.5 mL/kg; more than 20 kg: 55 mL/m^2. Given IV through a central line with arginine. Patients not responsive will require hemodialysis.

somatropin, rDNA origin

Zorbtive

Drug class and indications
Human growth hormone

Treatment of short-bowel syndrome in patients receiving specialized nutritional support.

Dosages and special alerts
Adults: 0.1 mg/kg/day subcutaneously to a maximum of 8 mg/day for a total of 4 wk. Swelling and arthralgias may limit use; reduce dose by 50%. Monitor for glucose intolerance and intracranial hypertension.

DANGEROUS DRUG

sorafenib tosylate

Nexavar

Drug class and indications
Kinase inhibitor, antineoplastic

Treatment of patients with advanced renal cell carcinoma, hepatocellular carcinoma.

Dosages and special alerts
Adults: 400 mg PO bid on an empty stomach (1 hr before or 2 hr after eating). Swallow tablets whole. Patients with adverse drug reactions: Temporarily stop drug, or reduce dose to 400 mg/day PO and monitor patient closely. Not recommended for pediatric patients. Monitor for skin reactions, hand-foot syndrome, hypertension.

streptomycin sulfate

Drug class and indications
Antibiotic

Treatment of tularemia, plague, subacute bacterial endocarditis (if less toxic agents are not appropriate).

Fourth drug in the treatment of TB.

Dosages and special alerts
Adults: 15 mg/kg/day IM, or 25–30 mg/kg IM 2 or 3 times a wk. Pediatric patients: 20–40 mg/kg/day IM or 25–30 mg/kg/IM 2 or 3 times a wk.
Tularemia: 1–2 g/day IM for 7–14 days.
Plague: 2 g/day IM in two divided doses for at least 10 days.
Tinnitus, dizziness, ringing in the ears, hearing loss are common. Monitor patient for renal toxicity, injection site infections.

DANGEROUS DRUG

streptozocin

Zanosar

Drug classes and indications

Alkylating drug, antineoplastic

Treatment of metastatic islet cell carcinoma of the pancreas.

Dosages and special alerts

500 mg/m^2 IV for 5 consecutive days every 6 wk, or 1,000 mg/m^2 IV once per wk for 2 wk, and then increase to 1,500 mg/m^2 IV each wk. Bone marrow suppression likely; monitor counts carefully and reduce dosage as needed. ⊗ ***Black box warning*** Monitor for renal and liver toxicity. Special handling of toxic drug required.

DANGEROUS DRUG

sunitinib

Sutent

Drug class and indications

Kinase inhibitor, antineoplastic

Treatment of GI stromal tumor if patient is intolerant to or tumor progresses after imatinib therapy.

Treatment of advanced renal cell carcinoma.

Dosages and special alerts

50 mg/day PO for 4 wk, followed by 2 wk of rest; repeat cycle. Monitor patient carefully for GI disturbances, bone marrow suppression; dosage adjustment may be needed.

talc, USP

Sterile Talc Powder

Drug class and indications

Sclerosing drug

To decrease the recurrence of malignant pleural effusion.

Dosages and special alerts

5 g in 50–100 mL sodium chloride injection injected into a chest tube after pleural fluid has been drained. Clamp chest tube and have patient change positions for 2 hr; unclamp chest tube and continue external suction. Acute respiratory distress syndrome, PE, MI, local reactions are common. Monitor patient closely.

tegaserod maleate

Zelnorm

Drug class and indications

5-HT$_4$ inhibitor

Treatment of IBS with constipation and chronic idiopathic constipation in women younger than 55 yr who meet specific criteria and who have no known pre-existing heart problems and are in critical need of the drug.

Available for restricted use only.

Dosages and special alerts

6 mg PO bid before meals for 4–6 wk; additional 4- to 6-wk courses may be considered. Patient must be made aware of drug's risks. Patient should be urged to report chest pain, severe headache.

telbivudine

Tyzeka

Drug class and indications

Nucleoside, antiviral

Treatment of chronic hepatitis B in adult patients with evidence of viral replication and either evidence of persistent elevations in serum aminotranferases (ALT or AST) or histologically active disease.

Dosages and special alerts

Adults older than 16 yr: 600 mg/day PO with or without food. Pediatric patients: Safety and efficacy not established. Patients with renal impairment: For creatinine clearance greater than 50 mL/min, no adjustment needed; for clearance of 30–49 mL/min, 600 mg PO every 48 hr; for clearance less than 30 mL/min, 600 mg PO every 72 hr; for end-stage renal disease, 600 mg PO every 96 hr. Monitor patient for myopathy, severe hepatic failure with steatosis, exacerbation of hepatitis B with discontinuation of drug.

DANGEROUS DRUG

temozolomide

Temodar

Drug class and indications

Antineoplastic

Treatment of refractory astrocytoma in patients at first relapse with disease progression on a drug regimen including a nitrosourea and procarbazine; treatment of advanced metastatic melanoma.

Treatment of adult patients with newly diagnosed glioblastoma multiforme with radiation therapy and then as maintenance therapy.

Dosages and special alerts

Anaplastic astrocytoma: Dose is based on body surface area. Taken for 5 consecutive days for a 28-day treatment cycle. Adjusted dose is based on neutrophil and platelet counts. Monitor bone marrow function closely. Especially toxic in women and the elderly.

Glioblastoma: 75 mg/m^2/day PO or IV for 42 days with focal radiation therapy, then 6 cycles: cycle 1—150 mg/m^2/day PO or IV for 5 days, 23 days rest; cycles 2–6—200 mg/m^2/day PO or IV for 5 days, 23 days rest.

DANGEROUS DRUG

temsirolimus

Torisel

Drug class and indications

Kinase inhibitor, antineoplastic

Treatment of advanced renal cell carcinoma.

Dosages and special alerts

30 min after giving prophylactic diphenhydramine 25–50 mg IV, give 25 mg IV infused over 30–60 min once per wk until disease progresses or unacceptable toxicity occurs. Monitor lung function, blood glucose level, bowel sounds, renal function. Assess patient for slowed healing. Do not give with vaccines. Do not give to pregnant women. Avoid giving with grapefruit juice, St. John's wort, numerous drugs.

teriparatide

Forteo

Drug class and indications

Parathyroid hormone, calcium regulator

Treatment of postmenopausal women with osteoporosis and high risk of fracture.

Treatment of men and women with osteoporosis associated with sustained systemic glucocorticoid therapy at high risk for fracture.

To increase bone mass in men with primary or hypogonadal osteoporosis at high risk for fracture.

Dosages and special alerts

20 mcg/day subcutaneously in thigh or abdominal wall; use for more than 2 yr is not recommended. ⊗ ***Black box warning*** Increased risk of osteosarcoma in rats; should not be use in patients with increased risk of osteosarcoma (Paget's disease, unexplained elevations in alkaline phosphatase level, open epiphyses, prior external beam or implant radiation therapy involving the skeleton). Not recommended for treatment of bone disease other than osteoporosis. May cause orthostatic hypotension; may increase risk of renal stones. Not for use by nursing mothers. Arthralgia, pain, and nausea are common.

thalidomide

Thalomid

Drug class and indications

Immune modulator

Treatment of erythema nodosum leprosum—painful inflammatory condition related to an immune reaction to dead bacteria following treatment of leprosy; newly diagnosed multiple myeloma; brain tumors; Crohn's disease; HIV-wasting syndrome; graft-host reaction in bone marrow transplant.

Dosages and special alerts

100–300 mg/day PO. Taken once daily with water at bedtime for at least 2 wk. Taper off in decrements of 50 mg every 2–4 wk. ⊗ ***Black box warning*** Associated with severe birth defects; women must have a pregnancy test and sign consent to use birth control to avoid pregnancy while on this drug (STEPS program).

tiludronate disodium

Skelid

Drug class and indications

Bisphosphonate

Treatment of Paget's disease in patients with alkaline phosphatase at least two times the upper limit of normal who are asymptomatic and at risk for future complications.

Dosages and special alerts

400 mg/day PO for 3 mo taken with 6–8 oz of plain water at least 2 hr before any other food or beverage. Monitor serum calcium closely; patient should increase intake of vitamin D and calcium; allow a 3-mo rest period if retreatment is needed.

tiopronin

Thiola

Drug class and indications

Thiol compound

Prevention of cystine kidney stone formation in patients with severe homozygous cystinuria with urine cystine levels exceeding 500 mg/day who are resistant to other therapy.

Dosages and special alerts

800 mg/day PO; increase to 1,000 mg/day in divided doses; take on an empty stomach. Monitor cystine levels at 1 mo and then every 3 mo. Patient should drink fluids liberally to 3 L/day.

tolazamide

Drug class and indications

Antidiabetic, first-generation sulfonylurea

Adjunct to diet and exercise to control blood glucose in patients with type 2 diabetes.

With insulin to control blood glucose levels and decrease the insulin dose in select patients with type 1 diabetes.

Dosages and special alerts

If fasting blood glucose is less than 200 mg/dL, 100 mg/day PO in the morning before breakfast. If fasting blood glucose is greater than 200 mg/dL, 250 mg/day PO. Do not exceed 1 g/day. Use caution with geriatric patients, who may be more sensitive to glucose-lowering effects. Adjust dosage based on patient response; switch to insulin in times of high stress. Be aware that patient may be at increased risk for CV events.

tolbutamide

Apo-Tolbutaminde (CAN), Orinase, Orinase Diagnostic

Drug class and indications

Antidiabetic, first-generation sulfonylurea, diagnostic agent

Adjunct to diet and exercise to control blood glucose level in patients with type 2 diabetes.

With insulin to control blood glucose levels and decrease insulin dose in select patients with type 1 diabetes.

To aid in diagnosis of pancreatic islet cell adenoma

Dosages and special alerts

1–2 g/day PO in the morning before breakfast; maintenance dose of 0.25–3 g/day PO based on patient response. Do not exceed 3 g/day. As a diagnostic agent: 20 mL IV infused over 2–3 min. Use caution with geriatric patients, who may be more sensitive to glucose-lowering effects; switch to insulin in times of high stress. Be aware that patient may be at increased risk for CV events.

tolvaptan

Samsca

Drug class and indications

Selective vasopressin receptor antagonist

Treatment of clinically significant hypervolemic or euvolemic hyponatremia, including patients with heart failure, cirrhosis, and SIADH.

Dosages and special alerts

15 mg PO once daily; may increase after at least 24 hr, based on patient response, to a maximum of 60 mg/day. ⊗ ***Black box***

warning Therapy should be initiated in a hospital setting, with close supervision of sodium and volume. Not for use when rapid correction of hyponatremia is needed. May cause fetal harm; do not give to nursing women. Dry mouth, constipation, increased blood glucose level, and polyuria are common.

DANGEROUS DRUG

topotecan hydrochloride

Hycamtin

Drug class and indications

Antineoplastic

Treatment of metastatic ovarian cancer after failure of traditional chemotherapy.

Treatment of small-cell lung cancer after failure of first-line treatment.

With cisplatin, for treatment of stage V recurrent or persistent carcinoma of the cervix when not amenable to surgery or radiation.

Dosages and special alerts

1.5 mg/m^2 IV over 30 min daily for 5 days, starting on day 1 of a 21-day course; minimum of 4 courses recommended (lung cancer, ovarian cancer).
0.75 mg/m^2 by IV infusion over 30 min on days 1, 2, 3 followed by cisplatin on day 1; repeat every 21 days (cervical cancer).
Provide analgesics. Suggest use of wig or head covering. Protect patient from exposure to infection. Barrier contraceptives should be urged. ⊗ ***Black box warning*** Monitor bone marrow carefully.

DANGEROUS DRUG

tositumomab and iodine I-131 tositumomab

Bexxar

Drug class and indications

Antineoplastic, monoclonal antibody

Treatment of CD20-positive, follicular non-Hodgkin's lymphoma in patients whose disease is refractory to rituximab and who have relapsed following chemotherapy.

Dosages and special alerts

Two-step treatment: 450 mg tositumomab IV in 50 mL 0.9% sodium chloride over 60 min, 5 mCi I-131 with 35 mg tositumomab in 30 mL sodium chloride IV over 20 min; then repeat as a therapeutic step, adjusting I-131 based on patient response. Drug is pregnancy category X. Risk of severe and prolonged cytopenia; hypersensitivity reactions including anaphylaxis have occurred.

tranexamic acid

Lysteda

Drug class and indications

Antifibrinolytic

Treatment of cyclic heavy menstrual bleeding.

Dosages and special alerts

1,300 mg PO tid for a maximum of 5 days during monthly menstruation. Reduce dosage with renal impairment. Increased risk of clots, stroke, and MI if combined with hormonal contraceptives, antihemophilic agents, or oral tretinoin. Visual changes or severe allergic reaction should lead to immediate discontinuation of drug. Cerebral infarct and cerebral edema have occurred. Most common adverse effects include pain, sinus and nasal symptoms, anemia, and fatigue.

trazodone hydrochloride

Apo-Trazodone (CAN), NuTrazadone (CAN)

Drug class and indications

Antidepressant

Treatment of depression in inpatients and outpatients and for depressed patients with or without anxiety.

Dosages and special alerts

150 mg/day PO in divided doses; may be increased to maximum of 400 mg/day PO in divided doses. For severe depresssion, maximum dosage 600 mg/day PO; adjust to a lower dosage as soon as possible. Geriatric patients should start at 75 mg/day PO in divided dos-

es with close monitoring. ⊗ ***Black box warning*** Limit quantities of drug in depressed and suicidal patients. Monitor patient for low BP. Discontinue drug if priapism occurs. Risk of suicidality is increased, especially in children, adolescents, and young adults.

trientine hydrochloride

Syprine

Drug class and indications

Chelate

Treatment of patients with Wilson's disease who are intolerant of penicillamine.

Dosages and special alerts

Adults: 750–1,250 mg/day PO in divided doses, maximum 2 g/day. Children: 500–750 mg/day PO; maximum, 1,500 mg/day. Interruption of therapy can lead to severe hypersensitivity reactions when drug is restarted. If iron supplements are taken, separate by at least 2 hr.

urofollitropin

Bravelle

Drug class and indications

Fertility drug

Sequentially with HCG to induce ovulation in patients who have previously received pituitary suppression.

Stimulation of multiple follicle development in ovulatory patients.

Dosages and special alerts

Patients who have received gonadotropin-releasing hormone agonist or antagonist suppression: 150 units daily subcutaneously or IM for the first 5 days of treatment. Subsequent dosing should be adjusted according to individual patient response, should not be made more frequently than once every 2 days, and should not exceed more than 75–150 units per adjustment. The maximum daily dose is 450 units; treatment beyond 12 days is not recommended. If patient response is appropriate, give HCG 5,000 to 10,000 units 1 day following the last dose of *Bravelle.* Monitor patient for ovarian overstimulation; warn patient of risk of multiple births.

ustekinumab

Stelara

Drug class and indications

Monoclonal antibody

Treatment of mild to moderate plaque psoriasis in adults who are candidates for phototherapy or systemic therapy.

Dosages and special alerts

100 kg or less: 45 mg subcutaneously, followed by 45 mg in 4 wk and then every 12 wk; more than 100 kg: 90 mg subcutaneously, followed by 90 mg in 4 wk and then every 12 wk. Risk of serious infections and malignancy. Do not use during active infection; if infection occurs, stop treatment. Most common adverse effects are headache, fatigue, and URI symptoms.

verteporfin

Visudyne

Drug class and indications

Ophthalmic drug

Treatment of age-related macular degeneration, pathologic myopia, ocular histoplasmosis.

Dosages and special alerts

6 mg/m^2 diluted in D_5W to total 30 mL IV into a free-flowing IV over 10 min at 3 mL/min using an inline filter and syringe pump. Laser light therapy should begin within 15 min of starting IV; may be repeated in 3 mo if needed. Protect patient from exposure to bright light for at least 5 days after treatment. Avoid use with hepatic impairment or sensitivity to eggs.

vigabatrin

Sabril

Drug class and indications

Antiepileptic, GABAase inhibitor

Monotherapy for children 1 mo–2 yr with infantile spasms.

Adjunctive therapy for adults with complex partial seizures not controlled by other therapy.

Dosages and special alerts
Children 1 mo–2 yr: 50 mg/kg/day PO bid oral solution to a maximum of 150 mg/kg/day PO bid. Adults: 500 mg PO bid to a maximum of 1.5 g PO bid with other antiepileptics. ⊗ ***Black box warning*** Risk of vision loss; limit dosage and duration of therapy and monitor patient's vision. Stop drug if vision changes occur. Risk of suicidal ideation; monitor patient accordingly. Causes anemia, somnolence, peripheral neuropathy, weight gain, edema. Taper dosage when discontinuing.

DANGEROUS DRUG

vorinostat

Zolinza

Drug class and indications
Histone deacetylase inhibitor, antineoplastic

Treatment of cutaneous manifestations in patients with cutaneous T-cell lymphoma who have progressive, persistent or recurrent disease on or following two systemic therapies.

Dosages and special alerts
400 mg PO once daily with food; continue until there is evidence of progression of disease or unacceptable toxicity. ⊗ ***Black box warning*** Monitor patient for increased bleeding, excessive nausea and vomiting, thromboembolic events. Encourage 2 L/day of fluid intake to prevent dehydration.

ziconotide

Prialt

Drug class and indications
N-type calcium channel blocker, analgesic

Management of severe chronic pain in patients who need intrathecal therapy and are intolerant or unresponsive to traditional therapy.

Dosages and special alerts
Initially 2.4 mcg/day by continuous intrathecal pump; may be titrated to a maximum 19.2 mcg/day (0.8 mcg/hr). Monitor for development of meningitis, psychotic behaviors, and neurological impairment.

Bibliography

Aschenbrenner, D., & Venable, S. *Drug Therapy in Nursing* (3rd ed). Philadelphia: Lippincott Williams & Wilkins, 2008.

Carpenito-Moyet, L.J. *Nursing Diagnosis: Application to Clinical Practice* (13th ed). Philadelphia: Lippincott Williams & Wilkins, 2009.

Drug Evaluations Subscription. Chicago: American Medical Association, 2010.

Drug Facts and Comparisons. St. Louis, MO: Facts and Comparisons, 2010.

Drug Facts Update: Physicians On-Line. Multimedia, 2010.

Fetrow, C.W., & Avila, J. *Professional's Handbook of Complementary and Alternative Medicines* (3rd ed). Springhouse, PA: Lippincott Williams & Wilkins, 2003.

Gilman, A.G., Hardman, J.G., & Limbird, L.E. (Eds). *Goodman and Gilman's The Pharmacological Basis of Therapeutics* (11th ed). New York: McGraw-Hill, 2006.

Griffiths, M.C. (Ed). *USAN and the USP 2006 Dictionary of Drug Names*. Rockville, MD: United States Pharmacopeial Convention, 2006.

Handbook of Adverse Drug Interactions. New Rochelle, NY: The Medical Letter, 2010.

Haynes, L., et al. *Nursing in Contemporary Society*. Upper Saddle River, NJ: Pearson Prentice Hall, 2004.

ISMP Medication Safety Alert! Huntington Valley, PA: Institute for Safe Medication Practices, 2010.

Karch, A.M. *Focus on Pharmacology* (5th). Philadelphia: Lippincott Williams & Wilkins, 2010.

Levine, R.R. *Pharmacology: Drug Actions and Reactions* (6th ed). Pearl River, NY: Parthenon Publishing Group, 2000.

The Medical Letter on Drugs and Therapeutics. New Rochelle, NY: Medical Letter, 2010.

PDR for Nonprescription Drugs. Oradell, NJ: Medical Economics Company, 2010.

PDR for Ophthalmology. Oradell, NJ: Medical Economics Company, 2010.

Physicians' Desk Reference (63rd ed). Oradell, NJ: Medical Economics Company, 2010.

Smeltzer, S.C., & Bare, B.G. *Brunner and Suddarth's Textbook of Medical-Surgical Nursing* (11th ed). Philadelphia: Lippincott Williams & Wilkins, 2006.

Tatro, D. S. (Ed). *Drug Interaction Facts*. St. Louis, MO: Facts and Comparisons, 2010.

Index

Generic names and **alternative therapies** are boldface in main entries. *Brand names* of drugs are in italics, followed by the generic name in parentheses. Brand names of Canadian drugs are followed by (CAN). Chemical or nonofficial names appear in regular typeface. **DRUG CLASSES** appear in bold capital letters with the drugs that fall in that class listed as official names under the class heading.

A

B

C

E

F

H

J

K

L

M

N

O

S

T

U

V

W

X

Y

Z